Radiology of the Liver, Biliary Tract, Pancreas and Spleen

GOLDEN'S DIAGNOSTIC RADIOLOGY

Volumes of Golden's Diagnostic Radiology Series published or in preparation

Bryan et al:	Diagnostic Neuroradiology
Campbell et al:	Radiologic, Ultrasonic, and Nuclear Diagnostic Methods in Obstetrics*
Castaneda:	Interventional Radiology
Clouse & Wallace:	Lymphatic Imaging—Lymphography, Computed Tomography and Scintigraphy
Cooley & Schreiber	Radiology of the Heart and Great Vessels*
Dreyfuss & Janower:	Radiology of the Colon*
Edeiken:	Roentgen Diagnosis of Diseases of Bone, *Fourth Edition*
Gottschalk, Hoffer, Berger, & Potchen	Diagnostic Nuclear Medicine, *Second Edition*
Hatfield & Wise:	Radiology of the Gallbladder and Bile Ducts*
Littleton:	Tomography—Physical Principles and Clinical Applications*
Martin:	Atlas of Mammography: Histologic and Mammographic Correlations
Rabin & Baron:	Radiology of the Chest*
Sussman & Newman:	Urologic Radiology*
Taveras & Wood:	Diagnostic Neuroradiology*

* Out of print

Radiology of the Liver, Biliary Tract, Pancreas and Spleen

Edited by
Arnold C. Friedman, M.D.
Associate Professor
Chief, Section of Abdominal Imaging
Department of Diagnostic Imaging
Temple University,
Philadelphia, Pennsylvania

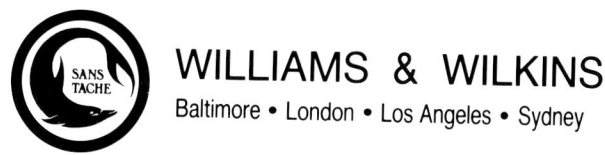

WILLIAMS & WILKINS
Baltimore • London • Los Angeles • Sydney

GOLDEN'S DIAGNOSTIC RADIOLOGY
JOHN H. HARRIS, JR., M.D., SERIES EDITOR

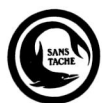

Senior Editor: Timothy H. Grayson
Associate Editor: Victoria M. Vaughn
Copy Editors: William Vinck, Kathleen Hull
Design: JoAnne Janowiak
Illustration Planning: Asterisk Group
Production: Raymond E. Reter

Copyright © 1987
Williams & Wilkins
428 East Preston Street
Baltimore, MD 21202, U.S.A.

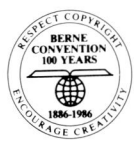

All rights reserved. This book is protected by copyright. No part of this book may be reproduced in any form or by any means, including photocopying, or utilized by any information storage and retrieval system without written permission from the copyright owner.

Accurate indications, adverse reactions, and dosage schedules for drugs are provided in this book, but it is possible that they may change. The reader is urged to review the package information data of the manufacturers of the medications mentioned.

Printed in the United States of America

Library of Congress Cataloging in Publication Data

Radiology of the liver, biliary tract, pancreas, and spleen.
   (Golden's diagnostic radiology)
   Includes bibliographies and index.
   1. Digestive organs—Radiography. 2. Digestive organs—Diseases—Diagnosis. I. Friedman, Arnold C. II. Series: Golden's diagnostic radiology series. [DNLM: 1. Biliary Tract—radiography. 2. Liver—radiography. 3. Pancreas—radiography. 4. Spleen—radiography. WI 141 R1293]
RC847.R33   1987   616.3'30757   86-7837
ISBN 0-683-03380-8

Composed and printed at the
Waverly Press, Inc.

87 88 89 90 91
10 9 8 7 6 5 4 3 2 1

To Wendy and Jeffrey for their inspiration and support

Series Editor's Foreword

It gives me great personal and professional pride and pleasure to introduce *Radiology of the Liver, Biliary Tract, Pancreas and Spleen*, edited and primarily authored by Arnold C. Friedman, M.D., Associate Professor and Chief of the Section of Abdominal Imaging at Temple University and Hospital in Philadelphia.

The scope of this text was specifically limited to what are considered to be the accessory organs of the alimentary tract to comply with the purpose and goal of the Golden Series which is to present contemporary, authoritative texts that will serve as reference sources for radiologists and others with particular interest in the title subject. This purpose and goal requires a comprehensive, in-depth review and discussion of the subject amply illustrated and annotated with a respectable bibliography of references that provide the reader with both historic and contemporary perspective of the subject. Because of the nearly exponential increase in the body of information pertinent to abdominal imaging that has resulted from the technologic and scientific advances in diagnostic and interventional procedures of abdominal imaging, we believe the Golden Series' philosophy can only be achieved, and yet have each book remain a useful, practical reference source, if the title subject is carefully defined.

The *Radiology of the Liver, Biliary Tract, Pancreas and Spleen* fulfills these criteria and so compliments other related titles in the Series. The extensive information contained in this text will make it a valuable supplement to others dealing with the broader subject of abdominal imaging and interventional radiology in which their very scope forces a less extensive discussion of the radiology of these critically important, complex organs that comprise the subject of this volume.

It is the tradition of the Golden Series that its authors be invited to prepare each text, which together, make the Series one of the most respected collections in Radiology. Because Dr. Friedman has earned, in a relatively short but intensively active career, a respected reputation as an abdominal imager with a primary interest in the gut and its accessory organs, he was a logical candidate to prepare this book. Consultations throughout the radiologic community revealed widespread recognition of Dr. Friedman as a clinical radiologist, researcher, and teacher. The notion that he be invited to author this text had unanimous support. Consequently, I was both delighted and excited when Dr. Friedman accepted the invitation to author the newest edition of The Golden Series.

Dr. Friedman has enlisted the aid of an impressive group of contributors, all of whom are well qualified to participate in this work and many of whom are well known in the field of abdominal imaging. Their individual experiences combined with the techniques and procedures of some of the most respected academic Radiology Departments in the country have been melded into a single authoritative compendium under Dr. Friedman's direction.

The organization of the subject matter into five distinct sections is simple, logical, and practical. The Contents also serves as a useful, quick index. The style of writing, established by Dr. Friedman and maintained throughout the book, is remarkably consistent, clear, direct, easy to follow, and free of intellectual ambiguities which tend to obfuscate.

The text is profusely illustrated with radiologic images of excellent quality that have been carefully selected to enhance the text. The liberal use of clear, accurate anatomic drawings and schematic representations of the salient aspect of ultrasound and computed tomographic (CT) images clarify otherwise difficult anatomic concepts and relationships and emphasize subtle or obscure radiologic images. Gross and microscopic pathologic illustrations provide direct radiologic-pathologic correlation. The references, which are conveniently located throughout each chapter, are comprehensive and authoritative and include those of classic or historic importance as well as appropriate references from the current literature.

I am very much aware of the truly remarkable advances that have been made in abdominal imaging and intervention during this decade. Even though I am neither an abdominal imager, nor an interventionalist, as I read the proof of the *Radiology of the Liver, Biliary Tract, Pancreas, and Spleen,* I found it to be a genuinely exciting book which more than does justice to these remarkable advances and which constitutes, in a single source, a comprehensive and authoritative discussion of the newest interventional procedures and imaging modalities, including magnetic resonance imaging (MRI), as they currently relate to the liver, biliary tract, pancreas, spleen and upper abdomen.

It has taken approximately 3 years for Dr. Friedman and his associates and Williams & Wilkins to bring this book to completion. The promise inherent in Dr. Friedman's agreement to write this text has come to fruition and far exceeds even my most optimistic expectations.

On behalf of Sara Finnegan, President of Williams & Wilkins, and all those members of Williams & Wilkins and Waverly Press who have contributed to the culmination of this project, I am proud to extend sincerest congratulations to Dr. Friedman and his contributors for adding luster to the already distinguished Golden Series of Diagnostic Radiology.

It is with the greatest enthusiasm that I recommend this text to you, the reader, as the definitive work on the *Radiology of the Liver, Biliary Tract, Pancreas and Spleen.*

John H. Harris, Jr., M.D., D.Sc.
Editor, Golden Series

Preface

For many years, the liver, spleen, and pancreas were relatively hidden organs. Diagnostic imaging was limited to plain films, radionuclide scans, and angiography, and mass lesions were inferred rather than directly depicted. The development of gray-scale ultrasound, computed tomography, and most recently, nuclear magnetic resonance imaging has made noninvasive demonstration of pathologic anatomy possible in these organs. More and more, diagnostic images resemble in vivo gross pathology, albeit in black and white. Simultaneously, refinements in sonography and percutaneous cholangiography and the development of iminodiacetic acid radionuclides have revolutionized biliary radiology. Angiography and cholangiography are now performed for therapeutic as well as diagnostic purposes. Percutaneous aspiration biopsy and drainage procedures have become commonplace.

With increasing frequency, radiologists are called upon to properly sequence a radiologic workup as well as to perform and interpret both diagnostic and therapeutic procedures. In order to carry out these functions well, the radiologist must be conversant with the clinical and pathologic aspects of diseases as well as their radiologic manifestations. The present text is an effort to correlate the radiologic manifestations of diseases of the liver, biliary tract, pancreas, and spleen with their clinical aspects and gross pathology.

Acknowledgments

I would like to thank all the contributors, without whom this book could not have been written. The secretarial assistance of Mrs. Thelma Estill, Ms. Pearl Mulraine, Ms. Barbara Hamer, Ms. Cathy Spiotta, Ms. Ellie Crissey, Mrs. Martha Ross, and Mrs. Milena Herman was vital for manuscript preparation. The line drawings were prepared by the Medical Illustration departments at Temple University, Walter Reed Army Medical Center, and the Armed Forces Institute of Pathology. The radiographic reproductions, which form the backbone of any radiology text, were ably performed by Mr. Milne Hewish of the Department of Diagnostic Imaging at Temple University, Mr. Henry Bacich of Medical Communications at Temple University, Medical Photography at the Uniformed Services University of the Health Sciences, and Mr. Robert Irving of the Radiology Department at George Washington University Hospital.

Special thanks must go to all the physicians who contributed their cases to the Department of Radiologic Pathology at the Armed Forces Institute of Pathology, and to Drs. David S. Hartman, Rebecca Glicksman, Pamela Murari, and Michael Reed for reviewing portions of the manuscript.

I am grateful to Jack Harris for giving me the opportunity to write this book, and to John Madewell and Joel Lichtenstein for encouraging me to undertake the task.

The staff at Williams & Wilkins has been unfailingly friendly, helpful, and cooperative throughout the entire preparation process.

Finally, saving the most important for the end, I thank my wife, Wendy, and my son, Jeffrey, for putting up with a less than full-time husband and father during the 4 years this book was in preparation. I hope to make it up to them in the next 4 years.

Contributors

David S. Ball, D.O.
Resident in Radiology, Temple University Hospital, Temple University, Philadelphia, Pennsylvania

Mark T. Birns, M.D.
Private practice of Gastroenterology and Endoscopic Biliary Surgery, Rockville, Maryland. Active Staff, Shady Grove Adventist Hospital, Maryland. Formerly Assistant Chief, Department of Gastroenterology, Walter Reed Army Medical Center, Washington, D.C. and Assistant Professor of Medicine, Uniformed Services University of the Health Sciences, Bethesda, Maryland

Leonard Bodner, M.D.
Formerly Assistant Professor, Department of Radiology, Montefiore Hospital and Medical Center, Albert Einstein College of Medicine, Bronx, New York. Currently New Brunswick Radiology Group, East Brunswick, New Jersey

Manuel L. Brown, M.D.
Associate Professor of Radiology and Associate Professor of Laboratory Medicine, Mayo Clinic Graduate School of Medicine, Rochester, Minnesota

Dina F. Caroline, M.D.
Assistant Professor of Radiology, Temple University, Department of Diagnostic Imaging, Temple University Hospital, Philadelphia, Pennsylvania

John Cavaluzzi, M.D.
Assistant Professor, Department of Radiological Sciences, The Johns Hopkins University School of Medicine. Chief, Sections of Angiography and Neuroradiology, Francis Scott Key Hospital, Baltimore, Maryland

Douglas M. Coldwell, M.D., Ph.D.
Assistant Professor, Departments of Radiology and Medical Oncology, George Washington University and George Washington University Hospital, Washington, D.C.

Abraham H. Dachman, M.D.
Assistant Professor of Radiology, Uniformed Services University, Bethesda, Maryland. Chief, Section of Abdominal Imaging, Walter Reed Army Medical Center, Washington, D.C.

Edward J. Farmlett, M.D.
Resident in Radiology, The Johns Hopkins University School of Medicine and The Johns Hopkins Hospital, Baltimore, Maryland

Darlene Fink-Bennett, M.D.
Clinical Assistant Professor of Radiology, Michigan State University. Attending Nuclear Medicine Physician, William Beaumont Hospital, Royal Oak, Michigan

Elliot K. Fishman, M.D.
Assistant Professor of Radiology, Department of Radiology and Radiological Sciences, The Johns Hopkins University School of Medicine. Co-director, Division of Computed Tomography, Department of Radiology, and the Johns Hopkins Hospital, Baltimore, Maryland

Dean L. Gain, M.D.
Southern California Radiology Medical Group, Glendale, California. Formerly Assistant Professor, Department of Radiology, The Johns Hopkins University School of Medicine and The Johns Hopkins Hospital, Baltimore, Maryland

Anne S. Giovannelli, M.D.
Fellow in Abdominal Imaging, Temple University Hospital, Temple University, Philadelphia, Pennsylvania

Michael C. Hill, M.B.
Associate Professor, Department of Radiology, George Washington University. Chief, Section of Ultrasound and CT, George Washington University Hospital, Washington, D.C.

Todd Johns, M.D.
Cpt. USMC, Chief, Section of Body Computed Tomography, Walter Reed Army Medical Center, Washington, D.C.

Adrian G. Krudy, Jr., M.D.
Division of Medical Imaging and Radiologic Sciences, Hillcrest Hospital, Mayfield Heights, Ohio. Formerly Chief, Section of Special Procedures, Department of Diagnostic Radiology, Clinical Center, National Institutes of Health, Bethesda, Maryland

David W. Levy, M.D.
Resident in Radiology, Temple University Hospital, Temple University, Philadelphia, Pennsylvania

Joel E. Lichtenstein, M.D.
Col. USAF, Chief, Division of Diagnostic Radiologic Pathology, Armed Forces Institute of Pathology, Washington, D.C. Presently Department of Radiology, Wilford Hall Hospital, San Antonio, Texas

Donna Magid, M.D.
Assistant Professor, Department of Radiology, The Johns Hopkins University School of Medicine and The Johns Hopkins Hospital, Baltimore, Maryland

Bruce M. Markle, M.D.
Associate Radiologist, Children's Hospital, National Medical Center, Associate Professor of Radiology and of Child Health and Development, George Washington University, Washington, D.C.

Alan H. Maurer, M.D.
Associate Professor of Radiology, Temple University School of Medicine, Director, Division of Nuclear Medicine, Department of Diagnostic Imaging, Temple University Hospital, Philadelphia, Pennsylvania

Donald G. Mitchell, M.D.
Fellow, CT/US/MRI, Hospital of the University of Pennsylvania, Philadelphia, Pennsylvania

Robert L. Pakter, M.D.
Instructor, Department of Radiology, The Johns Hopkins University School of Medicine and The Johns Hopkins Hospital, Baltimore, Maryland

Paul D. Radecki, M.D.
Assistant Professor of Radiology, Temple University, Department of Diagnostic Imaging, Temple University Hospital, Philadelphia, Pennsylvania

Steve Rindsberg, M.D.
Resident in Radiology, Temple University Hospital, Temple University, Philadelphia, Pennsylvania

Leora Sachs, M.D.
Clinical Assistant Professor, Department of Radiology, George Washington University Hospital, and George Washington University, Washington, D.C.

Roger C. Sanders, M.D.
Associate Professor, Department of Radiology, The Johns Hopkins University School of Medicine. Chief, Section of Ultrasound, The Johns Hopkins Hospital, Baltimore, Maryland

John C. Scatarige, M.D.
Assistant Professor of Radiology, Department of Radiology and Radiological Sciences, The Johns Hopkins Hospital, Baltimore, Maryland

Thomas H. Shawker, M.D.
Chief, Section of Ultrasound, Department of Diagnostic Radiology, Clinical Center, National Institutes of Health, Bethesda, Maryland

John L. Sherman, M.D.
The Neurology Center, Chevy Chase, Maryland. Formerly Major, US Army MC, and Chief of Diagnostic Radiology, Walter Reed Army Medical Center, Washington, D.C.

James G. Smirniotopoulos, M.D.
Chief, Section of Neurologic and ENT Radiologic Pathology, Armed Forces Institute of Pathology, Washington, D.C.

Seymour S. Sprayregen, M.D.
Professor of Radiology, Albert Einstein College of Medicine. Chief, Section of Vascular and Interventional Radiology, Montefiore Hospital and Medical Center, Bronx, New York

Heidi S. Weissmann, M.D.
Associate Professor, Department of Nuclear Medicine and Radiology, Albert Einstein College of Medicine. Adjunct Attending, Department of Nuclear Medicine, Montefiore Hospital and Medical Center, Bronx, New York

Contents

Series Editor's Foreword vii
Preface ix
Acknowledgments xi
Contributors xiii

Section I. LIVER

Chapter 1 Embryology, Anatomy, Histology, and Variations 3
Anne S. Giovannelli and Arnold C. Friedman

Embryology 3
Liver Anatomy 4
Histology 6
Plain Film Examination 7
Vascular Anatomy 8
Normal Liver Angiography 13
Normal Ultrasound of the Liver 15
Computed Tomography of the Normal Liver 22
Normal Radionuclide Imaging of the Liver 27
Emission Computed Tomography and the Liver 31
Anatomic Variants 35

Chapter 2 Anomalies, Congenital Disorders, and Pediatric Neoplasms 37
Arnold C. Friedman, Bruce M. Markle, Abraham H. Dachman, and Robert L. Pakter

Glycogen Storage Diseases 37
Cystic Fibrosis 39
Chronic Granulomatous Disease of Childhood 40
Mesenchymal Hamartoma 41
Infantile Hemangioendothelioma 43
Hepatoblastoma 48
Undifferentiated (Embryonal) Sarcoma 52

Chapter 3 The Plain Film of the Liver 55
Dina F. Caroline

Hepatomegaly and the Effects of Liver Size Alteration on Other Structures 55
Effects on Other Structures 60

Chapter 4 Cirrhosis, Other Diffuse Diseases, Portal Hypertension, and Vascular Diseases 69
Arnold C. Friedman, Todd Johns, David W. Levy, Steve Rindsberg, and Bruce M. Markle

Cirrhosis 69
Causes of Portal Hypertension Other than Cirrhosis 88
Other Diffuse Diseases 105
Vascular Diseases 134

Chapter 5	**Focal Diseases**		**151**
	Arnold C. Friedman, Elliot K. Fishman, Paul D. Radecki,		
	John C. Scatarige, John L. Sherman, Edward J. Farmlett,		
	Bruce M. Markle, Abraham H. Dachman, and Robert Pakter		
	Pyogenic Liver Abscess		151
	Hepatic Candidiasis		157
	Amebic Abscess		158
	Echinococcal Disease		164
	Congenital Simple Cysts		171
	Cavernous Hemangioma		173
	Focal Nodular Hyperplasia		183
	Hepatic Adenoma		188
	Biliary Cystadenoma and Cystadenocarcinoma		193
	Metastatic Disease in the Liver		199
	Hepatocellular Carcinoma		220
Chapter 6	**Magnetic Resonance Imaging of the Liver**		**265**
	Arnold C. Friedman		
	Normal Anatomy and Technique		265
	MRI in Diffuse Liver Diseases		267
	Cirrhosis		268
	Fatty Infiltration (Steatosis)		268
	Hepatic Iron Overload		270
	Copper Disease States		270
	Hepatic Masses		271
	Summary		281
Chapter 7	**Hepatic Trauma**		**283**
	Arnold C. Friedman		
	Clinical Findings		283
	Treatment		283
	Pathology		283
	Radiology		283
	Nuclear Medicine		283
Chapter 8	**Transcatheter Management of Hepatic Neoplasms**		**293**
	Douglas M. Coldwell		
	Rationale		293
	Radiologic Technique		294
	Chemotherapy		295
	Hepatic Arterial Embolization		298
Chapters 1–8	**Liver Angiography**		
	John Cavaluzzi		
	Nuclear Medicine of the Liver		
	Darlene Fink-Bennett, Heidi S. Weissmann, and Alan H. Maurer		

Section II.	**THE GALLBLADDER AND BILIARY TRACT**		
Chapter 9	**Embryology, Anatomy, Histology, and Radiologic Anatomy**		**305**
	Arnold C. Friedman and Leora Sachs		

	Embryology	305
	Anatomy	305
	Histology	309
	Normal Oral Cholecystogram and Barium Contrast Examination	311
	Normal Imaging of the Gallbladder and Biliary Tract	312

Chapter 10 Endoscopic Retrograde Cholangiopancreatography: General Considerations and the Role of the Radiologist — 333
Mark T. Birns

- ERCP: The Procedure ... 333
- ERCP as a Therapeutic Procedure ... 338
- Experimental Uses ... 347

Chapter 11 Anomalies and Congenital Disorders — 351
Bruce M. Markle, Arnold C. Friedman, and Leora Sachs

- Anomalies of the Gallbladder and Biliary Tract ... 351
- Neonatal Jaundice, Hepatitis, Extrahepatic Biliary Atresia, and Bile Duct Paucity ... 356
- Hepatobiliary Cystic Malformations (Polycystic Liver Disease, Congenital Hepatic Fibrosis, Caroli's Disease, Choledochal Cyst) ... 362
- Common Bile Duct Diverticulum (Type II Choledochal Cyst) ... 381
- Choledochcele (Type III Choledochal Cyst) ... 383

Chapter 12 Cholelithiasis and Cholecystitis — 387
Leora Sachs, Joel E. Lichtenstein, Arnold C. Friedman, Mark T. Birns, and James G. Smirniotopoulos

- Cholelithiasis ... 387
- Acute Cholecystitis ... 409
- Acalculous Cholecystitis ... 428
- Emphysematous Cholecystitis ... 431
- Chronic Cholecystitis ... 435
- Porcelain Gallbladder ... 439
- Milk of Calcium Bile ... 442
- Hydrops of Gallbladder ... 446
- Biliary Fistula ... 447
- Gallstone Ileus ... 451
- Mirizzi Syndrome ... 457

Chapter 13 Hyperplastic Cholecystoses and Benign and Malignant Gallbladder Tumors — 463
Leora Sachs, Joel E. Lichtenstein, Arnold C. Friedman, and James G. Smirniotopoulos

- The Hyperplastic Cholecystoses ... 463
- Benign Tumors ... 478
- Gallbladder Carcinoma ... 483

Chapter 14 Radiology of Jaundice Including, Choledocholithiasis and Biliary Neoplasms — 497
Arnold C. Friedman, Leora Sachs, and Mark T. Birns

- Jaundice ... 497
- Choledocholithiasis ... 515
- Biliary-Enteric Anastomoses ... 529

	Cholangiocarcinoma	535
	Miscellaneous Bile Duct Tumors	544
Chapter 15	**Inflammatory Cholangitis, Parasitic Diseases, Primary Biliary Cirrhosis, and Papillary (Ampullary) Stenosis**	**549**
	Mark T. Birns, Arnold C. Friedman, and Leora Sachs	
	Acute (Ascending) Cholangitis	549
	Recurrent Pyogenic Cholangitis	552
	Biliary Ascariasis and Other Miscellaneous Parasites	556
	Primary Sclerosing Cholangitis and Pericholangitis	559
	Pericholangitis Associated with Inflammatory Bowel Disease	566
	Primary Biliary Cirrhosis	569
	Papillary (Ampullary) Stenosis	572
Chapter 16	**Trauma to the Gallbladder and Biliary Tract**	**579**
	Arnold C. Friedman, David S. Ball, and Leora Sachs	
	Biliary Tract	579
	Biloma (Biliary Cyst)	586
	Gallbladder	589
Chapter 17	**MRI of the Gallbladder and Biliary Tract**	**593**
	Arnold C. Friedman	
	Normal Anatomy	593
	Gallbladder Disease	595
	Biliary Obstruction	597
Chapter 18	**Interventional Biliary Radiology**	**601**
	Douglas M. Coldwell	
	Benign Strictures	601
	Malignant Strictures	602
	Other Biliary Conditions	605
	Technique of Percutaneous Transhepatic Cholangiography	606
	Other Biliary Special Procedures	610
Chapters 9–18	**Nuclear Medicine of the Gallbladder and Biliary Tract** *Manuel L. Brown and Heidi S. Weissmann*	

Section III. THE PANCREAS

Chapter 19	**Embryology, Anatomy, Histology, and Physiology**	**619**
	Arnold C. Friedman and Mark T. Birns	
	Embryology	619
	Anatomy	620
	Radiologic Anatomy	623
	Histology	639
	Pancreatic Exocrine Function	640
Chapter 20	**Anomalies and Congenital Disorders**	**643**
	Bruce M. Markle, Arnold C. Friedman, and Mark T. Birns	
	Pancreatic Arteriovenous Fistula	643
	Pancreas Divisum	643
	Annular Pancreas	645

	Schwachman-Diamond Syndrome	650
	Cystic Fibrosis	651
Chapter 21	**Pancreatitis**	**657**
	Michael C. Hill, Mark T. Birns, Arnold C. Friedman, Donald G. Mitchell, Leonard Bodner, and Seymour S. Sprayregen	
	Acute Pancreatitis	657
	Chronic Pancreatitis	681
	Complications of Pancreatitis	713
	Pancreatic Pseudocyst	722
	Pancreatic Trauma	741
	Fat Replacement	746
Chapter 22	**Pancreatic Neoplasms**	**749**
	Arnold C. Friedman, Adrian G. Krudy, Jr., Thomas H. Shawker, Donald G. Mitchell, Mark T. Birns, Leonard Bodner, and Seymour S. Sprayregen	
	Duct Cell Origin: Cystic Neoplasms	751
	Duct Cell Origin: Solid	765
	Acinar Cell Origin	851
	Indeterminate Origin	853
	Connective Tissue Tumors	854
	Metastases, Lymphoma, and Leukemia	854
	Islet Cell Tumors	861
Chapter 23	**Magnetic Resonance Imaging of the Pancreas**	**887**
	Arnold C. Friedman	
	Normal Anatomy	887
	Inflammatory Disease	889
	Hemochromatosis	891
	Neoplasms	892
	Summary	895

Section IV. THE SPLEEN

Chapter 24	**Normal Anatomy and Radiology**	**899**
	Abraham H. Dachman	
	Embryology	899
	Gross and Microscopic Anatomy	900
	Physiology	902
	Radiologic Anatomy and Technique	903
Chapter 25	**Anomalies and Congenital Disorders**	**917**
	Abraham H. Dachman	
	Wandering Spleen/Splenic Torsion	917
	Accessory Spleen	919
	Splenic Band	922
	Splenic-Gonadal Fusion	922
	Asplenia	923
	Polysplenia	925
Chapter 26	**Trauma and Nontraumatic Rupture**	**931**
	Abraham H. Dachman	
	Trauma	931

	Splenosis	942
	Nontraumatic Splenic Rupture	943
Chapter 27	**Focal Diseases**	**947**
	Abraham H. Dachman and Donna Magid	
	Cysts	947
	Splenic Abscess	955
	Lymphoma	965
	Hemangioma	971
	Angiosarcoma	972
	Hamartoma	973
	Lymphangiomatosis	975
	Metastases	976
Chapter 28	**Diffuse Diseases**	**985**
	Abraham H. Dachman and Donna Magid	
	Splenomegaly	985
	Infections	992
Chapter 29	**Vascular Disease**	**997**
	Abraham H. Dachman	
	Arteriosclerosis and Occlusion of Splenic Artery	997
	Fibromuscular Hyperplasia	997
	Splenic Artery Aneurysm	998
	Arteriovenous Fistula	1000
	Splenic Artery Embolization	1001
	Solitary Splenic Vein Thrombosis	1002
	Rupture of Splenic Vein	1004
	Splenic Infarct	1005
	Splenorenal Shunt	1011
	Splenic Vascular Changes in Pancreatic Disease	1011
	Peliosis of the Spleen	1012
Chapter 30	**Miscellaneous Disorders**	**1015**
	Abraham H. Dachman	
	Dense or Opacified Spleen	1015
	Sickle Cell Anemia	1017
	Diaphragmatic Herniation	1028
	Gastric Ulcers Penetrating into Spleen	1028
	Inflammatory Pseudotumor	1028
Chapter 31	**Magnetic Resonance Imaging of the Spleen**	**1031**
	Arnold C. Friedman	
	Normal Anatomy	1031
	Splenic Pathology	1033
Chapters 24–30	**Nuclear Medicine of the Spleen**	
	Darlene Fink-Bennett and Heidi S. Weissmann	

Section V.	**BIOPSY AND DRAINAGE PROCEDURES IN THE UPPER ABDOMEN**	
Chapter 32	**Percutaneous Abscess and Fluid Drainage in the Upper Abdomen**	**1041**
	Dean L. Gain and Roger C. Sanders	
	Background	1041
	Imaging	1042
	Technique	1043
Chapter 33	**Guided Percutaneous Biopsy in the Upper Abdomen**	**1065**
	John C. Scatarige	
	Cytopathology	1065
	Imaging Modalities Available for Biopsy Guidance	1066
	Needle Selection	1068
	Indications	1071
	Contraindications	1079
	Mortality and Morbidity	1079
	Summary and Future Prospects	1081
	Index	**1085**

Color Plates

Figures shown in color are
also reproduced in black and white in their
respective chapters.

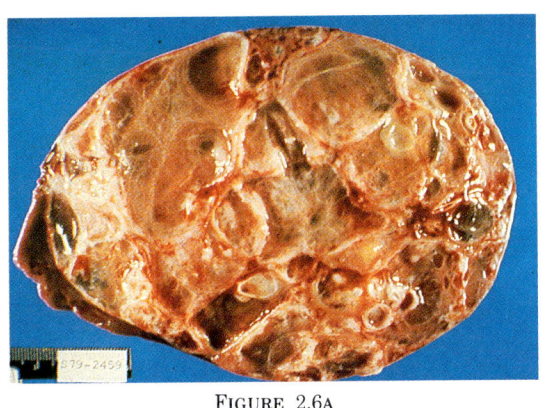

Figure 2.6a

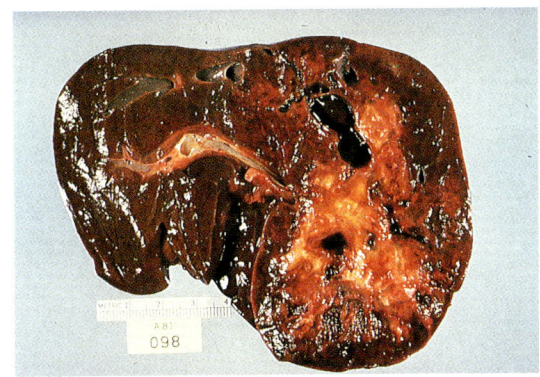

Figure 2.7

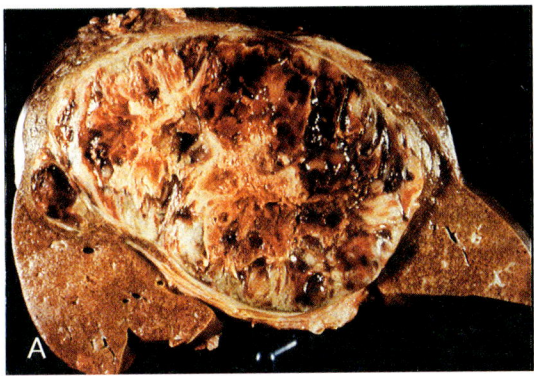

Figure 2.21a

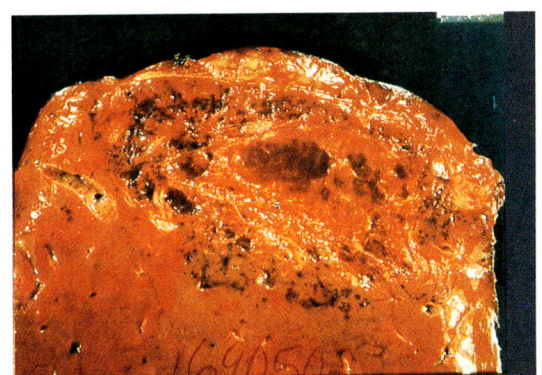

Figure 5.27

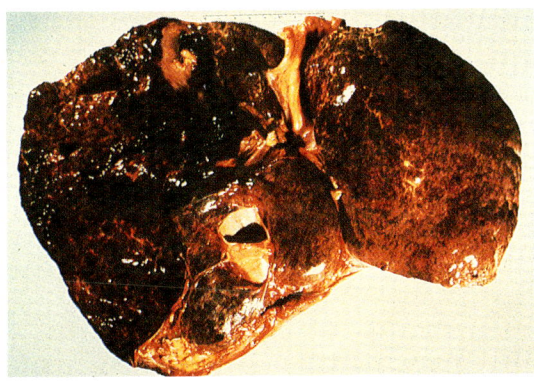

Figure 5.105

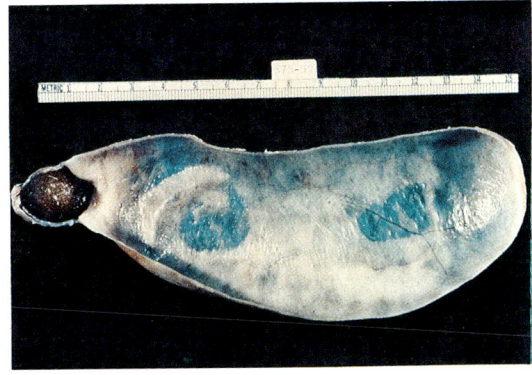

Figure 12.50

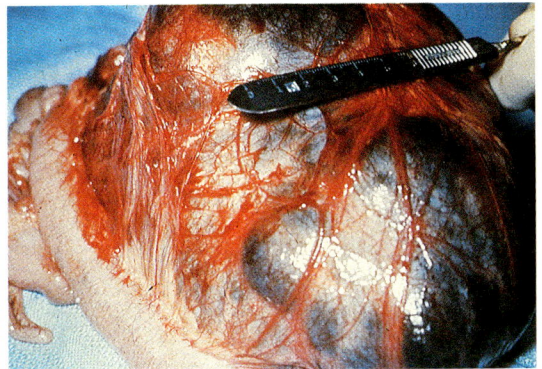

Figure 22.2

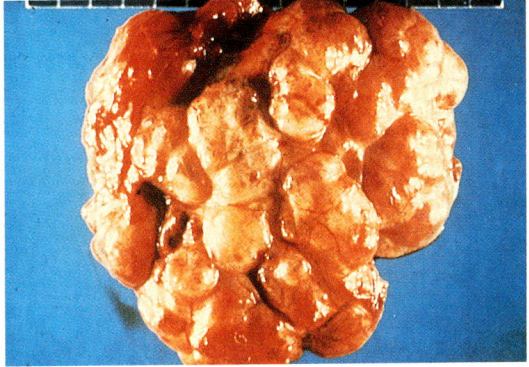

Figure 22.4a

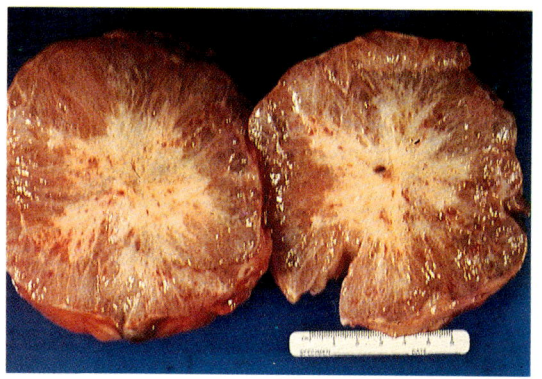

FIGURE 22.4b

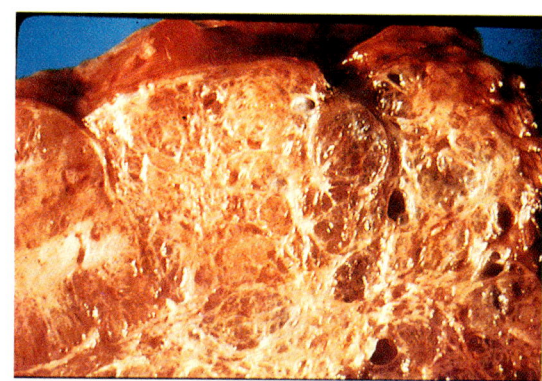

FIGURE 22.4c

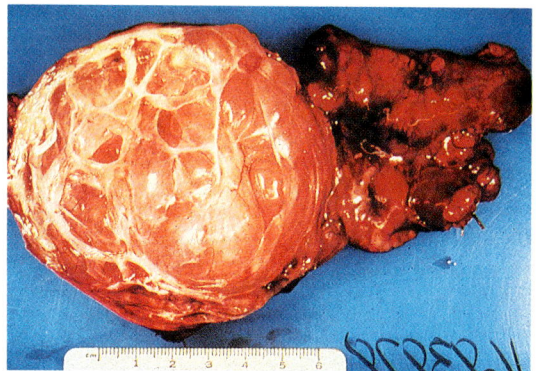

FIGURE 22.10a

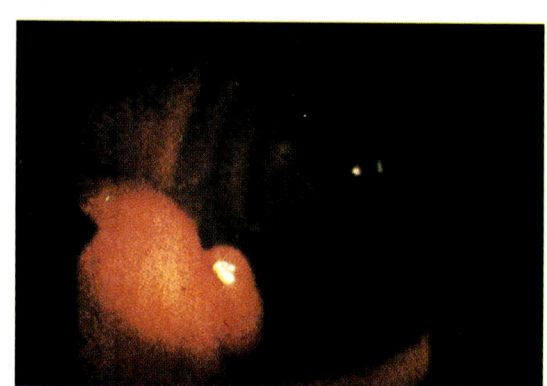

FIGURE 22.24b

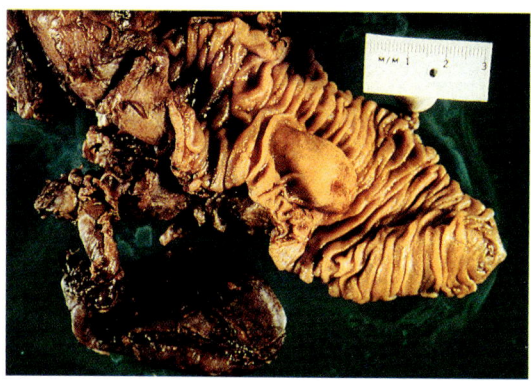

FIGURE 22.42b

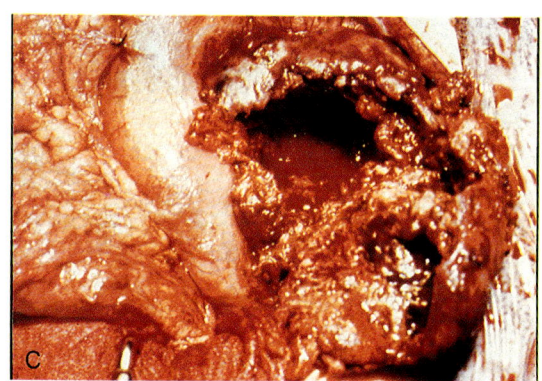

FIGURE 22.81c

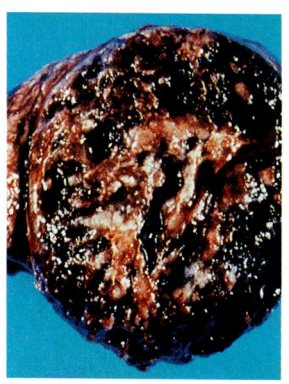

FIGURE 22.91f

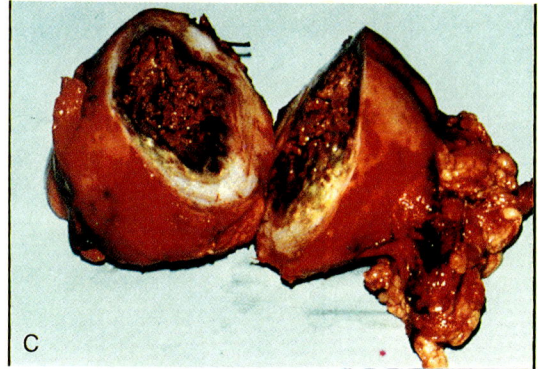

FIGURE 22.92c

SECTION I
The Liver

INTRODUCTION

It was not too many years ago that the only imaging procedures available for direct study of the liver were the plain radiograph, the radionuclide scintigram, and angiography. The former two suffered from lack of specificity and a relative lack of sensitivity. Angiography, although fairly sensitive and somewhat specific, is invasive and not without risk. Clinicians were often reluctant to request angiography and thus mass lesions often were undetected until they had reached quite a large size. Blind liver biopsy was often done to exclude the presence of metastases. Today, gray scale sonography and computerized tomography (CT) are extremely sensitive detectors of space-occupying liver disease. Although they are not that specific, they are used to guide percutaneous aspiration biopsies so that a specific diagnosis can be made with a minimal risk. Magnetic resonance imaging (MRI) has recently emerged on the scene and may become the best noninvasive imaging method for the liver. Currently it is hampered by motion-induced artifacts and prolonged imaging times. Only time will tell to what extent MRI will supplant sonography and CT.

No matter what hepatic imaging test is performed, proper interpretation is impossible without a thorough knowledge of liver anatomy, and of gross and sometimes microscopic pathology. I hope that this section imparts enough basic knowledge to make not only the findings of current imaging modalities in hepatic disease processes understood, but those of future modalities as well.

1
Embryology, Anatomy, Histology, and Variations

ANNE S. GIOVANNELLI, M.D., AND ARNOLD C. FRIEDMAN, M.D.

EMBRYOLOGY

The earliest appearance of what is to become the liver is a thickening of endoblastic epithelium in the 2.5-mm 18-day-old embryo (1). On the 22nd day the 3-mm embryo develops a diverticulum at the distal end of the foregut (1). On the 28th day (3.6 mm) this mass of tissue invaginates into the adjacent mass of splanchnic mesoderm called the septum transversum located between the primitive heart and the yolk sac (Fig. 1.1) (1). The leading edge of this hepatic bud subsequently divides into right and left branches from which columns of endodermal cells grow out into the vascular mesoderm. These cells grow, arborize, and anastomose with one another. Meanwhile, the paired vitelline veins and the umbilical vein element which course through the septum transversum become fragmented by these invading columns of cells to become the hepatic sinusoids. The intrahepatic bile ducts are thought to arise from dedifferentiation of partially differentiated hepatic parenchymal cells (1).

Hence, the columns of endodermal cells become the parenchymal liver cells, the vascular vitelline and umbilical vein elements become the sinusoids and the septum transversum mesoderm becomes the fibrous capsule and connective tissue elements of the liver. Later, some of the cells lining the sinusoids differentiate into larger macrophages, (Kupffer cells), the reticuloendothelial substance of the liver (2).

The left and right terminal branches of the main hepatic bud canalize to become the common hepatic, right and left hepatic ducts. With further canalization and arborization the ductal system eventually joins the bile capillaries. During the 5th month of development the liver cells begin to secrete bile. The gallbladder itself develops from the posterior edge of the original hepatic diverticulum (3).

Review of the embryogenesis of the hepatic vascular system may provide insight into the anomalies frequently encountered. Because of an inadequate yolk, vascular differentiation begins early in the human embryo in order to supply oxygen and nutrients. The rudiments of the blood vessels appear as aggregates of mesenchymal cells called angioblasts (3). Angioblasts organize into a flat epithelium surrounding a lumen in a capillary network (3). Alternatively blood vessels may develop in the form of sinuses, large irregular spaces surrounded by endothelium. Many of the larger veins are formed in this way (3).

Subsequent development of individual canals depends on the amount and direction of flow. Channels receiving the most flow enlarge, while channels receiving less flow remain as capillaries or involute (3).

At approximately 4 weeks, the embryologic abdominal arterial system is represented by paired dorsal aortas which give rise to paired vitelline artery branches in the cervical thoracic area. Over time, these vessels migrate caudally. The vitelline arteries fuse and the 10th pair of arteries form the celiac trunk, the 13th pair forms the superior mesenteric artery, and the 21st or 22nd pair form the inferior mesenteric artery. The frequently encountered variations of the celiac and superior mesenteric arteries can thus be traced to persistence of primitive vitelline artery anastomoses. Variations in caudal migration and gut rotation during development can also alter the position of the arterial origins (4).

The early embryologic venous system consists of the umbilical veins from the chorion, the vitelline veins from the yolk sac, and the cardinal veins in the body of the embryo itself. With further development of the embryo, these vessels undergo profound changes. The fates of the vitelline and umbilical veins are germane to the liver.

The dual vitelline veins accompany the yolk stalk into the body, then course cranially along-

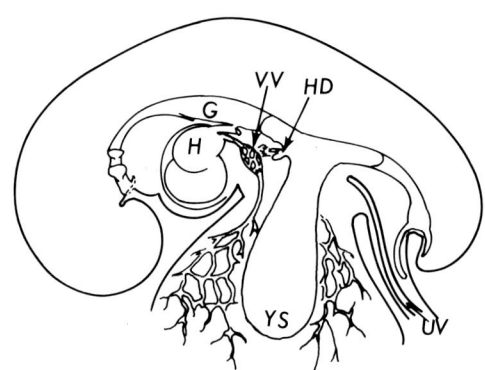

FIGURE 1.1. HUMAN EMBRYO, 28 DAYS
G, gut; *H*, heart; *HD*, hepatic diverticulum; *UV*, umbilical vein; *VV*, vitelline vein. Septum transversum is between the heart and yolk sac (*YS*).

side the foregut to the septum transversum and into the sinus venosus. It is within this intersection that the hepatic bud grows, fragmenting the vitelline veins and incorporating them into what will become the right and left lobe sinusoids. Cephalad to this sinusoidal complex is a short segment which returns blood to the sinus venosus. The distal portions become the portal vein, the sandwiched sinusoidal complex of the liver persists, and the proximal segment becomes the hepatic vein. Under the influence of flow changes induced by the developing gut, the portal vein assumes its S-shaped configuration. The superior mesenteric vein arises de novo in the dorsal mesentery of the intestinal loop and supercedes the vitelline veins (5).

The umbilical veins return blood from the placenta via the umbilical cord. They drain into the sinus venosus. Later, with development and prominence of the nearby hepatic sinusoidal system, the blood of the umbilical vein preferentially follows the sinusoids and the entire right and proximal left umbilical veins atrophy. The distal left umbilical vein shifts toward the midline and comes to occupy the free edge of the falciform ligament (5).

The ductus venosus develops as a conduit from the left umbilical vein to the common hepatic vein and later the inferior vena cava. The umbilical vein does, however, make contributions to the sinusoids to form an anastomosis with the portal system (5).

REFERENCES

1. DuBois AM: The Embryonic Liver. In Rouiller CH (ed): *The Liver-Morphology, Biochemistry, Physiology*. New York, Academic Press, 1963, pp 1–32.
2. Kelly DE, Wood RL, Enders AC: *Bailey's Textbook of Microscopic Anatomy*. Baltimore, Williams & Wilkins, 1984, pp 590–593.
3. Balinsky BI: *An Introduction to Embryology*, Ed 4. Philadelphia, W. B. Saunders, 1975, pp 459–460.
4. Reuter SR, Redman HC: *Gastrointestinal Angiography*. Philadelphia, W. B. Saunders, 1977, pp 31–65.
5. Arey LB: *Developmental Anatomy: A Textbook and Laboratory Manual of Embryology*. Philadelphia, W. B. Saunders, 1965, pp 255–259.

LIVER ANATOMY

The adult liver is the largest visceral organ of the body. It occupies the right upper quadrant with a variable portion extending transversely across the midline.

Anteriorly, beneath the right lobe lies the hepatic flexure of the colon. Directly posterior to the hepatic flexure of the colon lies the right kidney. Medial to these structures lie the gallbladder anteriorly and the duodenum in a slightly more posterior position (1).

The lesser curvature and anterior wall of the stomach lie adjacent to the inferior surface of the left lobe of the liver. The posterior aspect of the left lobe of the liver is grooved by the distal esophagus.

The superior surface of the liver lies below the right lung, but the more peripheral portions of the superior surface of the right lobe lie adjacent to the abdominal wall. The left lobe of the liver lies partially below the heart and to a variable extent below the left lung laterally (1).

The liver is covered by peritoneum except for: the fossa for the inferior vena cava, the fossa for the gallbladder, and the bare area, where the liver is in direct contact with the diaphragm just to the right of the inferior vena cava (Fig. 1.2).

The falciform ligament is a thin fibrous sheet extending from the umbilicus to the superior surface of the liver (Fig. 1.2). The falciform ligament contains the ligamentum teres or remnant of the umbilical vein. At the superior surface of the liver the falciform ligament separates and its reflections extend laterally to become the anterior leaf of the coronary ligament of the liver, the anterior boundary of the bare area. The posterior boundary of the bare area is the posterior leaf of the coronary ligament, where the peritoneum is reflected off the liver to the diaphragmatic area of the posterior abdominal wall (2).

On the right, the coronary ligament separates the right subphrenic space from the right sub-

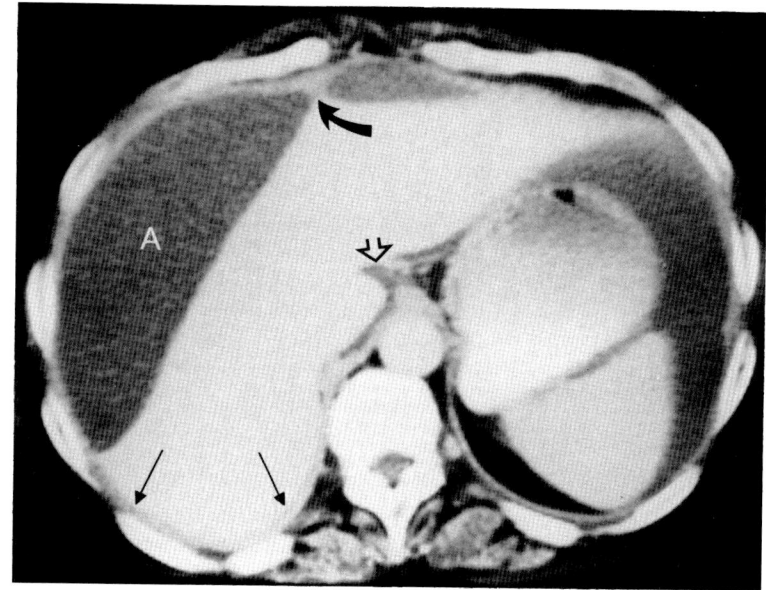

FIGURE 1.2. LIVER ANATOMY
Ascites (*A*) outlining the falciform ligament (*curved arrow*), interrupted at the bare area (*arrows*), and extending into a recess of the lesser sac (*open arrow*) anterior to the caudate lobe.

hepatic space (Morrison's pouch) (Fig. 1.3). The coronary ligament on the left separates the left subphrenic space into an anterior and a posterior compartment (Fig. 1.4).

The omentum between the liver and the stomach is named the gastrohepatic ligament and that between the liver and the duodenum is named the hepatoduodenal ligament. The gastrohepatic ligament (lesser omentum) divides the left subhepatic space into an anterior and posterior (lesser sac) compartment (Fig. 1.4). The hepatoduodenal ligament contains the common bile duct, the hepatic artery, the portal vein, nerves, and lymphatics (2).

The liver is held in position by its attachments

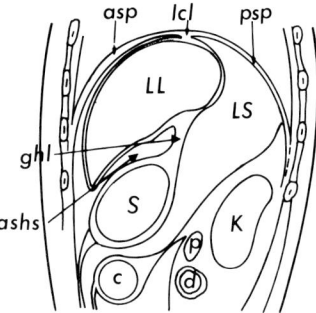

FIGURE 1.4. SAGITTAL SECTION THROUGH LEFT LOBE
Sagittal section through the left lobe of the liver (*LL*): *asp*, anterior subphrenic space; *lcl*, left coronary ligament; *psp*, posterior subphrenic space; *LS*, lesser sac; *ghl*, gastrohepatic ligament; *ashs*, anterior subhepatic space; *S*, stomach; *K*, kidney; *c*, colon; *p*, pancreas; *d*, duodenum.

to the diaphragm and to the anterior abdominal wall by the aforementioned ligaments. Posteriorly the inferior vena cava and the hepatic veins support the liver in place (2).

The traditional anatomic division of the liver is based on external landmarks on the visceral surface of the liver which have a roughly H-shaped configuration. Using this approach the lateral limb of the H is formed by a line connecting the gallbladder fossa and the sulcus for the inferior vena cava. The more medial limb of the H is formed by the fissure for the ligamentum venosum. The cross bar of the H consists of the porta hepatis, its vessels and ducts. Thus divided, the right lobe of the liver extends from the right lateral margin of the liver laterally to the sulcus

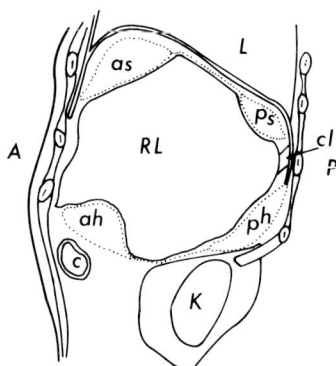

FIGURE 1.3. SAGITTAL SECTION THROUGH RIGHT LOBE
Sagittal section through the right lobe of the liver (*RL*): *as*, anterior subphrenic space; *ps*, posterior subphrenic space; *cl*, coronary ligament; *ph*, posterior subhepatic space; *ah*, anterior subhepatic space; *c*, colon; *K*, kidney; *L*, lung; *A*, anterior; *P*, posterior.

for the inferior vena cava dorsally and the gallbladder ventrally. The left lobe lies wholly to left of the falciform ligament and the fissures for the ligamentum teres and the ligamentum venosum. The quadrate lobe is anterior to the porta hepatis between the gallbladder fossa and the fissure for the ligamentum teres. The caudate lobe lies on the visceral surface of the liver between the sulcus for the inferior vena cava and the fissure for the ligamentum venosum (3). Surgical and angiographic considerations dictate a separate nomenclature for the anatomy of the liver based on the intrahepatic distribution of vessels and ducts (see ultrasound section).

REFERENCES

1. Gelfand, DW: Anatomy of the liver. *Radiol Clin North Am* 18:187, 1980.
2. McNulty JA: *Radiology of the Liver*. Philadelphia, W. B. Saunders, 1977, pp 1–26.
3. Kane RA: Ultrasound anatomy of the liver and biliary tree. *Semin Ultrasound* 1:87, 1980.

HISTOLOGY

The hepatocyte is the basic cellular element of the liver. Hepatocytes comprise approximately 70% of the liver by volume. Each hepatocyte measures approximately 30 μm in diameter and is polygonal in shape. The single or infrequently multiple nuclei divide by mitosis. The life expectancy of the hepatocyte is approximately 150 days. Hepatocytes have no basement membranes and can be considered to have three surfaces: one facing a sinusoid and space of Disse, one facing a bile canaliculus, and the third facing a neighboring hepatocyte (1).

Classically the lobule was described as the organizational unit of the liver. The lobule was that unit of parenchyma surrounding a central hepatic venule defined at its periphery by hexagonally arranged portals triads. Each portal triad consists of a portal branch vein, a branch of the hepatic artery, and a bile ductule as well as their accompanying lymphatic and neural elements (2).

Elegant studies performed by Rappaport and Bilbey reported in 1960 revised this conceptual arrangement. By injecting the main portal vein branches and the entire hepatic venous system with differently colored vinyl acetate and subsequently removing the hepatic parenchyma, it was shown that the area surrounding each central vein was supplied by blood from different sources and hence the tissue around each central vein could not be considered as a structural unit (2). Expanding on this, Rappaport proposed the hepatic acinus, an irregularly shaped but roughly triangular parenchymal mass with portal triad at its center, as the more appropriate organizational unit (Fig. 1.5). Each acinus lies between two or more terminal (central) hepatic veins. The width of an acinus is twice the length of a radicle sinusoid (2). Circulatory zones within the acini dividing hepatocytes into those closest to, midway, and most distal to the parent portal vein have also been defined (2). Hepatocytes in

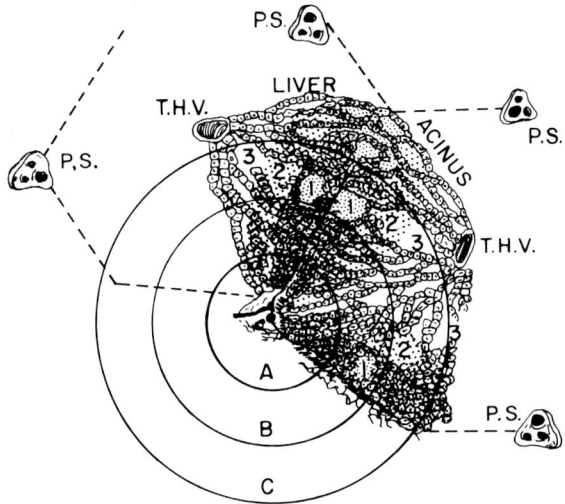

FIGURE 1.5. LIVER ACINUS AND ZONAL ARRANGEMENT OF CELLS

The liver acinus and zonal arrangement of cells: *1, 2, 3,* zones of first, second, and third order quality blood supply; *PS*, portal space; *THV*, terminal hepatic vein. Circles *B* and *C* represent peripheral circulatory areas around the "periportal" area, *A*, at whose center lies a portal triad. (Modified from Rappaport AM: Acinar units and the pathophysiology of the liver. In Rouiller CH (ed): *The Liver: Morphology, Biochemistry, Physiology*. Academic Press, New York, 1963, pp 266–320.)

the zone closest to the feeding vessels receive the freshest, most oxygenated, and nutrient richest blood (2). These hepatocytes are metabolically the most active as well as the most resilient; they are the last to die and the first to regenerate (2). Conversely, the more peripheral a hepatocyte is, the poorer the quality of the blood reaching it and the more susceptible it is to damage (2).

Despite the myriad functions performed by the liver as an organ, only one cell, the hepatocyte, is metabolically functional (1). It has been postulated that morphologic and functional differences exist among the hepatocytes in the various circulatory zones described above (2). Cells in the various zones are subject to different environments with regard to pressure, flow dynamics and supply of nutrients and oxygen (2). Certain enzymes will predominate in the various hepatocytes along the circulatory cascade (2).

Kupffer cells, cells of the reticuloendothelial system, constitute approximately 30% of the liver mass. These flat cells are intermittently arranged along the walls of the sinusoids and function in the production of immune bodies, phagocytosis, and blood formation.

REFERENCES

1. Kelly DE, Wood RL, Enders AC: *Bailey's Textbook of Microscopic Anatomy.* Baltimore, Williams & Wilkins, 1984, pp 590–593.
2. Rappaport AM: Acinar Units and the Pathophysiology of the Liver. In Rouiller CH (ed): *The Liver-Morphology, Biochemistry, Physiology.* New York, Academic Press, 1963, pp 266–320.

PLAIN FILM EXAMINATION

The plain film examination of the liver is somewhat limited by the fact that the liver is a soft tissue structure (radiological water density) and blends into adjacent soft tissue structures unless outlined by air or fat. These real borders (outlined by fat) or apparent borders (outlined by gas in adjacent organs) can provide helpful clues to the plain film interpretation (1).

Extraperitoneal fat invests the parietal peritoneum and surrounds the abdomen. Usually it is more prominent in the lateral and posterior abdomen but it is also present anteriorly and superiorly. It is this fat which defines the lateral, superior and posteroinferior surfaces of the right lobe of the liver on plain films of the abdomen. The right lateral margin of the liver is outlined by the extraperitoneal (properitoneal) fat which is continuous with the posterior pararenal space. Usually the right lateral margin of the liver has a smooth interface with this fat but with sufficient fat the costal grooves can be defined (2).

Riedel's "lobe," a common anatomical variant frequently seen in women, is merely a prominent tongue of the right lobe which extends inferiorly interposed between the right colon and the properitoneal fat (Fig. 1.6) (3).

The superior margin of the liver is usually defined by the apparent border of the right diaphragm, the basilar pleura and the aerated right lung (1). However, the superior margin of the liver is covered by a variable amount of extraperitoneal fat, again continuous with the posterior pararenal space. This lies between the undersurface of the right diaphragm and the parietal peritoneum and can occasionally be seen as an arcuate radiolucency between the diaphragm and the liver, mimicking either a pneumoperitoneum or a pneumoretroperitoneum (2).

The left superior surface of the liver cannot be distinguished on the plain film, probably because the heart superiorly has the same "water" density as the liver. The extreme left superior border of the liver, like its right counterpart may be de-

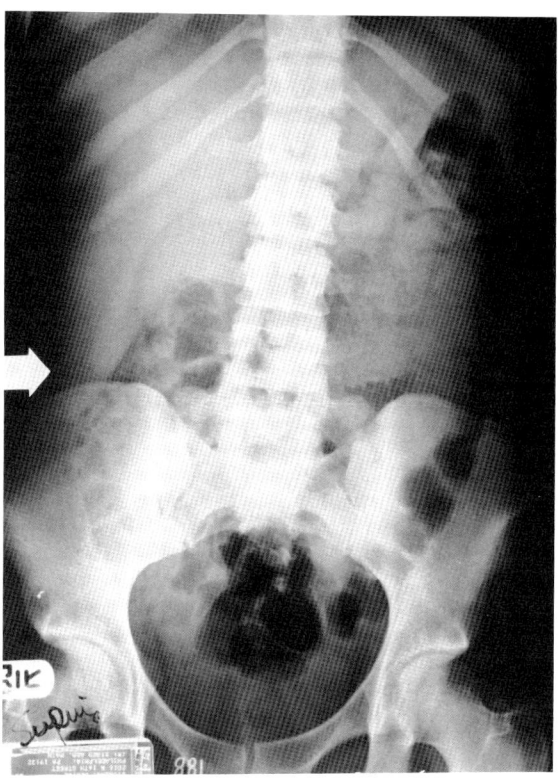

FIGURE 1.6. RIEDEL'S LOBE
Normal liver with a Riedel's lobe (*arrow*) in a young woman.

fined at the apparent border of the left diaphragm (1).

The inferior margin of the liver has a complicated topography but the same radiological principles apply (Fig. 1.6). Anteriorly, inferior to the right lobe lies the hepatic flexure of the colon. Posterior to the hepatic flexure lies the right kidney. Medial to these two organs lie the gallbladder anteriorly and the duodenum posteriorly. The anterior wall of the stomach and the lesser curvature of the stomach lie adjacent to the inferior surface of the left lobe. Much of the inferior surface of the liver lies in contact with retroperitoneal fat, pericolic fat, or fat in the greater omentum. The inferior border of the left lobe of the liver can be outlined by air in the stomach. Similarly, air in the duodenal bulb may produce an apparent border with the inferior central portion of the liver (1).

Fat is also present in the porta hepatis where it invests the common bile duct, hepatic artery, and the portal vein, as well as their accompanying neural and lymphatic elements. Periportal fat can be recognized occasionally on plain films of the abdomen as a curvilinear, sometimes branching, lucency in the right subphrenic space. Periportal fat can mimic air in the biliary tree (2).

Evaluation of the liver size by plain film is less accurate than either isotopic studies or ultrasound, however, gross hepatomegaly or focal enlargement can be recognized by displacement of adjacent structures from their expected positions (4).

REFERENCES

1. Gelfand DW: Anatomy of the liver. *Radiol Clin North Am* 18:187, 1980.
2. Mindelzun R, McCort JJ: Hepatic and perihepatic radiolucencies. *Radiol Clin North Am* 18:221, 1980.
3. McNulty JB: *Radiology of the Liver*. Philadelphia, W. B. Saunders, 1977, pp 28–59.
4. Gelfand DW: The liver: plain film diagnosis. *Semin Roentgenol* 10: 177, 1975.

VASCULAR ANATOMY

The liver has a dual blood supply: the hepatic artery usually arising from the celiac axis of the aorta provides arterial blood and the portal vein returns venous blood from the intestines and the spleen. Together, the portal vein and the hepatic artery enter the liver, with the common bile duct at the portal hepatis, a fissure deep in the inferior surface of the right lobe of the liver.

The celiac axis of the aorta is usually located between the lower half of T12 and the T12–L1 interspace. The celiac axis extends caudally approximately 1–2 cm and then ventrally. The usual branches of the celiac axis are the left gastric, the splenic, and the common hepatic arteries (Fig. 1.7). This "classic" arrangement is present in 55–65% of patients. The inferior phrenic arteries may also arise from the celiac artery either separately or as a single trunk in 55% of patients. When they arise from the celiac trunk they are the first branch or branches. Occasionally, the dorsal pancreatic artery arises from the celiac artery (1).

The common hepatic artery is smaller than the splenic artery and courses to the right and anteriorly giving off the gastroduodenal artery and sometimes the dorsal pancreatic artery (Fig. 1.7B). After giving off the gastroduodenal artery the common hepatic artery becomes the proper hepatic artery. The proper hepatic artery is usually short in length and, after entering the porta hepatis, divides into a right, left and occasionally a middle hepatic branch (Fig. 1.7). Both the left and right hepatic arteries come from the proper hepatic only about half the time. In the remainder of cases one or more branches of the hepatic artery have a partially or totally replaced origin (1). Rarely, the entire hepatic blood supply is replaced to the superior mesenteric artery (1).

The right hepatic artery early on gives rise to the cystic artery and then supplies the right lobe of the liver (Fig. 1.7B). In 45% of patients the left hepatic artery gives rise to the middle hepatic artery. In 25% of patients the left hepatic artery has a partially or totally replaced origin from the left gastric artery (1).

The middle hepatic artery arises from the proper hepatic artery in only about 10% of cases. Usually it is a branch of either the right or the left hepatic artery. The middle hepatic artery is the main supply to the quadrate lobe and may supply the caudate lobe and the gallbladder (1).

It should be remembered that the arteries to the liver are end-arteries. Multiple collaterals exist between the arterial branches in the hepatic hilum and sometimes more peripherally. These collateral pathways are seen more often when some part of the circulation to the liver has been compromised.

As described above, a simple common hepatic artery injection will demonstrate the entire arterial supply in only 55–65% of patients. While numerous anomalous circulations exist, the statistically important variations (Fig. 1.8) are: (a) left hepatic artery from the left gastric, 25%; (b) right hepatic artery completely replaced to the superior mesentery artery, 14%; and (c) right hepatic artery partially replaced to the superior mesentery artery, 8%. Only rarely does the right hepatic artery arise directly from the aorta. Occasionally the left hepatic artery may arise from

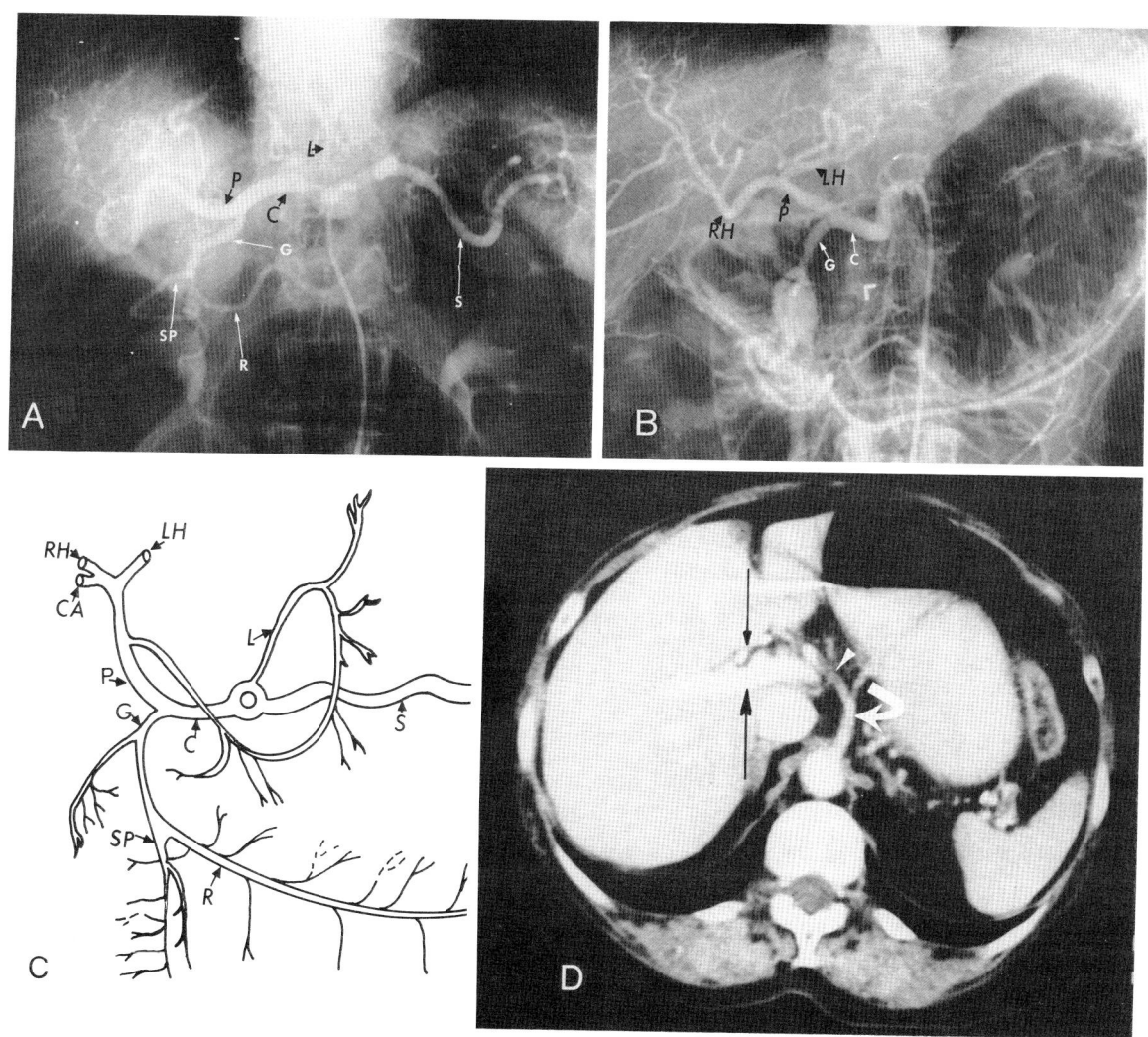

FIGURE 1.7. VASCULAR ANATOMY

A: Classic celiac axis: celiac arteriogram. *B:* Normal common hepatic arteriogram. *C:* Diagrammatic representation of *A* and *B:* *S*, splenic artery; *G*, gastroduodenal artery; *R*, right gastroepiploic artery; *SP*, superior pancreaticoduodenal artery; *C*, common hepatic artery; *L*, left gastric artery; *P*, proper hepatic artery; *RG*, right gastric artery; *CA*, cystic artery; *LH*, left hepatic artery; *RH*, right hepatic artery. *D:* Normal celiac artery (*curved arrow*), common hepatic artery (*white arrowhead*), right hepatic artery (*small arrow*), and portal vein (*large arrow*). (Air bolus augmented rapid infusion scan.)

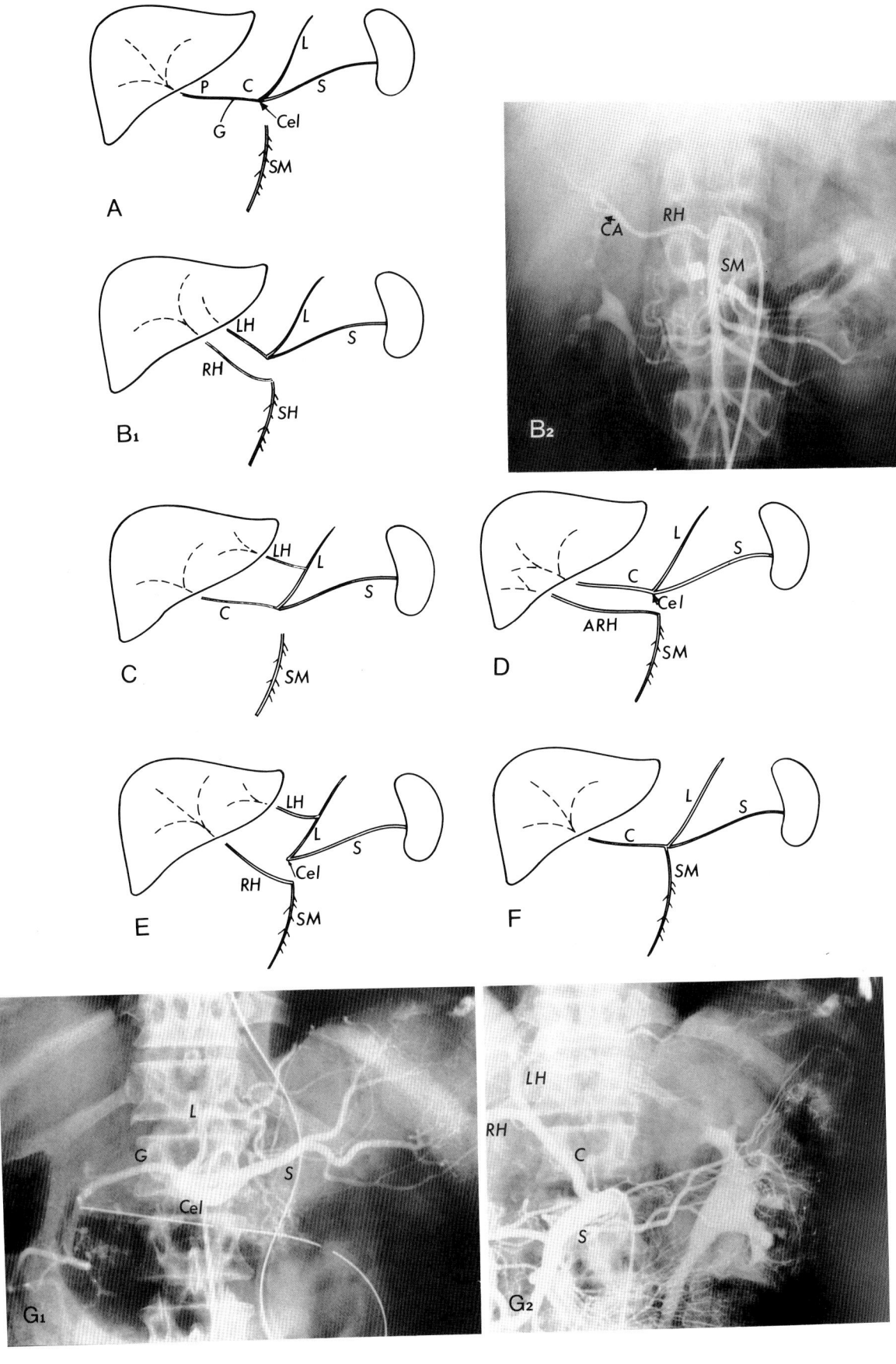

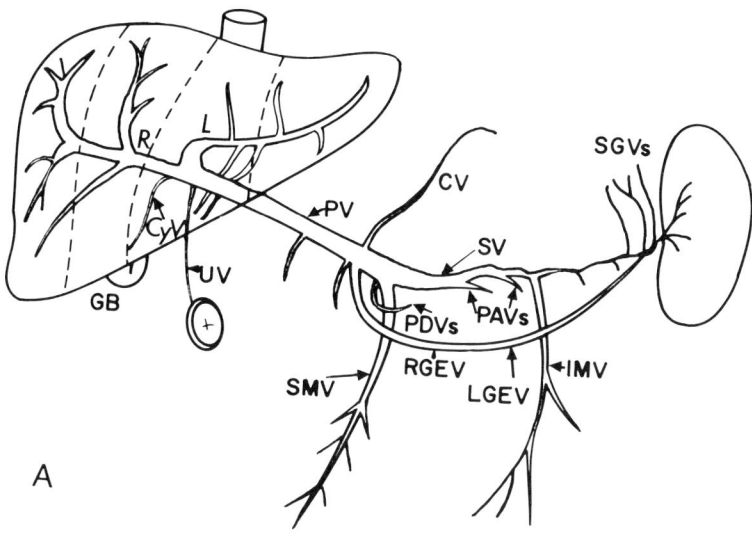

FIGURE 1.9. PORTAL VENOUS SYSTEM

A: Diagram. *B:* Venous phase of a splenic artery injection. *C* and *D:* Venous phases of priscoline-augmented inferior mesenteric artery (*C*) and superior mesenteric artery (*D*) injections, respectively. *SV*, splenic vein; *CV*, coronary vein; *PV*, portal vein; *SGVs*, short gastric veins; *SMV*, superior mesenteric vein; *IMV*, inferior mesenteric vein; *RGEV*, right gastroepiploic vein; *LGEV*, left gastroepiploic vein; *PDVs*, pancreaticoduodenal veins; *UV*, umbilical vein; *PAVs*, pancreatic veins; *CyV*, cystic veins; *L*, left portal vein; *R*, right portal vein; *GB*, gallbladder. *E, F:* Left portal vein in the intersegmental fissure (*arrow, E*) and origin of the left portal vein slightly caudad (*arrow, F*). Main portal vein extending into the right portal vein is shown in Figure 1.7D. (*E* and *F* are air bolus augmented rapid infusion scans.) *G:* Normal portal venous anatomy illustrated by an umbilical venogram.

the aorta or the superior mesenteric artery. Alternatively, the entire hepatic artery may arise from the superior mesenteric artery (1).

The portal vein, the other afferent supply to the liver is formed behind the neck of the pancreas by the junction of the superior mesenteric vein and the splenic vein (Figs. 1.7D and 1.9). The main portal vein ascends cephalad and to the right in the free edge of the lesser omentum. It enters the porta hepatis with the hepatic artery and the common bile duct, where it divides into the right and left branches (1). The right portal vein courses horizontally in the right lobe before dividing into an anterior and posterior branch (1).

The right portal vein and its branches tend to be constant in their appearance and location. The left portal vein tends to be smaller than the right and follows a longer, straighter course as it runs superiorly, anterior to the caudate lobe before making an abrupt anterior turn into the left intersegmental fissure where it gives off branches to the medial and lateral segments of the left lobe. The ligamentum teres (the remnant of the umblilical vein) arises from the anterior margin of the left portal vein (2).

The hepatic veins lie between the hepatic segments and are useful for describing intrahepatic segmental anatomy (Fig. 1.10). The right hepatic vein runs an oblique course in the intersegmental fissure between the anterior and posterior segments of the right lobe. It is usually the largest hepatic vein. The middle hepatic vein marks the junction between the true right and left lobes of the liver. The left hepatic vein runs in the left intersegmental fissure between the medial and lateral segments of the left lobe. The hepatic veins all drain obliquely cephalad and medially to enter the inferior vena cava close to its entry into the right atrium. While the hepatic veins

FIGURE 1.8. VARIATIONS IN THE CELIAC AXIS

A: Classical pattern. *B1:* Complete replacement of the right hepatic artery from the superior mesenteric artery. *B2:* Superior mesenteric arteriogram: replaced right hepatic artery and cystic artery. *C:* Left hepatic artery from left gastric artery. *D:* Accessory right hepatic artery from superior mesenteric artery. *E:* Right hepatic artery from superior mesenteric artery and left hepatic artery from left gastric artery. *F:* Common celiac/mesenteric trunk. *G:* Common hepatic from superior mesenteric. *1)* celiac injection opacifies splenic artery and left gastric artery. *2)* superior mesenteric injection opacifies common hepatic artery which branches into left and right hepatic arteries: *S*, splenic artery; *C*, common hepatic artery; *L*, left gastric artery; *SM*, superior mesenteric artery; *RH*, right hepatic artery; *LH*, left hepatic artery; *ARH*, accessory right hepatic artery; *Cel*, celiac artery; *CA*, cystic artery; *G*, gastroduodenal artery; *P*, proper hepatic artery.

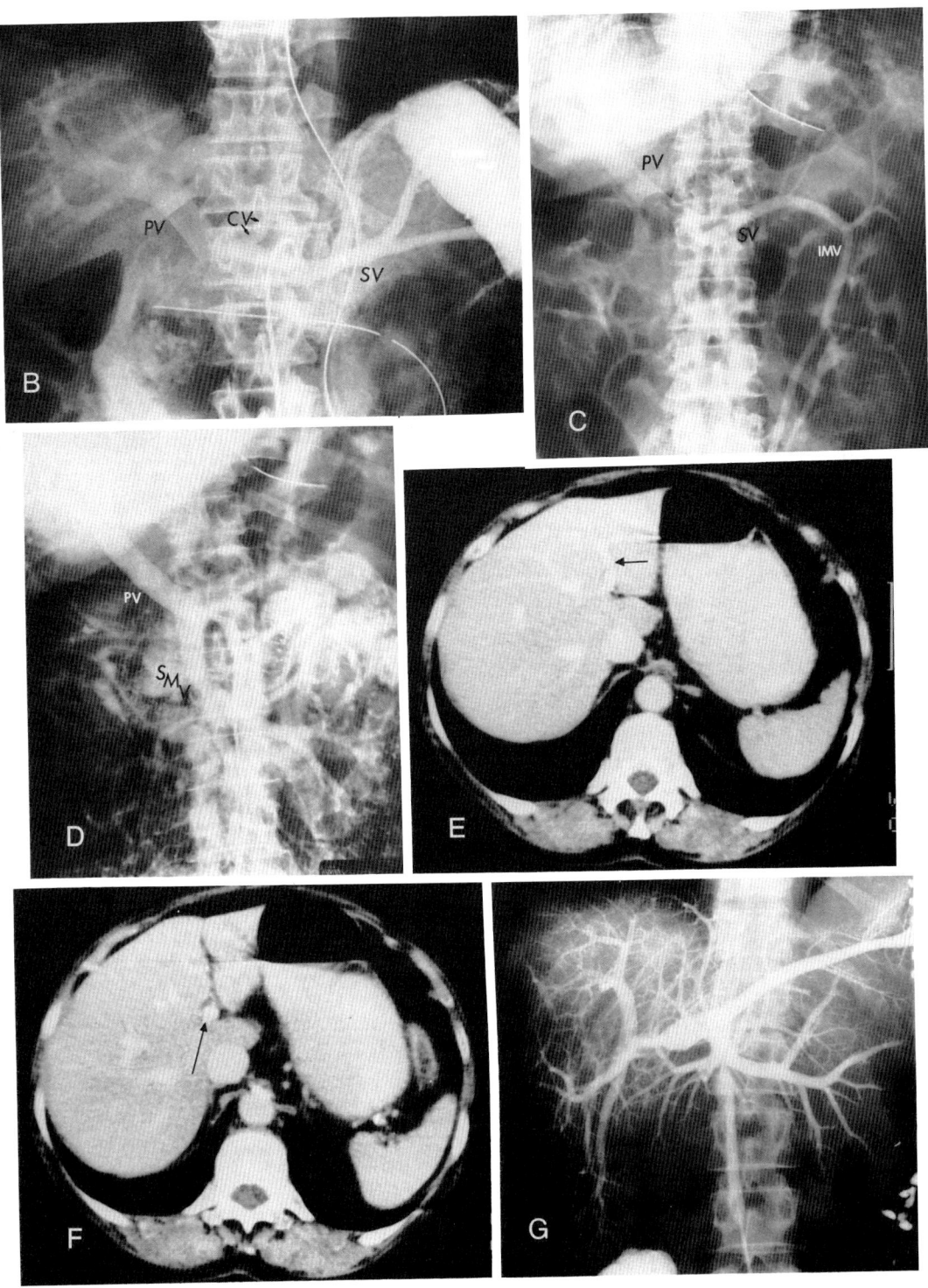

FIGURE 1.9*B–G.*

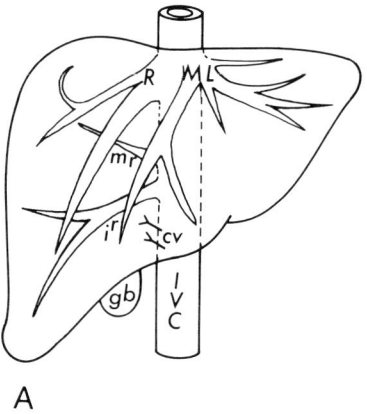
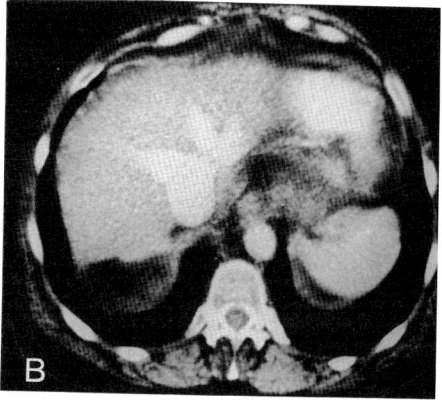
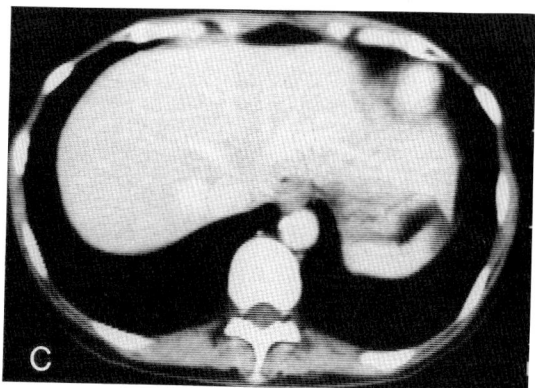

FIGURE 1.10. THE HEPATIC VEINS

A: Diagram of hepatic veins: *IVC*, inferior vena cava; *R*, right hepatic vein; *M*, middle hepatic vein; *L*, left hepatic vein; *mr*, middle right hepatic vein; *ir*, inferior right hepatic vein; *cv*, caudate lobe veins; *gb*, gallbladder. *B* and *C*: CT of two different patients showing the hepatic veins converging on the inferior vena cava. Note the normal variation in diameter. (*B* and *C* are air bolus augmented rapid infusion scans.)

may enter the inferior vena cava as a single trunk, more commonly the right hepatic vein enters separately and the middle and left veins form a conjoined trunk before entering the inferior vena cava (2).

Several small hepatic veins emptying the caudate lobe and portions of the right lobe usually enter the inferior vena cava separately. Occasionally a separate inferior right hepatic vein drains directly into the inferior vena cava (3).

REFERENCES

1. Reuter SR, Redman HC: *Gastrointestinal Angiography*. Philadelphia, W. B. Saunders, 1977, pp 31–65.
2. Pagani JJ: Intrahepatic vascular territories shown by computed tomography (CT). *Radiology* 147:173–178, 1983.
3. Makuuchi M, Hasegawa H, Yamakazo S, Bandai Y, Watanabe G, Ito T: The inferior right hepatic vein: ultrasonic demonstration. *Radiology* 148:213–217, 1983.

NORMAL LIVER ANGIOGRAPHY

The first angiographic examination usually performed in a patient with known or suspected hepatic disease is celiac and superior mesenteric arteriography which will delineate both hepatic arterial and portal venous anatomy. A routine celiac arteriogram might be performed with an injection of 40–50 ml of contrast material at 10–12 ml/sec. A typical filming sequence is 1 per sec for 7 sec and then 1 every 3 sec for 15 sec (1). If the splenic and portal veins are not well seen, superior mesenteric arteriography is done after injection of a vasodilator, usually tolazoline, to improve venous opacification. If the right hepatic artery is partially or totally replaced, the superior mesenteric arteriogram must be done without vasodilation (1). Improved detection of mass lesions can be obtained with the technique of infusion hepatic arteriography (1, 2).

Types of Hepatogram and Relevance to Detection of Space-Occupying Disease

The hepatogram is the diffuse parenchymal opacification observed during the late phase of any type of liver angiogram. Because of the dual blood supply of the liver, the hepatogram after a celiac injection is different from that after a selective hepatic injection (1). A pure arterial

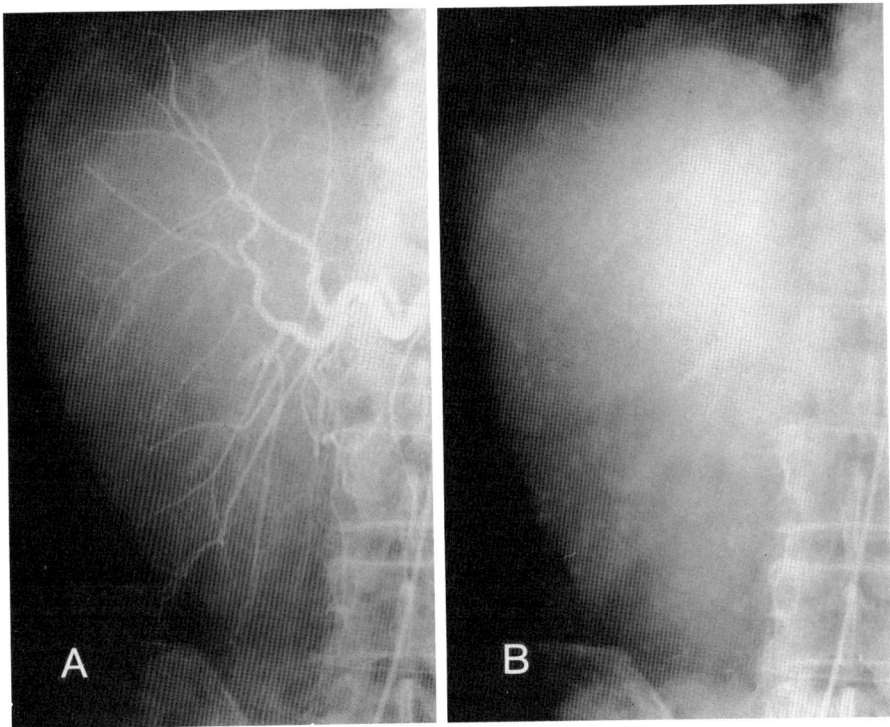

FIGURE 1.11. HEPATOGRAM

A: Normal arterial phase, replaced right hepatic catheterized off the superior mesenteric artery. *B:* Arterial hepatogram with spotted pattern more prominent than usual.

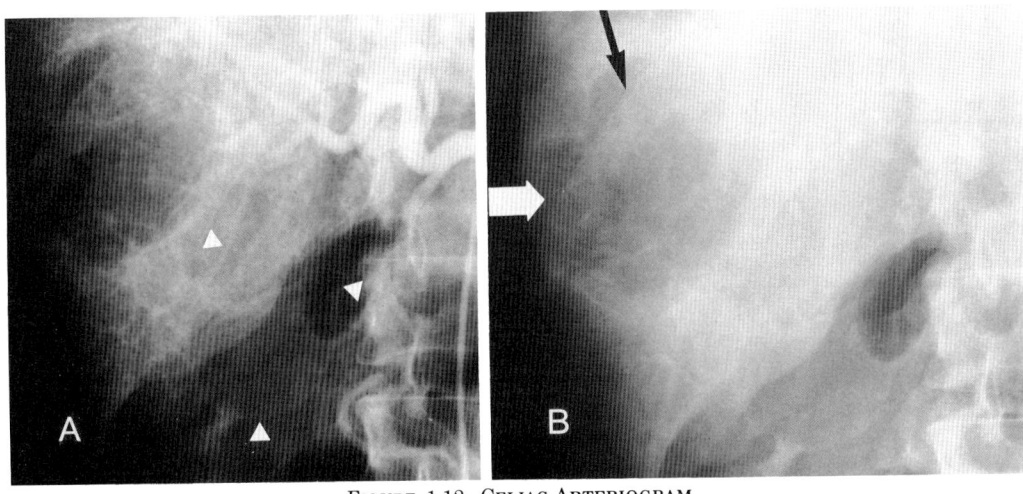

FIGURE 1.12. CELIAC ARTERIOGRAM

A: Speckled arterial hepatogram; the intrahepatic lucency is a hematoma. Note the normal gallbladder (*arrowheads*). *B:* The portal hepatogram is smoother; the hematoma (*arrows*) is still visible.

hepatogram is that resulting from arterial flow alone, as in a selective proper hepatic, right hepatic, or mid-hepatic arteriogram. Frequently an arterial hepatogram is spotted due to innumerable 1 mm densities throughout to represent opacified hepatic lobules (Figs. 1.11 and 1.12).

A pure portal hepatogram results from opacification of solely portal flow, as in splenic or superior mesenteric arteriography (no replaced hepatic artery) and direct portography (either via the spleen or the liver). The portal hepatogram is usually smooth and homogeneous (Fig. 1.12) (1).

A mixed hepatogram is observed in celiac arteriography or superior mesenteric arteriography when the right hepatic artery is replaced. The first portion of contrast material reaches the parenchyma via arterial flow, producing an initial arterial hepatogram, and the second portion reaches the parenchyma via portal flow, producing a slightly delayed portal hepatogram. Details of arterial morphology and the hepatogram are inferior to those obtainable with selective hepatic injection.

As opposed to the dual supply of normal parenchyma, neoplasms and other mass lesions are supplied almost exclusively by the hepatic artery and are almost always hypovascular during portography. This difference in blood supply can be exploited by selective hepatic arteriography. On the selective study, both normal parenchyma and tumors are initially opacified because both have arterial flow. Later, however, a tumor stands out as an opacified mass because the parenchymal stain is washed out by unopacified portal flow (1).

On a celiac injection, only half of the bolus arrives via the common hepatic artery and opacification of both parenchyma and tumor is suboptimal. When the second half arrives via the portal vein, parenchymal density continues to increase and tumors with minimal neovascularity become relatively hypovascular in the hepatogram phase. Since the eye is more sensitive to small increases in radiologic density than to decreases, the pure arterial hepatogram is superior to the portal hepatogram and the mixed hepatogram in detecting space-occupying disease. Many tumors less than 1 cm, and even as small as 1–2 mm, can be detected by infusion hepatic arteriography (3–5). Even "hypovascular" hepatocellular carcinoma and "hypovascular" metastases (hypovascular and difficult to detect on celiac injection) exhibit some degree of stain on infusion hepatic arteriography (1) and can be detected.

Transhepatic portography is discussed in the section on interventional radiology of the liver, and hepatic venography is discussed in the sections on cirrhosis and portal hypertension.

REFERENCES

1. Chuang VP: Hepatic tumor angiography: a subject review. *Radiology* 148:633–639, 1983.
2. Takashima T, Matsui O: Infusion hepatic angiography in the detection of small hepatocellular carcinomas. *Radiology* 136:321–325, 1980.
3. Wirtanen GW: A new angiographic technique in the diagnosis of liver tumor. *Radiology* 108:51–54, 1973.
4. Rosch J, Freeny P, Antonovic R, Gutierrez OH: Infusion hepatic angiography in diagnosis of liver metastases. *Cancer* 38:2278–2286, 1976.
5. Freeny PC, Antonovic R, Gutierrez OH, Rosch J: Diagnostic effectiveness of infusion hepatic angiography: a comparison with the conventional technique. *ROFO* 124:534–541, 1976.

NORMAL ULTRASOUND OF THE LIVER

On ultrasound, the parenchyma of the liver demonstrates a homogenous, moderately echogenic pattern, equal to or slightly less echogenic than the pancreas and more echogenic than normal renal cortical tissue (Fig. 1.13) (1).

The normal hepatic artery and bile ducts are not routinely visualized above the level of the porta hepatis. Interspersed within the parenchyma of the liver are tubular, fluid-filled structures representing the portal and hepatic venous circulations. Differentiation of the portal and hepatic veins can be accomplished in various ways. Tracing the vein of interest back to either the porta hepatis or the inferior vena cava is an obvious but tedious solution. Because the portal veins are encased in a collagenous sheath, their walls appear thicker and have marginal echoes more pronounced than those of the hepatic veins (Figs. 1.13*A, B* and 1.14*A*). The branching angles of the portal and hepatic veins have different orientations: the apex of an angle of portal branching will be oriented horizontally toward the porta hepatis, whereas the apex at the bifurcation of a hepatic vein is longitudinally oriented toward the inferior vena cava (Fig. 1.14). Also, the caliber of an hepatic vein increases progressively as it courses toward the diaphragm while a portal venous channel is largest in the porta hepatis (2).

The main portal vein arises just to the right of midline at the junction of the splenic and superior mesenteric vein. From here it courses cephalad and rightward into the porta hepatis where it lies anterior to the inferior vena cava before it bifurcates into right and left branches which then penetrate the liver substance (Fig. 1.15) (3).

The common hepatic artery arises from the celiac axis just cephalad to the body of the pancreas (Fig. 1.16*A*). From its origin the common hepatic artery courses to the right and, in the area of the neck of the pancreas, gives off the gastroduodenal artery. The gastroduodenal artery is seen approximately 30% of the time on ultrasound examination on the anterior surface of the neck of the pancreas. Continuing on now

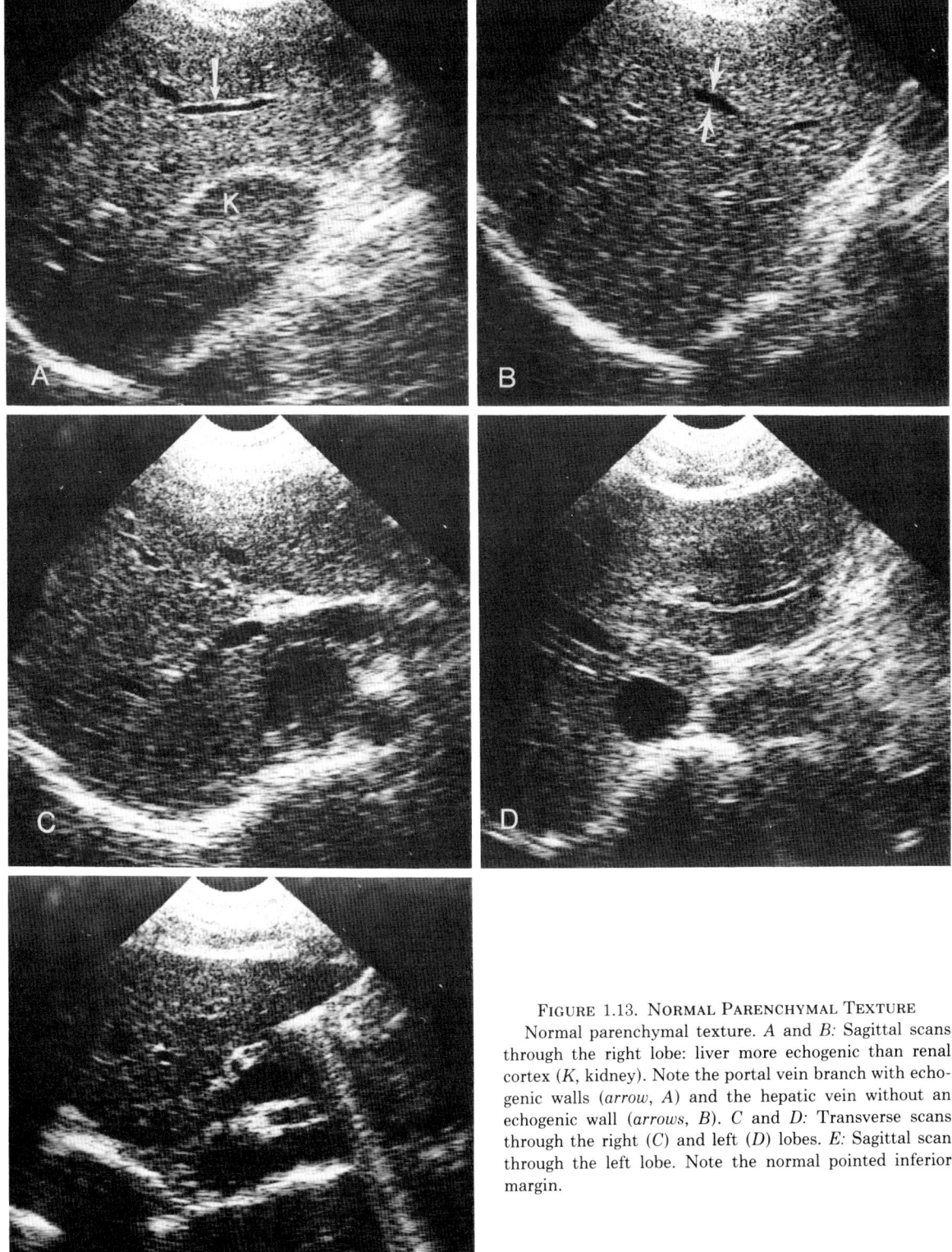

FIGURE 1.13. NORMAL PARENCHYMAL TEXTURE

Normal parenchymal texture. *A* and *B:* Sagittal scans through the right lobe: liver more echogenic than renal cortex (*K*, kidney). Note the portal vein branch with echogenic walls (*arrow, A*) and the hepatic vein without an echogenic wall (*arrows, B*). *C* and *D:* Transverse scans through the right (*C*) and left (*D*) lobes. *E:* Sagittal scan through the left lobe. Note the normal pointed inferior margin.

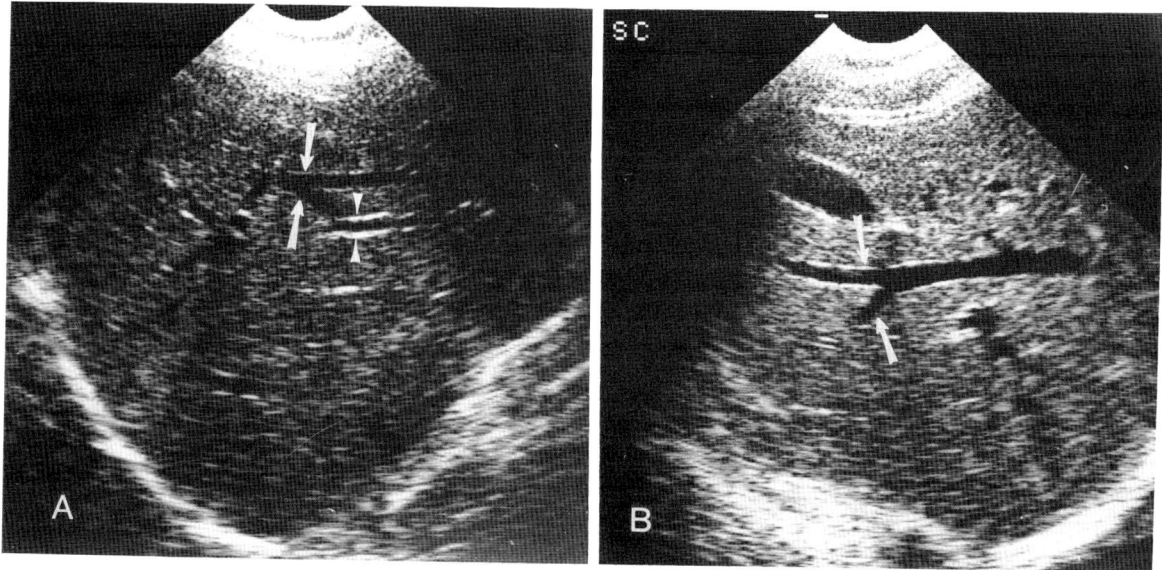

FIGURE 1.14. PORTAL AND HEPATIC VEINS
A: Longitudinally oriented hepatic venous bifurcation (*arrows*) pointing towards the hepatic venous confluence (sagittal scan, right lobe). Hepatic veins have relatively anechoic walls, whereas the portal veins have echogenic walls (*arrowheads*). *B:* Transversely oriented portal venous bifurcation (*arrows*) pointing towards the porta hepatis (transverse scan).

as the proper hepatic artery it turns anteriorly and cephalad to run along the hepatoduodenal ligament toward the porta hepatis with the common hepatic and common bile duct. Usually the proper hepatic artery lies anterior to the portal vein and to the left of the common bile duct in the hepatoduodenal ligament (Figs. 1.15C and 1.16B) (4).

Within the porta hepatis the proper hepatic artery bifurcates or trifurcates, giving rise to a large right and smaller left and middle hepatic arteries. The right hepatic artery turns laterally and enters the liver via the right intersegmental fissure, usually posterior to the bile duct, between the duct and the portal vein.

The other branches of the proper hepatic artery are less consistently imaged than the right hepatic artery. When seen, the middle hepatic artery runs in the left intersegmental fissure where it runs lateral to the ligamentum teres. The left hepatic artery is infrequently seen on ultrasound but can be seen ascending adjacent to the left portal vein when running into the left intersegmental fissure medial to the ligamentum teres (4).

There is much variation in the anatomy of the hepatic artery. Approximately 55–65% of patients have a classic configuration as described above. Ultrasonographically recognizable variations include the 25% or so of patients with right hepatic artery variants. In these patients either all (replaced right hepatic artery) or part (accessory right hepatic artery) of the right hepatic arterial supply arises from the superior mesenteric artery (Fig. 1.16C, D). The replaced accessory or right hepatic artery may course anterior or posterior to the superior mesenteric vein as it runs to the porta hepatis. A variant variety may be entirely retropancreatic or may course through the pancreatic head (4).

The intrahepatic ligaments and the fissures (Figs. 1.17 and 1.18) are rich in collagen and fat which render them highly reflective relative to the liver substance. The falciform ligament courses over the anterior surface of the liver and is in continuity with the ligamentum teres. It can be recognized to the right of the midline on transverse scans as a rounded hyperechoic density within the substance of the liver (Figs. 1.15A, B and 1.18A) (5). The falciform ligament and the ligamentum teres define the border between the lateral and medial segments of the left lobe.

The interlobar or major fissure of the liver runs along a plane connecting the sulcus for the inferior vena cava and the fossa for the gallbladder (Fig. 1.17). Portions of the fissure may be seen as a hyperechoic line owing to the presence of fat and collagen.

The fissure for the ligamentum venosum, which contains the hepatogastric ligament, is identified as an echogenic line coursing from the porta hepatis transversely deep within the liver

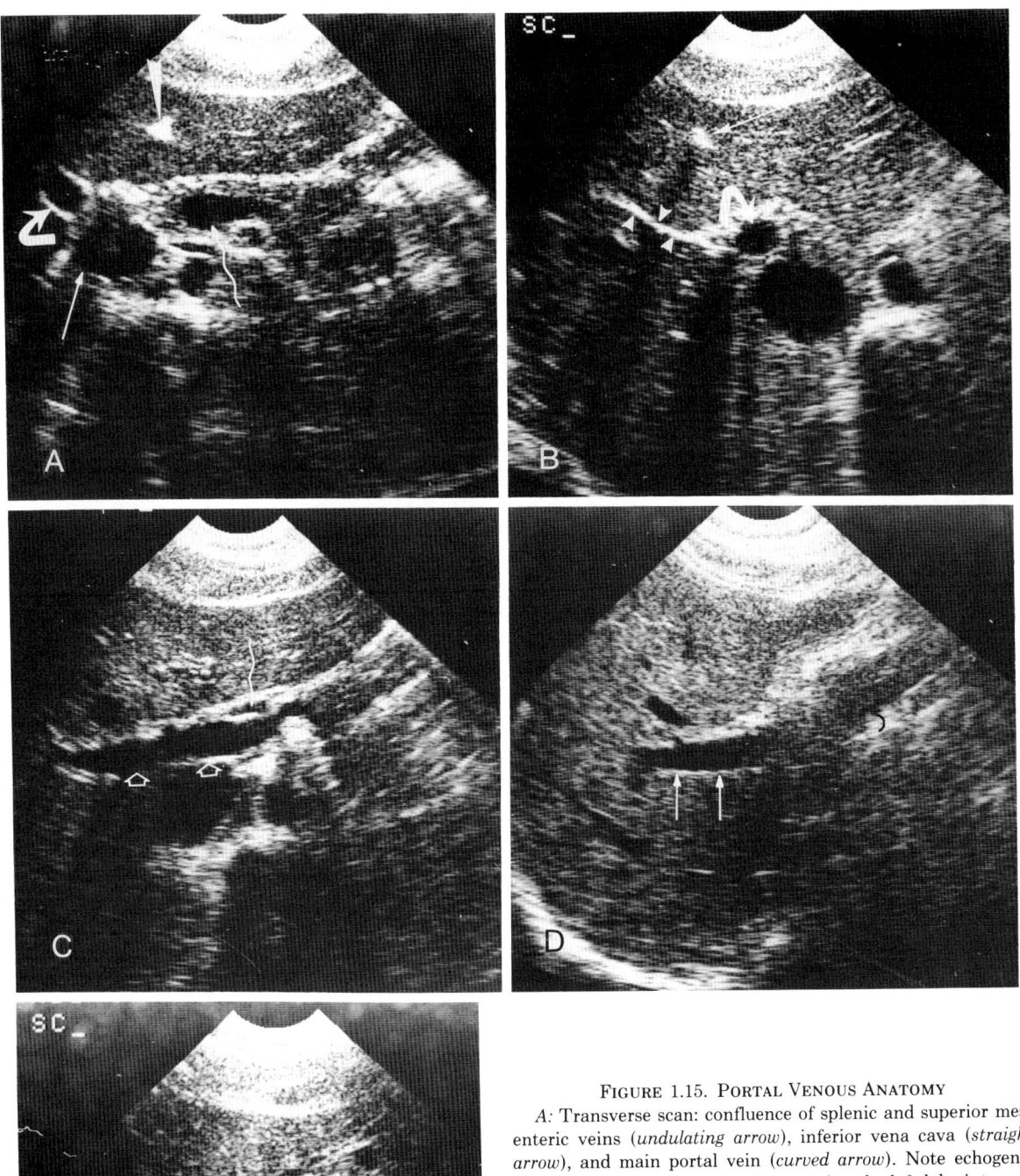

FIGURE 1.15. PORTAL VENOUS ANATOMY

A: Transverse scan: confluence of splenic and superior mesenteric veins (*undulating arrow*), inferior vena cava (*straight arrow*), and main portal vein (*curved arrow*). Note echogenic ligamentum teres (*arrowhead*) separating the left lobe into medial and lateral segments. *B:* Transverse scan cephalad to *A:* main portal vein (*curved arrow*) in the hepatoduodenal ligament anterior to the inferior vena cava. Note the major fissure (*arrowheads*) and the shadowing ligamentum teres (*arrow*). *C:* Angled transverse view laying out the main portal vein (*arrows*) anterior to the inferior vena cava. Note a portion of the proper hepatic artery (*undulating arrow*). *D* and *E:* Transverse views of the right (*arrows, D*) and left (*arrows, E*) portal veins. *E* is cephalad to *D*.

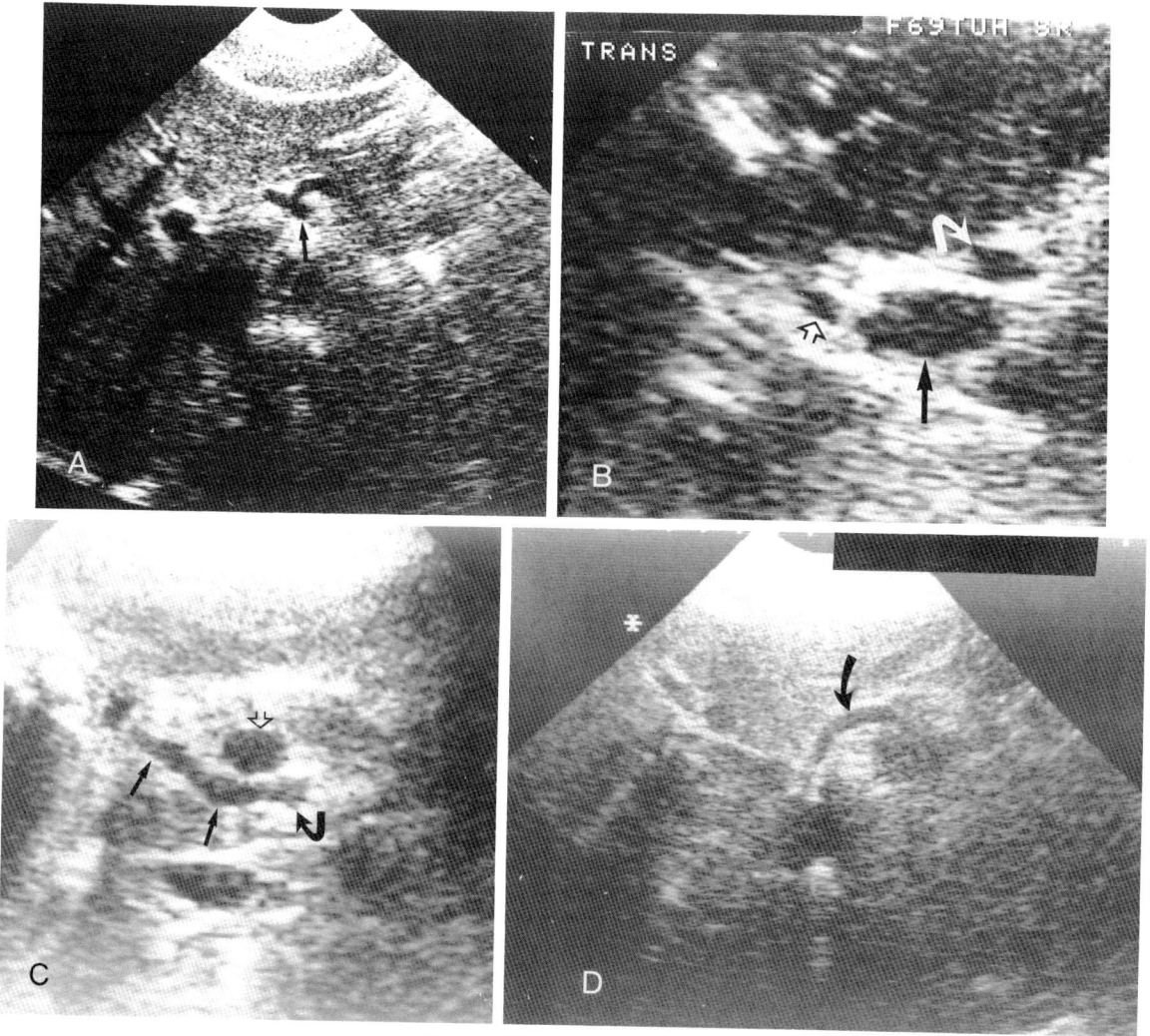

FIGURE 1.16. ARTERIAL SCANS

A: Transverse scan: celiac artery (*arrow*) bifurcating into the common hepatic and splenic arteries. *B:* Magnified transverse scan through the hepatoduodenal ligament: hepatic artery (*curved arrow*) anteromedial to the portal vein (*closed arrow*). Also seen is the common duct (*open arrow*). This is known as the "Mickey Mouse" sign in the hepatoduodenal ligament. *C* and *D:* Replaced right hepatic artery. Transverse sonogram (*C*) shows the replaced right hepatic artery (*arrows*) emanating from the superior mesenteric artery (*curved arrow*) and coursing behind the superior mesenteric vein (*open arrow*). A high transverse scan (*D*) shows the splenic artery (*arrows*) coming off the celiac and no visible hepatic artery.

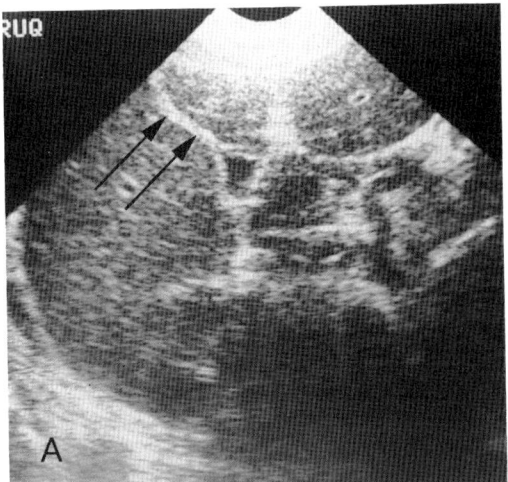

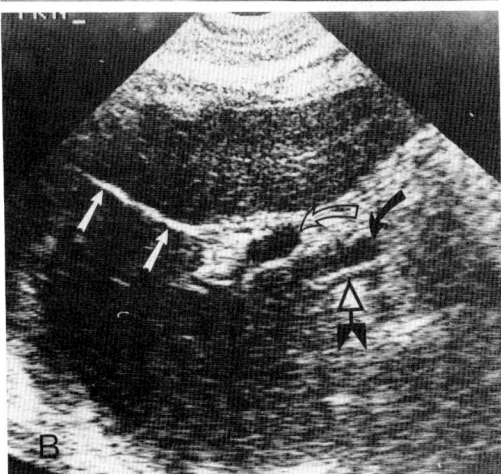

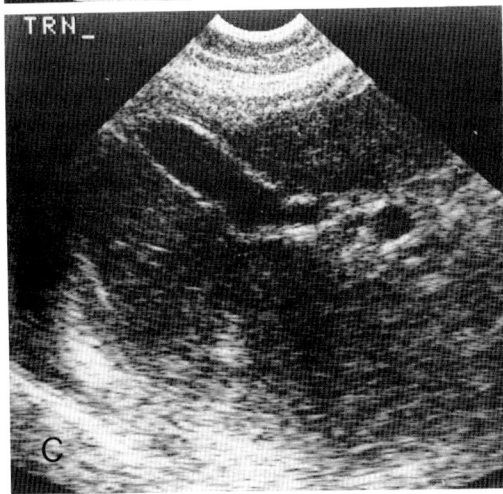

FIGURE 1.17. SONOGRAPHIC APPEARANCE OF THE MAJOR FISSURE

A and *B:* Transverse scans in different patients, showing different locations of the major fissure (*arrows*) due to different relative lobe sizes. Note portal vein (*open curved arrow*) and inferior vena cava (*tailed arrow*) and papillary process of the caudate lobe (*curved arrow*) in *B. C:* a trans-

substance. This fissure marks the border between the lateral segment of the left lobe and the caudate lobe (Fig. 1.18) (6).

The lobes of the liver as defined by surgical considerations are demarcated by the hepatic veins that course between them and form the boundaries of the various hepatic segments and lobes (Fig. 1.19). In contradistinction to the hepatic veins, the portal veins generally lie within hepatic segments. The proximal left portal vein is a notable exception as it partially divides the medial from the lateral segment of the left lobe.

The right and left hepatic lobes are separated by the major fissure of the liver (Fig. 1.17). Although the major fissure may be identified on most ultrasound exams it is often an incomplete boundary.

The left segmental (intersegmental) fissure divides the medial segment from the lateral segment of the left lobe. The lateral segment of the left lobe abuts against the caudate lobe, separated from it by the fissure of the ligamentum venosum (a remnant of the fetal ductus venosus which acted as a shunt for oxygenated blood from the umbilical vein to the inferior vena cava).

Although the hepatic veins form ideal segmental boundaries within the liver they are often identified only on the most superior ultrasound (Fig. 1.19) or CT cuts and therefore other landmarks that lie within the plane of the hepatic veins must be used to identify segmental anatomy in cross-section. The right lobe is separated into anterior and posterior segments by the right hepatic vein on cephalad scans. At lower levels the hepatic vein is no longer a constant landmark and the segmental boundary becomes an arbitrary division between the anterior and posterior branches of the right portal vein.

The right lobe of the liver is separated from the left lobe by somewhat more constant landmarks. On superior transverse sections the middle hepatic vein divides the lobes. On more inferior sections the major fissure, filled with a variable amount of fat, and the gallbladder act as the lobar boundary.

The left hepatic vein forms the most superior border between the medial and lateral segments of the left lobe. It parallels and briefly crosses the intersegmental fissure which forms the major caudad boundary. At a more caudad level the left portal vein acts as the intersegmental boundary. This is unusual in that the hepatic veins usually

verse scan just caudad to *B* to show the location of the gallbladder just beneath the major fissure.

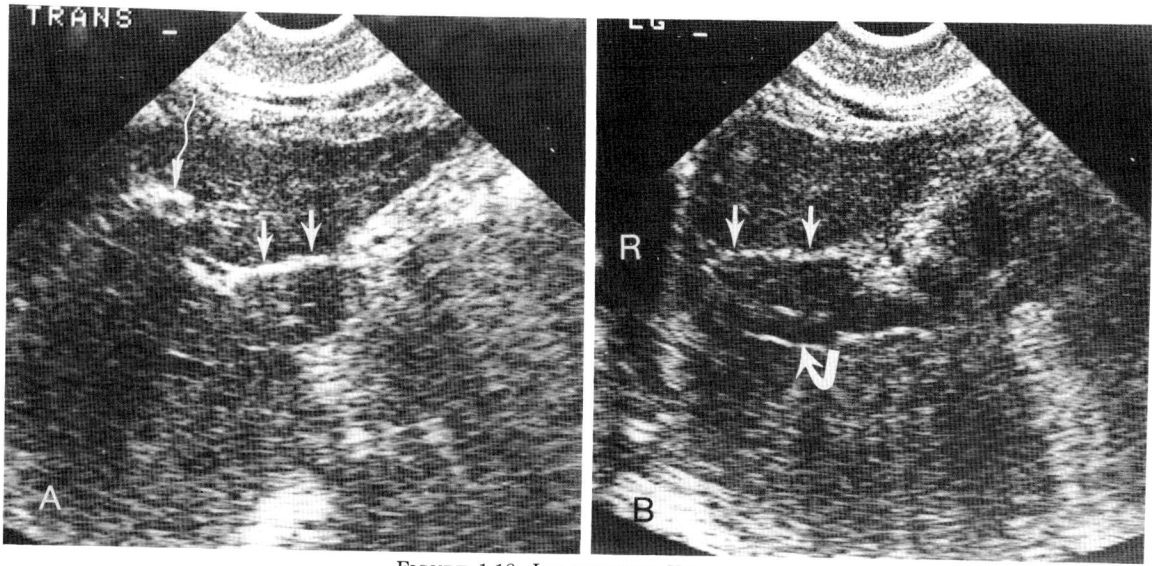

FIGURE 1.18. LIGAMENTUM VENOSUM
A and *B:* Transverse (*A*) and parasagittal scans (*B*) of the fissure of the ligamentum venosum (*arrows*) separating the left lobe from the more posterior caudate lobe. Note ligamentum teres (*undulating arrow*) in *A* as well as the normal pointed lateral tip of the left lobe (*R*, right atrium; *curved arrow*, inferior vena cava).

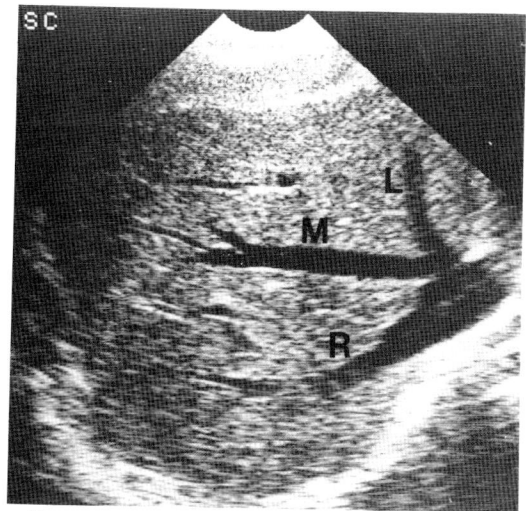

FIGURE 1.19. HEPATIC VEINS ON SONOGRAPHY
Transverse scan at the confluence of the hepatic veins showing left (*L*), middle (*M*), and right (*R*) hepatic veins.

act as segmental boundaries. On the most caudad sections obtained the ligamentum teres, surrounded by fat, acts as the segmental division (7).

Sonographic Determination of Liver Size

Several attempts have been made at sonographic measurement of liver size. Livers measuring 13.0 cm or less in the midhepatic line (sagittal dimension) are said to be of normal size 93% of the time, whereas a measurement of 15.5 cm or greater indicates hepatomegaly in 75%. Unfortunately, 25% in this study fell into the borderline zone (13–15.5 cm) (8). Another study compared cross-sectional area measurements to measurements of the sagittal length of the liver in the right midclavicular line and the midline, and found no advantage to the former. Normal ranges plus or minus two standard deviations for the sagittal lengths in a second study were 10.5 ± 3 cm and 8.1 ± 3.8 cm, respectively, in 915 healthy subjects (9). Liver volumes can be calculated from serial transverse scans by point integration (10); however, this is tedious.

In addition to a sagittal measurement, we rely on subjective assessment of liver size by the physician performing the real-time examination and find rounding of the normally tapered lateral edge of the left lobe on transverse scans to be a helpful sign of hepatomegaly.

REFERENCES

1. Kane, RA: Sonographic anatomy of the liver. *Semin Ultrasound* 3:190–197, 1981.
2. Hill MC, Sanders RC: Sonography of the upper abdominal venous system. In Sanders RC, Hill MC (eds): *Ultrasound Annual 1983*. New York, Raven Press, 1983, pp 271–313.
3. Callen PW, Filly RA, DeMartini WJ: The left portal vein: A possible source of confusion on ultrasound. *Radiology* 130:205–256, 1979.
4. Ralls PW, Quinn MF, Rogers WF, et al: Sonographic anatomy of the hepatic artery. *AJR* 136:1059–1063, 1981.

5. Hillman BJ, D'Orsi CJ, Smith EH, Bartrum RJ: Ultrasonic appearance of the falciform ligament. *AJR* 132:205–206, 1979.
6. Brown BM, Filly RA, Callen PW: Ultrasonographic anatomy of the caudate lobe. *J Ultrasound Med* 1:189–192, 1982.
7. Sexton CC, Zeman RK: Correlation of computed tomography, sonography and gross anatomy of the liver. *AJR* 141:711–718, 1983.
8. Gosink BB, Leymaster CE: Ultrasonic determination of hepatomegaly. *J Clin Ultrasound* 9:37–41, 1981.
9. Niederau C, Sonnenberg A, Muller JE, Erckenkbrecht JF, Scholten T, Fritsch WP: Sonographic measurments of the normal liver, spleen, pancreas, and portal vein. *Radiology* 149:537–540, 1983.
10. Fritschy P, Robotti G, Schneekloth G, Vock P: Measurement of liver volume by ultrasound and computed tomography. *J Clin Ultrasound* 11:299–303, 1983.

COMPUTED TOMOGRAPHY OF THE NORMAL LIVER

Normal hepatic parenchymal tissue is homogeneous, although variations in density exist from patient to patient. Without contrast enhancement, the liver usually measures between 40 and 70 Hounsfield units (HU), usually equal to or greater than the density of intravascular blood and other visceral structures such as the spleen (1). When the density of the liver is greater than that of flowing blood the larger intrahepatic vessels will appear as low attenuation structures within the liver (Fig. 1.20). Most of the intrahepatic vessels seen on CT are veins, recognizable by their round, oval, or linear branching patterns.

The hepatic veins are the most prominent in the upper portion of the liver where they converge to enter the inferior vena cava and in the intersegmental fissures where they serve as intrahepatic lobar delineators. The remainder of the vessels seen on CT are the portal vein branches emanating from the porta hepatis. The corresponding branches of the hepatic artery and bile ducts are smaller and are not seen in normal patients.

The hepatic fissures are usually well depicted on CT as fat-containing lines between denser hepatic parenchyma. The ligamentum teres is a circular density in the fat-containing falciform ligament (Fig. 1.21). The surgical lobar anatomy of the liver is shown well by CT, and its description as well as a description of the fissures is found in the ultrasound section. One difference is that the major fissure is often not depicted well on CT, and the boundary between right and left lobes below the level of the middle hepatic vein is approximated by a line connecting the gallbladder and the inferior vena cava (Fig. 1.22). An anatomic feature deserving mention here is the papillary process of the caudate lobe. The caudate lobe is on the posterosuperior surface of the liver, separated from the rest of the liver anteriorly by the fissure for the ligamentum venosum and posterolaterally by the inferior vena cava. At the level of the porta hepatis, the caudate lobe is connected to the right lobe by the caudate process, extending laterally between the inferior vena cava and the portal vein. The papillary process protrudes to the left, sometimes anteriorly and inferiorly. It may appear separate from the liver on transverse sections, mimicking an extrahepatic mass (2).

Intravenous Contrast Material in Hepatic CT

The effects of intravenous contrast material on the CT appearance of the liver depend on the relative concentration of iodinated material within the vascular and extravascular compartments at the time of the exposure. This relative concentration in turn depends on the amount of contrast material given, the rate of administration, and the time elapsed between contrast administration and the performance of the scan itself.

Approximately 20 sec after an intravenous bolus, the hepatic artery is opacified. Shortly thereafter there is opacification of the portal veins. Maximal enhancement of normal parenchyma occurs at 45–60 sec, coinciding with relatively dense portal and hepatic venous enhancement (3). Most lesions are best seen at this time as low density regions (because of the preponderance of hepatic arterial supply versus portal venous supply in tumors, the opposite of normal parenchyma). Over the next several minutes the density of vessels decreases, whereas that of the parenchyma is relatively stable as contrast material accumulates in the extravascular compartment. At 4–6 hr postcontrast, hepatic parenchyma is enhanced relative to other structures because of active hepatocyte accumulation prior to biliary secretion (4).

CT of the liver is usually performed after bowel opacification with oral contrast material. Scans may be performed without intravenous contrast for follow-up of known disease or prior to enhanced scans for a tailored liver examination, but most routine studies are performed with contrast only. The worst results are to be ex-

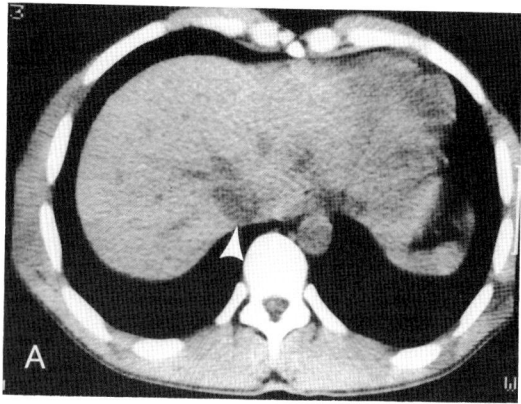

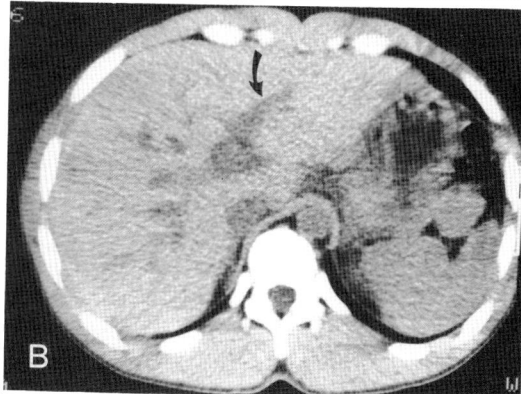

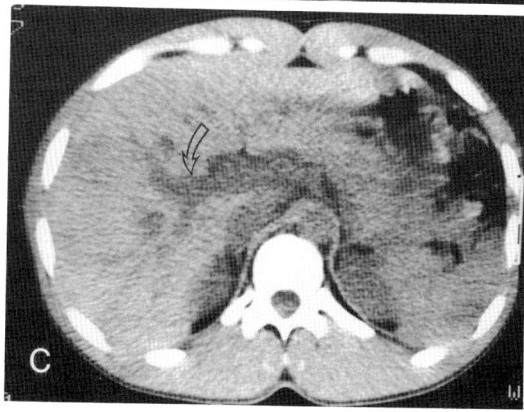

FIGURE 1.20. NORMAL NONCONTRAST CT
A: Level of the confluence of the hepatic veins, which are seen as tubular lucencies heading toward the inferior vena cava (*arrowhead*). *B* and *C:* Levels of left (*closed arrow*) and right (*open arrow*) main portal veins. Smaller portal radicles are seen as lucencies at these levels.

pected if scanning is delayed until after a contrast infusion is over, as masses can be rendered isodense. A bolus injection followed by an infusion that is continued for the duration of the examination will maintain high plasma iodine levels and usually avoids this problem. A multiple bolus technique is even better, but cumbersome (5). A compromise that we use successfully

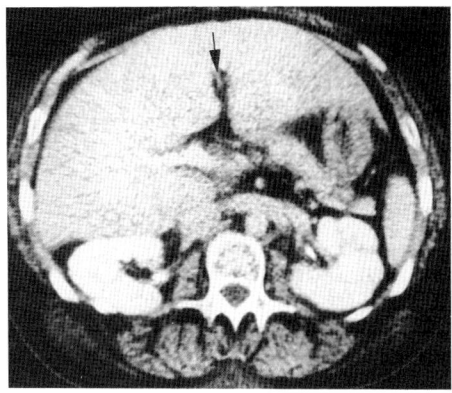

FIGURE 1.21. UMBILICAL VEIN IN THE LIGAMENTUM TERES (*arrow*) WITHIN FALCIFORM LIGAMENT

is a rapid infusion (augmented by injecting the bottle with 75–100 cc of air) throughout the scan of 150 cc of 60% contrast material (Fig. 1.23).

Dynamic Scanning

Dynamic scanning refers to giving a rapid bolus of contrast and obtaining scans as rapidly as possible to utilize the vascular phase of the bolus. The sodium salt of a contrast medium is preferable to its meglumine counterpart, due to significantly lower viscosity. The scanning may be done at a single level to better characterize a known lesion or at sequential levels using table incrementation (Fig. 1.24). This latter technique has been referred to as computed angiotomography when especially rapid scans are performed during breath holding to visualize vascular structures at multiple levels (6). This technique is limited, however, by tube cooling requirements, and the rapid scanning time necessary may markedly reduce resolution due to photopenic images.

High resolution survey dynamic scanning may be performed using conventional scan times on modern third or fourth generation equipment. In this technique, a large dose of contrast material (e.g., 50–70 g of iodine) is injected over 2–3 min, while the area of interest is scanned sequentially. Foley et al. (7), used this method to evaluate the liver in 56 patients with suspected hepatic metastases and noted that the average density difference between liver and lesion was 20 HU before contrast and 60 HU after.

Intra-arterial techniques, due to their invasive nature, are not commonly used for CT studies. They have usually been performed on patients with intra-arterial chemotherapy pumps (8), or as an adjunct to conventional angiography (9, 10).

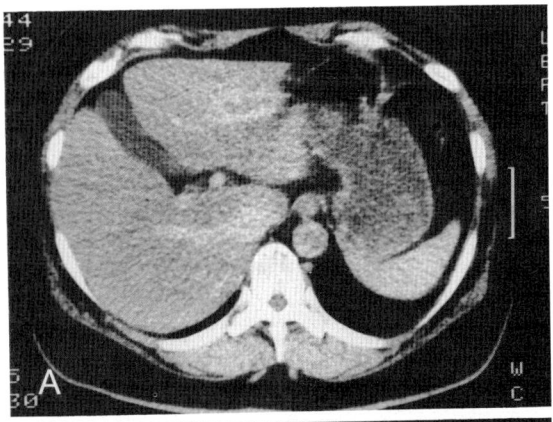
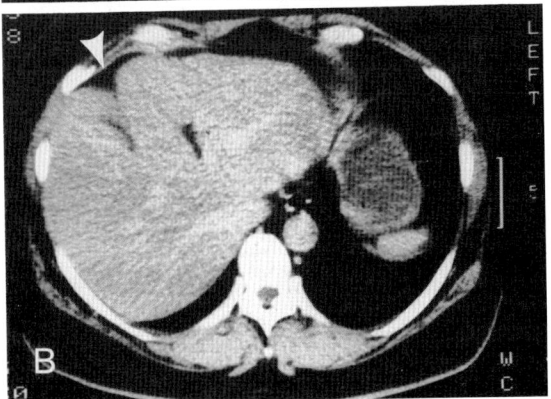
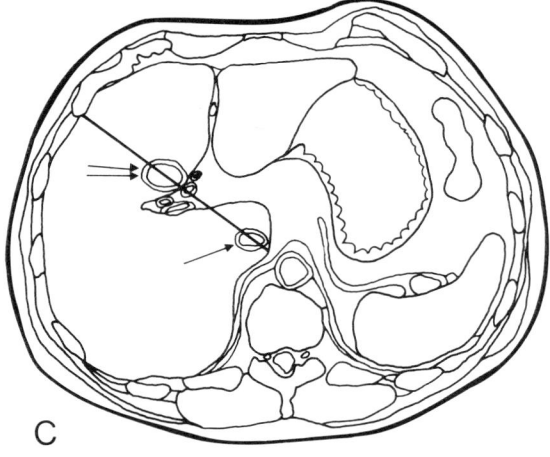

FIGURE 1.22. MAJOR HEPATIC FISSURE ON CT

A and *B:* Scans through (*A*) and just above (*B*) the gallbladder. The gallbladder is lying in the fissure surrounded by fat and part of the fissure is still seen (*arrowhead*) just cephalad to the gallbladder. *C:* Illustration of method of major fissure localization using a line connecting the gallbladder (*double arrows*) to the inferior vena cava (*single arrow*). This line is then drawn in the same place on scans at other levels.

FIGURE 1.23. NORMAL LIVER CT WITH AIR BOLUS AUGMENTED RAPID INFUSION

Normal liver CT with air bolus augmented rapid infusion. This is purposely a representative case, not a superb one; sometimes vascular anatomy is shown better (see normal vascular anatomy section). *A* and *B:* Cephalad portion of liver: small hepatic vein branches barely visible as radiodense lines. *C* and *D:* Fissure for the ligamentum venosum (*arrow*) dividing caudate lobe from the left lobe. A lesser sac recess is in this location. The left portal vein is well opacified (*curved arrow*). *E* and *F:* Fat-containing porta hepatis (*arrows*) anterior to the caudate lobe with enhanced left portal vein (*open arrow*) and right portal vein (*open curved arrow*) demonstrated. *G* and *H:* Lower cuts show a few branching opacified veins as well as the gallbladder (*arrow*) and confluence of the splenic and superior mesenteric veins (*arrowhead*). *I:* Scan through the porta hepatis at the tail end of a routine drip infusion CT. Intrahepatic vessels cannot be discerned.

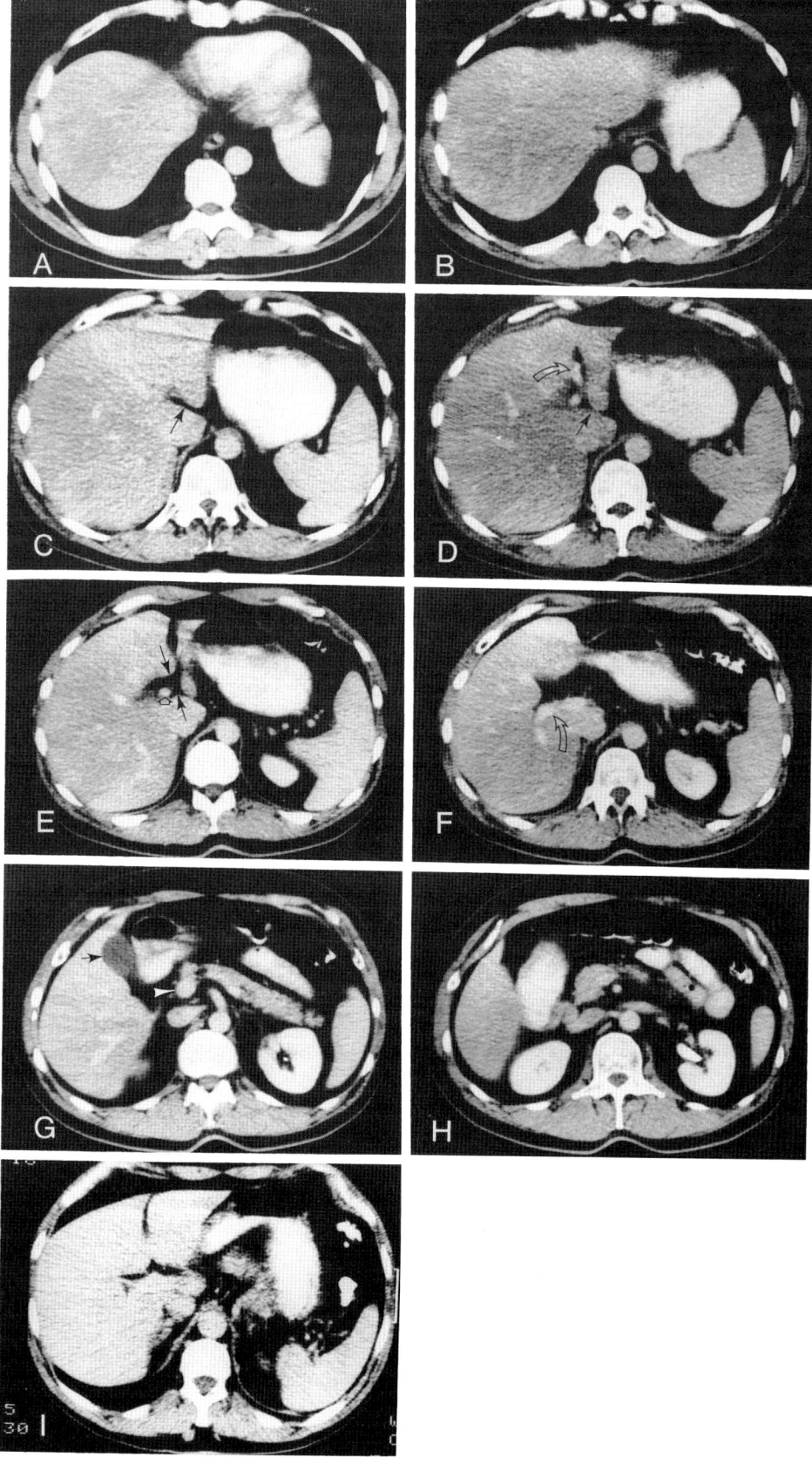

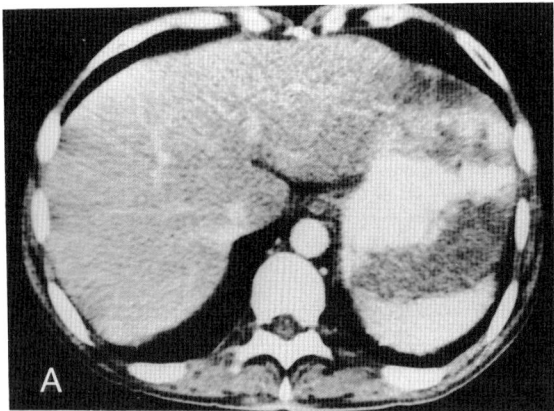

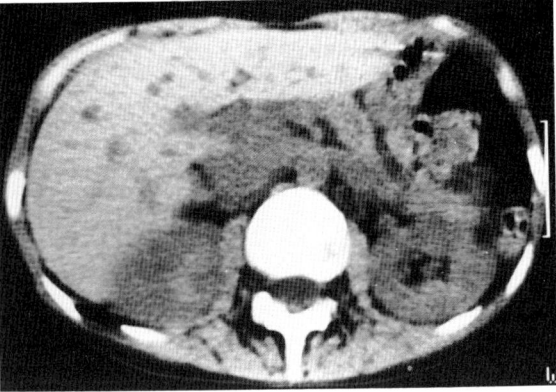

FIGURE 1.25. ENHANCED LIVER THE MORNING AFTER ADMINISTRATION OF TELEPAQUE FOR AN ORAL CHOLECYSTOGRAM

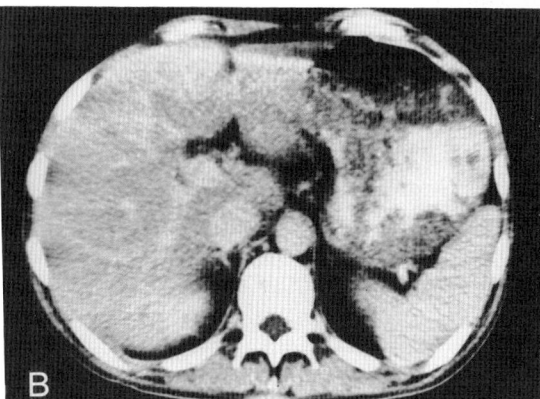

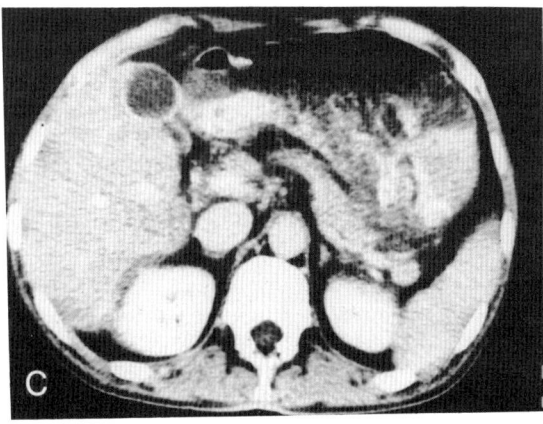

FIGURE 1.24. A–C: DYNAMIC SCAN WITH AUTOMATIC TABLE INCREMENTATION: NOTE GOOD DEPICTION OF INTRAHEPATIC VESSELS AND INTENSE GALLBLADDER WALL ENHANCEMENT.

Dynamic scanning may be performed using selective infusion of contrast material into the hepatic artery, referred to as CT angiography (CTA). Contrast can be injected at 3–5 ml/sec by a power injector or manually as a 10–25-ml bolus (8, 9, 10). Neoplasms, which receive their primary blood supply from the hepatic artery, will be enhanced to a greater extent than normal liver tissue. This technique may be especially valuable for detecting lesions in the left lobe, an area problematic for both ultrasound and conventional angiography.

Another approach to visualizing liver tumors is CT portography. In this method, 70–100 ml of contrast material are infused into the superior mesenteric or splenic artery at a rate of 0.4–0.6 ml/sec (11) or 25–30 ml at a rate of 3.0–6.0 ml/sec (10), enhancing normal liver tissue via the portal vein and leaving lesions without portal supply unenhanced. This method may be even more sensitive than CTA, although more contrast material is needed. For hypervascular nodules less than 0.5 cm, however, angiography is more sensitive. This is consistent with the finding that small experimentally implanted hepatic tumors may be perfused partly by the portal vein before generating a new arterial supply from the hepatic system (12).

Cholecystographic and Cholangiographic Contrast Materials

Neither oral cholecystographic nor intravenous cholangiographic contrast material has enjoyed widespread use in clinical liver CT (Fig. 1.25).

Liver Size by CT

Liver size can be determined by measurements as discussed in the ultrasound section. Liver volume can be measured by adding area measurements in successive transverse scans (13, 14), and normal volume is 1500 ± 230 cm^3 (one standard deviation) (13). Most physicians still assess hepatomegaly on CT subjectively.

REFERENCES

1. Haaga JR and Alfidi RJ: *Computed Tomography of the Whole Body.* St. Louis, C. V. Mosby, 1983, pp 575–579.
2. Auh YM, Rosen H, Rubenstein WA, Engel IA, Whalen JP, Kazam E: CT of the papillary process of the caudate lobe of the liver. *AJR* 142:535–538, 1984.
3. Marchal GY, Baert AL, Wilms GE: CT of noncystic liver lesions: bolus enhancement. *AJR* 135:57–65, 1980.
4. Rauschkolb EN, Steinberg RM, Sandler CM, et al: Delayed computed tomography of the liver following intravenous contrast. Presented at the 68th Annual Meeting of the RSNA, Chicago, Nov. 1982.
5. Rossi P, Baert A, Marchal W, et al: Multiple bolus technique versus single bolus infusion of contrast medium to obtain prolonged contrast enhancement of the pancreas. *Radiology* 144:929–931, 1982.
6. Moss AA, Dean PB, Axel L, Goldberg HI, Glazer GM, Friedman MA: Dynamic CT of hepatic masses with intravenous and intraarterial contrast material. *AJR* 138:847–852, 1982.
7. Foley WD, Berland LL, Lawson TL, Smith DF, Thorsen MK: Contrast enhancement technique for dynamic computed tomographic scanning. *Radiology* 147:797–803, 1983.
8. Prando A, Wallace S, Bernardino ME, Lindell MM: CT arteriography of the liver. *Radiology* 130:697–701, 1979.
9. Freeny PC, Marks WM: Computed tomographic arteriography of the liver. *Radiology* 148:193–197, 1983.
10. Nakao N, Miura K, Wada Y, Miura T: CT arteriography in hepatocellular carcinoma. *J Comput Assist Tomgr* 7:780–787, 1983.
11. Clark RA, Matsui D: CT of liver tumors. *Semin Roentgenol* 18:149–162, 1983.
12. Ackerman NB, Lien WM, Kondi ES, Silverman NA: The blood supply of experimental liver metastasis. I. The distribution of hepatic artery and portal vein blood to "small" and "large" tumors. *Surgery* 66:1067–1072, 1969.
13. Henderson JM, Heymsfield SB, Horowitz J, Kutner MH: Measurement of liver and spleen volume by computed tomography. *Radiology* 141:525–527, 1981.
14. Fritschy P, Robotti C, Schneekloth G, Vock P: Measurement of liver volume by ultrasound and computed tomography. *J Clin Ultrasound* 11:299–303, 1983.

NORMAL RADIONUCLIDE IMAGING OF THE LIVER

Liver scintigraphy utilizes radioactive isotopes coupled to various compounds to provide insight into functional anatomy. The two most frequently used agents are ^{99m}Tc-labeled sulfur colloid, for the visualization of the reticuloendothelial system, and ^{99m}Tc-labeled iminodiacetic acid derivatives for assessment of the hepatocyte-biliary system. The hepatobiliary scintigram is discussed in detail in the biliary section. Other agents such as gallium citrate and ^{99m}Tc-labeled red cells may also contribute useful information (1).

The liver contains the bulk of the body's reticuloendothelial cells (80–90%), with the remaining portion divided almost evenly between the spleen and the bone marrow. The hepatic reticuloendothelial cells (Kupffer cells) are distributed along the linings of the hepatic sinusoids.

Techniques for Liver Scintigraphy

A ^{99m}Tc-sulfur colloid liver-spleen scan is easy to perform. No patient preparation is necessary, and no adverse reactions to the radiopharmaceutical agents have been reported. The usual adult dose ranges from 2 to 10 mCi, with an average recommended dose of 5 mCi. The dose for children is 70 µCi/kg of body weight, with a minimum dose of 500 µCi. For rapid sequential flow studies (radionuclide angiography), 5–10 mCi of ^{99m}Tc-sulfur colloid are necessary. Radiation exposure is low, 0.2–0.3 rad/mCi (2).

Technetium-99m sulfur colloid particles range in size from 100–300 mµ. They are inert, inorganic colloids which do not undergo biologic turnover once within the Kupffer cells. The particles have a blood half-life ($t_{1/2}$) of approximately 2 min, and essentially all are cleared by the reticuloendothelial system. Normally, 80–90% of the ^{99m}Tc-sulfur colloid is trapped by the Kupffer cells of the liver, 5–10% by the spleen, and a smaller amount by the bone marrow.

Twenty to thirty minutes following the intravenous administration of ^{99m}Tc-sulfur colloid, 500–700K count scintiscans are obtained in the supine and/or upright position in anterior, right-anterior oblique, right-lateral, posterior, left-anterior oblique, and left-lateral projections utilizing a standard or large field of view gamma camera set at a photopeak of 140 keV and a 20% window with a low energy parallel hole collimator. An additional image is obtained in the anterior projection with a marker of known size, such as a lead bar or radioactive ruler, superimposed on the liver. The marker is placed over the inferior rib, allowing the liver's position in relation to this rib to be established, as well as an estimate of its size. Thus, a low lying or inferiorly displaced liver can be distinguished from hepatomegaly.

If a radionuclide angiogram is being performed, anterior sequential 2–3 sec images of the liver are obtained following the bolus injection of the radiotracer. Images can be recorded by computer for later display or on film. Radionuclide ^{99m}Tc-sulfur colloid angiography reflects regional blood flow. The liver receives 75–80% of its blood supply from the portal circulation and 20–25% from the systemic circulation via the hepatic artery. Thus, liver visualization lags 8–12 sec behind the kidney and spleen (3).

If radionuclide blood pool angiography is to be employed, the patient is injected with 15 mCi of ^{99m}Tc-labeled red blood cells. Anterior sequential 2-sec images of the liver are obtained for 1 min followed by immediate and 1–2 hr delayed anterior, right-lateral and posterior liver scans. The rapid sequence flow images reflect regional blood flow, while the immediate and delayed scans reflect the distribution of the liver's sinusoidal vasculature, i.e., a parameter most important when evaluating the degree of vascularity of an intrahepatic space-occupying lesion (3, 4).

Direct hepatic artery injection of radiopharmaceuticals such as ^{99m}Tc macroaggregated albumin can be employed to assess intrahepatic tumor accessibility to intra-arterial chemotherapy. If the radiopharmaceutical is identified within the tumor deposits (photopenic areas on technetium sulfur colloid liver scan), then direct instillation of chemotherapeutic agents can be employed (5, 6).

The sensitivity of the liver spleen scan for space-occupying disease can be improved by the use of single photon emission computed tomography. However, false-positive findings can occur because of misinterpretation of focal defects due to normal vessels (7, 8) and the cost and complexity of the study is increased.

Gallium-67 citrate is frequently used as an adjuvant imaging agent in the evaluation of liver disease. More often it is used to identify inflammations or abscesses and less commonly to identify neoplasms (9); 3–10 mCi of ^{67}Ga-citrate are injected intravenously where it becomes bound to blood proteins, principally to transferrin and also, possibly, to haptoglobin. By 48 hr after injection, approximately 90% of the ^{67}Ga-citrate has been extracted from the blood. Gallium images are then obtained (10). In a normal patient, gallium will concentrate in the liver, kidney, salivary glands, and mammary glands. Splenic uptake is variable. The major routes of excretion of gallium are divided between the kidneys and the colon.

While some abscesses can be imaged as early as 2 hr postinjection, most departments image at 6–8 hr and again at 24 hr postinjection (11). When needed, 48-hr imaging can be performed.

Several caveats exist in gallium scanning. Gallium is taken up in areas of granulation tissue formation and, hence, accumulates at the incision site for up to 1 week in the recent postoperative patient. In the postoperative and bedridden patient with bowel stasis, intracolonic gallium may cause interpretive difficulty (11). Occasionally, bowel catharsis can improve the quality of the study. Activity within the urine-filled bladder may mask existing pelvic disease (11).

Because ^{67}Ga-citrate is concentrated by the hepatocytes and not the Kupffer cells, gallium can provide a useful complement to the conventional liver spleen scan (11).

Abscesses within or around the liver will usually concentrate gallium. However, unusually thick walled, poorly vascularized abscesses may be gallium negative. Amebic abscesses of the liver are often gallium avid but the activity tends to accumulate in the hypervascular rim that surrounds the cavity. This "rim sign" is not specific for amebic abscess however (11).

Evaluation of patients with cirrhosis using gallium after focal defects are found on the sulfur colloid liver spleen scan is often helpful. Because hepatic pseudotumors and hepatomas can appear similar on the sulfur colloid scan it is helpful to know that approximately 90% of hepatomas are ^{67}Ga avid while less than 10% of cirrhotic pseudotumors accumulate gallium (11).

Questionable defects in the sulfur colloid image, especially along the inferior margin of the liver, in the region of the gallbladder may be better characterized and defined by hepatobiliary scintigraphy (12).

Other agents which can be helpful in the evaluation of hepatic disease include ^{99m}Tc polyphosphate compounds. Focal uptake within the liver has been commonly reported with metastatic mucinous adenocarcinoma of the colon and rectum, and, rarely in breast carcinoma, squamous cell carcinoma of the esophagus, oat cell carcinoma of the lung and malignant melanoma. Rarely cholangiocarcinoma of the liver may demonstrate focal activity. Diffuse hepatic necrosis and amyloidosis may demonstrate a generalized uptake (13).

Xenon-133, frequently used for ventilation studies of the lung, is lipophilic and may concentrate subdiaphragmatically in a fat infiltrated liver.

Perfusion scans with macroaggregated albumin (MAA) particles, 20–80 μm in size, in patients with cirrhosis-induced lung disease may reveal abnormal activity in the liver and spleen due to small pulmonary arteriovenous shunts (14).

The Normal Liver Scan

Evaluation of sulfur colloid liver-spleen scans should be systematic with attention to the size, shape, and position of the liver. Any extrinsic

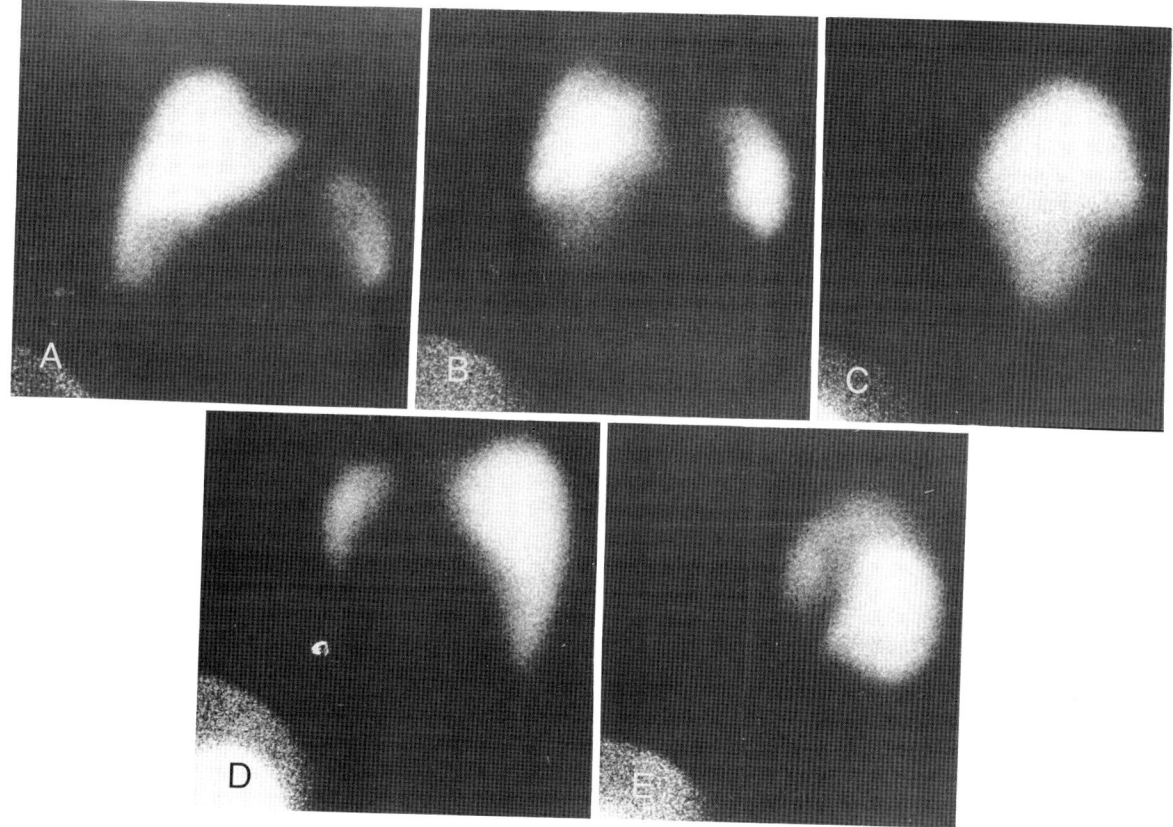

FIGURE 1.26. NORMAL SULFUR COLLOID SCAN
A: Anterior. B: LAO. C: R lateral. D: Posterior. E: L lateral.

compression on or focal defects within the liver should be noted. Attention should be paid to the distribution of colloid within the liver itself, as well as in the remainder of the body (15) and the clearance rate (amount of liver uptake versus activity remaining in the blood pool).

The normal ^{99m}Tc-sulfur-colloid liver scan (Fig. 1.26) should reveal a homogeneous distribution of radiocolloid throughout the liver. The liver should be located within the right upper quadrant with its superior surface abutting the diaphragm and its ventral surface adjacent to the anterior abdominal wall. Liver margins should be well defined.

The size of the liver is easily evaluated when calibrated rib markers are used. Usually in adults a vertical span in the midclavicular line of greater than 15–17 cm is considered abnormal. The size of the spleen should also be noted. In children, the maximal vertical dimension is equal to 8.8 + 0.46 × age/yr, and the ratio of its maximal vertical height to width is between 0.7:1 and 1.1:1 (3, 16).

Frequently, a liver-spleen scan is ordered because the physical examination suggests an enlarged liver. Again, rib markers can be of aid in demonstrating the exact position of the dome of the liver. Often, an apparently enlarged liver found by physical examination is shown to be normal in size but unusually low in position (15).

Liver shapes are varied. Mould et al. described 39 and McAfee has described 12 "normal variations" (3). The right lobe is always larger than the left, and if it extends into the pelvis, a Riedel's lobe configuration is present; if it extends into the chest (elevated right hemidiaphragm) there is a chapeau de gendarme's configuration (8).

Areas which normally do not accumulate ^{99m}Tc-sulfur colloid include the region of the porta hepatis, the gallbladder fossa, the incisura, the confluence of the hepatic veins and inferior vena cava, and the renal fossa. The porta hepatis is found midway between the superior and inferior borders of the liver immediately lateral to the incisura (the site of the falciform ligament). On anterior and lateral scintiscans, it appears as an area of photopenia, as no Kupffer cells are located within this region. The hepatic veins and inferior vena cava create a photopenic defect at the junction of the dome of the liver and the concavity of the liver's upper border (cardiac

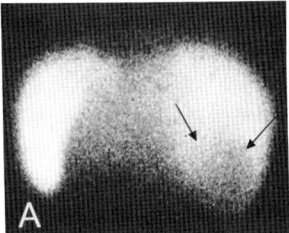 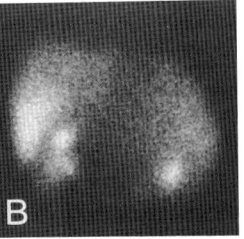

FIGURE 1.27. NORMAL RENAL FOSSA MIMICKING A MASS
A: Posterior view, sulfur colloid scan: apparent mass (*arrows*). *B:* Posterior view: filling in of defect after DTPA administration.

notch). On the anterior view, the gallbladder fossa is located along the inferior border of the right lobe of the liver; on the right lateral view it is located anteriorly and inferiorly. Spine attenuation accounts for the central band of decreased activity identified on the posterior projection and the kidney creates the concave defect posteromedially (Fig. 1.27).

Artifactual areas of diminished activity that can manifest themselves on liver-spleen scintigraphy include breast attenuation which characteristically creates a uniform area of decreased activity limited to the dome of the liver, photon attenuation resulting from a plaster spica, barium within the hepatic flexure, a contracted upper extremity, and fingers and/or metallic objects external to the liver (Fig. 1.28). If a well defined and concave defect is identified anterolaterally in obese patients or in patients with mild hepatomegaly, a rib artifact should be suspected (2, 3).

When evaluating focal defects on the liver-spleen scans it is essential to remember that an area devoid of sulfur colloid is devoid of functioning Kupffer cells. Little or no additional specificity can be inferred from the image without clinical correlation. Conversely, regions of pathology containing a normal complement of Kupffer cells will appear normal on the liver spleen scan.

The amount of ^{99m}Tc-sulfur colloid within the liver should always exceed that in the spleen (3). If there is a reversal of colloid distribution (particle uptake), hepatocellular disease and/or a primary splenic abnormality such as metastatic melanoma is present.

Assessment of the distribution of colloid within the liver itself is important. A reduction in the functioning Kupffer cell population per unit volume of liver will demonstrate decreased activity on the scan. Pathological processes affecting the liver diffusely can produce deviations in the distribution of the sulfur colloid and differentiation between extensive diffuse and early multifocal disease is not always possible. Additionally, alterations in blood flow within the liver can also produce alterations in the access of the sulfur colloid to the Kupffer cells and hence produce an inhomogeneous uptake pattern, hot spots or even focal defects (17, 18).

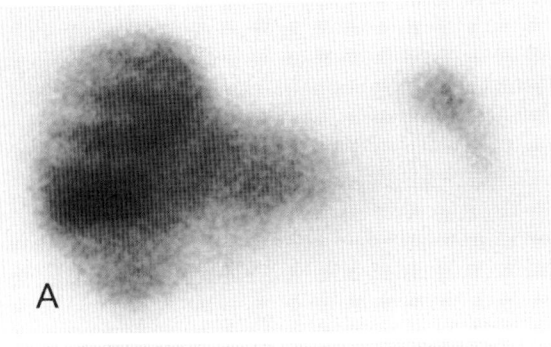
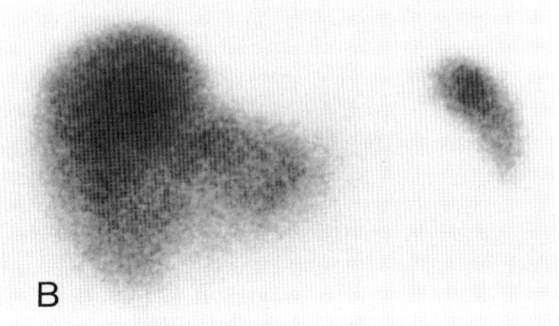

FIGURE 1.28. FINGER ATTENUATION, SULFUR COLLOID SCAN, ANTERIOR VIEW
A: Four linear defects, superolateral right lobe. *B:* Normal scan after removal of the patient's hand from the field.

Differentiation of Extrahepatic Masses from Intrinsic Hepatic Disease

Extrahepatic masses that can mimic liver enlargement clinically include tumors of the kidney (renal cell carcinoma, Wilms' tumor), pancreas, adrenal glands, and retroperitoneum. An abscess and/or empyema of the gallbladder may also mimic an enlarged liver on physical examination. By administering ^{99m}Tc-sulfur colloid, the liver's size and configuration can be easily assessed, and hepatomegaly readily confirmed or excluded as the etiology of the clinically palpable right upper quadrant mass. If an extrahepatic mass is creating the palpable abnormality, it may manifest itself as an extrinsic defect. Renal and adrenal mass pressure defects are best visualized on the posterior and/or lateral scintiscan. Gallbladder empyema and/or pancreatic lesions are

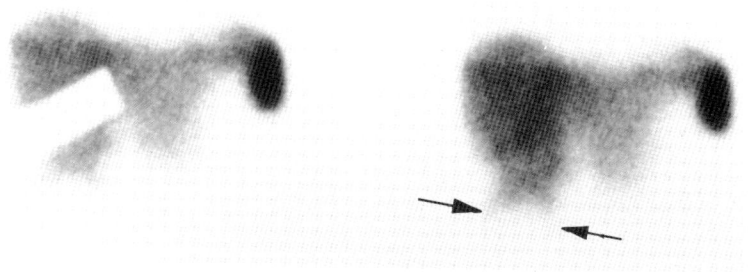

FIGURE 1.29. "SHOULDER SIGN" OF AN INTRAHEPATIC MASS (*arrows*)

best identified on the anterior view (Fig. 1.22). An extrahepatic mass can be differentiated from an intrahepatic mass by the presence of the "shoulder sign" (3). If the defect on liver scan is enclosed by Kupffer cells (shoulders), then an intrahepatic mass is present (Fig. 1.29). Shielding over the normal liver is frequently helpful to depict this sign. The absence of shoulders is most suggestive of an extrahepatic mass. A subphrenic abscess located between the liver and right hemidiaphragm may manifest itself as a superior surface indentation or inferior medial displacement of the liver. Gallium-67-citrate- or ^{111}In-labeled white cell scintigraphy is useful in the detection of subphrenic, as well as subhepatic, abscesses.

Today, sonography and/or CT are used for further specificity in differentiating extrahepatic from intrahepatic lesions, supplanting scintigraphy almost completely for this indication.

REFERENCES

1. Chervu LR et al: Radiopharmaceuticals for hepatobiliary imaging. *Semin Nucl Med* 12:5, 1982.
2. Alavi A, Arger P: *Abdomen—Multiple Imaging Procedures, Vol 3*, New York, Grune & Stratton, 1980.
3. Freeman L, Johnson P: *Clinical Scintillation Imaging, Second Edition*, New York, Grune & Stratton, 1975.
4. Front D, Royal HD, Israel O, et al: Scintigraphy of hepatic hemangiomas: the value of ^{99m}Tc labeled red blood cells: concise communication. *J Nucl Med* 22:684–687, 1981.
5. Ziessman HA, Thrall JH, Gyves JW, Ensminger WD, Niederhuber JE, Tuscan M, Walker S: Quantitative hepatic arterial perfusion scintigraphy and starch microspheres in cancer chemotherapy. *J Nucl Med* 24:871–875, 1983.
6. Miller DL, Schneider PD, Gianola FJ, Willis M, Vermess M, Doppmann JL: Assessment of perfusion patterns during hepatic artery infusion chemotherapy: EOE-13 CT and ^{99m}Tc-MAA scintigraphy. *AJR* 143:827–831, 1984.
7. Pettigrew FI, Witztum KF, Perkins SC, Johnson LL, et al: Single photon emission computed tomograms of the liver: normal vascular intrahepatic structures. *Radiology* 150:219–223, 1984.
8. Gottschalk A, Potchen J: Diagnostic nuclear medicine. In *Golden's Diagnostic Radiology*. Baltimore, Williams & Wilkins, 1976.
9. Johnson GS, Jones AE: *Atlas of Gallium-67 Scintigraphy*. New York, Plenum, 1973, pp 1–5.
10. Hauser MF, Gottschalk A: Comparison of the Anger tomographic scanner and the 15″ scintillation camera in gallium imaging. *J Nucl Med* 18:603, 1977.
11. Hauser MF, Alderson PO: Gallium-67 imaging in the abdomen. *Semin Nucl Med* 8:251, 1978.
12. Rao BK, Pastakla B, Lieberman LM: Evaluation of focal defects on technetium-99m sulfur colloid scans with new hepatobiliary agents. *Radiology* 136:497–499, 1980.
13. Hansen S, Stadalnik RC: Liver uptake of 99m Tc pyrophosphate. *Semin Nucl Med* 12:89, 1982.
14. Swett HA, Greenspan RH: Thoracic manifestations of liver disease. *Radiol Clin North Am* 18:269, 1980.
15. Ashare AB: Radiocolloid liver scintigraphy. *Radiol Clin North Am* 18:315, 1980.
16. Naftalis J, Leevy CM: Clinical estimation of liver size. *Dig Dis Sci* 8:236, 1963.
17. Waxman AD: Scintigraphic evaluation of diffuse hepatic disease. *Semin Nucl Med* 12:75, 1982.
18. Drum DE: Current status of radiocolloid hepatic scintigraphy for space occupying disease. *Semin Nucl Med* 12:64, 1982.

EMISSION COMPUTED TOMOGRAPHY AND THE LIVER

The ultimate goal of nuclear medicine imaging is to create an accurate, three-dimensional map of the radiopharmaceutical distribution within a patient. In conventional planar scintigraphy (PS) there is no information about depth. The standard scintillation camera provides only a two-dimensional image of a three-dimensional distribution of activity. Multiple views of the patient are usually obtained in order to better estimate the true three-dimensional shape of activity within an organ of interest.

Lesion contrast and edge detection is degraded in conventional imaging because of the superimposition of activity in surrounding tissues.

True quantification of activity in conventional images is complicated by the presence of background activity. With the ability to perform tomographic reconstructions, true volume measurements can be obtained using slices of known thickness and absolute tracer concentrations can then be calculated. Theoretically therefore nuclear medicine's ability to perform tomographic imaging with metabolically active tracers should provide better anatomic resolution and ultimately quantification of in vivo physiologic processes.

Emission computed tomography may be divided into two forms: single photon emission computed tomography (SPECT) and positron emission tomography (PET). SPECT uses conventional radiopharmaceuticals labeled with isotopes such as ^{99m}Tc or ^{123}I. The availability of these agents has practical advantages in the potential application of SPECT in most hospitals.

PET imaging requires the use of the unique 180° angular orientation of the annihilation photons produced by positron emitting radionuclides. Attenuation correction is not a significant problem with these radioisotopes. They usually have short half-lives and can be given in large quantities with minimal patient radiation burden. Their significance, however, lies in the fact that they can be produced as the key elements in organic compounds that are fundamental to body metabolism (e.g., carbon, oxygen, and nitrogen). A cyclotron or linear accelerator, however, is needed for their production and because of their short half-lives these facilities must be available at the imaging site. Since small hospital-based cyclotrons currently cost from 1 to 2 million dollars excluding the cost of a dedicated PET camera, financial considerations ultimately limit the widespread availability of PET imaging.

Both forms of emission CT lack sensitivity because of the difficulty of obtaining adequate counts in a short period of time. PET cameras are inherently more sensitive than SPECT systems since two γ-rays are emitted simultaneously in opposite directions. Sensitivity is further increased since the coincidence detection of annihilation photons determines location without the need for collimation.

SPECT camera systems are becoming more widely used since the same cameras can be used for conventional imaging. SPECT systems use a conventional scintillation camera which is modified to rotate 360° around the subject. Similar to x-ray computed tomography, filtered back projection is used for the reconstruction of images. There are theoretical limitations to the use of this method. Attenuation correction is essential for absolute quantification since single photon radioisotopes have lower energies and are more subject to tissue attenuation than positron

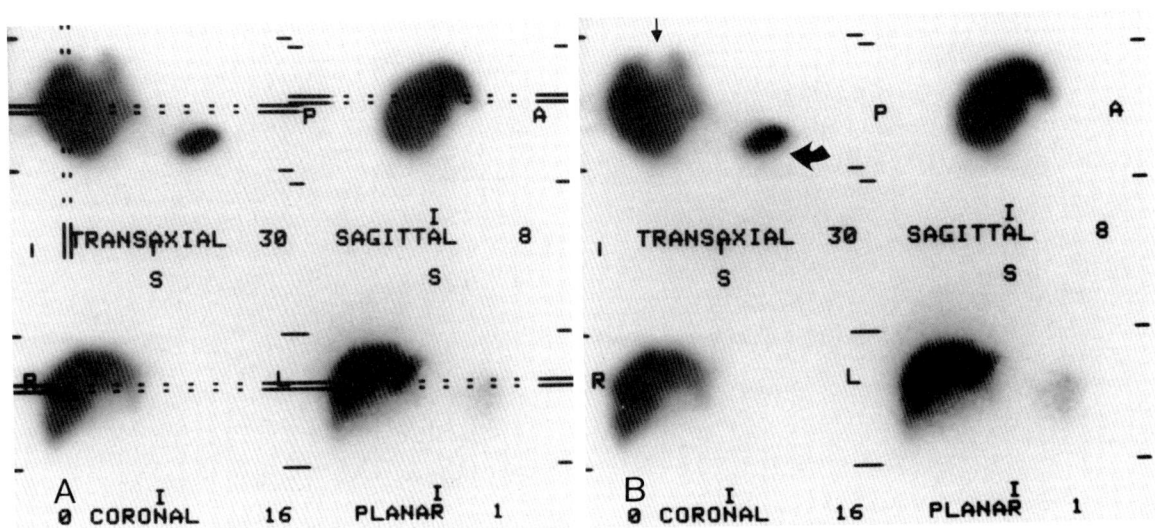

FIGURE 1.30. AXIAL, CORONAL, AND SAGITTAL RECONSTRUCTIONS

A: The dotted lines demonstrate the plane of reconstruction in each of three imaging planes. The transaxial slice level is demonstrated in the planar (*anterior view*) of the liver and spleen. The sagittal and coronal positions are indicated by the dotted lines in the transaxial plane. *B:* These same sections are shown again without superimposition of the lines which demonstrate the level of the plane of reconstruction. This normal study shows a truncated left lobe of the liver and a prominent separation between the right and left lobes (*small arrow*). The spleen is seen in its posterior location in the transaxial view (*curved arrow*).

isotopes. Spatial resolution with SPECT is dependent on the cube of the count rate as compared to the second power with standard scintigraphy. This in practice can lead to a substantial increase in imaging time. Since attenuation increases toward the center of an object methods still need to be devised to correct for changes in attenuation as a function of depth.

SPECT Techniques

Acquisition time for SPECT liver imaging is not significantly greater than that for conventional planar imaging. Typically, the camera acquisition is performed over 360° of rotation using 128 stops. At each stop an image is acquired for a preset time. For a 5 mCi dose of ^{99m}Tc-sulfur colloid images of 10–15 sec will typically result in 50,000–75,000 counts per stop. With 15 sec per image this result in a total acquisition time of 32 min which is comparable to the time required for a conventional 8 view liver-spleen study with PS.

Reconstructions can then be obtained in the axial, coronal, and sagittal planes (Fig. 1.30). Typically, spatial filtering of the SPECT images is performed. A Ramp-Hanning filter with a 0.5 cut-off may be used. Images are usually reconstructed with a 1.0 pixel width. At present no

TABLE 1.1.
ANATOMIC VARIATIONS CAUSING FALSE-POSITIVE STUDIES WITH SPECT AND PLANAR SCINTIGRAPHY

1. Thinning of the left lobe of liver
2. Renal impression
3. Gallbladder fossa
4. Prominent porta hepatis
5. Right costal rib impression
6. Hepatic veins
7. Falciform ligament
8. Dilated intrahepatic ducts

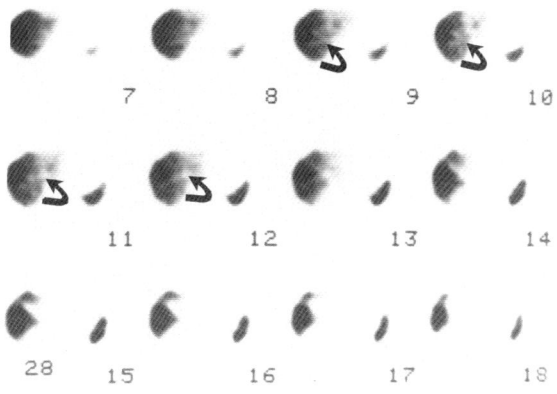

FIGURE 1.31. NORMAL INTRAHEPATIC VESSELS ON AXIAL SPECT

Normal intrahepatic vessels on axial SPECT: normal intrahepatic vessels can create confusing photopenic regions on SPECT. In order to differentiate these defects from space-occupying lesions, it is helpful to identify a linear, branching pattern on multiple slices (arrows, 9 and 10) extending toward the porta hepatis (arrows, 11 and 12), corresponding most often to portal veins. In difficult cases, labeled red cells can be used to further define vascular anatomy.

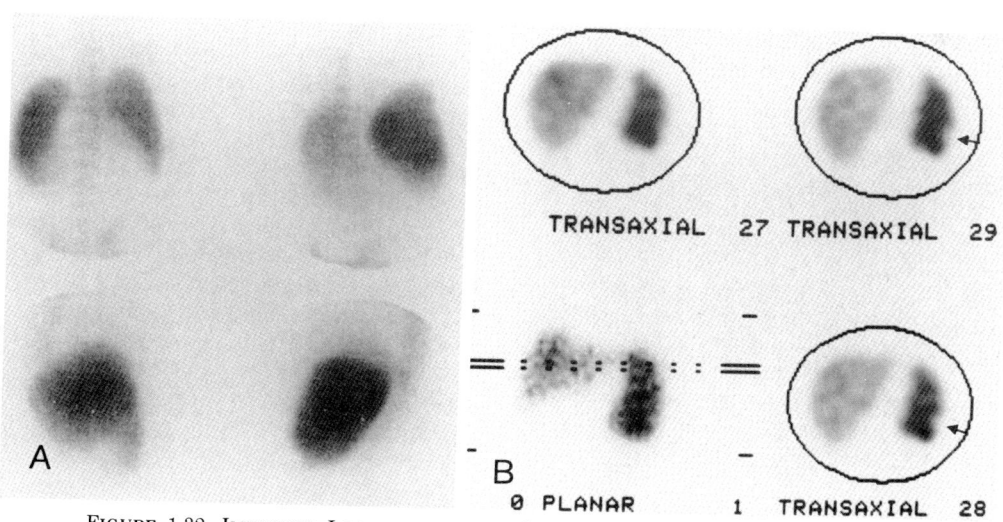

FIGURE 1.32. IMPROVED LOCALIZATION OF A SPLENIC DEFECT WITH SPECT IMAGING
A: Planar scintigraphy with ^{99m}Tc sulfur colloid in this patient with chronic leukemia shows hepatosplenomegaly and marked shift of colloid to the bone marrow indicating advanced parenchymal liver disease which may be related to the patient's chemotherapy. The patient developed left upper quadrant pain and the planar images fail to demonstrate any evidence for a splenic infarct. B: The transaxial images of the spleen clearly demonstrate a peripheral wedge shaped defect in the lateral border of the spleen (arrow) consistent with a splenic infarct.

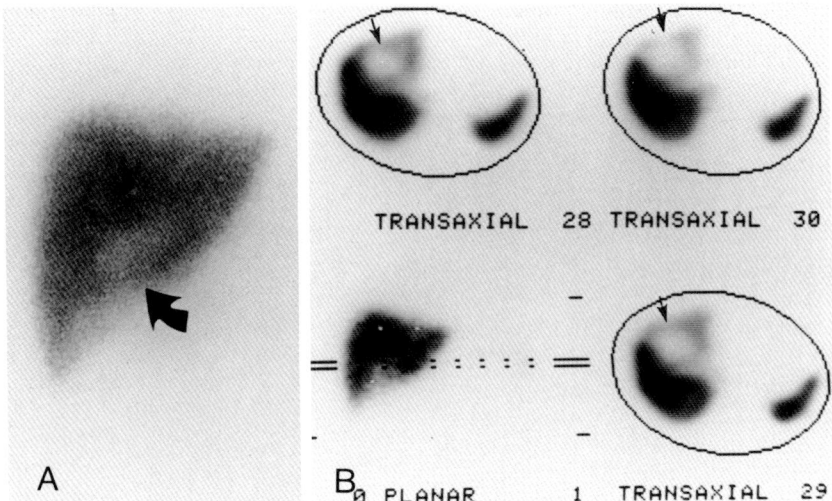

FIGURE 1.33. DETECTION OF SPACE-OCCUPYING DISEASE IN THE REGION OF THE PORTA HEPATIS WITH SPECT IMAGING
A: Conventional planar scintigraphy demonstrates prominent absence of radiotracer localization in the region of the porta hepatis (*curved arrow*). This can be a normal finding. *B:* Tomographic reconstructions in the transaxial plane demonstrate a large space-occupying lesion in the region of the porta hepatis which is clearly not related to vascular structures (*straight arrow*).

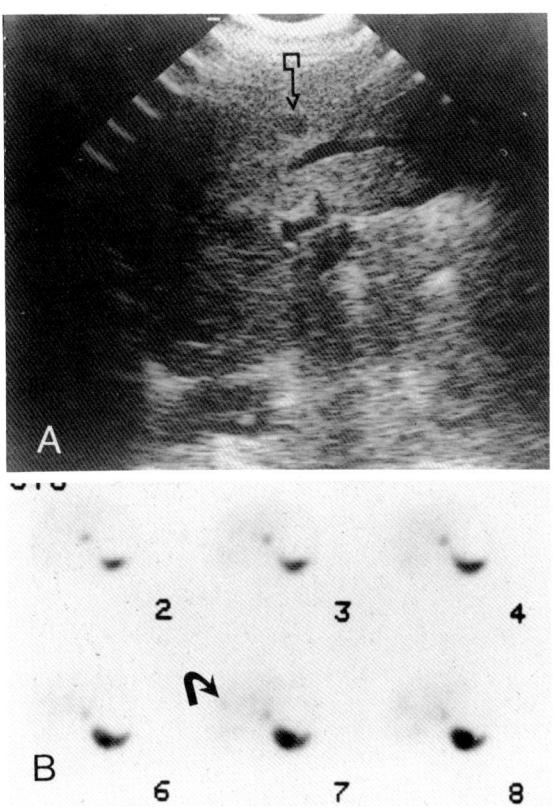

FIGURE 1.34. SPECT IN THE DIAGNOSIS OF CAVERNOUS HEMANGIOMA
A: Transverse sonogram shows a 1-cm diameter hypoechoic mass in the anterior portion of the right lobe of the liver (*arrow*), suspicious for metastasis. *B:* SPECT labeled red cell scintigram at 2 hr postinjection: focal accumulation of activity (*arrow*) in identical location diagnostic of hemangioma. Planar images were equivocal.

standardized technique for attenuation correction is available.

Results of SPECT Imaging

A recent study compared CT imaging with SPECT imaging and PS for detecting focal hepatic disease. CT had a higher sensitivity (91%) and specificity (96%) than either PS or SPECT alone, or the combination of PS and SPECT. SPECT alone had a sensitivity of 85% and a specificity of 90%. While these differences were not statistically different, receiver-operator curve (ROC) analysis showed that CT performance was best (1). In a similar study comparing PS and SPECT, SPECT has a sensitivity of 94% compared to 81% for PS (2).

While SPECT has increased sensitivity over PS, confusion with normal variants which are common on PS also can occur (Table 1.1). ROC analysis shows that SPECT yields higher false-positive ratios at low criteria levels (e.g., equivocal or uncertain responses). Particular care in interpreting SPECT imaging must be taken in defining normal intrahepatic structures which are not routinely seen on PS. The appearance of branching vascular or ductal structures seen on multiple sections is helpful for confirming normal anatomic structures (Fig. 1.31). Some investigators have suggested that the vascular structures be identified by labeling the patient's red blood cells (3).

The increase in sensitivity of SPECT imaging of the liver results from better visualization of small space-occupying lesions not well seen in PS (Figs. 1.32–1.34).

While SPECT imaging of the liver does not offer the precise anatomic resolution of CT or ultrasound it offers the advantage of improved resolution for scintigraphy particular with radiopharmaceuticals which have tissue and therefore diagnostic specificity (e.g., labeled red cells for hemangioma and labeled antibodies for tumor localization) (4).

REFERENCES

1. Brendel AJ, Lecca F, Drovillard J, SanGalli F, Eresue J, Wynchank S, Barat JL, Pucassov D: Single photon emission computed tomography (SPECT) planar scintigraphy, and transmission computer tomography: A comparison of accuracy in diagnosing focal hepatic disease. *Radiology* 153:527–532, 1984.
2. Strauss L, Bostel F, Clorius JH, Ekaterini R, Wellman H, George P: single photon emission computed tomography (SPECT) for assessment of hepatic lesions. *J Nucl Med* 23:1059–1065, 1982.
3. Pettigrew RI, Witztum KF, Perkins GC, Johnson ML, Burks RN, Verba JW, Halpern SE: Single photon emission computed tomography of the liver: Normal vascular intrahepatic structures. *Radiology* 150:219–223, 1984.
4. Rabinowitz SA, McKusiak KA, Strauss HW: ^{99m}Tc-red blood cell scintigraphy in evaluating liver lesions. *AJR* 143:63–68, 1984.

ANATOMIC VARIANTS

Riedel's lobe is quite common, especially in women. It is a downward tongue-like projection of the right lobe of the liver and not an accessory lobe (Fig. 1.35). The liver of the pig, dog, and camel is divided into many distinct and separate lobes by connective tissue strands. Occasionally the human liver may be similarly organized, and up to sixteen lobes have been reported. The accessory lobes are small and usually on the undersurface of the liver and are without clinical significance (1). Rarely, accessory lobes are intrathoracic. Even more rarely, an accessory lobe may have its own mesentery and undergo torsion, requiring operative intervention (2). Ectopic liver nodules are formed when an accessory lobe loses its continuity with the liver, and may be attached to the gallbladder, located within the gastrohepatic ligament, umbilical cord, adrenals, pancreas, splenic capsule, or thoracic cavity (3).

Congenital absence of the left lobe is an unusual anomaly thought to occur because of extension of the obliterative process that closes the ductus venosus to the left branch of the portal vein (Fig. 1.36). It must not be confused with acquired atrophy due to obstruction of the left branch of the portal vein, hepatic artery, or biliary tree by malignancy or stones. In acquired atrophy a shrunken lobe is detectable by CT and ultrasound. In congenital absence, the stomach and duodenal bulb are displaced to the left and cephalad and the stomach is folded on itself (4). On ultrasound and CT there is no liver to the left of the major fissure (4). The stomach fills the resultant void. An entity called "bipartite liver" has been described in which there is a large separation of left and right lobes simulating a mass lesion on radionuclide scans (3). The

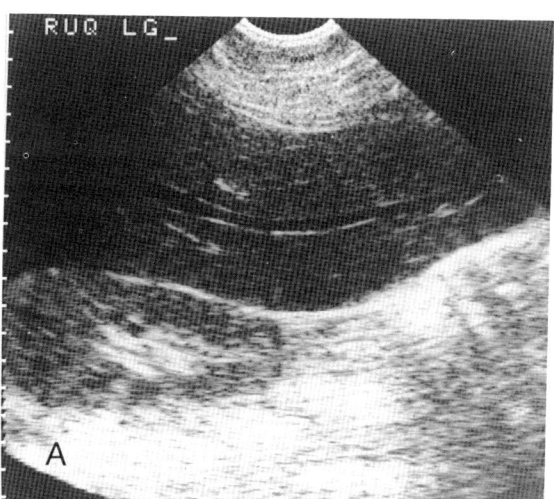

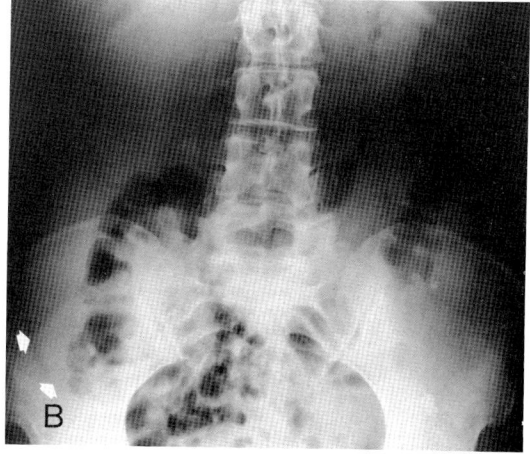

FIGURE 1.35. RIEDEL'S LOBE
A: Sagittal sonogram of a Riedel's lobe extending inferiorly way beneath the right kidney. B: Corresponding plain film: Riedel's lobe extending below the iliac crest (*arrows*).

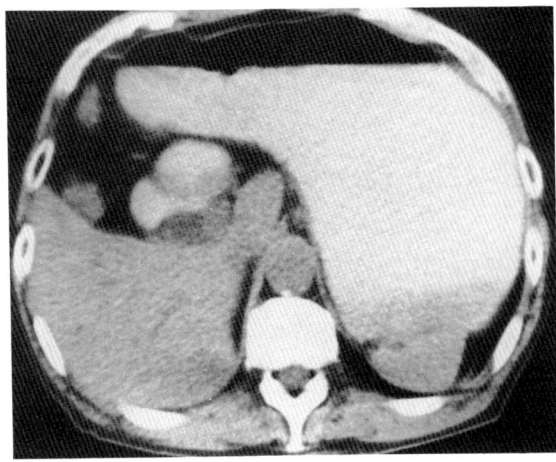

FIGURE 1.36. CT: CONGENITAL ABSENCE OF THE LEFT LOBE; THE STOMACH OCCUPIES THE REGION NORMALLY OCCUPIED BY THE LEFT LOBE

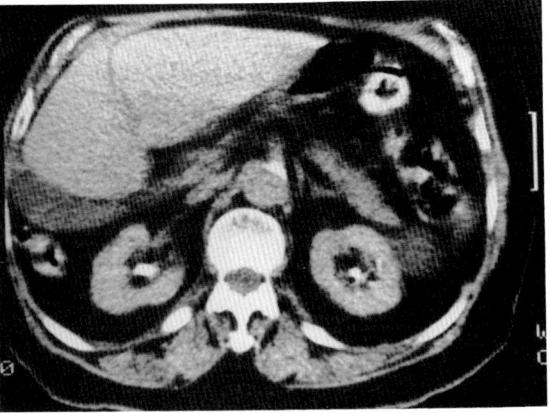

FIGURE 1.37. CT: CONGENITAL ABSENCE OF THE RIGHT LOBE; NOTE POSITION OF THE GALLBLADDER WHICH IS MORE POSTERIOR THAN USUAL

"empty space" is occupied by bowel, mesentery, and omentum. In fact, this anomaly may be absence of the medial segment of the left lobe. Congenital absence of the right lobe is exceedingly rare (Fig. 1.37).

REFERENCES

1. Fraser CG: Accessory lobes of the liver. *Ann Surg* 135:127, 1952.
2. Pujari BD, Deodhare SG: Symptomatic accessory lobe of the liver with review of the literature. *Postgrad Med J* 52:234–236, 1976.
3. Li YP, Morin ME, Tan A: Bipartite liver as a cause of ^{99m}Tc liver scan defect. *Applied Radiology*, pp. 97–98, July/Aug, 1982.
4. Belton RL, Van Zandt TF: Congenital absence of the left lobe of the liver: a radiologic diagnosis. *Radiology* 147:184, 1983.

2

Anomalies, Congenital Disorders, and Pediatric Neoplasms

ARNOLD C. FRIEDMAN, M.D., BRUCE M. MARKLE, M.D.,
ABRAHAM H. DACHMAN, M.D., AND ROBERT L. PAKTER, M.D.

GLYCOGEN STORAGE DISEASES

The glycogen storage diseases are a group of inherited metabolic disorders, most of which have an abnormality in the breakdown of glycogen to glucose which is reflected in abnormal structure or concentration of glycogen. Classification by type depends on the specific enzyme defect and/or distinct clinical presentation (1). In type I disease (von Gierke disease) absent or deficient glucose-6-phosphatase in the liver and kidneys leads to impaired breakdown of stored glycogen causing glycogen accumulation in hepatocytes and proximal tubules (2). Glucose synthesis is impaired and there is hypoglycemia, hyperglucagonemia, and elevated serum levels of triglycerides, cholesterol, and uric acid (1). Hepatic adenomas and hepatocellular carcinomas are seen just in type I disease. The latter are thought to result from malignant degeneration of the former and have occurred in at least three type I patients (1). Hepatomegaly can occur in types I, III, IV, and VI, and splenomegaly can occur in types I, IV, and VI (3). Cirrhosis develops only in types III and IV (1). Hepatic adenomas are thought to develop as a result of chronic hormonal stimulation secondary to the chronic hypoglycemia with decreased insulin and increased glucagon levels. They occur in childhood

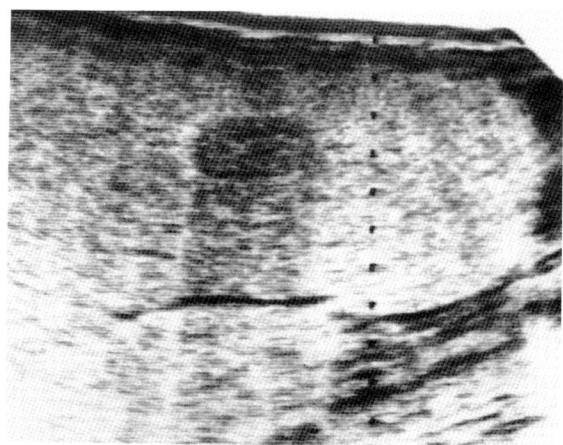

FIGURE 2.1. HEPATIC ADENOMA IN GLYCOGEN STORAGE DISEASE: LONGITUDINAL SONOGRAM

Longitudinal sonogram of a 22-yr-old woman with hepatic adenoma in glycogen storage disease: well circumscribed, uniformly echo-dense mass with enhanced through transmission and refractile shadowing within the caudal portion of the right lobe of an enlarged, attenuating liver. An incomplete hypoechoic rim is present. Centimeter markers are seen to the right of the umbilicus. (From Bowerman RA, Samuels BI, Silver TM: Ultrasonographic features of hepatic adenomas in type I glycogen storage disease. *J Ultrasound Med* 2:51–54, 1983.)

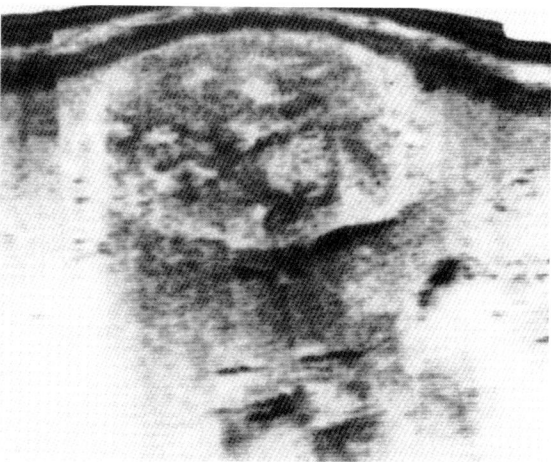

FIGURE 2.2. HEPATIC ADENOMA IN GLYCOGEN STORAGE DISEASE: TRANSVERSE SONOGRAM

Transverse sonogram of a 20-yr-old woman with hepatic adenoma in glycogen storage disease: multiple hypoechoic foci within an otherwise echogenic mass with a hypoechoic rim. Twenty months prior to this scan, the mass was uniformly echogenic as in *A*. The hypogenic regions represent hemorrhage. (From Bowerman RA, Samuels BI, Silver TM: Ultrasonographic features of hepatic adenomas in type I glycogen storage disease. *J Ultrasound Med* 2:51–54, 1983.)

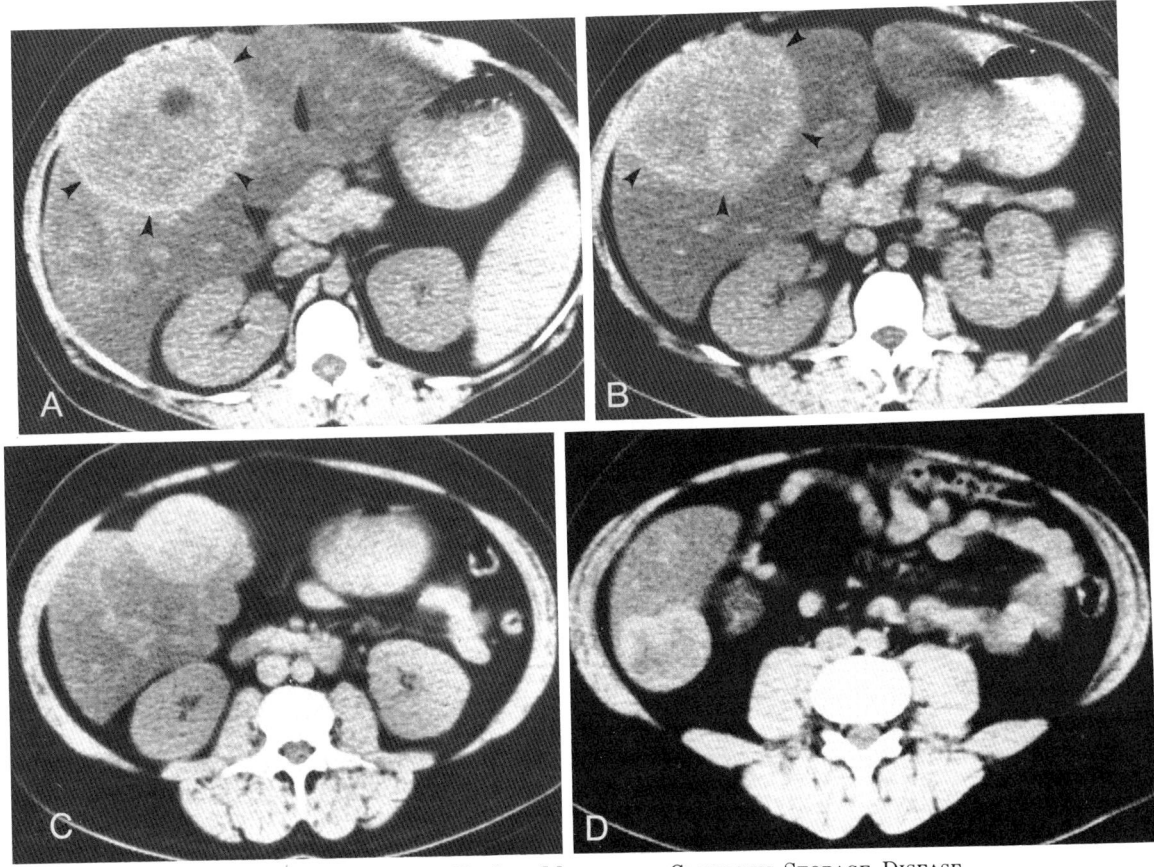

FIGURE 2.3. CT OF A 21-YR-OLD MALE WITH GLYCOGEN STORAGE DISEASE

A–D: Multiple masses, with some central low density (except for *C*), probably representing adenomas in a liver that is otherwise infiltrated with fat (noncontrast scan). (From Doppman JL, Cornblath M, Dwyer AJ, Adams AJ, Girton ME, Sidbury S: Computed tomography of the liver and kidneys in glycogen storage disease. *J Comput Assist Tomogr* 6:67–71, 1982.)

or adulthood (1). Treatment of type I disease is continuous nocturnal high carbohydrate feeding via nasogastric tube or gastrostomy and frequent meals and snacks during the day. If high serum glucose levels can be maintained, growth improves, chemistries normalize, adenomas may regress, and patients can lead fairly normal lives (1).

Radiology

Plain films of the abdomen may detect hepatosplenomegaly. The earliest finding on ^{99m}Tc-sulfur colloid liver-spleen scans is hepatomegaly which is followed by colloid shift to the spleen with patchy liver uptake. Minimal to marked splenomegaly is common at this point, but increased bone marrow accumulation is uncommon (1, 4). Adenomas are usually photopenic areas sometimes surrounded by a rim of increased uptake possibly representing compressed parenchyma. Rarely, adenomas are small regions of relatively increased uptake (1). Dynamic flow studies demonstrate hypervascularity in some adenomas (1). Rapid enlargement of a photopenic region suggests malignant transformation.

Sonographically, the liver is enlarged with increased echogenicity and sound attenuation probably from fatty infiltration, but conceivably from excess glycogen storage (1, 5). The liver is hyperechoic compared to the kidney, and nephromegaly may be present (1–3). Adenomas when small are homogeneous, well-demarcated echogenic solid masses that may be hyperechoic or hypoechoic compared to the abnormally echogenic liver (Fig. 2.1) (1, 5). Larger adenomas are heterogeneous with hypoechoic areas probably representing hemorrhage and/or necrosis (Fig. 2.2) (1, 5). Some are reported to have a thin, hypoechoic rim (possibly compressed parenchyma or a capsule) (5). A recently described feature of hepatic adenomas in type I glycogen storage disease not found in other hepatic adenomas is enhanced sound transmission with refractile shadowing at the tumor margins. This can be explained by a relative paucity of lipid and glycogen in the adenoma compared to the rest of the liver (5). On follow-up scans, adenomas are stable or slow growing. A rapid increase in size or loss of a smooth, well-defined border suggests malignant degeneration (1, 4).

CT of the liver is unique in that the liver can be hypodense, of normal density, or hyperdense, depending on the relative amounts of glycogen and fat. The former tends to elevate the CT number whereas the latter tends to lower it (2). In addition to hepatosplenomegaly, nephromegaly with a dense cortex from glycogen deposition may be detected (2). Hepatic adenomas in type I glycogen storage disease have similar CT characteristics to the other hepatic adenomas (hypodense to normal liver on unenhanced scans) except that they may appear spuriously hyperdense when there is fatty infiltration (Fig. 2.3) (2). Ring enhancement has been reported in one case (6).

Angiographic features of adenomas in type I glycogen storage disease are the same as other hepatic adenomas. Periodic sonography is the preferred imaging modality for following patients with type I glycogen storage disease (1).

REFERENCES

1. Wilkinson RH, Coleman RA, Rosenberg EK, Grossman H: Radionuclide and ultrasound imaging in glycogen storage disease. Exhibit, American Roentgen Ray Society Meeting, Las Vegas, Nevada, April, 1984.
2. Doppmman JL, Cornblath M, Dwyer AJ, Adams AJ, Girton ME, Sidbury J: Computed tomography of the liver and kidneys in glycogen storage disease. *J Comput Assist Tomogr* 6:67–71, 1982.
3. Miller JH, Stanley PP, Gates GF: Radiography of glycogen storage diseases. *AJR* 132:379–387, 1979.
4. Grossman H, Ram PC, Coleman RA, Gates G, Rosenberg ER, Bowie JD, Wilkinson RH: Hepatic ultrasonography in type I glycogen storage disease (von Gierke disease). Detection of hepatic adenoma and carcinoma. *Radiology* 141:753–756, 1981.
5. Bowerman RA, Samuels BI, Silver TM: Ultrasonographic features of hepatic adenoma in type I glycogen storage disease. *J Ultrasound Med* 2:51–54, 1983.
6. Biondetti PR, Fiore D, Muzzio PC: Computed tomography of the liver in von Gierke's disease. *J Comput Assist Tomogr* 4:685–686, 1980.

CYSTIC FIBROSIS

Liver and biliary tree abnormalities are present in 20–50% of patients with cystic fibrosis, but infrequently cause clinically recognized disease. Biliary cirrhosis is symptomatic in 2–3% of patients and is not seen in patients with no pancreatic involvement. Gallstones are an infrequent source of morbidity. Rarely, a biliary obstructive picture resembling biliary atresia may present in the newborn period (1–3).

Pathology

In patients who come to autopsy, fatty infiltration, hemosiderosis and focal areas of biliary cirrhosis are the most common histologic findings. Fatty infiltration is massive in 15% of cases. In older children the focal zones of cirrhosis may coalesce and 5% of children develop multilobular biliary cirrhosis and fibrosis. Histologic centrilobular atrophy due to right heart failure is sometimes superimposed (2).

Newborns show several patterns: (*a*) diffuse cholestasis, (*b*) periportal inflammation, fibrosis and proliferation of bile canaliculi, and (*c*) periportal changes without intrahepatic cholestasis (2). Some of these changes may be due to the effects of concomitant obstructive gastrointestinal disease or the effects of fasting and hyperalimentation (4). An uncommon but distinctive pattern is that of focal areas of excess biliary mucus in the lumen and epithelium of the large intrahepatic ducts (4). Rarely, mucus can obstruct the extrahepatic ducts (2).

The cystic duct may be stenotic or atretic, with mucosal hyperplasia and inspissated mucus in the residual lumen. The gallbladder may be atrophic and may contain both biliary sludge and calculi.

Clinical Symptomatology

Biliary cirrhosis may rarely be the clinical presentation of cystic fibrosis, symptoms being icterus, ascites, hematemesis, and hypersplenism (Fig. 2.4). Signs and symptoms of cholecystitis and cholelithiasis may present in the second decade of life. Newborn infants may present with persistent unexplained neonatal jaundice (1, 3).

Radiology

In one survey of 24 adolescent and adult cystic fibrosis patients, half of the patients had an abnormal appearing liver by ultrasonography: irregularly increased echogenicity. One eighth had a visibly large portal vein and splenomegaly. Fifteen of the 24 patients had a small gallbladder (most with calculi) or an unidentified gallbladder, while 8 of the 24 were normal (5).

Retrograde cholangiograms may demonstrate

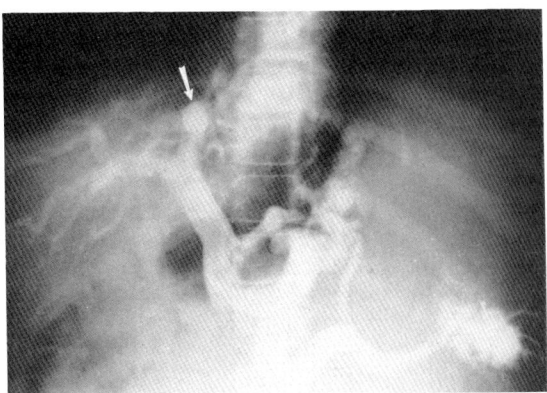

FIGURE 2.4. BILIARY CIRRHOSIS DUE TO CYSTIC FIBROSIS
A 12-yr-old girl with biliary cirrhosis due to cystic fibrosis. Splenomegaly and bleeding varices were present. Splenoportogram: enlarged coronary vein feeding gastroesophageal varices. Recanalized umbilical vein (*arrow*).

multiple filling defects, irregularity of ducts or even focal dilatation of some intrahepatic ducts (6).

Newborn infants with extensive mucus plugging of the hepatic ducts may show a pattern of complete biliary obstruction on hepatobiliary scans with ^{99m}Tc-IDA agents, thereby mimicking biliary atresia. The correct diagnosis is made at surgery when a mucus and bile filled biliary tree is encountered and operative cholangiography shows a patent biliary tree following aspiration of the contents of the ducts (7).

CT can show liver abnormalities in children and adolescents with cystic fibrosis even when liver disease is not suspected clinically (8). Reported findings include abnormalities in size, shape, or contour consistent with cirrhosis, abnormally low density consistent with fatty infiltration, and/or markers of portal hypertension such as splenomegaly and enlargement of the splenic and superior mesenteric veins. When liver disease is present on CT, pancreatic fat replacement is a likely concomitant finding.

REFERENCES

1. Doershuk CF, Boat TF: Cystic fibrosis. In: Berman RE, Vaughn VC, Nelson WE (eds): *Textbook of pediatrics.* Philadelphia, W.B. Saunders, 1983, pp 1086–1099.
2. Oppenheimer EH, Esterly JR: Pathology of cystic fibrosis. Review of the literature and comparison with 146 cases. *Perspect Pediatr Pathol* 2:241–278, 1975.
3. Park RW, Grand RJ: Gastrointestinal manifestations of cystic fibrosis: a review. *Gastroenterology* 81:1143–1161, 1981.
4. Witzleben CL: Neonatal liver disease. In Naeye RL, Kissane JM, Kaufman N (eds): *Perinatal Diseases.* Baltimore, Williams & Wilkins, 1981, pp 346–368.
5. Willi UV, Reddish JM, Teele RL: Cystic fibrosis: its characteristic appearance on abdominal sonography. *AJR* 134:1005–1010, 1980.
6. Bass S, Connon JJ, Ho CS: Biliary tree in cystic fibrosis. *Gastroenterology* 84:1592–1596, 1983.
7. Altman RP, Abramson S: Potential errors in the diagnosis and surgical management of neonatal jaundice. *J Pediatr Surg* (in press).
8. Cunningham DG, Churchill RJ, Reynes CJ: Computed tomography in the evaluation of liver disease in cystic fibrosis patients. *J Comput Assist Tomogr* 4:151–154, 1980.

CHRONIC GRANULOMATOUS DISEASE OF CHILDHOOD

Chronic granulomatous disease of childhood is characterized by a diminished ability of leukocytes to carry out normal bactericidal activity on engulfed bacteria. The condition is due to a congenital deficiency of the enzyme nicotinamide-adenine dinucleotide oxidase, which normally converts the reduced form of coenzyme NAD to the oxidized form, thus producing hydrogen peroxide. Failure to form hydrogen peroxide is felt to be responsible for the impaired ability of leukocytes to kill bacteria (1).

The trait is usually seen in males, being X-linked recessive, although occasionally it is seen in females, in which case it is transmitted as an autosomal recessive (2).

The disease is characterized clinically by recurrent infections primarily involving the paranasal sinuses, lungs, bones, lymph nodes, and liver. Typical bacterial species are *Staphylococcus aureus* or *S. epidermidis, Serratia,* or *Aerobacter* (3). *Aspergillus* organisms may also be present (4). The pathological response in patients with chronic granulomatous disease is similar to the granulomatous response in normal patients to acid-fast bacilli, brucella, or listeria.

Lymphadenopathy, hepatosplenomegaly, and hilar lymph node enlargement with pulmonary consolidation occur soon after antibiotics have been discontinued from a previous exacerbation. Staphylococcal abscesses may involve the liver, and osteomyelitis occurs of both small bones of the hands and feet and also of the long bones.

Liver involvement with chronic granulomatous disease may range from ill-defined granulomatous tissue to frank abscess formation. Old, healed granulomas can be detected as multiple intrahepatic calcifications, and chronic granulomatous disease should be strongly suspected in

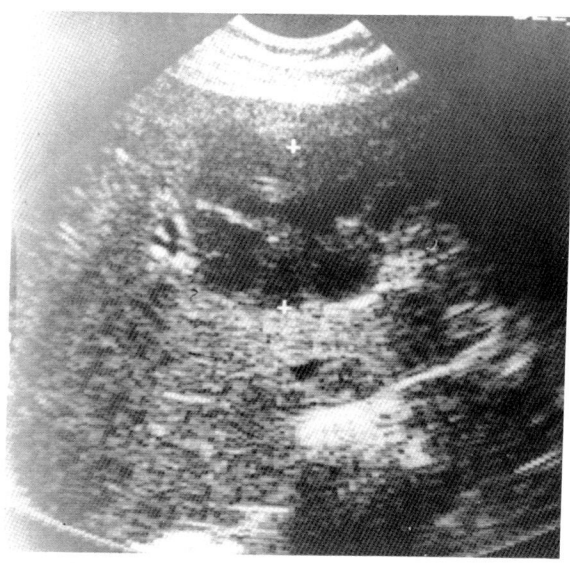

FIGURE 2.5. INTERMEDIATE PHASE BETWEEN GRANULOMA AND FRANK ABSCESS
Transverse sonogram shows a complex, partially liquefied solid mass (cursors) with minimally increased through transmission.

any male child with multiple hepatic calcifications. Ultrasound has been a useful modality for determining the type and extent of liver involvement in these patients (4). Granulomatous tissue is hypoechoic with poorly defined margins with respect to the normal liver tissue. No posterior enhancement is present. A frank abscess, on the other hand, shows a well defined, fluid-filled lesion with good through transmission (5). Affected livers may show a spectrum of findings between the granulomatous tissue and frank abscess (Fig. 2.5).

Early recognition of granulomatous disease should prompt early therapy. Percutaneous biopsy or aspiration via ultrasound or computed tomography may be very useful to document previously undiscovered disease in the liver, drain any abscess that may be present, and identify the proper organism so as to choose the appropriate antibiotic regimen.

REFERENCES

1. Markowitz M: Immunity, allergy, and related diseases. In: Behrman RE, Vaughan VC, Nelson WE (eds): *Textbook of Pediatrics.* Philadelphia, W. B. Saunders, 1983, p 475.
2. Quie PG, Kaplan EL, Page AR, Gruskay FL, Malawista SE: Defective polymorphonuclear-leukocyte function and chronic granulomatous disease in two female children. *N Engl J Med* 278:976, 1968.
3. Quie PG: Chronic granulomatous disease of childhood. In: Sulman I (ed): *Advances in Pediatrics.* Chicago, Year Book, 1969, pp 287–300.
4. Garel LA, Pariente DM, Nezelof C, Barnal VJ, Aboulker C, Sauvegrain J: Liver involvement in chronic granulomatous disease: the role of ultrasound in diagnosis and treatment. *Radiology* 153:117–121, 1984.
5. Newlin N, Silver T, Stuck K, Sandler MA: Ultrasonic features of pyogenic liver abscesses. *Radiology* 139:155–159, 1981.

MESENCHYMAL HAMARTOMA

Mesenchymal hamartoma is a rare cystic liver tumor that is probably developmental in origin and not a true neoplasm (1, 2). About 70 cases have been reported, with the majority occurring in children less than 3 yr old (1, 3). Although cases have been reported in older children and teenagers, embryonal sarcoma should be suspected in older children as it has a similar gross appearance and typically presents after infancy (3–5).

Clinical Features

Mesenchymal hamartoma usually presents as a painless, gradually enlarging abdominal mass in an otherwise healthy child (4, 6). Although the reported age range is newborn to 19 yr, the average age is 15–22 months (1, 3). There is a 2:1 male to female ratio (1, 7). Rapid enlargement may occur as fluid accumulates in degenerating tissue (1, 4, 8). Physical exam reveals a protuberant abdomen with a smooth or slightly bosselated, firm, nontender mass (1). There are no consistent laboratory abnormalities (1). As there are no reported instances of postoperative recurrence or malignant transformation, the surgical approach should be conservative. If the tumor is too large for easy resection, partial excision or incision and drainage of cysts is adequate (1, 2, 4).

Pathology

The right lobe is involved 6 times as often as the left and both lobes are involved in about 10% of cases (1). About 20% are pedunculated (1). Mesenchymal hamartomas are well demarcated but unencapsulated and average 16 cm or more in largest diameter (1, 7). They are round, ovoid, or irregular masses often with red, blue, or gray cysts bulging from the surface (Fig. 2.6A) (1). Cysts are present grossly in 80%. One, few, or

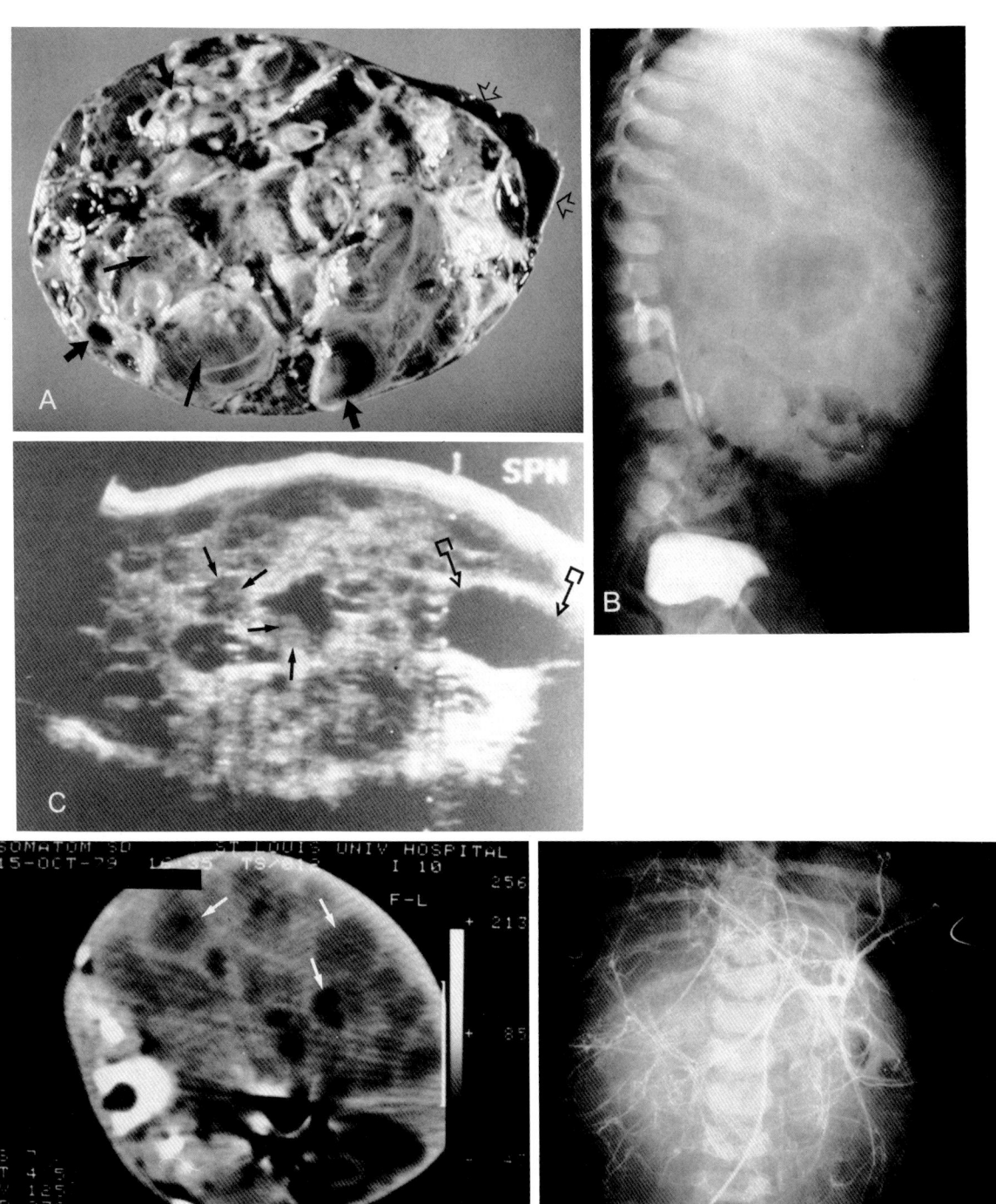

FIGURE 2.6. MESENCHYMAL HAMARTOMA

A 13-month-old boy with a 2-week history of abdominal distention and a palpable mass: mesenchymal hamartoma. *A:* Cut section of gross specimen: multiple cysts are present, some containing gelatinous material (*long arrows*) while others are fluid-filled (*short arrows*). The line of resection included a portion of the uninvolved left lobe (*open arrows*). *B:* Excretory urogram: large mass displacing the kidneys inferiorly. Multiple lucencies are present by virtue of the total body opacification effect. *C:* Longitudinal sonogram through the large mass: solid mass with numerous cystic spaces some with enhanced through-transmission (*large arrows*). Many have internal echoes (*smaller arrows*). *D:* CT (enhanced): Multiple lucencies of variable size and attenuation throughout the mass. *E:* Celiac arteriogram: intrahepatic arterial branches are splayed and distorted by the large mass. Some patchy regions of fine neovascularity are present, but overall the mass is hypovascular. (*A* and *D*) from Donovan AT, Wolverson MK, deMello D, Craddock T, Silberstein M: Multicystic mesenchymal hamartoma of childhood: computerized tomography and ultrasound characteristics. *Pediatr Radiol* 11:163–165, 1981.)

many may be present and their size ranges from a few mm in diameter up to 14 cm (1). The cysts can be round and discrete or irregular and multiloculated. The lining can be smooth or ragged and the contents are fluid or gelatinous and yellow to amber, not hemorrhagic or necrotic (1). Solid regions have varying amounts of loose yellow myxoid material intermingled with white fibrous bands and parenchymal nodules. At the junction with normal liver there may be satellite nodules (1). Microscopically, there is a mixture of cysts, bile ducts, vessels, hepatocytes, and mesenchyme (1, 2, 7, 8). Foci of extramedullary hematopoiesis and inflammatory cell infiltrates are present near bile ducts or vessels near the periphery of the lesion (1). The tumor probably originates from primitive mesenchymal tissue in the portal tracts (1, 2). The virtual absence of mitotic activity other than in the hematopoietic cells suggests that the major proliferative activity occurs before or shortly after birth (1). Growth in infancy is probably the result of fluid accumulation in the cysts (1, 7).

Radiology

Plain films may show a soft tissue mass but no calcification (5). Excretory urography can demonstrate round lucencies within the mass corresponding to cystic spaces and displacement of the kidney or ureter (Fig. 2.6B) (1, 6). Sulfur colloid liver-spleen scans generally show one or more areas of diminished uptake, but can be falsely negative when mesenchymal hamartomas are pedunculated (1). Sonography demonstrates many rounded hypoechoic areas within an echogenic background (4, 6). Some regions are echo-free and well defined with good transmission (serous fluid), others have scattered internal echoes with poor sound transmission (gelatinous fluid) (Fig. 2.6C) (4). Occasionally, multicystic hamartomas are solid, especially in younger infants (1). In one case, CT has shown a mass with multiple round variably sized low density regions that did not appreciably enhance after intravenous contrast administration (Fig. 2.6D) (6). Angiography shows displacement and stretching of vessels by a hypovascular mass (Fig. 2.6E) (3, 6). Patchy areas of fine neovascularity may be seen (6).

REFERENCES

1. Stocker JT, Ishak KG: Mesenchymal hamartoma of the liver: report of 30 cases and review of the literature. *Pediatr Pathol* 1:245–267, 1983.
2. Dehner LP, Ewing SL, Sumner HW: Infantile mesenchymal hamartoma of the liver. Histologic and ultrastructural observations. *Arch Pathol Lab Med* 99:379–382, 1975.
3. Grases PJ, Matos-Villalobos M, Arcia-Romero F, Lecuna-Torres V: Mesenchymal hamartoma of the liver. *Gastroenterology* 76:1466–1469, 1979.
4. Rosenbaum DM, Mindell HJ: Ultrasonographic findings in mesenchymal hamartoma of the liver. *Radiology* 138:425–427, 1981.
5. Stocker JT, Ishak KG: Undifferentiated (embryonal) sarcoma of the liver. *Cancer* 42:336–348, 1978.
6. Donovan AT, Wolverson MK, deMello D, Craddock T, Silberstein M: Multiple hepatic mesenchymal hamartoma of childhood. Computerized tomography and ultrasound characteristics. *Pediatr Radiol* 11:163–165, 1981.
7. Ishak KG, Rabin L: Benign tumors of the liver. *Med Clin North Am* 59:1011–1013, 1975.
8. Schonland MM, Millward-Sadler GH, Wright DH, Wright R: Hepatic tumors. In Wright R, Alberti KGMM, Karran S, and Millward-Sadler GH (eds): *Liver and Biliary Disease*. London, WB Saunders, 1979, pp 914–915.

INFANTILE HEMANGIOENDOTHELIOMA

Infantile hemangioendothelioma is the most common symptomatic vascular liver tumor of infancy (1–4). It is considered a benign tumor; however, aggressive behavior is occasionally seen microscopically, and rarely distant metastases have been reported (5). Greater than 85% of patients with hepatic hemangioendotheliomas present before 6 months (2, 6). The female to male ratio is 2:1. No racial predilection or genetic transmission is known. The tumor tends to grow rapidly after presentation and then regresses gradually over several months if the child can be supported without surgical intervention (1, 7, 8). Rarely, it persists into adulthood.

The exact incidence of infantile hemangioendothelioma is difficult to determine because often it has been either misdiagnosed or mislabeled in the literature as cavernous hemangioma (1, 7, 8). Cavernous hemangioma is the most common primary liver tumor in older age groups but is rarely found in infants as a clinically significant tumor. When found in infants, it is usually an incidental small focus at autopsy.

Clinical Features

The most common presenting features are a palpable mass, hepatomegaly or diffuse abdominal enlargement. Levick and Rubie (9) were the first to recognize an association between hemangioendothelioma of the liver and congestive heart failure (CHF), and there were subsequent reports substantiating this association (9, 10). However, in a review of 27 cases from the Armed Forces Institute of Pathology (AFIP) by Dachman et al. only one case presented with CHF and three additional patients developed CHF during their hospital course (11). Thus, CHF is less common a feature of infantile hemangioendothelioma than is generally thought. Cutaneous hemangiomas may be present in up to 45% of cases. Rarely, a murmur can be heard over the liver and jaundice may be present (11).

The serum alpha-fetoprotein is usually normal but can be moderately elevated. Elevation is probably due to persistence of fetal alpha-fetoprotein in these young patients rather than tumor production. If followed, levels will diminish.

Pathology

Hemangioendotheliomas may be round and smooth or multilobular and irregular. Although they have no true capsule, they tend to be well demarcated from surrounding liver tissue since they grow by compression rather than invasion. Pedunculated lesions are uncommon. The tumor is reddish-brown or white and is relatively soft and spongy. Central areas of large lesions tend to show evidence of infarction, hemorrhage, fibrosis, and foci of dystrophic calcification (Fig. 2.7). The calcification is often only microscopic and thus not always radiographically evident. Although small tumors are theoretically less likely to precipitate congestive heart failure, there is no good correlation between tumor size and congestive heart failure; localized or multicentric tumors may be associated with congestive heart failure.

Two histologic subtypes of infantile hemangioendothelioma have been reported (2). Type I consists of variable-sized vascular spaces lines by relatively immature, plump endothelial cells, sometimes in multiple layers with a distinctive tufting or budding appearance (Fig. 2.8). The endothelial cells are supported on a prominent reticulin network. The supporting stroma is fibrous, but foci of less well differentiated myxomatous tissue may occasionally be seen. Bile ducts are scattered between vascular spaces which may contain some hematopoietic cells (Fig. 2.8). Type II has more immature, bigger, pleomorphic cells with more hyperchromatic nuclei and reflects the more aggressive end of a spectrum in the behavior of this lesion (2). In the central areas of large lesions, foci resembling cavernous hemangioma may be found, adding to the confusion in terminology.

Histologically, the type II hemangioendothelioma may mimic hemangioendothelial sarcoma, but the latter is generally a disease of older adults. In addition to the difference in age, the sarcoma of adults typically demonstrates intrasinusoidal spread and invasion of central and portal veins, features not seen in infantile hemangioendothelioma. Nevertheless, the infantile lesion may have some limited malignant potential; it may behave aggressively and rare cases of metastases have been described (5), although it is difficult to document whether these represent true metastases or multifocal tumors.

In contrast, hemangiomas are characterized

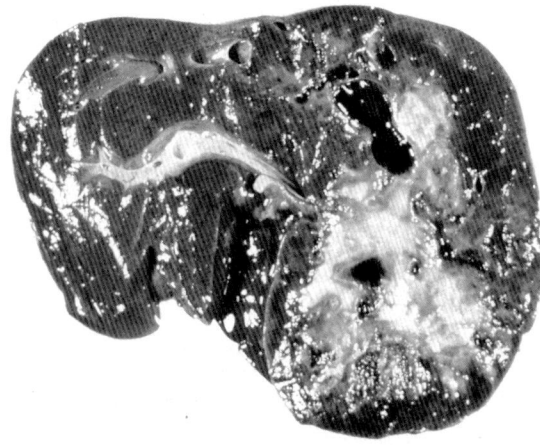

FIGURE 2.7. HEMANGIOENDOTHELIOMA GROSS SPECIMEN

Cut gross specimen of infantile hemangioendothelioma replacing most of the left lobe of liver. Note hemorrhagic central areas.

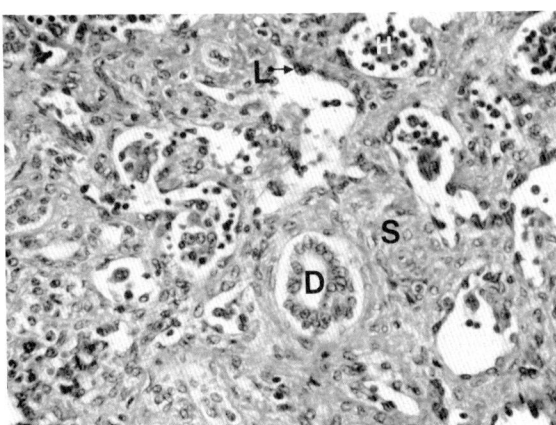

FIGURE 2.8. HIGH POWER MICROSCOPIC FIELD FROM HEMANGIOENDOTHELIOMA

Undifferentiated stroma (S), immature lining cells (L), hematopoiesis (H), bile ducts (D).

by varying sized vascular spaces lined by a single layer of mature, flat endothelial cells. The supporting stroma is scanty and composed of mature fibrous tissue, although more extensive areas of fibrosis and rarely dystrophic calcification may occasionally be seen, usually in elderly patients (12). Bile ducts are absent.

Radiology

Plain films of the abdomen may show a soft-tissue mass, hepatomegaly, or speckled calcification (Fig. 2.9). While calcification is suggestive of a hemangioendothelioma in children younger than 1 yr, it is nonspecific and may be seen in hepatoblastoma (the major differential diagnostic consideration), as well as hamartoma and metastatic neuroblastoma. Chest x-ray may show cardiomegaly and pulmonary venous hypertension if CHF is present.

Sonography is useful in localizing the mass to the liver and in hemangioendothelioma may show a hypoechoic, complex, or hyperechoic lesion (Fig. 2.10). Lesions may be single or multiple, discrete or poorly delineated. In at least one reported case hypoechoic lesions were nearly anechoic and mimicked cysts (11). If large cystic components are found, then the rare mesenchymal hamartoma becomes a likely consideration. Sonography can be used to follow hemangioendotheliomas. The lesions tend to regress slowly becoming increasingly hyperechoic and shrinking over a period of months (13).

Unenhanced CT of hemangioendothelioma shows one or more masses of lower density than surrounding liver tissue. Using bolus intravenous contrast material with both dynamic scanning and delayed scans CT may show focal areas of

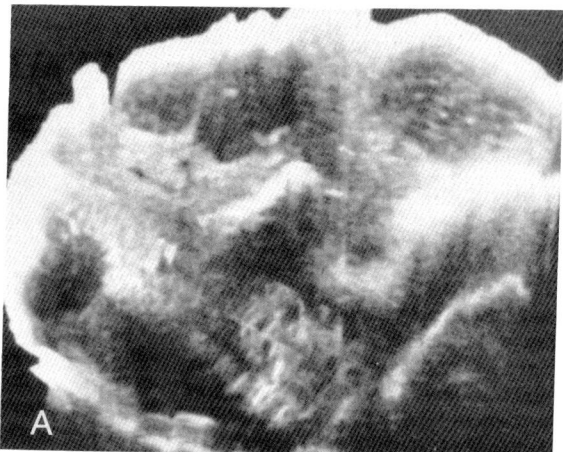
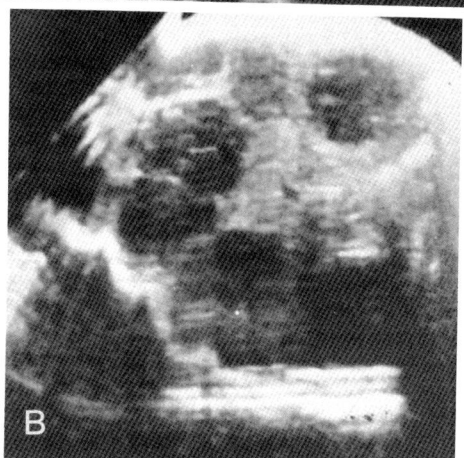

FIGURE 2.10. SONOGRAPHY OF MULTIFOCAL HEMANGIOENDOTHELIOMA

A: Transverse sonogram. B: Sagittal sonogram. Multiple discrete, hypoechoic, solid masses.

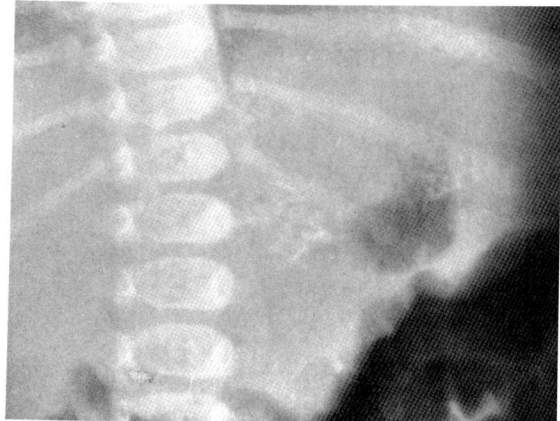

FIGURE 2.9. PLAIN FILM OF SPECKLED CALCIFICATION IN INFANTILE HEMANGIOENDOTHELIOMA IN LEFT LOBE OF LIVER

low attenuation that exhibit early peripheral enhancement after a bolus of contrast material with variable delayed central enhancement (Fig. 2.11A–C). This pattern is similar to that of cavernous hemangioma in adults as described by Barnett (14). This would be expected in the hemodynamically less active hemangioendotheliomas. Current data are insufficient to establish the reliability and specificity of this finding.

Liver scintigraphy is occasionally a useful adjunct to sonography and CT in demonstrating the hepatic origin of a lesion. Radionuclide angiography combined with pool studies can show the vascular nature of the mass (Fig. 2.11D, E) (15, 16).

Angiography confirms the vascular nature of the mass, but may be particularly useful in delineating the extent of the lesion when liver involvement is diffuse or as a preoperative guide (Fig. 2.12). A decreased caliber of the aorta distal to

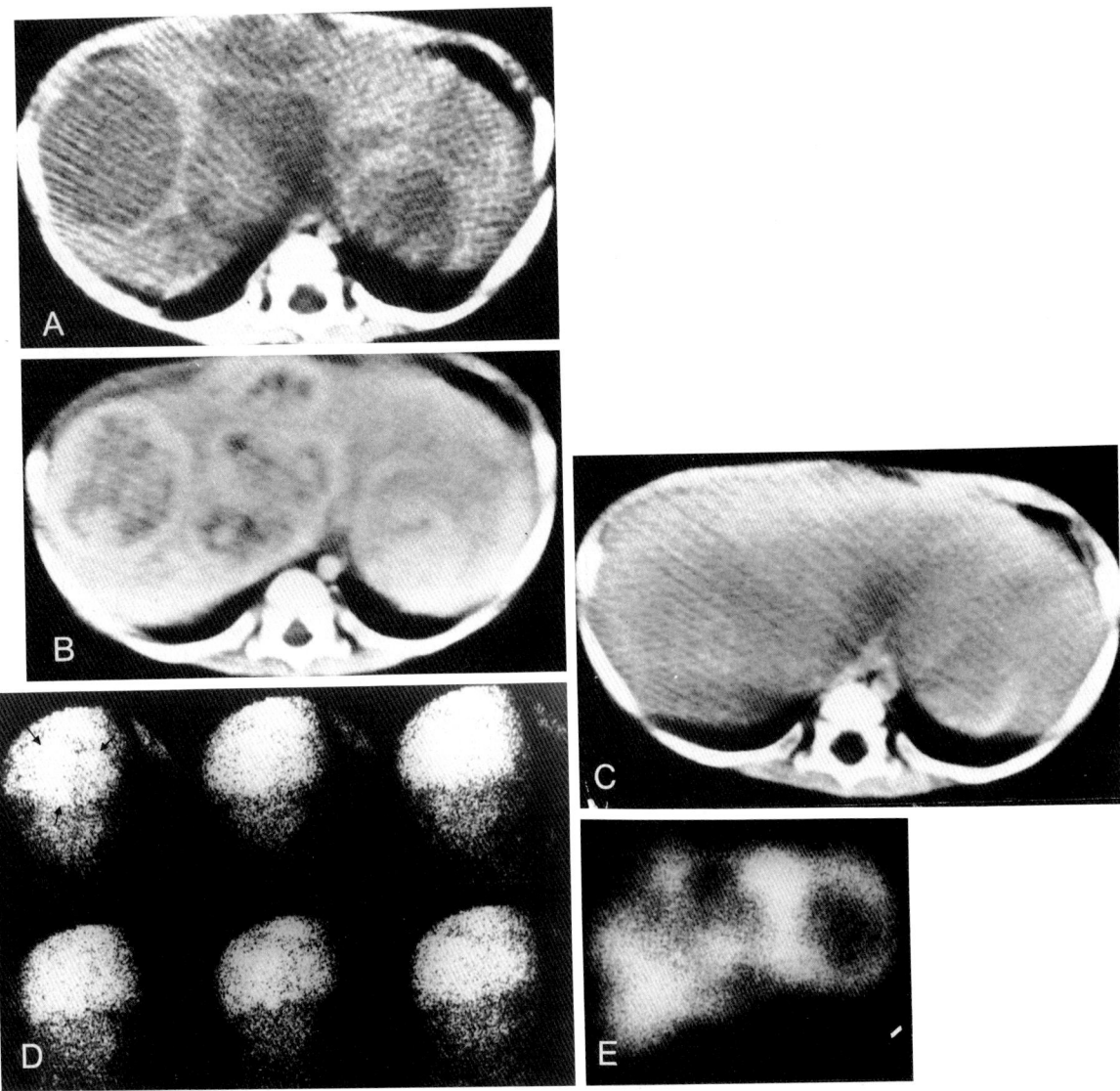

FIGURE 2.11. DYNAMIC CT OF MULTIFOCAL HEMANGIOENDOTHELIOMA

A: Precontrast CT: multiple, well demarcated masses of lower density than surrounding liver. *B:* Immediate postbolus CT: early edge enhancement of all lesions. *C:* Delayed postcontrast CT: tumor is nearly isodense with surrounding liver. *D:* Radionuclide angiography using ^{99m}Tc-labeled sulfur-colloid in the same patient. The angiogram shows increased arterial flow to the masses (*top left, arrows*). *E:* The static scan shows multiple cold intrahepatic masses.

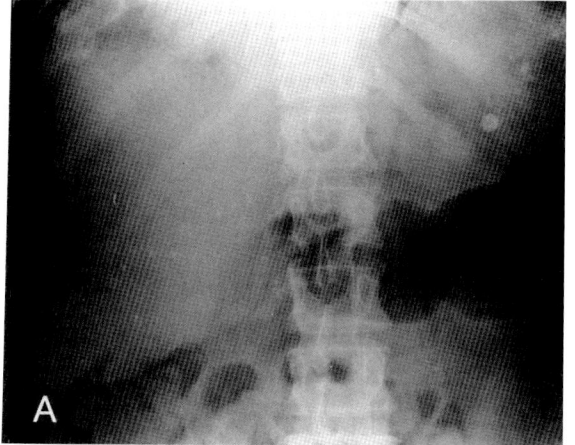
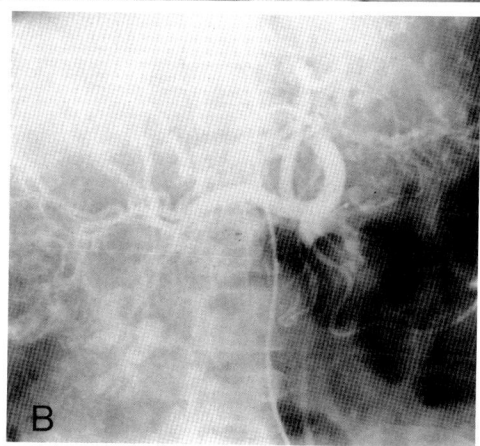
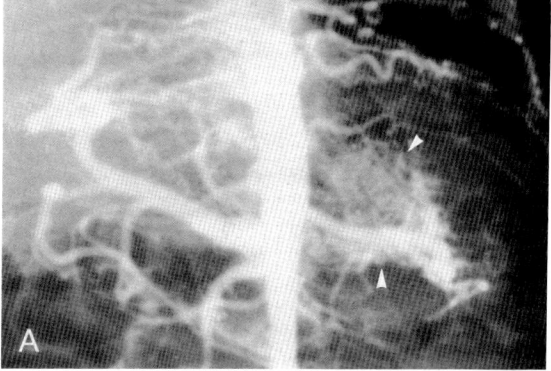
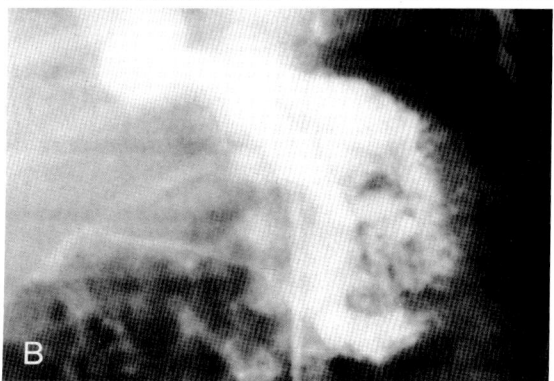

FIGURE 2.13. HEMANGIOENDOTHELIOMA WITH CONGESTIVE HEART FAILURE

A: Aortogram: tumor vascularity in left lobe of liver (*arrowheads*), decreased caliber of distal abdominal aorta occasionally seen in vascular liver tumors. *B:* Venous phase, selective hepatic artery injection with arteriovenous shunting to hepatic veins, an uncommon finding in hemangioendothelioma.

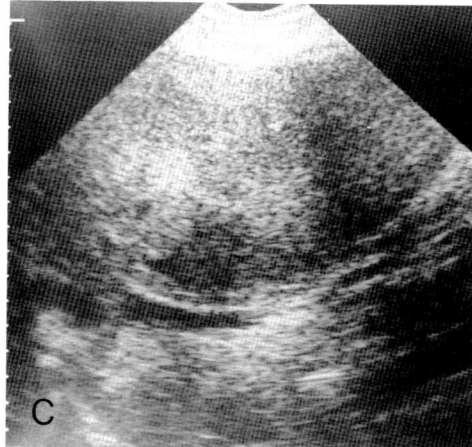

FIGURE 2.12. DIFFUSE HEMANGIOENDOTHELIOMATOSIS

Diffuse hemangioendotheliomatosis in an adult female presenting with hepatomegaly, ascites, and weight loss. Probably congenital. *A:* Plain film. Hepatomegaly displacing the stomach and phlebolith-like calcifications in the left lobe of the liver. *B:* Hepatic arteriogram. Multiple hypervascular lesions scattered throughout the liver. *C:* Parasagittal sonogram through the left lobe of the liver: hepatomegaly with an abnormal, inhomogeneous parenchymal architecture without depiction of well-defined masses.

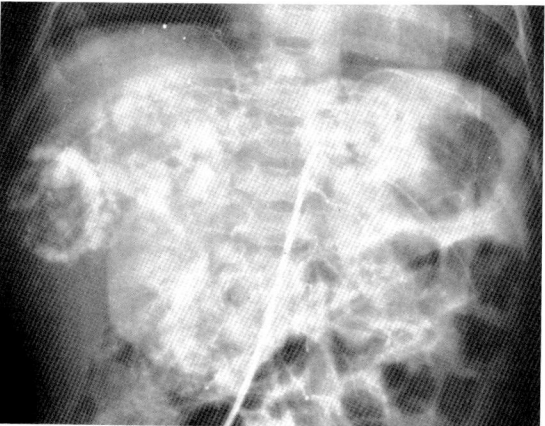

FIGURE 2.14. CELIAC ARTERIOGRAM, LATE ARTERIAL PHASE, MULTIFOCAL HEMANGIOENDOTHELIOMA

Multifocal tumors with large tortuous feeding vessels. Large lesions have areas of diminished vascularity centrally.

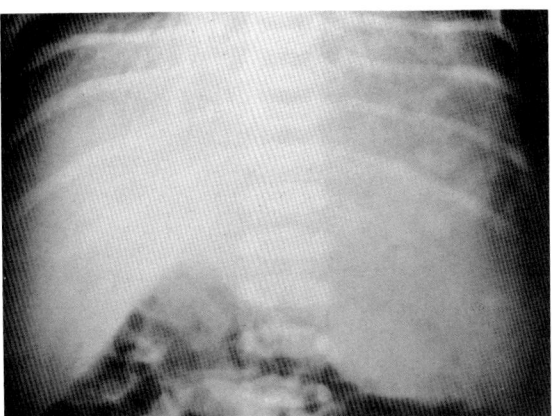

FIGURE 2.15. EXCRETORY UROGRAM OF HEMANGIOENDOTHELIOMA
Total body opacification phase, excretory urogram. Mottled pattern of increased density within a hemangioendothelioma. Scout film demonstrated a mass in the left lobe of the liver.

the origin of the hepatic artery and enlarged tortuous feeding vessels which do not taper normally may be seen (Fig. 2.13A) (17). There is often prolonged pooling of contrast material in vascular lakes or large areas of the tumor (Fig. 2.14). Early arteriovenous shunting together with enlarged tortuous feeding vessels may be the angiographic-pathophysiologic correlation to those few cases with high-output CHF (Fig. 2.13) (3, 11, 17). (In contrast, cavernous hemangiomas usually have normal sized feeding vessels and arteriovenous shunting is rare.) If an excretory urogram is performed, the total body opacification phase may demonstrate densities within the liver corresponding to vascular regions of the tumor correlating with dilated vascular lakes seen on angiography (Figs. 2.14 and 2.15) (3).

REFERENCES

1. Braun P, Ducharme JC, Riopelle JL, Davignon A: Hemangiomatosis of the liver in infants. *J Pediatr Surg* 10:121–126, 1975.
2. Dehner LP, Ishak KG: Vascular tumors of the liver in infants and children. *Arch Pathol* 92:101–111, 1971.
3. Slovis TL, Berdon WE, Holler JO, Casarella WJ, Baker DH: Hemangiomas of the liver in infants. *AJR* 123:791–801, 1975.
4. Leonidas JC, Strauss L, Beck AR: Vascular tumors of the liver in newborns. *Am J Dis Child* 125:507–510, 1973.
5. Ishak KG: Primary hepatic tumors in childhood. In: Popper H, Schaffner F (eds): *Progress in Liver Diseases*, Chap 28. New York, Grune & Stratton, 1976, pp 636–667.
6. Cleland RS: Benign and malignant tumors of the liver. *Pediatr Clin North Am* 6:427–447, 1959.
7. McLean RH, Moller JH, Warwick WJ: Multinodular hemangiomatosis of the liver in infancy. *Pediatrics* 49:563–573, 1972.
8. Berdon WE, Baker DH: Giant hepatic hemangioma with cardiac failure in the newborn infant. *Radiology* 92:1523–1528, 1962.
9. Levick CB, Rubie J: Hemangioendothelioma of the liver simulating congenital heart disease in an infant. *Arch Dis Child* 28:49–51, 1953.
10. Winters RW, Robinson SJ, Bates G: Hemangioma of the liver with heart failure: a case report. *Pediatrics* 14:117–119, 1954.
11. Dachman AH, Lichtenstein JE, Friedman AC, Hartman DS: Infantile hemangioendothelioma of the liver: a radiologic-pathologic-clinical correlation. *AJR* 140:1091–1096, 1983.
12. Ishak KG, Rabin L: Benign tumors of the liver. *Med Clin North Am* 59:995–1013, 1975.
13. Pardes JG, Bryan PJ, Gauderer MWL: Spontaneous regression of infantile hemangioendotheliomatosis of the liver. *J Ultrasound Med* 1:349–353, 1982.
14. Barnett PH: Computed tomography in the diagnosis of cavernous hemangioma of the liver. *AJR* 134:439–447, 1980.
15. Weiner SN, Parulekar SG: Scintigraphy and ultrasonography of hepatic hemangioma. *Radiology* 132:149–153, 1979.
16. Okuda K, Lio M: *Radiologic Aspects of the Liver and Biliary Tract. X-ray and Radioisotope Diagnosis.* Chicago, Year Book, 1976, pp 316–317.
17. Moss AA, Clark RE, Palubinskas AJ, Deborimier AA: Angiographic appearance of benign and malignant hepatic tumors in infants and children. *AJR* 113:61–69, 1971.

HEPATOBLASTOMA

Hepatoblastoma is the most common symptomatic liver tumor in children under the age of five (1). The term hepatoblastoma was coined by Willis to describe a group of tumors of embryonal origin histologically distinct from hepatocellular carcinoma of childhood (2). As complete surgical resection is crucial in successful outcome of therapy, proper radiologic evaluation is mandatory.

Hepatoblastoma most commonly occurs in the first 3 yrs of life, while hepatocellular malignancies in patients older than 5 yr tend to be morphologically similar to those found in adults (3–5). Hepatoblastoma affects infants at a younger age than Wilms' tumor. In a study by Gonzalez-Crussi et al., 52% of a total of 21 patients with hepatoblastoma were infants under 1 yr of age (5). In a national survey of pediatric surgeons almost half of 129 hepatoblastoma patients were

18 months of age or younger (6). Eleven were under 6 weeks and 3 were newborn. Cremin et al. reported a case of calcified congenital hepatoblastoma (7). There are several reported instances of hepatoblastoma in older children and the oldest child in the survey by the surgical section of the American Academy of Pediatrics was 15 (6). Cases have also been reported in siblings and in adults (8, 9). The male/female ratio is 3-2:1 (3, 10).

Clinical Features

Children usually present with hepatomegaly or a palpable abdominal mass. Weight loss, fever, nausea, vomiting and adenopathy may be present, and pathologic fracture from bone metastasis may occur. The alpha-fetoprotein is often persistently and markedly elevated. Anemia, leukocytosis, and abnormal function tests may also be noted.

Pathology

Grossly the hepatoblastoma most commonly forms a single mass within the right lobe of the liver (5). Less commonly multiple nodules may be present in which case both lobes are usually involved. Least common is diffuse tumor involvement of the entire liver parenchyma.

Hepatoblastomas are usually roughly spherical sharply circumscribed neoplasms. In most cases, hepatic parenchyma located distant to the site of compression is normal (5). Externally most hepatoblastomas are nodular and a portion usually bulges from one edge of the liver surface.

In a retrospective review of 35 cases of hepatoblastoma at the AFIP in 1967, 16 were classified as epithelial, that is predominantly containing epithelial cells of varying degrees of maturity and 19 as mixed epithelial and mesenchymal type, tissues of mesenchymal derivation in addition to epithelial elements being present (4). Other series have shown a predominance of the epithelial type. However, all reported cases of hepatoblastoma in adults have been of the mixed type (1). Controversy exists as to whether these adult cases are truly hepatoblastomas. The epithelial elements are subdivided into the embryonal and fetal type based on the degree of differentiation and cellular pattern.

Gonzalez-Crussi et al. describe a subtype of the fetal epithelial form with nests of tissue having features most typical of hepatocellular carcinoma (5). These tumors acted more aggressively with bone metastases in 2 patients out of 21. However, other studies have concluded that the fetal subtype has a better prognosis than other subtypes. A higher degree of anaplasia conveys a worse prognosis (1).

Radiology

The most common modality used in the past for the initial radiologic evaluation of patients with hepatoblastoma is the plain film of the abdomen. With the development of more advanced radiologic imaging techniques initial evaluation employs ultrasound concurrently with plain film imaging. In the study by Exelby et al. 85% of patients with hepatoblastoma showed some plain film abnormality, most commonly hepatomegaly (6). Sixty-two of sixty-five patients with various hepatic tumors had plain film abnormalities in a study by Miller et al. (11). In a retrospective study by Dachman et al. 10 of 18 patients demonstrated plain film calcifications, the majority which were of the mixed type, confirming the impression by others that calcification is more common in the mixed type (Fig. 2.16) (12). Since the masses are frequently large, often there is deviation of the kidney on urography and of the bowel on upper and lower gastrointestinal studies. Nuclear scintigraphy usually shows a nonspecific hepatic defect with ^{99m}Tc-sulfur colloid or a hepatobiliary agent. However, two cases have been reported in which colloid uptake was present within the mass and one also had IDA uptake (13). Gallium scans may or may not show avidity.

Ultrasound shows a large inhomogeneously echogenic mass, sometimes with calcification evident (Fig. 2.17A) (12, 14). Less often small anechoic foci are seen within the mass. This may

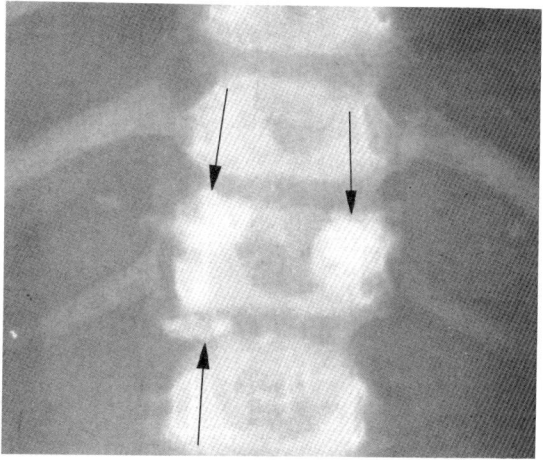

FIGURE 2.16. CALCIFICATIONS (*arrows*) IN A HEPATOBLASTOMA

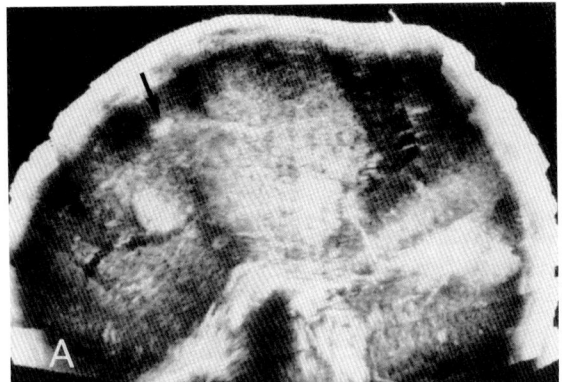

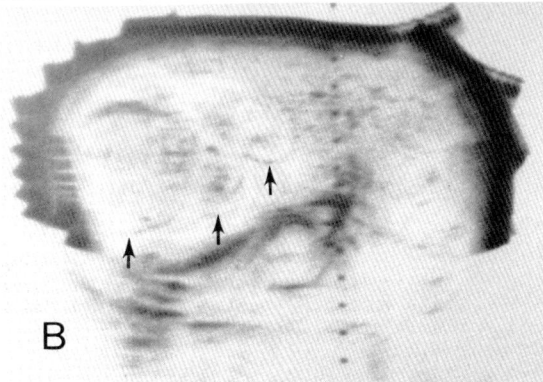

FIGURE 2.17. SONOGRAM OF HEPATOBLASTOMA
A: Large echogenic mass with foci of calcification present (*arrow*). This is the same case as Figure 2.18. B: Less common pattern of tumor lobulation makes this single mass appear almost as three separate nodules (*arrows*).

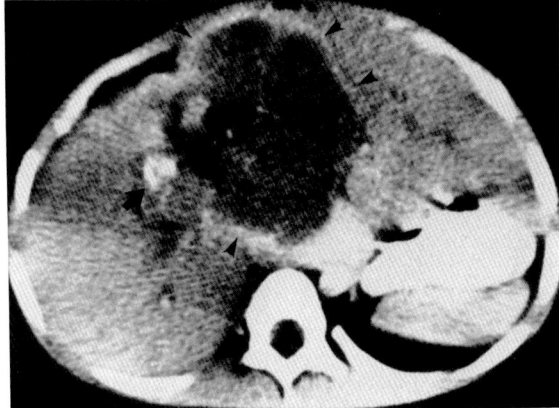

FIGURE 2.18. CT OF HEPATOBLASTOMA
Large solid low density mass with peripheral enhancement (*arrows*) on dynamic scanning. The focus of calcification (*large arrow*), correlates with the sonogram, Figure 2.17A.

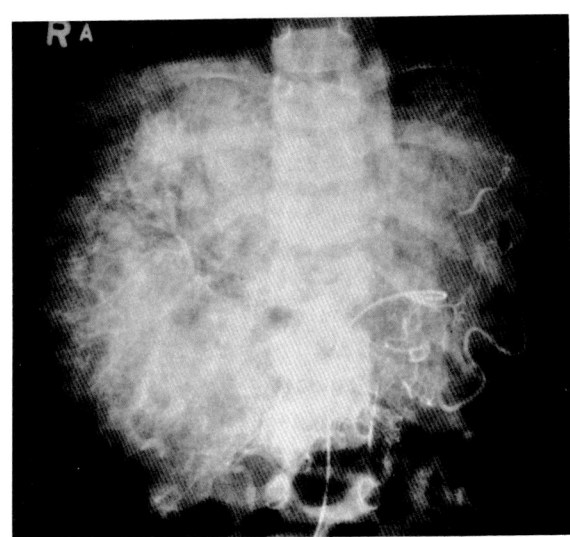

FIGURE 2.19. ANGIOGRAM OF THE PARENCHYMAL PHASE OF HEPATOBLASTOMA
The mass is hypervascular with some relatively hypovascular areas.

be due to tumor necrosis, or possibly areas of extramedullary hematopoiesis (12, 15). A lobular pattern due to sepatation within the tumor may be depicted on sonography (Fig. 2.17B) (12). Four cases of "cystic hepatoblastoma" have been described sonographically in which septae were seen in the cystic sonolucent masses (16). Careful review of the pathologic description leads me to believe that these were probably mesenchymal hamartomas, not hepatoblastomas.

Although hepatoblastoma can usually be detected on either precontrast or postcontrast CT scans, the tumor is best defined following the infusion of contrast material. The tumor will enhance slightly although to a degree far less than the normal liver parenchyma. A peripheral rim of enhancement may be seen if a dynamic series of images is obtained (Fig. 2.18). The rim is best seen in the arterial phase of the study. Involvement of the portal vein and/or inferior vena cava will be best defined following contrast enhancement.

The presence of coarse calcification is strongly suggestive of hepatoblastoma (12). These dystrophic zones may contain osseous matrix. Hemangioendotheliomas may also contain calcification but in these cases it is usually a fine granular calcification. This is the explanation of why the calcifications of hepatoblastoma are commonly seen on plain films of the abdomen while those secondary to hemangioendothelioma are usually not noted. Hepatocellular carcinoma may also present with coarse calcifications but this is usually seen in the fibrolamellar subtype or in patients with previous treatment with chemotherapy or radiation therapy.

LIVER ANOMALIES AND CONGENITAL DISORDERS

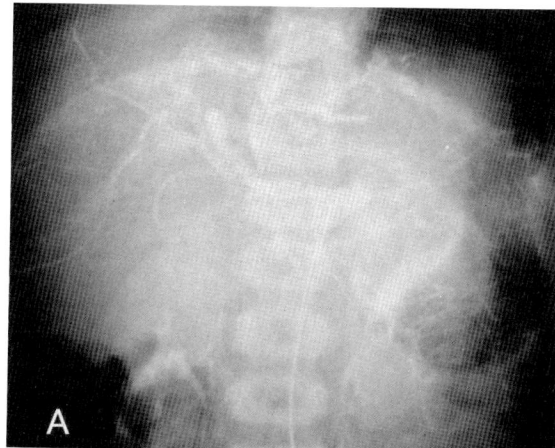

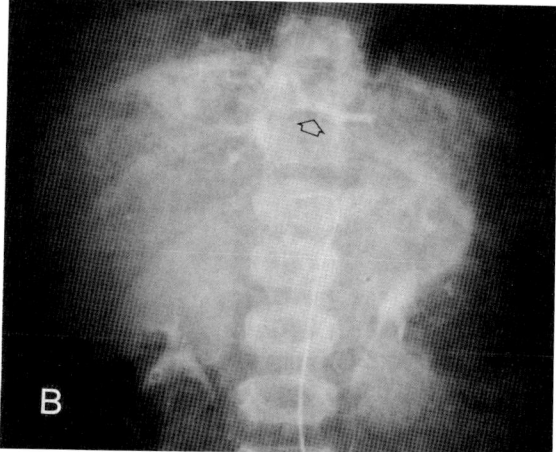

FIGURE 2.20. HEPATOBLASTOMA
Selective hepatic arteriogram on this 2-yr-old child demonstrates the large hypervascular mass involving predominately the right lobe of the liver with extension to the left lobe. The angio-architecture is bizarre with neovascularity and persistent opacification of venous structures on the late phase (*B, arrow*).

On angiography the tumor is usually hypervascular (Figs. 2.19 and 2.20). Neovascularity, puddling of contrast material, and stretched vessels may be seen. A spokewheel pattern has also been reported (12). Inferior vena caval compression or invasion may be seen.

While the findings are not pathognomonic they are strongly suggestive of the diagnosis. The major differential considerations are hemangioendothelioma, metastatic neuroblastoma, mesenchymal hamartoma, and (rarely) hepatocellular carcinoma. Many hemangioendotheliomas are predominantly hypoechoic and calcification when present is fine and fibrillary. The clinical features of neuroblastoma and an elevated vanillylmandelic acid are clues to its diagnosis. Mesenchymal hamartomas show large cystic spaces rather than small ones which may be seen in hepatoblastoma. Hepatocellular carcinoma is rare under the age of 5 yr.

REFERENCES

1. Lack IE, Neave C, Vawter GF: Hepatoblastoma: a clinical and pathologic study of 54 cases. *Am J Surg Pathol* 6:693–705, 1982.
2. Willis RA: The pathology of the tumors of children. In Cameron R, Wright GP (eds): *Pathological Monographs.* London, Oliver & Boyd, 1962, pp 57–61.
3. Weinberg AG, Finegold MJ: Primary hepatic tumors of childhood. *Hum Pathol* 6:512–537, 1983.
4. Ishak KG, Glunz PR: Hepatoblastoma and hepatocarcinoma in infancy and childhood: report of 47 cases. *Cancer* 20:396–422, 1967.
5. Gonzalez-Crussi F, Upton MP, Maurer HS: Hepatoblastoma: attempt at characterization of histologic subtypes. *Am J Surg Pathol* 7:599–612, 1982.
6. Exelby PR, Filler RM, Grewfeld JL: Liver tumors in children in the particular reference to hepatoblastoma and hepatocellular carcinoma: American Academy of Pediatrics Surgical Section Survey-1974. *J Pediatr Surg* 10:329–337, 1975.
7. Cremin BJ, Nuss D: Calcified hepatoblastoma in a newborn. *J Pediatr Surg* 9:913–915, 1974.
8. Napoli VM, Campbell W, Jr.: Hepatoblastoma in an infant sister and brother. *Cancer* 39:2647–2650, 1977.
9. Frasmeni JF Jr., Rosen PJ, Hull EW, Barth RF, Shapiro SR, O'Connor JF: Hepatoblastoma in infant sisters. *Cancer* 24:1086–1090, 1969.
10. Iwafuchi M, Muto T, Ohsawa Y, Yamashita Y, Matsuda Y, Yoshida K: Hepatoma in children: a clinical analysis on 15 cases. *Jpn J Surg* 11:454–459, 1981.
11. Miller JH, Gates GF, Stanley P: The radiologic investigation of hepatic tumors in childhood. *Radiology* 124:451–458, 1977.
12. Dachman AH, Pakter RL, Ros PR, Fishman EK, Goodman Z: Hepatoblastoma: a pathologic radiologic correlation of 41 cases (submitted for publication).
13. Diament MJ, Parvey LS, Tonkin ILD, Johnson KD, Bernstein R, Webber B: Hepatoblastoma: technetium sulfur colloid uptake simulating focal nodular hyperplasia. *AJR* 139:168–171, 1982.
14. Bellina PV Jr., Lang EK, Pisco JM, Handenmann M: Multidisciplinary approach to the diagnosis of hepatoblastoma: ultrasound, nuclear medicine and angiography. *South Med J* 73:1085–1087, 1980.
15. Isdale JM, Beck WP, Chappell JS: The radiological investigation of hepatocellular carcinoma in children. *S Afr Med J* 62:688–690, 1982.
16. Miller JH: The ultrasonographic appearance of cystic hepatoblastoma. *Radiology* 138:141–143, 1981.

UNDIFFERENTIATED (EMBRYONAL) SARCOMA

Malignant mesenchymal tumors of the liver are fairly uncommon. Differentiated monomorphic sarcomas such as rhabdomyosarcoma, leiomyosarcoma, fibrosarcoma, and liposarcoma occur rarely in the elderly and are usually unresectable. Pathologically they are large, hemorrhagic, and partially necrotic (1). There has been little radiologic experience reported with these tumors. Sarcomas of the ligamentum teres occur occasionally in younger patients and are more often resectable (1).

Undifferentiated (embryonal) sarcomas, although still uncommon, are the fourth most frequent hepatic tumor in the pediatric age group

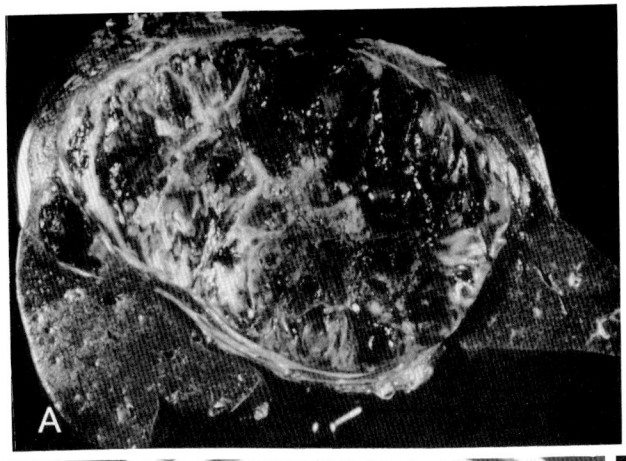

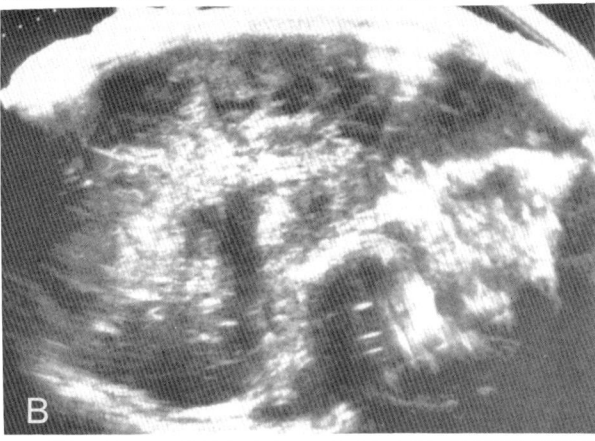

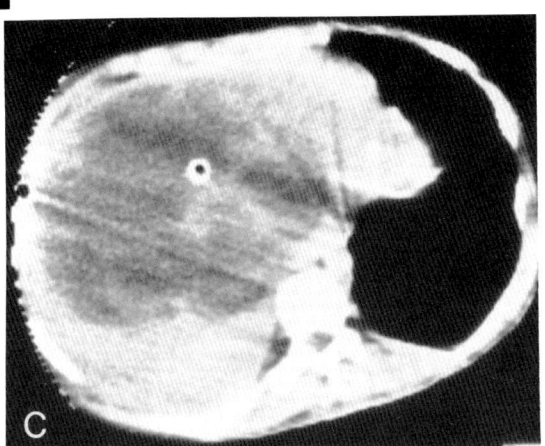

FIGURE 2.21. MOSTLY SOLID UNDIFFERENTIATED SARCOMA

A: Cut gross specimen: solid encapsulated mass with several dark regions of hemorrhagic necrosis. *B:* Transverse sonogram: large solid echogenic right-lobe mass. *C:* CT with contrast: large hypodense solid mass. Central apparent calcification is an artifact. *D:* Arteriogram: stretching and splaying of arteries with a few scattered regions of abnormal vascularity and early filling of bizarre veins (*arrows*), predominately hypovascular mass. *E:* Hepatogram: large lucent mass with abnormally walled veins.

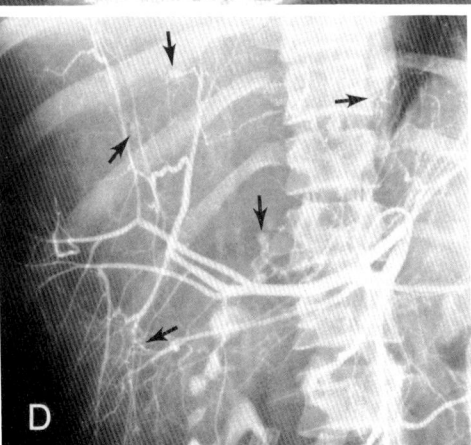

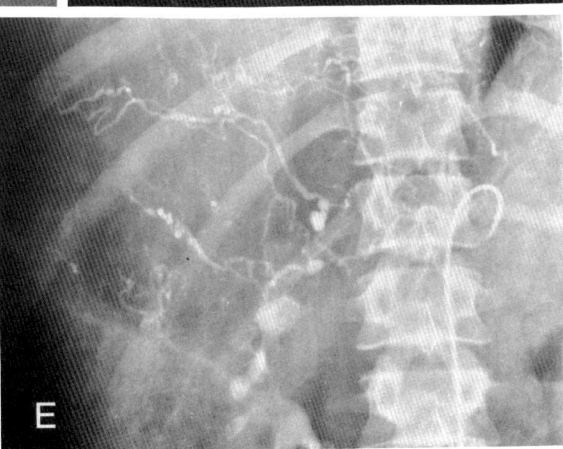

in the files of the AFIP (2). The absence of differentiated components prevents designation of this tumor by cell type. For example, leiomyosarcomas are identified by the presence of long, cigar-shaped nuclei and demonstration of myofribils, fibrosarcomas by elongated tumor cells closely invested by collagen fibers, and rhabdomyosarcomas by cross-striations in the malignant cells' cytoplasm (2). Approximately 65 cases of undifferentiated sarcoma have been reported, some under the names embryonal rhabdomyosarcoma, malignant mesenchymoma, embryonal sarcoma, fibromyosarcoma, and simply sarcoma (3).

Clinical Features

Approximately 90% occur in children up to the age of 15, the remaining 10% occur between the ages of 15 and 30 (3). Fifty-two percent occur between the ages of 6 and 10, and only 5% occur in the first 2 months of life (3). Patients generally present with an abdominal mass with or without abdominal pain. Fever, probably due to hemorrhage and necrosis, is prominent in about 5% and acute abdomen from spontaneous rupture can occur. Jaundice is absent at presentation. The duration of symptoms is usually a few days to one month but can be as long as 2 years (3).

On physical examination a right upper quadrant or epigastric mass is present. Laboratory data include a mild leukocytosis and anemia in about 50%, normal alpha-fetoprotein, and elevated liver enzymes in approximately 33% (3).

Treatment is surgical excision when feasible. Despite resection, chemotherapy, and radiation therapy, most patients are dead within 12 months of the diagnosis. One patient is alive and without evidence of recurrence 52 months after surgery, but the next longest survival is 19 months (3).

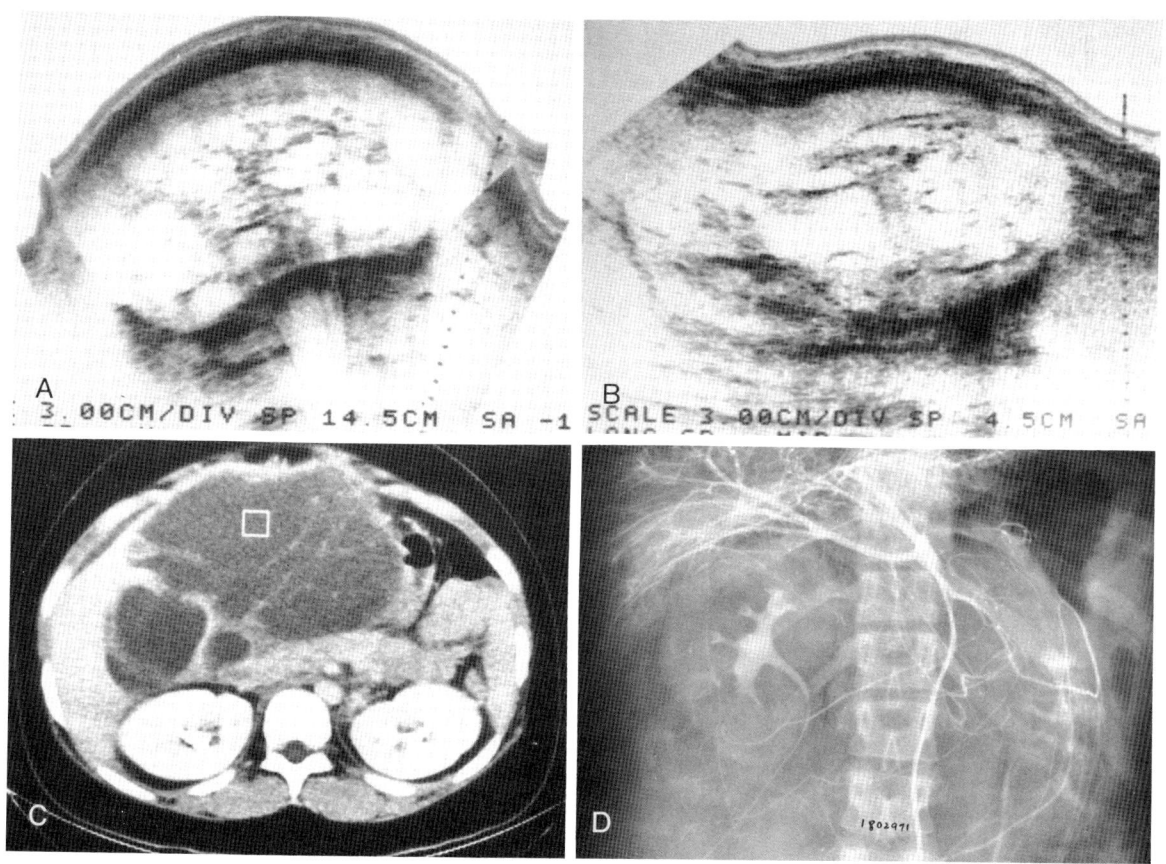

FIGURE 2.22. CYSTIC UNDIFFERENTIATED SARCOMA

A and *B:* Transverse and parasagittal sonograms through the large mass: multiple cystic spaces scattered among solid regions of tumor. *C:* Enhanced CT: large intrahepatic mostly cystic mass with a few septations. The sonogram gives a more accurate representation of internal architecture. *D:* Angiogram: huge hypovascular mass with splaying and stretching of arteries.

Pathology

Undifferentiated sarcoma is confined to the right lobe in 75%, the left lobe in 10%, and grows from the right into the left in 17%. Pedunculation is rare. Extension outside the liver and metastases may be present at presentation. The maximum diameter is generally between 10 and 20 cm. Grossly, undifferentiated sarcomas are globular, well-demarcated, and soft (Fig. 2.21A). The cut surface is yellow-gray to tan. More than 50% have multiple cystic areas with necrotic debris, clotted blood, or gelatinous material. A fibrous pseudocapsule of varying thickness usually surrounds the tumor, partially separating it from normal but compressed parenchyma. Multiple vessels, mostly thin-walled veins, are scattered throughout (Fig. 2.21E) (3).

Microscopically, the major component is stellate or spindle-shaped sarcomatous cells, closely packed and arranged in whorls and sheets, or scattered in a ground substance rich in acid mucopolysaccharide. Reticulin and collagen fibers are present among the cells. Foci of hematopoiesis are present in approximately 50%. The few epithelial elements present are in the periphery and thought to be trapped. The sarcomatous cells have round, elongated or highly irregular nuclei and numerous mitotic figures. Some cells have eosinophilic PAS-positive globules that are neither alpha–1-antitrypsin nor alpha-fetoprotein. There are no cross-striations (3). Undifferentiated sarcoma and mesenchymal hamartoma have the same tissue of origin—mesenchymal tissue. Mesenchymal hamartoma is an anomaly of development without malignant potential that usually presents in infants. Undifferentiated (embryonal) sarcoma is a true neoplasm most frequently presenting in older children (4).

Radiology

Plain films of the chest and abdomen may show hepatomegaly and diaphragmatic displacement but no calcification. Contrast examination of the gastrointestinal tract often shows displacement of the stomach, duodenum, ascending or transverse colon. Excretory urography may show inferior displacement of the right kidney. Sulfur colloid liver-spleen scans invariably show a defect (4).

Sonography and CT show large intrahepatic masses in which large cystic, low density regions are often present, corresponding to regions of hemorrhage and necrosis (Figs. 2.21 and 2.22). The degree of vascularity seen angiographically will vary from hypervascular to hypovascular, again depending on the degree of hemorrhage and necrosis (Figs. 2.21 and 2.22) (3). Intrahepatic vessels are stretched and separated by the mass, and there are scattered foci of neovascularity without prolonged pooling of contrast material (5). Radiologic findings do not permit differentiation from mesenchymal hamartoma; this differentiation cannot be made by gross inspection either. Mesenchymal hamartoma is more likely in children under three and undifferentiated (embryonal) sarcoma is more likely in older children (4).

REFERENCES

1. Schonland MM, Millward-Saddler GH, Wright DH, Wright R: Hepatic tumors. In Wright R, Alberti KGMM, Karran S, Millward-Sadler GH (eds): *Liver and Biliary Disease, Pathophysiology, Diagnosis, Management.* London, W.B. Saunders, 1979, pp 901–911.
2. Edmondson HA, Peters RL: Tumors of the liver: pathologic features. *Semin Roentgenol* 13:75–83, 1983.
3. Stocker JT, Ishak KG: Undifferentiated (embryonal) sarcoma of the liver. Report of 31 cases. *Cancer* 42:336–348, 1978.
4. Stocker JT, Ishak KG: Mesenchymal hamartoma of the liver: report of 30 cases and review of the literature. *Pediatr Pathol* 1:245–267, 1983.
5. Stanley RJ, Dehner LP, Hesker LP: Primary malignant mesenchymal tumors (mesenchymoma) of the liver in childhood. *Cancer* 32:973–984, 1973.

3

The Plain Film of the Liver

DINA F. CAROLINE, M.D.

HEPATOMEGALY AND THE EFFECTS OF LIVER SIZE ALTERATION ON OTHER STRUCTURES

Hepatomegaly

In normal adults, the liver, which is the largest solid organ in the body, weighs approximately 1500 g, or about 2.5% of total body weight. Linear maximum dimensions in the normal liver are approximately 12 cm anteroposterior, 22 cm transverse, and 17 cm longitudinal. There is a wide range in normal liver contour as well as variability dependent on sex, body habitus, and relation to other organs (1).

Imaging modalities have been applied in multiple attempts to evaluate liver size. Abdominal radiographs were found to correlate poorly with liver size (2). However, subjective description of hepatomegaly, or lack thereof on the basis of an abdominal radiograph is relatively accurate (3). Routine measurement of liver size on radiographs has proven too tedious to attain widespread acceptance (1). However, linear measurements can be made directly on computed tomography or ultrasonography. Radioisotope scanning (4), ultrasound (5), and CT (6), have been found to be quite accurate in determining liver volume, but volume alone is of limited clinical value.

Hepatomegaly is assessed on plain abdominal radiographs by the relationship of the liver to

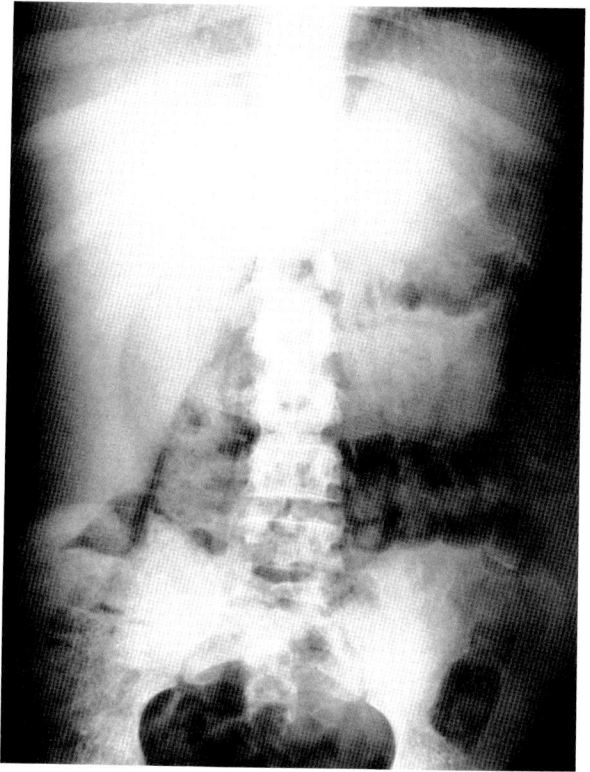

FIGURE 3.1. DIFFUSELY ENLARGED LIVER IN PATIENT WITH THALASSEMIA

The increased density secondary to iron content accentuates the border forming edges with right kidney (fat plane), stomach, and ascending colon (air within the viscus).

adjacent structures which may be appreciated as differences in density between soft tissue, air, and fat planes (Fig. 3.1). Frequently, the effect that enlargement or displacement of the liver has on adjacent organs is clinically important.

Generalized hepatomegaly may occur in multiple pathologic states some of which are listed in Table 3.1. When the liver enlarges uniformly, it tends to displace adjacent structures medially, downward, and to the left according to the vector principle described by Whalen et al. (7) (Figs. 3.2 and 3.3). The same vector principle applies when there are discrete masses within the liver, some causes of which are listed in Table 3.2. Outward growth from the epicenter of a mass is a major determinant of which structures will be affected and in which direction. This is modified to a considerable extent by individual anatomic variations in liver contour and in relationships between the liver and other abdominal and retroperitoneal organs (8, 9).

Focal enlargement of the liver may be simulated by multiple factors including masses within adjacent organs (Table 3.3) (Figs. 3.4 and 3.5). Planes between the intrinsically normal liver and the extrahepatic mass may be obscured on cross-sectional images; however, the vector principle is frequently useful in ascertaining the origin of the mass. Aberrant liver lobes, regenerated liver tissue, diaphragmatic herniation, or normal variants such as the Riedel's lobe, a prominent caudal extension of the right lobe, may also mimic liver masses (Fig. 3.6). Large intrahepatic plain film calcifications suggest the presence of an intrahepatic mass lesion; this too may be misleading (Fig. 3.7).

Various extrahepatic processes may also displace organs adjacent to the liver in a manner similar to that caused by diffuse hepatomegaly. Space-occupying processes in the right subpulmonic, subphrenic, or subhepatic recesses, massive ascites and diaphragmatic eventration, herniation, and phrenic nerve paralysis may be included in this category.

In contrast to liver enlargement, decrease in liver size, usually as a result of severe cirrhosis, may permit displacement of adjacent intra-abdominal organs to the right and cephalad. Diaphragmatic hernia or eventration may also permit adjacent organs to fill in the area vacated by the displaced liver.

Kattan (10) has used conventional radiographs to demonstrate the effect of diffuse or focal liver enlargement, relying on fat planes which outline either the true radiographic border or air within an adjacent viscus which forms an apparent border with the liver (1). Interpretation of true liver size and the relationships of the liver to its adjacent organs may be difficult using plain films alone. Appreciation of the liver's size and position as well as its relationship and effect on

TABLE 3.1.
CONDITIONS CAUSING DIFFUSE LIVER ENLARGEMENT

Passive congestion	Amyloid
Early cirrhosis	Wilson's disease
Fatty infiltration	Chronic granulomatous disease of childhood
Hepatitis	
Lymphoma	Gaucher's disease
Metastases	Leptospirosis
Diffuse hepatocellular carcinoma	Van Gierke's disease
	Niemann-Pick disease
Angiosarcoma	Weber-Christian disease
Mononucleosis	Galactosemia
Malaria	
Miliary TB, histoplasmosis or sarcoid	
Syphilis	

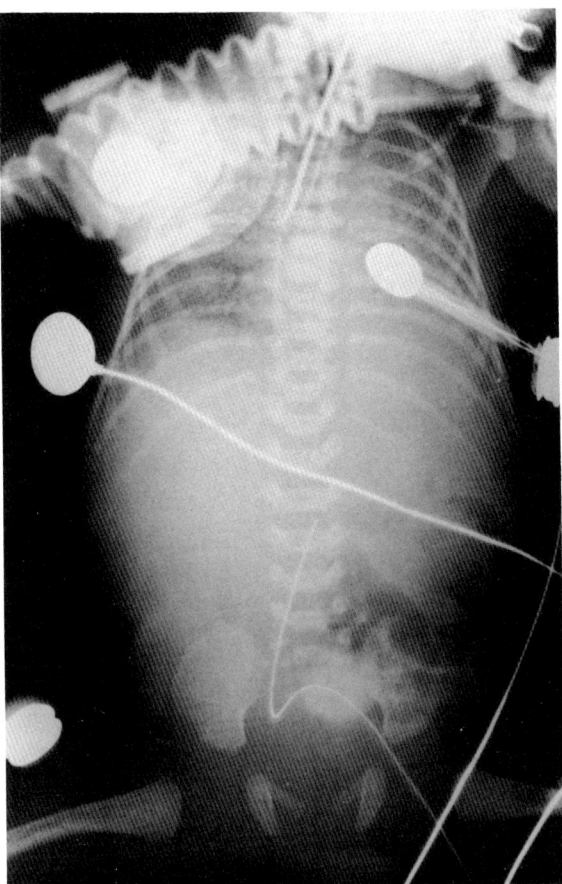

FIGURE 3.2. DIFFUSELY ENLARGED LIVER IN NEONATE DISPLACING ALL VISIBLE BOWEL GAS INTO LEFT LOWER QUADRANT

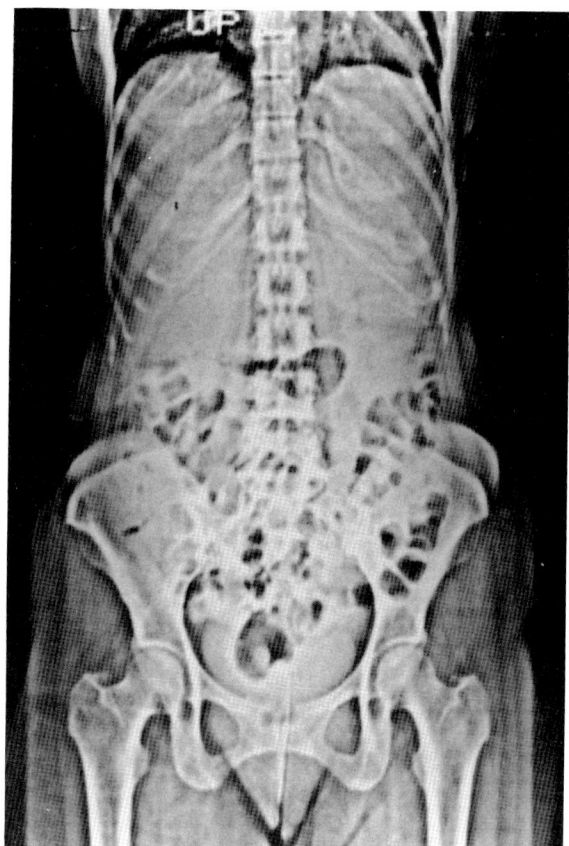

FIGURE 3.3. DOWNWARD DISPLACEMENT OF STOMACH AND BOWEL GAS IN PATIENT WITH DIFFUSELY ENLARGED LIVER FROM METASTATIC DISEASE

TABLE 3.3.
CONDITIONS WHICH MAY MIMIC HEPATOMEGALY

> Diaphragmatic eventration or herniation
> Phrenic nerve paralysis
> Massive ascites
> Subphrenic abscess
> Subpulmonic effusion
> Masses in adjacent organs including:
>   Colon
>   Renal
>   Stomach
>   Gallbladder
>   Pancreas
>   Adrenal

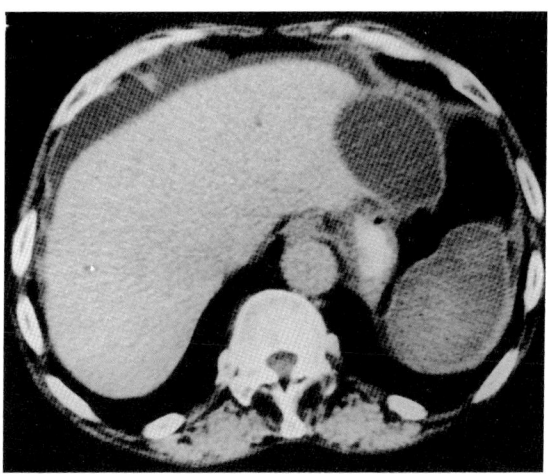

FIGURE 3.4. SPLENIC HEMATOMA, A PORTION OF WHICH MIMICS AN INTRAHEPATIC MASS

TABLE 3.2.
CONDITIONS CAUSING FOCAL HEPATIC ENLARGEMENT

> Anomalous lobes
> Metastases
> Cirrhosis
> Regenerative nodules
> Primary neoplasm (benign or malignant)
>   Adenoma
>   Focal nodular hyperplasia
>   Hepatocellular carcinoma
> Vascular tumors
>   Hemangioma
>   Hemangioendothelioma
> Cysts
>   Simple
>   Polycystic disease
>   Traumatic
>   Parasitic
> Abscess
>   Amebic
>   Pyogenic

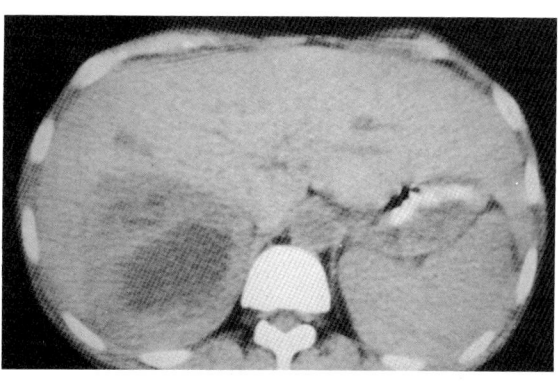

FIGURE 3.5. RIGHT ADRENAL TUMOR (PHEOCHROMOCYTOMA) WHICH APPEARS TO BE A MASS IN THE RIGHT LOBE OF THE LIVER

This patient also has a congenitally large left lobe (normal variant) which causes an extrinsic impression on the lesser curvature of the stomach, thereby mimicking another intrahepatic mass.

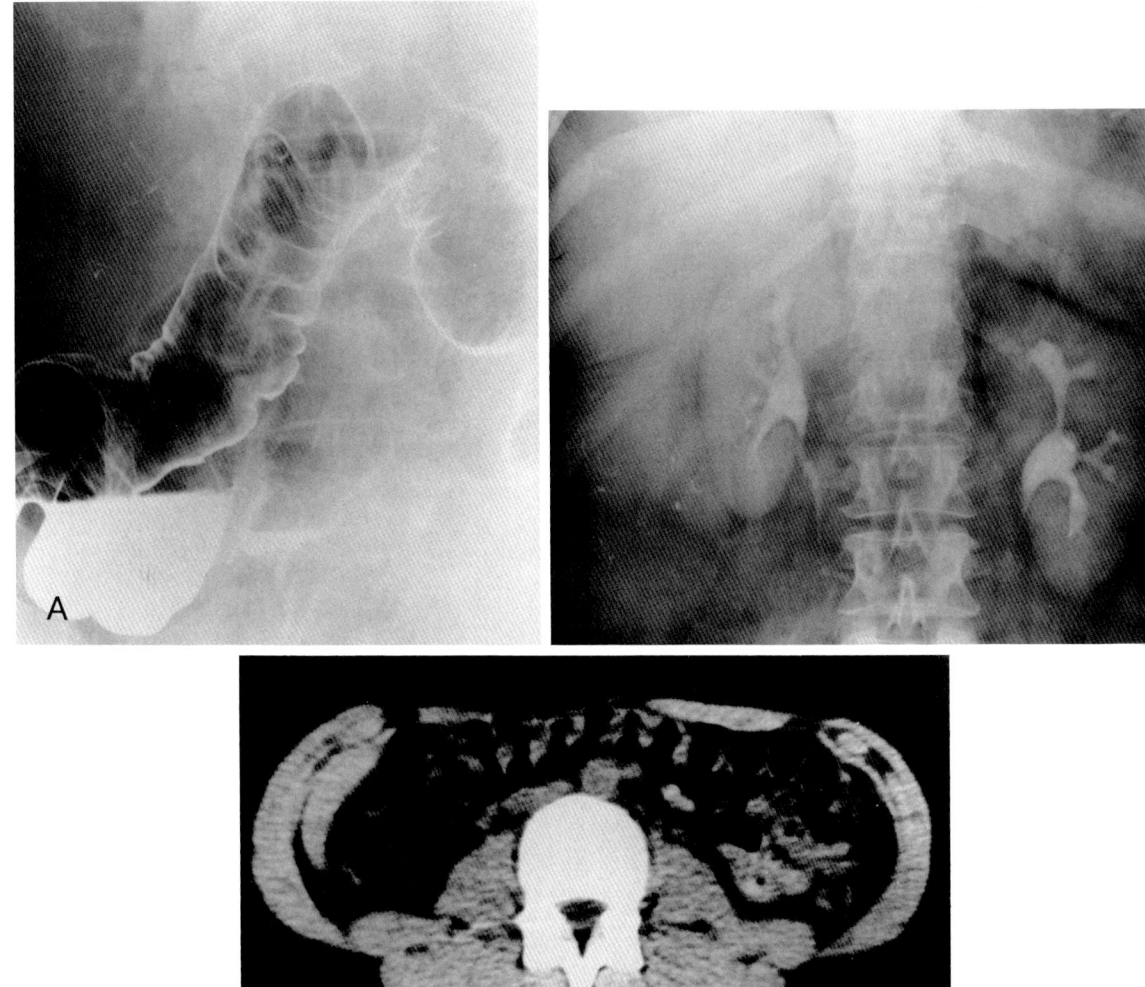

FIGURE 3.6. MIMICS OF HEPATIC ENLARGEMENT

A–C: Riedel's lobe mimicking hepatomegaly. *A:* Hepatic flexure, relating to the lateral and anterior portions of the inferior surface of the liver, is depressed. *B:* Right kidney, which relates more posteromedially to the visceral surface of the liver, is not displaced. *C:* Axial section of Riedel's lobe showing inferior extension of liver to just above iliac crest. *D–G:* Herniation of part of the liver through right hemidiaphragm mimicking a focal hepatic mass, even to the extent of growth under observation. (*D* and *E:* PA and lateral chest, showing apparent mass. *F* and *G:* follow-up, 5 yr later, shows increased size of "mass.")

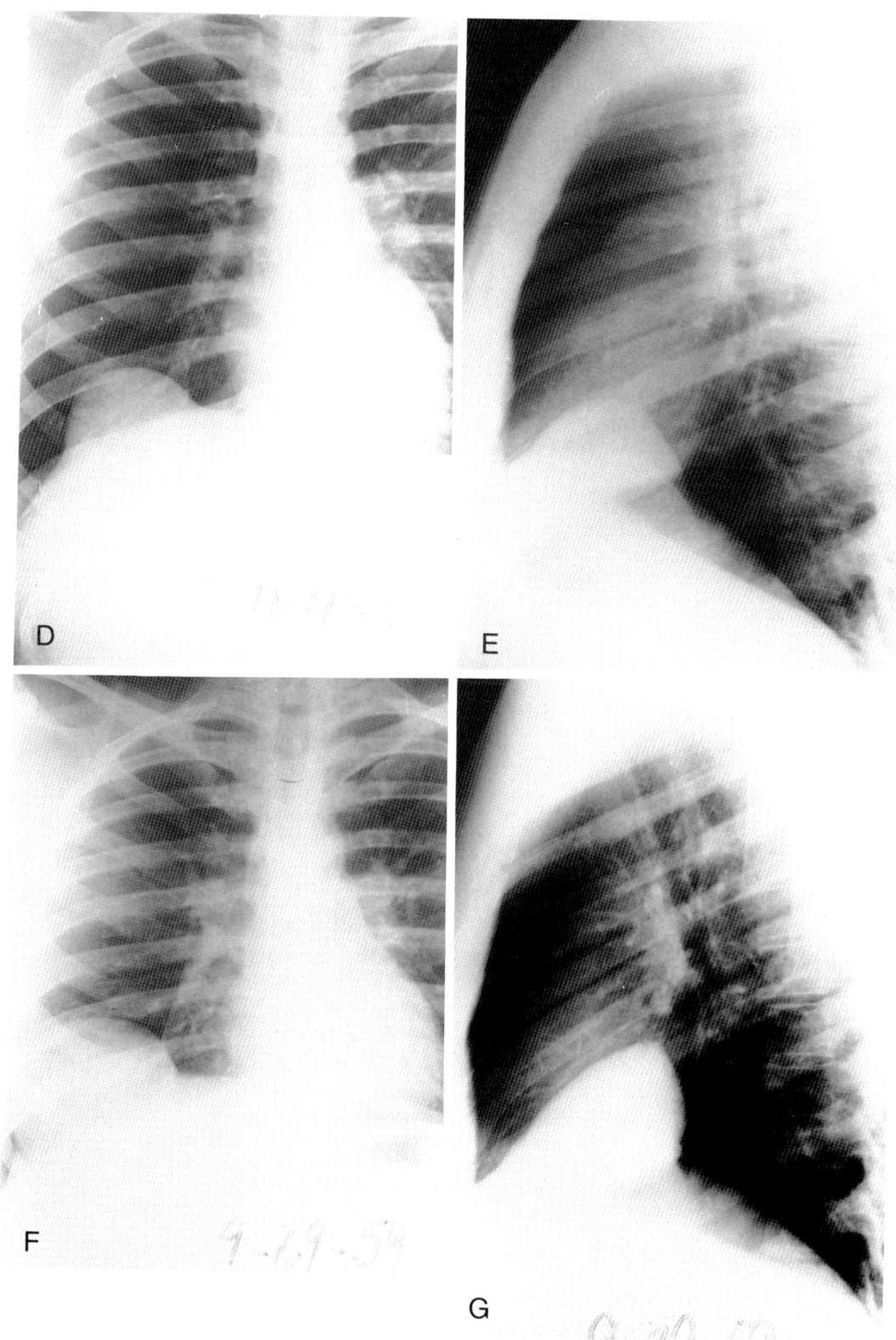

Figure 3.6D–G

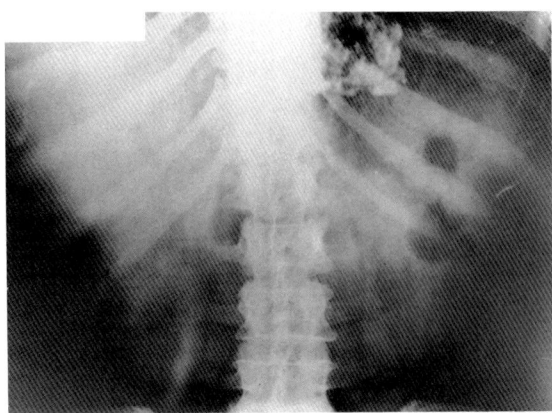

FIGURE 3.7. CALCIFIED GUMMA DUE TO SYPHILIS REPLACING LEFT LOBE OF LIVER

adjacent structures both in normal and abnormal states is enhanced by the use of other imaging modalities, specifically CT. A more complete understanding of the vector principle and its exposition regarding hepatomegaly may thus be attained.

EFFECTS ON OTHER STRUCTURES

Structures with direct relationship to the liver which may be displaced by the liver include the stomach, duodenum, hepatic flexure of the colon, gallbladder, right kidney, and diaphragm. Rarely, the esophagus, which courses directly behind the left lobe, may be affected (11). Of retroperitoneal structures in proximity to the liver, only the right kidney, by virtue of its being embedded in a large amount of fat, is mobile enough to actually be displaced by a large liver. The perirenal fat forms the border with the posterior aspect of the visceral surface of the liver which is frequently seen as the liver margin on plain films. Large vessels which are theoretically retroperitoneal are displaced by liver enlargement in conjunction with the organs to which they relate (Figs. 3.8 and 3.9). Other retroperitoneal structures are not sufficiently mobile to be displaced by an enlarged liver but may be indented, scalloped, or invaded by it. Scalloping of the spine by hepatomegaly in glycogen storage disease is such an example (12).

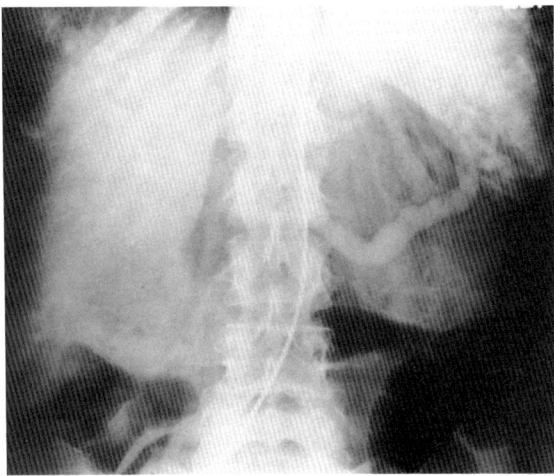

FIGURE 3.8. DEPRESSION OF SPLENIC VEIN IN PATIENT WITH DIFFUSE HEPATIC ENLARGEMENT SECONDARY TO METASTASES
This is the same patient as shown in Figures 3.3, 3.9, and 3.12.

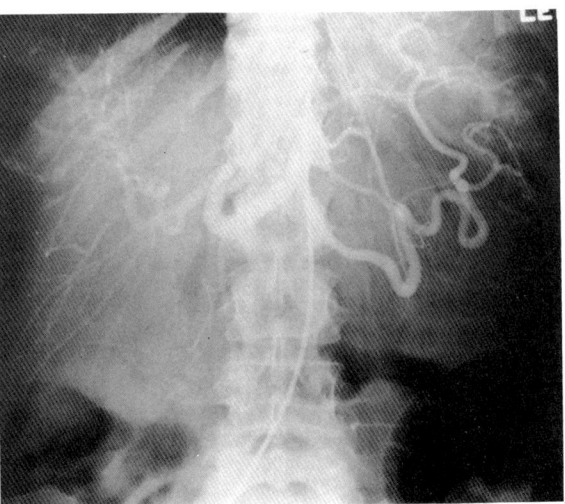

FIGURE 3.9. STRETCHING AND DEPRESSION OF LEFT GASTRIC ARTERY
The left lobe of the liver is enlarged by metastatic lesions.

The neck and body of the pancreas are often separated from the left lobe of the liver only by the lesser omentum and thus may be affected by a contiguous process in the liver (8).

Diaphragm

Nearly the entire right hemidiaphragm is related to the convex surface of the liver. The left lobe of the liver usually extends to about the mid-portion of the left hemidiaphragm; however, due to countereffects by the heart above, changes in diaphragmatic position due to hepatic size change are usually seen on the right. Generalized hepatomegaly causes elevation of the right hemidiaphragm (Fig. 3.10). An unusual contour of the superior surface of the liver may indent only a portion of right hemidiaphragm simulating an

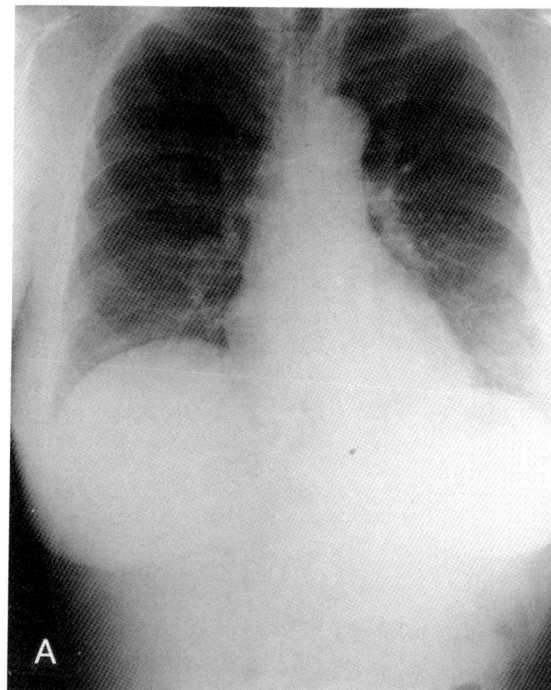
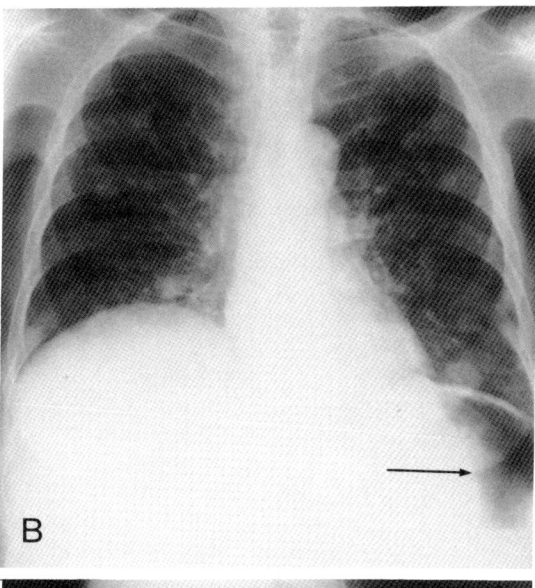
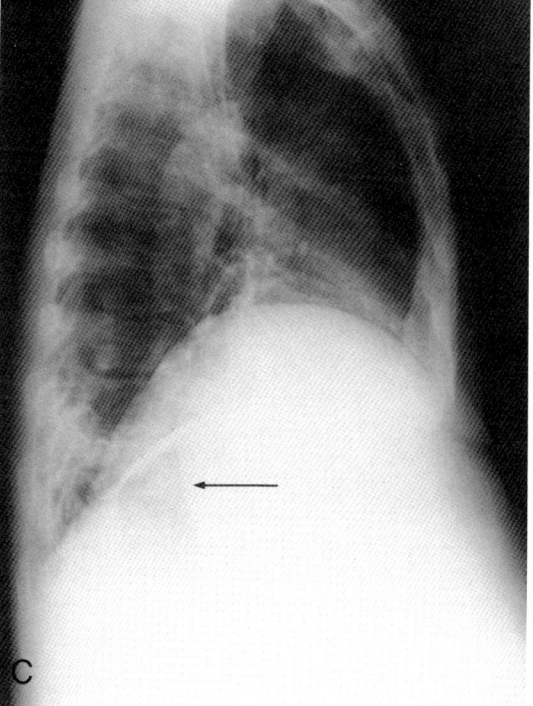

FIGURE 3.10. ELEVATION OF RIGHT HEMIDIAPHRAGM IN A PATIENT WITH CARCINOMA OF THE COLON WHO DEVELOPED DIFFUSE LIVER AND LUNG METASTASES OVER A 1-YR PERIOD
A: 6/83, hepatomegaly; *B:* 7/84, elevated right hemidiaphragm; 6/84, elevated right hemidiaphragm on lateral view (*C*). Note the posterior (*C*) and lateral (*B*) displacement of the gastric air bubble by the enlarged liver (*arrow*).

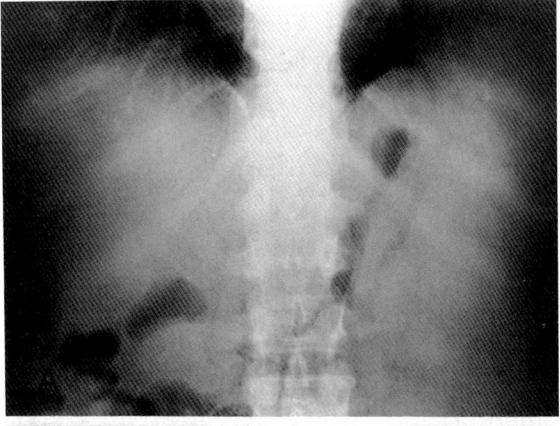

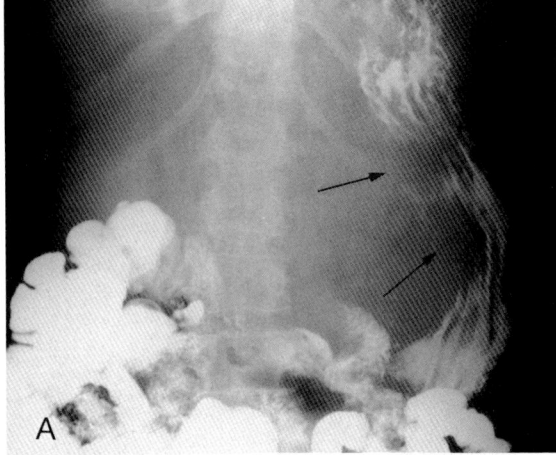

FIGURE 3.11. DIFFUSE HEPATOSPLENOMEGALY
A: Frontal view, and *B:* axial view. The patient has diffuse hepatosplenomegaly due to sarcoid demonstrating compression of the stomach between the liver and spleen.

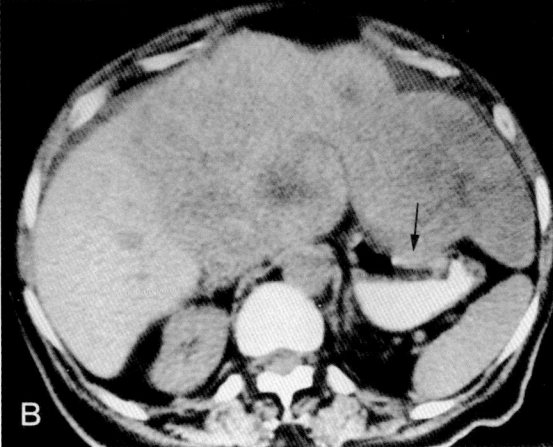

FIGURE 3.13. UPPER GI AND CT OF MASS EFFECT ON STOMACH
A: Upper GI showing stomach displaced to left and inferiorly with focal areas of impression on lesser curvature (*arrows*). *B:* axial scan demonstrating replacement of left lobe with metastases and focal protrusion (*arrow*) indenting lesser curvature of stomach.

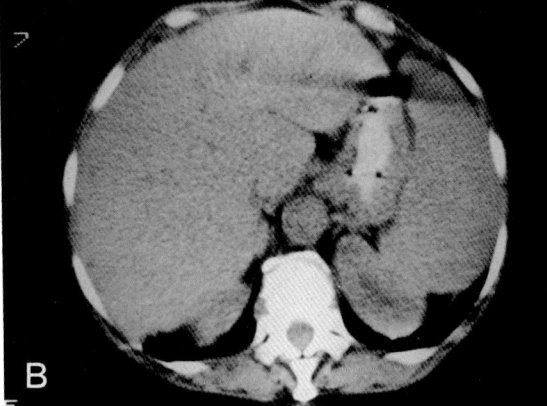

FIGURE 3.12. CT OF GASTRIC DISPLACEMENT
Axial section demonstrating marked caudal displacement of the body of the stomach. (This is the same patient as in Figure 3.3.)

eventration (C. D. Schneck, personal communication). With true eventration, the lower edges of the liver will be higher than expected. Sub-

pulmonic and subphrenic collections are frequently mimics of hepatomegaly by virtue of the resultant elevation of the right hemidiaphragm.

Stomach

On routine radiographs, the stomach is probably the most common organ seen to be displaced by hepatomegaly. This is because of the long common border between the two organs as the stomach moves posterior to anterior (from the fundus to the antrum) and then posterior again to the retroperitoneal fixation of the duodenum. Uniform enlargement of the liver displaces the stomach downward, to the left and posteriorly.

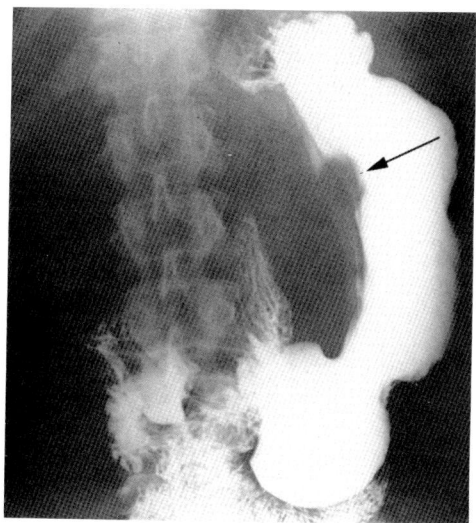

FIGURE 3.14. LIVER CYST MIMICKING GASTRIC MASS
Patient with polycystic disease and what seems to be a mural mass in lesser curvature (*arrow*). At laparotomy, this was shown to be due to a cyst in the left lobe of the liver.

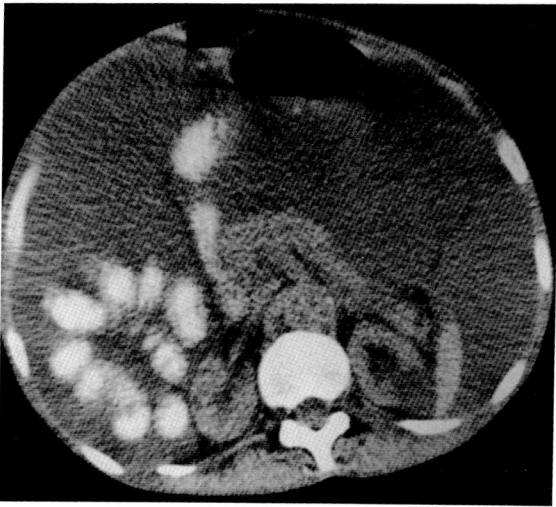

FIGURE 3.16. CIRRHOTIC PATIENT WITH TINY LIVER AND MARKED ASCITES
Antrum and duodenum are in normal position.

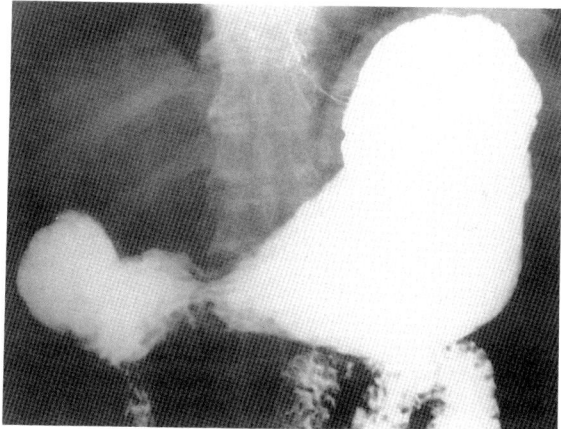

FIGURE 3.15. CIRRHOTIC PATIENT WITH SMALL LIVER
Antrum and duodenum are displaced cephalad and to the right.

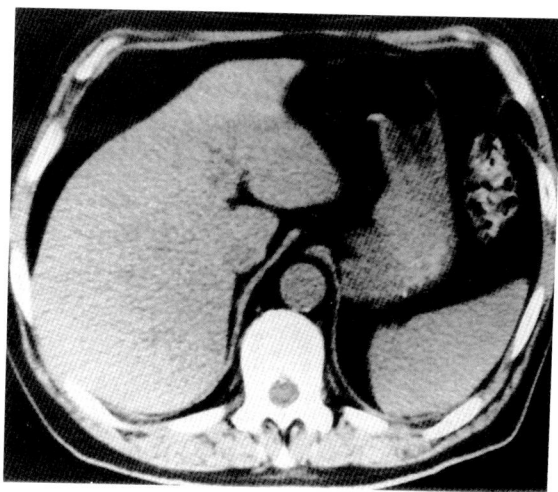

FIGURE 3.17. CONGENITALLY SMALL LATERAL SEGMENT OF LEFT LOBE WITH PROMINENT QUADRATE AND CAUDATE LOBES
Stomach is more medially placed filling space normally occupied by left lobe.

(Figs. 3.1, 3.3, and 3.10). The anteriorly placed left lobe of the liver is responsible for the posterior displacement. Conditions causing diffuse hepatosplenomegaly have counteracting forces on the stomach compressing rather than displacing it (Fig. 3.11). Enlargement of the sections of the right lobe produce directions of force in a roughly semicircular configuration around the porta hepatis and account for the displacement of the body and antrum down and to the left (Fig. 3.12). Focal masses within the liver, whatever their etiology, may displace only a portion of the stomach depending on the location of the mass and the specific vectors generated by it (Figs. 3.13 and 3.14).

Small livers, a result of end-stage cirrhosis, permit movement inversely to an enlarged liver, i.e. anteriorly, to the right and up, filling in some of the space vacated by the liver (Fig. 3.15). Severe cirrhosis is often accompanied by ascites which can fill the void created by the small liver and counteract any potential gastric displacement (Fig. 3.16). Since there is a tremendous amount of variability in liver morphology, presence of anomalous lobes and absence of all or part of a lobe may cause indentation or displacement of the stomach (13, 14) (Fig. 3.17).

Duodenum

There is a complex relationship between the duodenum and the liver since the two structures lie in close proximity through the anterior to posterior excursion of the duodenum. On a routine PA film with barium, the duodenal bulb lies between T12 and the upper portion of L3 in the vast majority of cases (15). Since the left lobe of the liver is anterior and the caudate lobe is posterior (and lateral) to the duodenum, focal space-occupying lesions will have opposite effects on the duodenum. The bulk of the right lobe is anterolateral and superior to the duodenum. With generalized hepatomegaly, the effect of the enlarged right lobe predominates and displaces the duodenum to the left and down (Figs. 3.18 and 3.19). As with the stomach, the duodenum may be displaced up and to the right if the liver is abnormally small (Fig. 3.15).

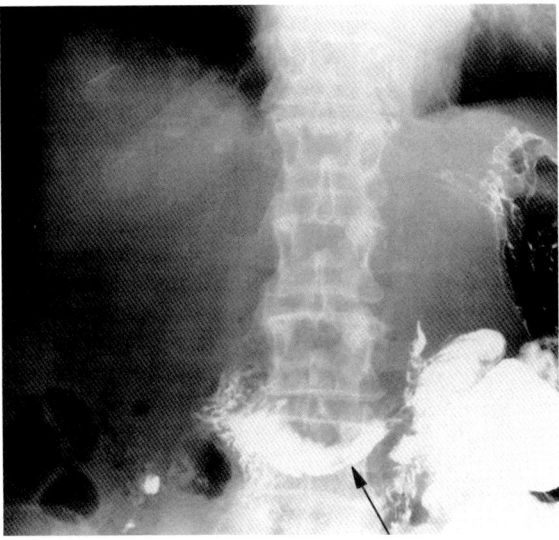

FIGURE 3.19. DISPLACEMENT OF DUODENAL BULB
Downward displacement of duodenal bulb (*arrow*) in patient with passive liver congestion due to cardiomyopathy.

Gallbladder

In the normal patient, there is enormous variability in the position of the gallbladder, which may be found anywhere from the subcostal re-

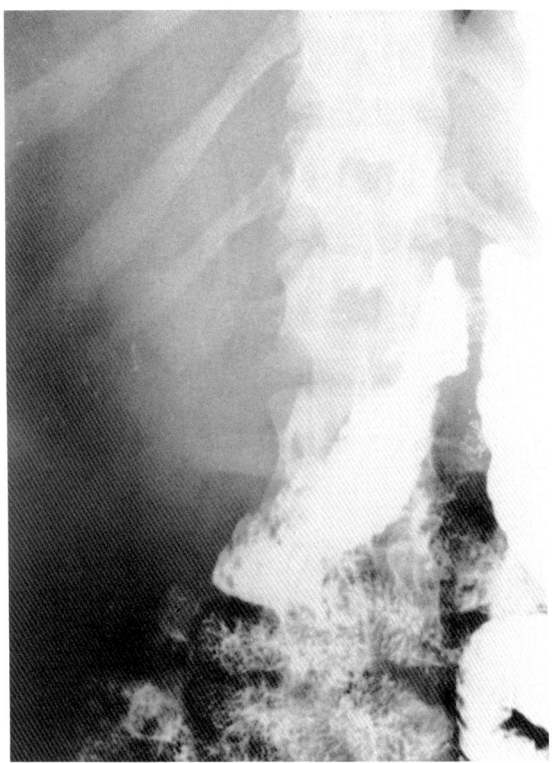

FIGURE 3.18. PORTIONS OF THE DUODENUM DISPLACED
First and second portions of the duodenum displaced to the left in patient with hepatoma. Note duodenal ulcer.

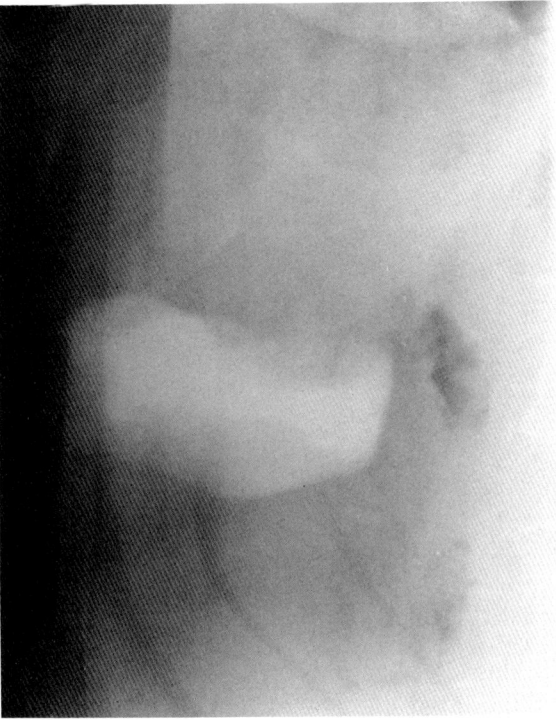

FIGURE 3.20. DEFORMITY OF THE GALLBLADDER
Patient with tertiary syphilis and hepar lobatum causing extrinsic compression of gallbladder. (From Fisher, MS: Hepar lobatum and other less exotic causes of gallbladder deformity. *Radiology* 91:308–309, 1968.)

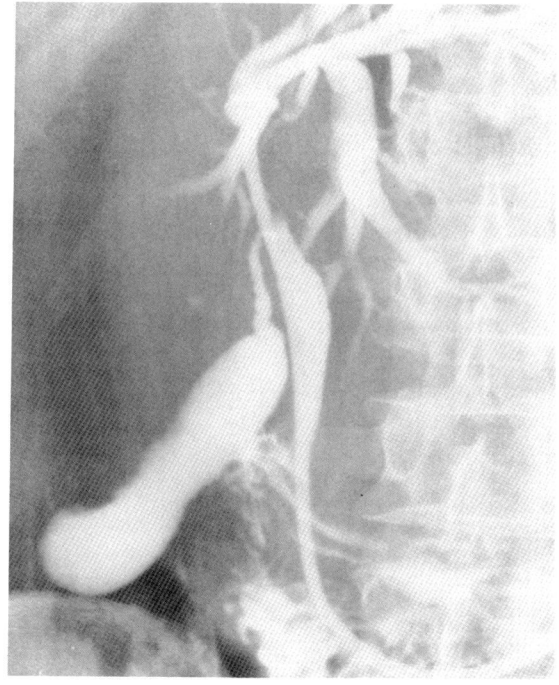

FIGURE 3.21. LIVER METASTASES CAUSING COMPRESSION AND INVASION OF GALLBLADDER

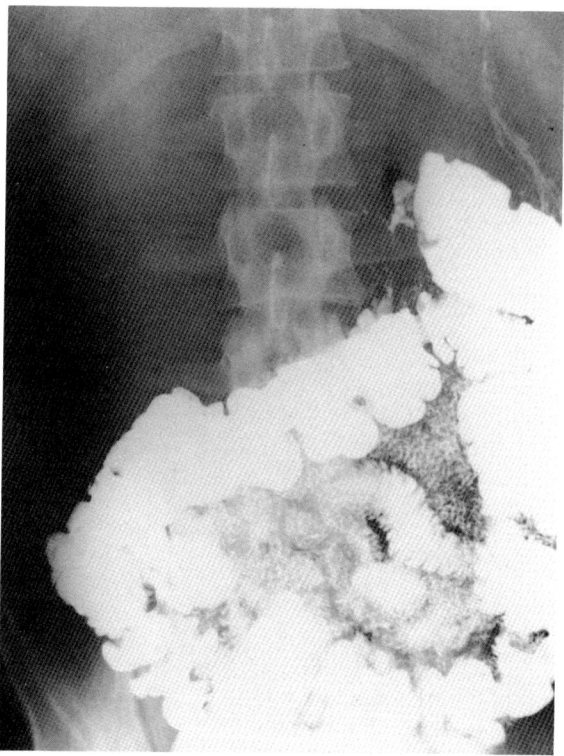

FIGURE 3.22. DEPRESSION OF HEPATIC FLEXURE IN THE SAME PATIENT AS FIGURE 3.18

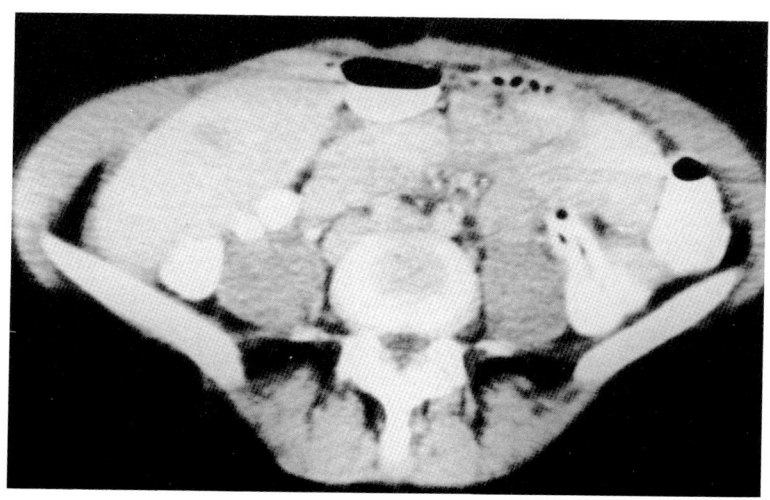

FIGURE 3.23. CT AT THE LEVEL OF THE AORTOILIAC BIFURCATION OF PATIENT WITH LIVER METASTASES AND MARKED CAUDAL DEPRESSION OF HEPATIC FLEXURE

gion to the pelvis on routine examinations. We thus rarely perceive displacement of a gallbladder due to hepatomegaly, although it obviously occurs nearly anytime there is diffuse liver enlargement. Indentations or deformity of the gallbladder are more likely to be observed and may be caused by any space occupying liver lesion adjacent to the gallbladder (16) (Figs. 3.20 and 3.21).

Colon

The hepatic flexure of the colon is closely related to the liver and causes an impression on the anterior aspect of the visceral surface of the right lobe. The intraperitoneal transverse colon retains a relationship with the liver for a variable, but generally short distance. Focal masses within the left lobe of the liver will therefore not

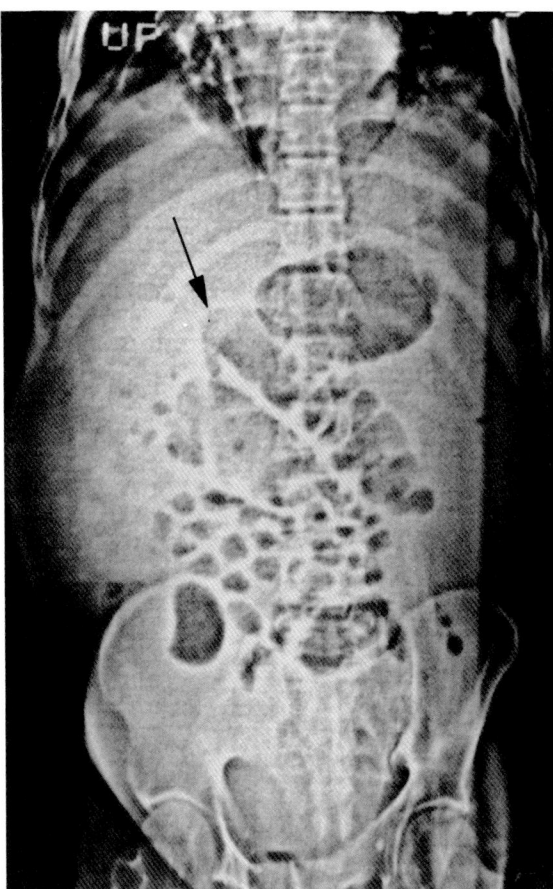

FIGURE 3.24. UPWARD DISPLACEMENT OF HEPATIC FLEXURE
Upward displacement of hepatic flexure is shown (*arrow*) in cirrhotic patient with small liver.

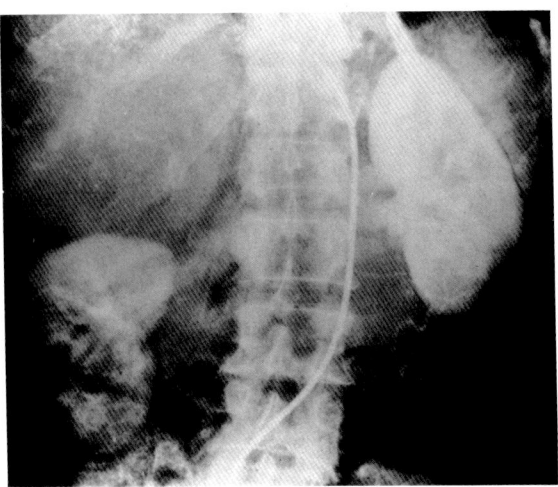

FIGURE 3.25. DOWNWARD DISPLACEMENT OF RIGHT KIDNEY
Downward displacement of right kidney in a patient with diffuse hepatoma. (Case courtesy of Dr. Howard M. Pollack.)

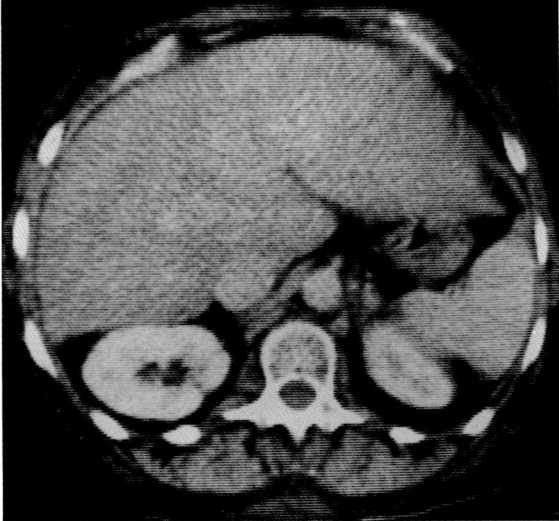

FIGURE 3.26. ROTATION OF AXIS OF RIGHT KIDNEY DUE TO HEPATOMEGALY CAUSED BY FATTY LIVER

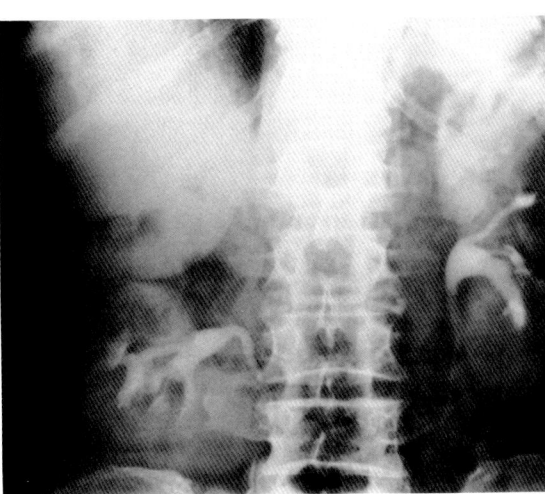

FIGURE 3.27. ROTATION AND DOWNWARD DISPLACEMENT OF KIDNEY
Lateral rotation and downward displacement of right kidney by prominent caudate lobe. (Case courtesy of Dr. Howard M. Pollack.)

be expected to affect the colon. Masses in the right lobe and generalized hepatomegaly will primarily displace the colon downward (Figs. 3.22 and 3.23). The hepatic flexure may be displaced cephalad when the liver is abnormally small (Fig. 3.24).

Right Kidney and Adrenal

Of all the retroperitoneal structures, the right kidney is the most mobile and most likely to be affected by hepatic enlargement. Normally, the right kidney abuts the posterior aspect of the

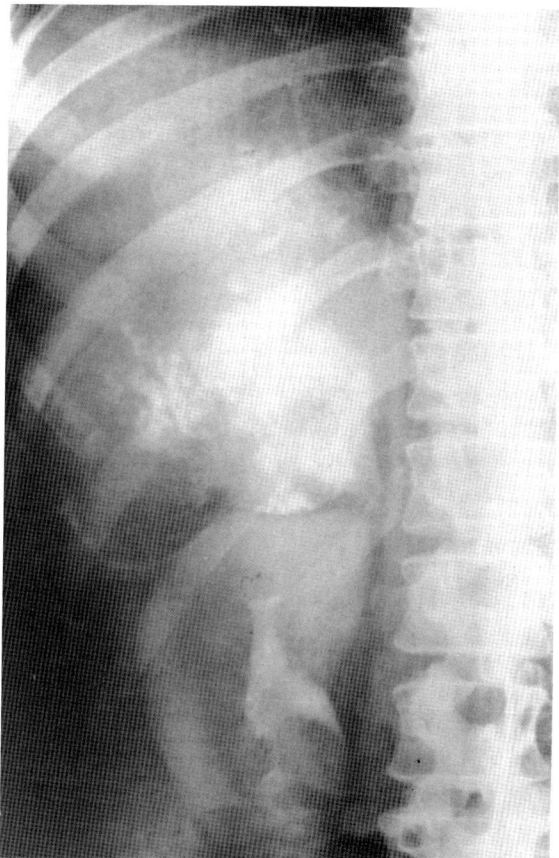

FIGURE 3.28. EFFACEMENT OF UPPER POLE OF RIGHT KIDNEY
Effacement of upper pole of right kidney by hemangioma. (From Fuselier HA: Case profile: a confusing suprarenal mass. *Urology* 6:512, 1975.)

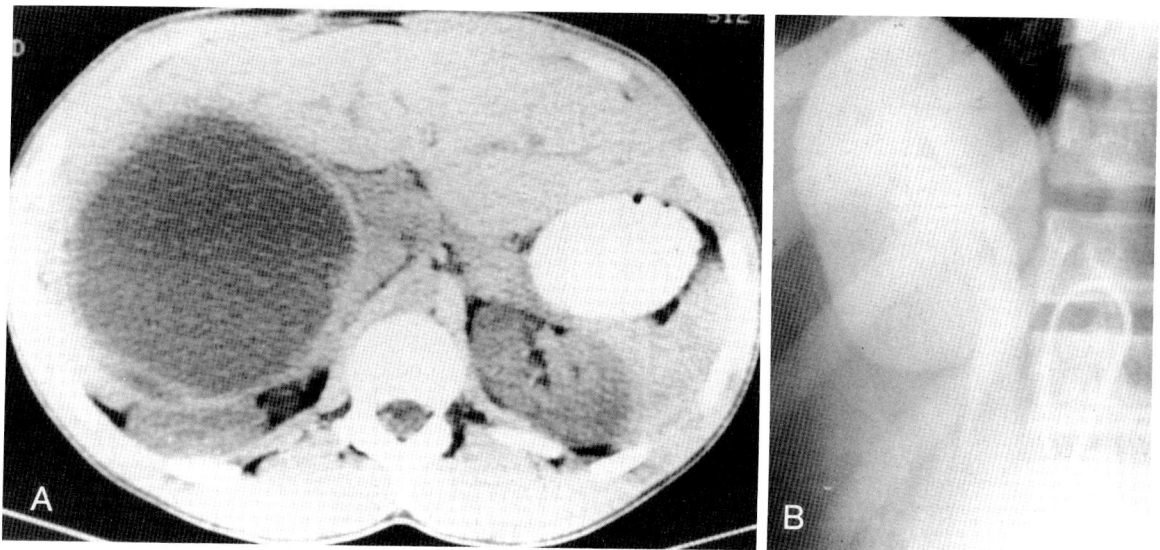

FIGURE 3.29. UPWARD DISPLACEMENT OF KIDNEY
A: large hematoma in the lower, posterior region of the right lobe. *B:* The right kidney is pushed up to a subdiaphragmatic location. (Case courtesy of Dr. Howard M. Pollack.)

visceral surface of the right lobe of the liver. The right adrenal may form an impression on the undersurface of the right lobe medial to that formed by the kidney and posterior to the duodenal impression. Enlargement of the liver generally causes downward displacement of the kidney (Fig. 3.25). Rotation may also be the sole effect of generalized hepatomegaly (Fig. 3.26), it may be combined with displacement (Fig. 3.27). Focal masses, depending on their location, may cause gross displacement or merely effacement of a surface of the kidney and simulate an adrenal mass (Fig. 3.28). An unusual occurrence is upward displacement of the kidney by a mass in the inferior portion of the right lobe (Fig. 3.29). Although liver enlargement sufficient to displace the right kidney might be expected to affect the right adrenal, we have not encountered such an example. This is likely at least partially because the normal adrenals were infrequently visualized prior to the availability of thin-section CT scans.

REFERENCES

1. Gelfand DW: Anatomy of the liver. *Radiol Clin North Am* 18:187–194, 1980.
2. Pfahler GE: The measurement of the liver by means of roentgen rays based upon a study of 502 subjects. *AJR* 16:558–564, 1926.
3. Riemenschneider PA, Whalen JP: The relative accuracy of estimation of enlargement of the liver and spleen by radiologic and clinical methods. *Radiology* 94:462–468, 1965.
4. Rollo FD, Deland FH: The determination of liver mass by radionuclide images. *Radiology* 91:1191–1194, 1968.
5. Rasmussen SN: Liver volume determination by ultrasonic scanning. *Br J Radiol* 45:579–585, 1972.
6. Henderson J, Heymsfield MSB, Horowitz J, Kutner MH: Measurement of liver and spleen volume by computed tomography. *Radiology* 141:525–527, 1981.
7. Whalen JP, Evans JA, Meyers MA: Vector principle in the differential diagnosis of abdominal masses. II. Right upper quadrant. *AJR* 115:318–333, 1972.
8. Schneck CD: The anatomical basis of abdominopelvic sectional imaging seminars. *Ultrasound* 11:13–41, 1983.
9. Netter FH: *Liver, Biliary Tract, Pancreas.* In The CIBA Collection of Medical Illustrations, Vol. 3, Digestive System, Part III. Summit, NJ., CIBA Pharmaceuticals, 1957, pp 5–6.
10. Kattan KR: The effect of changes in liver volume on the adjacent viscera. *Radiol Clin North Am* 18:195–207, 1980.
11. Kenneweg DJ, Cimmino CV: Esophageal obstruction and dysphasia caused by hepatomegaly. *Radiology* 91:783–784, 1968.
12. Miller J, Stanley P, Gates G: Radiography of glycogen storage disease. *AJR* 132:379–387, 1979.
13. Battle WM, Laufer I, Moldofsky PJ, Trotman BW: Anomalous liver lobulation as a cause of perigastric masses. *Dig Dis Sci* 24:65–69, 1979.
14. Meyers HI, Jacobson G: Displacements of the stomach and duodenum by anomalous lobes of the liver. *AJR* 79:789–792, 1958.
15. Kattan KR, Moskowitz M: Position of the duodenal bulb and liver size. *AJR* 119:78–84, 1973.
16. Fisher MS: Hepar lobatum and other less exotic causes of gallbladder deformity. *Radiology* 91:308–309, 1968.

4

Cirrhosis, Other Diffuse Diseases, Portal Hypertension, and Vascular Diseases

ARNOLD C. FRIEDMAN, M.D., TODD JOHNS, M.D., DAVID W. LEVY, M.D., STEVE RINDSBERG, M.D., AND BRUCE M. MARKLE, M.D.

CIRRHOSIS

Characterized by nodular parenchyma and widespread fibrosis with septa linking portal tracts and central canals, cirrhosis of the liver results from abnormal reconstruction of preexisting lobular architecture that was destroyed by some insult. Often the disease is advanced so far that the underlying cause cannot be determined pathologically. Cirrhosis is conventionally considered an irreversible scar end stage, but this can be disputed. Regression of iron overload cirrhosis has been described.

Etiology

By far, the most common cause of cirrhosis in the United States is alcoholic liver disease, which is micronodular in its early stages (accompanied by steatosis) (1). Subsequently, large nodules and broad septa develop. A useful differential diagnostic feature is the presence of alcoholic hepatitis, which is initially centrilobular and characterized by hydropic hepatocytes containing fat droplets and alcoholic hyaline. Other causes of cirrhosis are given in Table 4.1.

Pathogenesis

Although usually slow and insidious in development, cirrhosis may occur rapidly (within 5 months) following alcoholic or viral hepatitis (1). The pathogenesis involves hepatocellular necrosis, inflammation, regeneration, and fibrosis, all of which are interrelated. The initiating hepatocyte injury leads to inflammation, structural collapse, and fibrogenesis. The resulting septa cause circulatory disturbances, portal hypertension, and intrahepatic cholestasis. A vicious cycle is set up whereby hepatocellular injury and inflammation lead to pericellular fibrosis, which interferes with cell nutrition, and septa, which disturb hemodynamics, causing further cellular injury.

Pathology

A simple gross classification of cirrhosis into micronodular and macronodular is useful although imperfect (1). Cirrhosis is frequently both micronodular and macronodular and it can change from the former to the latter over time. The micronodular form has approximately equal-sized nodules up to 3 mm in diameter associated with septa of approximately equal width (up to 2 mm). The macronodular form is characterized by variably sized nodules, many greater than 3 mm and some as large as 3 cm or more, associated with irregular septa of varying width (often broad). Steatosis can develop in either form, and either may occur in an enlarged or a shrunken liver.

Cirrhosis is diagnosed by liver biopsy, the interpretation of which is improved by the use of connective tissue stains. Major diagnostic features in decreasing order of certainty are as follows: nodules surrounded by septa with or without portal and central canals, hepatic vein tributaries in contact with septa, and the presence of connective tissue septa linking central and portal canals. Parenchymal nodules are round portions of parenchyma (either portions of many lobules or one lobule) surrounded by connective tissue. They may have normal architectural arrangement, but usually the cytologic

TABLE 4.1.
CAUSES OF CIRRHOSIS

1. Alcoholic liver disease
2. Viral hepatitis, often macronodular
3. Drug induced (prolonged methotrexate, oxyphenisatin, α-methyldopa, nitrofurantoin, isoniazid)
4. Biliary obstruction (focal in adolescents with cystic fibrosis proximal to dilated bile ducts obstructed by inspissated PAS$^+$ material)
5. Congestive (prolonged congestive heart failure, hepatic venoocclusive disease)
6. Nutritional (intestinal bypass, severe steatosis, abetalipoproteinemia)
7. Iron overload, hemochromatosis or hemosiderosis, usually micronodular
8. Hereditary (Wilson's disease, $α_1$-antitrypsin deficiency, galactosemia, Type IV glycogen storage disease, hereditary fructose intolerance, tyrosinemia, hereditary tetany, Osler-Weber-Rendu syndrome, familial cirrhosis)
9. Multifactorial (inflammatory bowel disease, alcohol, viral, and congestive added to other causative factors)
10. Unknown etiology:
    a. Cryptogenic with female subgroup having lupus-like syndrome (lupoid)
    b. Primary biliary cirrhosis
    c. Obstructive infantile cholangiopathy (neonatal giant cell hepatitis ± intra- or extrahepatic biliary atresia or hypoplasia)

and architectural features of regeneration are present. Septa are connective tissue membranes of various widths resulting from either collapse of preexisting parenchyma or formation of new connective tissue fibers. They cause functional derangement when they connect central veins with portal canals and contain vessels permitting the short circuit of blood flow. The following conditions resemble cirrhosis but do not fulfill the above criteria: (a) Precirrhotic stages in biliary cirrhosis (either primary or obstructive), congestive fibrosis prior to nodule formation, fibrosis from sarcoidosis, and central hyaline sclerosis in alcoholic liver injury; (b) hepatic fibrosis with presinusoidal portal hypertension: schistosomiasis, myeloproliferative disease with splenomegaly, arteriovenous fistula, extrahepatic portal vein thrombosis, idiopathic portal hypertension, biliary dysplasia (Meyenburg complexes, Caroli's disease, congenital hepatic fibrosis); (c) hepatic fibrosis from toxins: Thorotrast, arsenicals, vinyl chloride, hypervitaminosis A, carbon tetrachloride; (d) radiation fibrosis; (e) Gaucher's disease; and (f) partial nodular transformation.

Pathophysiology

Several mechanisms are responsible for portal hypertension. Impaired drainage of blood from the liver is caused by compression of hepatic vein tributaries by regenerating nodules or fibrosis (1). Perisinusoidal fibrosis also impairs drainage of blood from the liver, as does portal tract scarring. Arteriovenous anastomoses in septa elevate portal pressure by bringing hepatic arterial pressure to bear on the portal vein. The decreased resistance to flow in an enlarged spleen causes an increase in blood flow via the splenic vein to the liver (whose vascular bed cannot expand in cirrhosis) causing an increase in portal vein pressure. All of the above factors lead to phlebosclerosis of the portal vein, higher pressures, and a vicious cycle. In response to portal hypertension, splanchnic venous blood is diverted from the liver by portosystemic anastomoses necessitating an increase in hepatic arterial flow. This causes enlargement and tortuosity of the hepatic artery. Hepatic arterial blood reaching the liver is diverted from the parenchyma by septal anastomoses between the afferent branches of the hepatic artery and both the portal vein and the efferent tributaries of the hepatic veins. Outflow block slows or reverses portal venous flow, and lobular distortion interferes with the intralobular microcirculation causing a diminution in liver function on a circulatory basis, independent of the status of the hepatocytes.

Additional features accompanying or caused by the altered hepatic circulation are: (a) decreased functional mass of hepatocytes even in enlarged livers; (b) ascites, caused by increased hepatic lymph flow and/or excess exudation from the peritoneal liver capsule and/or hypoalbuminemia; (c) altered bile flow (cholestasis can occur from periductal scarring, or excess secretion from elevated sinusoidal pressure. Prolonged cholestasis may cause copper deposition, which is mainly periportal, and usually occurs in primary biliary cirrhosis, other cholestatic cirrhoses, or $α_1$-antitrypsin deficiency); and (d) excess iron storage in periportal hepatocytes, either spontaneously or following shunt surgery.

REFERENCES

1. Popper H: Pathologic aspects of cirrhosis. A review. *Am J Pathol* 87:228–258, 1977.
2. Galambos J: The cirrhoses. In Bockus HL (ed): *Gastroenterology.* Philadelphia, W. B. Saunders, 1976, pp 366–416.

Ultrasound

A small, shrunken liver is seen only in advanced cases of cirrhosis. Liver size is either enlarged or normal in earlier stages. Criteria for

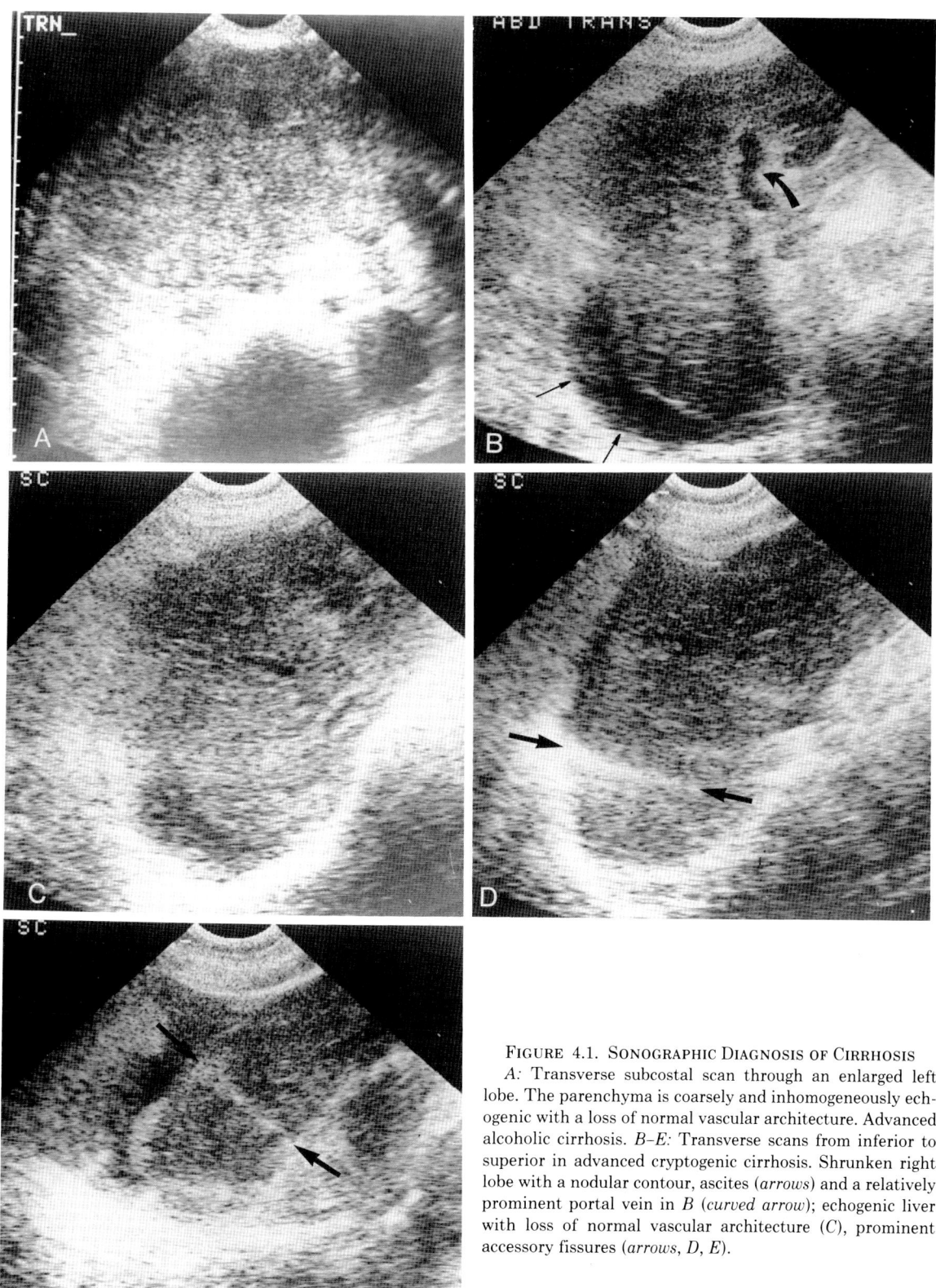

FIGURE 4.1. SONOGRAPHIC DIAGNOSIS OF CIRRHOSIS
A: Transverse subcostal scan through an enlarged left lobe. The parenchyma is coarsely and inhomogeneously echogenic with a loss of normal vascular architecture. Advanced alcoholic cirrhosis. *B–E:* Transverse scans from inferior to superior in advanced cryptogenic cirrhosis. Shrunken right lobe with a nodular contour, ascites (*arrows*) and a relatively prominent portal vein in *B* (*curved arrow*); echogenic liver with loss of normal vascular architecture (*C*), prominent accessory fissures (*arrows*, *D*, *E*).

the sonographic diagnosis of cirrhosis include increased parenchymal echogenicity, decreased beam penetration through the liver, and poor depiction of intrahepatic vessels, especially smaller branches (Fig. 4.1). Using the above criteria, cirrhosis could be diagnosed by ultrasound in 80% and 65% (true positive) in two series (1, 2). Unfortunately, a 20% false-positive rate was noted as well as the inability to distinguish fatty infiltration from cirrhosis (1). Identical findings to those observed in cirrhosis have been encountered in chronic hepatitis (3, 4). The decreased beam penetration and increased parenchymal echogenicity can be explained by collagen and/or fat deposition. Inability to see portal vein walls may be due to the increased surrounding parenchymal echogenicity "silhouetting" these normally echodense structures. Ancillary findings in cirrhosis include splenomegaly and ascites (1, 2). In advanced cases of cirrhosis accentuation of the fissures, contour indentations and nodularity, and, occasionally, large regenerating nodules are depicted (Fig. 4.1). The latter have approximately the same echo texture as the parenchyma, in contrast to hepatocellular carcinomas which are usually not isoechoic (Fig. 4.2). The left and caudate lobes are relatively preserved and are large compared to the shrunken right lobe.

Modern, real-time sonography's most clinically useful contribution to the care of patients with cirrhosis is the noninvasive evaluation of portosystemic collateral circulation. The advent of abdominal Doppler scanning may enhance the above. It has been asserted that a portal vein diameter larger than 13 mm in diameter is characteristic of portal hypertension in the appropriate clinical setting (5). Normal portal vein diameters have been reported in the range of 0.64–1.21 cm, contrasted to an average diameter of 1.2 cm in cirrhotics (6, 7). Using angiography, others have concluded that no significant difference in portal vein diameter exists between cirrhotics and controls and that portal vein caliber remains

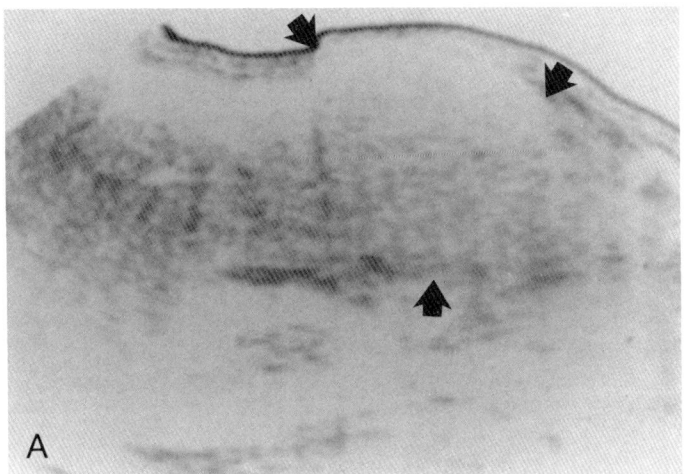

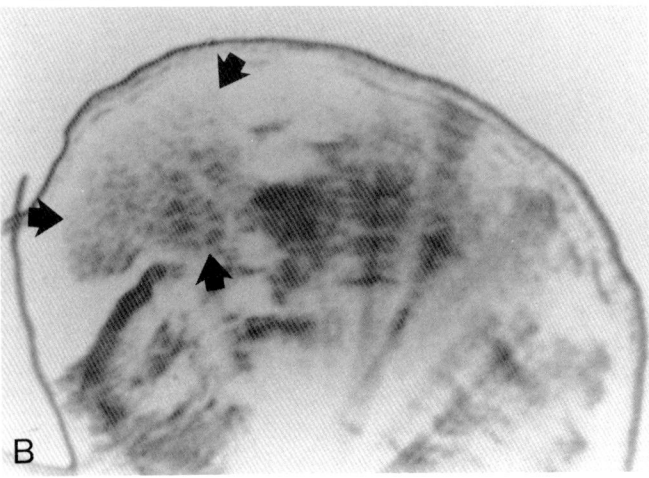
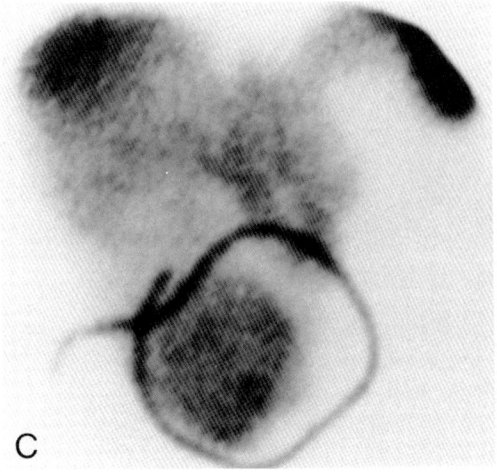

FIGURE 4.2. REGENERATING NODULE

A and B: Parasagittal and transverse scans, respectively, through the clinically palpable mass (*arrows*) at the tip of the right lobe, showing echo texture identical to the remainder of the liver. C: Hot marker encircling the palpable mass on a sulfur-colloid scan. The mass has uptake equal to or greater than the rest of the liver, diagnostic of regenerating nodule in the clinical context of cirrhosis.

constant or even diminishes with an increasing portohepatic gradient (because of the diversion of blood flow to collaterals) (8). Our experience with subjective assessment of portal (and splenic) vein size indicates that portal vein enlargement is insensitive to cirrhosis and portal hypertension, but when present it is a fairly accurate indicator of portal hypertension (Fig. 4.3E). In normal patients, the portal venous system distends with deep inspiration because of diaphragmatic descent and compression of the hepatic venous outflow. No dilatation can occur in portal hypertension since the veins are already maximally distended (9). Assessment of the sizes of the superior mesenteric and coronary veins is useful. The superior mesenteric vein is never larger than the portal vein in normal subjects, and a coronary vein larger than 0.4 cm in internal diameter is a useful sign of portal hypertension (10, 11) (Fig. 4.3B–D). A coronary vein larger than 0.7 cm usually indicates a portohepatic gradient larger than 10 mm Hg (8) which makes variceal bleeding likely.

Potential portosystemic collaterals in portal hypertension (Fig. 4.3A) are listed in Table 4.2.

Often the easiest collateral to identify sonographically is the coronary vein and its associated gastroesophageal varices. After identifying the origin of the coronary vein on longitudinal scans from either the splenic vein or the portal vein, varices can be seen as circular and tubular sonolucencies by angled longitudinal scans in the region of the gastroesophageal junction and lesser curvature of the stomach (Fig. 4.4) (10, 11). Esophageal varices can occasionally be depicted on cranially angled transverse subcostal scans through the left lobe of the liver. The umbilical vein connects the left portal vein to the systemic circulation via superficial epigastric veins radiating from the umbilicus (caput medusa, the Cruveilhier-Baumgarten syndrome). On transverse scans a recanalized umbilical vein is seen as a round sonolucency in the left intersegmental fissure surrounded by the echogenic fat in the falciform ligament (Fig. 4.5) (10, 11, 13). By scanning longitudinally, it can be followed caudally towards the umbilicus as a tubular sonolucency. Recent pathologic correlation indicates that it is not the umbilical vein itself that is recanalized, but rather that paraumbilical veins in the falciform ligament open up (14). The finding is specific for portal hypertension and excludes presinusoidal causes. A dilated inferior mesenteric vein can be identified sometimes by scanning along the inferior margin of the splenic vein to the left of the midline. Gastrorenal and splenorenal collateral veins can be seen by scanning coronally through the spleen and left kidney. The proximal splenic vein and its tributaries from the spleen can be identified in the splenic hilum and short gastric collaterals are medial to the spleen above the hilum (Fig. 4.6). Gastroepiploic varices are depicted along the greater curvature of the stomach and in the adjacent mesentery (11). Other sonographically detectable varices include paraduodenal veins, periportal veins, and collaterals in the pelvis (Fig. 4.7) (11). Enlarged cholecystic and pericholecystic veins have been described in patients with cirrhosis and portal hypertension, gallbladder carcinoma, and portal vein thrombosis (15). Preoperative mapping of collaterals is important prior to contemplated shunt surgery. The surgeon generally wishes to ligate coronary collaterals and any other large collateral system in order to maintain hepatopedal portal blood flow and avoid encephalopathy (16). If a splenorenal shunt is contemplated, demonstration of the splenic and left renal veins and exclusion of a retroaortic left renal vein is useful information to the surgeon. Failure to demonstrate the portal vein is strong evidence of occlusion: the empty porta hepatis is a broad, diamond-shaped band of high level echoes (13). Aneurysms of the portal vein can form, either proximally at the junction of the superior mesenteric vein and the splenic vein or more distally (6). They are thought to be either congenital or acquired secondary to portal hypertension. Parenchymal liver abnormalities are sometimes associated, but their developmental sequence is unclear (7). Most patients present with gastrointestinal bleeding, and shunt surgery can be helpful (7). Rupture can occur into the peritoneal cavity, the biliary tree, or the retroperitoneum and is often fatal (7).

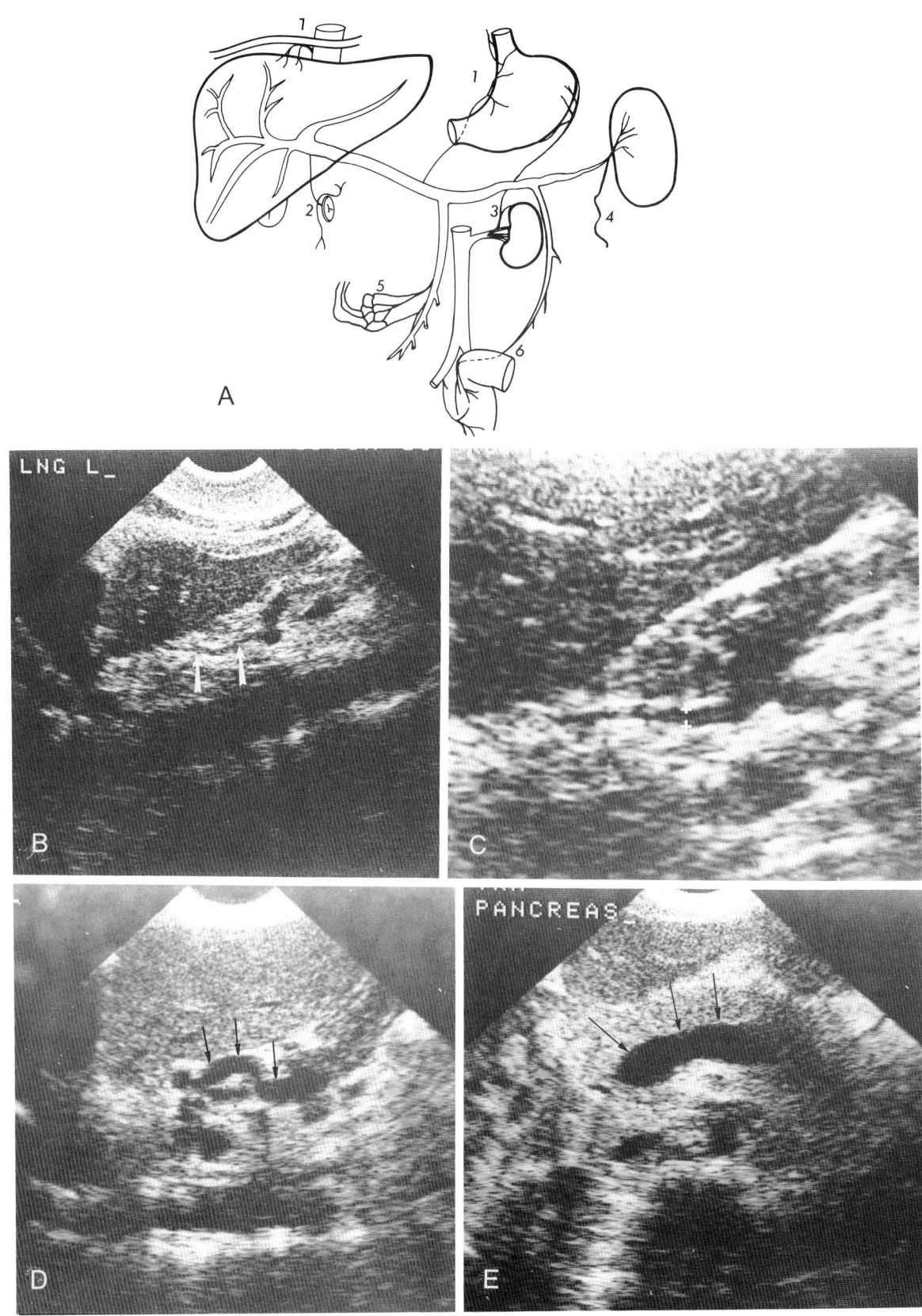

TABLE 4.2.
PORTASYSTEMIC COLLATERALS (12)

1. Transhepatic (portal vein to coronary vein, vertebral plexus, inferior vena cava, hemiazygos vein)
2. Gastroesophageal collaterals (varices)
3. Paraesophageal (coronary vein to azygos, hemiazygos, vertebral plexus)
4. Gastrorenal (gastric varices to left renal vein)
5. Portocoronary to pulmonary vein, gastroesophageal varices to left pulmonary vein
6. Splenorenal (splenic to left renal vein)
7. Splenocaval
8. Splenoazygos (hemiazygos, posterior abdominal wall)
9. Inferior mesenteric vein to hemorrhoidal (inferior and middle)
10. Pancreaticoduodenal to hemiazygos at the ligament of Treitz
11. Plexiform retroperitoneal (posterior abdominal wall, colic and mesenteric to inferior vena cava)
12. Pleuropericardial/peritoneal
13. Paraumbilical
14. Superior mesenteric to right renal vein
15. Intrahepatic (portal to hepatic vein)

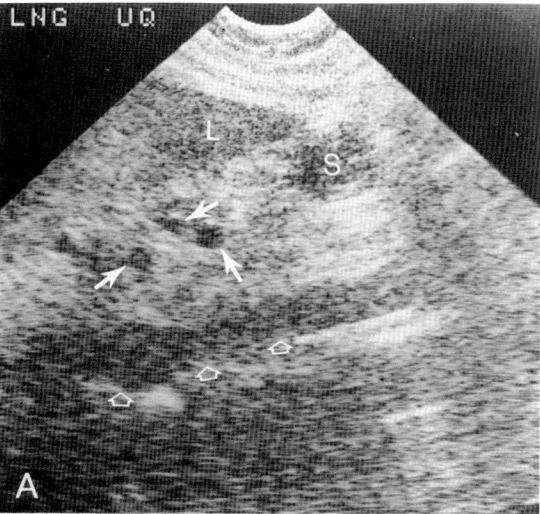

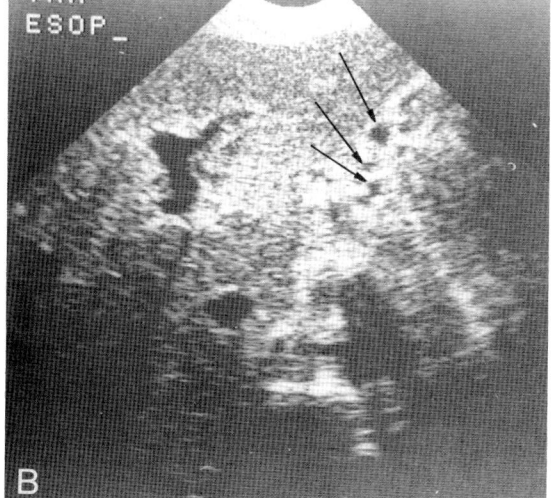

FIGURE 4.4. GASTROESOPHAGEAL VARICES
A: Parasagittal scan through the aorta (*open arrows*), left lobe of liver (*L*), and stomach (*S*) showing gastroesophageal varices (*arrows*) along the lesser curve of the stomach near the gastroesophageal junction. *B:* Transverse scan through the left lobe of the liver shows small, anechoic gastroesophageal varices (*arrows*) in the lesser omentum.

FIGURE 4.3. PORTOSYSTEMIC PATHWAYS
A: Diagrammatic representation of portosystemic collateral pathways: 1, gastroesophageal; 2, umbilical/epigastric or iliac; 3, gastric/adrenal and splenorenal; 4, splenic/retroperitoneal; 5, superior mesenteric/retroperitoneal; 6, inferior mesenteric and rectal-internal iliac (hemorrhoidal); 7, transcapsular. *B* and *C:* Sagittal scan through the aorta and the left lobe of the liver: normal coronary vein (*arrows*), measured 3.5 cm on magnification view (*C, cursors*). *D:* Sagittal scan of a patient with portal hypertension and varices in comparable plane: dilated coronary vein (*arrows*), about 1 cm in diameter. Adjacent sonolucencies are varices. *E:* Massively dilated splenic vein and portal venous confluence (*arrows*) posterior to the pancreas, transverse scan.

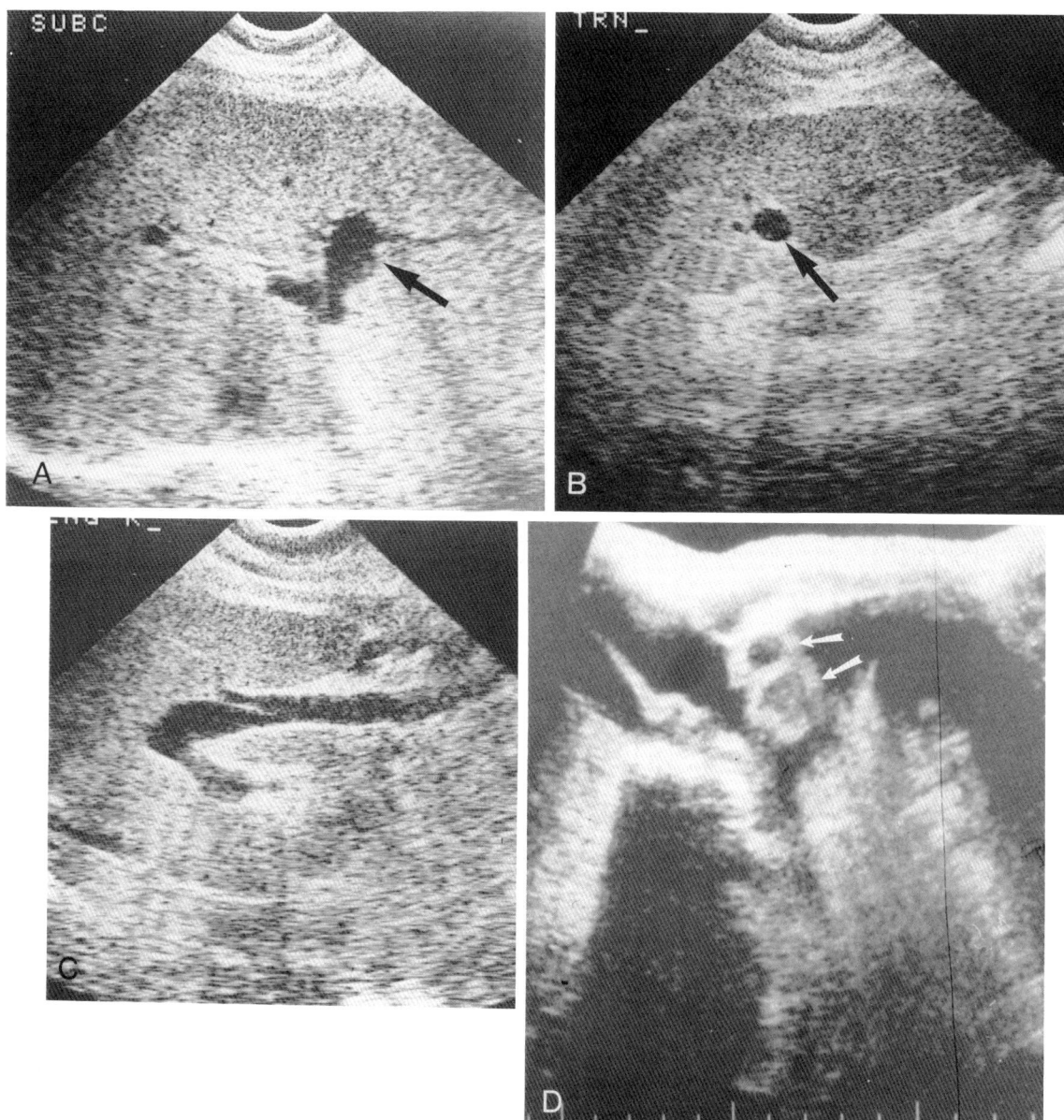

FIGURE 4.5. RECANALIZED UMBILICAL VEIN

A and *B:* Transverse scans at the confluence of the umbilical vein with the left portal vein (*arrow, A*) and slightly caudad in the falciform ligament showing the vein in cross-section (*arrow, B*). *C:* Parasagittal scan in the same patient as (*A, B*) shows the vein as a tubular lucency. It could be traced caudally towards the anterior abdominal wall. *D:* Two paraumbilical veins in cross-section (*arrows*) in the falciform ligament surrounded by ascites.

FIGURE 4.7. OTHER SONOGRAPHICALLY DETECTABLE VARICES

A–C: Advanced cirrhosis and unusual retroperitoneal collaterals: *A* and *B:* Transverse scans through right lobe, (*A*) cephalad to (*B*) show unusual collaterals (*arrows*). Liver (*L*) is bizarrely lobulated with abnormal echo texture and prominent echogenic septations. Caudate lobe (*C*) is prominent. *K*, kidney; *i*, inferior vena cava. *C:* Parasagittal scan shows one of the collaterals (*arrow*) between the lobulated liver and kidney (*K*). Compare to Figure 4.13, CT section, same case. *D:* Transverse scan in a different patient: pancreaticoduodenal collaterals (*arrows*) in the hepatoduodenal ligament just cephalad to the head of the pancreas.

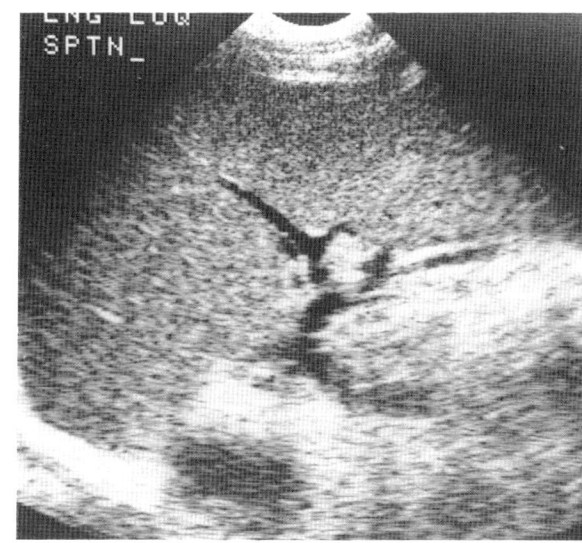

FIGURE 4.6. CORONAL SCAN THROUGH THE SPLEEN
Coronal scan through the spleen: massive splenomegaly and prominent proximal splenic vein with more than the usual number of branches visualized (collaterals).

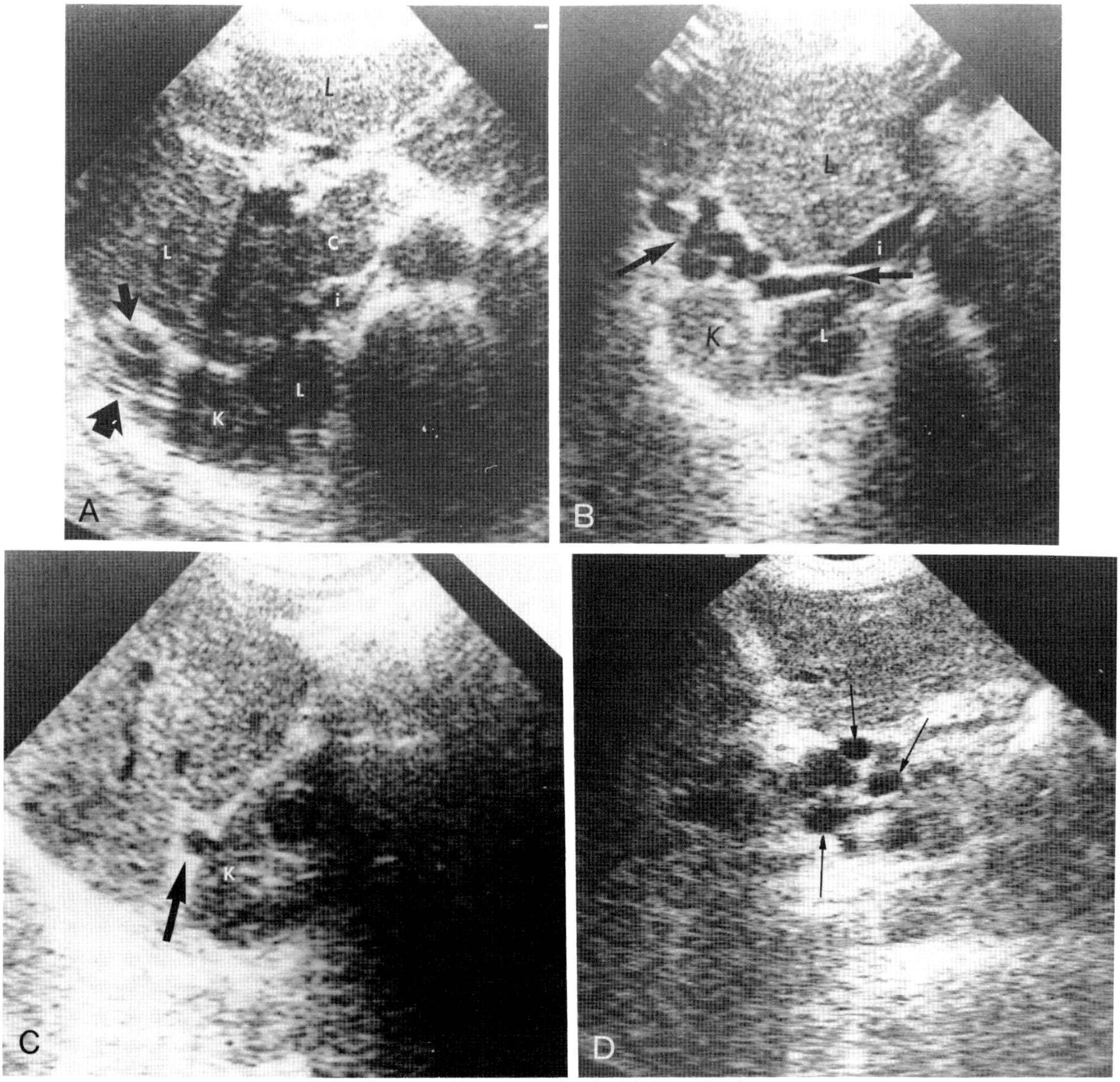

REFERENCES

1. Gosink BB, Lemon SK, Scheible W, Leopold GR: Accuracy of ultrasonography in diagnosis of hepatocellular disease. *AJR* 133:19–23, 1979.
2. Dewbury KC, Clark B: The accuracy of ultrasound in the detection of cirrhosis of the liver. *Br J Radiol* 52:945–948, 1979.
3. Kurtz AB, Rubin CS, Cooper HS, Nisenbaum HL, Cole-Beuglet C, Medoff J, Goldberg BB: Ultrasound findings in hepatitis. *Radiology* 136:717–723, 1980.
4. Blane CE, Jongeward RH Jr, Silver TM: Sonographic features of hepatocellular disease in neonates and infants. *AJR* 141:1313–1316, 1983.
5. Weinreb J, Kumari S, Phillips G, Pochaczevsky R: Portal vein measurements by real-time sonography. *AJR* 139:497–499, 1982.
6. Niederau C, Sonnenberg A, Muller J, Erckenbrecht JF, Scholten T, Fritsch WP: Sonographic measurements of the normal liver, spleen, pancreas, and portal vein. *Radiology* 149:537–540, 1983.
7. Vine HS, Sequeira JC, Widrich WC, Sacks BA: Portal vein aneurysm. *AJR* 132:557–560, 1979.
8. LaFortune M, Marleau D, Breton G, Viallet A, Lavoie P, Huet P: Portal venous system measurements in portal hypertension. *Radiology* 151:27–30, 1984.
9. Bolondi L, Gandolfi L, Arienti V: Ultrasonography in the diagnosis of portal hypertension: diminished response of portal vessels to respiration. *Radiology* 142:167–172, 1982.
10. Dach JL, Hill MC, Pelaez JC, LePage JR, Russell E: Sonography of hypertensive portal venous system: correlation with arterial portography. *AJR* 137:511–517, 1981.
11. Hill MC and Sanders RC: Sonography of the upper abdominal venous system. In Sanders RC, Hill MC (eds): *Ultrasound Annual 1983*. New York, Raven Press, 1983, pp. 290–300.
12. Doehner GA, Ruzicka FF, Rousselot LM, Hoffman G: The portal Venous system: on its pathological roentgen anatomy. *Radiology* 66:206–217, 1956.
13. Kane RA and Katz SG: The spectrum of sonographic findings in portal hypertension: a subject review and new observations. *Radiology* 142:453–458, 1982.
14. Lafortune M, Constantin A, Breton G, Legare AG, Lavoie P: The recanalized umbilical vein in portal hypertension: a myth. *AJR* 144:549–553, 1985.
15. Marchal GJF, Van Holsbeeck M, Tshibwabwa-Ntumba E, et al: Dilatation of the cystic veins in portal hypertension: sonographic demonstration. *Radiology* 154:187–189, 1985.
16. Nordlinger BM, Nordlinger DF, Fulenwider JT, Millikan WJ, Sones PJ, Kutner M, Steele R, Bain R, Warren WD: Angiography in portal hypertension: clinical significance in surgery. *Am J Surg* 139:132–141, 1980.

Computed Tomography

Fatty infiltration of the liver (steatosis) is the most characteristic CT feature of early cirrhosis, especially in alcoholic liver disease (1). Corresponding histology is the presence of clear intracytoplasmic vacuoles (fat) in hepatocytes. Although most commonly diffuse and uniform, fatty infiltration can be multifocal or focal. Normally, the liver is 6–12 HU denser than the spleen but this relationship is reversed in fatty infiltration. CT numbers are low in regions of fatty infiltration, but not necessarily negative (1, 2). Hepatomegaly is a frequent finding, but liver contour is normal. Hepatomegaly in early cirrhosis can also be due to hepatitis. Fatty infiltration is discussed more completely elsewhere under "Other Diffuse Diseases."

In the later stages of cirrhosis, an overall decrease in liver volume is seen accompanied by right lobe atrophy and relative hypertrophy of the left and caudate lobes (Fig. 4.8) (1, 3). Regenerating nodules and nonuniform atrophy/hypertrophy cause lobulation of the liver contour (Fig. 4.9). Regenerating nodules are isodense both before and after contrast enhancement and are isoechoic on ultrasound (1). The hepatic fissures and porta hepatis are wider and more prominent than usual because of parenchymal atrophy (1, 3). Nonuniform attenuation, at times very striking, can be present because of either chronic fatty infiltration or fibrosis (Fig. 4.10) (1). Intrahepatic veins may be poorly visualized (3). A caudate lobe to right lobe size ratio has been proposed as an accurate objective means of diagnosing cirrhosis on either ultrasound or CT (Fig. 4.11) (3). Three lines are drawn as follows: line 1 is parasagittal through the right lateral wall of the main portal vein at a level just caudad to its bifurcation, line 2 is parallel to line 1 through the most medial margin of the caudate lobe, and line 3 is perpendicular to lines 1 and 2 drawn midway between the main portal vein and the inferior cava, extended to the right abdomi-

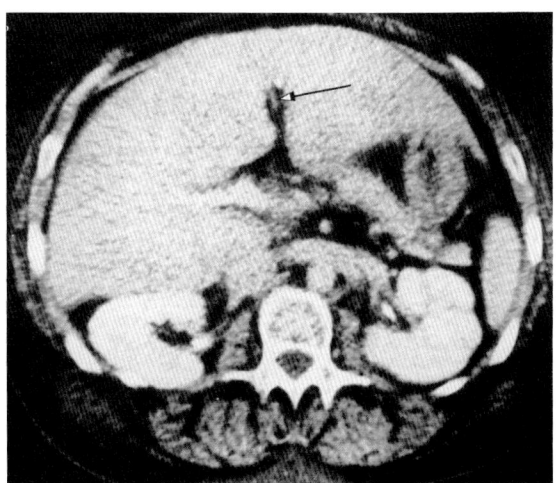

FIGURE 4.8. EARLY CIRRHOSIS
Early cirrhosis with enlarged left lobe, mildly prominent caudate lobe (but caudate lobe to right lobe ratio of 0.33 (false negative)) and recanalized umbilical vein (*arrow*).

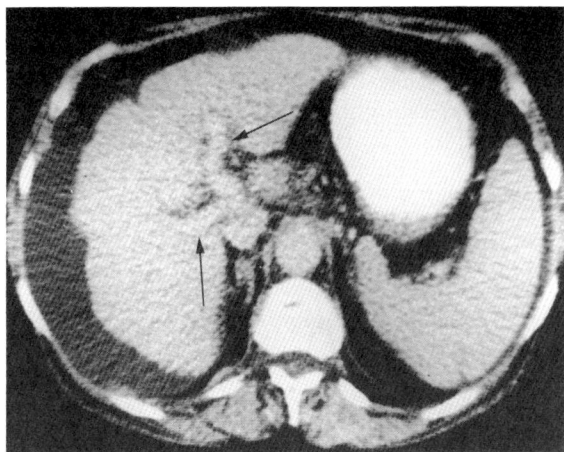

FIGURE 4.9. ADVANCED CIRRHOSIS
Small, lobulated liver, prominent portal vein (*arrows*) ascites and splenomegaly in advanced cirrhosis.

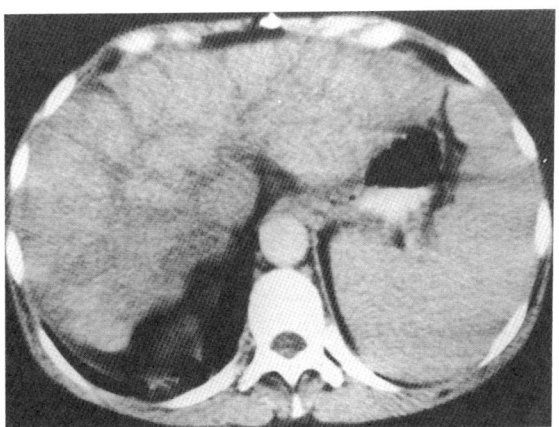

FIGURE 4.10. ADVANCED CIRRHOSIS
Extensive scarring, enlarged left lobe, and splenomegaly in advanced cirrhosis.

nal wall. The distance from the right abdominal wall to line 1 is Y and the distance between lines 1 and 2 is X (measurements made along line 3). The caudate lobe to right lobe size ratio is X/Y. According to published data, if this ratio exceeds 0.65, cirrhosis is present with a 96% confidence level and if it exceeds 0.73 the confidence level is 99%. Conversely, if it is less than 0.6, cirrhosis is present in only 13% (3). The increase in size of the caudate lobe relative to the right lobe is due to both enlargement of the caudate and fibrotic shrinkage of the right lobe. The enlarged caudate can cause constriction of the inferior vena cava, which may be contributory to the development of ascites and the hepatorenal syndrome. The hepatic arteries and portal veins supplying the caudate lobe have a shorter intrahepatic course than those supplying the right

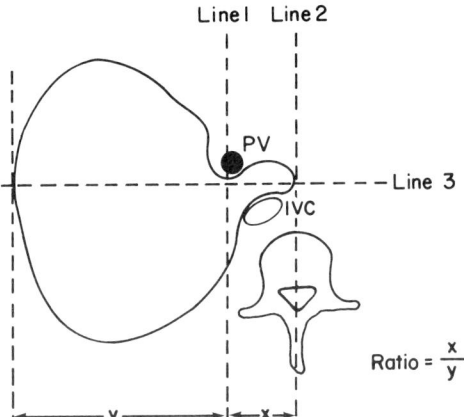

FIGURE 4.11. CALCULATION OF CAUDATE LOBE TO RIGHT LOBE RATIO

lobe and therefore undergo less distortion by cirrhosis, explaining the relative preservation and even hypertrophy of the caudate lobe in cirrhosis. Caudate lobe enlargement is absent early in cirrhosis and roughly parallels the degree of cirrhosis thereafter (3). Additional features seen on CT in cirrhosis are ascites, splenomegaly, and evidence of portasystemic collateral circulation.

CT in Portal Hypertension

The collaterals discussed in the ultrasound section can also be evaluated by CT. Portal and/or splenic vein enlargement is easily detected, as is portal vein aneurysm (Fig. 4.9). Portal vein thrombosis is seen as lucent clot surrounded by enhanced vessel wall on contrast enhanced scans. Enhancement within the clot is indicative of tumor extension into the portal vein, usually due to hepatocellular carcinoma. Periportal collaterals are depicted as numerous worm-like enhancing veins traversing the porta hepatis. Esophageal and/or gastric varices can be suggested on CT when marked contrast enhancement is seen in the thickened wall of the appropriate viscus (Fig. 4.12) (4). Portosystemic collaterals are tortuous, tubular, or round soft-tissue attenuation masses on unenhanced scans, and scans after bolus injection of contrast are often necessary to confirm their vascular nature (Fig. 4.13). Azygos, hemiazygos, and paraesophageal collaterals can mimic mediastinal masses, and retroperitoneal varices can mimic adenopathy or renal/adrenal masses (1, 4). Finally, the recanalized umbilical vein is readily depicted as a rounded or tubular enhancing opacity surrounded by fat in the falciform ligament coursing

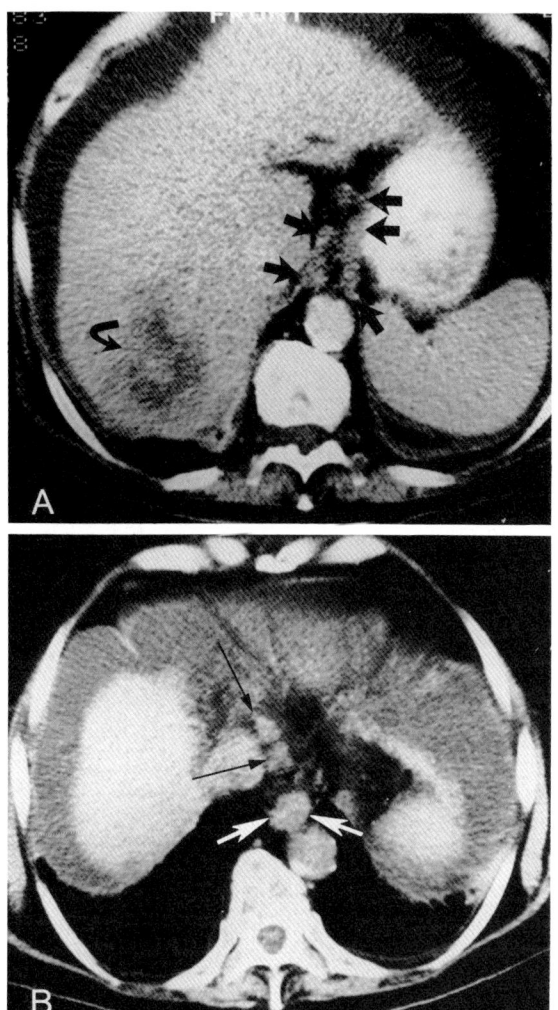

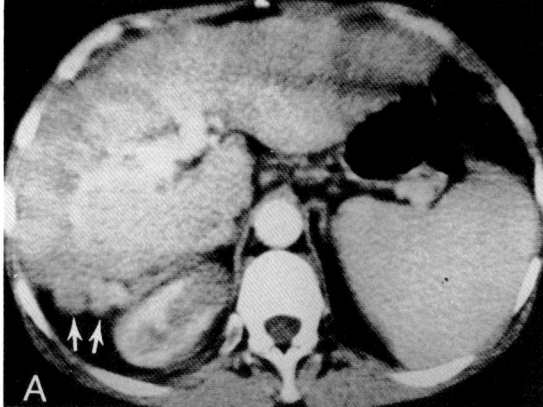

FIGURE 4.12. ADVANCED CIRRHOSIS
A and B: Gastroesophageal collaterals (*arrows*), ascites, small right lobe, large left lobe and caudate lobe, thickened esophageal wall from varices (*white arrows*), and hepatocellular carcinoma (*curved arrow*) in advanced cirrhosis.

caudally toward the abdominal wall, and sometimes terminating in a caput medusa (Fig. 4.8).

CT is more sensitive than arterial portography in detecting recanalization of the umbilical vein (Fig. 4.14) (5). Retroperitoneal collaterals and perisplenic mesenteric collaterals are also detected more reliably with CT (Fig. 4.14), and CT sometimes demonstrates more collaterals in the coronary venous system than arterial portography. On the other hand, angiography is more reliable than CT in demonstrating cavernous transformation of the portal vein and peripancreatic collaterals (5).

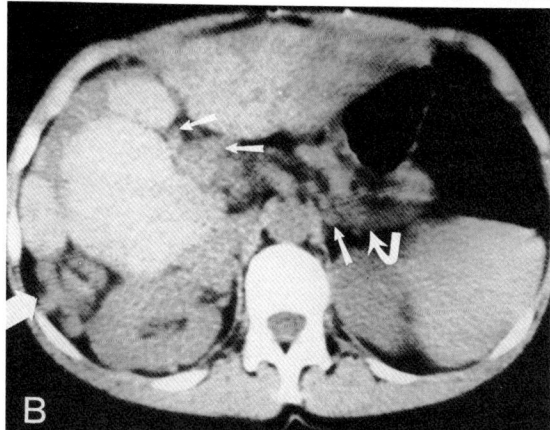

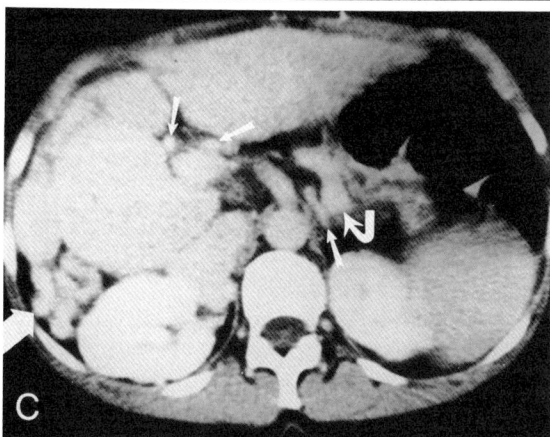

FIGURE 4.13. ADVANCED CIRRHOSIS WITH UNUSUAL COLLATERALS
Advanced cirrhosis with unusual collaterals. (See Fig. 7 ultrasound for same case.) A: Enlarged caudate and left lobes. Caudate-lobe to right-lobe ratio of 0.67. Enhancing collaterals between liver and kidney (*arrows*). B and C: Scans at nearly the same level before (B) and after (C) bolus injections of contrast showing multiple enhancing collaterals (*arrows*) and enlarged splenic vein (*curved arrow*). Note bizarre liver lobulation, nodularity, and attenuation inhomogeneity.

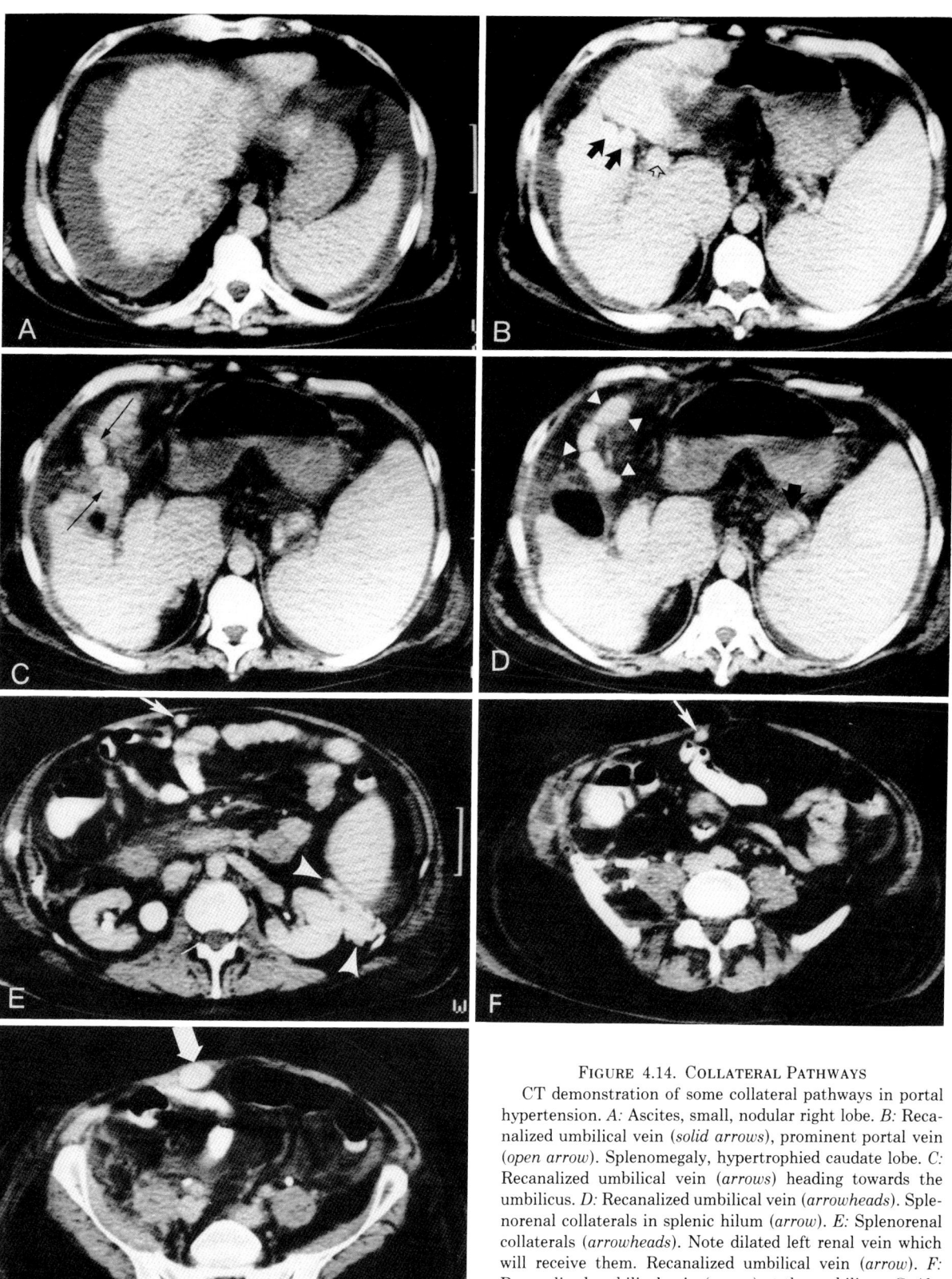

FIGURE 4.14. COLLATERAL PATHWAYS

CT demonstration of some collateral pathways in portal hypertension. *A:* Ascites, small, nodular right lobe. *B:* Recanalized umbilical vein (*solid arrows*), prominent portal vein (*open arrow*). Splenomegaly, hypertrophied caudate lobe. *C:* Recanalized umbilical vein (*arrows*) heading towards the umbilicus. *D:* Recanalized umbilical vein (*arrowheads*). Splenorenal collaterals in splenic hilum (*arrow*). *E:* Splenorenal collaterals (*arrowheads*). Note dilated left renal vein which will receive them. Recanalized umbilical vein (*arrow*). *F:* Recanalized umbilical vein (*arrow*) at the umbilicus. *G:* Abdominal wall collateral (*arrow*) caudad to the umbilicus joining the caput medusa.

REFERENCES

1. Waller RM III, Oliver TW Jr, McCain AH, Sones PJ Jr, Bernardino ME: Computed tomography and sonography of hepatic cirrhosis and portal hypertension. *Radiographics* 4:677–714, 1984.
2. Mulhern CB Jr, Arger PH, Coleman BG, Stein GN: Nununiform attenuation in computed tomography study of the cirrhotic liver. *Radiology* 132:399–402, 1979.
3. Harbin WP, Robert NJ, Ferrucci JT Jr: Diagnosis of cirrhosis based on regional changes in hepatic morphology. A radiological and pathological analysis. *Radiology* 135:273–283, 1980.
4. Ishikawa T, Tsukune Y, Ohyama Y, Fujikawa M, Sakuyama K, Fujii M: Venous abnormalities in portal hypertension demonstrated by CT. *AJR* 134:271–276, 1980.
5. McCain AH, Bernardino ME, Sones PJ Jr, Berkman WA, Casarella WJ: Varices from portal hypertension: correlation of CT and angiography. *Radiology* 154:63–69, 1985.

Barium Contrast Examinations in Portal Hypertension

The characteristic appearance of esophageal varices from portal hypertension is the thickening of distal esophageal folds on esophagography (Fig. 4.15). Distention of the lumen with barium or gas will partially or completely obliterate varices. Fluoroscopic skill is necessary for detecting small varices. Useful techniques include left anterior oblique (LAO) supine filming, videotape recording, Valsalva maneuver, coating the mucosa with barium paste, and anticholinergic drugs (1, 2).

Gastric varices in portal hypertension are usually predominantly fundal. Gastric varices without esophageal varices suggest splenic vein obstruction. They are multiple, smooth lobular filling defects (thickened, lobular folds) (Fig. 4.16). They are best demonstrated on double contrast views, and can be partially obliterated by overdistention (3, 4). Since gastric varices are often subserosal, the radiographic study may be positive in the face of negative or equivocal endoscopy.

Duodenal varices produce diffuse, serpiginous

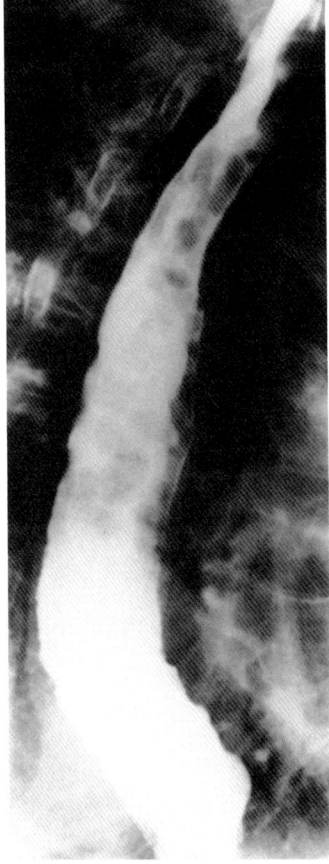

FIGURE 4.15. ESOPHAGEAL VARICES
Extensive esophageal varices: lobular, serpiginous filling defects proximally and scalloped contour defects distally.

thickening of folds, and are almost always associated with esophageal varices (4). When isolated, the usual cause is superior mesenteric vein obstruction. Jejunal or ileal varices are extremely rare, as are colonic varices. Rectal varices are radiographically quite similar to esophageal varices, and range in appearance from prominent hemorrhoids to serpiginous submucosal masses extending up into the distal sigmoid colon.

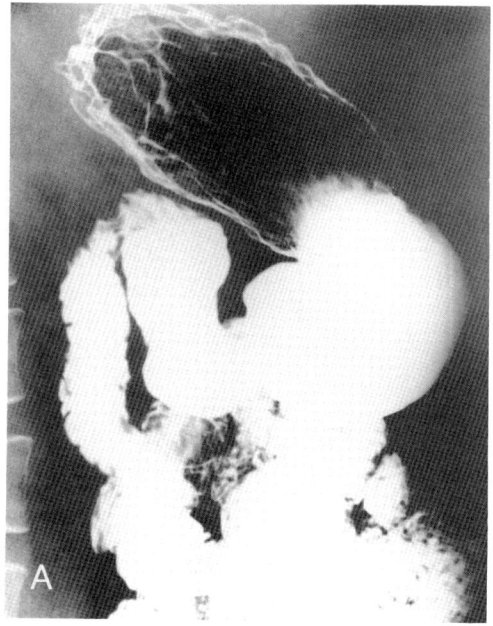
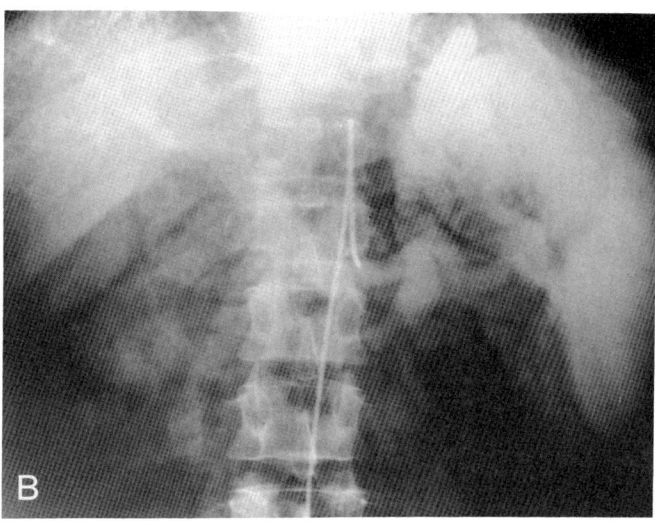
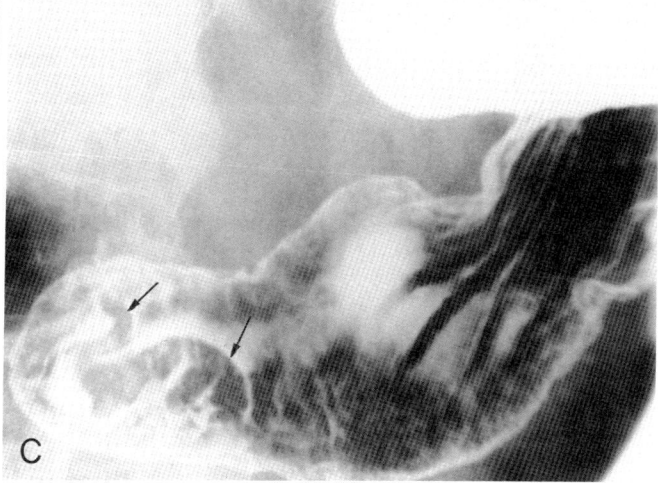

FIGURE 4.16. GASTRIC VARICES
A: Fundal varices: lobulated, thickened folds isolated to the fundus. B: Diagnosis of varices confirmed by the venous phase of a celiac arteriogram. C: Antral varices: lobulated, thickened fold in the antrum (arrows).

REFERENCES

1. Cockerill EM, Miller RE, Chernish SM et al: Optimal visualization of esophageal varices. AJR 126:512–523, 1976.
2. Nelson SW: The roentgenologic diagnosis of esophageal varices. AJR 77:599–611, 1957.
3. Sos T, Meyers MA, Baltaxe HA: Nonfundic gastric varices. Radiology 105:579–580, 1972.
4. Bateson EM: Duodenal and antral varices. Br J Radiol 42:744–747, 1969.

Angiography

The angiographic characteristics of cirrhosis are related to the pathophysiology discussed above (Figs. 4.17 and 4.18). Early findings consist only of stretched hepatic artery branches and a mottled parenchymal phase probably due to fatty infiltration. Moderate cirrhosis will manifest arterial corkscrewing and a slight increase in hepatic arterial flow. Severe cirrhosis causes contraction of liver volume, widespread corkscrewing of arteries and increased arterial flow, and occasionally shunting between the hepatic artery and the portal vein (Fig. 4.17D) (1, 2). Another finding that may occur is delayed emptying with persistence of contrast in the hepatic arteries out into the venous phase.

Macroregenerating nodules can be difficult to differentiate from neoplasm. They have fewer arterial branches than adjacent liver and exert a mass effect, stretching surrounding vessels (Fig. 4.17). They do not have arteriovenous shunting, tumor vascularity, vascular encasement, or serration. Hepatic venography will usually show patent hepatic veins within the "tumor" and portal veins can be seen to traverse the mass without thrombosis on portography (3).

Arterial portography is used to evaluate the portal venous system in cirrhosis less invasively than via percutaneous transhepatic portography

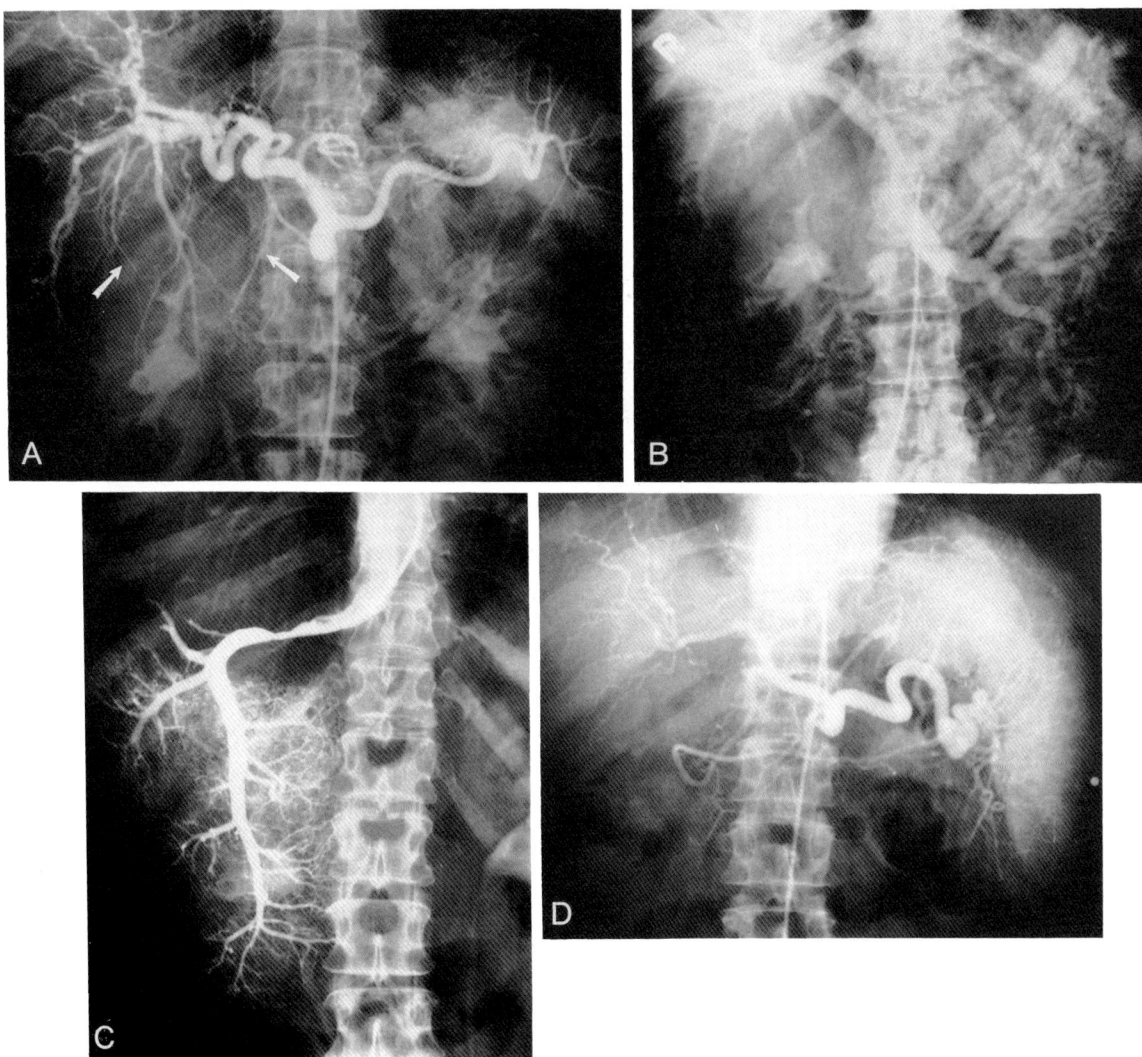

FIGURE 4.17. MACROREGENERATING NODULE IN CIRRHOSIS

A: Arteriogram shows corkscrewing and crowding of vessels in the upper portion of the right lobe consistent with cirrhosis. A mass is suggested by displacement and stretching of vessels in the inferior portion of the right lobe (*arrows*). However, there is no evidence of neovascularity, encasement or early venous opacification. *B:* Portal veins are elongated and displaced in the same region. *C:* A free hepatic venogram shows some stretching and straightening of 1st and 2nd order hepatic vein branches in the inferior portion of the right lobe without evidence of tumor invasion. *D:* Severe cirrhosis in a different patient: the celiac arteriogram shows splenomegaly and a small liver with corkscrewing of arteries.

or splenoportography (Fig. 4.18). High dose celiac and superior mesenteric angiography can usually demonstrate the portal vein when it is patent. Hepatofugal flow and portosystemic collaterals can be depicted. Collaterals commonly demonstrated are esophagogastric connecting the coronary vein to the azygos system, splenorenal, retroperitoneal, abdominal wall, and bowel wall via mesenteric veins. Occasionally direct channels to the inferior vena cava can be seen via splenocaval, mesocaval, and transhepatic veins.

Important structural and hemodynamic information can be obtained by the use of hepatic venography (4).

Catheterization of the hepatic veins may be obtained via either an antecubital or femoral vein approach. Both free and wedged hepatic venograms can be obtained as well as pressure recordings in the inferior vena cava and main hepatic vein (free hepatic vein pressure). The wedged hepatic venous pressure (portal pressure) can be measured via an end-hole catheter wedged in the peripheral portion of a hepatic vein. The

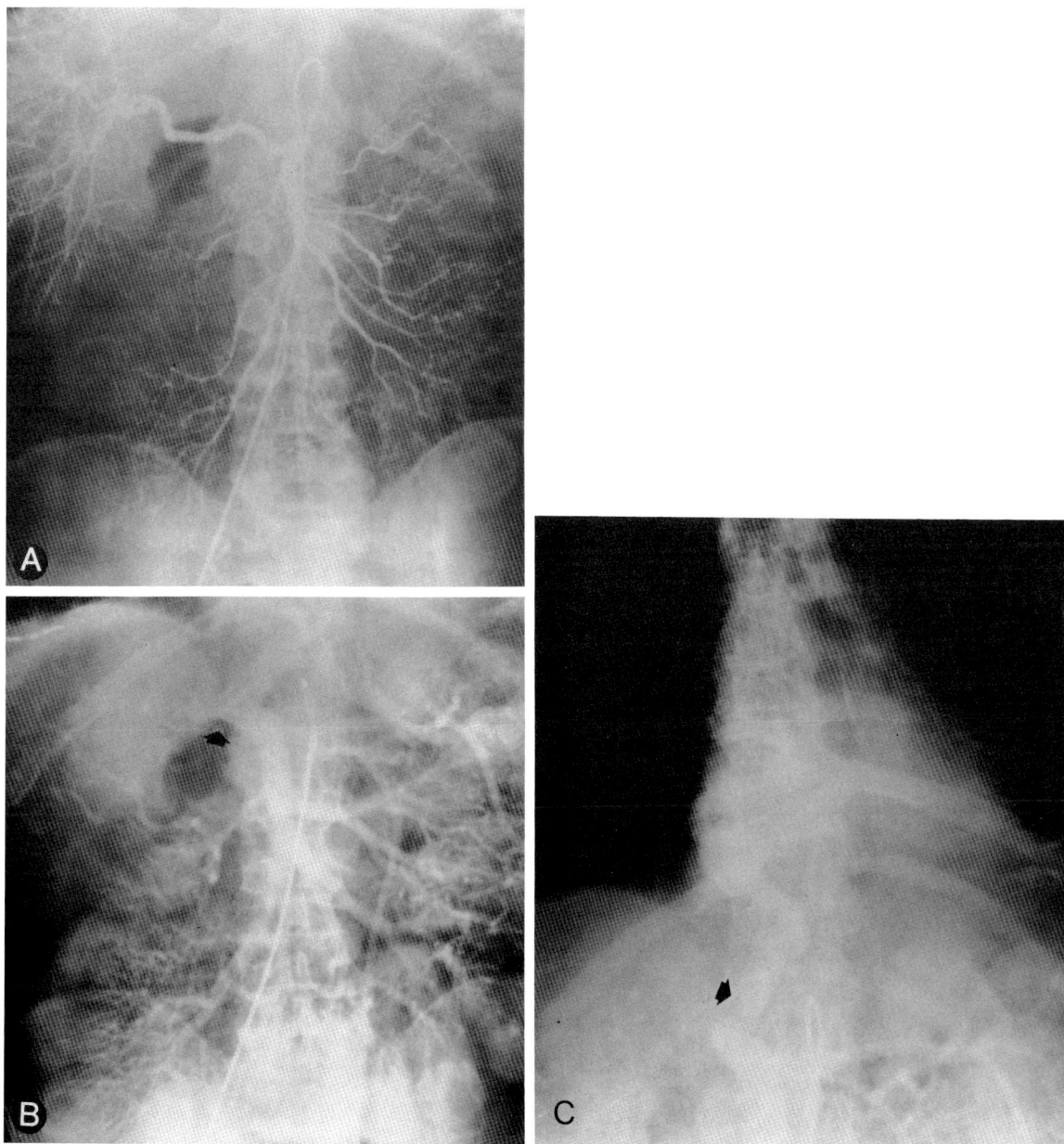

FIGURE 4.18. CIRRHOSIS WITH THROMBOSIS OF THE PORTAL VEIN AND ESOPHAGEAL VARICES

A: High-dose superior mesenteric angiogram: replaced right hepatic artery, mild corkscrewing. *B* and *C:* Venous phase: abrupt termination of the portal vein from thrombosis (*arrow*). Repeat injection with centering on the lower chest: hepatofugal flow filling the enlarged coronary vein (*arrow*) leading to esophageal varices (*C*).

normal free hepatic venogram shows fifth-order branching beyond the injected hepatic vein (or zero-order branch) (Fig. 4.19) (3). In fatty liver, spreading of hepatic vein branches occurs without loss of branching. Loss of branching accompanies fibrosis. Mild changes are defined as failure to visualize fifth-order branches beyond the injected vein. Loss of fourth- or third-order branches is considered moderate change, while loss of first- and second-order hepatic vein branches constitutes severe change. Extrinsic indentations of the opacified hepatic veins can be caused by large regenerating nodules. Corrected wedge pressures are obtained by subtracting the inferior vena cava pressure from the wedged hepatic vein pressure. Normal is 0–5 mm Hg, mild portal hypertension is 5–10 mm Hg, and over 15 mm Hg constitutes severe portal

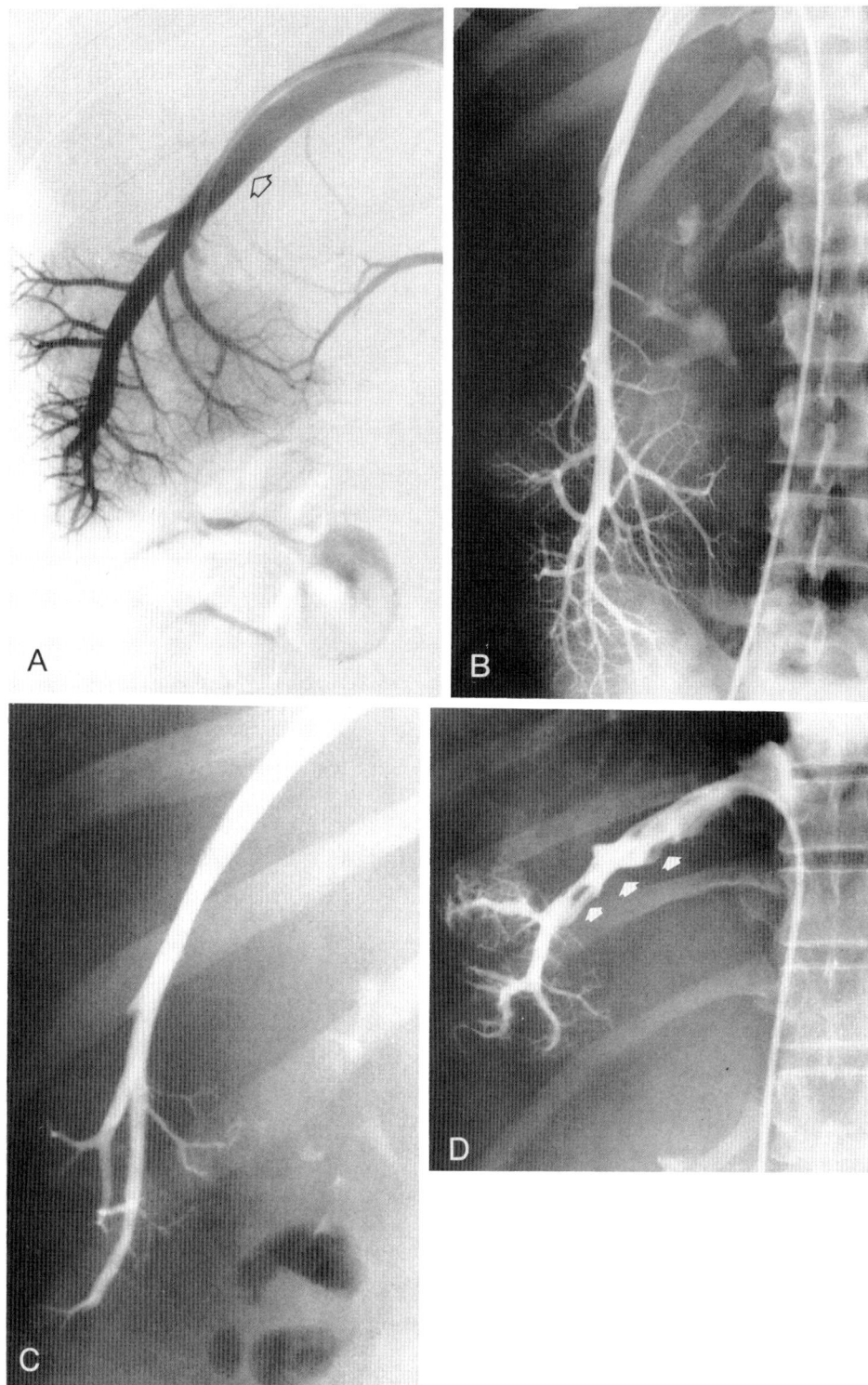

FIGURE 4.19. HEPATIC VENOGRAM
A: Normal free hepatic venogram showing 5th-order branches beyond the zero-order branch (*arrow*). An accessory hepatic vein is seen to the right of the figure. *B:* Fatty liver: normal branching with hepatomegaly. *C:* Severe cirrhosis: marked pruning, loss of 1st- and 2nd-order branches. *D:* Postnecrotic cirrhosis: severe pruning and extrinsic indentations (*arrows*) on the zero-order branch from macronodular regeneration.

hypertension. In general, pruning of hepatic vein branches on the free hepatic venogram correlates well with hepatic fibrosis and corrected hepatic vein wedge pressures in patients with alcoholic cirrhosis, alcoholic hepatitis, and postnecrotic cirrhosis. However, wedged hepatic vein pressures tend to vary, whereas free hepatic venogram changes remain constant over short periods of time. Free hepatic venography and pressure recording are useful alternatives to liver biopsy in patients with clotting disorders in which liver biopsy is contraindicated. However, manometric pressure determination is not useful in either determining the type of portasystemic shunt surgery or predicting its likelihood of success (5, 6). Retrograde filling of portal vein branches after wedged hepatic vein injection can document reversal of portal flow, supporting findings on the venous phase of superior mesenteric arteriography (Fig. 4.20) (7).

REFERENCES

1. Viamonte M, Warren WD, Fomon JJ: Liver panangiography in the assessment of portal hypertension in cirrhosis. *Radiol Clin North Am* 8:147–167, 1970.
2. Clemett AR: Roentgenology of the liver and bile ducts. In Margulis AR, Burhenne HJ (eds): *Alimentary Tract Roentgenology*. St. Louis, C. V. Mosby, 1973, pp 1230–1258.
3. Rabinowitz JG, Kinkabwala M, Ulreich S: Macroregenerating nodule in the cirrhotic liver. *AJR* 121:401–411, 1974.
4. Cavaluzzi J, Sheff R, Harrington DP, Kaufman SL, Barth K, Maddrey WR, White RI Jr: Hepatic venography and wedge hepatic vein pressure measurements in diffuse liver disease. *AJR* 129:441–446, 1977.
5. Smith GW: Use of hemodynamic selection criteria in the management of cirrhotic patients with portal hypertension. *Ann Surg* 179:782–790, 1974.
6. Reynolds T: Role of hemodynamic measurements in portasystemic shunt surgery. *Arch Surg* 108:276–281, 1974.
7. Nordlinger BM, Nordlinger DF, Fulenwider JT, Millikan WJ, Sones PJ, Kutner M, Steele R, Bain R, Warren WD: Angiography in portal hypertension. Clinical significance in surgery. *Am J Surg* 139:132–141, 1980.

Cholangiography in Cirrhosis

Direct cholangiography (usually ERCP) is sometimes indicated in patients with cirrhosis to

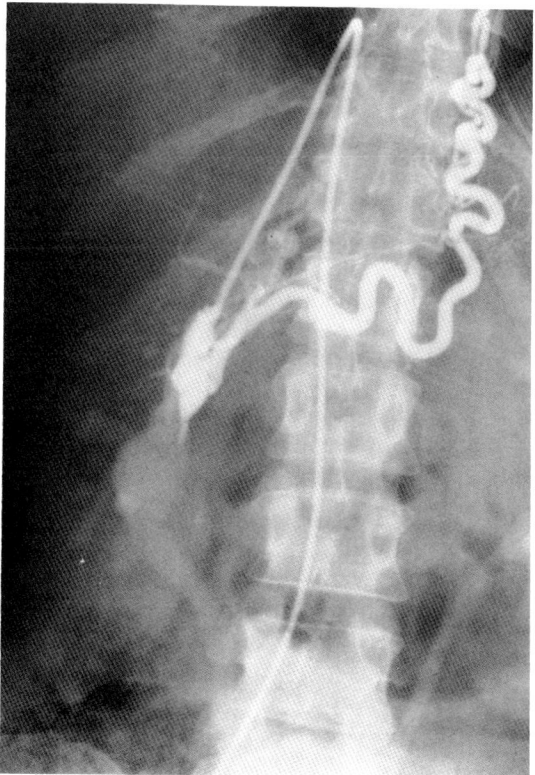

FIGURE 4.20. WEDGED HEPATIC VENOGRAM: MARKED HEPATOFUGAL FLOW WITH RAPID AND DENSE OPACIFICATION OF ESOPHAGEAL VARICES

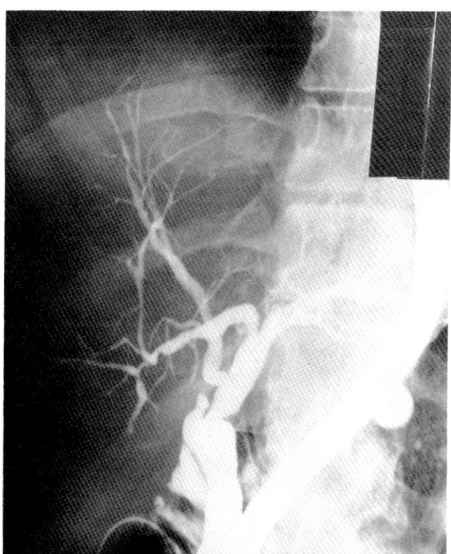

FIGURE 4.21. ERCP: SMALL LIVER IS DISPLACED FROM LATERAL ABDOMINAL WALL
Note the variably attenuated, undulating intrahepatic biliary tree with some stretching from nodular regeneration.

exclude mechanical biliary obstruction. When fatty infiltration predominates early in the course of the disease, one may see straightening, elongation, and separation of intrahepatic ducts. These findings are identical to those of any infiltrative liver disease (i.e., diffuse lymphoma). The cholangiogram is normal in milder cases of fatty infiltration. As the liver shrinks with increasing fibrosis, the intrahepatic ducts become crowded together. Corkscrewing, tortuosity, and mild changes in caliber may or may not be present (Fig. 4.21). Larger regenerating nodules will smoothly displace and splay adjacent ducts (1, 2).

REFERENCES

1. Falkenstein DB, Riccobono C, Sidhu G, et al: The endoscopic intrahepatic cholangiogram. Clinicopathologic correlation with postmortem cholangiograms. *Invest Radiol* 10:358–365, 1975.
2. Larsen CR, Scholz FJ, Wise RE: Diseases of the biliary ducts. *Semin Roentgenol* 11:259–267, 1976.

CAUSES OF PORTAL HYPERTENSION OTHER THAN CIRRHOSIS

Most cases of portal hypertension are fairly straightforward with a clear cut history of alcohol abuse leading to cirrhosis or viral hepatitis leading to postnecrotic cirrhosis. These patients have sinusoidal or postsinusoidal obstruction and an elevated wedge pressure. Occasionally the situation is not straightforward, and sophisticated hepatic angiography and venography are necessary both to establish whether the site of obstruction is postsinusoidal or presinusoidal and to determine an etiology. Presinusoidal portal hypertension is documented when a normal corrected hepatic wedge pressure is obtained in the face of portal hypertension. Extrahepatic causes of postsinusoidal hypertension such as constrictive pericarditis and congestive heart failure are usually diagnosed by other means, but elevated systemic venous pressures obtained during hepatic venography may be useful in corroborating a clinical diagnosis. Angiographic techniques are vital in the diagnosis of obstructions and/or stenoses of the inferior vena cava and/or hepatic veins.

Presinusoidal Portal Hypertension

The major cause of presinusoidal hypertension in the United States is portal vein thrombosis. Usual causes include neonatal omphalitis, complications of pancreatitis, neoplastic invasion, and stasis in cirrhosis. Unusual causes are intraabdominal infections such as appendicitis, diverticulitis, or inflammatory bowel disease, trauma, coagulopathy, and idiopathic (1). Portal venous thrombosis can be intraheptic or extrahepatic, partial, or complete.

Radiology of Portal Venous Thrombosis

Very rarely, calcification can be seen in either clot in the portal vein or in its wall (Fig. 4.22)

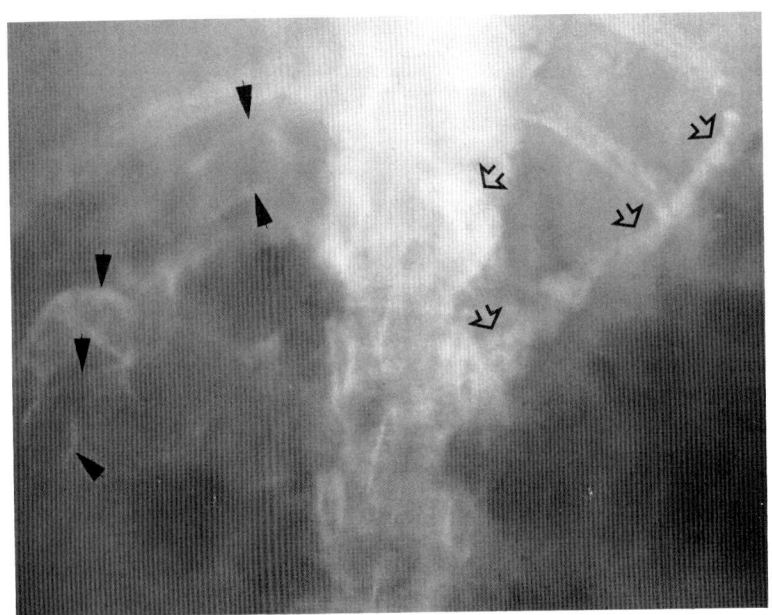

FIGURE 4.22. CALCIFIED PORTAL VEIN, SPLENIC VEIN AND CORONARY VEIN
Note solid calcification consistent with clot (*open arrows*) and tram-track wall calcification (*arrows*).

(2, 3). Portal vein wall calcification is seen as parallel radiodense lines directed along the course of the portal vein. They are often discontinuous and slightly irregular. Calcified portal vein clot, on the other hand, has calcification throughout without marginal density accentuation. The presence of either type of calcification implies portal vein obstruction, which is usually but not necessarily complete.

Sonography can demonstrate portal vein thrombosis quite reliably in the main portal vein or its larger branches as echogenic material within the vascular lumen (Figs. 4.23 and 4.24).

On occasion, when the obstruction is complete and the lumen is entirely filled, one may have difficulty identifying the vein at all (1), and a diamond-shaped echogenic band will be seen instead of the expected tubular lucency in the porta hepatis (4). With chronic portal vein thrombosis, the thrombus may become organized and ultimately recanalized. Multiple collateral channels may be formed (Fig. 4.25). Sonographically, the diagnosis is suggested when the following triad of findings is present: (a) nonvisualization of the extrahepatic portal vein, (b) a bright echogenic band representing either thrombus or periportal

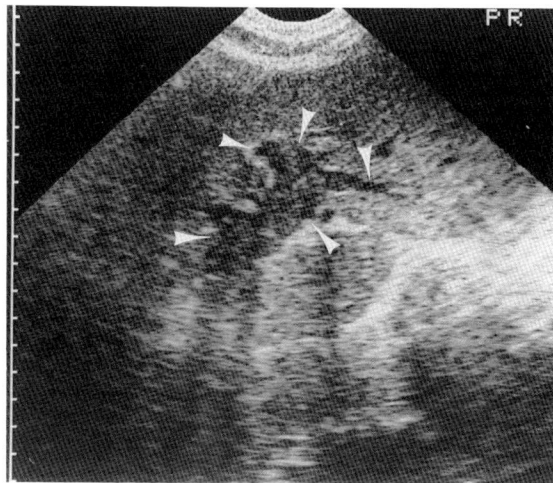

FIGURE 4.23. TUMOR THROMBUS FILLING THE PORTAL VEIN AND ITS LARGER BRANCHES (arrows): HEPATOCELLULAR CARCINOMA

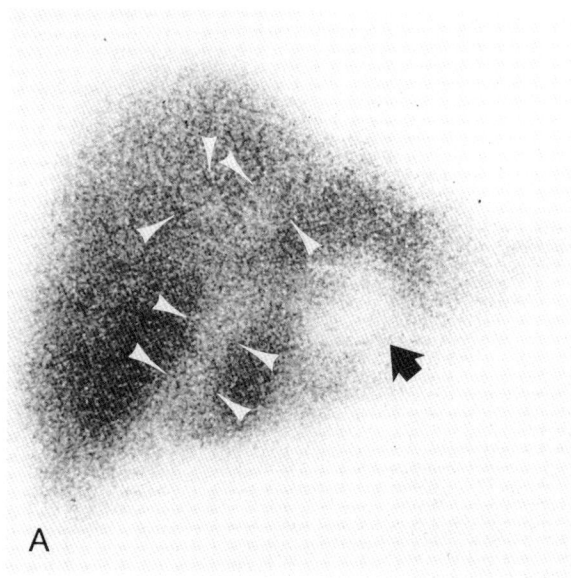
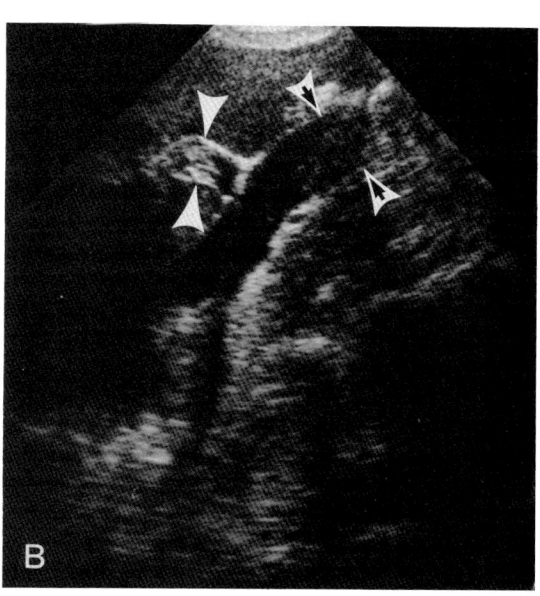

FIGURE 4.24. PORTAL VEIN TUMOR THROMBUS FROM HEPATOCELLULAR CARCINOMA

A: Sulfur colloid scan: central branching region of decreased activity (*arrowheads*) representing enlarged, tumor-filled portal venous system. The round cold region is the primary hepatocellular carcinoma (*black arrow*). *B:* Corresponding sonogram: portal vein partially filled with tumor thrombus (*arrowheads*). Tumor thrombus in inferior vena cava as well (*black on white arrows*).

fibrosis in the region of the portal vein, and (c) periportal collaterals appearing as multiple serpiginous, tubular vascular channels in the region of the portal vein (Fig. 4.25F, G) (5–7). Doppler studies of the collateral channels will detect flow patterns characteristic of portal veins (8). The

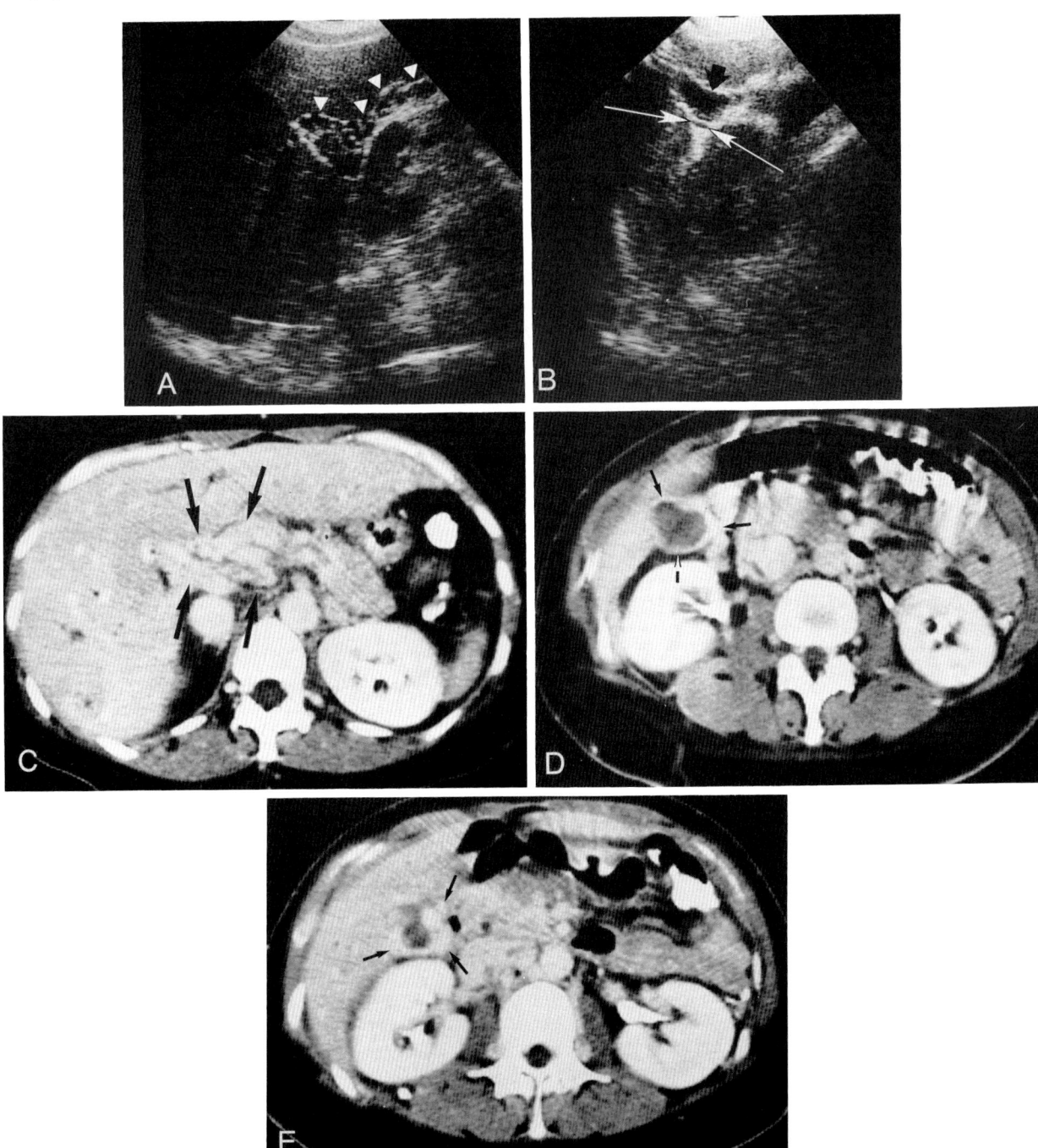

FIGURE 4.25. SONOGRAPHIC DEMONSTRATION OF COLLATERALS IN PORTAL VEIN THROMBOSIS

A: Serpiginous periportal collaterals (*arrowheads*). B: Pericholecystic collateral (*white arrows*) beneath the gallbladder (*black arrow*). C: CT corresponding to A: tubular, densely enhanced periportal collaterals (*arrows*). D and E: CT scans corresponding to B: Densely enhanced thickened gallbladder "wall." Some of the enhancement (*arrows*) is due to pericholecystic collateral veins. F and G: Cavernous transformation of the portal vein in a child. Transverse (F) and parasagittal (G) scans show tubular, serpiginous peripancreatic collaterals (*arrowheads*) extending up into the portal hepatis. (Case courtesy of William Scheible, M.D., University of California, San Diego.)

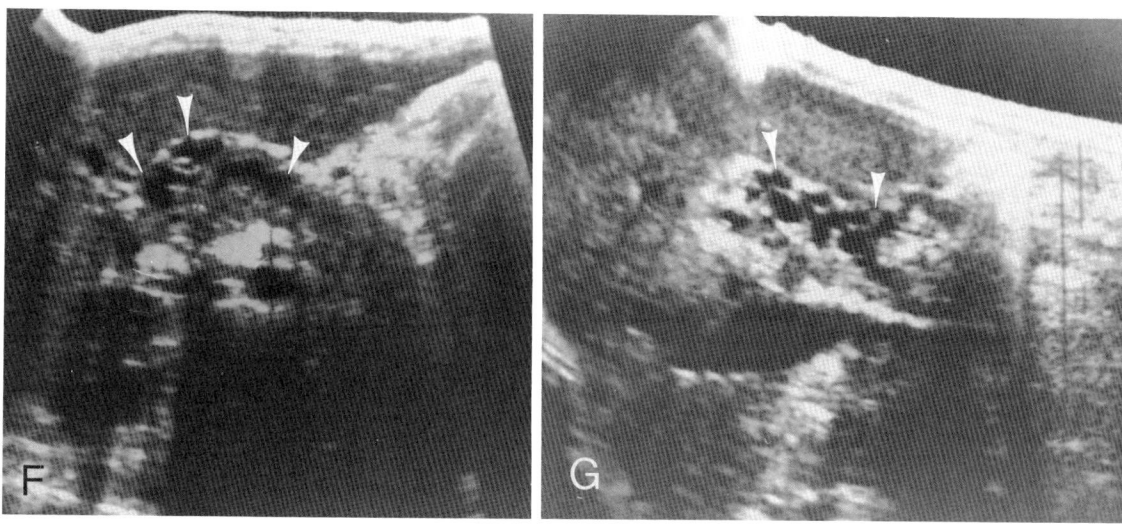

FIGURE 4.25F and G

portal venous system demonstrates continuous flow with little or no cardiac or respiratory variation compared to the systemic circulation.

Contrast-enhanced CT will show portal venous thrombosis as a low density center surrounded by an enhanced periphery. Some controversy exists as to whether the peripheral enhancement is flow around clot or enhancement of the wall due to the vasa venorum. Conceivably either can occur. When the vein is both occluded and enlarged, either by sonography or CT, the chances are great that there is tumor thrombus present. Hepatocellular carcinoma, cholangiocarcinoma, pancreatic carcinoma, and gastric carcinoma are the common offenders. The correlate to the angiographic "thread and streaks" sign of tumor thrombosis on ultrasound is the presence of numerous small lucencies within the echogenic clot. The corresponding CT finding is streaky contrast enhancement of the clot. An indirect CT sign of portal venous obstruction is lobar hypodensity on either noncontrast scans or CT scans after a contrast infusion into the superior mesenteric artery (CT portography). The former is probably from fatty infiltration due to ischemia, whereas the latter is analogous to a perfusion defect on pulmonary scintigraphy. Another indirect CT sign of portal occlusion is arterioportal shunting on dynamic CT in which opacification of the involved portal branch occurs prematurely in the arterial phase (simultaneously with aortic opacification) (9, 10). A more detailed description of CT and sonography of portal vein involvement by neoplasm can be found in the section on hepatocellular carcinoma.

Patients with presinusoidal portal vein obstruction have no increased resistance to hepatic venous outflow. Some portal collateral flow occurs, but most of the blood supply to the liver must come from the hepatic artery. The liver tends to be small in size and portasystemic collaterals develop (11). Celiac arteriography will show dilatation of the hepatic artery and its branches and sometimes a small liver. The splenic artery will be enlarged if there is splenomegaly. If the thrombosis is due to hypervascular tumor such as hepatocellular carcinoma, streaky enhancement of the tumor thrombus can be seen, the "thread and streaks" sign (12). Collaterals of the coronary and inferior mesenteric veins are seen in the venous phase. The venous phase of a superior mesenteric injection is best in demonstrating portal-portal collaterals through the head of the pancreas, gallbladder, and common bile duct to the intrahepatic portal vein branches (cavernous transformation) (Fig. 4.26). Transhepatic portography or splenoportography may be necessary to actually depict the occlusion (Figs. 4.27 and 4.28).

Intrahepatic causes of presinusoidal hypertension include schistosomiasis, hepatoportal fibrosis, partial nodular transformation of the liver, sarcoidosis, and fibrosis due to vinyl chloride exposure, Thorotrast, viral hepatitis, congenital hepatic fibrosis, and the precirrhotic stages of biliary cirrhosis. Hepatoportal fibrosis and partial nodular transformation will be discussed here as the other entities are discussed elsewhere in this book.

Hepatoportal fibrosis or sclerosis refers to intrahepatic portal vein obstruction in the absence of cirrhosis or other known specific causes of portal vein obstruction (Fig. 4.29) (13). The ter-

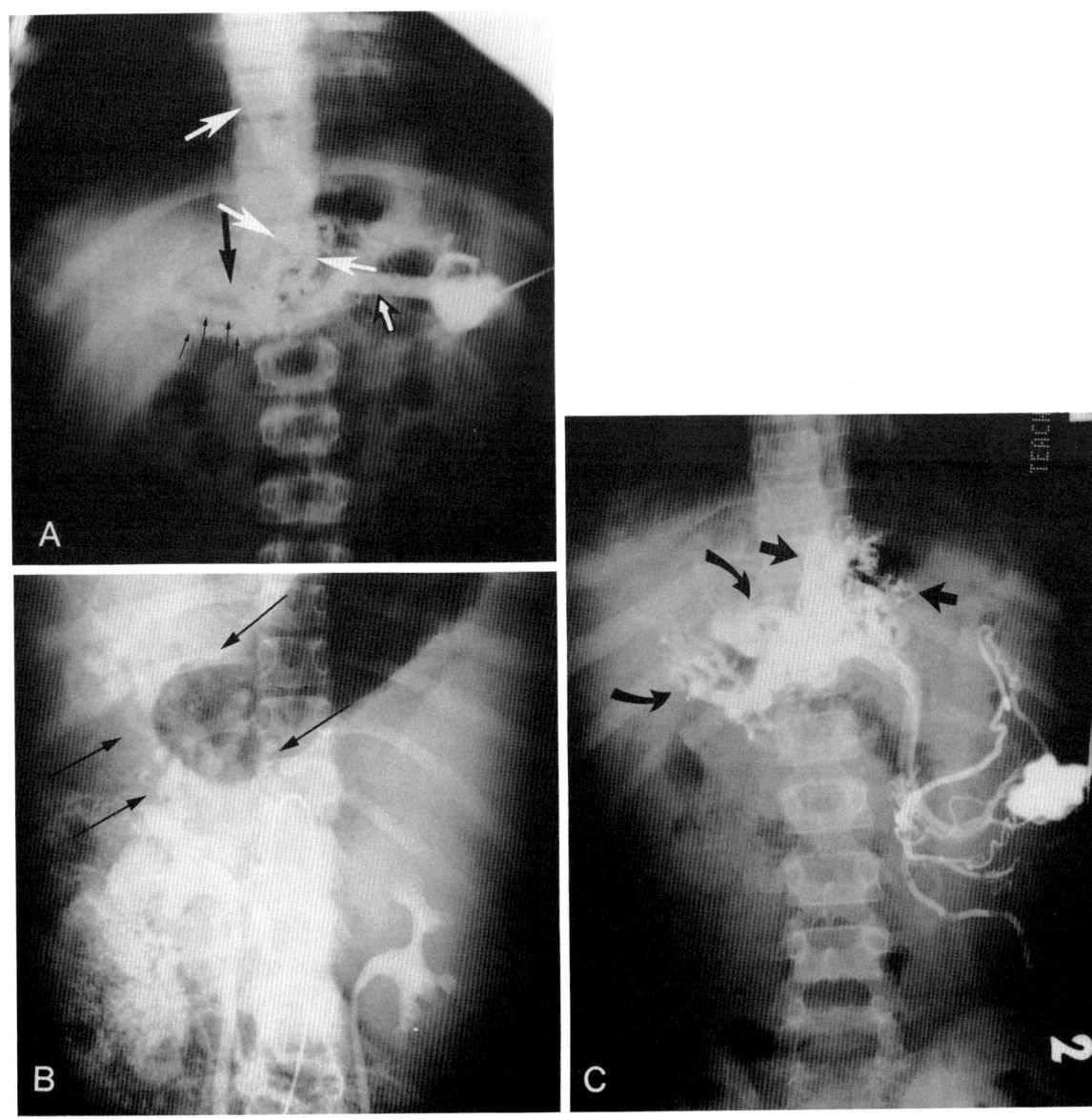

FIGURE 4.26. ANGIOGRAPHY OF CAVERNOUS TRANSFORMATION OF THE PORTAL VEIN

A: Cavernous transformation of the portal vein in a child, splenoportogram: bridging collaterals (*black arrows*), varices (*white arrows*) and splenic vein (*white on black arrow*). *B:* Venous phase of a superior mesenteric injection in another child with cavernous transformation of the portal vein: multiple periportal serpiginous collaterals (*arrows*) and splenomegaly. *C:* A 9-yr-old with unexplained splenomegaly since infancy. Splenoportogram: anastomotic vessels to the abdominal wall, gastroesophageal varices (*straight arrows*) and cavernous transformation of the portal vein (*curved arrows*).

minology in the literature is confusing with the entity being referred to as: idiopathic portal hypertension, primary portal hypertension, noncirrhotic intrahepatic portal hypertension, noncirrhotic portal fibrosis, intrahepatic portal hypertension, and obliterative portal venopathy. The extent of portal fibrosis is variable, although usually minor. The etiology of the intrahepatic portal vein phlebitis and sclerosis is thought to be previous intraabdominal infection. Arterial portography or direct portography usually shows abrupt obstructions in the intrahepatic portal veins (14).

A similar group of patients has been described in which the sites of occlusion are the very small, distal intrahepatic portal vein branches. Portal fibrosis may be present but in a pattern different from and not suggestive of congenital hepatic

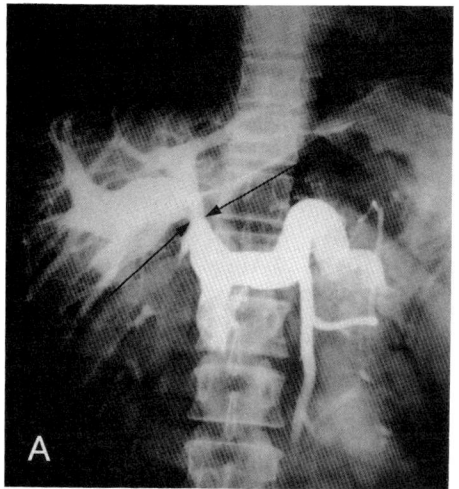
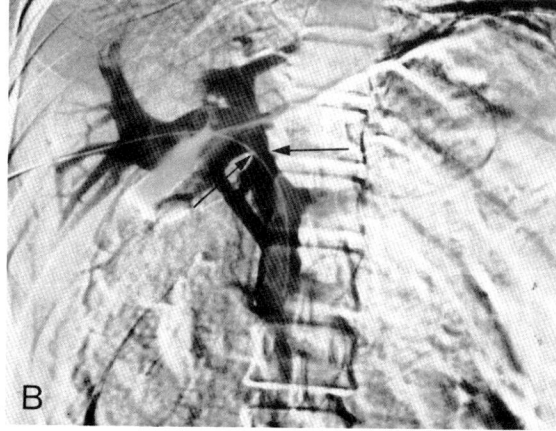

FIGURE 4.27. TRANSHEPATIC PORTOGRAM SHOWING A PORTAL VEIN WEB, AN EXTREMELY UNUSUAL CAUSE OF PORTAL HYPERTENSION
A: Portal system is dilated proximal to the web (*arrows*). B: Guidewire traversing the web (*arrows*) which was perforate prior to angioplasty. (Case courtesy of Michael Huggins, M.D., Brooke Army Medical Center, San Antonio, Texas.)

fibrosis. Extrahepatic portal veins are patent and portal pressure is elevated with a gradient between it and the wedge hepatic vein pressure (Fig. 4.29). Free hepatic venograms in these patients show narrow angles between the large veins and their tributaries, the "weeping willow" appearance. This is in contrast to the wide angles seen in cirrhotics (15). This group of patients may not, in fact, be considered anything more than a subset of patients with hepatoportal fibrosis diagnosed at an earlier stage.

Partial nodular transformation of the liver is a disease of adults that presents with portal hypertension, splenomegaly, and bleeding varices (16). Biopsy of the liver shows nodular transformation of the liver parenchyma with scant fibrosis without cirrhosis or inflammation. Angiographic findings include portal vein pressure elevation with patency but a grossly abnormal intrahepatic portal vein architecture due to distortion and stretching by the liver nodules. Overall liver size is usually within normal limits.

Finally, a rare but surgically correctible cause of presinusoidal portal hypertension is increased flow due to arteriovenous fistulas between mesenteric or hepatic arteries and the major tributaries of the portal vein or the portal vein itself (17). Underlying etiologies include hepatic or abdominal trauma, surgery such as gastrectomy (Fig. 4.30) or bowel resection, percutaneous liver biopsy, rupture of a visceral artery aneurysm into the portal venous system, or arteriovenous shunting due to a hypervascular tumor in the mesentery (Fig. 4.31). Patients can present either with variceal bleeding or generalized nonspecific complaints such as weight loss and malaise. An epigastric or periumbilical bruit may be present. Cross-sectional imaging studies may suggest the correct diagnosis, but visceral angiography is definitive, and can be therapeutic if the fistula can be embolized.

Postsinusoidal Portal Hypertension

Extrahepatic postsinusoidal portal hypertension is caused by such entities as prolonged tricuspid incompetence, chronic congestive heart failure, constrictive pericarditis (Fig. 4.32), as well as thrombosis of the posthepatic portion of the inferior vena cava and/or hepatic veins (Budd-Chiari syndrome). The latter is of major interest to radiologists and will be discussed in detail.

Budd-Chiari Syndrome

This rare syndrome, resulting from obstruction to hepatic venous drainage, was first described by Budd in 1845 and then further elucidated by Chiari in 1899 (18). Although the majority of cases are idiopathic, many underlying conditions can cause the syndrome: hypercoagulable states, especially polycythemia vera and oral contraceptive use; neoplasms of the liver, kidneys, adrenals, and inferior vena cava; trauma; pregnancy; and fibrous webs or membranes of the inferior vena cava and/or hepatic veins (18, 19). Progressive thrombotic occlusion of small centrilobular veins occurs more frequently in the West Indies and Middle East than elsewhere and is associated with consumption of herbal teas containing senecio (bush tea) (19). A pseudo–Budd-Chiari syndrome in which an en-

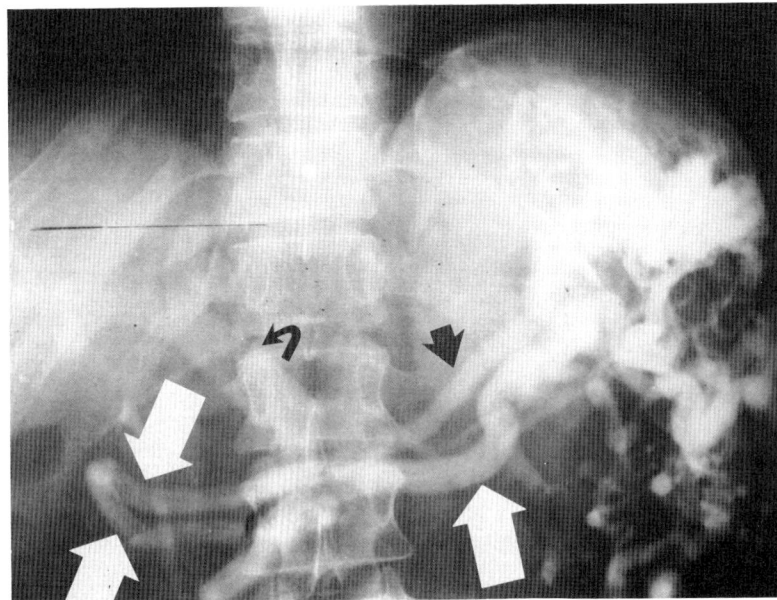

FIGURE 4.28. SPLENIC VEIN OBSTRUCTION PRESENTING WITH VARICEAL BLEEDING
Splenoportography in this patient with a proximal splenic vein occlusion shows large perisplenic varices and reconstitution of the portal vein (*curved arrow*) by meandering collaterals (*arrows*). Arterial portography was inconclusive.

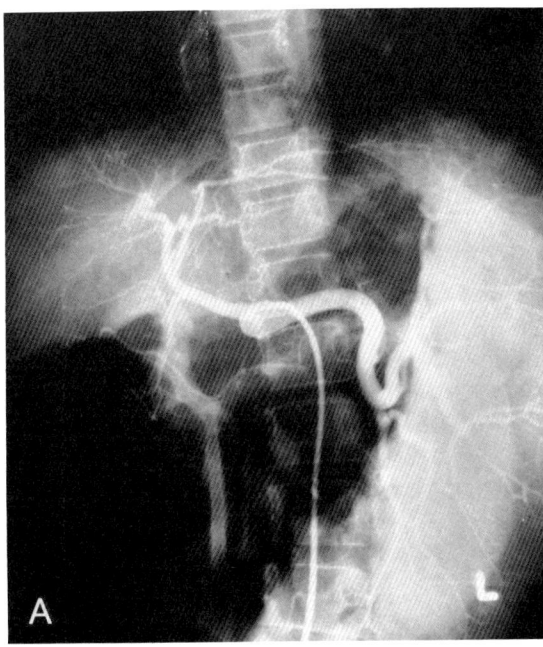
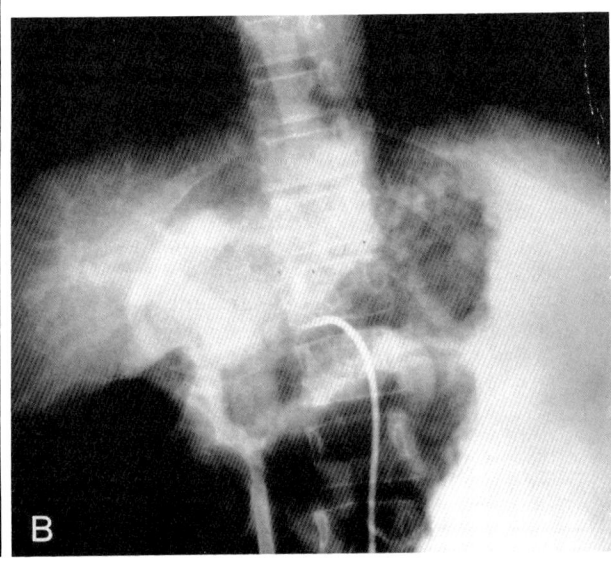

FIGURE 4.29. POSSIBLE HEPATOPORTAL FIBROSIS
An 11-yr-old boy with splenomegaly, leukopenia, thrombocytopenia, and anemia. UGI: varices. *A:* Celiac arteriogram shows a large spleen and a small hepatic artery with small branches. *B:* The portal venous phase shows a patent portal vein and normal branches. Liver biopsy showed minimal portal tract fibrosis with patent portal venules. A major differential consideration is congenital hepatic fibrosis. If variceal bleeding becomes a problem, response to splenorenal shunting is usually good.

larged left lobe impedes hepatic venous outflow has been described (18).

Clinical

Patients usually experience an insidious onset of nonspecific symptoms followed by abdominal pain (secondary to liver capsule distention), hepatomegaly, and ascites. Liver function tests are usually abnormal but quite nonspecific. The most common misdiagnosis is cirrhosis with portal hypertension, and congestive heart failure with hepatic congestion can cause a similar pic-

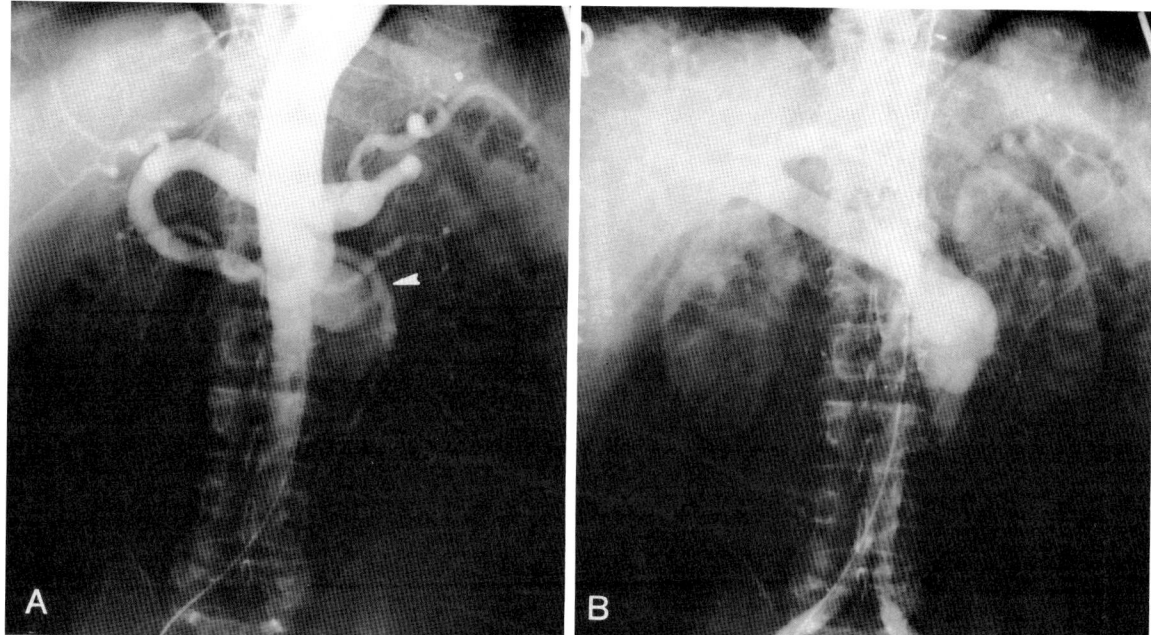

FIGURE 4.30. EXTRAHEPATIC ARTERIOVENOUS FISTULA

Extrahepatic arteriovenous fistula causing portal hypertension in a 62-yr-old man following partial gastrectomy. A: Aortogram shows greatly enlarged common hepatic and gastroduodenal arteries with rapid filling of a mesenteric vein. There is enlargement of the portal vein tributary at the site of the arteriovenous fistula which is displacing the superior mesenteric artery (*arrowhead*) to the left. B: Filling of the main portal vein and its intrahepatic branches is quite dramatic later in the arterial phase.

ture. Infrequently the disease is fulminant with a rapidly downhill, fatal course (18, 19).

Medical management consists of diuretics, salt restriction, and treatment of any underlying condition. Anticoagulants and systemic fibrinolytics have not been successful. A portoatrial shunt appears to provide effective treatment. Lysis of webs, either surgical or via angioplasty, is the treatment of choice in selected cases, as is liver transplantation (18, 19).

Pathology

The Budd-Chiari syndrome may be classified into three main groups based on the distribution of venous disease: (*a*) occlusion of the inferior vena cava with or without secondary occlusion of hepatic veins, (*b*) primary occlusion of the major hepatic veins, either right or left, or both, with or without occlusion of the inferior vena cava, and (*c*) veno-occlusive disease of the liver, a progressive thrombotic occlusion of small centrilobular veins.

Liver biopsy is usually non-specific, showing only hepatic congestion. In some cases the following constellation of highly suggestive findings have been reported: centrilobular congestion with dilated and empty central lobular and sublobular veins and compressed sinusoids containing few red cells. Towards the periphery of the lobules, the sinusoids are widely dilated and trabeculae packed with red cells are seen. This is thought to reflect a collateral circulation whereby blood leaves the central sinusoids and enters the space of Disse becoming intermingled with the cells of the liver plates (18).

Radiology

Nuclear Medicine

Hepatic scintigraphy may demonstrate a characteristic pattern in Budd-Chiari syndrome: a central region of normal activity (appearing hot) surrounded by the rest of the liver which has greatly diminished activity (Figs. 4.33A and 4.34E, F) (20–23). In addition, a colloid shift to an enlarged spleen and the bone marrow is usually present as well. The hot caudate lobe is posterior, an important differentiating point from the anterior hot spot that can be seen in superior vena cava occlusion. The characteristic pattern is seen only when the veins draining the caudate lobe (which enter separately into the inferior vena cava) are spared. When all hepatic veins are affected, nonspecific findings of hepa-

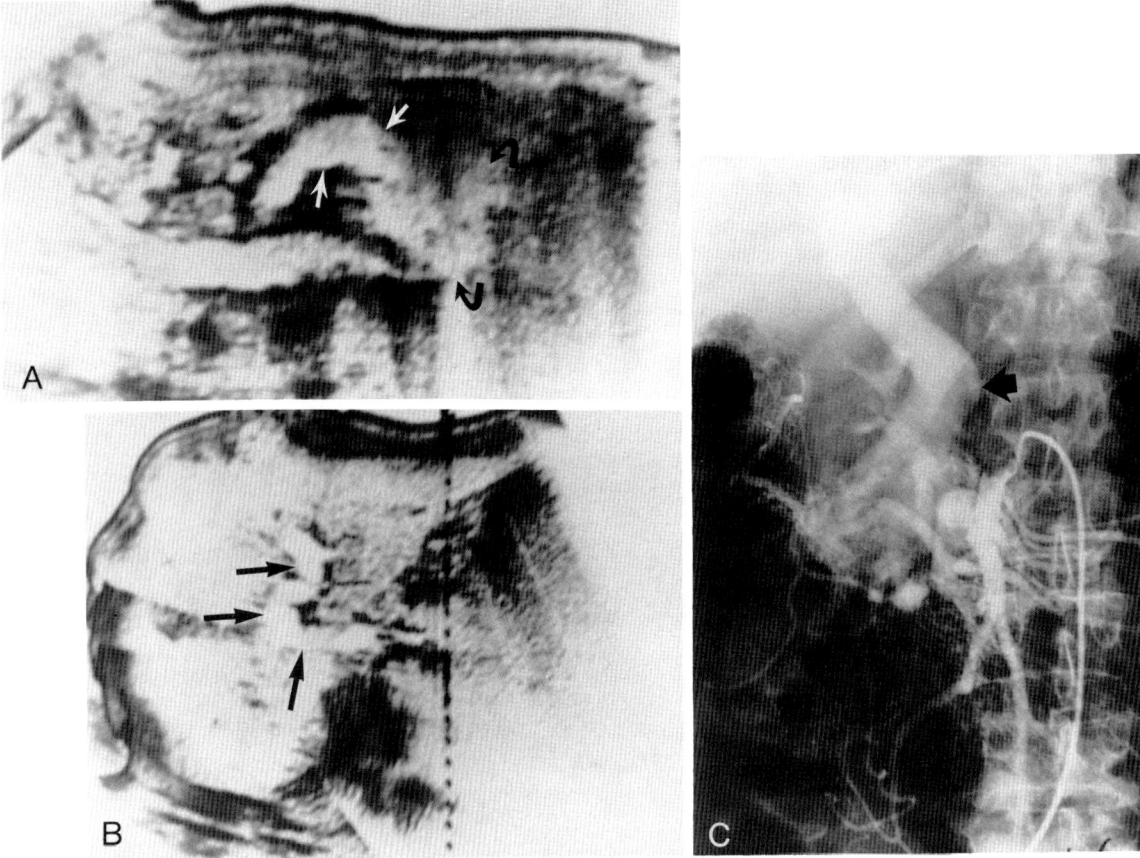

FIGURE 4.31. MESENTERIC SARCOMA CAUSING EXTRAHEPATIC ARTERIOPORTAL SHUNTING AND PORTAL HYPERTENSION
Elderly male presenting with anemia. UGI showed varices. *A* and *B:* Parasagittal and transverse sonograms show dilatation of the portal vein (*arrows*) and a mass that proved to be in the root of the mesentery (*curved arrows*). *C:* Superior mesenteric arteriogram shows tumor stain and rapid shunting into the portal vein (*arrow*).

tomegaly with patchy diminished uptake and colloid shift are seen (Fig. 4.35) (18, 19). Wedge-shaped focal peripheral defects suggesting infarcts may be present. Cases have been reported in which a nonspecific pattern is seen initially with progression over time to the hot caudate lobe configuration (24).

Sonography

In patients with hepatic veno-occlusive disease, if the main hepatic vein is uninvolved the only sonographic finding may be enlargement of the caudate lobe with atrophy of the remainder of the liver (25). Sometimes collateral veins from the obstructed segments to the relatively spared caudate lobe can be depicted by ultrasound as comma-shaped or curled-tubular lucencies (26). With thrombosis of one or more of the main hepatic veins, echogenic clot within their lumina may be seen (Fig. 4.33C, D), but sometimes the only findings are reduced size or nonvisualization of the hepatic veins (Fig. 4.36D) (18, 26–29). In patients with Budd-Chiari syndrome from tumor compression of the hepatic veins or inferior vena cava, the diagnosis can be suspected from the sonographic depiction of a mass compressing venous structures (22). However, sonography is not definitive in this situation because masses can compress veins without invading them or producing obstruction (1). When the etiology is membranous obstruction of the inferior vena cava, the cava appears to disappear either at an intrahepatic level or between the liver and the right atrium (1, 25). The web itself is not depicted. When the obstruction is intrahepatic, additional sonographic findings are communicating collateral veins between the right and/or middle hepatic veins and the inferior hepatic vein and enlarged inferior right hepatic veins. If the obstruction is suprahepatic, additional sonographic findings will be limited to depiction of portal and systemic collaterals with patent hepatic veins (1).

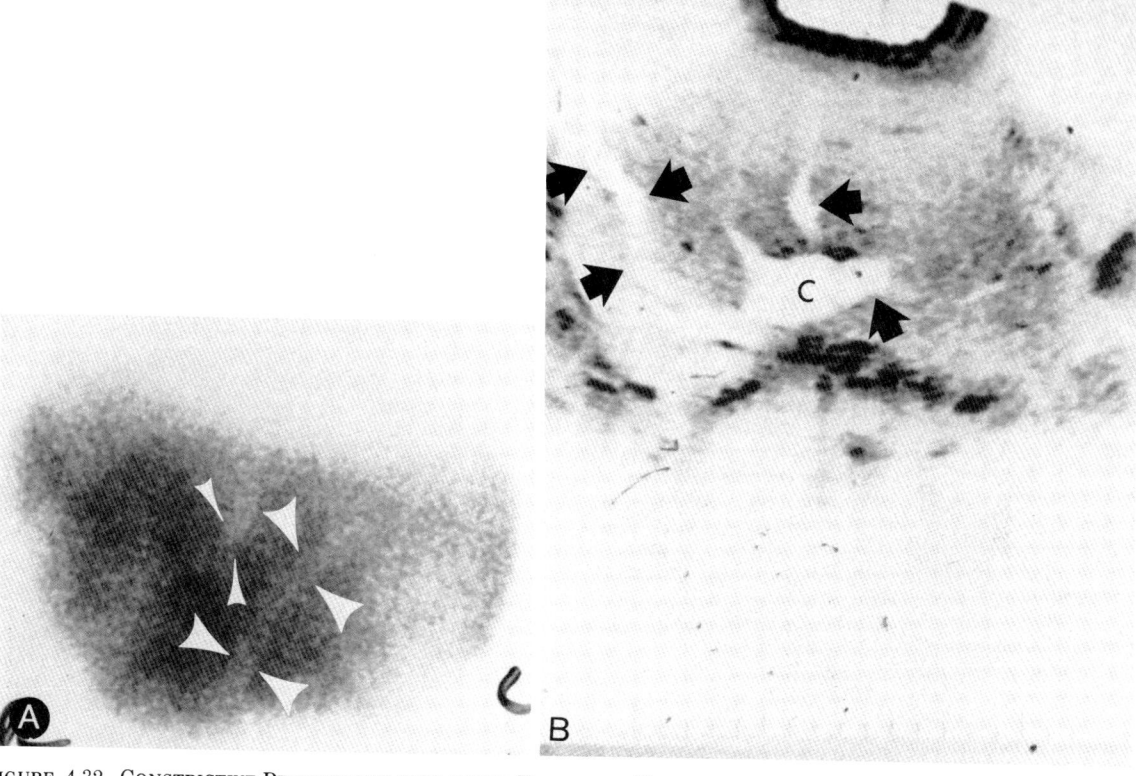

FIGURE 4.32. CONSTRICTIVE PERICARDITIS FOLLOWING TRAUMATIC HEMOPERICARDIUM CAUSING PORTAL HYPERTENSION
A: Sulfur colloid scan: multiple photopenic regions, several were tubular in at least one projection (*arrowheads*). *B:* Transverse sonogram: dilated hepatic veins (*arrows*) are responsible for most of the scintigraphic abnormalities. Their presence correctly suggests elevated right heart pressure. Other scans showed dilated portal veins as well. Note the hepatic venous confluence (*C*).

Computed Tomography

CT typically demonstrates caudate lobe enlargement with patchy enhancement of the rest of the liver and lack of visualization of the hepatic veins (26, 28, 30). Occasionally there is marked caudate lobe enhancement due to preferential flow from obstructed segments to the relatively unobstructed caudate (Figs. 4.34*B* and *C* and 4.36*A*) (28, 31). Frank infarcts can occur as large or small hypodense nonenhancing regions difficult to differentiate from tumors (Figs. 4.34*B–D* and 4.36*C*). With partial Budd-Chiari (obstruction of a single vein) the affected liver segment is hypodense simulating a mass lesion (30, 32). In patients with membranous inferior vena cava obstruction, CT can show narrowing or occlusion of the inferior vena cava above the web and sometimes thrombus below it (25). Enlarged retroperitoneal collaterals will also be seen (25, 33).

Angiography

If the correct diagnosis is not suspected prior to angiography, the first examination will be from the arterial side. Celiac and hepatic angiography reveal an enlarged, swollen liver and spleen with marked stretching and bowing of the hepatic arteries (Fig. 4.36*E*). The hepatogram is dense, prolonged and sometimes inhomogeneous (Fig. 4.36*F, G*). With chronic disease the hepatic arteries may dilate, and retrograde flow into the portal veins with portosystemic collaterals may occur. Arterial portography can demonstrate patency of the splenic and portal veins with sluggish and hepatofugal flow. This picture is nonspecific.

Characteristic findings occur during hepatic venography, which is done in conjunction with studies of the inferior vena cava and its junction with the right atrium (11, 18, 19). Cavography may demonstrate occlusion at the level of the

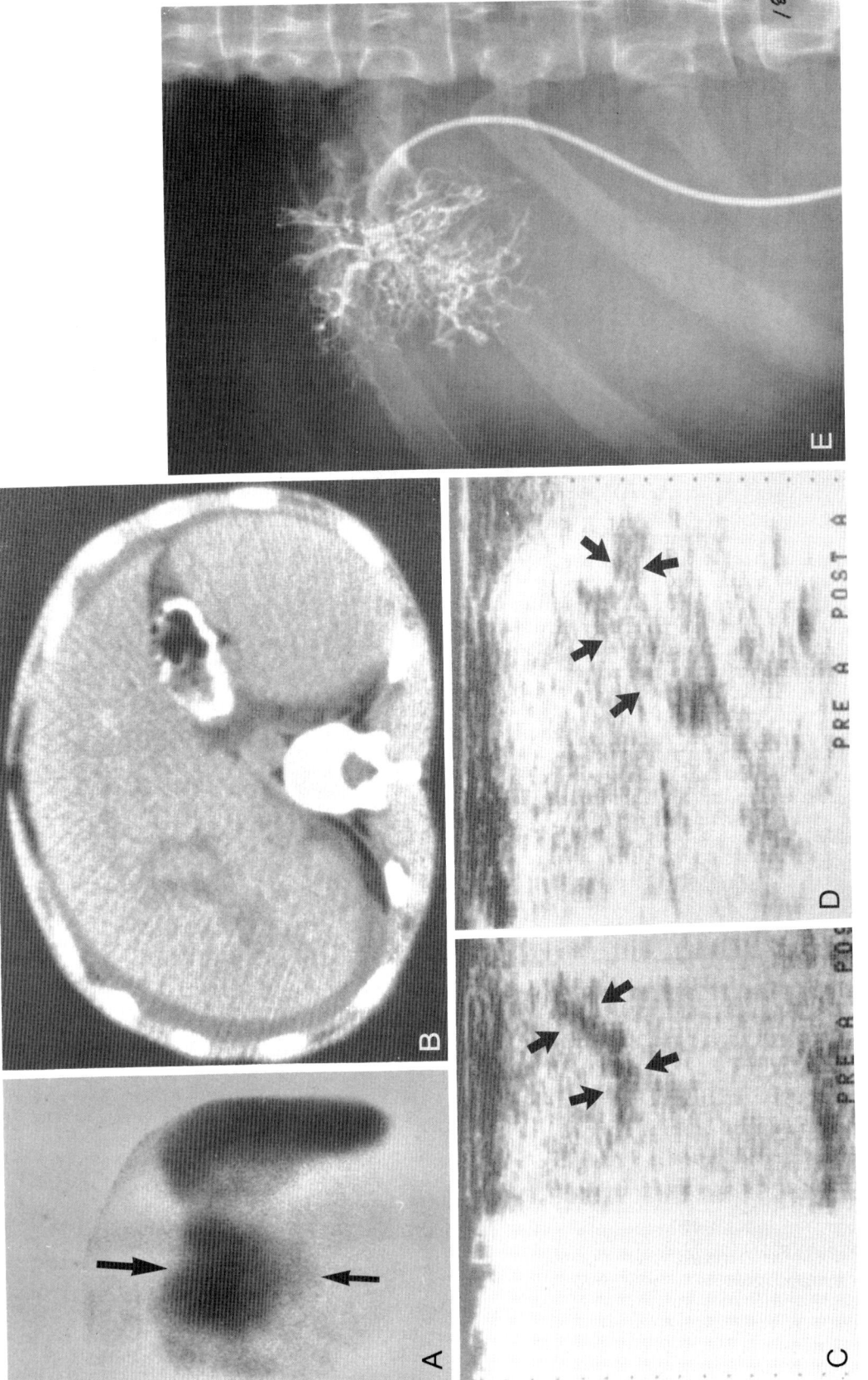

FIGURE 4.33. BUDD-CHIARI SYNDROME

Budd-Chiari syndrome in a 36-yr-old female patient with insidious onset of abdominal pain and increased girth. Hepatomegaly was present on physical examination. *A*: Sulfur colloid scan: hot, enlarged caudate lobe (*arrows*) with little activity in the rest of the liver. Splenomegaly with colloid shift to the spleen and bone marrow. *B*: CT scan: nonspecific hepatosplenomegaly and ascites. Later generation equipment and bolus contrast injection might have been more informative. *C* and *D*: Real-time sonography: branching echogenicities representing clot in hepatic veins (*arrows*) and inability to identify normal hepatic veins. *E*: Hepatic venogram: spiderweb network of collaterals.

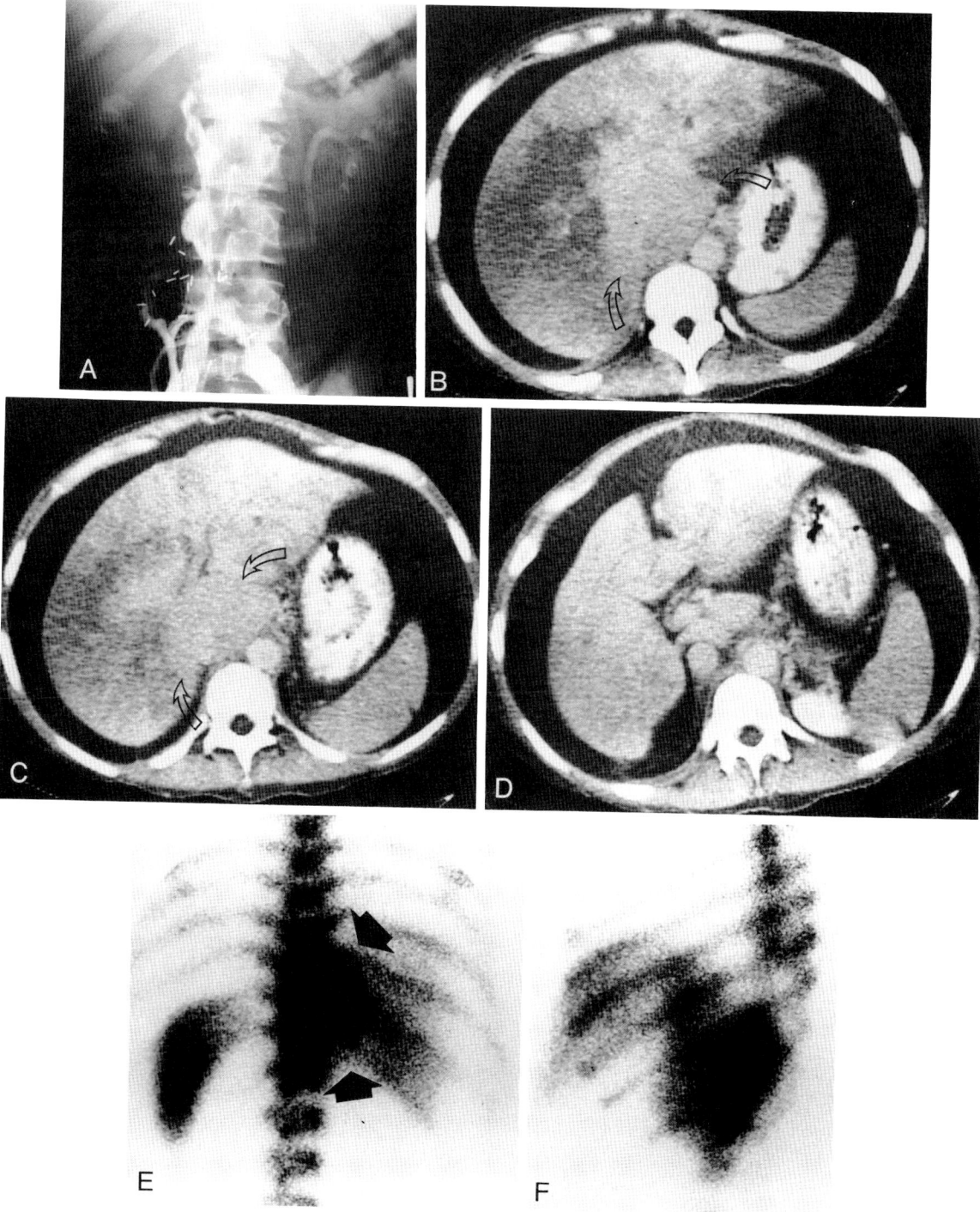

FIGURE 4.34. INFERIOR VENA CAVA THROMBOSIS PRESENTING AS BUDD-CHIARI SYNDROME

A: Cavogram: thrombi, attempted recanalization, and collateral flow. *B–D:* Hepatic contrast-enhanced CT: multiple peripheral regions of low attenuation consistent with infarction. Hypertrophied caudate lobe (*arrows*). Note massive ascites. *E:* Posterior sulfur colloid scan: liver and spleen displaced from abdominal wall by ascites. Colloid shift to spleen and marrow. Small liver with relatively increased uptake centrally (*arrows*). *F:* The left lateral view shows that the central increased hepatic uptake is posterior, corresponding to the caudate lobe.

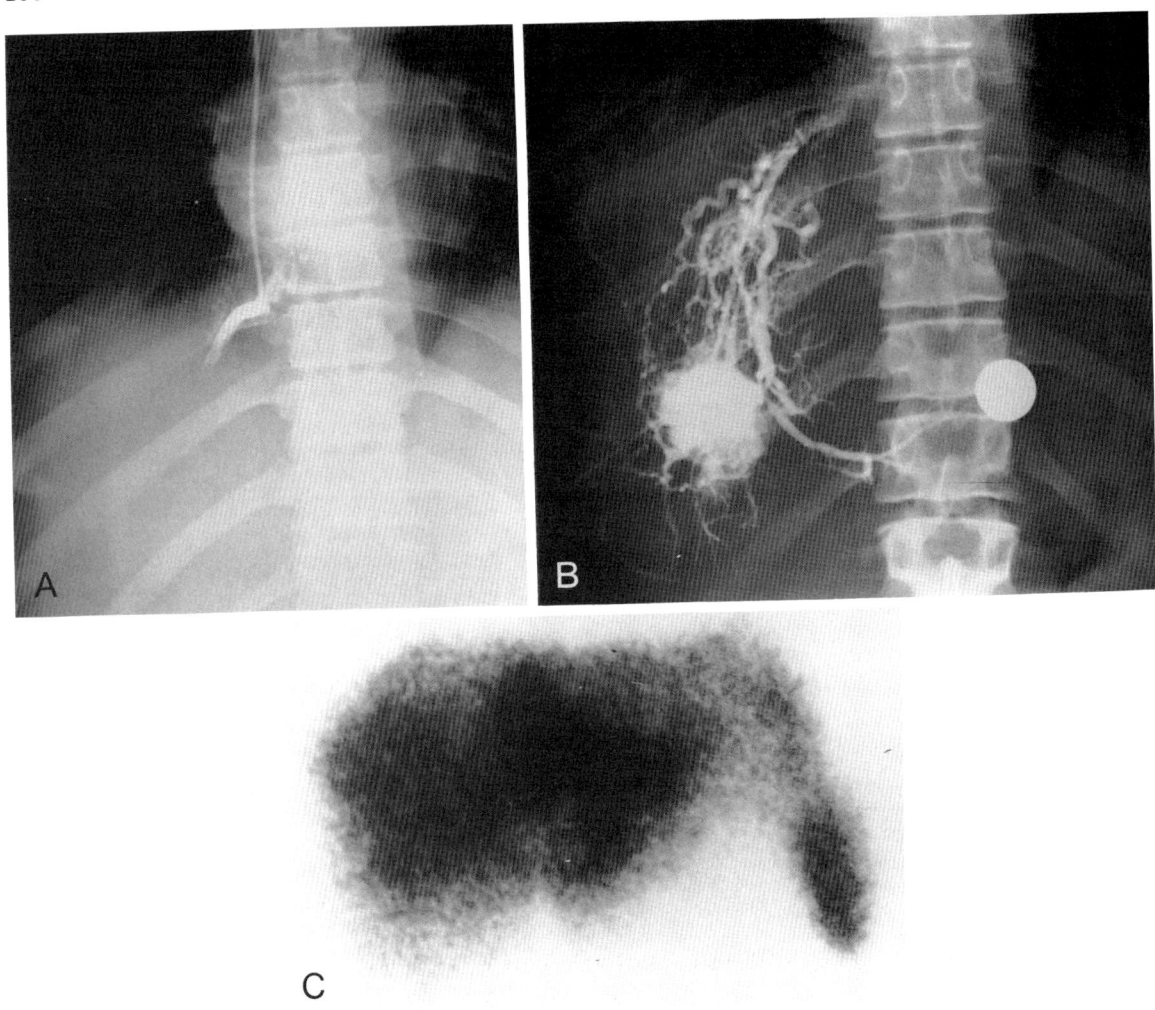

FIGURE 4.35. BUDD-CHIARI SYNDROME

A: Inferior vena cava not patent, hepatic vein catheterization from above showed occlusion. *B:* Percutaneous parenchymal injection opacifies a collateral venous network. *C:* Anterior sulfur colloid scan: patchy liver uptake. Central relatively hot region was not posterior on oblique views (not shown). Mild colloid shift (spleen is as hot as liver on anterior view).

renal or hepatic veins with tumor extension into the cava or impairment of flow due to compression by an extrinsic mass (which sometimes is the enlarged caudate lobe) (Fig. 4.34A). Caval webs studied from below are concave obstructions with small central openings. They are best demonstrated when the catheter is placed just below them because flow in the obstructed cava may be reversed. Study from above may be needed. If the cava is not occluded the hepatic veins must be selectively catheterized and wedged hepatic venography performed (Fig. 4.35A). This study will demonstrate a spiderweb network pattern of collateral veins and/or lymphatics with absence of sinusoidal filling (Figs. 4.33E and 4.36I). A coarse network of collateral veins flowing toward the entrances of the major hepatic veins into the inferior vena cava indicates anastomoses between hepatic and systemic veins along the surface of the liver. Narrowing of the hepatic veins near their ostia due to webs may be demonstrated by venography. If the cava is occluded, the hepatic veins may be studied from above via the right atrium. When the hepatic veins cannot be catheterized, cavography with Valsalva maneuver demonstrating no reflux into the hepatic veins gives a presumptive diagnosis of hepatic vein occlusion (Fig. 4.36H). Alternatively, a percutaneous transhepatic contrast injection into the hepatic parenchyma will fill collateral channels and demonstrate the spiderweb pattern (9) (Fig. 4.35B).

When thrombosis is limited to one or more lobar hepatic veins arteriography can be quite

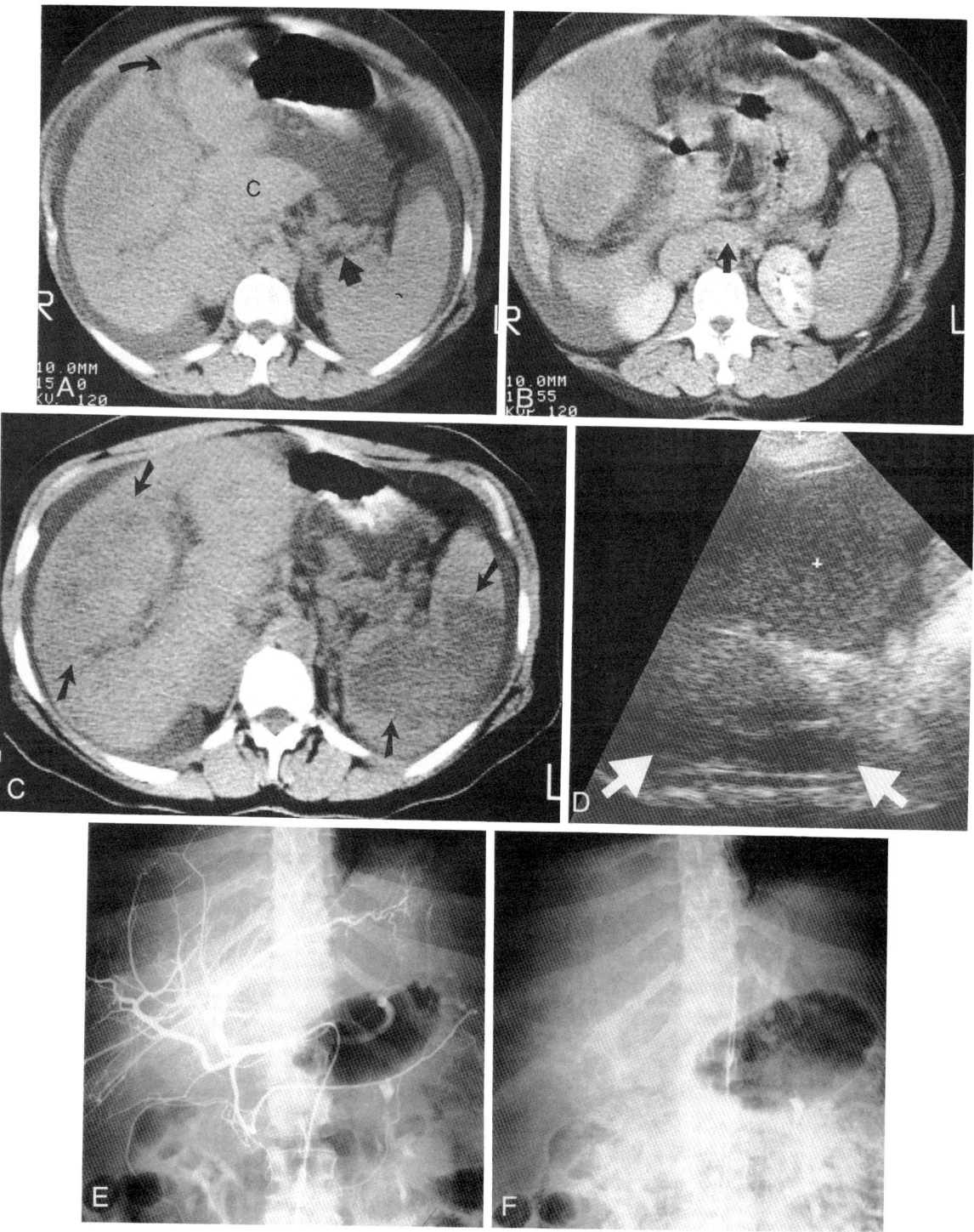

FIGURE 4.36. YOUNG WOMAN WITH BUDD-CHIARI DUE TO POLYCYTHEMIA VERA

A and *B:* CT shows ascites, splenomegaly, prominent fissures, caudate enlargement (*c*), a spontaneous splenorenal shunt (perisplenic varices that could be followed to the dilated left renal vein (*arrows*), and a recanalized umbilical vein (*curved arrow*). *C:* Repeat CT six months later: low density hepatic and splenic infarcts (*arrows*). *D:* Parasagittal sonogram: no hepatic veins entering the inferior vena cava (*arrows*). *E:* Selective hepatic arteriogram: stretched arteries with some curvilinear displacement. No neovascularity or encasement. *F* and *G:* Late films from the selective hepatic (*F*) and a superior mesenteric injection *(G):* prolonged hepatogram and persistent opacification of bizarre venous structures. *H:* Inferior vena cavogram with Valsalva: no reflux into hepatic veins. *I:* Hepatic venogram: spider web collaterals.

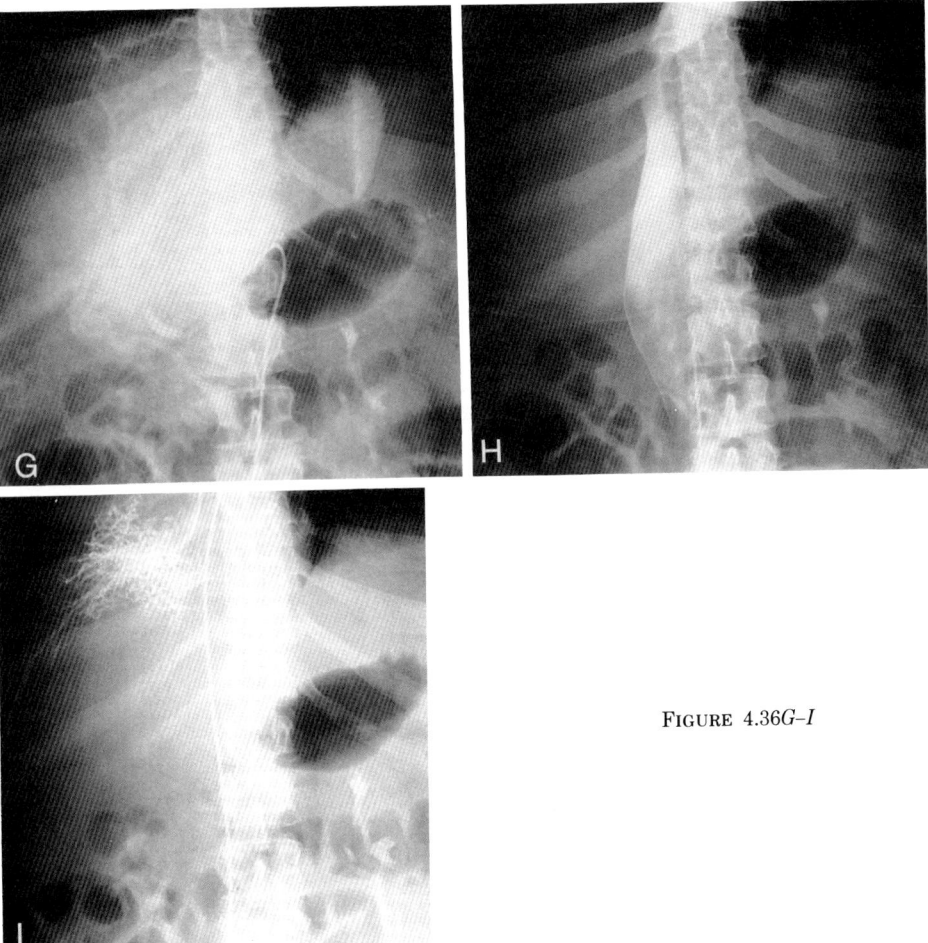

FIGURE 4.36G–I

confusing (Fig. 4.37) (34, 35). In this condition (partial Budd-Chiari) blood is diverted from the obstructed lobe (or lobes) which atrophies to other lobes which hypertrophy. The vessels in the obstructed lobe (or lobes) are crowded and constricted, whereas they are displaced and stretched elsewhere. Retrograde portal flow and sinusoidal puddling can occur in the venooccluded lobe. The arteriographic appearance of a shrunken lobe next to an enlarged hyperperfused lobe with stretched vessels together with arterioportal flow is easily misinterpreted as hepatocellular carcinoma in the normal hyperperfused lobe superimposed upon a cirrhotic liver (veno-occluded shrunken lobe(s)). Hepatic venography will demonstrate collaterals from the occluded lobe to the rest of the liver and will be diagnostic.

Angioplasty and Membranes

Congenital membranes or webs are a rare cause of obstruction of the inferior vena cava and major hepatic veins, but they are a common cause of Budd-Chiari syndrome and portal hypertension in Japan (19, 36). Caval membranes are usually directly above the entrance of the right hepatic vein and below the diaphragm and usually below the entrance of the left hepatic vein. The latter may be partially or completely occluded with an old thrombus or have a small ostium or a web. Solitary hepatic vein webs do not occur without inferior vena cava webs (36). Caval membranes are considered to be congenital and may result from an abnormal extension of the perinatal obliterative process that causes closure of the ductus venosus. They are valve-like and usually <5 mm thick and histologically similar to the wall of the inferior vena cava. Occasionally the obstruction in the inferior vena cava is segmental rather than membranous (37). It is therefore important to opacify both sides of the web to evaluate its thickness and search for the presence of any associated thrombus. A jet of contrast material will be seen in those cases in which a perforation is present.

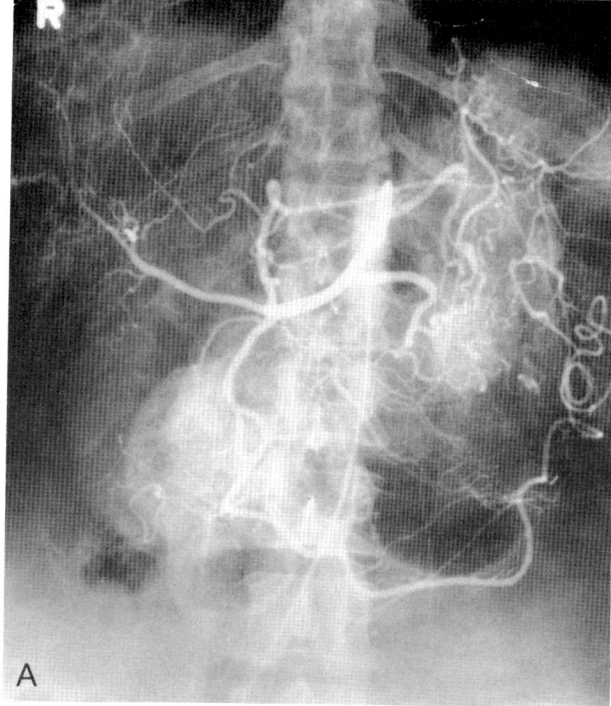
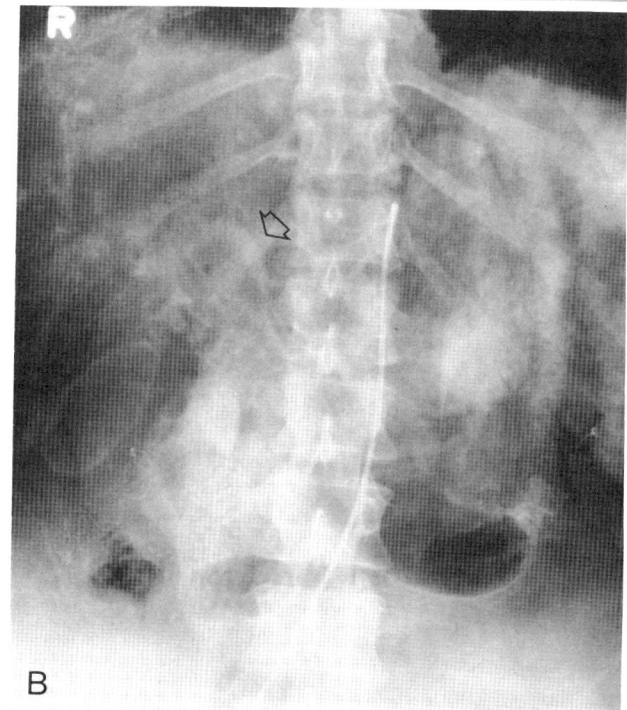
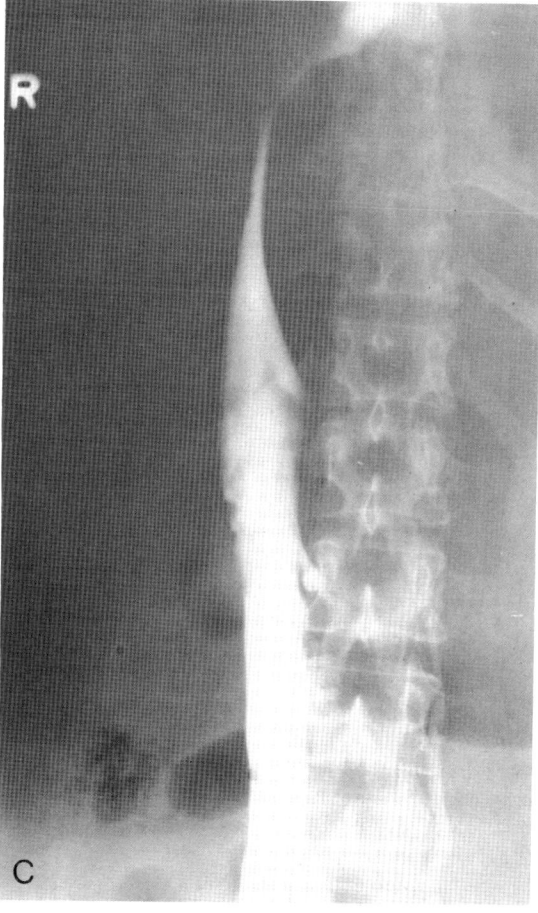

FIGURE 4.37. PARTIAL BUDD-CHIARI–RIGHT HEPATIC VEIN THROMBOSIS WITH ATROPHY OF THE RIGHT LOBE AND HYPERTROPHY OF THE LEFT LOBE
A: Celiac angiogram: crowded, corkscrewed arteries in the right lobe, enlargement of the left hepatic artery with stretching and displacement of its branches. *B:* Persistent opacification of venous structures (*arrow*) on a capillary phase film. *C:* Inferior vena cavogram: compression of the intrahepatic portion of the cava by an enlarged left lobe. Hepatic veins could not be entered.

Current treatment of choice for both caval webs and segmental obstruction is Gruntzig balloon angioplasty (36–38). Formerly most cases were treated with thoraco-abdominal surgery with mixed results although some were treated with finger fracture via the right atrium or Fogarty balloon rupture via the saphenous vein (36).

The majority of membranes or webs in the hepatic veins and their branches are probably acquired and may be the residual of thrombophlebitis or some other inflammatory disease.

They are multiple, involve smaller branches, and are not amenable to surgery (19). Angioplasty may have a role to play in this condition because successful dilatation of one major vein with restoration of patency can be therapeutic in terms of Budd-Chiari syndrome even when all three are initially occluded (38). Thrombolytic therapy with streptokinase or urokinase may also be helpful (39).

REFERENCES

1. Hill MC, Sanders RC: Sonography of the upper abdominal venous system. In Sanders RC, Hill MC (eds): *Ultrasound Annual 1983*. New York, Raven Press, 1983, pp 271–313.
2. Baker SR, Broker MH, Charnsangavej C, Sitron AP: Calcification in the portal vein wall. *Radiology* 152:18, 1984.
3. Haddow RA, Kemp-Harper RA: Calcification in the liver and portal system. *Clin Radiol* 18:225, 1967.
4. Webb LJ, Berger LA, Sherlock S: Gray-scale ultrasonography of the portal vein. *Lancet* 2:675–677, 1977.
5. Marx M, Scheible W: Cavernous transformation of the portal vein. *J Ultrasound Med* 1:167–169, 1982.
6. Kauzlaric D, Petrovic M, Barnier E: Sonography of cavernous transformation of the portal vein. *AJR* 142:383–384, 1984.
7. Van Gansbeke D, Avni EF, Delcour C, Engelholm L, Struyven J: Sonographic features of portal vein thrombosis. *AJR* 144:749–752, 1985.
8. Weltin G, Taylor KJW, Carter AR, Taylor CR: Duplex Doppler: identification of cavernous transformation of the portal vein. *AJR* 144:999–1001, 1985.
9. Mathieu D, Grenier P, Larde D, Vasile N: Portal vein involvement in hepatocellular carcinoma: dynamic CT features. *Radiology* 152:127–132, 1984.
10. Matsui O, Takashima T, Kadoya M, Kitagawa K, Kamimura R, Itoh H, Suzaki M, Ida M: Segmental staining on hepatic arteriography as a sign of intrahepatic portal vein obstruction. *Radiology* 152:601–606, 1981.
11. Reuter SR, Redman HC: *Gastrointestinal Angiography*. Philadelphia, W. B. Saunders, 1977, pp 340–345.
12. Okuda K, Musha H, Yoshida T et al: Demonstration of growing casts of hepatocellular carcinoma in the portal vein by celiac angiography: the thread and streaks sign. *Radiology* 117:303, 1975.
13. Clemett AR: Roentgenology of the liver and bile ducts. In Margulis AR, Burhenne HJ (eds): *Alimentary Tract Roentgenology*. St Louis, C. V. Mosby, 1973, pp 1230–1258.
14. Talner LB, Boyer JL, Clemett AR: Intrahepatic portal vein occlusion: a cause of portal hypertension. *Radiology* 92:1265–1270, 1969.
15. Futagawa S, Fukazawa M, Musha H, Isomatsa T, Koyama K, Ito T, Horisawa M, Makayama S, Sugiura M, Kameda H, Okuda K: Hepatic venography in non-cirrhotic idiopathic portal hypertension. *Radiology* 141:303–309, 1981.
16. Sherlock S, Feldman CA, Moran B, Scheuer PJ: Partial nodular transformation of the liver with portal hypertension. *Am J Med* 40:195–203, 1966.
17. Rossi P, Carillo FJ, Alfidi RJ, Ruzicka FF Jr: Iatrogenic arteriovenous fistulas. *Radiology* 111:47–51, 1974.
18. Floyd JL: The radiographic gamut of Budd-Chiari syndrome. *Am J Gastroenterol* 76:381–387, 1981.
19. Tisnado J, Cho S-R, Carithers RL Jr., Goldschmidt RA, Vines FS, Amendola M: The Budd-Chiari syndrome: angiographic pathologic correlation. *Radiographics* 3:155–180, 1983.
20. Thijs LG, Heidendal GAK, Huijgens PC et al: The use of nuclear medicine procedures in the diagnosis of Budd-Chiari syndrome. *Clin Nucl Med* 3:389–392, 1978.
21. Tavill AS, Wood EJ, Kreel MSL: The Budd-Chiari syndrome: correlation between hepatic scintigraphy and the clinical, radiological, and pathological findings in 19 cases of hepatic venous outflow obstruction. *Gastroenterology* 68:509, 1975.
22. Meindols H, Langer B: Liver scan in Budd-Chiari syndrome. *J Nucl Med* 17:365, 1976.
23. Stadalnik RC: "Hot spots" in liver imaging. *Semin Nucl Med* 9:220–221, 1979.
24. Lisbona R, Katz S, Mishkin S: Serial radionuclide liver imaging in Budd-Chiari syndrome. *J Can Assoc Radiol* 32:175–177, 1981.
25. Makuuchi M, Hasegawa H, Yamazaki S, Moriyama N, Takayasu K, Okazaki M: Primary Budd-Chiari syndrome: ultrasonic demonstration. *Radiology* 152:775–779, 1984.
26. Harter LP, Gross BH, St. Hilaire J, Filly RA, Goldberg HI: CT and sonographic appearance of hepatic vein obstruction. *AJR* 139:176–178, 1982.
27. Blickman JG, McArdle CR: Budd-Chiari syndrome. *J Comput Assist Tomogr* 5:409–410, 1981.
28. Yang PJ, Glazer GM, Bowerman RA: Budd-Chiari syndrome: computed tomographic and ultrasonographic findings. *J Comput Assist Tomogr* 7:148–150, 1983.
29. Weill FS, Le Mouel A, Bihr E, Rohmer P, Zeltner F, Perrisney G: Ultrasonic patterns of acquired Budd-Chiari's syndrome. *Europ J Radiol* 1:236–237, 1981.
30. Rossi P, Sposito M, Simonetti G, Sposato S, Cusumano G: CT diagnosis of Budd-Chiari syndrome. *J Comput Assist Tomogr* 5:366–369, 1981.
31. Cho KJ, Geisinger KR, Shields JJ, Forrest ME: Collateral channels and histopathology in hepatic vein occlusion. *AJR* 139:703–709, 1982.
32. Nakamura H, Tanaka T, Hori S, Yoshioka H, Kuroda C: Partial Budd-Chiari syndrome. *J Comput Assist Tomogr* 6:833–835, 1982.
33. Baert AL, Fevery J, Marchal G, Goddeeris P, Wilms G, Ponette E, De Groote J: Early diagnosis of Budd-Chiari syndrome by computed tomography and ultrasonography: report of five cases. *Gastroenterology* 84:587–595, 1983.
34. Galloway S, Casarella WJ, Price JB: Unilobar veno-occlusive disease of the liver. *AJR* 119:89–94, 1973.
35. Maguire R, Doppman J: Angiographic abnormalities in partial Budd-Chiari syndrome. *Radiology* 122:629–635, 1977.
36. Meier WL III, Waller RM III, Sones PJ Jr: Budd-Chiari web treated by percutaneous transluminal angioplasty. *AJR* 137:1257–1258, 1981.
37. Yamada R, Sato M, Kawabata M, Nakasuka H, Nkamura K, Nobuyuki K: Segmental obstruction of the hepatic inferior vena cava treated by transluminal angioplasty. *Radiology* 149:91–96, 1983.
38. Uflacker R, Francisconi CF, Rodriguez MP, Amaral NM: Percutaneous transluminal angioplasty of the hepatic veins for treatment of Budd-Chiari syndrome. *Radiology* 153:641–642, 1984.
39. Greenwood LH, Yrizarry JM, Hallett JR Jr, Scoville GS Jr: Urokinase treatment of Budd-Chiari syndrome. *AJR* 141:1057–1059, 1983.

OTHER DIFFUSE DISEASES

Although diverse in nature, the liver diseases discussed below all have in common hepatomegaly, hepatocellular dysfunction, and the potential for scarring and portal hypertension.

Fatty Liver

While fatty liver (fatty infiltration of the liver, hepatic steatosis) has been associated with a variety of clinical disorders (Table 4.3), alcoholic liver disease is the most common cause in North America (1–3). Fatty liver is not only the most frequent abnormality discovered on liver biopsy in alcoholic patients, but also occurs in over 50% of alcoholic patients in whom there is no clinical or laboratory evidence of liver disease (3). Fatty liver seems to be prevalent in the nonalcoholic population as well. Fatty change has been noted in up to 50% of adult patients with diabetes mellitus (2). Further, a recent epidemiological study reported histological evidence of fatty liver at autopsy in 25% of a nonalcoholic previously healthy adult male population meeting accidental death (4).

Pathogenesis

Fatty liver is defined as an excessive accumulation of triglyceride, appearing as small or large vacuoles, within the cytoplasm of hepatocytes. Triglycerides, fatty acids, phospholipids, cholesterol, and cholesterol esters comprise about 5% of the weight of a normal liver; severe fatty liver may produce a liver nearly 40–50% triglyceride by weight (1, 2).

Fatty liver represents either a nonspecific response to hepatocyte injury or one facet of a more generalized metabolic derangement (2). The hepatocyte plays a central role in the metabolism of fatty acids and the production of triglycerides and lipoproteins. Alteration or disruption of one or more of the many steps in hepatic lipid metabolism may result in excess accumulation of triglyceride in hepatocytes (5). Possible mechanisms include the following: (*a*) excessive mobilization of fatty acids from adipose tissue with large quantities entering hepatocytes (ethanol abuse, starvation, corticosteroids); (*b*) increased hepatic esterification of fatty acids to triglyceride (ethanol); (*c*) decreased synthesis of apoprotein for coupling and eventual transport with triglyceride, with consequent accumulation of cytoplasmic triglyceride (CCl_4, phosphorus, tetracycline (high dose)); and (*d*) impaired lipoprotein transport from hepatocytes.

TABLE 4.3.
CLINICAL DISORDERS ASSOCIATED WITH FATTY LIVER

Common
1. Alcoholic liver disease
2. Diabetes mellitus
3. Obesity
4. Protein-calorie malnutrition
5. Chronic illness (tuberculosis, inflammatory bowel disease, congestive heart failure)
6. Severe hepatitis
7. Endogenous and exogenous corticosteroids
8. Parenteral nutrition
9. Intestinal bypass for obesity
10. Hepatotoxins (CCl_4, phosphorus, chemotherapy)

Uncommon
1. Cystic fibrosis
2. Trauma
3. Reye's syndrome
4. Acute fatty liver of pregnancy
5. Glycogen storage disease
6. Massive tetracycline therapy
7. Enzymatic deficiency (glycogen synthetase)

Clinical Features

Fatty liver may exhibit several clinical patterns. First, the clinically "silent" fatty liver may be manifest as an asymptomatic slightly enlarged liver detected on routine examination of an obese or diabetic patient (1). In this group, liver function tests are often normal. Second, vague right upper quadrant pain and tenderness with associated hepatomegaly may indicate fatty liver in the alcoholic (1) and nonalcoholic patient (6); serum transaminase and alkaline phosphatase levels may be elevated in this group (3). Finally, acute fatty liver may rarely present with jaundice, acute hepatic failure, and encephalopathy (exposure to hepatotoxins, acute fatty liver of pregnancy) (7–8).

Historically, the diagnosis of hepatic steatosis has required the histological demonstration of large cytoplasmic fat vacuoles with peripheral displacement of the hepatocyte nucleus. A 0 to +4 histological grading system for fatty liver has been described and used clinically (3). The amount of cytoplasmic fat does not appear to correlate well with the severity of serum enzyme abnormalities (2).

Radiological Imaging in Fatty Liver

Because of the varied and nonspecific nature of the clinical findings, the prevalence of fatty liver, and the increasing frequency of hepatobiliary imaging procedures, the radiologist is frequently the first to suggest the presence of fatty liver. Fatty change may be diagnosed by several radiological imaging modalities.

Plain Film Diagnosis. In 1954, Steinbach et al. (9) noted scattered hepatic radiolucencies on an abdominal film of a child with known cystic fibrosis, and postulated cirrhosis with fatty infiltration as the cause. These diagnoses were histologically confirmed on subsequent open liver biopsy. Twenty years later, Swischuk (10) recognized the "radiolucent liver sign" in two infants subsequently proven to have marked fatty change. In each case, the liver, which normally is of similar radiodensity to abdominal wall muscles and clearly separable from properitoneal fat, was enlarged and uniformly radiolucent (Fig. 4.38). Additional reports have validated these plain film obervations in infants and children (11–13). In a series of 19 patients, Yousefzadeh et al. (13) added additional findings of fatty liver including a fat-fluid interface of intraperitoneal ascites and the lateral border of the radiolucent liver, and suggested that blurring of the normally sharp medial border of the right properitoneal fat stripe was the earliest plain film finding of fatty liver.

Radionuclide Imaging. ^{99m}Tc-sulfur colloid liver scans are frequently abnormal in fatty change. Geslien et al. (14) studied the utility of sulfur colloid liver scans in diffuse liver disease in a series of 109 patients, 22 of whom had biopsy-proven fatty liver. The liver scan was intepreted as abnormal in 19 of 22 (86% sensitivity). Diffuse, nonhomogeneous radionuclide uptake was the most frequently scintigraphic observation in 15 of 22 (68%); other findings included reversal of the liver-spleen uptake ratio in 9 of 22 (41%), and increased bone marrow uptake in 9 patients (41%) (Fig. 4.39). Some overlap in the constellation of scintigraphic findings for cirrhosis and fatty liver was noted, however.

The localization of ^{133}Xe in liver during ventilation imaging appears to be more specific for fatty liver (Fig. 4.40). Carey et al. (15) noted ^{133}Xe activity in the right upper quadrant during ventilation imaging in 38% of patients in a small series, and postulated that, due to its high fat solubility, ^{133}Xe liver retention indicated fatty change. Ahmad et al. (16) studied hepatic ^{133}Xe uptake in rats with ethanol-induced fatty liver and in human subjects undergoing ^{133}Xe ventilation scans. In general, good correlation was noted between ^{133}Xe liver activity and the quantity of liver fat in the rat model, and the ^{133}Xe activity and suspected fatty change based on clinical data in the human subjects. The above authors suggested the use of ^{133}Xe as a screening and follow-up procedure for hepatic steatosis.

Ultrasound. Fatty tissue is very echogenic on B-mode ultrasound examination (17). The sonographic findings of diffuse fatty liver include increased fine parenchymal echogenicity, impaired visualization of the borders of intrahepatic vessels, increased attenuation of sound with poor visualization of the deeper portions of the right lobe and diaphragm, and hepatomegaly (17, 18) (Fig. 4.41). Attempts to grade the sever-

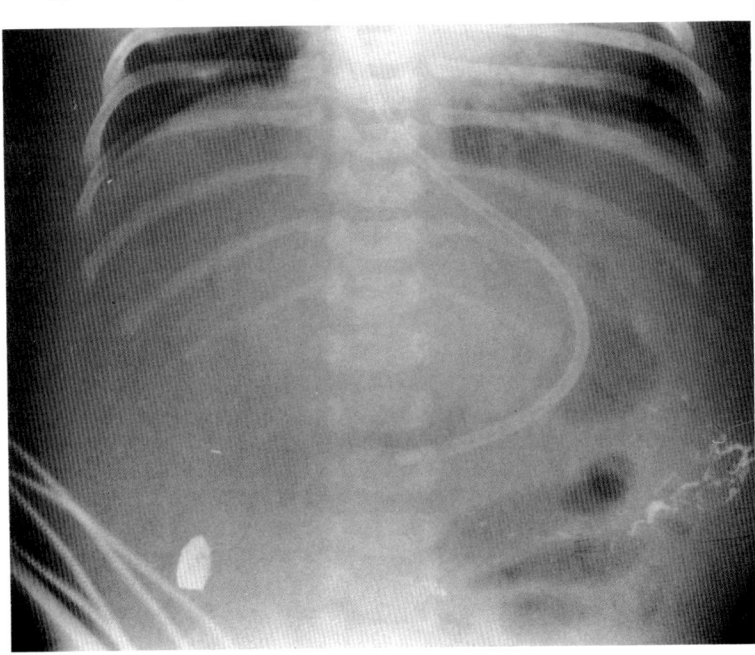

FIGURE 4.38. ENLARGED LIVER FROM FATTY INFILTRATION

Plain film of an infant with cystic fibrosis and severe malnutrition from malabsorption shows a lucent, enlarged liver from fatty infiltration.

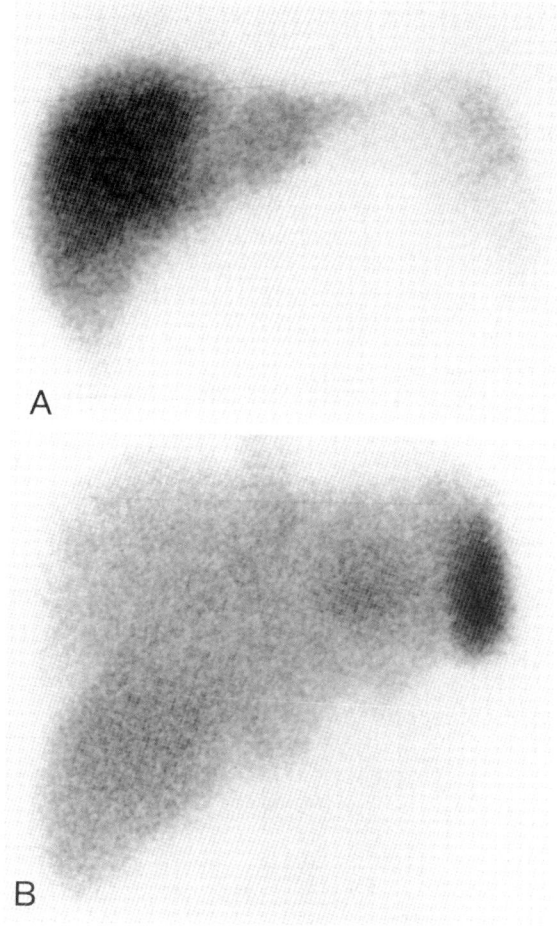

FIGURE 4.39. ^{99m}Tc-Sulfur Colloid Liver Imaging in Fatty Liver

A: Anterior image of a normal patient shows uniform radionuclide distribution in a liver of normal size. *B:* Biopsy-proven fatty change. Anterior scan reveals nonhomogeneous radionuclide distribution in a markedly enlarged liver and increased splenic activity. Bone marrow uptake is also present and was better appreciated on posterior views.

ity of fatty change based on sonographic criteria have been made (18).

The reported accuracy of the B-mode sonographic diagnosis of fatty liver has been variable. Foster et al. (19) noted a 60% sensitivity for the sonographic detection of biopsy-proven fatty liver, while other reports have documented accuracies of 85% (18) and 97% (20). The difficulty of sonographic discrimination between fatty liver and cirrhosis has been addressed by several authors, and may reflect overlap in sonographic criteria and/or coexistence of both processes in the same patient (17, 18, 21). There are currently no published reports documenting the accuracy of diagnosing fatty liver with real-time instruments.

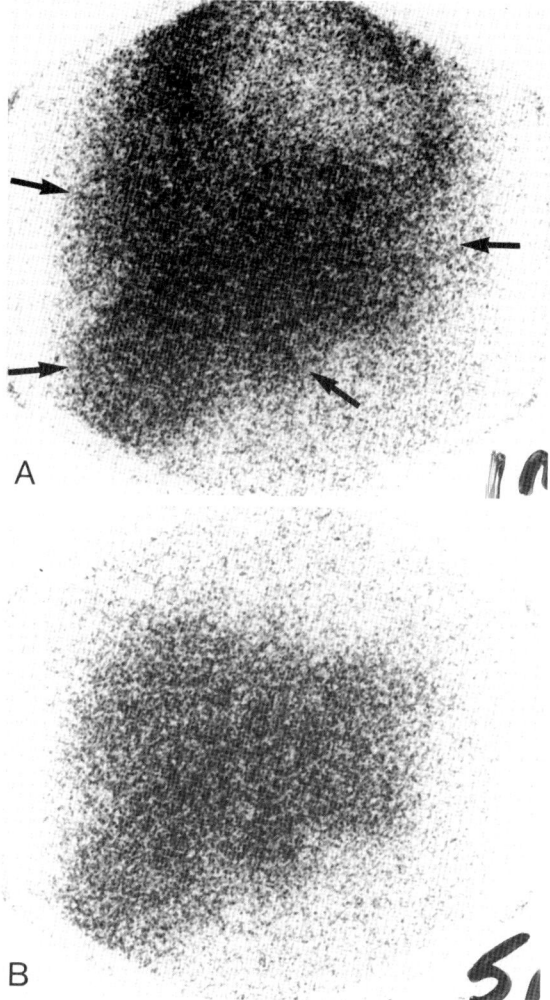

FIGURE 4.40. Xenon Scan

Anterior ^{133}Xe ventilation scans of the lower chest and upper abdomen in the same patient as in Fig. 4.39B. *A:* Xenon has localized in the liver (*arrows*) on the 1-min image. Note also residual xenon in the lung bases. *B:* Five-minute delayed anterior image shows persistent, diffuse xenon localization in the liver, and xenon clearance from the lung bases.

Computed Tomography. The development of body CT has permitted the unambiguous diagnosis of fatty liver (22); indeed, CT has become the "gold standard" for the imaging of fatty change. Marked fatty metamorphosis presents a striking CT pattern of liver parenchymal attenuation reduced below that of the normal portal vein and vena cava (Fig. 4.42A) (22). In this situation, liver attenuation values at or below those of water are common. Since attenuation values of normal liver average about 8 HU above those of spleen (23), milder degrees of fatty liver can be confidently diagnosed by CT when this

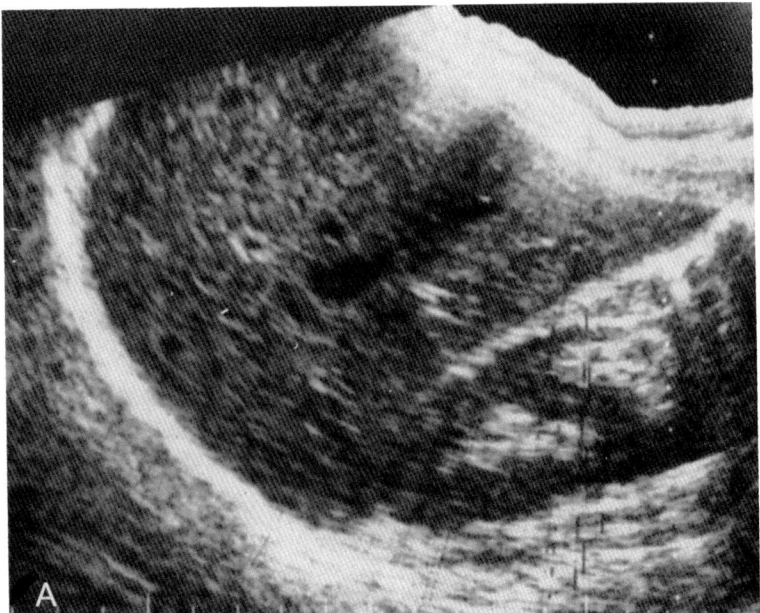

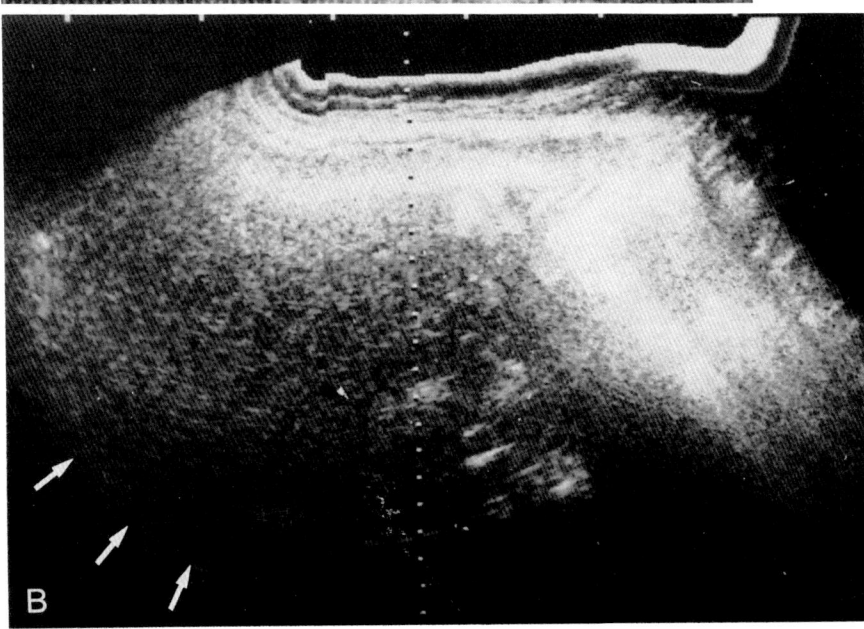

FIGURE 4.41. B-MODE SONOGRAPHIC FINDINGS IN FATTY LIVER
A: Sagittal liver sonogram in a normal patient demonstrates uniform parenchymal echoes and good visualization of the intrahepatic vessels, diaphragm and right kidney. *B:* Sagittal right upper quadrant sonogram of a patient with fatty infiltration. Parenchymal echogenicity and sound attenuation are increased, and there is impaired visualization of the intrahepatic vessel borders, right hemidiaphragm (*arrows*) and right kidney. (Both images produced by a 3.5 MHz medium-focus transducer.)

normal liver/spleen relationship is reversed (Fig. 4.42C).

Excellent correlation between the level of hepatic triglyceride on biopsy and CT attenuation coefficient has been reported in both animal models (24, 25) and in human clinical studies (26, 27). So close has been the correlation, in fact, that CT has been proffered as a simple, noninvasive and quantitative modality for diagnosis and follow-up of patients with suspected fatty liver (25, 26).

Magnetic Resonance Imaging. Preliminary experience with magnetic resonance imaging (MRI) of the liver has revealed no characteristic alterations in fatty change (28–30). However, one recent report suggests that MRI may succeed in distinguishing acute hepatocellular inflammation from cirrhosis and fatty liver (29).

Unusual Features and Radiological Significance

Focal Fatty Change. Traditionally viewed as a diffuse process, fatty infiltration of the liver may also be patchy or nonuniform in its distribution on radiological imaging (31, 32). The study of postmortem livers has suggested that

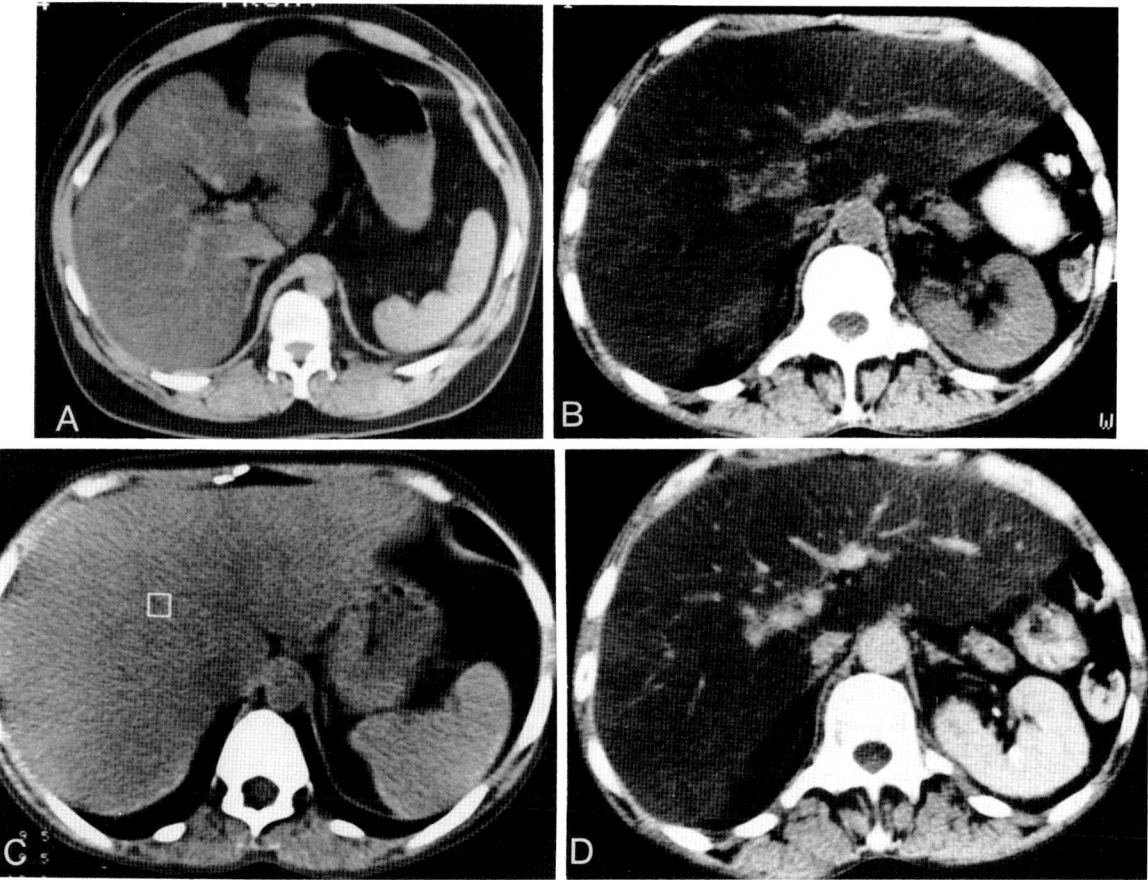

FIGURE 4.42. FATTY LIVER CHANGES

A: Diffuse fatty liver. *B:* Severe fatty change with marked reduction of liver parenchymal attenuation highlighting the portal veins and inferior vena cava. *C:* Mild fatty infiltration showing the liver attenuation slightly less than spleen. Mean attenuation within the cursor was 19.2 HU. *D:* Same case as *B* at nearly the same level with contrast enhancement.

focal fatty change may, in fact, be a common lesion occurring in association with a number of clinical problems (33). Although the precise mechanism for development of focal fatty change is not understood, regional hepatic ischemia in patients predisposed to fatty liver may play an important role (33).

CT has provided the most complete imaging data on focal fatty change. Patterns of fatty change have been classified as: (*a*) complete, (*b*) nearly complete (sparing a portion of one lobe), (*c*) geographic (large confluent areas), (*d*) multifocal, and (*e*) patchy (Fig. 4.43) (34). Localized fatty infiltration is typically nonspherical, poorly marginated, fan-shaped, and produces no mass effect or alteration of hepatic contour (35). Preservation of the normal portal vasculature has been cited as an important feature differentiating regional fatty change from space-occupying mass lesions such as abscess or neoplasm (34). Measurement of absolute attenuation values in focal fatty change is less helpful due to a very wide range of variability and overlap with expected values for metastatic tumor and other hepatic masses (34, 35). A sulfur colloid scan can be helpful if it shows no focal mass. This happens because enough functioning Kupffer cells are present despite the focal fatty infiltration (Fig. 4.43*F, G*).

Rapid Appearance and Disappearance. CT has also shown that diffuse or regional changes in lipid content of the liver may occur rapidly. Marked fatty change appeared within a 2-week interval following institution of L-asparaginase treatment for lymphoblastic lymphoma (36). Similar rapid events could be expected following initiation of parenteral nutrition. Fatty infiltration may also resolve promptly. Dramatic reduction in focal and diffuse fatty liver occurred within 6 and 19 days, respectively, in two alcoholic patients following hospitalization and improvement of nutritional status (37). Sawada et

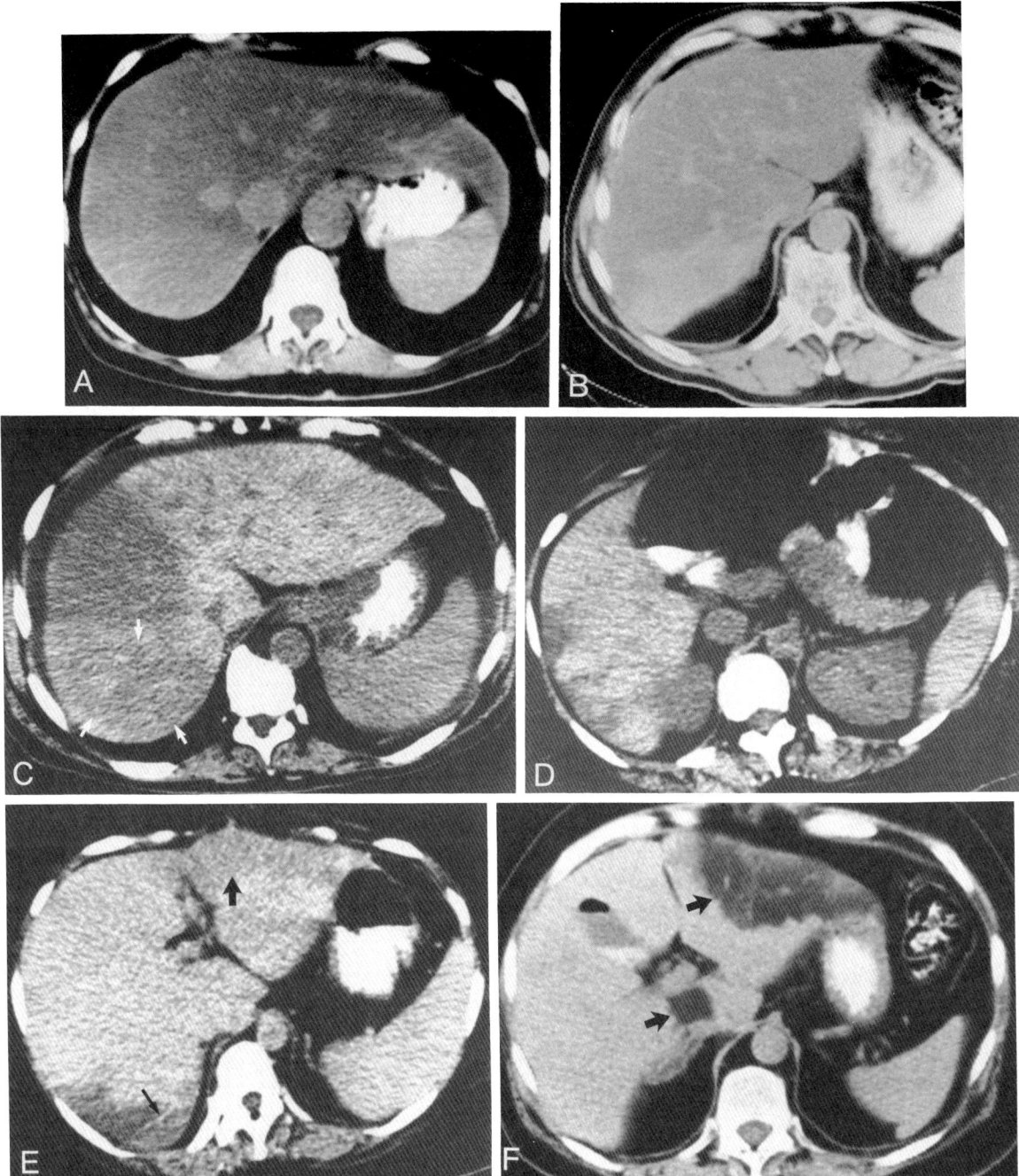

FIGURE 4.43. VARIETY OF PATTERNS OF FOCAL FATTY CHANGE, DEMONSTRATED ON COMPUTED TOMOGRAPHY

A: Nearly complete, sparing the lateral portion of the left lobe and posterior right lobe. *B:* CT shows fatty infiltration with focal sparing in the posterior right lobe. The patient was referred because of an outside ultrasound that suggested a hypoechoic mass in the posterior right lobe. *C:* Geographic involvement, with a sharply defined zone of fatty change in the anterior segment of the right lobe, and poorly marginated zone in the posterior right lobe (*arrows*). *D:* Multifocal involvement with small, peripheral scalloped zones of fatty change in the right lobe. *E:* Similar findings in the right lobe and left lobe (*large arrow*). Note the small hepatic vessel within the posterior right lobe low attenuation zone (*small arrow*), excluding a mass effect. *F* and *G:* Multifocal fatty infiltration involving the left lobe and the caudate lobe (*arrows*). Note the normal vessels in the affected region of the left lobe. The patient has Cushing's syndrome and abnormal liver function tests. The sulfur colloid scan (*G*) shows no evidence of a mass, further excluding neoplasm.

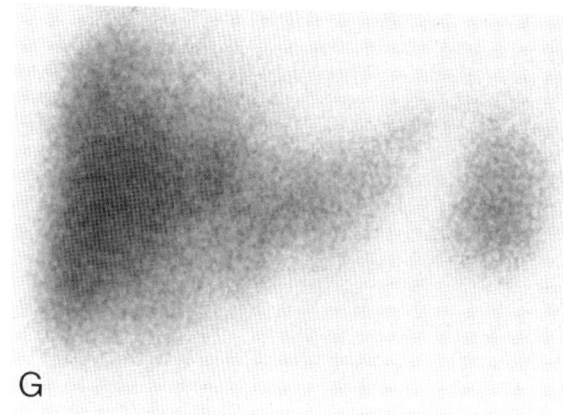

FIGURE 4.43G

al. (38) noted complete regression of focal fatty change over a 3-month interval.

Significance of Fatty Liver. As previously noted, fatty change is a nonspecific response of the liver to a variety of metabolic derangements or hepatotoxins. Particularly when diffuse in distribution, the radiological diagnosis of fatty liver presents no problem. However, recognition and the correct diagnosis of fatty liver is clinically important in several specific situations.

1. The "silent" fatty liver: The detection of fatty change by ultrasound or CT may provide useful and reassuring clinical information in the obese or diabetic patient with unexplained hepatomegaly or abnormal liver function tests discovered on routine examinations.

2. Differentiating focal fatty change from a more significant space occupying mass (Figs. 4.44 and 4.45): Although the CT criteria for focal fatty change described by Gale et al. (34) and Halvorsen et al. (35) will usually permit correct diagnosis, occasions will arise when abscess or tumor exclusion will not be possible. In such cases, correlation of the CT abnormality with ^{99m}Tc-sulfur colloid (35) or ^{133}Xe (39) liver imaging may be very helpful in resolving the issue (Figs. 4.43F, G and 4.44). Guided percutaneous biopsy of focal fatty liver has been successfully performed with 22-gauge or, preferably, 18-gauge needles (40, 41) and should be reserved for difficult or equivocal cases (34).

The difficulty in diagnosing focal fatty infiltration by sonography has been addressed by several authors (32, 35, 42). Focal fatty infiltration is depicted as an echogenic mass with greater than normal attenuation of sound. Because of gain manipulation, focally spared normal parenchyma in a diffusely infiltrated liver is often falsely depicted as a sonolucent mass (Fig. 4.46).

3. Coexistence of diffuse fatty change and space-occupying mass lesion(s): The diagnosis of benign or malignant space-occupying masses in the patient with diffuse fatty liver may be extremely difficult (35, 42, 43). Spherical areas with attenuation values greater than surrounding fatty liver may represent a significant mass or simply an "island" of uninvolved normal liver (Fig. 4.47) (35, 44). If the mass(es) possesses low attenuation values similar to the surrounding fatty change, the presence of such masses may be underestimated or missed altogether. Under these circumstances, the more invasive procedures of guided percutaneous biopsy, selective hepatic angiography, or computed angiotomography may be necessary (43).

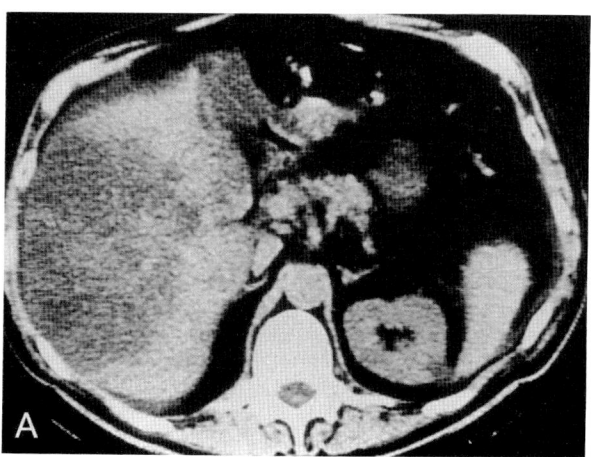
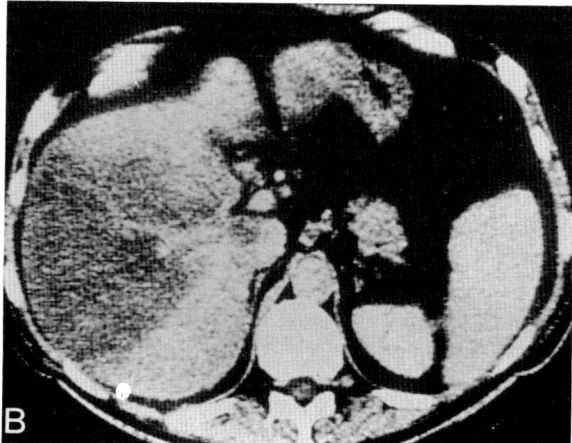

FIGURE 4.44. FOCAL FATTY INFILTRATION SIMULATING HEPATOCELLULAR CARCINOMA, USE OF BIOPSY

A and *B:* Noncontrast and contrast enhanced (drip infusion) scans showing a low density right lobe mass in an alcoholic male patient. Needle biopsy was done because of the nonspecific appearance and showed fatty infiltration. (Case courtesy of Joseph P. Finizio, M.D., Southern Maryland Hospital Center.)

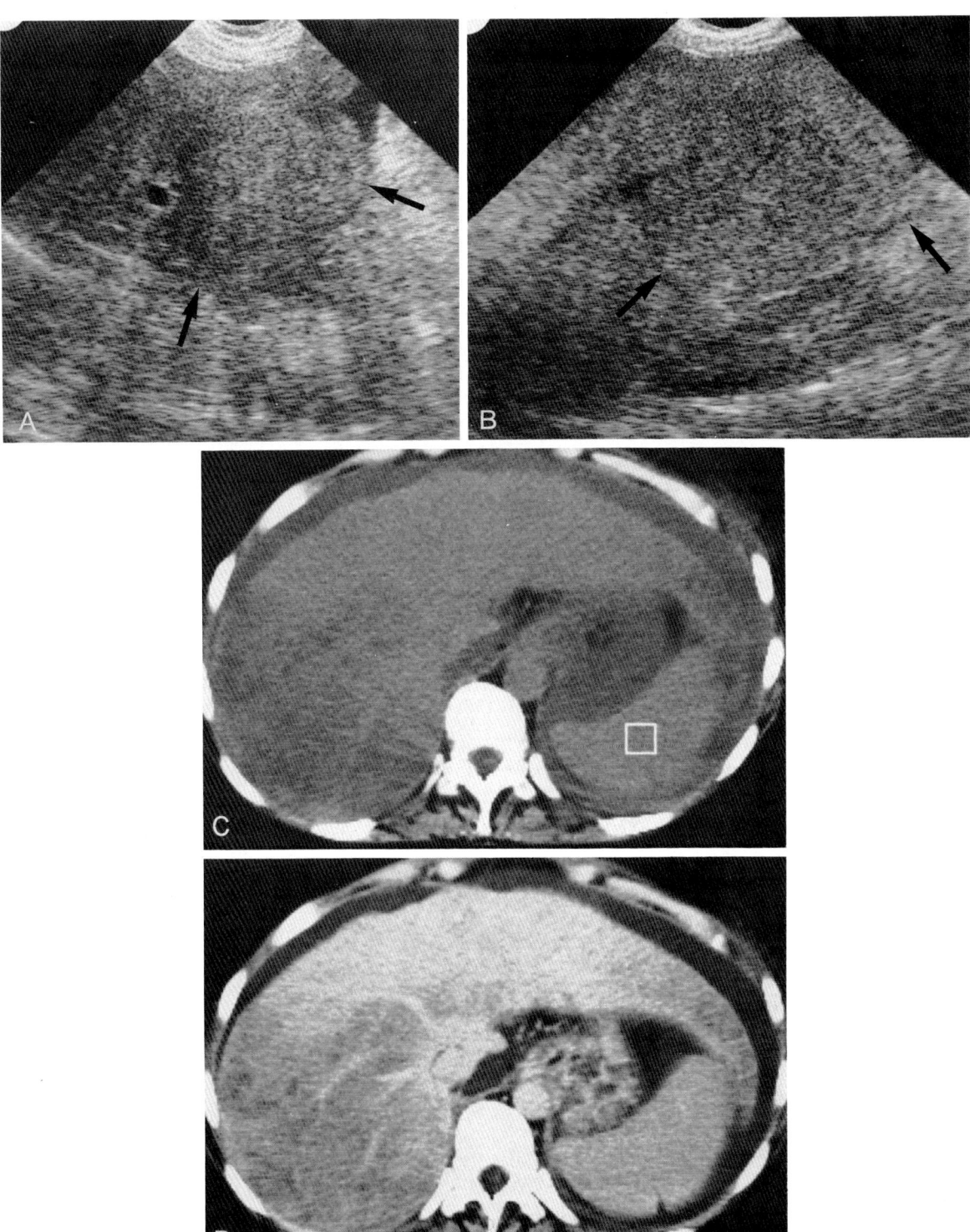

FIGURE 4.45. FOCAL FATTY INFILTRATION SIMULATING HEPATOCELLULAR CARCINOMA, USE OF DYNAMIC CT

A and *B:* Transverse and parasagittal sonograms of an alcoholic female suggesting a mass (*arrows*). Note the poor sound penetration and lack of vascular architecture. *C:* Unenhanced CT shows hepatomegaly, diffuse low hepatic density and focal areas of further diminished density in the posterior right lobe and the lateral left lobe. *D:* Dynamic CT in the portal venous phase showing normal vessels in the posterior right lobe suggesting focal fatty infiltration. The patient died from acute alcoholic hepatitis and autopsy confirmed fatty infiltration. *E:* Sulfur-colloid liver spleen scan shows spleen and marrow uptake and almost no liver uptake consistent with severe hepatocellular disease. *F:* HIDA scan shows hepatomegaly, poor liver uptake and increased renal excretion consistent with severe hepatocellular disease. Nuclear imaging also excluded neoplasm.

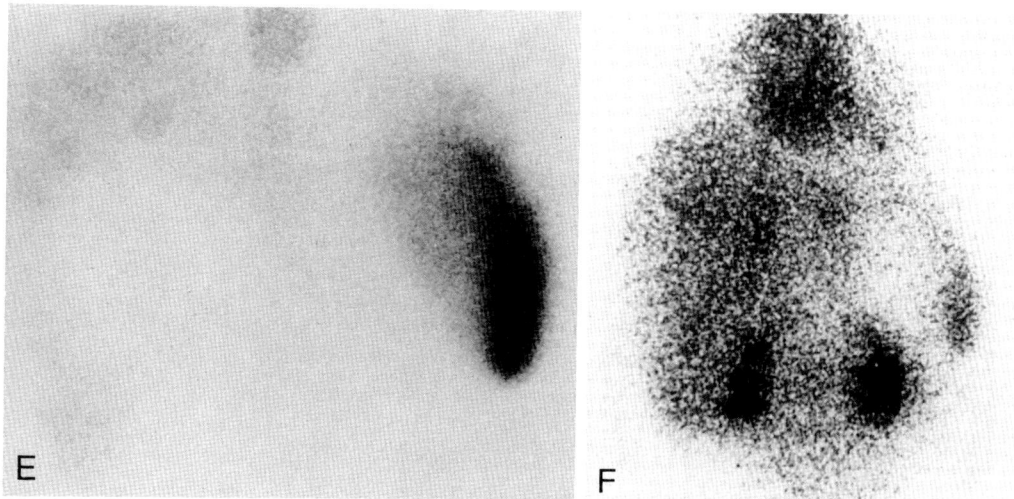

FIGURE 4.45E and F

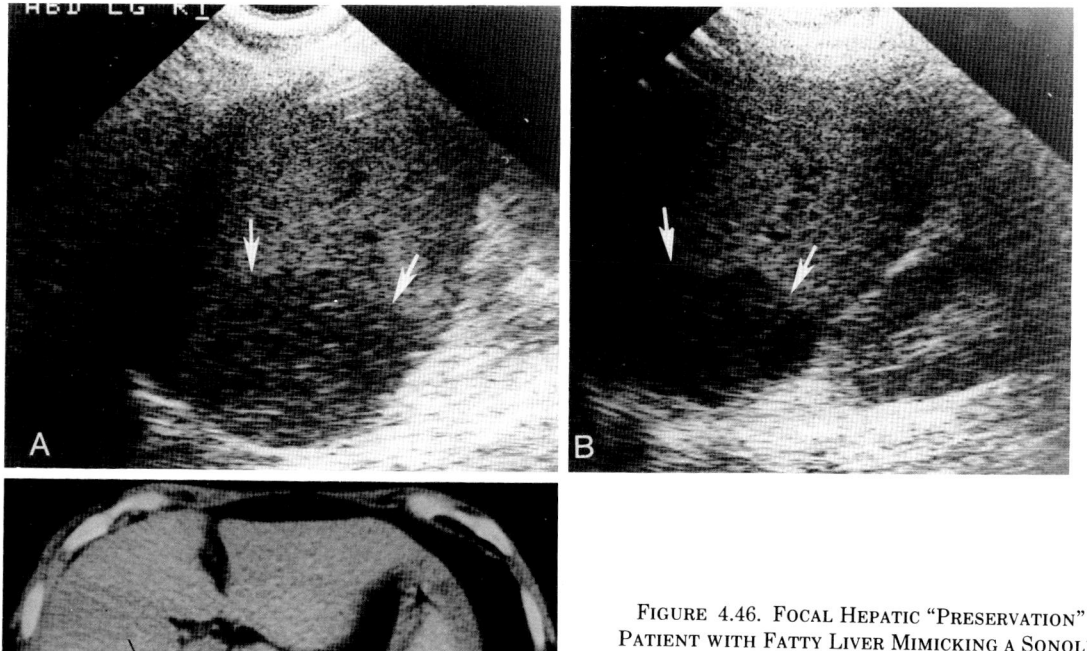

FIGURE 4.46. FOCAL HEPATIC "PRESERVATION" IN A PATIENT WITH FATTY LIVER MIMICKING A SONOLUCENT MASS LESION

A and *B:* Sagittal and transverse scans: apparent sonolucent mass (*arrows*) in the suprarenal portion of the posterior right lobe. *C:* Noncontrast CT: the mass corresponds to focally preserved parenchyma (*arrows*).

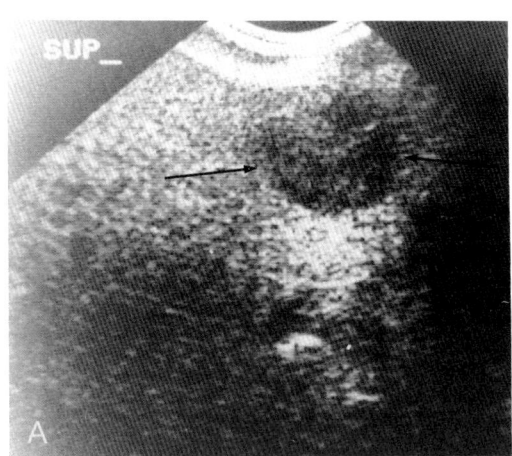
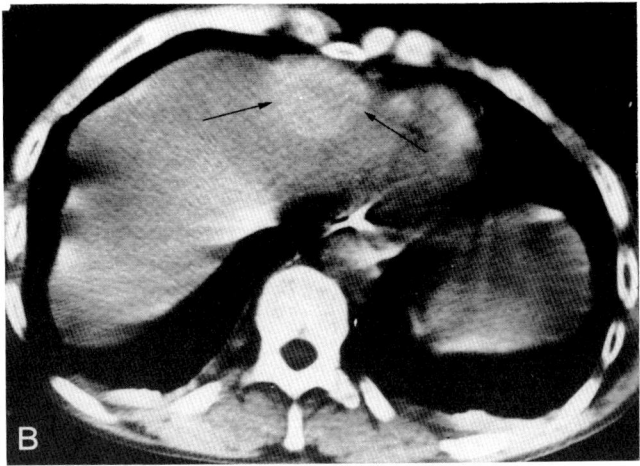

FIGURE 4.47. INCIDENTAL MASS DISCOVERED IN AN ALCOHOLIC WITH A FATTY LIVER

A: Sonolucent mass (arrows) with more through transmission than adjacent fat infiltrated parenchyma. B: Apparently hyperdense mass (arrows). "Roundness" and lack of straight margins suggest mass rather than focal parenchymal preservation. Needle biopsy showed hepatocellular carcinoma.

REFERENCES

1. Isselbacher KJ, LaMont JT: Infiltrative and metabolic diseases affecting the liver. In Petersdorf RG, Adams RD, Braunwald E, Isselbacher KJ, Martin JB, Wilson JD (eds): *Harrison's Principles of Internal Medicine.* New York, McGraw-Hill, 1983, pp 1818–1821.
2. Alpers DH, Sabesin M: Fatty liver: biochemical and clinical aspects. In Schiff L, Schiff ER (eds): *Diseases of the Liver.* Philadelphia, J. B. Lippincott, 1982, pp 813–845.
3. Pimstone NR, French SW: Alcoholic liver disease. *Med Clin North Am* 68:39–56, 1984.
4. Ground KEU: Prevalence of fatty liver in healthy male adults accidentally killed. *Aviat Space Environ Med* 55:59–61, 1984.
5. Robbins SL, Cotran RS: *Pathological Basis of Disease.* Ed 2, Philadelphia, WB Saunders, 1979, pp 22–54.
6. Moran JR, Ghishan FK, Halter SA, Greene HL: Steatohepatitis in obese children: a cause of chronic liver dysfunction. *Am. J. Gastroenterol* 78:374–377, 1983.
7. Hague WM, Duncan SLB, Slater DN: Acute fatty liver of pregnancy. *J R Soc Med* 76:652–659, 1983.
8. Pockros PJ, Peters RL, Reynolds TB: Idiopathic fatty liver of pregnancy: findings in ten cases. *Medicine* 63:1–11, 1984.
9. Steinbach HL, Crane JT, Bruyn HB: The Roentgen demonstration of cirrhosis of the liver with fatty metamorphosis: report of a case due to congenital fibrocystic disease. *Radiology* 62:858–861, 1954.
10. Swischuk LE: A new and unusual roentgenographic finding of fatty liver in infants. *AJR* 122:159–164, 1974.
11. Griscom NT, Capitanio MA, Wagoner ML, Culham G, Morris L: The visibility fatty liver. *Radiology* 117:385–389, 1975.
12. Melhem RE: The radiolucent liver. *Pediatr Radiol* 4:153–156, 1976.
13. Yousefzadeh DK, Lupetin AR, Jackson JH: The radiographic signs of fatty liver. *Radiology* 131:351–355, 1979.
14. Geslien GE, Pinsky SM, Poth RK, Johnson MC: The sensitivity and specificity of ^{99m}Tc-sulfur colloid liver imaging in diffuse hepatocellular disease. *Radiology* 118:115–119, 1976.
15. Carey JE, Purdy JM, Moses DC: Localization of ^{133}Xe in liver during ventilation studies. *J Nucl Med* 15:1179–1181, 1974.
16. Ahmad M, Witztum KF, Fletcher JW, Hendelshott LR, Klos D, George EA, Donati RM: Xenon-133 accumulation in hepatic steatosis. *J Nucl Med* 18:881–885, 1977.
17. Behan M, Kazam E: The echographic characteristics of fatty tissues and tumors. *Radiology* 129:143–151, 1978.
18. Scatarige JC, Scott WW, Donovan PJ, Siegelman SS, Sanders RC: Fatty infiltration of the liver: ultrasound and computed tomographic correlation. *J Ultrasound Med* 3:9–14, 1984.
19. Foster KJ, Dewbury KC, Griffith AH, Wright R: The accuracy of ultrasound in the detection of fatty infiltration of the liver. *Br J Radiol* 53:440–442, 1980.
20. Weiss H: Die Stellung der Sonographie im Rahmen der Leberdiagnostik. *Med Klin* 74:154–160, 1979.
21. Gosink BB, Lemon SK, Scheible W, Leopold GR: Accuracy of ultrasonography in diagnosis of hepatocellular disease. *AJR* 133:19–23, 1979.
22. Stephens DH, Sheedy PF, Hattery RR, MacCarty RL: Computed tomography of the liver. *AJR* 128:579–580, 1977.
23. Piekarski J, Goldberg HI, Royal SA, Axel L, Moss AA: Difference between liver and spleen CT numbers in the normal adult: its usefulness in predicting the presence of diffuse liver disease. *Radiology* 137:727–729, 1980.
24. Ducommun JC, Goldberg HI, Korobkin M, Moss AA, Kressel HY: The relation of liver fat to computed tomography numbers: a preliminary experimental study in rabbits. *Radiology* 130:511–513, 1979.
25. Kawata RYO, Sakata K, Kunieda T, Saji S, Doi H, Nozawa Y: Quantitative evaluation of fatty liver by computed tomography in rabbits. *AJR* 142:741–746, 1984.
26. Bydder GM, Chapman RWG, Harry D, Bassan L, Sherlock S, Kreel L: Computed tomography attenuation values in fatty liver. *Comput Tomogr* 5:33–35, 1981.
27. Yajima Y, Narui T, Ishii M, Abe R, Ohtsuki M, Goto Y, Endo S, Yamada K, Ito M: Computed tomography in the diagnosis of fatty liver: total lipid content and computed tomography numbers. *Tohoku J Exp Med* 136:337–342, 1982.

28. Young IR, Bailes DR, Burl M, Collins AG, Smith DT, McDonnel MJ, et al: Initial clinical evaluation of a whole body nuclear magnetic resonance (NMR) tomograph. *J. Comput Assist Tomogr* 6:1-18, 1982.
29. Stark DD, Goldberg HI, Moss AA, Bass NM: Chronic liver disease: evaluation by magnetic resonance. *Radiology* 150:149-151, 1984.
30. Doyle FH, Pennock JM, Banks LM, McDonnel MJ, Bydder GM, Steiner RE, et al: Nuclear magnetic resonance imaging of the liver: initial experience. *AJR* 138:193-200, 1982.
31. Mulhern CB, Arger PH, Coleman BG, Stein GN: Nonuniform attenuation in computed tomography study of the cirrhotic liver. *Radiology* 132:399-402, 1970.
32. Scott WW, Sanders RC, Siegelman SS: Irregular fatty infiltration of the liver: diagnostic dilemmas. *AJR* 135:67-71, 1980.
33. Brawer MK, Austin GE, Lewin KJ: Focal fatty change of the liver, a hitherto poorly recognized entity. *Gastroenterology* 78:247-252, 1980.
34. Gale ME, Gerzof SG, Robbins AH: Portal architectures: a differential guide to fatty infiltration of the liver on computed tomography. *Gastrointest Radiol* 8:231-236, 1983.
35. Halvorsen RA, Korobkin M, Ram PC, Thompson WM: CT appearance of focal fatty infiltration of the liver. *AJR* 139:277-281, 1982.
36. Wenzel DJ, Batist G: Implications of rapid uniform density changes on hepatic computed tomography. *J Comput Assist Tomogr* 7:209-214, 1983.
37. Bashist B, Hecht HL, Harley WD: Computed tomographic demonstration of rapid changes in fatty infiltration of the liver. *Radiology* 142:691-692, 1982.
38. Sawada S, Kawa S, Murata T, Tanaka Y, Koishi T, Fukagae N: Localized fatty infiltration of the liver: CT demonstration of its disappearance on treatment. *Acta Radiol Diagn* 24:359-361, 1983.
39. Patel S, Sandler CM, Rauschkolb EN, McConnel BJ: [133]Xe uptake in focal hepatic fat accumulation: CT correlation. *AJR* 138:541-544, 1982.
40. Pagani JJ: Biopsy of focal hepatic lesions: Comparison of 18 and 22 gauge needles. *Radiology* 147:673-675, 1983.
41. Haaga JR, LiPuma JP, Bryan PJ, Balsara VJ, Cohen AM: Clinical comparison of small- and large-caliber cutting needles for biopsy. *Radiology* 146:665-667, 1983.
42. Wilson SR, Rosen IE, Chin-sang HB, Arenson AM: Fatty infiltration of the liver—an imaging challenge. *J Can Assoc Radiol* 33:227-232, 1982.
43. Lewis E, Bernardino ME, Barnes PA, Parvey HR, Soo C, Chuang VP: The fatty liver: pitfalls in the CT and angiographic evaluation of metastatic disease. *J Comput Assist Tomogr* 7:235-241, 1983.
44. Lamki N, Raval B: Computed tomographic diagnosis of hepatic metastases in fatty infiltration. *J Comput Assist Tomogr* 7:227-228, 1983.

Hepatitis

Hepatitis is a diffuse inflammation of the liver which can be divided into acute and chronic forms. The latter form can be subdivided into persistent and active categories. Pathologically, acute hepatitis shows hepatocellular necrosis and diffuse disarray without portal or periportal abnormalities. In chronic persistent hepatitis there is periportal inflammation but preserved lobular architecture. Chronic active hepatitis has more extensive inflammation, piecemeal necrosis and, often, fibrosis (1).

Ultrasound

Acute hepatitis, when severe enough, may cause decreased parenchymal echogenicity and increased brightness and demonstrability of portal vein radicle walls (2). Identical findings have

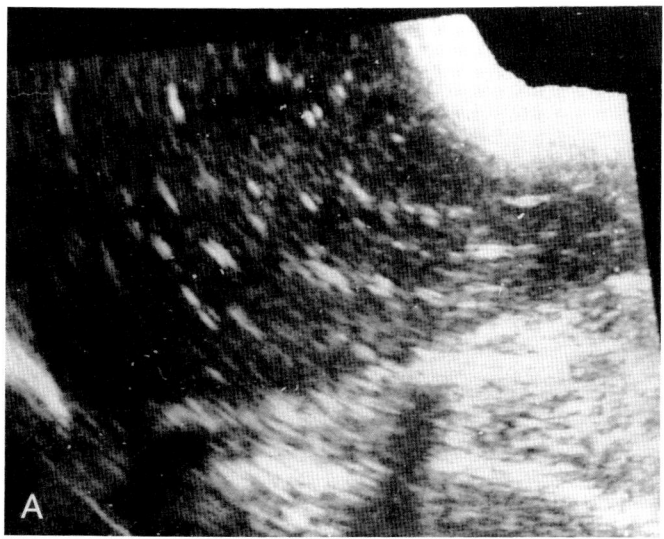
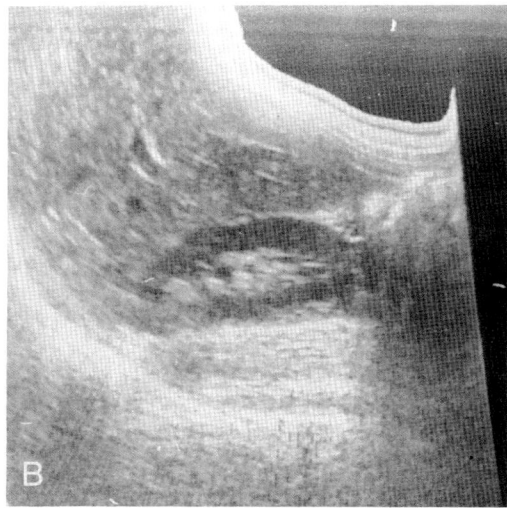

FIGURE 4.48. TOXIC SHOCK SYNDROME
A: Toxic shock syndrome in a young woman. Sagittal sonogram through the right lobe during the acute illness shows decreased hepatic parenchymal echogenicity and accentuation of portal vein radicle wall echoes. *B:* A repeat sagittal scan 6 months later when the patient was well was normal. (From Lieberman JM, Bryan PJ, Cohen AM: Toxic shock syndrome: sonographic appearance of the liver. *AJR* 137:606-607, 1981.)

been reported in toxic shock syndrome, leukemia, and diabetic ketoacidosis (Fig. 4.48) (2, 3). Increased periportal echogenicity has been seen in cytomegalovirus (CMV) infection, biliary atresia, nesidioblastosis, α_1-antitrypsin deficiency, microabscesses, and idiopathic neonatal jaundice (4). This sonographic pattern may be due to hepatocyte swelling or other factors changing the acoustic properties of the liver parenchyma.

Chronic hepatitis, when sufficiently severe, causes coarsening of parenchymal texture and some increased echogenicity with consequent "silhouetting" of the portal vein radicle walls. This results in decreased demonstrability of portal vein branches (2). These findings can be explained on the basis of the inflammatory infiltrate and increased amount of fibrous tissue surrounding the hepatic lobules (2). Fatty infiltration, chronic congestive heart failure, diffuse hepatocellular carcinoma, lymphoma and diffuse metastatic disease, biliary atresia, nesidioblastosis and ascending cholangitis have been reported to show the same findings, with fatty infiltration probably the most common (2, 4).

The main role of ultrasound in acute or chronic hepatitis is to exclude biliary obstruction as the cause of the liver disease.

Computed Tomography

Unless fatty infiltration is present, the attenuation of the liver is generally not altered in the above diseases so that a change in liver size, if present, is the only finding.

REFERENCES

1. De Groote J, Gedigk P, Popper H et al: A classification of chronic hepatitis. *Lancet* 2:626–628, 1978.
2. Kurtz AB, Rubin CB, Cooper HS, Nisenbaum HL, Cole-Beuglet C, Medoff J, Goldberg BB: Ultrasound findings in hepatitis. *Radiology* 136:717–723, 1980.
3. Lieberman JM, Bryan PJ, Cohen AM: Toxic shock syndrome: sonographic appearance of the liver. *AJR* 137:606–607, 1981.
4. Blane CE, Jongeward RH Jr, Silver TM: Sonographic features of hepatocellular disease in neonates and infants. *AJR* 141:1313–1316, 1983.

Hemochromatosis

Hemochromatosis is a disorder characterized by excess iron deposition in several organs of the body; specifically, the liver, spleen, lymph nodes, pancreas, gastrointestinal tract, kidneys, heart, and endocrine glands (1). Iron overload in the liver often leads to cirrhosis with portal hypertension. Hemochromatosis is classified into two types, primary or idiopathic, and secondary. Primary hemochromatosis is an inherited condition and develops as a result of a mucosal defect in the intestinal wall allowing an increased absorption of ingested iron (2, 3). The early stages of idiopathic hemochromatosis are characterized by a high plasma iron concentration, a high percentage saturation of plasma transferrin, and increasing deposits of hemosiderin in the liver and other organs with the passage of time (4). Only after the accumulation of a markedly increased concentration of storage iron does pathologic, biochemical, and clinical evidence of organ damage appear.

Secondary hemochromatosis develops as a result of multiple blood transfusions (generally greater than 100 pints) (5) with secondary iron overload in patients with thalassemia, sideroblastic anemia, or other chronic anemias. It also occurs in congenital transferrin deficiency disorders, cirrhosis, in patients who ingest excessive dietary iron, porphyria cutanea tarda, and as a sequela of portacaval shunts (4). Hemosiderosis is a term reserved for increased iron deposition without associated organ damage (5).

Clinical Features

The presenting clinical features of hemochromatosis reflect the chronic and insidious nature of the disorder. Patients with primary hemochromatosis do not usually develop signs and symptoms until the fourth or fifth decades of life. Many years pass before the usual 20–40 g of iron have accumulated at the time of diagnosis (4). This is in contrast to patients with secondary hemochromatosis who may present at an earlier age (6). The earlier onset may be due to the presence of an unusually high amount of available dietary iron coupled with a more severe metabolic defect (4). Fully developed hemochromatosis develops primarily in males in a ratio of 10:1. The diminished frequency of the disorder occurring in females is thought to be due to the loss of iron by normal menstruation, pregnancy, and lactation.

The initial manifestations of hemochromatosis include diabetes mellitus (30%), hyperpigmentation (90%), and abdominal symptoms, such as dull abdominal pain, nausea, vomiting, diarrhea, and hematemesis. Symptoms related to the onset of diabetes mellitus include weight loss, lassitude, and weakness. Although it was earlier assumed that diabetes mellitus occurred in patients with hemochromatosis on the basis of pancreatic islet failure, recent investigations have suggested a more complicated mechanism with at least three factors of primary importance: familial predisposition to develop diabetes, impaired glucose tolerance owing to cirrhosis, and pancreatic insufficiency (4). Pigmentation of the skin appears as diffuse bronze, slaty, or metallic tint to the skin. The color changes in some patients are minimal (7).

Enlargement of the liver is found in over 90% of patients with hemochromatosis, and is the most common physical finding. The liver is firm in consistency and has a smooth surface on palpation. Liver function tests remain surprisingly normal, provided the patient does not ingest excessive amounts of alcohol. Hepatocellular carcinoma is an important late complication in patients with hemochromatosis, occurring in about 14% of cases (8). The development of a hepatocellular carcinoma is suggested by unexplained weight loss, fever, nodular enlargement of the liver, jaundice, and ascites in a patient with previously well-controlled hemochromatosis.

Endocrine dysfunction is a common feature of hemochromatosis. Loss of libido, impotence, loss of body hair, amenorrhea, and testicular atrophy are common and almost constantly seen in young patients. Pituitary insufficiency has been seen in a certain number of affected patients (9).

Right and left sided cardiac decompensation and arrhythmias are seen in approximately 15% of patients with hemochromatosis (4). Congestive heart failure may occur with ventricular dilatation, and frequently responds poorly to conventional therapy (5). The presence of cardiac arrhythmias portend a poor prognosis (4). The most common arrhythmias are ventricular extrasystoles, but supraventricular and ventricular tachycardias, ventricular fibrillation, and varying degrees of heart block may also occur.

Arthropathy is now a recognized feature associated with the signs and symptoms of hemochromatosis. Arthralgia and arthritis occur in about 50% of patients. Although it may be confined to the hands and wrists, it usually progresses to involve the larger joints. Patients in whom the onset of hemochromatosis appears after 50 years of age are more likely to develop arthritis than those who manifest the disease earlier in life. Chondrocalcinosis is commonly associated with hemochromatosis in as many as two thirds of patients (1). Small subchrondral cyst-like rarefactions located in the metacarpal heads, and predilection for the second and third metacarpal joints are characteristic features. Frequently uniform narrowing of cartilage is present. In contrast to rheumatoid arthritis, there are no marginal erosions, synovial thickening, ulnar deviation or subcutaneous nodules.

Pathology

The pathologic findings in hemochromatosis reflect the accumulation of excess iron over an extended period of time. In the fully established disease, the total amount of iron stored in the body varies between 25 and 50 g in contrast to 3.5–4.5 g in a 70-kg healthy adult male (5). Iron deposits are greatest in the liver and pancreas where they can be 50–100 times the normal amount (10).

The most characteristic and diagnostically important findings of hemochromatosis are seen in the liver. The two most important features of liver involvement include extensive pigmentation and fibrosis. In the early stages, the liver may show only portal zone fibrosis with deposition of iron in the periportal liver cells, and, to a lesser extent, in the Kupffer cells (11). Dense, fibrous septa later develop forming a network surrounding groups of lobules. The hemosiderin deposits gradually are distributed throughout the lobules as well as in biliary duct epithelium, Kupffer cells, and connective tissue. Fatty change within the liver is unusual, and the glycogen content of the liver cells is normal (11). Ultimately, a fully established cirrhosis develops with nodularity typically micronodular. The liver is greatly enlarged, weighing over 2000 g. The cut surface has a reddish brown color with a firm consistency.

Radiology

Rarely, plain films may demonstrate a homogeneous increased hepatic radiopacity but this finding is uncommon and difficult to appreciate when present. Ultrasound does not show any significant abnormality unless cirrhosis or hepatocellular carcinoma supervenes. Radionuclide scintigraphy likewise shows no significant abnormality.

CT has aided greatly in the noninvasive diagnosis of hemochromatosis. While liver biopsy with its array of complications was the primary mode of diagnosing hemochromatosis in the past, extensive work has been done demonstrating the value of CT in making the correct diagnosis in suspected patients (12–21).

Hemochromatosis can be readily diagnosed when an overall homogeneous increase in density

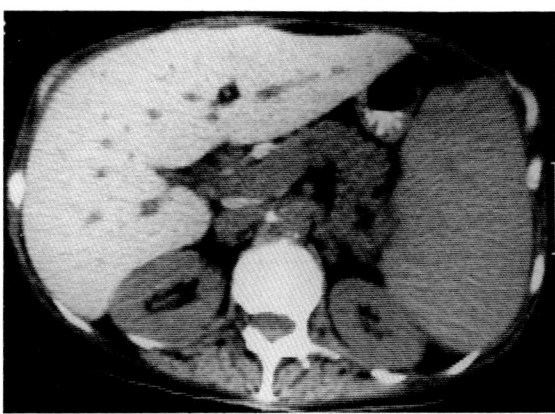

FIGURE 4.49. SIDEROBLASTIC ANEMIA AND TRANSFUSIONAL OVERLOAD HEMOSIDEROSIS
Elderly woman with sideroblastic anemia for many years and transfusional overload hemosiderosis. Radiodense liver and peripancreatic lymph nodes.

of the hepatic parenchyma is demonstrated (Fig. 4.49). The CT numbers of normal unenhanced liver average 30–60 Hounsfield units (12, 16). Using scanning energies of 120 kvp, the average CT density of the liver in patients with hemochromatosis averages 75–130 Hounsfield units. As a result of the overall increase in density of the liver parenchyma, intrahepatic veins stand out against the background of the hyperdense liver. A similar appearance can be seen in glycogen storage disease and after hyperalimentation treatment of malnutrition (acute massive protein deposition) (21).

By using dual energy scanning techniques, CT has been found useful in quantitating the amount of iron stores in the liver (19). Changing the scanning energy from 120 kvp to 80 kvp will result in a change of the CT number of the liver if an excessive amount of high atomic number element such as iron is present. Experimental work has shown that there is in fact a constant relationship between a change in CT attenuation value for each gram of iron present in the liver.

CT is also able to demonstrate, if present, increased density in the spleen, pancreas, lymph nodes, and adrenal glands (Fig. 4.49).

REFERENCES

1. Jensen PS: Hemochromatosis: a disease often silent but not invisible. *Radiology* 126:343, 1976.
2. Finch SC, Finch CA: Idiopathic hemochromatosis, an iron storage disease. *Medicine* 34:381–430, 1955.
3. Grace ND, Powell LW: Iron storage disorders of the liver. *Gastroenterology* 67:1257–1283, 1974.
4. Bothwell TH, Carlton RW: Hemochromatosis. In Schiff L (ed): *Diseases of the Liver.* Philadelphia, J. B. Lippincott, 1982, pp 1003–1042.
5. Priest RJ, Berk JE. Hemochromatosis. In Bockus HL et al (eds): *Gastroenterology.* Philadelphia, W. B. Saunders, 1976, pp 451–470.
6. Byrd RB, Cooper T: Hereditary iron-loading anemia with secondary hemochromatosis. *Ann Intern Med* 55:103, 1961.
7. Cawley EP, Hsu YT, Wood BT et al: Hemochromatosis and the skin. *Arch Dermatol* 100:1, 1969.
8. Williams R et al: Venesection therapy in idiopathic hemochromatosis: an analysis of 40 treated and 18 untreated patients. *Q J Med* 31:1, 1969.
9. Stocks AE, Martin FR: Pituitary function in hemochromatosis. *Am J Med* 45:839, 1968.
10. Powell LW: Hemochromatosis and related iron storage disease. In Wright R et al (eds): *Liver and Biliary Disease.* Philadelphia, W.B. Saunders, 1979, pp 788–804.
11. Sherlock S: *Diseases of the Liver and Biliary System.* Oxford, Blackwell Scientific, 1981, pp 346–356.
12. Mills SR, Doppman JL, Nienhuis AW: Computed tomography in the diagnosis of disorders of excessive iron storage of the liver. *J Comput Assist Tomogr* 1:101, 1977.
13. Houang MTW, Skalicka A, Arozena X, Huens ER, Shaw DG: Correlation between computed tomographic values and liver iron contents in thalassemia major with iron overload. *Lancet* 1:322, 1979.
14. Chapman RWG, Williams G, Bydder G, Dick R, Sherlock S, Kreel L: Computed tomography for determining liver iron content in primary hemochromatosis. *Br Med J* 280:440, 1980.
15. Long JA, Doppman JL, Nienhuis AW, Mills SR: Computed tomographic analysis of beta-thalassemic syndromes with hemochromatosis: pathologic findings with clinical and laboratory correlations. *J Comput Assist Tomogr* 4:159–165, 1980.
16. Howard JM, Ghent CN, Cavey LS, Flanagan PR, Valberg LS: Diagnostic efficacy in the detection of body iron overload. *Gastroenterology* 84:209–215, 1983.
17. Mitnick JS, Bosniak MA, Megibow AJ, Karpatkin M, Feiner HD, Kutin N, Natta FN, Piomelli S: CT in beta-thalassemia: iron deposition in the liver, spleen, and lymph nodes. *AJR* 136:1191–1194, 1981.
18. Berger PE, Kuhn JP: Computed tomography of the hepatobiliary system. *Radiol Clin North Am* 19:436–438, 1981.
19. Goldberg HI, Cann CE, Moss AA, Ohto M, Brito A, Federle M: Non-invasive quantitation of liver iron in dogs with hemochromatosis using dual energy CT scanning. *Invest Radiol* 17:375–380, 1982.
20. Goldberg HI: Recognition of hepatocellular disorders by computed tomography. In Moss AA, Goldberg HI, Norman D (eds): *Interventional Radiologic Techniques: Computed Tomography and Ultrasonography.* New York, Academic Press, 1981, pp 265–274.
21. Royal SA, Beiderman BA, Goldberg HI, Koerper MM, Thaler MM: Detection and estimation of iron, glycogen and fat in liver of children with hepatomegaly using computed tomography. *Pediatr Res* 13:408, 1979.

Wilson's Disease

Wilson's disease, also known as hepatolenticular degeneration, is a rare, autosomal recessive inherited disorder of copper metabolism. Patients present with acute, subacute, or chronic liver disease, a disorder of the nervous system involving the motor cortex of the brain, and, occasionally, severe psychiatric disorders. Once nervous system damage has occurred, the Kayser-Fleischer ring, a characteristic corneal pigment, is invariably present (1).

The liver is the organ most commonly affected in this disorder and also is the site for the biochemical abnormalities leading to increased concentrations of copper in the body. The basal ganglia is another site affected by increased copper deposition.

The primary defect in Wilson's disease appears to be related to impaired biliary excretion of copper. The excessive absorption of copper from the gut and increased excretion of copper in the urine appear to be secondary. Impaired biliary excretion of copper may be related to the fact that hepatic lysosomes lack the normal mechanism to excrete into bile the copper that has been cleared from ceruloplasmin, a copper containing plasma glycoprotein. Although this defect may be associated with diminished production of ceruloplasmin, the exact role of ceruloplasmin is unclear, as some patients with Wilson's disease have normal or near normal levels of the protein (1).

During the initial stage of the disease, copper accumulates in the liver until all the hepatic binding sites are filled. Copper then gradually accumulates to a toxic level in other organs, specifically the brain, kidney, and eye.

Clinical Findings

Wilson's disease usually affects children, adolescents, or young adults. Patients over the age of 40 rarely present with symptoms of Wilson's disease. Clinical manifestations of copper excess are rare before age 6, and one-half of untreated patients remain asymptomatic to age 16. Wilson's disease occurs in Jews of Eastern European origin, Arabs, southern Italians, Japanese, Chinese, Indians, and any community having a high intermarriage rate.

In children, liver disease predominates, and patients present with a variety of clinical disorders. They may have progressive jaundice, ascites, or fulminant hepatitis. Acute intravascular hemolysis may be due to destruction of erythrocytes by a sudden flux of copper from the necrotic hepatocytes. Chronic active hepatitis presents at 10–30 years of age with jaundice, high transaminase levels, and hypergammaglobulinemia. The picture closely resembles other forms of chronic active hepatitis. The patient may also present with insidiously developing cirrhosis. Vascular spiders, splenomegaly, ascites, and portal hypertension may be present.

Neuropsychiatric changes become increasingly important in the older child. Patients presenting after the age of 20 usually have neurological symptoms arising from basal ganglia dysfunction. Resting and intention tremors, spasticity, rigidity, chorea, drooling, dysphagia, and dysarthria are common. Sensory changes are extremely rare. Dystonia carries a very poor prognosis. Psychiatric disturbances range from neuroses to manic depressive and other psychoses. Some patients may show only a slow deterioration of personality (1).

Pathology

Pathological evidence of accumulated copper occurs first in the liver. The characteristic liver lesion is a postnecrotic necrosis, although all grades of change from periportal fibrosis to a coarse, macronodular cirrhosis may be seen. This develops slowly over the years and presumably is related to the rate of copper deposition.

Abnormal fat and glycogen deposits are the earliest findings seen by light microscopy. Liver cells show multiple nuclei, clumped glycogen, and glycogen vacuolization of the nuclei. Later, fat becomes more prominent and early fibrosis can be seen spreading from the portal triads. Copper is usually periportal in distribution and associated with atypical lipofucsin deposits. The rate and mode of progression from this initial steatosis and fibrosis to cirrhosis are variable. Modest infiltrates of mononuclear cells are not uncommonly associated with abnormal collagen deposits. In other instances, a clinical and histological picture of chronic active hepatitis with piecemeal necrosis, erosion of marginal plates, and parenchymal collapse develops. This florid hepatitis may subside spontaneously, with progression toward postnecrotic cirrhosis, or escalate suddenly to fulminant hepatitis.

The swollen, fatty cells are eventually replaced by inflammatory cells and fibrous tissue leading to portal hypertension, splenomegaly, and esophageal varices. In the final stages of untreated disease, the liver is composed of few remaining hepatocytes, consisting of fat-laden, copper-rich cells (1).

The brain shows changes primarily in the basal ganglia. The pathologic changes involve principally the lentiform nucleus and to a lesser extent the cortex, cerebellum, subthalamic nucleus, red nucleus, dentate nucleus, substantia nigra, and thalamus. There is disruption of the spongy tissue and glycogen granules in the brain cells. Disintegration of cortical nerve cells proceeds in some cases to actual cavitation of the basal ganglia. Computed tomography has been useful in demonstrating the brain lesions in patients with Wilson's disease (2).

The Kayser-Fleischer ring is due to brownish-green pigment in Descemet's membrane lining the posterior surface of the cornea (1).

The kidney shows fatty and hydropic change with copper deposition in the proximal convoluted tubules. Increased copper in the kidney, however, does not usually alter kidney function. Hematuria, proteinuria, the Fanconi syndrome, and renal tubular acidosis rarely occur (1).

Radiology

Liver CT and MRI may be disappointing in Wilson's disease as the picture may not be differentiable from cirrhosis (3). Fatty infiltration and excess copper can cancel each other out in advanced disease, so that high CT density may not be seen. The asymptomatic heterozygote carrier state for Wilson's disease may be detected incidentally on abdominal CT. In these instances excess copper in the liver causes increased hepatic attenuation identical to hemochromatosis (4). Perhaps dual energy scanning will be able to quantify hepatic copper in Wilson's disease. MRI is discussed further in the chapter on MRI of the liver. Skeletal changes are seen in patients with Wilson's disease and include demineralization of bone, premature osteoarthritis, Schmorl's nodes of the spine, osteochondritis dissecans, and periosteal reaction about the trochanters (5). A high incidence of cholelithiasis is present in patients with Wilson's disease, probably due to a combination of hemolysis of red cells damaged by copper and hypersplenism in those patients with portal hypertension (6). Radionuclide scanning and sonography do not show findings other than those of chronic liver disease.

REFERENCES

1. Walshe JM: Wilson's disease (hepatolenticular degeneration). In Bockus HL (ed): *Gastroenterology*. Philadelphia, W. B. Saunders, 1976, pp 492–497.
2. Kvicala V, Vymazal J, Nevsimalova S: Computed tomography of Wilson's disease. *AJNR* 4:429, 1983.
3. Lawler GA, Pennock JM, Steiner RE, Jenkins WJ, Sherlock S, Young IR: Nuclear magnetic resonance (NMR) imaging in Wilson's disease. *J Comput Assist Tomogr* 7:18, 1983.
4. Mayer DP, Kressel HY, Soloway RS: Asymptomatic carrier state in Wilson's disease. *J Comput Assist Tomogr* 7:146–147, 1983.
5. Mindelzun R, Elkin M, Schienberg IH et al: Skeletal changes in Wilson's disease: a radiological study. *Radiology* 94:127–132, 1970.
6. Girdany B: The abdomen and gastrointestinal tract. In Silverman FN (ed): Caffey's Pediatric X-ray Diagnosis. Chicago, Year Book, 1985, p 1378.

Granulomatous Diseases of the Liver

Granulomatous disease of the liver denotes the presence of a focal inflammatory process in the liver substance with histologic features of a granuloma. The term granulomatous hepatitis has also been used to describe this condition, but it is not accurate since the lesion is not a hepatitis and hepatocellular dysfunction is not commonly associated (1).

Granulomas of the liver may be found in patients of any age, sex, or race. Presenting complaints are often vague and nonspecific: fever, weight loss, malaise, and anorexia. Presenting signs include hepatomegaly, splenomegaly, jaundice, lymphadenopathy, and skin lesions. It is important to elicit historical information such as contact with or previous treatment for tuberculosis, syphilis or other infections, exposure to drugs or chemicals, contact with animals or ticks, or travel to tropical locations where unusual parasites are endemic.

Pathology

A host of causes of granulomatous disease of the liver has been elucidated, including viral, bacterial, fungal, and parasitic infections, chronic granulomatous disease of childhood, sarcoidosis, Wegener's granulomatosis, and toxic reactions to a variety of drugs and chemicals (sulfonamides, phenylbutazone, halothane, allopurinol, hydralazine, quinidine, beryllium). The granulomas are nodules that are usually well circumscribed and distinct from the surrounding liver tissue. They consist of a vascularized aggregate of histiocytes and hypertrophied fibroblasts that form a round or oval shape. The granuloma may remain intact or undergo caseous, suppurative, or granulomatous necrosis (2). Specific diagnosis of the disease process producing the granulomatous reaction in the liver by histologic appearance is often impossible. Some diseases, however, produce a fairly specific granulomatous reaction. In sarcoidosis there is minimal or central necrosis in contrast to the caseating necrosis caused by tuberculosis. At least 20% of the time, no specific etiology for granulomas of the liver is found (3).

Tuberculosis

The liver is almost always seeded during the hematogenous phase of tuberculosis but in most instances there are few clinical abnormalities (4). Usually the only residuum is one or several small granulomas. Liver involvement is common in miliary tuberculosis with clinical hepatomegaly and sometimes jaundice. The miliary tubercle consists of a mass of epithelioid cells, lymphocytes and giant cells, and acid fast bacilli may be seen. Miliary tubercles may coalesce to form larger tuberculomas. Early in the course of miliary TB a biopsy may disclose only small, noncaseating granulomas difficult to differentiate from sarcoidosis (5).

Radiology

The appearance of multiple, small intrahepatic calcifications due to old tuberculous granulomas is familiar to all, whether on plain film or CT. On ultrasound they are small, shadowing echogenicities. Miliary tuberculosis generally has no hepatic radiologic abnormalities. We have seen one case of miliary tuberculosis in which a gallium scan showed multiple hot spots in the liver and other imaging modalities were noncontributory (Fig. 4.50).

Sarcoidosis

Noncaseating granulomatous lesions of the liver occur in all stages of sarcoidosis. Epithelioid and giant cells with portal triad predilection is found in two-thirds. In a minority of patients with sarcoid, hepatic signs and symptoms dominate the clinical picture. Hepatomegaly, jaundice, presinusoidal portal hypertension, and even hepatic failure can occur (Fig. 4.51) (5, 6).

In cases of hepatic sarcoid with portal hypertension, the hepatic vein wedge pressure is normal or slightly increased with an increased portal vein or intrasplenic pressure suggesting presinusoidal portal hypertension. The free hepatic venogram will either be normal or show minimal abnormalities (Fig. 4.52) (7). Portography will show a normal portal vein.

Histoplasmosis

The liver is second only to the spleen in the abdomen in frequency of involvement by *Histoplasma capsulatum* (1). There are no specific signs or symptoms, although hepatomegaly is not infrequent. Fever, oropharyngeal or laryngeal ulceration, pulmonary disease, or adrenal insufficiency suggest widely disseminated disease (4). Definitive diagnosis of hepatic histoplasmosis depends on demonstration of fungi in Kupffer cells. Often a nonspecific granuloma (sometimes caseating) is the only histologic finding. The radiologic appearance of granulomas in the liver due to histoplasmosis is the same as that due to tuberculosis (Fig. 4.53).

Brucellosis

Hepatic granulomas usually form in *Brucella abortus* infection although *Brucella suis* is a more invasive organism that causes hepatic suppuration occasionally followed by calcification in the liver and spleen (1). There are no specific clinical features to suggest hepatic brucellosis, and the hepatic lesions bear no relation to the severity of the infection or the patient's overall clinical status (1). Slight hepatomegaly may occur. Progression to liver fibrosis and cirrhosis has been demonstrated on rare occasions (2). The hepatic granulomas are composed of epithelioid cells and round cells and are located both within the lobule and the portal triad (5). Aspiration biopsy usually gives positive results. Precise diagnosis depends on elevation of agglutinins or complement fixation titers or culturing the organism. Radiologic examination may reveal calcification(s) in the liver or spleen.

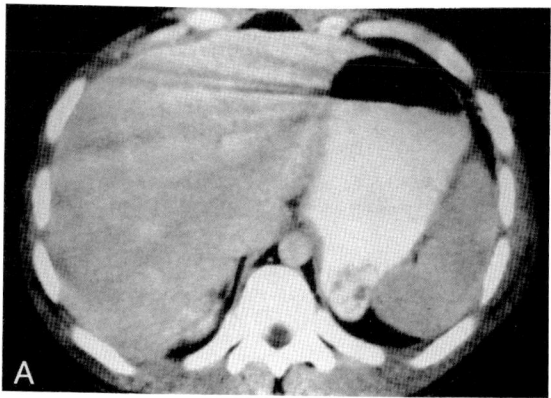
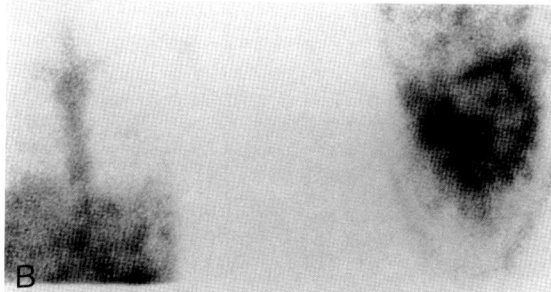

FIGURE 4.50. GALLIUM SCAN FOR MILIARY TUBERCULOSIS
A: Contrast-enhanced CT shows a normal appearing liver and spleen. Note the enhanced peritoneum. *B:* The 48-hr gallium scan with chest and upper abdomen on the left and abdomen and pelvis on the right: multiple foci of increased uptake in the liver and spleen as well as the mesentery. Tuberculous peritonitis, mesenteritis, and hepatitis in a young male patient with fever of unknown origin.

Leptospirosis

Leptospirosis is transmitted to humans by polluted water or contact with infected tissue. An

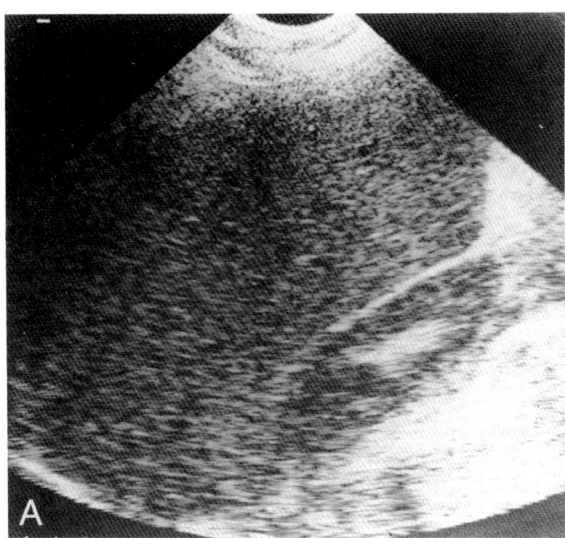
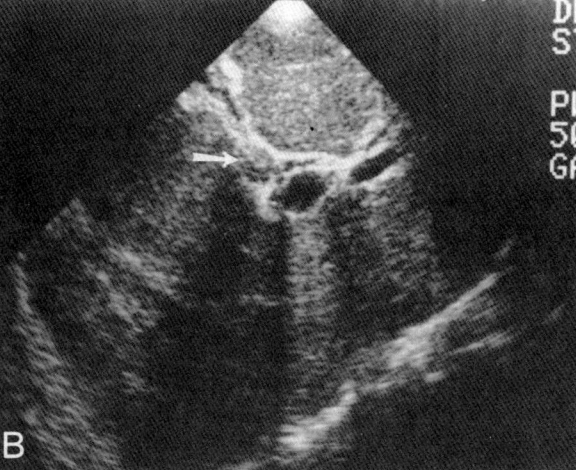
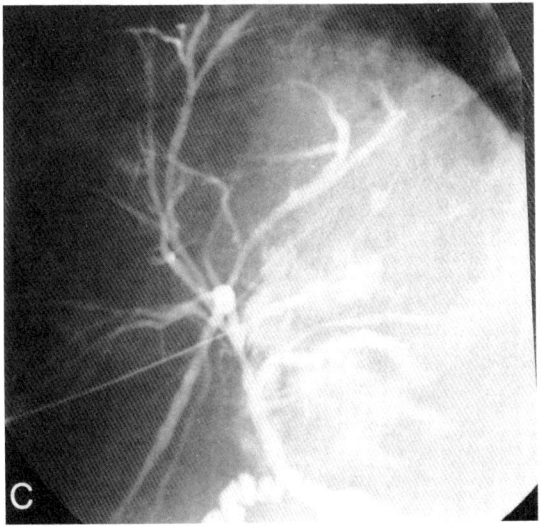

FIGURE 4.51. SARCOIDOSIS
A: Sagittal sonogram in a patient with chronic granulomatous hepatitis and portal hypertension due to sarcoid liver disease: hepatomegaly with a decrease in visibility of vascular architecture. B: Periportal adenopathy (*arrow*) on this transverse sonogram of a patient with chronic sarcoid hepatitis. Not an infrequent finding, this adenopathy can become prominent enough to cause biliary obstruction. C: ERCP (same patient as B), performed to exclude biliary tract obstruction as a contributing factor to the patient's liver disease. Splayed and stretched intrahepatic ducts, compatible with an infiltrative liver disease. Undulating right hepatic and common bile ducts, correlating well with adjacent adenopathy.

abrupt onset of high fever, headache, nausea, and vomiting are common presenting symptoms. Jaundice is present in as many as 75% of patients with *Leptospira icterohemorrhagicae* infection, but less than 10% when other leptospira organisms are the offending agents (4), and hepatomegaly and liver tenderness are usually present when there is jaundice. A bleeding tendency occurs in 30–50% of patients and hemorrhage can be severe. Leptospirosis produces focal hepatic necrosis and/or cholangitis. A diffuse, nonspecific degeneration of hepatocytes and usually Kupffer cells occurs. Identification of leptospira organisms in systemic infection is made by culture and/or serologic study with antibodies against leptospiral serotypes. Liver involvement is confirmed by the presence of leptospira organisms on histologic examination. Ultrasound would be expected to show findings similar to those in acute viral hepatitis (hypoechoic liver

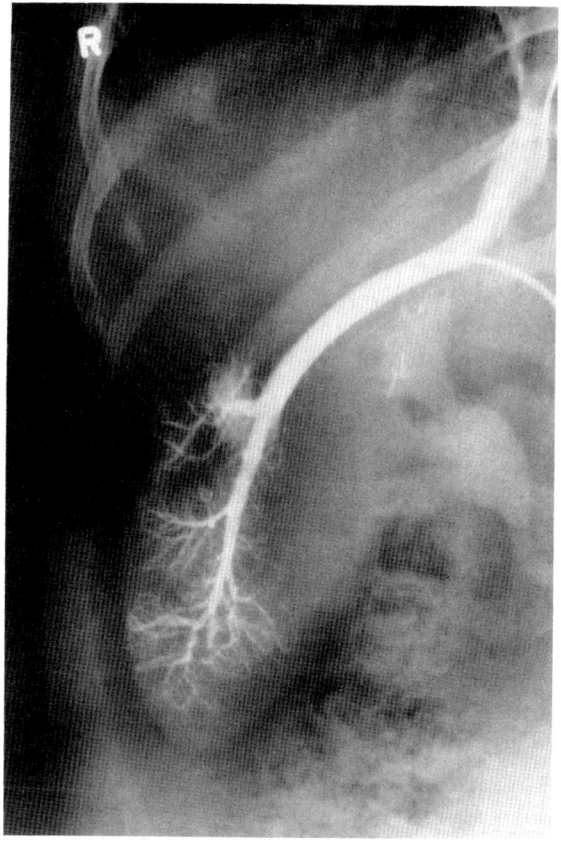

FIGURE 4.52. SARCOID LIVER DISEASE
Free hepatic venogram showing loss of fifth-order branches which is considered a mild abnormality. The patient had presinusoidal portal hypertension. (From Cavaluzzi JA, Sheff R, Harrington DP, Kaufman SL, Barth K, Maddrey WC, White RI Jr: Hepatic venography and wedge hepatic vein pressure measurements in diffuse liver disease. *AJR* 129:441–446, 1977.)

parenchyma and bright portal venous walls) in acute leptospirosis.

REFERENCES

1. Sherlock S: *Diseases of the Liver and Biliary System.* Oxford, Blackwell Scientific, 1981, pp 418–423.
2. Berk JE, Cohen M: Granulomas of the liver. In Bockus et al. (eds): *Gastroenterology.* Philadelphia, W. B. Saunders, 1976, pp 288–298.
3. Spiro HM: *Clinical Gastroenterology.* New York, Macmillan, 1977, p 1120.
4. Leevy CM: *Diseases of the Liver and Biliary Tract.* Chicago, Yearbook, 1976, pp 33–41.
5. Edmondson HA, Schiff L: Needle biopsy of the liver. In Schiff HL (ed): *Diseases of the Liver.* Philadelphia, J. B. Lippincott, 1975, pp 262–263.
6. Maddrey WC, Johns CJ, Boitnott JK, Iber FL: Sarcoidosis and chronic hepatic disease. *Medicine* 49:375–395, 1970.
7. Cavaluzzi JA, Sheff R, Harrington DP, Kaufman SL,

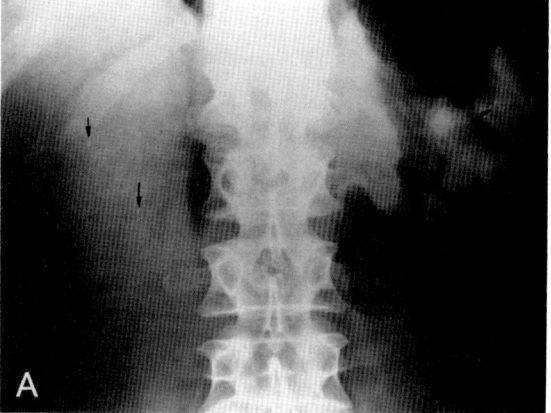

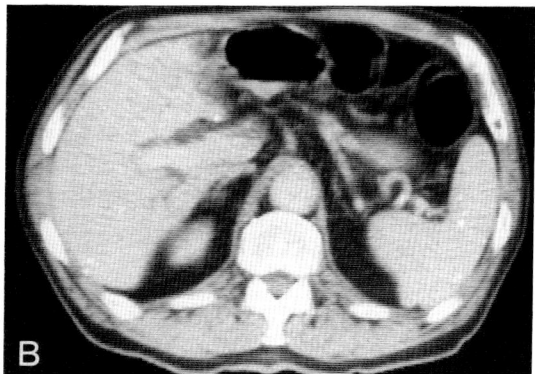

FIGURE 4.53. LIVER AND SPLEEN CALCIFICATIONS CONSISTENT WITH PRIOR TUBERCULOSIS OR HISTOPLASMOSIS
A: Plain film. *B:* Computed tomography.

Barth K, Maddrey WC, White RI Jr: Hepatic venography and wedge hepatic vein pressure measurements in diffuse liver disease. *AJR* 129:441–446, 1977.

Schistosomiasis

One of the most common and most serious parasitic diseases in man, schistosomiasis is estimated to affect 150–200 million people with a prevalence of 70% in endemic areas (1, 2). *Schistosoma mansoni* occurs in Africa, the Middle East, South America, and the West Indies, *Schistosoma japonicum* occurs in China, the Philippines, and Japan, and *Schistosoma haematobium* occurs mostly in North Africa and the Middle East. Hepatic involvement is one of the severest clinical forms of schistosomiasis, and although identical in the three types of schistosomiasis, it is much more likely to occur in *S. japonicum* or *S. mansoni* than *S. haematobium*.

Life Cycle and Pathophysiology

The larvae shed by snails (intermediate host) into fresh water enter through the intact skin or buccal mucosa of man (definitive host) into lymphatic channels. They migrate into the mesenteric and portal veins, where, as adults, they deposit ova which embolize distally in the portal system. The host reacts to the ova with a granulomatous inflammation, which becomes replaced by fibrous tissue leading to periportal fibrosis (1, 2). Heavy, chronic infestations lead to progressive intrahepatic portal vein occlusion. presinusoidal portal hypertension, varices, and splenomegaly. Schistosomiasis is the most common cause of portal hypertension in the world.

Clinical Findings

Since parenchymal destruction occurs very late in the course of the disease, if at all, clinical and laboratory signs of hepatocellular dysfunction are usually absent, and the chief problem is portal hypertension and bleeding varices. Treatment is directed toward control of variceal hemorrhage.

Pathology

On gross examination, the cut surface of the liver shows thickened, fibrotic portal tracts extending from the porta hepatis toward the periphery. Slight external depressions are visible on the surface of the uncut specimen, marking the underlying fibrosis (1). This macroscopic appearance of periportal fibrosis, termed "clay-pipestem fibrosis," is pathognomonic for hepatic schistosomiasis. Histologically, ova can be seen within the fibrotic bands in varying numbers (1). Thick, newly formed capillary networks surround the portal venules giving an angiomatous appearance to the granulomas and the fibrosis (2). These capillaries probably form intrahepatic portasystemic shunts (2).

Plain Films and Contrast Examinations

A liver containing more than 100 million eggs demonstrates advanced fibrosis and calcification dense enough to be detectable on conventional radiographs (3). However, in most cases of hepatic schistosomiasis, calcification is too faint to be detected on plain films. Splenomegaly is frequent. A barium meal will demonstrate esophageal and sometimes gastric varices when hepatic schistosomiasis has advanced far enough to cause portal hypertension.

Ultrasound

Densely echoic thick bands replace the normal portal venous system radiating from the porta hepatis to the liver periphery (Fig. 4.54). These bands are more numerous and larger centrally and are about 5–20 mm in cross-sectional diameter (1, 2). When imaged longitudinally the bands are tubular and they are round to oval in cross-section. A "bird's claw" appearance is present at bifurcation points (1). Within the bands a central lucency representing the enclosed portal vein (either patent or filled with fresh clot) is often seen (1, 2). The lucency can be either circular and central, ovoid and eccentric, or linear depending on the plane of section (2). Although probably pathognomonic of schistomiasis in the proper clinical context, failure to find these sonographic features of pipestem fibrosis does not exclude the diagnosis (2). Associated findings include small, normal or large size with smooth contour (liver), splenomegaly, ascites, portasystemic collaterals, and occasionally cholelithiasis (1).

Computed Tomography

Corresponding to the bands of periportal fibrosis seen sonographically and pathologically, CT can demonstrate curvilinear bands of increased attenuation within the liver extending to its periphery and indenting its surface (3). The high density of these bands is probably due to dystrophic calcification.

Angiography

Hemodynamics are those of presinusoidal block and essentially the same as those of portal vein thrombosis: normal hepatic venous outflow, decreased portal blood flow and compensatorily increased hepatic arterial flow (4). Pre-hepatic portal vein pressures are elevated but the wedge hepatic pressure is normal or only slightly elevated. Therefore, celiac arteriography will demonstrate dilatation of the hepatic artery and its branches and possibly varices involving the left gastric and inferior mesenteric veins. The venous phases of celiac and superior mesenteric angiography will show a patent portal vein and intrahepatic portal vein branches and hepatic venography is normal. Angiography has the same two roles to play in schistosomiasis as in other causes

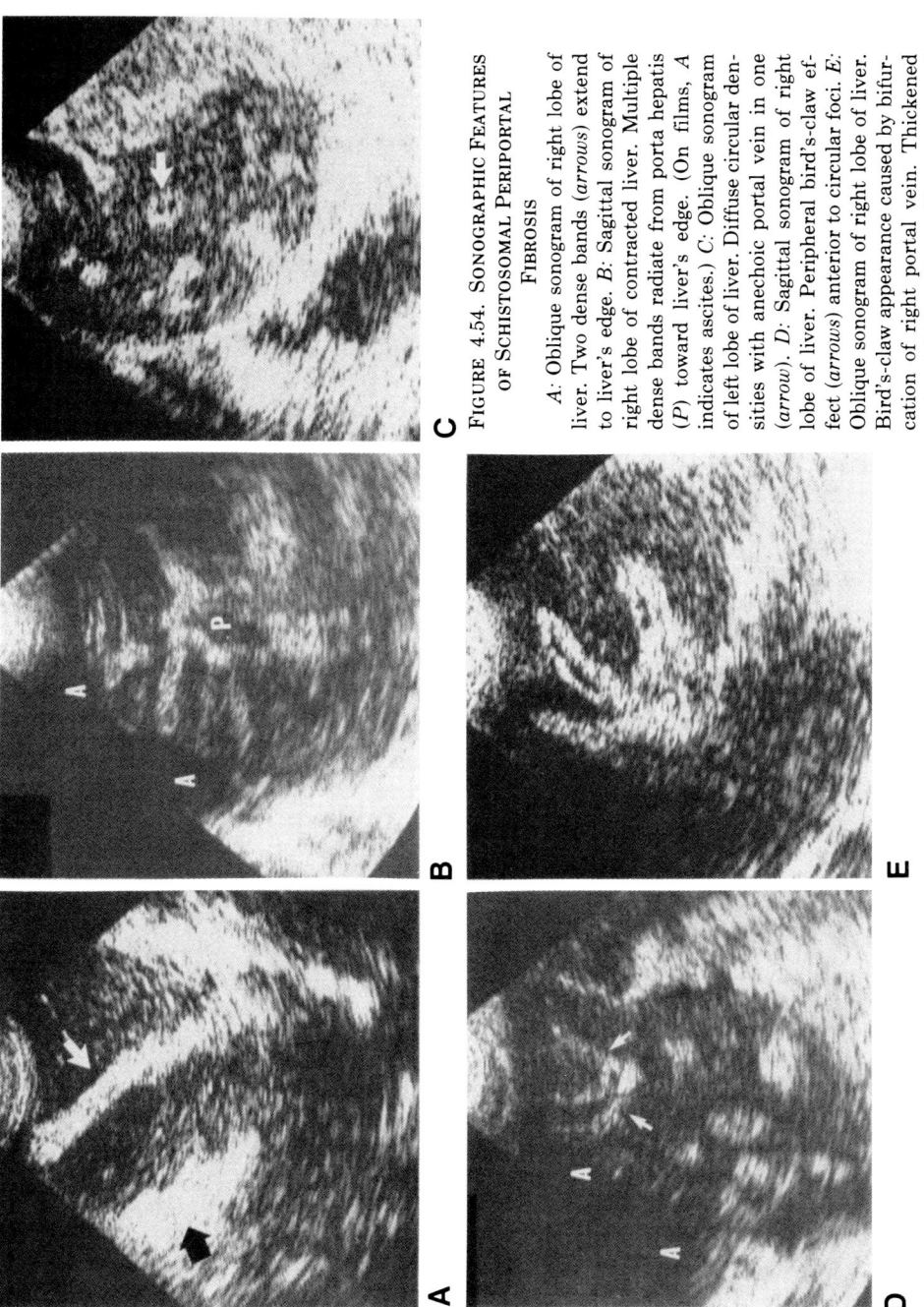

FIGURE 4.54. SONOGRAPHIC FEATURES OF SCHISTOSOMAL PERIPORTAL FIBROSIS

A: Oblique sonogram of right lobe of liver. Two dense bands (*arrows*) extend to liver's edge. *B*: Sagittal sonogram of right lobe of contracted liver. Multiple dense bands radiate from porta hepatis (*P*) toward liver's edge. (On films, *A* indicates ascites.) *C*: Oblique sonogram of left lobe of liver. Diffuse circular densities with anechoic portal vein in one (*arrow*). *D*: Sagittal sonogram of right lobe of liver. Peripheral bird's-claw effect (*arrows*) anterior to circular foci. *E*: Oblique sonogram of right lobe of liver. Bird's-claw appearance caused by bifurcation of right portal vein. Thickened periportal tissue is readily seen around two anechoic portal vein branches. (From Fataar S, Bassiony H, Satyanath S, Vassileva J, Hanna RM: Characteristic Sonographic Features of Schistosomal Periportal Fibrosis. *AJR* 143:69–71, 1984.)

of portal hypertension: delineating of vascular anatomy prior to shunt surgery and, occasionally, as a temporizing measure, percutaneous variceal obliteration.

REFERENCES

1. Fataar S, Bassiony H, Satyanath S, Vassileva J, Hanna RM: Characteristic sonographic features of schistosomal periportal fibrosis. *AJR* 143:69–71, 1984.
2. Hussain S, Hawass ND, Zaidi AJ: Ultrasonographic diagnosis of schistosomal periportal fibrosis. *J Ultrasound Med* 3:449–452, 1984.
3. Hamada M, Ohta M, Yasuda Y, Fukae S, Fukushima M, Nakayama S, Akagawa H, Ohtake H: Hepatic calcification in schistosomiasis japonica. *J Comput Assist Tomogr* 6:76–78, 1984.
4. Reuter SR, Redman HC: *Gastrointestinal Angiography.* Philadelphia, W. B. Saunders, 1977, pp 340–343.

Thorotrast-Induced Disease in the Liver and Spleen

Thorotrast is a 20% colloidal solution of thorium dioxide in aqueous dextran introduced by Bluhbaum et al. (1) in Germany in 1928 as a radiographic contrast agent. The high atomic number of thorium made it an excellent contrast material. It was used primarily for cerebral angiography. Ninety percent of the estimated 50,000 to 100,000 patients who received it were studied for this purpose. Thorotrast was also used for hepatosplenography, peripheral angiography, and visualization of various body cavities. Nineteen years after its introduction, MacMahon et al. (2) reported the first case of a Thorotrast-induced angiosarcoma of the liver. Since that time numerous studies have reported additional cases of this association, as well as other Thorotrast-related neoplasms, in particular, cholangiocarcinoma and hepatocellular carcinoma.

^{232}Th is produced when ^{236}U decays by emission of α particles. Its physical half-life is 1.4×10^7 years. In the process of its decay to stable ^{208}Pb, thorium and its daughter products emit 6 α particles and 4 β particles as well as several γ rays. The energy emitted per second for each gram of thorium is 1.7×10 MeV. This value increases to 1.5×10^5 MeV as the daughter decay products establish equilibrium. The biological half-life is 400 years as excretion of thorium is nearly negligible. Typically, a 15–75-ml dose (3–15 g) of Thorotrast was administered for angiography (3).

Thorotrast particles of 3–10 μm are phagocytized by the reticuloendothelial cells of the liver, spleen, and bone marrow with slow redistribution to the lymphatics. The liver absorbs 70% of the injected dose, the spleen 20%, and the remaining dose is shared primarily by the bone marrow and lymph nodes.

Several authors have tried to estimate the radiation dose involved in a typical diagnostic study using Thorotrast. Kaul and Noffz (4) stated that a 25-ml dose of Thorotrast will, over a 30-year period, yield a mean dose of 750 rads to the liver, 2100 rads to the spleen, and 270 rads to the bone marrow. Looney (5), Kato et al. (6) and Janower et al. (7) have suggested similar figures. All point out that there is great variability in any given patient and the dosage figures may vary by as much as a factor of 1000. In view of the high radiation burden to the liver and spleen, it is not at all surprising that increasing numbers of patients exposed to Thorotrast have developed hepatic angiosarcoma as well as cholangiocarcinoma and hepatocellular carcinoma (8, 9). The latency period from Thorotrast exposure to the development of liver cancer is 26 years (3); however, this ranges from 3 to 40 years (10). Kato et al. (6) found that some radiation effects were dose dependent, in particular a decreased latency with an increased dose rate. The discovery of Thorotrast-induced cancers (as well as the severe soft-tissue fibrotic reaction caused by its extravasation) led to the discontinuation of Thorotrast in the 1950s.

Plain Radiography

Radiographs obtained shortly after the administration of thorium dioxide show uniform and smooth distribution throughout the liver and spleen, corresponding to the location of reticuloendothelial cells (Fig. 4.55).

Radiographs obtained years later reveal a different, but characteristic pattern (Figs. 4.56–4.59) (5, 8, 11). The initial homogeneous hepatic pattern develops a lacy, reticular appearance as Thorotrast slowly migrates to the lymphatic system. The reticular pattern is most apparent in the periphery of the right lobe, especially at the inferior margin. The spleen becomes markedly dense and small over time due to superimposition of punctate opacities. As Thorotrast migrates to the lymphatics, regional lymph nodes accumulate thorium dioxide. Deposits are greatest in peripancreatic and periportal nodes, although involvement of perisplenic nodes does occur. The lymph nodes are metallic density, and irregularly shaped. In addition, small linear densities extending from the nodes may be seen, representing opacified lymphatic channels. When the ho-

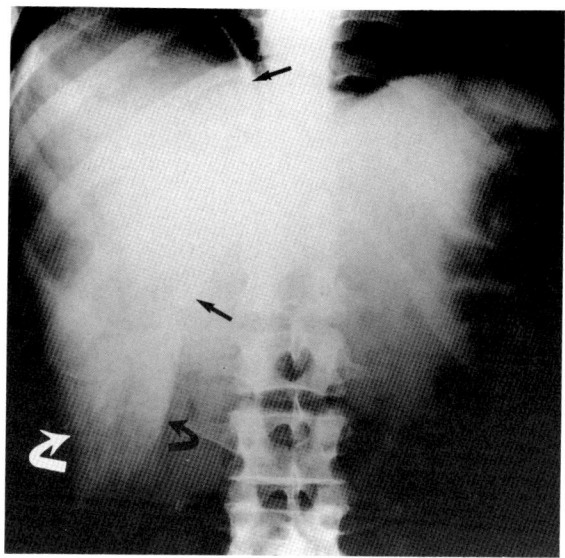

FIGURE 4.55. DIAGNOSTIC THOROTRAST HEPATOGRAM
About 24 h after injection, a large lucent liver mass (*arrows*) is seen. Remaining parenchyma at the tip of the right lobe is radiodense (*curved arrows*) save for tubular lucencies representing unopacified portal veins. No contrast in lymph nodes yet.

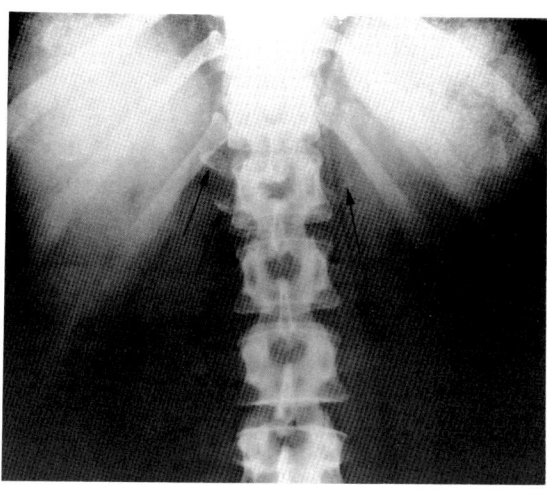

FIGURE 4.56. EARLY MIGRATION PATTERN
Early migration pattern: slightly dense liver with punctate opacities (hard to reproduce). Dense, punctate normal-sized spleen. Opaque lymph nodes (*arrows*).

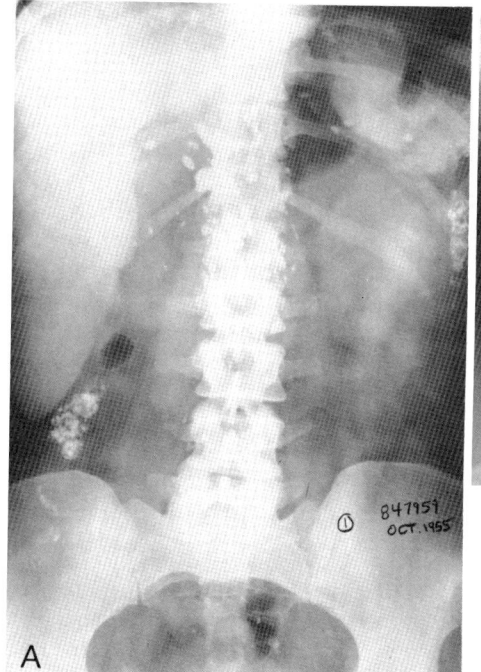

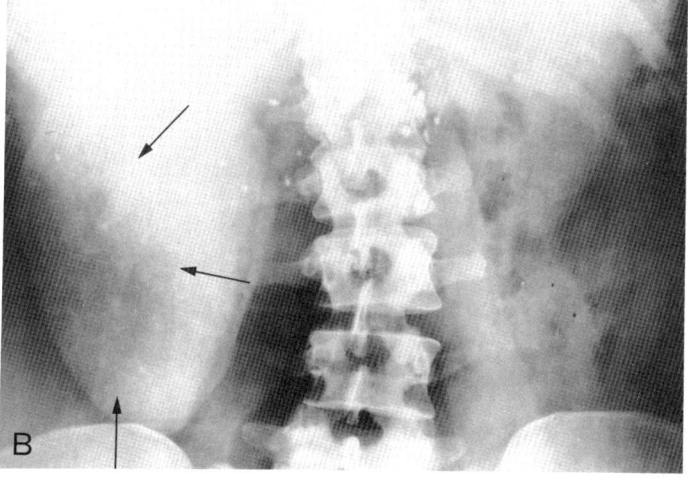

FIGURE 4.57. SEVERAL YEARS AFTER THOROTRAST ADMINISTRATION
A: Several years after injection: uniformly radiodense liver, punctate density in spleen, many opacified nodes. Film is from an oral cholecystogram. *B:* Coned-down view of right lobe of liver 2 yr after (*A*). Ill-defined lucency (*arrows*) within dense finely punctate liver represents cholangiocarcinoma.

mogeneous increased hepatic density disappears, detection of hepatic masses by plain radiography is nearly impossible. Some splenic masses will be visible as filling defects in the Thorotrast-laden spleen (Fig. 4.59).

Pathology

Light and electron microscopy have demonstrated thorium dioxide in the Kupffer cells and macrophages, both free within the cytoplasm and

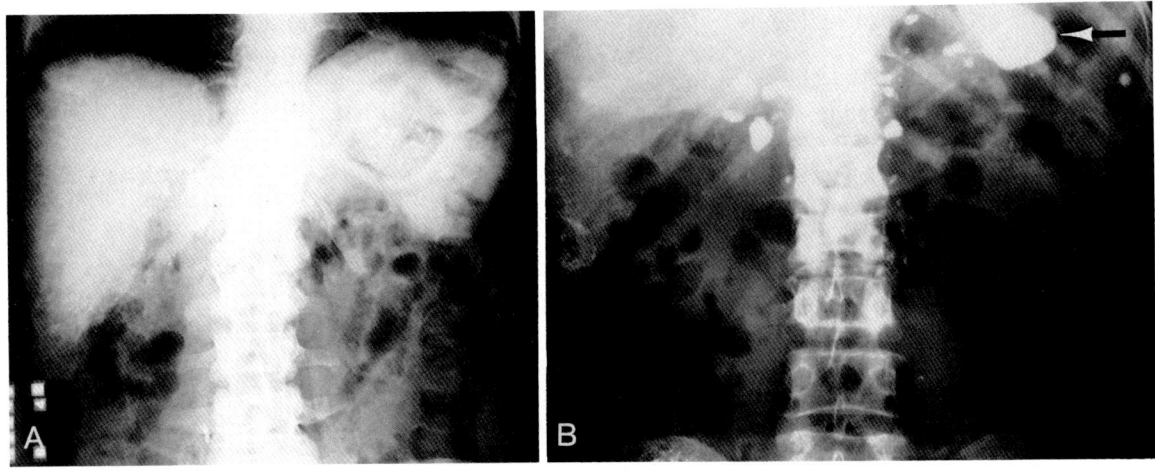

FIGURE 4.58. LATE THOROTRAST

A: Densely reticulated liver. Spleen dense but normal size. Many opaque nodes. *B:* Small liver with reticular pattern most prominent at tip of right lobe. Spleen (*arrows*) very radiodense and small. Many opaque nodes.

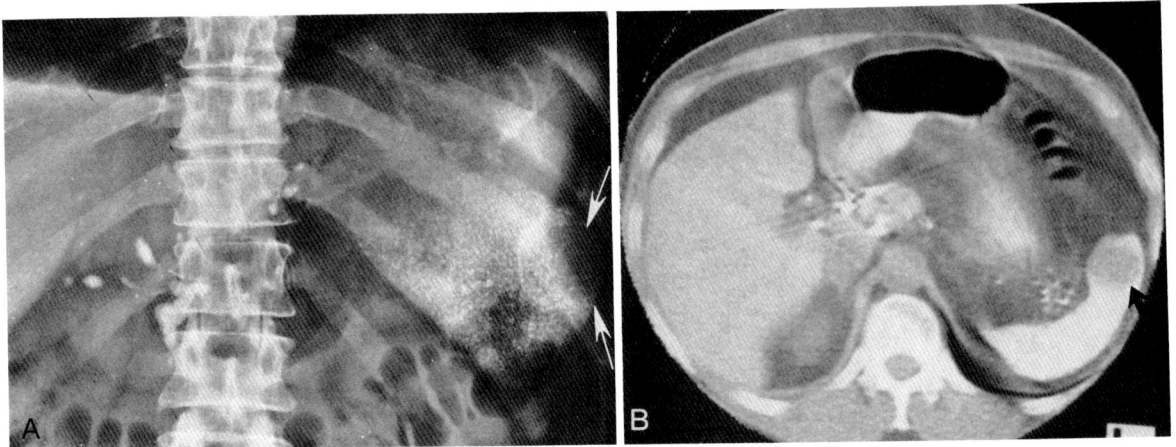

FIGURE 4.59. PRIMARY SPLENIC ANGIOSARCOMA

A: Punctate densities in spleen displaced by a filling defect (*arrows*). *B:* Corresponding CT. Tumor (*arrows*) is a defect in the nearly homogeneously dense appearing spleen. Adjusting the window width and center would bring out the punctate opacities. Note calcified nodes and normal hepatic attenuation.

within phagosomes (Fig. 4.60). The macrophages and Kupffer cells gradually transfer thorium to the portal triads. Direct thorium uptake by hepatocytes has been documented followed by excretion into bile. Small particles have been observed in hepatocytes as long as 30 years after injection (12). Pathologic studies have shown that fibrosis occurs to variable degrees around the portal triads as well as the centrilobular veins (12, 13). Thorium-containing brown granules are scattered throughout the liver, surrounded by collagen bundles in the portal triads.

Hepatic veno-occlusive disease producing postsinusoidal obstruction and portal hypertension has been observed (13). Although the pathogenesis is not clear, it is felt to be secondary to radiation-induced endothelial injury to the central vein with subsequent fibrosis. Peliosis hepatis has been reported to occur in Thorotrast exposure. Okuda et al. (14) suggested that a weakness in the reticular framework leads to sinusoidal dilatation with formation of large blood-filled cystic collections.

Most reports have described angiosarcomas accounting for 50% of the Thorotrast-associated neoplasms, while cholangiocarcinoma and hepatocellular carcinoma accounted for the remaining half (7). A study in Japan found that half of the Thorotrast-associated malignancies were cholangiocarcinomas and the remaining half

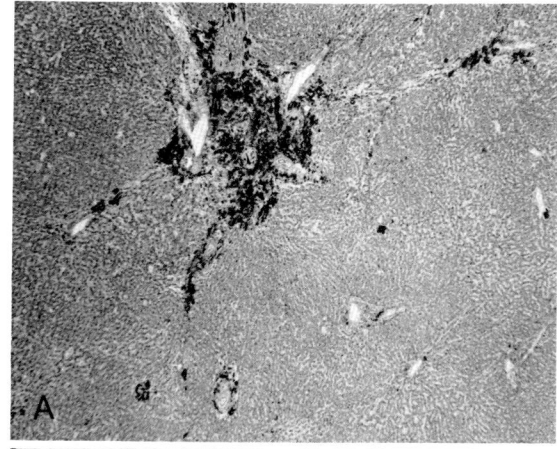
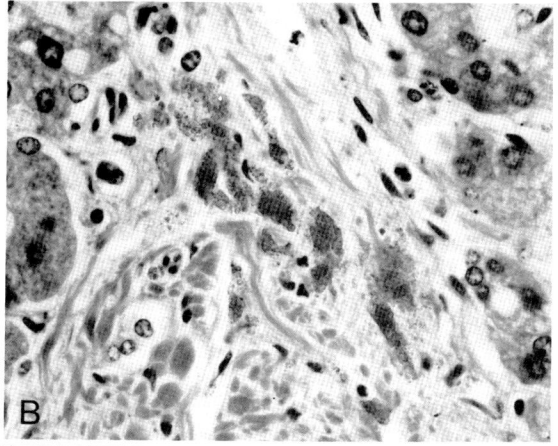
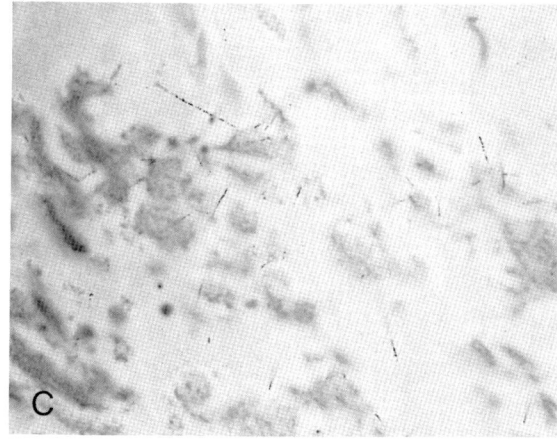

FIGURE 4.60. ELECTRON MICROSCOPY DEMONSTRATING THOROTRAST

A: Low power photomicrograph showing Thorotrast (dark material) predominantly in portal macrophages, and also in small clusters of Kupffer cells (AFIP negative 85-9111, ×25). *B:* High power photomicrograph showing granular aggregates of Thorotrast in center of field (AFIP negative 85-9109, ×630). *C:* Autoradiograph showing alpha tracks in photographic emulsion overlying Thorotrast (AFIP negative 85-9110, ×630).

were divided between angiosarcomas and hepatocellular carcinomas (15). A possible explanation for this discrepancy may be related to the smaller doses used in Japan. Dahlgren (16) has enumerated the three following criteria for implicating Thorotrast: (*a*) thorium particles must be found in the immediate vicinity of the tumor, (*b*) the latency period must be long (greater than 20 years), and (*c*) the radiation dose must be sufficiently high.

Angiosarcoma

Angiosarcomas are exceedingly rare tumors. The reported incidence of this neoplasm varies from 0.14 per million to 0.25 per million (17). Epidemiological studies in New York confirmed that Thorotrast-induced angiosarcoma was increasing in the 1970s (18). In Japan the incidence of angiosarcoma is still increasing. The longer latency period is probably due to the smaller doses employed in Japan. It is estimated that 7–10% of all hepatic angiosarcomas are Thorotrast-related (9).

Clinically, patients with angiosarcoma present with epigastric pain, jaundice, weakness, nausea, malaise, and occasionally catastrophic hemoperitoneum (19, 20). Liver function tests are abnormal. In particular, the γ-glutamyl transpeptidase, as well as alkaline phosphatase, is almost always elevated (21). Angiosarcomas are frequently multinodular, occasionally solitary, and often red-purple from hemorrhage (2, 9, 17). Histologically, precursor stages can be identified consisting of regions of combined hyperplasia of hepatocytes and a variety of sinusoidal and presinusoidal cells associated with an excess of reticulin and sinusoidal dilatation (9). (See section on angiosarcoma of the liver for further details.)

Cholangiocarcinoma

Patients with cholangiocarcinoma present with symptoms similar to other hepatic tumors, complaining of vague right upper quadrant pain, nausea, vomiting, weight loss, weakness, and jaundice.

As with the Thorotrast-associated angiosarcomas, the γ-glutamyl transpeptidase and alkaline phosphatase are usually elevated. Pathologically, Thorotrast-associated cholangiocarcinomas are similar to other cholangiocarcinomas except that Thorotrast-associated hepatic fibrosis coexists (22). Interestingly, half of the patients in one series had associated thyroid disease (hypothyroidism and/or malignancy) (22).

Hepatocellular Carcinoma

Clinically, symptoms and signs are no different than in hepatocellular carcinomas associated with cirrhosis.

Splenic Angiosarcoma

Only about 55 cases of splenic angiosarcoma have been reported (23). They have an extremely poor prognosis with only 20% of patients surviving 6 months after diagnosis. Seventy percent metastasize to liver and about 33% undergo spontaneous rupture (21). There has only been one report of splenic angiosarcoma associated with Thorotrast (24). If angiosarcoma is present in both liver and spleen, the liver is assumed to be the primary site when precursor lesions are present in the liver (9). The low incidence of Thorotrast-induced angiosarcoma of the spleen may be explained by the underlying pathologic process in Thorotrast exposure. Fibrous replacement of the red pulp occurs, while in white pulp only arteries are recognizable. Thus, there is often complete replacement of normal splenic tissue with fibrous tissue, and therefore no normal splenic tissue remains to undergo malignant change (25). The two spleens that we have personally seen in which malignancy was present were normal or near normal in size (Fig. 4.59).

Role of Computed Tomography

As anticipated, CT is superior to plain radiography in its depiction of the presence and distribution of Thorotrast in the liver and spleen (Fig. 4.61). Ultrasound is often hampered in these patients by fibrosis and poor beam penetration. Soft tissue masses representing neoplasms in the liver, spleen, and lymph nodes (sometimes surrounding Thorotrast, due to metastatic disease) are far more likely to be detected by CT than by plain films (Figs. 4.62, 4.63). Invasion of contiguous soft-tissue structures is only shown by CT. Interestingly, Thorotrast deposition in the liver is usually of little or no help in my experience in detecting space-occupying disease because of its usually reticular, irregular distribution, whereas its more regular distribution in the spleen does facilitate mass detection. For the most part, CT detects hepatic Thorotrast-induced neoplasms as hypodense mass(es) replacing parenchyma, and splenic masses as filling defects in the Thorotrast-laden spleen. Splenic CT can depict the

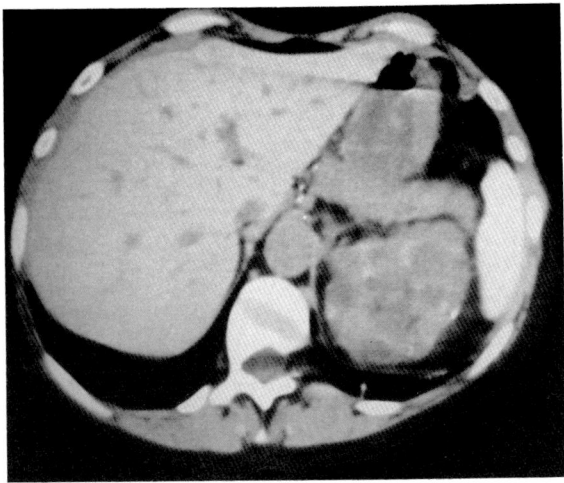

FIGURE 4.61. HOMOGENEOUSLY OPAQUE LIVER
Punctate nature of splenic opacity is barely discernible. Incidental polycystic kidneys. Plain film showed no hepatic abnormality.

spleen as homogeneously dense when plain radiography shows innumerable punctate densities; this is a function of window width and level during photography.

Differentiation among regenerating nodule(s), peliosis hepatis, and malignancy when space-occupying disease is seen in the liver in a Thorotrast patient is probably not strictly possible by CT unless ancillary findings such as adenopathy or dilated bile ducts are present. Sulfur colloid scans are likely to be contributory only if a region in question on CT is hot, suggesting regenerative nodule. Angiography may be able to differentiate between angiosarcoma and peliosis hepatis as the cause of CT-demonstrated space-occupying masses (the former classically has peripheral tumor staining in the late arterial phase; the latter does not), but more advanced cases of angiosarcoma need not demonstrate this finding (26). Dynamic CT is not likely to help, as there may be considerable overlap between CT enhancement characteristics of angiosarcoma, peliosis hepatis, and cavernous hemangioma. As far as differentiating among angiosarcoma, cholangiocarcinoma, and hepatocellular carcinoma, some CT findings suggest a specific diagnosis. Splenic metastases favor angiosarcoma, and dilated bile ducts favor cholangiocarcinoma. Spontaneous hemoperitoneum favors angiosarcoma. Prognosis is dismal with all three malignancies. A splenic space-occupying mass in a Thorotrast patient is likely to be either metastatic or primary angiosarcoma.

While cases of Thorotrast-induced malignancies peaked in the late 1970s and early 1980s,

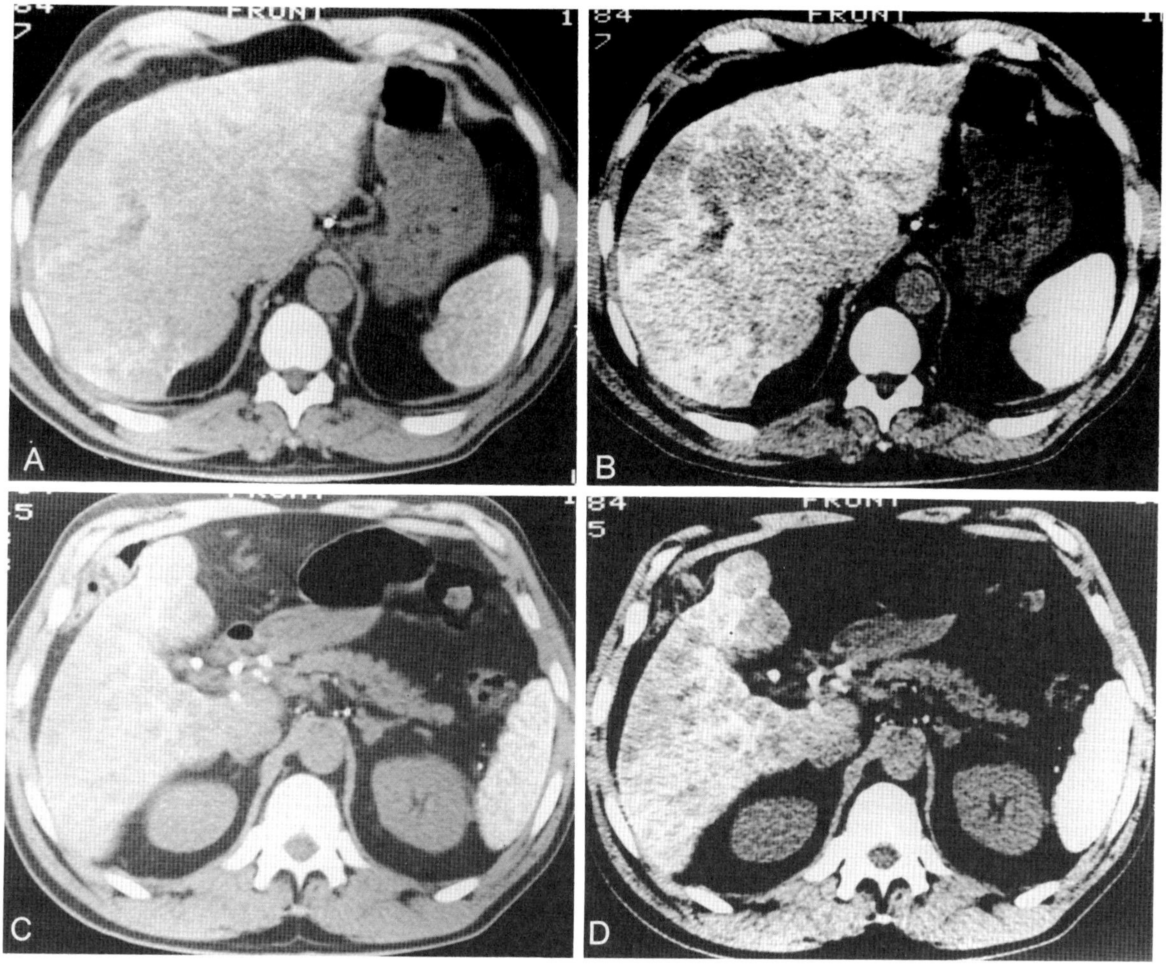

FIGURE 4.62. MULTIFOCAL HEPATOCELLULAR CARCINOMA FROM THOROTRAST
A and *C:* Window width 426, center 21: reticular hepatic densities peripherally. Punctate spleen. Radiolucent tumor in liver barely seen. *B* and *D:* Window width 100, center 43, same scans as *A* and *C*, hypodense tumor in liver seen to better advantage. Spleen now appears homogeneous.

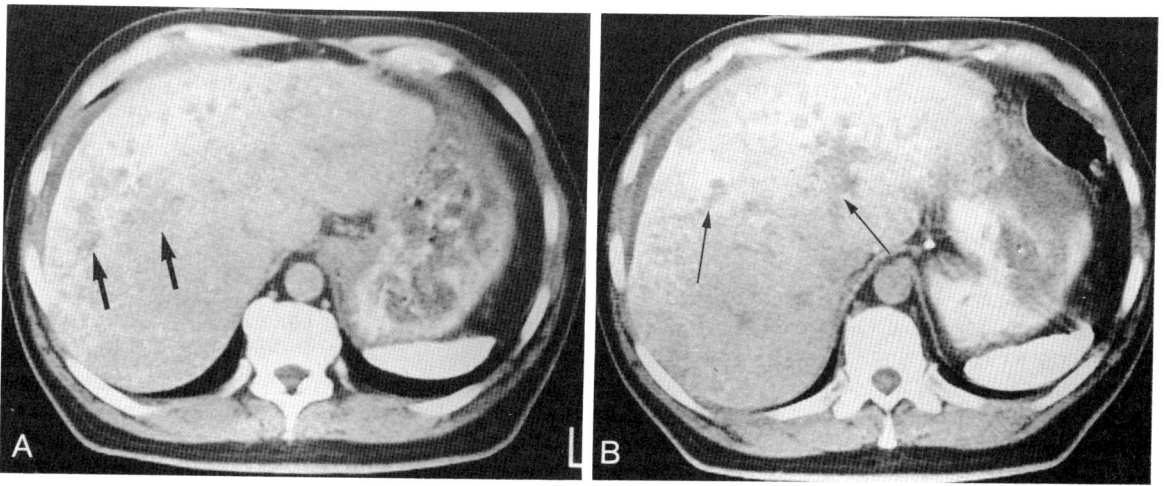

FIGURE 4.63. MULTIFOCAL CHOLANGIOCARCINOMA FROM THOROTRAST
A: Remaining hepatic thorotrast is peripheral. Hypodense region (*arrows*) represents tumor. Some lucencies are dilated ducts. *B:* Lower cut: Dilated ducts (*arrows*). Homogeneously dense spleen and ascites on *A* and *B*.

continued awareness by clinicians and radiologists will be required for some time yet to come.

REFERENCES

1. Bluhbaum T, Frik K, Kalkbrenner H: Eine neuve Anwendungsart der Kolloide in der Rontgendiagnostik. *Forschr Roentgenstr* 37:18–29, 1928.
2. MacMahon HE, Murphy AS, Bates MI: Endothelial-cell sarcoma of liver following Thorotrast injections. *Am J Pathol* 23:585–611, 1947.
3. Lightfoote JB, Heitz Jr CJ, Smolin MF: CT appearance of reticuloendothelial Thorotrast deposition with hepatic angiosarcoma. CT Clinical Symposium, Vol. 7. Milwaukee, General Electric Medical Systems, 1984.
4. Kaul A, Noffz W: Tissue dose in Thorotrast patients. *Health Phys* 35:113–121, 1978.
5. Looney WB: An investigation of the late clinical finding following Thorotrast (thorium dioxide) administration. *AJR* 83:163–185, 1960.
6. Kato Y, Mori T, Kumatori T: Estimated absorbed dose in tissues and radation effects in Japanese Thorotrast patients. *Health Phys* 44:273–279, 1983.
7. Janower ML, Miettinen OS, Flynn MJ: Effects of long-term Thorotrast exposure. *Radiology* 103:13–20, 1972.
8. Silverman PM, Ram PC, Korobkin M: CT appearance of abdominal Thorotrast deposition and Thorotrast-induced angiosarcoma of the liver. *J Comput Assist Thomogr* 4:655–658, 1983.
9. Popper H, Thomas LB, Telles NC, Falk H, Selikoff IJ: Development of hepatic angiosarcoma in man induced by vinyl chloride, Thorotrast, and arsenic. *Am J Pathol* 92:349–369, 1978.
10. Christensen P, Madsen MR, Jensen OM: Latency of Thorotrast-induced renal tumours. *Scand J Urol Nephrol* 17:127–130, 1983.
11. Gondos B: Late clinical roentgen observations following Thorotrast administration. *Clin Radiol* 24:195–203, 1973.
12. Irie H, Mori W: Long term effects of thorium dioxide (Thorotrast) administration on human liver. *Acta Pathol Jpn* 34(2):221–223, 1984.
13. Dejgaard A, Krogsgaard K, Jacobsen M: Veno-occlusive disease and peliosis of the liver after Thorotrast administration. *Virchows Arch (Pathol Anat)* 403:87–94, 1984.
14. Okuda K, Omata M, Itoh Y, et al.: Peliosis hepatis as a late and fatal complication of Thorotrast liver disease. Report of five cases. *Liver* 1:110–122, 1981.
15. Seiji Y, Syun H, Hiroo T, Choichiro K, Shinji T: Survey of Thorotrast-associated liver cancers in Japan. *JNCI* 70:31–35, 1983.
16. Dahlgren S: Late effects of thorium dioxide on liver of patients in Sweden. *Ann NY Acad Sci* 145:718, 1967.
17. Vianna NJ: Tumors in patients with angiosarcoma of the liver. *Ann Intern Med* 95:185–186, 1981.
18. Vianna NJ, Brady JA, Cardamone AT: Epidemiology of angiosarcoma of liver in New York State. *NY State J Med* 895–899, 1981.
19. Tavares MH, Saracoca A, Oliveria EA, et al.: Thorium dioxide and the liver up-date clinical and bio-chemical findings. *Environ Res* 18:173–7, 1979.
20. Mahony B, Jeffrey RB, Federle MP: Spontaneous rupture of hepatic and splenic angiosarcoma demonstrated by CT. *AJR* 183:965–966, 1982.
21. Kendo K, Yosmihiro A, Yoshihiki M, et al.: Resection of Thorotrast-induced cholangiocarcinoma. *Am J Gastroenterol* 78:429–433, 1983.
22. Rubel LR, Ishak KG: Thorotrast-associated cholangiocarcinoma. *Cancer* 50:1408–1415, 1982.
23. Chen KT, Bolles CG, Gilbert EF: Angiosarcoma of the spleen. *Arch Pathol Lab Med* 103:122–128, 1979.
24. Gardner DL, Ogilivie RF: The late results of injection of Thorotrast: 2 cases of neoplastic disease following contrast angiography. *J Pathol Bacteriol* 78:133–144, 1959.
25. Burroughs AK, Bass NM, Wood J, Sherlock S: Absence of splenic uptake of radiocolloid due to Thorotrast in a patient with Thorotrast-induced cholangiocarcinoma. *Br J Radiol* 55:598–600, 1982.
26. Whelan JG Jr, Creech JL, Tamburro CL: Angiographic and radionuclide characteristics of hepatic angiosarcoma in vinyl chloride workers. *Radiology* 118:549–557, 1976.

Amyloidosis

Amyloidosis is a pathologic process of uncertain etiology characterized by the deposition of an extracellular fibrous protein in one or more sites in the body. The diagnosis is made by examination of appropriately stained tissue obtained by biopsy. The liver is often affected in patients with amyloidosis, and hepatomegaly can be a presenting sign.

Nuclear Medicine

Radionuclide scanning of the liver can offer useful information in hepatic amyloid, whereas other imaging studies will show nonspecific abnormalities that may be quite difficult to interpret (Fig. 4.64). Bone-scanning radiopharmaceuticals concentrate in amyloid-containing organs with ^{99m}Tc-pyrophosphate giving better results than ^{99m}Tc-methylene diphosphonate (1). Gallium scanning gives inconsistent results, and sulfur colloid scans for hepatic amyloid have been disappointing (1). A poor correlation exists between liver function tests and hepatic amyloid, and pyrophosphate scans can be positive in the face of normal liver function tests (1). Mechanisms of pyrophosphate uptake in amyloid are poorly understood; possibilities include binding of calcium, and therefore pyrophosphate, during the process of extracellular amyloid fibril deposition and transchelation of ^{99m}Tc from pyrophosphate to the amyloid protein molecule in the extracellular space (1).

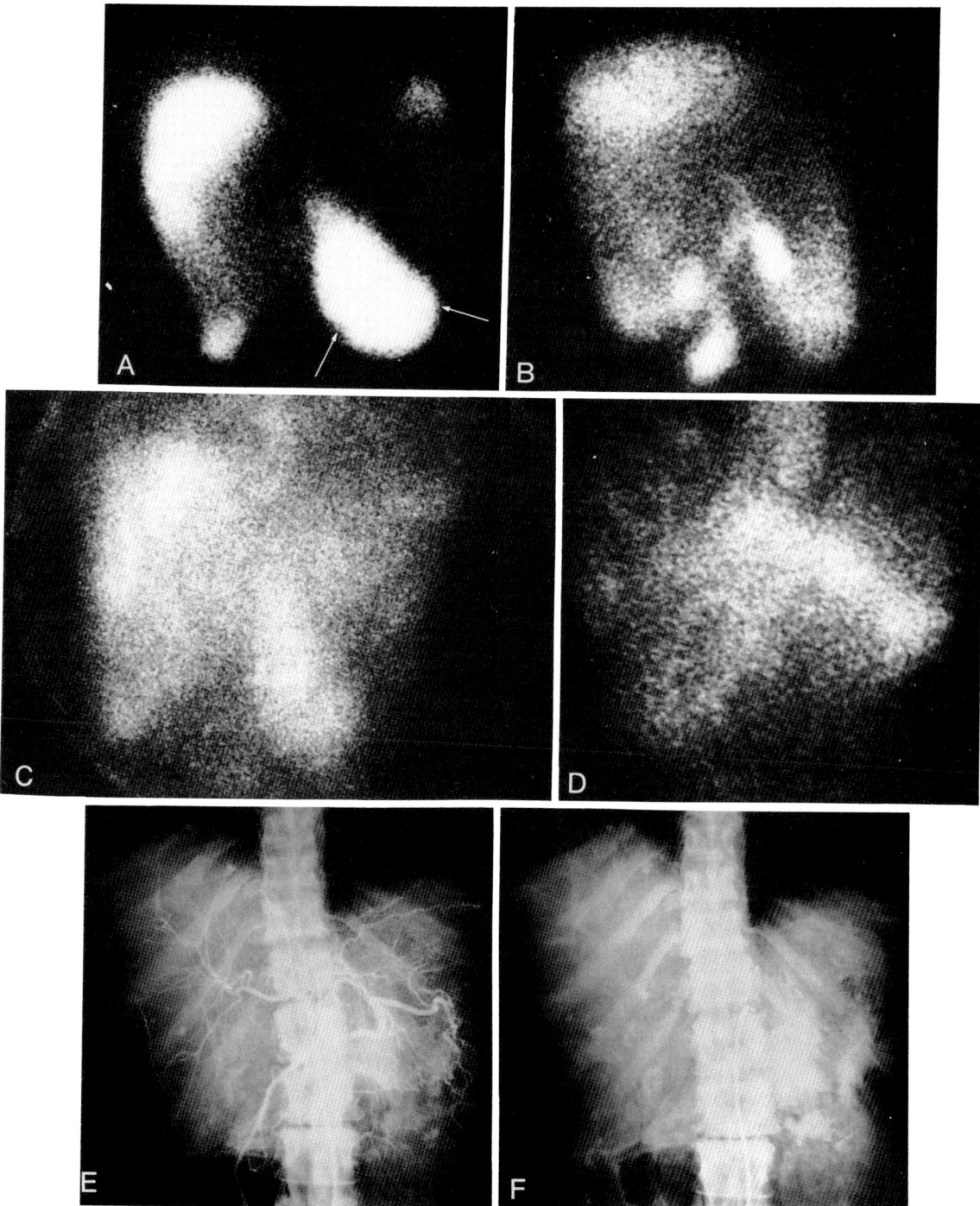

FIGURE 4.64. HEPATIC AMYLOIDOSIS

Elderly woman with hepatomegaly, weight loss, and abnormal liver enzymes. Hepatic amyloidosis. *A:* Sulfur colloid scan: large regions of absent activity and a hypertrophied portion of left lobe in left mid-abdomen (*arrows*). Faint left upper quadrant activity in the spleen. *B:* HIDA scan, 35 min: distorted biliary tree. Hepatocyte uptake corresponds to regions of colloid uptake. Regions of decreased activity are seen in the same location as *A*. *C:* Gallium scan: greatest uptake corresponds to the regions of normal reticuloendothelial and hepatocyte function, but some gallium is present in the regions that were devoid of sulfur colloid and HIDA. *D:* Technetium pyrophosphate scan gives mirror-image of *A* and *B*: activity concentrated in the poorly functioning portions of the liver containing the most amyloid, quite suggestive of the correct diagnosis. *E* and *F:* Arterial and venous phase of a celiac arteriogram, respectively. Hepatomegaly with splaying and stretching of intrahepatic arteries. Marked distortion of veins and mottled parenchymogram. Nonspecific findings. A second generation CT with a drip infusion of contrast revealed nothing other than hepatomegaly (not shown).

REFERENCES

1. Lee VW, Caldarone AG, Falk RH, Rubinow A, Cohen AS: Amyloidosis of heart and liver: comparison of ^{99m}Tc-pyrophosphate and ^{99m}Tc-methylene diphosphonate for detection. *Radiology* 148:239–242, 1983.

VASCULAR DISEASES

Hepatic artery aneurysms, Osler-Weber-Rendu disease, periportal sinusoidal dilatation and peliosis hepatis, liver infarction and portal venous gas will be discussed under this heading.

Hepatic Artery Aneurysm

The first case of hepatic artery aneurysm was reported by autopsy in 1809 (1). Since then approximately 250 cases have been reported (2). Etiologies, in descending order of frequency, are systemic infections, arteriosclerosis, cholecystitis, trauma, syphilis, tuberculosis, polyarteritis nodosa, liver abscess, cystic medial necrosis, and congenital (1–4). In recent years, trauma and arteriosclerosis have been the leading causes with infections less frequent (5). Hepatic artery infusion chemotherapy and percutaneous biliary procedures are causes increasing in frequency.

Clinical Findings

Diagnosis prior to surgery or autopsy is uncommon (1–7). Prior to rupture, symptoms are nonspecific or absent (2). Pain, either epigastric or in the right upper quadrant, is the most common symptom, present in two-thirds (7). A classic triad of abdominal pain, jaundice, and gastrointestinal bleeding (suggesting hemobilia) is present in about one-third (1, 5). When the above are accompanied by an abdominal bruit or pulsatile mass the diagnosis of hepatic artery aneurysm should be suspected (5). The reported age range is 10–83 years (mean 38) with a 2–3:1 male to female ratio (1, 4). Rupture can occur into the peritoneal cavity, extrahepatic biliary duct, duodenum, gallbladder, portal vein, or stomach in descending order of frequency (2, 4). Jaundice may be due to intrabiliary clots or extrinsic compression (1). Hepatic artery aneurysms are usually fatal if untreated or treated after rupture (6). Since 1950, 45% of those operated have survived surgery; prior to that time survival was uncommon (5). Treatment most often consists of hepatic artery ligation with or without resection (7). Recently, transcatheter Gelfoam embolization for small aneurysms and Gianturco coil occlusion of the hepatic artery for large aneurysms have been successful (7).

Pathology

The extrahepatic arteries are involved 4 times as often as the intrahepatic, with the main hepatic artery the most common site (1, 4). Extrahepatic aneurysms are larger than intrahepatic aneurysms (1, 4). Fibrous adhesions to surrounding structures are common (4).

Radiology

Ring-like calcification in the right upper quadrant that does not involve the gallbladder or kidney should suggest the diagnosis (Fig. 4.65) (1–6). However, often such calcification is not detectable on plain films (4). Large aneurysms may produce mass effects on adjacent viscera on barium contrast examination (1). Sonography, CT, and angiography of hepatic artery aneurysms demonstrate findings similar to those seen with aneurysms in the aorta and elsewhere. Aneurysms of the proximal hepatic artery, which passes quite close to the pancreas, may mimic cystic pancreatic masses (Fig. 4.66). Dynamic scanning with a large contrast bolus may be necessary to avoid misdiagnosis. Hepatic artery aneurysms in polyarteritis nodosa and other vasculitides are usually small, multiple, intrahepatic, and associated with vascular irregularity.

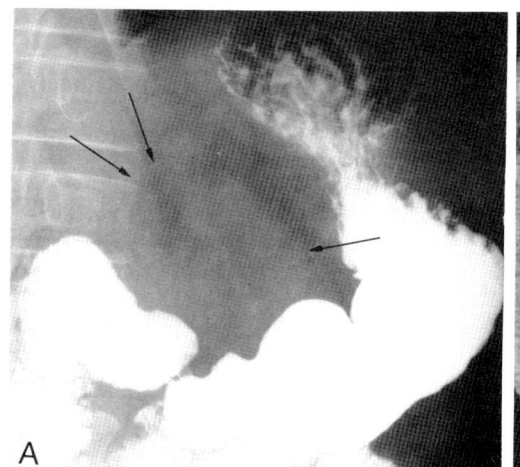
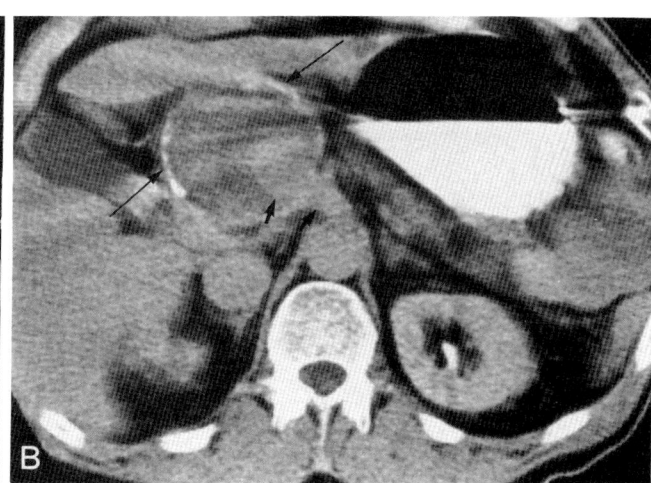
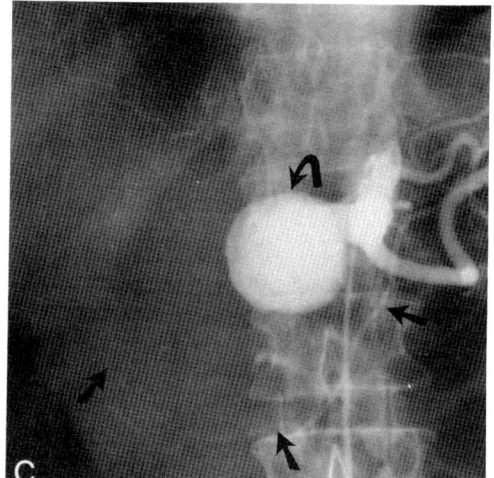

FIGURE 4.65. HEPATIC ARTERY ANEURYSM: ASYMPTOMATIC
Asymptomatic 62-yr-old male patient: atherosclerotic hepatic artery aneurysm. *A:* Retrogastric soft tissue mass with faint wall calcification, appreciated only in retrospect. *B:* CT five years later, done for follow-up of hemochromatosis: partially calcified mass (*arrows*). Central higher intensity area represents the patent portion and is continuous with the celiac artery (*small arrows*). *C:* Celiac arteriogram: slow flow into patent eccentric lumen (*curved arrow*). Aneurysm itself outlined by stretched artery (*arrows*). The hepatic artery was reconstituted distal to the aneurysm by collaterals via the superior mesenteric artery.

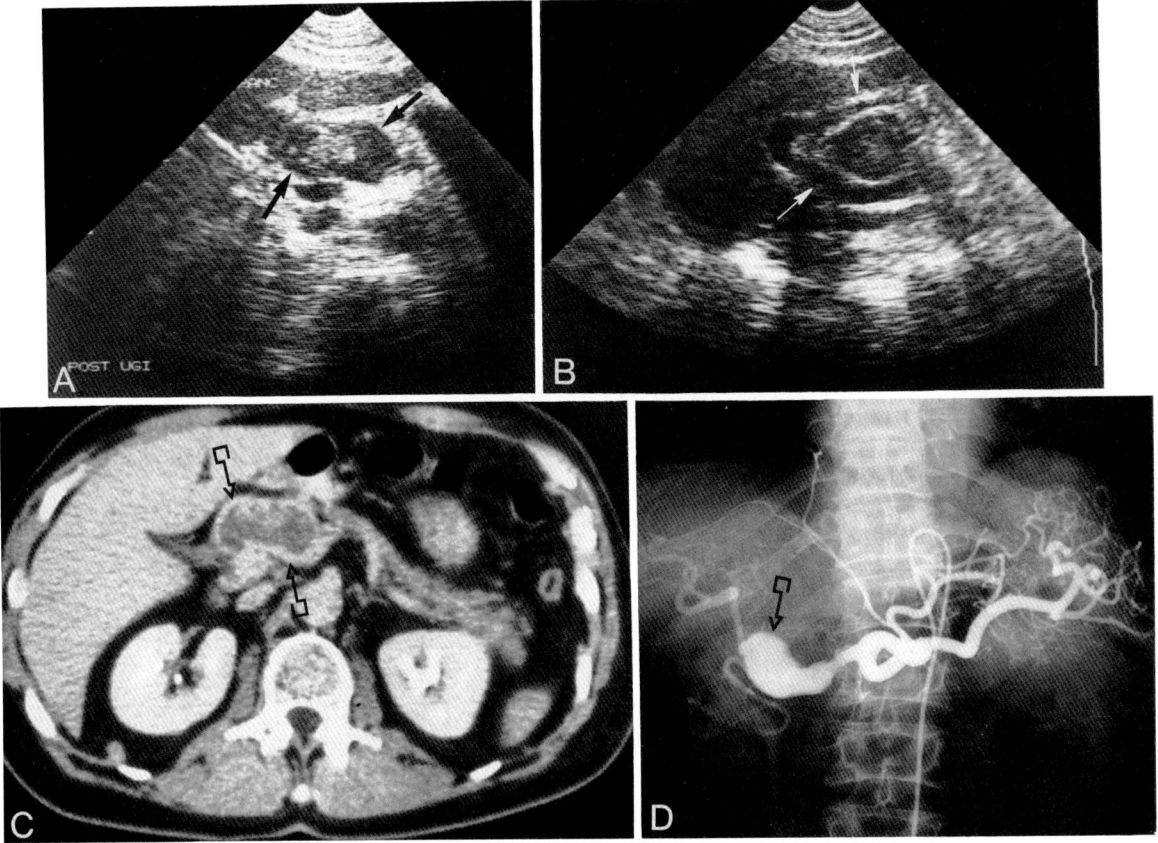

FIGURE 4.66. HEPATIC ARTERY ANEURYSM: MINIMALLY ASYMPTOMATIC
Hepatic artery aneurysm in a minimally symptomatic middle-aged man mimicking a pancreatic mass. A and B: Transverse and parasagittal scans of a complex mass (arrows) in the region of the neck of the pancreas. C: Low density mass with rim enhancement apparently of pancreatic origin (arrows). D: Celiac arteriogram diagnostic of hepatic artery aneurysm (arrow).

REFERENCES

1. Guida PM, Moore SW: Aneurysm of hepatic artery. Report of five cases with a brief review of the previously reported cases. Surgery 60:299–310, 1966.
2. Erskine JM: Hepatic artery aneurysm. Vasc Surg 7:106–125, 1973.
3. Quinn JL, Martin JF: Hepatic artery aneurysm. AJR 87:284–286, 1962.
4. Jarvis L, Hodes PJ: Aneurysm of the hepatic artery demonstrated roentgenographically. AJR 72:1037–1040, 1954.
5. Winchester DP, Seed RW, Bergan JJ, Conn J: Jaundice, hemobilia and hemoperitoneum, consequences of rupture of hepatic artery aneurysm. Am J Surg 120:384–387, 1970.
6. Sutton D, Lawton G: Angiographic diagnosis of aneurysms involving the hepatic artery. Clin Radiol 24:43–48, 1973.
7. Jonsson K, Bjernstad A, Eriksson B: Treatment of a hepatic artery aneurysm by coil occlusion of the hepatic artery. AJR 134:1245–1247, 1980.

Osler-Weber-Rendu Disease (Hereditary Hemorrhagic Telangiectasia)

Hereditary hemorrhagic telangiectasia (HHT) was characterized for a long time by the triad of epistaxis, multiple telangiectases of the mucous membrane and skin, and dominant inheritance. Gradually, it has been recognized that nearly all organ systems may be involved. Telangiectases, aneurysms, and/or arteriovenous shunts have been found in the lung, the entire gastrointestinal tract, the liver, spleen, kidney, genital tract, brain, aorta, bones, conjunctiva, and retina (1). HHT is a rare disease with an incidence of about 1–2:100,000. The ensuing discussion is confined to hepatic manifestations of HHT.

Clinical Findings

Three subgroups of hepatic disease in HHT have been described: (a) HHT with liver telangiectases, fibrosis and/or cirrhosis; (b) HHT with cirrhosis and no liver telangiectases; and (c) HHT with liver telangiectases but no fibrosis or cirrhosis (1). The average age at presentation with liver disease is 57 with a preponderance of postmenopausal women (1). Groups a and b have right upper quadrant pain, anemia, hepatomegaly, and often splenomegaly. Thrills or bruits may be present over the liver. Portal hypertension and encephalopathy may occur, even in group c. Liver function is usually fairly well preserved; elevated alkaline phosphatase and slight hyperbilirubinemia are usually the only abnormalities (1, 2).

Pathology

All cases of cirrhosis in HHT have certain features in common. The cirrhosis is usually macronodular with broad areas of fibrosis and irregular septum formation. The fibrotic bands usually contain many telangiectases of varying size. Cavernous hemangiomas, hepatic artery aneurysms, and both hepatoportal and hepatohepatic arteriovenous fistulas have been demonstrated by either angiography or corrosion casts (1). In group c the derangement is purely vascular.

Radiology

Ultrasound can demonstrate enlargement of the hepatic artery with lack of normal tapering when arteriovenous fistula is present (Fig. 4.67A, B) (3, 4). The actual malformation itself can be depicted as dilated, serpiginous tubular structures with echogenic walls and prominent pulsations (Fig. 4.67A, B) (3). Sonographic findings of cirrhosis, when present, are similar to those seen in other causes of cirrhosis (3). In addition to discrete vascular malformations within the liver, angiography can demonstrate uniformly dilated and tortuous hepatic arteries, a moderately dense and slightly mottled hepatogram, and early but not immediate hepatic vein opacification (Fig. 4.67C) (4, 5). These findings suggest arteriocapillary-venous shunting in the liver. The chest x-ray may provide an important clue to the diagnosis by showing cardiomegaly and mild pulmonary plethora suggesting a hyperdynamic state. Vascular lesions elsewhere in the body should be sought by angiography as clinically indicated.

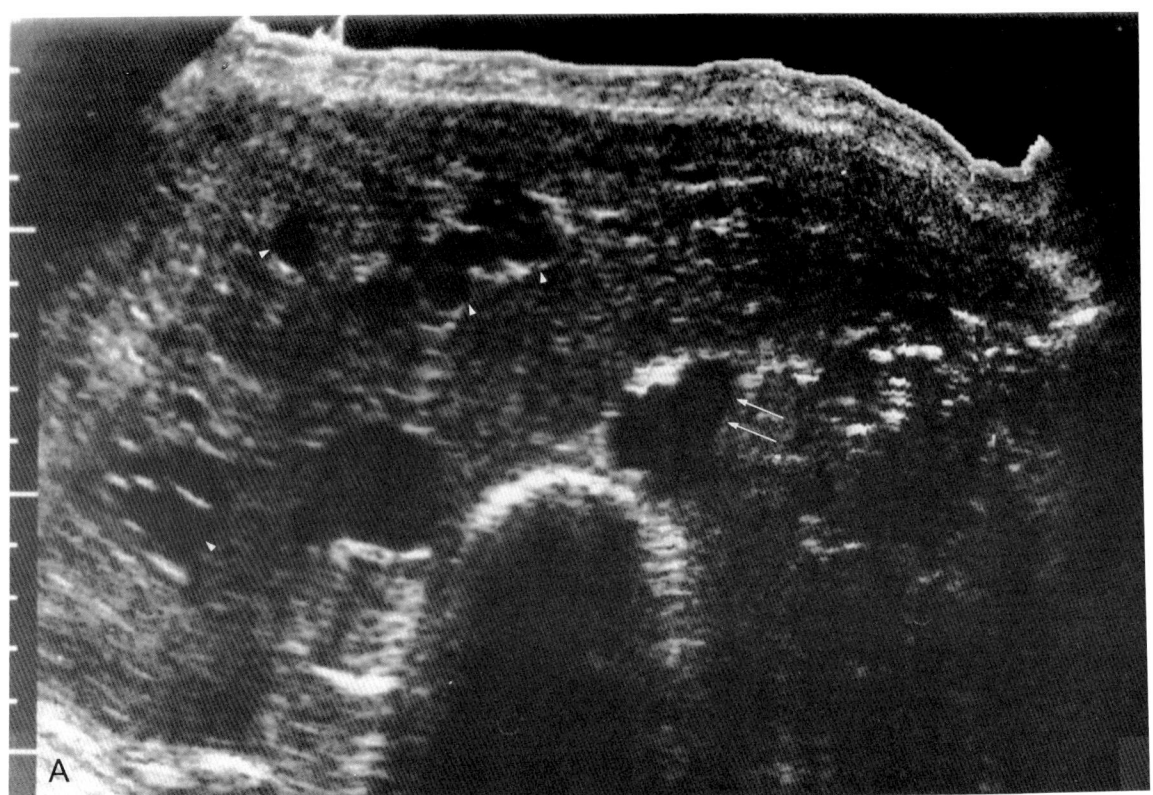
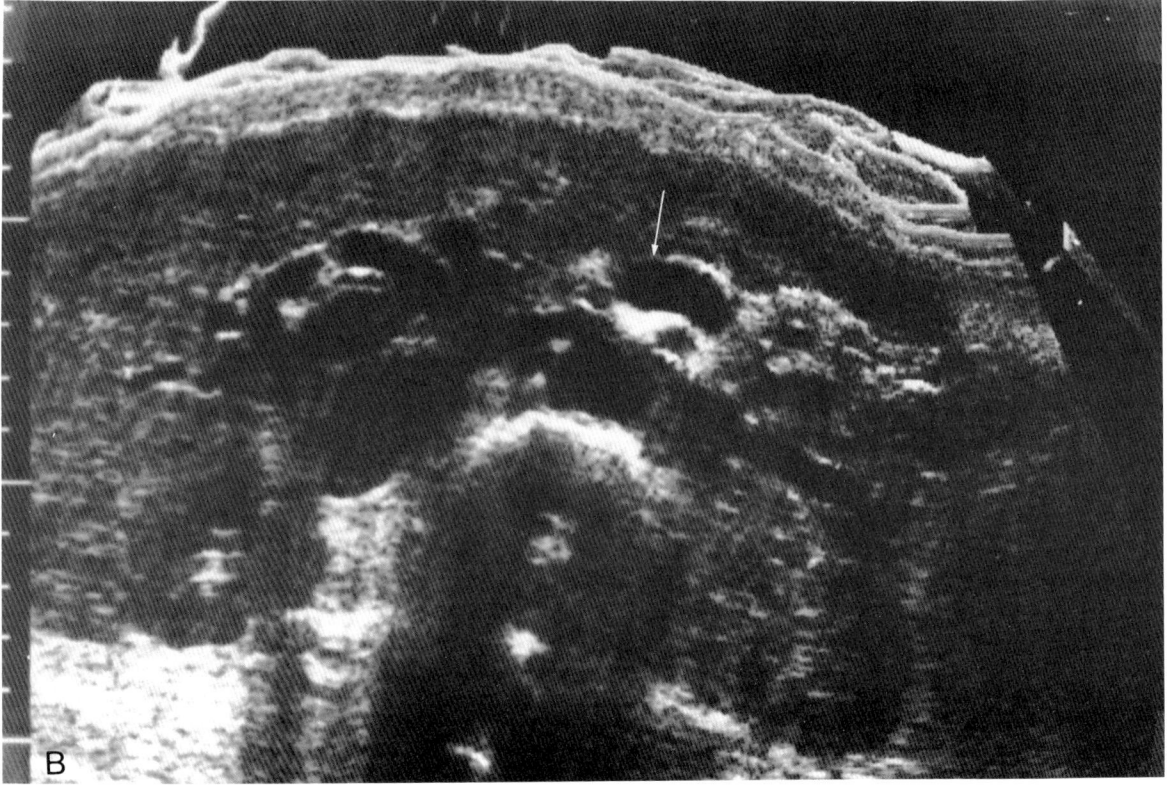

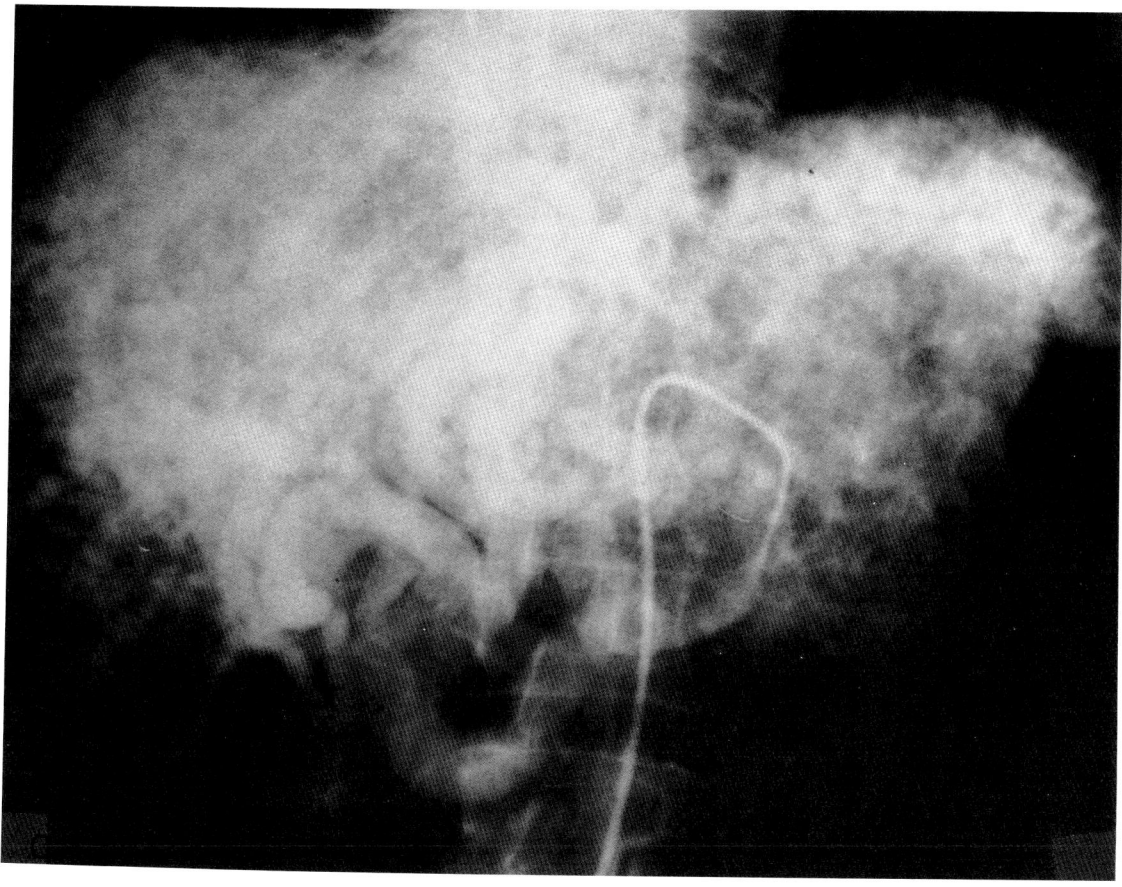

Figure 4.67C

REFERENCES

1. Martini GA: The liver in hereditary haemorrhagic telangiectasia: an inborn error of vascular structure with multiple manifestations: a reappraisal. *Gut* 19:531–537, 1978.
2. Feizi O: Hereditary hemorrhagic telangiectasia presenting with portal hypertension and cirrhosis of the liver. *Gastroenterology* 63:660–664, 1972.
3. Clooogman HM, DiCapo RD: Hereditary hemorrhagic telangiectasia: sonographic findings in the liver. *Radiology* 150:521–522, 1984.
4. Danchin N, Thisse JY, Neimann JL, Faivre, G: Osler-Weber-Rendu disease with multiple intrahepatic arteriovenous fistulas. *Am Heart J* 105:856–859, 1983.
5. Jaques P, Delaney D: Hepatic angiography in hereditary hemorrhagic telangiectasia. *Gastrointest Radiol* 2:149–152, 1977.

Periportal Sinusoidal Dilatation and Peliosis Hepatis

Periportal sinusoidal dilatation and peliosis hepatis are vascular disorders of the liver induced by steroids. The former is associated with oral contraceptive steroids and the latter primarily with androgenic, anabolic steroids (1, 2). Although some believe these lesions are part of a

---

FIGURE 4.67. HEREDITARY HEMORRHAGIC TELANGIECTASIA
A 74-yr-old woman with family history of Osler-Weber-Rendu disease admitted for acute congestive heart failure (high output). *A:* Transverse sonogram through the celiac axis: dilated celiac artery at its take-off from the aorta (*arrows*). Multiple intrahepatic arteriovenous malformations (*arrowheads*). *B:* Transverse scan through the porta hepatis: multiple enlarged vascular structures mimicking dilated bile ducts. Enlarged common hepatic artery (*arrow*). *C:* Hepatic arteriogram, arterial phase: enlarged hepatic artery, numerous arteriovenous malformations, and early draining hepatic veins. Autopsy showed hepatic fibrosis and cirrhosis in addition to multiple telangiectasias of the GI tract, lung and liver. (From Cloogman HM, DiCapo RD: Hereditary hemorrhagic telangiectasia: sonographic findings in the liver. *Radiology* 150:521–522, 1984.)

spectrum of a single pathophysiologic entity (3), a distinction between the two is probably appropriate (1).

Clinical Findings

Presenting signs and symptoms in patients with periportal sinusoidal dilatation are variable except that hepatomegaly and elevated erythrocyte sedimentation rate are consistent (1, 2). One-fifth have abdominal pain, probably from distention of the liver capsule (1). Liver function tests are either normal or mildly elevated (1, 2). After cessation of oral contraceptives, there is a clinical and biochemical improvement (2).

Peliosis hepatis traditionally has occurred in patients with underlying debilitating diseases such as carcinomatosis, tuberculosis, diabetes, and chronic renal disease (1–3). Recently it has been associated with anabolic androgenic and contraceptive steroids (1–4). However, when it occurs as a complication of oral contraceptives it is always located adjacent to adenomas (1). Hepatomegaly is common, and jaundice and severely impaired liver function may be seen (1, 3). It is unclear whether the abnormal liver function is a result of the peliosis or a manifestation of underlying illness (3). Presentation with severe abdominal pain due to rupture of a peliotic lake into abdominal cavity can occur (1, 4). Death may result from shock or liver failure (1). Peliosis can be reversed if the underlying illness is successfully treated or the steroids are discontinued (5).

Pathology

The external surface of the liver in periportal sinusoidal dilatation has been described as having brown or bluish discoloration or as being normal (1). Microscopically, there are dilated sinusoids lined by endothelial and Kupffer cells predominantly in the periportal zones (1, 2).

Examination of the external liver surface in peliosis hepatis reveals multiple blue-black projections of variable size (1). Microscopically, there are blood-filled lacunar spaces lined by hepatocytes (1). These lakes may communicate with adjacent sinusoids or hepatic vein tributaries (1).

Radiology

Sulfur colloid scans of the liver have been reported to show hepatomegaly and, in two instances, focal defects suggesting mass in patients with periportal sinusoidal dilatation (1). It is not clear how a focal defect is produced although intrahepatic hematoma is a possibility. Hepatic venography in two cases was normal. Hepatic arteriography in two cases has shown multiple small accumulations of contrast varying in size from barely perceptible to 1 cm in diameter (Fig. 4.68). These first appear in the late arterial phase and become more prominent in the parenchymal and venous phases (1, 3). One of these cases was reported as peliosis hepatis although the microscopy showed periportal sinusoidal dilatations (3).

Angiography in peliosis hepatis should show findings similar to those of periportal sinusoidal dilation (Fig. 4.69). One case has been reported in which most peliotic spaces failed to opacify and were small lucencies in the hepatogram (6). Splenoportography in a case of peliosis in a child showed small opacities corresponding to the peliotic lakes (5). Differential diagnosis of periportal sinusoidal dilatation and peliosis on hepatic arteriography would include primarily multiple, small hemangiomas and the multiple telangiectasias of Osler-Weber-Rendu syndrome (3). Wedged hepatic venography in one case of peliosis hepatis secondary to anabolic steroids demonstrated clusters of 6-mm spherical spaces opacifying prior to sinusoidal staining. Four months after drug withdrawal a repeat study showed regression of the spherical spaces with residual 0.5-mm hepatoportal channels thought to represent persistently dilated sinusoids (6).

One case of peliosis hepatis has been reported in which sonography was contributory. The true diagnosis probably was periportal sinusoidal dilatation, as the underlying etiology was oral contraceptives. Sonography was performed because a sulfur colloid scan showed multiple filling defects even though liver function tests were normal. The sonogram showed hepatomegaly with a nonspecific heterogeneous parenchymal echo texture (both echopenic and echogenic regions) most prominent in the right lobe. Angiography and biopsy were "compatible with the diagnosis of peliosis hepatis" (7).

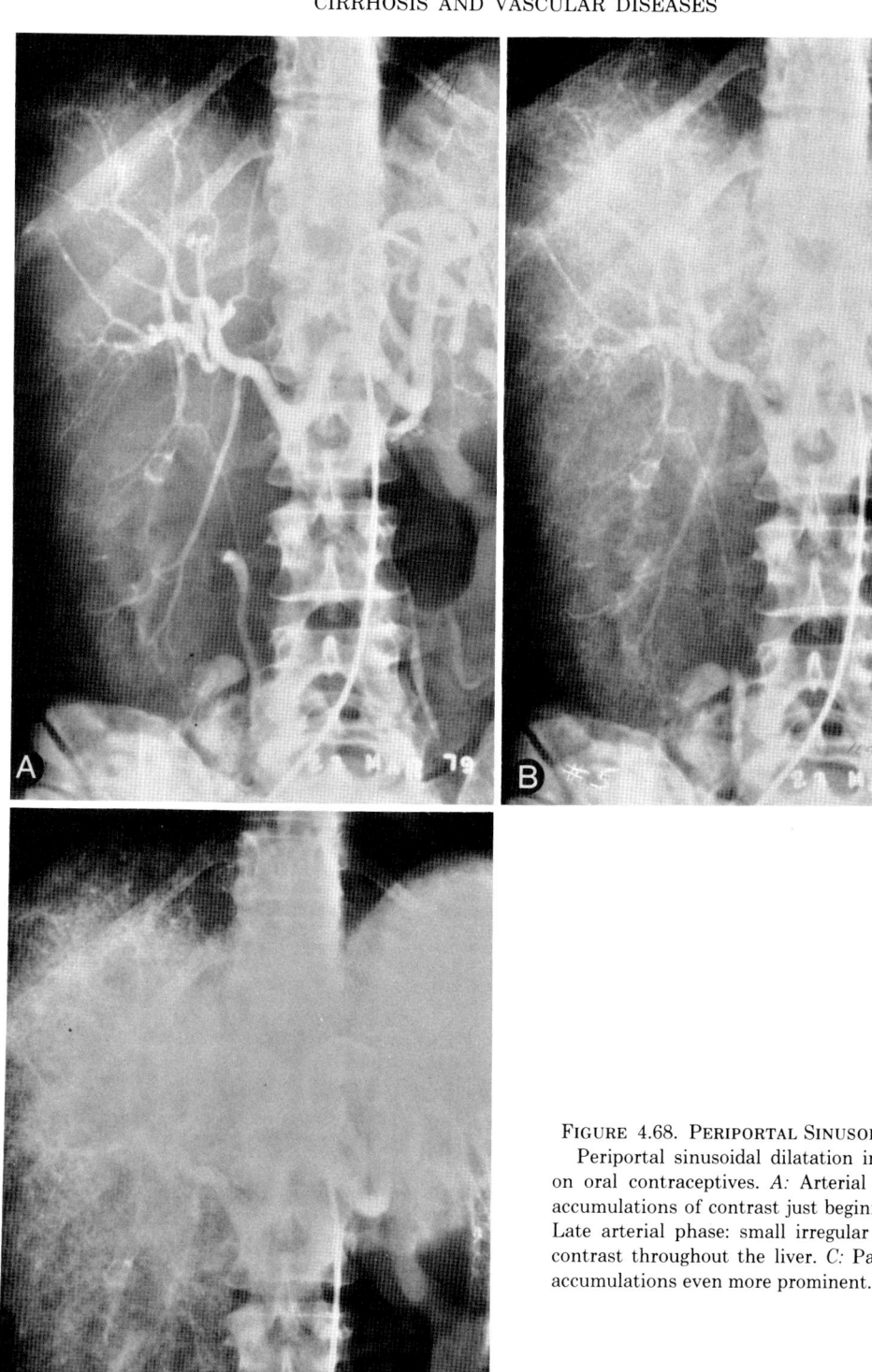

FIGURE 4.68. PERIPORTAL SINUSOIDAL DILATATION
Periportal sinusoidal dilatation in a young woman on oral contraceptives. *A:* Arterial phase: peripheral accumulations of contrast just beginning to appear. *B:* Late arterial phase: small irregular accumulations of contrast throughout the liver. *C:* Parenchymal phase: accumulations even more prominent.

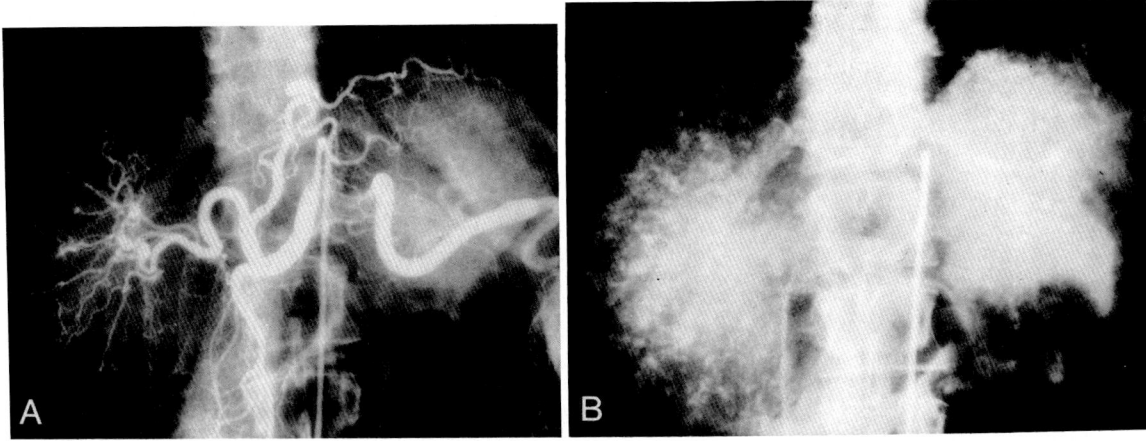

FIGURE 4.69. PELIOSIS HEPATITIS
Peliosis hepatis: middle-aged man with unknown underlying chronic liver disease. A: Arterial phase: corkscrewing of arteries and small liver consistent with cirrhosis. B: Parenchymal phase: irregular contrast accumulations scattered throughout the liver, similar to but larger than (A). (Case courtesy of Lennard Nadalo, M.D.)

REFERENCES

1. Scully RE, Mark EJ, McNeely BU: Case records of the Massachusetts General Hospital. N Engl J Med 307:934–941, 1982.
2. Winkler, K., Poulsen H: Liver disease with periportal sinusoidal dilatation. A possible complication to contraceptive steroids. Scand J Gastroenterol 10:699–704, 1975.
3. Plisken M: Peliosis hepatis. Radiology 114:29–30, 1975.
4. Zimmerman HJ: Peliosis hepatis. In Farber E, Fisher MM (eds): Toxic Injury of the Liver. New York, Marcel Dekker, 1980, pp 713–714.
5. Odievre M, Chaumont P, Gautier M, Vermes JM: Reversible peliosis in the liver of a child. Arch Fr Pediatr 34:654–658, 1977.
6. Lyon J, Bookstein JJ, Cartwright CA, Romano A, Heeney DJ: Peliosis hepatis: diagnosis by magnification wedged hepatic venography. Radiology 150:647–649, 1984.
7. Lloyd RL, Lyons EA, Levi CS, Bristowe JR, Schollenberg J: The ultrasonographic appearance of peliosis hepatis. J Ultrasound Med 1:293–294, 1984.

Hepatic Infarction

Hepatic infarction is relatively rare and usually not diagnosed until autopsy. The dual blood supply of the liver is thought to be protective. Hepatic infarction is usually secondary to hepatic arterial occlusion, but evidence exists that infarction can occur after occlusion of the portal vein only or even one of its branches (1).

Clinical Findings

Patients generally have severe abdominal or back pain, leukocytosis, and elevated liver enzymes. Fever or hypothermia is frequently present, simulating infection (1).

Common causes of hepatic infarction are atherosclerotic occlusion of the hepatic artery, hepatic artery thrombosis, embolus or aneurysm, polyarteritis nodosa, neoplastic encasement of the hepatic artery (carcinoma of the pancreas), polycythemia vera and oral contraceptives (thrombosis), and low flow secondary to biliary disease, anesthesia, or shock (1). Diseases of the superior mesenteric artery may result in hepatic infarction when the right hepatic artery is replaced. In part, this may explain the predilection of infarction for the right lobe. Tumors of the liver and cirrhosis both appear to diminish the liver's susceptibility to infarction, probably secondary to an increase in anastomoses and collaterals between the hepatic artery and the portal vein (1).

Pathology

Infarcts are usually wedge-shaped and sharply distinct from adjacent normal parenchyma (1). Endothelial-lined bile-filled cysts (bile lakes) that communicate with biliary tree and are surrounded by fibrous tissue can be seen near occluded vessels (2, 3). The mechanism for bile cyst production is postulated to be ischemic necrosis of bile duct epithelium leading to biliary extravasation (3). Such events may be pathogenetic in Caroli's disease (3).

Histologically, infarcts typically show centrilobular zonal parenchymal necrosis and a peripheral zone of surviving portal tracts, hepatic veins, and interlobular stroma. Random areas of necrosis involving deep and superficial liver substance are often present (1).

Ultrasound

The sonographic appearance of hepatic infarction should vary with the age of the infarct. Acute infarcts are difficult to detect until sufficient edema and round cell infiltration occur to render them hypoechoic. As the necrotic tissue is resorbed and/or if bile lakes form, cystic changes will be observed (Fig. 4.70A, B). If the patient survives, bile cysts indistinguishable from simple

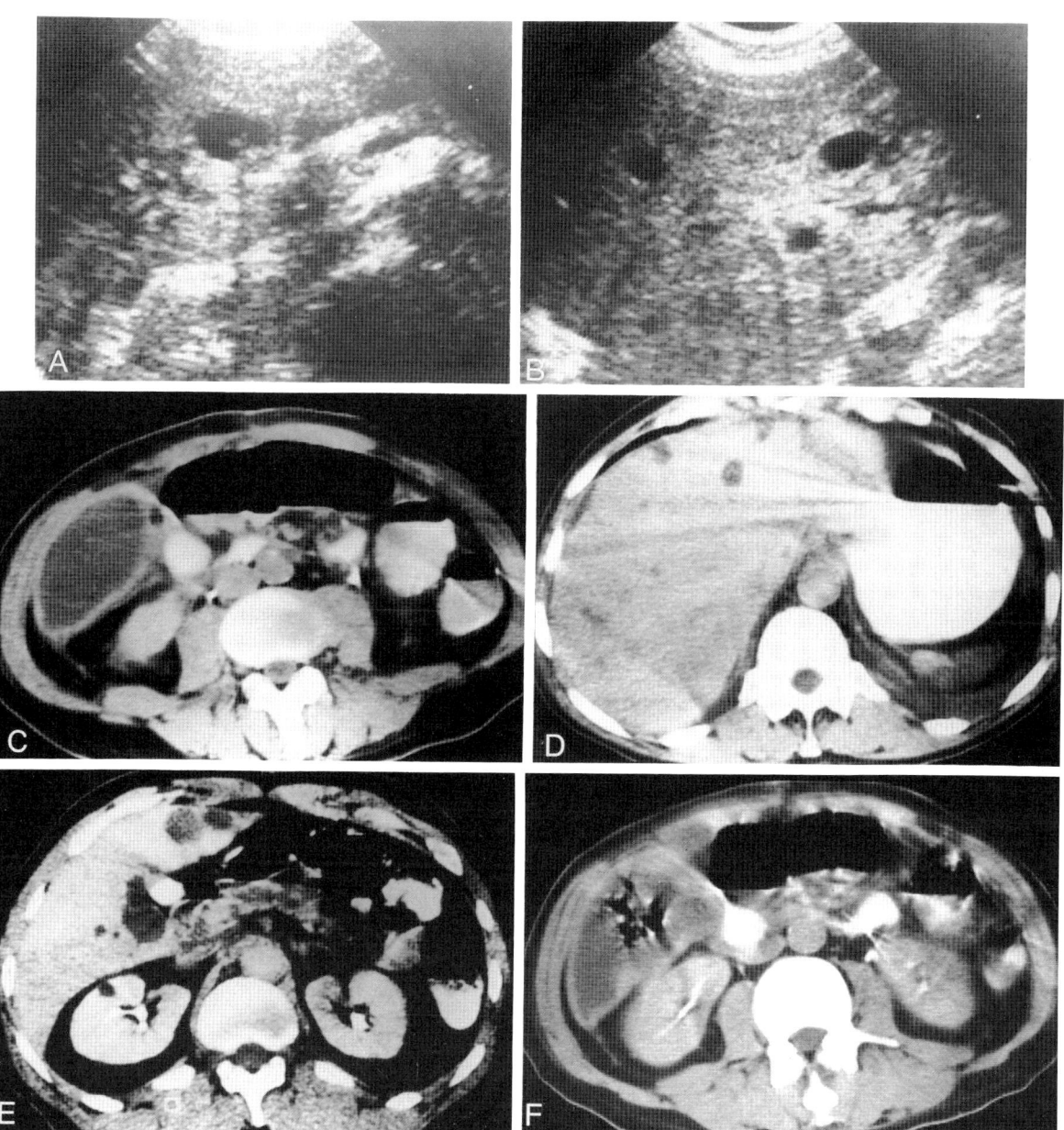

FIGURE 4.70. HEPATIC INFARCTION

A 64-yr-old man presented with abdominal pain and diarrhea. Initial evaluation suggested mesenteric ischemia. Right upper quadrant pain, and fever developed and he had abnormal liver function tests. Angiography showed superior mesenteric artery occlusion. Surgery was unsuccessful and the patient died after a long hospital course. Autopsy confirmed liver infarction without infection. A: Transverse sonogram depicting an infarct as a target lesion with an echogenic excrescence and a cystic periphery. B: Later in the patient's course more cysts developed as the infarcts evolved. C: Contrast enhanced CT shows a peripheral low density infarct in the right lobe with rim enhancement. D: Multiple target infarcts on CT corresponding to A. E: Multiple cysts corresponding to B. F: Later in the patient's course gas was produced in the large infarct shown in C. Aspiration yielded only necrotic material; gram stain and culture were negative.

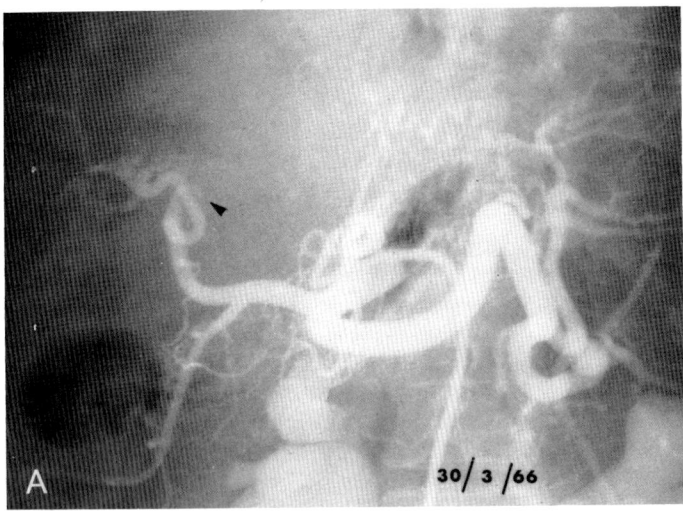
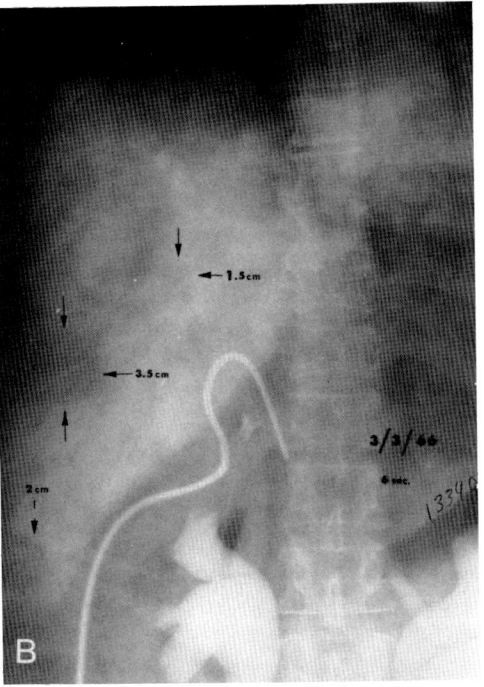

FIGURE 4.71. HEPATIC INFARCTION
Middle-aged woman with hepatic infarction from polycythemia vera and hepatic artery thrombosis. *A:* Celiac injection shows hepatic arterial branch occlusions (*arrowhead*). *B:* Parenchymal phase shows multiple defects in the right lobe representing infarcts.

liver cysts can be seen. Echogenic scarring and indentation of the liver contour are theoretically possible.

Computed Tomography

In the acute stage, infarcts can be isodense or hypodense on unenhanced scans. Due to lack of perfusion, they are low density lesions on contract enhanced scans (1). Infarcts are well-circumscribed and often wedge-shaped extending to the periphery. A thin high attenuation subcapsular rim may be present secondary to collateral perfusion (Fig. 4.70C) (1). As the infarct evolves, hypodense target lesions from necrosis are depicted (Fig. 4.70D). If the patient survives, bile lake formation can occur with an appearance indistinguishable from simple cyst (Fig. 4.70E). Gas may be produced in the absence of infection (Fig. 4.70F). Infarcts in other organs, such as kidney, spleen, or bowel may be seen, depending on the underlying disease process.

As is obvious from the above discussion, infarcts are indistinguishable by sonography and CT from more common conditions such as abscesses and metastases. Close clinical correlation and, often, needle aspiration are necessary to make the correct diagnosis.

Angiography

Hepatic arteriography is very useful in selected instances to demonstrate surgically correctible causes of hepatic infarction. When the diagnosis is obscure after clinical and noninvasive imaging evaluation, the angiographic depiction of hepatic arterial occlusion can be crucial in reaching the correct diagnosis (Fig. 4.71).

Nuclear Medicine

Focal hepatic necrosis from any cause will give rise to photon deficient regions on both sulfur colloid and hepatobiliary scans. Infarction should be considered when peripheral, wedge-shaped, sharply defined defect(s) are seen on scintiscans. The defects will correspond in distribution to the occluded hepatic vasculature. Scintigraphy may be more sensitive than sonography and CT for detecting these changes (4, 5).

Focal or diffuse regions of hepatic necrosis may show avidity for bone-scanning agents (6). Cholescintigraphy can demonstrate communicating bile lakes.

REFERENCES

1. Adler DD, Glazer GM, Silver TM: Computed tomography of liver infarction. *AJR* 142:315–318, 1984.
2. Peterson IM, Neumann CH: Focal hepatic infarction with bile lake formation. *AJR* 142:1155–1156, 1984.

3. Doppman JL, Dunnick NR, Girton M, Fauci AS, Popovsky MA: Bile duct cysts secondary to liver infarction: report of a case and experimental production by small vessel hepatic artery occlusion. *Radiology* 130:1–5, 1979.
4. Drum DE: Current status of radiocolloid hepatic scintigraphy for space-occupying disease. *Semin Nucl Med* 12:64–74, 1982.
5. Chen V, Hamilton J, Qizilbash A: Hepatic infarction: a clinicopathologic study of seven cases. *Arch Pathol Lab Med* 100:32–36, 1976.
6. Lyons KP, Kuperus J, Green HW: Localization of ^{99m}Tc-pyrophosphate in the liver due to massive liver necrosis: case report. *J Nucl Med* 18:550–552, 1977.

Portal Venous Gas

Intrahepatic portal venous gas is most often associated with bowel infarction. Other causes include ulcerative colitis, necrotizing enterocolitis, small bowel obstruction, intraabdominal abscess, gastric ulcer, and pneumonia. The prognosis upon recognition of portal venous gas is not necessarily as grim as was originally thought (1).

Plain Films

The radiologic hallmark of portal venous gas is the detection of branching linear gas densities within the liver, seen predominantly in smaller peripheral branches (Fig. 4.72). Gas in the biliary tree, on the other hand, tends to collect centrally in the larger bile ducts. This difference is explained by the centrifugal flow of portal venous blood as contrasted to the centripetal flow of bile (1). Ancillary plain film findings seen in patients with portal venous gas include gas in the mesenteric vessels and/or intestinal walls.

Sonography

Sonography may detect portal venous gas in infants with necrotizing enterocolitis when the abdominal radiograph is still normal (2). The appearance of gas in the portal venous system is similar to that elsewhere in the body. Bright linear or confluent echoes with or without acoustical shadowing, are present in the main portal vein, its peripheral radicles or in the superior mesenteric vein (Fig. 4.73). On sonography as well as on radiography, portal gas is predominantly peripheral due to the direction of blood flow, while biliary gas usually remains central (3, 4). Early on, the gas may be appreciated on real-time examination only as intermittently flowing, highly echogenic, inconstantly shadowing microbubbles within the portal veins. Coordination of bursts of bubbles with intestinal peristalsis may be observed. The microbubbles can also be seen passing from the peripheral vessels preferentially into nondependent portions of the hepatic parenchyma (2). It is important to distinguish portal venous gas from normal, rapidly flowing echoes that are commonly seen in large vessels. These normal echoes are generally of low amplitude and appear to flow continuously (3). They arise from aggregates of red blood cells.

Computed Tomography

Rarely used in a specific search for portal venous gas, CT may be used in differentiating portal venous gas from pneumobilia when doubt

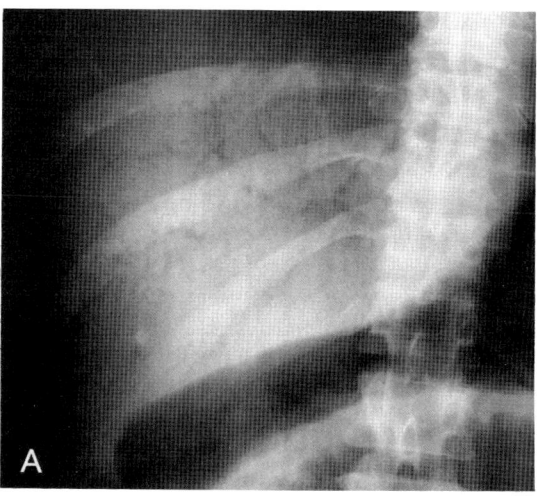
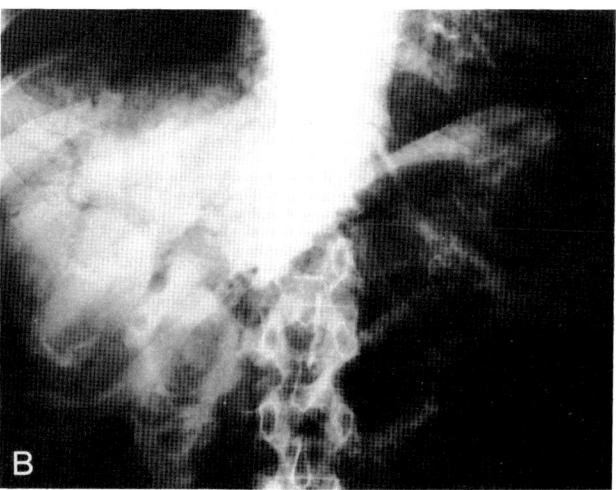

FIGURE 4.72. RADIOLOGIC HALLMARK OF PORTAL VENOUS GAS

A: Coned down view of the right upper quadrant: linear branching intrahepatic lucencies representing portal venous gas in a patient with leukemia and small bowel pneumatosis. The patient died shortly after this film was taken. *B:* Postmortem film in a different patient: air within the entire portal venous system. The patient died from small bowel infarction.

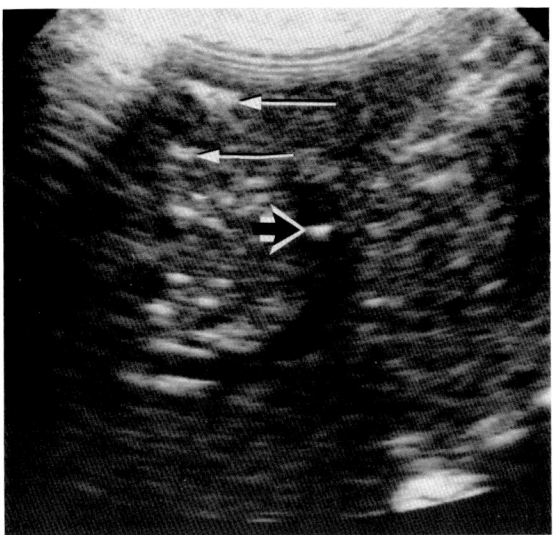

FIGURE 4.73. SONOGRAPHIC APPEARANCE OF GAS IN PORTAL VENOUS SYSTEM

Linear echogenicities (*arrows*) collecting fairly superiorly in the liver representing portal venous gas on this transverse scan of a neonate with necrotizing enterocolitis. (From Merritt CRB, Goldsmith JP, Sharp MJ: Sonographic detection of portal venous gas in infants with necrotizing enterocolitis. *AJR* 143:1059–1062, 1984.)

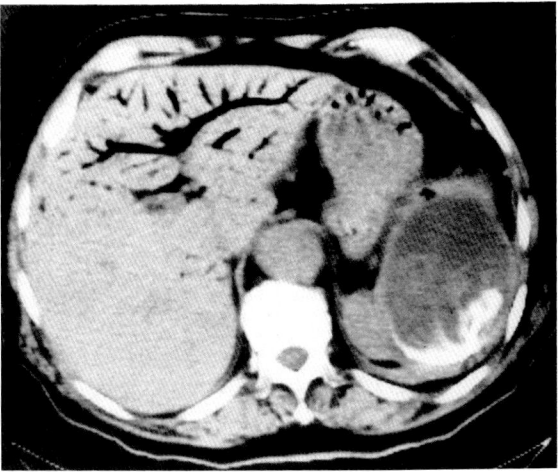

FIGURE 4.74. EXTENSIVE PORTAL VENOUS GAS ON CT

Note preferential involvement of anterior portion of liver. Lower cuts showed gas within the splenic vein. The etiology was the large splenic abscess, which is present in the left upper quadrant, partially opacified by contrast as part of a percutaneous drainage procedure. The patient did well after drainage.

REFERENCES

1. Wiot JF, Felson B: Gas in the portal venous system. *AJR* 86:920–929, 1961.
2. Meritt CRB, Goldsmith JP, Sharp MJ: Sonographic detection of portal venous gas in infants with necrotizing enterocolitis. *AJR* 143:1059–1062, 1984.
3. Laing FC, Rego JD Jr., Jeffrey RB: Ultrasonographic identification of portal vein gas. *J Clin Ultrasound* 12:512–514, 1984.
4. Gosink BB: Intrahepatic gas: differential diagnosis. *AJR* 137:763–767, 1981.

exists after plain film study (Fig. 4.74). CT will of course, be more sensitive than radiography in the demonstration of gas in the portal veins as well as other associated locations (mesenteric vessels and/or bowel wall).

DIFFUSE LIVER DISEASE AND NUCLEAR MEDICINE

The diffuse liver diseases all manifest themselves by abnormal liver function studies and sometimes a palpably enlarged liver. They can be subdivided into the broad categories of cirrhosis, viral disease, metabolic disease, granulomatous disease, and other miscellaneous infiltrative disorders. They all share many scintigraphic features in common.

Cirrhosis

A number of patterns of sulfur colloid scan findings are possible in cirrhosis, depending on the stage and severity of the disease. In early disease, fatty infiltration may predominate and scan findings are limited to hepatomegaly sometimes with a mild inhomogeneity of tracer within the liver and a mild colloid shift to the bone marrow and spleen. As the disease progresses, the liver shrinks, redistribution of colloid becomes more pronounced, and splenomegaly develops (Fig. 4.75A, B). Scans taken early after injection may show a high blood pool concentration secondary to slow clearance (Fig. 4.76A, B). In end-stage disease, the liver is small and contracted with little or no activity present; consequently there is intense activity in bone marrow, spleen, and sometimes lung (Fig. 4.76A). Lung activity implies sepsis or other conditions that stimulate the hepatic reticuloendothelial system and is a poor prognostic sign. Ascites may be suggested when the liver and spleen are displaced from the abdominal wall (Fig. 4.75A, B). The cirrhotic liver will often show relative preservation of reticuloendothelial function in and hypertrophy of the left lobe compared to the right lobe. Mottling of uptake within the cirrhotic liver is sometimes severe enough to mimic space-occupying disease (pseudotumors) (Fig. 4.76A). The basis of this appearance is a local relative decrease in Kupffer cell volume due to shunting,

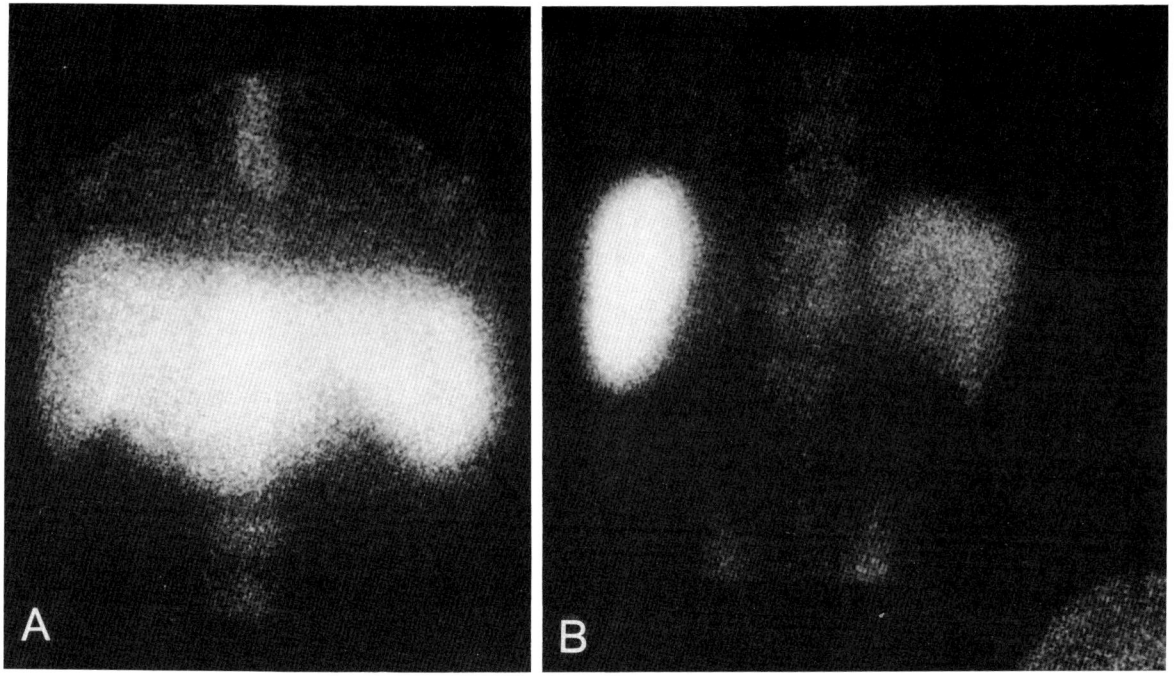

FIGURE 4.75. SCINTIGRAPHIC CHANGES OF CIRRHOSIS

Anterior (A) and posterior (B) sulfur colloid liver spleen scans demonstrating scintigraphic changes of cirrhosis. Note prominent left lobe, small right lobe, colloid shift, bone marrow uptake, and liver displacement away from the lateral body wall by ascites.

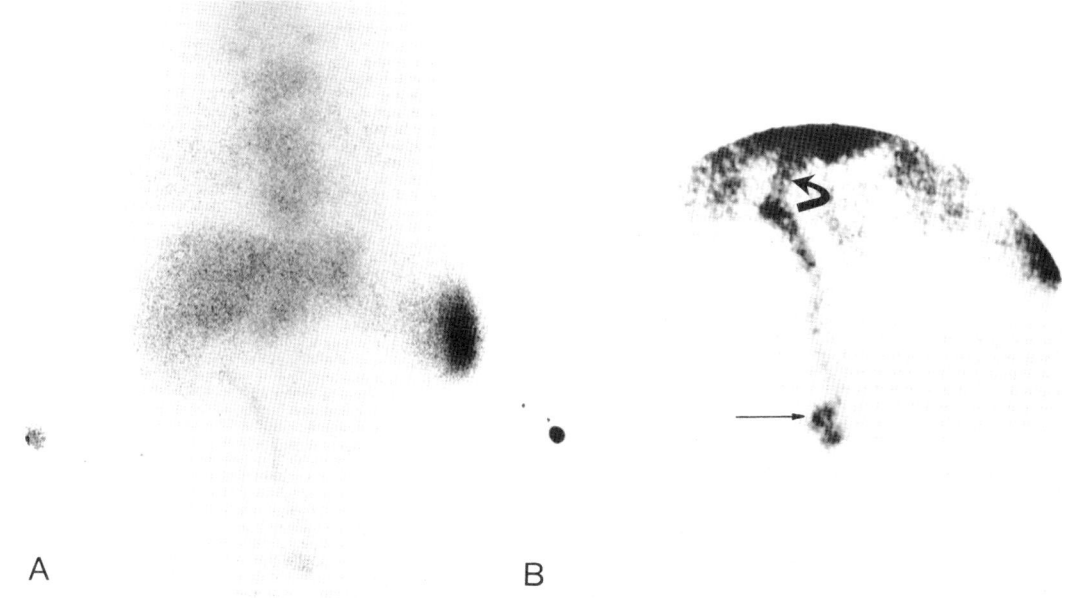

FIGURE 4.76. END-STAGE CIRRHOSIS WITH VISUALIZATION OF RECANALIZED UMBILICAL VEIN

A: Anterior view: colloid shift to spleen, mottled liver, marrow, lung and blood pool activity. Unusual linear activity extending from umbilical region towards liver. B: Frame from a radionuclide angiogram proving that the linear activity in (A) is a recanalized umbilical vein. Note caput medusa (*arrow*) and left portal vein (*curved arrow*).

necrosis, severe inflammation, scarring or regenerating nodules without Kupffer cell activity. Filling in of these hypoactive regions on Tc-IDA scans may occur, a feature helpful in ruling out neoplasm. Care must be taken to avoid confusing the hot, enlarged spleen from congestive splenomegaly associated with severe hepatocellular disease with a primary splenic disease. Radionuclide angiography will show earlier than normal arrival of activity in the liver secondary to increased hepatic arterial flow as a result of portal hypertension (1).

The sulfur colloid scan findings in cirrhosis are not specific by themselves, but they can be used to characterize the chronicity and severity of the disease process in the appropriate clinical setting. A normal liver spleen scan does not completely exclude cirrhosis (1).

Alcoholic Liver Disease

Early alcoholic liver disease with minimal fatty infiltration will show a normal scan. Severe fatty infiltration will be manifest as hepatomegaly and colloid redistribution, and alcoholic hepatitis will often have depression of sulfur colloid uptake in addition to hepatomegaly and colloid shift. Severe acute alcoholic hepatitis may show no liver uptake. However, a normal scan does not completely exclude alcoholic hepatitis (1).

Viral Hepatitis

Patients with mild viral hepatitis will have a normal scan or mild hepatomegaly with or without mildly patchy uptake. These changes result from interstitial edema, and will revert to normal as the disease subsides (Fig. 4.77). Splenomegaly

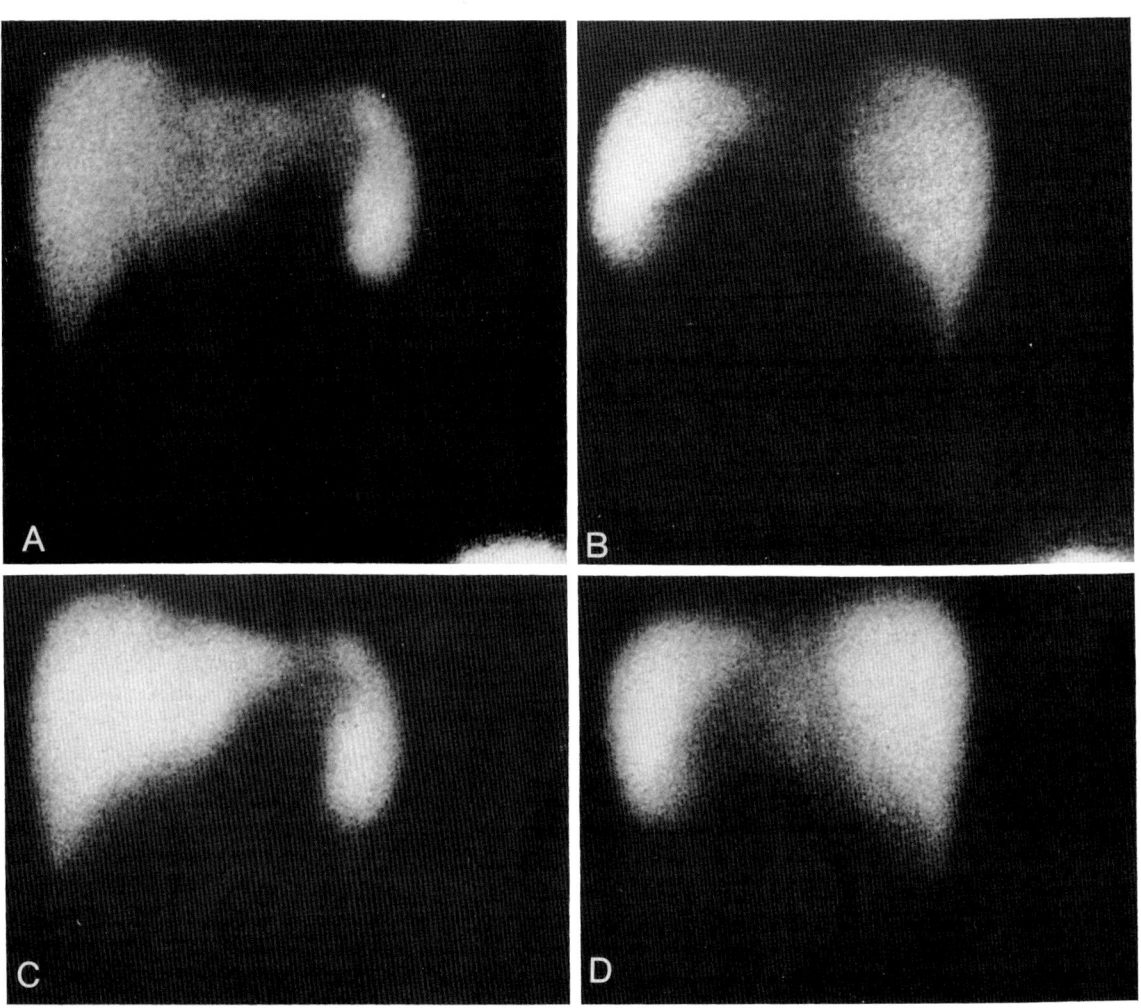

FIGURE 4.77. MILD TO MODERATE VIRAL HEPATITIS
A and *B:* Anterior and posterior views, sulfur colloid scan: colloid shift and patchy left lobe. *C* and *D:* Reversion to normal 1 month later.

is sometimes seen in association with viral hepatitis, and rarely, there will be a focal defects simulating mass lesions.

In fulminant viral hepatitis, liver size can be enlarged, normal, or small, and uptake will be faint. Small liver size on the scan carries a poor prognosis, as does the presence of pulmonary uptake. Patients with fulminant hepatitis will have significant colloid redistribution, poor isotope clearance and some splenomegaly (1).

Metabolic, Granulomatous, and Infiltrative Diseases

These diseases most commonly result in hepatosplenomegaly with an irregular distribution of colloid within the liver and, at times, a colloid shift. The size of the liver and the degree of irregular radiopharmaceutical distribution within the liver is proportional to the amount of fat, glycogen, neoplasm, or granulomatous change (depending on the disease in question) distributed within the liver. Regions of significant patchy reduction of uptake are good sites for biopsy when the etiology of the disease is unknown. Hepatic fat content can be quantitated by determining the amount of radioxenon accumulated within it. Xenon-133 is fat soluble and its retention within an organ is proportional to that organ's lipid content (3).

Differentiation between Hepatocellular Disease and Metastases

Heterogeneity of hepatic uptake, splenomegaly, and bone marrow uptake are good identifiers (high sensitivity) of hepatocellular disease. Only bone marrow uptake, however, is a good discriminator (high specificity); splenomegaly has some value as a discriminator. The presence of focal demarcated photopenic regions is a good discriminator for metastatic disease (4).

Comparison of the Sulfur Colloid Scan and the IDA Hepatobiliary Scan in Hepatocellular Disease

In general, the hepatocyte phase of the hepatobiliary scan gives information equivalent to that of the sulfur colloid scan. However, a disease process that affects the function of the reticuloendothelial cells and the hepatocytes unequally or disturbs their relative numbers will result in the two radionuclides producing discordant scans. This discordance may occur in hepatocellular disease depending on: the nature and severity of the disease process, the amount of intrahepatic shunting, the relative saturation of the reticuloendothelial system by viral particles or cellular debris, the extent of involvement of each cell type by the disease process, and the relative ischemia of each cell type.

Hepatic reticuloendothelial colloid clearance is decreased in cirrhosis. Hepatic reticuloendothelial phagocytic function is increased in chronic hepatitis but decreased in alcoholic hepatitis. In cirrhosis and alcoholic hepatitis, therefore, there may be regions of little or no uptake on the sulfur colloid scan that have normal activity on the IDA scan. In nonmetastatic hepatic dysfunction produced by renal cell carcinoma (Stauffer syndrome), there is Kupffer cell hypertrophy and hepatocyte dysfunction; therefore the colloid scan will be normal but the IDA scan abnormally cold (5).

Radiation Injury to the Liver

Hepatic injury from external beam ionizing radiation (3000–4000 rads within 6 weeks) can cause diminished activity on radionuclide liver scans. This may be transient, with recovery within 3 months. Usually, hepatic radiation is unintentional, occurring when the liver is included in the treatment portal for lymphoma, or renal, breast, and esophageal carcinoma. Early in the treatment, the sulfur colloid scan may be normal with a region of diminished activity on the IDA scan because the hepatocytes are more sensitive than the Kupffer cells. Later, after hepatocyte regeneration has taken place, there will be a region of diminished activity on the sulfur colloid scan with a normal or near normal IDA scan. The characteristic defect of radiation injury is rectangular and well-delineated, corresponding to the portal (Fig. 4.78) (5). Scintigraphy is the screening procedure of choice for radiation injury to the liver as changes may be inapparent on sonography and CT (6).

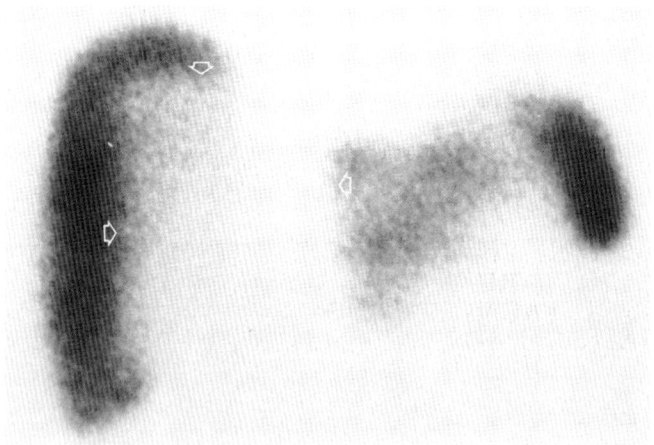

FIGURE 4.78. RADIATION INJURY
Sharply demarcated defect bounded by straight lines corresponding to the radiation port (*arrows*): radiation injury, sulfur-colloid scan.

REFERENCES

1. Waxman AD: Scintigraphic evaluation of diffuse hepatic disease. *Semin Nucl Med* 12:75–88, 1982.
2. Sternlieb I, Scheinberg IH: Radiocopper in diagnosing liver disease. *Semin Nucl Med* 2:176, 1972.
3. Ahmad M, Witzhum K, Fletcher J et al: Xenon accumulation in hepatic steatoses. *J Nucl Med* 18:881–885, 1977.
4. Simon TR, Neumann RL, Gorelick F, Riely C, Hoffer P, Gottschalk A: Scintigraphic diagnosis of cirrhosis: a receiver operator characteristic analysis of common interpretative criteria. *Radiology* 138:723–726, 1981.
5. Lamki L: A dichotomy in hepatic uptake of ^{99m}Tc-IDA and ^{99m}Tc-colloid. *Semin Nucl Med* 12:92–94, 1982.
6. Freeman L, Johnson P: *Clinical Scintillation Imaging.* New York, Grune & Stratton, 1975.

5

Focal Diseases

ARNOLD C. FRIEDMAN, M.D., ELLIOT K. FISHMAN, M.D.,
PAUL D. RADECKI, M.D., JOHN C. SCATARIGE, M.D.,
JOHN L. SHERMAN, M.D., EDWARD J. FARMLETT, M.D.,
BRUCE M. MARKLE, M.D., ABRAHAM H. DACHMAN, M.D., AND
ROBERT L. PAKTER, M.D.

PYOGENIC LIVER ABSCESS

Pyogenic abscess, a focal suppurative lesion of the liver caused by bacteria, is now the commonest cause of hepatic abscess in developed countries. Delay in diagnosis of this well-known but uncommon condition contributes to a relatively high mortality rate ranging from 20 to 80% (1–3). Mortality is higher in cases of multiple abscesses. The use of radionuclide scanning, ultrasound, and computerized tomographic imaging has resulted in earlier diagnosis and has helped to reduce the mortality in recent years. The incidence as a percentage of hospital admissions has ranged from 0.004 to 0.016% (4). The age range is broad and the mean has gradually increased and pyogenic liver abscess is now seen most frequently in the sixth and seventh decades. Some investigators have reported an incidence greater in men than in women (2).

Etiology and Pathogenesis

The source of infection in pyogenic hepatic abscess can be divided into seven groups:

1. Obstructive biliary tract disease with associated cholangitis.
2. Portal pyemia secondary to suppurative appendicitis, diverticular disease, or rarely, colitis or other inflammatory disease in the portal drainage area. Aggressive surgical treatment of appendicitis and the use of antibiotics have caused a decline in the incidence of hepatic abscess of this etiology.
3. Direct spread from a contiguous organ, e.g., cholecystitis, peptic ulcer, subphrenic and perinephric sepsis.
4. Trauma, with direct contamination of the liver through rupture or laceration.
5. Infarction after embolism or complicating sickle cell disease.
6. Arterial dissemination of bacteria can occur in patients with indwelling arterial catheters for arterial infusion chemotherapy (5).
7. Cryptogenic hepatic abscesses are thought to arise from invasion of dead space (e.g., cysts) or dead tissues (infarcts, necrotic tumor) by pyogenic intestinal flora that either are not cleared in a normal manner or saturate the clearance mechanism, as in rupture of a diverticulum into the portal system (1, 4).

Bacteria commonly cultured from hepatic abscesses include *Escherichia coli* and other Enterobacteriaceae, aerobic streptococci and *Staphylococcus aureus*. Anaerobic bacteria are the causative agents in 45% and are probably responsible for many of the so-called "sterile" liver abscesses, reflecting the lack of adequate anaerobic transport and culture techniques (6). Immunosuppressed patients tend to have infections from unusual organisms and multiple small abscesses disseminated throughout the liver and spleen (7, 8). Patients with chronic granulomatous disease are also more susceptible to abscesses.

Pyogenic liver abscesses are multiple in 50–67% of patients, involving both lobes of the liver in 50% of these patients. The right lobe is involved in more than 75% of cases, most often in the posterior portion. This distribution has been explained on the basis of two-current blood flow in the portal vein. It is suggested that the superior mesenteric vein drains to the right lobe and the inferior mesenteric vein drains to the left lobe of the liver (9). Only 25% of abscesses are peripheral and contiguous with the liver capsule, unlike the majority of amebic abscesses (10).

Pathology

In the acute stage, an abscess consists of a focal accumulation of white cells in a region of parenchymal necrosis. In the subacute stage, the central collections of white cells become necrotic and neovascularity with fibroblastic proliferation occurs around the periphery. In the chronic stage, the abscess becomes walled off by the intense fibroblastic proliferation (11).

Clinical Findings

The classical presentation is with abdominal pain, swinging pyrexia, night sweats, vomiting, and malaise. Seventy-nine percent of patients present with pyrexia, 68% with pain, 43% with nocturnal sweating, 39% with vomiting or malaise (9). Jaundice is reported in 0–20% of cases, particularly when there is complicating biliary tract disease and usually indicates suppurative cholangitis and multiple abscess formation. Sixty-seven percent of patients presenting with pain complain of pain in the right upper quadrant, classically in the right subhepatic area. This pain is due to direct peritoneal irritation by the inflammatory process. About 28% of patients with pain either present with generalized abdominal pain or report a period of generalized abdominal pain followed by a pain-free interval of 1–5 weeks. This pain is probably generated by the stretching of the hepatic capsule and the pain-free interval is possibly due to a slowing of the cellulitic phase of the abscess formation. One-third of patients have no pain at the time of presentation (3), and some of these patients may present with a fever of unknown origin. Examination of the patient's abdomen is usually nonspecific. Tender hepatomegaly is found in fewer than half the patients; however, abdominal tenderness and rigidity can be marked. Patients may also present with symptoms of complications of pyogenic liver abscess such as rupture of the abscess into the chest, pericardium, or abdomen.

Radiology

Plain Films

The roentgen signs of liver abscess usually are too indefinite to permit a diagnosis from plain roentgenograms. Abdominal films may demonstrate hepatomegaly or gas-fluid levels within the liver (12) and fluoroscopy may demonstrate restricted motion of the right hemidiaphragm. Calcifications may be seen in the liver as a result of healed pyogenic abscesses (13). Findings on chest radiographs, although frequently seen, are nonspecific and include areas of discoid atelectasis, a right pleural effusion, and elevation and/or fixation of the right hemidiaphragm. Gas within the hepatic parenchyma, with or without an air-fluid level, is the only reliable sign of an intrahepatic abscess on a radiograph.

Urography

Tomograms of the liver taken during the total body opacification phase of excretory urography can reveal a hepatic abscess as a sharply defined radiolucent mass (Fig. 5.1).

Ultrasound

Most hepatic abscesses are seen in the chronic stage and are hypoechoic lesions with round or ovoid irregular margins (Fig. 5.2) (10, 14). Thick walls and increased echogenicity around the abscess are additional signs of chronicity (15, 16); however, the walls are usually well-defined and mildly echogenic but not thick. Occasionally, elliptical, lenticular, bilobate, or other shapes may be seen. Distal acoustic enhancement of variable degree is usually seen and is frequently a very prominent feature. Internal echogenicity

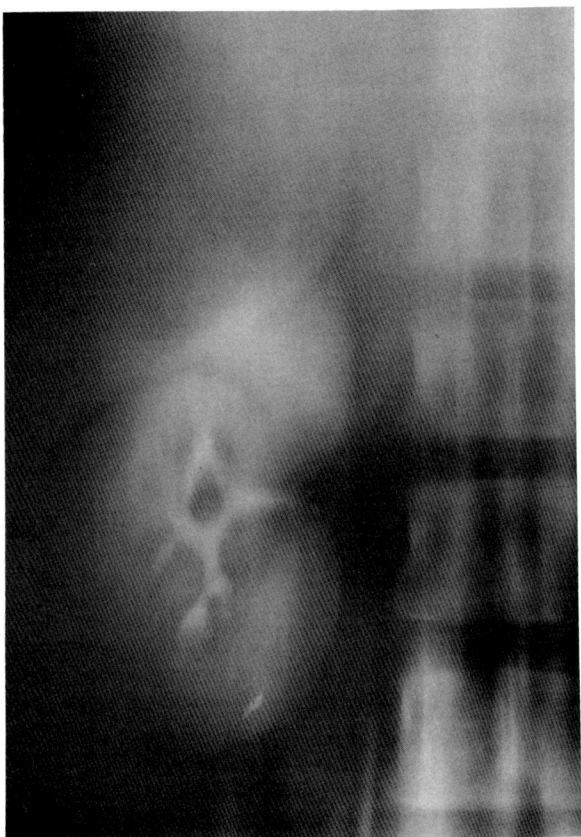

FIGURE 5.1. PYOGENIC ABSCESS
Nephrotomogram: sharply delineated radiolucent mass within the liver representing a pyogenic abscess.

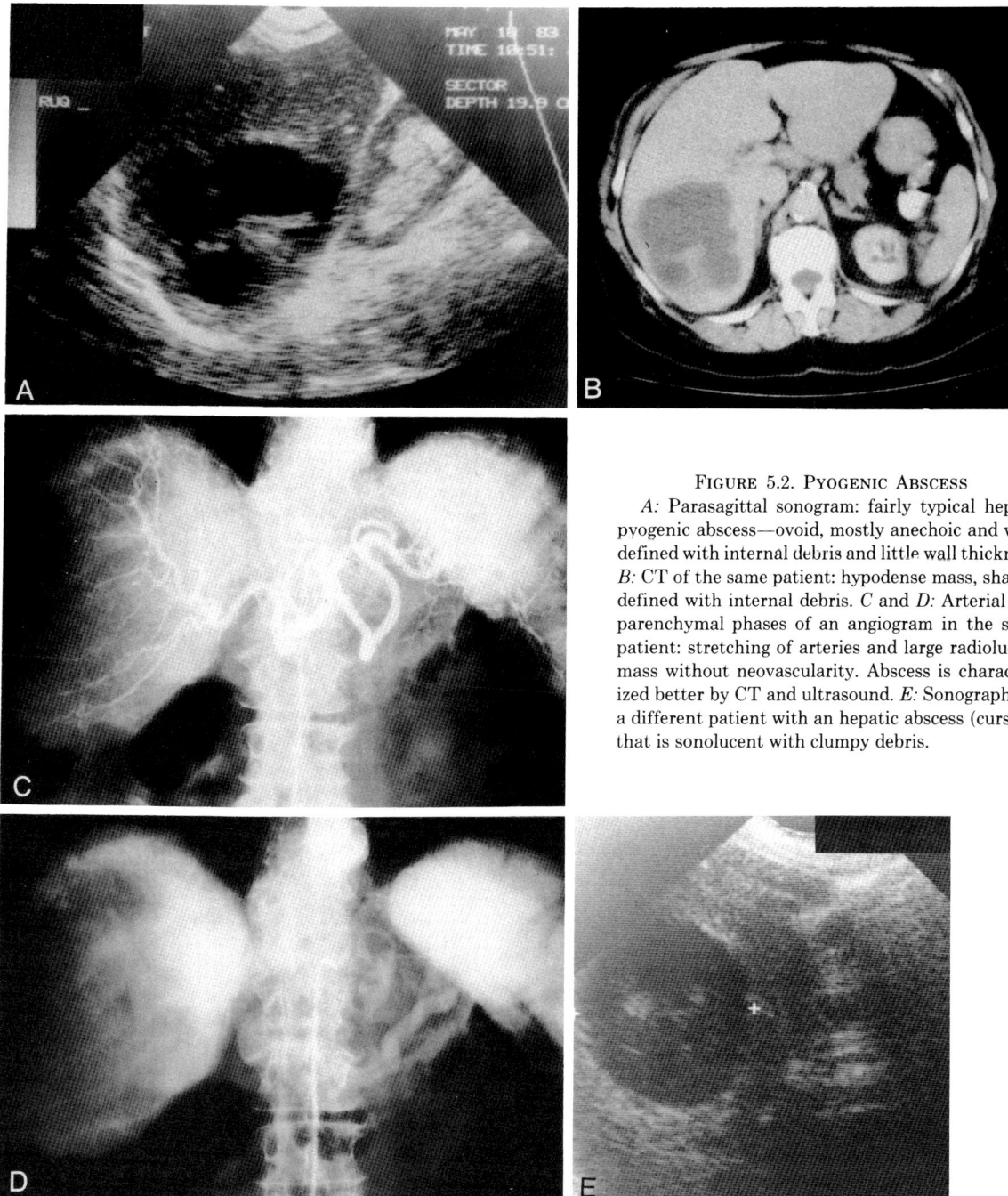

FIGURE 5.2. PYOGENIC ABSCESS
A: Parasagittal sonogram: fairly typical hepatic pyogenic abscess—ovoid, mostly anechoic and well-defined with internal debris and little wall thickness. B: CT of the same patient: hypodense mass, sharply defined with internal debris. C and D: Arterial and parenchymal phases of an angiogram in the same patient: stretching of arteries and large radiolucent mass without neovascularity. Abscess is characterized better by CT and ultrasound. E: Sonography of a different patient with an hepatic abscess (cursors) that is sonolucent with clumpy debris.

is very variable ranging from low-level echoes to coarse, clumpy debris and occasionally a fluid-debris level is seen (Fig. 5.2) (10, 17). Gas-containing abscesses are intensely echogenic with strong posterior reverberations and acoustic shadowing in some cases (15), while in others no distal acoustic shadowing is present (Fig. 5.3) (18). Acute abscesses are poorly demarcated focal regions of slightly increased echogenicity, whereas subacute abscesses are better demarcated with occasionally small central anechoic foci reflecting early development of a wall and neutrophil necrosis, respectively (Figs. 5.4 and 5.5) (11). Hepatic microabscesses due to S. au-

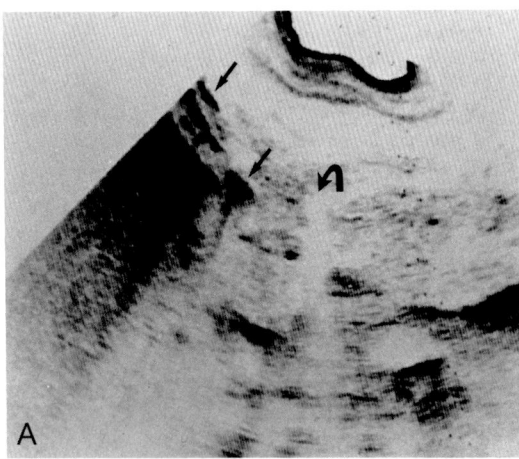
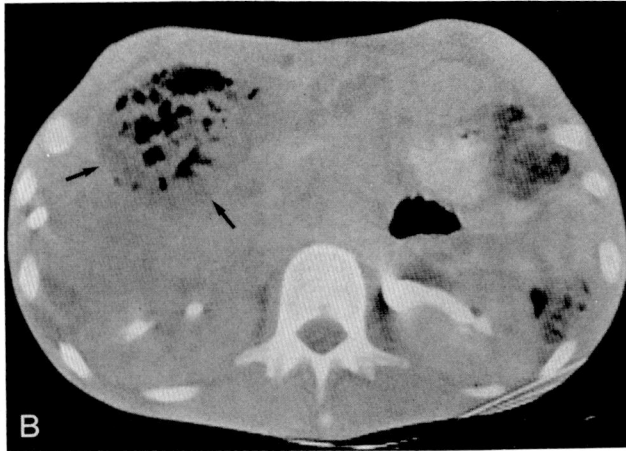

FIGURE 5.3. GAS-CONTAINING ABSCESS

A: Strong echoes and reverberations (*arrows*) and one area of shadowing (*curved arrow*) on a single-pass contact scan through a gas-containing hepatic abscess. B: CT of the same patient photographed at lung settings demonstrating the gas-containing abscess (*arrows*).

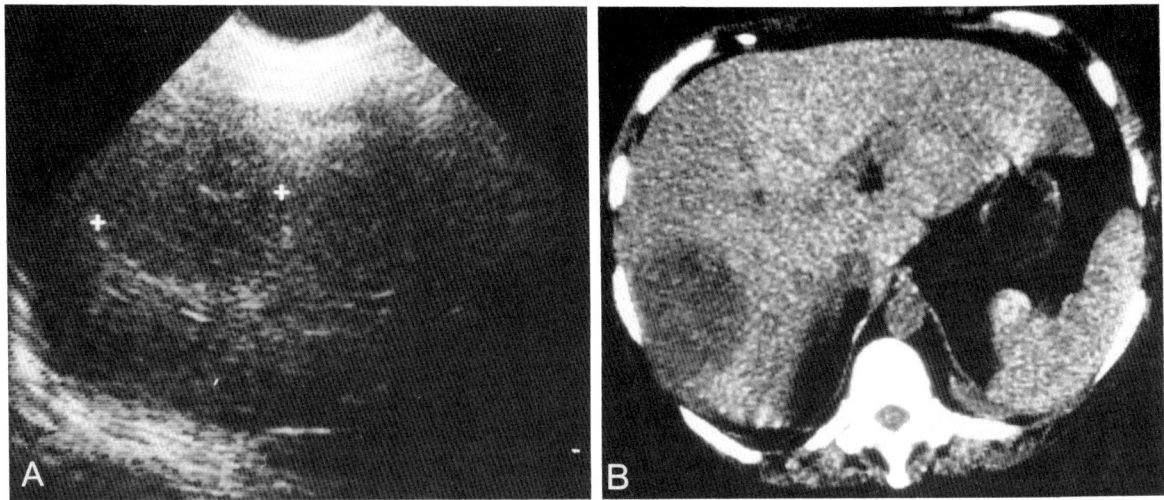

FIGURE 5.4. ISOECHOIC ACUTE ABSCESS

A: Isoechoic abscess between the cursors, detectable only by virtue of an echogenic wall. B: CT of the same patient (noncontrast): the abscess is hypodense compared to the liver but isodense with the inferior vena cava. Its contents have not yet liquefied.

reus in immunocompetent patients are indistinguishable from hepatic candidiasis (multiple small target lesions).

Computed Tomography

There is no characteristic CT appearance of pyogenic hepatic abscess although all are hypodense compared to adjacent liver (19, 20). A hepatic abscess may appear as a multiloculated single cavity or as multiple contiguous cavities (Figs. 5.2B, 5.3B, and 5.6). Most are inhomogeneous (19), but some hepatic abscesses are sufficiently well-circumscribed and have low enough density to be mistaken for cysts (20). In general, gas is present less often in hepatic abscesses than in abdominal abscesses (Fig. 5.3B) (19). Intravenous contrast administration increases the density difference between the abscess and the hepatic parenchyma allowing easier detection of the abscess. The wall of the abscess may demonstrate some increase in density, depending on the method of injection. Staphylococcal microabscesses in immunocompetent patients have the same CT appearance as hepatic candidiasis.

Dynamic CT densitometry reveals an abscess-

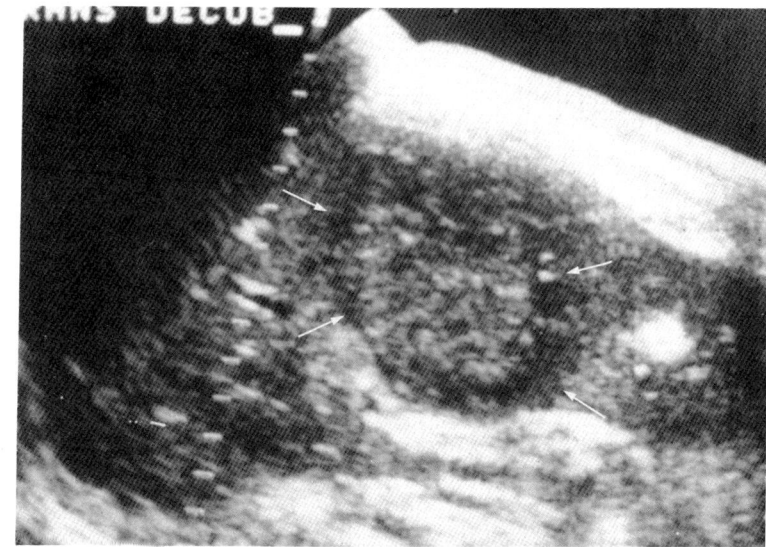

FIGURE 5.5. PYOGENIC ACUTE ABSCESS
Transverse sonogram: slightly hyperechoic abscess with a thick, hypoechoic wall (outlined by *arrows*).

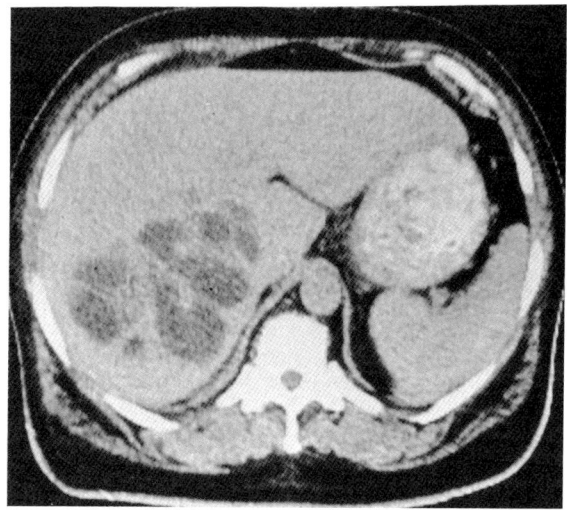

FIGURE 5.6. UNUSUAL MULTILOCULAR PYOGENIC ABSCESS
CT of an unusual multilocular pyogenic abscess mimicking an echinococcal cyst except for the lack of a defined wall.

liver density difference curve in which the curve ascends rapidly and descends quickly in a pattern of peripheral enhancement (21). A "double target sign" consisting of a hypodense central area surrounded first by a hyperdense ring and then a hypodense zone on dynamic CT is highly suggestive of pyogenic abscess and was found in 30% in one series (21). Dynamic CT may also show surrounding parenchymal arterial phase lobar hyperdensity possibly due to arterioportal shunting (21). Rarely, CT may not detect a small abscess. This is more likely to occur in a patient in which the overall liver density is decreased secondary to diffuse fatty infiltration or hepatic edema (19, 20).

Radionuclide Imaging

Scintigraphically, liver abscesses are depicted as photopenic lesions on liver-spleen, hepatobiliary, blood flow and blood pool images, as they displace and or destroy parenchymal tissue and are avascular lesions.

Technetium-99m sulfur colloid examinations of the liver are less sensitive and less specific than either computed tomography or ultrasound (22). Abscesses are shown as photon-deficient areas, as are other space-occupying lesions in the liver. Acute abscesses may not be detected because of lack of displacement of Kupffer cells (11). Liver abscesses are avid accumulators of gallium-67 citrate. Approximately 80% of these lesions will demonstrate ^{67}Ga-citrate uptake equal to or greater than surrounding liver parenchyma. It is important to note that a ^{67}Ga-citrate study of the liver should never be interpreted without a corresponding ^{99m}Tc-sulfur colloid study. Failure to correlate these two studies can result in false negative gallium studies, i.e., the hypoactive lesions on the ^{99m}Tc-sulfur colloid appearing isoactive on the ^{67}Ga-citrate study. In such an instance, correlation of the two studies clearly demonstrates the lesions to be ^{67}Ga-avid despite the apparent uniform distribution of the ^{67}Ga-citrate. ^{67}Ga-citrate is not helpful in differential diagnosis since it shows positive uptake in some benign and malignant tumors of the liver as well as abscesses. The use of indium-111 white

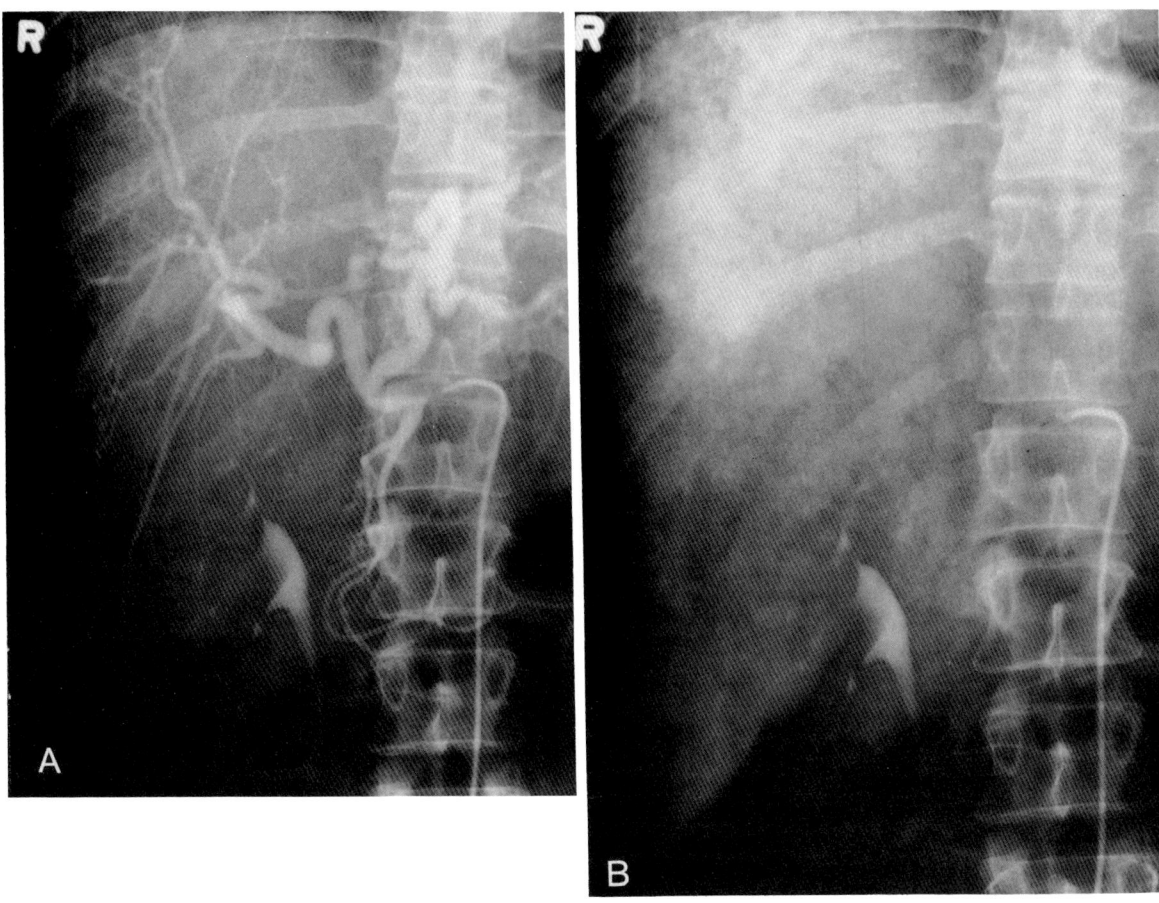

FIGURE 5.7. ANGIOGRAM OF A HEPATIC ABSCESS
A and B: Arterial and parenchymal phases of an angiogram showing stretching and displacement of intrahepatic arteries and mottled lucent parenchymogram in the right lobe. No neovascularity or early draining veins.

blood cells is useful in some patients to help differentiate abscess from other lesions when combined with sulfur colloid imaging. This technique has a high degree of specificity for lesions that have polymorphonuclear infiltration, and in general, solid tumors will not show uptake (23). Unfortunately, hepatic abscesses less than 2 cm are not detected by ^{111}In tagged white blood cells.

Angiography

The role of angiography in the diagnosis of hepatic abscess is limited, as the aforementioned techniques are more sensitive and specific (24). Most pyogenic abscesses studied angiographically are chronic and are avascular focal masses with vessel displacement and a hypervascular periphery (Figs. 5.2C and D, and 5.7A and B) (11). Acute or subacute abscesses can have increased vascularity within the abscess, irregular surrounding vessels, and, rarely, arteriovenous shunting (either portal or hepatic) (11). Very early abscesses can have intense hypervascularity without any associated mass effect (11).

REFERENCES

1. Buchman TG, Zuidema GD: The role of computerized tomographic scanning in the surgical management of pyogenic hepatic abscess. *Surg Gynecol Obstet* 153:1–9, 1981.
2. Barbour GL, Juniper K Jr: A clinical comparison of amebic and pyogenic abscess of the liver in sixty-six patients. *Am J Med* 53:323–333, 1972.
3. Young AE: The clinical presentation of pyogenic liver abscess. *Br J Surg* 63:216–219, 1976.
4. McFee AS, Franklin ME Jr, Aust JB: Pyogenic liver abscess. In Sabiston DC (ed): *Davis-Christopher Textbook of Surgery*. Philadelphia, W. B. Saunders, 1981, pp 1194–1201.
5. D'Orsi CJ, Ensminger W, Smith EH, Lew M: Gasforming intrahepatic abscess: a possible complication of arterial infusion chemotherapy. *Gastrointest Radiol* 4:157–161, 1979.
6. Sabbaj J, Sutter VL, Finegold SM: Anaerobic pyogenic liver abscess. *Ann Intern Med* 77:629–738, 1972.
7. Callen PW, Filly RA, Marcus FS: Ultrasonography and

computed tomography in the evaluation of hepatic microabscesses in the immunosuppressed patient. *Radiology* 136:433–434, 1980.
8. Sty JR, Starshak RJ: Comparative imaging in the evaluation of hepatic abscesses in immunocompromised children. *J Clin Ultrasound* 11:11–15, 1983.
9. Holdstock G, Balasegaram M, Millward-Sadler GH, Wright R: The liver in infection. In Wright R, Alberti KGMM, Karran S, Millward-Sadler GH (eds): *Liver and Biliary Disease.* Philadelphia, W. B. Saunders, 1979, p 1157.
10. Newlin N, Silver TM, Stuck KJ, Sandler MA: Ultrasonic features of pyogenic liver abscesses. *Radiology* 139:155–159, 1981.
11. Freeny PC: Acute pyogenic hepatitis: sonographic and angiographic findings. *AJR* 135:388–391, 1980.
12. McNulty JG: *Radiology of the Liver.* Philadelphia, W. B. Saunders, 1977, pp 253–262.
13. Darlak JJ, Moskowitz M, Kattan KR: Calcifications in the liver. *Radiol Clin North Am* 18:211, 1980.
14. Taylor KJW, Rosenfield AT: Ultrasound (Chapter 14). In Margulis AR, Burhenne HJ (eds): *Alimentary Tract Radiology.* St. Louis, C. V. Mosby, 1979, pp 183–207.
15. Kuligowska E, Connors SK, Shapiro JH: Liver abscess: sonography in diagnosis and treatment. *AJR* 183:253–257, 1982.
16. Yeh HC, Rabinowitz JG: Ultrasonography and computed tomography of the liver. *Radiol Clin North Am* 18:321–338, 1980.
17. Cunningham JJ: In vitro gray scale echography of protein-lipid fluid collection in liver tissue. *J Clin Ultrasound* 14:255–258, 1976.
18. Gosink BB: Intrahepatic gas: differential diagnosis. *AJR* 137:763–767, 1981.
19. Halvorsen RA, Korobkin M, Foster WL, Silverman PM, Thompson WM: The variable CT appearance of hepatic abscesses. *AJR* 141:941–946, 1984.
20. Rubinson HA, Isikoff MB, Hill MC: Diagnostic imaging of hepatic abscesses: a retrospective analysis. *AJR* 135:735–740, 1980.
21. Mathieu D, Vasile N, Fagniez P-L, Segui S, Grably D, Larde D: Dynamic CT features of hepatic abscesses. *Radiology* 154:749–752, 1985.
22. Grossman ZD, Wistow BW, Bryan PJ, Dinn WM, McAfee JG, Kieffer SA: Radionuclide imaging, computed tomography, and gray-scale ultrasonography of the liver: a comparative study. *J Nucl Med* 18:327–332, 1977.
23. Fawcett HD, Lantieri RL, Frankel A, McDougall IR: Differentiating hepatic abscess from tumor: combined In-111 white blood cell and ^{99m}Tc liver scans. *AJR* 135:53–56, 1980.
24. Gutierrez OH, Rosch J: Limitations of angiographic differential diagnosis in major hepatic processes. *ROFO* 127:1–8, 1977.

HEPATIC CANDIDIASIS

The liver is an unusual site for candidiasis to develop; hepatic candidiasis occurs nearly exclusively in immunosuppressed individuals. Common clinical settings are: children and adults with leukemia, chronic granulomatous disease of childhood, renal transplant recipients, and patients undergoing chemotherapy for myeloproliferative disorders (1–3). The diagnosis is difficult because of the nonspecific nature of the presenting signs and symptoms (fever, abdominal pain, tenderness to palpation of the liver, and hepatomegaly) (1). Hepatomegaly may be due to concomitant fatty infiltration rather than the candidiasis per se (4). Pathologic examination of the liver generally reveals multiple microabscesses or small granulomas which often contain both mycelia and yeast.

Radiology

Technetium-99m sulfur colloid scans will show hepatomegaly with either uniform uptake or focal photopenic regions due to abscesses (1). Gallium scans show regions of diminished uptake that correspond to those seen on the sulfur colloid scan. Possible explanations for this unusual gallium appearance include: low grade white cell response to the infection, paucity of white cells in the host, or inability of gallium to get into the lesion because of infarction (1). Similar findings have been reported in gallium imaging of actinomycosis and other anaerobic infections (1).

The sonographic findings are characteristic and consist of multiple small hypoechoic masses with echogenic centers giving a target or bull's-eye appearance (Fig. 5.8) (1–3). The hypoechoic

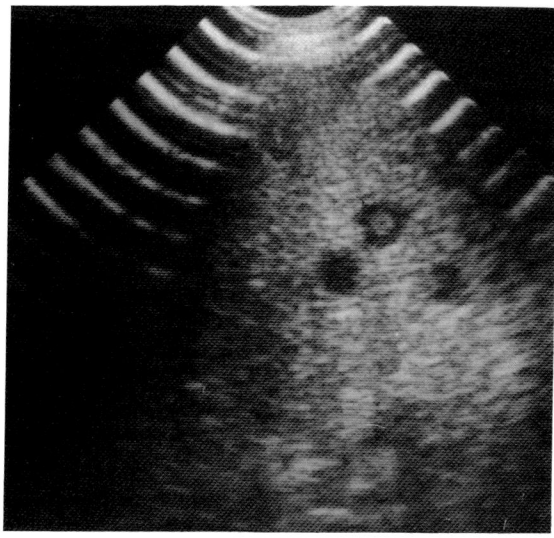

FIGURE 5.8. HEPATIC CANDIDIASIS
Real-time sonogram showing three hypoechoic microabscesses from hepatic candidiasis. Only one has a target appearance (one should not expect each microabscess to have a target appearance).

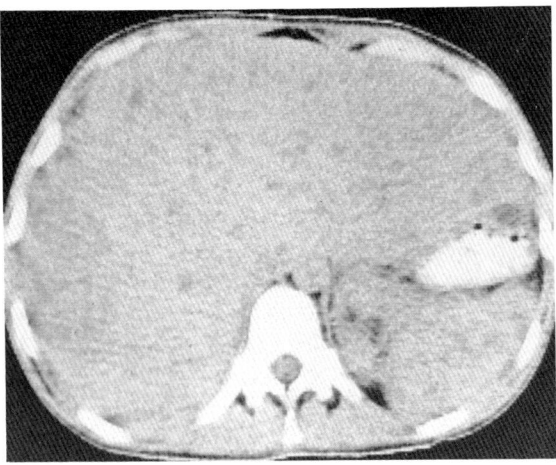

FIGURE 5.9. HEPATIC CANDIDIASIS
CT of the same patient as in Figure 5.8. The microabscesses are innumerable poorly defined low density lesions. The spleen is also affected.

region is composed of necrotic debris and pus and the bright central echo is probably a mycelial core (3).

CT can demonstrate multiple small low density lesions but is not as likely as ultrasound to show a target appearance (a central dot of higher attenuation) (Fig. 5.9) (3). The partial volume effect is probably the culprit.

Differential diagnosis on sonography and CT must include metastatic disease, lymphoma and leukemia (5, 6), other unusual or opportunistic infections and septic emboli. Culture and histologic examination of a percutaneous aspirate obtained with guidance by either modality can give a definitive diagnosis of candidiasis (3).

REFERENCES

1. Miller HM, Greenfield LD, Wald BR: Candidiasis of the liver and spleen in childhood. *Radiology* 142:375–380, 1982.
2. Callen PW, Filly RA, Marcus FS: Ultrasonography and computed tomography in the evaluation of hepatic microabscesses in the immunosuppressed patient. *Radiology* 136:433–434, 1980.
3. Ho B, Cooperberg PL, Li DKB, Mack L, Naiman SL, Grossman L: Ultrasonography and computed tomography of hepatic candidiasis in immunosuppressed patients. *J Ultrasound Med* 1:157–159, 1982.
4. Holdstock G, Balasegaram M, Millward-Sadler GH, Wright R. The liver in infection. In Wright R, Alberti KGMM, Karran S, Millward-Sadler CH (eds): *Liver and Biliary Disease*, Philadelphia, W. B. Saunders, 1979, pp 1137–1179.
5. Scheible W, Gosink BB, Leopold GR: Gray scale echographic patterns of hepatic metastatic disease. *AJR* 129:983–987, 1977.
6. Ginaldi S, Bernardino ME, Jing BS, Green B: Ultrasonographic patterns of hepatic lymphoma. *Radiology* 136:427–431, 1980.

AMEBIC ABSCESS

Amebic abscess of the liver is caused by the parasite *Entamoeba histolytica*. Although the major manifestations of amebiasis are enteric in location, the organism is not limited to the intestinal tract. The liver is the most common extraintestinal organ affected (1–25% of patients). Amebic abscess of the liver is a complication, which, if left untreated, often proceeds to a fatal outcome (1).

Clinical Findings

Formerly believed to occur principally in tropical and subtropical regions, amebiasis is now recognized to be endemic in areas of the United States with poor sanitation, especially the South (2). For unknown reasons, males are affected more often than females in a 4:1 ratio (1, 2). Amebiasis is most common in adults, especially in the third, fourth, and fifth decades (1, 2).

Amebic abscess of the liver may present in a variety of ways (3, 4). Amebic abscess may accompany an acute attack of intestinal amebiasis or may present weeks to months or even years after the initial intestinal infection. Often there is no clue as to when the bowel disease occurred. Onset may be insidious with vague right upper quadrant pain or very rapid with fever, chills, rigor, and sharp stabbing pain. The pain is usually located over the liver, although it may be located anteriorly below the right costal margin, or posteriorly over the twelfth rib. The pain may be pleuritic in nature, worsened by deep breathing or coughing or it may be referred to the right shoulder due to involvement of the diaphragm. Pain and tenderness are greatest when the lesion is expanding rapidly (3). Anorexia, weight loss, nausea, vomiting, and fatigue are accompanying symptoms.

The most common finding on physical examination is an enlarged, tender liver. The spleen is not enlarged, and if it is, other diagnoses should be entertained. The right hemidiaphragm may be elevated to percussion and exhibit poor excursion. Fever is usually present but may be low grade.

Characteristically a moderate leukocytosis is found in hepatic amebic abscesses versus a more pronounced leukocytosis in a pyogenic liver abscess. Mild anemia is common (4). Eosinophilia is not a feature of amebic abscess of the liver as opposed to other parasitic infections. Liver function tests are nonspecifically elevated. Jaundice is rare. Even after careful examination, less than half of patients show evidence of trophozoites or cysts in the stools. Serologic tests are positive in nearly all patients with proven amebic liver abscess. Because of persistence of elevated antibody titers months to years after cure, serology in endemic areas is of most value in excluding the diagnosis.

Thoracic involvement occurs in 10–35% of patients with hepatic amebiasis (4). Rupture may occur into the pleura or lungs causing an empyema or pulmonary abscess. A hepato-bronchial fistula may develop and present as expectoration of dark chocolate brown material (1). Rupture into the pericardium (usually fatal) or lesser sac may occur in abscesses involving the left lobe (3). Intraperitoneal rupture causes acute peritonitis. Rupture into the portal vein, bile ducts, or gastrointestinal tract is rare. Rupture into the bronchial tree or the gastrointestinal tract may lead to spontaneous cure.

Chloroquine and metronidazole are effective in eradicating amebic liver abscesses. Drainage, although usually unnecessary, is indicated in impending perforation or failure to respond to drug therapy. Adequate drainage can usually be accomplished by needle alone (4). A therapeutic trial of metronidazole in suspected amebic liver abscess may cause serious error, as this drug inhibits anaerobic bacteria, a major cause of pyogenic liver abscess (4).

Pathology

E. histolytica gains access to the portal system through the intestinal walls and thereby enters the liver. Actual invasion and growth of the amebae in the liver are more likely if an overwhelming number of parasites with relatively increased virulence enter the liver, or if host resistance is lowered. It is thought that the amebae lodge in small portal radicles in sufficient numbers to cause thrombosis and infarction of parenchyma. Amebic cytolytic activity causes tissue destruction and abscess formation. It is uncertain whether an inflammatory amebic hepatitis actually precedes the frank suppurative abscess cavity (1). The infection may cease by itself with healing by connective tissue replacement and scar formation, or it may go on to form a large abscess cavity. The outcome depends on the virulence of the organisms and the host resistance (2). During the early phase of abscess formation, amebae are found in the center of focal necrosis. However, as the abscess enlarges and matures, the amebae are more likely to be found in the peripheral zone of necrotic tissue. The right lobe of the liver is most commonly affected, usually near the dome of the diaphragm. Although amebic abscess is usually solitary, multiple abscesses develop in about 25% (1, 2, 4). The right lobe is affected much more often than the left lobe (4). The gross appearance is an enlarged liver with single or multiple abscesses usually between 2 and 12 cm in diameter (5). Aspiration typically yields an opaque reddish, dirty brown, or pink material which is thick in new abscesses and becomes thinner with age (4). *E. histolytica* can sometimes be demonstrated by direct microscopy or culture of the aspirated fluid.

Radiology

Plain film findings include elevation of the right hemidiaphragm with decreased mobility, obliteration of the right costophrenic angle by pleural effusion, and right lower lobe atelectasis and/or infiltrate (Fig. 5.10) (4). Well defined basal opacities can be seen in contiguity with the diaphragm after transdiaphragmatic spread. Loculated pleural densities representing empyemas result after intrapleural rupture (Fig. 5.11) (4). The appearance of pericardial effusion often heralds rupture into the pericardium (4).

Intravenous infusion hepatotomography can depict amebic abscesses as radiolucencies surrounded by a relatively thick opaque band (5).

Scintigraphically, amebic abscesses, like pyogenic abscesses, appear as photopenic areas on liver/spleen, hepatobiliary, blood flow and blood pool imaging (Fig. 5.12A). They too displace and/or destroy liver parenchymal cells, and thus produce photopenic areas on isotopic images (6). If gallium-67 citrate is administered, amoebic abscesses are sometimes manifested as a photopenic area surrounded by a rim of radiotracer, i.e., the rim of increased activity representing the inflammatory reaction produced by the amoebic abscess (corresponding to the photopenic area) itself (Fig. 5.12B) (7). Unfortunately, pyogenic abscesses may look similar. Amebic abscesses are not as well detected on gallium scans as are pyogenic liver abscesses.

The sensitivity of sulfur colloid liver scintigraphy in the detection of amoebic abscess is approximately 98%. Thus, it can be extremely useful in aiding in the establishment of the ap-

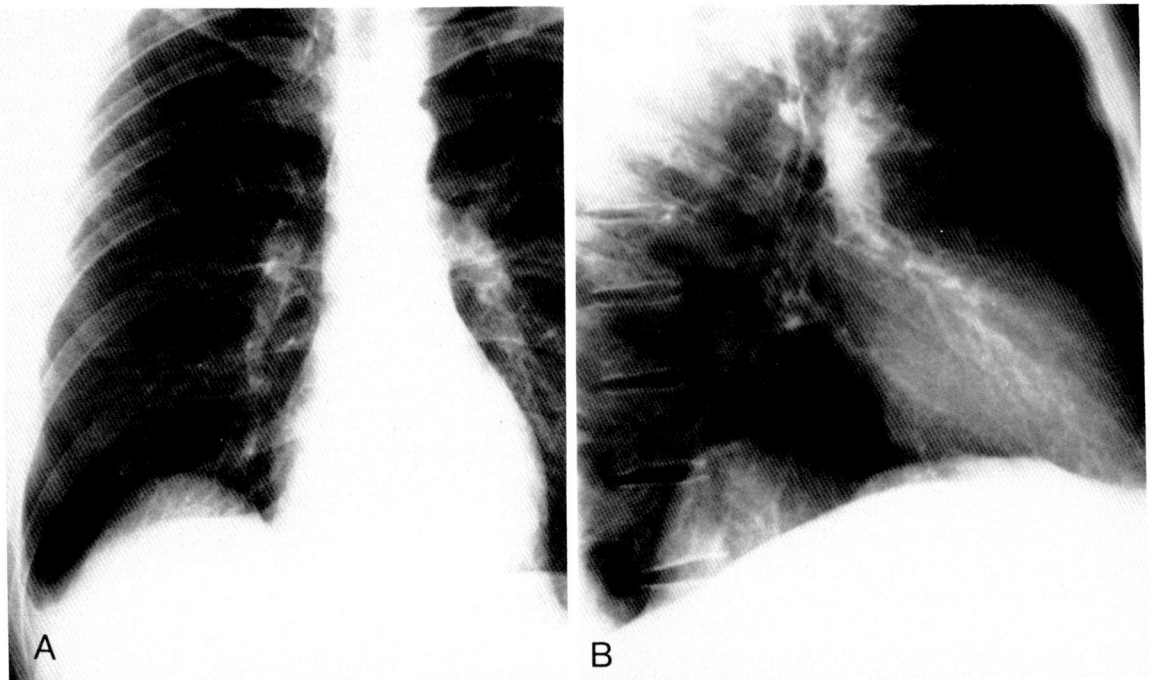

FIGURE 5.10. AMEBIC ABSCESS

A and *B:* Posteroanterior and lateral chest films: focal elevation of the right hemidiaphragm from an amebic abscess in the right lobe of the liver.

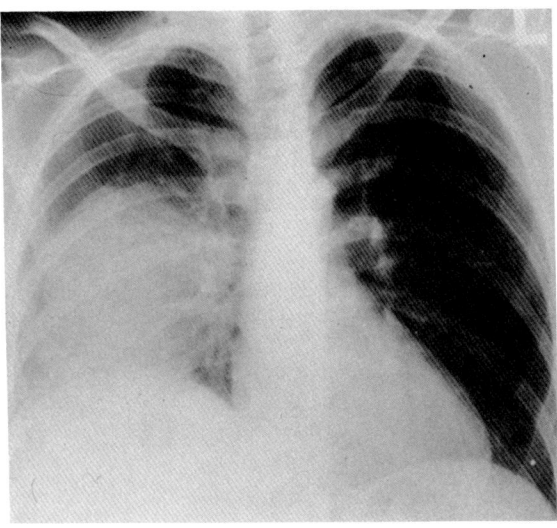

FIGURE 5.11. ELEVATED RIGHT HEMIDIAPHRAGM AND LARGE LOCULATED PLEURAL EFFUSION FROM A RUPTURED AMEBIC ABSCESS

propriate diagnosis. Additionally, it can also be used to monitor the patient's response to therapy. If appropriately treated, abscesses may disappear within 2–5 months post-therapy.

The sonographic appearance of an amebic abscess is variable and usually nonspecific (Fig. 5.13) (5, 7–11). The usual pattern is that of a homogeneously hypoechoic area with well-defined smooth thin walls. Prior to liquefaction a relatively new amebic abscess can mimic an echogenic mass (Fig. 5.14). In general, the older the lesion the smoother the wall and the fewer the echoes, findings that correlate well with pathologic observations of debris resorption and thinning of abscess content with age (Fig. 5.15) (5). Other manifestations on ultrasound are fluid-fluid levels, a complex mixture of cystic and highly echogenic components, target lesions with a dense echogenic center and a hypoechoic periphery, lesions with increased through transmission and lesions with a surrounding thick, echogenic halo. One finding that strongly suggests an amebic abscess is diaphragmatic disruption suggestive of rupture of the abscess into the pleural space (Fig. 5.16) (11). Post-therapy follow-up of patients with hepatic amebic abscesses have shown that the abscesses disappear over a 1½-month to 2-yr interval leaving normal or minimally altered liver parenchyma sonographically. There is no tendency for larger abscesses to take a longer time to resolve (12). Cysts may be permanent residua and indistinguishable from simple liver cysts (12). During the first few weeks of drug therapy, the size of the abscess may

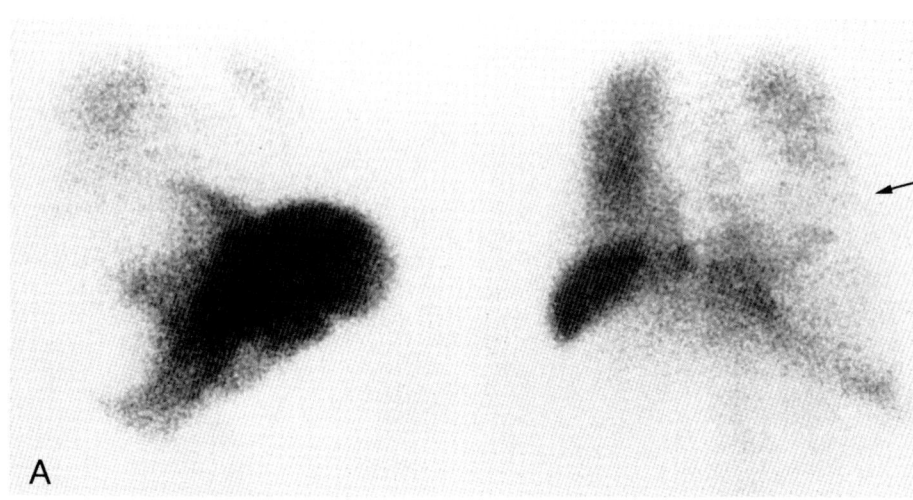

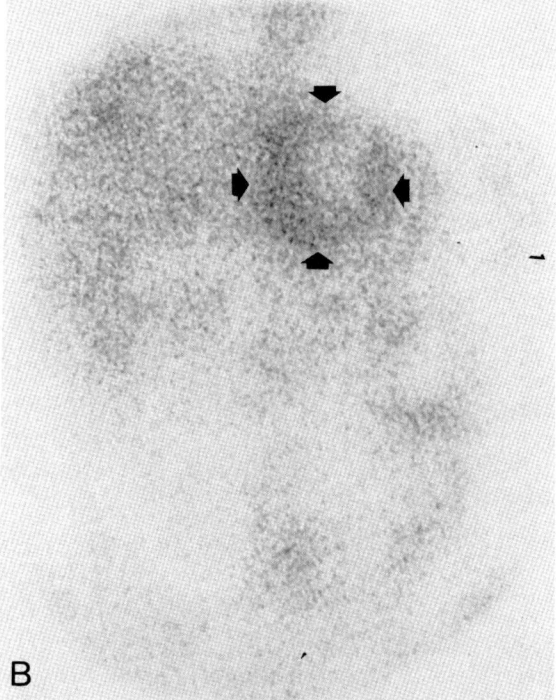

FIGURE 5.12. AMEBIC ABSCESS
A: Anterior (*left*) and posterior (*right*) liver/lung scan (sulfur-colloid and ^{99m}Tc-MAA) shows large hepatic defect representing a large amebic abscess. Note separation of liver dome and lung base (*arrow*) indicating transdiaphragmatic spread. *B:* Gallium scan of an amebic abscess: thick rim of uptake (*arrows*) surrounding a central photopenic region. (From Rubinson HA, Isikoff MB, Hill MC: Diagnostic imaging of hepatic abscesses: a retrospective analysis. *AJR* 135:735–740, 1980.)

increase, decrease or remain the same (Fig. 5.15). Initial changes include enlarging anechoic areas and production of multiple foci of high amplitude echoes. Initial enlargement on sonography does not imply treatment failure if there is clinical improvement. Later the amebic abscess shrinks and fills in with echoes resembling normal parenchyma (12). Some successfully treated abscesses may calcify rather than shrink (Fig. 5.17) (11). Ultrasound is very useful as guidance if needle aspiration of the abscess is deemed necessary.

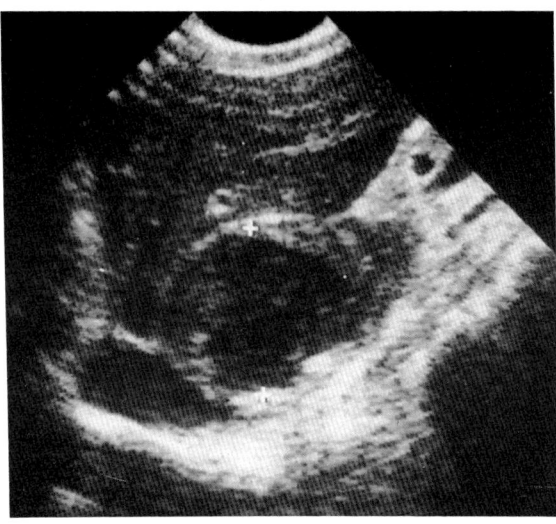

FIGURE 5.13. AMEBIC ABSCESS
Parasagital sonogram: hypoechoic amebic abscess in the caudate lobe (*cursors*). The abscess is fairly young, as evinced by the large number of internal echoes and thick internal contents.

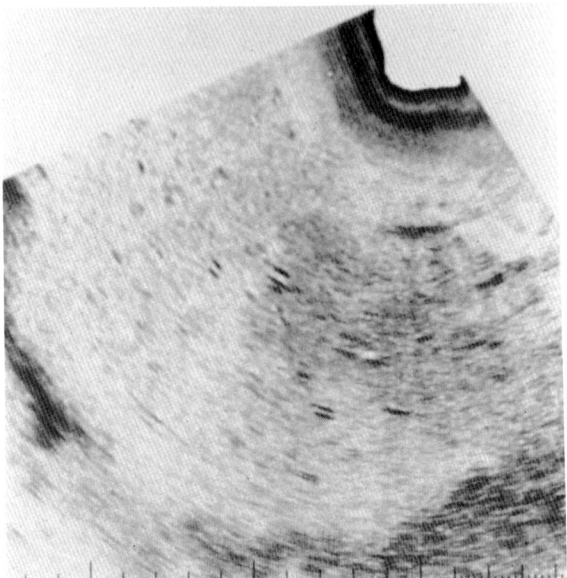

FIGURE 5.14. SOLID AMEBIC ABSCESS
Parasagittal sonogram: ill-defined hyperechoic solid amebic "abscess" scanned very early, prior to liquefaction.

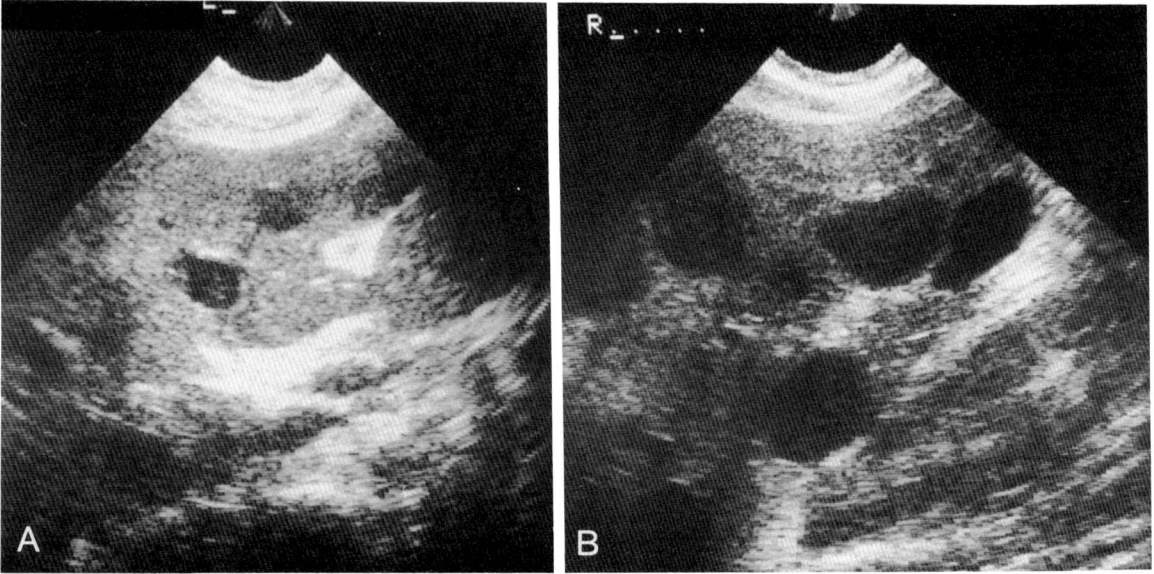

FIGURE 5.15. RESPONSE OF AMEBIC ABSCESS TO TREATMENT
A: Baseline scan: three hypoechoic abscesses with considerable numbers of internal echoes and poor through-transmission.
B: Two weeks later, despite good clinical response, the abscesses have increased in size and number. They have liquefied to a greater extent as well.

CT has also been utilized to evaluate patients with suspected amebic abscesses (10). Number, size, and location of amebic abscesses can easily be evaluated by CT. A nonspecific, well-defined lesion of attenuation lower than the surrounding normal parenchyma is generally found (Fig. 5.18). Early lesions may have densities similar to a solid tumor. Present at times is a thin crescentic or circumferential zone of low density parallel to and just beyond the wall. Its pathologic correlate is unknown although it could represent inflamed parenchyma (13). Contrast enhancement may occur peripherally in the wall but does not occur centrally (13). Although CT is sensitive in demonstrating hepatic amebic abscesses, it usually does not provide any significant information beyond what is obtained by liver scintigraphy and ultrasound.

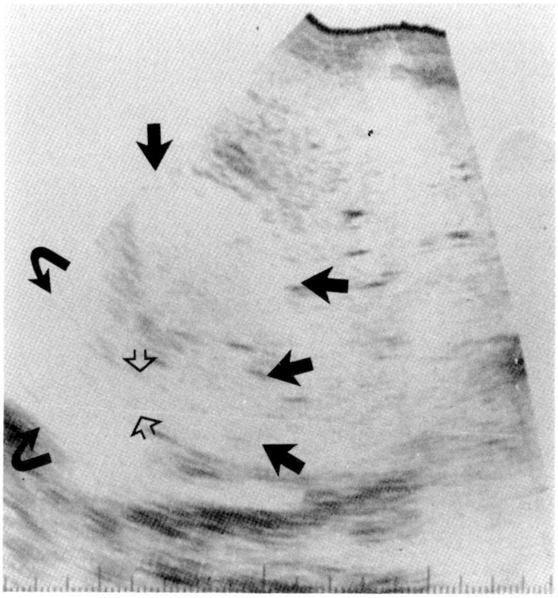

FIGURE 5.16. RUPTURED AMEBIC ABSCESS
Parasagittal scan of an amebic abscess (*arrows*) that has ruptured through the diaphragm (*open arrows* define the breach) and has caused an empyema (*curved arrows*).

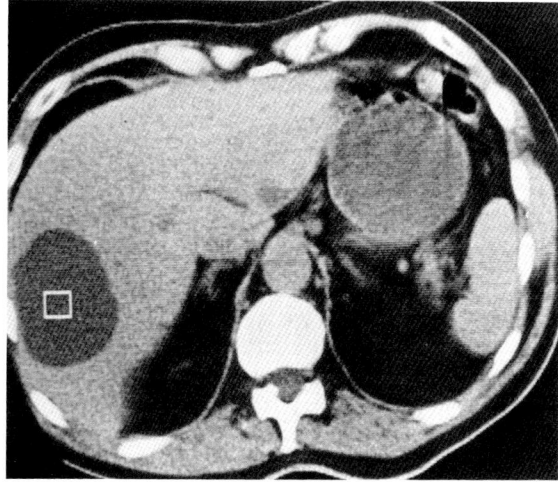

FIGURE 5.18. CT OF AN AMEBIC ABSCESS: NONSPECIFIC LOW ATTENUATION MASS

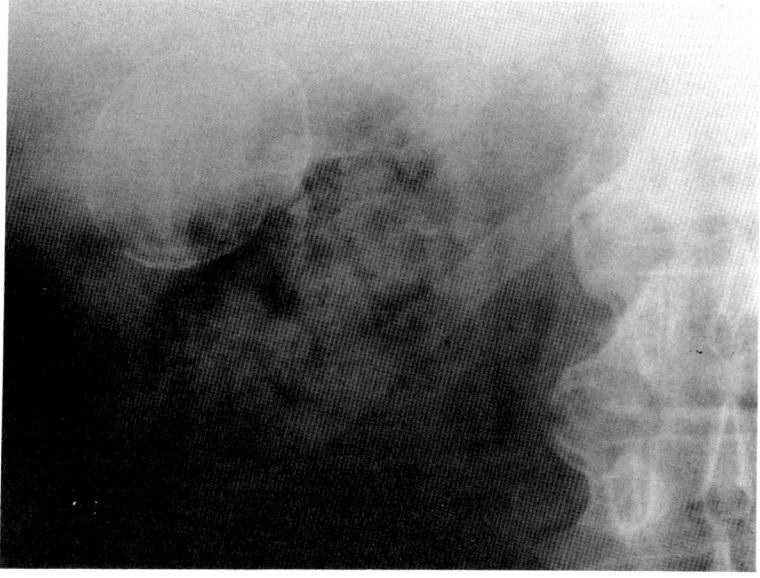

FIGURE 5.17. CONED DOWN VIEW OF THE RIGHT UPPER QUADRANT: CALCIFICATION IN THE WALL OF A HEALED AMEBIC ABSCESS

REFERENCES

1. Curtis KJ, Sleisenger MH: Amebic abscess of the liver. In Sleisenger MH, Fordtran JS (eds): *Gastrointestinal Disease.* Philadelphia, W. B. Saunders, 1978, pp 1700–1705.
2. DeBakey ME, Jordan GL: Hepatic abscess. In Schiff L (ed): *Diseases of the Liver.* Philadelphia, J. B. Lippincott, 1975, pp 1103–1136.
3. Adams EB, MacLeod IN: Invasive amebiasis. *Medicine* 56:325–334, 1977.
4. Sherlock S: *Diseases of the Liver and Biliary System.* Oxford, Blackwell Scientific, 1981, pp 431–435.
5. Boultbee E, Simjee AE, Rooknoodeen F, Engelbrecht HE: Experiences with gray scale ultrasonography in hepatic amebiasis. *Clin Radiol* 30:683–689, 1979.
6. McCready VR: Scintigraphic studies of space-occupying liver disease. *Semin Nucl Med* 2:111–116, 1972.
7. Rubinson HA, Isikoff MB, Hill MC: Diagnostic imaging of hepatic abscesses: a retrospective analysis. *AJR* 135:735–740, 1980.
8. Ralls PW, Colletti PM, Quinn MF, Halls J: Sonographic findings in hepatic amebic abscess. *Radiology* 145:123–126, 1982.
9. Ralls PW, Meyers HI, Lapin SA, Rogers W, Boswell MD, Halls J: Gray-scale ultrasonography of hepatic amebic abscesses. *Radiology* 132:125–129, 1979.
10. Sukov RJ, Cohen LJ, Sample WF: Sonography of hepatic amebic abscess. *AJR* 134:911–914, 1980.
11. Landay MJ, Setiawan H, Hirsch G, Christensen EE, Conrad MR: Hepatic and thoracic amebiasis. *AJR* 135:449–454, 1980.
12. Ralls PW, Quinn MF, Boswell WD Jr, Colletti PM, Radin DR, Halls J: Patterns of resolution in successfully treated hepatic amebic abscess: sonographic evaluation. *Radiology* 149:541–543, 1983.
13. Stephens DM, Sheedy PF II: The liver. In Haaga JR, Alfidi RJ (eds): *Computed Tomography of the Whole Body.* St. Louis, C. V. Mosby, 1983, pp 589–590.

ECHINOCOCCAL DISEASE

Epidemiology

Echinococcal (hydatid) disease is a parasitic tapeworm infection caused by the larvae of either *Echinococcus granulosus* or *Echinococcus multilocularis (alveolaris)*. *E. granulosus*, the most common form, is endemic in sheep raising countries of South America, the Near and Middle East, East and South Africa, Central Europe, Australia, New Zealand, Alaska and Western Canada. In the United States it is rare but found most often in Utah, California, New Mexico, Arizona, and the lower Mississippi River Valley (1, 2).

Echinococcus granulosus

The liver is the organ most commonly infected by the parasite (approximately 70% of all hydatid cysts are located in the liver), and worldwide, the most common cyst of the liver is the echinococcal cyst (1). Hydatid cysts are also known to occur in the brain, lung, kidney, and bone.

Humans are infected secondarily by ingestion of food or water contaminated by dog feces containing the eggs of the parasite. Once the intermediate host ingests the eggs, the outer capsule of the egg is dissolved by digestive juices and the released oncosphere passes through the duodenal mucosa into the portal circulation and lodges in the liver, either to die and disintegrate or grow into an echinococcal cyst (3, 4). The cyst may attain a size up to 20 cm (5). The right lobe of the liver is the most common location in which cysts are found, presumably due to the greater amount of portal venous flow to that portion of the liver (3).

Clinical Findings

Most echinococcal cysts go undetected throughout an infected person's life and the only complaint may be a vague upper abdominal fullness or pain due to the enlarging cyst encroaching on adjacent organs. Often a mass is felt unexpectedly by the patient or physician. If complications develop, the patient may experience dramatic symptoms. Cysts near the liver hilum may compress biliary ducts and vessels, causing jaundice and lobar atrophy, or portal hypertension with splenomegaly (5). Growth of the cyst may encroach upon, erode through, and finally rupture into the biliary system, expelling the contents of the cyst into the bile ducts and causing obstructive jaundice (6). Rupture of the cyst into the biliary tract occurs in 5–10% of cases with liver involvement, and may be minute and occult or massive and frank (7). Harris described a triad of symptoms and signs typical of rupture into the biliary tract which included biliary colic with or without an allergic reaction in adolescents or young adults, jaundice, and laminated membranes of the cyst in feces (8). Symptoms may mimic those of cholecystitis exactly, and the diagnosis can be suspected only if there are other signs of hydatid disease. In one series, rupture occurred most often into the right hepatic duct (55%), followed by the left hepatic duct (29%), the bifurcation (9%), the gallbladder (69%) and the common bile duct (1%) (9).

Sudden abdominal pain followed by urticaria and fever with or without anaphylactic shock occurs when a cyst suddenly ruptures into the peritoneal cavity (1, 3). Peritoneal implants may occur (Fig. 5.19). Intrathoracic rupture may be

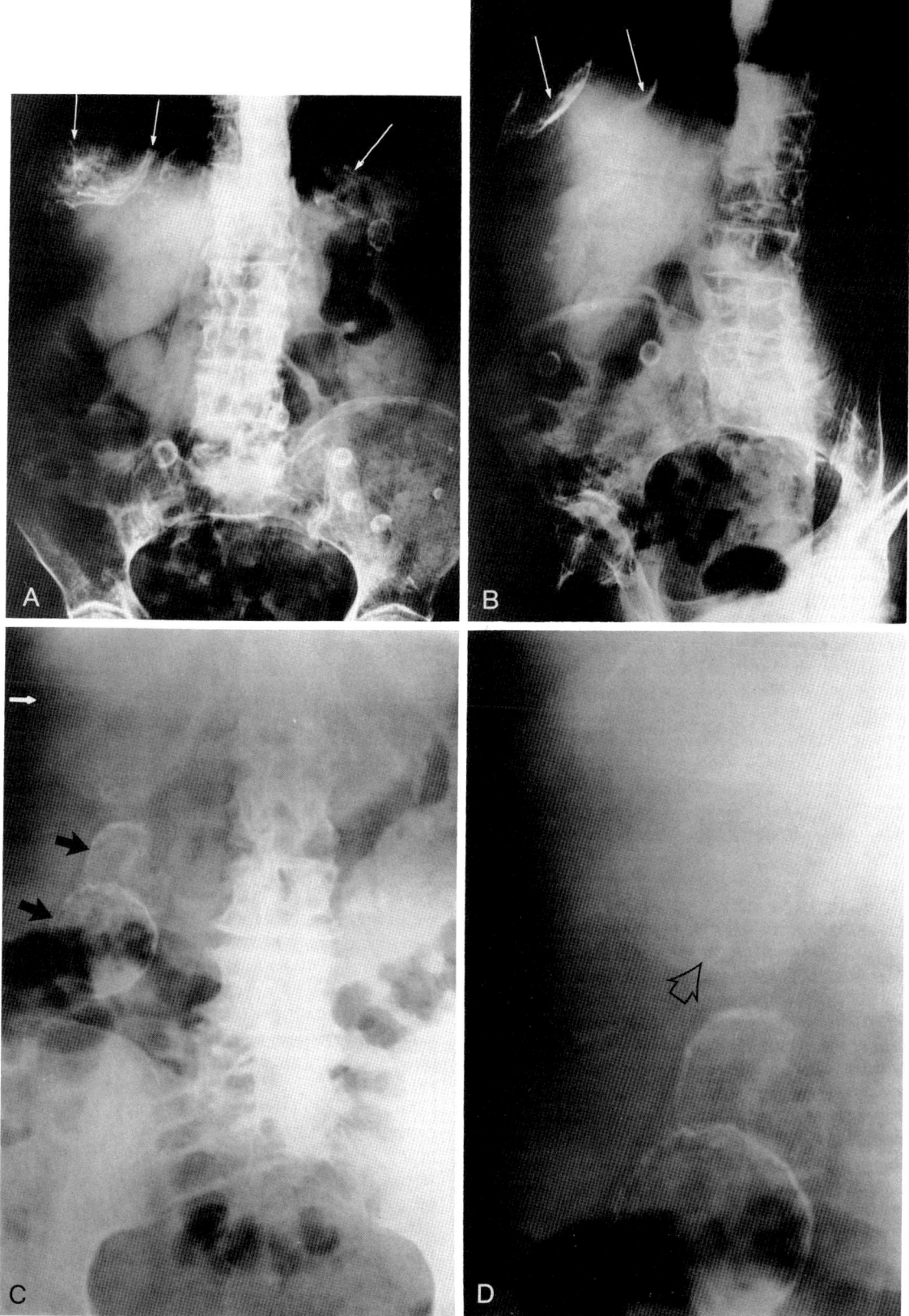

FIGURE 5.19. ECHINOCOCCAL DISEASE

A and *B:* Frontal (*A*) and oblique (*B*) films of the abdomen demonstrate calcified collapsed hydatid cysts in the right and left lobes of the liver (*arrows*) after intraperitoneal rupture. The multiple round calcifications are daughter cysts in the peritoneal cavity. *C* and *D:* Abdominal film showing three calcified hydatid cysts (*arrows*). (*C*). Blow-up (*D*) shows daughter cyst (*arrow*) to better advantage.

acute or chronic and is also characterized by severe pain, as well as dyspnea and coughing when rupture has occurred into the bronchus (3). Occasionally a Budd-Chiari syndrome may develop due to vascular compression by an enlarging cyst.

An eosinophil count over 5% is seen in about 50% of the patients and above 7% in 25% of infected patients (1). Eosinophil counts tend to be much higher in patients with rupture (20–25%) than in patients with uncomplicated intrahepatic cysts. Leukocytosis is usually seen when there is an infected cyst. Liver function testing is usually not helpful (1). The intradermal test of Casoni is helpful but gives false positives in other helminthic diseases. Five laboratory studies are currently used in the preoperative diagnosis of hydatid cyst: complement fixation, double diffusion, immunoelectrophoresis, indirect hemagglutination, and latex agglutination (10). The first three are the most specific and are positive in 70–90% of patients with abdominal hydatid disease. Conventional wisdom is that percutaneous needle aspiration for diagnosis or therapy is contraindicated in suspected hydatid cyst because of the danger of anaphylactic reaction or dissemination of cyst contents. However, a review of 222 cases of inadvertent needling or rupture of hepatic echinococcal cysts revealed only one anaphylactic death and six cases of "asthma" (11). One case of curative percutaneous drainage of a hepatic hydatid cyst has been reported. In properly selected cases, percutaneous drainage may be the treatment of choice (11). Prolonged administration of mebendazole kills the germinative layer and has been especially effective against peritoneal and pulmonary hydatid cysts since they have less surrounding fibrotic reaction than their hepatic counterparts. Intracystic instillation of mebendazole may be a useful adjunct to percutaneous therapy (11).

Surgery is usually performed once the diagnosis of hydatid cyst of the liver has been made, with the possible exception of the asymptomatic, completely calcified cyst. Complete resection is the preferred surgical treatment.

Pathology

Hydatid cysts are usually single at first, but with time, daughter cysts may develop by fragmentation of the original cyst. About 20% of patients have multiple cysts (5). Each cyst consists of an endocyst formed by elements of the parasite itself which includes the inner germinative layer which gives rise to the brood capsules and scolices and an external membrane composed of a laminated chitin-like substance surrounded by an outer membrane or pericyst, which is formed by host granulation tissue and fibrosis in reaction to the parasite (4). The cysts grow slowly and may not become symptomatic until adulthood, many years after the initial infection which often occurs during childhood.

The fluid within the cyst is usually clear, unless the cyst becomes secondarily infected. Bile-stained fluid is seen in cysts which have ruptured into the biliary system, and old cysts may contain a thick, gelatinous material (1). Cysts implanted near the liver edge are often bilocular or pedunculated and encircled by adhesions to the diaphragm or peritoneum.

Radiology

Plain Films. The plain film of the abdomen is positive in about 35% of cases (6). Hepatomegaly is valuable only when circumscribed with a round border corresponding to the protruding part (6). Complete peripheral calcification in the pericyst is said to imply inactivity or death (6). However, it is probably more a reflection of chronicity rather than lack of viability. Polycyclic rim calcification in both mother and daughter cysts or the crushed eggshell calcification from cyst rupture and collapse can give a fairly specific plain film diagnosis (Fig. 5.19). Rounded, thin white lines surrounding the cyst due to a compressed pericyst caused by rapid growth have been described (6). Pneumobilia and/or air in the cysts can occur secondary to biliary rupture and incompetence of the sphincter of Oddi. Air fluid levels and floating membranes and vesicles may be seen as well (6). Pericystic gas bubbles imply superinfection (6). Elevation and deformity of the right hemidiaphragm may be seen on a chest film. Pleural effusion can be seen in cases of transdiaphragmatic perforation as well as chest wall masses, and bronchobiliary fistula can cause pneumobilia (6).

Intravenous Hepatotomography. This procedure is described as plain film hepatotomography performed 10 minutes after intravenous administration of urographic contrast material and was 83% accurate in one series (6). Findings are similar to those seen in the parenchymal phase of arteriography: round radiolucencies sometimes surrounded by a halo of increased density secondary to contrast accumulation in the pericyst. Haloes are 2–3 mm thick in uncomplicated cysts and may be thicker if there is superimposed bacterial infection.

Nuclear Medicine. Scintigraphically, hydatid cysts and amoebic abscesses are identical. Both organisms usually reach the liver via the right lobar portal trunk creating an intrahepatic mass, manifested as a photopenic area on technetium sulfur colloid liver scan which elicits an inflammatory reaction, manifested as a rim of increased activity on gallium-67 citrate study.

Ultrasound. Several sonographic appearances have been described (3, 5, 12, 13). The hydatid cyst may be a well-defined anechoic mass indistinguished from a simple cyst. Septations are frequently seen. Daughter cysts are depicted as small cysts internally tangent to the mother cyst (Fig. 5.20). Floating membranes or vesicles can be seen. Punctate shadowing and internal echogenicities are due to small calcifications. Thickening, shagginess and shadowing involving the wall is caused by peripheral calcification. Internal echogenic regions without shadowing or layering are sometimes demonstrated and suggest superinfection. Cysts may be multiple and oriented in a horizontal, vertical or diagonal array. Sometimes multiple cysts together with some echogenic areas are enclosed within a single capsule termed a "racemose" appearance. Rarely, hydatid cysts will have a predominantly solid or completely solid appearance. This appearance may be due to a high rate of activity of the germinative membrane, creating numerous daughters which are crammed together causing a solid appearance (14). When intrabiliary rupture has occurred (Fig. 5.21A), hydatid sand can be seen in dilated ducts and has the appearance of low level layering echoes, similar to sludge in the gallbladder (9).

Computed Tomography. Hydatid cysts are low density, well demarcated, round masses with or without internal septations (Figs. 5.20C and 5.22) (2, 4, 6, 9, 15, 16). Septa and the cyst wall enhance after intravenous contrast administration. Daughter cysts with their own walls may be depicted in the interior of the mother cyst. Calcifications are crescentic or ring-shaped usually in the reactive portion of the cyst wall (Fig. 5.22). After intrabiliary cyst rupture, high density material may be seen in a dilated common bile duct (9). Cyst septal enhancement after cholangiographic contrast material infusion has also been reported after intrabiliary rupture (9).

Cholangiography. Direct cholangiography can demonstrate filling defects in dilated bile ducts from membranes, scolices or hydatid sand after intrabiliary rupture. Biliary radicles will be displaced and/or distorted by the cyst itself (Fig. 5.23) (6).

Angiography. Intrahepatic arteries are splayed around an avascular area representing the cyst. During the hepatogram phase there is often a halo of increased density around the cyst (Fig. 5.24) (17).

Hepatic Alveolar Echinococcosis (*Echinococcus multilocularis*)

Echinococcal disease caused by *E. multilocularis* is rarer than that caused by *E. granulosus*. There is no distinct encompassing shell of reactive host tissue, and the disease process tends to become diffuse and infiltrative, resembling a malignancy both clinically and radiologically (18, 19). The embryos invade the liver and form small cysts which in turn form innumerable tiny daughter cysts. The gelatinous nature of the cysts can lead to an erroneous diagnosis of mucinous adenocarcinoma.

The fox is the main host of the adult parasite; less commonly, dogs or cats serve as hosts. The usual intermediate hosts are wild rodents, who are infected by eating feces-contaminated berries. The fox is infected by ingesting infested rodents. Humans can be infected via two routes: intake of contaminated wild berries, other plants, or water, and contact with foxes. The chief endemic regions are central Europe, the Soviet Union, Iran, Afghanistan and Japan, Alaska, Canada, and the north central United States (20).

Clinical Findings

Antiparasitic drugs are presently not efficacious, and the only hope for cure is complete surgical extirpation, therefore early diagnosis and anatomic staging are critical. Initial diagnosis is usually immunologic, but sonography and CT can be used for screening, verification of indeterminate immunologic studies and guided biopsy (21).

Pathology

Grossly, the liver lesion is usually a solitary mass sometimes with peripheral satellite extensions. The process is infiltrative without any limiting membrane and can extend to large regions of the liver. The mass is composed of innumerable cysts the larger of which are 1–10 mm in diameter (21). In a fashion identical to an infiltrative neoplasm, the mass expands causing stenoses of intrahepatic bile ducts and hepatic and portal veins, resulting in obstructive jaundice and portal hypertension. Central necrosis can occur. Preterminal events include infec-

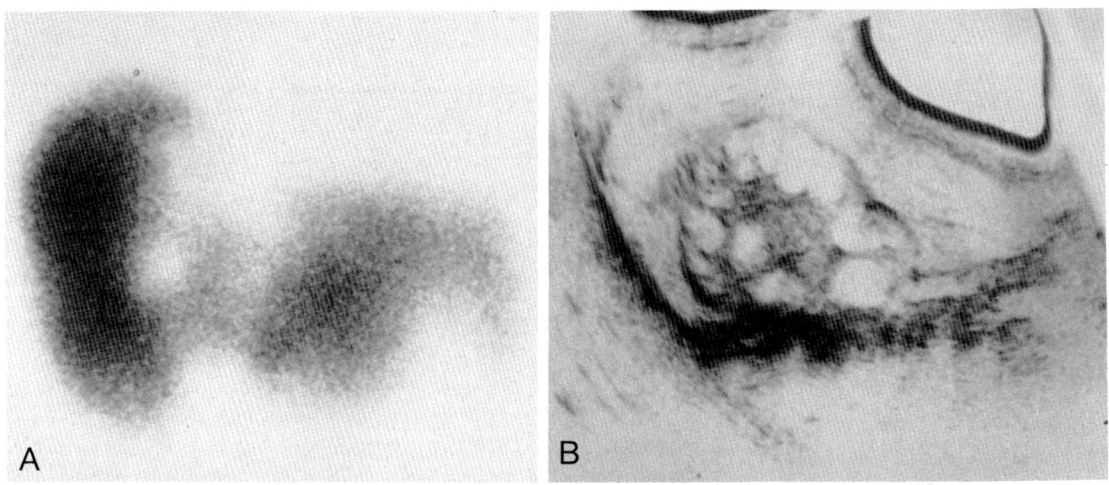
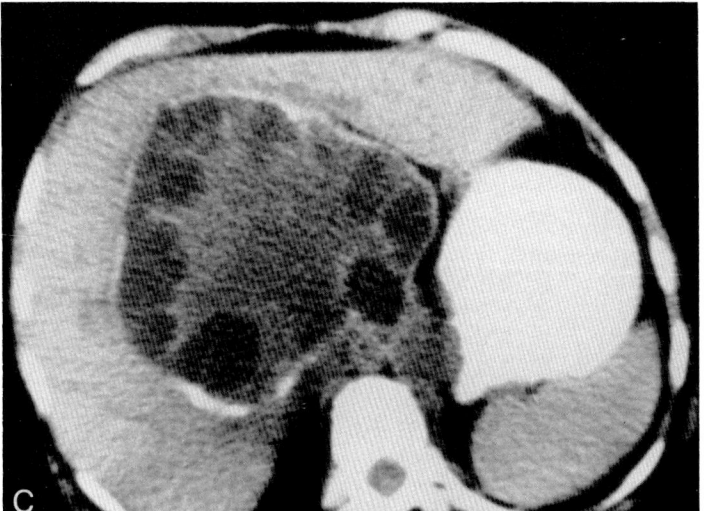

FIGURE 5.20. ECHINOCOCCAL DISEASE
A: Sulfur colloid scan shows an irregular region of diminished uptake in the right lobe. *B:* Parasagittal sonogram of the same patient shows a well-demarcated polycystic mass suggesting hydatid cyst. *C:* Contrast enhanced CT of the same patient shows the hydatid cyst to be partially calcified with a thin, enhancing rim. *D* and *E:* Cystogram after percutaneous puncture of the hepatic hydatid cyst demonstrating loculations and communication with the biliary tree. The procedure was uneventful. Low power view of aspirate showing brood capsule and scolices (*E*). (Case courtesy of Bruce Rubin, M.D., Holy Cross Hospital, Silver Spring, MD.)

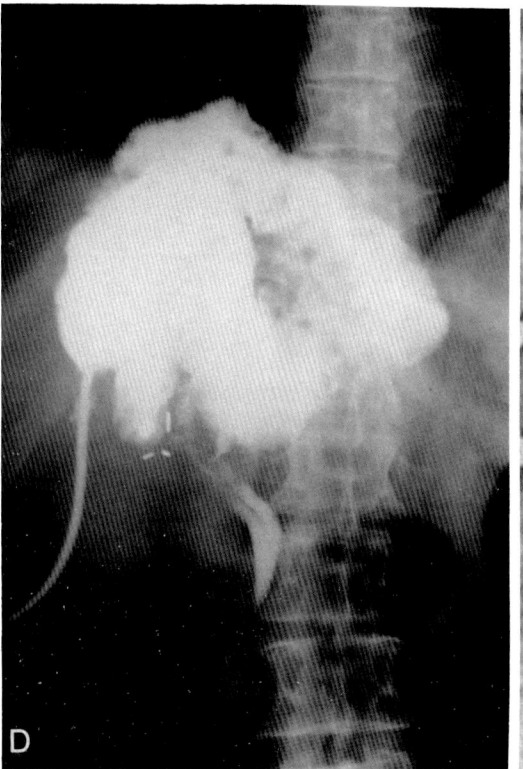
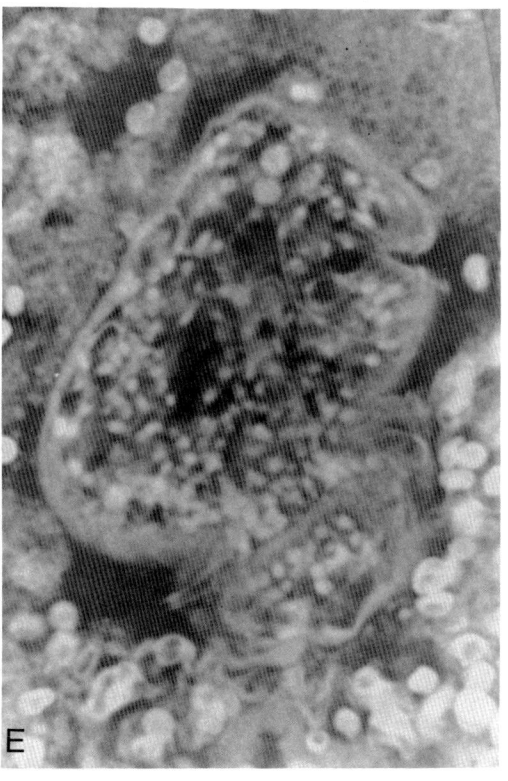

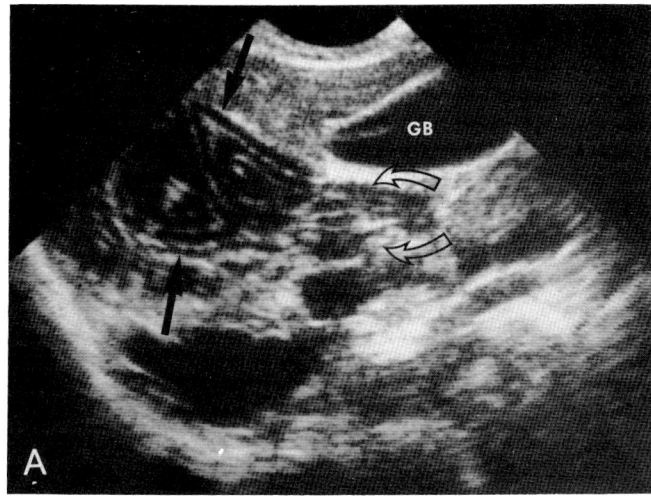
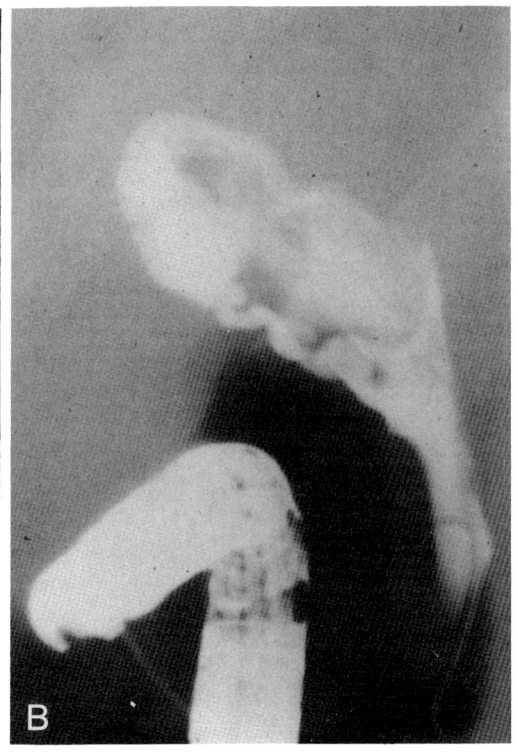

FIGURE 5.21. ECHINOCOCCAL DISEASE
A: Parasagittal sonogram reveals multiple layers in a hydatid cyst (*arrows*) which has collapsed into the common duct (*curved arrows*) (*GB:* gallbladder) *B:* ERCP in the same patient shows complete obstruction by a filling defect.

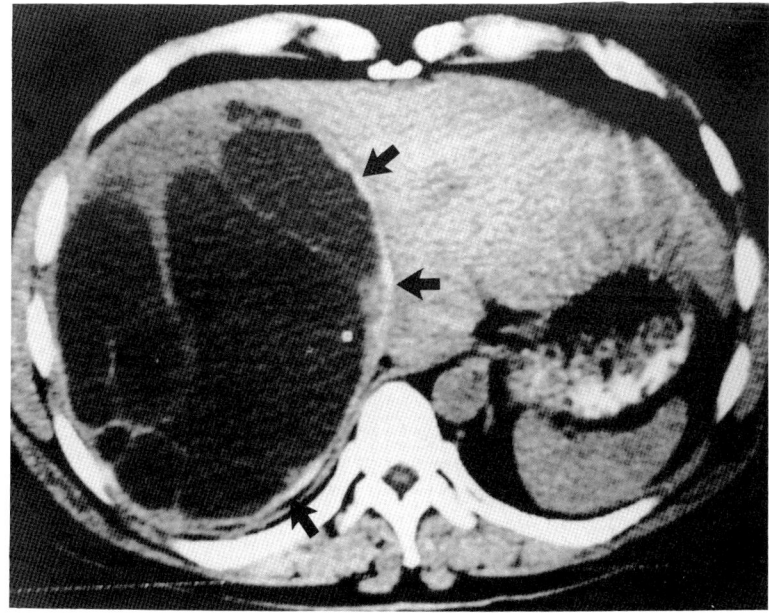

FIGURE 5.22. ECHINOCOCCAL DISEASE
Unenhanced CT: Large septated low density hepatic hydatid cyst with partial wall calcification (*arrows*). Major differential consideration is biliary cystadenoma/cystadenocarcinoma.

tion, abscess, cholangitis, septicemia, gastrointestinal hemorrhage, and parasitic metastasis to heart, lung and brain (21).

Radiology

Plain Films. Plain films, when positive, show multiple nodular intrahepatic calcifications.

Ultrasound. Parasitic masses are echogenic and ill-defined, single or multiple, with a propensity to spread to the liver hilum. Individual cysts are too small to be imaged. Regions of relatively sonolucent necrosis with or without debris are frequently present. Shadowing echogenic microcalcifications are often seen within the masses. Associated findings that may be present depend-

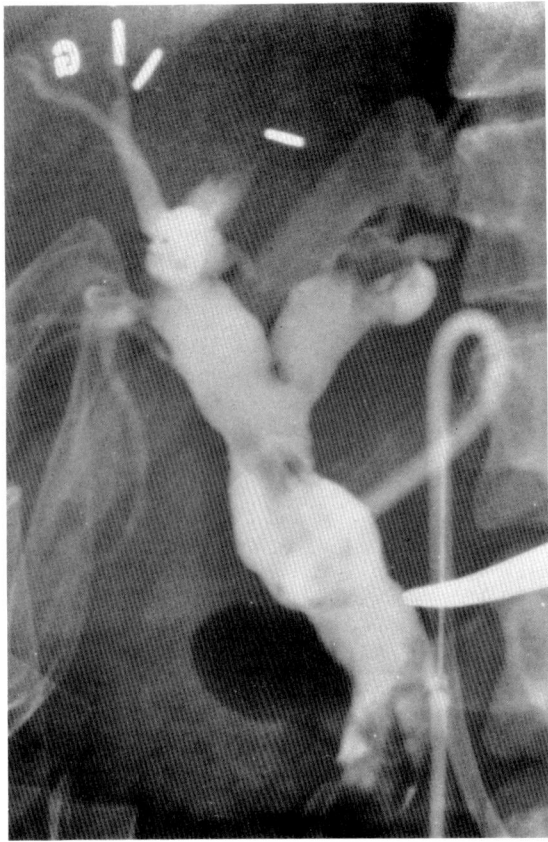

FIGURE 5.23. ECHINOCOCCAL DISEASE
Operative cholangiogram shows filling defects in the biliary tree as a result of intrabiliary rupture of an echinococcal cyst.

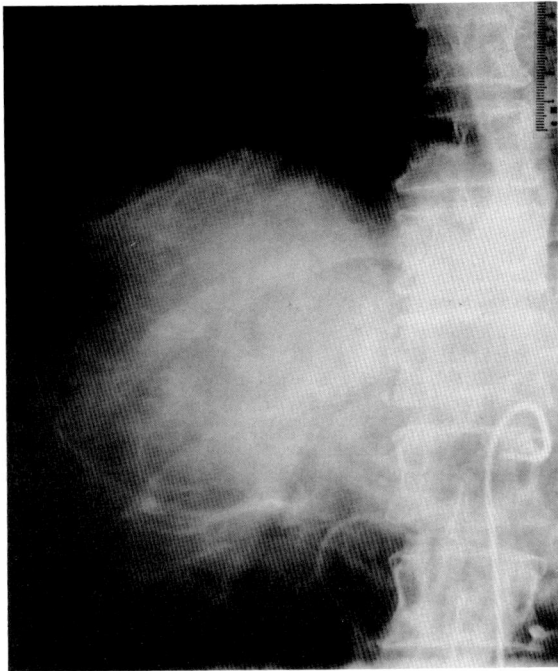

FIGURE 5.24. ECHINOCOCCAL DISEASE
This hepatogram phase of a hepatic arteriogram shows a multiseptate radiolucent mass representing an echinococcal cyst.

ing on the stage of the disease include: dilated bile ducts, portal hypertension and collaterals, portal vein thrombosis, parasitic involvement of the spleen, hepatic vein occlusion, inferior vena cava occlusion, and abdominal lymphadenopathy (21).

Computerized Tomography. Lesions are heterogeneous, hypodense, and poorly marginated. Little or no enhancement occurs after bolus injection of contrast material. Microcalcifications within the lesion are demonstrated with a high degree of sensitivity. Pseudocystic necrotic regions of near water density (0–10 Hounsfield units (HU)) can be seen surrounded by the hypodense (30–40 HU) solid component. Hilar invasion and biliary tract dilatation are frequent. Liver CT can demonstrate all the associated findings listed in the ultrasound section; in addition metastases in the lung bases or heart can be picked up (21).

Angiography. Although necessary only as a preoperative road map, arteriography will show rather suggestive changes of intrahepatic arterial tapering and obstruction caused by the infiltrative neoplasm-like mass.

Summary

Echinococcal disease may resemble a variety of space-occupying lesions of the liver, namely, simple cyst, polycystic liver disease, abscess, metastasis, chronic hematoma, and biliary cystadenoma/cystadenocarcinoma. Obtaining a history (often remote) of travel to endemic areas of hydatid disease is important in considering the proper diagnosis. Simple cysts and polycystic liver disease may be excluded by virtue of the rim enhancement which often occurs with hydatid disease and not the former (2). When daughter cysts are present within the larger parent cyst, the diagnosis of *E. granulosus* can be suggested by sonography and CT. Exclusion of a primary or secondary malignant tumor of the liver is often difficult, especially with *E. multilocularis*, and positive serologic tests are vital in arriving at the correct preoperative diagnosis (2).

REFERENCES

1. Vilardel E: Echinococcal (hydatid) cysts of the liver. In Bockus HL et al (eds): *Gastroenterology*. Philadelphia, W. B. Saunders, 1976, pp 570–575.
2. Scherer U, Weinzierl M, Sturm R, Schildberg F, Zrenner

2. M, Lissner J: Computed tomography in hydatid disease of the liver, a report on 13 cases. *J Comput Assist Tomogr* 2:612–617, 1978.
3. Hadidi A: Sonography of hepatic echinococcal cysts. *Gastrointest Radiol* 7:349–354, 1982.
4. Choliz J, Olaverri FJL, Casas TF, Zubieta SO: Computed tomography in hepatic echinococcosis. *AJR* 139:699–702, 1982.
5. Babcock DS, Kaufman L, Cosnow I: Ultrasound diagnosis of hydatid disease (echinococcosis) in 2 cases. *AJR* 131:895–897, 1978.
6. Gonzalez LR, Marcos J, Illanas M, Hernandez-Mora M, Pena F, Picouto JP, Cienfuegos JA, Alvarez JLR: Radiologic aspects of hepatic echinococcosis. *Radiology* 130:17–21, 1979.
7. Macris GJ, Galanis NN: Rupture of echinococcus cyst of the liver into the biliary ducts. *Am Surg* 32:36, 1966.
8. Harris JD: Rupture of hydatid cysts of the liver into the biliary tracts. *Br J Surg* 52:210, 1965.
9. Subramanyam BR, Balthazar EJ, Naidich DP: Ruptured hydatid cyst with biliary obstruction: diagnosis by sonography and computed tomography. *Gastrointest Radiol* 8:314–343, 1983.
10. Chemtal AK, Bowry TR, Ahmad Z: Evaluation of five immunodiagnostic techniques in echinococcus patients. *Bull WHO* 59:767–772, 1981.
11. Mueller PR, Dawson SL, Ferrucci JT Jr, Nardi GL: Percutaneous drainage of hepatic echinococcal cyst. Presented at the annual meeting of the Society of Gastrointestinal Radiology, Napa Valley, Calif., October, 1984.
12. Gharbi HA, Hassine W, Brauner MW, Dupuch K: Ultrasound examination of the hydatid liver. *Radiology* 139:459–463, 1981.
13. Hadidi A: Ultrasound findings in liver hydatid cysts. *J Clin Ultrasound* 7:365–368, 1979.
14. Barriga P, Cruz F, Lepe V, Lathrop R: An ultrasonographically solid, tumor-like appearance of echinococcal cysts in the liver. *J Ultrasound Med* 2:123–125, 1983.
15. Newmark H, Smith JJ, Burrows R, Silberman EL: Echinococcal cyst of the liver seen on computed tomography. *J Comput Assist Tomogr* 2:231–232, 1978.
16. Kirschner LP, Ferris RA, Mero JH, Moss ML: Hydatid disease of the liver evaluated by computed tomography. *J Comput Assist Tomogr* 2:229–230, 1978.
17. Baltaxe HA, Fleming RJ: The angiographic appearance of hydatid disease. *Radiology* 97:559–604, 1970.
18. Bonakdarpour A: Echinococcus disease. Report of 112 cases from Iran and a review of 611 cases from the United States. *Radiology* 99:660–667, 1967.
19. Reeder MM, Palmer PES: *Radiology of Tropical Diseases with Epidemiologic Pathologic, and Clinical Correlation.* Baltimore, Williams & Wilkins, 1981, pp 157–222.
20. Kasai Y, Koshino I, Kawanishi N, Sakamoto H, Sasaki E, Kumagai M: Alveolar echinococcosis of the liver. Studies on 60 operated cases. *Ann Surg* 191:145–152, 1980.
21. Didier D, Weiler S, Rohmer P, Lasseguc A, Deschamps JP, Vuitton D, Miguet JP, Weill F: Hepatic alveolar echinococcosis: correlative US and CT study. *Radiology* 154:179–186, 1985.

CONGENITAL SIMPLE CYSTS

Thought to represent embryologic malformations, congenital simple cysts were found in 0.17% of abdominal operations in a large surgical series (1). It was conceded that small cysts were not detected. Since the advent of high resolution grey-scale ultrasound and CT, hepatic simple cysts are detected with considerable frequency (2).

Clinical Findings

Simple cysts occur slightly more often in females and usually come to attention in the 5th through 7th decade. In a large surgical series, symptoms initiated exploration in only approximately 17% of patients (1). Common presentations in symptomatic patients were abdominal mass (55%), hepatomegaly (40%), pain (33%), and jaundice (9%). Rarely, simple cysts present as an emergency because of torsion, rupture into the peritoneum, or intracystic hemorrhage (1, 3). Asymptomatic simple cysts can be observed or percutaneously aspirated for diagnosis. Aspiration is sometimes advised to exclude metastases when a primary tumor is present. If hydatid disease is a possibility based on travel history, a negative serologic complement fixation test should be obtained prior to aspiration (2). As simple cysts recur after percutaneous aspiration, sometimes as rapidly as in 2 weeks (4), symptomatic cases often require surgical excision for cure (1, 2, 4). However, in a recent report six simple hepatic cysts were successfully ablated by injection of 95% ethanol through an aspiration catheter. One quarter of the cyst volume is replaced with the alcohol (5). Contrast injection is recommended prior to ethanol injection to rule out communication with the biliary tree or extravasation outside the cyst. Carcinoma arising in the lining of a cyst wall has been reported but is very rare (1).

Pathology

Solitary simple cysts are usually unilocular and average 4.3 cm in diameter but may reach as large a diameter as 20 cm (1, 3). Cuboidal epithelium usually lines the wall and bile duct epithelium is present in the lining with ductal elements in the wall in about 50% (1). Cyst fluid is usually clear and colorless or yellow with negative cystology (1, 2).

Radiology

Plain films and gastrointestinal contrast examinations can demonstrate a mass if the cyst is sufficiently large (3). Rarely there is dystrophic wall calcification (3). Excretory urography may demonstrate an intrahepatic radiolucency. Radionuclide liver scans show photon deficient areas. Sonographic criteria for a simple hepatic cyst are the same as those elsewhere in the body: lack of internal echoes, smooth walls, strong back wall, and good through transmission (2). CT characteristics of a simple hepatic cyst are sharp demarcation, lack of contrast enhancement, homogeneity, and CT numbers between 0 and +20 H (Fig. 5.25). Angiography is rarely performed for simple hepatic cyst; the features reported are stretching of arteries and veins around a well-demarcated avascular mass which is radiolucent in the hepatogram phase (Fig. 5.26) (3). Congenital hepatic cysts do not communicate with the biliary tree and will not fill on cholangiography.

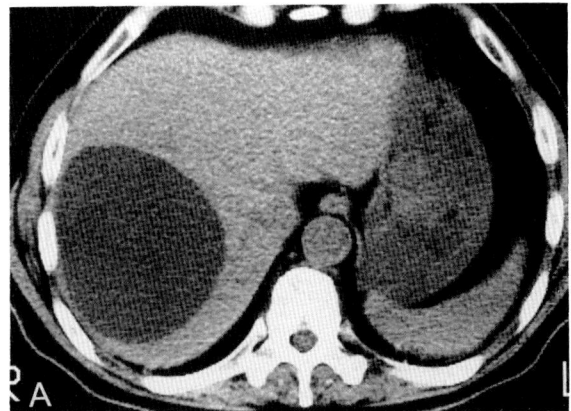
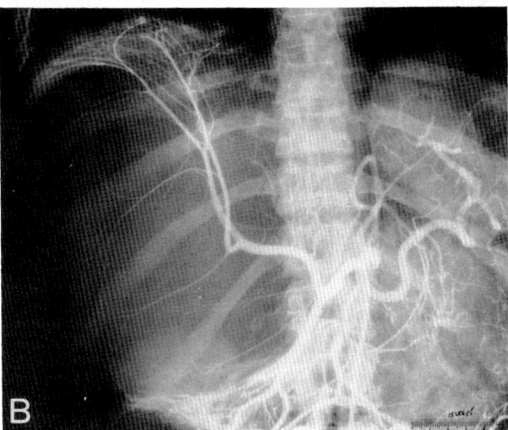
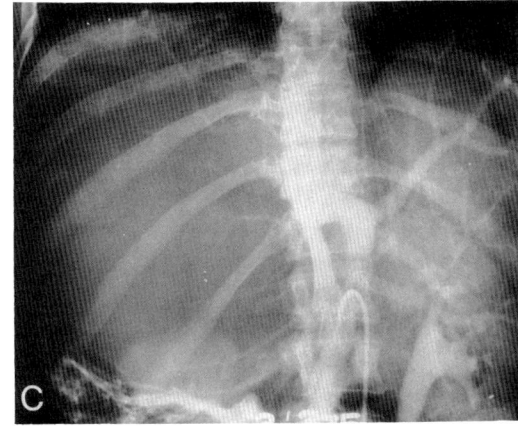

FIGURE 5.26. LARGE SIMPLE CYST
A: Large simple cyst on CT. *B:* Arteriogram shows stretched arteries and arc-like displacement. *C:* The cyst is radiolucent on the venous phase as well. The portal veins are affected in a similar manner to the arteries.

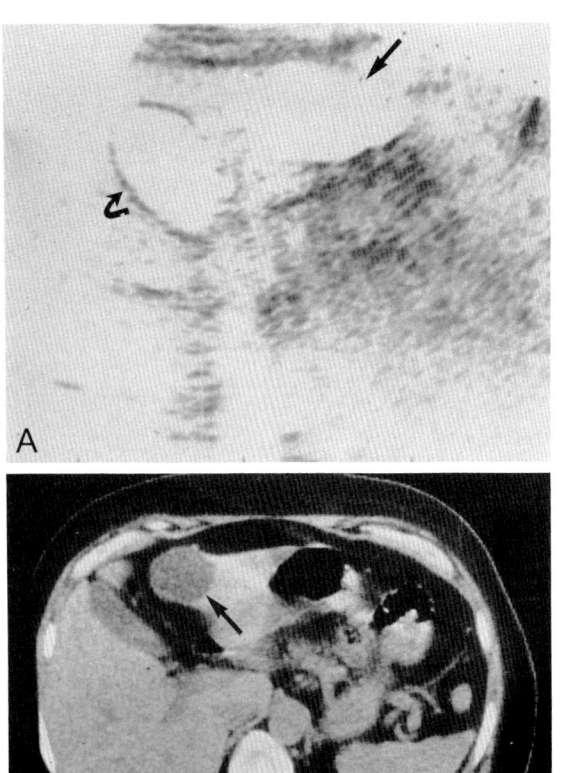

FIGURE 5.25. ANECHOIC SIMPLE CYST
A: Transverse sonogram: anechoic simple cyst (*arrow*) with sharp back wall and sonic enhancement. Compare to gallbladder (*curved arrow*). *B:* Corresponding CT: homogeneous mass (*arrow*) with same attenuation as gallbladder.

REFERENCES

1. San Felippo PM, Beahrs OH, Weiland LH: Cystic disease of the liver. *Ann Surg* 179:922–925, 1974.
2. Roemer CE, Ferrucci JT Jr., Mueller PR, Simeone JF, Van Sonnenberg E, Wittenberg J: Hepatic cysts: diag-

nosis and therapy by sonographic needle aspiration. *AJR* 136:1065–1070, 1981.
3. McNulty JG: *Radiology of the Liver*. Philadelphia, W. B. Saunders, 1977, pp 167–172.
4. Saini S, Mueller PR, Ferrucci JT Jr., Simeone JF, Wittenberg J, Butch RJ: Percutaneous aspiration of hepatic cysts does not provide definitive therapy. *AJR* 141:559–560, 1983.
5. Bean WJ, Rodan BA: Hepatic cysts: treatment with alcohol. *AJR* 144:237–241, 1985.

CAVERNOUS HEMANGIOMA

Cavernous hemangioma is the most common benign liver tumor; its autopsy incidence is 0.4–7.3% (1–3). There is no sex predilection for hemangiomas found at autopsy or incidentally, but in symptomatic patients, a female preponderance of 4–9:1 has been reported (1, 2, 4). A hormonal influence on the growth of hemangiomas has been postulated to explain the increased incidence of symptomatic hemangiomas in multiparous females (1, 2). Although the majority of hemangiomas are incidental findings, rupture with intra-abdominal hemorrhage has been reported in 4.5% (1). Other symptoms and signs include sudden, severe pain from thrombosis, palpable mass, abdominal bruit, symptoms from adjacent organ compression, thrombocytopenia, and hypofibrinogenemia (1–4). Minor trauma often precipitates the episodes of hemorrhage (4). Symptomatic cavernous hemangiomas usually occur in middle-aged patients and almost never in patients less than 2 years old (2). Symptoms almost never occur in hemangiomas less than 4 cm in diameter (5).

Needle biopsy using 22 or 20 gauge needles is usually uneventful. Significant bleeding can occur after biopsy with larger gauge needles (6). Fine-needle biopsies of hemangiomas are likely to yield only blood and some endothelial cells making exclusion of malignancy difficult at best. Cores obtained with larger needles are more diagnostic, but are obtained at greater risk. The appearance at peritoneoscopy may be diagnostic if the mass is on the liver surface (3). Hemangiomas do not recur after complete excision (3).

Pathology

Cavernous hemangiomas are usually solitary and less than 2 cm in size (1–3). Ten percent are multiple. Symptomatic hemangiomas are larger and may exceed 30 cm in diameter (1, 3). Hemangiomas are commonly subcapsular, 20% are peduculated and mobile (1, 3). The right lobe is more frequently involved than the left (1, 3). Hemangiomas are soft, reddish-purple or blue masses separated from the surrounding parenchyma by a fibrous pseudocapsule (Fig. 5.27) (1–3). Gross thrombosis, fibrosis or calcification may be present (1). Microscopically, the tumor consists of fairly large vascular channels lined by a single row of flattened endothelial cells (1, 2). The supporting fibrous stroma is usually scanty, but may be dense and hyalinized and rarely calcified or even ossified (1, 2). The vascular spaces communicate with each other in an intricate pattern and may be thrombosed (7). Calcified phleboliths are extremely uncommon (8). The tendency toward fibrosis increases as the patient gets older. The rare true hemangioma differs from the common cavernous hemangioma

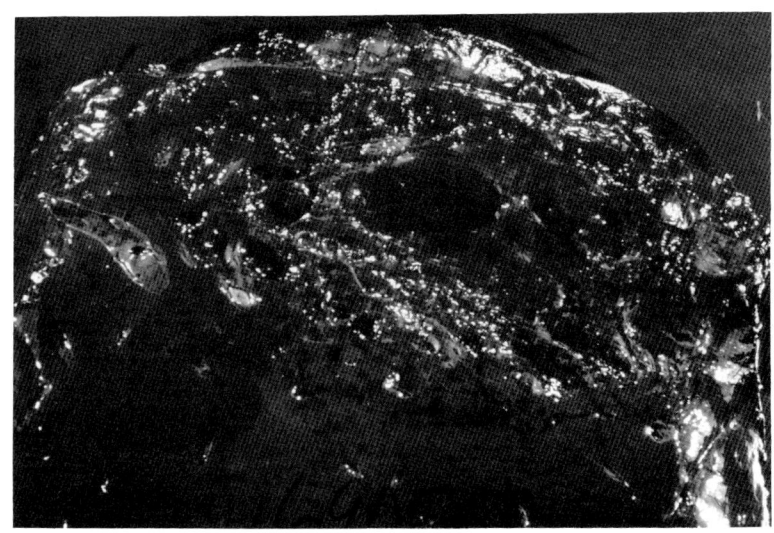

FIGURE 5.27. TYPICAL CAVERNOUS HEMANGIOMA
Cut gross specimen showing the typical spongy appearance of a cavernous hemangioma.

in that it is a proliferation of vascular embryonic tissue remnants (3).

Radiology

Plain Films

Large cavernous hemangiomas may be appreciated as soft-tissue masses. Contrast examinations can show displacement of the gastrointestinal tract. Calcification is unusual; when it occurs it is usually in the fibrous stroma and consists of one or more radiating trabeculae or spicules (Fig. 5.28) (7, 9, 10). Calcified phleboliths are very rare (1, 9).

Sonography

Cavernous hemangiomas can present many ways sonographically, but most have been reported to be hyperechoic (Figs. 5.29A and 5.30A and B) (11–14). Mixed patterns with hyperechoic and large hypoechoic or anechoic regions are seen in larger hemangiomas that have undergone internal hemorrhage or necrosis (Figs. 5.31 and 5.32A) (10). Sharply defined back walls and increased through transmission may be seen in the anechoic regions correctly indicating fluid. Central echogenic septa can be seen in those lesions that have developed central scars following necrosis (Fig. 5.31) (10). Acoustic enhancement distal to uniformly echogenic hemangiomas can be seen because of an increased blood content compared to hepatic parenchyma (15). The finding of a small, well-defined uniformly echoic liver mass suggests the diagnosis of hemangioma; however, metastasis and primary hepatic malignancy have to be excluded and other benign liver tumors should be considered.

Computed Tomography

Cavernous hemangiomas are spherical or ovoid well-demarcated hypodense masses on unenhanced scans (Fig. 5.29B, top left) (16). Calcification is quite unusual and is central when it occurs. The enhancement pattern after drip infusion of contrast is nonspecific, and hemangiomas often become isodense in this situation. A characteristic enhancement pattern does occur

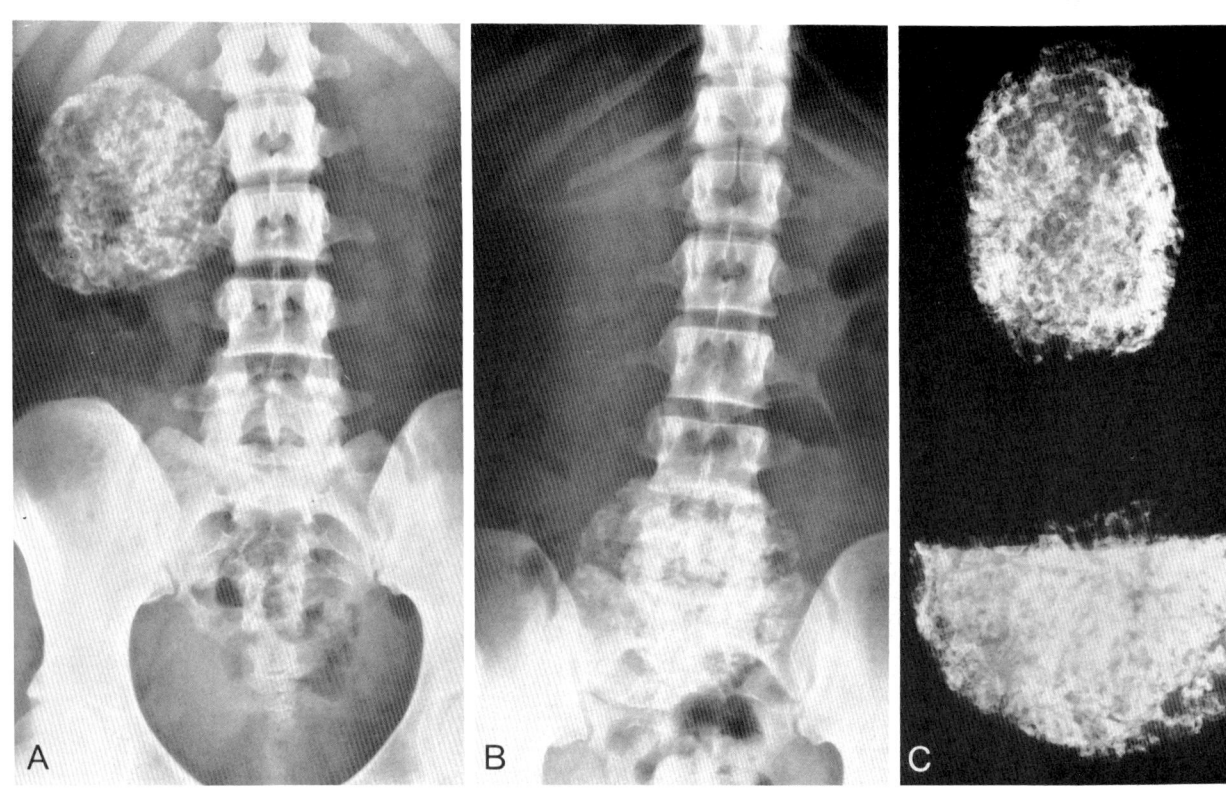

FIGURE 5.28. MOBILE CALCIFIED ABDOMINAL MASS

Young female patient with a mobile calcified abdominal mass due to a pedunculated degenerated cavernous hemangioma. *A* and *B:* Supine and erect films demonstrate mobility and dystrophic calcification. *C:* Specimen radiograph confirms extensive calcification in fibrous tissue.

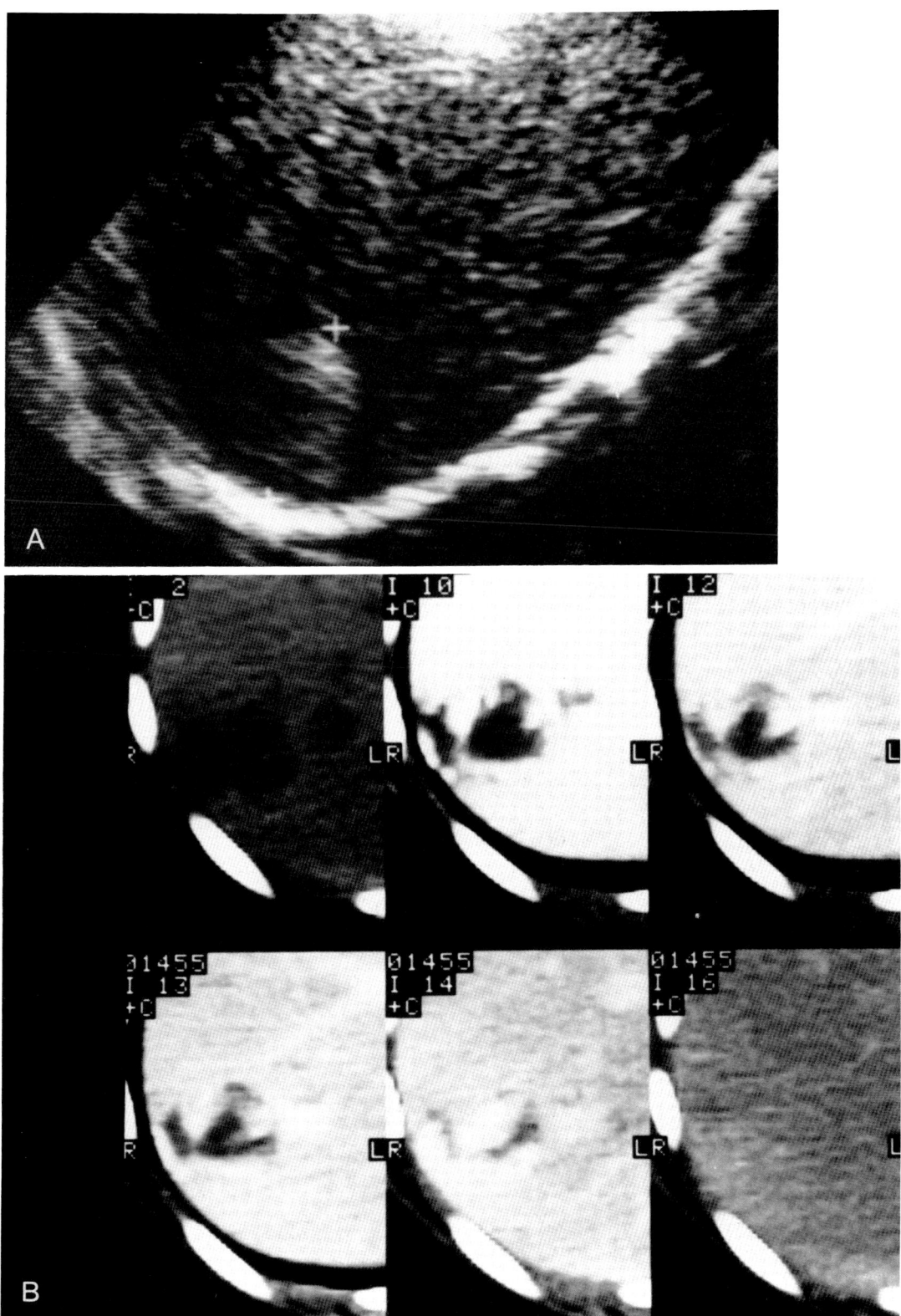

FIGURE 5.29. HEMANGIOMA
A: Parasagittal sonogram shows a small echogenic hemangioma. *B:* Typical CT pattern in the same case. Times after contrast bolus injection: (*Top*) Left-to-right noncontrast, 40 sec, 80 sec. (*Bottom*) Left-to-right 100 sec, 120 sec, and 8 min.

after bolus injection (100 cc) of contrast material using dynamic scanning (Fig. 5.29B). About 15 seconds after contrast injection, dense and thick peripheral enhancement occurs with centripetal fill-in progressing towards isodensity over the next few minutes up to one hour. Regions of fibrosis or thrombosis may remain hypodense (Fig. 5.32B) (11, 16–19). A typical CT pattern of hemangioma with intense peripheral contrast enhancement and isodense fill-in was seen in 69% of hemangiomas and only 5% of metastases in one series, and the probability of a lesion having this pattern being a hemangioma was 93% in patients without a known primary (20). However, if a patient has a primary malignancy, the odds of a liver mass being a metastasis increase dramatically and the probability of a lesion with the hemangioma pattern being a hemangioma drops to about 80% (20).

Nuclear Medicine

Scintigraphy with ^{99m}Tc-sulfur colloid depicts hemangiomas as nonspecific focal regions of decreased activity (Fig. 5.30). One case has been reported with sulfur colloid avidity (21). Delayed (1–2 hr) blood pool images obtained after injection of ^{99m}Tc-labeled red cells characteristically show increased activity in hemangiomas, which, coupled with decreased activity seen on a flow study, is diagnostic of hemangioma (Fig. 5.30) (22–25). The decreased flow is an important differential from hepatocellular carcinoma, which may have increased blood pool activity but not in conjunction with decreased flow. The occasional cavernous hemangioma will have increased flow on the radionuclide angiogram, but it will be even hotter on the delayed blood pool images. Blood pool images in hemangiomas showed increased activity by 15 min in one series (25), but further delayed imaging is still recommended. Some hemangiomas will not demonstrate these characteristic scintigraphic findings because of fibrosis. Optimal blood pool scintigraphy of the liver for hemangioma requires careful patient positioning and knowledge of the lesion's location from prior sonography or sulfur-colloid scans. Our experience with this technique has been rewarding. We feel that it is at least as specific as CT if not more so, and it is cheaper, less dangerous, and easier to perform than bolus-enhanced dynamic CT. We have seen cases in which the radionuclide method not only correctly diagnosed a mass discovered on ultrasound as a hemangioma when the CT was nonspecific, but also discovered other hemangiomas that were not seen with CT or sonography. We have reliably detected hemangioma 2–3 cm in size using stand-

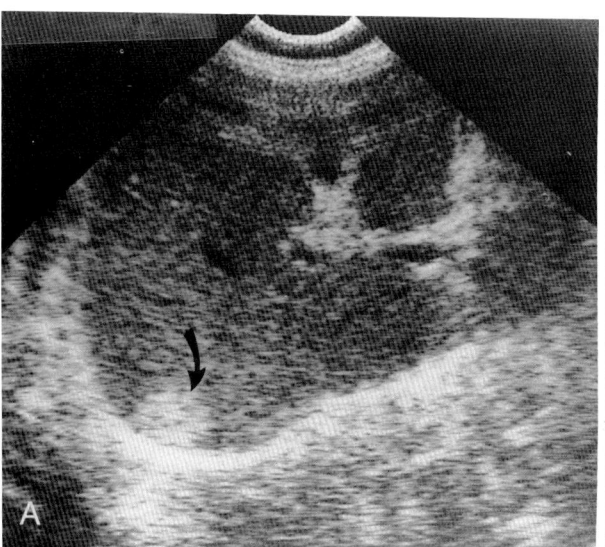
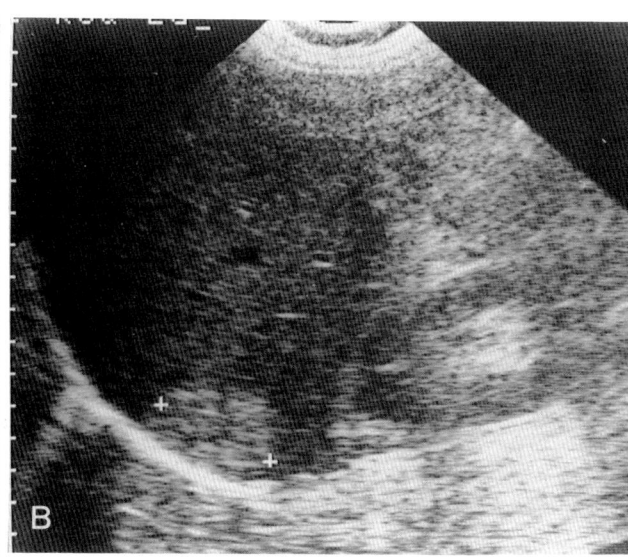

FIGURE 5.30. HEMANGIOMA

A and B: Transverse and parasagittal sonograms show a 3 cm echogenic mass (arrow, cursors) in the right lobe of a 43-yr-old woman. C: Posterior sulfur colloid scan shows a corresponding photopenic region (arrow). D–F: Labeled red-cell scintigraphy at 15 min, 30 min, and 2 hr shows progressively increasing activity corresponding to the hemangioma (arrows). Flow studies showed no increased activity (not shown). All views are posterior. G–I: Sulfur colloid and 30-min labeled red cell scintigrams, respectively, in a young woman. The multiple hemangiomas are cold on the colloid scan (G) and hot on the red cell scan (H). The arterial phase of the radionuclide angiogram showed no increased flow, and the venous phase (I) shows defects corresponding to the hemangiomas.

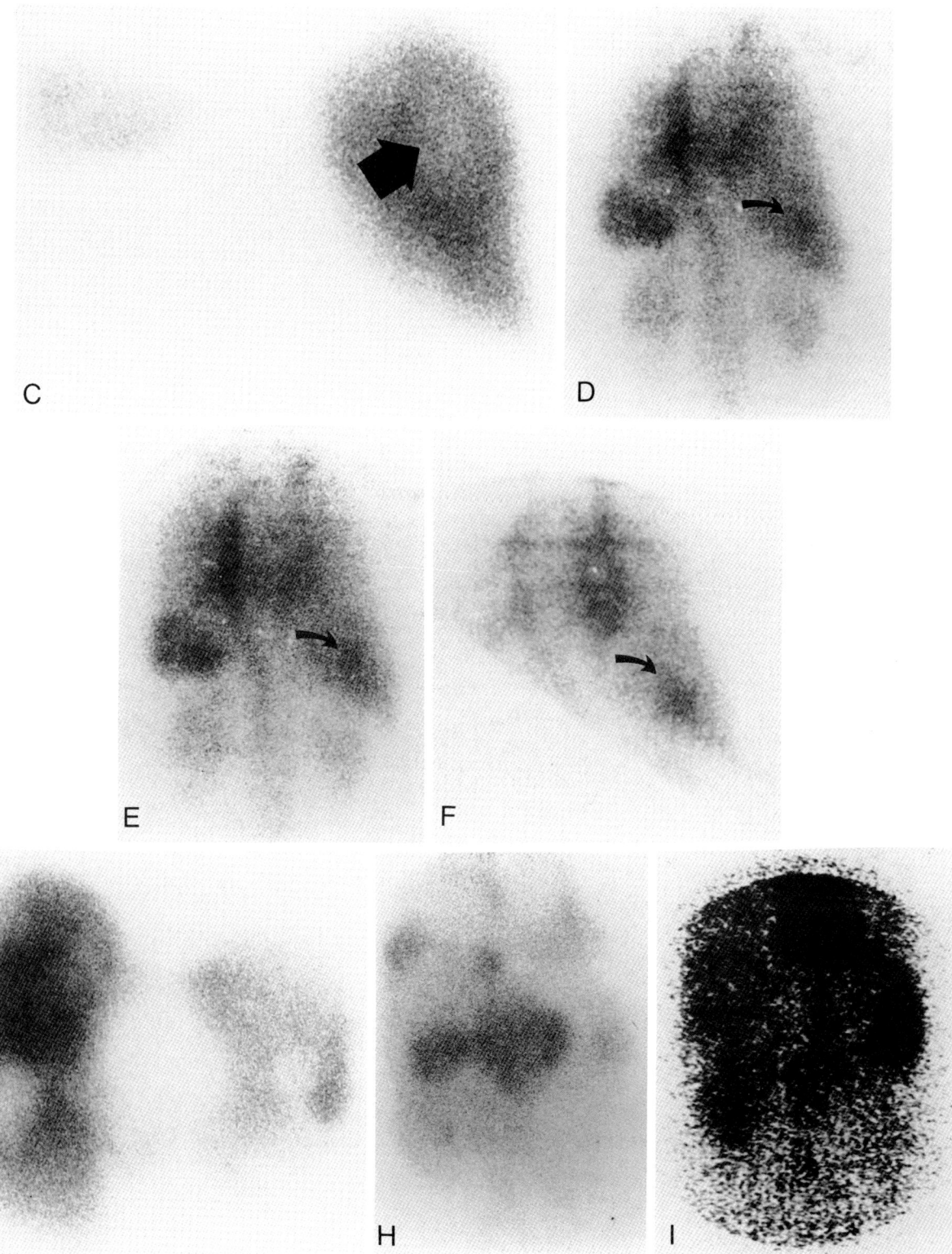

FIGURE 5.30C–I

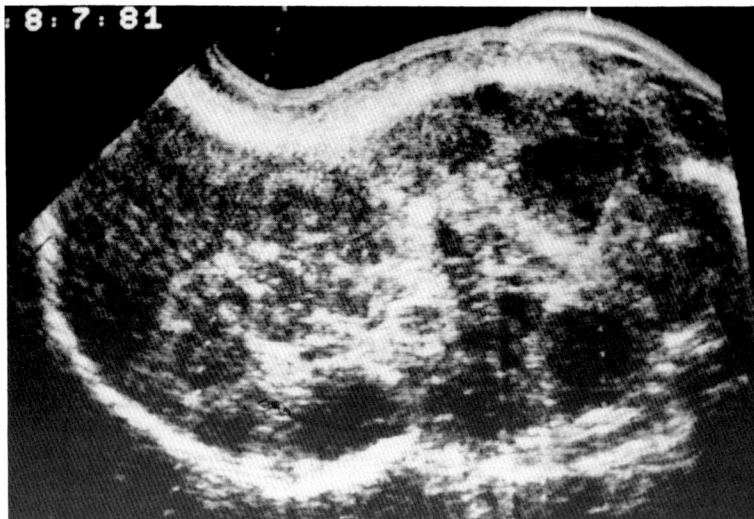

FIGURE 5.31. LARGE COMPLEX HEMANGIOMA
Large complex hemangioma with hypoechoic and nearly isoechoic nodules. The central hyperechoic regions correspond to fibrosis.

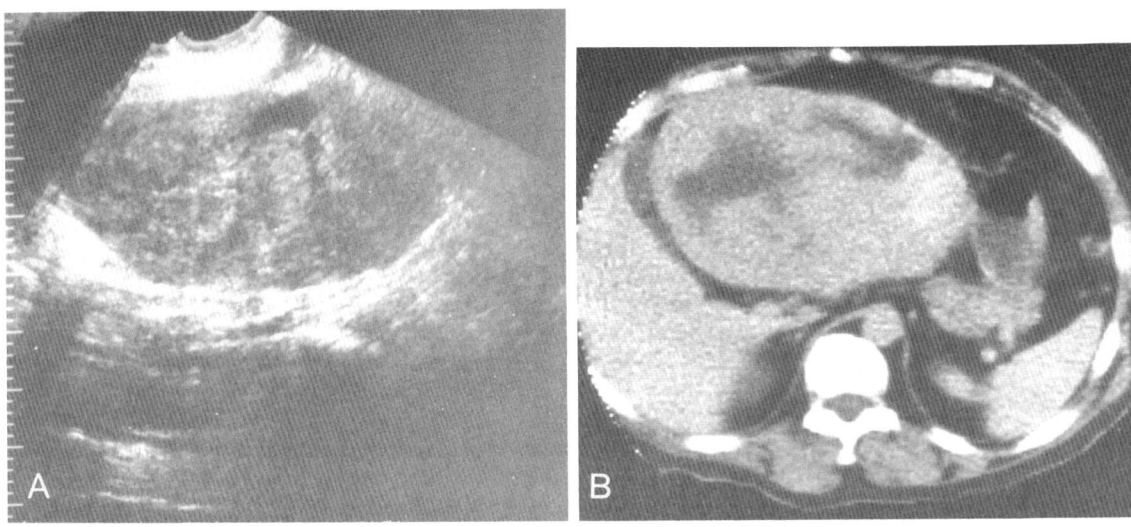

FIGURE 5.32. LARGE COMPLEX HEMANGIOMA
A: Transverse sonogram of a large complex hemangioma replacing the left lobe. *B:* Corresponding drip-enhanced CT showing central stellate regions of subacute hemorrhage. The patient had experienced epigastric pain.

ard planar scintigraphy. SPECT has been quite useful in our hands for lesions 1–2 cm in size when planar images are negative. It is important to carefully correlate the SPECT image with sonography and/or CT to separate the hemangioma from normal vessels. We have yet to encounter a metastasis that we misdiagnosed as a hemangioma on scintigraphy.

Angiography

The hepatic artery and its branches larger than 1 mm in diameter supplying a cavernous hemangioma are normal except in massive tumors when their size may be slightly increased (Fig. 5.33) (7). Arteries smaller than 1 mm may be more tortuous than normal and they opacify vascular spaces singly or in clusters (7). Arterial branches are displaced away from the center of the mass (Fig. 5.34), and there is no vascular encasement, invasion, neovascularity or rapid circulation (16, 25). Punctate lakes of contrast material, either single or multiple appear very early in the arterial phase and become denser and more diffuse over the first 10–12 sec (7, 16, 26) (Fig. 5.34). Arterioportal shunting has been reported, but is quite rare (27). In small hemangiomas the stain becomes homogeneous, whereas in larger ones it may be ring- or C-shaped due to slow opacification of the center or central fibro-

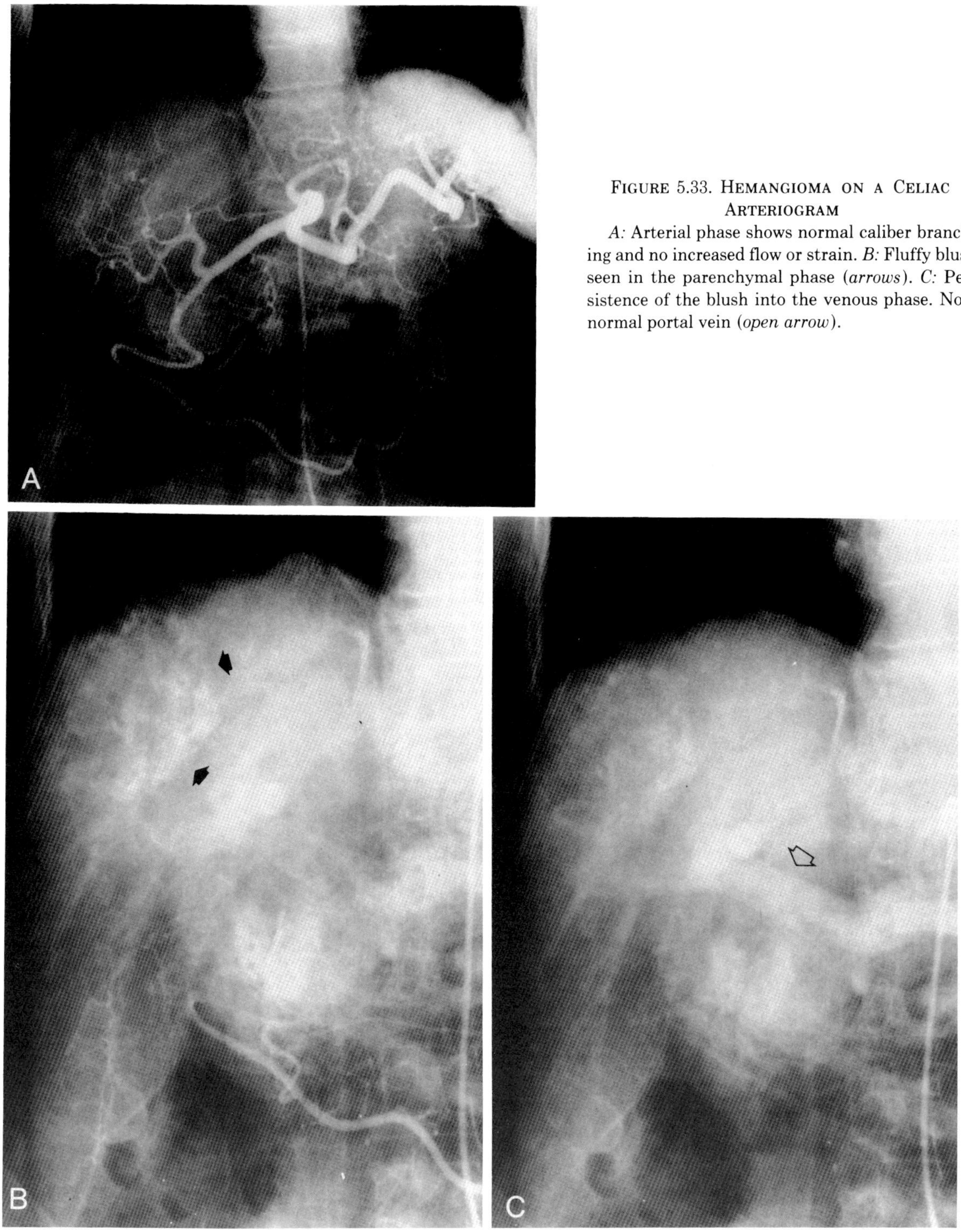

FIGURE 5.33. HEMANGIOMA ON A CELIAC ARTERIOGRAM
A: Arterial phase shows normal caliber branching and no increased flow or strain. *B:* Fluffy blush seen in the parenchymal phase (*arrows*). *C:* Persistence of the blush into the venous phase. Note normal portal vein (*open arrow*).

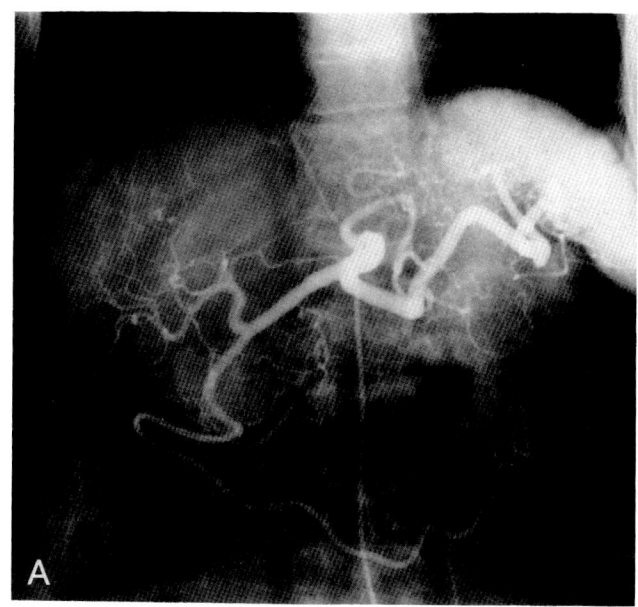

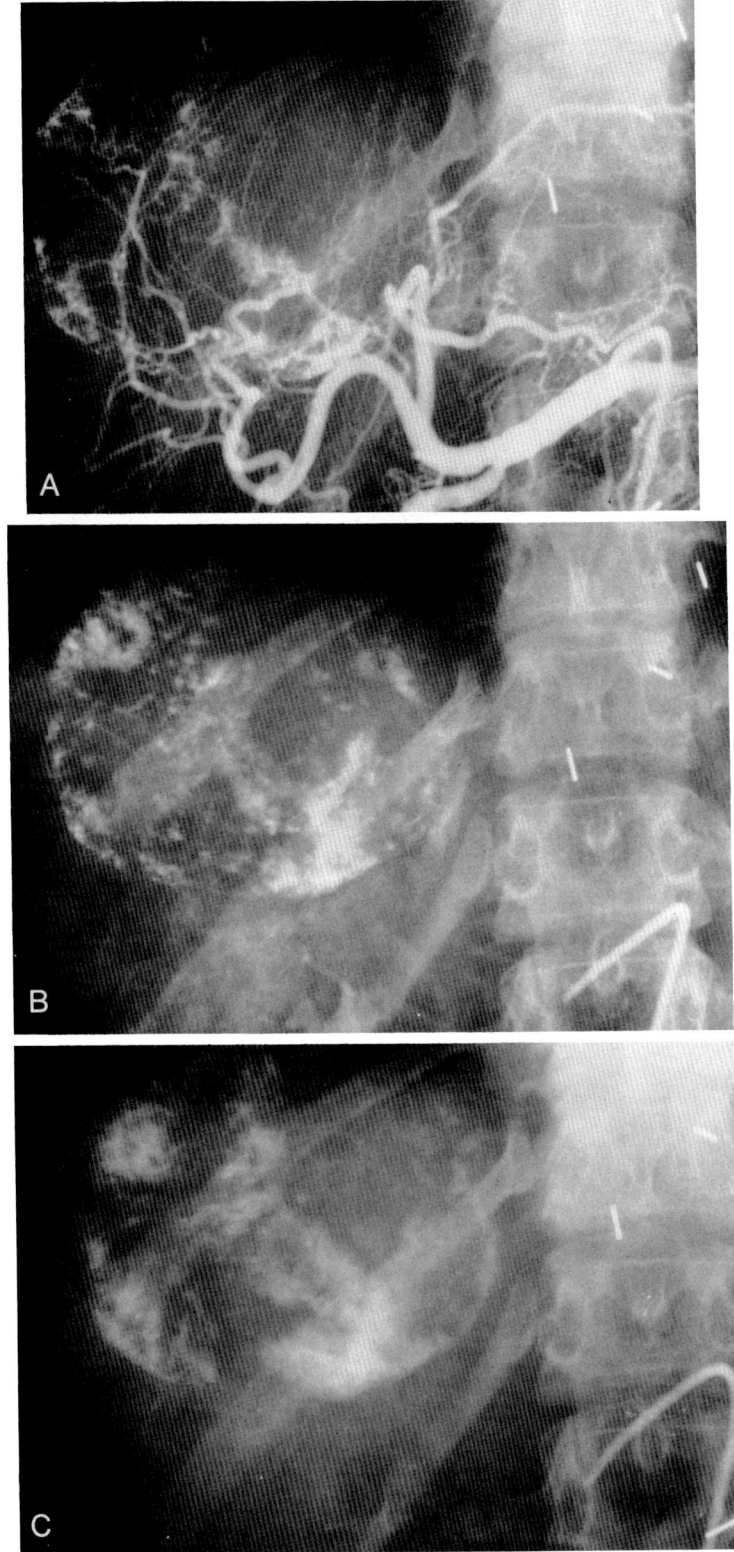

FIGURE 5.34. HEMANGIOMA

A: Hepatic arteriogram of a hemangioma showing stretched arteries and early, peripheral, punctate staining. *B:* Parenchymal phase shows punctate staining which is beginning to diffuse. *C:* Persistence of the blush which is now diffusing into the center of the mass.

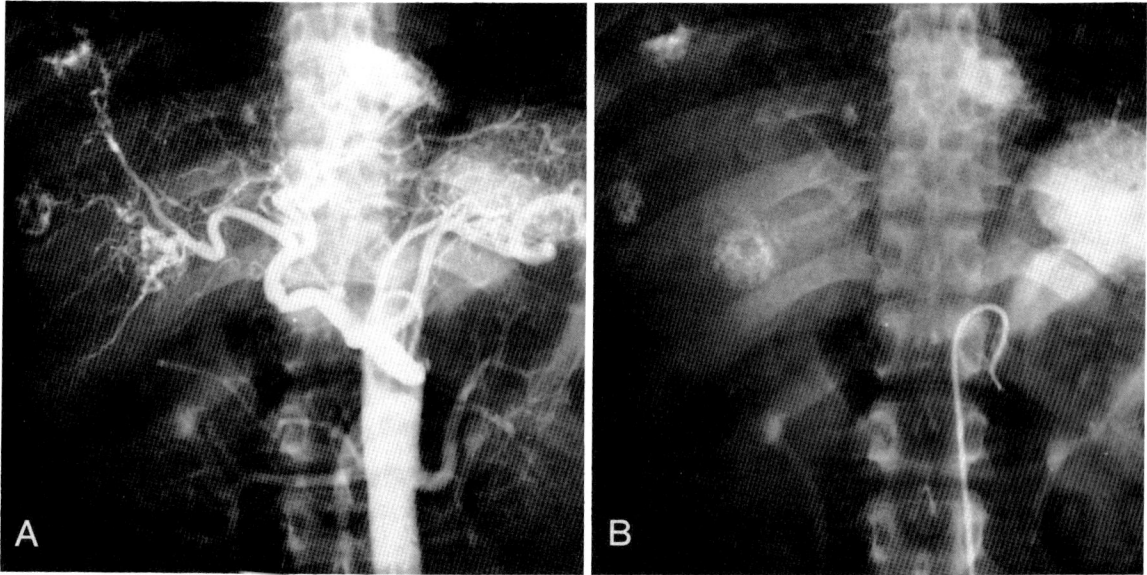

FIGURE 5.35. HYPERVASCULAR LIVER MASSES

A and *B:* Fifty-two-year-old woman with right lower quadrant pain and fever. CT showed multiple low density lesions. Angiography reveals multiple bilobar, small, well-defined hypervascular liver masses (*A*). The initially lucent centers filled in late in the parenchymal phase and blushes persisted well into the venous phase (*B*). Because of the difficulty in excluding vascular metastatic disease, laparotomy with needle and wedge biopsies was performed. The masses were impalpable at surgery. Multiple hemangiomas.

sis/thrombosis (28). Opacification persists well into the venous phase often up to 30–45 sec, and delayed filming is mandatory. It is this delayed opacification that is diagnostic of hemangioma, due to contrast material cycling through tortuous vascular channels in addition to puddling in partially thrombosed vascular spaces (7). If portography is performed, cavernous hemangiomas will not opacify from the portal vein and the portal vein is usually normal (Fig. 5.33). Hypervascular metastasis (such as renal or thyroid carcinoma, carcinoid-islet cell tumor, melanoma, choriocarcinoma, mucinous cystic neoplasm of the pancreas) can be a difficult angiographic differential diagnosis, but contrast accumulation usually does not persist as it does in hemangioma (Fig. 5.35).

Summary

Cavernous hemangioma of the liver commonly presents incidentally as an echogenic mass on ultrasound. In these circumstances when the sonographic appearance is typical no further workup is usually needed. If the same sonographic findings are present in a symptomatic patient or in a patient with a known primary or if the sonogram is atypical for hemangioma, further workup with labelled red cell scintigraphy is advisable (Fig. 5.36). If the diagnosis is in doubt after the scintigram, depending on institutional preferences and clinical considerations, one might proceed with fine-needle aspiration, dynamic CT, guided core biopsy, peritoneoscopy with or without biopsy, or angiography.

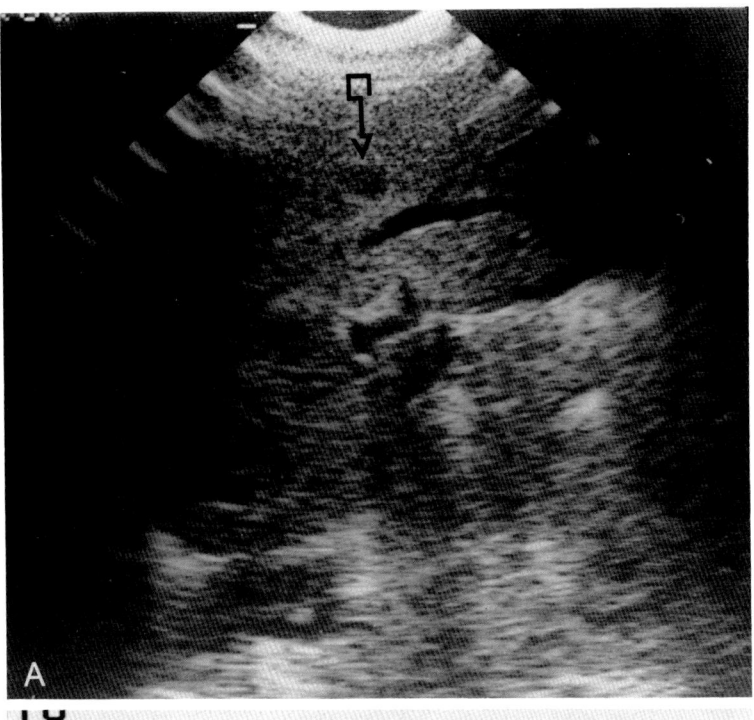
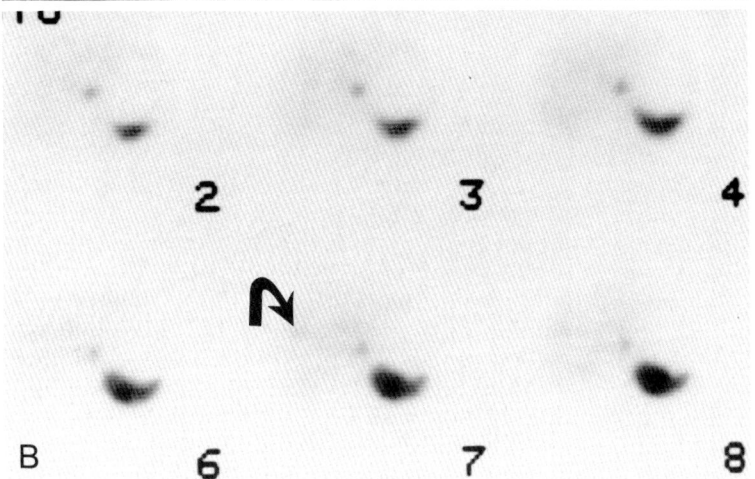

FIGURE 5.36. SPECT IN THE DIAGNOSIS OF CAVERNOUS HEMANGIOMA
A: Transverse sonogram shows a 1 cm diameter hypoechoic mass in the anterior portion of the right lobe of the liver (arrow), suspicious for metastasis. B: SPECT-labeled red cell scintigram at 2 hr postinjection: focal accumulation of activity (arrow) in identical location diagnostic of hemangioma. Planar images were equivocal.

REFERENCES

1. Ishak KG, Rabin L: Benign tumors of the liver. Med Clin North Am 59:995–1013, 1975.
2. Schonland MM, Millward-Sadler GH, Wright DH, Wright R: Hepatic tumors. In Wright R, Alberti KGMM, Karran S, Millward-Sadler GH (eds): Liver and Biliary Disease. Philadelphia, W. B. Saunders, 1979, pp 911–913.
3. Sherlock S: Diseases of the Liver and Biliary System. Oxford, Blackwell Scientific, 1981, pp 469–470.
4. Schiff L: Hepatic neoplasia—selected clinical aspects. Semin Roentgenol 18:71–74, 1983.
5. Adam YG, Huvos AG, Fortner JG: Giant hemangiomas of the liver. Ann Surg 172:239–245, 1970.
6. Wittich GR, van Sonnenberg E, Mueller PR, Haaga JR, Ferrucci JT Jr, Brandtner W, Bernardino ME, Cooperberg P, Lee T: Fine needle biopsy of cavernous hemangioma of the liver. Presented at the 10th Scientific Assembly and Annual Meeting, RSNA, Washington, D.C., November 25–30, 1984.
7. Olmstead WW, Stocker JT: RPC from the AFIP. Radiology 117:59–61, 1975.
8. Edmondson MA, Peters RL: Tumors of the liver: pathologic features. Semin Roentgenol 18:17–83, 1983.
9. Darlak JJ, Moskowitz M, Kattan KR: Calcifications in the liver. Radiol Clin North Am 18:209–219, 1980.
10. Gore RM, Goldberg HI: Plain film and cholangiographic findings in liver tumors. Semin Roentgenol 18:87–93, 1983.
11. Freeny PC, Vimont TR, Barnett DC: Cavernous hemangioma of the liver: ultrasonography, arteriography and computed tomography. Radiology 132:143–148, 1979.

12. McArdle CR: Ultrasonic appearance of a hepatic hemangioma. *J Clin Ultrasound* 6:122–123, 1978.
13. Wiener SN, Parulekar SG: Scintigraphy and ultrasonography of hepatic hemangioma. *Radiology* 132:149–153, 1979.
14. Bree RL, Schwab RE, Neiman HL: Solitary echogenic spot in the liver: is it diagnostic of a hemangioma? *AJR* 140:41–45, 1983.
15. Taboury J, Porcel A, Tubiana JM, Monnier JP: Cavernous hemangioma of the liver studied by ultrasound: enhancement posterior to a hyperechoic mass as a sign of hypervascularity. *Radiology* 149:781–785, 1983.
16. Johnson MC, Sheedy PF, Stanson AW, et al: Computed tomography and angiography of cavernous hemangiomas of the liver. *Radiology* 138:115–121, 1981.
17. Araki T, Itai Y, Furui S, et al: Dynamic CT densitometry of hepatic tumors. *AJR* 135:1037–1043, 1980.
18. Barnett PH, Zerhoni EA, White RI, Siegelman SS: Computer tomography in the diagnosis of cavernous hemangioma of the liver. *AJR* 134:439–447, 1980.
19. Itai Y, Ohtomo K, Araki T, Furui S, Iio M, Atomi Y: Computed tomography and sonography of cavernous hemangioma of the liver. *AJR* 141:315–320, 1983.
20. Freeny PC, Marks WM: Patterns of contrast enhancement of benign and malignant hepatic neoplasms during bolus dynamic CT scanning. Presented at the 70th Scientific Assembly and Annual Meeting, RSNA, Washington, D.C., November 25–30, 1984.
21. Volpe JA, Johnson GS: "Hot" hepatic hemangioma: a unique radiocolloid concentrating liver scan lesion. *J Surg Oncol* 2:373–377, 1970.
22. Front D, Royal HD, Israel O, Parker JA, Kolodny GM: Scintigraphy of hepatic hemangiomas the value of ^{99m}Tc-labeled red blood cells: concise communication. *J Nucl Med* 22:684–687, 1981.
23. Engel MA, Marks DS, Sandler MA, Shetty P: Differentiation of focal intrahepatic lesions with ^{99m}Tc-red blood cell imaging. *Radiology* 146:777–782, 1983.
24. Wilcox NE, Joo KG: Sluggish perfusion in hepatic hemangioma. *Clin Nucl Med* 5:465–467, 1980.
25. Rabinowitz SA, McKusick KA, Strauss HW: ^{99m}Tc red blood cell scintigraphy in evaluating focal liver lesions. *AJR* 143:63–68, 1984.
26. Abrams RM, Beranbaum ER, Santos JS, Lipson J: Angiographic features of cavernous hemangioma of the liver. *Radiology* 92:308, 1969.
27. Winograd J, Palubinskas AJ: Arterial-portal venous shunting in cavernous hemangioma of the liver. *Radiology* 122:331–332, 1977.
28. McLaughlin MJ: Angiography in cavernous hemangioma of the liver. *AJR* 113:50–55, 1971.

FOCAL NODULAR HYPERPLASIA

The considerable confusion in the literature regarding this entity is reflected by the number of names it has: hepatic pseudotumor, focal cirrhosis, lobar cirrhosis, isolated regenerative hyperplasia, partial nodular transformation, benign hepatoma, hepatic hamartoma, parenchymal hamartoma (1–5). Current theory is that focal nodular hyperplasia (FNH) is either a congenital hamartomatous malformation or a reparative process in one or more areas of focal injury possibly secondary to a vascular anomaly (1, 4, 5).

In 1973, Baum et al. (6) described an association between oral contraceptives and hepatic adenomas, a finding which has been supported by other authors since then. Unfortunately, much confusion has been generated by the inconsistent application of pathologic criteria in the differentiation of hepatic adenoma and focal nodular hyperplasia, which has limited a careful analysis of the literature. Despite continued controversy, most authors feel there is no etiologic relationship between oral contraceptives and focal nodular hyperplasia (1, 7). There is, however, support for the observation that oral contraceptives increase the propensity for focal nodular hyperplasia to present with hemoperitoneum. Klatskin (8) found that only 1% of patients with focal nodular hyperplasia who were not taking oral contraceptives presented with rupture and hemoperitoneum, whereas 14% of those with focal nodular hyperplasia who had used oral contraceptives presented with these complications. This increased hemorrhagic tendency is postulated to be a direct effect of the oral contraceptives on the vasculature supplying the tumor (1, 3, 7–9).

Clinical Findings

Age range at presentation of patients with focal nodular hyperplasia is from 7 months to 75 yr, with most cases between the third and fifth decades of life (1). There is a 2:1 female preponderance (1). Only 20% are symptomatic; common signs and symptoms are abdominal mass, pain, or discomfort (1). Portal hypertension can be present in patients with multiple nodules (1). Most patients have normal liver function tests (1). When focal nodular hyperplasia presents in infancy or childhood, symptoms and signs such as abdominal enlargement and vomiting are usually present (4). Surgical resection for pedunculated or otherwise easily resected lesions is recommended, and biopsy alone rather than radical surgery for extensive tumors is probably the best course as there is no evidence of malignant potential (1, 2, 4, 8, 9).

Pathology

The right lobe is affected twice as often as the left (1). Focal nodular hyperplasia is solitary in about 80% with two or more nodules present in about 20% (1, 3). Most are subcapsular although occasionally focal nodular hyperplasia is pedunculated (5%) or deep within the liver (1, 2).

In a large series of all ages, 85% were 5 cm or less in diameter (1), although in infants and children they are usually 7 cm or larger in diameter (4). This discrepancy is probably because only symptomatic cases are discovered in children.

Grossly, focal nodular hyperplasia is well-demarcated but usually unencapsulated, lobulated, and lighter than the rest of the liver. Characteristically there is a central stellate mass of connective tissue radiating towards the periphery (Fig. 5.37D). Large veins and arteries are present at the periphery and in the deep stellate scar. There are numerous bile ductules and smaller vessels in the radiating septa (1–3).

Histologically, the lesion is composed of nodules of hepatocytes and Kupffer cells, which lack central veins or portal triads, and are separated by fibrous septae. Bile duct proliferation within these fibrous septa or between hepatocytes is a constant finding (1–3).

Biopsy differentiation from fibrolamellar hepatocellular carcinoma is easiest with a wedge biopsy, rather than aspiration cytology or core biopsy.

Radiology

No calcification is present on plain films (4, 5). Gastrointestinal contrast examinations may show displacement and/or indentation of the gallbladder, stomach, or hepatic flexure.

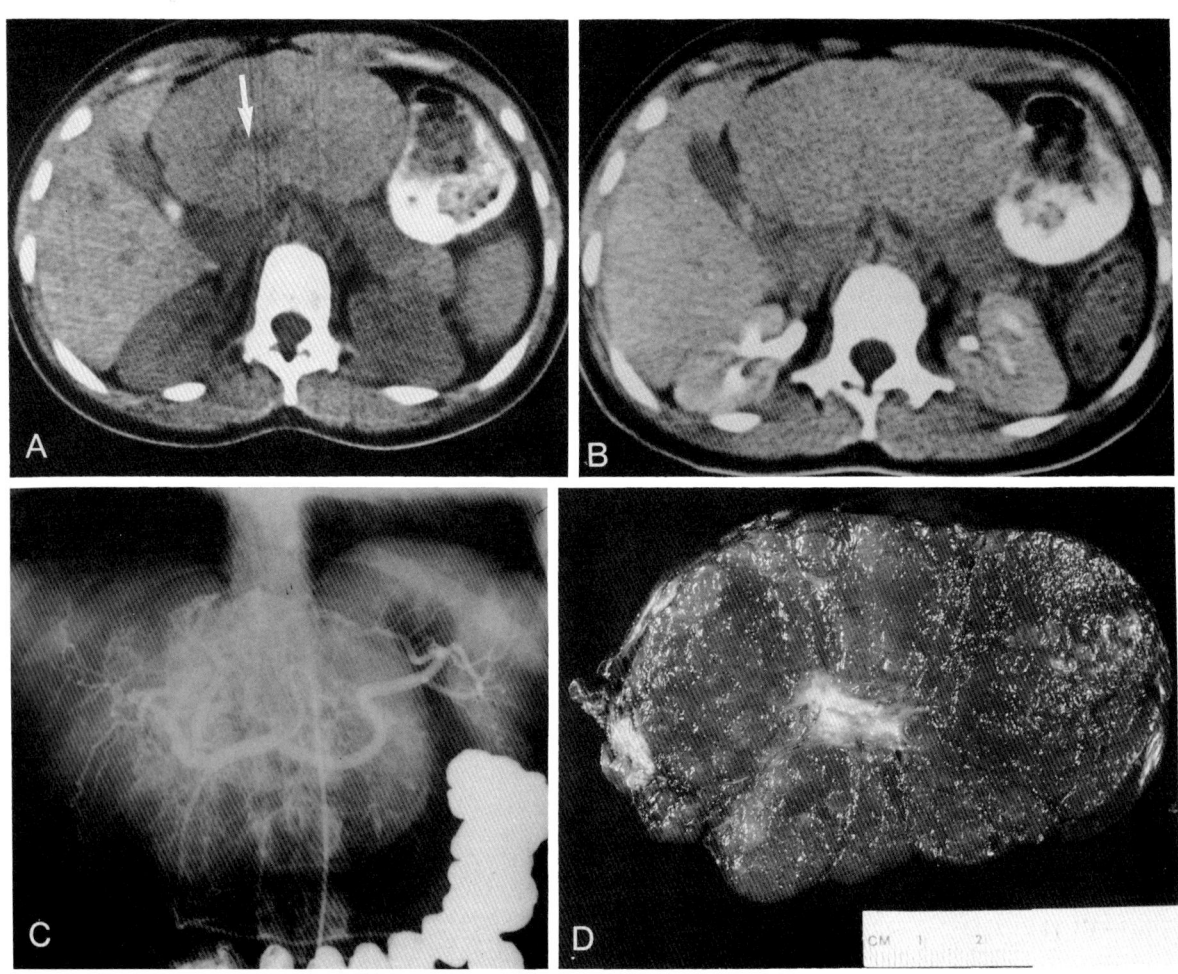

FIGURE 5.37. FOCAL NODULAR HYPERPLASIA

A 30-yr-old woman with abdominal pain and a palpable epigastric mass: focal nodular hyperplasia. *A:* Unenhanced CT: well-defined hypodense mass replacing part of the left lobe of the liver. A central scar (*arrow*) is noted. *B:* Enhanced CT: the lesion is now isodense and the central scar is no longer seen. *C:* Angiogram: hypervascular mass supplied by a network of dilated hepatic artery branches. A diffuse tumor blush was seen in the hepatogram phase (not shown). *D:* Cut gross specimen, obvious central scar. (From Fishman EK, Farmlett E, Kadir S, Siegelman SS: Computed tomography of benign hepatic tumors. *J Comput Assist Tomogr* 6:472–481, 1982.)

Ultrasound

The sonographic features of focal nodular hyperplasia are highly variable. Typically focal nodular hyperplasia is a well-defined subcapsular mass with echogenicity either greater or less than that of the surrounding liver. The presence of a central linear stellate group of echoes has been reported to correspond closely to the fibrotic scar seen pathologically in focal nodular hyperplasia and is suggestive of this lesion (Fig. 5.38C) (10). However, the central scar seen sometimes in fibrolamellar hepatocellular carcinomas can be identical in sonographic appearance. This find-

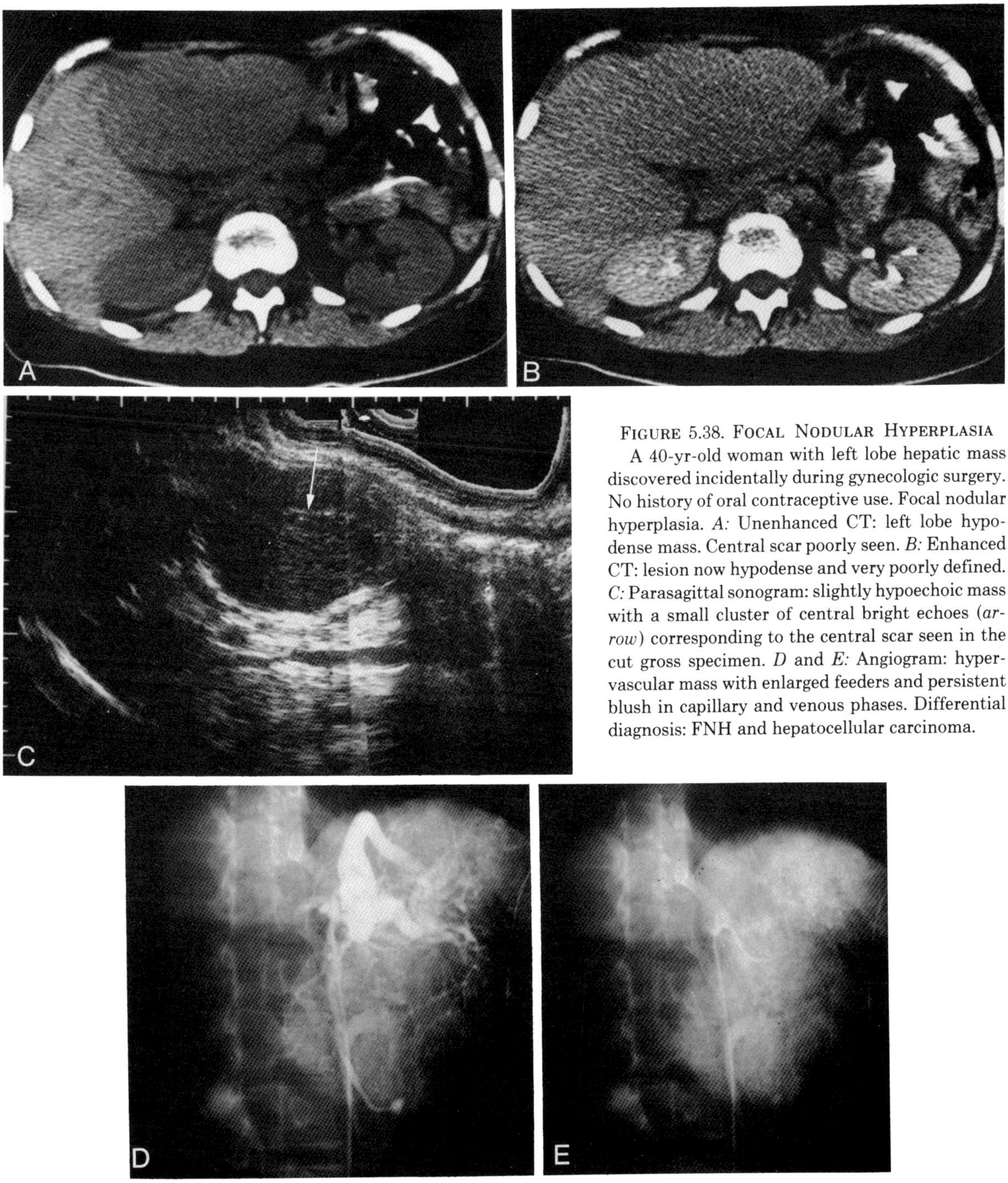

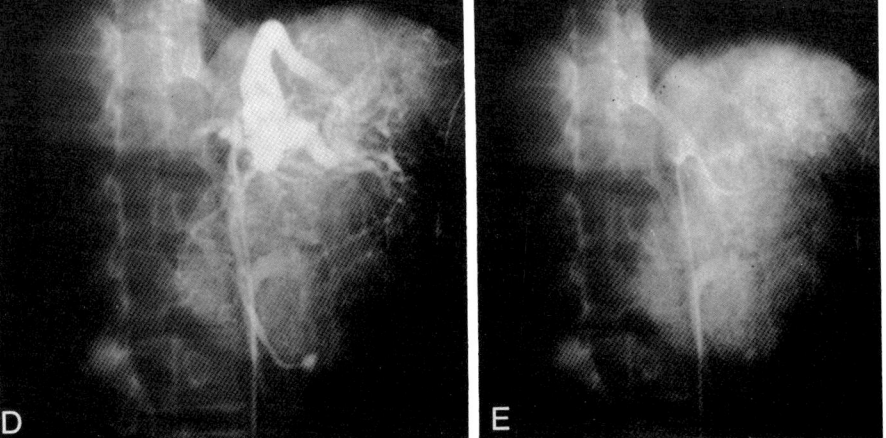

FIGURE 5.38. FOCAL NODULAR HYPERPLASIA
A 40-yr-old woman with left lobe hepatic mass discovered incidentally during gynecologic surgery. No history of oral contraceptive use. Focal nodular hyperplasia. *A:* Unenhanced CT: left lobe hypodense mass. Central scar poorly seen. *B:* Enhanced CT: lesion now hypodense and very poorly defined. *C:* Parasagittal sonogram: slightly hypoechoic mass with a small cluster of central bright echoes (*arrow*) corresponding to the central scar seen in the cut gross specimen. *D* and *E:* Angiogram: hypervascular mass with enlarged feeders and persistent blush in capillary and venous phases. Differential diagnosis: FNH and hepatocellular carcinoma.

ing of a central scar has also been reported one other time as an unusual variant of hepatic lymphoma by Wenzel and Winters (11).

Computed Tomography

On noncontrast scans, focal nodular hyperplasia characteristically presents as a low attenuation lesion (20–40 HU), although this feature is neither constant nor specific (Fig. 5.38A and B). When seen, the presence of a central cleft-like radiolucency on a noncontrast scan which corresponds to the central scar seen pathologically, is strongly suggestive of focal nodular hyperplasia (Fig. 5.37A and B) (12). This central low density may disappear after contrast enhancement. Fibrolamellar hepatocellular carcinomas can have a similar central low density scar. However, this scar is seen best on contrast-enhanced scans and may be partially calcified, so that differentiation may still be possible from focal nodular hyperplasia, in which calcification has not been seen to our knowledge. Wenzel and Winters (11) reported a low density cleft in a patient with hepatic lymphoma, but in that one case the border of the lesion was ill-defined as opposed to the usual well-defined border of focal nodular hyperplasia. Hemorrhage is much less common in focal nodular hyperplasia than in hepatic adenoma so its presence favors hepatic adenoma over focal nodular hyperplasia.

In most cases of focal nodular hyperplasia, the lesions become isodense with the surrounding parenchyma following enhancement by bolus technique (Fig. 5.37B). This underscores the need for both contrast and noncontrast scans to avoid the possibility of a false negative diagnosis if only contrast enhanced scans are obtained. Although the vascularity of hepatic adenomas is variable, hepatic adenomas usually do not enhance to the same extent as surrounding normal liver, thus allowing differentiation from focal nodular hyperplasia in some cases.

Angiography

Classically, focal nodular hyperplasia is a hypervascular mass with a dense tumor blush in the capillary and portal venous phases (Figs. 5.37C, 5.38D and E, and 5.39). Lucent septations within the stain may be seen, corresponding to radiating fibrous septa. In large tumors, the feeding arteries sometimes penetrate the mass and then divide into smaller radiating branches giving a spokewheel appearance (Fig. 5.39) (13, 14). No encasement, neovascularity, or arteriovenous shunting occurs (13, 14). Regions of hemorrhage or necrosis are unusual, as opposed to hepatic adenoma. A recent review showed approximately one-third of FNH tumors having the classic pattern of a central feeder with spokewheel vessels radiating towards the periphery, whereas two-thirds had feeders entering from the periphery (15). When FNH tumors are small, large feeding arteries are not seen; rather a reticular pattern of small vessels inside the lesion is usually demonstrated.

Nuclear Medicine

The scintigraphic appearance of focal nodular hyperplasia is variable on sulfur colloid scans. About 60% of cases will show uptake in the mass equal to that of normal parenchyma, so that the scan could be read as normal if other imaging modalities are not available for comparison (Fig. 5.39). Thirty to forty percent will be relatively photopenic and about 10% will show hyperconcentration of the radionuclide (Fig. 5.40) (15). No other hepatic masses except for regenerating nodules contain sufficient numbers of Kupffer cells to show uptake equal to or greater than normal parenchyma (16). Case reports of focally increased sulfur colloid uptake due to hemangioma, hepatoblastoma, liver herniation, and within hepatocellular carcinoma exist, but are sufficiently rare so as not to merit serious consideration (17, 18). Other considerations when a hot spot is seen on sulfur colloid scintigraphy include superior or inferior vena cava obstruction (anterior), and hepatic venoocclusive disease (posterior); these entities can be included or excluded based on clinical history and results of other imaging examinations. The mechanism of hyperconcentration of sulfur colloid within focal nodular hyperplasia can be either an increase in number of Kupffer cells per unit volume, an increase in function of the cells themselves, or a relative increase in blood flow to the tumor (17). Focal nodular hyperplasia may or may not concentrate gallium-67 citrate (16, 17, 19). In the past, normal (compared to the rest of the liver) or decreased activity has been seen within focal nodular hyperplasia on Rose Bengel scans, with the latter more likely (12, 20). Technetium-99m IDA scans likewise may occasionally show slightly increased or normal activity compared to the normal parenchyma, but are more likely to show photopenia (20). Focal nodular hyperplasia tends to be hot on both radionuclide angiography and blood pool scintigraphy.

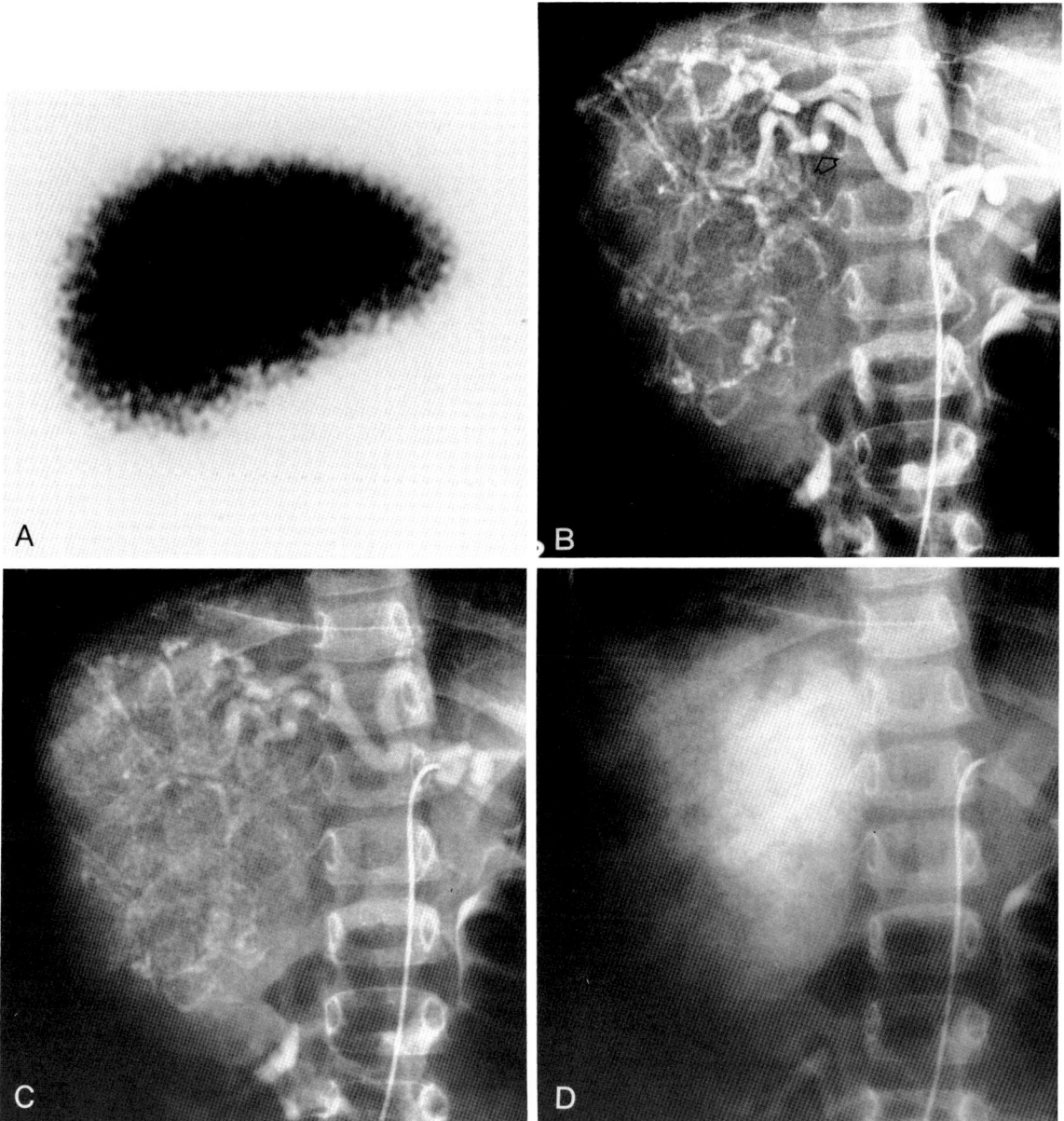

FIGURE 5.39. FOCAL NODULAR HYPERPLASIA IN A CHILD

A: ^{99m}Tc-sulfur colloid scan: normal uptake in right lobe of the liver where a mass was palpable. A gallium scan failed to demonstrate any galliophilic areas within the mass (not shown). *B:* Celiac arteriogram: enlarged right hepatic artery supplying a well-circumscribed highly vascular mass in the right lobe of the liver. Some vessels appear to supply a prominent circumferential set of arteries which send many penetrating branches to the tumor. Second hypertrophied hepatic artery branch appears to enter the tumor (*arrow*) and then supply radiating branches as well. *C:* Late arterial phase: no early draining veins, vascular encasement, or venous laking. *D:* Parenchymal phase: sharply marginated mass with a dense blush. No venous laking or vascular encasement.

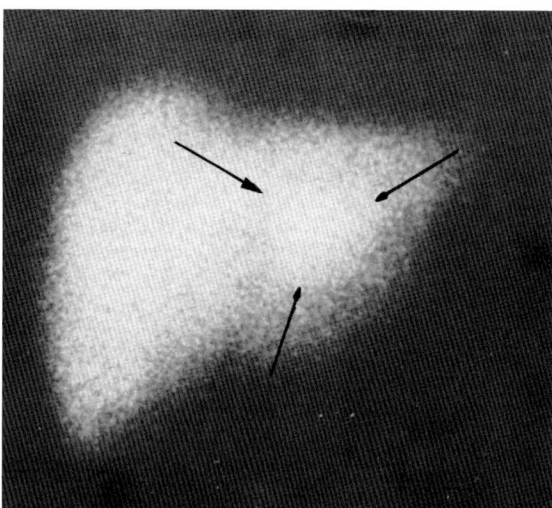

FIGURE 5.40. COMPARED TO NORMAL PARENCHYMA, SLIGHTLY INCREASED UPTAKE IN FOCAL NODULAR HYPERPLASIA IN THE LEFT LOBE (arrows)

REFERENCES

1. Ishak KG, Rabin L: Benign tumors of the liver. Med Clin North Am 59:996–999, 1975.
2. Edmonson HA: Differential diagnosis of tumors and tumor-like lesions of the liver in infancy and childhood. J Dis Child 91:169–171, 1956.
3. Schonland MM, Millward-Sadler GH, Wright DH, Wright R: Hepatic tumors. In Wright R, Alberti KGMM, Karran S, Millward-Sadler CH (eds): Liver and Biliary Disease. Philadelphia, W. B. Saunders, 1979, pp 904–905.
4. Tate RC, Chacko MV, Singh S, Ogden L: Parenchymal hamartoma of the liver in infants and children. Am J Surg 123:346–350, 1972.
5. Siebert JJ, Soper RT: Preoperative diagnosis of benign hepatic hamartoma by correlation radioisotopic and angiographic studies. Pediatr Radiol 4:149–152, 1976.
6. Baum JK, Holtz F, Bookstein JJ, Klein EW: Possible association between benign hepatomas and oral contraceptives. Lancet 2:926–927, 1973.
7. Fechner RE, Roehm JOF Jr: Angiographic and pathologic correlations of hepatic focal nodular hyperplasia. Am J Surg Pathol 1:217–224, 1977.
8. Klatskin G: Hepatic tumors: possible relationship to the use of oral contraceptives. Gastroenterology 73:386–394, 1977.
9. Knowles DM II, Wolff M: Focal nodular hyperplasia of the liver—a clinicopathologic study and review of the literature. Hum Pathol 7:533–545, 1976.
10. Scatarige JC, Fishman EK, Sanders RC: The sonographic "scar sign" in focal nodular hyperpliasia of the liver. J Ultrasound Med 1:275–278, 1982.
11. Wenzel D, Winters C Jr: The scar sign in hepatic neoplasia. J Ultrasound Med 2:160–168, 1983.
12. Fishman EK, Farmlett E, Kadir S, Siegelman SS: Computed tomography of benign hepatic tumors. J Comput Assist Tomogr 6:472–481, 1982.
13. Goldstein HM, Neiman HL, Mena E, Bookstein JJ, Appelman HD: Angiographic findings in benign liver cell tumors. Radiology 110:339–343, 1974.
14. Casarella WJ, Knowles DM, Wolff M, Johnson PM: Focal nodular hyperplasia and liver cell adenoma: radiologic and pathologic differentiation. AJR 131:393–402, 1978.
15. Rogers JV, Mack LA, Freeny PC, Johnson ML, Sones PJ: Hepatic focal nodular hyperplasia: angiography, CT, sonography, and scintigraphy. AJR 137:983–990, 1981.
16. Sandler MA, Petrocelli RD, Marks DS, Lopez R: Ultrasonic features and radionuclide correlation in liver cell adenoma and focal nodular hyperplasia. Radiology 135:393–397, 1980.
17. Piers DA, Houthoff HJ, Krom RAF, Schuur KH, Sikkens H, Weits J: Hot spot liver scan in focal nodular hyperplasia. AJR 135:1289–1292, 1980.
18. Diament MJ, Parvey LS, Tonkin ILD, Johnson KD, Bernstein R, Webber B: Hepatoblastoma: technetium sulfur colloid uptake simulating focal nodular hyperplasia. AJR 139:168–171, 1982.
19. Atkinson GO Jr, Kodroff M, Sones PJ, Gay BB Jr: Focal nodular hyperplasia of the liver in children: a report of three new cases. Radiology 137:171–174, 1980.
20. Biersack HJ, Thelen M, Torres JF, Lackner K, Winkler CG: Focal nodular hyperplasia of the liver as established by ^{99m}Tc sulfur colloid and HIDA scintigraphy. Radiology 137:187–190, 1980.

HEPATIC ADENOMA

Despite some continuing controversy, most authors agree that oral contraceptives are related both to the development of hepatic adenomas and to factors increasing their tendency to bleed (1–3). Although hepatic adenomas are reported predominantly in females their occurrence has also been noted in the male population. In these cases, however, a history of steroid use (androgens) is frequent. Patients with Type I glycogen storage disease (von Gierke's disease) have a propensity for the development of multiple hepatic adenomas.

Clinical Findings

Patients with hepatic adenoma usually present with a right upper quadrant mass and abdominal pain, which often is secondary to hemorrhage within the tumor and/or rupture with hemoperitoneum. They can be asymptomatic with hepatomegaly discovered as an incidental finding. Klatskin (4) found that 41% of patients with hepatic adenoma who used oral contraceptives developed hemoperitoneum, and 39% were found later to be ruptured. Of those who did not use oral contraceptives, 15% developed hemoperitoneum and 14% were later found to be ruptured.

The common complications of hemorrhage, hemoperitoneum, and rupture as well as the persistently unresolved question of malignant potential, have lead most authorities to recommend surgical resection as the treatment of choice for hepatic adenomas (4, 5). This underscores the necessity for diagnostic accuracy in differentiating this tumor from focal nocular hyperplasia and other lesions such as hemangiomas which would often be treated conservatively. Regression of hepatic adenomas after cessation of oral contraceptives is rare (6).

Pathology

Hepatic adenoma is a benign epithelial tumor which is usually a solitary smooth mass that is frequently partially or completely encapsulated (2). Adenomas are frequently subcapsular and of quite large size (6–30 cm in diameter) at diagnosis (6). The tumor is composed of cells resembling hepatocytes, but having a vacuolated glycogen-rich cytoplasm. Hepatic adenomas lack the Kupffer cells, nodularity, septations, and central fibrous scar of focal nodular hyperplasia. Proliferating bile ducts are not found except near the capsule of the adenoma. These tumors are usually richly vascularized with thin-walled, endothelial-lined vessels dispersed among the hepatocytes. Foci of hemorrhage and necrosis are found in up to 50% of patients. In order to make the diagnosis of a hepatic adenoma and exclude a well-differentiated hepatocellular carcinoma, aspiration cytology or core biopsy may not be sufficient; a wedge biopsy is often necessary.

Ultrasound

Hepatic adenomas are solid masses that are usually echogenic but sometimes hypoechoic (Fig. 5.41A). In symptomatic patients, sonolucent regions within the solid mass representing hemorrhage and necrosis can be depicted (Fig. 5.42) (7). In the proper clinical context, these findings are quite suggestive of hepatic adenoma. Sonography can detect fluid in the peritoneal cavity in instances of intraperitoneal rupture.

Computed Tomography

Although isodense hepatic adenomas have been reported (8), these lesions characteristically present as low density lesions on noncontrast scans, a finding, which by itself, is nonspecific. The low density cleft seen in some cases of focal nodular hyperplasia is not seen in hepatic adenomas. Hepatic adenomas have a variable degree of vascularity and thus enhance following contrast injection to a variable degree. However, in our experience, the lesion does not enhance to the same extent as normal liver parenchyma (Fig. 5.41B) (9). Most hemangiomas may be distinguished from adenomas by their pattern of enhancement with filling in of the lesion from the periphery to the center. Areas of intratumoral hemorrhage are a common finding on CT of hepatic adenomas and strongly suggest the diagnosis (Figs. 5.42B and 5.43). Hemoperitoneum can be detected and sometimes specifically diagnosed appearing as high density ascites.

Arteriography

Angiography is useful both in the diagnosis and in planning the surgical approach to the patient with hepatic adenoma. Hepatic adenomas are commonly hypervascular, but the arteries are not as tortuous nor as densely concentrated as those of focal nodular hyperplasia. They also lack the characteristic septated capillary blush, having a more homogeneous tumor stain. Nonetheless, hypervascular hepatic adenomas are very difficult to distinguish from focal nodular hyperplasia (Fig.5.41D and E). The vascular supply in most cases of hepatic adenoma is circumferential with feeding vessels coursing towards the center of the lesion (Fig. 5.41D) (10, 11). This finding is suggestive of hepatic adenoma, but can be seen in focal nodular hyperplasia as well (10). Casarella et al. (10) reported that 50% of adenomas studied angiographically were hypovascular with displacement and draping of hepatic arteries (Fig. 5.42C). In one-third of these cases, subcapsular hemorrhage and ischemic central necrosis were observed. Thus, a hypovascular mass, the presence of hemorrhage and necrosis, or a hypervascular mass with a circumferential arterial supply is suggestive but not specific for hepatic adenoma. Occasionally the angiographic appearance of hepatic adenomas may simulate a hepatocellular carcinoma and biopsy would be necessary for differentiation. Hepatic adenomas are often indistinguishable from hepatocellular carcinomas despite the use of multiple imaging modalities. In fact, in a recent series of 23 cases of hepatic adenoma from the Mayo Clinic, two showed malignant changes on microscopic examination (12).

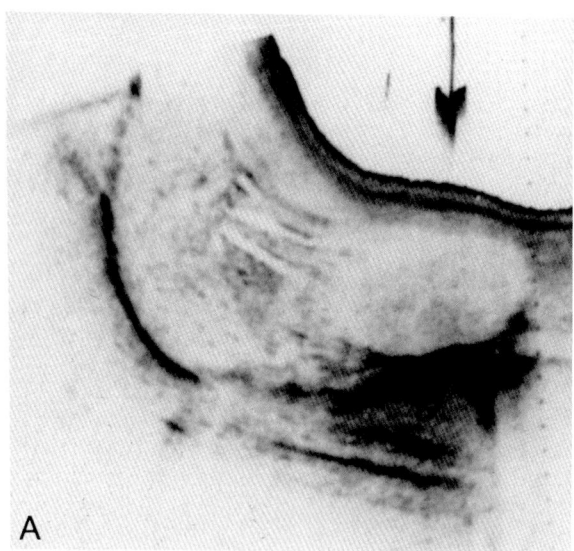
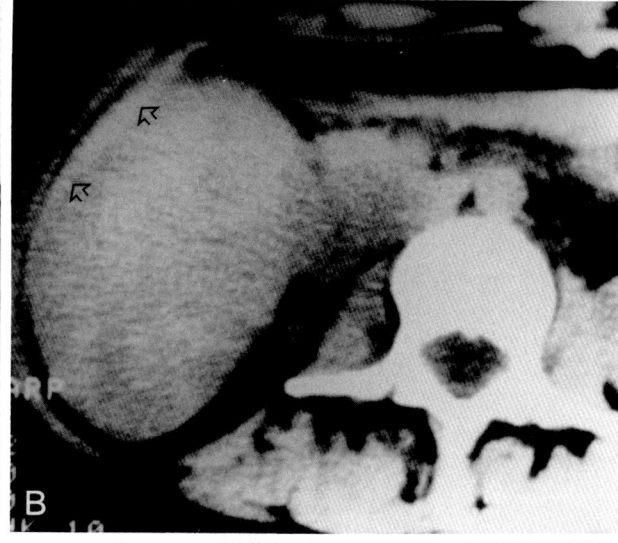
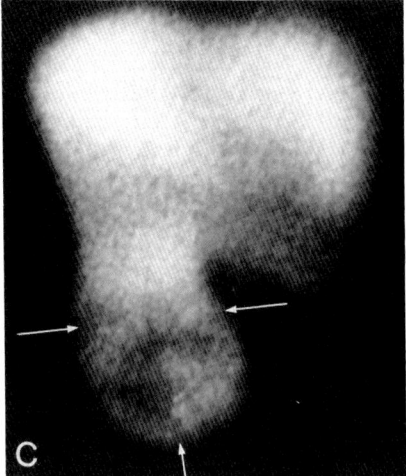

FIGURE 5.41. ADENOMA WITHOUT HEMORRHAGE

Asymptomatic woman with history of oral contraceptive use. *A:* Parasagittal sonogram: nearly isoechoic solid hepatic mass. *B:* Enhanced CT: mass enhances slightly less than normal parenchyma: a rim of normal parenchyma is seen (*arrows*) anterolaterally to the mass. *C:* RAO sulfur colloid scan: some colloid uptake is present within the mass (*arrows*), but less than normal parenchyma. *D:* SMA arteriogram, replaced right hepatic artery: hypervascular mass with an enlarged feeding artery. Arterial supply is from multiple arteries branching centrally off a peripheral capsular vessel (*arrows*). *E:* Parenchymal phase: Well-circumscribed intense tumor blush.

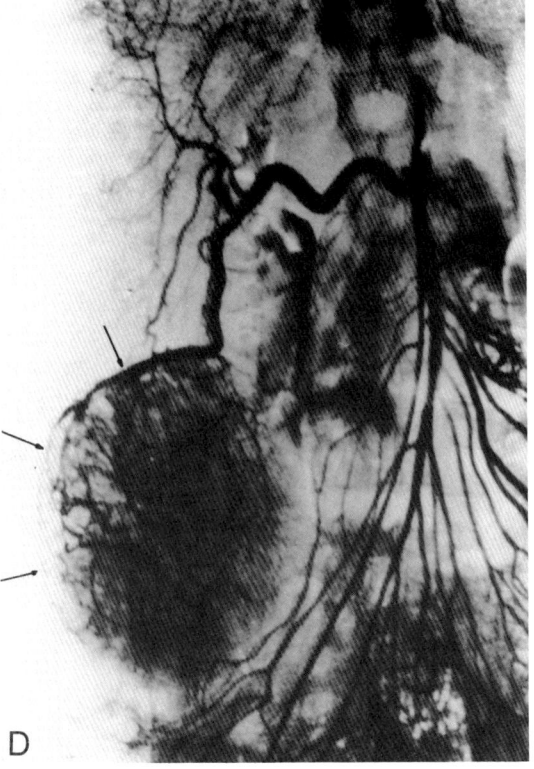
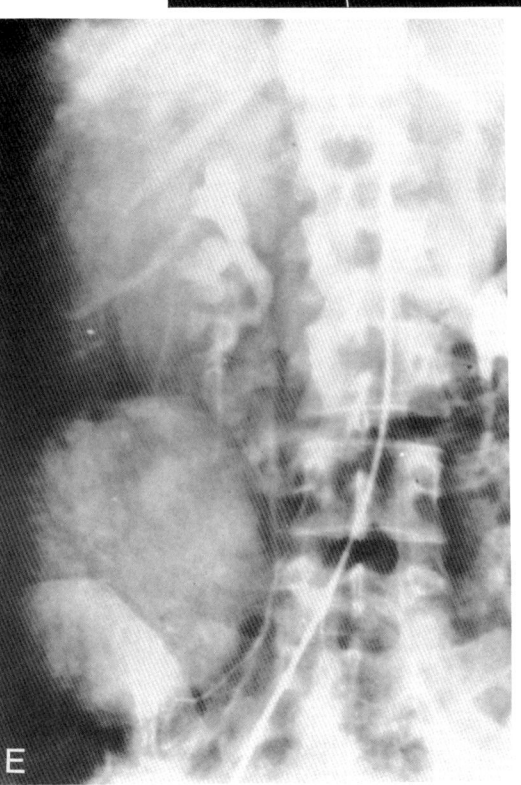

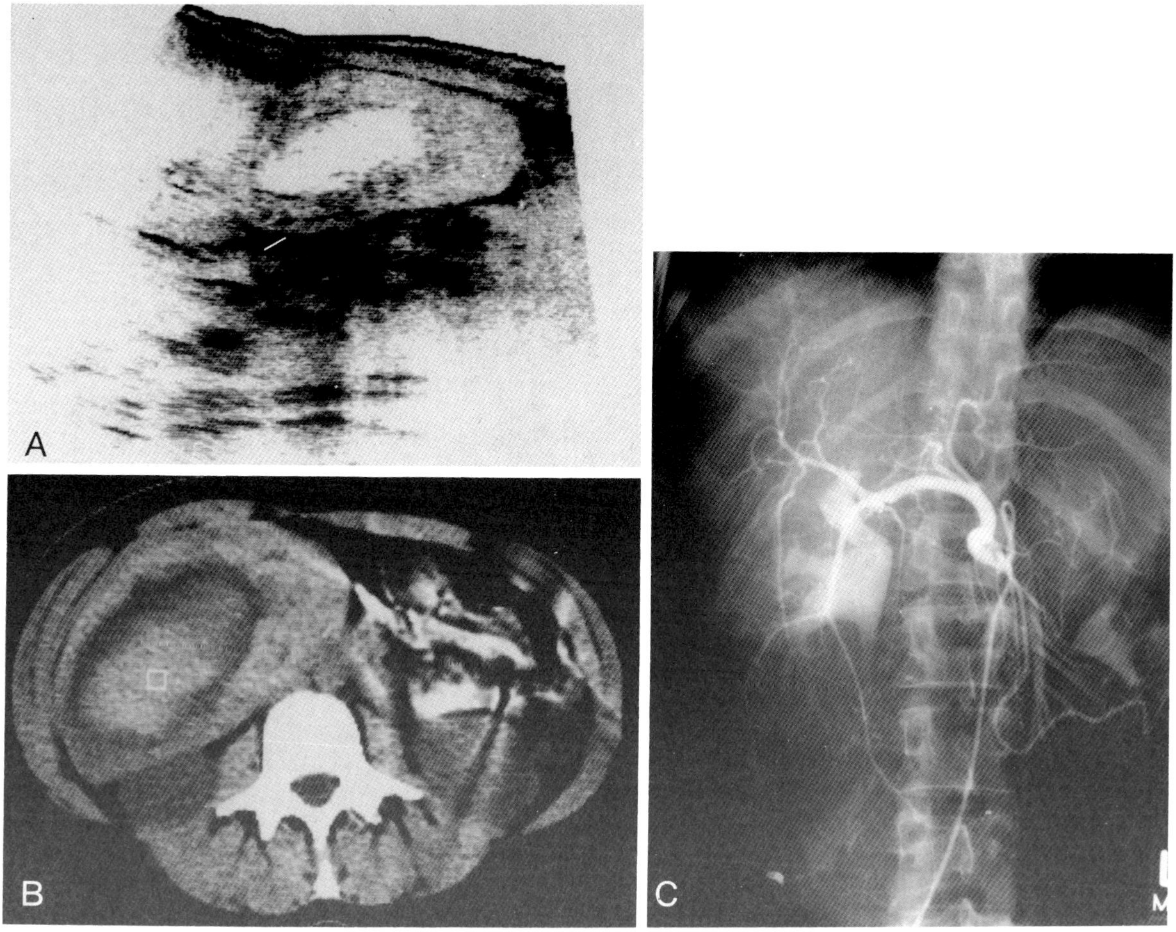

FIGURE 5.42. HEPATIC ADENOMA
A 24-yr-old woman with sudden onset of right upper quadrant pain. Oral contraceptive use for 5 yr. *A:* Parasagittal sonogram: moderately echogenic mass with a large central sonolucency due to hemorrhage. *B:* Unenhanced CT: low density hepatic mass with central high attenuation region (90 HU, cursor) corresponding to hemorrhage. *C:* Hepatic arteriogram: hypovascular inferior right lobe mass with stretching and splaying of arteries and no neovascularity.

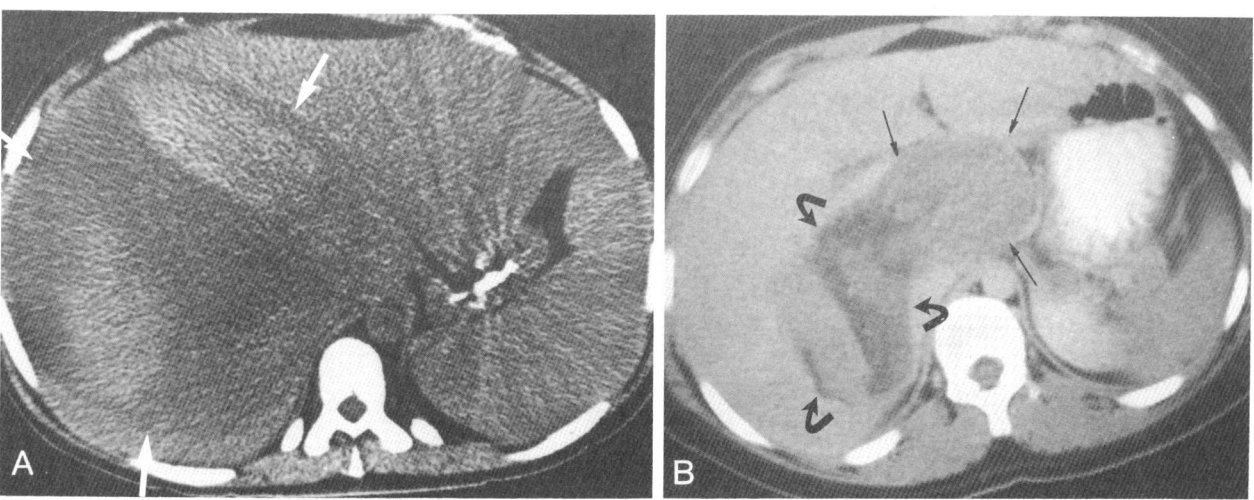

FIGURE 5.43. TWO CASES OF MASSIVE HEMORRHAGE FROM HEPATIC ADENOMAS
A: A 26-yr-old man with severe right upper quadrant pain and no history of steroid use. Unenhanced CT: 17-cm hypodense mass (*arrows*) with large dense regions of hemorrhage. *B:* Young female patient with history of oral contraceptive use who presented in the ER with pain and shock. Emergency surgery was required. Enhanced CT: Adenoma replacing and enlarging the caudate lobe (*arrows*). Large hematoma (*curved arrows*).

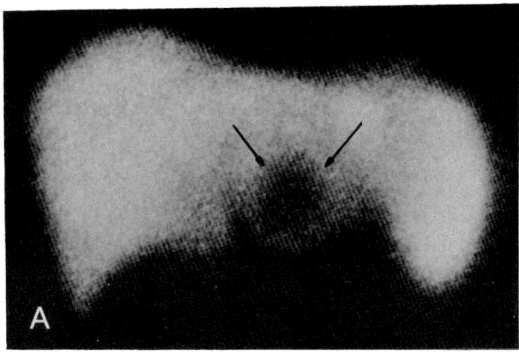
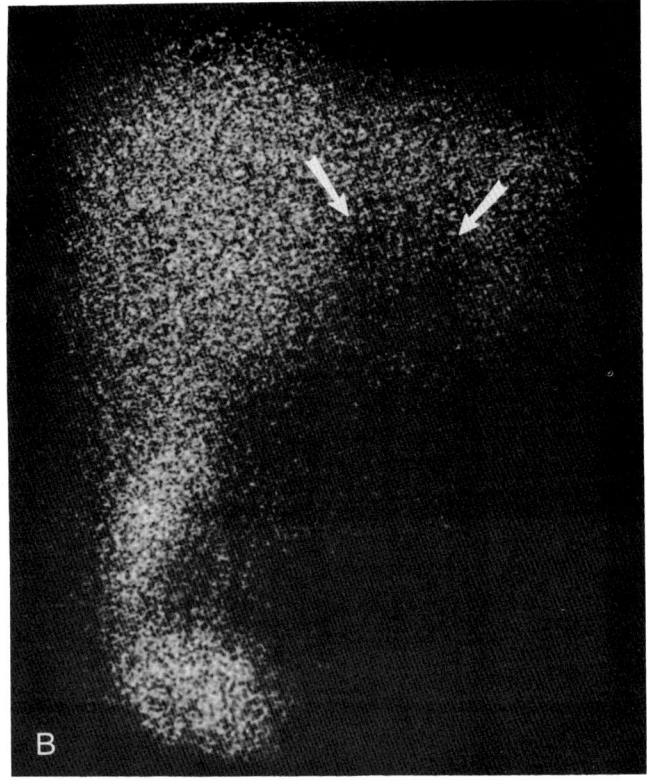

FIGURE 5.44. SCINTIGRAPHY OF HEPATIC ADENOMA
A: Sulfur colloid scan: cold mass (arrows). B: A 24-hr delayed hepatobiliary scan: no uptake (arrows).

Nuclear Medicine

Adenomas are likely to present as photopenic lesions during sulfur colloid scintigraphy since they are essentially devoid of Kupffer cells (7, 9). In theory, delayed ^{99m}Tc-IDA scanning might frequently show activity within the neoplasm via a similar mechanism to that operating in hepatocellular carcinoma (see Nuclear Medicine section on hepatocellular carcinoma). Cases of hepatic adenoma with IDA uptake on early images have been reported (13). Hepatic adenomas with extensive internal hemorrhage will be either cold on IDA scintigraphy, or conceivably, show peripheral uptake and central photopenia. The majority of hepatic adenomas are not hot on radionuclide angiography and blood pool studies, although some that are hypervascular will be (Fig. 5.44).

REFERENCES

1. Fechner RE, Roehm JOF Jr: Angiographic and pathologic correlations of hepatic focal nodular hyperplasia. Am J Surg Pathol 1:217–224, 1977.
2. Ishak KG, Rabin L: Benign tumors of the liver. Med Clin North Am 59:995–1013, 1975.
3. Baum JK, Holtz F, Bookstein JJ, Klein EW: Possible association between benign hepatomas and oral contraceptives. Lancet 2:926–929, 1973.
4. Klatskin G: Hepatic tumors: possible relationship to the use of oral contraceptives. Gastroenterology 73:386–394, 1977.
5. Knowles DM II, Wolff M: Focal nodular hyperplasia of the liver—a clinicopathologic study and review of the literature. Hum Pathol 7:533–545, 1976.
6. Schonland MM, Millward-Saddler GH, Wright DH, Wright R: Hepatic tumors. In Wright R, Alberti KGMM, Karran S, Millward-Sadler GH (eds): Liver and Biliary Disease. Philadelphia, W. B. Saunders, 1979, pp 902–904.
7. Sandler MA, Petrocelli RD, Marks DS, Lopez R: Ultrasonic features and radionuclide correlation in liver cell adenoma and focal nodular hyperplasia. Radiology 135:393–397, 1980.
8. Havrilla TR, Pep RG, Alfidi RJ, Haaga JR: Benign hepatic tumors and cysts in women using oral contraceptive agents. Cleve Clin Q 44:41–47, 1977.
9. Fishman EK, Farmlett EJ, Kadir S, Siegelman SS: Computed tomography of benign hepatic tumors. J Comput Assist Tomogr 6:472–491, 1982.
10. Casarella WJ, Knowles DM, Wolff M, Johnson PM: Focal nodular hyperplasia and liver cell adenoma: radiologic and pathologic differentiation. AJR 131:393–402, 1978.
11. Goldstein HM, Neiman HL, Mena E, Bookstein JJ, Appelman HD: Angiographic findings in benign liver cell tumors. Radiology 110:339–343, 1974.
12. Kerlin P, David GL, McGill DB et al: Hepatic adenoma and focal nodular hyperplasia: clinical, pathological and radiologic features. Gastroenterology 84:994–1002, 1983.
13. Vincent LM, Rho TH, McCartney WH, Mauro MA: Hepatic adenoma demonstration of discordant uptake with Tc-99m sulfur colloid and ^{99m}Tc DISIDA. Clin Nucl Med 9:415–416, 1984.

Bile Duct Hamartoma (Adenoma)

These rare benign liver tumors are generally encountered serendipitously in middle-aged patients, usually males, at laparotomy or autopsy (1). Their primary clinical significance is that they are easily confused with metastatic carcinoma on gross inspection. Microscopic findings are characteristic: they are composed of small duct-like structures separated by moderate amounts of mature connective tissue stroma. They often contain medium-sized arteries and veins. They are usually small (<1 cm) pale, firm circumscribed nodules, often subcapsular, and solitary or multiple. The angiographic appearance has been described as a small region of abnormal vascularity appearing in the mid to late arterial phase and persisting into the venous phase. The blush may be ring-like. Tumor vessels, laking, and arteriovenous shunting are not present (2).

Bile duct adenomas, if large enough, are manifested as well-defined regions of decreased activity on sulfur colloid scans.

REFERENCES

1. Schonland MM, Millward-Sadler GH, Wright DH, Wright Ralph: Hepatic tumors. In Wright R, Alberti KGMM, Karran S, Millward-Sadler GH (eds): *Liver and Biliary Disease*, Philadelphia, W. B. Saunders, 1979. p 907.
2. McLaughlin MJ, Phillips MJ: Angiographic findings in multiple bile-duct hamartomas. *Radiology* 116:41–43, 1975.

BILIARY CYSTADENOMA AND CYSTADENOCARCINOMA

Biliary cystadenoma and cystadenocarcinoma are rare tumors that arise in the liver or, less frequently, the extrahepatic biliary tree. They bear a resemblance to mucinous cystic neoplasms of the pancreas, and are thought to be of developmental origin from bile ducts with very slow growth (1).

Clinical Findings

Eighty percent of cystadenomas occur in women and 81.5% are seen in patients older than 30 (1). Patients with intrahepatic cystadenoma present with abdominal swelling and/or mass of weeks to years in duration (1). Pain is present in 60% and nonspecific complaints, such as dyspepsia, anorexia, nausea, and vomiting are present less frequently (1). Jaundice occasionally occurs due to duct compression. There has been one report of intraperitoneal and retroperitoneal rupture (1). Rarely intrahepatic biliary cystadenomas are incidental findings at laparotomy or autopsy (1). Extrahepatic biliary cystadenomas have nonspecific early symptoms and signs such as nausea, vomiting, and right upper quadrant pain (2). Palpable mass is rare. Jaundice is always present and is often fluctuating, suggesting a ball-valve effect. Surgical treatment of cystadenoma has consisted of aspiration, drainage, marsupialization, enucleation, and excision. In view of the potential for malignant transformation, wide local excision is advisable, and recurrence after complete excision is uncommon (1). Biliary cystadenocarcinomas have a 5:3 female to male predominance, and a similar mode of presentation to cystadenoma (1). They are though to arise in previously benign cystadenomas (1). While biliary cystadenocarcinomas are capable of spread beyond the liver and distant metastasis, long-term survival is possible with complete excision and prognosis is better than with intrahepatic cholangiocarcinoma (1).

Pathology

Cystadenomas involve the right lobe in 50%, both lobes in about 30%, and the left lobe in about 20% (1). The majority are large, frequently exceeding 10 cm in maximum diameter with a reported range of 3.5–25 cm (1, 2). They have a smooth external surface with outward bulge (1). Almost all are grossly multilocated; only two unilocular ones have been reported (1). Gross papillary excrescences projecting inwards off the walls are common. The cyst fluid may be mucinous, serous, contain hemosiderin, cholesterol, or necrotic material (1, 2). Connections to large intrahepatic ducts have been reported but are unusual. A mural nodule may then prolapse and cause intermittent jaundice (1). Location is intrahepatic in 85% and extrahepatic in 15% (2).

Microscopically the locules are lined by a single layer of biliary-type epithelium with papillary projections but no atypia or mitotic figures (1). Both cytoplasm and cyst fluid stain positively for mucin. The supporting stroma is compact and cellular resembling ovarian stroma (1).

Cystadenocarcinomas are grossly similar to cystadenomas except that excrescences are more common and solid areas may be present (1). The cyst fluid is more likely to be blood stained, frankly hemorrhagic, or chocolate colored (1). Microscopically, the locules are lined by both benign and malignant epithelium. The latter is multilayered with numerous papillary projections (1). There are breaks in the basement membrane and invasion of the underlying stroma (1).

Radiology

Biliary cystadenoma and cystadenocarcinoma cannot be differentiated radiologically, although large solid areas other than papillary projections suggest malignancy. Nonspecific soft-tissue masses and organ displacement are seen on plain films (1). One cystadenocarcinoma with peripheral wall calcification has been reported (1). Excretory urograms can show radiolucencies corresponding to the cystic regions (Fig. 5.45).

Cystadenomas and cystadenocarcinomas are nonspecific photopenic masses on sulfur colloid and gallium scintigraphy as well as radionuclide angiography and blood pool imaging.

Sonographically, biliary cystadenomas and cystadenocarcinomas are ovoid cystic masses with irregular margins, single or multiple septations, and sometimes papillary excrescences and/or fluid-fluid levels (Figs. 5.46–5.49) (3–5). The CT appearance is also similar to mucinous cystic neoplasms of the pancreas: near water density mass with septations and sometimes excrescences (Figs. 5.46 and 5.47) (3–5). Angiographically, both mucinous cystic neoplasm of the pancreas and biliary cystadenoma/cystadenocarcinoma are avascular with small clusters of peripheral abnormal vessels and a thin blush in the wall and septa (Figs. 5.46*D* and 5.50) (3, 4). Vessels are stretched and splayed around the mass. Papillary excrescences, when present, can be demonstrated as foci of abnormal vessels with mild tumor blush in the parenchymal phase.

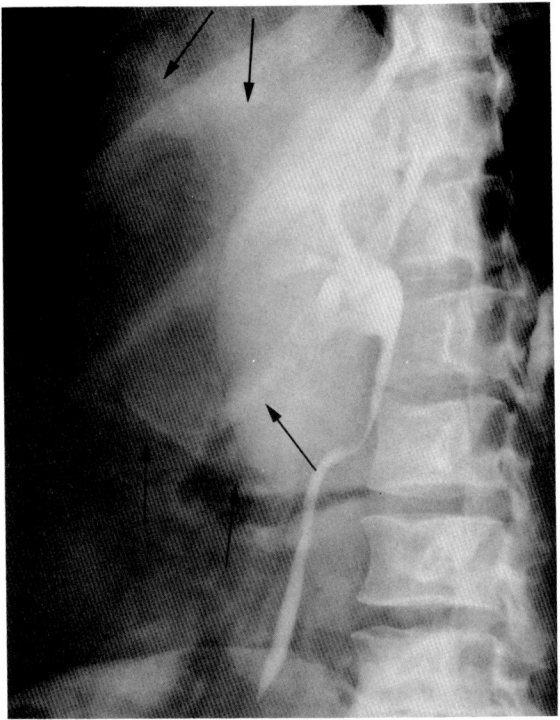

FIGURE 5.45. EXCRETORY UROGRAM OF CYSTADENOMA
Biliary cystadenoma shown as a multiseptated radiolucent mass (*arrows*) anterior to the right kidney by virtue of total body opacification.

ERCP or percutaneous cystography can demonstrate rare findings such as intraductal prolapse or communication with the biliary tree (Fig. 5.48) (5). The latter can probably be excluded by a negative ^{99m}Tc-IDA derivative scan.

Direct cholangiography in cases of extrahepatic biliary cystadenoma or cystodenocarcinoma shows ductal dilation proximal to a partially obstructing extraluminal mass. Streaming of contrast material around a smooth intraluminal component can be shown (Fig. 5.49) (2).

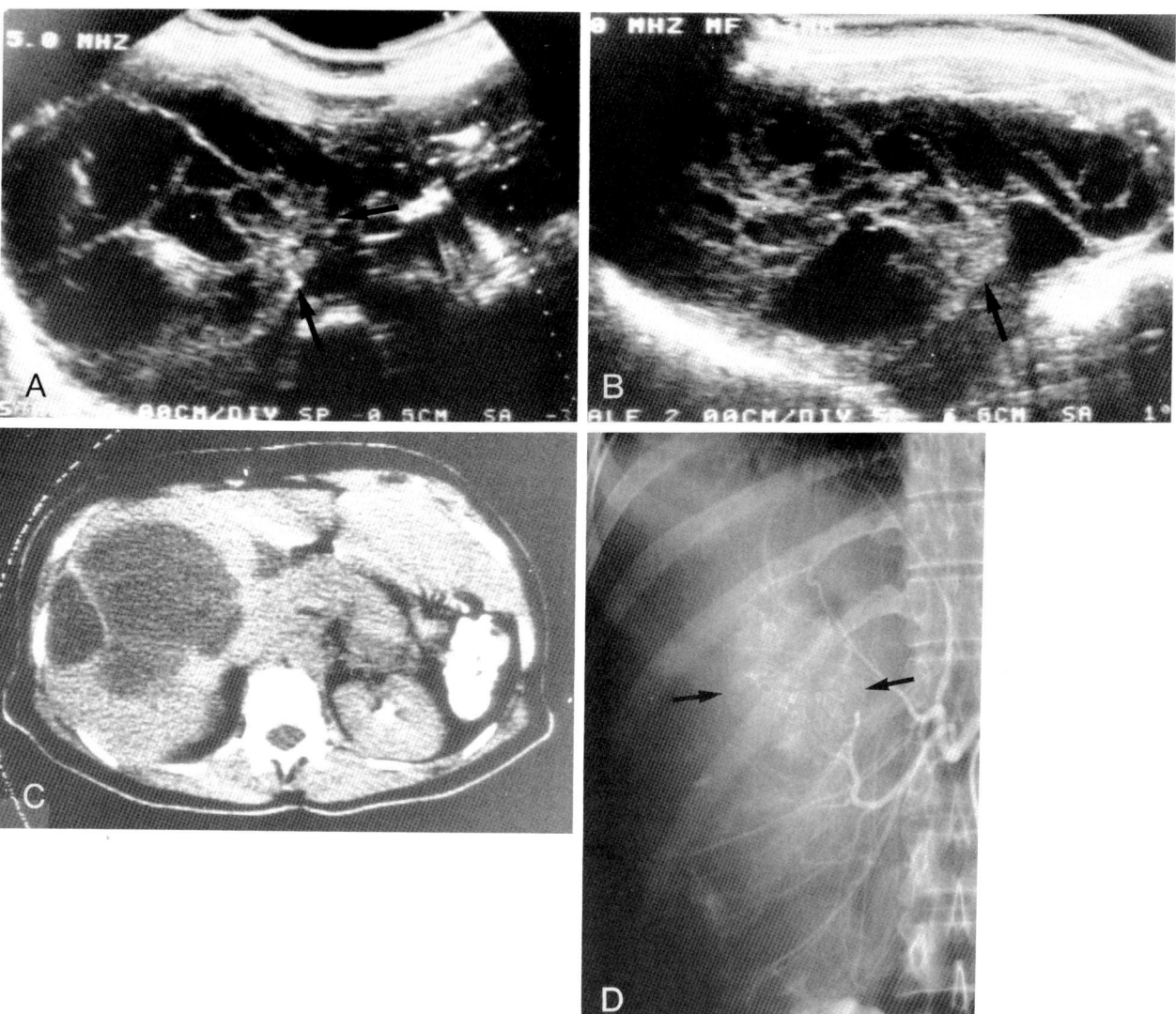

FIGURE 5.46. MULTISEPTATED BILIARY CYSTADENOMA WHOSE INTERNAL ARCHITECTURE IS DEPICTED BETTER BY ULTRASOUND THAN CT

A and *B:* Transverse and parasagittal scans: large mass with multiple cystic spaces many of which contain solid nodules. Relatively solid region medially in the central portion of the mass (*arrows*). *C:* Representative enhanced CT slice: cystic spaces of slightly differing attenuation, but less septations than sonography. *D:* Hepatic arteriogram: Splaying of arteries around this huge, mostly hypovascular mass. Nodule of hypervascularity (*arrows*) corresponds to solid region seen on sonography.

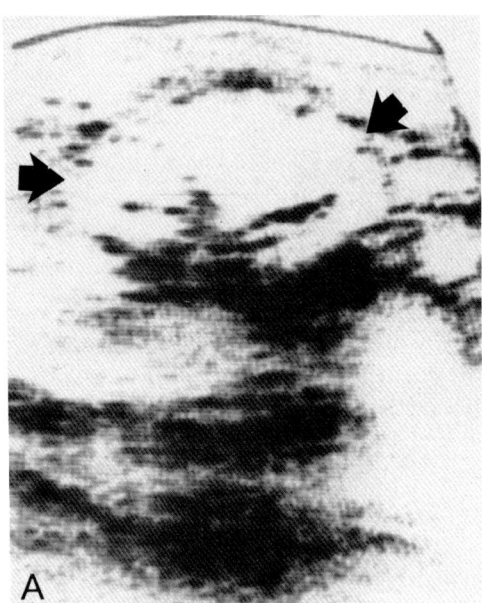
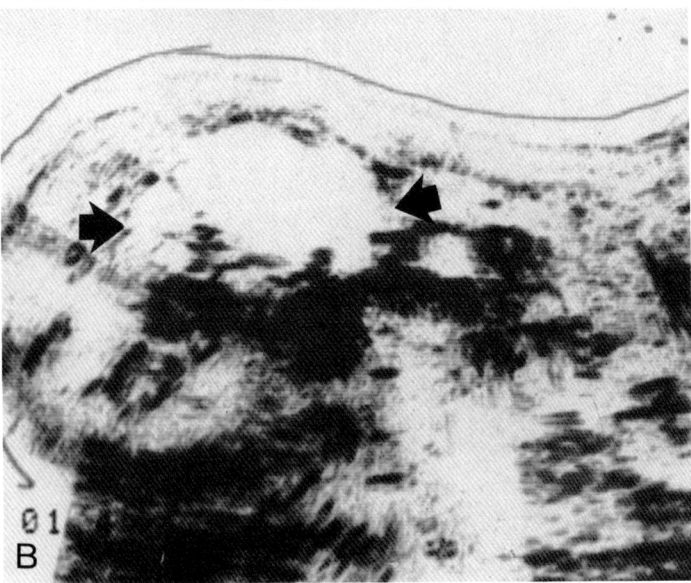
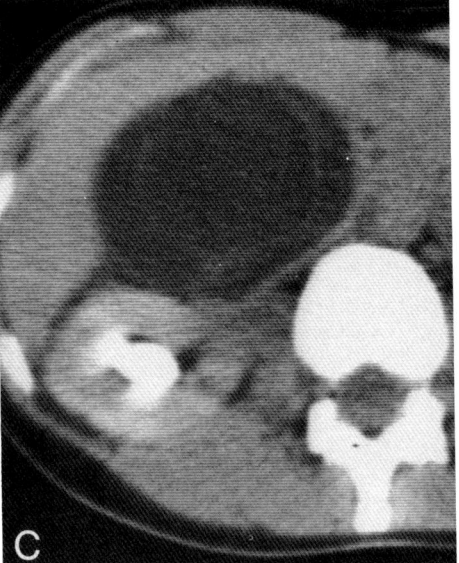

FIGURE 5.47 A 36-YR-OLD WOMAN WITH PAINFUL EPIGASTRIC MASS: BILIARY CYSTADENOMA. THE INTERNAL ARCHITECTURE IS SHOWN BETTER WITH SONOGRAPHY

A and *B:* Transverse and longitudinal scans respectively: thick-walled cystic mass with nodules and septations (*arrows*). *C:* CT: mural nodule and septations barely visible. (From Frick MP, Feinberg SB: Biliary cystadenoma, *AJR* 139:393–395, 1982.)

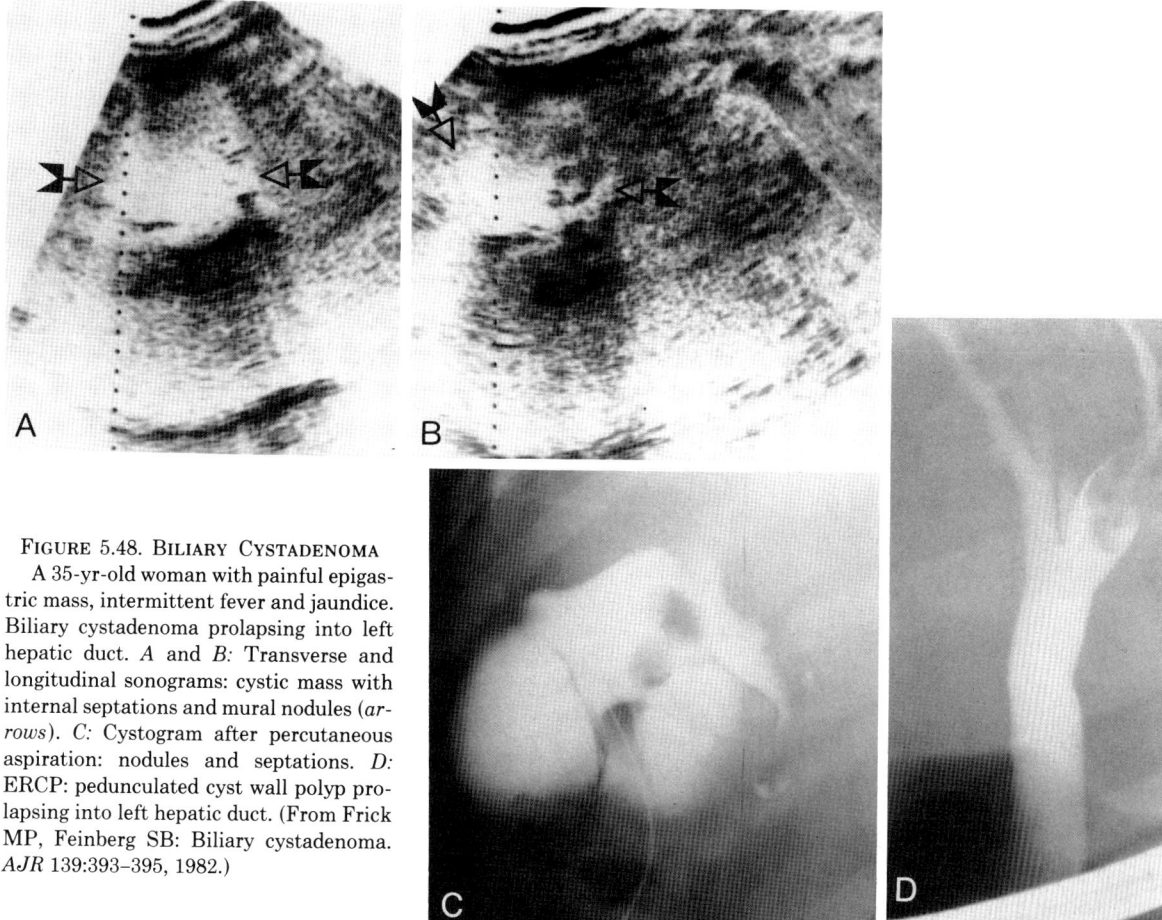

FIGURE 5.48. BILIARY CYSTADENOMA
A 35-yr-old woman with painful epigastric mass, intermittent fever and jaundice. Biliary cystadenoma prolapsing into left hepatic duct. *A* and *B:* Transverse and longitudinal sonograms: cystic mass with internal septations and mural nodules (*arrows*). *C:* Cystogram after percutaneous aspiration: nodules and septations. *D:* ERCP: pedunculated cyst wall polyp prolapsing into left hepatic duct. (From Frick MP, Feinberg SB: Biliary cystadenoma. *AJR* 139:393–395, 1982.)

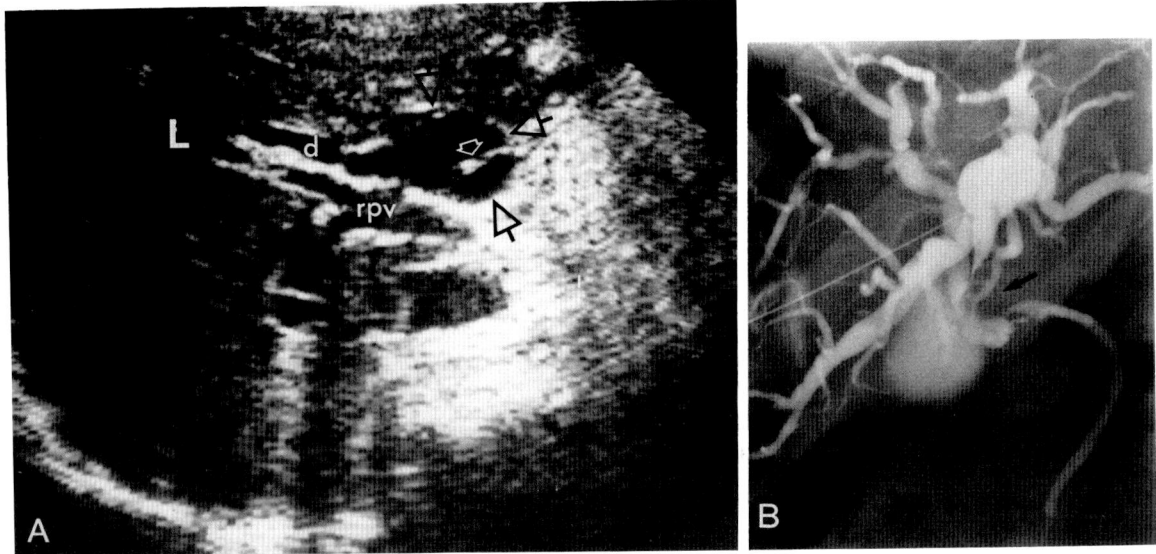

FIGURE 5.49. CYSTADENOMA OF THE PROXIMAL COMMON HEPATIC DUCT

A 54-yr-old woman with intermittent pruritus and jaundice. *A:* Transverse sonogram of liver (*L*) at porta hepatis: 4 cm cystic mass (*black arrows*) of proximal bile duct with thick internal septum (*white arrow*) (*rpv*, right portal vein; *d*, dilated right hepatic bile duct). *B* and *C:* Films from transhepatic cholangiogram: intrahepatic bile duct dilatation proximal to partially obstructing extraluminal mass (*arrow*) arising from proximal common hepatic duct just caudad to the bifurcation (*B*). Streaming of contrast around well-circumscribed lobule (*arrow*) that protrudes into a proximal hepatic duct. (From Nagorney DM, LeSage GD, Charboneau JW, McGough PF: Cystadenoma of the proximal common hepatic duct: the use of ultrasonography and transhepatic cholangiography in diagnosis. *Mayo Clin Proc* 59:118–121, 1984.)

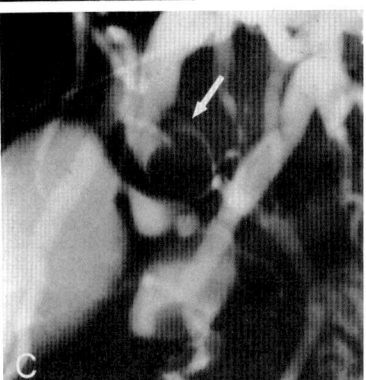

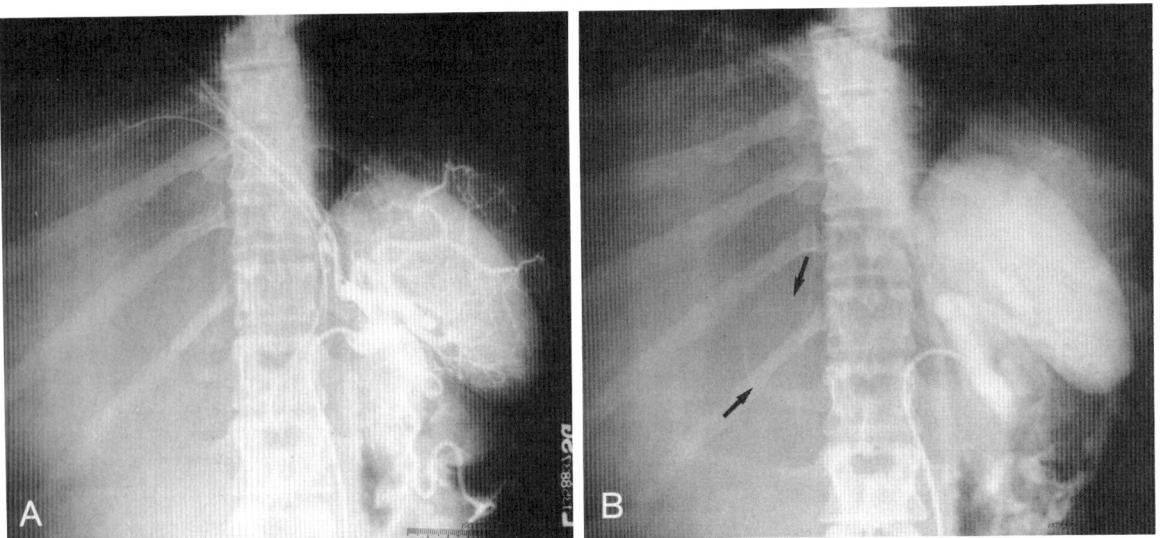

FIGURE 5.50. DAUGHTER CYST IN BILIARY CYSTADENOMA ON ANGIOGRAPHY MIMICKING HYDATID CYST

A: Arterial phase of celiac injection: huge mass splaying hepatic arteries. *B:* Hepatogram: radiolucent mass with "daughter cyst" (*arrows*).

REFERENCES

1. Ishak KG, Willis GW, Cummins SD, Bullock AA: Biliary cystadenoma and cystadenocarcinoma. Report of 14 cases and review of the literature. *Cancer* 39:322–338, 1977.
2. Nagorney DM, LeSage GD, Charboneau JW, McGough PF: Cystadenoma of the proximal common hepatic duct. The use of abdominal ultrasonography and transhepatic cholangiography in diagnosis. *Mayo Clin Proc* 59:118–121, 1984.
3. Stanley J, Vujic I, Schabel SI, Gobien RP, Reines HD: Evaluation of biliary cystadenoma and cystadenocarcinoma. *Gastrointest Radiol* 8:245–248, 1983.
4. Forrest ME, Cho KJ, Shields JJ: Biliary cystadenoma: sonographic-angiographic-pathologic correlation. *AJR* 139:723–727, 180.
5. Frick MP, Feinberg SB: Biliary cystadenoma. *AJR* 139:393–395, 1982.

METASTATIC DISEASE IN THE LIVER

The liver is second only to regional lymph nodes as a site for metastatic disease. It is estimated that 25–50% of all patients dying of cancer will have metastatic disease in the liver at autopsy (1). The most frequent primary sites are colon, lung, breast, and pancreas. Detection of disease in the liver will significantly change the patient's staging and therapy. Metastatic disease in the liver usually indicates advanced disease and a poor prognosis.

Signs and symptoms of liver disease occur in 50% of patients with hepatic metastases. Hepatomegaly is the most common finding. Ascites and jaundice are also frequently seen. Biochemical hepatic function tests can be misleading and may be elevated in numerous benign abnormalities; liver enzymes are normal in the presence of hepatic metastases as frequently as 25–50%. Therefore, liver function studies are not very useful in detecting metastatic disease and evaluation by an imaging procedure is necessary.

Radionuclide liver/spleen scanning has significant false-negative and false-positive rates ranging from 15 to 25% with respect to metastases. Lesions less than 2 cm are rarely detected by these scans and central lesions considerably greater than 2 cm can frequently be missed. Computed tomographic and realtime ultrasonography are more sensitive in identifying small masses in the liver (2, 3).

Computed Tomography

Computed tomography is an extremely accurate means of detecting small focal masses in the liver. Diffuse microscopic metastatic disease can be impossible to detect, however. With improved technology since the introduction of CT, resolution has considerably improved so that discrete lesions less than 1.0 cm can usually be detected with proper technique. Scan thickness, scan interval and the use of intravenous contrast all influence lesion detection (Fig. 5.51).

Metastatic hepatic disease has a variety of CT appearances. Lesions can be multiple or solitary, well defined or poorly delineated and of varying size. Calcifications may be identified in certain lesions (Fig. 5.52). Most masses are solid focal areas with decreased attenuation relative to normal hepatic parenchyma. Most lesions are identifiable on unenhanced scans, however, due to the fairly wide ranges of attenuation with occasional overlaps, water soluble iodinated contrast is used to separate out neoplastic tissue, blood vessels and normal hepatic parenchyma (Fig. 5.53).

The key to CT diagnosis of hepatic metastasis is to increase contrast between an abnormal mass and the normal hepatic parenchyma. Several methods of using water-soluble iodinated contrast in improving the detection of hepatic metastasis have been proposed (4–9). Contrast enhancement is time dependent. Intravenously injected contrast material given as a bolus injection arrives in the liver in two separate peaks, initially the arterial peak and then the portal venous peak. The double afferent circulation of the liver is 25% arterial and 75% portal venous inflow. The largest differences in attenuation values between lesions and adjacent normal structures will generally occur shortly before or shortly after peak normal parenchymal enhancement. Since the liver receives most of its contrast enhancement through the portal venous circulation, peak contrast enhancement in the liver parenchyma usually occurs 10–20 sec after peak contrast enhancement in organs with solely arterial inflow, such as the spleen and kidneys. Peak contrast enhancement in hepatic malignant lesions, which receive most of their blood supply from the hepatic arterial system will occur some 10 to 20 seconds before normal liver enhancement (4). There is a small contribution to hepatic malignancies by the portal venous blood supply (10).

Several methods of using water-soluble contrast have been examined including intravenous drip infusions, intravenous drip infusions pre-

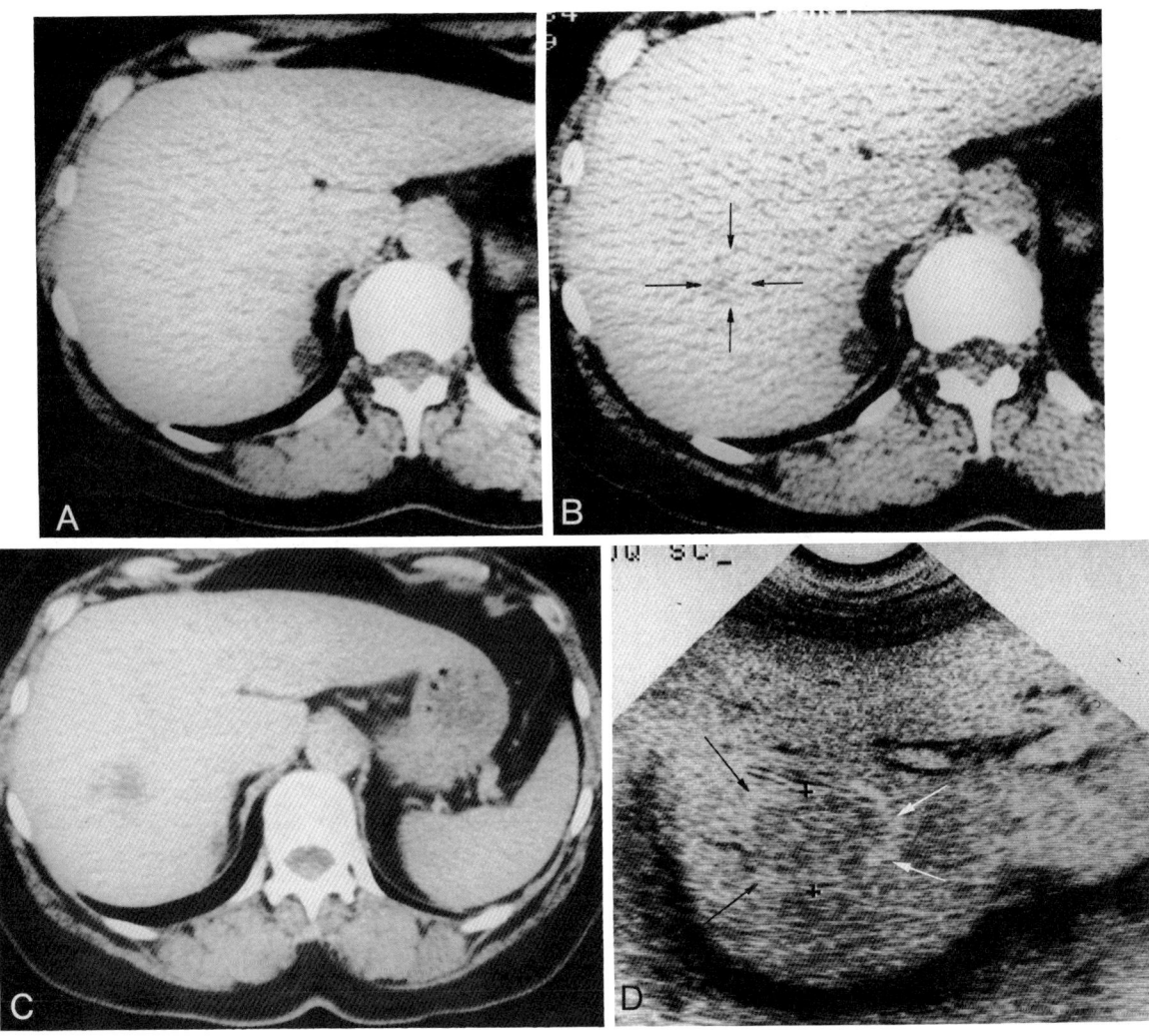

FIGURE 5.51. COLON CARCINOMA METASTASIS DETECTED ONLY ON 4-MM THICK SLICE
A: A 8-mm thick slice (contrast-enhanced): small hepatic cyst in posteromedial right lobe. *B:* 4-mm thick slice performed to better evaluate the cyst shows a subtle metastasis (*arrows*). *C:* Repeat CT 7 months later: obvious metastasis. The cyst is unchanged. *D:* Sonogram (transverse) corresponding to (*C*): nearly isoechoic mass (*cursors*), seen by virtue of hypoechoic halo (*arrows*).

ceded by a bolus, direct hepatic arterial injections and single large volume bolus venous injections. A rapid decrease in arterial opacification begins at about 20–30 sec after a bolus peripheral venous injection because of extravascular diffusion and spread of the bolus throughout the total blood volume. Maximum venous opacification occurs about 45 sec after the bolus. Equilibration of intra- and extravascular components is reached in 5 min. Maximal liver parenchymal enhancement does not occur during the arterial phase, but later during the equilibrating phase reflecting the double afferent circulation of the liver. Contrast enhancement is accentuated by intravenous bolus administration and rapid sequence scans while differential enhancement is less apparent if a drip infusion technique is used (9).

Most hepatic metastases are hypovascular and hypodense and liver to tumor contrast is maximized by rapid scanning following high dose contrast material delivery (Figs. 5.54 and 5.55). Hypodense lesions on CT that become isodense with normal hepatic parenchyma over 5–15 min following contrast administration have been described (6), and support the use of a post-contrast incremental dynamic scan following a rapid large contrast infusion. Lesions with a necrotic center and a vascular rim should also be detected by dynamic postcontrast scans, although the vas-

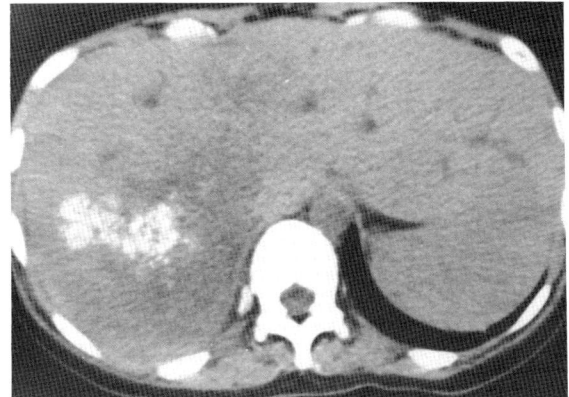

FIGURE 5.52. NONCONTRAST CT: CALCIFICATIONS WITHIN A HYPODENSE MASS-MUCINOUS ADENOCARCINOMA OF THE COLON METASTASIS

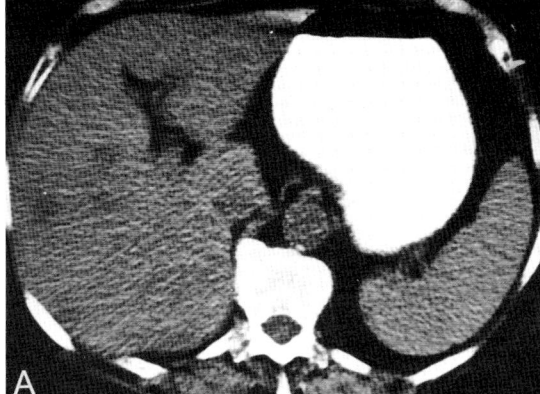

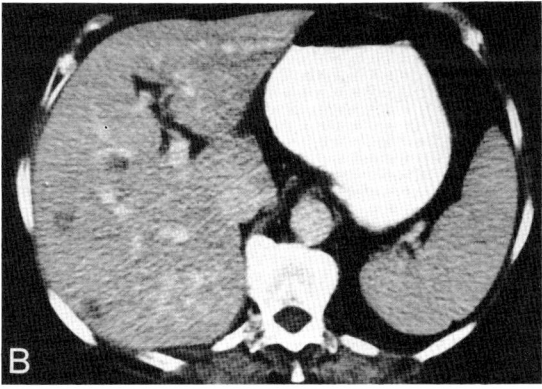

FIGURE 5.54. METASTATIC MELANOMA
Improved visualization after contrast using the same technique as Figure 5.53. *A:* Unenhanced scan: suggestion of multiple low density lesions. *B:* Much clearer depiction after contrast.

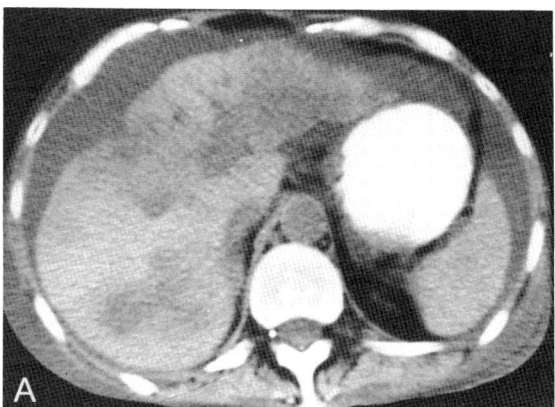

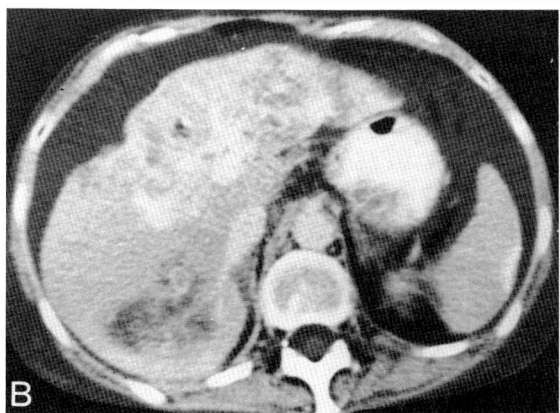

FIGURE 5.53. METASTATIC OVARIAN CARCINOMA
High-dose rapid infusion of 150 ml 60% meglumine diatrizoate did not add information above that in the unenhanced scan. *A:* Unenhanced scan: ascites and multiple low density masses in the liver. *B:* Irregular enhancement of the metastases.

cular periphery can become isodense with hepatic parenchyma (Figs. 5.56 and 5.57). Enhanced rims of neovascularity are best demonstrated during the arterial phase of single level dynamic scanning performed after selective hepatic artery injection.

Computed tomographic arteriography maximizes differential contrast enhancement in the detection of metastatic liver disease. This is an expensive and invasive procedure but is justified in evaluating patients prior to major hepatic resection, and, using it, Freeny found additional hepatic lesions in 55% of patients who were considered candidates for surgery based on intravenous bolus enhanced CT scans of the liver (8). CT arteriography is also time consuming and should be reserved for those patients evaluated for hepatic resection (Fig. 5.58).

Initial CT examination of a suspected hepatic metastatic or primary malignancy should be performed without intravenous or arterial contrast. If multiple masses are present, then there is little need to perform a postcontrast scan. If no focal lesions are present on a precontrast study, or only a single hepatic lesion is identified and further clinical information is desired, then a postcontrast incremental dynamic scan should

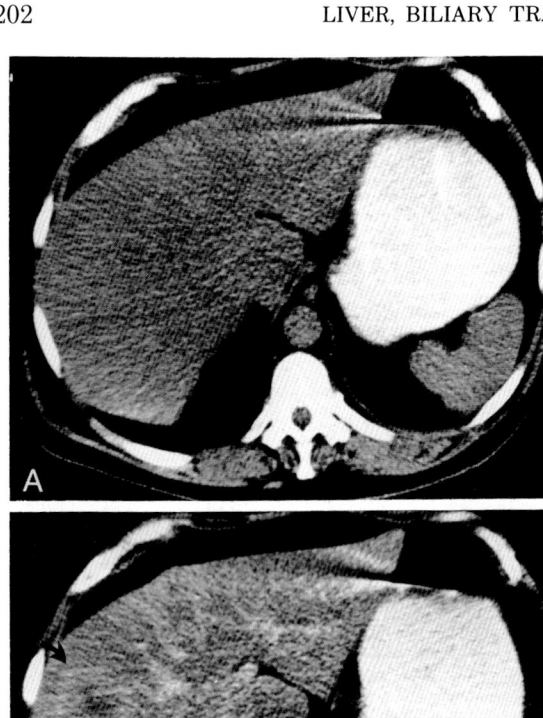
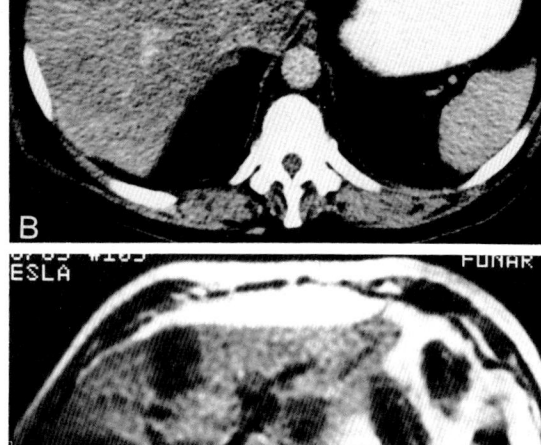
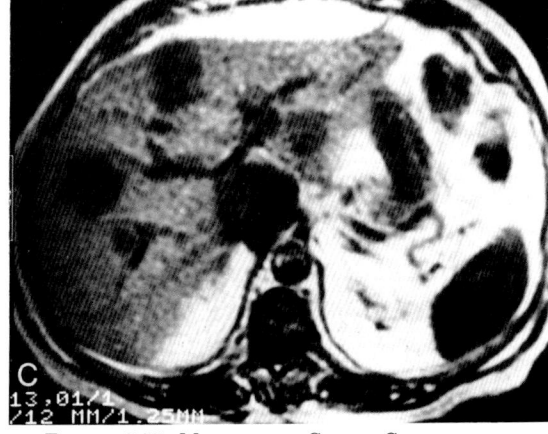

FIGURE 5.55. METASTATIC COLON CARCINOMA
Use of contrast and MRI. *A:* Unenhanced CT: no discrete mass. *B:* Enhanced scan, same technique as in Figures 5.53 and 5.54: only one definite metastasis (*arrow*). In retrospect, there is lobulation along the anterior margin of the liver, and the caudate lobe is prominent and inhomogeneous. *C:* IR 310/1500 MRI performed at 0.3T: multiple, low intensity metastases now apparent. Inversion recovery or short TE spin echo and chemical shift imaging are currently the best MR sequences for detecting liver metastases. The role of MRI in liver metastasis is evolving and uncertain.

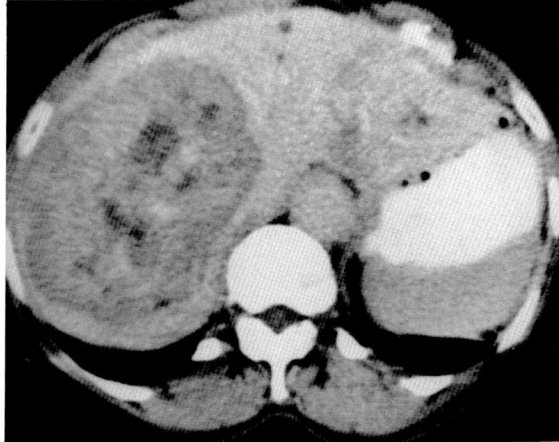

FIGURE 5.56. LARGE RECTAL CARCINOMA METASTASES IN THE RIGHT AND LEFT LOBES SHOWING IRREGULAR CONTRAST ENHANCEMENT
The left lobe mass has become almost isodense.

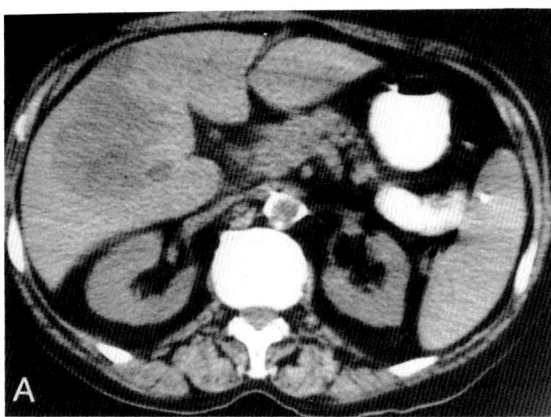
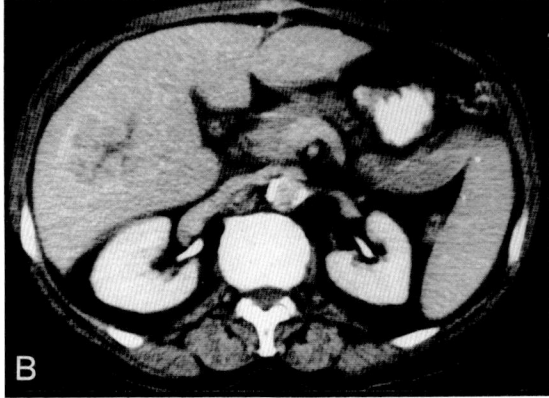

FIGURE 5.57. CONTRAST ENHANCEMENT CAUSING DIMINISHED VISIBILITY OF A SQUAMOUS CELL LUNG CARCINOMA METASTASIS
A: Precontrast and *B:* postcontrast scans. When following a known lesion to assess change in size in response to therapy, it is important to standardize quantity and method of contrast administration. The lesion appears smaller in (*B*) than in (*A*) merely because contrast was given.

be obtained. Lesion number and size are best assessed with the postcontrast technique. Single level dynamic scans to characterize temporal phases of contrast enhancement should be reserved to evaluate cases in which there is a high index of suspicion for hemangioma.

Calcifications in metastatic foci are easily identified and can be small punctate focal areas or more confluent areas of increased attenuation. The most common metastatic tumor to demonstrate calcification is mucinous carcinoma of the colon (Fig. 5.52); metastatic papillary serous ovarian cystadenocarcinoma, medullary carcinoma of the thyroid, renal cell carcinoma, and gastric malignancies also may demonstrate focal calcifications.

Organ-specific contrast agents may significantly increase CT visualization of metastatic hepatic disease (Fig. 5.59). Ethiodized oil emulsions (EOE) consisting of 1–4 μm globules of iodinated esters of poppy seed oil in an aqueous solution with surfactants and a buffer can freely pass through the pulmonary capillary bed following slow intravenous infusion. The particles are of a size selectively phagocytosed by the reticuloendothelial cells in the liver and the spleen. This permits high iodine concentration in these organs with a relatively low iodine dose (50 mg/

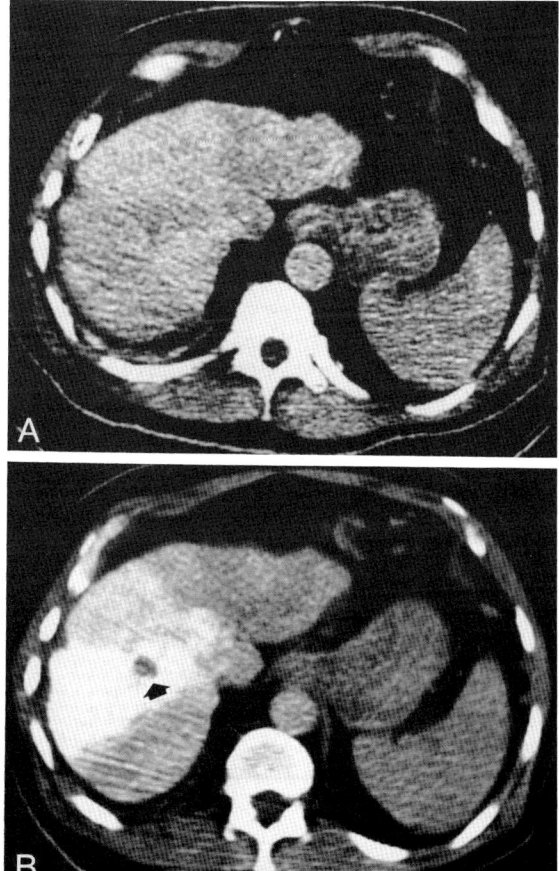

FIGURE 5.58. CT ANGIOGRAPHY FOR RECTAL CARCINOMA METASTASIS

A: Conventional enhanced CT: mottled attenuation in right lobe, no focal mass. Abnormal liver function tests were present. *B:* CT angiogram, contrast injected through a catheter in the right hepatic artery: hypovascular metastasis (*arrow*).

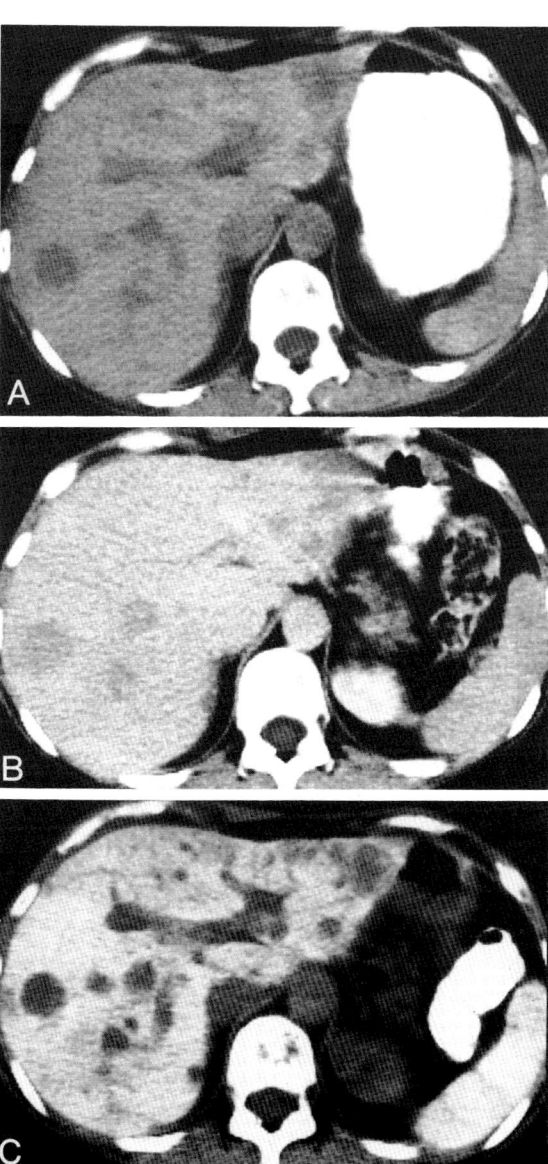

FIGURE 5.59. USE OF EOE FOR METASTATIC DISEASE

A and *B:* Pre- and postcontrast scans show multiple liver metastases. *C:* EOE-enhanced scan demonstrates smaller metastases than (*A*) and (*B*), and shows the larger ones with greater clarity. (Case courtesy of John Vermess, M.D., National Institutes of Health, Bethesda, MD.)

kg, or 3.5 g for a 70-kg man, using a 7-ml EOE dose) allowing marked increase in attenuation of these organs without an appreciable change in tumor attenuation. The average increase in attenuation is 30 HU for the liver and 55 of the spleen. The liver and spleen remain opacified for hours after the EOE infusion. Within 48 hr, 90% of the contrast has been eliminated from the liver and spleen.

The sensitivity of EOE CT liver scans is significantly greater than CT with iodinated water soluble contrast or liver scintigraphy (11, 12). Histologic specificity is not improved over standard CT criteria. Although the incidence of adverse reactions is greater with EOE than with water soluble contrast, these are usually minor and the potential benefits in clinical management of cancer patients are great, as single small lesions are the most important to detect for potential surgical resection. EOE is not available at this time for routine clinical use. Other contrast agents such as heavy metal particulates, radio-opaque liposomes and iodinated starch particles have also been investigated in allowing better detection of hepatic metastatic disease but these agents have had little investigational use in humans (13–16).

REFERENCES

1. Gilbert HA, Kagan AR: Metastases: incidence, detection and evaluation. In Weiss L (ed): *Fundamental Aspects of Metastasis*. New York, Elsevier, North-Holland, 1976.
2. Djang WT, Young SW, Castellino RA, Lantieri R: Computed tomography of the liver: evaluating focal defects on radionuclide liver-spleen scans. *AJR* 937–940, 1984.
3. Alderson PO, Adams DF, McNeil BJ, Sanders R, Siegelman SS, Finberg JH, Hessel SJ, Abrams HL: Computed tomography, ultrasound, and scintigraphy of the liver in patients with colon or breast carcinoma: a prospective comparison. *Radiology* 149: 225–230, 1983.
4. Axel L, Dean PB, Moss AA, Stansberry RT: Functional imaging of the liver—information from dynamic CT. *Invest Radiol* 19:23–29, 1984.
5. Moss AA, Dean PB, Axel L, Golberg H, Glazer GM, Friedman MA: Dynamic CT of hepatic masses with intravenous and intra-arterial contrast material. *AJR* 138:847–852, 1982.
6. Marchal GJ, Baert AL, Wilms GE: CT of noncystic liver lesions: bolus enhancement. *AJR* 135:57–65, 1980.
7. Araki T, Itai Y, Furui S, Tasaka A: Dynamic CT densitometry of hepatic tumors. *AJR* 135:1037–1043, 1980.
8. Freeny PC, Marks WM: Computed tomographic arteriography of the liver. *Radiology* 148:193–197, 1983.
9. Foley WD, Berland LL, Lawson TL, Smith DF, Thorsen MK: Contrast enhancement technique for dynamic hepatic computed tomographic scanning. *Radiology* 147:797–803, 1983.
10. Lin G, Hagerstrand I, Lunderquist A: Portal blood supply of liver metastases. *AJR* 143:53–55, 1984.
11. Miller DL, Rosenbaum RC, Sugarbaker PH, Vermess M, Willis M, Doppman JL: Detection of hepatic metastases: comparison of EOE-13 computed tomography and scintigraphy. *AJR* 141:931–935, 1983.
12. Miller DL, Vermess M, Doppman JL, Simon RM, Sugarbaker PH, O'Leary TJ, Grimes G, Chatterji DG, Willis M: CT of the liver and spleen with EOE-13: review of 225 examinations. *AJR* 143:235–253, 1984.
13. Havron A, Davis MA, Seltzer SE, Paskins-Hurlburt A, Hessel SJ: Heavy metal particulate contrast materials for computed tomography of the liver. *J Comput Assist Tomogr* 4:642–648, 1980.
14. Havron A, Seltzer SE, Davis MA, Shulkin P: Radiopaque liposomes: a promising new contrast material for computed tomography of the spleen. *Radiology* 140:507–511, 1981.
15. Cohen Z, Seltzer SE, David MA, Hanson RN: Iodinated starch particles: new contrast material for computed tomography of the liver and spleen in lymphoma. *J Comput Assist Tomogr* 5:843–846, 1981.
16. Caride VJ, Sostman HD, Twickler J, Zacharis H, Orphanoudakis SC, Jaffe CC: Brominated radiopaque liposomes: contrast agent for computed tomography of liver and spleen—a preliminary report. *Invest Radiol* 17:381–385, 1982.

Ultrasound in Metastatic Disease

High resolution real-time ultrasound is the most sensitive imaging modality in detecting small hepatic masses when compared to computed tomography or radionuclide imaging (1). The diagnostic efficacy of ultrasound depends to a large degree on the skill of the sonographer. Sonography should be the first diagnostic procedure of choice to screen for possible hepatic metastatic involvement and it can also evaluate the spleen, kidneys, pancreas, and the remainder of the upper abdomen. The radionuclide scan has been considered the initial diagnostic procedure to evaluate hepatic lesions and in some comparative studies was found to be more sensitive than sonography (2, 3), but these studies are out of date, were performed without realtime equipment, and were also performed with less sonologist involvement than is currently the standard of care. If the ultrasound is technically suboptimal due to intestinal bowel gas or body habitus, then computed tomography should be performed. Realtime scanning eliminates the need for static B-scanning.

Despite its ability to detect small masses, ultrasound is relatively restricted for precise diagnosis in that lesions can usually only be characterized as cystic, isoechoic with hepatic parenchyma or more or less echogenic than surrounding hepatic parenchyma. The appearance is nonspecific and, in most cases, biopsy is necessary for definitive histological diagnosis.

Several studies have attempted to correlate the ultrasonic appearance of hepatic metastasis with the site of origin. Metastatic adenocarcinoma from the colon and pancreas tends to be hyperechoic relative to normal hepatic parenchyma (4). Large masses tend to have a hypoechoic center, probably reflecting tumor necrosis, and sequential scans of large metastatic foci following treatment may show the development of a hypoechoic center, supporting this impression. Factors other than specific cell type are also important in determining the sonographic appearance of hepatic metastasis. Hemorrhage produces lesions of greater echogenicity than normal renal parenchyma and this could be expected in the liver as well. Fibrous tissue, collagen and mucin content also affect echogenicity. Marchal correlated sonographic patterns in liver metastasis with histology and microangiography and concluded that real tumor vascularity as well as the extravascular circulation are both important in the echogenic appearance in some liver metastases (5). Sonolucent lesions (Fig. 5.60) correspond to rather homogeneously cellular masses, and strongly reflective lesions usually demonstrate a very irregular histologic configuration due to either hypervascularity or an irregular pattern of fibrosis or calcification (Figs. 5.61–5.63).

A thin poorly echoic rim is sometimes seen surrounding liver metastases (halo) and indicates the presence of tissue of a different acoustic impedance (Fig. 5.51D) (6). This could be either tumoral or extratumoral in origin. Extratumoral possibilities would include peritumoral liver parenchymal alterations such as parenchymal compression and/or fibrosis or peritumoral venous hyperemia. Tumoral causes would include necrosis and vascularization or fatty infiltration. Microangiopathic and histologic correlation suggest that peritumoral parenchymal compression is probably a common cause of this halo detected sonographically in liver metastasis (7).

Perfluoroctylbromide has been described as an ultrasound contrast material in tumor imaging. This organic compound produces an echogenic rim around induced hepatic malignancies in rabbits and also produces increased attenuation around intrahepatic tumors detectable by computed tomography (8). The clinical usefulness of this substance in humans has not been determined.

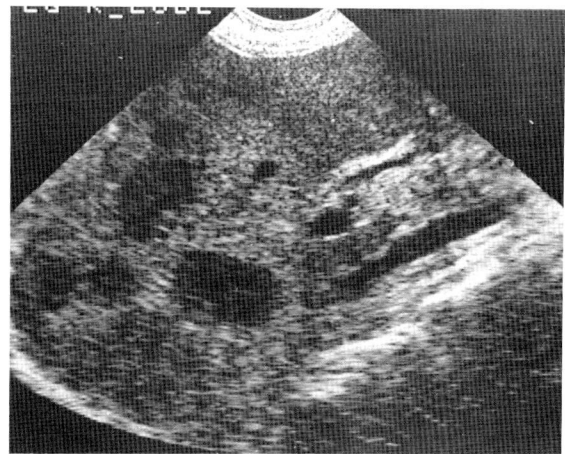

FIGURE 5.60. MULTIPLE HYPOECHOIC BREAST CARCINOMA METASTASES: PARASAGITTAL SONOGRAM

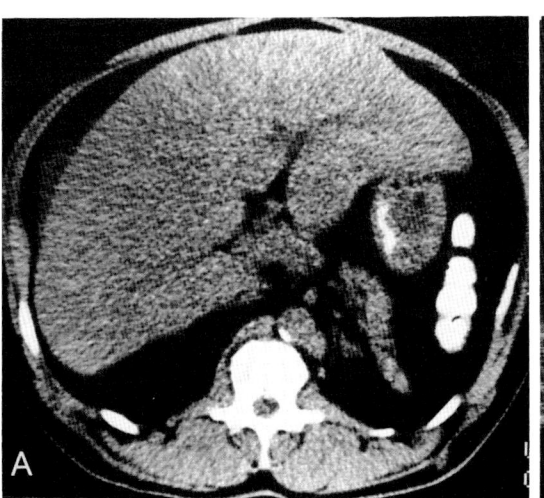 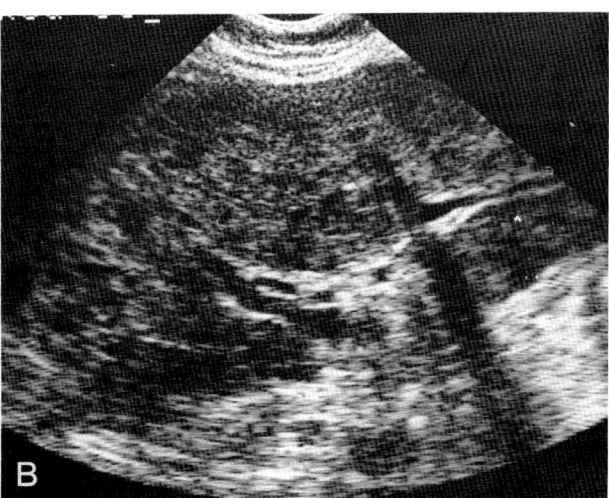

FIGURE 5.61. ANAPLASTIC CARCINOMA
Unknown primary, sonographic depiction of metastases superior to CT. *A:* CT: unenhanced scan shows an inhomogeneous hepatic attenuation but no focal mass. Enhanced scan (not shown) was not more revealing. *B:* Transverse sonogram, RAO position: innumerable confluent echodensities due to metastases.

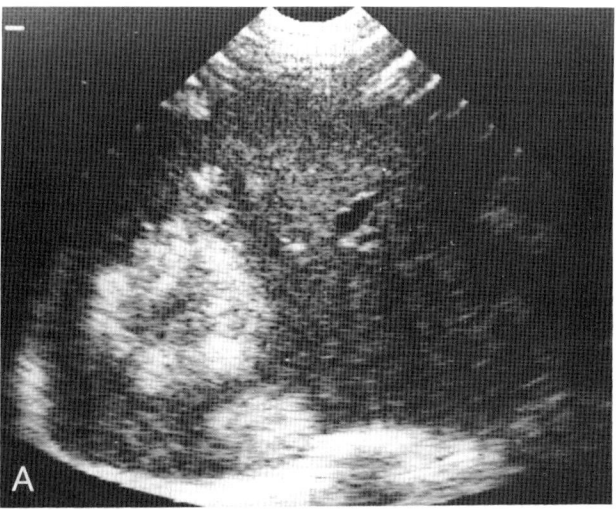 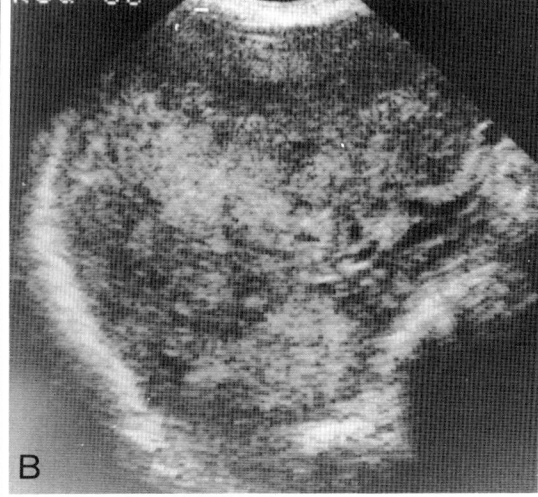

FIGURE 5.62. CALCIFIED METASTASES
Calcified metastases, echogenic but nonshadowing (individual calcifications too small to shadow). *A:* Transverse scan, mucinous adenocarcinoma of the colon. (Same case as shown in Fig. 5.52.) *B:* Transverse scan, papillary serous ovarian carcinoma.

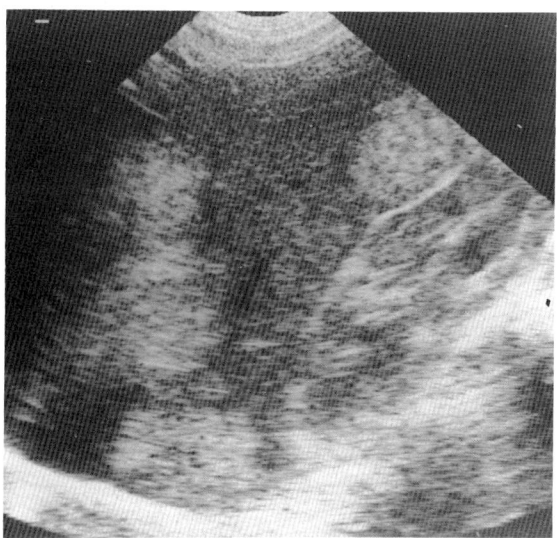

FIGURE 5.63. MUCINOUS ADENOCARCINOMA
Parasagittal scan, mucinous adenocarcinoma of the colon. Echogenic noncalcified metastases seen here are hard to differentiate from calcified metastases.

REFERENCES

1. Sheu J-C, Sung J-L, Chen D-S, Yu J-Y, Wang T-H, Su C-T, Tsang Y-M: Ultrasonography of small hepatic tumors using high-resolution linear-array real-time instruments. *Radiology* 150:797–802, 1984.
2. Bryan PJ, Dinn WM, Grossman ZD: Correlation of CT, gray scale ultrasonography and radionuclide imaging of the liver in detecting space-occupying processes. *Radiology* 124:387–393, 1977.
3. Snow JH, Goldstein HM, Wallace S: Comparison of scintigraphy, sonography and computed tomography in the evaluation of hepatic neoplasms. *AJR* 132:915–921, 1979.
4. Hillman BJ, Smith EH, Gammelgaard J, Holm HH: Ultrasonographic-pathologic correlation of malignant hepatic masses. *Gastrointest Radiol* 4:361–368, 1979.
5. Marchal G, Tshibwabwa-Tumba E, Oyen R, Pylser K, Goddeeris R: Correlation of sonographic patterns in liver metastases with histology and microangiography. *Invest Radiol* 20:79–84, 1985.
6. Scheible W, Gosink BB, Leopold GR: Gray scale echographic patterns of hepatic metastatic disease. *AJR* 129:983–987, 1977.
7. Marchal GJ, Pylyser K, Tshibwabwa-Tumba EA, Verbeken EK, Oyen RH, Baert AL, Lauweryns JM: Anechoic halo in solid liver tumors: sonographic, microangiographic, and histologic correlation. *Radiology* 156:479–483, 1985.
8. Mattrey RF, Scheible FW, Gosink BB, Leopold GR, Long DM, Higgins CB: Perfluoroctylbromide: A liver/spleen-specific and tumor-imaging ultrasound contrast material. *Radiology* 145:759–762, 1982.

Computed Tomography and Ultrasound in Lymphoma and Leukemia

Primary hepatic lymphoma is rare. Secondary liver involvement is not uncommon and autopsy series have demonstrated liver involvement in 60% of patients with Hodgkin's disease and 50% of those with non-Hodgkin's lymphoma (1, 2). Adequate liver biopsy specimens are the most reliable method of determining the presence of hepatic lymphoma despite a relatively high false negative rate. It has been reported that percutaneous needle biopsy may have up to a 50% false negative rate (3, 4), laparoscopic biopsy up to a 20% false negative rate (5, 6) and laparotomy a 15% false negative rate.

The most common type of intrahepatic involvement of Hodgkin's disease is a diffuse distribution throughout the hepatic parenchyma. The Hodgkin's lesions appear to arise from the Kupffer cells in the parenchyma and to produce granulomas which may grow or coalesce to form the nodules which may become grossly evident at autopsy. Bile ducts are usually preserved. Although some enlargement of the liver is not unusual, massive enlargement is rare, and hepatomegaly is a nonspecific clinical finding and is not a good predictor of hepatic involvement in Hodgkin's or non-Hodgkin's lymphoma (1). Periportal lymph nodes are frequently enlarged but they seldom produce jaundice by compressing the biliary ductal system.

Focal nodular lesions are less frequent than an infiltrative pattern, and a combination of diffuse and nodular lesions occur in only 3% of Hodgkin's patients with hepatic involvement. Autopsy in non-Hodgkin's lymphoma reveals that diffuse hepatic involvement is found as frequently as tumor nodules of varying size, which can resemble metastatic carcinoma. Malignant lymphomas make up to 20% of postrenal transplant malignancies (7).

Computed Tomography

The CT pattern in most cases of hepatic lymphoma is not specific and mimics metastatic disease and primary hepatic neoplasms. The diffuse infiltrative forms of lymphoma can produce irregular decreased attenuation scattered throughout the entire liver, but this is difficult to differentiate from cirrhosis and fatty infiltration. Calcifications are uncommon, and if present suggest a nonlymphomatous process, such as metastatic mucinous adenocarcinoma. The most common described finding on CT is relatively

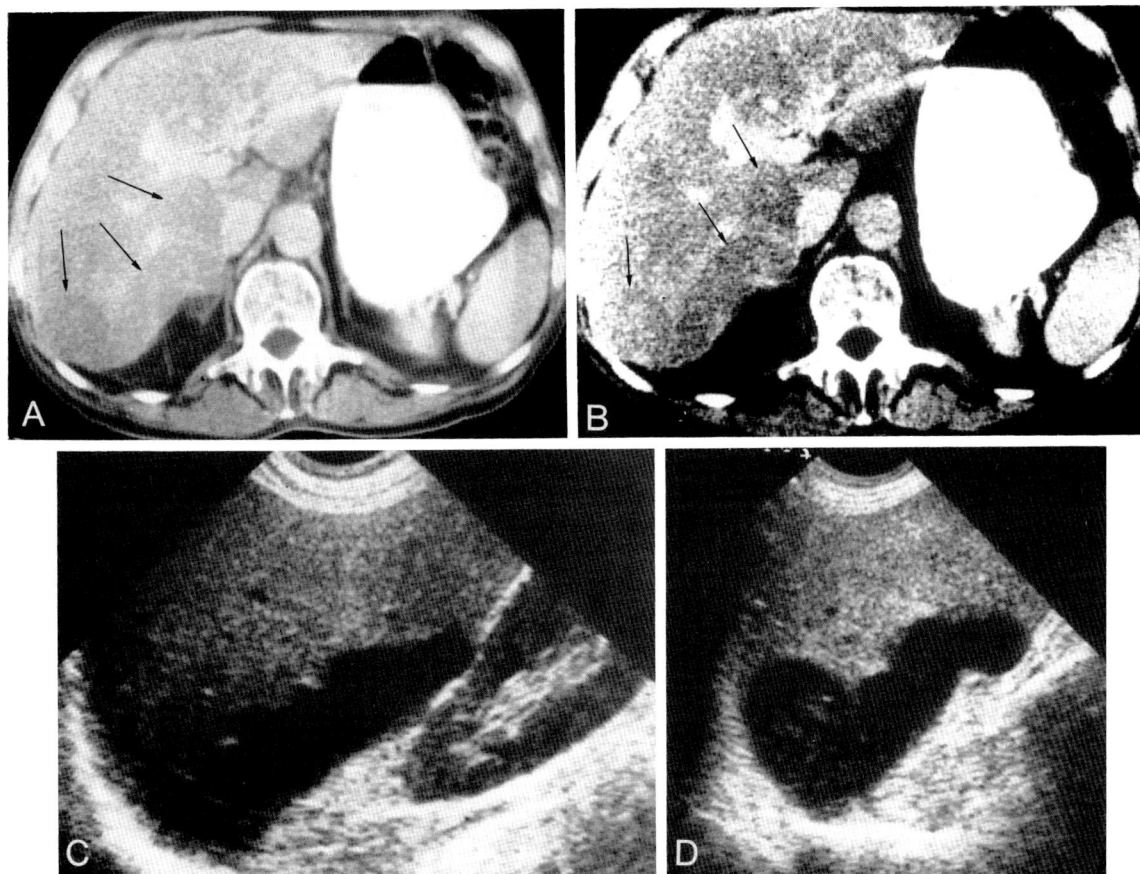

FIGURE 5.64. HEPATIC LYMPHOMA DEMONSTRATED TO BETTER ADVANTAGE BY SONOGRAPHY

A and *B:* Conventional and narrow window settings: barely perceptible low density mass (*arrows*). *C* and *D:* Parasagittal and transverse sonograms: obvious anechoic but solid mass, very suggestive of lymphoma. (From Charboneau JW, James EM, Reading CC: Sonography case of the day. *AJR* 142:1075–1079, 1984.)

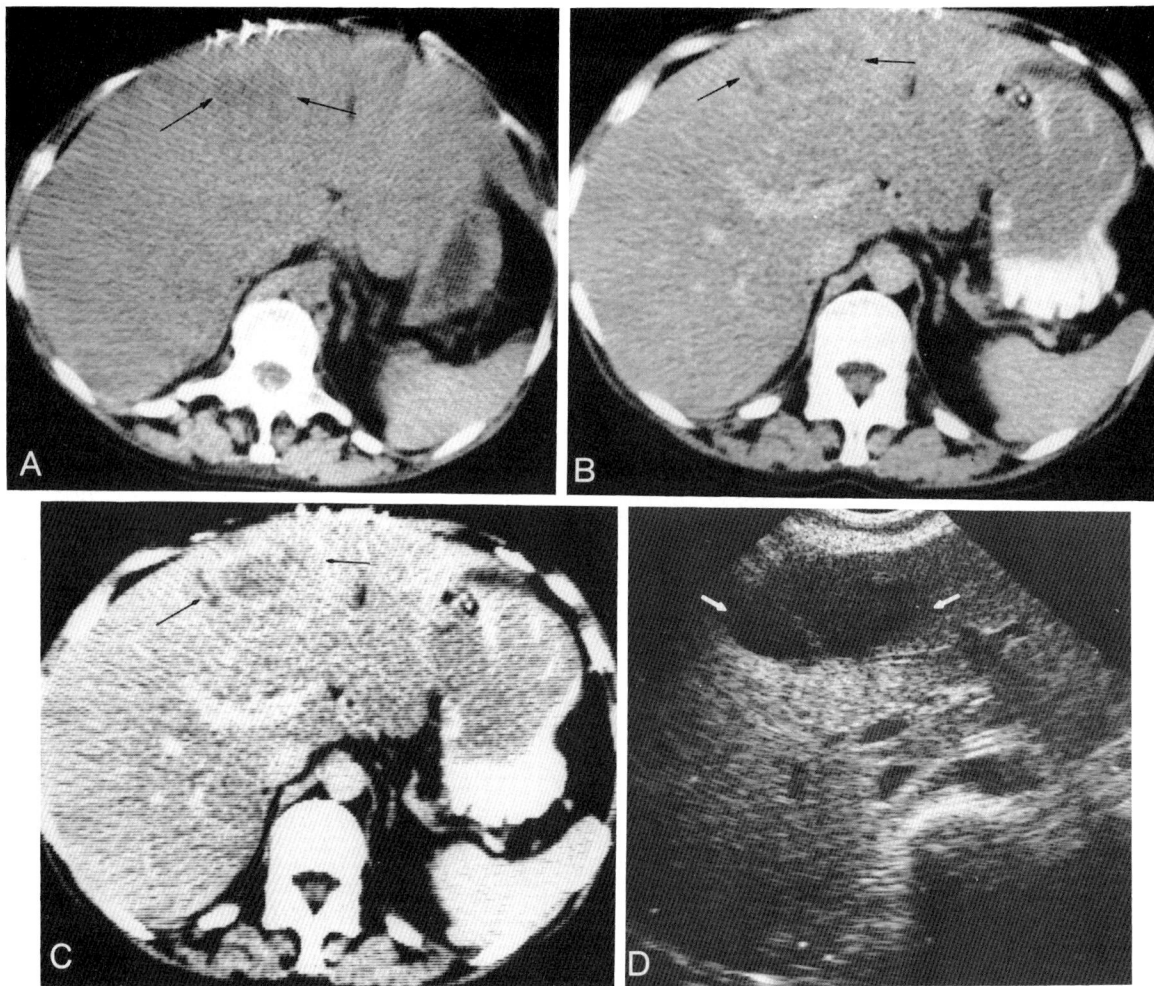

FIGURE 5.65. HISTIOCYTIC LYMPHOMA

A: Unenhanced CT: poorly defined low attenuation mass (*arrows*), hepatomegaly. *B* and *C:* Mass is more obvious after contrast (*B*), especially with narrow windows (*C*). *D:* Transverse sonography depicts the hypoechoic mass to best advantage (*arrows*).

homogeneous areas of decreased attenuation, some with irregular margins which merge imperceptibly with normal hepatic parenchyma (Figs. 5.64A and B, and 5.65A–C) (8, 9). Lymphomatous hepatic lesions rarely enhance significantly relative to normal liver parenchyma following intravenous contrast. As diffuse disease is much more common than focal masses, the relative ineffectiveness of computed tomographic diagnosis of hepatic lymphoma is not unexpected, and minimal disease is not likely to be detected. Hepatic involvement with lymphoma in postrenal transplant patients has been characterized by rapidly growing solitary or multiple intrahepatic masses as well as intraperitoneal and retroperitoneal masses with a central zone of low density related to central necrosis (7).

Ethiodol-Oil-Emulsion-13 is a selective hepatosplenic imaging agent composed of the iodinated ethyl ester of the fatty acid of poppy seed oil. An intravenous infusion of this substance raises the attenuation coefficients of the liver and spleen. Most side effects with this agent are minor. Initial results of EOE-13 demonstrate significant diagnostic improvement in the evaluation of lymphomatous involvement of the liver and spleen (10). This has been described in both early stage Hodgkin's disease and late stage non-Hodgkin's patients. Lesions greater than 0.5 cm were consistently imaged. Therefore, EOE-13 may be useful in the detection of hepatosplenic lymphomatous abnormalities particularly when minimal differences in attenuation exist between them and normal parenchymal tissue. A normal

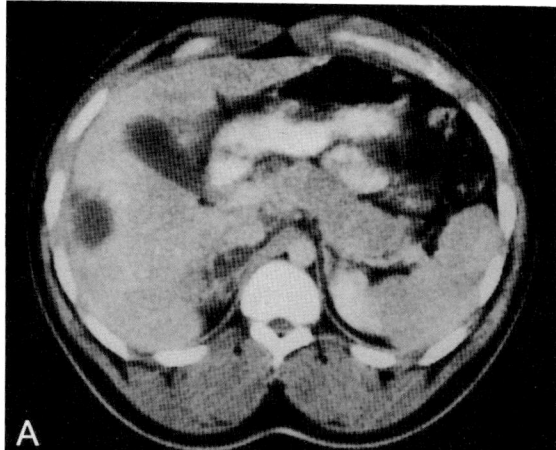

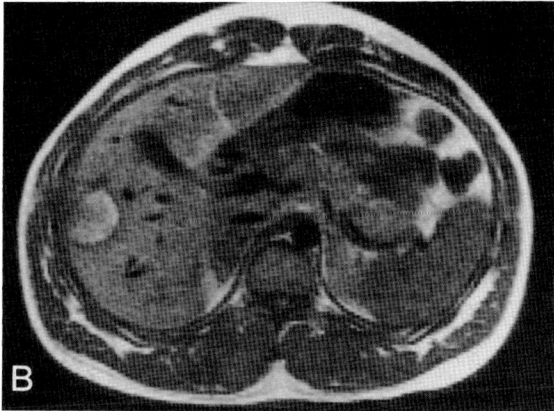

FIGURE 5.66. LYMPHOMA SHOWN BY MRI
A: Low density mass in the lateral right lobe. B: Hyperintense mass, SE 28/500. The findings are probably due to old hemorrhagic necrosis. (From Weinreb JC, Brateman L, Maravilla KR: Magnetic resonance imaging of hepatic lymphoma. AJR 143:1211–1214, 1984.)

EOE-13 examination does not exclude the presence of small lesions (less than 0.5 cm in size), and diffuse microscopic disease may also be imperceptible with this agent.

Magnetic resonance imaging and computed tomography have been compared in evaluating histologically proven hepatic lymphomatous involvement (Fig. 5.66) (11). CT and MRI were positive in one out of thirteen patients. Future technical upgrades of magnetic resonance imaging may improve the ability of MR especially relative to computed tomography and ultrasound in detecting hepatic involvement.

Ultrasound

Various ultrasound patterns of hepatic lymphoma have been described. Hypoechoic relatively well-defined masses without sound transmission are most commonly described (Figs. 5.64C and D and 5.65D), followed by a diffuse alteration of the usual homogeneously echogenic hepatic parenchyma (12, 13). Although most lesions are hypoechoic, echogenic masses simulating metastatic disease or primary hepatocellular carcinoma or cirrhosis can occasionally be found. Gross disease must be present before it is detected by sonography. Thus, a negative hepatic sonogram does not mean a disease-free liver while a positive sonogram does indicate significant hepatic involvement. Hypoechoic hepatic masses are non-specific as they can be seen in Hodgkin's lymphoma, non-Hodgkin's lymphoma and various other abnormalities.

Although leukemic involvement of the liver is uncommon it is usually found in patients with acute myelogenous or lymphocytic leukemias and usually takes the form of microscopic infiltration. In these cases hepatic sonography would be normal or may show nonspecific hepatomegaly and a nonspecific alteration of normal hepatic echo texture. Focal hepatic leukemic infiltrates (chloromas) appearing as multiple well-defined virtually anechoic masses without sound transmission involving both hepatic lobes have been described (13). Many of these lesions contain central, punctate hyperechoic regions giving a "bulleye" appearance.

REFERENCES

1. Levitan R, Diamond HD, Craver LF: The liver in Hodgkin's disease. *Gut* 2:60–71, 1971.
2. Rosenberg SA, Diamond HD, Jaslowitz B, et al: Lymphosarcoma: a review of 1,269 cases. *Medicine* 40:31–84, 1961.
3. Bagley CM Jr, Roth JA, Thomas LB et al: Liver biopsy in Hodgkin's disease: clinicopathologic correlations in 127 patients. *Ann Intern Med* 76:219–225, 1972.
4. Scheuer PJ: *Liver Biopsy Interpretation.* Baltimore, Williams & Wilkins, 1973.
5. Coleman M, Lightdale CJ, Vinciguerra VP et al: Peritoneoscopy in Hodgkin's disease: confirmation of results by laparotomy. *JAMA* 236:2634–2636, 1976.
6. Beretta G, Spinelli P, Rilke F et al: Sequential laparoscopy and laparotomy combined with bone marrow biopsy in staging Hodgkin's disease. *Cancer Treat Rep* 60:1231–1237, 1976.
7. Tubman DE, Frick MP, Hanto DW: Lymphoma after organ transplantation: radiologic manifestations in the central nervous system, thorax, and abdomen. *Radiology* 149:625–631, 1983.
8. Zornoza J, Ginaldi S: Computed tomography in hepatic lymphoma. *Radiology* 138:405–410, 1981.
9. Weinreb JC, Brateman L, Maravilla KR: Magnetic resonance imaging of hepatic lymphoma. *AJR* 143:1211–1214, 1984.
10. Ginaldi S, Bernardino ME, Jing B-S, Green B: Ultrasonographic patterns of hepatic lymphoma. *Radiology* 136:427–431, 1980.

11. Thomas JL, Bernardino ME, Vermess M, Barnes PA, Fuller LM, Hagemeister FB, Doppman J, Fisher RI, Longo DL: EOE-13 in the detection of hepatosplenic lymphoma. *Radiology* 145:629–634, 1983.
12. Charboneau JW, James EM, Reading CC: Sonography case of the day. *AJR* 142:1075–1079, 1984.
13. Lepke R, Pagani JJ: Sonography of hepatic chloromas. *AJR* 138:1176–1177, 1982.

Nuclear Medicine for Metastases

The liver is the most frequent site of blood borne metastatic disease. Metastatic deposits have been found in 10% of unselected postmortem livers and in 50% of livers of patients dying of cancer. They represent the most common cause of any space-occupying lesions within the noncirrhotic liver. In the cirrhotic liver, metastases occur infrequently (1% if biliary cirrhosis is excluded) (1).

Metastases represent the most common hepatic malignancy to create space-occupying lesions on liver/spleen scintigraphy. Appropriately, their detection represents the most frequent indication for the performance of this study. Tumors which tend to metastasize to the liver arise in the colon, rectum, stomach, pancreas (hematogenous spread via the portal system), kidney, breast, lung, uterus, cervix, ovary, skin (melanoma), prostate, and bladder. In children, neuroblastoma and Wilms' tumors also metastasize to the liver, as do the hematological malignancies (leukemia, lymphoma).

When metastases disseminate to the liver, they are usually found to involve both the right and left lobes (77%), are both superficial and deep in location (70%), are rarely solitary (2%), and are often greater than 2 cm in diameter (70%). Hepatomegaly is frequently present (70%), and if one lobe is involved, it is more often the right (20%) than left (3%). Of interest, up to 11% of liver metastases are neither grossly visible nor detectable by palpation (2).

Scintigraphically, metastases are manifested as one or more discrete focal areas of decreased activity (strict criteria positive) or by an inhomogeneous distribution of technetium-99m sulfur colloid within a normal or enlarged liver (liberal criteria positive). Tumors from breast, lung, and hematologic neoplasms result in liberal criteria positive liver scans secondary to tiny tumor deposits disseminated throughout the liver parenchyma; those from the gastrointestinal and genitourinary tracts result in strict criteria positive scintiscans due to bulk lesions which displace 1.5 cm or more of liver tissue (Figs. 5.67A and B and 5.68A and B). When both the liver and spleen are affected, lymphoma or melanoma should be suspected.

The accuracy of liver/spleen scintigraphy in detecting verified liver metastases is 80–85%. Sensitivities as high as 90–95% are achieved in patients with primary sites of metastases that produce large space-occupying lesions which are greater than 1.5 cm in size and located either superficially or within the left lobe of the liver (optimal resolution criteria (2–4)).

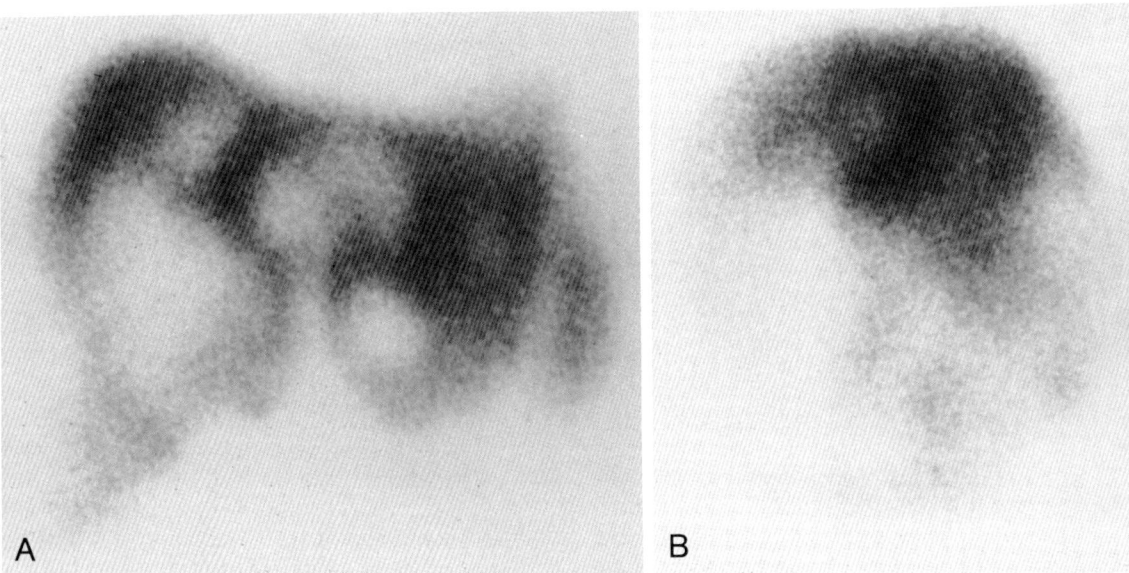

FIGURE 5.67. METASTATIC COLON CARCINOMA
A: Anterior and *B:* right lateral views from a sulfur-colloid scan: multiple space-occupying masses: metastatic colon carcinoma.

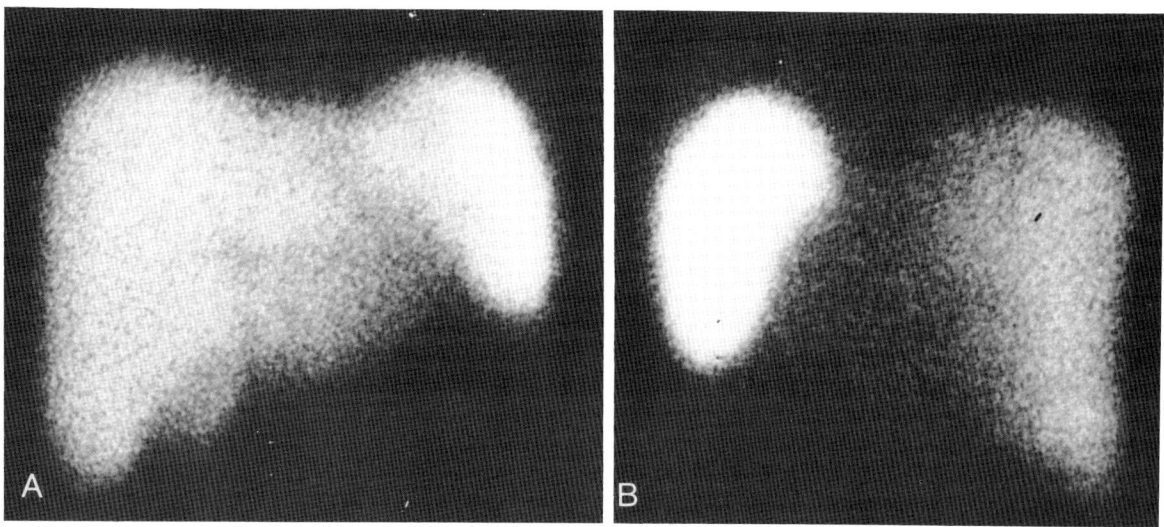

FIGURE 5.68. BREAST METASTASES
A: Anterior and *B:* posterior views from a sulfur-colloid scan: colloid shift and inhomogeneous tracer activity in the liver due to breast metastases (liberal criteria positive).

Patients with gastric carcinoma, stage IV uterine carcinoma, stage III melanoma, and small cell lung carcinoma should routinely undergo perioperative liver/spleen scintigraphy (or other liver imaging), as there is a high incidence of liver involvement at the time of initial diagnosis. Liver function studies may be normal and the patients asymptomatic. Perioperative routine liver/spleen scans (or other liver imaging) need not be performed, however, in patients with carcinoma of the colon, rectum, breast, stage I-III uterine, bladder, prostate, or renal carcinoma, stages I and II melanoma, or bronchogenic carcinoma, unless there is an elevated alkaline phosphatase, SGOT and/or clinical evidence (hepatomegaly, weight loss, malaise, lassitude, fever, jaundice) of metastases. In the absence of these abnormal parameters, true positive yields are low, false positives high, and the examination unrewarding. If liver/spleen scans are performed in "symptomatic" or high risk patients (stage III melanoma, gastric carcinoma, stage IV uterine carcinoma, and small-cell lung carcinoma), liver metastases will be found at the time of initial diagnosis in up to 26% (5). An abnormal liver scan even in conjunction with normal liver function tests should be interpreted as indicative of, but not pathognomonic for, metastases, and the patient should undergo sonography or CT with fine needle biopsy to confirm the presence of metastases if unnecessary chemotherapy is to be avoided.

Gallium scintigraphy and blood pool imaging can aid occasionally in the detection of intrahepatic metastases. Forty percent of gastrointestinal metastases are gallium-avid. Hypervascular metastases can arise from renal cell carcinoma, carcinoid tumor, choriocarcinoma, adrenal carcinoma, colonic carcinoma, breast carcinoma and melanoma; hypovascular metastases can originate from the stomach, colon, pancreas and lung. Hypervascular tumors appear as areas of increased activity on blood pool imaging, hypovascular tumors as photopenic areas (Fig. 5.69*A–C*) (3).

In view of the potential for false positive interpretation of liver scintigrams, hepatic sonography should be employed to differentiate a "prominent porta hepatis" from a true space-occupying lesion (6) and a nonhomogeneous distribution of radiotracer within the liver due to chemotherapy from liberal criteria positive metastatic disease (7). It is well to note that chemotherapeutic liver changes are transient in nature, lasting no longer than 6 months in duration and a significant number (10 of 40) of patients with a prominent porta scintigraphically have liver metastases (4).

Occasionally, hepatic metastases will be detected serendipitously as hot spots on a bone scan by virtue of accumulation of the bone-seeking radiopharmaceutical (Fig. 5.69*D*). Reported primaries include: breast, colon, oat cell of the lung, melanoma, and squamous cell of the esophagus (8, 9). Iodine-131 imaging may be used with excellent sensitivity and specificity for identification of hepatic metastases from functioning thyroid cancers (10).

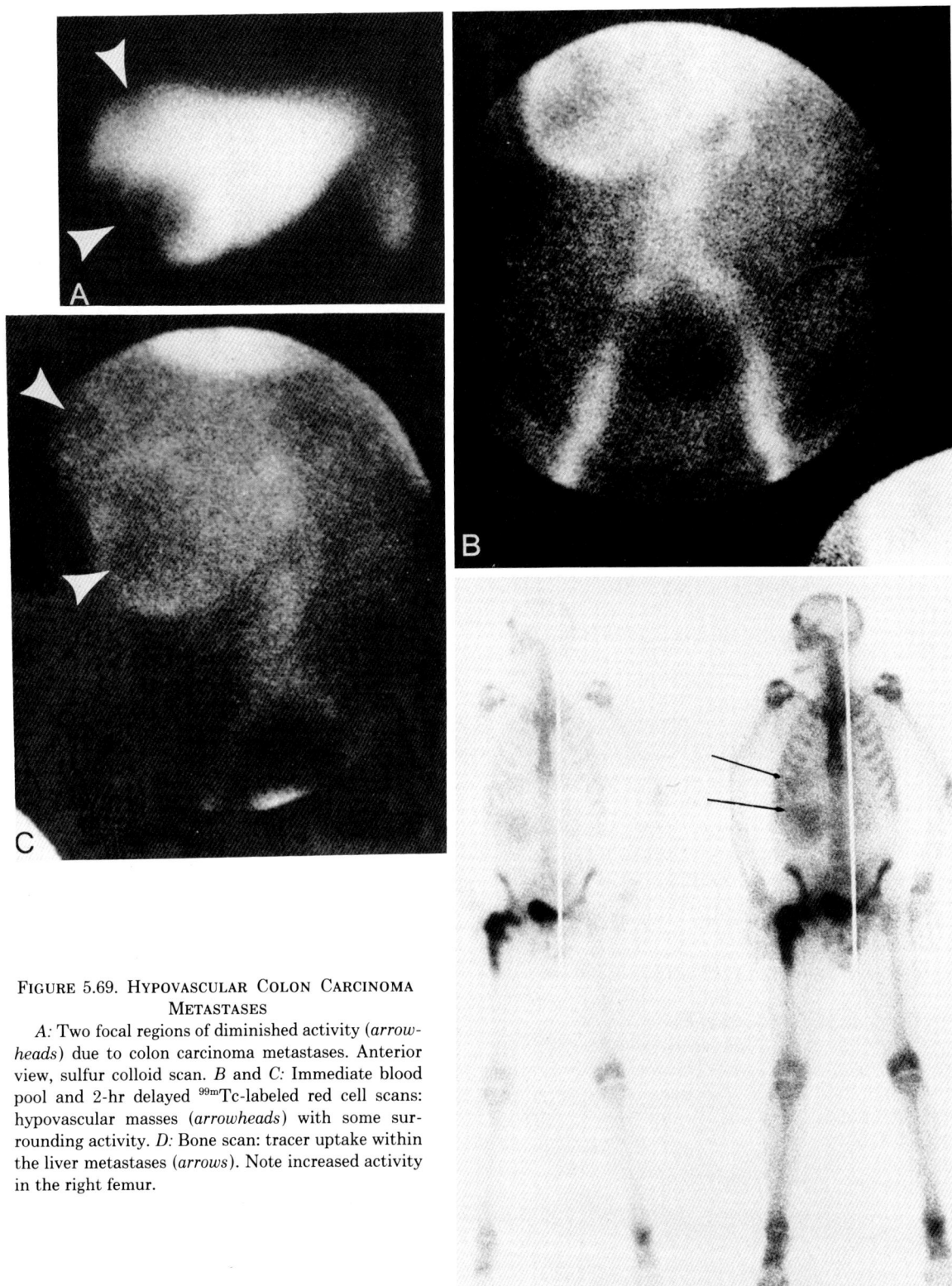

FIGURE 5.69. HYPOVASCULAR COLON CARCINOMA METASTASES

A: Two focal regions of diminished activity (*arrowheads*) due to colon carcinoma metastases. Anterior view, sulfur colloid scan. *B* and *C:* Immediate blood pool and 2-hr delayed ^{99m}Tc-labeled red cell scans: hypovascular masses (*arrowheads*) with some surrounding activity. *D:* Bone scan: tracer uptake within the liver metastases (*arrows*). Note increased activity in the right femur.

REFERENCES

1. Wright, GD: *Atlas of Liver Pathology*, Vol 4. Philadelphia, J. B. Lippincott, 1982.
2. Freeman L, Johnson P: *Clinical Scintillation Imaging*, Ed 2. New York, Grune & Stratton, 1975.
3. Siegel B, Alazraki N, Alderson P et al: *Nuclear Radiology Syllabus*, Series 2, Chicago, American College of Radiology, 1978.
4. Drum DE: Detection of hepatic space-occupying lesions by nuclear medicine techniques. *Postgrad Radiol* 2:305–317, 1982.
5. Harbert J: Efficacy of bone and liver scanning in malignant disease: facts and opinions. In Freeman L, Weissmann H (eds): *Nuclear Medicine Annual 1982*. New York, Raven Press, 1982.
6. Takayasu K, Moriyama N, Suzuki M, Yamada T, Fukutake T, Shima Y, Kobayashi C, Musha H, Okuda K: False-positive liver scans due to portal hypertension: correlation with percutaneous transhepatic portograms in 33 patients. *Radiology* 147:211–214, 1983.
7. Abramson SJ, Barash FS, Seldin DW, Berdon WE: Transient focal liver scan defects in children receiving chemotherapy (pseudometastases). *Radiology* 150:701–702, 1984.
8. Hansen S, Stadalnik RC: Liver uptake of ^{99m}Tc-pyrophosphate. *Semin Nucl Med* 12:89, 1982.
9. Baumert JE, Lantieri RL, Horning S, McDougall IR: Liver metastases of breast carcinoma detected on ^{99m}Tc-methylene diphosphonate bone scan. *AJR* 134:389–391, 1980.
10. Woolfenden JM, Waxman AD, Wolfstein RS et al: Scintigraphic evaluation of liver metastases from thyroid carcinoma. *J Nucl Med* 16:669–671, 1975.

Nuclear Medicine for Lymphoma and Leukemia of the Liver

Hepatomegaly and splenomegaly are nonspecific findings on sulfur colloid scans in patients with lymphoma or leukemia; they may or may not indicate hepatosplenic neoplasia. An inhomogeneous radiotracer distribution in the liver and spleen with decreased splenic uptake may be seen but is also nonspecific. Occasionally, discrete photopenic regions are seen which are fairly reliable indicators of neoplastic involvement. A prominent porta hepatis often indicates portal nodes in this patient population (1).

As lymphoma is often gallium avid, gallium scintigraphy is useful in determining the nature of colloid scan photopenic regions in patients with lymphoma.

REFERENCE

1. Waxman AD: Scintigraphic evaluation of diffuse disease. *Semin Nucl Med* 12:75–88, 1982.

Screening for Metastatic Disease to the Liver

The medical literature is replete with articles comparing the relative efficacy of radionuclide scintigraphy, ultrasound, and CT in detecting liver metastases. Because of rapid technologic advances in CT and sonography, most of these review articles were out of date when they were published. Different groups reach different conclusions (1–4). The study of choice depends on factors such as availability (scheduling delays), cost, and local equipment and expertise in addition to relative sensitivities and specificities. At Temple University, we use high resolution real-time sonography as the initial screening technique because of its rapidity, availability, and high resolution. In a small percentage of patients, the scan is suboptimal because of a high subcostal liver or grossly obese body habitus. In those patients, we perform 3-sec scan time CT both unenhanced and with a 150 ml air injection augmented rapid infusion of 60% contrast. All patients with potentially resectable liver metastases on sonography receive CT as well for staging. Although advocates of hepatic scintigraphy can cite specificity and sensitivity essentially equal to sonography and CT (1), we feel that scintigraphy has important disadvantages. If a mass is detected on a scintigram, our clinicians still want sonography and/or CT to determine whether it is cystic or solid, to search for additional abnormalities, and often to perform a guided biopsy. They are also reluctant to stop at a normal scintigram when their clinical suspicion of metastasis is high. Finally, a considerable number of false positive such as gallbladder, renal fossa, and porta hepatis defects are generated by scintigraphy which must be resolved by additional imaging. We reserve scintigraphy for suspected hemangiomas, adenomas, focal nodular hyperplasia, and difficult cases of fatty infiltration. Often several radionuclides are needed to solve these difficult problems. The efficacy of SPECT in screening for metastases has yet to be extensively evaluated, but SPECT adds to the cost of scintigraphy, increases its complexity, and may also generate false positives.

REFERENCES

1. McClees EC, Gedgaudas-McClees RK: Screening for diffuse and focal liver disease: the case for hepatic scintigraphy. *J Clin Ultrasound* 12:75–81, 1984.
2. Lewis E: Screening for diffuse and focal liver disease: the case for hepatic sonography. *J Clin Ultrasound* 12:67–73, 1984.
3. Berland LL: Screening for diffuse and focal liver disease: the case for hepatic computed tomography. *J Clin Ultrasound* 12:83–89, 1984.
4. Alderson PO, Adams DF, McNeil BJ, Sanders R, Siegelman SS, Finberg HJ, Hessel SJ, Abrams HL: Computed tomography, ultrasound, and scintigraphy of the liver in patients with colon or breast carcinoma: a prospective comparison. *Radiology* 149:225–230, 1983.

Plain Films for Liver Metastases

Plain films are rarely of any use in evaluating metastatic disease to the liver as they are often normal. The most common abnormality seen is a nonspecific hepatomegaly. Liver metastases infrequently calcify. The most common primary that causes calcified liver metastases is mucinous adenocarcinoma of the gastrointestinal tract especially colon and rectum (1). The calcifications characteristically are punctate; they may be stippled, amorphous, granular, trabecular, or flaky (Fig. 5.70) (2). Calcified liver metastases have also been noted from primary carcinomas of the thyroid (frequently medullary carcinoma) (Fig. 5.71), lung, kidney, breast, adrenal, testis, and ovary (frequently papillary serous cystadenocarcinoma) as well as sarcomas such as melanoma and mesenchymal sarcomas (3). Any liver metastasis can calcify after successful chemotherapy or radiation therapy.

The right upper quadrant should be scrutinized on excretory urographic tomograms, as occasionally liver metastases can be incidentally

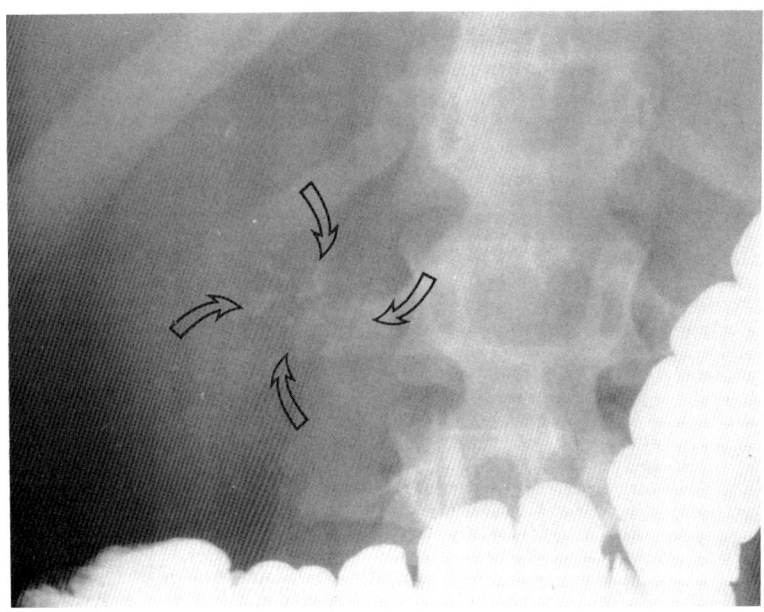

FIGURE 5.70. PUNCTATE AND FLAKY CALCIFICATIONS DUE TO A CALCIFIED COLON METASTASIS (*ARROWS*)

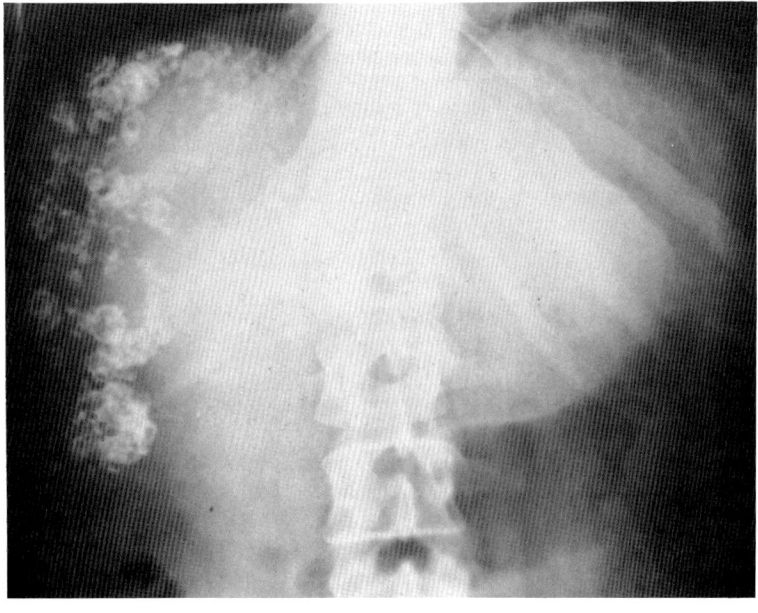

FIGURE 5.71. SPHERICAL CALCIFICATIONS FROM METASTATIC MEDULLARY CARCINOMA OF THE THYROID (*UNTREATED*)

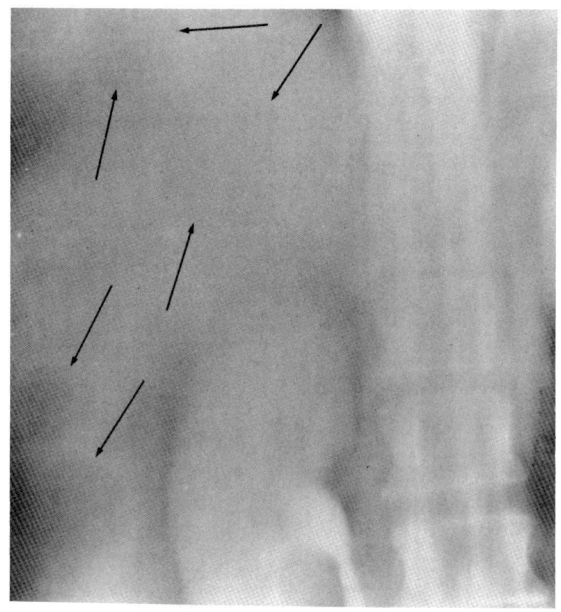

FIGURE 5.72. TOMOGRAM DURING AN EXCRETORY UROGRAM SHOWING LIVER METASTASES
Hepatomegaly and four round lucencies (*arrows*) representing metastases from gastric carcinoma. The two more cephalad lesions are only faintly seen. Liver cysts would look the same.

detected as radiolucencies by virtue of the total body opacification effect (Fig. 5.72).

REFERENCES

1. Khilnani MT: Calcified liver metastases from carcinoma of the colon. *Dig Dis Sci* 6:229, 1961.
2. Miele AJ, Edmonds HW: Calcified liver metastases: a specific roentgen sign. *Radiology* 80:779, 1963.
3. Darlak JJ, Moskowitz M, Kattan KR: Calcifications in the liver. *Radiol Clin North Am* 18:209–219, 1980.

Cholangiography of Metastatic Disease and Lymphoma/Leukemia

Opacification of the biliary tree is rarely attempted or clinically indicated in the evaluation of metastatic disease. If performed, the findings will often be striking, but not specific.

Diffuse neoplastic infiltration of the liver can produce duct stretching, attenuation, and diminished branching resembling cirrhosis and steatosis. In addition to metastases and lymphoma or leukemia, primary liver neoplasms such as hepatocellular carcinoma, cholangiocarcinoma, or angiosarcoma can cause a nearly identical appearance. Unifocal or multifocal metastases, lymphomatous nodules or chloromas commonly smoothly displace and splay ducts. Partial or even complete obstruction is not uncommon (Figs. 5.73 and 5.74). Ulceration or filling of a necrotic metastasis is distinctly unusual. Again, differentiation from a hepatic primary is not possible.

Angiography of Hepatic Metastases and Lymphoma

Metastases

Classically, liver metastases have been separated into hypovascular and hypervascular groups angiographically (1). This has been based primarily on comparison of tumor stain to the parenchymal blush in the hepatogram phase of a celiac injection. Hypervascular metastases include: renal cell carcinoma, choriocarcinoma, carcinoids and islet cell tumors, ovarian cystadenocarcinomas, melanoma and other sarcomas such as leiomyosarcoma. Adenocarcinomas of the colon, stomach, jejunum, ileum, gallbladder, and pancreas are usually hypovascular. It must be remembered that almost all metastases of any substantial size have greater arterial than portal

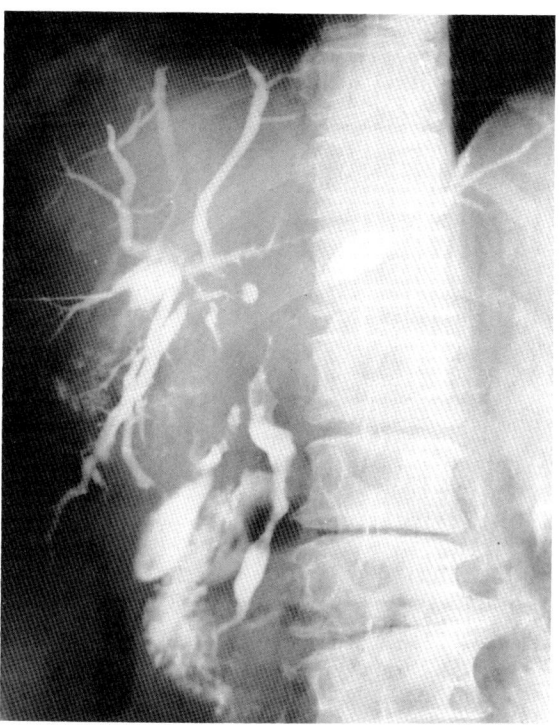

FIGURE 5.73. CHOLANGIOGRAPHY OF LIVER METASTASES
PTC shows stretching and diminished branching of ducts in the superior portion of the right lobe. The metastases from colon carcinoma have also encased the bifurcation in the porta hepatis and produced extensive extrahepatic duct abnormalities probably due to peribiliary nodes.

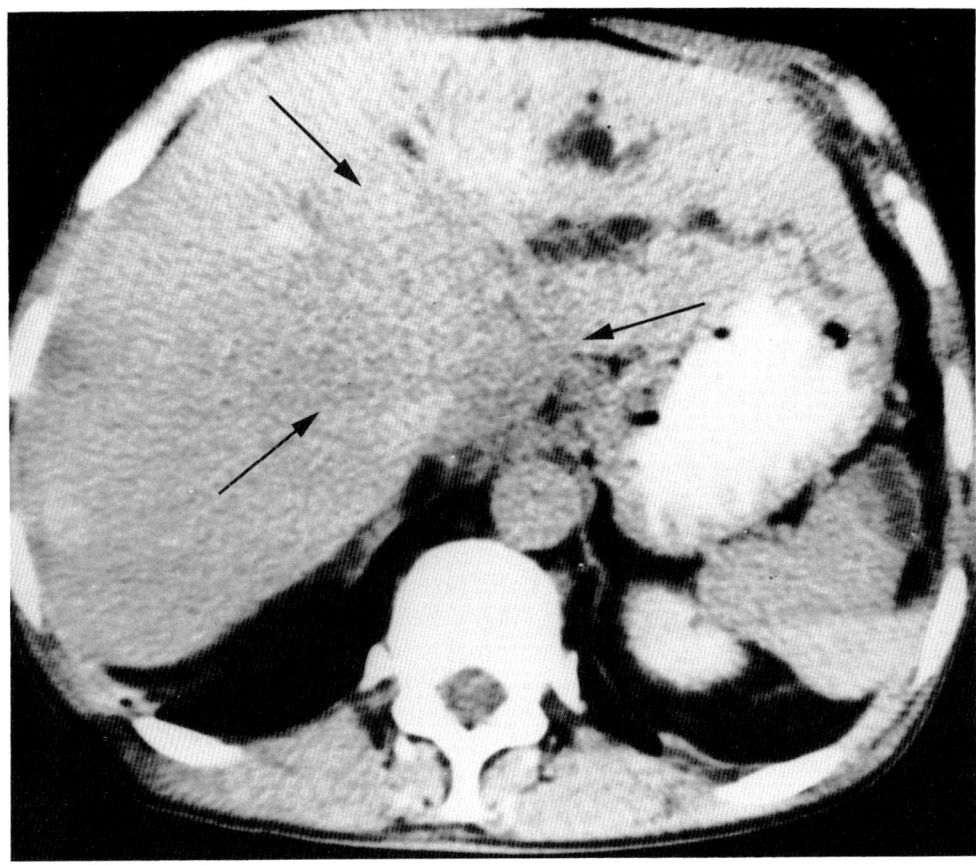

FIGURE 5.74. METASTATIC ADENOCARCINOMA
Contrast-enhanced CT of a case similar to that shown in Figure 5.73. Metastatic adenocarcinoma is producing a barely visible hypodense mass (*arrows*) but causing obvious obstruction of the ducts draining the left lobe.

supply, and this fact can be used to render them "hypervascular" with appropriate technique (see below). Liver metastases are usually multiple and peripheral in distribution (1).

Hypervascular metastases stand out as rounded areas of increased radiodensity in the hepatogram phase of the injection (Fig. 5.75). Larger metastases may have neovascularity and splay intrahepatic arteries. Extremely vascular metastases can have enlarged feeding arteries and even arteriovenous shunting. Necrosis or intratumoral hemorrhage is seen as a central radiolucency within the tumor stain. Metastases from primary cystic neoplasms such as mucinous cystic neoplasms of the pancreas often have cystic metastases (hypervascular rim and radiolucent center) (Fig. 5.76). Hypervascular metastases on the order of 0.5–1.0 cm in diameter can be identified. Hypovascular metastases, on the other hand, are filling defects in the hepatogram, and must be at least 2–3 cm in diameter to be detected by celiac arteriography. Larger masses will displace intrahepatic arteries (Fig. 5.77) (1). The weaknesses of celiac arteriography in the detection of metastases are caused by the dual blood supply of the liver. Contrast-laden portal blood overwhelms the arterial portogram and can obscure the tumor stain (which is arterial) of metastases which would otherwise be vascular, and hypovascular metastases have to be fairly large and quite hypovascular to be seen as negative defects in the portal hepatogram phase (Fig. 5.78). In the current era of high-quality sonography and CT, celiac arteriography is rarely useful for evaluating liver metastases.

On the other hand, selective hepatic arteriography does have a role to play in certain clinical circumstances. Its use in planning arterial infusion chemotherapy is discussed in detail in the chapter devoted to that subject. When surgical resection is contemplated for suspected isolated metastatic disease, infusion hepatic arteriogra-

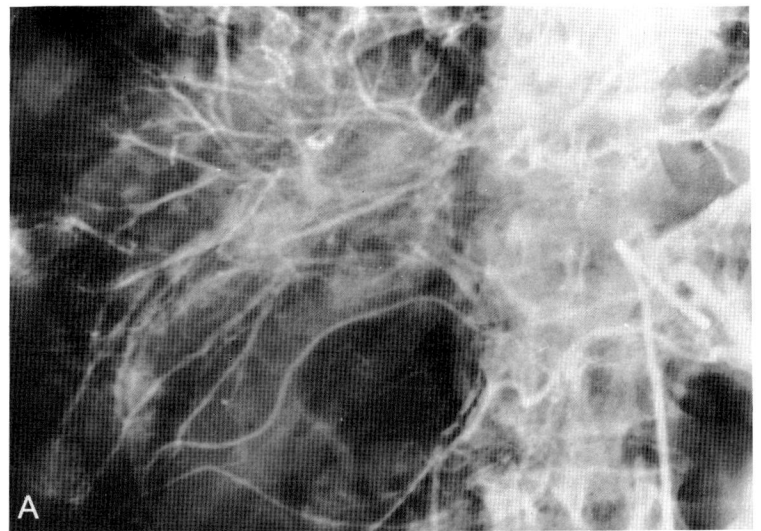

FIGURE 5.75. SELECTIVE HEPATIC ARTERIOGRAM

A and *B:* Late arterial and hepatogram phases of a selective hepatic arteriogram: innumerable hypervascular metastases from metastatic islet cell tumor of the pancreas.

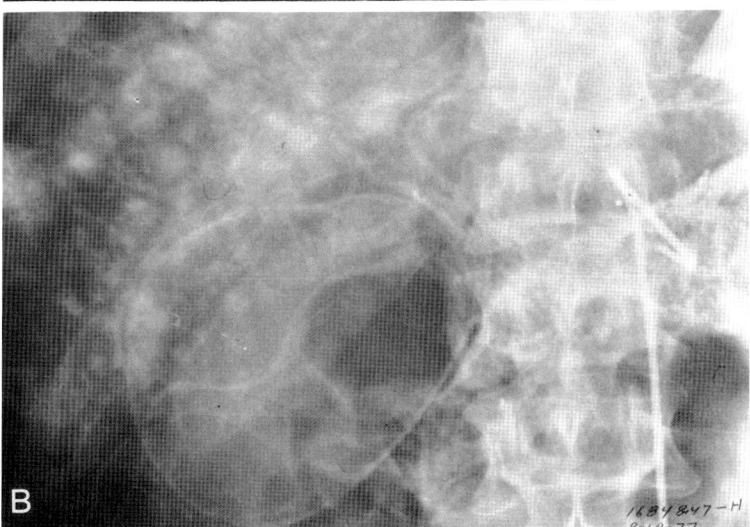

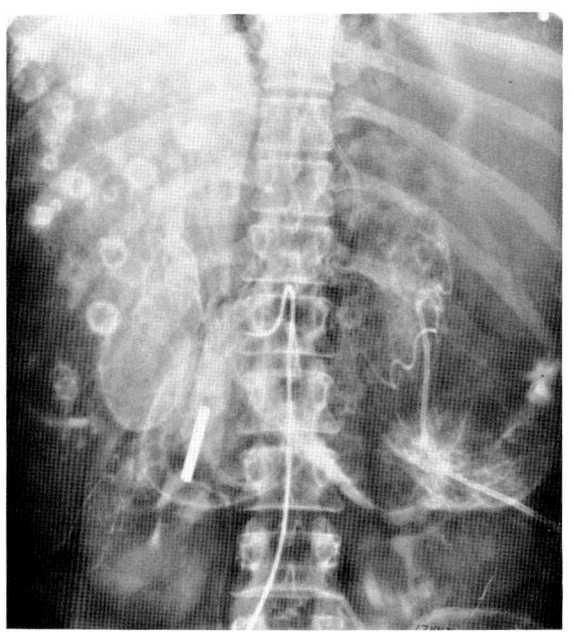

FIGURE 5.76. CYSTIC METASTASES FROM MUCINOUS CYSTIC NEOPLASM OF THE PANCREAS (CYSTADENOCARCINOMA)

Hepatogram phase of a selective hepatic arteriogram.

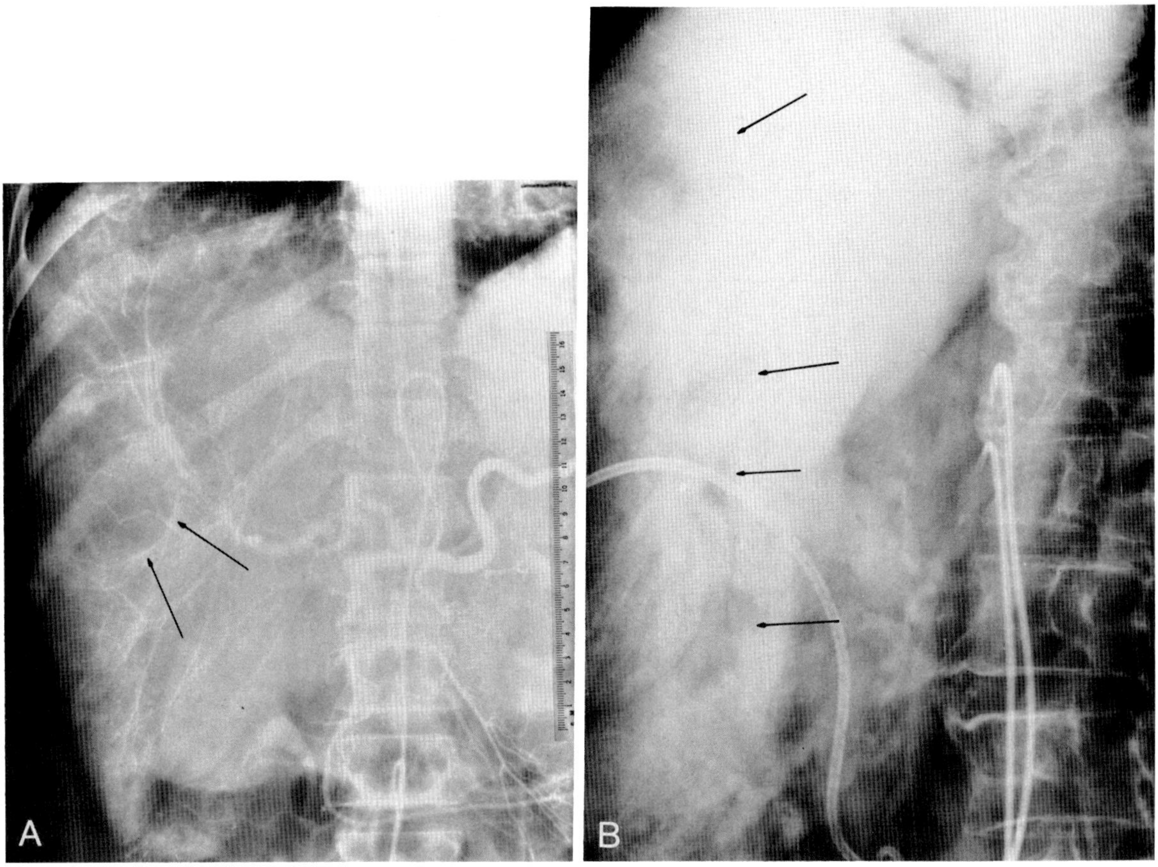

FIGURE 5.77. HYPOVASCULAR METASTASES
A: Arterial splaying (*arrows*) by a large hypovascular metastasis. *B:* Portal hepatogram phase of a combined celiac and superior mesenteric injection: several filling defects (*arrows*) representing hypovascular pancreatic carcinoma metastases.

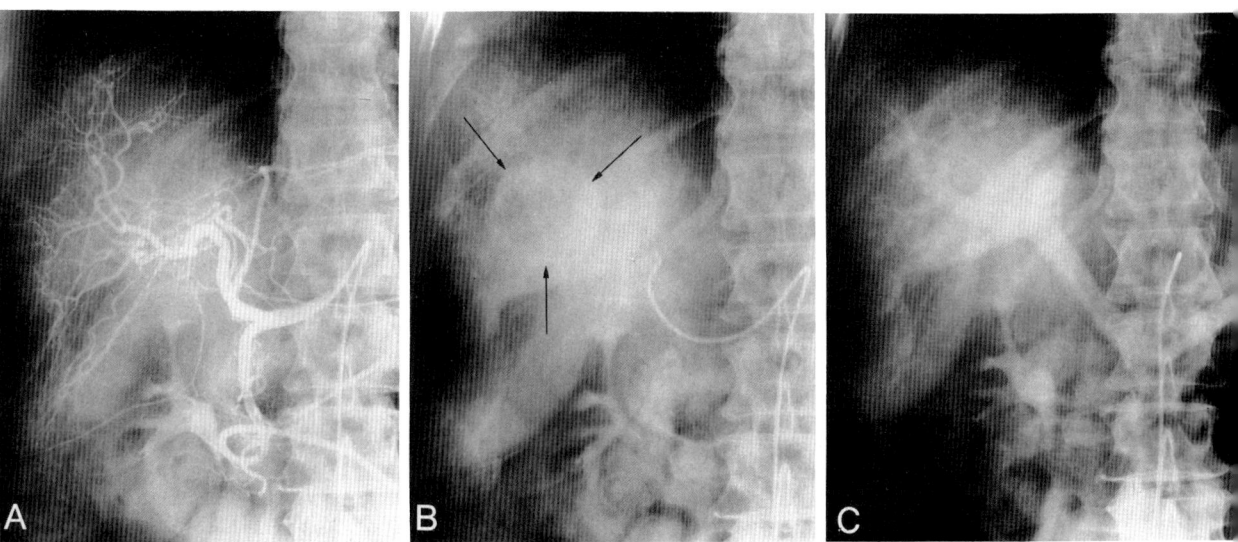

FIGURE 5.78. METASTATIC COLON CANCER SEEN BY SELECTIVE HEPATIC ARTERIOGRAPHY; MISSED BY CELIAC ARTERIOGRAPHY
A: Arterial phase of hepatic injection-mass lesion not diagnosable. *B:* Ring enhancing mass on ensuing hepatogram phase (*arrows*). *C:* No diagnosable mass on hepatogram phase of celiac injection.

phy followed by CT arteriography or portography as needed is more sensitive than conventional CT and sonography in detecting additional lesions. These techniques can detect reliably even hypovascular metastases on the order of 1 cm or less in diameter, and are far superior in evaluating the left lobe (Fig. 5.79). Their use and its theory are discussed in detail in the section on normal liver angiography and the section on staging of hepatocellular carcinoma. If EOE-13 or a similar hepatosplenographic CT contrast material becomes available for general use, all forms of angiography will probably become obsolete for staging liver metastases.

Lymphoma

Angiography is rarely indicated and rarely performed in patients with hepatic lymphoma. Find-

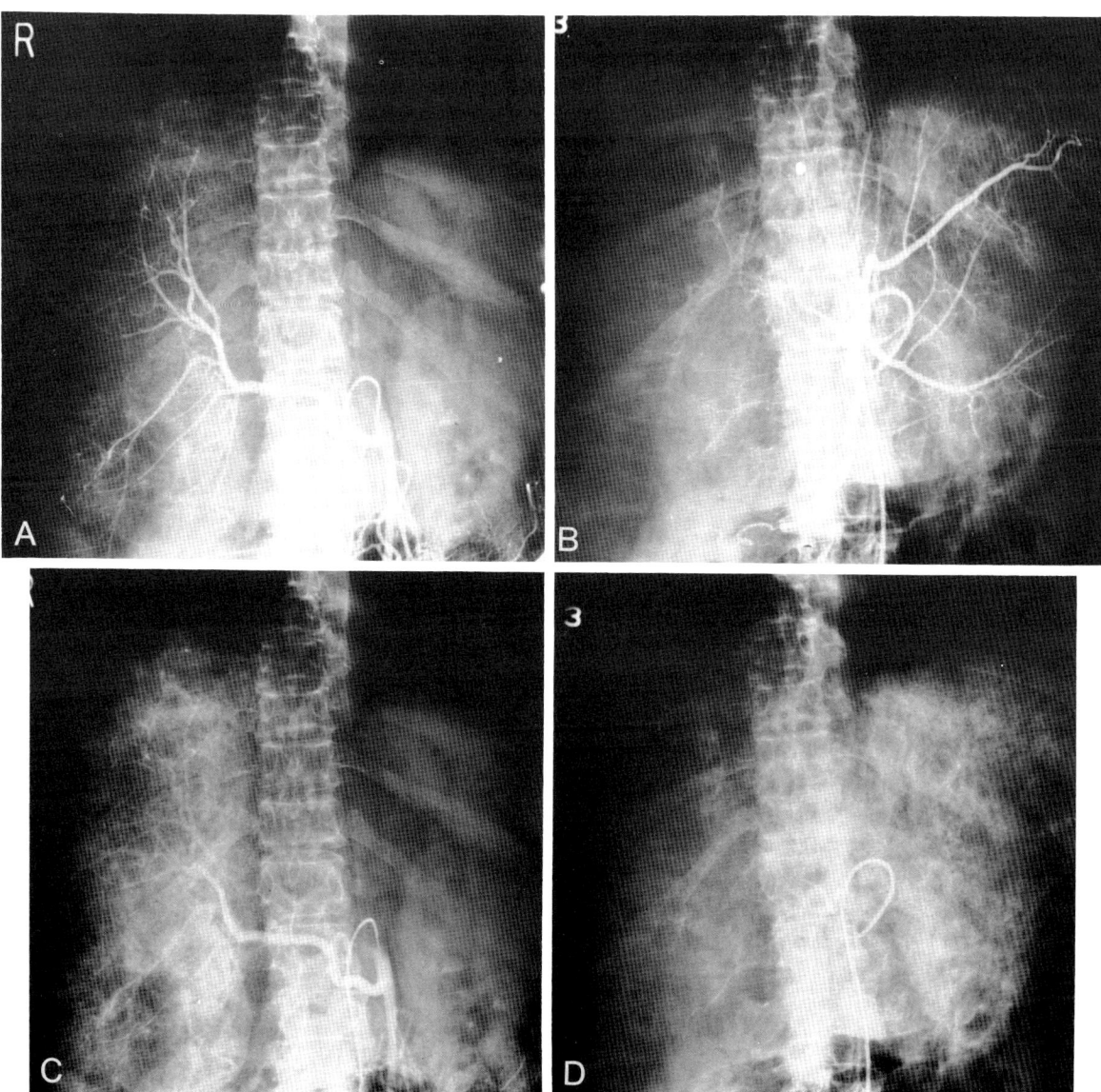

FIGURE 5.79. HYPOVASCULAR BREAST METASTASES DEMONSTRATED BY SELECTIVE HEPATIC ARTERIOGRAPHY
A and *B:* Right hepatic (replaced) and left hepatic arterial phases: arterial stretching and splaying. *C* and *D:* Hepatogram phases: innumerable small and large filling defects.

ings consisting of primarily arterial displacement around single or multiple intrahepatic masses have been reported. Sometimes there are moderate numbers of tumor vessels, but feeders do not dilate. The masses are seen as filling defects in the hepatogram phase. When lymphoma involves the liver diffusely, the only findings are nonspecific hepatomegaly and vascular spreading (1).

REFERENCE

1. Reuter SR, Redman HC: *Gastrointestinal Angiography*, Philadelphia, W. B. Saunders, 1977, pp 153–161.

HEPATOCELLULAR CARCINOMA

Hepatocellular carcinoma (formerly termed hepatoma), comprises about 90% of all primary liver malignancies (1). In the United States and Europe, hepatocellular carcinoma is an uncommon tumor with an autopsy incidence of 0.2–0.77%, but in Asia and Africa the incidence is 5.5% (2). In some endemic areas of Asia and Africa, the incidence is as high as 10–20% (2). The age of affected patients peaks in the 3rd and 4th decades in high incidence areas and in the 6th and 7th decades in low incidence areas (1–3). Males are affected five times as often as females when hepatocellular carcinoma arises in a cirrhotic liver, but there is no sex predilection for those hepatocellular carcinomas arising in previously normal livers (4).

Etiology and Pathogenesis

Etiologic factors can be divided into three categories: cirrhosis, chronic hepatitis B virus infection, and carcinogens (1–6).

Cirrhosis

Eighty percent of hepatocellular carcinomas occur in livers with preexisting cirrhosis (2). They are most likely to occur in the macronodular (postnecrotic) type in which they develop with a frequency of 13–24% and the micronodular cirrhosis of hemachromatosis (7–22%) (2, 5). Alcoholics who develop hepatocellular carcinoma frequently have stopped drinking and their cirrhosis has progressed from the micronodular type to the macronodular type (5). Hepatocellular carcinoma complicates alcoholic cirrhosis in approximately 3.2% (2), but seldom occurs in other types (cardiac, biliary, Wilson's disease, metabolic) (5). Hepatocellular carcinomas have been reported to occur with increased frequency in α_1-antitrypsin deficiency (2). The overall incidence of hepatocellular carcinoma in cirrhotics in the United States is 5%, but is 40–50% in Africa and Southeast Asia (2, 5). The difference is probably due to the higher incidence of alcoholic micronodular cirrhosis in the United States (2). The development of hepatocellular carcinoma in cirrhosis is thought to be secondary to active regeneration going out of control with a time course of eight months to fourteen years from onset of cirrhosis to the diagnosis of hepatocellular carcinoma (2). There is a high incidence of hepatocellular carcinoma associated with membranous obstruction of the inferior vena cava in South America and Japan (5).

Chronic Hepatitis B Virus Infection

Hepatitis B surface antigen is more prevalent in hepatocellular carcinoma patients than the rest of the population, and antihepatitis B core antigen (suggesting continued replication) is present to even a greater degree (2). Forty-five to 50% of patients dying with cirrhosis from chronic viral hepatitis have hepatocellular carcinoma (4).

Carcinogens

A strong correlation between dietary aflatoxin content and hepatocellular carcinoma exists in southeast Asia and Africa (2). Aflatoxin is a mycotoxin produced by Aspergillus fumigatus which grows on improperly stored peanuts, corn, and other grains (2). Also implicated as dietary factors are cycasin from cycad nuts and akaloids from a variety of plants in endemic areas in Africa, South America and Asia (2). Siderosis caused by high dietary levels of iron (from local beer) is thought to be a factor in the high incidence of hepatocellular carcinoma among the Bantu in Africa (1). Oral contraceptive and anabolic androgenic steroids have been implicated as causative factors by circumstantial evidence (4, 7). Doubt has recently been case on the theory that oral contraceptives are causative agents (7). Hepatocellular carcinomas occur after Thorotrast administration, but less commonly than angiosarcoma (2). We have seen hepatocellular carcinomas develop in areas of the liver included in radiation portals for Wilms' tumor.

Hepatocellular carcinoma in childhood is rare, but when it does occur, it is often associated with preexisting liver disease, including giant cell hepatitis, tyrosinosis, galactosemia, glycogen storage disease, and biliary atresia. Children over five years of age are most often affected.

Clinical Findings

The mode of presentation can be divided into six groups in descending order of frequency (1, 5, 6): (*a*) frank carcinoma—malaise, anorexia, weight loss, abdominal pain, tender hepatomegaly; (*b*) icteric—mechanisms are tumor infiltrating liver, lymph node compression of bile ducts, tumor necrosis and hemobilia, intrahepatic mass compressing ducts, or tumor growing into ducts and extending intraluminally. Stool is hemepositive in 70% (8); (*c*) occult—obscured by cirrhosis and discovered at laparotomy or autopsy; (*d*) acute—catastrophic hemoperitoneum secondary to rupture of a mass or erosion of a surface vessel; (*e*) febrile—chills, high fever, and severe pain and tenderness in the liver from central tumor necrosis and/or hemorrhage; and (*f*) metastatic disease—metastasis to lung, bone, or brain as presenting feature.

Hepatocellular carcinoma must be suspected in any patient with cirrhosis who decompensates without obvious cause (5, 6). Miscellaneous signs and symptoms include Budd-Chiari syndrome (5), hypoglycemia (1, 5), hypercalcemia (1, 5), erythrocytosis (1, 5), hyperlipidemia (5), sexual precocity or gynecomastia (1), and bruit or friction rub over the liver (1, 3).

Liver function tests are abnormal, but may not be helpful in those patients with underlying cirrhosis. Alpha-fetoprotein levels are elevated above 400 ng/ml in greater than 90% of patients with hepatocellular carcinoma (1–6). Alpha-fetoprotein is synthesized in fetal life by both the liver and yolk sac. After the age of two, alpha-fetoprotein is barely detectable in normals (<30 ng/ml) (2). Elevated levels may occur in nonmalignant liver diseases, but levels greater than 1000 ng/ml strongly suggest hepatocellular carcinoma (2).

Prognosis is grim; once the diagnosis is made, average survival is 6 months (1–6). Hepatocellular carcinomas in childhood are more often resectable (3). Patients die from cachexia, liver insufficiency, tumor rupture, or bleeding varices (6). One-third of patients show response to Adriamycin (3).

Pathology

There are three patterns of tumor growth. Nodular and massive are the most common, and diffuse is the least common (1, 2, 4, 6). The nodular pattern consists of multiple variably sized nodules up to 5 cm in diameter. Each nodule has an arterial branch supplying it (4).

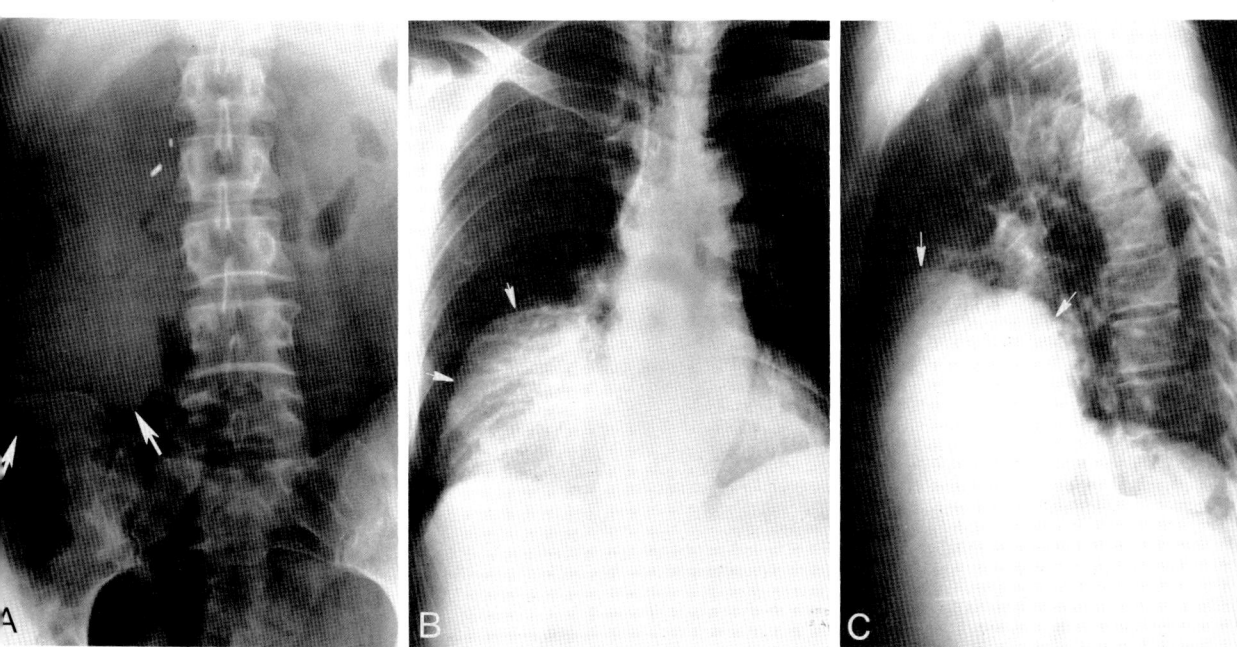

FIGURE 5.80. HEPATOCELLULAR CARCINOMA

A: Plain film of a hepatocellular carcinoma: soft-tissue mass projecting off the inferior right lobe (*arrows*). *B* and *C:* PA and lateral chest films: localized elevation of the right hemidiaphragm due to a large hepatocellular carcinoma in the right lobe (*arrows*).

Confusion with metastases and cirrhotic nodularity can occur. The massive pattern consists of a large mass usually in the right lobe which may have one or several small satellite nodules. A small percentage of large solitary hepatocellular carcinomas are encapsulated and more amenable to resection (4). The diffuse infiltrative type consists of tiny indistinct nodules and its appearance is hard to differentiate grossly from cirrhosis. The major blood supply to the tumor is from the hepatic artery (4). Portal vein invasion is present grossly in 25–40%, and hepatic vein invasion in 16% at autopsy. Invasion into the inferior vena cava and even growth into the right atrium can occur (1).

Histologically, cells in hepatocellular carcinomas resemble hepatocytes but have cytologic features of malignancy—large hyperchromatic nuclei and mitotic figures (2). The cells form cords or trabeculae sometimes separated by a blood-filled sinusoidal stroma (2, 6). In better differentiated hepatocellular carcinomas, tumor cells elaborate bile, a diagnostic feature when present (2, 6). Each cluster of tumor cells is covered by a layer of flat endothelium. Poorly differentiated hepatocellular carcinomas may be composed of large bizarre anaplastic giant cells (2, 6). Other patterns include acinar and clear cells (6). There is little fibrous stroma in the usual hepatocellular carcinoma (2). A recently described variant is sclerosing hepatocellular carcinoma, characterized by intense fibrosis in which neoplastic tubular structures are embedded (7). This tumor occurs in a middle-aged to elderly population and is strongly associated with hypercalcemia. It is frequently misdiagnosed as metastatic adenocarcinoma and is difficult to differentiate from cholangiocarcinoma (7). The other hepatocellular carcinoma with fibrous stroma is the fibrolamellar variant, discussed under its own heading.

Radiology

Plain Films

Generalized hepatomegaly or a localized bulge in the liver contour due to hepatocellular carcinoma may be seen (Fig. 5.80A) (8–10). The localized bulge in the diaphragm (usually the right) is hard to differentiate from normal variants, however, a rapid change in size and configuration will provide a clue (Fig. 5.80B and C) (8). Splenomegaly from portal hypertension may be present.

It has been reported in many articles and reviews that calcification in hepatocellular carcinomas is unusual and more common in children than adults (9–15). Critical review of this literature reveals that the calcified primary malignant liver tumors in adults were either cholangiocarcinomas, or mixed cholangio-hepatocellular carcinomas, or hepatocellular carcinomas in noncirrhotic young adults. The latter probably are fibrolamellar hepatocellular carcinomas. In children under the age of five, most calcified liver tumors are either hepatoblastomas or hemangioendotheliomas. Review of case material at the Armed Forces Institute of Pathology (AFIP) showed that radiographically calcified adult hepatocellular carcinomas were fibrolamellar hepatocellular carcinomas. Calcification in the usual hepatocellular carcinomas that develops in cirrhotics would have to be of the dystrophic type. Although these hepatocellular carcinomas do undergo hemorrhage and necrosis, patients generally do not live long enough untreated for calcification to develop. Therefore, a calcified (plain film) liver tumor is not likely to be a conven-

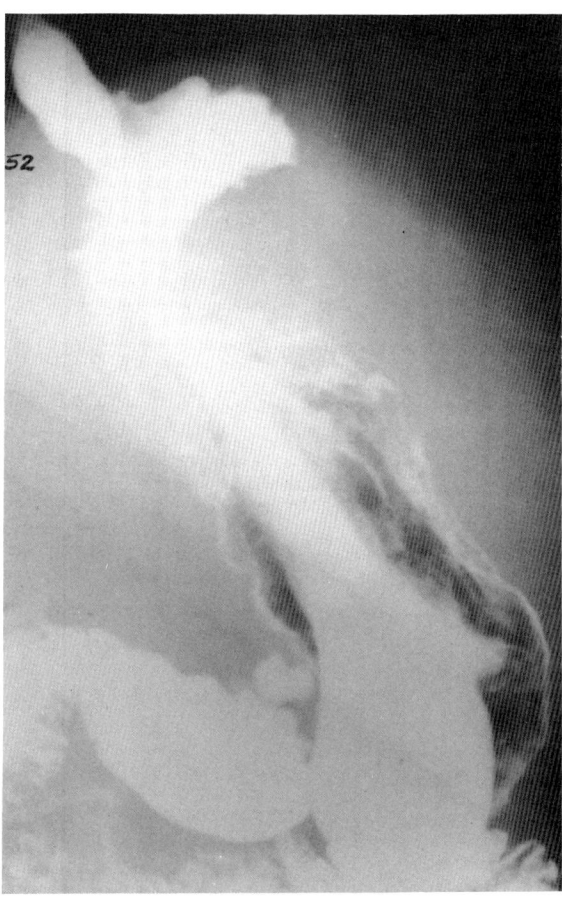

FIGURE 5.81. HEPATOCELLULAR CARCINOMA
Lateral film from a barium meal: extrinsic mass indenting the anterior wall of the stomach—hepatocellular carcinoma in the left lobe.

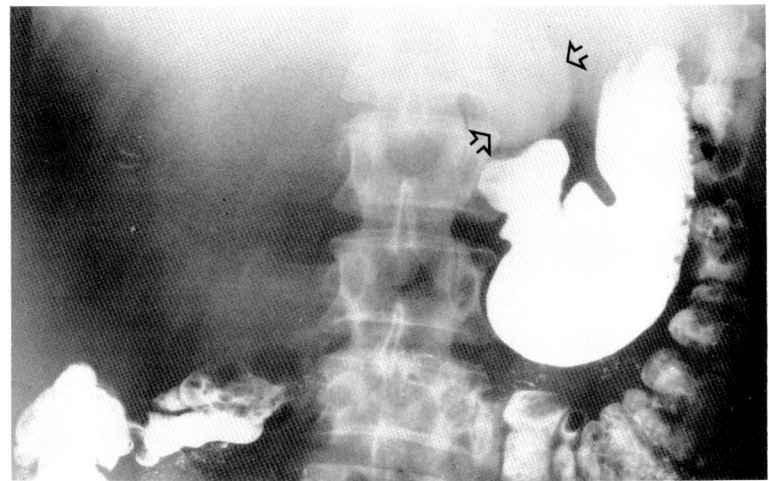

FIGURE 5.82. HEPATOCELLULAR CARCINOMA
Displaced gallbladder (*arrows*) and stomach by a large hepatocellular carcinoma in the right lobe.

tional hepatocellular carcinoma. Conceivably, the sclerosing variety of hepatocellular carcinoma could be sufficiently calcified to demonstrate plain film calcification.

Barium Contrast Studies

Displacement of the opacified gastrointestinal tract by an enlarged liver or focal displacement of the stomach, duodenum or colon by a localized liver mass can be seen (Figs. 5.81 and 5.82) (8, 11). Esophageal varices are often present in patients with underlying cirrhosis or hepatocellular carcinoma-induced portal vein obstruction (8).

REFERENCES

1. Shonland MM, Millward-Sadler GH, Wright DH, Wright R. Hepatic tumors. In Wright R, Alberti KGMM, Karran S, Millward-Sadler GH (eds): *Liver and Biliary Disease*. Philadelphia, W. B. Saunders, 1979, pp 886–894.
2. Robbins SL, Cotran RS: *Pathologic Basis of Disease*. Philadelphia, W. B. Saunders, 1979, pp 1065–1068.
3. Sherlock S: *Diseases of the Liver and Biliary System*. Oxford, Blackwell Scientific, 1981, pp 456–469.
4. Edmondson HA, Peters RL: Tumors of the liver: pathologic features. *Semin Roentgenol* 18:75–83, 1983.
5. Schiff L: Hepatic neoplasia: selected clinical aspects. *Semin Roentgenol* 18:71–74, 1983.
6. Tien-yu L: Tumors of the liver. In Bockus HL et al (eds): *Gastroenterology*. Philadelphia, W. B. Saunders, 1976, pp 522–531.
7. Goodman ZD, Ishak KG: Hepatocellular carcinoma in women: probable lack of etiologic association with oral contraceptive steroids. *Hepatology* 2:440–444, 1982.
8. Van Sonnenberg E, Ferrucci JT: Bile duct obstruction in hepatocellular carcinoma—clinical and cholangiographic characteristics. *Radiology* 130:7–13, 1979.
9. McNulty JG: *Radiology of the Liver*. Philadelphia, W. B. Saunders, 1977, pp 44, 367–378.
10. Gore RM, Goldberg HI: Plain film and cholangiographic findings in liver tumors. *Semin Roentgenol* 18:87–93, 1983.
11. Omata M, Peters RL, Tatter D: Sclerosing hepatocellular carcinoma: relationship to hypercalcemia. *Liver* 1:33–49, 1981.
12. Darlak JJ, Moskowitz M, Kattan KR: Calcifications in the liver. *Radiol Clin North Am* 18:214, 1980.
13. Karras BG, Cannon AH, Zanon B: Hepatic calcifications. *Acta Radiol* 57:458, 1962.
14. Boijsen E, Abrams HL: Roentgenologic diagnosis of primary carcinoma of the liver. *Acta Radiol (Diagn)* 3:257–277, 1965.
15. Haddow RA, Kemp-Harper RA: Calcification in the liver and portal system. *Clin Radiol* 18:225–236, 1967.

Ultrasound

The accuracy of ultrasound in the detection of hepatocellular carcinoma is generally reported to be between 65 and 80% (1, 2); however, a recent study claimed 94% sensitivity in detecting hepatocellular carcinomas less than 3 cm in diameter with high resolution equipment (3). The ultrasonic appearance of hepatocellular carcinoma is variable but can be divided into three major categories which correlate well with the reported pathologic data (4). The most common finding is a discrete lesion (either solitary or multiple) (Fig. 5.83). These lesions are usually hyperechoic or hypoechoic but are sometimes isoechoic and detected chiefly by virtue of a thin radiolucent halo corresponding to the tumor capsule (Fig. 5.84*B* and *C*). The second pattern is diffuse parenchymal involvement with disorganization of the normal echo pattern. Multiple areas of increased and decreased echogenicity are present throughout the distorted liver without distinct masses (Fig. 5.83). The third appearance is a combination of the discrete and diffuse hepatic patterns. Unfortunately, these ultrasonic patterns can also be seen with metastases to the

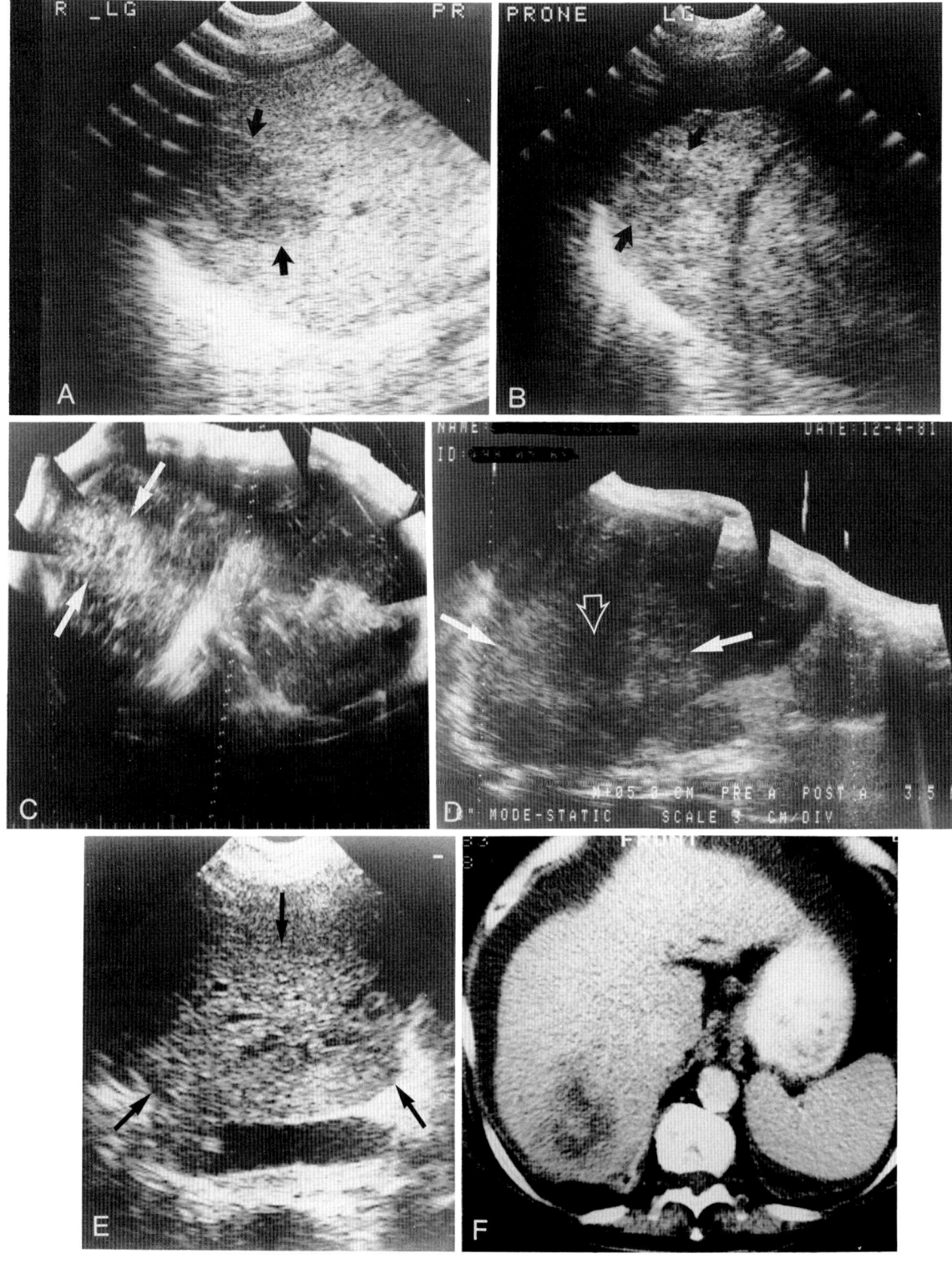

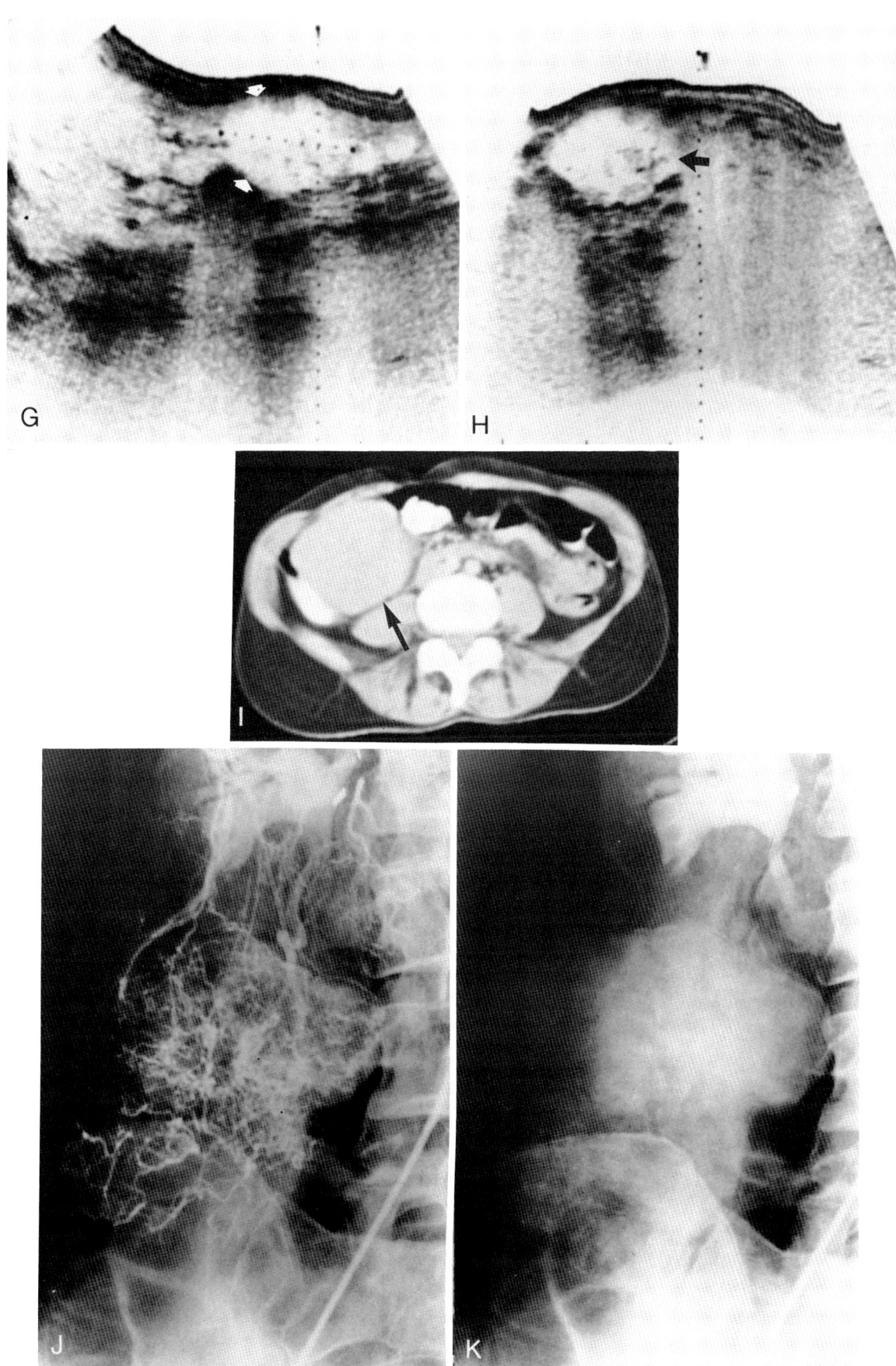

FIGURE 5.83H–K

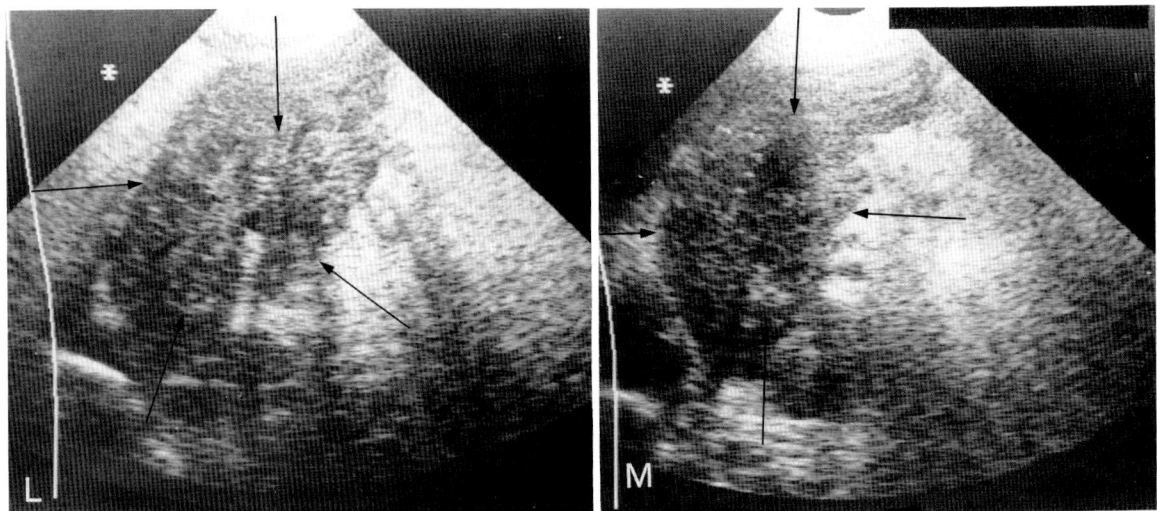

FIGURE 5.83. HEPATOCELLULAR CARCINOMA: SONOGRAPHY

A and *B:* Hypoechoic hepatocellular carcinoma, underlying cirrhosis. *A:* Sagittal scan through the dome of the liver reveals poorly defined hypoechoic mass (*arrows*). *B:* Adjacent sagittal scan through a region of the tumor that is only slightly hypoechoic with a very coarse texture and still poorly marginated (*arrows*). *C:* Transverse scan of a hyperechoic hepatocellular carcinoma (*arrows*). *D:* Longitudinal scan of a hyperechoic hepatocellular carcinoma (*white arrows*) with a central hypoechoic zone from either hemorrhage or necrosis (*open arrow*). *E:* Coronal scan of a nearly isoechoic hepatocellular carcinoma (*arrows*) with an irregular central hypoechoic region. *F:* Rapid drip infusion CT of the same patient as in *E:* poorly defined mostly hypodense solid solitary mass. Note varices anterior to the aorta and medial to the stomach and ascites. *G* and *H:* Parasagittal and transverse sonograms of a hypoechoic hepatocellular carcinoma (*arrows*) which was solid without necrosis. *I:* Corresponding CT scan (drip infusion): isodense tumor visible because of contour bulge only (*arrow*). *J* and *K:* Corresponding late arterial and capillary phases of an arteriogram: marked bizarre hypervascularity and intense tumor stain. *L* and *M:* Parasagittal scans through the left lobe: nearly isoechoic hepatocellular carcinoma (*arrows*).

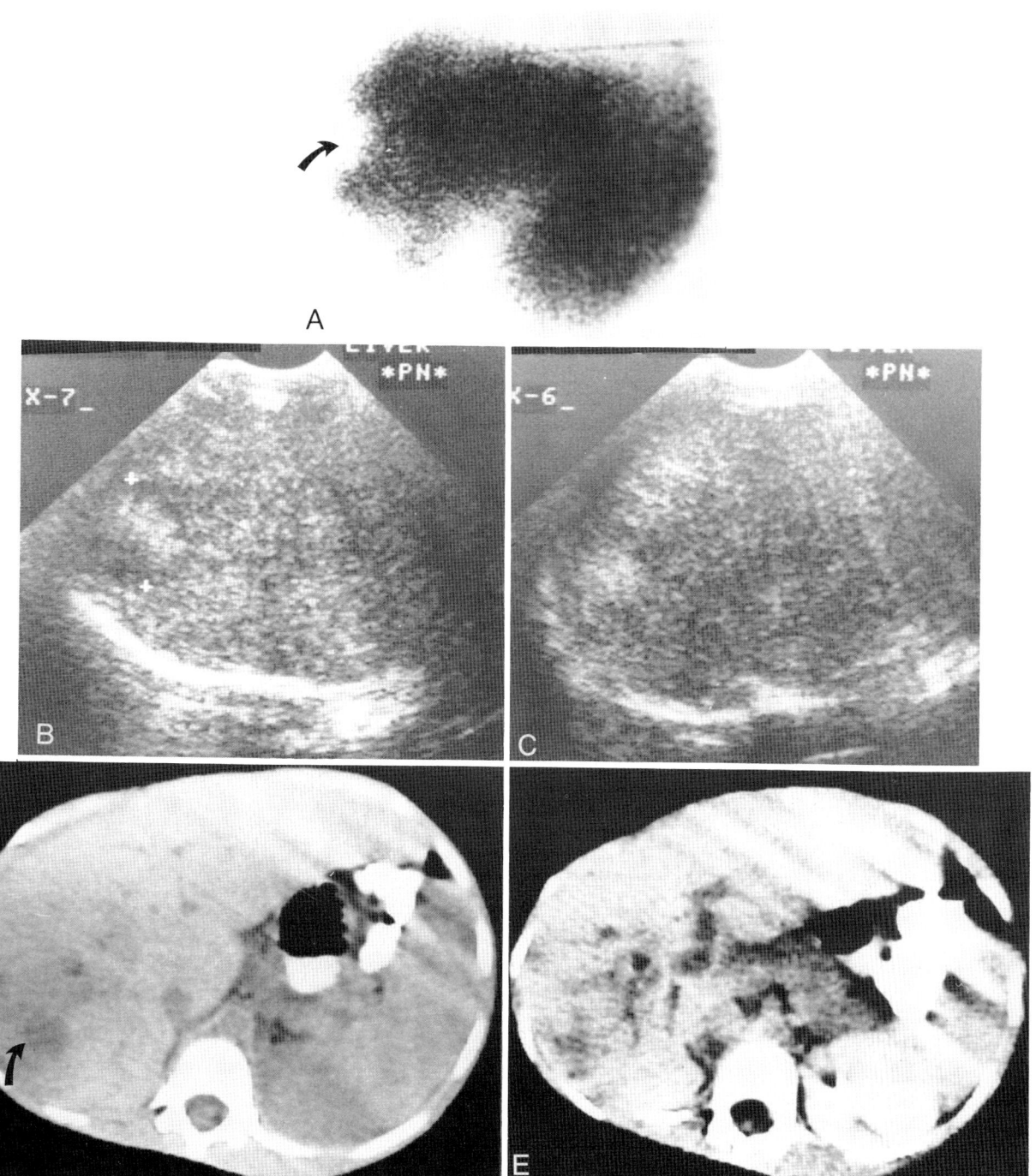

FIGURE 5.84. ANGIOGRAPHIC STAGING

Hepatocellular carcinoma in a 22-yr-old woman status postnephrectomy and radiation for Wilm's tumor as a child. *A:* Sulfur colloid scan, RAO: small posterolateral defect. *B* and *C:* Transverse sonograms through right lobe: well-defined hyperechoic mass with halo (*cursors, B*). Poorly defined hyperechoic region just cephalad, *C.* Tumor or cirrhosis? *D:* Noncontrast CT shows extensive infiltration by hypodense neoplasm. *Arrow* points to region seen as well-defined mass on sonogram. *E:* Enhanced CT: dilated ducts in addition to mass. Patient had heme+ stools and intermittent jaundice due to hemobilia. *F–H:* Right hepatic arteriogram: very hypervascular infiltrative mass with neovascularity involves entire right lobe. *I:* Left hepatic arteriogram. Medial segment of left lobe is involved and lateral segment is spared. In this case angiography was superior to noninvasive methods. Possibly dynamic CT could have done better. *J–M:* Infusion hepatic arteriography and CT arteriography in staging hepatocellular carcinoma. *J:* Conventional contrast enhanced CT shows only one mass in the left lobe (cursor). *K–M:* Infusion hepatic arteriogram: satellite (*arrow*) in the right lobe, tumor is unresectable. CT arteriogram shows large left lobe mass densely enhancing (*L*) as well as enhancing satellite (*arrow, M*).

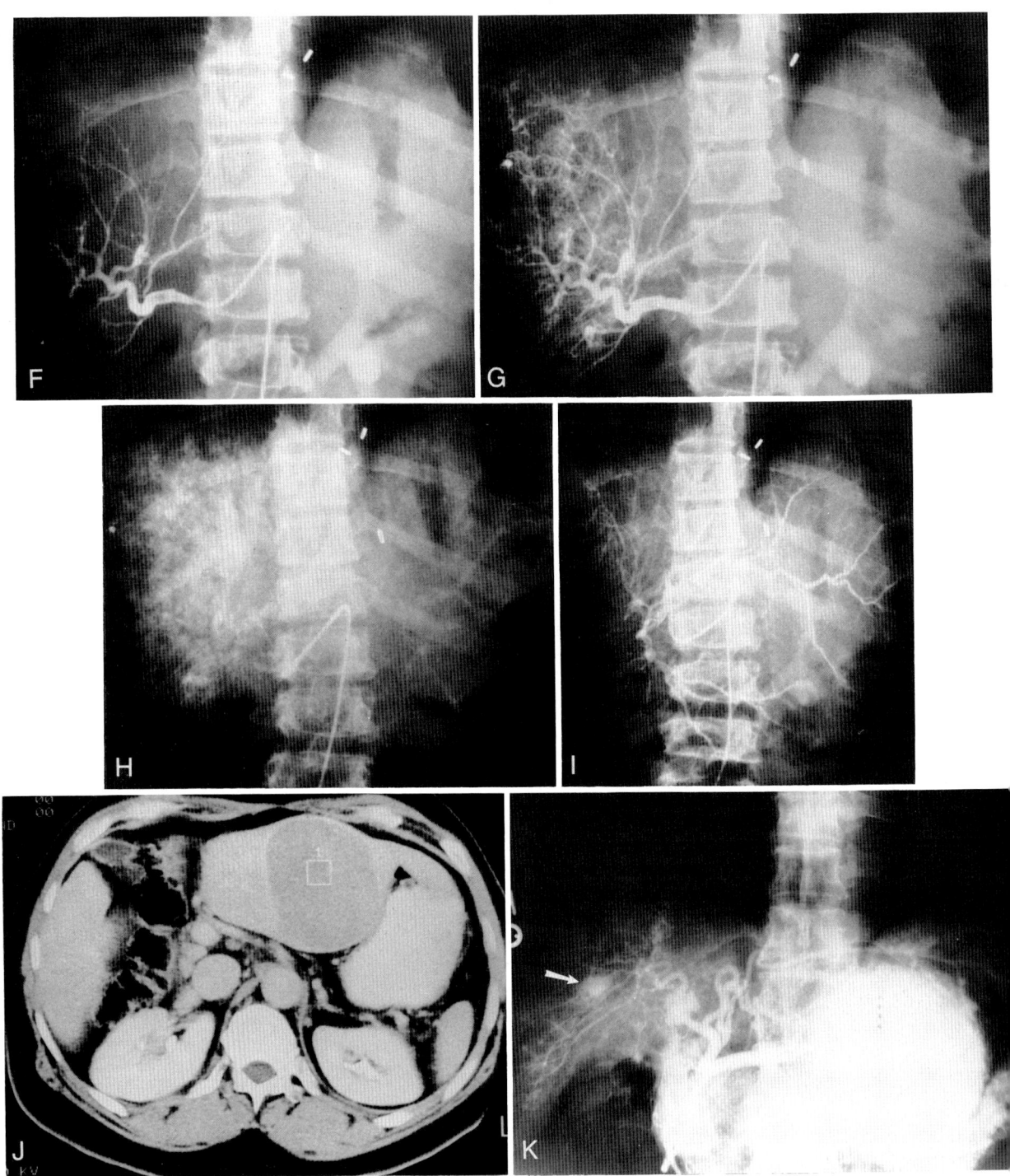

FIGURE 5.84*F–K*

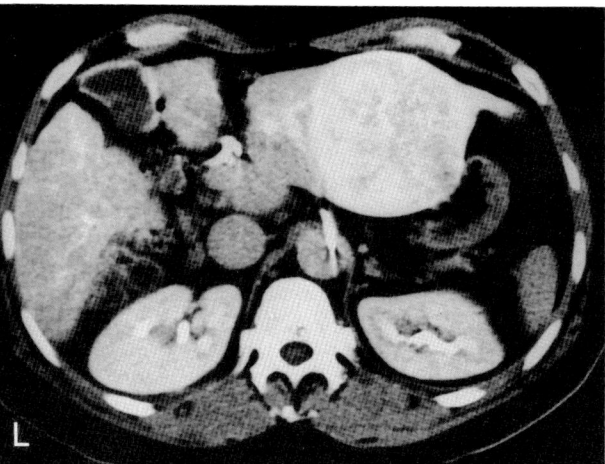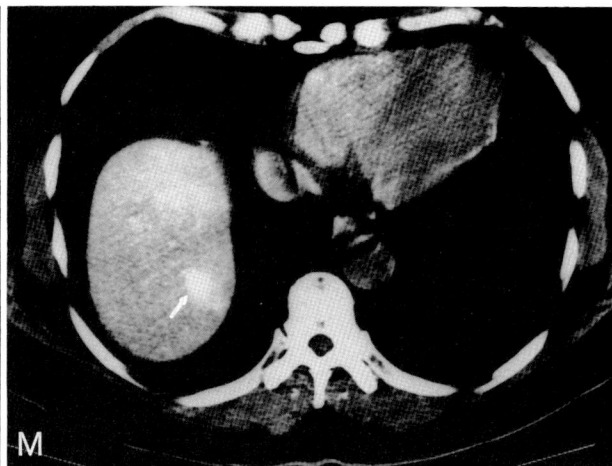

FIGURE 5.84L and M

liver; therefore, biopsy is required for definitive tissue diagnosis. The biopsy can be done under ultrasonic or CT guidance.

The diffuse pattern of hepatic involvement in hepatocellular carcinoma can also be stimulated by lymphoma, cirrhosis or hemochromatosis. In the light of the relatively common occurrence of hepatocellular carcinoma in patients with cirrhosis, the overlapping ultrasound pattern is a potential problem. Cottone et al. (5) evaluated 100 cirrhotic patients with clinical suspicion of hepatocellular carcinoma. Ultrasound was diagnostic with 27 of 30 patients (sensitivity 90%) with proven hepatocellular carcinoma. There were five false positive examinations (specificity of 93%). The difficulty in such cases arises where a focal hyperechoic zone is due to a cirrhotic nodule and not to hepatoma.

The variability of the hepatic echo pattern in patients with hepatocellular carcinoma has been shown to correlate with tumor morphology (6). A hypoechoic lesion corresponds to a solid tumor without evidence of tissue necrosis (Fig. 5.83H-K). On the other hand, a hyperechoic lesion is caused by either fatty metamorphosis within the tumor or severe sinusoidal dilatation. Lesions with a mixed echo pattern are partially necrotic.

Small hepatocellular carcinomas are usually hypoechoic, whereas most that are larger than 2–3 cm are hyperechoic compared to the hepatic parenchyma (3).

Secondary signs of hepatocellular carcinoma including ascites and hepatomegaly can also be detected by the ultrasonic examination (7, 8). Unfortunately, these findings can be detected in numerous other conditions and are nonspecific.

Hepatocellular carcinoma can invade the portal vein and/or the hepatic veins, with or without extension into the inferior vena cava (Fig. 5.85A). Intraluminal tumor or clot is depicted as echoes either partially or completely filling the lumen (9). Enlargement of veins in addition to intraluminal mass suggests tumor thrombus rather than bland thrombus. Hepatocellular carcinoma invades the vein draining the segment in which it is located and can extend hepatofugally: from left portal vein to umbilical vein, right portal vein to main and left portal vein, or right hepatic vein to inferior vena cava (9). Documentation of venous involvement by ultrasound favors hepatocellular carcinoma over metastatic disease (9). Intraoperative ultrasound has been shown to be useful in localizing impalpable hepatocellular carcinomas (3).

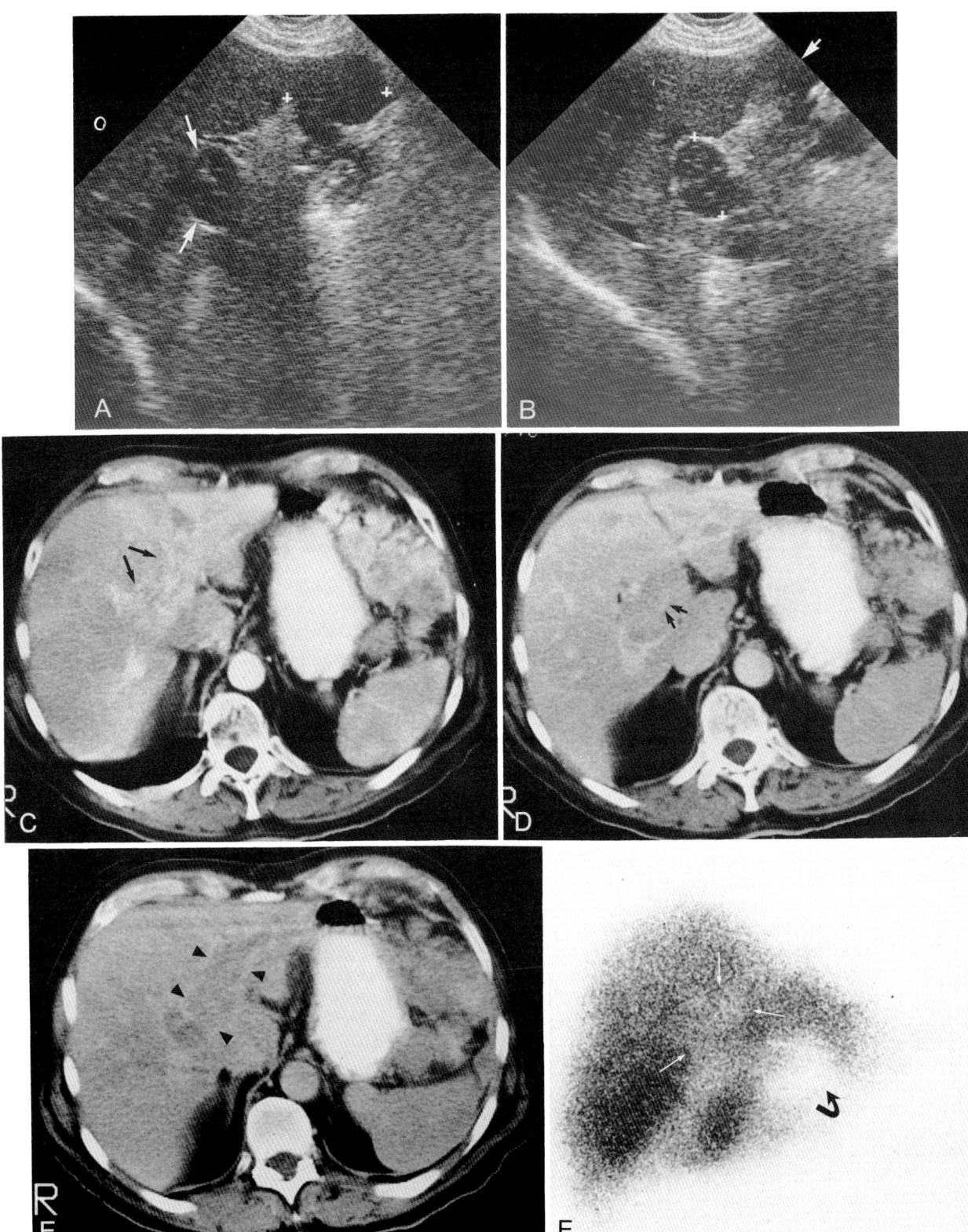

FIGURE 5.85. UNUSUAL HEPATOCELLULAR CARCINOMA PRESENTING AS PALPABLE INTRAPERITONEAL MASSES
Intrahepatic mass not seen on ultrasound or CT, but shown on radionuclide scan. *A:* Parasagittal sonogram: mass beneath the liver with same texture as liver (*cursors*). Portal vein is enlarged and filled with tumor (*arrows*). *B:* Slightly different sagittal scan showing mass (*arrow*) and tumor in portal vein (*cursors*). *C–E:* Dynamic CT: Arterial phase (*C*) demonstrates streaky enhancement in the region of the portal vein (*arrows*) simultaneously with dense aortic opacification, indicating arterioportal shunting. Note enhancing intraperitoneal mass lateral to the stomach. Venous phase (*D*) shows minimal tumor thrombus enhancement (*arrows*). Delayed scan (*E*) shows linear enhancement around the portal vein (*arrowheads*) consistent with enhancement via vasa vasorum. *F:* Sulfur colloid scan: central branching defects (*arrows*) from the enlarged tumor-filled portal veins. Intrahepatic mass (*curved arrow*) is probably the primary hepatocellular carcinoma.

REFERENCES

1. Taylor KJW, Carpenter DA, Hill CR, McCready VR: Gray scale ultrasound imaging. *Radiology* 119:415-423, 1976.
2. Broderick TW, Gosink B, Menuck L, Harris R, Wilcox J: Echographic and radionuclide detection of hepatoma. *Radiology* 135:149-151, 1980.
3. Shen JC, Sung JL, Chen DS, Yu JY, Wang TH, Su CT, Tsang YM: Ultrasonography of small hepatic tumors using high resolution linear-array real-time instruments. *Radiology* 150:797-802, 1984.
4. Edmondson HA, Steiner PA: Primary carcinoma of the liver. *Cancer* 7:462, 1954.
5. Cottone M, Marceno MP, Maringhini A, Rinaldi F, Russo G, Sciarrino E, Turri M, Pagliaro L: Ultrasound in the diagnosis of hepatocellular carcinoma associated with cirrhosis. *Radiology* 147:517-519, 1983.
6. Tanaka S, Kitamura T, Imaoka S, Saskaki Y, Taniguchi H, Ishiguro S: Hepatocellular carcinoma: sonographic and histologic correlation. *AJR* 140:701-707, 1983.
7. Kamin PD, Bernardino ME, Green B: Ultrasound manifestations of hepatocellular carcinoma. *Radiology* 131:459-461, 1979.
8. Boultbee J: Gray scale ultrasound in hepatocellular carcinoma. *Clin Radiol* 30:547-552, 1979.
9. Subramanyam BR, Balthazar EJ, Hilton S, LeFleur RS, Horii SC, Raghavendra BN: Hepatocellular carcinoma with venous invasion: sonographic-angiographic correlation. *Radiology* 150:793-796, 1984.

Computed Tomography

The CT appearance of hepatocellular carcinoma (Table 5.1) can be divided into three categories: solitary mass, multiple masses, or diffuse parenchymal involvement (Figs. 5.83F and 5.86). On unenhanced scans the solitary mass is often well defined and distinct from normal liver parenchyma. The lesion usually is 20-30 HU lower in attenuation than the adjacent normal liver (1-4). Foci of calcification (see fibrolamellar section below), hemorrhage or necrosis may be detected within the lesion (Figs. 5.83F and 5.86E and F).

The frequency with which calcification is seen on CT within hepatocellular carcinoma is somewhat controversial. Successfully treated (radiation or chemotherapy) lesions routinely calcify (see section on therapeutic nuclear medicine). Many series in the literature do not compulsively differentiate intrahepatic cholangiocarcinoma and mixed cholangiohepatocellular carcinomas from hepatocellular carcinomas. Few series separate out fibrolamellar carcinomas and sclerosing hepatocellular carcinomas, the former known to be prone to calcify and the latter suspected to be. In our experience, coarse, chunky, trabecular central calcification occupying a small portion of the tumor indicates either fibrolamellar hepatocelular carcinoma, cholangiocarcinoma or a mixed tumor. Fine, punctate, sand-like calcification distributed within a large portion of the tumor suggests metastatic disease or possibly the sclerosing variant of hepatocellular carcinoma. The usual hepatocellular carcinoma associated with cirrhosis rarely calcifies *prior to therapy*, and is more likely to have the punctate pattern when it does calcify. Careful examination of Table 5.1 reveals that the apparently high incidence of calcification (similar to some reports in the literature) can be explained by: (a) young patients with high incidence of fibrolamellar, (b) low incidence of known cirrhosis, and (c) unknown number of cases of the sclerosing variant or mixed cholangiocellular-hepatocellular carcinomas because of limited biopsy material.

Following bolus contrast enhancement, the lesion may or may not be better delineated. Most hepatocellular carcinomas will enhance due to their hypervascularity but will still have lower CT attenuation than enhanced normal liver (the latter often enhances to a greater degree). More peripheral portions of large lesions and small tumor nodules may be obscured by contrast enhancement as they become isodense with surrounding liver. Unfortunately the solitary hepatocellular carcinoma cannot be reliably differentiated from a liver metastasis or other primary liver tumors by CT alone, although demonstration of venous invasion favors hepatocellular carcinoma strongly versus metastasis. Contrast enhancement facilitates detection of portal venous or vena caval invasion by tumor (3-6).

The presentation of hepatocellular carcinoma as multiple discrete masses (Fig. 5.86B) on CT may also be simulated by metastatic disease (1). The number and size of the tumor masses will vary though most masses are in the range of 2-4 cm.

Diffuse tumor involvement is the third pattern of hepatocellular carcinoma seen on CT scans. At times it is difficult to distinguish between diffuse tumor involvement and extensive multifocal masses. It may be difficult to detect a diffuse hepatocellular carcinoma in patients with underlying cirrhosis of the liver (see Fig. 5.93).

Finally, hepatocellular carcinoma may appear as a relatively hyperdense mass in patients with fatty infiltration (Fig. 5.86G).

In a series of 225 cases of hepatic masses evaluated by CT Itai et al. (1) noted that hepatocellular carcinoma was suggested by the following: masses either isodense or slightly hypodense compared to surrounding liver on plain scans, a circular zone of radiolucency surrounding the mass (capsule); bulging of the tumor from the liver surface; and decreased density of an entire

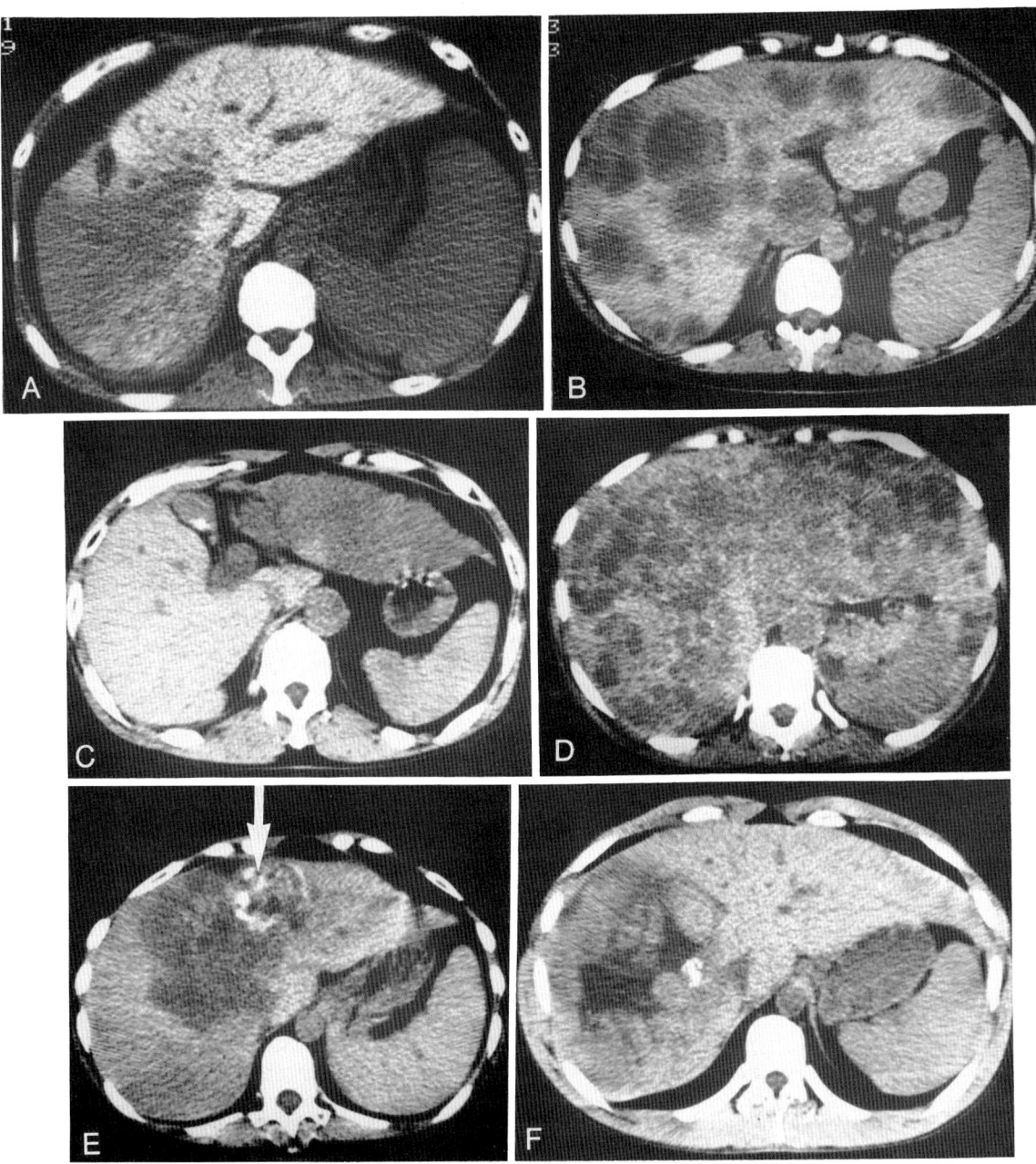

FIGURE 5.86. HEPATOCELLULAR CARCINOMA: CT

A: Poorly demarcated hypodense right lobe hepatocellular carcinoma with a posterior infiltrative component. Noncontrast CT. Note dense liver due to hemochromatosis, splenomegaly and ascites. *B:* Noncontrast CT: multifocal hypodense hepatocellular carcinoma mimicking metastatic disease. *C:* Noncontrast CT: hypodense hepatocellular carcinoma diffusely infiltrating the left lobe. *D:* Noncontrast CT: hypodense hepatocellular carcinoma with multiple small nodules and regions of diffuse infiltration. *E* and *F:* Atypical hepatocellular carcinomas, noncontrast CT: *E* shows hypodense solitary mass with calcification (*arrow*). Could this really be a mixed cholangiocellular-hepatocellular tumor? *F* shows solitary hypodense mass with central region of hemorrhage and small calcification. Could this be a fibrolamellar or mixed cholangiohepatocellular tumor? *G:* Noncontrast CT: hyperdense (relatively) hepatocellular carcinoma (*arrowheads*) in a patient with a fatty liver.

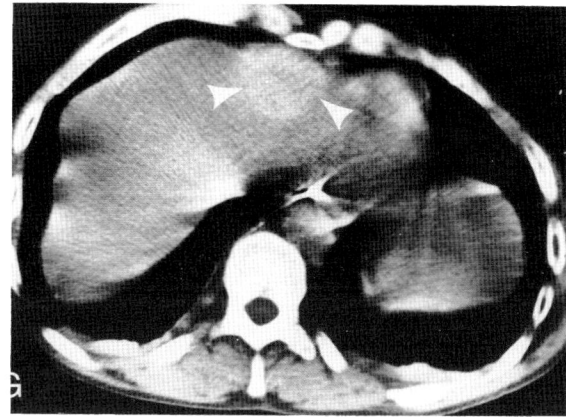

FIGURE 5.86G

TABLE 5.1.
RESULTS OF CT EVALUATION OF 117 PATIENTS WITH HEPATOCELLULAR CARCINOMA AT JOHNS HOPKINS HOSPITAL

Patient population
  117 patients
    81 male
    36 female
    50.3 yr average age (range: 11–79 yr)
CT findings
  Solitary lesion: 26 (size range of 2 × 3 × 1 cm to 18 × 18 × 15 cm)
  Multiple lesions: 32
    <5 cm: 11
    > 5 and <10 cm: 6
    >10 cm: 15
  Diffuse parenchymal involvement: 59
    <50% liver: 44
    >50% liver: 15
  Calcification in tumor: 27 (23%)
  Underlying cirrhosis: 13 (11.1%)

lobe with diffuse enhancement following bolus contrast injection. Seventy-five percent of their hepatocellular carcinomas had an intense, diffuse, imhomogeneous blush following bolus injection. Cirrhosis was present or suspected on CT in 62% of patients with hepatocellular carcinoma versus less than 10% of patients with metastatic disease to the liver in their series.

The diagnostic accuracy of CT in detecting hepatocellular carcinoma is a function of both scanning technique and scanner resolution. Most large series have a reported accuracy of over 80% (1, 4). Takashima et al. (8) evaluated 7 hepatomas less than 2 cm in size and found CT accurate in 1 case (14%) but angiography accurate in 6 of the 7 cases (86%). A potential source of error in their CT scans was that patients were examined only with contrast enhancement and these smaller lesions may have become isodense. Optimal CT technique employing pre- and post-bolus contrast scans should detect most hepatocellular carcinomas 1 cm or more in size. Inamoto et al. (2) divided the CT appearance of hepatoma into four groups based on their visualization both before and after contrast enhancement. (a) group 1 (40%)—both contrast enhanced (C^+) and non-contrast (C^-) scans were positive and equally good. Most solitary masses were in this category; (b) group 2 (30%)—the C^+ scan was best and the tumor was poorly seen with the C^- scan; (c) group 3 (25%)—the C^- scan was better and on the C^+ scan the tumor was isodense or appeared smaller; and (d) group 4 (5%)—both the C^+ and C^- scans were negative. Groups 2, 3, and 4 were comprised mostly of multinodular or diffuse tumor types.

CT also is useful for the early detection of metastases from hepatocellular carcinoma. The most common site of metastasis is to the lung. Metastases to the adrenal glands, lymph nodes, and skeleton are also readily demonstrated with CT scanning.

The technical approach to CT scanning of the liver varies from institution to institution. Practical factors such as scanner availability and patient load often will result in an abbreviated study. At the Johns Hopkins Hospital a strict scanning protocol is followed in the patient with a suspected liver mass. An unenhanced scan is performed first with consecutive scans at 1 cm intervals through the entire liver. If one or more lesions are detected the patient is repositioned in the scanner at that level. 1 ml/kg of Hypaque-60 is then injected via a bolus technique. Rapid sequential images are then obtained to evaluate the vascularity of the lesions. Such a sequential imaging technique following bolus injection helps differentiate hepatic neoplasms from hemangiomas. The rest of the liver is then re-scanned at 1 cm intervals in order to detect any other lesions brought out by enhancement. Table 5.1 summarizes findings in 117 patients with hepatocellular carcinoma using the above CT technique.

Staging with Ultrasound and CT

At most institutions, surgical resection is undertaken for hepatocellular carcinoma whenever possible. Carcinoma limited to one lobe can theoretically be cured by lobectomy. If the median segment of the left lobe is involved in addition to the right lobe, a trisegmentectomy can be performed. If all segments are affected, curative resection is not possible unless transplantation is feasible. Relative contraindications to curative surgery vary among institutions and include ascites, severe liver failure or profound jaundice, tumor invasion of the distal main portal vein or bifurcation of the right and left portal veins and local extrahepatic extension (9). Absolute contraindications are proven metastatic disease and tumor involvement of the inferior vena cava or main portal vein.

Conventional CT is somewhat better than ultrasound in assessing distribution of hepatocellular carcinoma within the liver, although combining both modalities will give greater accuracy than either alone. Ultrasonography is somewhat better than routine CT in evaluating the possibility of tumor involving the inferior vena cava and portal veins. CT is superior in detecting extrahepatic extension, adenopathy and distant metastatic disease. Ascites and biliary obstruction are seen quite well with either modality (9). Unfortunately, some patients will be called resectable on both ultrasound and routine CT who are not (either because of involvement of all lobes or major veins) if special studies such as dynamic CT, CT arteriography, CT portography, digital subtraction angiography, or arteriography are not performed.

Dynamic CT

Early enhancement of hepatocellular carcinoma is related to its tumor vascularity which is derived from the hepatic artery. Delayed enhancement is a result of slow diffusion of contrast into an abnormality large extravascular space. The use of dynamic scanning probably improves detection rate versus non-dynamic techniques. Inamoto et al. (10) detected 81% of hepatocellular carcinomas <5 cm in diameter and 70% of those <2 cm in diameter. During the arterial phase 80% of their tumors enhanced either partially or completely. At 40-60 sec there was frequently a hyperdense periphery and a hypodense center. Delayed scans showed disappearance of the lesion in 10%. Although the surgical specimen showed a capsule in 67% of their cases, it could be detected on CT in only 6% as either a low density rim on noncontrast scans or an enhanced ring on postcontrast scans. One case has been reported in which dynamic CT demonstrated an otherwise isodense hepatocellular carcinoma by showing distorted intrahepatic vasculature (11).

Dynamic CT is a useful adjunct to arteriography in determining resectability (12, 13). Performed as a separate study to evaluate venous involvement, dynamic CT can be done at the level of the tumor, the level of the main portal vein (Fig. 5.85C-E) and the dome of the liver (hepatic veins and inferior vena cava). Endovenous tumor is usually persistently lucent although arterial phase enhancement can occur due to tumor vascularity (Fig. 5.85D) (13-15). Frequently, however, there is linear, periportal, arterial phase hypervascularity (tram-track) secondary to enhancement via the portal vasa vasorum (Fig. 5.85E) (13, 16). At times an invaded lobar portal vein is nonvisualized and replaced by poorly defined arterial hypervascularity (correlate of angiographic thread and streaks) (Fig. 5.85C) (13). Another sign of portal vein occlusion is lobar hypodensity on precontrast scans (possibly from fatty infiltration secondary to ischemia) (13, 17). Arterioportal shunting occurs distal to an occluded portal vein branch and is manifested by contrast appearing in the portal vein in the arterial phase (4, 17, 18). Finally, the following also suggest tumor in the portal vein: portal vein density 20-30 HU < the aorta after contrast, main portal vein diameter >3 cm (normal 2 ± 0.4 cm) and dilatation of a lobar portal vein branch >2 cm (normal 1.4 ± 0.4 cm (13)). Differentiation of tumor thrombus from bland thrombus is difficult unless the thrombus enhances. However, in the clinical setting of known hepatocellular carcinoma, thrombus in one or more of the portal veins is nearly always due to tumor, especially when the affected vein is enlarged.

Dynamic CT or CT arteriography is useful in documenting the presence of a disease-free lateral segment of the left lobe (often a challenge for conventional arteriography). Surgical planning is facilitated by good demonstration of the hepatic veins by dynamic CT as these veins demarcate hepatic segments and surgical planes (19). A discussion of the CT findings in hepatocellular carcinoma invading the hepatic veins and or inferior vena cava can be found under the heading "Budd-Chiari syndrome."

Several institutions have begun to evaluate the use of CT arteriography (CTA) for increased accuracy in the detection of hepatocellular carcinoma. CTA is a technique whereby contrast is infused with a pump at the rate of 1-5 ml/sec or injected manually as a 10-25-ml bolus through an intrahepatic arterial catheter with dynamic scans being obtained in the arterial and portal phase (20). Early reports by Prando et al. (21) and Freeny and Marks (14) showed significant improvement over conventional enhancement technique. Prando evaluated 12 patients and in 10 of them CTA improved tumor detection. In 6 of the 10 patients it was the only method that accurately detected the full extent of disease. Of the 12 patients one had a hepatocellular carcinoma which was well seen with CTA but not detected on noncontrast or standard infusion scans. Freeny and Marks evaluated 22 patients with CTA and in 12 cases (55%) additional tumor nodules were detected. Nakao et al. (22) evaluated 32 patients with hepatocellular carcinoma with CTA. The contrast material was infused into both the hepatic and superior mesenteric arteries. CTA was successful in detecting both the primary tumor and early infiltration of the portal vein. All authors agree that CTA should be reserved for those patients in whom hepatic lobectomy is contemplated, or in whom there is a discrepancy between different imaging modalities (14, 20–22).

CT portography (23, 24) is a variation of CTA and is performed with contrast infusion into the mesenteric artery at 0.4–0.6 ml/sec. The infusion is begun 30 seconds prior to scanning and is continued throughout the scanning time. Dynamic sequential CT with automatic table incrementation is necessary to cover the entire liver and takes 2–3 min of scanning time and 70–100 ml of contrast material. Lesions as small as 0.5 cm in diameter can be detected as lucencies surrounded by enhanced hepatic parenchyma. The techique enhances normal parenchyma maximally and masses are enhanced minimally. It may be the most sensitive means of detecting invasion of the liver hilum and portal vein.

Regions of hepatic parenchyma without a portal blood supply (distal to an obstructed portal vein) must not be confused with neoplasm. The former are wedge-shaped segmental low density regions extending from the liver hilum to its surface or a segmental boundary, similar to perfusion defects seen on lung scans in patients with pulmonary embolism (24).

In the future, CT of the liver using EOE-13 may prove to be the most sensitive CT method of detecting and staging hepatocellular carcinoma.

REFERENCES

1. Itai Y, Nishikawa J, Tasaka A: Computed tomography in the evaluation of hepatocellular carcinoma. *Radiology* 131:165–170, 1979.
2. Inamoto K, Sugiki K, Yamasaki H, Nakao N, Miura T: Computed tomography and angiography of hepatocellular carcinoma. *J Comput Assist Tomogr* 4:832–839, 1980.
3. Moss AA, Schrumpf J, Schnyder P, Korobkin M, Shimshak RR: Computed tomography of focal hepatic lesions: a blind clinical evaluation of the effects of contrast enhancement. *Radiology* 131:427–430, 1979.
4. Kunstlinger F, Federle MP, Moss AA, Marks W: Computed tomography of hepatocellular carcinoma. *AJR* 134:431–437, 1980.
5. Dunnick NR, Ihde DC, Doppman JL, Bates HR: Computed tomography in primary hepatocellular carcinoma. *J Comput Assist Tomogr* 4:59–62, 1980.
6. Hosoki T, Chatani M, Mori S: Dynamic computed tomography of hepatocellular carcinoma. *AJR* 193:1099–1106, 1982.
7. Itai Y, Araki T, Ferui S, Tasaka A: Differential diagnosis of hepatic masses on computed tomography with particular reference to hepatocellular carcinoma. *J Comput Assist Tomogr* 5:834–842, 1981.
8. Takashima T, Matsui O, Suzuki M, Ida M: Diagnosis and screening of small hepatocellular carcinomas. *Radiology* 145:635–638, 1982.
9. LaBerge JM, Laing FC, Federle MP, Jeffrey RB Jr, Lim RC Jr: Hepatocellular carcinoma: assessment of resectability by computed tomography and ultrasound. *Radiology* 152:485–490, 1984.
10. Inamoto K, Tanaka S, Yamazaki H, Okamoto E: Computed tomography in the detection of small hepatocellular carcinomas. *Gastrointest Radiol* 8:321–326, 1983.
11. Itai Y, Araki T, Furui S, Tasaka A: Differential diagnosis of hepatic masses on CT with particular reference to hepatocellular carcinoma. *J Comput Assist Tomogr* 5:834–842, 1981.
12. Marks WM, Jacobs RP, Goodman PC, Lim RC Jr: Hepatocellular carcinoma: clinical and angiographic findings and predictability for surgical resection. *AJR* 132:7–11, 1979.
13. Mathieu D, Grenier P, Larde D, Vasile N: Portal vein involvement in hepatocellular carcinoma: dynamic CT features. *Radiology* 152:127–132, 1984.
14. Freeny PC, Marks WM: CT arteriography of the liver. *Radiology* 148:193–197, 1983.
15. Suzuki M, Itoh H, Konishi H, Ida M, Matsui O, Takashima T: Hepatocellular carcinoma involving the portal vein. *J Comput Assist Tomogr* 6:831–832, 1982.
16. Vigo M, DeFuveri D, Biondetti PR, Benedetti L: CT demonstration of portal and superior mesenteric vein thrombosis in hepatocellular carcinoma. *J Comput Assist Tomogr* 4:627–629, 1980.
17. Inamoto K, Tanaka S, Yamazaki H, Hayashi T, Hidaka H, Miura K: Arterioportal fistula in hepatocellular carcinoma. *J Comput Assist Tomogr* 7:1251–1253, 1983.
18. Foley WD, Varma RR, Lawson TL, Berland LL, Smith DF, Thorsen MK: Dynamic CT and duplex ultrasonography: adjuncts to arterial portography. *J Comput Assist Tomogr* 7:77–82, 1983.
19. Pagani JJ: Intrahepatic vascular territories shown by CT: the value of CT in determining resectability of hepatic tumors. *Radiology* 147:173–178, 1983.
20. Clark RA, Matsui O: CT of liver tumors. *Semin Roentgenol* 18:149–162, 1983.
21. Prando A, Wallace S, Bernardino ME, Lindell NM Jr: Computed tomographic arteriography of the liver. *Radiology* 130:697–701, 1979.
22. Nakao N, Mirua K, Takayaso Y, Wada Y, Miura T: CT arteriography in hepatocellular carcinoma. *J Comput Assist Tomogr* 7:780–787, 1983.
23. Clark RA, Matsui D: CT of liver tumors. *Semin Roentgenol* 18:149–162, 1983.
24. Matsui O, Takashima T, Kadoya M, Kitagawa K, Kamimura R, Itoh H, Suzuki M, Ida M: Segmental staining on hepatic arteriography as a sign of intrahepatic portal vein obstruction. *Radiology* 152:601–606, 1984.

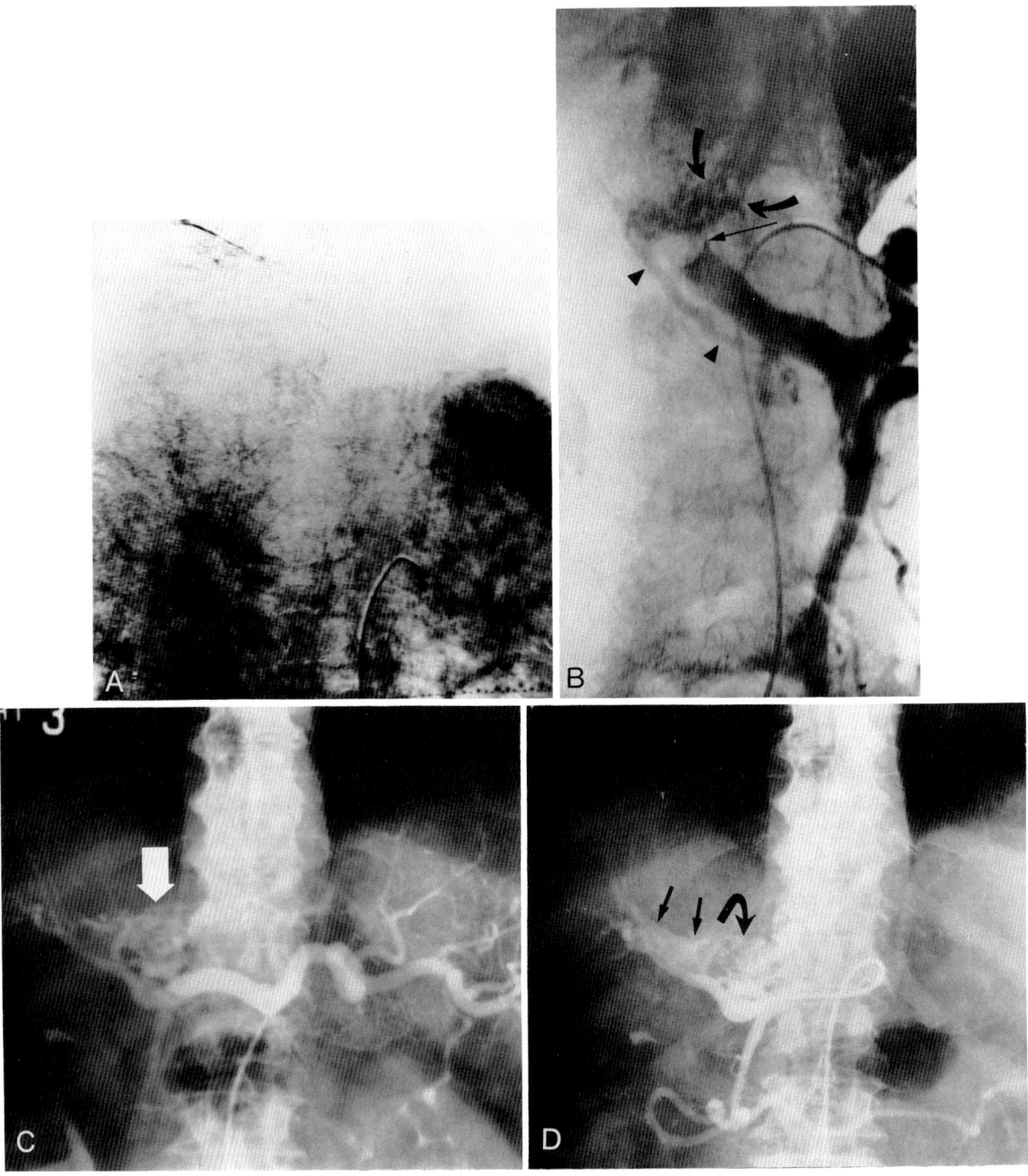

FIGURE 5.87. DIFFUSE HEPATOCELLULAR CARCINOMA WITH PORTAL INVASION

A: Subtraction print shows tumor stain throughout the liver. *B:* Venous phase shows portal vein occlusion (*arrow*), a portal-portal collateral (*arrowheads*), and the thread and streaks sign of tumor thrombus in the left portal vein (*curved arrows*). *C–G:* Rapid A-V shunting in another patient with portal vein invasion. Celiac angiogram shows irregular portal opacification in the arterial phase (*C, arrow*). Selective hepatic injection shows rapid portal filling (*D, straight arrows*) and thrombus within the vein (*D, curved arrow*). Superselective injection shows hypervascular tumor in the right lobe (*E* and *F, arrows*). CT showed extensive tumor (*G, arrows*).

Angiography

Diagnostic Features

Classically, angiography of hepatocellular carcinoma shows a hypervascular mass with tumor angioneogenesis, marked tumor blush, sometimes enlarged feeding arteries, arteriovenous shunting with rapid clearing (Fig. 5.87C and D), some puddling, and early draining veins (Figs. 5.83, 5.84, 5.88, and 5.89). Serration of artery walls can be seen, corresponding to encasement by tumor (Fig. 5.90). Invasion into portal and/or hepatic veins can occur with subsequent development of portal hypertension (Fig. 5.87). Tumor thrombus within major veins is usually demonstrated during the venous phase, but it is sometimes itself hypervascular, appearing in the arterial phase (thread and streaks sign) (1–4). Optimal evaluation of the portal system often requires arterial portography with injection of a vasodilator prior to injection of contrast material. The better differentiated tumors are highly vascular while the more anaplastic ones are poorly vascularized (5). A small percentage of hepatocellular carcinomas are hypovascular-to-avascular compared to the liver parenchyma (5) (Fig. 5.90). Percentage quoted varies due to dif-

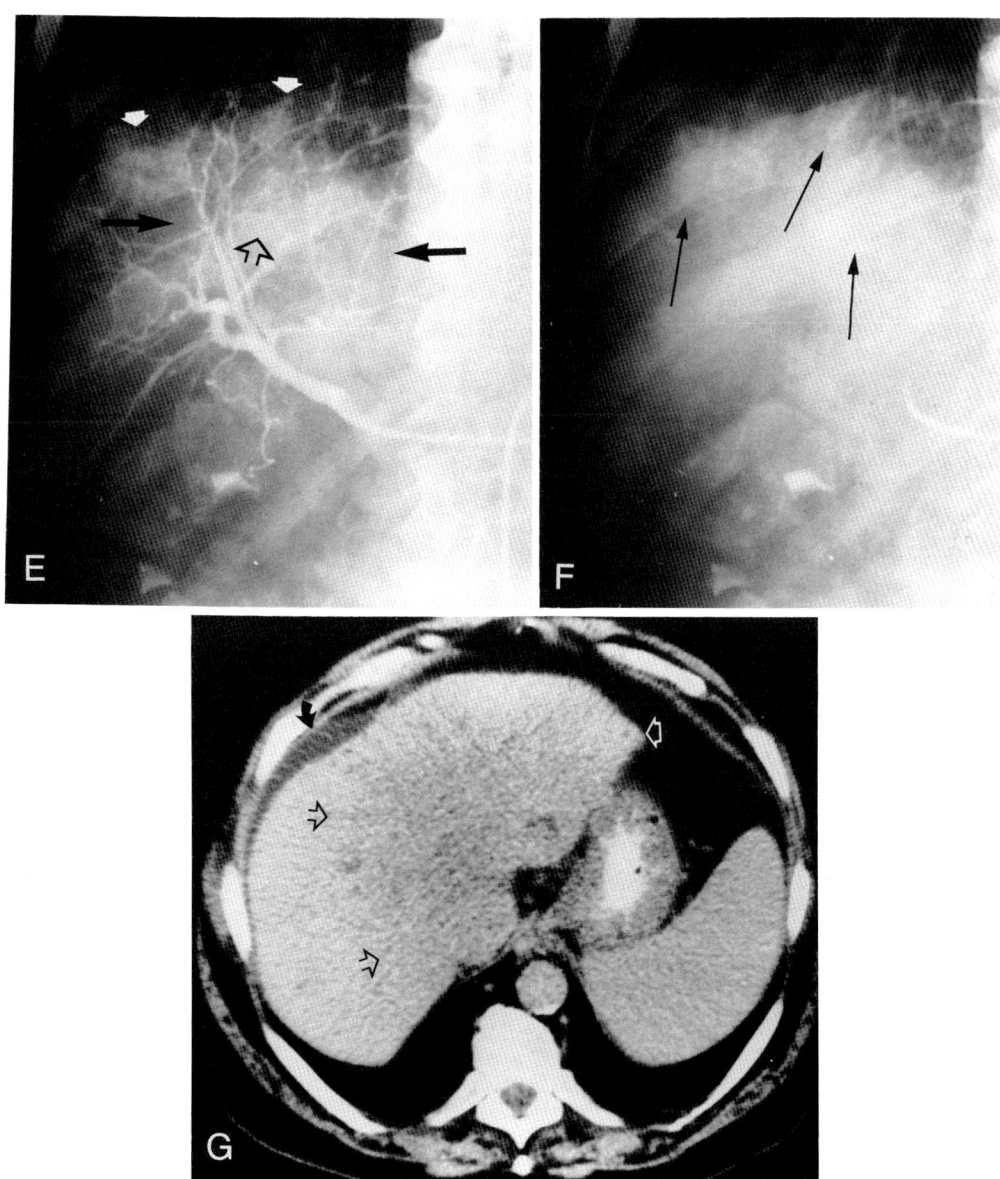

FIGURE 5.87E–G

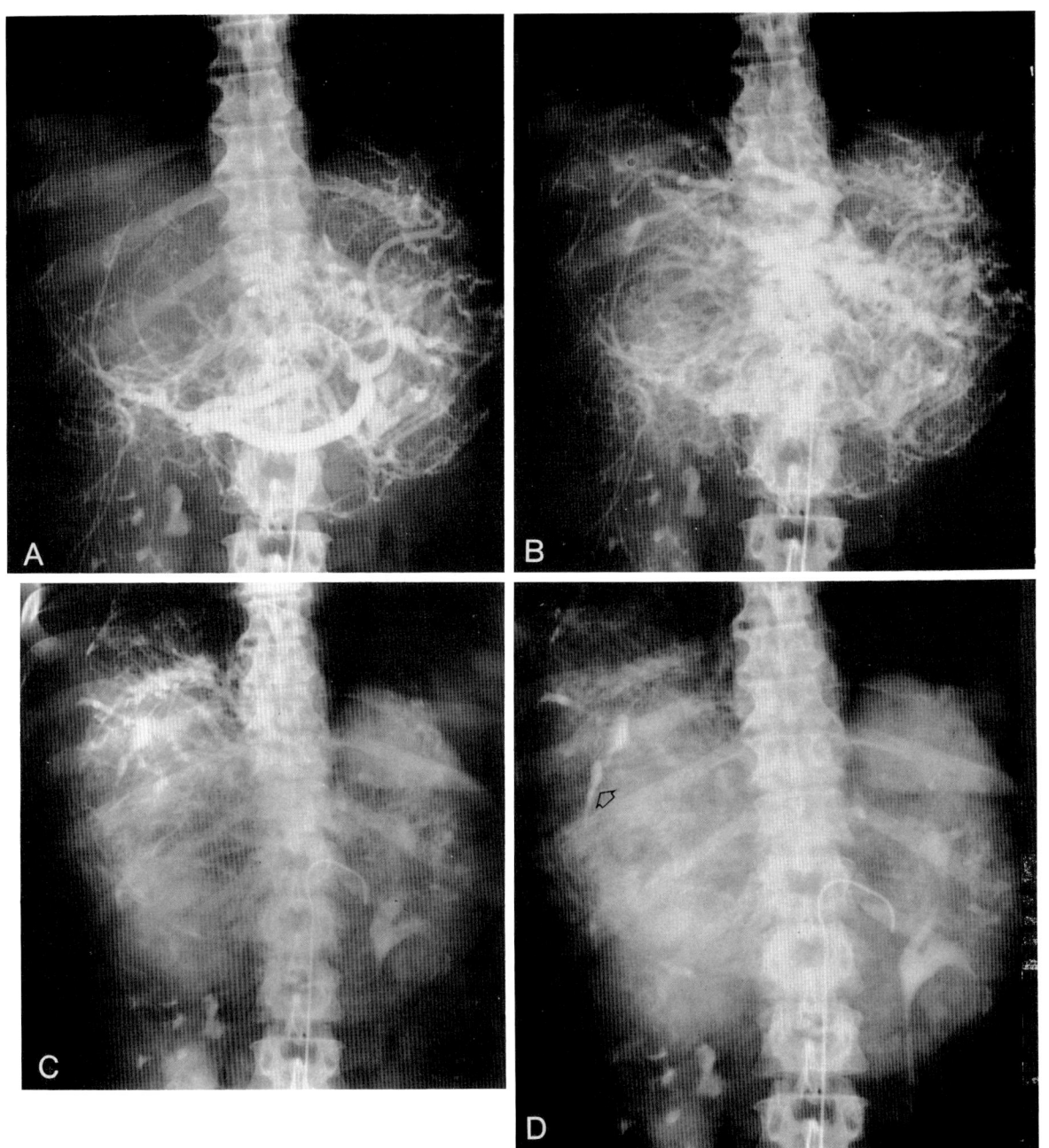

FIGURE 5.88. HYPERVASCULAR HEPATOCELLULAR CARCINOMA

Hypervascular hepatocellular carcinoma: Celiac angiogram demonstrates a large, hypervascular mass involving both lobes of the liver with hypertrophied arterial branches, tumor neovascularity (A and B), and bizarre venous opacification with persistence of contrast media in abnormally dilated veins (C and D).

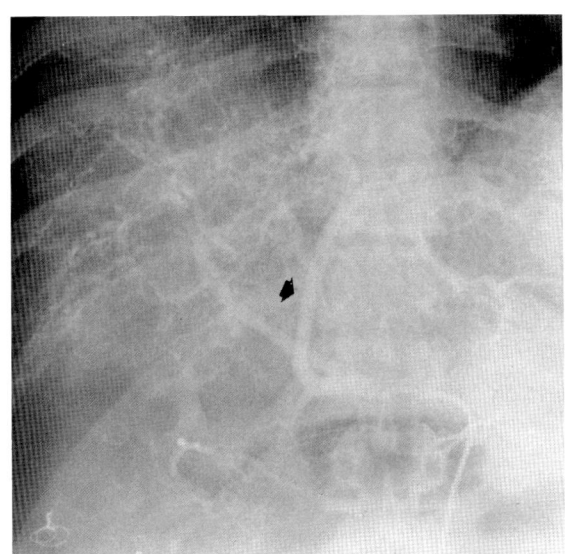

FIGURE 5.89. DIFFUSE NEOVASCULARITY IN HEPATOCELLULAR CARCINOMA

Right common hepatic arteriogram shows corkscrewed vessels compatible with cirrhosis and diffuse neovascularity of peripheral branches consistent with hepatocellular carcinoma. The enlarged left hepatic artery (*arrow*) and the left lobe neovascularity indicate that the neoplasm is diffuse throughout the liver.

ferences in population and technique and different definitions of vascularity, but 5–10% is a reasonable estimate (3, 5). Some hepatocellular carcinomas have a vascular rim surrounding a central avascular region corresponding to intratumoral hemorrhage (5).

Multicentric hepatocellular carcinomas (usually hypervascular, occasionally hypovascular) are difficult to distinguish from metastatic disease by angiography. Appropriate clinical setting and vascular invasion suggest hepatocellular carcinoma. Diffuse hepatocellular carcinoma, which may be anaplastic and hypovascular, is often difficult to diagnose angiographically especially when superimposed upon cirrhosis (as is usually the case in the diffuse form). This problem is further exacerbated by the possible presence of macroregenerating nodules in cirrhosis which can mimic hypovascular hepatocellular carcinoma angiographically (6). When possible, correlation of the angiographic mass with a region of increased uptake on a sulfur colloid scan is quite helpful in reaching a correct diagnosis of regenerating nodule.

Staging

Using celiac and/or selective hepatic injections, most disease will be uncovered (Fig. 5.84*A–I*). Superselective catheterization may be necessary to ascertain whether the vascular supply of the tumor(s) crosses intralobar segments and to detect satellite nodules (5). Injection of the main hepatic artery or its branches allows the detection of hypervascular nodules on the order of 1 cm in size, but hypovascular lesions less than 2 cm may well escape detection (7, 8). Arterial portography will show tumor thrombi in the portal veins when present as occlusions, and a corresponding perfusion defect will be seen in the portal hepatogram.

Infusion hepatic angiography (IHA) employs the injection of 50 ml of contrast into the hepatic artery over 10 sec as compared to 15–20 ml in 2–3 sec in conventional arteriography (CHA) (7). Filming is extended to 40 seconds as opposed to 20 sec in CHA. Small hypovascular foci less than 2 cm in diameter can be detected in the capillary phase of IHA that are invisible in the arterial phase of IHA and invisible on CHA. Tumor foci are stained with contrast material during IHA and normal liver parenchyma is "washed out" by unopacified portal blood allowing superior detection of disease. The same principle can be used in CT arteriography (Fig. 5.84*J–M*) (7, 9). IHA will probably improve evaluation of the left lobe, which is a difficult area for CHA. A potential pitfall in IHA is segmental staining, which is staining of a hepatic segment whose portal supply is occluded (10). This is always accompanied by increased visualization of small peripheral arterial branches and sometimes by retrograde filling of the obstructed portal veins(s) (10). Although a useful sign of portal vein obstruction, segmental staining can obscure actual depiction of the hepatocellular carcinoma responsible for the portal vein occlusion. Segmental staining is thought to caused by shunting, either transsinusoidal or peripheral arterioportal. It occurs only rarely with CHA.

Angiographic evaluation of the hepatic veins and inferior vena cava for possible invasion by hepatocellular carcinoma is described under the "Budd-Chiari Syndrome."

Once the diagnosis is histologically established, sonography and CT should be performed (if they have not already been done) in an attempt to establish unresectability. Biopsy proof of lymph nodes or liver masses to prove unresectability is advisable as adenopathy could be reactive and a hepatic nodule could be an incidental hemangioma. If the hepatocellular carcinoma is still considered resectable after these and other conventional staging procedures (chest x-ray, bone scan, etc) dynamic CT should prob-

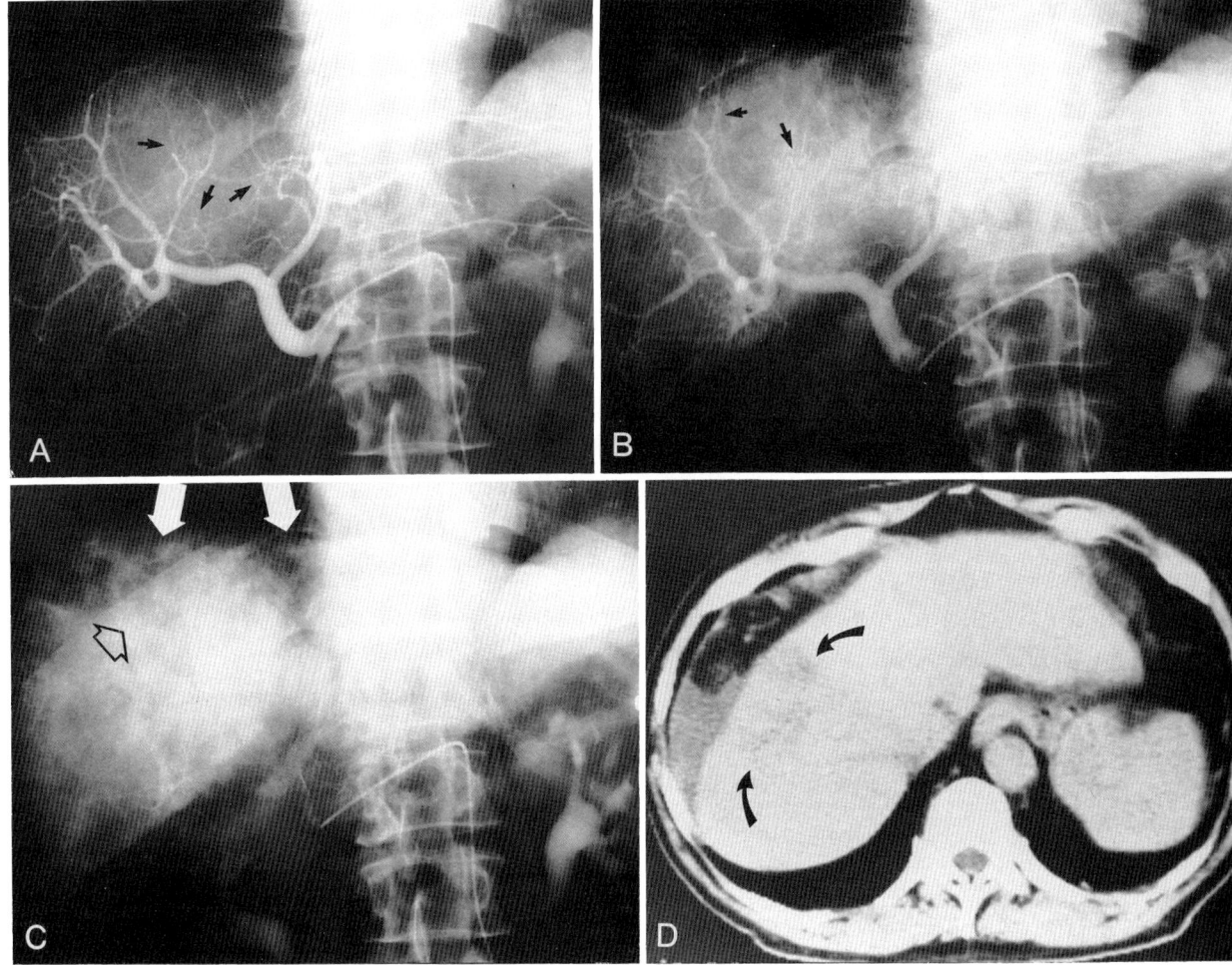

FIGURE 5.90. HYPOVASCULAR HEPATOCELLULAR CARCINOMA
Hypovascular hepatocellular carcinoma, macronodular cirrhosis: displaced and stretched arteries in right lobe by regenerating nodules with encased, serrated arteries (*arrows*) in regions of tumor (*A* and *B*). The hepatogram shows multiple smooth defects from regenerating nodules and defects from infiltrating tumor (*arrows*) in both right and left lobes (*C*). Extent of tumor was not shown as well by CT (*arrows*, *D*), but technique was not optimal (low dose contrast).

ably be done next. Finally, angiography, especially IHA and if feasible, CT arteriography/portography can show unresectability even when all non-invasive studies suggest the opposite.

REFERENCES

1. Reuter SR, Redman HC, Siders DB: The spectrum of angiographic findings in hepatoma. *Radiology* 94:89–94, 1970.
2. Kido C, Sasaki T, Kaneko M: Angiography of primary liver cancer. *AJR* 113:70–82, 1971.
3. Chuang VP: Hepatic tumor angiography: a subject review. *Radiology* 148:633–639, 1983.
4. Okuda K, Musha H, Yoshuda T, Kanda Y, Yamakazo T, Jinnouchi S, Moriyama M, Kawaguchi S, Kubo Y, Shimokawa Y, Kojiro M, Kuratonii S, Sakamoto K, Nakashima T: Demonstration of growing casts of hepatocellular carcinoma in the portal vein by celiac angiography: the thread and streaks sign. *Radiology* 117:303–309, 1975.
5. Marks WM, Jacobs RP, Goodman PC, Lim RC Jr: Hepatocellular carcinoma: clinical and angiographic findings and predictability for surgical resection. *AJR* 132:7–11, 1979.
6. Rabinowitz JG, Kinkabwala M, Ulreich S: Macroregenerating nodule in the cirrhotic liver. *AJR* 121:401–411, 1974.
7. Tashashima T, Matsui O: Infusion hepatic angiography in the detection of small hepatocellular carcinomas. *Radiology* 136:321–325, 1980.
8. Baum S: Hepatic arteriography. In Abrams HL (ed): *Angiography: Vascular and Interventional Radiology.* Boston, Little, Brown, 1983, pp 1492–1497.
9. Chuang V: Pitfalls of CT in the detection of hepatic masses and indication for hepatic arteriography. Presneted at the 14th Annual Meeting and Postgraduate Course of the Society of Gastrointestinal Radiologists, Napa, California, September 29 to October 3, 1984.
10. Matsui O, Takashima T, Kadoga M, Kitagawa K, Kanumura R, Itoh H, Suzuki M, Ida M: Segmental staining on hepatic arteriography as a sign of intrahepatic portal vein obstruction. *Radiology* 152:601–606, 1984.

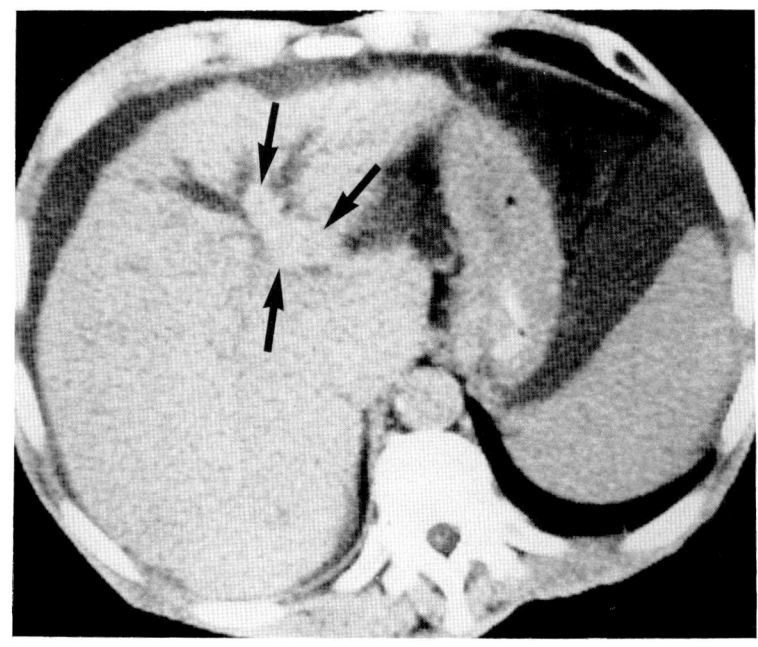

FIGURE 5.91. ISOLATED LEFT DUCTAL OBSTRUCTION BY HEPATOCELLULAR CARCINOMA
Obstruction limited to the left lobe ducts by an enhancing hepatocellular carcinoma (*arrows*). Slight liver hyperdensity due to hemochromatosis, and ascites.

Cholangiography

Mechanisms for hepatocellular carcinoma-induced biliary obstruction include: pedunculated tumor extension into the extrahepatic ducts, plugging by clot or tumor debris, direct invasion of the intrahepatic ducts, and metastatic lymph node compression of duct(s) in the porta hepatis (1). Careful examination of biliary debris and "mud" may yield a cytologic diagnosis. Hepatocellular carcinoma can also cause localized intrahepatic duct obstruction with proximal dilatation (Fig. 5.91) (2). Such patients may not be jaundiced due to the functional reserve of the liver.

Findings on direct cholangiography most commonly consist of bulky, smooth or lobulated and slightly irregular obstructing intraluminal mass(es) in the proximal extrahepatic duct (Fig. 5.92) (1). Distal common duct filling defects, when seen, usually represent clot or tumor debris. The degree of obstruction can be total or there may be only mild to moderate proximal dilatation. Occasionally intra or extrahepatic ducts are displaced by mass effect, but marked stenosis in such cases is uncommon (1). Obstruction by metastatic lymph nodes from hepatocellular carcinoma in the porta hepatis is rarely distinguishable by cholangiography from other causes of lymphadenopathy in the porta (Fig. 5.93).

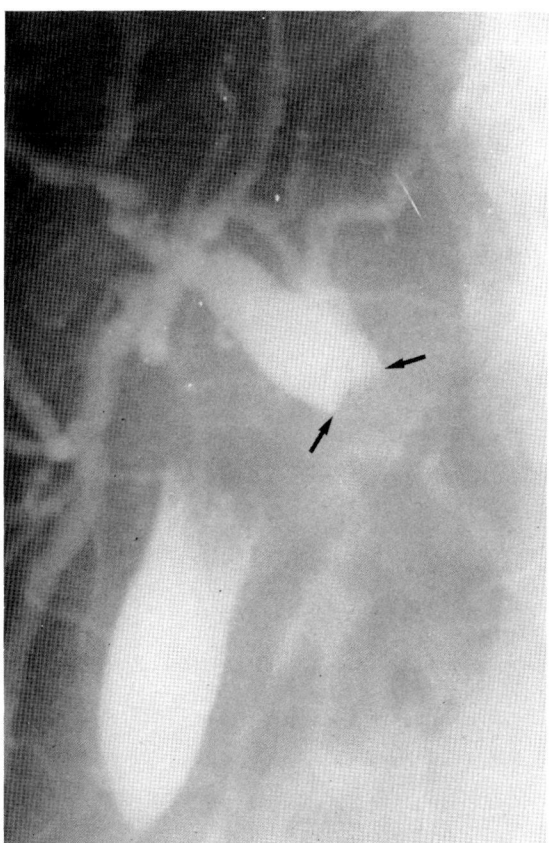

FIGURE 5.92. TRANSHEPATIC CHOLANGIOGRAM
Transhepatic cholangiogram: obstruction of the common duct by hepatocellular carcinoma (*arrows*).

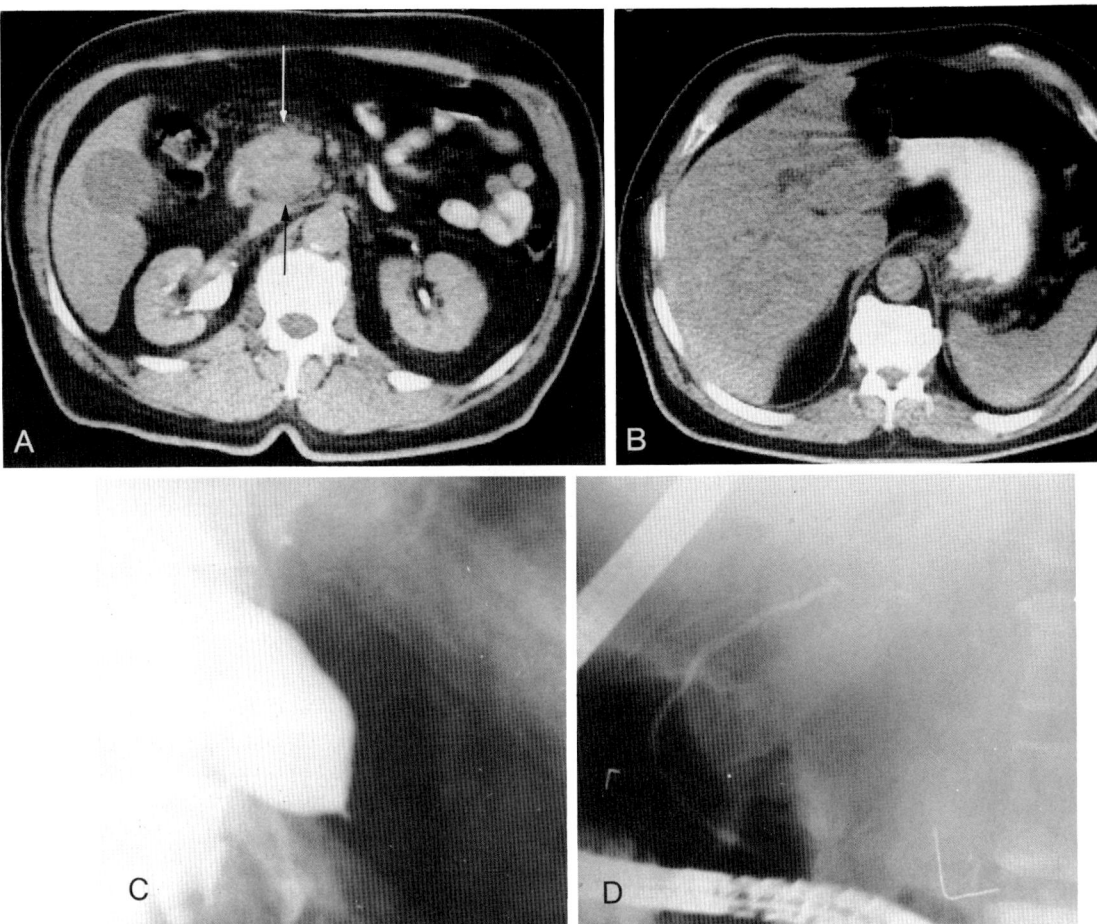

FIGURE 5.93. DIFFUSELY INFILTRATIVE HEPATOCELLULAR CARCINOMA
Diffusely infiltrative hepatocellular carcinoma invisible on CT presenting as common bile duct obstruction from peripancreatic adenopathy in an alcoholic. A and B: Drip infusion CT shows a mass in the head and uncinate process of the pancreas (arrows) and dilated intrahepatic ducts. No liver parenchymal abnormalities were seen. C: Transhepatic cholangiogram shows complete obstruction of the suprapancreatic common bile duct mimicking carcinoma of the pancreas. D: Normal endoscopic pancreatogram. The liver was diffusely infiltrated by hepatocellular carcinoma at surgery. Dynamic CT might have shown intrahepatic tumor.

REFERENCES

1. vanSonnenberg E, Ferrucci JT Jr: Bile duct obstruction in hepatocellular carcinoma (hepatoma)-clinical and cholangiographic characteristics. Radiology 130:7–13, 1979.
2. Araki T, Itai Y, Tasaka A: Computed tomography of localized dilatation of the intrahepatic bile ducts. Radiology 141:733–736, 1981.

Digital Subtraction Angiography

Early experience suggests that intraarterial digital subtraction arteriography (IA-DSA) can detect and stage hepatocellular carcinomas with the same accuracy as conventional arteriography (1, 2). Advantages of IA-DSA include use of smaller volumes of contrast material, superb arterial portography, improved evaluation of the left lobe because of removal of overlapping bone, and reduced film cost. Disadvantages include limited field of view and inability to evaluate arteries less than 1 mm. in diameter because of reduced spatial resolution. The role, if any, of IA-DSA vis-à-vis conventional arteriography in the radiologic evaluation of hepatocellular carcinoma awaits the results of larger series for definition.

REFERENCES

1. Flannigan BD, Gomes AS, Stambuk EC, Lois JF, Pais SO: Intraarterial digital subtraction angiography: comparison with conventional hepatic arteriography. Radiology 148:17–21, 1983.

2. Ariyama J: Intraarterial digital subtraction angiography. Presented at the fourteenth annual meeting and postgraduate course, Society of Gastrointestinal Radiologists, Sept. 29–Oct. 3, 1984.

Lipiodol-CT Studies

When 2–5 ml of Lipiodol (Andre-Gelbe Laboratories, France) are dripped into the common or proper hepatic artery after arteriography, plain films show immediate opacification of large hepatocellular carcinomas. CT scans shortly afterwards demonstrate diffuse hepatic opacification (not necessarily uniform) with greater opacification in and around tumors. CT 7–10 days later shows excellent contrast between normal parenchyma and neoplasm, as the contrast has cleared from the former to a large extent. It is still recognizable within the latter for periods up to one year, making the technique useful for follow-up. The Lipiodol-CT scan can detect hepatocellular carcinomas as small as 3.7 mm in diameter. In one large series, it detected many more satellite nodules than sonography, conventional and dynamic CT, and angiography (11). It may prove to be an invaluable technique for staging. The proposed mechanism for the marked difference in tissue clearance between hepatic parenchyma and hepatocellular carcinoma is the lack of lymphatics and Kupffer cells in hepatocellular carcinomas (1). Patterns of retention in cavernous hemangiomas and metastatic lesions appear different, suggesting some usefulness in differential diagnosis. Small fibrotic or necrotic hepatocellular carcinomas may go undetected by Lipiodol-CT because of the inability of the contrast to get into the tumor (1).

Transcatheter Gelfoam embolization following arterial infusion of Lipiodol mixed with chemotherapeutic agents has shown promise as palliative therapy in hepatocellular carcinoma (1, 2).

REFERENCES

1. Yumoto Y, Jinno K, Tokuyama K, Araki Y, Ishimitsu T, Maeda H, Konno T, Iwamoto S, Ohnishi K, Okuda K: Hepatocellular carcinoma detected by iodized oil. *Radiology* 154:19–24, 1985.
2. Ohishi H, Uchida H, Yoshimura H, Ohue S, Ueda J, Katsuragi M, Matsuo N, Hosogi Y: Hepatocellular carcinoma detected by iodized oil. *Radiology* 154:25–29, 1985.

Nuclear Medicine

Hepatocellular carcinomas are usually manifest as a single photopenic region on a liver/spleen scan (about 70%); other less common appearances include multiple space-occupying defects (15–20%) (Fig. 5.94) and a heterogeneous distribution of tracer throughout the liver (about 10%). It is extremely unusual for Kupffer cells to be present within the tumor in a quantity sufficient to cause sulfur colloid avidity (1–3). About 70–90% of hepatocellular carcinomas are gallium avid (Fig. 5.94). Uptake is reduced in less vascular tumors and in those with marked necrosis, and moderately to well-differentiated tumors show the strongest uptake (4). The gallium scan should be interpreted in conjunction with a sulfur colloid scan to better appreciate a small degree of uptake in the former by comparison to the cold region on the latter.

Radionuclide angiography using ^{99m}Tc-labeled red cells usually reveals augmented flow in sizable hepatocellular carcinomas. Delayed blood pool images (1–2 hr) are usually cold, but occasionally show increased activity. Even in the latter instance, there is not increased blood pool activity out of proportion to the flow as there is in cavernous hemangioma (5, 6).

Until recently, there were only scattered case reports of Tc-IDA or related tracer uptake in hepatocellular carcinomas (7), most lesions being cold. A small series recently reported uptake in four of four cases, however (8). Delayed scans were necessary to demonstrate Tc-IDA uptake. The findings of Lee and coworkers (8) were as follows: the hepatogram phase of hepatobiliary scintigraphy (5–15 min) shows the tumor as a cold region relative to the surrounding normal parenchyma. Delayed scans from 30 min to 4 hr disclose increased tumor activity compared to the diminishing activity in the normal liver. Pulmonary metastases accumulated activity as well. The postulated mechanism is that hepatocellular carcinomas that concentrate hepatobiliary tracers are well-differentiated enough to make some bile but are unable to rapidly excrete it due to a lack of functioning biliary ducts. Therefore they are cold relative to normal parenchyma initially, but gradually become relatively hot as the normal liver excretes its activity. If Lee's results can be duplicated, hepatobiliary scintigraphy could become an important tool in differential diagnosis of hepatic mass lesions and staging of hepatocellular carcinomas. A caveat should be noted: the finding of a mass lesion that is hot on IDA and cold on sulfur colloid has a differential diagnosis that includes hepatic adenoma, regenerating nodule, and breast metastasis (9). Conversely, a normal IDA scan cannot rule out hepatocellular carcinoma, as the latter

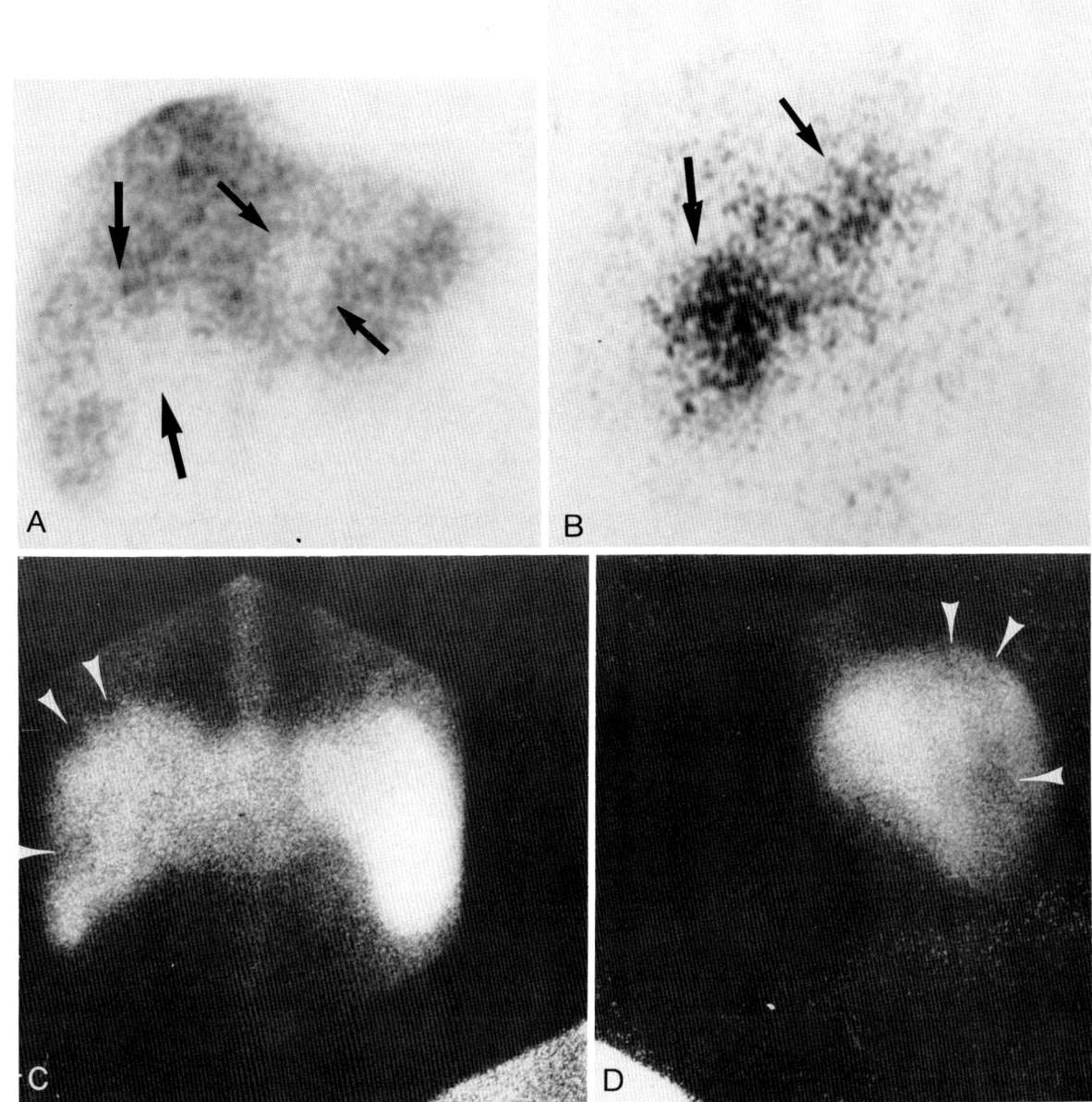

FIGURE 5.94. MULTIFOCAL HEPATOCELLULAR CARCINOMA

A and *B:* Multifocal hepatocellular carcinoma, cold on sulfur colloid scan (*arrows, A*) and hot on gallium scan (*arrows, B*). The patchy and poor uptake seen on the colloid scan is due to underlying cirrhosis. *C* and *D:* Hepatocellular carcinoma superimposed on cirrhosis. Anterior (*C*) and lateral (*D*) views from a sulfur colloid scan show two space-occupying peripheral lesions (*arrowheads*). Note colloid shift and bone marrow uptake.

could be isointense (unless delayed images are obtained) (9).

^{99m}Tc-labeled bone scanning agents may, on occasion, be taken up by hepatocellular carcinomas (10). The exact mechanism is unknown but radiologically or even histologically demonstrable calcification is not a prerequisite.

Radioimmunoglobulin Therapy

^{131}I-Antiferritin IgG is preferentially bound by hepatocellular carcinoma. This agent has induced remissions in 40% of hepatocellular carcinoma patients for up to 3 yr (11). CT scans are useful adjuncts for determining liver and tumor

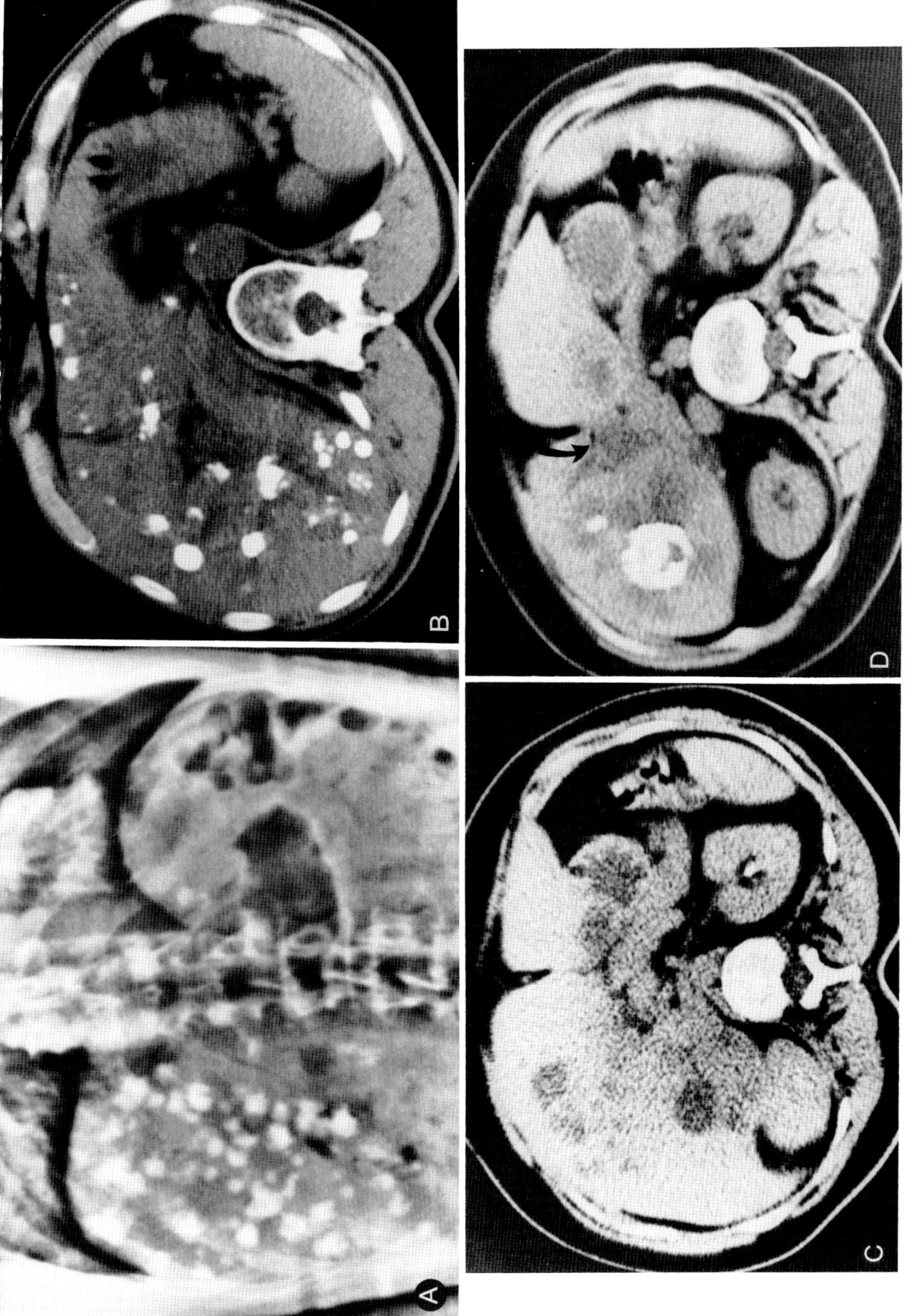

FIGURE 5.95. CT MONITORING OF RADIONUCLIDE RADIOTHERAPY

A and B: Completely calcified, successfully treated multifocal hepatocellular carcinoma. Topogram (A) and scan (B). C and D: Recurrence. Scan in 1979 (C) shows extensive disease. Two years later (D) one region has extensively calcified, the lesion in the lateral segment of the left lobe is unchanged, but a new lesion is present in the medial segment of the left lobe (arrow) adjacent to the intersegmental fissure.

volumes prior to treatment and for monitoring the success of the therapy (12). Disappearance of visible tumor and/or extensive tumor calcification appear to be good prognostic signs (Fig. 5.95).

REFERENCES

1. Alavi A, Arger P: *Abdomen-Multiple Imaging Procedures,* Vol 3, New York, Grune & Stratton, 1980.
2. Freeman L, Johnson P: *Clinical Scintillation Imaging.* New York, Grune & Stratton, 1975.
3. Siegel B, Alazraki N, Alderson P et al: *Nuclear Radiology Syllabus* (second series). Chicago, American College of Radiology, 1978.
4. Waxman AD, Richmond R, Juttner H, Siemsen JK, Heffelinger MJ, Fink E: Corelation of contrast angiography and histologic pattern with gallium uptake in primary liver-cell carcinoma: noncorrelation with alpha-feto protein. Concise communication. *J Nucl Med* 21:324–327, 1980.
5. Rabinowitz SA, McKusick KA, Strauss HW: ^{99m}Tc red blood cell scintigraphy in evaluating focal liver lesions. *AJR* 143:63–68, 1984.
6. Engel MA, Marks DS, Sandler MA, Shetty P: Differentiating focal intrahepatic lesions with ^{99m}Tc-red blood cell imaging. *AJR* 146:777–782, 1983.
7. Utz JA, Lull RJ, Anderson JH, Lambrecht RW, Brown JM, Henry W: Hepatoma visualization with ^{99m}Tc-pyridoxylidene glutamate. *J Nucl Med* 21:747–749, 1980.
8. Lee VW, O'Brien MJ, Devereux DF, Morris PM, Shapiro JH: Hepatocellular carcinoma: uptake of ^{99m}Tc-IDA in primary tumor and metastasis. *AJR* 143:57–61, 1984.
9. Vincent LM, Renner JB: Uptake of hepatobiliary agents by hepatocellular carcinoma (1). *AJR* 143:1119–1120, 1984.
10. Desai AG, Schaffer B, Park CH: Accumulation of bone-scanning agents in hepatoma. *Radiology* 149:292, 1983.
11. Order SE: Radioimmunoglobulin therapy of cancer. *Compr Ther* 10:9–18, 1984.
12. Leichner PK, Klein JK, Garrison JB, Jenkins RE, Nickoloff EL, Ettinger DS, Order SE: Dosimetry of ^{131}I-labeled anti-ferritin in hepatoma: a model for radioimmunoglobulin dosimetry. *Int J Radiat Oncol Biol Phys* 7:323–333, 1981.

Fibrolamellar Hepatocellular Carcinoma

This recently described neoplasm has been confused both with focal nodular hyperplasia and hepatic adenoma (1, 2). It has epidemiologic, clinical, and pathological features distinct from other hepatocellular carcinoma (1–6).

Clinical Findings

Age range is 5–35 yr with a mean of 23 yr and no sex predilection (1, 2). Patients do not have underlying cirrhosis nor are there any known predisposing risk factors (1, 2). Presenting symptoms include abdominal pain, malaise, hepatomegaly, and jaundice (1, 2). α-Fetoprotein is normal, whereas it is usually over 1000 ng/ml in the usual hepatocellular carcinoma (1). Liver function tests are nonspecifically elevated (1). Prognosis is considerably better than for the usual hepatocellular carcinoma associated with cirrhosis: 32 months vs. 6 months average survival, 48% vs. 17% resectability, 63% vs. 30% 5-yr survival after successful resection (3). Isolated metastases may be successfully extirpated (2). Accurate diagnosis and staging is, therefore, essential. Patterns of spread are the same as in conventional hepatocellular carcinoma.

Pathology

Most often the tumor is a solitary large mass 4–17 cm in diameter which may have satellite nodules (1, 2). Masses are partially or completely encapsulated and may even be pedunculated (1, 2). A prominent depressed central fibrous scar with bulging margins may be present reminiscent of focal nodular hyperplasia (Fig. 5.96) (2). Large, thin-walled veins are seen in the capsule and fibrous septa. Large areas of necrosis are absent (3).

Major distinctive histologic features are deeply eosinophilic, polygonal hepatocytes, and abundant fibrous stroma arranged in thin parallel bands around the tumor cells (Fig. 5.97) (1–3). Mitotic figures are rare and the tumors are medium-grade without highly anaplastic areas (1–3). The fibrous stroma comprises layers of hyalinized bands which may coalesce into thick scars (1).

Radiology

The major radiologic clue to the diagnosis is the presence of central stellate or trabecular calcification, which is seen in roughly 40% of plain films and CT scans (Fig. 5.98A–C). The region of calcification is small compared to overall tumor size. It has been reported in many articles and reviews that calcification in untreated hepatocellular carcinoma is unusual and more common in children than adults (4, 5, 7–14). After treatment it is not unusual for hepatocellular carcinoma to undergo calcification. Critical review of this literature reveals that the calcified primary hepatic malignancies in adults were either cholangiocarcinomas, mixed cholangiohepatocellular carcinomas, or hepatocellular carcinomas in young, noncirrhotic adults. The latter probably were fibrolamellar hepatocellular carcinomas. In children under the age of five, most calcified liver tumors are either hepatoblastomas or hemangioendotheliomas. Sclerosing hepatocellular carcinoma is an unusual pri-

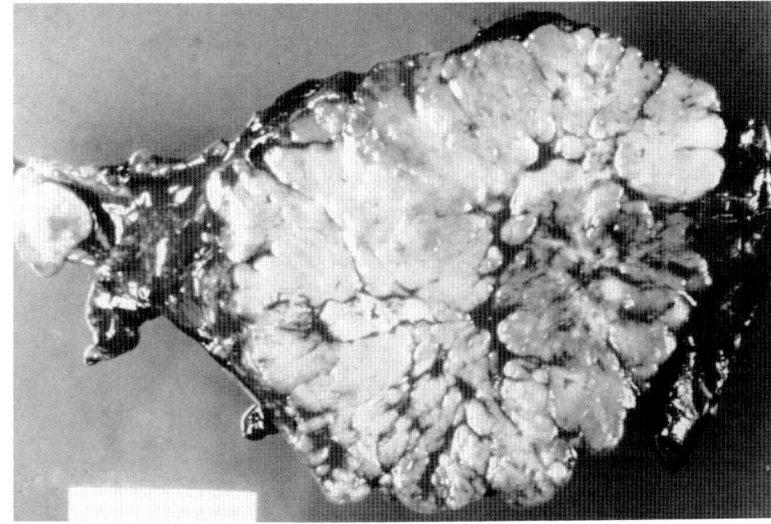

FIGURE 5.96. FIBROLAMELLAR HEPATOCELLULAR CARCINOMA
Cut gross specimen of a fibrolamellar HCC shows a central scar and compartmentalization.

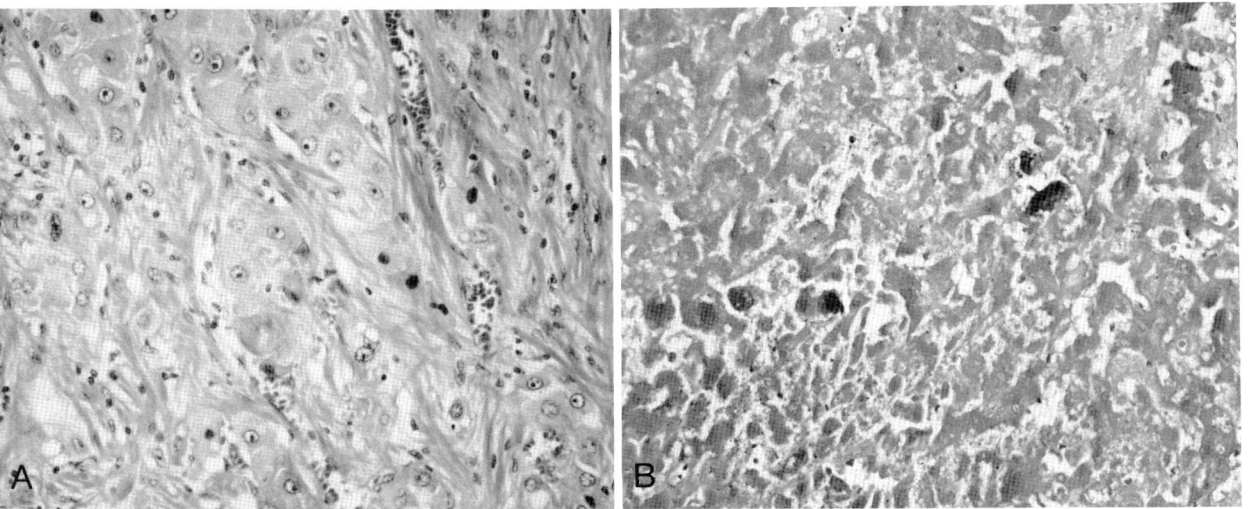

FIGURE 5.97. FIBROLAMELLAR HEPATOCELLULAR CARCINOMA
A: Microscopic section of fibrolamellar HCC demonstrates large, polygonal, granular, eosinophilic tumor cells and abundant fibrous stroma (H&E, ×250). B: Region of tumor necrosis with dark-staining microcalcification (H&E, ×250).

mary liver carcinoma characterized by intense fibrosis in which calcification could conceivably occur. However, sclerosing hepatocellular carcinoma occurs in an older age group than fibrolamellar hepatocellular carcinoma (mean 63) (15). Review of accessioned hepatocellular carcinomas in the AFIP Department of Radiologic Pathology showed no radiographically calcified hepatocellular carcinomas that were not fibrolamellar. A large liver mass in a young adult with a small amount of central calcification with or without satellite masses and a normal α-fetoprotein level is likely to be either a fibrolamellar hepatocellular carcinoma or partially calcified hemangioma or an intrahepatic cholangiocellular carcinoma. Fibrolamellar hepatocellular carcinomas are cold on sulfur-colloid scintigraphy (Fig. 5.98F), fairly echogenic and well-demarcated on ultrasound and nearly always hypervascular on angiography (Figs. 5.98D, E, G, and H and 5.99C) (7). They are typically well-demarcated, homogeneous and hypodense on unenhanced or drip infusion CT (Figs. 5.99B and 5.100C) (7). Contrast enhancement can be shown by bolus enhanced CT, which should be performed prior to angiography for staging (Fig. 5.98). The occasional demonstration of compartmentalization by fibrous septa on angiography and CT, although interesting, is not specific since similar appearances have been reported in

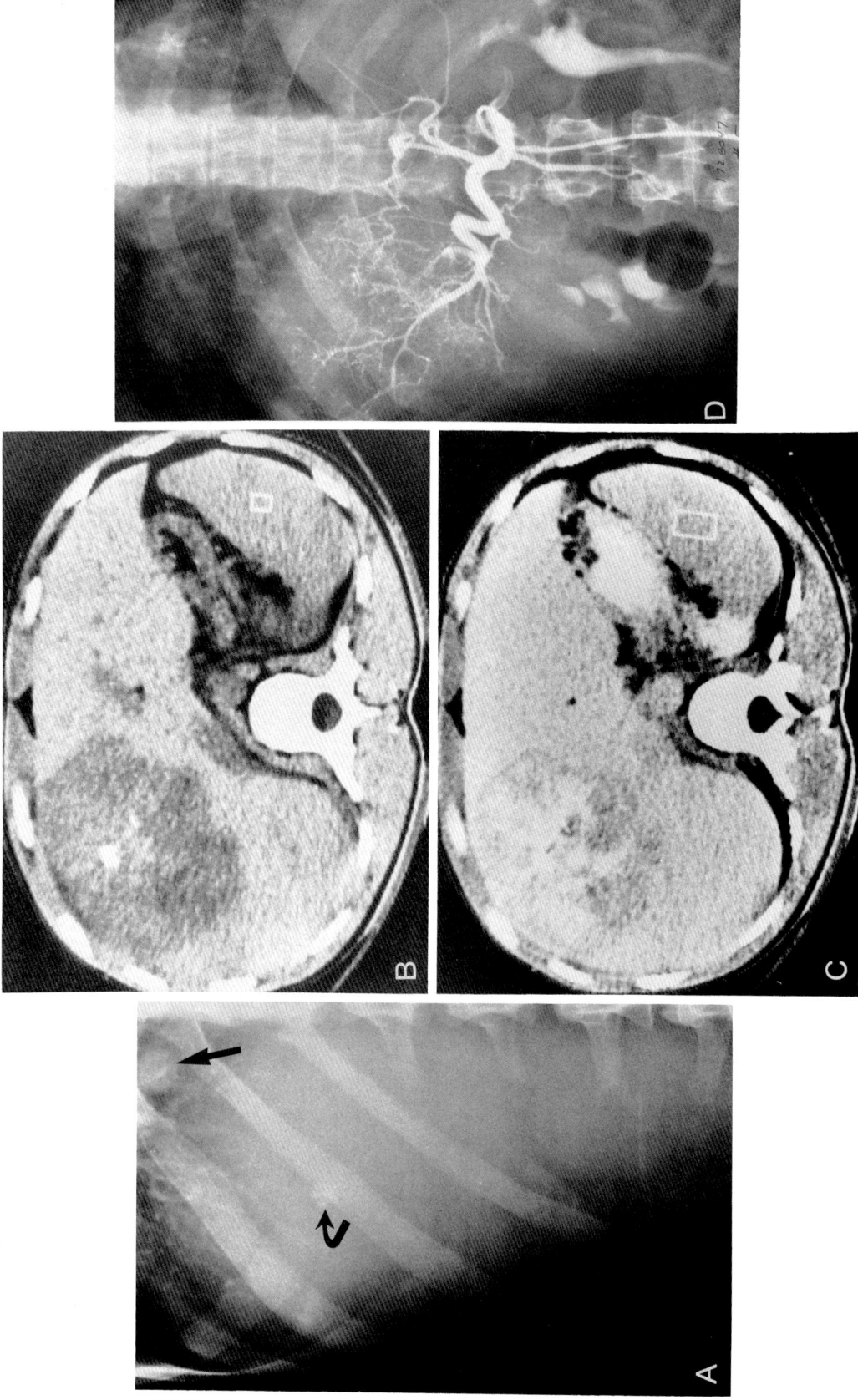

FIGURE 5.98 FIBROLAMELLAR HEPATOCELLULAR CARCINOMA

A: Plain film calcification (*curved arrow*) is present in this 20-yr-old man with fibrolamellar HCC. Note metastasis in right lower lobe (*arrow*). *B*: Unenhanced CT shows central calcification within a well-demarcated mass. *C*: Dynamic scan after bolus injection of contrast shows marked enhancement and a suggestion of compartmentalization. *D* and *E*: Hepatic arteriogram demonstrates hypervascularity, neovascularity, and a dense tumor stain with compartmentalization. Note the satellite nodule (*arrow*). *F–H*: Left lobe fibromellar HCC. Sulfur colloid scan (*F*) shows a large, cold mass. Hepatic arteriography (*G* and *H*) shows a hypervascular mass with neovascularity.

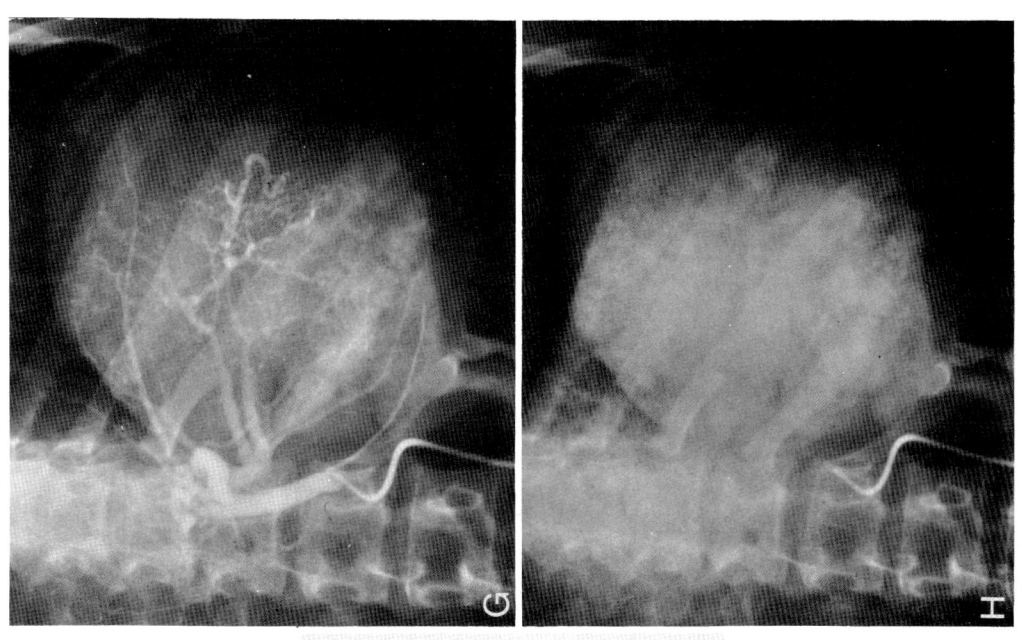
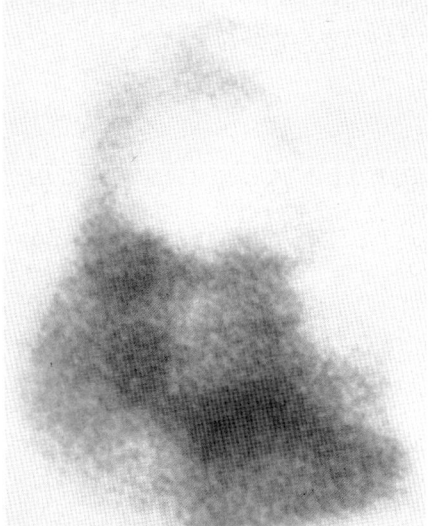
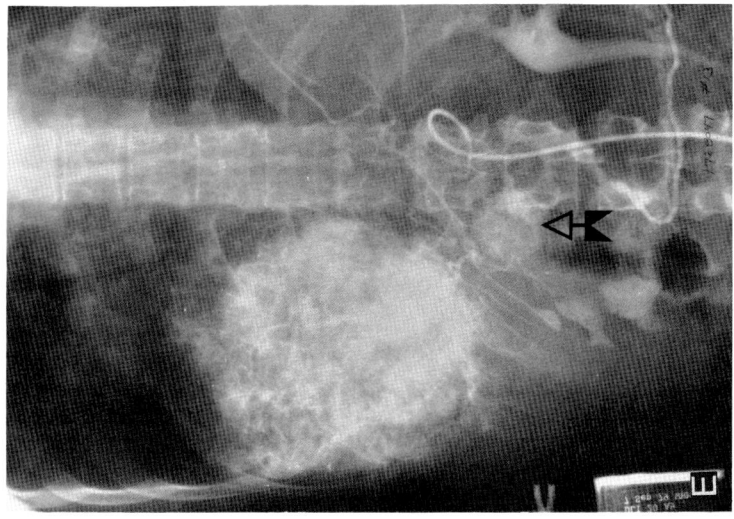

FIGURE 5.98*E–H*

249

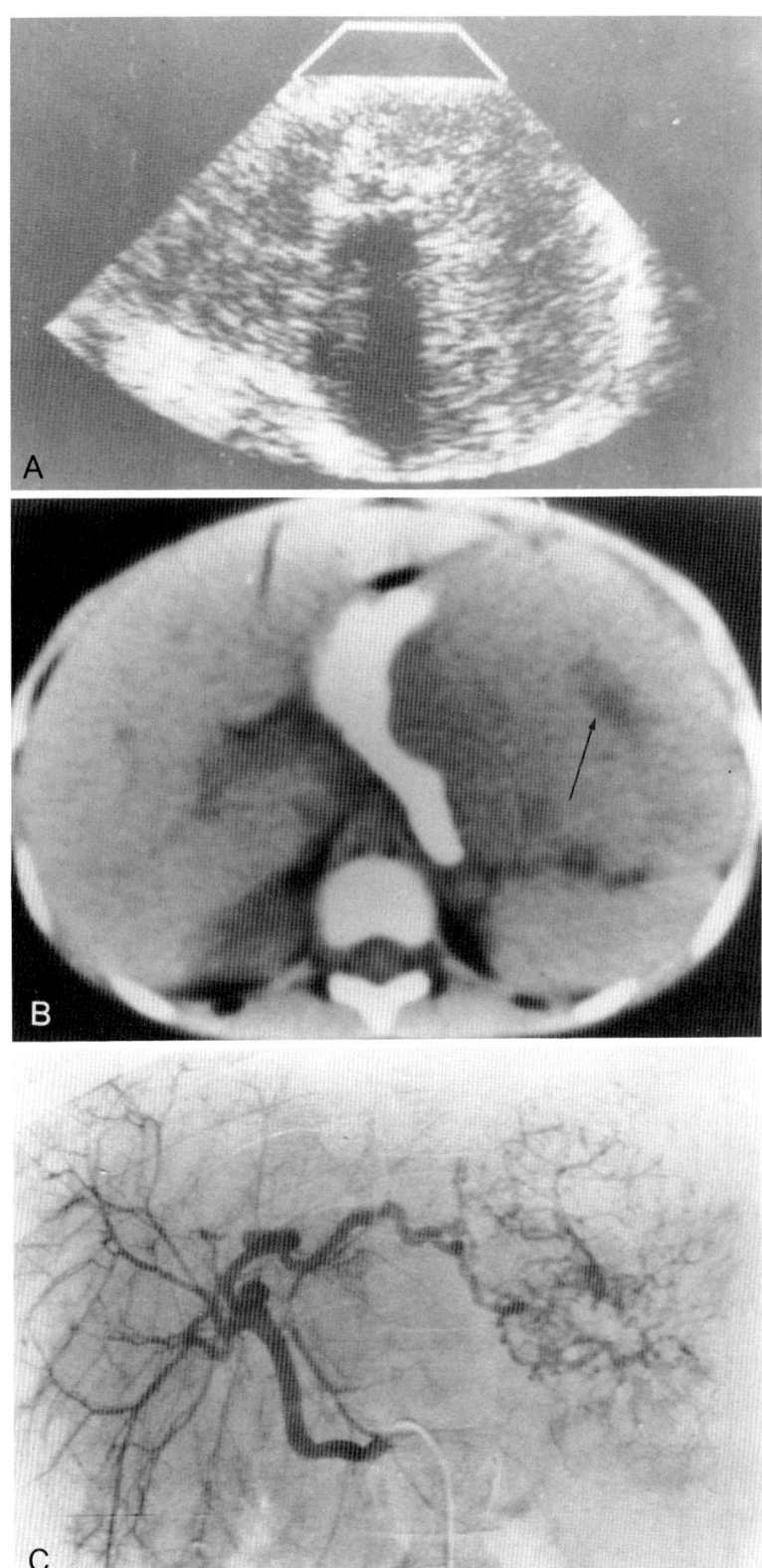

FIGURE 5.99. FIBROLAMELLAR HEPATOCELLULAR CARCINOMA

Ten-year-old girl with fibrolamellar HCC (same case as in Fig. 5.96). *A:* Real-time sonogram shows a well-demarcated left upper quadrant moderately echogenic mass with a densely echogenic shadowing central scar. *B:* The mass is hypodense and well-demarcated with a low density central scar (*arrow*) on unenhanced CT. *C:* Arteriography shows a hypervascular mass with an enlarged feeder and neovascularity.

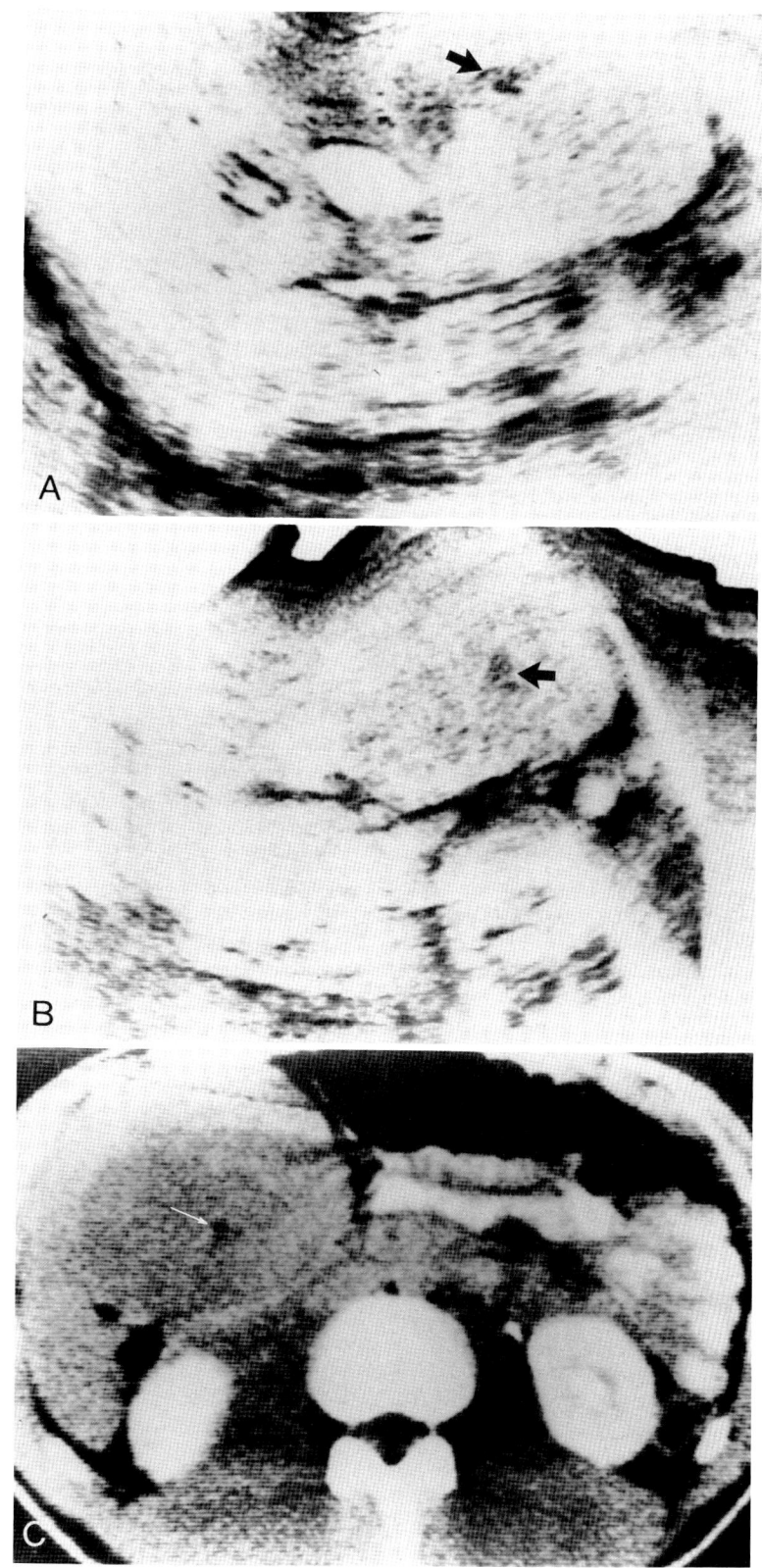

FIGURE 5.100. FIBROLAMELLAR HEPATOCELLULAR CARCINOMA

Fibrolamellar HCC in a 20-yr-old man. *A* and *B:* Parasagittal and transverse sonograms show a well-demarcated moderately echogenic mass with an echogenic central scar (*arrows*). *C:* The mass is hypodense, and sharply demarcated with a small central low density scar (*arrow*) on a CT scan performed during drip infusion of contrast.

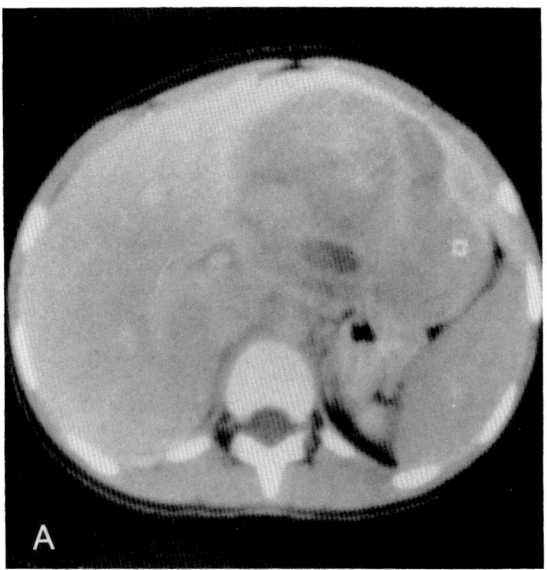 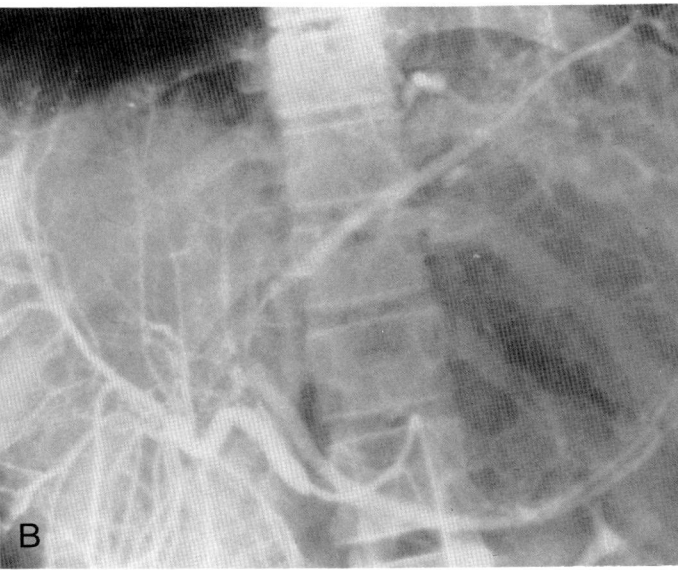

FIGURE 5.101. HEMORRHAGE INTO A FIBROLAMELLAR HEPATOCELLULAR CARCINOMA
A: Enhanced CT shows a large left lobe mass with a complex architecture: both high and low density regions are present, consistent with hemorrhage into a mass. *B:* Celiac angiogram: predominantly hypovascular mass. Note, however, the enlarged left hepatic artery and the hypervascularity in the periphery, consistent with hemorrhage into a preexisting hypervascular mass.

focal nodular hyperplasia (Fig. 5.98C-E) (16-18). Occasionally central small, shadowing echodensities are seen on sonography which correlate with CT central low density regions and represent central fibrous scars (Figs. 5.99 and 5.100) (7). This is the same central region that may undergo calcification. Central echogenic scars that are hypodense on unenhanced CT have been described in focal nodular hyperplasia (16, 18). However, these scars may enhance and disappear after contrast infusion. Scarring can also occur in hemangiomas after hemorrhage and/or necrosis. Occasional atypical fibrolamellar hepatocellular carcinomas are hypovascular on angiography. One explanation is bleeding into the tumor which can also cause an atypical variegated appearance on CT (Fig. 5.101). Coupled with one instance of spontaneous rupture with hemoperitoneum that we have seen, this suggests a propensity for fibrolamellar hepatocellular carcinoma to bleed. It will not be possible to suggest a correct diagnosis radiologically in those tumors that undergo hemorrhage, and confusion with hepatic adenoma may occur. The staging sequence suggested for conventional hepatocellular carcinoma can be applied to fibrolamellar hepatocellular carcinoma, but more agressive surgery is often indicated.

Differential diagnosis of a well-demarcated, homogeneous moderately echogenic and hypodense liver mass in a teenager or young adult would include hemangioma, hepatic adenoma, focal nodular hyperplasia, cholangiocarcinoma, and hepatocellular carcinoma, both the usual variety and fibrolamellar.

Features favoring fibrolamellar hepatocellular carcinoma are: (*a*) negative α-fetoprotein, (*b*) lack of underlying liver disease, (*c*) central small calcification and/or central stellate scar with or without septation, and (*d*) positive gallium scan. However, lack of the latter two cannot be used to exclude fibrolamellar hepatocellular carcinoma. If characteristic features of hemangioma cannot be demonstrated by radionuclide blood pool scans, dynamic CT, or angiography and no uptake of sulfur colloid to suggest focal nodular hyperplasia is present, the only definitive way to exclude fibrolamellar hepatocellular carcinoma is by obtaining tissue. Since small cores or needle aspirates of fibrolamellar hepatocellular carcinoma could look like hepatic adenoma or focal nodular hyperplasia, multiple core biopsies from different regions of the tumor done percutaneously or laparascopically are the minimum needed. One may have to resort to surgical wedge biopsy or resection depending on clinical considerations.

REFERENCES

1. Craig JR, Peters RL, Edmonson HA, Omata M: Fibrolamellar carcinoma of the liver: a tumor of adolescents and young adults with distinctive clinicopathologic features. *Cancer* 46:372–379, 1980.

2. Berman MM, Libbey NP, Foster JH: Hepatocellular carcinoma. Polygonal cell type with fibrous stroma—an atypical variant with a favorable prognosis. Cancer 46:1448–1455, 1980.
3. Wong LK, Link DP, Frey CF, Ruebner BH, Tesluk H, Primstone NR: Fibrolamellar hepatocarcinoma: radiology, management, and pathology. AJR 139:172–175, 1982.
4. Farhi DC, Shikes RH, Murari PJ, Silverberg SG: Hepatocellular carcinoma in young people. Cancer 52:1516–1525, 1983.
5. Lack EE, Neave C, Vawter GF: Hepatocellular carcinoma. Review of 32 cases in childhood and adolescence. Cancer 52:1510–1515, 1983.
6. Giacomantonio M, Ein SH, Mancer K, Stephens CA: Thirty years of experience with pediatric primary liver tumors. J Pediatr Surg 19:523–526, 1984.
7. Friedman AC, Lichtenstein JE, Fishman EK, Goodman Z, Siegelman SS, Dachman AH: Fibrolamellar hepatocellular carcinoma. Radiology 157:583–587, 1985.
8. McNulty JG: Radiology of the Liver. Philadelphia, W. B. Saunders, 1977, pp 44, 367–378.
9. Gore RM, Goldberg HI: Plain film and cholangiographic findings in liver tumors. Semin Roentgenol 18:87–93, 1983.
10. Darlak JJ, Moskowitz M, Kattan KR: Calcifications in the liver. Radiol Clin North Am 18:214, 1980.
11. Karras BG, Cannon AH, Zanon B: Hepatic calcifications. Acta Radiol (Diagn) 57:458, 1962.
12. Boijsen E, Abrams HL: Roentgenologic diagnosis of primary carcinoma of the liver. Acta Radiol (Diag) 3:257–277, 1965.
13. Haddow RA, Kemp-Harper RA: Calcification in the liver and portal system. Clin Radiol 18:225–236, 1967.
14. Kunstlinger F, Federle MP, Moss MA, Marks W: Computed tomography of hepatocellular carcinoma. AJR 134:431–437, 1980.
15. Omata M, Peters RL, Tatter D: Sclerosing hepatic carcinoma: relationship to hypercalcemia. Liver 1:33–49, 1981.
16. Scatarige JC, Fishman EK, Sanders RC: The sonographic scar sign in focal nodular hyperplasia of the liver. J Ultrasound Med 1:275–278, 1982.
17. Rogers JV, Mack LA, Freeny PC, Johnson ML, Sones PJ: Hepatic focal nodular hyperplasia: angiography, CT, sonography, and scintigraphy. AJR 137:983–990, 1981.
18. Fishman EK, Farmlett E, Kadir S, Siegelman SS: Computerized tomography of benign hepatic tumors. J Comput Assist Tomogr 6:472–481, 1982.

Intrahepatic Cholangiocarcinoma

Cholangiocarcinoma may arise from either the intrahepatic or extrahepatic ducts. The former will be discussed below, whereas the latter is described in the section on the biliary tree.

Clinical Findings

As opposed to hepatocellular carcinoma, cholangiocarcinoma is distributed fairly evenly throughout the world and is not strongly associated with cirrhosis, hepatitis B virus or hemochromatosis (1). An increased incidence is present in patients with Caroli's disease, sclerosing cholangitis and inflammatory bowel disease, and in patients with clonorchiasis or opisthorchiasis (1–4). These entities all have in common chronic biliary obstruction and infection. Thorotrast is an unusual predisposing factor in the development of cholangiocarcinoma (1). In general, intrahepatic cholangiocarcinoma occurs only about 10% as often as hepatocellular carcinoma, and only 25% arise in a cirrhotic liver (4).

Peripheral intrahepatic cholangiocarcinomas present clinically with abdominal pain, anexoria, and weight loss (1). Jaundice only occurs if both right and left ducts are obstructed or if there is massive parenchymal replacement. Prognosis and patterns of spread are similar to that of hepatocellular carcinoma. Current treatment modalities include hepatic resection for localized disease, chemotherapy, both systemic and intraarterial, and hepatic artery occlusion (1).

Pathology

Grossly, cholangiocarcinoma is gray-white and firmer than hepatocellular carcinoma because of its fibrous stroma (1–5). Growth patterns are similar to hepatocellular carcinoma—either massive (with or without satellite nodules), multinodular, or diffuse (1). Sometimes polypoid or papillary tumors arise from the larger peripheral bile ducts. On occasion, cholangiocarcinomas arising from the hilum extend along the intrahepatic bile ducts fanning out into the liver such that the site of origin cannot be defined. The sclerosing cholangitis type frequently has no gross tumor at surgical inspection with diagnosis made by demonstrating microscopic spread diffusely along the biliary tree (6). It is unknown whether the sclerosing cholangitis type develops from preexisting sclerosing cholangitis, is malignant from its onset and initially very slow growing and difficult to diagnose as malignant, or both. Extensive invasion of larger vessels as seen in hepatocellular carcinoma does not occur as frequently in cholangiocarcinoma (1, 7).

Cholangiocarcinoma histologically is usually a sclerosing adenocarcinoma, but it can be less well-differentiated (1–5). Characteristically, an abundant fibroblastic stroma is present (1–5). Mucin may be produced, but there is no bile secretion (1–5). Tumor cells are usually arranged in tubules resembling bile ducts (5, 6). Sometimes there is a papillary pattern (6). Cell type is columnar or cuboidal with nuclei smaller and less variable in size than in hepatocellular carcinoma (5, 6). Differential diagnosis from metastatic adenocarcinoma or sclerosing hepatocellular carcinoma is, at times, difficult (1, 3). Cholangiohepatocellular carcinoma, a rare variant, has histological features of both cholangiocellular carcinoma and hepatocellular carcinoma (1, 3, 5).

Radiology

Plain Films. Intrahepatic cholangiocarcinoma rarely will demonstrate dystrophic calcification in necrotic regions (8–12). The calcification is punctate or linear, located centrally, and small compared to the overall size of the tumor (Fig. 5.102) (13). Occasionally opaque calculi are present in biliary radicals obstructed by cholangiocarcinoma (8).

Sonography and CT. *Massive or Nodular.* There are no cross-sectional imaging features of the massive or nodular forms of intrahepatic cholangiocarcinoma that distinguish it from the more common metastatic disease and hepatocellular carcinoma other than the fact that cholangiocarcinoma is more likely to be associated with dilated bile ducts than the latter two diseases. Sonographically, one or more masses may be detected. They may be hypoechoic, isoechoic or hyperechoic and either homogeneous or inhomogeneous (Fig. 5.103A and B). Usually biliary tree dilatation accompanies the mass(es) (Fig. 5.103A and B). Echoes within the dilated biliary tree can be produced by excess mucin (nonshadowing) or calculi proximal to the obstruction (shadowing). The biliary dilatation can be diffuse including intrahepatic and extrahepatic ducts or focal and contiguous to the mass. Diffuse dilatation is probably caused by excess mucin secretion into the ductal system. Involvement of the major venous structures can be detected (Fig. 5.103A and C).

Two CT appearances have been described (6, 14). The first, correlating with a papillary morphology, is a well-defined round to oval hypodense mass with a slightly denser internal component on non-contrast scans (Fig. 5.103D). Bolus injection of contrast produces prominent enhancement of the large internal component (Fig. 5.103E). The second appearance is that of a hypodense mass with only slight contrast enhancement (Fig. 5.104A and C). Either of the above may be well or poorly marginated. Satellite masses may be present (Fig. 5.104B), and biliary dilatation as described above is frequently present (Fig. 5.103F). Mucin or calculi in the biliary tree are depicted as small, relatively high attenuation foci within dilated ducts. Involvement of portal veins and inferior vena cava can be detected (Fig. 5.103E and F).

Diffuse (Sclerosing Cholangitis Type). In general no mass will be detected although the affected ducts may have bright walls on sonography and thickened walls on CT. Dilated ducts may be mainly confined to one lobe or segment with or without dilatation of the extrahepatic biliary tree (6). Foci of high density or increased echoes in the biliary tree may be present due to mucin or stones. Loss of liver volume in affected lobes is frequent (6).

Cholangiography. *Massive or Nodular.* Cholangiography is not usually necessary for management of these tumors unless surgical or interventional radiologic procedures to palliate jaundice are contemplated. When performed, opacified ducts are typically draped around a bulky mass which is obstructing other duct(s). Intraluminal mass (with or without ulceration) or an irregular, eccentric stricture is present at the point of obstruction (6, 9). Intraluminal filling defects elsewhere in the biliary tree can be present due to mucin, tumor, or stones (6).

Diffuse (Sclerosing Cholangitis Type). Beaded strictures or longer segment constrictions are found either focally or diffusely in the biliary tree. Differentiation from sclerosing cholangitis is often not possible by cholangiography and must be made using clinical and pathologic data. Clues to the correct diagnosis of cholangiocarcinoma are patterns of distribution atypical for sclerosing cholangitis or the presence of any masses.

Angiography. As opposed to hepatocellular carcinoma, cholangiocarcinoma generally does not have large hypervascular tumor vessels, arteriovenous shunts or venous tumor thrombi (6). Fine tumor neovascularity may be seen along with irregular, encased or obstructed small arteries (Fig. 5.104D and E) (15–17). Arterioarterial collaterals along the course of the bile ducts have been described in association with arterial obstruction (15). Poorly marginated regions of mild tumor blush may be seen (18). Dilated bile ducts may be depicted as branching tubular lucencies in the hepatogram phase and encasement of portal vein branches may be seen during arterial portography (18). Arteriography is usually reserved for additional staging of those multinodular or massive cholangiocarcinomas that appear resectable on ultrasound and CT.

Nuclear Medicine. Peripheral intrahepatic cholangiocarcinomas present scintigraphically as one or more photopenic space-occupying lesions within the liver on sulfur-colloid scans. Segmental biliary obstruction can be demonstrated, if present, by hepatobiliary scintigraphy. The mass lesion itself is cold on the hepatogram phase of ^{99m}Tc-IDA scintigrams. Rarely, bone scan agents can be taken up by an intrahepatic cholangiocarcinoma (19). Intrahepatic cholan-

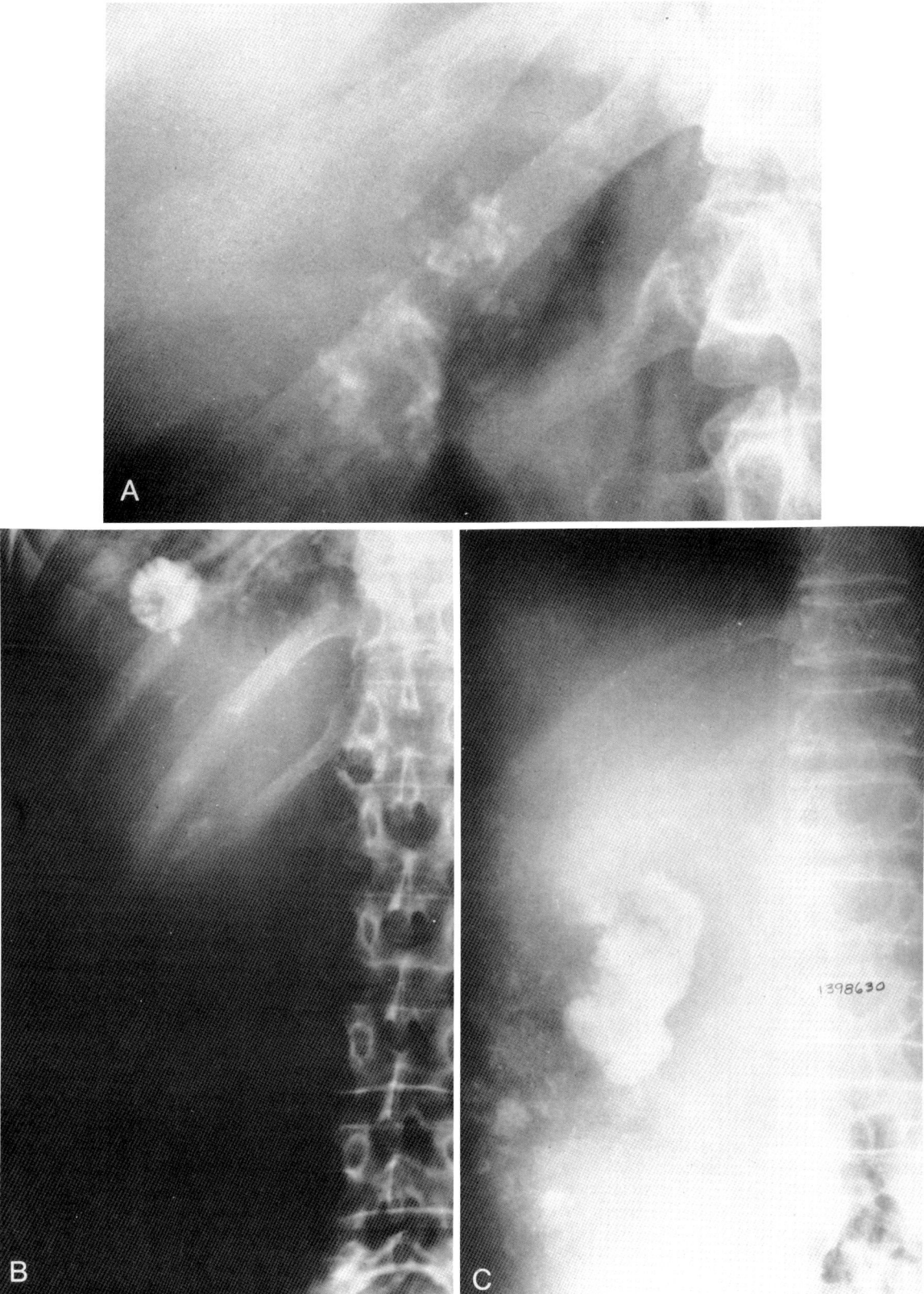

FIGURE 5.102. CALCIFICATION IN CHOLANGIOCARCINOMA
A: Close-up of coalescing irregular shaped calcifications. *B:* Dense, nearly uniform spherical calcification. *C:* Extensive coalescing punctate calcification and a large dense irregularly shaped calcification in a mixed cholangiohepatocellular carcinoma.

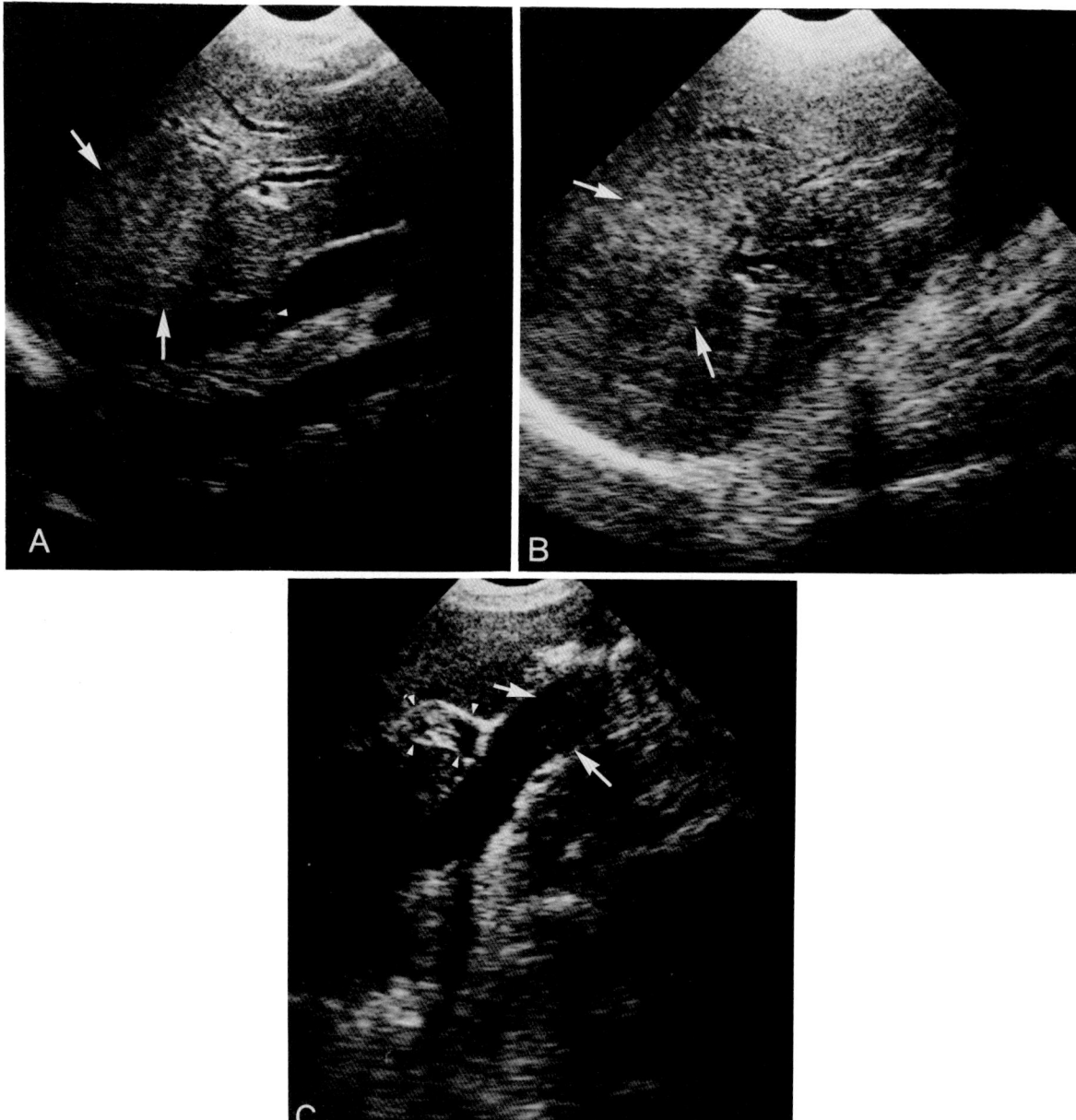

FIGURE 5.103. HUGE SOLITARY INTRAHEPATIC CHOLANGIOCARCINOMA INVADING THE PORTAL VEIN AND THE INFERIOR VENA CAVA IN A 35-YR-OLD WOMAN

A and *B:* Longitudinal sonograms showing a slightly hyperechoic mass (*arrows*) and dilated intrahepatic ducts. Note mass in inferior vena cava (*arrowhead*). *C:* Oblique scan shows tumor in inferior vena cava (*arrows*) and portal vein (*arrowheads*). *D:* Noncontrast CT: Large low density mass, slightly denser central component. *E:* Dynamic scan, slightly higher level: irregular enhancement within the tumor, nonvisualization of the inferior vena cava and large hemiazygous vein (*white arrow*) suggesting inferior vena cava involvement. Note wedge-shaped lucency peripheral to tumor (*black arrows*) due to portal perfusion defect. *F:* Lower level: Numerous enhanced tubular structures in region of portal vein are periportal collaterals from portal vein obstruction. Round and tubular lucencies in the liver are dilated ducts. Inferior vena cava is dilated below its point of obstruction. *G:* Two-hour delayed same level as (*D*): vicarious excretion of contrast by hepatocytes gives somewhat better appreciation of true tumor margins.

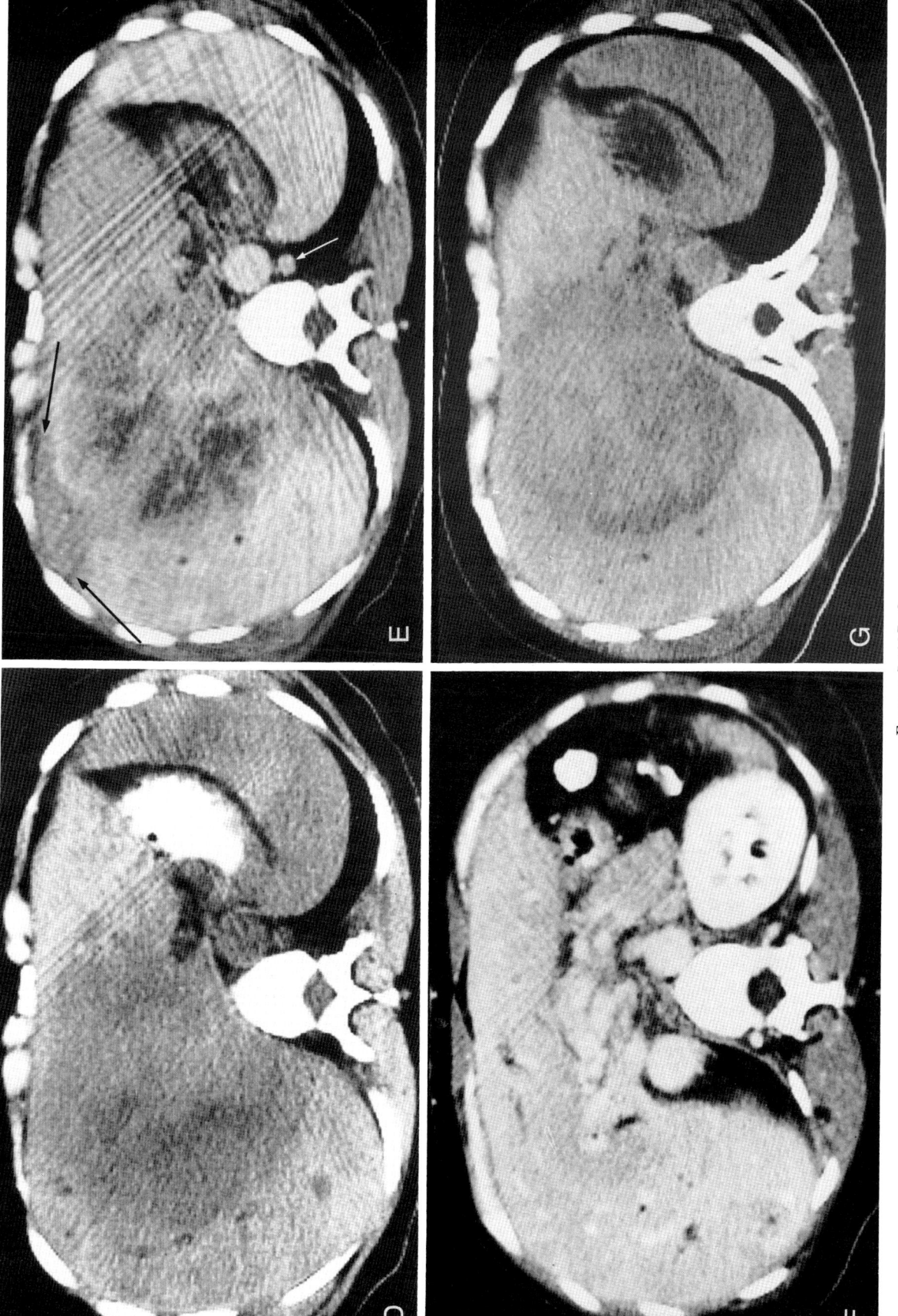

FIGURE 5.103D–G

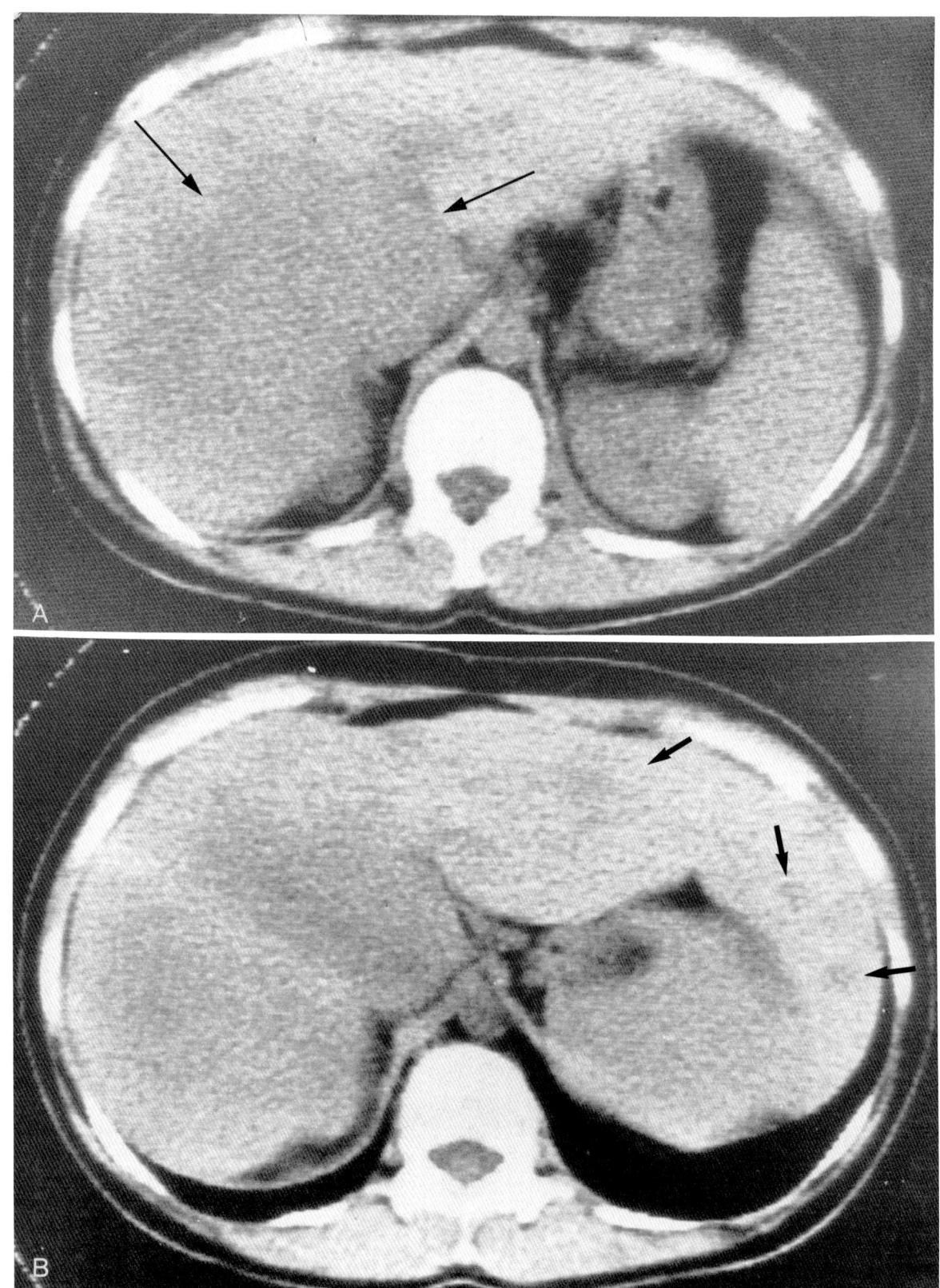

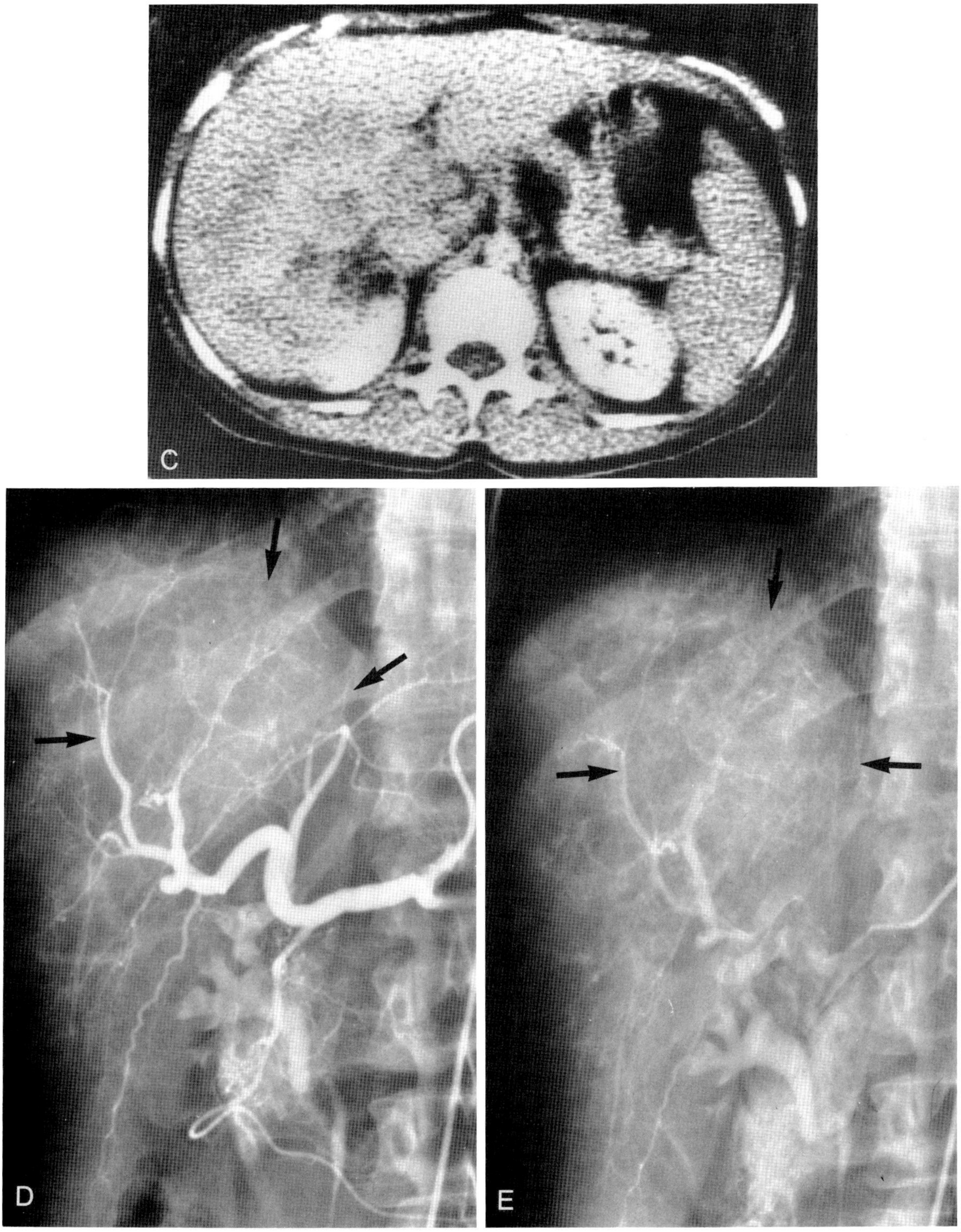

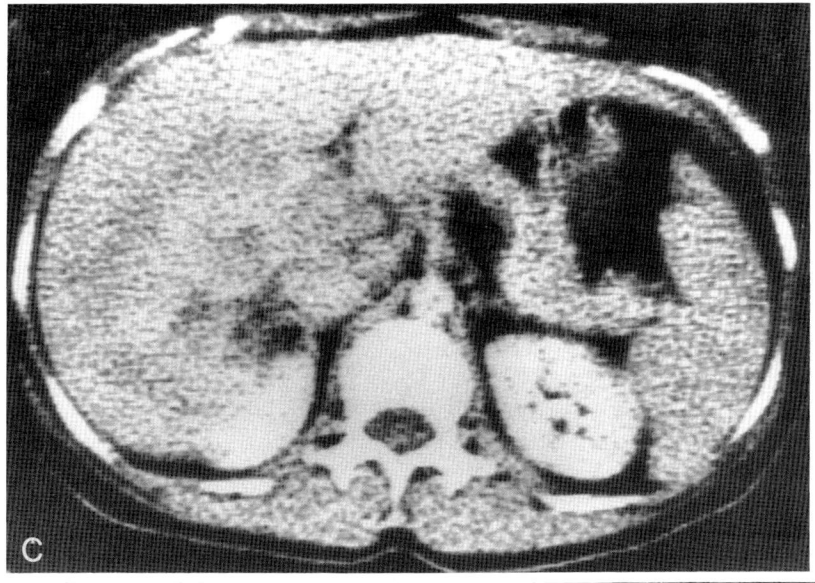

FIGURE 5.104C–E

FIGURE 5.104. CHOLANGIOCARCINOMA: CT AND ANGIOGRAPHY

A and *B:* Noncontrast scans: large poorly marginated low density mass (*arrows*) involves right lobe, caudate lobe and medial segment of left lobe (*A*). Satellite nodules in the lateral segment of the left lobe (*B*) (*arrows*). Second patient (*C, D, E*). *C:* Contrast-enhanced scan, narrow window: moderate enhancement of the tumor. *D* and *E:* Arterial phase, right hepatic injection: stretched and encased arteries and poorly marginated mild blush (*arrows* outline tumor).

giocarcinomas are generally not hot on radionuclide angiography and blood pool studies or gallium scans.

REFERENCES

1. Schonland MM, Millward-Sadler GH, Wright DH, Wright R: Hepatic tumors. In Wright R, Alberti KGMM, Karran S, Millward-Sadler GH (eds): *Liver and Biliary Disease.* Philadelphia, W. B. Saunders, 1979, pp 897–899.
2. Plorde JJ: Other trematodes of flukes. In Thorn GW, et al (eds): *Harrison's Principles of Internal Medicine.* New York, McGraw-Hill, 1977, pp 1112–1113.
3. Robbins SL, Cotran RS: *Pathologic Basis of Disease.* Philadelphia, W. B. Saunders, 1979, pp 1066–1067.
4. Edmondson HA, Peters RL: Tumors of the liver: pathologic features. *Semin Roentgenol* 18:78–79, 1983.
5. Tien-yu L: Tumors of the liver. In Bockus HL et al (eds): *Gastroenterology.* Philadelphia: W. B. Saunders, 1976, p 524.
6. Itai Y, Araki T, Furui S, Yashiro N, Ohtomo K, Iio M: Computed tomography of primary intrahepatic biliary malignancy. *Radiology* 147:485–490, 1983.
7. Gold JA, Sostman HD, Burrell MI: Cholangiocarcinoma with portal vein obstruction. *Radiology* 130:15–20, 1979.
8. Sherlock S: *Diseases of the Liver and Biliary System.* Oxford, Blackwell Scientific, 1981, pp 459–460.
9. Gore RM, Goldberg HI: Plain film and cholangiographic findings in liver tumors. *Semin Roentgenol* 18:87–93, 1983.
10. Allen RW, Holt AH: Calcification in primary liver carcinoma. *AJR* 99:150–152, 1967.
11. Karras BG, Cannon AH, Zanon B: Hepatic calcifications. *Acta Radiol (Diagn)* 57:458–468, 1962.
12. Darlak JJ, Moskowitz M, Kattan KR: Calcifications in the liver. *Radiol Clin North Am* 18:209–220, 1980.
13. Haddow RA, Kemp-Harper RA: Calcification in the liver and portal system. *Clin Radiol* 18:225–236, 1967.
14. Clark RA, Matsui O: CT of liver tumors. *Semin Roentgenol* 18:149–162, 1983.
15. Walter JF, Bookstein JJ, Bouffard EV: Newer angiographic observations in cholangiocarcinoma. *Radiology* 118:19–23, 1976.
16. Reuter SR, Redman HC, Bookstein JJ: Angiography in carcinoma of the biliary tract. *Br J Radiol* 44:636–641, 1971.
17. Kaude J, Rian R: Cholangiocarcinoma. *Radiology* 100:573–580, 1971.
18. Freeny PC: Angiography of hepatic neoplasms. *Semin Roentgenol* 18:114–122, 1983.
19. Guiberteau MJ, Potsaid MS, McKusick KA: Accumulation of ^{99m}Tc-disphosphonate in four patients with hepatic neoplasms: case reports. *J Nucl Med* 17:1060–1061, 1976.

Angiosarcoma of the Liver (Hemangioendothelial Sarcoma, Kupffer Cell Sarcoma, Hemangiosarcoma)

Etiology

Original reports of this rare tumor were in European vineyard workers exposed to arsenicals in insect sprays and dusts (1, 2). Angiosarcoma is the most common liver tumor resulting from exposure to Thorotrast, developing after a latent period of 15–24 yr (1–4). More recently, angiosarcoma has been reported in male polyvinyl chloride workers after a latent period of 4–28 yr (1–3). Patients in any of these three categories may develop precursor lesions consisting of patchy capsular and subcapsular fibrosis, portal fibrosis, and atypia of the cells lining the sinusoids (2). Some cases have no known etiology, but these may merely represent faulty history or as yet undiscovered carcinogens.

Clinical Findings

Presenting signs and symptoms are nonspecific, including malaise, anorexia, weight loss, hepatosplenomegaly, and right upper quadrant pain. Jaundice and ascites are late features (1). Microangiopathic hemolytic anemia and platelet sequestration within the tumor have been reported (1, 4). Catastrophic hemoperitoneum may occur any time in the course of the disease because of rupture of a superficial nodule. Patients with hepatic angiosarcoma generally have a rapidly downhill course from the time of diagnosis, usually dying within a year of presentation (1–4).

Pathology

Angiosarcoma is usually multinodular, occasionally it occurs as a solitary nodule. Even then, satellite nodules are usually present. Nodules are gray-white or red-purple from hemorrhage (1–3) (Fig. 5.105). The bulk of the liver eventually becomes diffusely replaced by tumor. Metastasis occurs to the lungs, spleen, porta hepatis nodes, portal vein, thyroid, peritoneal cavity, and bone marrow (1, 2).

Histologically, precursor stages can be identified consisting of regions of combined hyperplasia of hepatocytes and a variety of sinusoidal and presinusoidal cells associated with an excess of reticulin and sinusoidal dilatation. The mixed hyperplasia of the various sinusoidal cells then proceeds to an overgrowth of angiosarcoma cells, presumably derived from endothelium. In early stages, the angiosarcoma cells remain in contact with hepatocytes. A trabecular arrangement then ensues due to loosening of the lobular plates by sinusoidal dilatation and primary peliosis. As hepatocytes disappear, various growth patterns develop, terminating in nodular, solid angiosarcoma composed of spindle or polyhedral cells that undergo hemorrhage and/or necrosis form-

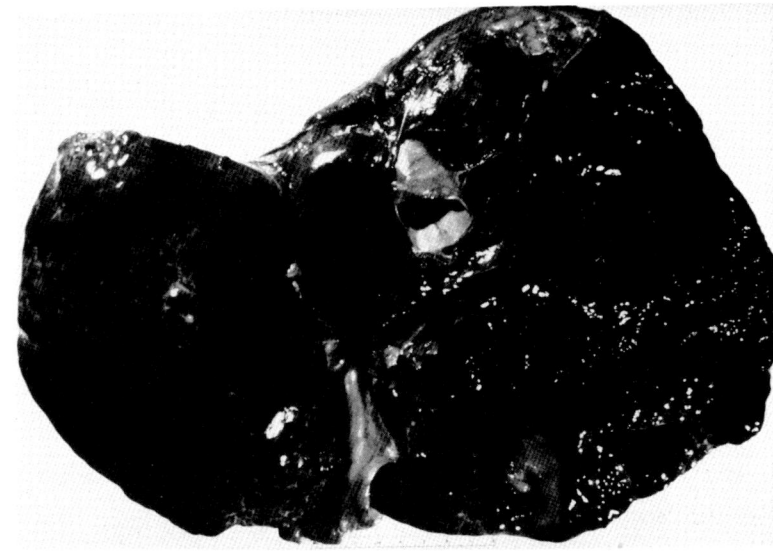

FIGURE 5.105. GROSS SPECIMEN OF AN ANGIOSARCOMA: MOST OF THE LIVER IS REPLACED BY THE BLUISH NEOPLASM

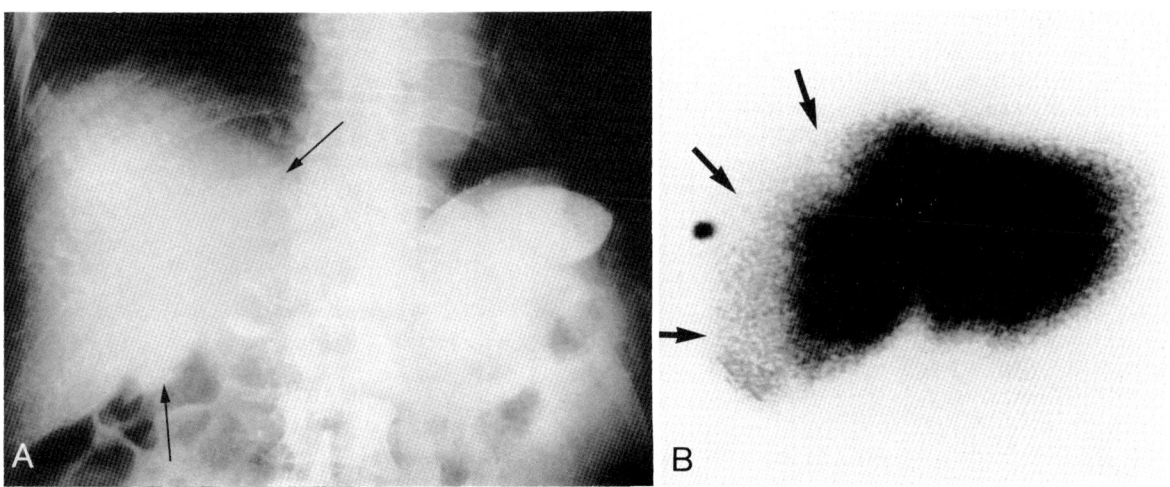

FIGURE 5.106. ANGIOSARCOMA FROM THOROTRAST
A: Plain film, same patient as in Fig. 5.105: Trabeculated pattern of residual Thorotrast in periphery of right lobe of liver. More medially there is a homogeneous increased density (*arrows*). Tumor cannot be diagnosed. Note small spleen and lymph nodes containing Thorotrast. *B:* Sulfur colloid scan shows photopenic region peripherally on the right (*arrows*). Fibrosis with no functioning reticuloendothelial cells or tumor? Biopsy showed both tumor and fibrosis.

ing secondary peliotic spaces (5). Extramedullary hematopoiesis is a regular feature of the tumor sinusoids (3).

Radiology

Plain Films. Although angiosarcoma does not calcify, at times the diagnosis can be suggested on plain films when the underlying cause is Thorotrast exposure. The tumor may be depicted as any radiolucent regions displacing or replacing otherwise opacified hepatic and/or splenic parenchyma (6). Large peliotic cysts have to be considered as a differential diagnostic possibility, as well as cholangiocarcinoma or hepatocellular carcinoma. Unfortunately, the increased density due to thorotrast is often reticulated, making plain film detection of a superimposed mass difficult if not impossible (Fig. 5.106).

Nuclear Medicine. Sulfur-colloid scans show cold defects corresponding to regions of neoplasm. The defects are often peripheral (Fig. 5.106) and may be hard to distinguish from anatomic variants, fibrosis or peliosis (7). Splenomegaly is often present in cases unassociated with thorotrast, and can be due to extensive tumor replacement of the liver, portal invasion, or stimulation of splenic cells with increased blood flow induced by vinyl chloride. Defects in the spleen, when seen, usually represent splenic metastases. Little experience is available with Gallium scans in angiosarcomas (7). Hot spots (increased vascularity) are often present on blood flow and blood pool scintiscans (5).

Ultrasound. Angiosarcomas can be either solid masses or mixed masses with both solid and anechoic components, the latter corresponding to regions of hemorrhage and necrosis (8). Relative echogenicity compared to the liver will be variable, depending on how much hepatic fibrosis is present. In fact, the tumor may be difficult or impossible to detect by ultrasound because of beam attenuation by a fibrotic liver (depending on location within the liver) (9). When the angiosarcoma has become diffuse it is impossible to differentiate tumor from destructive parenchymal liver disease.

Computed Tomography. Unenhanced CT depicts angiosarcomas as hypodense masses (Fig. 5.107). When the etiology is Thorotrast exposure, the displacement and replacement of Thorotrast-laden parenchyma can be helpful (Fig. 5.108) (6, 8, 9). Masses in the spleen representing metastases may be seen (Figs. 5.107 and 5.108) (6). Regions of hemorrhage into the tumor are depicted as high density regions when fresh and low density regions when older. When the angiosarcoma has progressed to diffusely permeate the liver it will be seen as low density replacement of parenchyma possibly difficult to distinguish from destructive peliosis or fatty infiltration. After bolus contrast administration there is striking peripheral enhancement of any focal angiosarcoma masses giving a similar appearance to that of cavernous hemangioma (8). This pattern may not be appreciable once the neoplasm has permeated large regions of the liver.

Angiography. The hepatic arteries supplying the tumor are of normal size, although enlargement of arteries supplying other portions of the liver may be enlarged, presumably on a compensatory basis (7). Arterial displacement is sometimes seen, but not encasement. Hypervascular changes are sometimes present around the periphery of any masses but not tumor vessels. A tumor stain appears around the periphery of the masses in the mid-arterial phase and character-

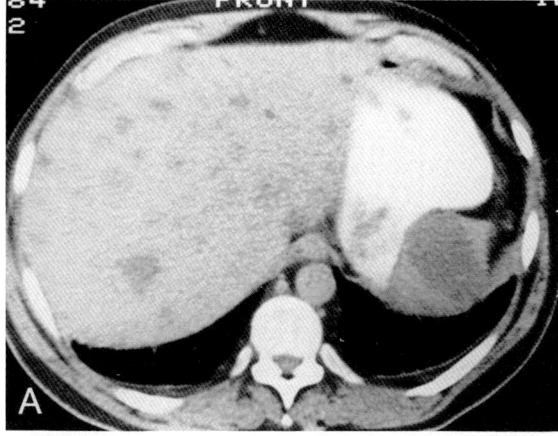
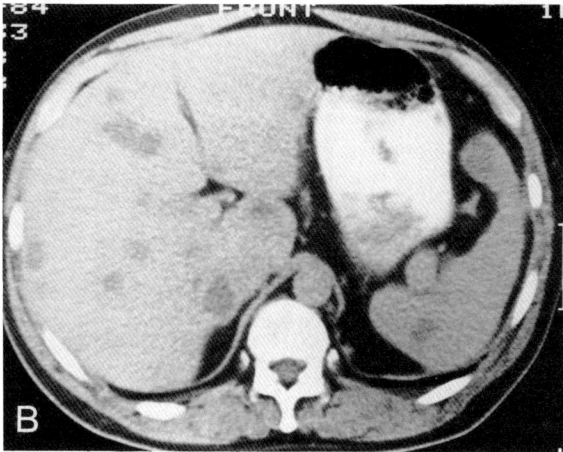

FIGURE 5.107. NON-THOROTRAST ANGIOSARCOMA
A and *B:* Multinodular low density neoplasm in liver with splenic metastases.

istically lasts for a prolonged period of time, up to 34 sec (7). Some degree of central hypovascularity is frequently present due to hemorrhage and/or necrosis, and some puddling can occur in the central hypovascular region (7). The maximal stain and/or puddling generally occurs prior to the portal venous phase of the study (on a celiac injection) (Fig. 5.109). Periportal sinusoidal dilatation or peliosis hepatis may be present elsewhere in the liver (see section describing these entities for a description of findings). The characteristic prolonged peripheral stain may not be present when the neoplasm has advanced to the point of extensive parenchymal replacement (Figs. 5.109 and 5.110).

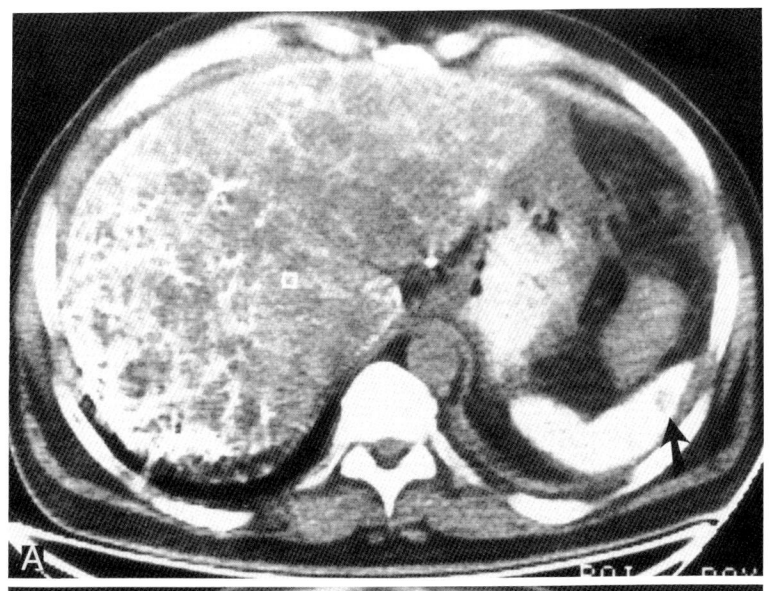

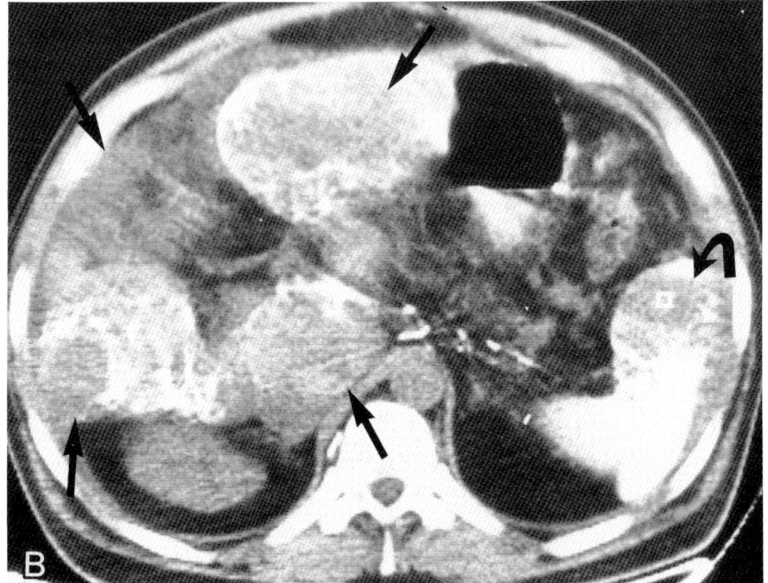

FIGURE 5.108. ANGIOSARCOMA FROM THOROTRAST, METASTASES TO SPLEEN

A: Trabeculated pattern of thorotrast in the liver with a large region relatively devoid of Thorotrast: infiltrative tumor vs. destructive parenchymal changes. Defect in spleen (*arrow*) from metastatic angiosarcoma. *B:* Lower cut: soft tissue masses unequivocally replacing Thorotrast-laden parenchyma and extending into the peritoneum (*arrows*). Splenic metastasis (*curved arrow, cursor*) also displacing Thorotrast and invading peritoneum.

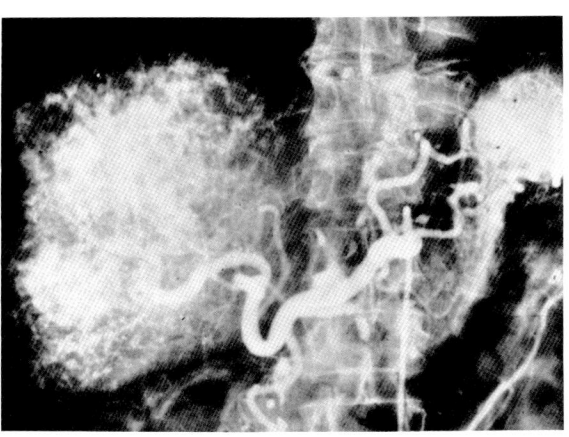

FIGURE 5.109. CELIAC ARTERIOGRAM, ANGIOSARCOMA
Multinodular hypervascular tumor in the mid-arterial phase infiltrating the right lobe.

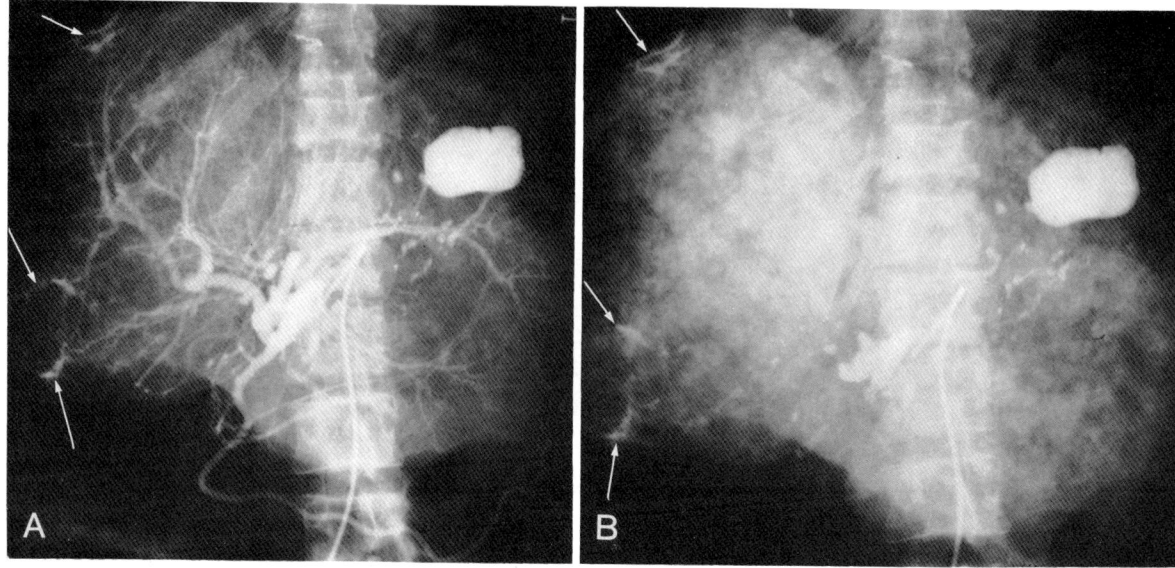

FIGURE 5.110. ANGIOSARCOMA FROM THOROTRAST

Angiosarcoma from Thorotrast replacing almost the entire liver. Note minimal residual hepatic Thorotrast (*arrows*) and Thorotrast in spleen and lymph nodes. *A:* Early arterial phase: note normal-sized but splayed intrahepatic arteries and little in the way of tumor stain and no encasement. *B:* Hepatogram: very mottled and the liver is misshapen. The more intensely staining regions seen throughout the liver correspond to the neoplasm.

REFERENCES

1. Schonland MM, Millward-Sadler GH, Wright DH, Wright R: Hepatic tumors. In: Wright R, Alberti KGMM, Karran S, Millward-Sadler GH (eds): *Liver and Biliary Disease.* Philadelphia, W. B. Saunders, 1979, pp 908–910.
2. Robbins SL, Cotran RS: *Pathologic Basis of Disease.* Philadelphia, W. B. Saunders, 1979, p 1068.
3. Edmondson HA, Peters RL: Tumors of the liver: pathologic features. *Semin Roentgenol* 18:80, 1983.
4. Sherlock S: *Diseases of the Liver and Biliary System.* Oxford, Blackwell Scientific, 1981, pp 468–469.
5. Popper H, Thomas LB, Telles NC, Falk H, Selikoff IJ: Development of hepatic angiosarcoma in man induced by vinyl chloride, thorotrast, and arsenic. Comparison with cases of unknown etiology. *Am J Pathol* 92:349–369, 1978.
6. Arbona GL, Lloyd TV, Lucas J, Sharma HM: Computed tomographic demonstration of angiosarcoma of the spleen. *South Med J* 75:348–349, 1982.
7. Whelan JG Jr, Creech JL, Tamburro CL: Angiographic and radionuclide characteristics of hepatic angiosarcoma found in vinyl chloride workers. *Radiology* 118:549–557, 1976.
8. Mahony B, Jeffrey RB, Federle MP: Spontaneous rupture of hepatic and splenic angiosarcoma demonstrated by CT. *AJR* 138:965–966, 1982.
9. Silverman PM, Ram PC, Korobkin M: CT appearance of abdominal thorotrast deposition and thorotrast-induced angiosarcoma of the liver. *J Comput Assist Tomogr* 7:655–658, 1983.

6

Magnetic Resonance Imaging of the Liver

ARNOLD C. FRIEDMAN, M.D.

NORMAL ANATOMY AND TECHNIQUE

The hepatic parenchyma has moderate intensity using spin echo (TE 28) and inversion recovery sequences. Against this gray background, normal vessels (hepatic and portal veins, inferior vena cava, and main hepatic artery) are depicted as low intensity structures because of their flowing blood (Fig. 6.1). With longer TEs (56 ms and higher) the parenchyma becomes darker and portal veins become bright, while other vessels remain dark (Fig. 6.1). Presumably, this is due to slower flow in portal veins. At field strengths ranging from 0.04T to 0.7T T1s have been reported from 155–397 ms and T2s from 40–96 ms (1). T1 is dependent on field strength and can be approximated by the formula T1 (liver) = $0.000534 \, f^{0.38} \pm 22\%$ where f is the Larmor frequency (42.58T, T = field strength in Tesla). T2 of the liver is relatively independent of field strength and has been reported from 40–96 ms (1). A recent report gave a normal T1 of 533 ± 136 ms (range 228–956 ms) and a normal T2 of 56 ± 8 ms (range 38–112 ms) using a 0.35T imager on 28 patients (2). Given the wide ranges and inherent inaccuracies of current methods of relaxation time calculations done with clinical MR imagers, only major trends can be spotted (1, 2).

The liver must be imaged with both T1-weighted and T2-weighted sequences for optimal sensitivity in detecting mass lesions. Spin echo sequences with short and long TEs/TRs are the most popular (2–7). Inversion recovery sequences (T1 and proton density weighted) with TIs of 400 and 277 ms and TRs of 1.0 or 1.8 sec have also proven useful (2, 7). Simple proton spectroscopic imaging, by exploiting the difference in the rate of precession between aqueous and aliphatic protons, has been shown in preliminary work to improve the detection of liver metastases and fatty infiltration (8).

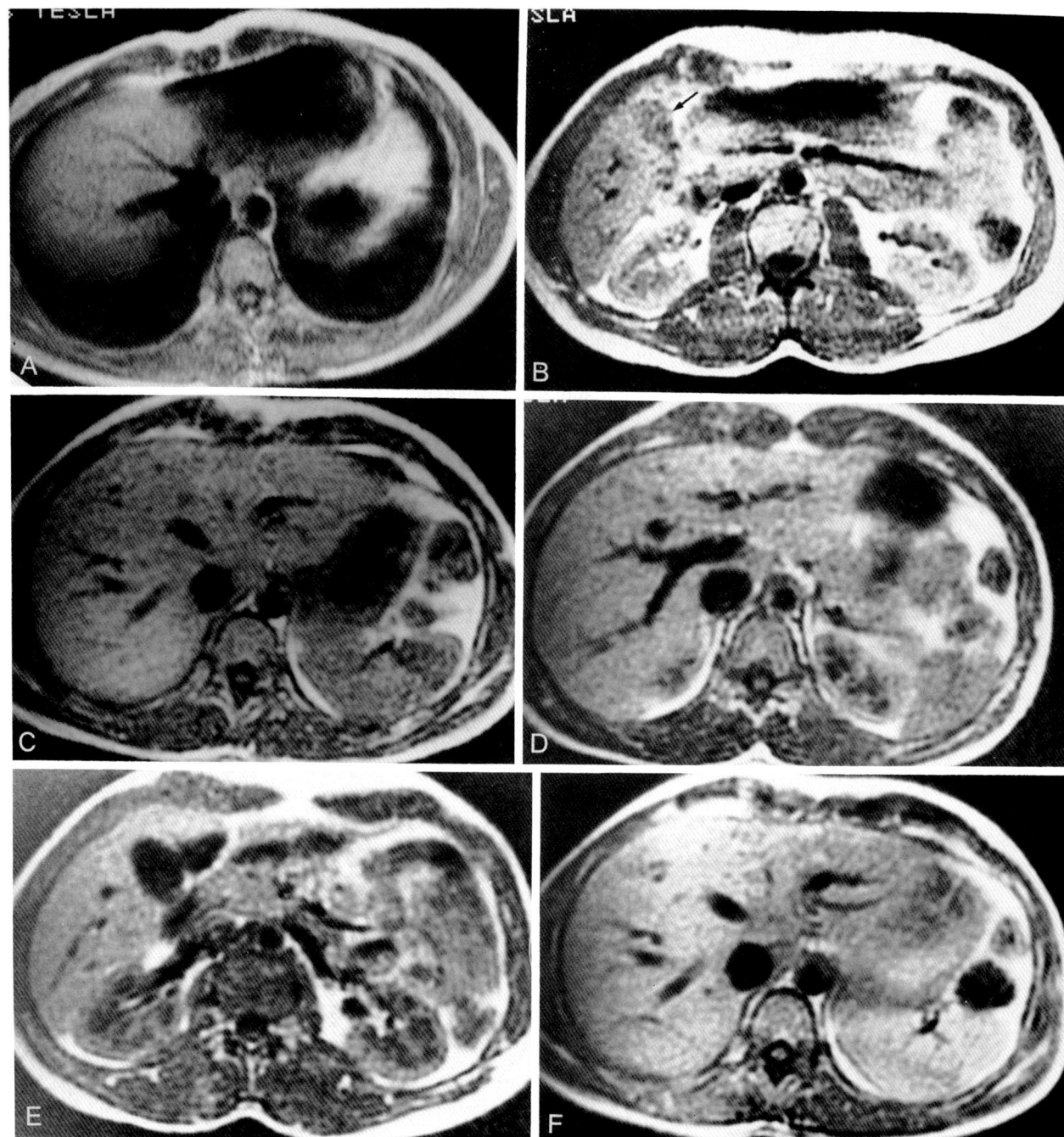

FIGURE 6.1. NORMAL ANATOMY

A: Confluence of the hepatic veins draining into the inferior vena cava (SE 28/500). *B*: Peripheral veins seen as dark branching structures at the level of the gallbladder (*arrow*). The hepatic parenchyma has moderate intensity (SE 28/500). *C–E*: Inferior vena cava, hepatic and portal veins have low intensity as does the gallbladder. The parenchyma has moderate intensity (IR 310/1500). *F* and *G*: Similar anatomy (SE 28/1000). *H–J*: SE 28/2000, similar anatomy, gallbladder is hyperintense (*arrow*). *K* and *L*: Images degraded somewhat by motion artifacts, portal veins (*arrows*) are hyperintense and parenchyma is less intense than on TE 28 images (SE 56/1000 and SE 56/2000).

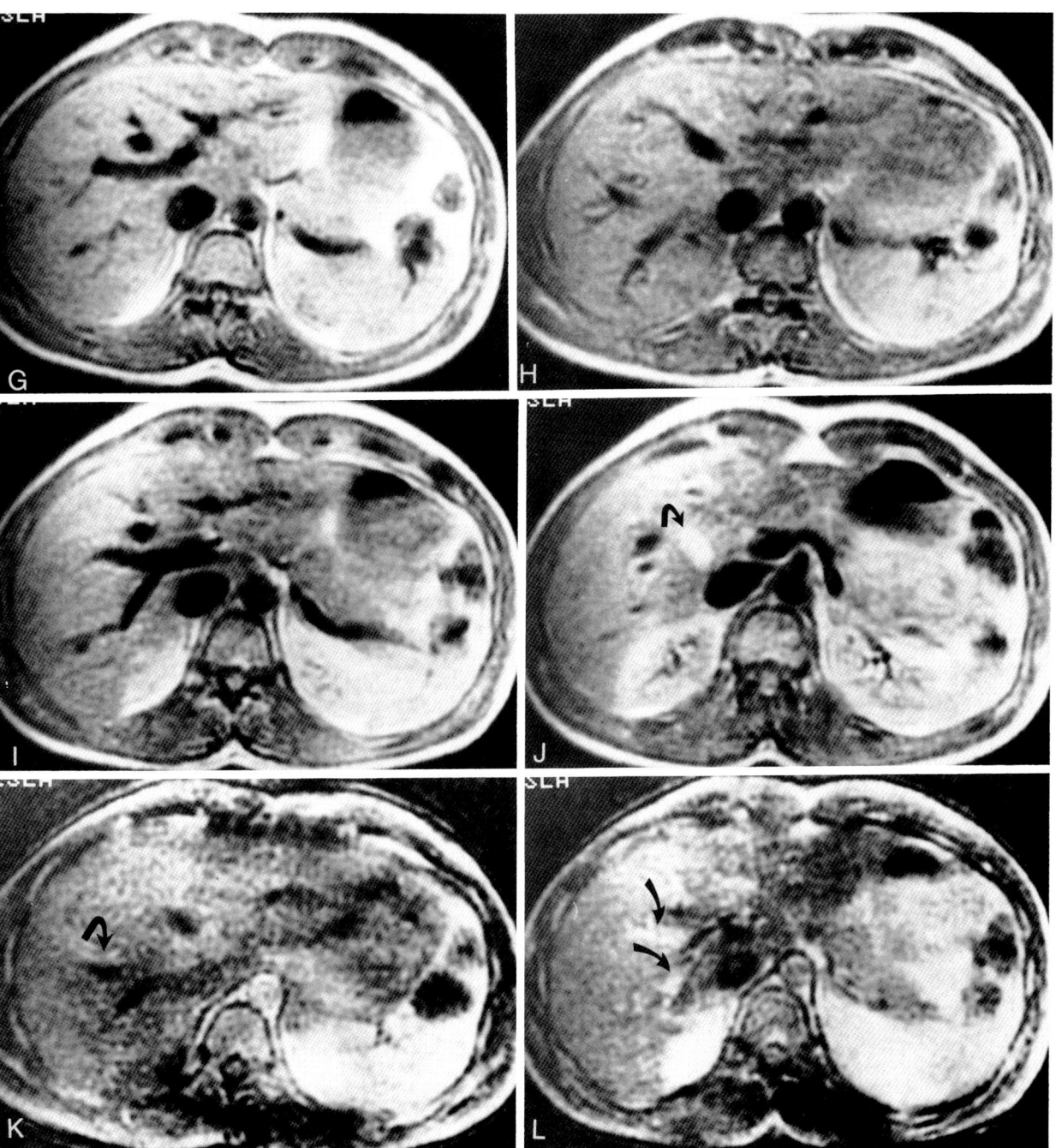

FIGURE 6.1G–L

MRI IN DIFFUSE LIVER DISEASES

Prolonged T1 and T2 values have been demonstrated in hepatitis as well as corresponding increased signal intensity (9, 10). The prolongation of T2 and the visual increased intensity appear to be more diagnostically useful than the lengthening of T1. MRI is extremely sensitive in detecting early changes associated with chemical hepatitis and may be clinically useful in detecting and quantifying hepatocyte damage due to hepatitis (9, 10).

CIRRHOSIS

Available data on the subject of MRI in cirrhosis are sparse and conflicting. Doyle et al. showed decreased intensity and prolongation of T1 in 10 cases of cirrhosis using T1-weighted sequences at 0.15T (T1 rose from 210–270 ms to 280–450 ms) (11). Smith et al. showed similar findings in 5 patients at a field strength of 0.04T (T1 rose from 140–170 ms to 180–300 ms) (12). However, Stark et al. maintained that cirrhosis alone, in the absence of hepatitis, does not markedly alter the MRI characteristics of the liver (10). Data published by Goldberg et al. showed no alterations in T1 or T2 induced by periportal fibrosis in cirrhotic rats (12). Patients with alcohol-induced cirrhosis, by far the most common type in this country, have components of hepatitis and steatosis in addition to fibrosis. The effects of these processes separately and together on the MR image need further study (13).

FATTY INFILTRATION (STEATOSIS)

Routine magnetic resonance imaging has not been sensitive to diffuse fatty infiltration of the liver (9, 12, 14) but one case of focal fatty infiltration did show a region of increased intensity on MR (15) (Fig. 6.2) and one series of 3 cases showed increased liver intensity despite no T1 change using saturation recovery and inversion recovery sequences at 0.15T (11). Experimentally produced fatty infiltration with massively increased hepatic triglyceride content showed no significant changes in T1 or T2 relaxation times and only a small increase in hepatic intensity (9), despite the short T1 and the prolonged T2 of fat. This was explained by the fact that when routine techniques are used, most of the signal comes from water protons in the liver which are unaffected by the infiltrated fat. A modified spin echo technique specifically designed to exploit the small difference in the rates of precession of aqueous and aliphatic protons (simple proton spectroscopic imaging) is sensitive to small changes in hepatic fat content and can separate fatty from normal liver (16) (Fig. 6.3). Signals sampled at a time when water and fat protons

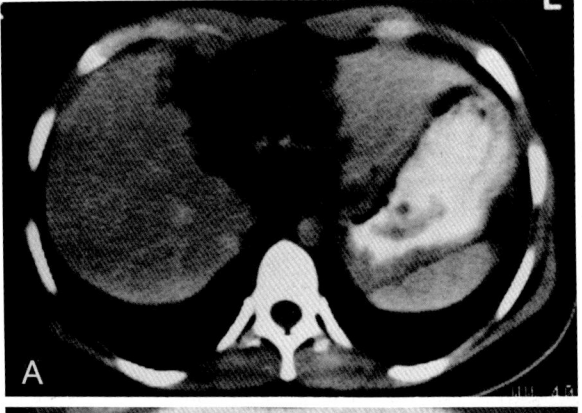
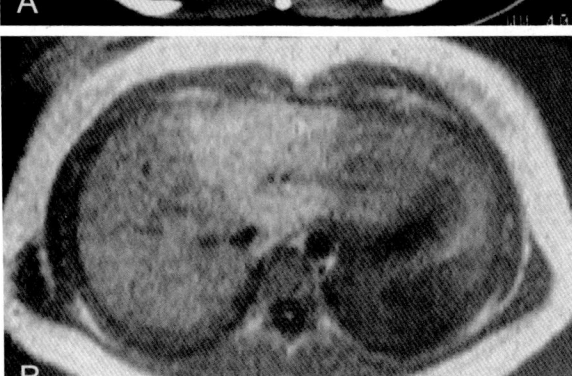
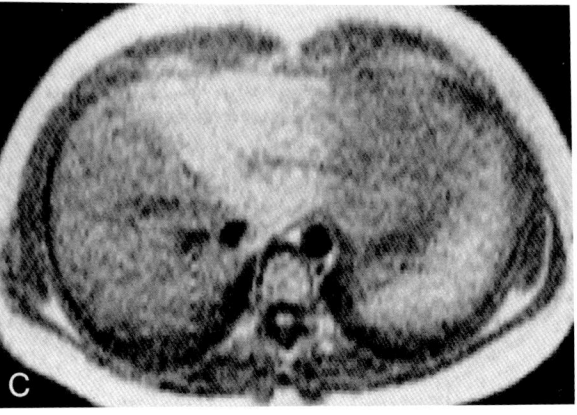

FIGURE 6.2. FOCAL FATTY INFILTRATION ON MRI WITH CT CORRELATION

A: Hypodense medial segment of left lobe with normal vessels coursing through, consistent with focal fatty infiltration. B and C: MRI: the fatty region is hyperintense with low intensity blood vessels within it. (B: inversion recovery, C: SE 30/1000). (From Wenker JC, Baker MK, Ellis JH, Glant MD: Focal fatty infiltration of the liver: demonstration by magnetic resonance imaging. AJR 143:573–574, 1984.)

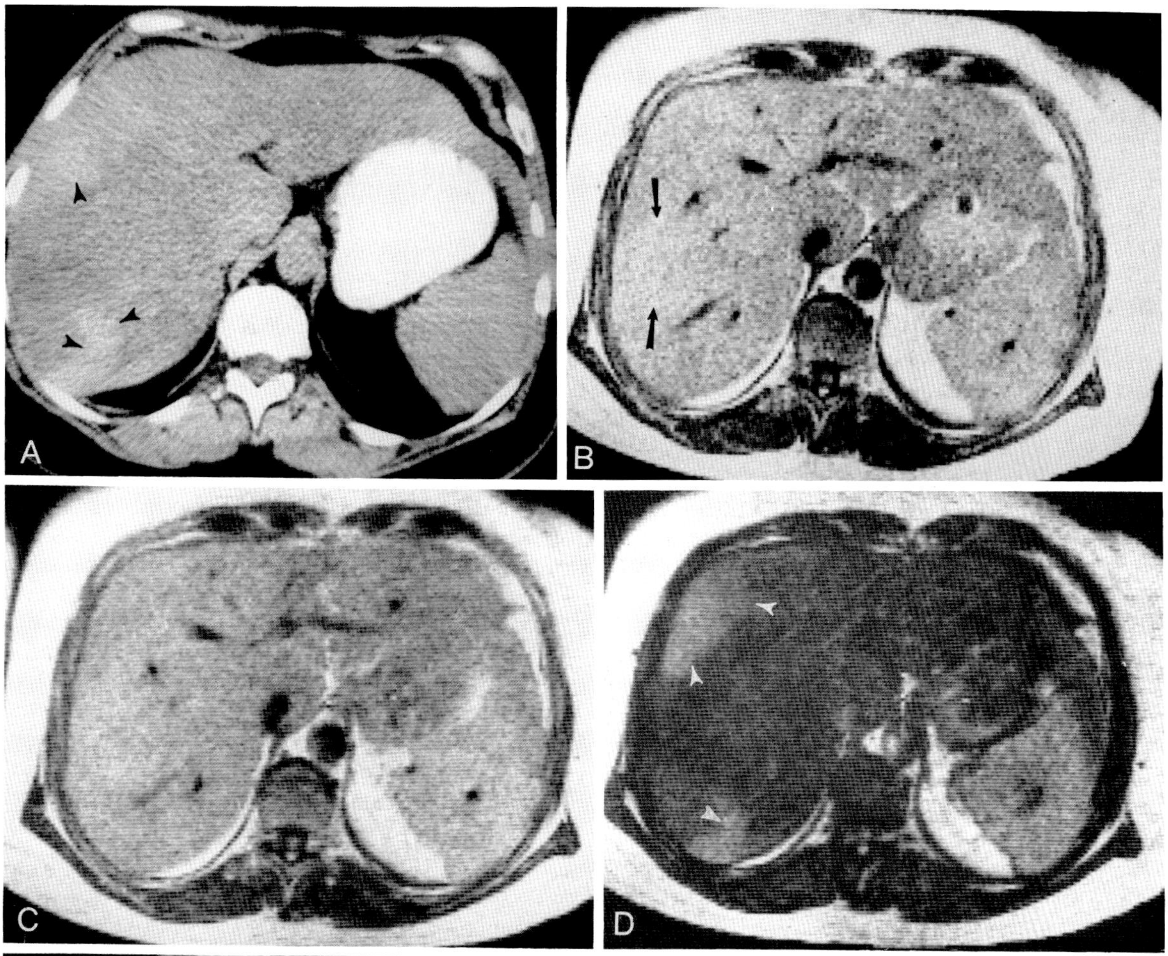

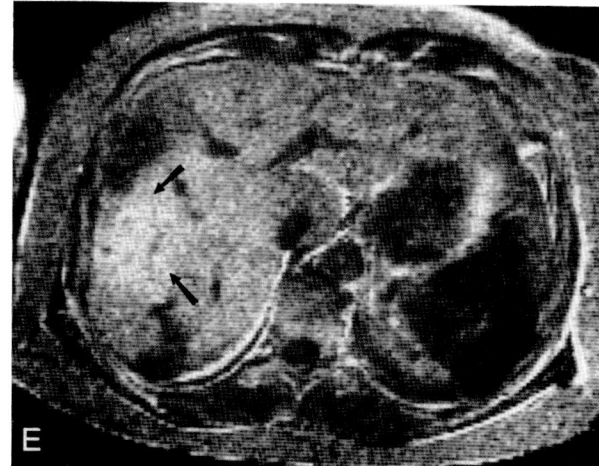

FIGURE 6.3. USE OF SIMPLE PROTON SPECTROSCOPIC IMAGING IN FATTY LIVER

A: Precontrast CT scan demonstrates the liver to have an inhomogeneous appearance. While most of the liver has a low attenuation value compatible with fatty infiltration, islands of normal liver tissue (*arrowheads*) can also be identified. *B*: NMR image obtained with a conventional spin echo technique using TR900/TE30 showed that only a small portion of the liver in the right lobe (*arrows*) has a higher signal intensity than the rest of the liver. However, the left lobe of the liver, which was clearly fatty on CT scan, has a similar signal intensity as islands of normal liver parenchyma. *C*: In-phase image. Note the similarity between in-phase and conventional spin echo image, as shown in *B* (TR900/TE40). *D*: Opposed image. Islands of normal liver (*arrowheads*) which have a higher signal intensity can be easily distinguished from the fatty liver, which has a similar signal intensity to paraspinal muscle. Demarcation between apparently uninvolved and fatty liver is as clear in the opposed image as in CT scan, (TR900/TE40). *E*: Lipid image. Three different intensities can be noted in the liver. While apparently uninvolved liver has very low signal intensity (similar to paraspinal muscle), the rest of the liver has a much higher intensity, representing a higher lipid content. Note that a small portion of the right lobe (*arrows*) is brighter than the left lobe suggesting that the former has an even higher lipid fraction although they have similar CT attenuation values. (TR900/TE40). (From Lee JKT, Dixon WT, Ling D, Levitt RG, Murphy WA: Fatty infiltration of the liver: demonstration by proton spectroscopic imaging—preliminary observations. *Radiology* 153:195–201, 1984.)

are pointing in opposite directions yield an "opposed" image, in which regions of fat are low intensity. Thus diffuse and focal fatty infiltrations are depicted as hypointense regions.

HEPATIC IRON OVERLOAD

Reticuloendothelial iron overload (mostly hemosiderin) occurs early in many conditions and does not cause significant tissue damage. Parenchymal (hepatocellular) iron overload (mostly ferritin) occurs later and leads to fibrosis and cirrhosis. The normal liver contains about 0.1 mg/g of iron, and a mean of 1.8 mg/g is present when pathologic examination shows excess hemosiderin deposits (17). Concentrations of hepatic iron as low as 1.2 mg/g have been detected as abnormal by MRI (9). Hemosiderin (the degradation product of ferritin) contains large amounts of ferric ion, which is paramagnetic and shortens T1 and T2 relaxation times of neighboring protons. Ferritin is also paramagnetic by virtue of its ferric ion content. It is possible that a cytoplasmic pool of low molecular weight iron is actually more responsible for the relaxation time shortening than the former two forms of iron (18). Using spin echo sequences, T1 shortening predominates and intensity increases at concentrations of ferric ion up to 5 mmol/liter, but at greater concentrations (which occur clinically) T2 shortening is dominant and intensity is markedly reduced (19) (Fig. 6.4).

Marked decreases in T2 and intensity and moderate decreases in T1 in both transfusional hemosiderosis and idiopathic hemochromatosis have been reported by several investigators (9, 11, 14, 17–19). The amount of iron overload can be quantified by in vitro MR since relaxation rates (1/T1 and 1/T2) are linearly related to hepatic iron concentration (correlation coefficients 0.84 and 0.93, respectively) (18). In vivo calculations of T1 and T2 cannot be done presently because of the extremely low intensities on spin echo images. The prolongation of T1 by fibrosis and cirrhosis is a potential confounding factor but has yet to cause clinical difficulty in interpreting MR images in patients with iron overload states. Similar to the liver, decreased intensity may be noted in the spleen and pancreas (18).

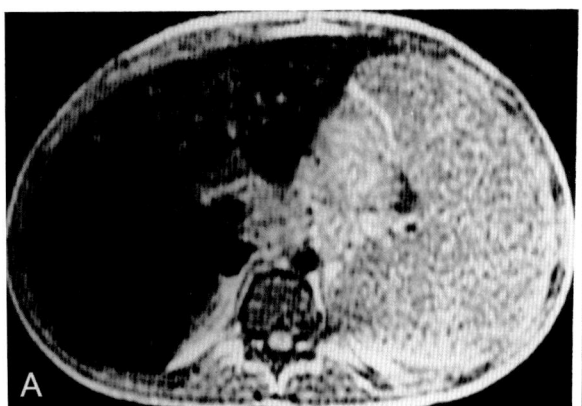 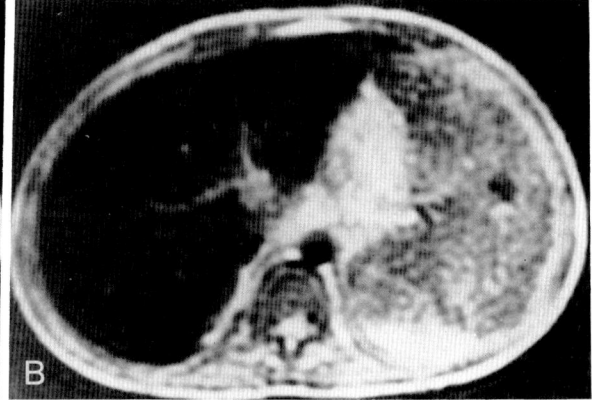

FIGURE 6.4. TRANSFUSION IRON OVERLOAD HEMOSIDEROSIS IN A 9-YR-OLD WITH SICKLE CELL ANEMIA
A: MRI shows extremely hypointense liver and splenomegaly, SE 28/500 (A) and SE 56/2000 (B).

COPPER DISEASE STATES

Copper disease states include Wilson's disease, long-standing biliary obstruction, primary biliary cirrhosis, and Hodgkin's disease. The normal range of hepatic copper concentration is 15–55 mg/g. Copper levels >250 mg/g in dry liver biopsy specimens are seen only in Wilson's disease and long-standing biliary obstruction (17). Levels as high as 700 mg/g have been seen in the former. High concentrations of copper have been seen in Hodgkin's disease, so it is possible that hepatic Hodgkin's disease can enter into the differential diagnosis of elevated hepatic copper (17). As does the ferric ion, the paramagnetic Cu^{2+} ion shortens both T1 and T2. Increased liver intensity and shortened T1 was seen with inversion recovery (T1-weighted) sequences in two patients with primary biliary cirrhosis and increased liver copper deposition and a long T1 with decreased intensity was seen in a patient with primary biliary cirrhosis and unknown liver copper content (0.15T) (11). At 0.15T, T1 seems to be shortened by elevated copper levels but lengthened by cirrhosis (fibrosis) and the result in any given patient is difficult to predict. The one patient with Wilson's disease in the same series had cirrhosis with a small nodular liver and both a normal T1 and a normal intensity (11, 20).

HEPATIC MASSES

Simple Cyst

Hepatic cysts are well-defined round regions of diminished intensity on T1-weighted spin echo sequences by virtue of their prolonged T1 (T1 = 1000 ms at 0.04T, normal liver 140–170 ms) (12) (Fig. 6.5). When TE and/or TR are lengthened, signal will increase in hepatic cysts by virtue of their prolonged T2. Hemorrhage into a cyst can cause increased intensity on T1-weighted sequences.

Hemangioma

Cavernous hemangiomas often have a very characteristic MR appearance and MR appears quite sensitive in their detection (5). They are round, homogeneous, well-circumscribed low intensity masses on spin echo images with short TE/TR and very high intensity on images with long TE/TR (2, 5, 21). Hepatic cyst is the only other hepatic mass that routinely has these MR characteristics but cysts are easily excluded by ultrasound. Metastases and hepatocellular carcinomas occasionally look similar, but usually are heterogeneous on at least one spin echo sequence if several TEs and TRs are used (5). Hemangiomas have a prolonged T1 (350–370 ms compared to normal liver values of 140–170 ms at 0.04T) (12), and prolonged T2 (100 ± 30 ms) (3, 6). They are best differentiated from other masses by hyperintensity on long TE/TR (T2-weighted) spin echo images (2, 3, 5, 6, 20). At short TRs they are hypo or isointense at TE 28 and somewhat hyperintense at TE 56 (5). About 10% of hemangiomas do not have the above typical appearance, probably due to hemorrhage, necrosis and/or fibrosis (Fig. 6.6) (3, 5, 6).

Focal Nodular Hyperplasia

We have seen one benign liver mass that probably is focal nodular hyperplasia in which MRI showed the central scar but did not really contribute to the diagnosis (Fig. 6.7).

Adenoma

The MRI appearance of hepatic adenoma in two reported cases was indistinguishable from that of hepatocellular carcinoma (2). T1 and T2 relaxation times were within the ranges observed for metastases and hepatocellular carcinoma. The internal architecture and capsule were depicted better by MR than CT, but the reverse was true for calcification (2).

Hepatocellular Carcinoma

Assigning T1 and T2 values to hepatocellular carcinomas is difficult because of marked slice-to-slice variations presumably due to hemor-

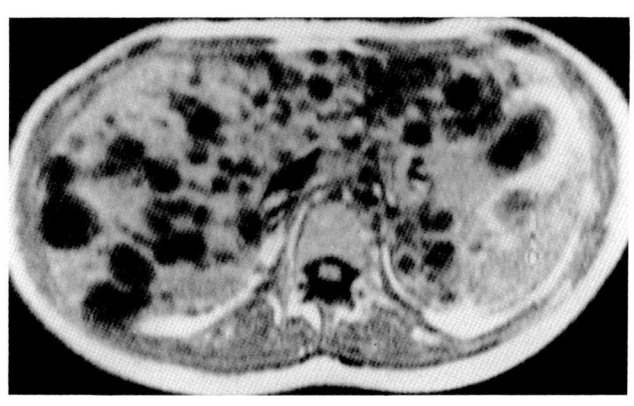

FIGURE 6.5. MULTIPLE LOW INTENSITY HEPATIC CYSTS IN A PATIENT WITH ADULT POLYCYSTIC KIDNEY DISEASE (SE 28/500)

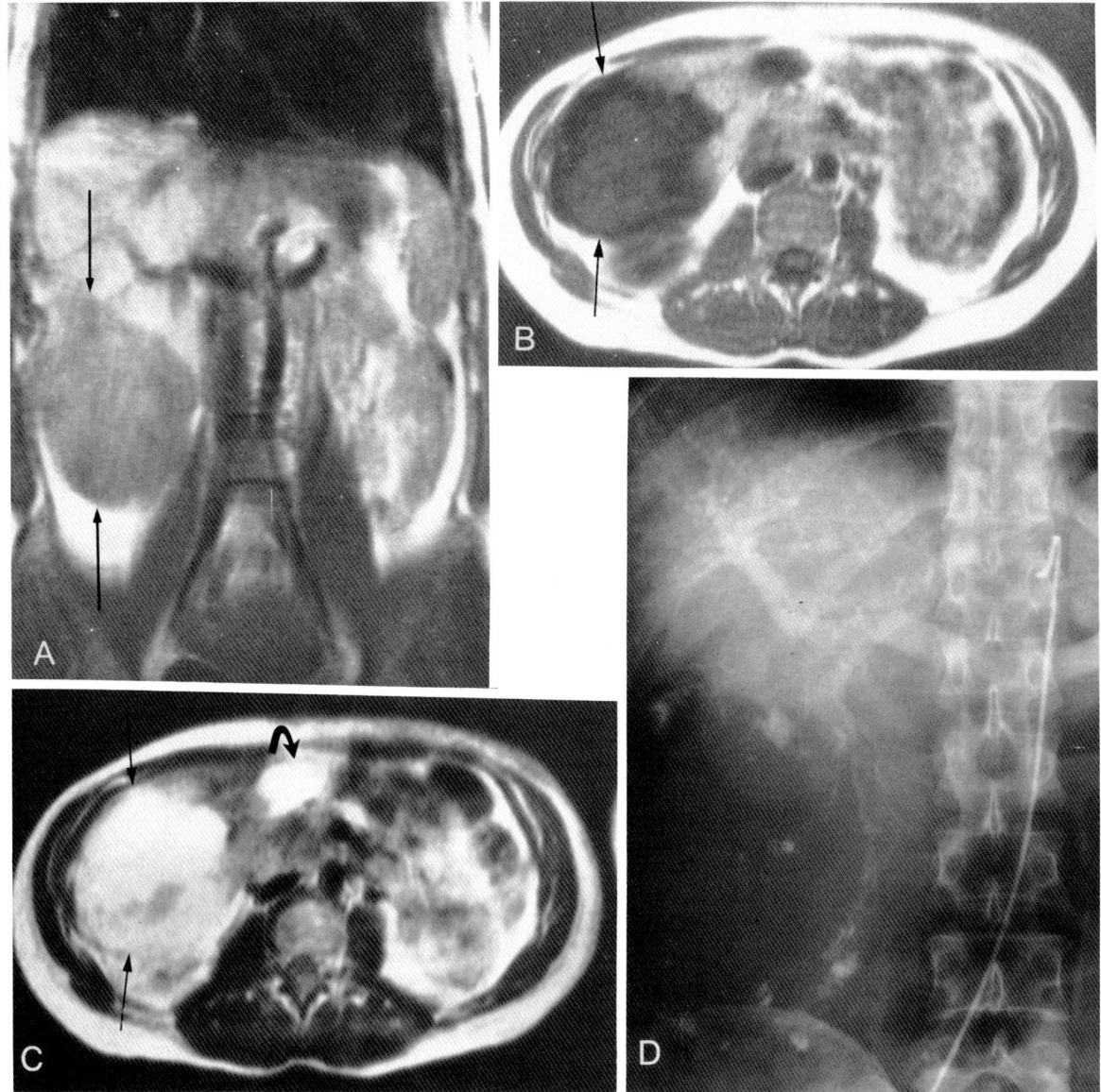

FIGURE 6.6. LARGE, SOMEWHAT ATYPICAL HEMANGIOMA

A and B: T1-weighted images, coronal and axial show a large, low intensity mass (*arrows*). C: The T2-weighted image shows a hyperintense mass (*arrows*) with internal inhomogeneity probably due to fibrosis. Note that the mass is almost as intense as the gallbladder (*curved arrow*). D: Confirmatory angiogram, venous phase. (Case courtesy of Joachim Seeger, M.D., University of Arizona Health Sciences Center, Tucson, AZ.)

rhage, necrosis, and fibrosis. Hepatocellular carcinomas have greater intensity than normal liver on T2-weighted spin echo sequences and lower intensity on inversion recovery and T1-weighted spin echo images (Fig. 6.8) (2). T1 and T2 relaxation times are generally both prolonged. T1s are reported as 300–450 ms (compared to normal liver of 140–170 ms, 0.04T) (12), and 460–530 ms (compared to normal liver 210–270 ms, 0.15T) (11). T2s are 60 ± 8 ms, only slightly longer than normal liver (56 ± 8 ms) (3, 6), but always <80 ms, differentiating hepatocellular carcinoma from hemangioma in most instances. The best contrast with spin echo technique is seen with a long TE. Some hepatocellular carcinomas are virtually isointense at short TE and short TR, and some are seen best on inversion recovery, especially with a long TR and a short TI (2). MRI can demonstrate either sharp or indistinct margins, internal septations and in-

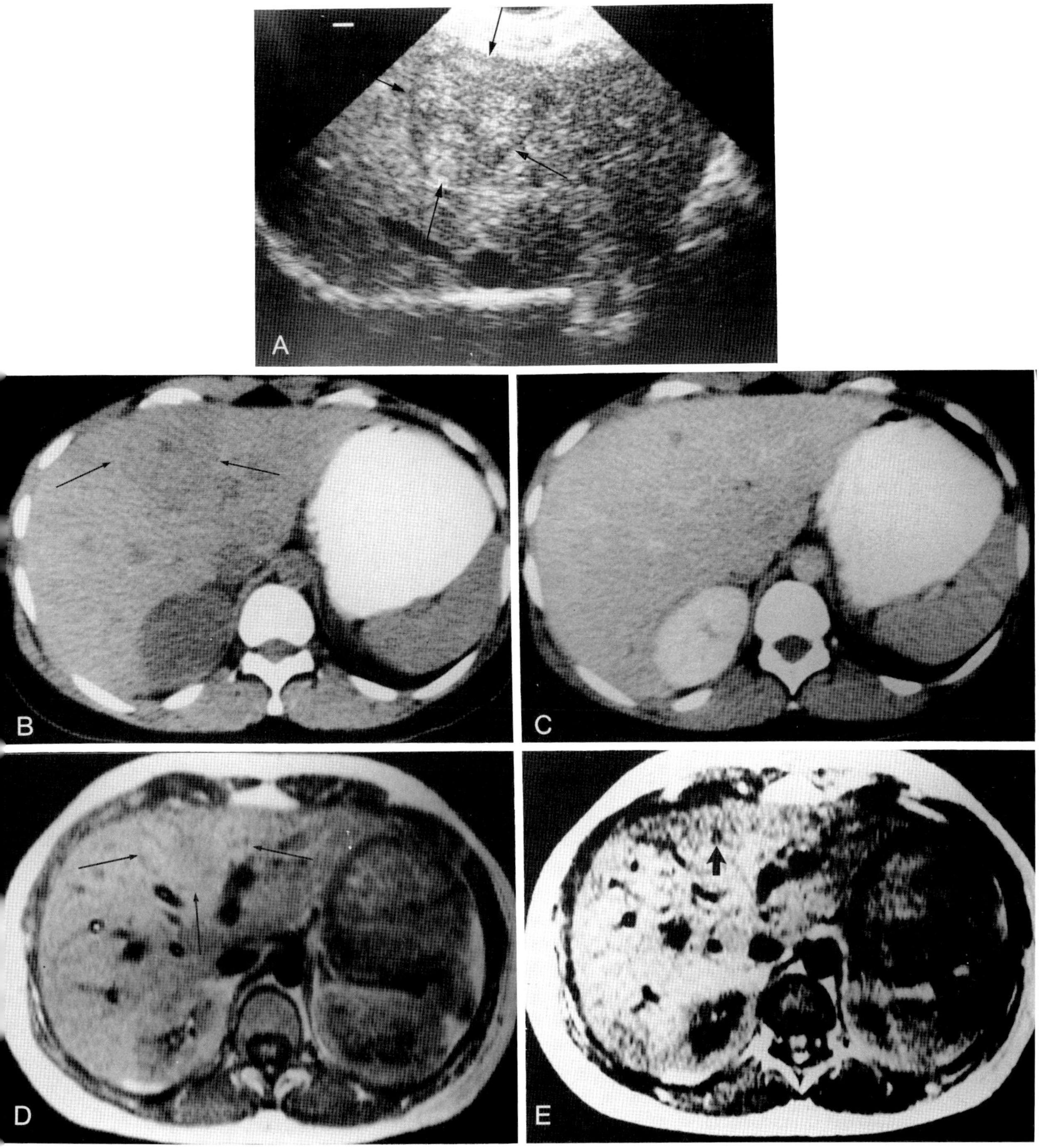

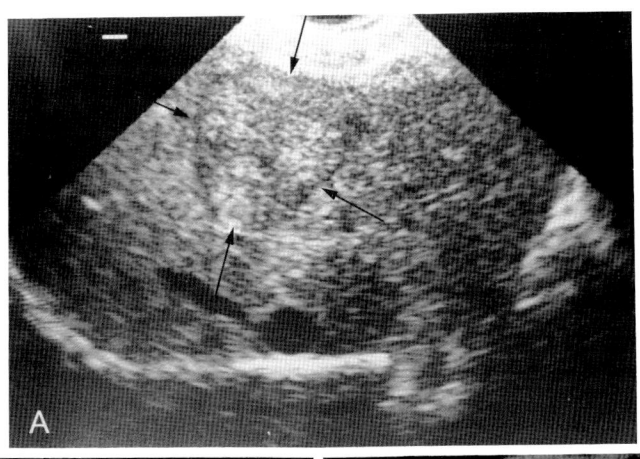

FIGURE 6.7. PROBABLE FOCAL NODULAR HYPERPLASIA

Probable focal nodular hyperplasia found incidentally on sonogram in a 22-yr-old woman with no history of oral contraceptive use. The MRI is nonspecific and somewhat inferior to CT and sonography. Radionuclide scans suggest the correct diagnosis. Biopsy refused, the mass is unchanged on serial sonography over one year. *A*: Transverse sonogram shows well demarcated mass (*arrows*), nearly isoechoic, surrounded by a thin hypoechoic rim. *B* and *C*: CT without (*B*) and with (*C*) contrast. Well demarcated hypodense mass (*arrows*) with lucent rim that enhances more than hepatic parenchyma except for a central, nonenhanced region (probably scar). *D*: Mass (*arrows*) barely detectable (SE 28/500). *E*: Slightly cephalad to (*D*), photographed at a narrow window to highlight hypointense central scar (*arrow*) (SE 28/500). *F* and *G*: respectively: mass (*arrows*) is more easily seen. Note gentle displacement of vein on (*G*) (SE 28/1000 and 28/2000). *H* and *I*: Sulfur-colloid scan (*H*) and HIDA scan (*I*): greater uptake of sulfur colloid than HIDA (*arrows*), favoring focal nodular hyperplasia. The mass was galliopenic (gallium scan not shown), mitigating against a hepatocellular carcinoma.

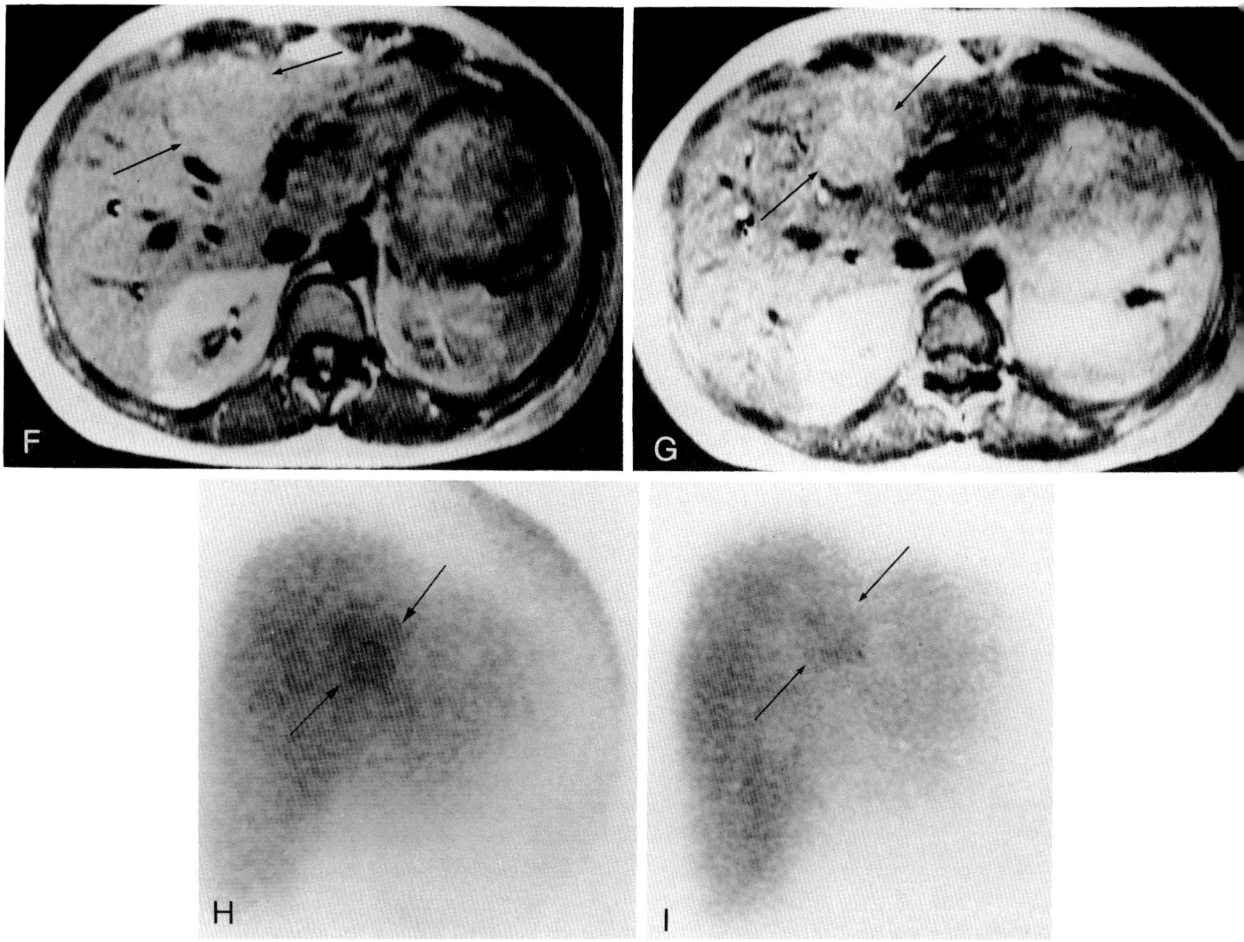

274   LIVER, BILIARY TRACT, PANCREAS, SPLEEN

FIGURE 6.7F–I

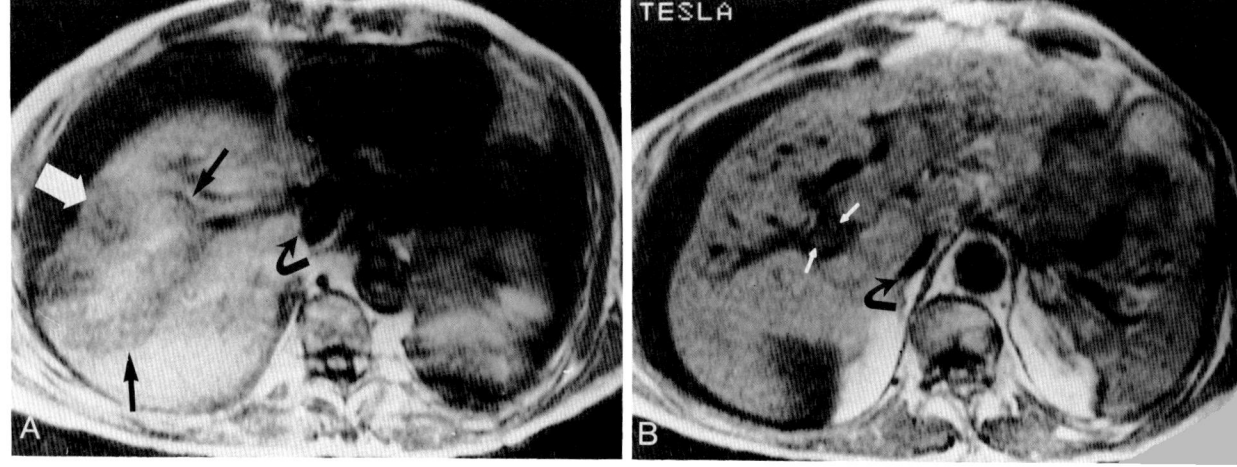

FIGURE 6.8. HEPATOCELLULAR CARCINOMA INVADING THE PORTAL VEIN (SE 28/500)
A: Mixed hypo and isointense mass (*arrows*) in right lobe just beneath diaphragm. Note hypointense ascites anterior to mass and intact IVC (*curved arrow*) with draining hepatic veins. *B*: Tumor thrombus in portal vein seen as intraluminal signal (*arrows*). IVC intact (*curved arrow*).

homogeneities, vascular displacement or invasion (Fig. 6.8), and biliary obstruction or invasion (2). As with CT, focal and multifocal hepatocellular carcinomas are well depicted and usually obvious, whereas the infiltrating diffuse variety is difficult to detect. MRI may show the presence of the latter by dint of diffusely altered liver intensity and loss of the normal hepatic vascular pattern (2).

Cholangiocarcinoma

Three cases of intrahepatic cholangiocarcinoma detected with MRI have been reported (12). Their T1s varied in a range (200–350 ms) that was lower than hepatocellular carcinoma or metastasis but higher than normal liver values (140–170 ms, 0.04T), but overlap was present. It is unlikely that intrahepatic cholangiocarcinomas can be differentiated from hepatocellular carcinomas by MRI (Fig. 6.9).

Metastatic Disease

Liver metastases always have a longer T1 than normal liver (280–450 ms, normal liver 140–170 ms, 0.04T (12); 560–810 ms, normal liver 210–270 ms, 0.15T (11); 428 ± 60 ms, normal liver 177 ± 60 ms, 0.15T (14); 40% longer, 0.35T (2)), and are, therefore, usually hypointense on T1-weighted spin echo images and inversion recovery images (2, 4). T2s have been quite inconsistent, one reported series calculated T2 at 14.5 ± 3 ms (normal 19.7 ± 10 ms) (14), whereas a more recent series calculated T2 for metastases at 64 ± 5 ms (3, 6) with 90% having a T2 < 80 ms which was felt to be a useful criterion to differentiate metastasis from hemangioma. A third series showed T2s on average 21% longer than normal liver, but 7% had shorter T2s (0.35T) (2). Currently, calculated T1 and T2 relaxation times are not that useful in metastatic disease because they vary among different tumors and even within the same tumor in a single patient (2).

Spin echo technique employing multiple TEs and TRs was thought to be equal in sensitivity to CT in detecting liver metastasis in a recent series (4). Metastases were usually hypointense on T1-weighted images and hyperintense on T2-weighted sequences, the latter usually giving the best demonstration of metastases. They can be isointense on one or two sequences but almost never on four. They are usually heterogeneous in internal architecture on at least 1 pulse sequence (5). Size measured by MR was slightly less on T1-weighted sequences than T2-weighted sequences, and the former may correlate better with true size (4). On inversion recovery sequences, metastases are usually low intensity (Fig. 6.10), but occasionally they may be high intensity. Shorter TIs and longer TRs give slightly better contrast (2). The center of a metastasis often has a longer T1 than its periphery, resulting in an appearance similar to rim enhancement on contrast-enhanced CT (2). Other techniques have been used: Young et al. reported that inversion recovery has greater contrast than partial saturation recovery in metastatic disease (20), and Alfidi et al. thought that inversion recovery and calculated T1 images were better than saturation recovery (22). Simple proton spectroscopic imaging promises to be superior to any other published MR technique in detecting liver metastases (8, 16). Gadolinium-DTPA has been studied as an MR intravenous contrast material in the liver (23). Normal liver parenchyma and portal veins were found to enhance after intravenous infusion of 0.1 mmol of Gd-DTPA. Eighteen of twenty hepatic tumors increased in intensity, with greatest increases seen in inversion recovery sequences. Unfortunately, this resulted in diminished difference between the originally hypointense tumors and the liver. Spin echo showed marked tumor intensity increase in nine, little increase in two, and none in nine (23).

Hepatic Lymphoma

MRI of 13 patients with hepatic lymphoma showed focal abnormalities in only one (24). Calculated T1 and T2 relaxation times were within one standard deviation of normal. Thus, diffuse lymphoma could not be detected. Conceivably, different imaging techniques or improved relaxation time calculations will be able to detect diffuse hepatic lymphoma in the future.

Portal Hypertension

We have found MRI to be quite informative in the evaluation of portasystemic collaterals in portal hypertension (Fig. 6.10). Dilated veins are nicely displayed as low intensity tubular structures. Although it is not likely to replace ultrasound for screening, MR may have a role (possibly replacing angiography) in preoperative (shunt surgery) planning (25). In addition to ascites (which is low intensity) MR often shows splenic enlargement and intensity change due to T1 and T2 prolongation in portal hypertension (2, 12). T1-weighted spin echo or inversion recovery images will show diminished intensity

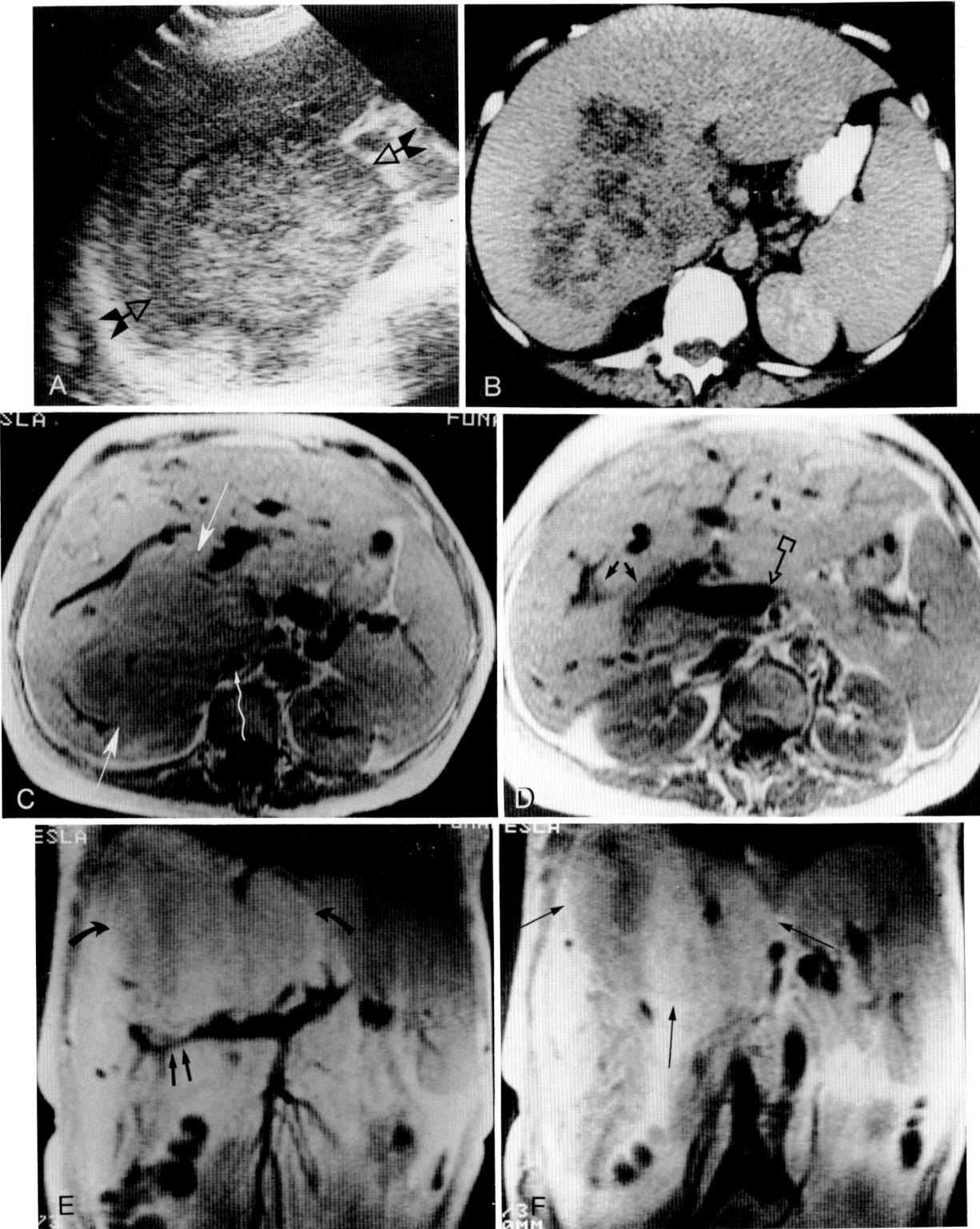

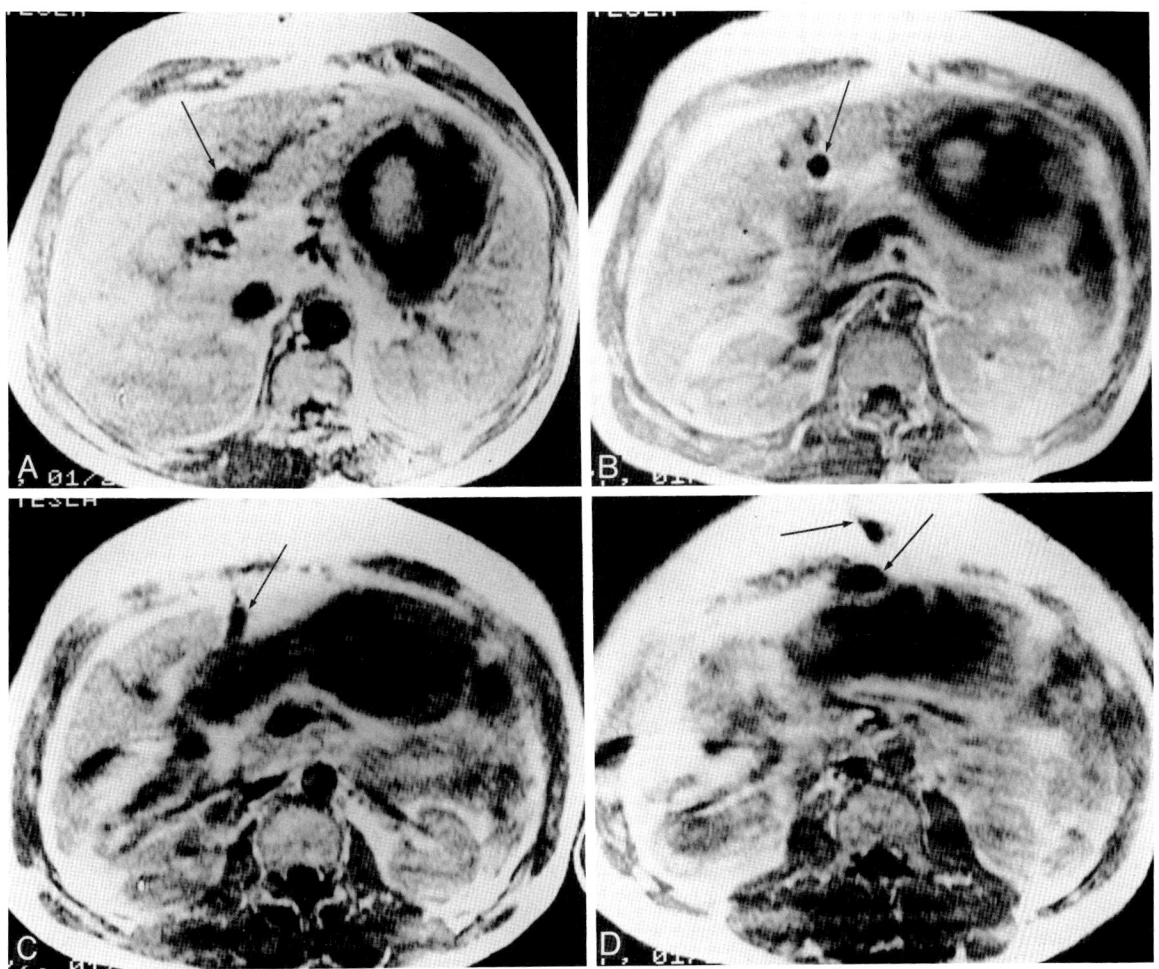

FIGURE 6.10. MRI IN PORTAL HYPERTENSION

A–D: Dilated umbilical vein (*arrows*) (SE 28/500). *E*: Dilated coronary vein (*white arrows*) and abdominal wall collateral (*black arrows*) (SE 28/500). *F–I*: Cavernous transformation of the portal vein: incidental finding in lymphoma workup. Patient is allergic to urographic contrast. *F* and *G*: Noncontrast CT: Nodular densities (*arrows*)—nodes or veins? *H* and *I*: MRI (SE 28/500): Collateral veins (*curved arrows*) corresponding to CT abnormality. Nonvisualization of main portal vein with porta hepatis collaterals (*small arrows*). *J–S*: Budd-Chiari Syndrome and cirrhosis, the former suggested by sonography and CT but confirmed by MRI. *J* and *K*: Contrast enhanced CT: very irregular liver parenchyma, enlarged left and caudate lobes consistent with macronodular cirrhosis, nonvisualization of intrahepatic IVC and hepatic veins, dilated azygos vein, splenomegaly, ascites. *L* and *M*: Transverse and sagittal sonograms, respectively: enlarged caudate lobe (*white arrow*) beneath stretched portal veins (*black arrow*), patent IVC (*open arrow*). Despite careful search, no hepatic veins could be found. *N–P*: Axial MRI. *N* and *O*: (SE 38/2000): Patent cava without any hepatic veins draining into it (*large white arrows*, note compression on *O*). Serpiginous, narrow black intrahepatic lines are collateral veins, the largest of which is part of the left hepatic vein (*arrowheads*). Dilated azygos vein is seen (*black arrow*) next to aorta. *P*: IR 310/1500: poorer resolution but better contrast. Heterogeneous signal from liver parenchyma corresponding to CT density differences seen in (*K*). Low intensity region in the right lobe may reflect regionally worse vascular congestion. Hypointense spleen reflecting vascular congestion from portal hypertension. *Q*: Coronal MRI (SE 28/500): Compressed but patent IVC (*arrow*). High intraluminal signal proximally (*curved arrows*) representing slow flow. No hepatic veins draining into IVC. MRI diagnosis: Budd-Chiari with hepatic venous occlusion. *R*: Cavagram with Valsalva: no reflux into hepatic veins. Patent IVC, but compressed just below right atrium. *S*: Hepatic venogram: middle hepatic vein is the only vein that could be catheterized. Collateral network is opacified, with filling of the left hepatic vein (arrow), corresponding to *N*.

FIGURE 6.9. INTRAHEPATIC CHOLANGIOCARCINOMA

MRI (SE 28/500) gave best depiction of intact portal vein, but added little else. *A*: Transverse sonogram: well-demarcated, mostly hyperechoic mass (*arrows*). *B*: Contrast-enhanced CT: Heterogeneous hypodense mass. *C*: Axial MRI: hypointense mass (*arrows*) displacing vessels. Intact IVC (*undulating arrow*). *D*: More caudad cut: intact portal vein (large arrow). Dilated ducts (*small arrows*). *E*: Coronal scan barely showing the tumor (*curved arrows*) but demonstrating intact but displaced portal vein (*arrows*) and superior mesenteric vein. *F*: Somewhat better tumor depiction more posteriorly (*arrows*).

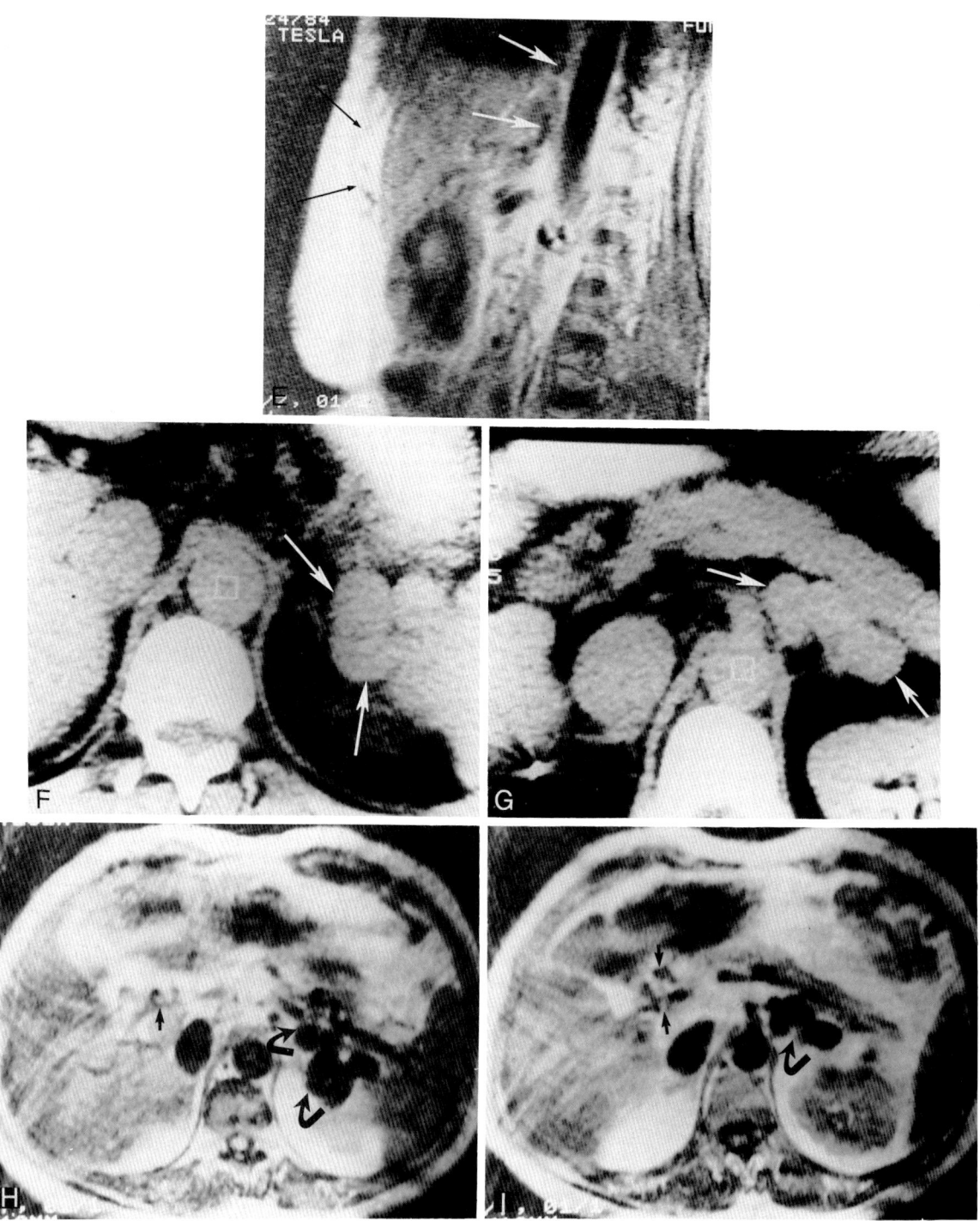

FIGURE 6.10E–I

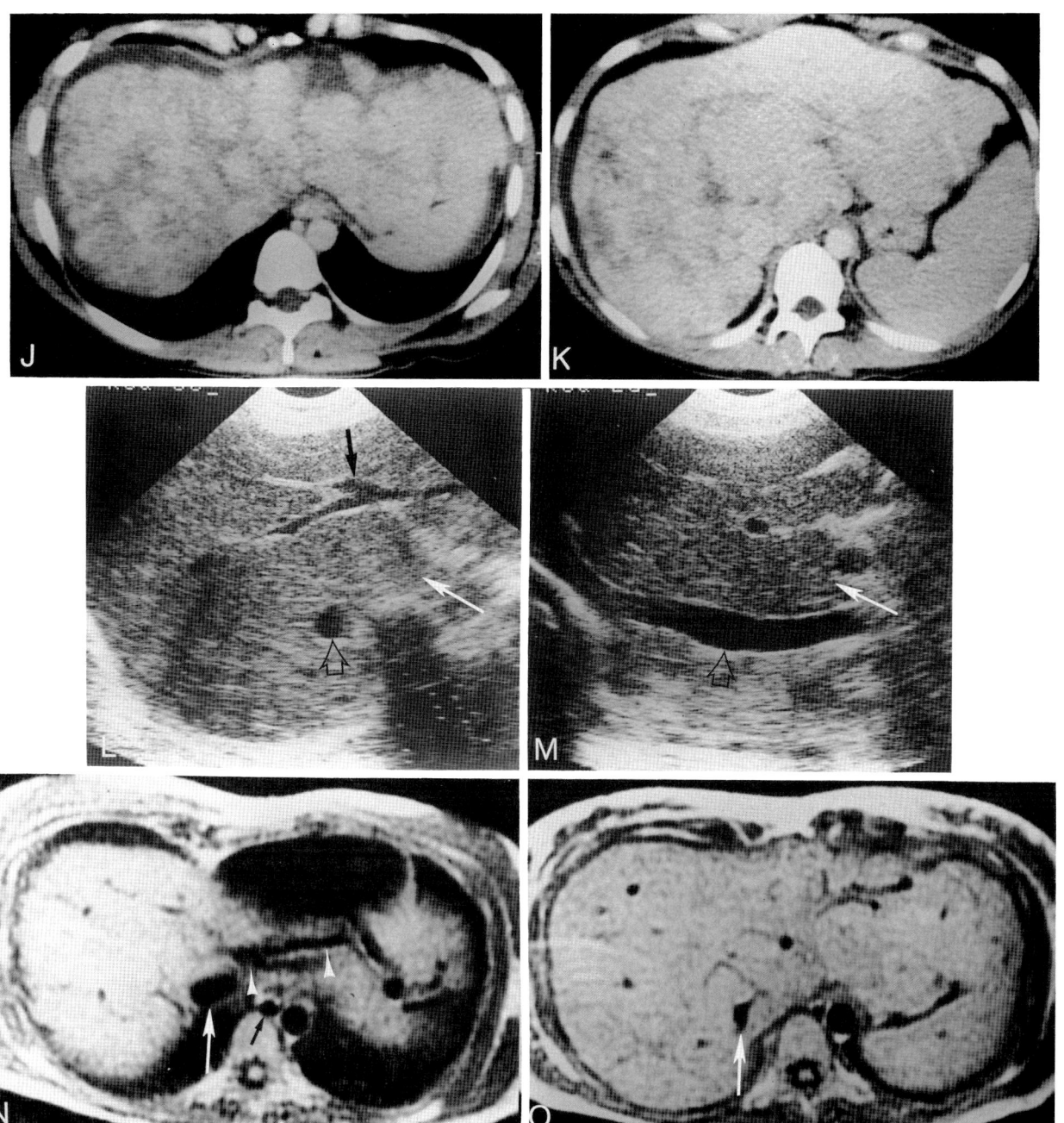

FIGURE 6.10*J–O*

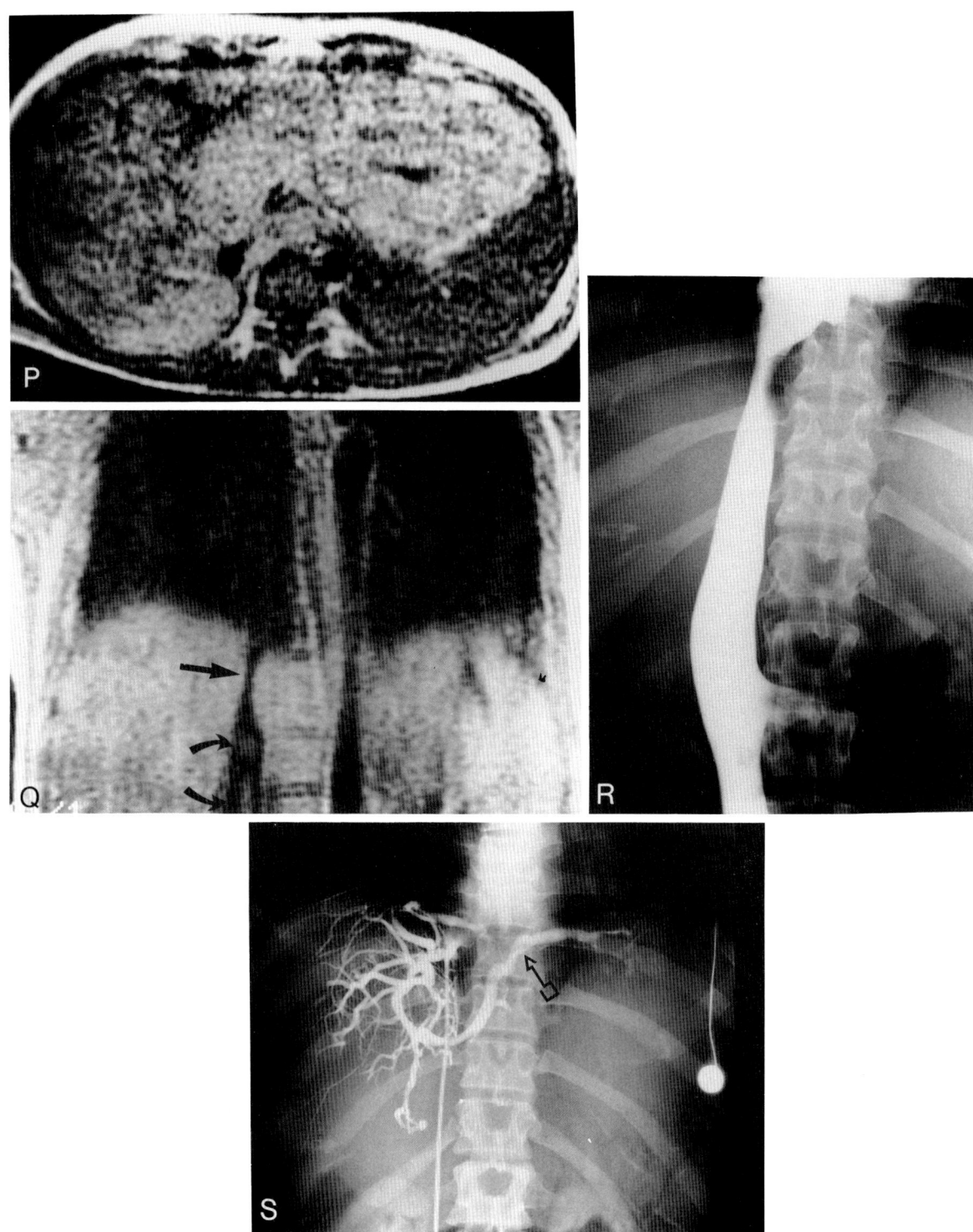

FIGURE 6.10P–S

(Fig. 6.10P) and T2-weighted spin echo images will show increased intensity. These findings may be due to splenic edema from venous congestion. The same findings can be seen in splenic vein occlusion due to pancreatic disease.

SUMMARY

Compared to CT, MRI of the liver offers better display of the internal architecture of tumors, better depiction of their relationship to regional blood vessels (25), better depiction of disease extent, and freedom from clip and other streak artefacts. CT depicts calcification much better and can assess tumor vascularity using intravenous contrast material and does not suffer from respiratory motion blurring. Potentially, MR will be able to assess tumor vascularity with MRI contrast agents and has the potential for superior display and diagnosis of diffuse liver diseases, although currently CT is superior for fatty infiltration. The multiplanar capability of MRI is useful in our experience only for evaluating the effects of masses on blood vessels and in studying collaterals in portal hypertension. Potentially, MR can detect neoplastic involvement of the liver earlier than CT because longer T1 and T2 relaxation times have been measured in histologically normal regions in neoplastically involved tissues (24).

REFERENCES

1. Bottomley PA, Foster TH, Argersinger RE, Pfeifer LM: A review of normal tissue hydrogen NMR relaxation times and relaxation mechanisms from 1–100 MHz: dependence on tissue type, NMR frequency, temperature, species, excision, and age. *Med Phys* 11:425–448, 1984.
2. Moss AA, Goldberg HI, Stark DB, Davis PL, Margulis AR, Kaufman L, Crooks LE: Hepatic tumors: magnetic resonance and CT appearance. *Radiology* 150:141–147, 1984.
3. Itai Y, Ohtomo K, Furui S, Iio M: Non-invasive diagnosis of small cavernous hemangioma of the liver: combined use of US, CT and MR. Presented at the 70th Scientific Assembly and Annual Meeting of RSNA, Washington, D.C., November 25–30, 1984.
4. Heiken JP, Lee JKT, Ling D, Glazer H: MR imaging of hepatic metastases. Presented at the 70th Scientific Assembly and Annual Meeting of RSNA, Washington, D.C., November 25–30, 1984.
5. Glazer GM, Aizen AM, Francis IR, Gyves JW, Lande I, Adler DD: MR imaging of hepatic cavernous hemangioma. Presented at the 70th Scientific Assembly and Annual Meeting of RSNA, Washington, D.C., November 25–30, 1984.
6. Ohtomo K, Itai Y, Furui S, Kukubo T, Yoshikawa K, Yashiro N, Iio M: MR imaging of hepatic tumors: differential diagnosis by T2. Presented at the 70th Scientific Assembly and Annual Meeting of RSNA, Washington, D.C., November 25–30, 1984.
7. Weinreb JC, Brateman L, Maravilla KR: Magnetic resonance imaging of hepatic lymphoma. *AJR* 143:1211–1214, 1984.
8. Dixon WT: Simple proton spectroscopic imaging. *Radiology* 153:189–194, 1984.
9. Stark DD, Bass NM, Moss AA, Bacon BR, McKerrow JH, Cann CE, Brito A, Goldberg HI: Nuclear magnetic resonance imaging of experimentally induced liver disease. *Radiology* 148:743–751, 1983.
10. Stark DD, Goldberg HI, Moss AA, Bass NM: Chronic liver disease: evaluation by magnetic resonance. *Radiology* 150:149–151, 1984.
11. Doyle FH, Pennock JM, Banks LM, McDonnell MJ, Bydder GM, Steiner RE, Young IR, Clarke GJ, Pasmore T, Gilderdale DJ: Nuclear magnetic resonance imaging of the liver: initial experience. *AJR* 138:193–200, 1982.
12. Smith FW, Mallard JR, Reid A, Hutchison JMS: Nuclear magnetic resonance tomographic imaging in liver disease. *Lancet* 963–966, (May) 1981.
13. Goldberg HI, Moss AA, Stark DD, McKerrow J, Engelstad B, Brito A: Hepatic cirrhosis: magnetic resonance imaging. *Radiology* 153:737–739, 1984.
14. Buonocore E, Borkowski GP, Pavlicek W, Ngo F: NMR imaging of the abdomen: technical considerations. *AJR* 141:1171–1178, 1983.
15. Wenker JC, Baker MK, Ellis JH, Glant MD: Focal fatty infiltration of the liver: demonstration by magnetic resonance imaging. *AJR* 143:573–574, 1984.
16. Lee JKT, Dixon WT, Ling D, Levitt RG, Murphy WA: Fatty infiltration of the liver: demonstration by proton spectroscopic imaging—preliminary observations. *Radiology* 153:195–201, 1984.
17. Runge VM, Clanton JA, Smith FW, Hutchison J, Mallard J, Partain CL, James AE: Nuclear magnetic resonance of iron and copper disease states. *AJR* 141:943–948, 1983.
18. Stark DD, Moseley ME, Bacon BR, Moss AA, Goldberg HI, Bass NM, James TL: Magnetic resonance imaging and spectroscopy of hepatic iron overload. *Radiology* 154:137–142, 1985.
19. Brasch RC, Wesbey GE, Gooding CA, Koerper MA: Magnetic resonance imaging of transfusional hemosiderosis complicating thalassemia major. *Radiology* 150:767–771, 1984.
20. Kressel HY, Mamourian A, Haggar A, Axel L, Gefter W, Soloway R: MR imaging of primary liver masses. Presented at the 70th Scientific Assembly and Annual Meeting of RSNA, Washington, D.C., November 25–30, 1984.
21. Young IR, Bailes DR, Burl M, Collins AG, Smith DT, McDonnell MJ, Orr JS, Banks LM, Bydder GM, Greenspan RH, Steiner RE: Initial clinical evaluation of a whole body nuclear magnetic resonance (NMR) tomograph. *J Comput Assist Tomogr* 6:1–18, 1982.
22. Alfidi RJ, Haaga JR, El Yousef SJ, et al.: Preliminary experimental results in humans and animals with a superconducting whole-body nuclear magnetic resonance scanner. *Radiology* 143:175–181, 1982.
23. Steiner RE, Carr DH, Bydder GM, Young IR: Use of Gadolinium-DTPA as an intravenous contrast agent in MR imaging of the liver and pancreas. Presented at the

70th Scientific Assembly and Annual Meeting of RSNA, Washington, D.C., November 25–30, 1984.

24. Bernardino ME, Small W, Goldstein J, Sewell CW, Sones PJ, Gedgaudas-McClees K, Galambos JT, Wenger J, Casarella WJ: Multiple NMR T2 relaxation values in human liver tissue. *AJR* 141:1203–1208, 1983.

25. Wall SD, Goldberg HI, Moss AA, Margulis AR, Amparo EG, Stark DD, Hricak H, Higgins CB: Effect of hepatic disease on hepatic vasculature, demonstration by MRI. Presented at the 70th Scientific Assembly and Annual Meeting of RSNA, Washington, D.C., November 25–30, 1984.

7
Hepatic Trauma

ARNOLD C. FRIEDMAN, M.D.

After the spleen and kidney, the liver is the third most common organ injured in abdominal trauma. Liver injury occurred in 3% of trauma patients in one series from a large shock trauma center (1). Formerly associated mostly with penetrating trauma, liver injury is now usually caused by blunt trauma because of the increase in high speed motor vehicle accidents (2). Most deaths from hepatic injuries occur within the first 24 hr after trauma from exsanguination, and most of these patients go directly to surgery without sophisticated radiologic study (3).

CLINICAL FINDINGS

Symptoms and signs include abdominal or right upper quadrant pain, shock, and peritoneal irritation. Other intra-abdominal organs are frequently seriously injured especially the kidneys and the pancreas, and thoracic injuries are commonly present (1). Currently, mortality from hepatic trauma is 10–20%, with half of deaths from the liver injury itself, and half from other associated injuries (1).

Routine laboratory studies may reveal an elevated white blood cell count, a decrease in hematocrit and elevation of SGOT and SGPT, although the latter enzymes usually are not elevated until several hours after trauma. Mild bilirubin elevation can occur on the third or fourth day after the hepatic trauma. Peritoneal lavage is highly sensitive in detecting the hemoperitoneum associated with hepatic injury; as little as 20 ml of blood results in a positive lavage. However, the source of the blood is not identified, and hepatic injuries without hemoperitoneum will not be detected.

TREATMENT

Shock and thoracic injuries are treated first (1). In dealing with the injured liver, bleeding is first controlled and then necrotic, devitalized tissue is removed and external drainage established (1). Although it is unusual for major hepatic dysfunction to be caused by hepatic artery injury, repair of a traumatized artery is generally attempted (1). Portal vein repair should be attempted even though ligation may be survived (3). Injuries to hepatic veins are a major factor in immediate mortality from hepatic trauma and are difficult to repair (1).

The presence of hepatic laceration alone does not require surgery. In one series, 80% of hepatic injuries required little or no surgical treatment of the liver although some patients needed surgery for other associated injuries (3). In the absence of other significant injuries, the need for surgery can be related to the size of the laceration and the amount of hemoperitoneum. If one or more of the following hepatic problems is present, surgery is needed: large laceration, medium to large hemoperitoneum, or growing hematoma (3). In a series from one institution, 60% of hepatic lacerations could be nonoperatively managed, with infection and continued bleeding less frequent in the group treated conservatively (4).

PATHOLOGY

Hepatic injuries range in extent from small lacerations confined to the interior of the liver with an intact capsule to large lacerations with intrahepatic hematoma, subcapsular hemorrhage, and capsular disruption (1, 5). When the capsule is disrupted, blood and bile can extravasate into the peritoneal cavity. The right lobe is affected much more often than the left lobe, possibly due to greater volume and greater proximity to ribs (1, 4). Injuries to the hepatic hilum are usually rapidly fatal, and patients do not survive long enough to undergo laparotomy. Parenchymal disruption can be complicated by hepatic parenchymal emboli to the right heart and lungs (1).

RADIOLOGY

Plain Films

Fractures of the right lower ribs are present in almost 50% of patients with liver trauma (6). Hemoperitoneum, hepatomegaly and irregularity of the liver margin, downward displacement of the hepatic flexure, and loss of the inferior liver-fat interface suggest liver injury (6). Hemoperitoneum is seen as fluid in the pelvis or in the flanks, displacing the colon away from the properitoneal fat stripes. Subcapsular hematoma may change the liver contour and displace adjacent viscera, and can be depicted as a crescentic radiolucency by total body opacification during excretory urography (6). Common chest film findings associated with hepatic trauma include elevation of the right hemidiaphragm, pleural effusion, hemothorax, diaphragmatic irregularity, pulmonary opacities from contusions, and pneumothorax (6).

Sonography

Although not used as frequently as CT in hepatic trauma, there is some evidence to suggest that sonography is nearly as accurate, especially in children (Fig. 7.1) (7). Sonography can detect fresh intrahepatic hematomas as small as 3–5 ml as rounded echogenic foci (Fig. 7.2) (8). Linear echogenic regions are seen when hematomas occur after percutaneous transhepatic cholangiography (8). Sonography has difficulty in detecting small lacerations in the dome of the right lobe. Subcapsular hematomas are anechoic, hypoechoic, or septated (depending on age) lenticular or curvilinear fluid collections (9). Blood in the peritoneal cavity does not usually clot, so that it is seen as an ovoid sonolucency in the pelvis, a lenticular curvilinear lucency in the subphrenic space, and a small, triangular sonolucency in Morrison's pouch (9).

Intrahepatic hematomas are frequently highly echogenic in the first 24 hr, and become fairly sonolucent by 96 hr after clotting (9). Septations and internal echoes develop in 1–4 weeks. Older hematomas are generally quite hypoechoic and can be either thin serosanguinous fluid or solid

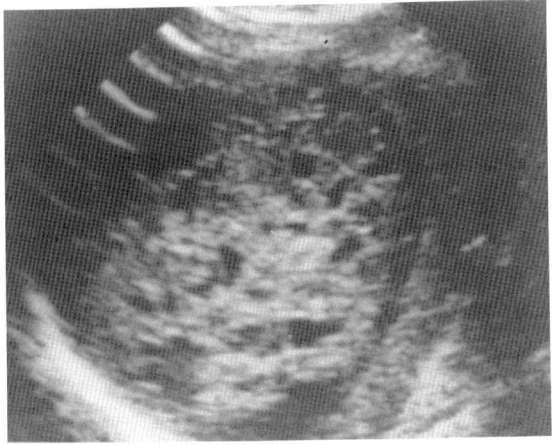

FIGURE 7.1. PARASAGITTAL SONOGRAM
Parasagittal sonogram showing a large mostly echogenic intrahepatic hematoma just beneath the diaphragm. The exam was done about two hours after the automobile accident.

and gelatinous (10). Transducer frequency is important: unclotted blood is echogenic at 7.5 MHz, and sonolucent at 3.5 MHz (9).

It is important to remember that left upper quadrant trauma can cause lacerations and hematomas in the right lobe, probably by a contrecoup mechanism (11), and scanning must not be confined to the spleen and left kidney in such situations. A major disadvantage of ultrasound compared to CT is the greater ability of CT to depict unsuspected injuries (7). Portable real-time examinations in children in the intensive care unit were less accurate in one series than examinations in the radiology department (7), somewhat negating one advantage of ultrasound.

Computed Tomography

Computed tomography is probably the radiologic examination of choice in hepatic trauma (4). Hepatic lacerations and both intrahepatic and subcapsular hematomas are detected. Hemoperitoneum can be diagnosed and quantified (Fig. 7.3). The retroperitoneum can be evaluated, and clinically unanticipated findings, which are

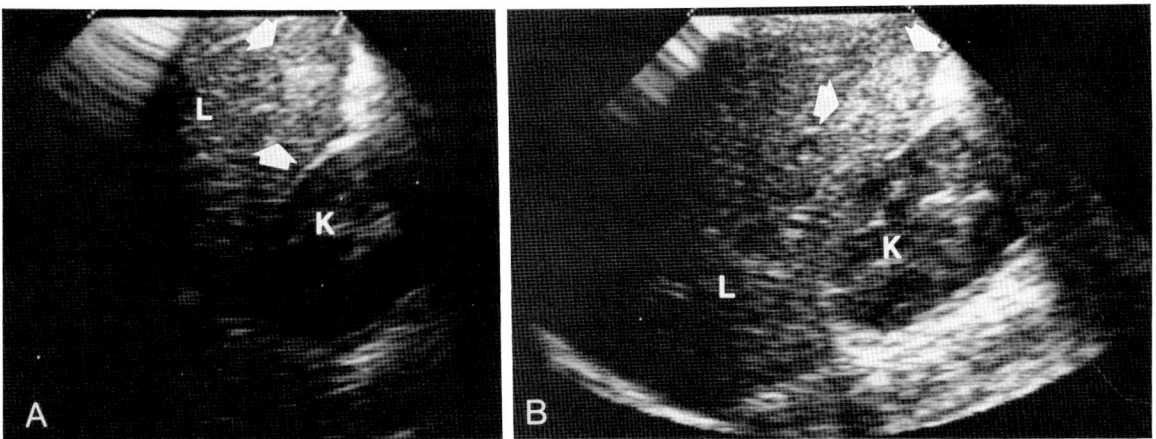

FIGURE 7.2. PARASAGITTAL AND TRANSVERSE SONOGRAMS

A and *B*: Parasagittal (*A*) and transverse (*B*) sonograms in a 2-yr-old girl with a small liver contusion. A small echogenic hematoma is present (*arrows*) in the liver (*L*) just anterior to the right kidney (*K*). (From Kaufman RA et al.: Upper abdominal trauma in children: imaging evaluation. *AJR* 142:449–460, 1984.)

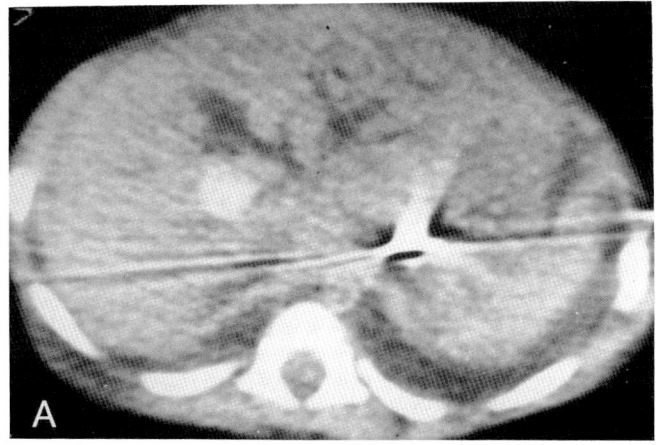

FIGURE 7.3. CT SCANS

A and *B*: CT scans both before (*A*) and after (*B*) contrast infusion in a child with hepatic lacerations. The hyperdense hematoma is best seen without contrast. On one or two scans, the branching lucent laceration could be confused with dilated bile ducts. The hemoperitoneum is depicted as low density fluid lateral to the liver and spleen. The streak artefacts are from a nasogastric tube. *C:* Hepatic trauma in a different patient: blood is seen around the liver and spleen and in the lesser sac recess medial and superior to the caudate lobe. In addition, thrombi are present (*arrows*) in the hepatic artery. These were not suspected clinically, and were confirmed by angiography. (Courtesy of Sandy Shultz, M.D., Washington, D.C.)

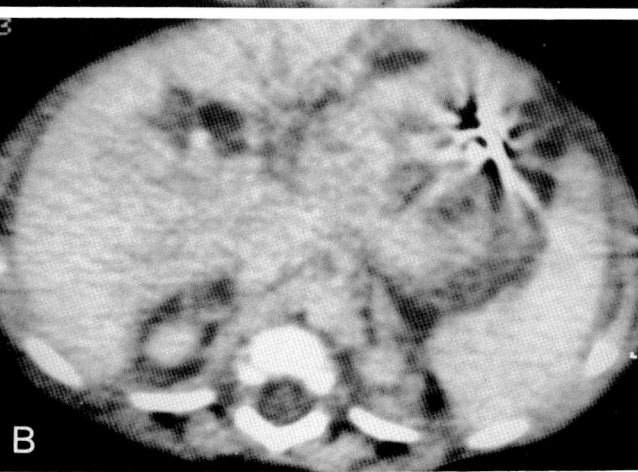

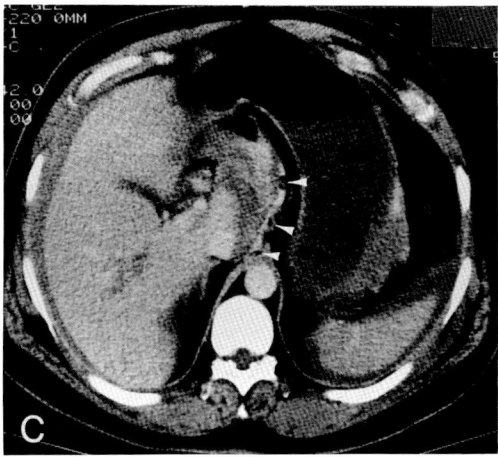

fairly common, are detected (Fig. 7.3C) (6). A baseline CT is valuable in the follow-up of patients who are subsequently scanned for suspected enlarging hematoma, liver infarction, biloma or infection (4, 5). Those patients who are relatively stable after blunt abdominal trauma or limited penetrating injury such as biopsy or minor stabbing are candidates for CT evaluation of suspected hepatic injury. Ideally, CT is performed prior to peritoneal lavage to insure that any intraperitoneal fluid detected is blood, not dialysate (4). Unstable patients or those with severe penetrating injuries should go to surgery or diagnostic and therapeutic angiography (3). Technical difficulties may be encountered with streak artifacts from gastric air-contrast levels and beam-hardening rib artifacts, but usually these do not pose clinically significant problems (4). Maximum information is obtained with closely spaced precontrast and postcontrast scans from the diaphragm through the lower poles of the kidney, followed by widely spaced postcontrast scans through the pelvis. Noncontrast scans are sometimes omitted to save time. Scanning the pelvis is important because seemingly trivial lacerations with small amounts of blood in the upper abdomen may be accompanied by surprisingly large amounts of blood in the pelvis (12).

Hepatic lacerations are the most common hepatic injury depicted by CT, and are linear, round, or branching low density regions (Fig. 7.3) (4). In the acute phase, they are slightly less dense than the parenchyma with poorly defined margins. As the interval between the injury and the scan increases, lacerations become lower in attenuation and more sharply defined (3, 5). A combination of blood and damaged parenchyma fills the cleft between lacerated fragments. Intrahepatic hematomas are usually hypodense (30–40 HU) with respect to normal parenchyma but may have hyperdense (70–100 HU) foci (Figs. 7.3A, 7.4A) (4, 5, 13). Sometimes intrahepatic hematomas can be round or oval space-occupying masses without true laceration being present (Fig. 7.4A). Subcapsular hematomas are usually associated with lacerations but may be isolated (5). They are well-circumscribed lenticular or oval low density fluid collections that typically flatten or indent the underlying hepatic parenchyma (Fig. 7.5) (4, 5). Again the longer the interval from injury, the lower the attenuation will be (3). Subcapsular or intrahepatic hematomas can be isodense or hyperdense if there is pre-existing fatty infiltration. Parenchymal fragmentation can be suggested when fragments of hepatic tissue are seen within fluid collections (Fig. 7.6) (4). Hyperdense hematoma can give the same appearance (2). Clotted blood tends to have very dense foci because of clot retraction, whereas unclotted blood (i.e. hemoperitoneum) may be difficult or impossible to differentiate from other fluid collections (such as ascites).

Postoperatively, the original laceration may be invisible after repair or it may still be depicted as a linear, poorly marginated lucency that returns to normal with healing (2). Traumatized parenchyma has been reported to undergo focal fatty infiltration temporarily producing an irregularly marginated region of negative CT numbers (14). More typically, as damaged hepatic tissue and hematoma is resorbed, the residual defect with central low attenuation becomes smoothly marginated and shrinks (15). Healing generally takes 3–4 weeks but may take longer (15). Calcification occurs occasionally.

Perihepatic and subcapsular fluid collections may be infected in the post-operative period and aspiration may be indicated. Without aspiration, abscess can be differentiated postoperatively from hematoma only if gas is present.

Angiography

Currently, angiography is rarely needed for the diagnosis of hepatic trauma, but it may be helpful in the occasional instance when the patient is stable and definitive diagnosis has not been made by noninvasive imaging. Angiographic findings soon after hepatic trauma are as follows. An intrahepatic hematoma will displace intrahepatic arteries (Fig. 7.7), whereas a subcapsular hematoma will compress and stretch intrahepatic arteries. Active bleeding is manifested by contrast material leaking into a laceration (Fig. 7.8B), or, less commonly, into the biliary tree. Arteriovenous fistulas are usually arterioportal because of the anatomic proximity of the hepatic arterial and portal branches (Figs. 7.8A, 7.9). Liver contusions cause a mottled hepatogram with delayed arterial emptying, and sometimes arterial collaterals bypassing occlusions are seen. Subcapsular hematomas compress normal parenchyma, appearing as sharply defined lucent defects against the densely staining compressed parenchyma. Intrahepatic lacerations and hematomas are radiolucent defects in the hepatogram; the former tend to be better defined than the latter (Fig. 7.7). Several days after trauma, angiography can still demonstrate hematomas and occluded arteries if they are present, but since lacerations tend to clot, active contrast

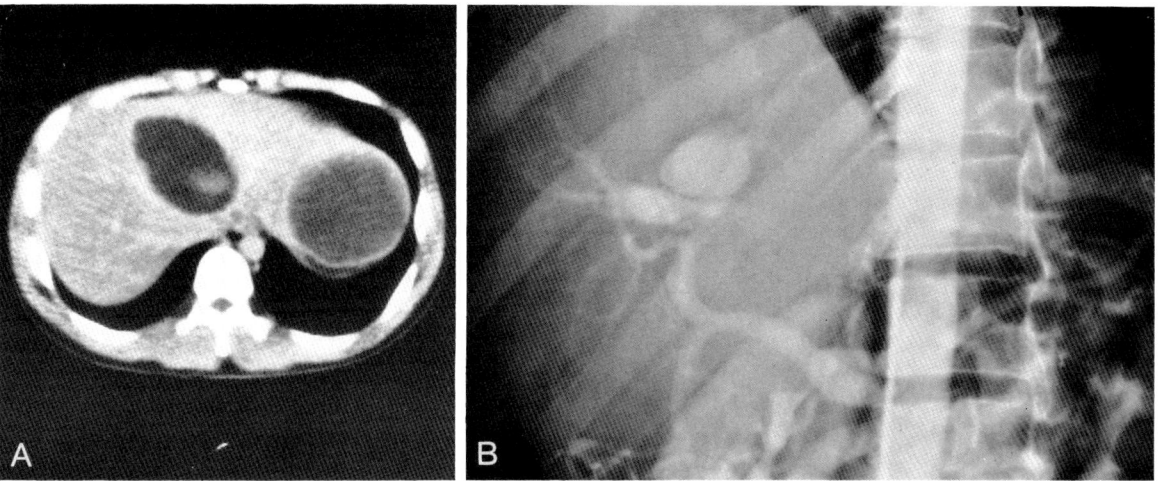

FIGURE 7.4. CONTRAST-ENHANCED CT AFTER TRAUMA

A and *B*: Contrast-enhanced CT (*A*) 11 days after trauma in a clinically stable 24-yr-old male outpatient shows a resolving hematoma in the lateral left lobe and a round density within a more medial hematoma, suggesting a pseudoaneurysm. Epigastric pain and elevated enzymes developed, and angiography (*B*) was performed 1 week later and proved the diagnosis of post-traumatic pseudoaneurysm.

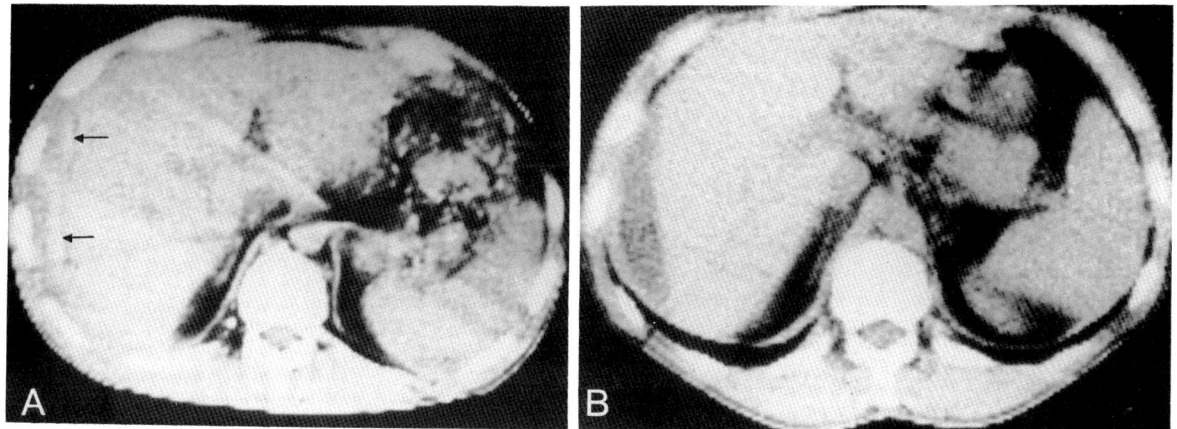

FIGURE 7.5. NONCONTRAST CT

A and *B*: Noncontrast CT scans of an acute, hyperdense subcapsular hematoma (*A*) (*arrows*) that became more typically low density after one week (*B*). Flattening of the underlying liver is better seen in *B*.

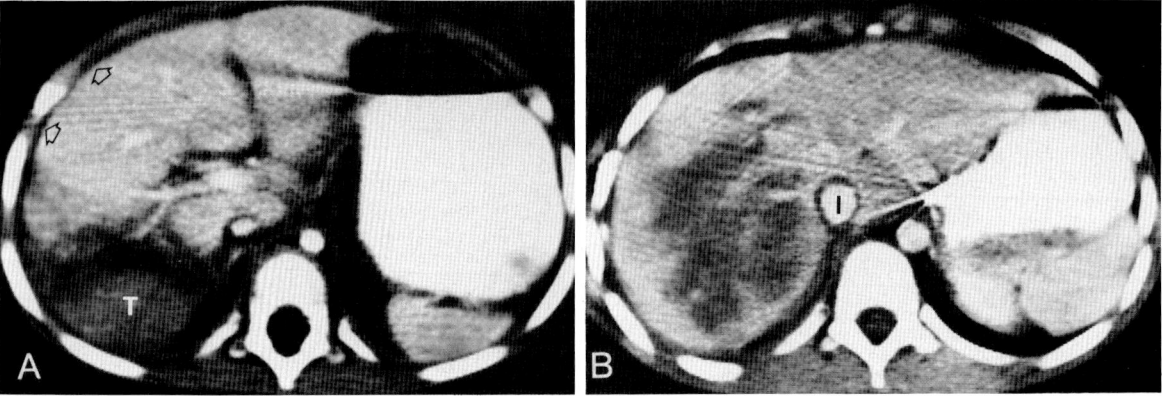

FIGURE 7.6. CT EVALUATION OF UPPER ABDOMINAL TRAUMA

A: Large fragment of the posterior right lobe is transsected (*T*) in a 3-yr-old girl. Hemoperitoneum surrounds the liver (*arrows*). *B*: Rupture of the liver with a halo of blood surrounding the inferior vena cava (*I*) in a 10-yr-old boy. Fragments of hepatic parenchyma are present within the large hematoma. (From Kaufman RA et al.: Upper abdominal trauma in children: imaging evaluation. *AJR* 142:449–160, 1984.)

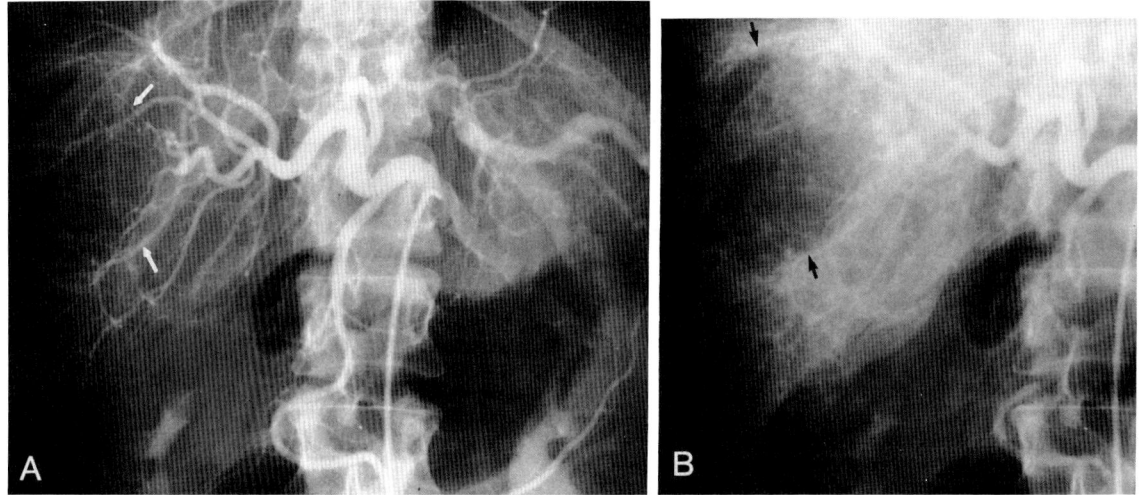

FIGURE 7.7. SELECTIVE HEPATIC ARTERIOGRAM OF AN INTRAHEPATIC HEMATOMA CAUSED BY LIVER BIOPSY

A: Arterial phase: stretched and splayed arteries (*arrows*). *B*: Hepatogram: the hematoma is a lucent defect (*arrows*).

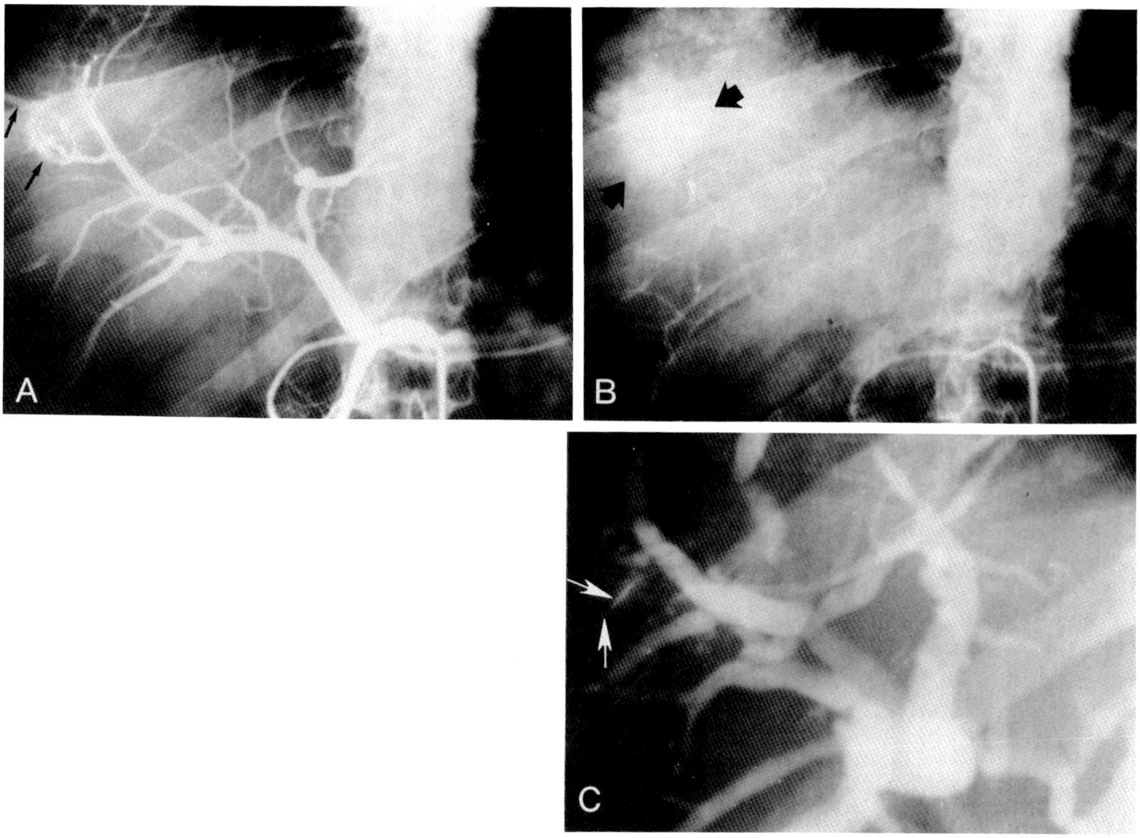

FIGURE 7.8. ARTERIOPORTAL FISTULA WITH ACTIVE BLEEDING (HEMOBILIA) 3 DAYS AFTER PERCUTANEOUS TRANSHEPATIC CHOLANGIOGRAM, TREATED WITH GELFOAM EMBOLIZATION
A: Arterial phase, hepatic arteriogram: opacification of portal vein branch (*arrows*) indicating arterioportal fistula. Flow was away from the hepatic hilum, indicating portal vein, not bile duct. *B*: Late arterial phase: contrast extravasation (*arrows*). *C*: Film from PTC showing needle (*arrows*) in the region of the arterioportal fistula.

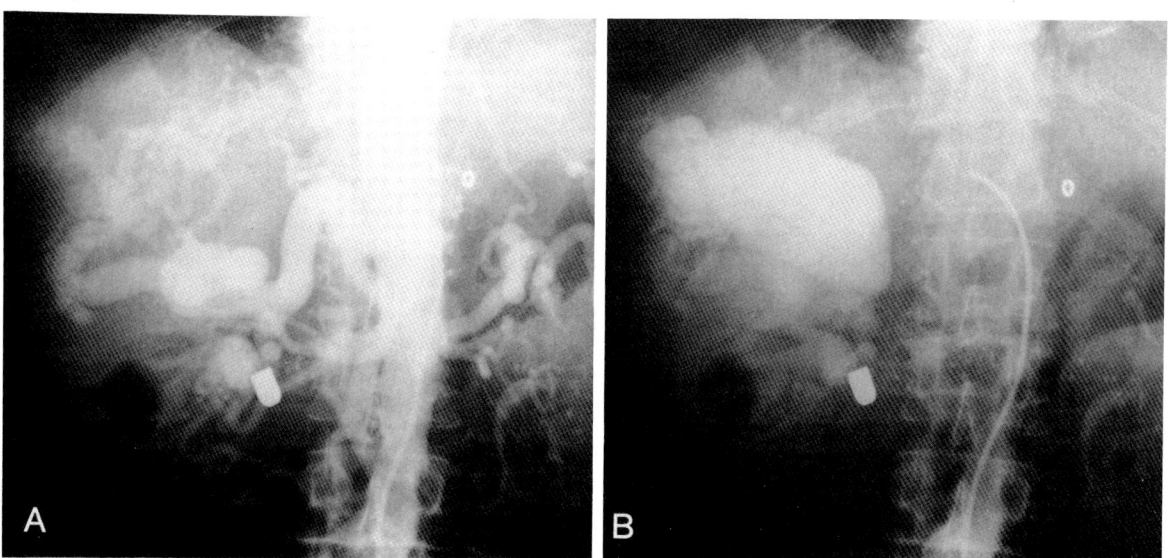

FIGURE 7.9. ARTERIOPORTAL FISTULA FROM A GUNSHOT WOUND
A: Aortogram: rapid filling of intrahepatic portal veins which course adjacent to arteries causing the arteries to appear duplicated. Note enlarged hepatic artery and bullet. *B*: Capillary phase: massively dilated portal vein.

leakage will have ceased making lacerations harder to identify. Traumatic arteriovenous fistulas and aneurysms often will disappear on their own over time (16). Therapeutic angiography is quite helpful in selected patients. Selective embolization with Gelfoam is effective in the management of free intraperitoneal hemorrhage or hemobilia (17). Traumatic hepatic artery aneurysms can be successfully treated with Gelfoam embolization or isobutyl-2-cyanoacrylate occlusion (17). Intrahepatic arterioportal fistulas are hard to treat surgically, but can be closed by detachable balloons or stainless steel coils (17).

NUCLEAR MEDICINE

Sulfur colloid scintigraphy can be used to assess the extent of hepatic injury and monitor its course. The spleen, of course, can be evaluated as well. Radionuclide angiography should be performed as part of the study as it may demonstrate abnormalities in the great vessels, heart and lung bases, renal arteries and other major abdominal vessels. The use of ^{99m}Tc-IDA scintigraphy in assessing the biliary tree is discussed in the biliary trauma chapter.

Hepatic abnormalities that can be demonstrated include early arterial perfusion of the liver and minimal hepatomegaly as well as subcapsular or intrahepatic hematomas. The latter are depicted as peripheral or central regions of diminished activity by virtue of their displacement of Kupffer cells (18). Compared to CT, false negatives tend to be small lesions, thin, linear lacerations, particularly those located deep to the surface, and injuries to the left lobe (7). Sources of false positives include rib impression, thinning in or small size of the left lobe, prominent porta hepatis, overlying breast tissue, large gallbladder impression, and prominent defect at the hepatic venous confluence (18).

Follow-up in those patients treated conservatively can be provided by scintigraphy (Fig. 7.10). A gradual regression over 3–4 months should be

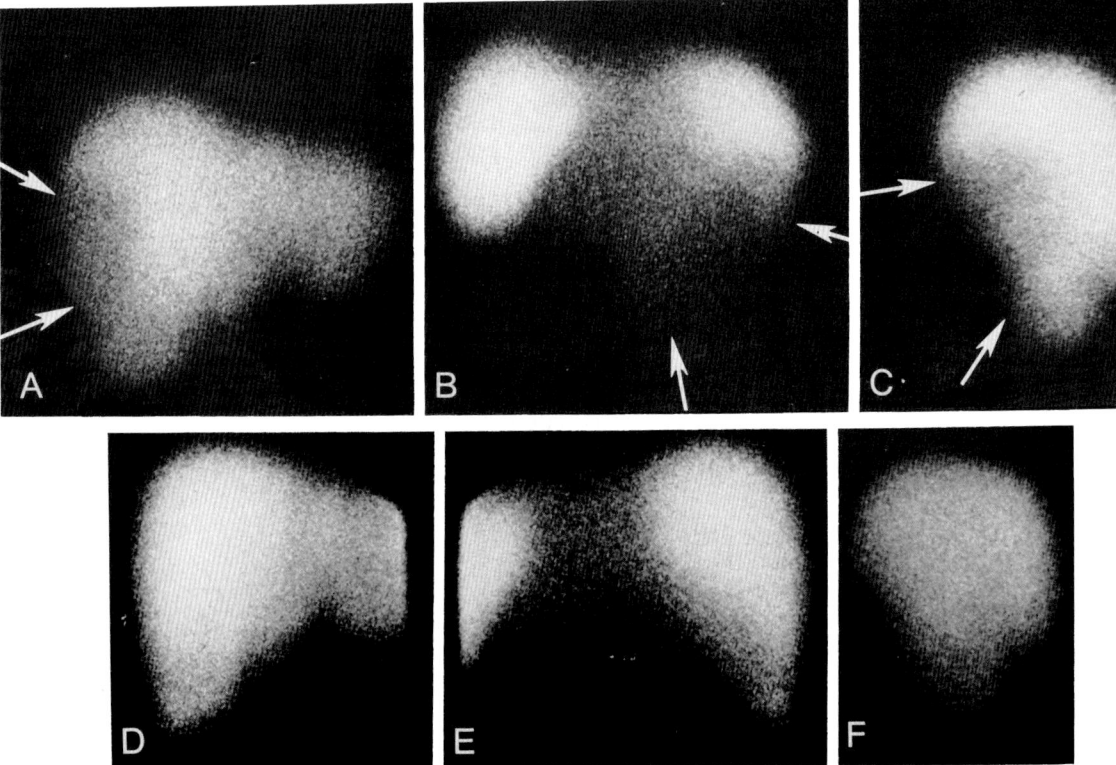

FIGURE 7.10. PERIPHERAL INTRAHEPATIC OR SUBCAPSULAR POST-TRAUMATIC HEMATOMA FOLLOWED TO RESOLUTION BY SCINTIGRAPHY
A–C: Anterior, posterior, and right lateral views from a sulfur colloid scan: posterolateral photon-deficient region (*arrows*). *D–F*: Corresponding views one month later are normal.

seen, although a completely normal appearance may never be regained. In those requiring resection, the regenerating liver may assume a globular shape, with resolution occurring over 6 months, and the uninvolved lobe may enlarge as a result of compensatory hypertrophy (18).

In adults, CT is generally preferable both because of its better accuracy and its ability to evaluate the entire abdomen. In young children, scintigraphy has several important advantages. It is easier to perform, requiring less sedation and no intravenous or oral contrast material. It is less affected by patient motion and can be done at the bedside. On the other hand, liver/spleen scintigraphy often must be supplemented by excretory urography or renal scintigraphy (7).

REFERENCES

1. Haney PJ, Whitley NO, Brotman S, Cunat JS, Whitley J: Liver injury and complications in the post-operative trauma patient: CT evaluation. *AJR* 139:271–275, 1982.
2. Schwartz SI: Liver. In: Schwartz SI, Shires GT, Spencer PC, Storer EH (eds): *Principles of Surgery*, Ed 3. New York, McGraw-Hill, 1979, pp 1269–1275.
3. Toombs BD, Sandler CM, Raushkolb EN, Strax R, Harle TS: Assessment of hepatic injuries with computed tomography. *J Comput Assist Tomogr* 6:72–75, 1982.
4. Federle MP: Computed tomography of blunt abdominal trauma. *Radiol Clin North Am* 21:461–475, 1983.
5. Moon KL, Federle MP: Computed tomography in hepatic trauma. *AJR* 141:309–314, 1983.
6. Mindelzun RE, McCort JJ: Upper abdominal trauma: conventional radiology. *Semin Roentgenol* 19:259–268, 1984.
7. Kaufman RA, Towbin R, Babcock DS, Gelfand MJ, Guice KS, Oldham KT, Noseworthy J: Upper abdominal trauma in children: imaging evaluation. *AJR* 142:449–460, 1984.
8. vanSonnenberg E, Simeone JF, Mueller PR, Wittenberg J, Hall DA, Ferrucci JT, Jr.: Sonographic appearance of hematoma in liver, spleen and kidney: a clinical, pathologic and animal study. *Radiology* 147:507–510, 1983.
9. Kuligowska E, Mueller PR, Simeone JF, Fine C: Ultrasound in upper abdominal trauma. *Semin Roentgenol* 19:281–295, 1984.
10. Wicks JD, Silver TM, Bree RL: Gray scale features of hematomas: an ultrasonic spectrum. *AJR* 131:977–980, 1978.
11. Froelich JW, Simeone JF, McKusick KA, Winzelberg GG, Strauss HW: Radionuclide imaging and ultrasound in liver/spleen trauma: a prospective comparison. *Radiology* 145:457–461, 1982.
12. Federle MP: CT of upper abdominal trauma. *Semin Roentgenol* 19:269–280, 1984.
13. Toombs BD, Lester RG, Ben-Menachem Y, Sandler CM: Computed tomography in blunt trauma. *Radiol Clin North Am* 19:17–35, 1981.
14. Pardes JG, Haaga JR, Borkowski G: Focal hepatic fatty metamorphosis secondary to trauma. *J Comput Assist Tomogr* 6:769–771, 1982.
15. Kaufman RA, Babcock DS: An approach to imaging the upper abdomen in the injured child. *Semin Roentgenol* 19:308–320, 1984.
16. Reuter SR, Redman HC: *Gastrointestinal Angiography*. Philadelphia, W. B. Saunders, 1977, pp 198–208.
17. Casarella WJ, Martin EC: Angiography in the management of abdominal trauma. *Semin Roentgenol* 321–327, 1984.
18. McConnell BJ, McConnell RW, Guiberteau MJ: Radionuclide imaging in blunt trauma. *Radiol Clin North Am* 19:37–51, 1981.

8

Transcatheter Management of Hepatic Neoplasms

DOUGLAS M. COLDWELL, M.D., PH.D.

Within the last two decades, the radiologist has become more and more involved in both the diagnosis and treatment of hepatic neoplasms. The advent of intra-arterial infusion and embolization techniques has led to these developments. An understanding of the basics of intra-arterial infusion, the drugs utilized, and embolization procedures and complications is essential. However, a close working relationship with the oncologist is the most important aspect of treatment of these neoplasms by radiologic techniques.

RATIONALE

The basic premise of intra-arterial chemotherapy infusion is that a higher local concentration of the agent will have a greater biological effect on the tumor compared to those concentrations achievable with intravenous infusion (1–4). This seems logical since most chemotherapeutic agents have a steep dose-response curve (5). That is, a small increase in increment of dose will yield a very great difference in the response of the tumor. This incremental increase in the available chemotherapeutic concentration may not be available with systemic infusions because of associated toxicities. With infusion of the systemic dose intra-arterially the local concentration will be higher than with systemic concentrations with toxicities certainly no higher than with intravenous infusion. In fact, the systemic concentration, and therefore the related toxicities, may be lower because of a "first pass" effect. The tumor may selectively extract the chemotherapeutic agent from the blood causing a lower concentration to be available to the systemic circulation. The higher local concentration will also result in a steeper concentration gradient than the systemic (intravenous) infusion would. Such a steep of gradient will force the chemotherapeutic agent into the tumor more effectively than the gradient available with systemic chemotherapy.

The local effectiveness of the chemotherapy is a function of sensitivity of the tumor to the administered drug, local conditions (pH, pCO2, pO2, blood flow), tumor vascularity (or lack of it), total tumor burden, tumor growth characteristics, and the condition of the remaining normal liver. The effectiveness of intra-arterial chemotherapy can only be judged empirically and usually often after a single trial (6). A previous trial of the drug administered intravenously without response is not adequate as the high local concentration cannot be duplicated. It may be that there is a therapeutic concentration level which is not reached by intravenous infusion (7).

Chen and Gross (8) have used a pharmacologically based, linear computer model to investigate intra-arterial and intravenous drug delivery. They found that the local concentrations were definitely increased with the former while the systemic drug availability was decreased. The observed increase depends on the local environment and the efficiency of the local tissues in removing the agent from the circulation. Sadee et al. (9) and Ensminger et al. (10) found that local extraction of cytotoxic drugs resulted in only 10–50% of the administered dose reaching the systemic circulation. Intra-arterial administration of 5-FU should, and did, show a decrease in the observed toxicities. Such effects have been shown with a variety of chemotherapeutic agents including *cis*-platinum, doxorubicin (Adriamycin), bleomycin, methotrexate, and melphalan (11, 12).

By increasing the contact time with the tumor, a greater tissue concentration of drug should be reached. Anderson et al. (13) demonstrated this in dogs by using a balloon to occlude the arterial flow to a hind limb while perfusing it with a chemotherapeutic agent. The observed tissue levels were 7–9 times higher than that seen with infusion alone. When a second catheter was then placed in the femoral vein occluding it, and the blood withdrawn in order to recirculate it via the femoral artery, the tissue levels were approximately 300 times that seen in infusion alone (14).

RADIOLOGIC TECHNIQUE

Selective catheterization is an absolute requirement for the placement of the catheter for infusion (15). In hepatic infusions, a celiac arteriogram is first performed in order to characterize the hepatic arterial anatomy. Good visualization of the left gastric, common hepatic, proper hepatic and left and right hepatic arteries is necessary. A convenient classification system is one developed by Michaels (16). This classifies the origin and course of the left and right hepatic arteries and their most common variations (Table 8.1) (17).

Selective injection into the left and right hepatic arteries is then performed using a slow rate of injection over long periods of time and extended filming. This infusion angiography is more sensitive and specific for detecting hepatic metastases then the usual high flow rate and short duration arteriograms. After selective right and left right hepatic arteriograms are performed, the catheter is then left in either hepatic artery. Usually the artery that supplies the majority of the lesions is utilized for infusion of the chemotherapy. Most times this is the right hepatic artery. Redistribution of the vascular flow within the liver to infuse the entire liver utilizing one catheter may be accomplished by placing a Gianturco stainless steel coil in the origin of the hepatic artery that is not used for infusion (17). Immediately after this coil is placed intrahepatic collateral vessels open and allow treatment of the entire liver via one catheter placed in a lobar artery (Fig. 8.1).

The initial catheter used is usually a simple curve 6.5 French catheter (Cook Industries, Bloomington, IN) inserted via a femoral approach. Selective catheterization also requires the use of hepatic, splenic, reverse curve, or cobra shapes. For younger patients or when using the axillary approach, a 5 French polyethylene catheter is utilized. Once selective catheterization of the required lobar artery is performed an exchange is made for a catheter which has been shaped to match the infused vessel. This individually formed catheter will remain in place more readily. To ensure correct placement of the catheter, daily upper abdominal radiographs should be performed in the Radiology Department. The catheters are secured to the skin using a clear air tight dressing (Tegaderm, 3M Corp, St. Paul, MN).

Since any foreign object in the vascular system will promote thrombus development a nonthrombogenic environment must be created (18, 19). Systemic heparinization is usually used with the patient receiving 10,000–20,000 units of heparin per day. The heparin may be administered intravenously or mixed with chemotherapy and administered through the arterial line. Another option is utilizing a Y-connector and administer-

TABLE 8.1.
HEPATIC ARTERIAL ANATOMY CLASSIFICATION

Type I	The right hepatic (RH) middle hepatic (MH), and left hepatic (LH) arteries are from the celiac artery (CA) (55%)
Type II	The RH and the MH are from the CA, replaced LH from the left gastric artery (LGA) (10%)
Type III	The MH and LH are from the CA, replaced RH from the superior mesenteric artery (SMA) (11%)
Type IV	The MH is from the CA, replaced RH from the SMA and replaced LH from the LGA (1%)
Type V	The RH, MH, and LH are from the CA, and an accessory RH is from the LGA (8%)
Type VI	The RH, MH, and LH are from the CA, and an accessory RH is from the SMA (7%)
Type VII	The RH, MH, and LH are from the CA. An accessory RH is from the SMA, and an accessory LH is from the LGA (1%)
Type VIII	Patterns are combined: (a) a replaced RH and an accessory LH (b) an accessory RH and a replaced LH (2%)
Type IX	Absent celiac hepatic artery. The entire hepatic trunk is from the SMA (4.5%)
Type X	Absent celiac hepatic artery. The entire hepatic trunk is from the LGA (0.5%)
Type X (variant)	Double celiac hepatic arteries (no common hepatic artery). The RH is from the proximal CA, the LH is from the distal end of the CA

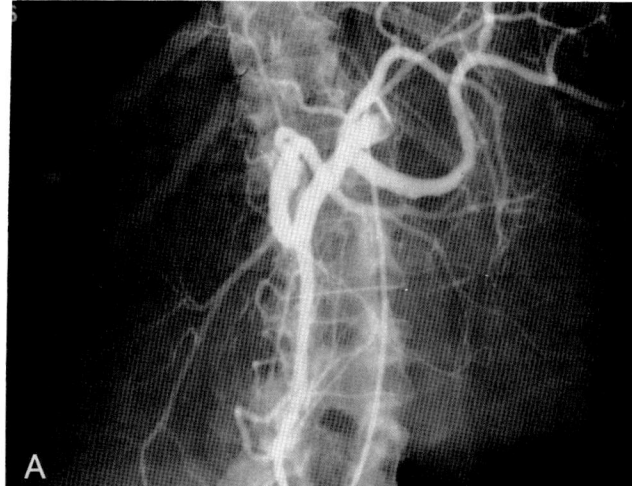
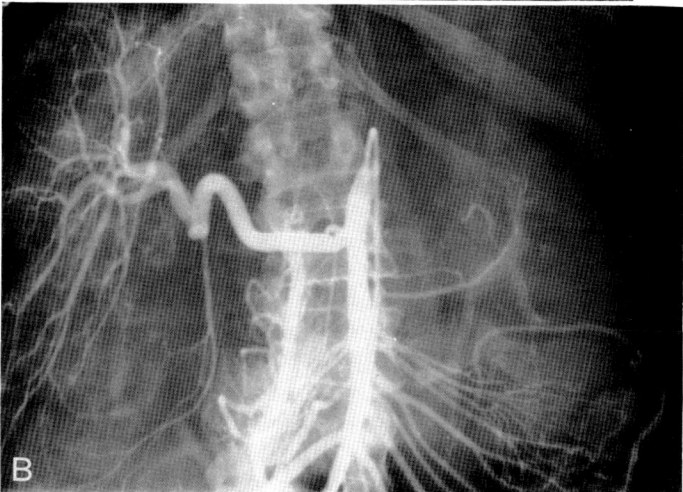
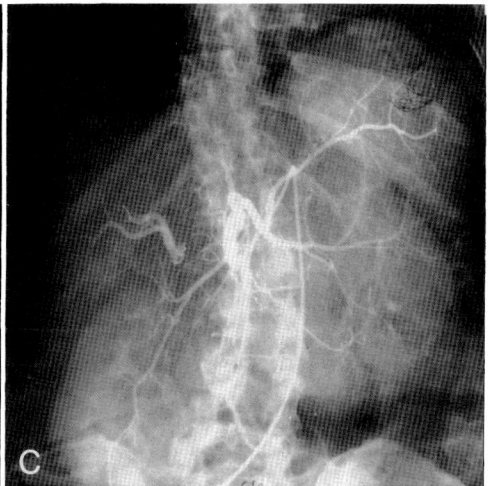

FIGURE 8.1. CELIAC ARTERIOGRAM

A: The celiac arteriogram demonstrates no evidence of a right hepatic artery. *B*: The right hepatic artery is originating from the SMA. *C*: In order to infuse a single artery, stainless steel coils were placed in the replaced right hepatic artery. This left hepatic arteriogram shows the intrahepatic collateral vessels filling the right hepatic circulation distal to the coils. This arteriogram was performed within ten minutes of the second (*B*), demonstrating the speed with which these vessels open. Hepatic metastases are present in both lobes from breast carcinoma.

ing the heparin again through the arterial catheter. It must be noted here that heparin is not compatible with doxorubicin and must be given via the intravenous route when this drug is utilized for infusion (20). The patient will have received some heparin during the angiographic procedure and is usually returned to his room with a pump (Life Care Pump, Abbott Labs, Chicago) infusing 10,000 units of heparin in 1 liter at a rate of 40 ml per hour. Such heparinization will allow the catheter to remain thrombus free until the chemotherapy is begun. The clotting time should be kept at 1.5–2 times normal during the infusion.

CHEMOTHERAPY

Chemotherapeutic agents inhibit DNA synthesis or function by acting on enzymes, substrates, or even on the DNA itself. The most "active" cells in the cell cycle are the ones which are the most sensitive to interference with their metabolism. These are the proliferating cells in the mitotic cycle. The most rapidly multiplying normal cells are in the bone marrow, gastrointestinal epithelium, hair follicles, and gonads. As expected, these areas also show the evidence of chemotherapeutic side effects most readily. Since tumor cells are, by definition, rapidly growing, they too should react to chemotherapy, and show more permanent effects since normal tissues have a greater capability for repair than neoplastic tissues. Unfortunately, toxicity is often the limiting factor in the treatment of tumors.

While the mode of action of many chemotherapeutic agents is unknown, many drugs act only on a certain phase of the cell cycle. The period of mitosis (M phase) is the time of actual cell division. This is followed by the first gap phase (G1 phase) which is followed by the DNA synthesis (S phase). The last phase which all cells enter is the G2 gap phase which is then followed by mitosis. A resting phase which some cells enter is the G0 phase; this may also represent the stem cell population.

The effectiveness of a specific agent is dependent on the interaction between the drug, the tumor, and the patient. The dose, route of administration, growth characteristics of the tumor, the portion of the cell cycle affected by the drug, drug pharmacokinetics, and patient age and condition all play a role in how effective a drug will be on a particular tumor. When drugs are used in combination, they should be individually active against the tumor. Ideally, the drugs should potentiate each other and not have the same toxicities.

The alkylating agents used most commonly in hepatic artery infusions are dimethyl-1-triazeno imidazole carboximide (DTIC) and cis-diamminedichloroplatinum (CDDP). DTIC interferes with purine metabolism and nucleic acid synthesis and has its major effect in G2 phase although its exact mechanism is not yet known. CDDP is an inorganic drug which inhibits DNA synthesis by cross-linking strands of DNA (21). RNA and protein synthesis are also disrupted by CDDP but to a lesser extent. CDDP is not cell cycle specific.

DTIC has a short plasma half-life and is excreted by the renal tubules and not reabsorbed. Its major toxicities are nausea, vomiting, and myelosuppression with thrombocytopenia and leukopenia. The myelosuppression is usually maximal approximately three weeks after administration. The average dose is 50 mg/m^2/day for 5 days. DTIC has been used in combination with doxorubicin and CDDP for malignant melanoma and other sarcomas metastatic to liver (22).

CDDP is initially rapidly cleared from the vascular system but remains present in the kidneys, liver, ovary and uterus for at least 6 days following intravenous injection. Thirty to forty-five percent of the drug is excreted in 5 days. Little work has been done on the pharmacokinetics of intra-arterial infusion of CDDP. The major toxicities seen with CDDP use are renal and otic. Decreased creatinine clearance is seen and is usually reversible after discontinuation of the drug (23). If renal function is diminished initially, the dose of CDDP may be decreased.

The need for a preinfusion creatine clearance, not merely a serum creatinine level, is clear. Hypomagnesemia, as another manifestation of renal tubular damage, may also be seen particularly in children. Ototoxicity with tinnitus and impaired hearing especially in the high frequency range is seen when high doses of CDDP are used. Nausea, vomiting, and mild myelosuppression may also be present. Hypersensitivity reactions, usually the formation of hives, are infrequently seen. The average dose of CDDP is 60–160 mg/m^2 infused over 2–24 hr. CDDP is qualitatively more effective when given intra-arterially. Its more frequent uses are in the treatment of hepatoma and hepatic metastases from melanoma, breast carcinoma (with vinblastine), colon carcinoma (with FUDR), renal carcinoma and metastatic tumors of unknown origin (with 5-FU, doxorubicin, and mitomycin C).

The antimetabolites 5-fluorouracil (5-FU) and floxuridine (FUDR) act on the biosynthetic pathway forming the pyrimidine base unique to DNA, thymine (5-methyluracil). They both are active in the S phase (24). These drugs concentrate in the tumor tissue and remain there longer than in normal tissues. Even though the drugs are metabolized in the liver, the major toxicities are seen in the gastrointestinal tract and the hematopoetic system. The symptoms seen are stomatitis, diarrhea, ulcerations, and bleeding (22). The myelosuppression presents as leukopenia and thrombocytopenia. Both drugs are administered as an infusion for 5 days at 100 mg/m^2/day for FUDR or 75–100 mg/m^2 day for 5-FU. FUDR and 5-FU have been used for both primary and secondary tumors of the liver. FUDR is combined with mitomycin C or CDDP for infusion of metastatic carcinoma of the colon (Fig. 8.2). Doxorubicin and mitomycin C are added to FUDR for the treatment of metastatic tumors of unknown origin and primary hepatomas.

Doxorubicin (Adriamycin) is an antitumor antibiotic which is a fermentation product of the fungus *Streptomyces peucetius*. It has a tetracycline ring structure with an unusual sugar, daunosamine, attached by glycosidic linkage. Doxorubicin intercalates daunosamine between adjacent base pairs on a DNA strand and prevents the template activity of DNA (25). Of particular interest is the ability of doxorubicin to attach very tightly to myocardial DNA and this accounts for its myocardial toxicity (26). It is rapidly absorbed from the plasma by the liver, heart, kidneys, and lungs, and spleen with a biphasic disappearance curve. Doxorubicin is cleared by

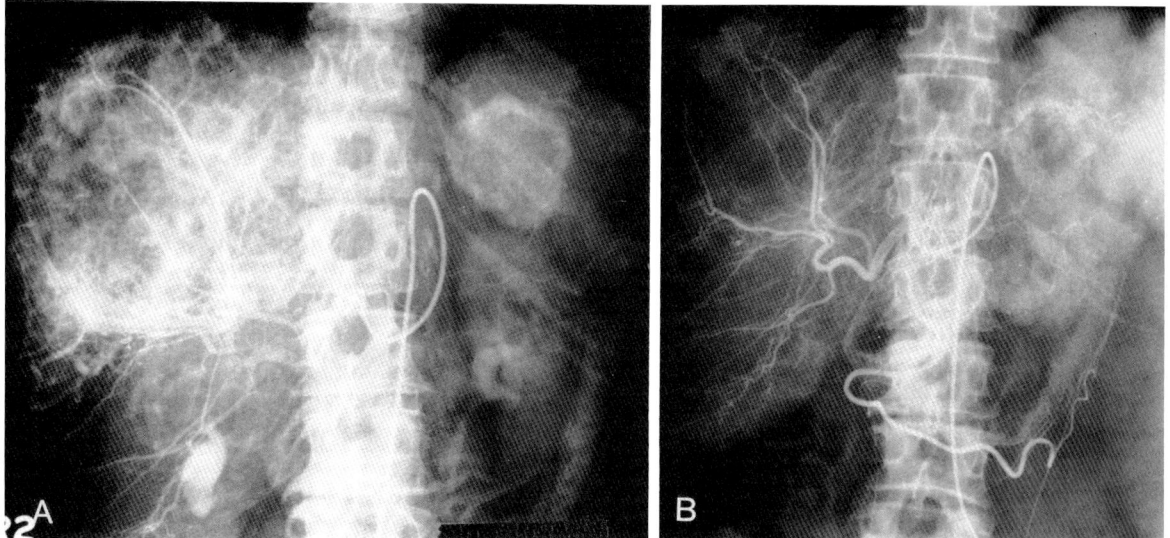

FIGURE 8.2. MULTIPLE HYPERVASCULAR HEPATIC METASTASES
A: Multiple hypervascular hepatic metastases from colon carcinoma are present on this initial right hepatic arteriogram. The CEA level is 50 ng/ml. B: After three courses of intra-arterial infusion of FUDR and mitomycin C, there is dramatic improvement. The CEA level now is 5 ng/ml.

the liver with little excretion by the kidneys. The initial half-life is about one hour with a delayed half-life of roughly seventeen hours. High plasma levels are markedly prolonged in patients with impaired hepatic function. Myelosuppression, primarily granulocytopenia, is the major dose limiting complication with the nadir reached by the second week and recovery by the fourth week after therapy. Cardiomyopathy is the other major toxic reaction and is demonstrated by congestive heart failure. This reaction is unusual if the total lifetime dose of doxorubicin is less than 550 mg/m^2 or 450 mg/m^2 when there has been mediastinal irradiation. Minor toxicities seen are mucositis, nausea, vomiting, and reversible alopecia. It should be noted that doxorubicin is incompatible with heparin and 5-FU and forms precipitates when they are mixed. The usual intra-arterial dose is 15–40 mg/m^2 administered over 2–4 hr. This dose is applicable when the catheter is in a larger artery (e.g., the proper hepatic artery) and the catheter tip in the center of the artery. When more selective infusions are performed, the dose of doxorubicin should be reduced due to the vesicant effects of the drug. Doxorubicin has shown activity against primary hepatomas (when combined with mitomycin C and floxuridine), cholangiocarcinomas, and metastases from an unknown primary.

Mitomycin C is another antitumor antibiotic and is a product of *Streptomyces caespitosus*. It is an alkylating agent and requires activation of a quinone by its reduction and loss of methoxy group. This drug is activated by the liver (27). The most significant toxicity is myelosuppression, primarily leukopenia and thrombocytopenia. Anemia, nausea, and vomiting are also observed. Mitomycin C is used in doses up to 15 mg/m^2 infused over 2 hours. Its primary use in the liver is in combination with doxorubicin and floxuridine for primary hepatomas, cholangiocarcinomas, and metastases from an unknown primary.

Vinblastine is one of the vinca alkaloids derived from the periwinkle plant. It is cell cycle specific and blocks mitosis with metaphase arrest. It binds with tubulin, a key protein in cellular microtubules, which may also explain some of its toxic effects (28). Bone marrow depression is the principal toxicity and is manifested by leukopenia. Neurologic toxicities, such as depression and paresthesias, are also seen. Vincristine appears to show less myelosuppression than vinblastine but more neurologial effects (22). Alopecia, nausea, and vomiting may also occur. The dose used is 1.6–2.0 mg/m^2/day for 5 days. Vinblastine has shown activity when combined with CDDP against breast carcinoma metastatic to the liver.

While it is not the purpose of this text to

HEPATIC ARTERIAL EMBOLIZATION

Occlusion of the peripheral arterioles may provide palliation in patients with localized neoplasms or those tumors which have not responded to intra-arterial chemotherapy. This technique produces tumor necrosis without destroying significant normal hepatic tissue (32, 33). Other uses for embolization lie in the redistribution of the hepatic vasculature so that a single infusion catheter may be utilized (17). This embolization employs stainless steel coils and more proximal placement.

Multiple agents are used in embolization: Gelfoam, polyvinyl alcohol foam (Ivalon), and stainless steel coils (34–36). Gelfoam sponge may be cut into 3–5 mm cubes or 2 × 5 mm pieces and delivered through a 1 ml tuberculin syringe into the catheter. Use of particles this large will only occlude proximally and temporarily as the Gelfoam will resorb. The Ivalon particles which are available measure 149–250, 150–590, 590–1000, and 1000–2000 µm in diameter. The particles are delivered in a nonsterile state and should be divided into doses of 200–250 mg and sterilized with ethylene oxide. It is suggested that dividing the doses into individual plastic syringes with paraffin occluding the end is a convenient method. These doses may then be suspended at the time of embolization with normal saline and contrast and injected. To achieve a more uniform suspension, the Ivalon should be injected back and forth through a tube or three-way stopcock between two syringes (34).

Stainless steel Gianturco coils made from 0.028-inch wire with Dacron fibers attached to the end may be used to occlude medium-sized arteries (37). The coils come in three sizes: 3, 5, and 8 mm in diameter. The size of the artery to be occluded determines the size of coil used. If too small a coil is used, it will float with the prevailing current and may lodge in an unexpected and untoward location. Collateral flow within the liver opens immediately after a proximal occlusion is made, as seen in surgical ligation. This property, however, may be used to advantage since intrahepatic collateral vessels make it possible to infuse the entire liver with only one catheter even when anomalous origins of the hepatic arteries are present.

Distal embolization of the liver with Ivalon particles for antitumor therapy is based on the finding that most (90%) of the blood supply to hepatic tumors is from the hepatic arteries even though they metastasize to the liver via the portal vein. Normal liver parenchyma receives only 15–20% of its blood supply from the hepatic artery. Therefore, by embolizing the hepatic artery, the tumor necroses and the normal tissue is protected by its portal venous supply. Obviously, portal vein patency should be demonstrated before commencing with embolization.

Hepatic arterial embolization (HAE) may be used as primary therapy or after infusion therapy has been unsuccessful, for control of pain, hemorrhage (e.g., after a liver biopsy or percutaneous transhepatic cholangiogram) or arteriovenous shunting or preoperatively to reduce blood loss during resection. Recent examination of a series of cases has shown that the contraindications to HAE are few and include involvement of 70% or more of the liver by tumor, and SGOT levels of 100, LDH levels of 450, bilirubin of 2. When all three are present, more than half of the patients have died from hepatorenal failure within 1 month (38). Another relative contraindication is previous duodenal surgery which disrupts peribiliary and periportal collateral vessels leading to increased risk of hepatic abscess formation. In patients with extensive hepatic metastases, selective embolization of a single lobe with chemotherapeutic infusion into the other is an option.

Both the clinician and the radiologist should be aware of the postembolization syndrome which includes nausea, vomiting, fever, and leukocytosis. This syndrome begins shortly after the embolization has begun and lasts from one to five days. Blood cultures are unrewarding and the patient should be treated symptomatically. During this time, the liver function tests will rise dramatically and then return to baseline, or below. The return of these values to lower levels will correspond to the patient's symptomatic recovery. To decrease the postembolization syndrome, single lobes are embolized at one sitting rather than the entire liver. The patient then returns in three to four weeks for the remaining liver to be embolized. After the first course, the

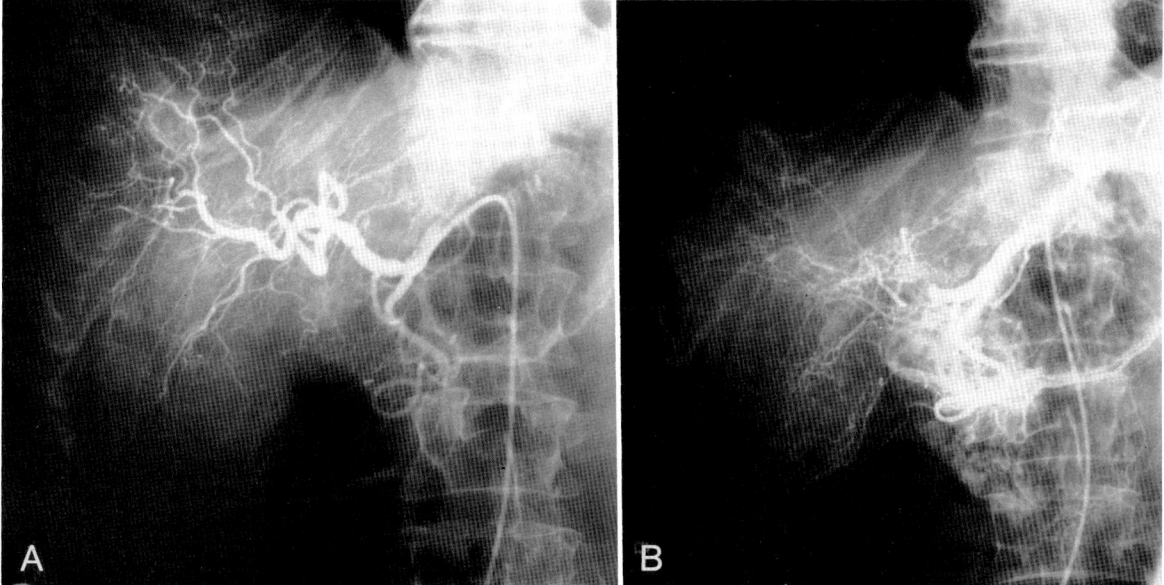

FIGURE 8.3. METASTASES FROM LEIOMYOSARCOMA
A: The initial right hepatic arteriogram demonstrates metastases from a leiomyosarcoma. B: After three embolizations with Ivalon, these metastases can no longer be seen. Periductal and peribiliary collateral vessels are present. There was great symptomatic relief after this procedure.

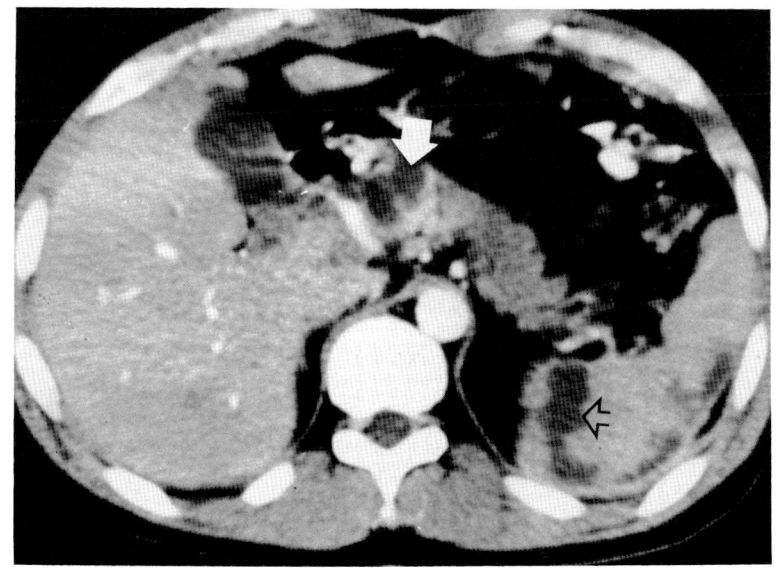

FIGURE 8.4. PANCREATIC AND SPLENIC INFARCTION

This CT scan of the upper abdomen demonstrates high attenuation areas within the liver which represent the Ivalon used to embolize the patient's metastatic melanoma. Low attenuation areas in the head of the pancreas (*solid arrow*) and in the spleen (*open arrow*) represent pancreatic and splenic infarction from overzealous embolization in inexperienced hands.

entire liver may then be embolized with only moderate symptoms. The patient is much more symptomatic after the first embolization than after any subsequent one. HAE should be repeated at monthly intervals for three complete embolizations of the liver. At that time, the patient should be re-evaluated and subsequent embolizations performed at longer intervals. It may not be possible to embolize more than 3–5 times because the large vessels may be completely occluded and only collateral vessels present (Fig. 8.3). Hepatic arterial infusion may then be considered.

The care needed to be taken during the embolization procedure cannot be overemphasized. Selective catheterization of the lobar arteries is necessary. The Ivalon slurry should be placed in the arteries using a dilute solution mixed with contrast and the catheter tip fluoroscoped during the embolization. In inexperienced hands, the results may be disastrous (Fig. 8.4). Embolization until stasis of contrast in the vessel is seen represents the end-point. If the catheter is to be used for other vessel injections, a Gelfoam plug should be injected through it in order to clear it. Postembolization arteriograms are not encouraged since the turbulence of the injection may dislodge some particles of Ivalon.

This technique has been utilized successfully in the treatment of APUDomas of the pancreas, melanomas, leiomyosarcomas, and nonreponsive colon and renal cell carcinoma metastases to the liver, and primary hepatomas (30, 40). HAE may be combined with embolization of the liver with chemotherapeutic agents mixed in a slurry, the so-called "chemoembolization" (41). The chemotherapy agents which have been used are CDDP and mitomycin C. For example, 50 mg of CDDP may be suspended in 5–10 ml of saline and mixed with the Ivalon slurry. This combination has been used in the treatment of metastatic melanoma to the liver with dramatic results. In a small series of patients, metastatic lesions in the liver have been observed to completely disappear (42).

REFERENCES

1. Klopp CT, Alford TC, Bateman J et al: Fractional intraarterial cancer chemotherapy. *Ann Surg* 132:811–832, 1950.
2. Cromer JK, Bateman JC, Bery GH et al: Use of intraarterial nitrogen mustard therapy in the treatment of cervical and vaginal cancer. *Am J Obstet Gynecol* 63:538–548, 1952.
3. Sullivan RD, Norcross JW, Watkins JE: Chemotherapy of metastatic liver cancer by prolonged hepatic artery infusion. *N Engl J Med* 270:321–327, 1964.
4. Ansfield FJ, Ramirez G, Skibba JL et al: Intrahepatic arterial infusion with 5-fluorouracil. *Cancer* 28:1147–1151, 1971.
5. Frei E III (ed): *Cancer Medicine*. Philadelphia, Lea & Febiger, 1973, pp 717–730.
6. Wallace S, Chuang VP: Liver tumors, diagnosis and management. In Herlinger H, Lunderquist A (eds): *Clinical Radiology of the Liver*. New York, Marcel Dekker, 1983, pp 715–864.
7. Patt YZ, Chuang VP, Wallace S et al: The palliative role of hepatic arterial infusion and arterial occlusion in colorectal carcinoma metastatic to the liver. *Lancet* 1:349–351, 1981.
8. Chen HSG, Gross JF: Intra-arterial infusion of anticancer drugs: theoretic aspects of drug delivery and review of responses. *Cancer Treat Rep* 64:31–40, 1980.
9. Sadee W, Finn C, Schwandt HJ et al: 5-Fluorouracil (5-FU) pharmacokinetics following various routes of administration. *Proc Am Assoc Cancer Res ASCO* 16:187, 1975.
10. Ensminger W, Rosowsky A, Raso V et al: A clinical-pharmacological evaluation of hepatic arterial infusions of 5-fluoro-2-deoxyuridine and 5-fluorouracil. *Cancer Res* 38:3784–3792, 1978.
11. Jaffe N, Knapp J, Chuang VP et al: Osteosarcoma; intra-arterial treatment of the primary tumor with *cis*-diamminedichloroplatinum II (CDP): angiographic, pathologic and pharmacologic studies. *Cancer* 51:402–407, 1983.
12. Fleishman GB, Yap HY, Chuang S et al: Intrahepatic arterial combination sequential *cis*-diamminedichloroplatinum (II) and vinblastine for refractory metastatic breast carcinoma regionally confined to the liver (abstract). *Proc Am Assoc Cancer Res*, 1982.
13. Anderson JH, Gianturco C, Wallace S: Experimental transcatheter intra-arterial infusion-occlusion chemotherapy. *Invest Radiol* 16:496–500, 1981.
14. Wright KC, Charnsangavej A, Wallace S et al: Regional isolation-perfusion: an experimental percutaneous approach tested and compared to arterial occlusion-infu
15. Chuang VP, Wallace S: Interventional approaches to hepatic tumor treatment. *Semin Roentgenol* 18:127–135, 1983.
16. Michaels NA: *Blood Supply and Anatomy of the Upper Abdominal Organs with a Descriptive Atlas*. Philadelphia, J. B. Lippincott, 1955, pp 372–373.
17. Chuang VP, Wallace S: Hepatic arterial redistribution for intraarterial infusion of hepatic neoplasms. *Radiology* 135:295–299, 1980.
18. Jaffee BM, Donegan WL, Watson F et al: Factors influencing survival in patients with untreated hepatic metastases. *Surg Gynecol Obstet* 127:1–11, 1968.
19. Watkins E Jr, Khazazei AE, Nahra KS: Surgical basis for arterial infusion chemotherapy of disseminated carcinoma of the liver. *Surg Gynecol Obstet* 130:581–605, 1970.
20. Angel JE: *Physicians' Desk Reference*. Oradell, N.J., Medical Economics Co., 1985.
21. Wheeler GP: Some biochemical effects of alkylating agents. *Fed Proc* 26: 885–892, 1967.
22. Goodman LS, Gilman A: *The Pharmacological Basis of Therapeutics*. New York, Macmillan, 1975.
23. Rosenberg B: Fundamental Studies with Cisplatin. *Cancer* 55:2203–2216, 1985.
24. Heidelberg C: Fluorinated pyrimidines and their nucleosides. In Sartorelli AC, Johns DG (eds): *Antineoplastic and Immunosuppressive Agents*, Part II. Berlin, Springer-Verlag, 1975, pp 193–231.
25. Pigram WJ, Fuller W, Hamilton LD: Stereochemistry of intercalation: interaction of daunomycin with DNA. *Nature New Biol* 235:17–19, 1972.
26. Le Frak EA, Pitha J, Rosenheim S, Gottlieb JA: A clinicopathologic analysis of Adriamycin cardiotoxicity. *Cancer, NY*, 32:302–314, 1973.
27. Crooke ST, Bradner WT, Mitomycin C: A review. *Cancer Treat Rev* 3:121–139, 1976.
28. Creasy WA: Vincaalkyloids and colchicine. In Sartorelli AC, Johns DG (eds): *Antineoplastic and Immunosuppressive Agents*, Part II Berlin, Springer-Verlag, 1975, pp 670–694.
29. Yap HY, Fleishman G, Fraschini G: Intra-arterial infusion for liver metastases from breast cancer. *Cancer Bull* 36:27.
30. Patt YZ, Mavligit GM, Chuang VP et al: Percutaneous hepatic arterial infusion of mitomycin C and floxuridine: An effective treatment for metastatic colorectal carcinoma in the liver. *Cancer* 46:261–265, 1980.
31. Patt YZ, Chuang VP, Wallace S et al: Hepatic arterial infusion of chemotherapy for primary or metastatic liver tumors. *Cancer* 51:1359–1363, 1983.

32. Chuang VP, Wallace S: Current status of transcatheter management of neoplasms. *Cardiovasc Intervent Radiol* 3:256–267, 1980.
33. Chuang VP, Wallace S: Arterial infusion and occlusion in cancer patients. *Semin Roentgenol* 16:13–25, 1981.
34. Chuang VP, Soo CS, Wallace S: Ivalon embolization in abdominal neoplasms. *AJR* 136:729–733, 1981.
35. Chuang VP, Wallace S, Swanson D: Technique and complications of renal carcinoma infarction. *Urol Radiol* 2:223–228, 1981.
36. Chuang VP, Wallace S, Gianturco C et al: Complications of coil embolization: Prevention and management. *AJR* 137:809–813, 1981.
37. Chuang VP, Wallace S, Gianturco C: A new improved coil for tapered-tip catheter for arterial occlusion. *Radiology* 135:507–510, 1980.
38. Charnsangavej C: Personal communication.
39. Wallace S, Chuang VP, Swanson D et al: Embolization of renal carcinoma: experience with 100 patients. *Radiology* 138:563–570, 1981.
40. Chuang VP, Wallace S: Hepatic artery embolization in the treatment of hepatic neoplasms. *Radiology* 142:546–547, 1982.
41. Kato T, Nemoto R, Mori H et al: Arterial chemoembolization with microencapsulated anticancer drug. *JAMA* 245:1123–1127, 1981.
42. Wallace S: Personal communciation.

SECTION II
The Gallbladder and Biliary Tract

INTRODUCTION

Most of the previous edition of the Golden's series devoted to the gallbladder and biliary tract dealt with intravenous cholangiography and oral cholecystography. Today, the latter is dead and the former is dying, supplanted for the most part by real-time sonography. In the intervening years, Tc-IDA compounds have replaced radioiodinated Rose Bengal for hepatobiliary scintigraphy, greatly expanding its clinical application. Percutaneous transhepatic cholangiography and ERCP have become commonplace, widely available procedures, and interventional biliary radiology offers an alternative to many surgical procedures. Exploratory laparotomy to differentiate obstructive from nonobstructive jaundice is a thing of the past.

CT has not had quite the impact on the gallbladder and biliary tract that it has had on other regions of the body, and it is likely that the same will be true for MRI.

Knowledge of anatomy, pathology, and clinical aspects of diseases is especially crucial for dealing with problems in the biliary tract and gallbladder both because of the necessity in the current economic climate for choosing wisely among the multitude of available tests and the often severe adverse consequences of mistakes. The text that follows is intended to be instructive in these aspects as well as diagnostic imaging per se.

9
Embryology, Anatomy, Histology, and Radiologic Anatomy

ARNOLD C. FRIEDMAN, M.D., AND LEORA SACHS, M.D.

EMBRYOLOGY

The origin of the gallbladder and extrahepatic ducts is separate and distinct from that of the intrahepatic ducts, preceding development of the latter by several weeks. At the 2.5-mm stage of embryonic development, a bud from the ventral margin of the primitive foregut forms two diverticula. The more cephalad of the two is responsible for formation of the liver and intrahepatic biliary tree, whereas the more caudad forms the gallbladder and extrahepatic ducts. At the 5-mm stage, the originally hollow gallbladder-common duct primordium becomes solid, but the common duct lumen is reestablished by the 7.5-mm stage and that of the gallbladder is reestablished somewhat later (1, 2). In the fetus, communications between the gallbladder and intrahepatic ducts (cystohepatic ducts, Luschka ducts) are present. These usually regress completely by adulthood, but large anomalous remnants are occasionally persistent which, if unrecognized at cholecystectomy, can be severed resulting in a postoperative bile leak (3).

Embryologic development of the ampulla of Vater and the choledochoduodenal junction is complex and will be briefly summarized. Initially multiple vacuoles form in the wall of the duodenum which coalesce into first two and finally one channel. The primitive ampullary component elongates displacing the junction of the pancreatic and common bile ducts farther from the duodenal lumen. This migration is then reversed to a varying degree in association with the development of the surrounding musculature. This variability accounts for marked differences in ampullary anatomy in the normal population (4).

Formation of the intrahepatic ducts is induced by a solid cord of cells extending from the junction of the cystic and common ducts toward the liver hilum at the point of contact of this solid cord with the hepatocytes. Intrahepatic duct development occurs after the 18-mm stage along the framework of the previously formed portal vein branches. The marked variation in configuration of intrahepatic ducts can be accounted for by the unpredictable manner in which they can wind around the preexisting portal veins (1, 2).

REFERENCES

1. Langman J: *Medical Embryology.* Baltimore, Williams & Wilkins, 1969, pp 262–264.
2. Elias H, Sherrick JC: *Morphology of the Liver.* New York, Academic Press, 1969.
3. Hayes MA, Goldenberg IS, Bishop CC: The developmental basis for bile duct anomalies. *Surg Gynecol Obstet* 107:447–456, 1958.
4. Schwegler RA Jr, Boyden EA: Development of pars intestinalis of common bile duct in human fetus, with special reference to origin of ampulla of Vater and sphincter of Oddi. *Anat Rec* 67:441–467, 68:17–41, 193–219, 1937.

ANATOMY

Gallbladder

The pear-shaped gallbladder is attached to the inferior surface of the liver at the major interlobar fissure. The gallbladder fossa (the impression in the liver in which it lies) also contains areolar tissue in which run blood vessels, lymphatics, and nerves. The remainder of the gallbladder is covered by peritoneum. The organ is usually about 10 cm long and 3–5 cm in diameter when

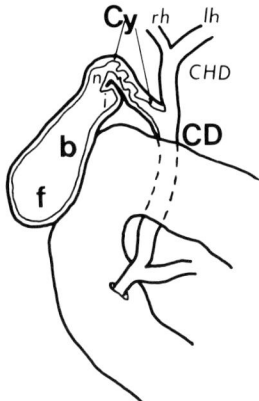

FIGURE 9.1. GALLBLADDER ANATOMY
Gallbladder anatomy: f = fundus, b = body, n = neck, i = infundibulum, Cy = cystic duct with valves of Heister, rh = right hepatic duct, lh = left hepatic duct, CHD = common hepatic duct, CD = common bile duct.

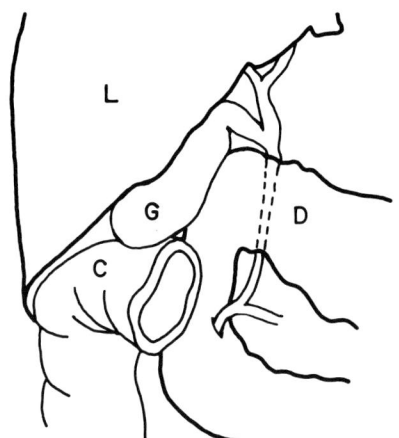

FIGURE 9.3. COMMON BILE DUCT
Coronal view of common bile duct coursing behind the duodenum (D) to join the pancreatic duct prior to entering the duodenum; L = liver, G = gallbladder, C = colon.

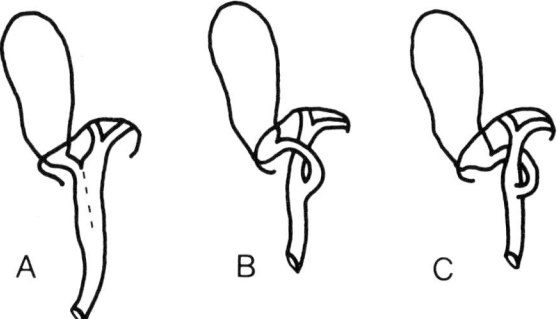

FIGURE 9.2. SOME VARIATIONS IN THE CYSTIC DUCT
A: Adherent to hepatic duct. B and C: anterior and posterior spirals, respectively, joining common hepatic duct on left side.

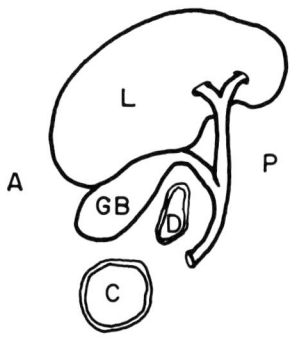

FIGURE 9.4. SAGITTAL SECTION OF THE COMMON DUCT
Sagittal section of the relationships of the common duct to adjacent structures; A = anterior, P = posterior, GB = gallbladder, D = duodenum, C = colon.

filled, and its capacity is about 50 ml. The fundus is the bulbous distal portion which may or may not project below the anterior inferior liver edge. The body of the gallbladder is the midportion which is in contact with the second portion of the duodenum and the colon. The infundibulum (Hartmann's pouch) bulges toward the cystic duct at the free edge of the lesser omentum, and the neck of the gallbladder is that portion between the body and the cystic duct (Fig. 9.1) (1).

The cystic duct varies in length from person to person but is usually 2–3 cm long. Its initial portion off the gallbladder is tortuous with mucosal flaps called the valves of Heister (Fig. 9.1). Its union with the common hepatic duct to form the common bile duct is variable, but almost always the cystic duct runs parallel with the common hepatic duct for at least a short distance (Fig. 9.2). The two may be encircled by a common connective tissue sheath. Thus some cystic duct remnant after cholecystectomy is a necessity. The cystic duct usually joins the right lateral aspect of the common hepatic duct but sometimes it opens into the anterior or even the medial aspect (spiraling around the common hepatic duct either anteriorly or posteriorly) (1–3). The latter arrangement may predispose towards Mirizzi syndrome (common hepatic duct obstruction by a gallstone in the cystic duct) (Fig. 9.2).

Biliary Tract

The right and left hepatic ducts emerging from the liver unite about 0.75–1.5 cm caudad to the liver to form the 2–3 cm long common hepatic duct which then combines with the cystic duct forming the 10–15 cm long common bile duct. The latter descends in the hepatoduodenal ligament behind the postbulbar duodenum and

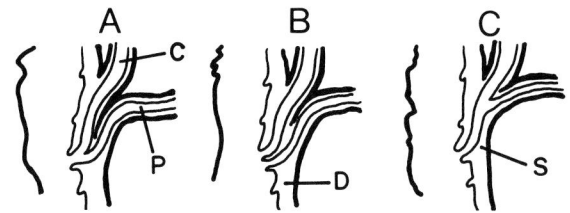

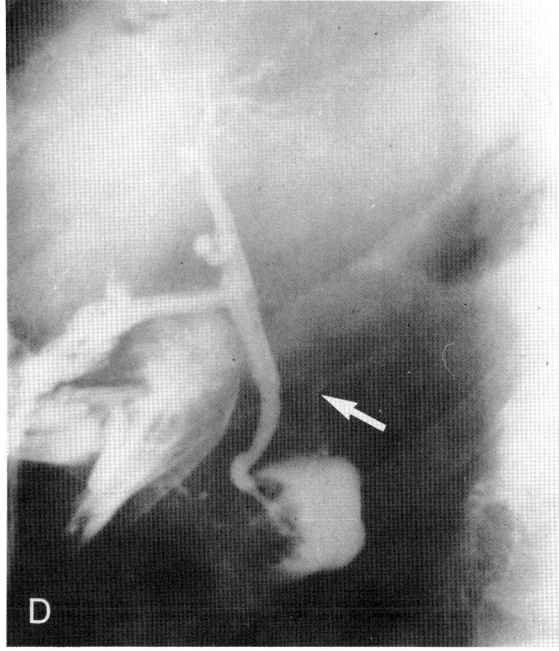

FIGURE 9.5. TYPES OF UNION OF COMMON BILE DUCT AND MAIN PANCREATIC DUCT

A: Short common channel. *B:* No common channel. *C:* Long common channel. C = common bile duct, P = main pancreatic duct, D = duodenal wall, S = sphincter. *D:* Drainage of common bile duct and pancreatic duct (*arrow*) into a duodenal diverticulum. This increases the difficulty of ERCP and related procedures.

stances each duct has its own opening into the duodenum. Lastly, the ducts may unite before entering the duodenum, resulting in a long common channel traversing the duodenal wall (1, 5). In their course through the submucosa of the duodenum, the pancreatic and common bile ducts are surrounded by layers of smooth muscle forming the sphincter of Oddi. A second sphincter, the sphincter choledochus (sphincter of Boyden) surrounds only the distal bile duct from its entrance into the duodenum to its junction with the pancreatic duct. These sphincters regulate bile flow into the duodenum (1, 6).

The distribution of the larger intrahepatic ducts is quite variable. The variations in the right lobe are more likely to be clinically significant (5). Usually the duct of the anterior segment of the right lobe appears to continue the smooth curve of the common hepatic duct with a cephalad orientation (Fig. 9.6). The posterior segmental duct, whose peripheral branches have a more caudal and lateral distribution, usually makes a sharp turn just distal to its origin as it courses around a major portal vein branch. Common variants include drainage of either the anterior or posterior right lobe segmental duct into the left hepatic duct. A low insertion of the right hepatic duct or a segmental or subsegmental branch into the common hepatic duct is not uncommon. Insertion into the cystic duct can occur, but is less common. Anomalous branches (subvesical ducts) may be found in the region of the gallbladder but almost never communicating with the latter (7).

Vascular and Lymphatic Anatomy

The cystic artery originates from the right hepatic artery near its origin from the common hepatic artery in about 66–75% of individuals. Otherwise, in rough descending order of frequency, it originates from the middle or left hepatic artery, the common hepatic artery, the gastroduodenal artery, the celiac artery or even directly from the aorta (1, 8, 9). Double cystic arteries are also frequent variations, occurring in 2–25% of the population (8). The cystic artery gives off two major branches 2–5 cm distal to its origin: the anterior (superficial right) branch to the free peritoneal surface of the gallbladder and the posterior (deep left) branch to the nonperitoneal surface of the gallbladder. Additional small intrahepatic branches of the right hepatic artery supply the gallbladder directly from the liver. Anastomoses exist between the cystic artery and the extrahepatic portion of the right

through the head of the pancreas inferiorly and slightly to the right to enter duodenum at the papilla of Vater (Figs. 9.3 and 9.4). The latter structure is usually located along the posteromedial margin of the descending limb of the duodenum. More distal insertion (junction of descending and transverse portions or into the transverse segment) is not uncommon, but higher insertion into the immediate postbulbar region or bulb itself is quite unusual (4, 5).

The exact union of the main pancreatic duct and the common bile duct varies individually (Fig. 9.5). Most frequently, the ducts join within the duodenal wall and have a short common portion. The ampulla of Vater is the dilated terminus of this common channel. In other in-

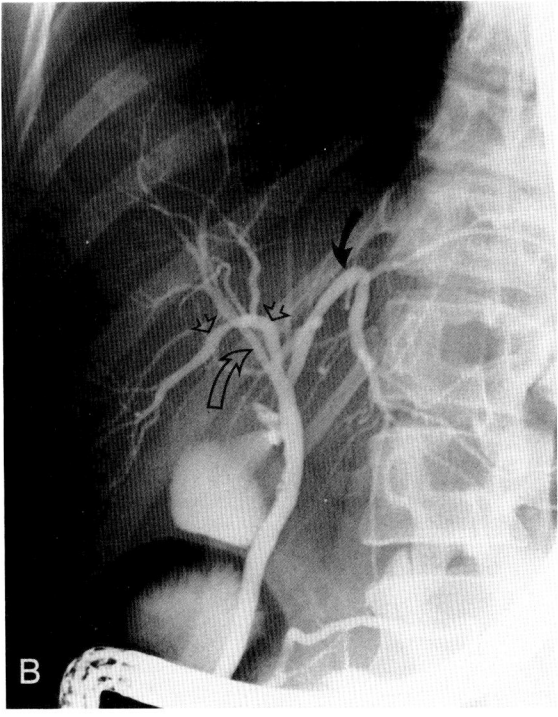

FIGURE 9.6. Usual Configuration of the Main Intrahepatic Ducts

A: Line drawing: *RHD* = right hepatic duct, *LHD* = left hepatic duct, *CHD* = common hepatic duct. *B:* ERCP: note the curve of the posterior segment of the right hepatic duct (*open arrows*). The courses of the left hepatic duct (*closed curved arrow*) and the anterior segment of the right hepatic duct (*open curved arrow*) are well demonstrated.

hepatic artery as well as arteries supplying the common bile duct. Venous drainage is directly into the liver via a complicated plexus or into the portal system via anastomoses with the choledochal and superior mesenteric veins (8, 9).

The common bile duct is supplied by branches of the hepatic, cystic, gastroduodenal, and pancreaticoduodenal arteries, with the principal supply coming from the posterior superior pancreaticoduodenal artery. Branches of the right gastric, suprarenal, and superior mesenteric arteries may also contribute to the arterial supply of the common bile duct. The common hepatic duct is supplied by small branches of the hepatic artery that anastomose with the cystic artery (8).

Most of the lymphatic drainage from the liver and the intrahepatic biliary tree collects in lymphatics around the intrahepatic branches of the portal vein. The accompanying bile ducts have a dense, sometimes subepithelial lymphatic network. Drainage is into several lymphatic vessels in the liver hilum which drain in turn into the hepatic lymph nodes around the common hepatic duct and the main portal vein. These lymphatics continue to chains of lymph nodes around the celiac axis and inferior vena cava. Some drainage from peripheral intrahepatic bile ducts is into lymphatics that pass through the hiatus for the inferior vena cava directly into the thoracic duct. Lymph vessels from the gallbladder and extrahepatic biliary tree drain to either the hepatic nodes or the superior pancreatic nodes in the region of the head and neck of the pancreas (1).

REFERENCES

1. Netter FH: *The Ciba Collection of Medical Illustrations,* Vol III, Digestive System, Part III, Liver Biliary Tract and Pancreas. Summit, NJ, Ciba Pharmaceutical Products, 1957, pp 22–24.
2. Hatfield PM, Wise RE: *Radiology of the Gallbladder and Bile Ducts.* Baltimore, Williams & Wilkins, 1976, pp 9–10.
3. Moosman DA, Coller FA: Prevention of traumatic injury to the bile ducts; study of structures of cysto-hepatic angle encountered in cholecystectomy and supraduodenal choledochostomy. *Am J Surg* 82:132–143, 1951.
4. Schwartz A, Birnbaum D: Roentgenologic study of the topography of the choledocho-duodenal junction. *AJR* 87:772–776, 1962.
5. Hatfield PM, Wise RE: Anatomic variation in the gallbladder and bile ducts. *Semin Roentgenol* 11:157–164, 1976.
6. Copenhaver WM, Bunge RP, Bunge MR: *Bailey's Textbook of Histology.* Baltimore, Williams & Wilkins, 1971, pp 477–479, 489–491.
7. Healey JE Jr, Schroy PC: Anatomy of the biliary ducts within the liver: analysis of prevailing patterns of branchings and the major variations of the biliary ducts. *Arch Surg* 66:599–616, 1953.
8. Kaude JV, Hawkins IF Jr: Angiography of the gallbladder and biliary tract. *Semin Roentgenol* 11: 191–195, 1976.
9. Deutsch V: Cholecysto-angiography. Visualization of the gallbladder by selective celiac and mesenteric angiography. *AJR* 101:608–616, 1967.

HISTOLOGY

The gallbladder wall is composed of three layers: mucosa, muscularis, and serosa. The mucosa is thrown into tiny folds that produce a honeycombed, pocketed surface ("areae cholecysticae") (1, 2). These folds disappear with extreme distention. The epithelium is composed of tall columnar cells. The tunica propria consists of richly vascularized connective tissue and a few scattered smooth muscle cells derived from the muscularis. Small mucous glands occur in the neck. Pocket-like invaginations of the surface epithelium extending down into the muscular and perimuscular layers are called Rokitansky-Aschoff sinuses. The muscular layer of the gallbladder is formed by interlacing longitudinal and circular smooth muscle fibers with interspersed elastic connective tissue. Just external to the muscularis are perimuscular and subserous layers of connective tissue. Aberrrant embryonic bile ducts are sometimes found in the serosa connecting to the liver but not the lumen of the gallbladder (Luschka ducts). They may serve as a pathway for the spread of infection. The gallbladder functions as a reservoir for the bile produced by the liver. It concentrates bile by reabsorbing water and solutes through its mucosal layer (1, 3).

The extrahepatic bile ducts are lined by high columnar epithelium which is sometimes thrown into irregular folds. The subepithelial connective tissue is rich in elastic fibers but very sparse in muscle fibers except in the cystic duct and the distal common bile duct (sphincter of Oddi). Mucus-producing glands in the deep layers are connected to the lumen by long ducts (1, 3).

The smallest branches of the intrahepatic duct system are the intralobular bile canaliculi, which form an intercommunicating network of channels between the cells of the hepatic plates, radiating outward from the central axis of the lobule. Most canaliculi drain into small interlobular bile ducts (cholangioles) found at the periphery of a lobule. Canals of Hering are short connections between hepatic cells and interlobular bile ducts lined by cuboidal cells. A few canaliculi empty into small intralobular bile ducts which extend to variable depths within the lobule. Each interlobular duct joins with others, forming progressively larger ducts lined by cuboidal or columnar epithelium. As the ducts increase in size towards the porta hepatis, the connective tissue layer becomes thicker with many elastic fibers and only few smooth muscle cells. Interlobular bile ducts always accompany branches of the portal vein and hepatic artery, with these structures together with interlobular connective tissue and lymphatics occupying the portal canal (1, 3).

REFERENCES

1. Copenhaver WM, Bunge RP, Bunge MR: *Bailey's Textbook of Histology.* Baltimore, Williams & Wilkins, 1985, pp 488–491.
2. Kotler RE, Louw JH: The mucosal pattern of the gallbladder ("areae cholecysticae"). *Br J Radiol* 57:289–291, 1984.
3. Netter FH: *The Ciba Collection of Medical Illustrations* Vol. III, Digestive System, Part III, Liver, Biliary Tract, and Pancreas. Summit, NJ, Ciba Pharmaceutical Products, 1957, p 22.

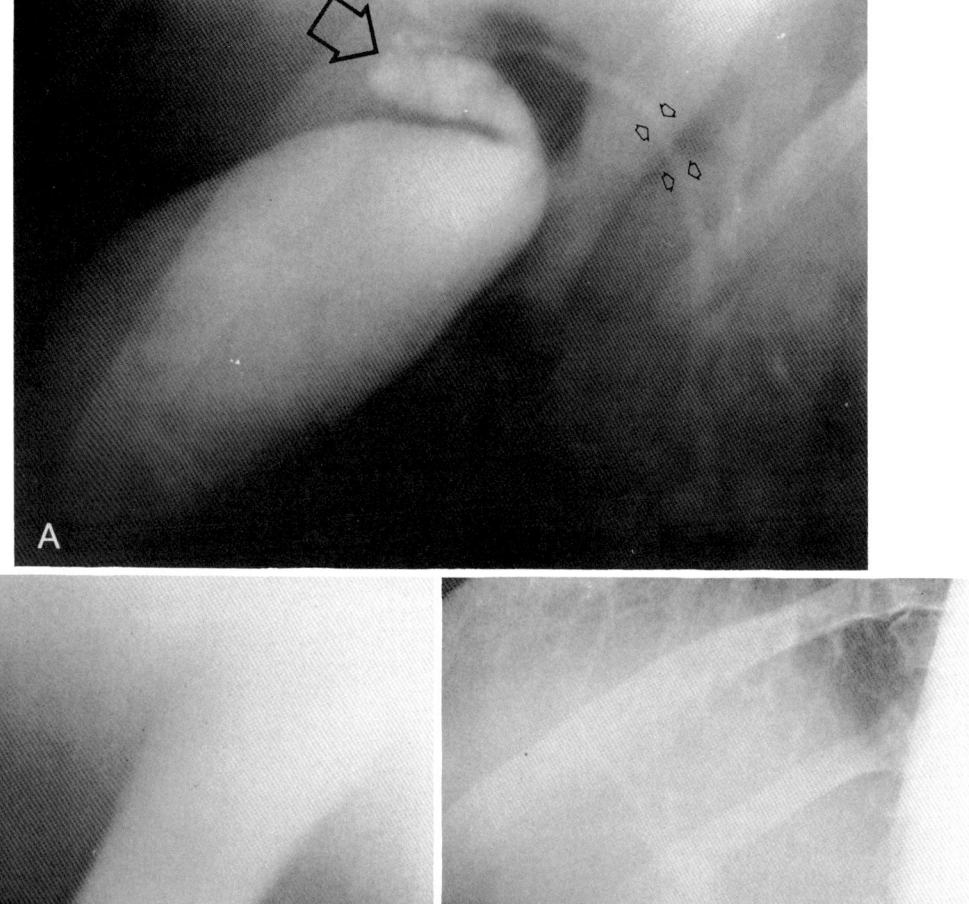
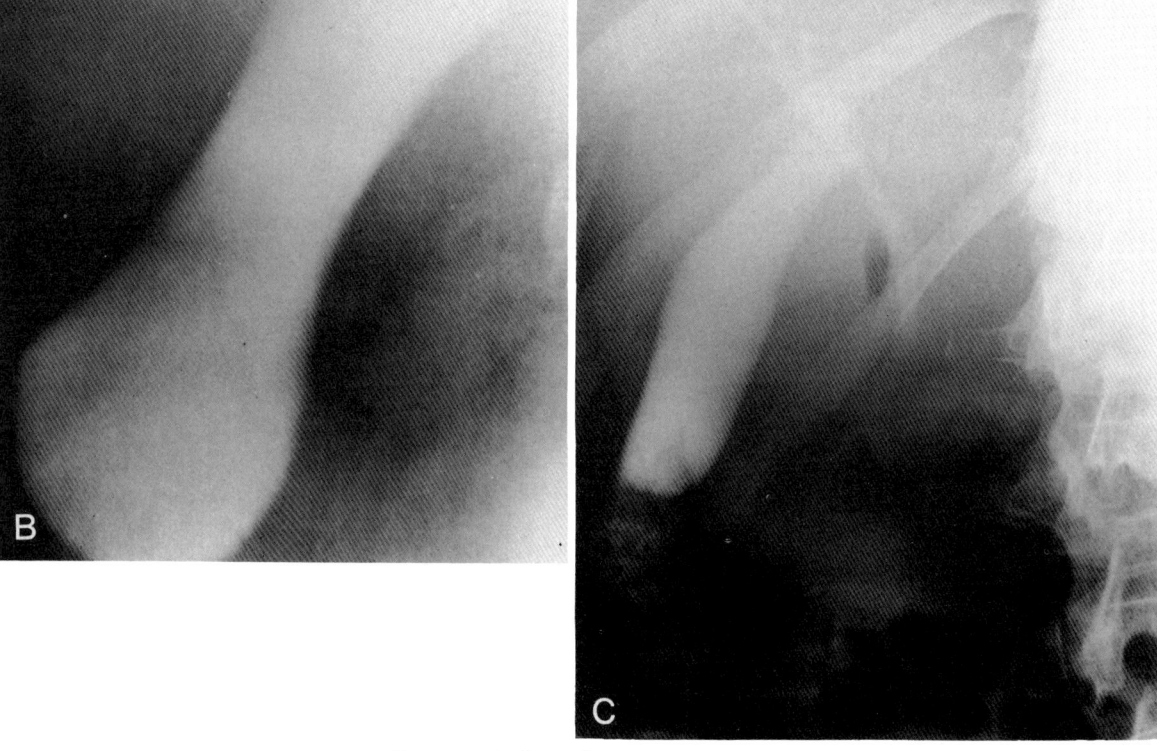

FIGURE 9.7. ORAL CHOLECYSTOGRAM

A: Normal oral cholecystogram: well-opacified gallbladder with visualization of cystic duct and valves of Heister (*large arrow*) as well as common bile duct (*small arrows*). *B* and *C:* Pre-fat normal spot film of the gallbladder (*B*). No ductal structures seen. Post-fat film (*C*) demonstrates filling of the intrahepatic biliary tree and common bile duct as well as a change in shape of the gallbladder.

NORMAL ORAL CHOLECYSTOGRAM AND BARIUM CONTRAST EXAMINATION

The technique of oral cholecystography is discussed in the section on cholelithiasis. A normally functioning gallbladder appears as an opaque, pear-shaped organ in the right upper quadrant on oral cholecystography. The neck of the gallbladder and the beginning of the cystic duct are seen best on supine films, whereas the fundus is seen best on erect films. Post–fatty meal films can, at times, show the entire cystic duct and the common bile duct, especially with tomography (Fig. 9.7).

The gallbladder is anterolateral to the first and second portions of the duodenum, and the neck of the gallbladder and cystic duct cross in front of the duodenum at the junction of the first and second portions. The common bile duct descends behind the duodenal bulb or postbulbar duodenum on its way to the ampulla. Thus, impressions by these structures on the duodenum are often seen during a barium meal examination. Quite uncommonly, barium will reflux for no apparent reason from the duodenum into the distal common bile duct (Fig. 9.8).

The papilla of Vater is an elevated mound of tissue about 8–10 mm in diameter that is frequently demonstrated on high quality double contrast films of the duodenum as a small submucosal mass along the posterior medial wall of the descending duodenum. 1.5 cm is an approximate upper limit of normal size on roentgenograms. The papilla's exact location can vary between the immediate postbulbar duodenum and the proximal transverse duodenum, so that the following landmarks are useful in excluding other causes of small submucosal masses: the promontory, straight segment and the longitudinal fold (Fig. 9.9). The promontory is a localized outward bulge of the lumen along the inner aspect of the mid-descending duodenum. The papilla is either just on the promontory or within a centimeter below it. The straight segment is a flat portion of the inner duodenal wall devoid of folds immediately distal to the promontory extending 2–3 cm distally. The longitudinal fold is a mucosal hood over the papilla that extends distally 2–3 cm parallel to the straight segment and perpendicular to the transversely oriented duodenal folds (Fig. 9.9) (1).

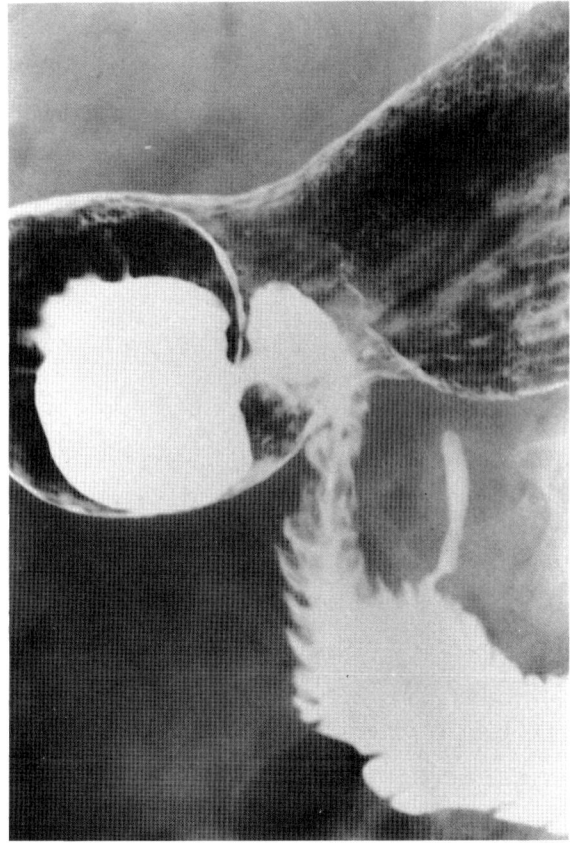

FIGURE 9.8. UGI: REFLUX OF BARIUM INTO THE DISTAL COMMON BILE DUCT

On occasion, the fundus of the gallbladder will cause an extrinsic mass effect upon the superior haustral row of the anterior hepatic flexure on a barium enema (2).

REFERENCES

1. Eaton SB Jr, Ferrucci JT Jr: *Radiology of the Pancreas and Duodenum*. Philadelphia, W. B. Saunders, 1973, pp 109–113.
2. Berk RN, Ferrucci JT Jr, Leopold GR: *Radiology of the Gallbladder and Bile Ducts, Diagnosis and Intervention*. Philadelphia, W. B. Saunders, 1983, pp 30–40, 83–90.

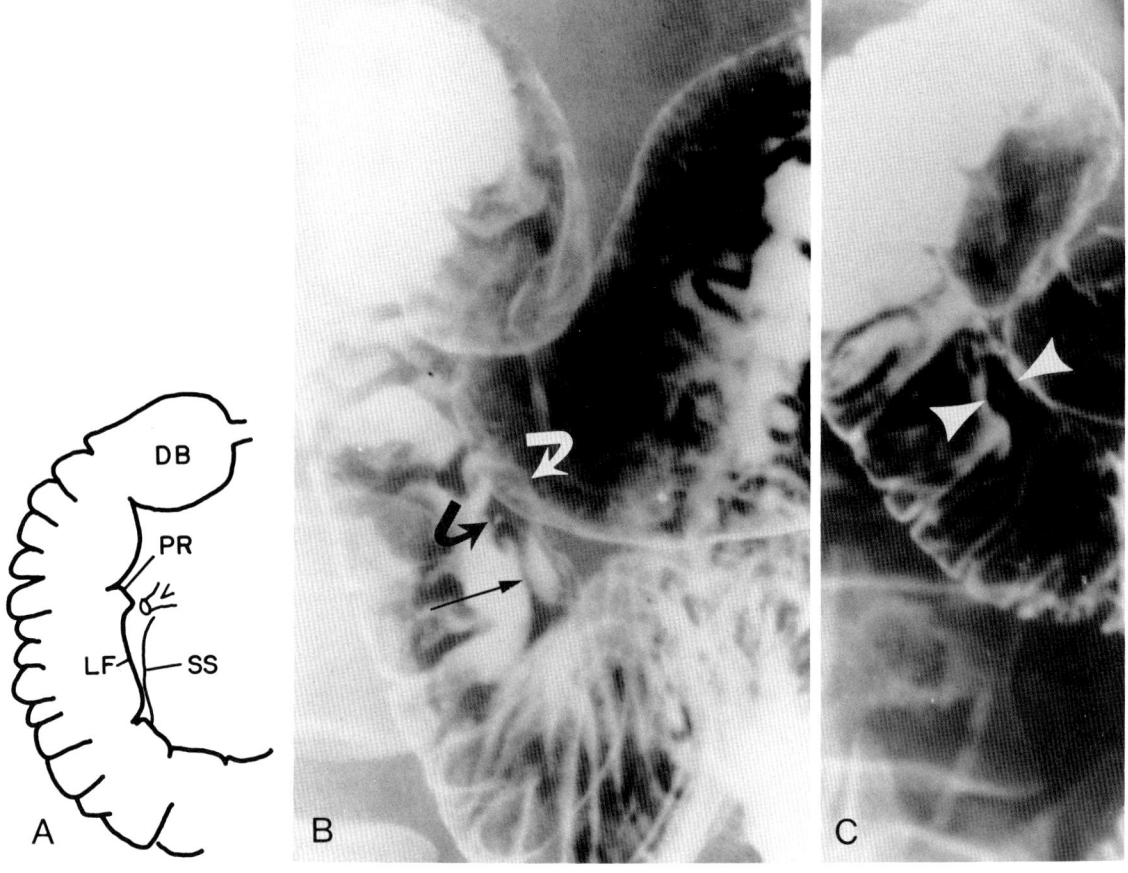

FIGURE 9.9. DUODENAL ANATOMY
A: Perivaterian duodenal anatomy: *DB* = duodenal bulb, *PR* = promontory, *LF* = longitudinal fold, *SS* = straight segment. *B:* Longitudinal fold (*arrow*) running upward forming a hood over the papilla (*curved arrows*). *C:* Papilla en face (*arrowheads*) with a central dot of barium in its opening mimicking an ulcerated submucosal mass.

NORMAL IMAGING OF THE GALLBLADDER AND BILIARY TRACT

Radiopharmaceuticals

The current class of biliary radiopharmaceuticals, the ^{99m}Tc-labeled iminodiacetic acid derivatives, has as its progenitor the iodinated dyes. Rose bengal (tetraiodotetra-chlorofluorescein) was first reported as an agent that could be used to study liver function by Delprat in 1923 (1). In a dog model Delprat showed that rose bengal is removed from the circulation at a constant rate and that the rate is slower in the chloroform-injured liver. Yuhl and colleagues (2) reported on the imaging of the gallbladder with ^{131}I-diiodofluorescein in 1953. In their work they injected 1 mCi of the agent, and using the new scintiscanner began scanning at 20 min. The gallbladder was identified in all their normal subjects. It was in 1955 that George Taplin and his associates (3) first reported on their work with radioiodinated rose bengal in animals and humans. Uptake and excretion rates were obtained by using a calcium tungstate γ-ray scintillation counter positioned over the liver but pointed away from the gallbladder. Their work showed a clear separation of normal from abnormal uptake-excretion patterns. Doctor Taplin, in his introduction, sets the stage for hepatobiliary imaging when he lists the advantages of the radioactive rose bengal test (3):

> First, it measures polygonal call function directly rather than by changes occurring in the blood (thereby eliminating repeated venipunctures); second, it registers graphically the rate of dye uptake and time necessary

for its excretion from the liver; third, it is the only dye test which can be used safely in the presence of biliary tract obstruction because of the minute quantities and low toxicity of the dye employed; fourth it gives information concerning liver circulation as well as patency of the biliary tract; and fifth, it appears to be many times more sensitive than nonradioactive dye tests.

Although a number of other agents were examined, ^{131}I-rose bengal remained the only commonly used hepatobiliary radiopharmaceutical until the mid-1970s. Nordyke (4) used a two probe system to detect tracer in the circulation (positioned against the head) and in the intestine (positioned below the liver slightly to the left of midline) and scanning to determine if gallbladder activity was present. He attempted to determine if there was biliary tract obstruction and, when the gallbladder visualized, to localize the obstruction to the distal common duct. In 1965 Eyler and associates (5) analyzed 75 scans in jaundiced patients with bilirubin levels above 1.0 mg/100 ml. A number of variables, including liver size, uniformity of tracer, gallbladder and/or bowel visualization and visualization of ducts was felt to be helpful in the differential diagnosis of jaundice. Burke and Halko (6) described the use of dynamic hepatobiliary studies using ^{131}I-rose bengal and a gamma camera. The use of the γ-camera removed the difficulties of probe position and collimation, and since more of the abdomen could be visualized, there was a greater sensitivity in monitoring biliary excretion of the tracer. ^{131}I-rose bengal has been used to differentiate neonatal hepatic cholestasis from biliary atresia by measuring the tracer excreted in the stool. If less than 10% of the activity administered was present in a 3-day stool collection (without significant urine contamination), the diagnosis of biliary atresia could be made (7, 8).

The use of ^{99m}Tc-labeled hepatobiliary agents started with ^{99m}Tc-penicillamine in 1972 (9) followed rapidly by ^{99m}Tc pyridoxylidene glutamate in 1974 (10) and ^{99m}Tc-dimethylacetanilido-iminodiacetate (HIDA) in 1975 (11). The new ^{99m}Tc compounds allowed much larger amounts of activity to be administered while maintaining acceptable patient exposure.

Pharmacology

All of the hepatobiliary imaging agents depend on active transport across the sinusoid-hepatocyte membrane and excretion into the biliary canaliculi. There is good evidence that several structural criteria are important for biliary excretion. Compounds with molecular weights between 300 and 1000 tend to be excreted in bile, while lower molecular weight compounds are excreted in urine. Compounds with both a strong polar group and a nonpolar portion tend to be favored by the biliary system. Compounds that are excreted in the bile also tend to be firmly bound by plasma proteins. This last function may prevent or impede glomerular filtration by the kidney or may be important for transfer to the membrane of the hepatocyte (12).

There are several carriers which bind compounds after entering the liver sinusoids. These carriers are specific for anions, cations, neutral substances and bile salts. It appears that the ^{99m}Tc IDA derivatives are competitively inhibited by anion dyes (13), and therefore are also influenced by the level of bilirubin. Once the tracer has been transported across the hepatocyte membrane, compounds may or may not be conjugated before being actively transported into the biliary canaliculi. The pharmacology and pharmacokinetics of the biliary agents are well covered in review chapters by Fritzberg (13) and Loberg et al. (14).

Various derivatives of iminodiacetic acid (IDA) have been formulated and tested. Loberg and colleagues (14) list the necessary structural features for the formation of ^{99m}Tc-IDA complexes with cholescintigraphic properties as: (a) diacetate substitution on the amine nitrogen; (b) a carbamoyl or similar electron-withdrawing substituent, β to the amine; and (c) a lipophilic group. Since their introduction the IDA compounds have been used almost exclusively for clinical studies.

The agents are now approved for general use and are easily obtained in kit form from radiopharmaceutical companies. The kits use stannous chloride as a reducing agent as well as the IDA derivative in lyophilized form in a sterile pyrogen-free vial. The user merely adds up to 100 mCi of ^{99m}Tc-pertechnetate (2–3 ml) to the vial, swirls the contents for 1–2 min and the

TABLE 9.1.
RADIATION ABSORBED DOSE (mrad/mCi) FOR DISIDA

Organ	Fasting	Whole Meal Gallbladder Stimulation
Liver	130	65
Gallbladder wall	2090	780
Small bowel	120	200
Upper large bowel	210	370
Lower large bowel	140	240
Ovary	42	72
Testes	3	4
Marrow	9	10
Whole body	17	17

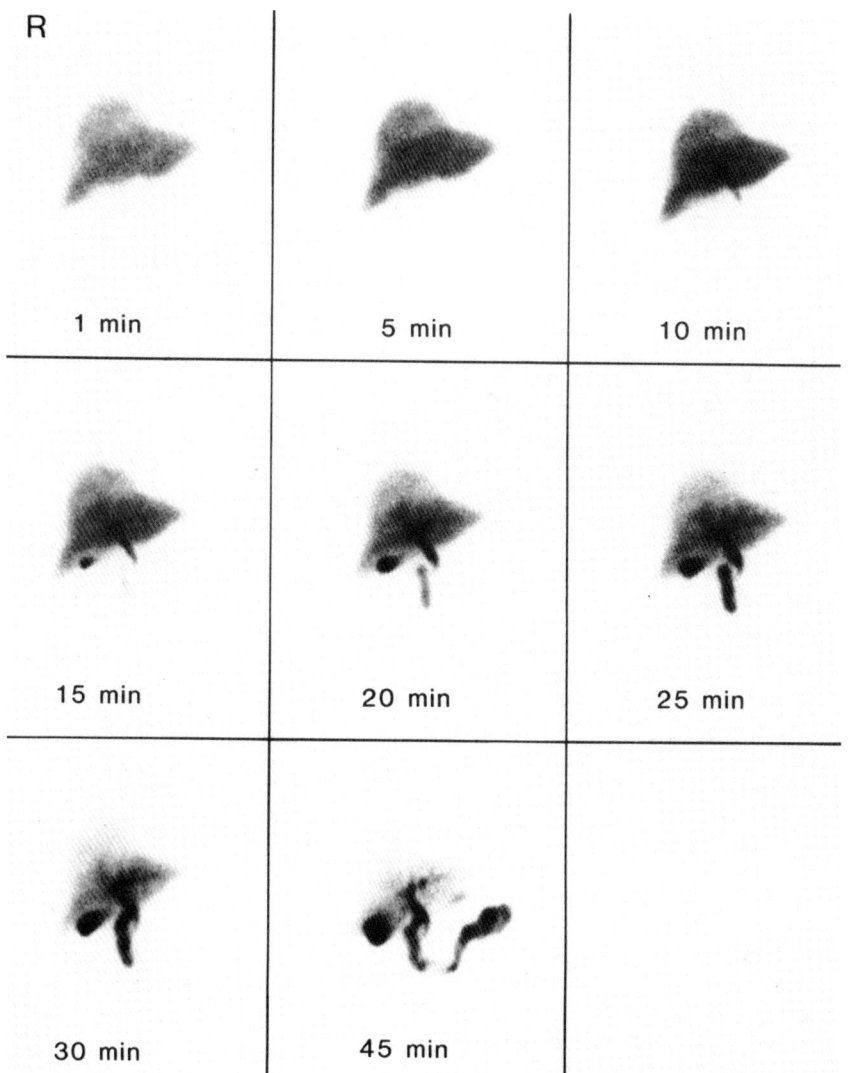

FIGURE 9.10. NORMAL ^{99m}Tc-DISIDA CHOLESCINTIGRAM

Excellent uptake of the radiotracer by the liver is followed by prompt excretion into the common duct, gallbladder and intestine.

^{99m}Tc-IDA is ready for patient administration. Although the agents are stable for up to 120 hr, the manufacturers and FDA state that the material should be used within 6 hr.

Radiation Exposure

Brown et al. (15), using serial γ camera and blood and urine samples, showed that in normal subjects between 5 and 20% of the administered activity was recovered in the urine during the first day. For the diisopropyl-IDA compound the half-lives for hepatic uptake and excretion were 4.8 ± 0.7 min and 18.8 ± 2.5 min, respectively with a 24-hr urinary excretion of 11.1 ± 1.5%. When normal fasting subjects and subjects in whom a whole meal was used for gallbladder stimulation were studied, the radiation exposure for diisopropyl-IDA (DISIDA) was as shown in Table 9.1. Agents other than DISIDA are reported on in the original article from an earlier work by this group (16). There is a change in the biodistribution and radiation exposure when there is an elevation of bilirubin and therefore greater renal excretion. They recommend using 3 mCi (111 MBq) in patients with normal levels of bilirubin and up to 8 mCi (300 MBq) in jaundiced patients. They also suggest considering gallbladder stimulation with milk after visualization in order to reduce the absorbed dose to the gallbladder; however, this of course will increase the absorbed dose to bowel and ovaries.

Patient Preparation

Patients should be fasting 2–4 hr before the start of the hepatobiliary scan. This allows the gallbladder to relax after the normal postprandial cholecystokinin stimulation. In patients who have been fasting for a prolonged period or in patients on total parenteral nutrition it may be helpful to administer Kinevac (Sincalide) (a CCK analog) ½ to 1 hr prior to the study. This agent is given by very slow intravenous administration (several minutes) in a dose of 0.2–0.4 µg/kg and causes gallbladder contraction followed by relaxation. Rapid administration can result in failure of a normal gallbladder to contract due to the induction of spasm of the cystic duct/neck of the gallbladder. With the patient lying supine beneath an Anger gamma camera, positioned to include the liver, biliary tree and proximal small bowel, 3–6 mCi of ^{99m}Tc-IDA are administered intravenously. Five hundred thousand to one million count images are obtained at 1 min and then every 5 min for 30 min. If necessary, 45-min, 60-min, and oblique or lateral projections are taken. Studies in which the gallbladder, common duct, or duodenum are not visualized by 1 hr are continued to 1½, 2, or 4 hr when necessary.

The Normal Scan

The image obtained at 1 min is primarily a blood pool image. Heart, liver, spleen, and kidneys and other vascular structures can be visualized. By the 5-min scan the liver should have taken up most of the tracer. Some renal excretion may be seen early (5–10 min) in individuals with normal hepatobiliary function. This route of excretion is more prominent in patients with hepatocellular disease. The early images are important to evaluate hepatic parenchyma, hepatic function, and to locate the kidneys. As the right kidney may approximate the position of the gallbladder, these early images are helpful to avoid any confusion in later scans. The biliary tract is usually seen at 10–20 min with visualization of the major intrahepatic ducts, common hepatic and common bile duct. Typically, the gallbladder is seen within 30–60 min and some activity reaches the small bowel by 1 hr. A normal hepatobiliary scan is shown in Figure 9.10.

Weissmann et al. (17) describe nonbiliary findings in the four phases of hepatobiliary scanning (Table 9.2).

In the vast majority of patients the parenchymal phase of the hepatobiliary scan shows a similar pattern to that seen on ^{99m}Tc-sulfur colloid liver images (17–19). Discordant images have been described in cirrhosis (19), hepatocellular carcinoma (20), hemochromatosis (21), hepatitis (22), and hypervitaminosis A (23).

TABLE 9.2.
FOUR PHASES OF HEPATOBILIARY FINDINGS[a]

A. Blood pool phase (1–5 min)
 1. Cardiac enlargement, aneurysm, pericardial effusions
 2. Hypervascular or hypovascular lesions (18)
 3. Splenic or renal enlargement
 4. Ascites
B. Hepatocyte phase (5–20 min)
 1. Focal liver lesions (tumors, abscesses, cysts, etc.)
 2. Contour defects (subcapsular hematoma, subphrenic abscesses, etc.)
C. Renal excretion phase (5–15 min)
 1. Nonvisualization of kidneys
 2. Enhanced renal visualization (hepatocellular disease, obstructive jaundice)
 3. Masses
 4. Positional changes
 5. Hydronephrosis
D. Intestinal phase (30–60 min)
 1. Malrotation
 2. Bowel displacement by abdominal masses
 3. Gastric reflux
 4. Postoperative displacement (diversionary shunts, bowel plication)
 5. Persistent loops of non filling of loops (pancreatitis, focal or generalized ileus

[a] Modified from Weissmann et al. (17).

REFERENCES

1. Delprat GD: Studies on liver function: rose bengal elimination from the blood as influenced by liver injury. Arch Intern Med 32:401–410, 1923.
2. Yuhl ET, Stirrett LA, Itill MR et al: The cholescintigram. A preliminary report. Surgery 34:724–727, 1953.
3. Taplin GV, Meredith OM, Kade H: The radioactive (^{131}I-tagged) rose bengal uptake-excretion test for liver function using external gamma-ray scintillation counting techniques. J Lab Clin Med 45:665–678, 1955.
4. Nordyke RA: Biliary tract obstruction and its localization with radioiodinated rose bengal. Am J Gastroenterol 33:563–573, 1960.
5. Eyler WR, Schuman BM, DuSault LA et al: The radioiodinated rose bengal liver scan as an aid in the differential diagnosis of jaundice. AJR 94:469–476, 1965.
6. Burke G, Halko A: Dynamic clinical studies with radioisotopes and the scintillation camera. II. Rose bengal ^{131}I-liver function studies. JAMA 198:608–618, 1966.
7. Sharp HL, Krivit W, Lowman ST: The diagnosis of complete extrahepatic biliary obstruction with rose bengal-^{131}I. J Pediatr 70:46, 1967.
8. Thaler MM, Gellis SC: Studies in neonatal hepatic and biliary atresia. Am J Dis Child 116:280, 1968.
9. Tubis M, Krishnamurthy GT, Edow JS: ^{99m}Tc-penicilamine: a new cholescintigraphic agent. J Nucl Med 13:652–654, 1972.
10. Baker RJ, Bellen JC, Ronai PM: ^{99m}Tc-pyridoxylideneglutamate: a new rapid cholescintigraphic agent. J Nucl Med 15:476, 1974.
11. Harvey E, Loberg MD, Cooper M: ^{99m}Tc-HIDA: a new

radio-pharmaceutical for hepatobiliary imaging. *J Nucl Med* 16:533, 1975.
12. Firnan G: Why do [99mTc] chelates work for cholescintigraphy? *Eur J Nucl Med* 1:137–139, 1976.
13. Fritzberg AR: The evaluation of hepatocyte function with radiotracers. In Billinghurst MW, Colombetti LG (eds): *Studies of Cellular Function Using Radiotracers.* Boca Raton, FL, CRC Press, 1982, pp 74–97.
14. Loberg MD, Nunn AD, Porter DW: Development of hepatobiliary imaging agents. In Freeman LM, Weissman HS (eds): *Nuclear Medicine Annual.* New York, Raven Press, 1981.
15. Brown PH, Krishnamurthy GT, Bobba VR et al: Radiation dose calculation for five [99mTc]-IDA hepatobiliary agents. *J Nucl Med* 23:1025–1030, 1982.
16. Brown PH, Krishnamurthy GT, Bobba VVR et al: Radiation dose calculation for Tc-99m HIDA in health and disease. *J Nucl Med* 22:177–183, 1981.
17. Weissmann HS, Sugarman LA, Frank MS et al: Serendipity in technetium-99m dimethyl iminoidiacetic acid cholescintigraphy. *Radiology* 135:449–454, 1980.
18. Makler PT, Velchik MG, Weingrad T et al: Unusual appearance of a highly vascular lesion on [99mTc]-DISIDA hepatobiliary scintigraphy. *Clin Nucl Med* 8:483–485, 1983.
19. Brown ML, Freitas JE, Wahner HW: Useful hepatic parenchymal imaging in hepatobiliary scintigraphy. *AJR* 136:893–895, 1981.
20. Lee VW, Shapiro JH: Specific diagnosis of hepatoma using [99mTc]-HIDA and other radionuclides. *Eur J Nucl Med* 8:191–195, 1983.
21. Knopf DR, McClees EC, Fajaman WA, et al.: Discordant hepatic uptake of [99mTc]-sulfur colloid and [99mTc]-DISIDA in hemochromatosis. *AJR* 141:563–564, 1983.
22. Lamki L: A dichotomy in hepatic uptake of [99mTc]-IDA and [99mTc]-colloid. *Semin Nucl Med* 12:94–95, 1982.
23. Vincent LN, McCartney WH, Mauro MA et al: Discordant hepatic uptake between [99mTc]-sulfur colloid and [99mTc]-DISIDA in hypervitaminosis A. *J Nucl Med* 25:207–208, 1984.

Sonography of the Gallbladder: Technique and Anatomy

Technique

More than any other imaging technique, ultrasound is operator dependent. Meticulous attention to technique is essential if accurate studies are to be produced. Only highly trained sonographers should perform scans. Physician supervision and participation increases the accuracy of the procedure. Real-time scanning is preferable to static scanning because of the infinite number of planes available and the shorter examination time. The only patient preparation required is an overnight (minimum 6 hr) fast to allow for maximal distention of the gallbladder. At the same time interference from bowel gas generated by swallowing will be minimized. Good quality scans of the gallbladder will be obtained in only 50% of nonfasting patients. The spurious wall thickening and poor stone visibility that result from lack of distention coupled with excess gas makes interpretation less accurate. In the emergency situation, adequate scans can usually be obtained because nausea and vomiting simulate the fasting state. The common hepatic duct can usually be depicted well with or without fasting (1).

The highest possible frequency transducer that provides adequate penetration should be used. In most adults this will be a 3.5 mHz transducer, but in thin patients a 5.0 mHz or even a 7.5 mHz transducer can be successfully employed for better resolution. The overall gain and TGC should be individually adjusted and varied during the examination. Settings for the gallbladder should be lower than those used for the liver as too high a gain can obliterate shadowing from calculi.

Scanning is started in the supine position subcostally. Suspended deep inspiration often is helpful in bringing liver and gallbladder to a more sonographically accessible position below the ribs. In patients with a high liver or excess gas, intercostal scanning may be necessary. Both longitudinal and transverse scanning is necessary. Patients are then examined in right anterior oblique and left lateral decubitus positions. These maneuvers are useful for unfolding kinks in the gallbladder, evaluating sludge, displacing gas-filled bowel loops, and detecting small stones which may become visible by virtue of motion. Erect views are even better for demonstrating shifting stones but the gallbladder may become obscured by gas in the hepatic flexure.

Anatomy

The gallbladder is a fluid-filled pear-shaped ovoid structure located in the right upper quadrant just beneath the liver in the gallbladder fossa (Fig. 9.11). The latter is an indentation on the inferior surface of the liver, medial to the right lobe, that can be either prominent or shallow and imperceptible. The size of the gallbladder is quite variable with upper limits of 8.0–10.0 cm in length and 4.0–5.0 cm in anteroposterior diameter. Large, yet unobstructed gallbladders are seen in alcoholism, diabetes, hyperalimentation and narcotic analgesia (diminished emptying) and in the WDHA syndrome (increased biliary excretion).

The main interlobar fissure (divides the liver into right and left lobes) is an important landmark which has a constant relationship to the gallbladder (Fig. 9.11C and D) (2). Peripancreatic fat extends into the fissure, causing it to appear as a highly reflective line. The cephalad portion of the fissure contains the proximal right portal vein and its caudad end abuts on the gallbladder neck. On transverse scans, the fissure is seen to run obliquely from an anterolateral location towards the porta hepatis, with the gallbladder lying in a similar oblique course at its caudad end. In some individuals, the fissure is short and the neck of the gallbladder is adjacent to the right or main portal vein. A poorly distended, hard to visualize gallbladder may be located by following the fissure.

When the gallbladder is distended and welldefined, the anterior wall is seen as a smooth, highly reflective layer not more than 2.0–3.0 mm thick. The entire thickness of the posterior wall is usually difficult to depict because of artifacts from underlying bowel gas. A characteristic double-walled appearance can be seen in the contracted, postprandial gallbladder. Three layers are present: a highly reflective outer layer, a sonolucent middle layer, and a poorly reflective inner layer. This appearance in the contracted gallbladder is important to recognize since a triple layered wall has been described as a sign of acute cholecystitis. However, the gallbladder is usually distended in acute cholecystitis rather than contracted (3).

Some gallbladders contain a fold in the posterior wall at the junction of the body and infundibulum which may protrude into the lumen and even exhibit weak shadowing, mimicking a stone Fig. 9.11E and F). Turning the patient into a left lateral decubitus position will usually cause the fold to disappear (4). The phrygian cap deformity, a normal variant in which the fundus is folded on the body, can be depicted sonographically in a similar fashion (Fig. 9.11G) (5). Very tiny acoustic shadows may originate from the edges of the gallbladder wall and the larger bile ducts in normals. They are caused by refraction of the sound beam at the interface of a medium of high velocity with one of lower velocity. Shadowing can also occur in the region of the neck of the gallbladder (Fig. 9.11B). These shadows may also be refractive although in the past they have been ascribed to the valves of Heister and/or the convoluted course of the cystic duct (6). A number of normal gas-containing structures adjacent to the gallbladder may simulate gallstones. The duodenum may be in direct contact with the medial wall of the gallbladder and mimic a gallstone when entirely filled with gas. A gas-filled viscus directly beneath the gallbladder such as the hepatic flexure or a loop of small bowel may produce a pseudostone appearance with a highly reflective surface layer and distal acoustic shadowing. The viscus may even indent the gallbladder wall and due to the tomographic nature of sonography the echo and shadow can appear to arise from an intraluminal location. Careful scanning in a variety of positions and planes will show that the echoes and shadows originate from outside the gallbladder (7).

Gallbladder Ectopia

Gallbladder ectopia is uncommon but a significant problem in differential diagnosis when the organ is diseased because of unusual pain patterns. Until recently, very few cases were diagnosed preoperatively. In descending order of frequency, the most common ectopies are: beneath the left lobe, intrahepatic, and retrohepatic (8). Other less common locations are within the falciform ligament, within the interlobar fissure, and within the anterior abdominal wall. Diagnosis of retrorenal gallbladder by ultrasound and CT has been reported (9). The gallbladder was depicted behind the right kidney by both modalities with no gallbladder seen in the expected location. The diagnosis was confirmed by CT following administration of iopanoic acid. Extremely rare is the suprahepatic gallbladder, in which the gallbladder is subdiaphragmatic and posterior just above an abnormally high hepatic flexure (10). This condition is thought to be secondary to hypoplasia of the right lobe of the liver. An acquired ectopy that may be seen on ultrasound is herniation of the gallbladder through the foramen of Winslow into the lesser sac with or without strangulation (10). Whenever the gallbladder cannot be found in its expected location and no surgery has been performed on the patient, agenesis must be considered. Other rare anomalies that may be encountered are gallbladder duplication and congenital diverticula which are not easy to differentiate from each other by ultrasound.

The Gallbladder in Pregnancy

Functional and morphologic changes in the gallbladder during pregnancy have only recently been studied with ultrasound. Two factors were implicated in the past to explain the increased incidence of gallstones in women who have been pregnant. The first is lithogenic bile (decreased bile salt concentration and increased cholesterol concentration). The second is gallbladder stasis due to smooth muscle inhibition by high levels of progesterone and estrogen.

According to sonographic studies (11–13), no increase in gallbladder size occurs in the first trimester. During the second and third trimesters, the gallbladder volume doubles but the lon-

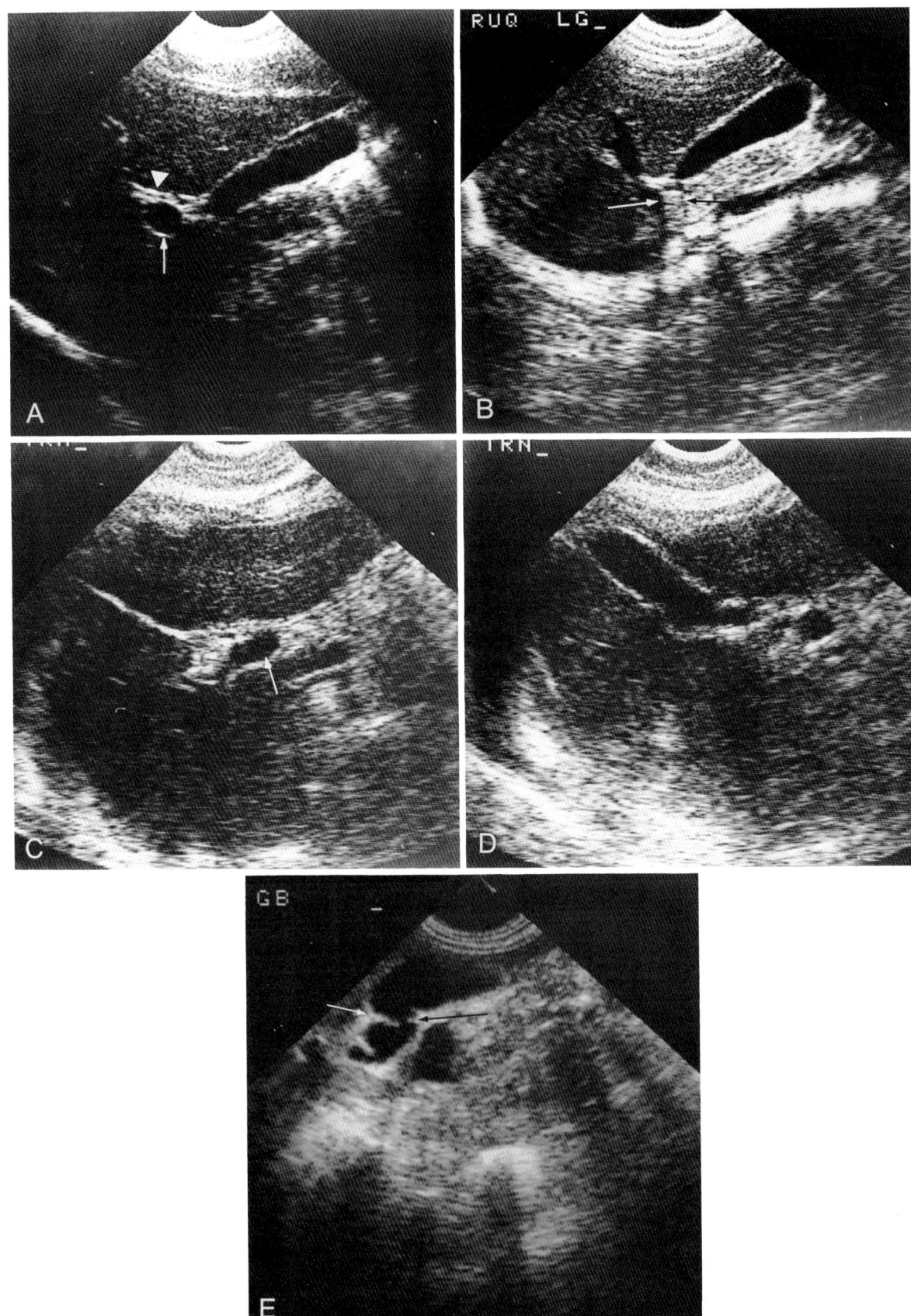

FIGURE 9.11. *A–E.*

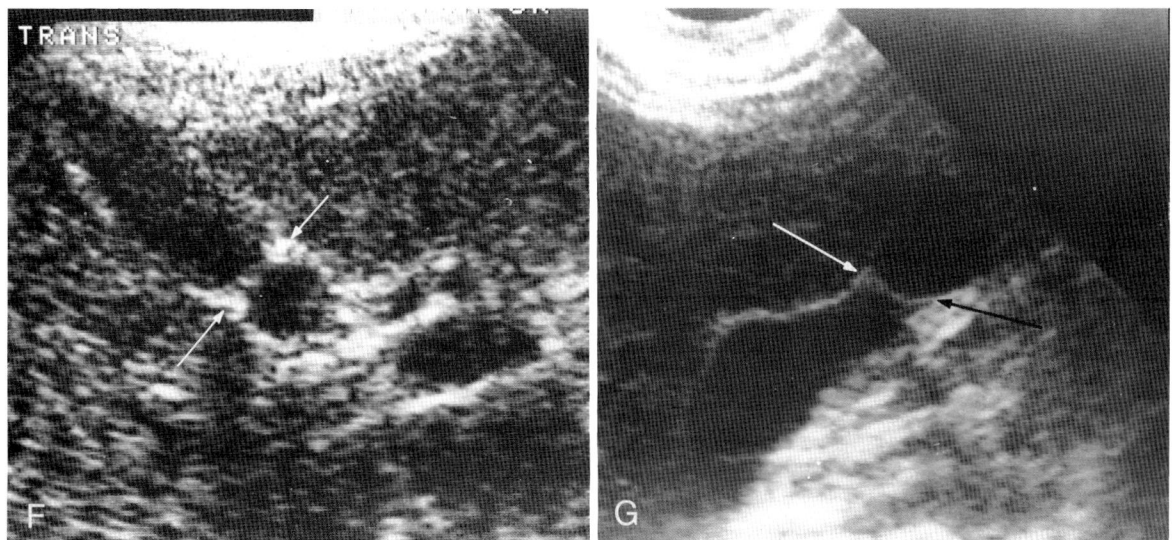

FIGURE 9.11. NORMAL GALLBLADDER SONOGRAPHY

A: Parasagittal scan: anechoic except for a few reverberation echoes anteriorly. Note the common duct (*arrowhead*) anterior to the portal vein (*arrow*) in the hepatoduodenal ligament just cephalad to the gallbladder. *B:* Parasagittal scan: refractive shadowing from the neck of the gallbladder (*arrows*). Normal study. *C:* transverse view of the major interlobar fissure (*echogenic line*). Note portal vein (*arrow*). *D:* Slightly caudad to (*C*) is the normal gallbladder seen transversely. *E:* Parasagittal section: normal posterior junctional fold (*arrows*). Folds in the gallbladder neck may simulate complete septa. *F:* Magnified transverse scan: fold at the neck of the gallbladder (*arrows*). *G:* Fold in gallbladder (*arrows*) representing phrygian cap. Parasagittal sonogram.

gitudinal diameter does not exceed the upper limit of normal (10.0 cm). In a study of 36 pregnant women (13), one-third developed gallbladder sludge which persisted until shortly after delivery, at which time gallbladder size and content returned to normal. Gallbladder contractility as demonstrated by rescanning after a fatty meal was normal. A 3.5–10% incidence of gallstones is present in the general obstetric population (11, 14, 15) and both de novo stone development and increase in number of stones during pregnancy has been documented by sonography. Cholestasis of pregnancy is a disorder in which serum bile acids, transaminases and alkaline phosphatase are elevated with associated pruritus (16). Although the common duct is normal sonographically, the gallbladder is, on average, 60% larger than in normal pregnancy.

REFERENCES

1. Hess ML, Cunningham JJ: Effect of examination time of day on the quality of real-time cholesonograms. *AJR* 143:251–253, 1984.
2. Callen PW, Filly RA: Ultrasonographic localization of the gallbladder. *Radiology* 133:687–691, 1979.
3. Marchal G, Van de Voorde P, Van Dooren W, Ponette E, Baert A: Ultrasonic appearance of the filled and contracted normal gallbladder. *J Clin Ultrasound* 8:439–442, 1980.
4. Sukov RJ, Sample WF, Sarti DA, Whitcomb MJ: Cholecystosonography—the junctional fold. *Radiology* 133:435–436, 1979.
5. Edell S: A comparison of the "Phrygian cap" deformity with bistable and gray scale ultrasound. *J Clin Ultrasound* 6:34–35, 1978.
6. Sommer FG, Minton MJ, Filly RA: Acoustic shadowing due to refractive and reflective effects. *AJR* 132:973–977, 1979.
7. McCune BR, Weeks LE, O'Brien TF, Martin JF: "Pseudostone" of the gallbladder ultrasound findings and case report. *Gastroenterology* 73:1149–1151, 1977.
8. Greaves FW, Nguyen KT, Sauerbrei EE: Retrohepatic gallbladder diagnosed by sonography and scintigraphy. *J Can Assoc Radiol* 34:319–320, 1983.
9. Ehman RL, Morrish HF: Retrorenal gallbladder, a case report. *J Can Assoc Radiol* 34:321–322, 1983.
10. Youngwirth LD, Peters JC, Perry MC: The suprahepatic gallbladder. An unusual anatomic variant. *Radiology* 149:57–58, 1983.
11. Bach DB, Satin R, Palayew M, Lisbona R, Tessler F: Herniation and strangulation of the gallbladder through the foramen of Winslow. *AJR* 142:541–542, 1984.
12. Stauffer RA, Adams A, Wygal J, Lavery JP: Gallbladder disease in pregnancy. *Am J Obstet Gynecol* 144:661–664, 1982.
13. Braverman DZ, Johnson ML, Kern F: Effects of pregnancy and contraceptive steroids on gallbladder function. *N Engl J Med* 302:362–364, 1980.
14. Bartoli E, Calonaci N, Nenci R: Ultrasonography of the gallbladder in pregnancy. *Gastrointest Radiol* 9:35–38, 1984.
15. Williamson SL, Williamson MR: Cholecystosonography in pregnancy. *J Ultrasound Med* 3:329–331, 1984.
16. Ylostalo P, Kirkinen P, Heikkinen J, Maentausta O, Jarvinen PA: Gallbladder volume and serum bile acids in cholestasis of pregnancy. *Br J Obstet Gynaecol* 89:59–61, 1982.

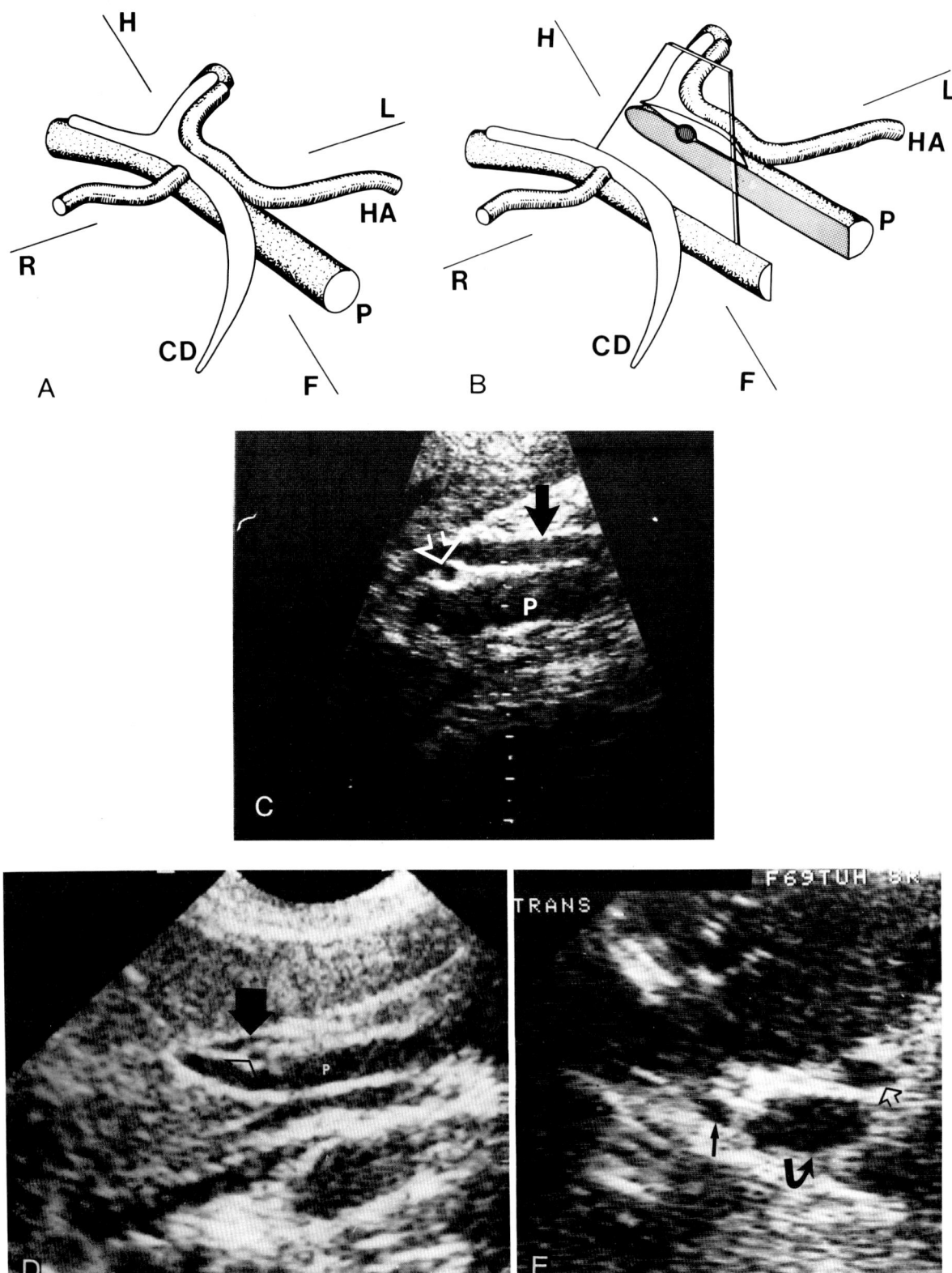

FIGURE 9.12.

Biliary Tract—Sonographic Anatomy

Technique

Patients are generally scanned in combinations of supine, right anterior oblique and left lateral decubitus positions, with the transducer placed subcostally. The beam is angled and rotated until the structures of the porta hepatis are identified. Ideally, the common duct, portal vein, and hepatic artery are depicted in both longitudinal and transverse projections. When possible, the common duct should be traced through the head of the pancreas. Overlying gas in the duodenum and hepatic flexure may preclude visualization of the most distal common duct. This may be partially or completely overcome by a change in positioning or filling the stomach and duodenum with water.

Anatomy

The common duct, portal vein and hepatic artery course together in the hepatoduodenal ligament which runs obliquely across the right upper quadrant (Figs. 9.12–9.15). As the cystic duct and its insertion into the common hepatic duct are variable in position and rarely depicted by sonography, common hepatic duct cannot be reliably distinguished from common bile duct and the term "common duct" is used. The portal vein is most posterior in location, the common duct is anterolateral, and the proper hepatic artery is anteromedial (Fig. 9.12E). This relationship holds true in most people until the vessels exit the hepatoduodenal ligament just cephalad to the head of the pancreas where the proper hepatic artery curves medially to form the common hepatic artery and the common duct curves laterally to enter the second portion of the duodenum at the ampulla of Vater. The common duct is tethered to the porta hepatis superiorly and inserts into the medial aspect of the duodenum inferiorly. The remainder of the common duct is relatively unfixed in its course along the lateral edge of the hepatoduodenal ligament (1). The common duct takes a sharp dorsal bend when it crosses over the portal vein. For this reason, it is not always possible to depict the entire common duct in one plane. Also, the course of the common duct may be altered by mass lesions. Bowing may become exaggerated when dilatation occurs (2).

A transverse segment in the mid-common duct has been described in 6% of the normal population and 18% of obstructed ducts (3). This transverse segment varies from 35–60 mm in length and may extend to or even across the midline. This variant is not likely to cause any problems in normals, but it may be confused with portal or splenic vein or pancreatic duct in an obstructed system. Failure to appreciate the true course of the common duct may prevent identification of the distal segment and the cause of the obstruction (Fig. 9.15).

The proper hepatic artery may either bifurcate or trifurcate in the porta hepatis into right, left and main hepatic arteries. Usually, only the right hepatic artery is identified at sonography (4). In 50–85% of patients, the right hepatic artery passes between the common duct and portal vein prior to entering the intersegmental fissure (Fig. 9.12C and D) (4, 5). In 15% it will cross anterior to the common duct (Fig. 9.13). As the common duct and the hepatic artery are frequently the same size, it can be difficult to distinguish the two. Occasionally, all three channels in the porta hepatis are parallel, compounding the problem (Fig. 9.14) (4). Twenty-five percent of patients have a hepatic artery variant (4), but only 3% are identified as such sonographically (4). The replaced or accessory right hepatic artery is seen as a tubular structure arising from the superior mesenteric artery coursing either anterior or posterior to the superior mesenteric vein, retro- or intrapancreatic, toward the porta hepatis (Fig. 9.16) (4).

Confusion may arise when the hepatic artery

FIGURE 9.12. NORMAL PORTA HEPATIS SONOGRAPHY

A: Normal vascular and ductal structures of the porta hepatis as viewed from right anterior oblique perspective. Common duct (CD) ventral to portal vein (P) until duct diverges to enter pancreatic head more dorsally and laterally. Hepatic artery (HA) originates medially, oriented transversely, then passes ventromedial to portal vein and parallels vein for a short distance. Right hepatic artery passes between duct and vein. (R = right; L = left; H = head; and F = feet. Same annotations in Figs. 9.12B, 9.13–9.15.) B: Same structures cut and separated to show approximate sonographic plane of section. Wedge-shaped sector corresponds roughly to sonogram. C: Corresponding oblique sonogram, marks 1 cm apart. Common duct (closed arrow) parallels and is ventral to portal vein (P). Hepatic artery (open arrow) seen in cross-section between duct and vein. D: Similar scan in a patient with a smaller caliber common duct. (Same annotations as 9.12C.) E: Magnified transverse view of the common duct (closed arrow), hepatic artery (open arrow) and portal vein (curved arrow) in the hepatoduodenal ligament. (From Berland LL, Lawson TL, Foley WD: Porta hepatis: sonographic discrimination of bile ducts from arteries with pulsed Doppler with new anatomic criteria. AJR 138:833–840, 1982.)

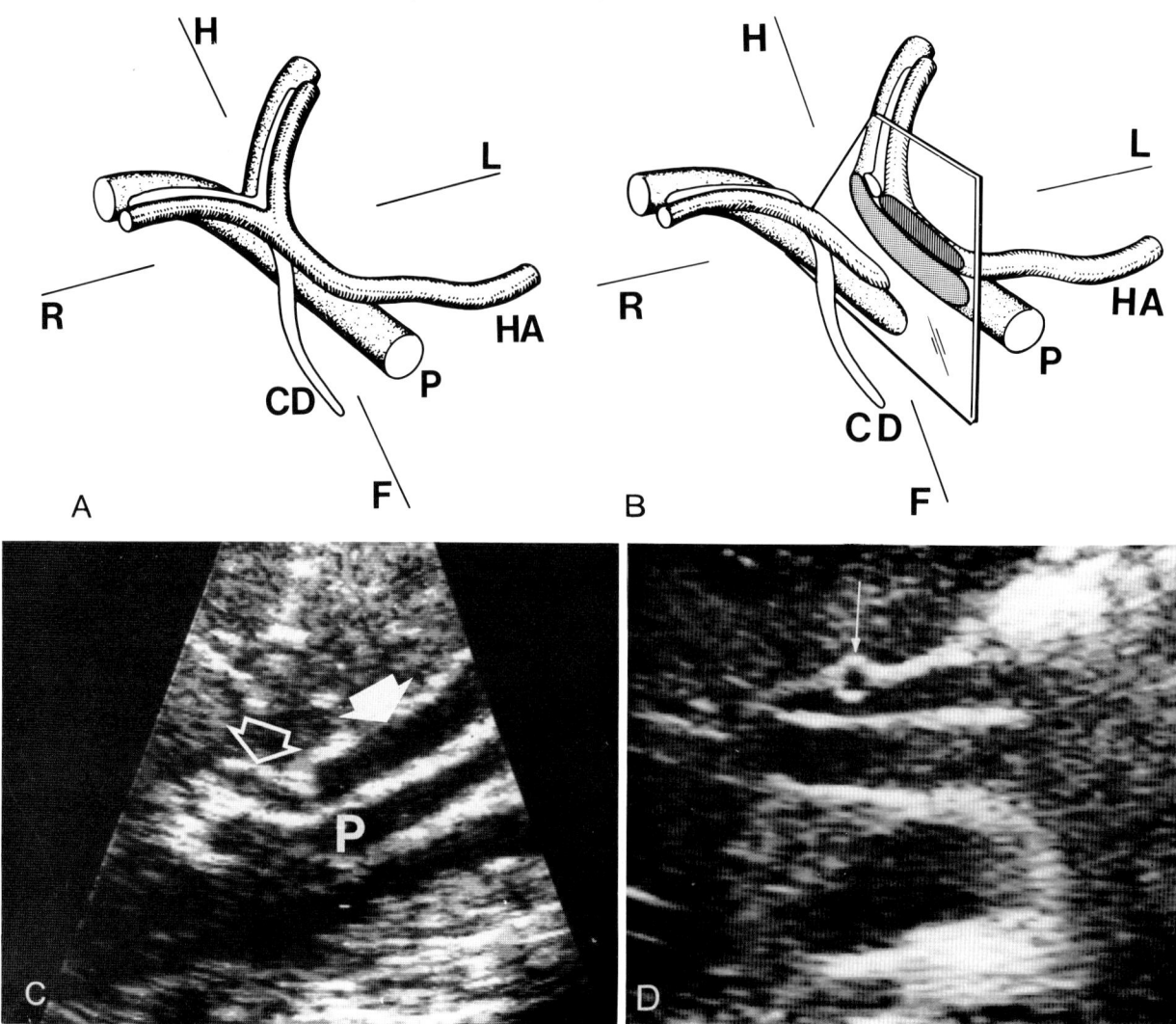

FIGURE 9.13. SONOGRAPHY OF VARIANTS IN THE PORTA HEPATIS

A: Porta hepatis in two individuals in whom artery is ventral to duct, which occurs in about 15% of patients. *B:* Structures cut and separated to indicate approximate plane of section of sonogram. *C:* Corresponding oblique sonogram. Hepatic artery (*closed arrow*) parallels portal vein (*P*) for several cms. Common duct (*open arrow*) smaller than hepatic artery, and duct was dorsal rather than ventral to artery. In this case, artery might have been confused with duct if high resolution real-time sonography and pulsed Doppler had not been used. *D:* Different patient: hepatic artery (*arrow*) anterior to common duct and portal vein. (From Berland LL, Lawson TL, Foley WD: Porta hepatis: sonographic discrimination of bile ducts from arteries with pulsed Doppler with new anatomic criteria. *AJR* 138:833–840, 1982.)

is tortuous. It may course in and out of the plane of section several times, either in front of or behind the common duct. Occasionally, the right hepatic artery will not be seen at all.

The use of real-time equipment and pulsed Doppler facilitates identification of vessels and ducts, which can be traced to their origins for definitive identification. Usually the common duct is parallel to the portal vein and the sagittal axis. The hepatic artery is usually transversely oriented. When it is in direct contact with the common duct, it will indent the wall of the latter. Intrinsic pulsation of the hepatic artery can be seen at times. The portal vein is continuous inferiorly with the superior mesenteric and splenic veins. Superiorly it bifurcates into right and left intrahepatic branches. The right portal vein divides into anterior and posterior segmental veins. The left portal vein veers in a sharp anterior direction where it is joined by the umbilical portion of the left portal vein (6). The common hepatic duct, intrahepatic ducts, and hepatic arteries run anterior to the portal venous structures. Normal intrahepatic ducts are smaller in caliber than adjacent portal veins and are not depicted.

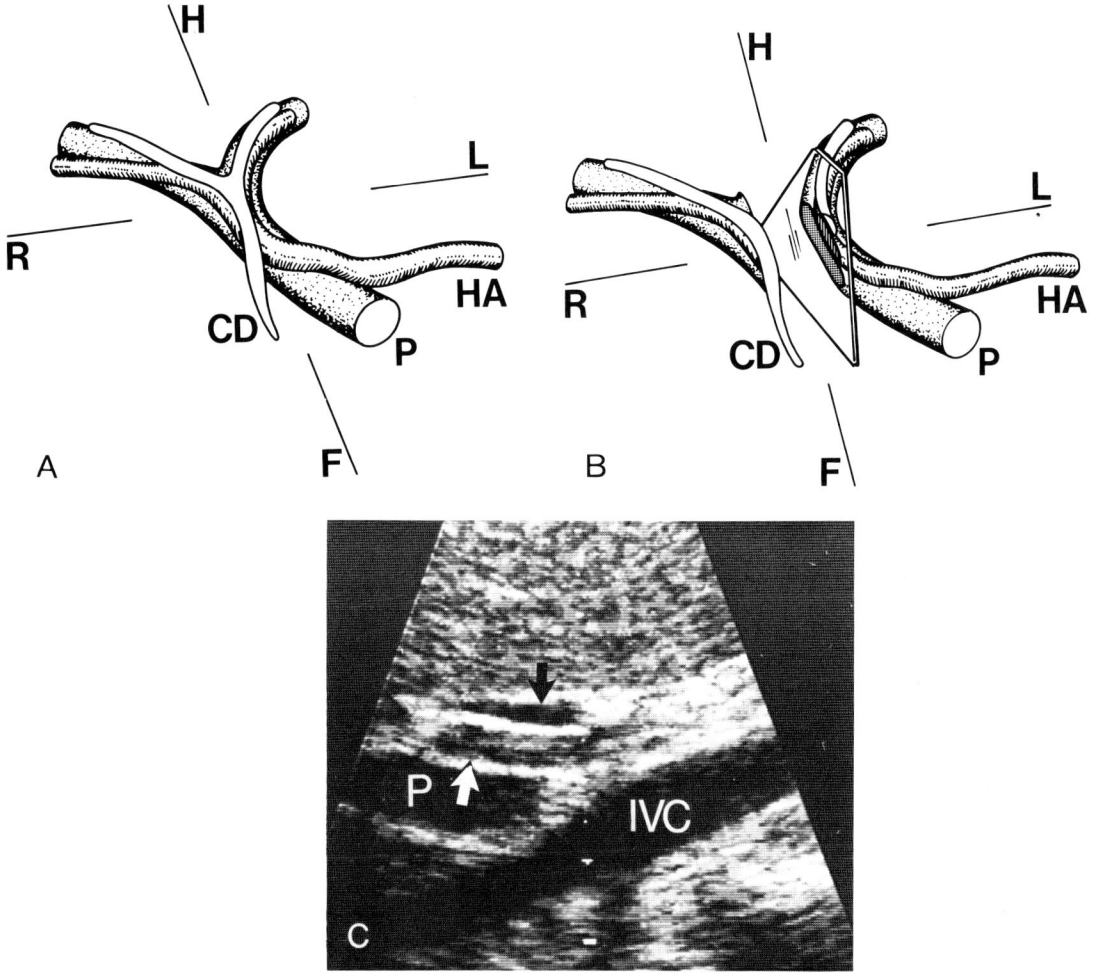

FIGURE 9.14. PORTA HEPATIS

A: Porta hepatis in patient in whom duct, artery, and vein all briefly travel in same vertical plane. *B:* Same structure cut and separated to demonstrate longitudinal plane of section. *C:* Corresponding sonogram. Common duct (*black arrow*), hepatic artery (*white arrow*), and portal vein (*P*) all in same plane of section ventral to inferior vena cava (*IVC*). Common duct varies slightly in caliber within this frame, while hepatic artery has uniform diameter. (From Berland LL, Lawson TL, Foley WD: Porta hepatis: sonographic discrimination of bile ducts from arteries with pulsed Doppler with new anatomic criteria. *AJR* 138:833–840, 1982.)

The Size of the Normal Common Duct

The diameter of the common duct is usually measured sonographically at the point where it crosses anterior to the right portal vein. Therefore, one is usually measuring the common hepatic duct. Measurements more distally (often of the common bile duct) tend to be slightly wider. Radiographic studies (intravenous and direct cholangiograms) placed the upper limits of the normal common duct at 10 mm with an average of 7–8 mm. Early sonographic studies agreed with these dimensions. More recent studies have lowered these parameters. Results of four recent series totaling over 1200 patients place the upper limits of the normal common duct at 4 or 5 mm measured from inner wall to inner wall, perpendicular to the walls (7–10). Of this normal population, 5% of asymptomatic patients will have common ducts measuring between 4 and 7 mm. As the common duct increases in size roughly 1 mm per decade over the age of 50, some elderly patients will have apparently enlarged common ducts (11). The following are causes of the discrepancy between sonographic and radiographic duct dimensions (12): radiographic methods involve magnification (about a factor of 1.3), choleresis from intravenous contrast material causes dilatation, injection of variable volumes with variable pressures causes variable measurements, underestimation by ultrasound due to artifactual wall thickening caused by "blooming"

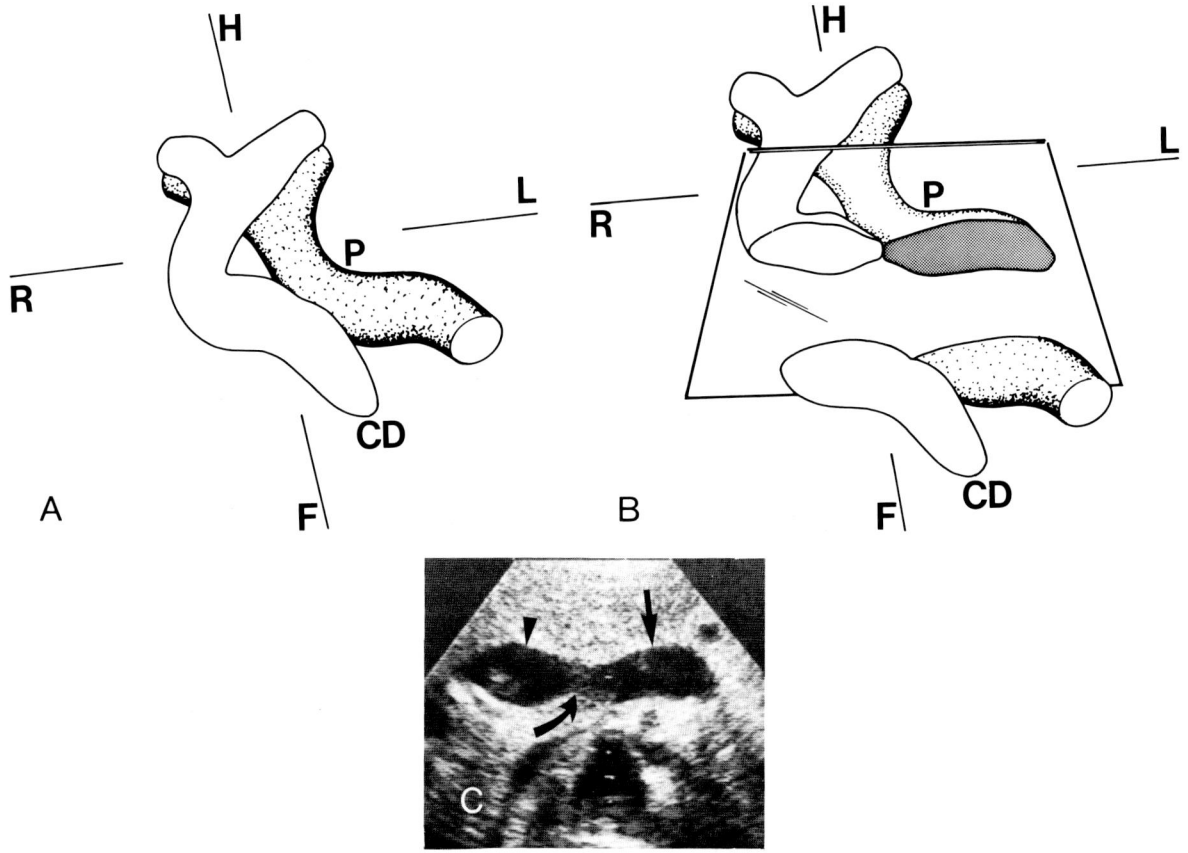

FIGURE 9.15. DILATED COMMON DUCT
A: Dilated common duct and portal and splenic vein. *B:* Structures cut and separated in transverse plane. *C:* 75° transverse sector scan. Transversely oriented common duct (*arrowhead*) initially mistaken for continuation of large splenic vein (*arrow*). Differentiation of these structures art at first appreciated because adjacent walls of duct and vein (*curved arrow*) were parallel to sound beam and thus did not provide strong specular reflector. Echoes within duct and vein were artifactual. (From Berland LL, Lawson TL, Foley WD: Portal hepatis: sonographic discrimination of bile ducts from arteries with pulsed Doppler with new anatomic criteria. *AJR* 138:833–840, 1982.)

of echoes, measurement of the transverse diameter radiographically and the sagittal diameter sonographically, and, finally, lack of distinction in some series between true normals and patients with previous surgery and/or preexisting obstruction.

The Post-Cholecystectomy Common Duct

The issue of whether or not the post-cholecystectomy common duct dilates has been debated in the literature since the 1890s when Oddi reported dilatation of the common duct in post-cholecystectomy dogs. The explanation for this phenomenon is that in the absence of the gallbladder the common duct dilates to function as a bile reservoir. Most studies of this issue have two major limitations. First, only post-cholecystectomy scans are available and there is no way to verify the size of the common duct preoperatively. Secondly, asymptomatic patients with mildly dilated ducts are assumed to be normal and not worked up further.

Four recent studies surveying post-cholecystectomy patients report mildly enlarged common ducts in 5, 10, and 58% of patients (10, 13, 14). Two studies compared common duct diameter pre and post cholecystectomy in the same patients. Post-surgical dilatation with no evidence of interval obstruction occurred in 1 out of 40 and 1 out of 67 patients (13, 14). Patients who had dilated ducts prior to surgery had either a diminution in size or no change after cholecystectomy. No correlation exists between common duct exploration and post-operative dilatation of the common duct. In summary, a common duct that is normal before surgery will generally remain so after surgery unless some pathology supervenes. Only a small minority of patients will have an unexplained increase in common

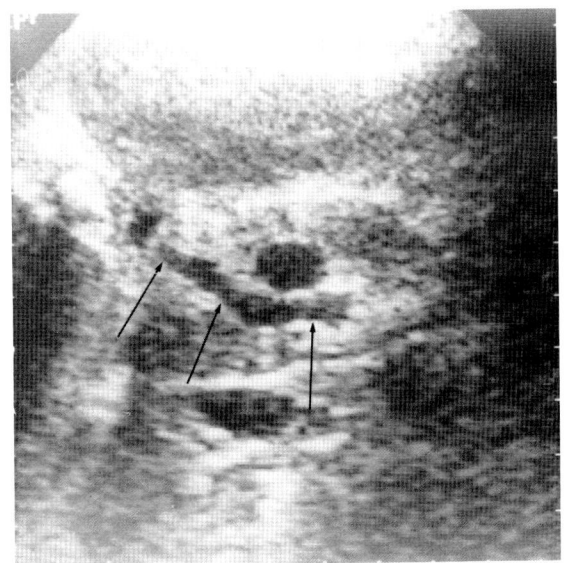

FIGURE 9.16. REPLACED RIGHT HEPATIC ARTERY
Replaced right hepatic artery (*arrows*) coming off the superior mesenteric artery and coursing behind the superior mesenteric vein through the pancreas toward the porta hepatis.

duct diameter. Once a duct is dilated, it may lose some elasticity and may never return to normal size. Therefore, some post-cholecystectomy patients will have dilated but nonobstructed common ducts.

The Fatty Meal in Common Duct Evaluation

Recent studies by Simeone et al (15, 16) have shown excellent results using a fatty meal to aid in the sonographic evaluation of the common duct because measurement of duct diameter alone is not always accurate in establishing the presence or absence of obstruction. Ingestion of a fatty meal initiates the release of cholecystokinin by intestinal mucosa. Cholecystokinin causes gallbladder contraction, increases bile flow from the liver and relaxes the sphincter of Oddi. The latter two functions persist in the post-cholecystectomy patient. The normal response to a fatty meal in pre and post cholecystectomy patients is for the common duct to either remain the same or decrease in size. The abnormal response, by the initially normal-sized duct, is an increase in caliber. When evaluating dilated or equivocal-sized ducts, an abnormal response is no change or an increase in size. If a dilated or equivocal-sized duct decreases to under 5 mm in diameter, it is probably not obstructed. The use of the fatty meal is most helpful in post-cholecystectomy patients, who frequently have dilated but unobstructed ducts. An abnormal response to the fatty meal was reported as the sole sonographic finding in multiple causes of obstruction such as cases of ampullary stenosis, choledocholithiasis, cholangiocarcinoma, pancreatitis and pancreatic carcinoma. Sensitivity was 84%, and all false negative patients had abnormal liver function tests. Despite these impressive figures, the fatty meal is not widely used in the sonographic evaluation of the common duct. In our institution, post-cholecystectomy patients with a high clinical index of suspicion for biliary obstructive pathology (elevated enzymes, suggestive symptoms) and normal ultrasound go on to ERCP. Those post-cholecystectomy patients with dilated ducts and no other findings either clinically or sonographically are usually followed or evaluated with biliary scintigraphy, and those with dilated ducts and other clinical or sonographic abnormalities go either to CT, PTC, ERCP, or surgery depending on the exact circumstances.

Bile Duct Distensibility

The walls of the human extrahepatic biliary tree are composed mainly of elastic fibers and connective tissue with little in the way of smooth muscle fibers. Biliary ducts expand and contract in response to fluctuating hydrostatic pressure due to their inherent elastic recoil. Dramatic changes in size can be observed fluoroscopically during direct cholangiography (17).

REFERENCES

1. Hatfield PM, Wise RE: Anatomic variation in the gallbladder and bile ducts. *Semin Roentgenol* 11:157–164, 1976.
2. Ralls PW, Quinn MF, Halls J: Biliary sonography: ventral bowing of the dilated common duct. *AJR* 137:1127–1129, 1981.
3. Jacobson JB, Brodey PA: The transverse common duct. *AJR* 136:91–95, 1981.
4. Berland LL, Lawson TL, Foley WD: Porta hepatis: sonographic discrimination of bile ducts from arteries with pulsed Doppler with new anatomic criteria. *AJR* 138:833–840, 1982.
5. Ralls PW, Quinn MF, Rogers W, Halls J: Sonographic anatomy of the hepatic artery. *AJR* 136:1059–1063, 1981.
6. Bandai Y, Makuuchi M, Watanabe G, Ito T, Sugiura M, Wada T: Sonographic differentiation between the umbilical portion of the left portal vein and intrahepatic bile ducts. *J Clin Ultrasound* 8:207–211, 1980.
7. Sample WF, Sarti DA, Goldstein LI, Weiner M, Kadell BM: Gray-scale ultrasonography of the jaundiced patient. *Radiology* 128:719–725, 1978.
8. Parulekar SG: Ultrasound evaluation of common bile duct size. *Radiology* 133:703–707, 1979.
9. Cooperberg PL, Li D, Wong P, Cohen MM, Burhenne HJ: Accuracy of common hepatic duct size in the evaluation of extrahepatic biliary obstruction. *Radiology* 135:141–144, 1980.

10. Niederau C, Muller J, Sonnenberg A et al: Extrahepatic bile ducts in healthy subjects, in patients with cholelithiasis, and in postcholecystectomy patients; a prospective ultrasonic study. *J Clin Ultrasound* 11:23–27, 1983.
11. Wu CC, Ho YH, Chen CY: Effect of aging on common bile duct diameter: a real-time ultrasonographic study. *J Clin Ultrasound* 12:473–478, 1984.
12. Sauerbrei EE, Cooperberg PL, Gordon P, Li D, Cohen MM, Burhenne HJ: The discrepancy between radiographic and sonographic bile-duct measurements. *Radiology* 137:751–755, 1980.
13. Mueller PR, Ferrucci JT, Simeone JF et al: Postcholecystectomy bile duct dilatation: myth or reality? *AJR* 136:355–358, 1981.
14. Graham MF, Cooperberg PL, Cohen MM, Burhenne HJ: The size of the normal common hepatic duct following cholecystectomy: an ultrasonographic study. *Radiology* 135:137–139, 1980.
15. Simeone JF, Mueller PR, Ferrucci JT et al: Sonography of the bile ducts after a fatty meal: an aid in detection of obstruction. *Radiology* 143:211–215, 1982.
16. Simeone JF, Butch RJ, Mueller PR et al: The bile ducts after a fatty meal: further sonographic observations. *Radiology* 154:763–768, 1985.
17. Mueller PR, Ferrucci JT, Simeone JF, van Sonnenberg E, Hall DA, Wittenberg J: Obstruction on the distensibility of the common duct. *Radiology* 142:467–472, 1982.

Computed Tomography of the Gallbladder

The normal gallbladder is an oval or elliptical low density organ located in its fossa beneath the liver at the junction of the right and left lobes. On transverse scans the gallbladder may appear to be intrahepatic; this is a result of the cross-sectional technique as the gallbladder is often surrounded on all sides save its inferior surface by liver. Bile in the gallbladder is normally of near water density (−5 to +15 HU). The gallbladder wall normally enhances after intravenous contrast administration, and this enhancement can be visually striking in wall segments that are inferior to the liver and bordered by fat (Fig. 9.17). Normal gallbladder wall thickness is difficult to evaluate on CT for several reasons. One is never certain that the wall is actually being cut perpendicularly as opposed to at an angle, and no special effort is made to distend the gallbladder prior to CT. The partial volume effect can also be a problem. Usually normal wall thickness is 2 mm or less if the organ is distended. Wall thickness over 4 mm is probably abnormal provided the gallbladder is not contracted. The contents of the gallbladder do not enhance on conventional postcontrast scans, however, if scans are performed 15–24 hr after urographic contrast has been administered intravascularly for other purposes the gallbladder will opacify on CT by virtue of the small percentage of hepatobiliary contrast excretion that occurs even with normal renal function (Fig. 9.18) (1–3).

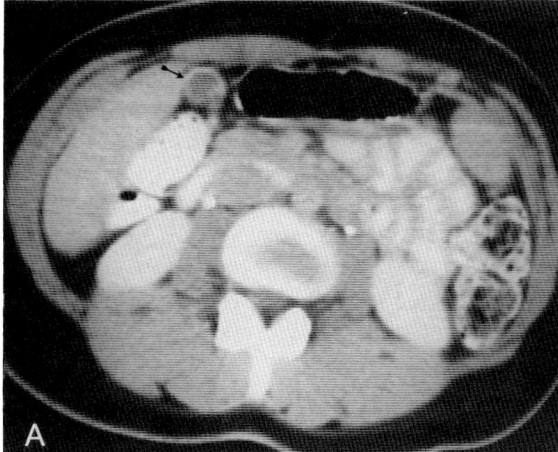
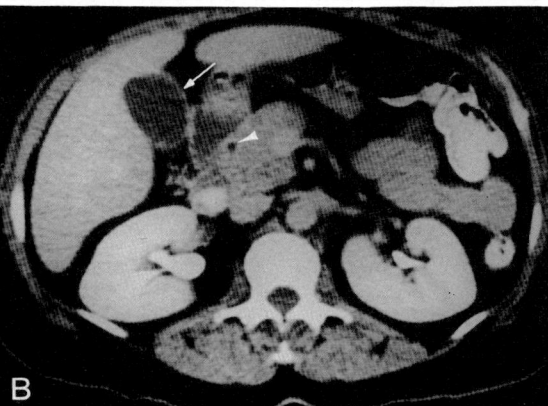

FIGURE 9.17. NORMAL ENHANCING GALLBLADDER WALL
Normal, thin, enhancing gallbladder wall (*arrow*), two examples (*A* and *B*). Note normal distal common bile duct (*arrowhead*) in the head of the pancreas (*B*).

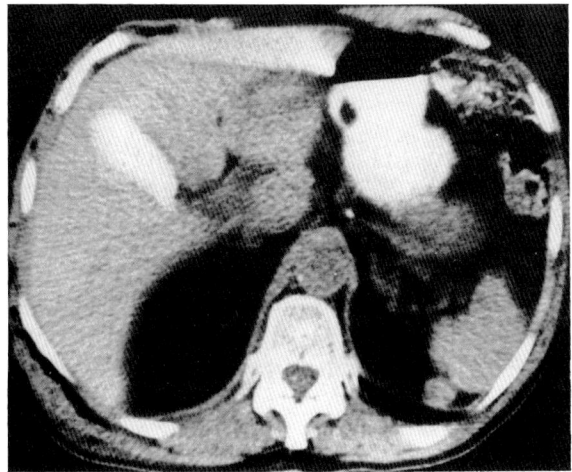

FIGURE 9.18. GALLBLADDER OPACIFICATION BY UROGRAPHIC CONTRAST MATERIAL
Intense gallbladder opacification on an abdominal CT performed 17 hr after a contrast-enhanced cranial CT.

REFERENCES

1. Havrilla TR, Reich NE, Haaga JR, Seidelmann FE, Cooperman AM, Alfidi RJ: Computed tomography of the gallbladder. *AJR* 130:1059, 1978.
2. Toombs BD, Sandler CM, Conoley PM: Computed tomography of the nonvisualizing gallbladder. *J Comput Assist Tomogr* 5:164, 1981.
3. Koehler RE, Stanley RJ: Computed tomography of the gallbladder and bile ducts. In Berk RN, Ferrucci JT Jr, Leopold GR (eds): *Radiology of the Gallbladder and Bile Ducts, Diagnosis and Intervention.* Philadelphia, W. B. Saunders, 1983, pp 244-245.

Normal CT of the Biliary Tract

The intrahepatic portions of the biliary tree are adjacent to portal veins and, when normal, are too small to see on CT (1). Even when opacified by intravenous cholangiographic contrast material (a technique with very limited indications), normal ducts are not visible proximal to the immediate periportal areas (2). Using high doses of intravenous urographic contrast material, the normal common hepatic and/or common bile duct can be depicted in about one third of patients in cross-section as a circular, water density structure 2-6 mm in diameter (Fig. 9.19). An anteroposterior measurement is more accurate than a transverse one as it is more likely to avoid obliquity (3). Sonographic measurement is generally considered more reliable. The common hepatic duct and proximal common hepatic duct usually form a fairly straight tube anterolateral to the portal vein at a 40° angle to the midline. A transverse segment is present in about 6% of normals and 18% of dilated ducts. The remainder of the common bile duct is either intrapancreatic or in a groove posterolateral to the head of the pancreas, running at an angle of

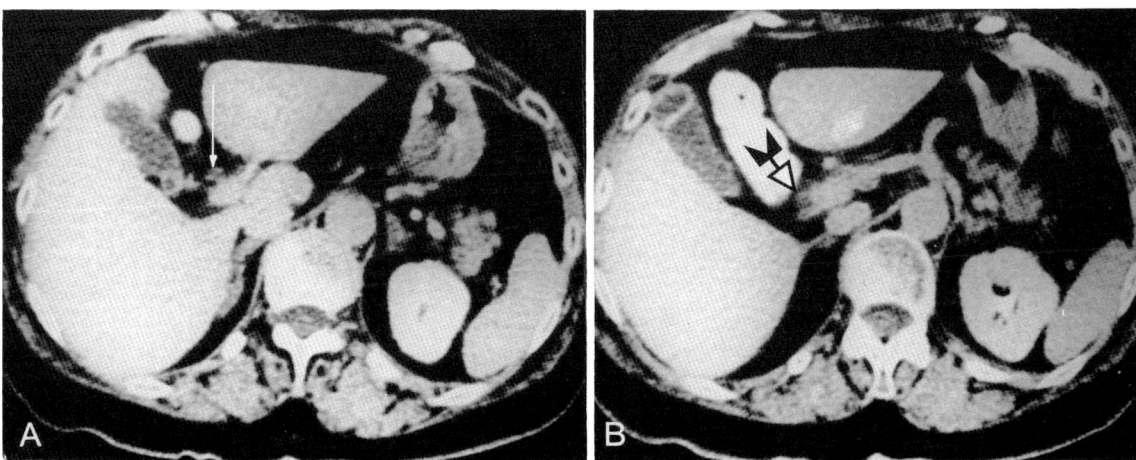

FIGURE 9.19. CT OF NORMAL BILIARY TREE
A: Normal common hepatic duct (*arrow*) anterolateral to the portal vein. *B:* More caudal cut: normal common bile duct (*arrow*) lateral to the portal vein.

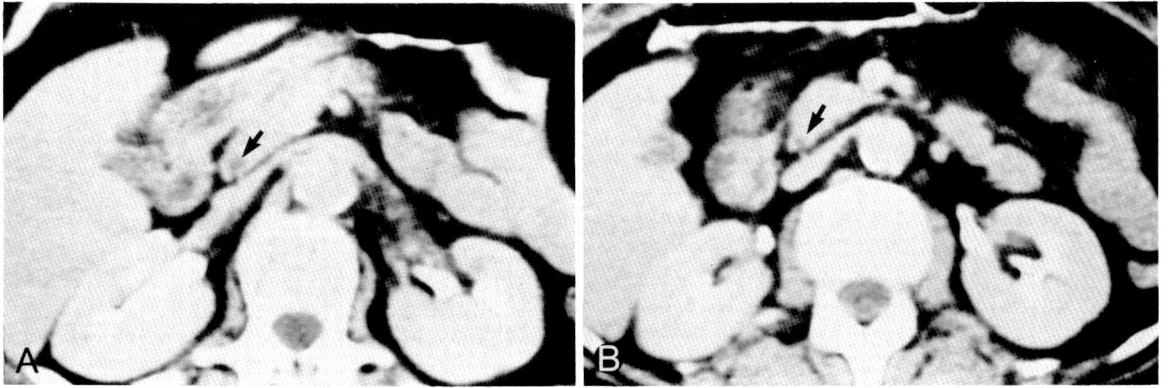

FIGURE 9.20. NORMAL DISTAL COMMON BILE DUCT
A and *B:* Normal preampullary distal common bile duct (*arrow*) in the head of the pancreas. See also Figure 9.17B.

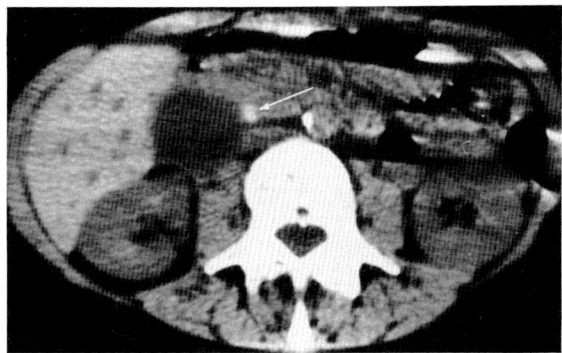

FIGURE 9.21. CT AFTER NONFUNCTIONING ORAL CHOLECYSTOGRAM
CT after a nonfunctioning oral cholecystogram: opacified distal common bile duct (arrow).

about 20 degrees to the midline (Fig. 9.20) (4). Oral cholecystographic contrast given 2 hours prior to CT with calcium ipodate (4), or the night before CT with iopanoic acid (5), opacifies at least some portion of the biliary tree, usually the common bile duct, in about 85–90% of normal patients. Normal measurements for the distal common bile duct using this technique are 4.7 ± 1.2 mm with gallbladder in and 6.8 ± 1.1 mm with gallbladder out (5). Although advocated for superior delineation of the anatomy in the region of the head of the pancreas, this technique has not gained widespread acceptance (Fig. 9.21).

REFERENCES

1. Koehler RE, Stanley RJ: Computed tomography of the gallbladder and bile ducts. In Berk RN, Ferrucci JT Jr, Leopold GR (eds): *Radiology of the Gallbladder and Bile Ducts, Diagnosis and Intervention.* Philadelphia, W. B. Saunders, 1983, p 244.
2. Arndt RD, Joyce PW, Gray RK, Haveson SB, Bos CJ: Iodipamide enhanced computed tomography of the pancreas. *Radiology* 139:491–493, 1981.
3. Foley WD, Wilson CR, Quiroz FA, Lawson TL: Demonstration of the normal extrahepatic biliary tract with computed tomography. *J Comput Assist Tomogr* 4:48–52, 1980.
4. Pretorius DH, Gosink BB, Olson LK: CT of the opacified biliary tract: use of calcium ipodate. *AJR* 138:1073–1075, 1982.
5. Greenberg M, Greenberg BM, Rubin JM, Greenberg IM: Computed-tomographic cholangiography. *Radiology* 144:363–368, 1982.

Cholangiography

If the gallbladder is filled during a transhepatic or endoscopic retrograde cholangiogram, it should be evaluated with erect compression spot films if information thus gained is likely to be of clinical significance. Other maneuvers, such as decubitus horizontal beam films, may have to be

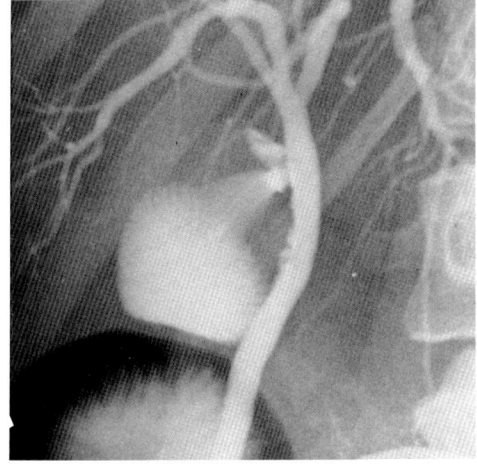

FIGURE 9.22. ERCP: NORMAL GALLBLADDER FOLDS SEEN AT ITS PERIPHERY

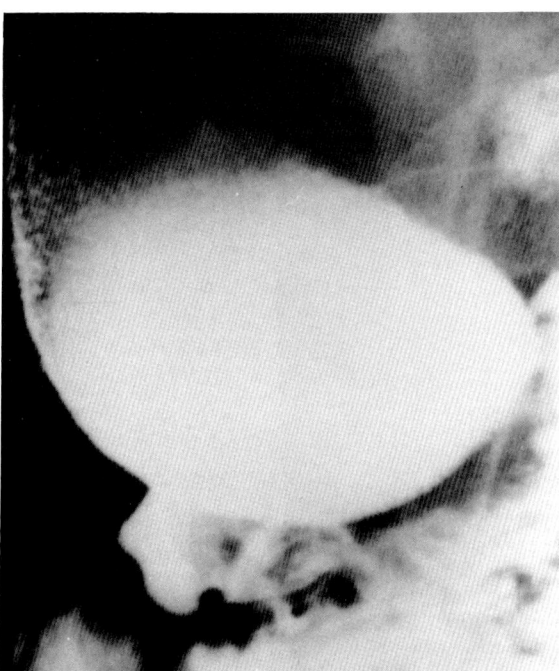

FIGURE 9.23. "BARIUM ON VELVET" GALLBLADDER, STATUS POST-CHOLEDOCHOJEJUNOSTOMY

resorted to if the patient cannot stand. Apparent filling defects seen on supine films must be distinguished from poor mixing of bile and contrast, which almost never causes problems during oral cholecystography. Horizontal beam films must be obtained to evaluate any filling defect. This phenomenon is well-known to those who used to perform intravenous cholangiography (1). "Mucosal relief" films during the early filling phase of retrograde cholangiography can demonstrate normal mucosal folds (Fig. 9.22). An appearance termed "barium on velvet" may be seen when barium refluxes into the gallbladder during a barium meal (barium cholangiogram) after a biliary-enteric anastomosis (Fig. 9.23). This represents radiographic depiction of "areae cholecysticae," the micromucosal pattern of the gallbladder, which should not be confused with pathology such as a strawberry gallbladder (2).

REFERENCES

1. Berk RN, Ferrucci JT Jr, Leopold GR: *Radiology of the Gallbladder and Bile Ducts, Diagnosis and Intervention.* Philadelphia, W. B. Saunders, 1983, p 126.

2. Kottler RE, Louw JH: The mucosal pattern of the gallbladder ("areae cholecysticae"). *Br J Radiol* 57:289–291, 1984.

Normal Cholangiography

Although this discussion will concern itself chiefly with normal cholangiographic anatomy obtained via the percutaneous and endoscopic routes, the radiographic appearance of the biliary tree described applies to operative and T-tube cholangiography as well. ERCP is successful in experienced hands in obtaining a cholangiogram in a normal patient about 90% of the time (1), whereas percutaneous transhepatic cholangiog-

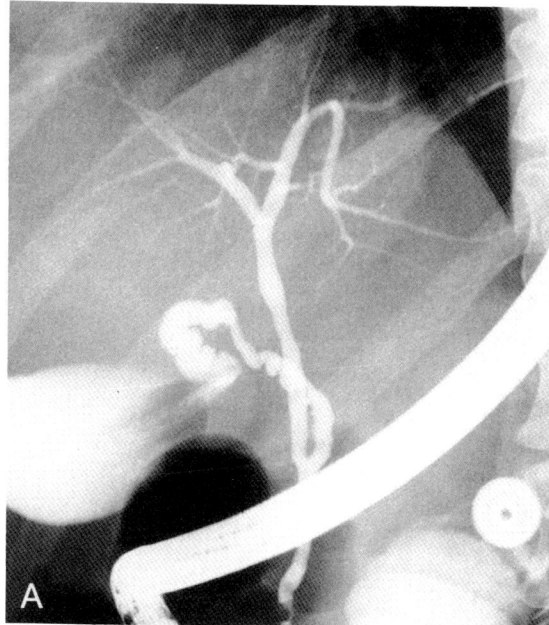
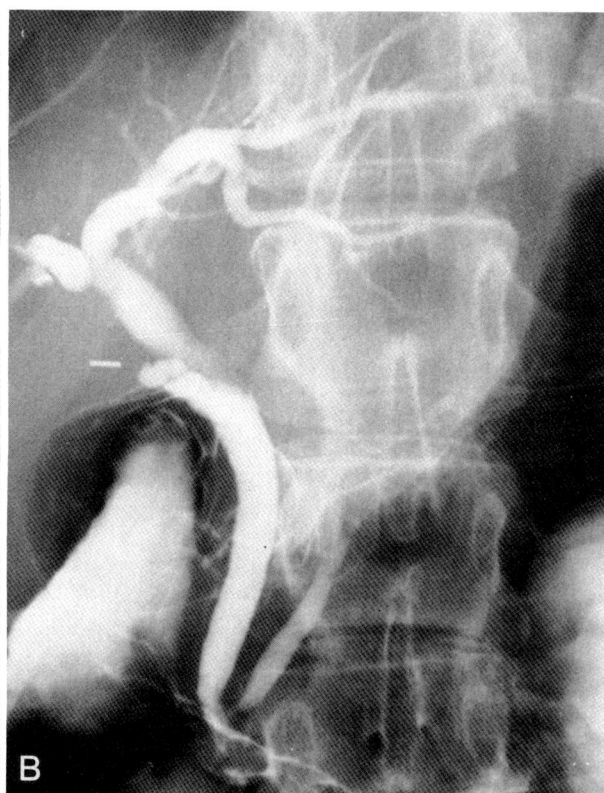
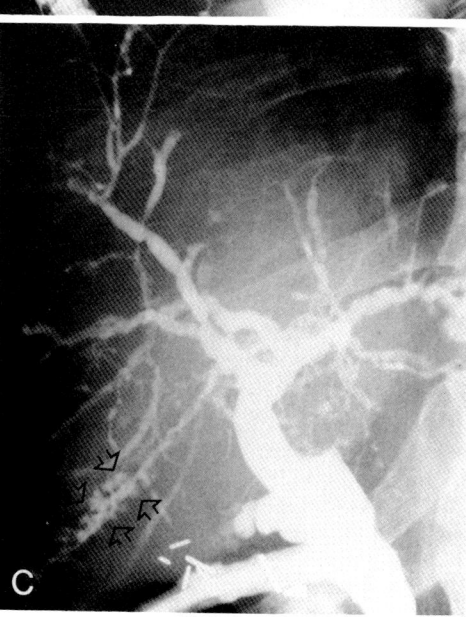

FIGURE 9.24. Normal ERCP
A: Gallbladder in and *B:* gallbladder out: common duct somewhat wider. *C:* T-tube cholangiogram: overinjection with opacification of too many peripheral radicles and parenchymal staining (*arrows*). Appearance is hard to distinguish from cholangitis.

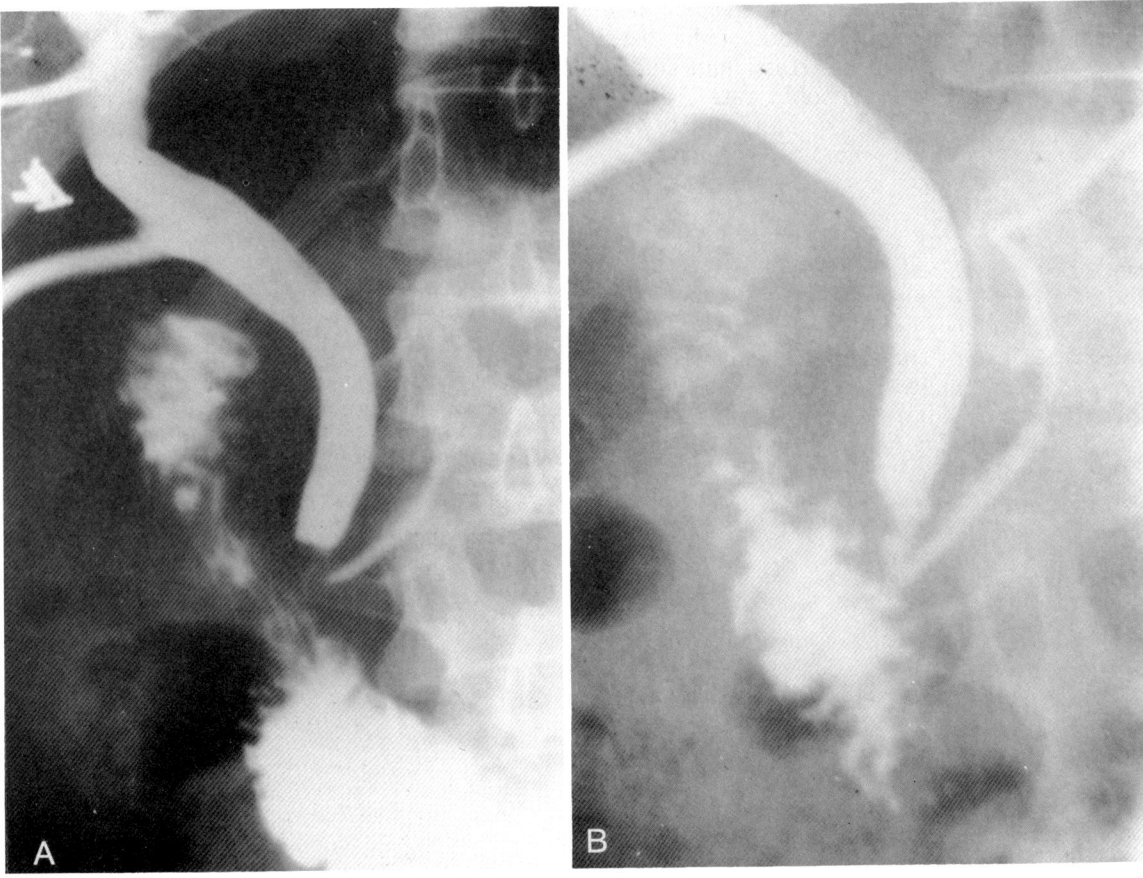

FIGURE 9.25. PSEUDOCALCULUS EFFECT: T-TUBE CHOLANGIOGRAM
A: Apparent obstruction by calculus-large amount of contrast in duodenum is a clue that obstruction is transient. *B:* After 1.0 mg glucagon IV: wavy distal common bile duct but free flow into duodenum without any stone.

raphy opacifies normal ducts in 70–80% based on multi-institutional studies of hundreds of patients (2–4). The success rate of PTC can be improved somewhat by more central but still intrahepatic needle placement and perseverance: making up to 15 passes does not increase the complication rate (3). Patient tolerance will generally not permit more attempts and one runs into diminishing returns beyond this point. Success rates for ERCP are lower in the face of biliary-enteric anastomosis or Billroth II partial gastrectomy.

In a study of 49 normal retrograde cholangiograms, the mean maximal duct width was 4.3 mm (range: 2.3–6.9 mm) for the intrapancreatic common bile duct, 4.9 mm (range: 2.3–8.5 mm) for the prepancreatic common bile duct, and 4.6 mm (range: 2.1–9.2 mm) for the common hepatic duct. Widths tended to increase with age. The prepancreatic portion of the common bile duct tended to be the widest segment, although in a considerable minority, either the intrapancreatic duct or the common hepatic duct was the widest.

The mean maximum width of the extrahepatic common duct was 4.6 mm with a standard deviation of 1.1 mm. This would give an upper limit of normal of 6.8 mm. However, the authors felt that 9 mm is more appropriate as an upper limit of normal. Often, normal common ducts are quite small (less than 4 mm in diameter). All of these measurements were corrected for magnification by comparison with the known diameter of the endoscope (5). Measurements during PTC should be comparable. Contrast should flow freely from the common duct into the duodenum fluoroscopically during a normal cholangiogram (Fig. 9.24A and B).

ERCP in normal patients usually results in synchronous opacification of the cystic duct and main intrahepatic ducts, followed by progressive opacification of the gallbladder and smaller intrahepatic ducts. If, after appropriate positioning, including right lateral decubitus and Trendelenburg, and prolonged injection time, the intrahepatic biliary tree is filled out to third-order branches and the gallbladder is not opacified, a pathologic process must be suspected (6). Possibilities include: obstructing lesions of the distal common bile duct producing stasis and sludge, and lesions that obstruct or obliterate the gallbladder and or cystic duct, such as stones, gallbladder carcinoma, or chronic cholecystitis.

Normal intrahepatic ducts are small, but actual size is dependent on technical factors such as injection pressure and runoff into the gallbladder. Second and third order branches can be shown fairly routinely, but overinjection with opacification of tiny peripheral branches is to be avoided because of the risk of cholangiovenous reflux and bacteremia (Fig. 9.24C) (7). The normal intrahepatic biliary tree branches regularly and smoothly. Splaying or crowding of ducts, caliber irregularities, strictures, and filling deflects are absent (Fig. 9.24A and B).

The Ampullary Sphincters and the Pseudocalculus Effect

The band of smooth muscle encircling the common bile duct just proximal to the sphincter of Oddi is the sphincter of Boyden. When partially relaxed, the sphincters of Boyden and Oddi can create a wavy and narrowed appearance to the distal common bile duct that can be mistaken for ampullary stenosis or even neoplasm (Fig. 9.25B (8). When contracted, the sphincters can transiently obstruct the flow of contrast material into the duodenum (the pseudocalculus effect) (9, 10). The upper border of the pseudocalculus is rounded, mimicking the meniscus of a calculus, and no lower border is seen (Fig. 9.25A). The pseudocalculus sometimes disappears spontaneously during further fluoroscopic filling. Intravenous administration of 1.0 mg of glucagon usually will abolish the pseudocalculus (Fig. 9.25B), which is rarely seen during ERCP since these patients are routinely given glucagon.

REFERENCES

1. Stewart ET, Geenen JE: Endoscopic retrograde cholangiography. In Berk RN, Ferrucci JT Jr, Leopold GR (eds): *Radiology of the Gallbladder and Bile Ducts, Diagnosis and Intervention.* Philadelphia, W. B. Saunders, 1983, pp 370, 381.
2. Harbin WP, Mueller PR, Ferrucci JT Jr: Complications and use patterns of fine needle transhepatic cholangiography: a multi-institutional study. *Radiology* 135:15, 1980.
3. Mueller PR, Harbin WP, Ferrucci JT Jr et al: Fine needle transheaptic cholangiography: refinements and reflections after 450 cases. *AJR* 136:85, 1981.
4. Cronan JJ: The imaging of biliary obstruction. *Semin Ultrasound CT MR* 5:376–398, 1984.
5. Lasser RB, Silvis SE, Vennes JA: The normal cholangiogram. *Dig Dis Sci* 23:586–590, 1978.
6. Rohrmann CA Jr, Ansel HJ, Protell RL, Silverstein FE, Silvis SE, Vennes JA: Significance of the nonopacified gallbladder in endoscopic retrograde cholangiography. *AJR* 132:191–195, 1979.
7. Berci G, Hamlin JA: Operative and post-operative cholangiography. In Berk RN, Ferrucci JT Jr, Leopold GR (eds): *Radiology of the Gallbladder and Bile Ducts, Diagnosis and Intervention.* Philadelphia, W. B. Saunders, 1983, pp 407–408.
8. Goldberg HI: Operative and postoperative cholecystocholangiography. *Semin Roentgenol* 11:203–211, 1976.
9. Beneventano TC, Schein CJ: The pseudocalculus sign in cholangiography. *Arch Surg* 98:731–733, 1969.
10. Mujahed, Evans JA: Pseudocalculus defect in cholangiography. *ARJ* 116:337–341, 1972.

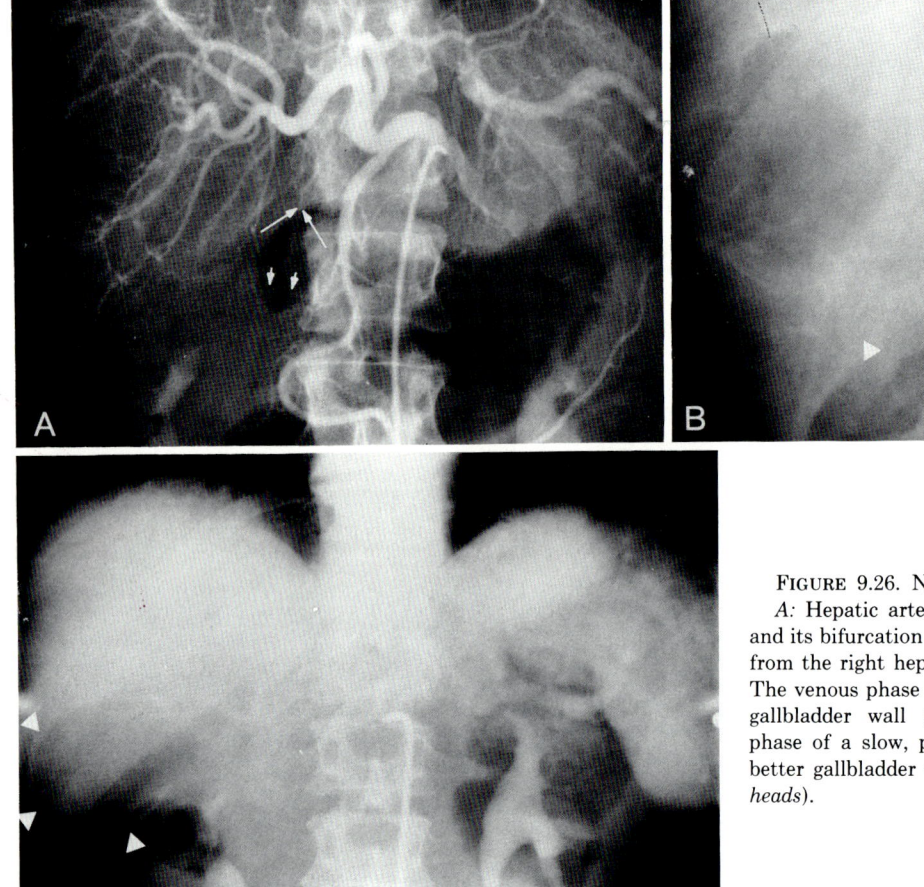

FIGURE 9.26. NORMAL ANGIOGRAPHY
A: Hepatic artery injection: cystic artery and its bifurcation (*small arrows*) originating from the right hepatic artery (*large arrows*). The venous phase B: shows the normal thin gallbladder wall (*arrowheads*). C: Venous phase of a slow, prolonged celiac injection: better gallbladder wall visualization (*arrowheads*).

Angiography

Before the advent of fine-needle cholangiography, ultrasound, and CT, angiography was used by some to evaluate malignant diseases of the gallbladder and extrahepatic biliary tree. The 2–3 mm thick gallbladder wall can be well-delineated during the capillary phase of celiac or hepatic arteriography, especially if slow, prolonged injection and/or tolazoline vasodilation is employed (Fig. 9.26) (1, 2). Extrahepatic bile duct walls are not normally seen, and neither are common duct arteries identifiable even with superselective injections (2).

REFERENCES

1. Deutsch B: Cholecysto-angiography. Visualization of the gallbladder by selective celiac and mesenteric angiography. *AJR* 101:608–615, 1967.
2. Kaude JV, Hawkins IF Jr: Angiography of the gallbladder and biliary tract. *Semin Roentgenol* 11:191–195, 1976.

10

Endoscopic Retrograde Cholangiopancreatography: General Considerations and the Role of the Radiologist

MARK T. BIRNS, M.D.

Endoscopic retrograde cholangiopancreatography (ERCP) has become an important diagnostic and therapeutic procedure in patients with diseases of the biliary tract and pancreas. By defining the ductal architecture it serves both as a confirmatory test for lesions suspected on sonography or CT and as a preoperative road map. It is the single best test for depicting the pancreatic duct and competes with percutaneous transhepatic cholangiography (PTC) for primacy in evaluation of the biliary ducts. Advances in technique as well as improvement in the design of fiberoptic systems have made ERCP a relatively safe, atraumatic procedure in the hands of skilled endoscopists.

ERCP has fairly recently become more than just a means of obtaining radiographs. Pancreatic and biliary secretions can be obtained for cytologic, chemical, serologic, and bacteriologic studies. Manometry of the sphincter of Oddi can be performed. Endoscopic sphincterotomy affords high risk patients nonoperative biliary surgery and offers post-cholecystectomy and post-biliary surgery patients with retained stones or recurrent disease an alternative to repeat laparotomy. Stents for obstructive biliary lesions, catheter placement for infusion of antibiotics or chemicals, and balloon dilatation of strictures are the newest therapeutic maneuvers available via ERCP.

This chapter deals with clinical and technical aspects of both diagnostic and therapeutic ERCP. Interpretive features are discussed under the various diseases covered throughout this book.

ERCP: THE PROCEDURE

Indications

Although originally intended to distinguish intra- from extrahepatic causes of jaundice, delineate pancreatic ductal disease, and complement other radiologic tests, acceptance for ERCP in experienced hands as a primary diagnostic modality is growing (1–8). Common indications for ERCP are listed in Table 10.1. Intravenous cholangiography, because of its low accuracy and frequent adverse contrast reactions, has been rendered obsolete even in patients with normal serum bilirubin (9).

ERCP has been used more recently to search for the etiology of chronic unexplained abdominal pain. In one series, ERCP demonstrated small gallstones in 25 of 32 patients with biliary-type pain and negative oral cholecystograms and sonograms (10). One must question the quality of the sonography in this report, however (Fig. 10.1). Other studies have revealed ERCP identifying pancreatic ductal abnormalities in 25% and retained calculi in 8% of patients with post-cholecystectomy pain (11). ERCP may often demonstrate an etiology in unexplained or "idiopathic" pancreatitis yielding such findings as pancreas divisum, ampullary stenosis, and biliary calculi which are amenable to surgical correction (12, 13). Patients with transient liver chemistry abnormalities and chronic recurrent abdominal pain may have biliary dyskinesia with sphincter of Oddi spasm or dysfunction demon-

TABLE 10.1.
INDICATIONS FOR ERCP[a]

1. Clinically substantiated suspicion of a pancreatic lesion
   A. Suspicion of chronic pancreatitis or chronic relapsing pancreatitis
   B. Suspicion of sequelae secondary to pancreatitis
   C. Suspicion of pancreatic carcinoma
2. Suspicion of benign or malignant papillary stenosis
3. Possible extrahepatic cholestasis
   A. Obstructive jaundice of unknown origin
   B. In cases of nonopacification of the gallbladder and cystic duct despite visualization of the extrahepatic biliary tree by other methods of cholangiography
   C. Suspicion of abnormalities of the intrahepatic biliary tree
   D. Suspicion of variant anatomy of the extrahepatic biliary tree based on studies via other modalities
   E. Suspicion of choledocholithiasis despite negative other radiologic noninvasive tests
4. Unclear upper abdominal pain in patients previously subjected to cholecystectomy or to cholangioenteric anastomosis
5. Patients with diabetes mellitus with weight loss and vague abdominal complaints
6. Metastatic adenocarcinoma, primary site undetermined, possibly biliary or pancreatic

[a] Adapted from Anacker H, Weiss HD, Kramann B: Indications, contraindications and complications in *Endoscopic Retrograde Pancreaticocholangiography (ERPC)*. New York, Springer-Verlag, 1977, pp 25–30.

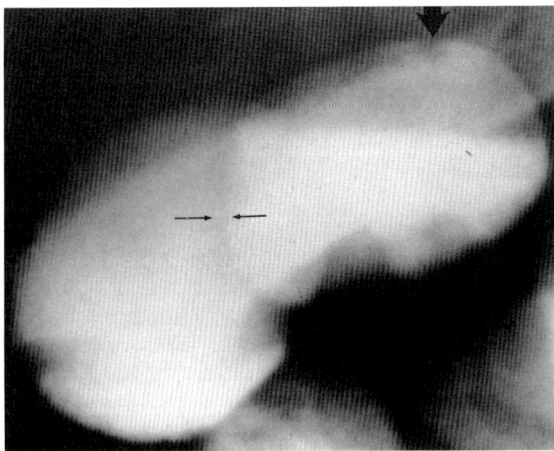

FIGURE 10.1. SMALL GALLBLADDER POLYP
ERCP demonstrates a small gallbladder polyp (*large arrow*) that most likely is a cholesterol polyp or an adenoma. Also seen is a septation (*thin arrows*). Although the latter was depicted by oral cholecystography and sonography, the former was not. The sonogram, however, was not a real-time examination.

strable by manometric studies performed via ERCP (14).

Contraindications

The contraindications to ERCP include those to upper gastrointestinal endoscopy in general. Although avoidance of patients with acute cholangitis or acute pancreatitis has been previously recommended (6, 8), current potential therapeutic endoscopic decompression tilts the risk/benefit ratio in favor of performing ERCP in an attempt to relieve the obstruction in cases of choledocholithiasis or gallstone pancreatitis (3–5). Generally, ERCP is deferred for 3–4 weeks following acute pancreatitis to avoid an exacerbation that might be induced by acinar filling (15). If a pancreatic pseudocyst or pancreatic fistula is suspected, ERCP can be performed if adequate surgical back-up is available (4, 8, 15).

ERCP can usually be performed safely in patients allergic to urographic contrast material using premedication with Benadryl and steroids, according to most authors (16). Although a nephrogram can be seen following ERCP due to contrast absorption through the pancreaticobiliary ductal epithelium, direct intravascular injection is unlikely as opposed to PTC in which some direct intravascular injection is frequent (17–19). Injection of sterile USP barium sulfate suspension for cholangiography should be considered in patients with documented prior severe contrast reactions.

When ERCP is needed in patients with serum positivity for hepatitis B surface antigen, gas sterilization of the equipment after the procedure is recommended and the personnel performing the procedure must take proper precautions (20–22).

Contrast material in the right upper quadrant or in the region of the pancreas from prior studies should be cleared prior to the performance of ERCP.

Complications

The complication rate in experienced hands is 2–3% (2). The incidence of complications seems to vary inversely with the skill and experience of the endoscopist. Inexperienced operators may have 4 times the failure rate and twice the complication rate of their experienced counterparts (8, 15). The most frequent complications are pancreatitis (1%) and cholangitic sepsis (0.8%) (4, 5, 15, 23). Mortality ranges betwen 0.01 and 0.8%, usually from sepsis (cholangitic or pancreatic abscess) (2, 4, 5, 15, 23). Although some advocate adding an aminoglycoside antibiotic to the contrast material (24), there are data to suggest that this practice is not efficacious in preventing infection (23, 25).

Asymptomatic hyperamylasemia may occur in up to 70% of patients after injection of the pancreatic duct (5, 23, 26). Serum lipase can become elevated asymptomatically in a similar percentage of patients. A decrease is usually seen in 24 hours with normalization within 48–96 hr (8). This chemical pancreatitis is probably due to acinarization as a result of slight overfilling (5, 8, 15, 23).

Clinical symptomatic pancreatitis occurs in 0.7–7.4% with recent figures on the order of 1% especially with experienced operators. A higher incidence of clinical pancreatitis is associated with acinarization coupled with urographic visualization but not acinarization alone (27). Trasylol (a trypsin inhibitor), antibiotics, and glucagon are all ineffective for the prevention of pancreatitis (2, 23).

Sepsis is most common in patients with common bile duct obstruction, especially malignant obstruction. The most common organisms are *Escherichia coli* and *Pseudomonas* (28). Injection into a pseudocyst runs the risk of conversion into a pancreatic abscess which carries prolonged morbidity, a 20% mortality, and usually necessitates a surgical procedure (26).

Naturally, ERCP carries with it the risks of upper gastrointestinal endoscopy; a complication rate of 0.1–0.2%, a mortality rate of 0.014–0.065%, which may include infection, perforation, bleeding, cardiopulmonary accident, and reaction to premedication (28, 29).

Failure of Cannulation

Surveys by the American Society of Gastroenterology and others show a success rate for ERCP of 92% (3, 8, 30). Reasons for cannulation failure are related more to the operator's technical skill rather than to any anatomic variant. The success rate rises from 56% during one's first 100 cases to 93% after 200 cases (8). Knowledge of anatomic landmarks and variants as well as the necessary changes in positioning the endoscope for cannulation is crucial to the success of the procedure. In a large survey, experienced workers had fewer examination failures and a 3% complication rate while inexperienced endoscopists and novices had a 62% failure rate and more than a 6% complication rate (31). Intravenous glucagon, which relaxes the duodenum and the sphincter of Oddi, facilitates cannulation, because instrumental manipulation, cannulation, contrast injection and its leakage into the duodenum all provoke increased motility and spasm.

Situations that truly present technical difficulties for ERCP (Table 10.2) include: duodenal diverticulum with an intradiverticular or juxtadiverticular insertion of the papilla, papillary spasm, papillary stenosis, pyloric stenosis, duodenal displacement, previous gastroduodenal surgery, and failure to obtain adequate duodenal paralysis. Pancreas divisum is an interesting anatomic challenge in which the duct of Wirsung may be cannulated at the same time as the common bile duct, but a separate cannulation of the accessory papilla (usually requiring a small metal-tipped catheter) is needed to opacify the duct of Santorini (Fig. 10.2A).

Finally, patients with subtotal gastrectomies present technical problems. Although seemingly less difficult than a Billroth II, the Billroth I is a particular anatomic challenge because of the small working distance between the stomach and the ampulla, since the ampulla is in a high position in the first portion of the duodenum (Fig. 10.2B). A side-viewing instrument may experience a blind spot in the region of the ampulla as it moves around the shortened duodenum. Patients with a Billroth II anastomosis are cannulated with a forward-viewing endoscope (32, 33). Cannulation and sphincterotomy may require special instruments because of reverse angulation and forward-viewing. The ampulla is approached from below as the endoscope ascends the afferent loop. Once familiarity with this altered anatomy is obtained, successful ERCP has been reported in 80% of Billroth II patients (8) (somewhat lower than this author's experience).

ERCP vs. PTC

In patients with jaundice and suspected biliary obstruction, PTC and ERCP are competitive means of opacifying the biliary tree. PTC is a less costly and simpler procedure, usually performed by a radiologist, whose success is dependent on two variables: the expertise of the operator, and the degree of biliary dilatation (34). Studies of PTC success rates show an overall success rate of 89% with up to six passes. The success rate is 97% in patients with dilated ducts, and 70.2% in patients with nondilated ducts if a maximum of 12 passes are made (34).

Although sepsis may occur after either PTC or ERCP, the risk of bile leakage and resultant bile peritonitis following PTC is greater (35). However, PTC has the advantage of more easily leaving a catheter in place to drain the obstructed system. Reinjection after several days of decompression by external drainage frequently better defines the obstructing lesion (36). Many authors from different centers around the world report that routine use of preoperative biliary drainage via PTC to lower the bilirubin level to less than 10 mg per cent improves surgical mortality figures (37–39). Opinions to the contrary do exist, however (40, 41). Permanent drainage, can of course, be established with percutaneous catheters or percutaneously inserted endoprostheses for patients judged not to be surgical candidates.

ERCP depicts the pancreatic duct as well as the biliary tree, so that in cases in which pancreatic disease may be the cause of the biliary obstruction ERCP may provide significant extra diagnostic information compared to PTC. Mucosal abnormalities in the stomach, duodenum, and ampullary region that can be revealed by ERCP are occasionally pertinent in the jaundiced patient. Internal or external drainage can also be accomplished endoscopically. However, ERCP is more expensive, more time-consuming, and far more technically dependent than PTC, with information obtained directly proportional to the skill of the examiner (8). Most authors consider PTC the procedure of choice when ducts are dilated on sonography or CT and ERCP the procedure of choice with nondilated ducts.

Endoscopic and Radiologic Technique

ERCP is performed in a fluoroscopy room equipped with a floating tilt table and a television image intensifier with spot film capability. The room needs to be large enough to accommodate the endoscopic equipment and the added personnel comprising the "ERCP team." The latter includes the endoscopist and an endoscopy technician, a radiologist and a radiographer. The endoscopist and his/her technician are responsible for monitoring the patient and controlling the events surrounding the cannulation. The radiologist follows the contrast material fluoroscopically and obtains spot films in appropriate positions. The radiographer assists the radiologist and obtains overheads when necessary. The endoscopist and the radiologist jointly determine the concentration of contrast material to be injected, adequacy of ductal filling, and the presence or absence of pathology requiring further

TABLE 10.2.
TECHNICAL DIFFICULTIES IN ERCP (7)

1. Papillary opening within a duodenal diverticulum
2. Papillary spasm impeding cannulation
3. Papillary stenosis, benign or malignant
4. Altered anatomy secondary to surgery with Billroth I or Billroth II anatomosis
5. Endoscopic problems: pyloric stenosis, post-operative displacement of duodenum, duodenal inflammation or hyperperistalsis, pancreatic inflammation or impingement
6. Common channel "flap": resultant inability to opacify second duct following successful cannulation and filling of primary duct

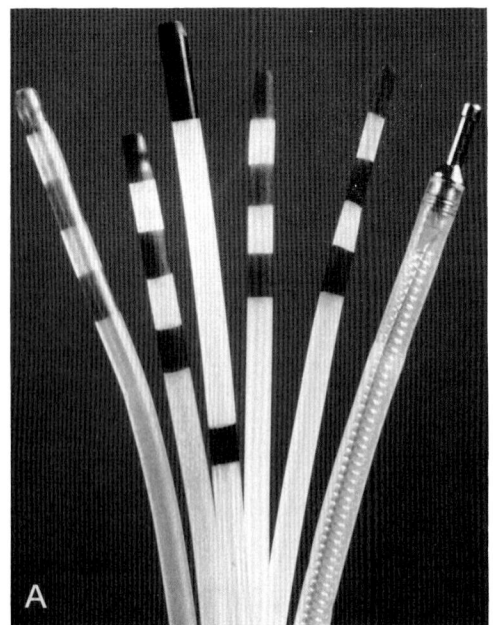
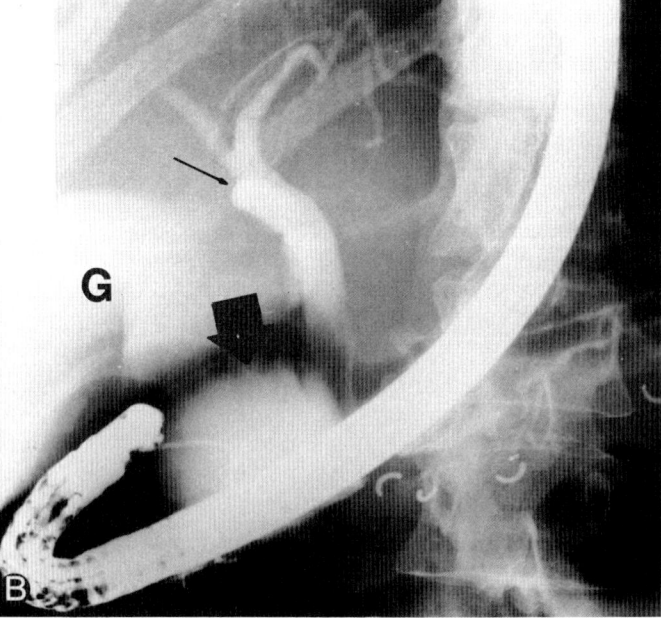

FIGURE 10.2. ERCP
A: Photographs of the tips of ERCP cannulas, courtesy of Olympus Corporation, Lake Success, NY. Note metal-tipped cannula at the far right. B: Normal endoscopic cholangiogram in a patient who is postsurgical Billroth I. Contrast in the neoduodenal bulb (*large arrow*) overlies the distal common bile duct. The gallbladder (G) and cystic duct (*small arrow*) are well filled.

projections or management. Because prolonged fluoroscopy may be required, all personnel in the room must be protected by thyroid shields and lead-impregnated glasses in addition to lead aprons. Prolonged fluoroscopy should be reserved for ductal filling only, as radiation causes deterioration of the fiberoptic bundles in the endoscope.

The patient is initially placed in a prone position and intravenous anesthesia (usually diazepam) is administered. The endoscope, although a side-viewing instrument, is passed through the oropharynx in the usual fashion and blindly advanced into the esophagus. The stomach is insufflated with air and the pylorus identified. The pyloric channel is first seen in the 12 o'clock position and the endoscope is straightened as it approaches the pyloric channel. This causes the pylorus to descend to 6 o'clock on the viewing screen. The endoscope is then advanced into the duodenal bulb and blindly around the post-bulbar duodenum to the descending duodenum where the papilla can be identified. The key to the ERCP is positioning the endoscope so that a catheter can be easily advanced into the papilla.

Cannula position determines which duct fills preferentially although sometimes both ducts will fill simultaneously. Sometimes, especially with common channel anatomy, overfilling of one duct will cause the shared wall to close off the other duct, making its opacification impossible. Therefore, the duct that is likely to provide the most information should be filled first.

Sixty percent meglumine diatrizoate is used for pancreatography. Some physicians like to warm the contrast to lessen its viscosity. The contrast is injected under fluoroscopic control and followed until the distal main pancreatic duct (which may bifurcate at its terminus in the tail) is adequately filled. Generally there is some radicle filling and minimal acinarization. We tend to avoid more than minimal acinarization in order to decrease post-ERCP pancreatitis, although some authors have advocated complete acinarization to further define parenchymal disease (42). To accomplish this safely, they add 50 mg of a nonionic surfactant, polyoxyethylene hydrogenated castor oil (containing vitamin K_2), to each 15 ml of sodium iothalamate. The nonionic surfactant increases the permeability of the duct walls to contrast material, allowing rapid parenchymal staining. With this method (parenchymography) the normal pancreas is smoothly contoured and homogeneously staining, carcinoma produces a field defect, and an irregularly contoured, inhomogeneously staining, small gland is seen in chronic pancreatitis. This technique has not gained widespread acceptance most likely because of improvements in CT. Endoscopic pancreatography is discussed in greater detail in the section in this book on the pancreas in the chapters on pancreatitis and pancreatic neoplasms.

Opacification of the biliary tree often requires the catheter to be brought upward almost parallel to the longitudinal fold by either maneuvers to "lift" the ampullary opening or by "bowing" the catheter to get the plane of the biliary tree in line with the catheter (43). Once opacification occurs, early filming is important for depicting filling defects, as even dilute contrast material can be too radiodense and obscure filling defects when the ductal system is completely filled. A streaming artefact produced by contrast layering along the dependent wall may initially give the erroneous impression of a narrowed common duct. The biliary tree should be filled in its entirety including the cystic duct and gallbladder when the latter are still present. The left hepatic duct and its branches will fill first by virtue of the patient's prone position, since the left ductal system is anterior. The patient is then repositioned supine to fill the right hepatic ducts. Tilting the head of the table down may help fill the most proximal radicles. If contrast flows preferentially into the gallbladder, intrahepatic filling will be unavoidably suboptimal. This needs to be kept in mind, as intepretation of underfilled ductal structures is hazardous. After good filling of all structures is achieved, multiple spot films are exposed with proper positioning to demonstrate the entire biliary tree. Liberal use of compression with a balloon paddle is recommended.

The endoscope is then withdrawn using suction to remove excess contrast from the stomach and duodenum and decompress these organs to prevent aspiration. The table is then tilted to a semierect position for evaluation of the distal common bile duct, assessment of the rate of emptying of the biliary tree, and compression spot filming of the gallbladder. Delayed films are obtained when necessary to document prolonged retention of contrast within the biliary tree. The normal post-cholecystectomy biliary tree should drain within 45 min, and delay beyond this time suggests anatomic or functional papillary stenosis (44).

ERCP AS A THERAPEUTIC PROCEDURE

One of the major advantages of ERCP is its ability to be a therapeutic procedure at the time of a diagnostic study. First introduced in 1973, endoscopic sphincterotomy (effectively endoscopic biliary surgery) has raised the endoscopist's capabilities close to those of the surgeon. With the advent of special equipment, imagination, and new techniques, therapeutic ERCP has proven to be a cost-effective alternative to surgery most significantly in high risk patients with retained common bile duct stones, recurrent stones, papillary stenosis, and bile duct malignancies.

Endoscopic Cytology and Collection of Fluids

Almost as a natural complement to diagnostic ERCP, following ductal opacification, aspirates of secretions from both the pancreatic and biliary tree may be obtained. The use of a bolus injection of secretin has helped in the collection of pancreatic secretion by siphonage (45). These samples can subsequently be sent for chemical as well as cytologic studies. In this manner, early pancreatic carcinoma may be detected by virtue of a decrease in both volume and bicarbonate (1, 45, 46).

Cytology brushes, now commercially available for the duodenoscope, can be used to obtain brushings from the inside of the pancreatic or biliary ducts, additionally aiding in early diagnosis of suspected malignant neoplasms. Cytology obtained via brushing may be crucial in distinguishing between sclerosing cholangitis and biliary ductal carcinoma as well as between chronic pancreatitis and pancreatic carcinoma (1, 4).

Intraductal forceps biopsy for histologic diagnosis of ductal lesions has also been used (1, 47). Insufficient data are available to comment on the relative safety of this procedure.

Lastly, transendoscopic needle aspiration biopsy to obtain cytologic specimens from the pancreatic parenchyma has been performed through the wall of the stomach or duodenum. When a submucosal lesion is suspected, aspiration cytology may be of value if malignant cells are found (1, 2). Tumor localization by ERCP, in concert with ultrasound or CT scan estimation of pancreatic mass-to-skin distance, has allowed percutaneous aspiration of pancreatic masses for pathologic diagnosis (48).

Sphincter of Oddi Manometry

To further understand and define the function of the sphincter of Oddi as well as assess its emptying patterns in response to stimuli, sphincter manometry can be performed to provide pressure measurements within the sphincter zone. Standard diameter teflon catheters with a side port and a water or saline perfused system can obtain pressure readings when attached to a pressure transducer and recorder; a second catheter may be attached to the outside of the endoscope for a duodenal pressure baseline. By pulling the perfused catheter back through the ampulla, a 2 mm high pressure zone can be found to correspond with suspected sphincter location (1, 2, 49). The normal bile duct to duodenal lumen gradient is less than 10 mm Hg. According to Geenen (49), normal contractions have a mean amplitude of 101 mg Hg, a wave duration of 4.3 sec, and a wave frequency of 4.1 per min.

Defining biliary dyskinesia as a cause of pain or the presence of papillary spasm may be best performed by manometry (50). The latter diagnosis may occasionally defy examination because of the inability to cannulate a tight sphincter. Once the diagnosis is made, endoscopic papillotomy may be performed to abolish the high pressure gradient present between the bile duct and duodenum (51, 52).

At present, however, sphincter manometry still remains more a research tool than a convincingly clinically useful modality (2).

Endoscopic Biliary Surgery

Endoscopic Electrosurgical Sphincterotomy

Indications and Contraindications. Endoscopic sphincterotomy is a technique indicated for the clinical situations described in Table 10.3. The most common indication (80–85%) is for removal of retained or recurrent common bile duct stones in patients post-cholecystectomy (5). Despite common bile duct exploration, between 4.3 and 14% of patients are found to have retained or recurrent common bile duct stones following surgery (53). The majority of patients may have had primary bile duct stones form months to years post-cholecystectomy. Patients with anatomic or functional papillary stenosis also may benefit from the procedure especially when the diagnosis is demonstrated manometrically (5, 51, 52) (see "Papillary Stenosis" in

TABLE 10.3.
INDICATIONS FOR ENDOSCOPIC SPHINCTEROTOMY

1. Biliary tract calculi
   A. Residual or recurrent calculi following cholecystectomy
   B. Calculi impacted at the papilla of vater or lowermost portion of the common bile duct with or without gallstone pancreatitis
   C. Calculi forming in distal aspect of common bile duct in patients post-choledochoduodenostomy ("sump syndrome")
   D. Intrahepatic biliary tract stones
2. Benign stenosis of the papilla of vater
3. Benign or malignant stricture of common bile duct
4. High pressure in the bile duct ("biliary dyskinesia")

TABLE 10.4.
CONTRAINDICATIONS FOR ENDOSCOPIC SPHINCTEROTOMY

1. Inexperience
2. Coagulation disorder
3. Incorrect positioning of electrode tip
4. Large stones, over 2.5 cm
5. Periampullary diverticula (relative to experience)
6. Acute pancreatitis (except with obstructing gallstones)
7. Long stricture of distal bile duct
8. Abnormalities of proximal bile duct (preventing passage of stones or drainage into distal duct)

Chapter 15). These patients account for 13–16% of endoscopic sphincterotomies. Contraindications are listed in Table 10.4.

Technique. Endoscopic sphincterotomy permits controlled enlargement of the papillary orifice by electrosurgical cutting. The cutting device that is able to perform this maneuver is called a sphincterotome which is composed of a wire externalized at the distal end of a plastic cannulating catheter that can be pulled taut and changed into a bowed position after introduction into the bile duct (Fig. 10.3). Application of current through the wire creates a cutting current which will then sever the fibers of the muscles in the sphincter of Oddi as well as the intraduodenal segment of the terminal bile duct. Typically, the first cut occurs 2–4 sec after blanching and dessication of the tissue. Thereafter, incremental cutting of one to three millimeters will lengthen the incision as necessary (54). The resultant incision may vary from 6 to 9 mm in a papillotomy allowing passage of a stone or extraction of stones up to 1 cm. For sphincterotomy, the incision may extend through the entire sphincter for a distance of 1.5–3.5 cm allowing spontaneous passage or extraction of stones up to 2.5 cm (4).

It is important to identify fluoroscopically proper insertion and placement of the sphincterotome in the opacified common bile duct to prevent injury to the pancreatic duct. Following the sphincterotomy, the size of the incision can be etimated with a flexed sphincterotome or an inflated balloon. If further cutting is necessary, the sphincterotomy is "sized to the stone" being removed making the cut of minimal length to just accommodate the calculus (2). In this manner, a terminal biliary fistula is created which heals within three to five days (4). Following the decrease in edema, the size of the incision may enlarge allowing spontaneous passage of stones. Over the next twelve months there is a 25–30% reduction in incisional length with no further significant reduction in length at 2 yr (52). Destruction of the sphincter mechanism and obliteration of the pressure gradient between common bile duct and duodenum remains unchanged for at least two years following sphincterotomy (52).

On occasion, the sphincterotomy may be staged: a papillotomy may be first performed to achieve drainage of the biliary tree or stone dislodgement when an associated gallstone pancreatitis is present. An additional full sphincterotomy may be performed at a later time semielectively or electively completing the stone extraction following the resolution of the edema and inflammation (4).

An uncomplicated sphincterotomy requires 24–48 hr of postprocedural hospitalization. In our center, the patient is given four doses of a third generation cephalosporin that achieves high biliary levels because of instrumentation of the bile duct. However, prophylactic antibiotics are no longer felt to be necessary in some European centers (54). In our experience, cholangitis has not occurred in patients treated with antibiotics following instrumentation. The patient is fasted initially but allowed to begin eating the following morning. Major complications of bleeding or pancreatitis usually will manifest themselves within the initial postoperative hours, although bleeding may occur as late as 7 days (54).

Complications. Endoscopic sphincterotomy is ideal for elderly patients either prior to cholecystectomy or post-cholecystectomy since it obviates the morbidity and mortality associated with major abdominal surgery. Unless problems are encountered during the sphincterotomy, the actual procedure itself is brief. No general anesthesia is required and the postoperative period is relatively short. Most patients are ambulatory

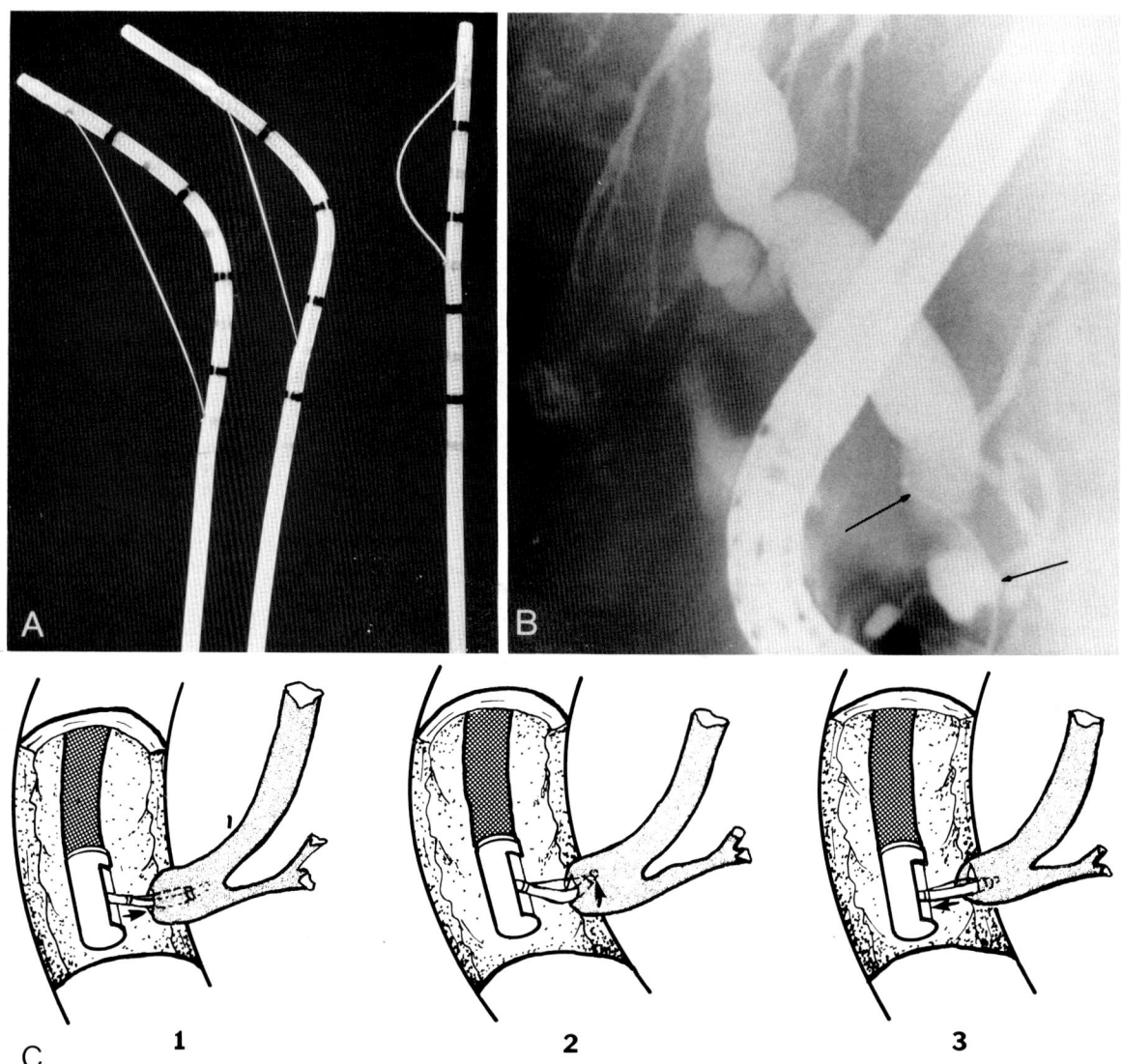

FIGURE 10.3. ENDOSCOPIC SPHINCTEROTOMY

A: Sphincterotomes, courtesy of Olympus Corporation, Lake Success, NY. *B:* Radiograph of a sphincterotome (*arrows*) in place. *C:* Artist's rendition of a papillotomy: (*1*) Insertion into papilla, (*2*) bowing of the catheter, current application and cutting, and (*3*) withdrawal. (Modified from Bedogni G, Oselladore D, Ricci E, Rossoni R: Endoscopic papillosphincterotomy. In: Operative Endoscopy of the Digestive Tract. Padova, Italy, Piccin Medical Books, 1984, p 117.)

TABLE 10.5.
COMPLICATIONS OF ENDOSCOPIC SPHINCTEROTOMY (5, 55)

Complications	Geenen (320 Patients, Unpublished Data)	Geenen (1250 Patients, United States)	Safrany (3618 Patients, Worldwide)	Neuhaus
Hemorrhage	8	29	90	10
Cholangitis	2	25	49	2
Pancreatitis	7	41	48	7
Perforation	1	14	40	3
Stone Impaction	3	—	27	3
Total	21 (6.6%)	109 (8.7%)	254 (7.0%)	27 (6.7%)
Mortality	2 (0.6%)	15 (1.2%)	50 (1.4%)	2 (0.5%)
Surgery		23 (1.8%)		5 (1.3%)

later the same day and no abdominal incision or drains are present requiring prolonged specialized hospital care. Usually patients can be discharged within 48–72 hr.

The current American and European experience of complications following endoscopic sphincterotomy is summarized in Table 10.5 (5). The author's experience as well as personal communications from close colleagues possessing significant experience in the procedure show these numbers to be somewhat high since they incorporate many centers with varying degrees of examiner experience. Three points to note are: (*a*) complications decrease with increasing experience, (*b*) the risk of bleeding is proportional to the size of the sphincterotomy incision and (*c*) most complications may respond to medical therapy alone.

Pancreatitis following ERCP is discussed previously in this chapter and is only slightly more frequent following sphincterotomy than ERCP alone (5).

The most prevalent complication following a sphincterotomy is bleeding (2, 4, 5, 54). The occurrence of bleeding appears to be related to incision length. Vascular anatomy in the region of the bile duct and sphincter is variable, and a large incision or malposition of the sphincterotome may sever vessels. A recognizable jet may be seen in such instances and significant intraduodenal bleeding would indicate that emergency surgery is required. A less traumatic bleed of a smaller arteriole may cease spontaneously and be manifest only by melena. Last, oozing from the edges of the severed mucosa may occur and can be eliminated by increasing the coagulation current. The latter two types of hemorrhage usually require at most one or two transfusions (54–56). Delayed bleeding as late as seven days following sphincterotomy has been reported and is presumably related to sloughing of the coagulum at the sphincterotomy site (54, 57). The many different techniques of sphincterotomy including different current settings seem to have no effect on overall rate of bleeding complications (54).

Retroperitoneal perforation which accounts for 0.8% of all complications usually manifests itself clinically by fever, leukocytosis, and back or abdominal pain. It may be first noted by contrast leakage around the common duct seen at the time of the closing cholangiogram (Fig. 10.4). It may respond to antibiotics, nasogastric suction, and parenteral nutrition alone provided adequate intraduodenal biliary drainage is assured endoscopically. By contrast, if an inadequate drainage of bile is observed, then emergency surgery is indicated (58).

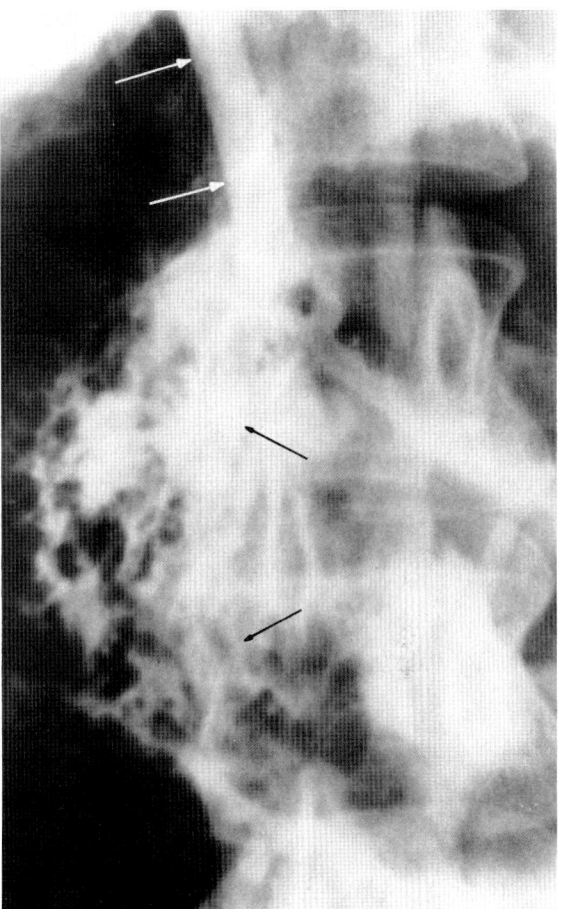

FIGURE 10.4. BILIARY PERFORATION
Spot film showing retroperitoneal air and contrast (*black arrows*) due to perforation of the distal common bile duct. The duct proximal to the obstruction (*white arrows*) is opacified.

Functionally, duodenobiliary reflux has been reported in 43–75% of cases following endoscopic sphincterotomy. However, clinical or subclinical cases of ascending cholangitis, pancreatitis, or chronic inflammatory changes of the bile ducts have not been recognized as late complications (59).

The morbidity and mortality rates of endoscopic procedures are still relatively low when compared to statistics on reexploration of the common bile duct and operative sphincteroplasty with the attendant 5.4–14.3% mortality expected for second operations (44, 60).

New advances in the endoscopic management of biliary obstruction due to stone disease with nasobiliary drains to avert cholangitis, as well as increasing success rates with sphincterotomy and stone extraction have reduced the incidence and severity of complications of choledocholithiasis dramatically (2–5, 44, 54, 56, 59–62).

Extraction of Common Bile Duct Stones with Balloon or Basket

When a sphincterotomy of presumed adequate size has been made, a balloon can be passed into the common bile duct and inflated (Fig. 10.5A). A radiograph is taken at that point with the inflated balloon in place in order to size the match of stone and sphincterotomy for delivery of the stone (Fig. 10.5B). Since the inflated balloon is of a known size, the stone size can be fairly accurately estimated, allowing for magnification (54). This is crucial, since the risk of hemorrhage from sphincterotomy is proportional to incision length (44, 54); impaction of the stone at the ampulla in patients with oversized stones may create a surgical emergency (55, 59). Following delivery of the stone, the balloon is reinserted and used to clear remaining debris from the duct.

For stones that will not pass with the balloon catheter, various grasping baskets have been devised (Fig. 10.6). These can grasp the stone and pull it through the opening. It is best not to tighten the basket down completely on the stone for fear of causing basket impaction as well. The incidence of impaction is greater with the use of the basket. In cases of impacted stone, recent novel approaches to undoing the problem and avoiding surgery have been designed by Neuhaus and Safrany (55) and Wurbs (61) and are described more in detail on pages 344–345.

For large stones that are unable to pass even through a sizeable sphincterotomy, lithotripsy can be instituted to crush the stone into several fragments which can be extracted through the opening or pass spontaneously. The stone is trapped in a reinforced steel Dormia basket, and a mechanical crushing force is achieved when the basket is contracted externally using a crank (44, 61 (Fig. 10.6E). Ultrasonic lithotripsy is another alternative.

Patients with Billroth II gastrectomy present technical problems from an anatomic standpoint that have currently been overcome with the de-

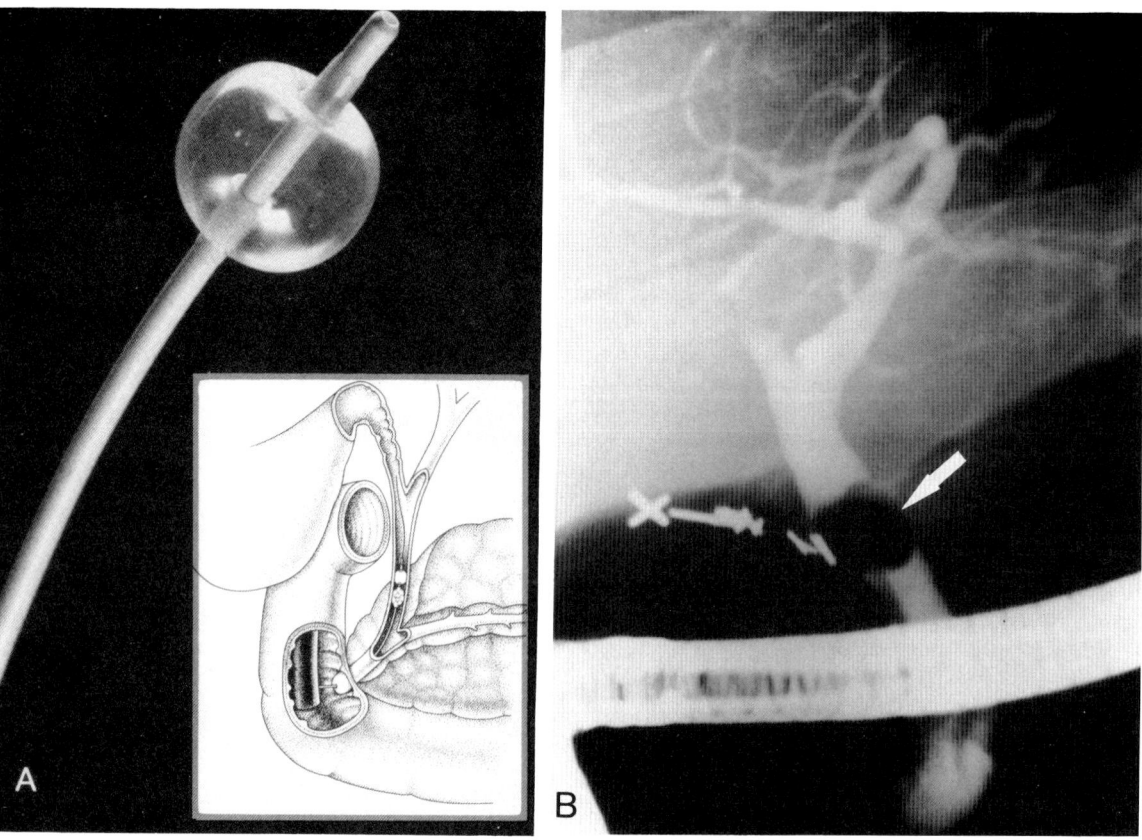

FIGURE 10.5. BALLOON EXTRACTION

A: Stone balloon catheter and diagram (*insert*). (Courtesy of Microvasive, 31 Maple Street, Milford, MA 01757.) *B:* Balloon (*arrow*) snugly fit into the common duct.

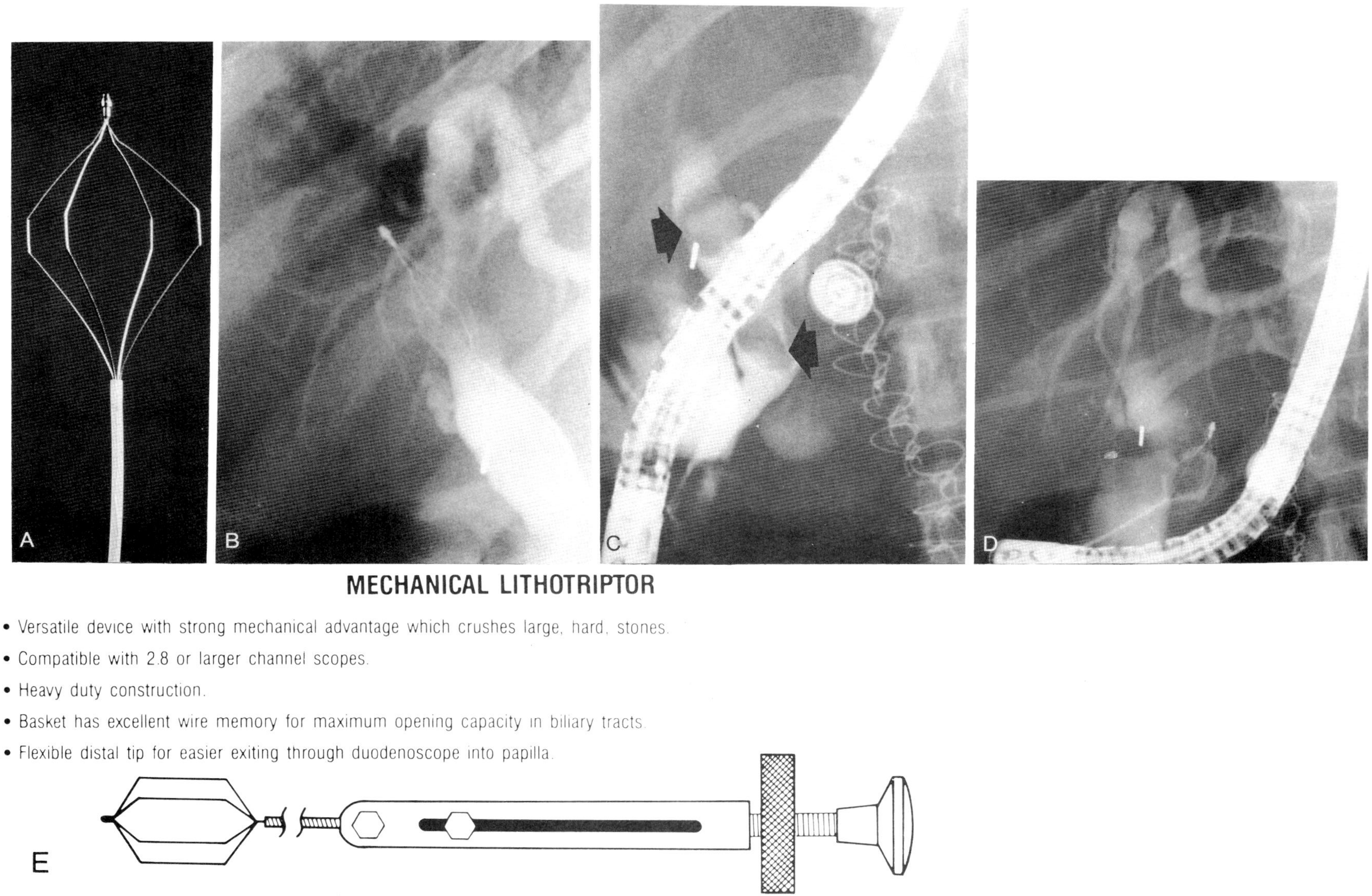

MECHANICAL LITHOTRIPTOR

- Versatile device with strong mechanical advantage which crushes large, hard, stones.
- Compatible with 2.8 or larger channel scopes.
- Heavy duty construction.
- Basket has excellent wire memory for maximum opening capacity in biliary tracts.
- Flexible distal tip for easier exiting through duodenoscope into papilla.

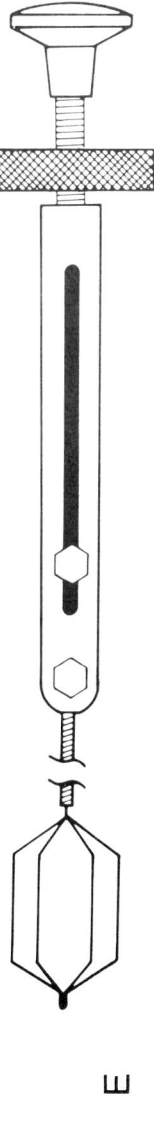

FIGURE 10.6. BASKET STONE EXTRACTION

A: Retrieval basket. (Courtesy of Olympus Corporation, Lake Success, NY) *B*: Radiographic appearance of a stone basket. *C*: Two common duct calculi (*arrows*). *D*: The second stone is trapped in the basket; the first has already been extracted. *E*: Mechanical lithotriptor. (Courtesy of American Endoscopy, 7150 Hart Street, Mentor, OH 44060.)

velopment of a Sohma (reverse) papillotome (63). Alternative techniques for performing sphincterotomy in this group of patients came with modifications of the endoscopic equipment and the development of a needle tip diathermic cutter which can create a choledochodenal fistula (Fig. 10.7). The needle tip diathermic cutter is introduced into the papillary opening and advanced in the proximal direction toward the biliary duct to create a sphincterotomy (32).

In patients with distal biliary obstruction from stones not allowing for introduction of the sphincterotome, a straight wire papillotome similar to the needle tip diathermic cutter described above has been devised to decompress the biliary tree by creating an endoscopic choledochoduodenostomy (64).

Stones may form following a choledochoduodenostomy or choledochojejunostomy when exclusion of bile flow by surgical diversion has created a distal, nonfunctioning limb of the common bile duct described by Siegel as the "sump syndrome" (65, 66). Accumulation of debris from the reflux of gastrointestinal contents thru the patent anastomosis as well as presence of lithogenic bile or sphincter dysfunction may result in cholangitis, pancreatic pain or cholestasis. Endoscopic sphincterotomy with extraction of stones and debris thru the ampulla is recommended as the primary treatment modality for this problem (65, 66) (Fig. 10.8).

The only instance for which endoscopic sphincterotomy is indicated during the acute phase of pancreatitis is in patients with gallstone-related acute pancreatitis. Emergency biliary decompression possibly requiring the use of a diathermic sphincterotomy previously described for impacted stones may result in prompt clinical and biochemical improvement (67–69).

Last, a recent interesting and nonsurgical approach to endoscopic removal of small and medium sized bile duct stones without the use of sphincterotomy was suggested by Staritz using a "medical sphincterotomy" (70). The intact papilla is dilated using glyceryl trinitrate administered as a sublingual spray, and Dormia basket extraction is performed. Some larger stones could be removed in this fashion after lithotripsy. Other stones too large to negotiate the papilla or requiring a dosage exceeding 3.6 mg of glyceryl trinitrate underwent conventional sphincterotomy (70).

Complications of Endoscopic Stone Extraction. With large stones the possibility of impaction is quite real. In cases of stone impaction, a multiquadrant papillotomy extension using a diathermic cutter has been suggested for extraction of the large impacted stone (71). Extraction of the stone with a Dormia basket can cause a combined impaction of both the basket and the stone, a rare but disconcerting complication. We find that keeping the basket from complete closure while grasping the stone may prevent this from happening. It can be treated conservatively (55) or by a second scope introduced to enlarge the papillotomy using a Mori knife (type of diathermic cutter) (61). Conservative treatment of impaction (either stone alone or stone plus basket) consists of passage of a nasobiliary drain to relieve the obstruction for several days during which edema subsides and

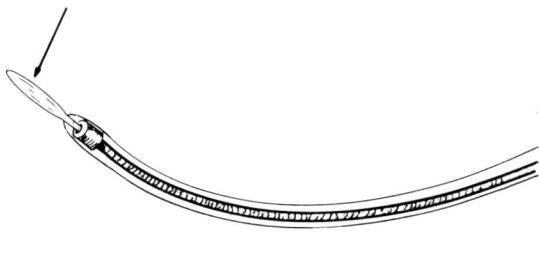

FIGURE 10.7. NEEDLE TIP DIATHERMIC CUTTER WITH THE CUTTING EDGE (*ARROW*) PUSHED OUT

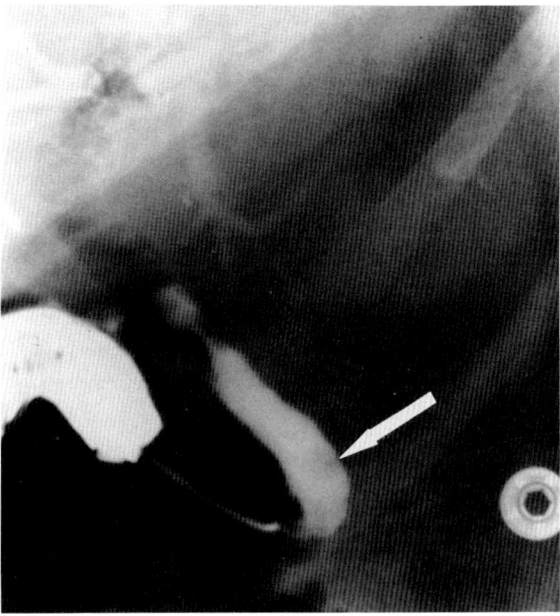

FIGURE 10.8. SUMP SYNDROME
Stone in distal common bile duct (*arrow*) in a patient who is postsurgical choledochoduodenostomy (note pneumobilia).

spontaneous passage of the stone may occur. Failure to pass the impacted object(s) would then require surgical intervention for removal (55).

Endoscopic Retrograde Stents and Drains

Biliary stents have come into wider use over the last few years. In cases of complete or near complete biliary obstruction from either pancreatic or biliary neoplasms or common bile duct strictures, stents placed into the biliary tree for internal drainage afford relief from the sequelae of obstructive jaundice. The stent allows bile from the obstructed proximal ducts to enter the proximal ports of the stent, bypass the obstruction with and drain out the distal ports of the stent into the duodenum. These stents may be removed and replaced when necessary (72–74).

There are several endoprosthetic configurations: double pigtail, single pigtail, and straight

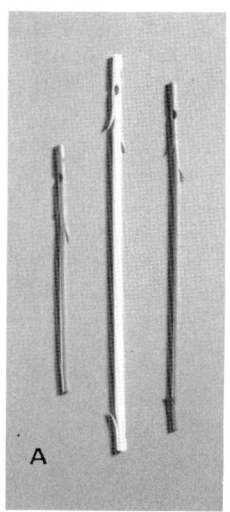
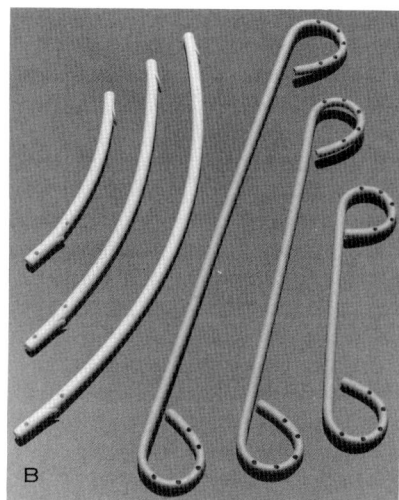

FIGURE 10.9. ENDOPROSTHESES
A: Different sizes of straight endoprostheses with side flaps. (Courtesy of Olympus Corporation, Lake Success, New York.) B: Different sizes of double-pigtail and straight endoprostheses with side flaps. (Courtesy of Microvasive Inc., 31 Maple Street, Milford, MA 01757.)

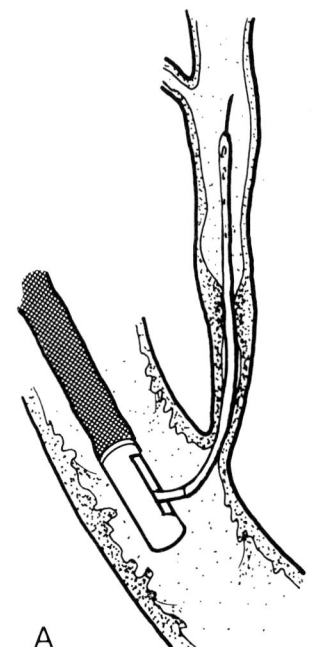
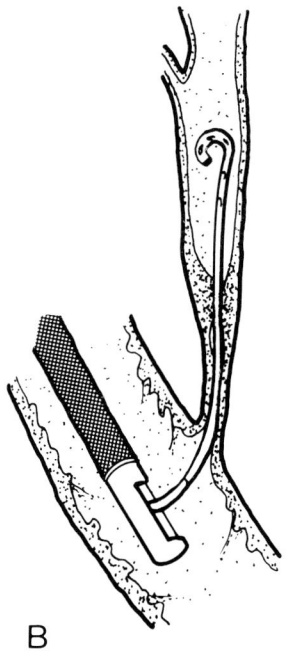
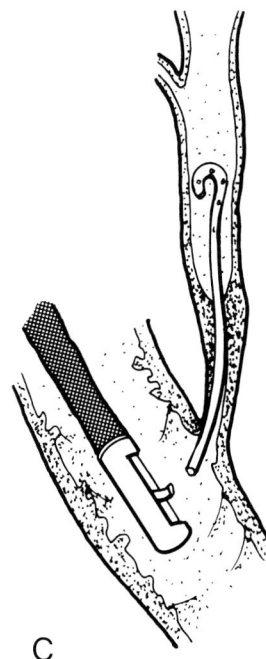

FIGURE 10.10. ENDOSCOPIC SINGLE PIGTAIL ENDOPROSTHESIS INSERTION
A: Prosthesis with guidewire passed across obstruction. B: Guidewire removed, pigtail formed. C: Pushing catheter removed. (Modified from Bedogni G, Oselladore D, Ricci E, Rossoni R: Endoscopic papillosphincterotomy. In: Operative Endoscopy of the Digestive Tract. Padova, Italy, Piccin Medical Books, 1984, p 151.)

(Fig. 10.9). The double pigtail stent assumes its configuration above and below the obstruction; the single pigtail has its curved end in the biliary tract; and the straight endoprosthesis employs side flaps to prevent dislodgement. Currently, the straight stent has gained popularity because of its ease of insertion and improved flow rate (74, 75). High strictures from sclerosing cholangitis or common bile duct tumor are somewhat more difficult to stent. Recently, the use of pancreatic stenting for both tumors and chronic pancreatitis has been advocated (74).

Insertion of a stent can be performed at the time of a diagnostic ERCP (Fig. 10.10). A guide wire is passed through the catheter once it is in good position, preferably past the obstruction, and the catheter is removed. A dilating catheter can then be used, if necessary, sliding it in over the guide wire and then again removing the catheter after adequate size has been achieved. The stent-pusher catheter complex is then threaded over the guide wire, and after the stent is pushed into its final position by the pusher catheter both the guide wire and pusher catheter are removed. Patency of the stent and successive drainage can be assessed almost immediately by seeing the return of fluid through the stent (5, 74, 76).

In a similar manner, a nasobiliary drain can be placed with the exception being that the drain, once inserted, is connected by a thin continuous catheter to an external port emerging from the nose. This is effected by first bringing the tube out of the mouth and withdrawing the endoscope, passing a nasogastric tube from the nose to the mouth, and then threading the drainage catheter through the nasogastric tube to its proximal outlet through the nares (5, 61, 72–74, 76).

External drainage is efficacious in cases of cholangitis or obstructions with viscid bile since saline and/or antibiotics can be infused until bile flows freely and/or the cholangitis clears. In addition, infusion of monooctanoin for dissolution of large common bile duct stones, reinjection of contrast for repeat cholangiography to observe tumor progress or stone passage, and drainage past large stone impaction following sphincterotomy with unsuccessful stone extraction are now feasible using the nasobiliary catheter (5, 50, 73, 74). The surgical literature has supported the use of preoperative biliary drainage in patients with obstruction (36–43), and such drainage can be accomplished via a nasobiliary catheter.

Balloon Catheter Dilation

As has been discussed in other chapters, papillary stenosis or biliary dyskinesia may be secondary to sphincteric motility dysfunction as measured by manometry. In the same manner as achalasia, balloon dilatation has been shown to be effective in decreasing sphincteric pressure and dilating the opening (5, 43). Additionally, for strictures of the common bile duct and more recently the pancreas, hydrostatic balloon dilatation may be effective therapeutically in improving bile or pancreatic flow rates and decreasing the incidence of recurrent cholangitis. There is evidence that strictures will recur after dilatation unless they are allowed to heal around a large stent (43). Currently, various types and sizes of through-the-scope balloons are available (Fig. 10.11).

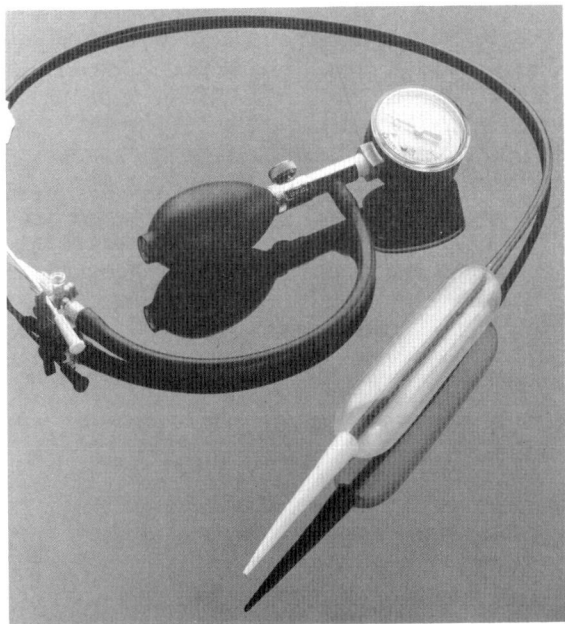

FIGURE 10.11. ENDOSCOPIC BALLOON DILATATION CATHETER
(Courtesy of Microvasive, 31 Maple Street, Milford, MA 01751.)

EXPERIMENTAL USES

Per Oral Transduodenal Pancreatocholangioscopy

The Japanese have pioneered a "mother and baby" instrument which consists of a fine fiberscope less than 3 mm in diameter which can be passed through the side-viewing instrument into the pancreatic and biliary duct systems (Fig. 10.12). Following sphincterotomy, the "baby" scope is easily passed into the biliary system and can be guided into the intrahepatic ducts. The bile is flushed out and replaced by saline or air to visualize the duct lumen, but control of the "baby" endoscopy tip is lacking (1, 77, 78). Nevertheless, its main use is in confirmation of suspected neoplastic processes; the capacity for adequate biopsy under direct vision using the technique is somewhat dubious. The potential research and practical applications of this procedure are significant.

Toposcopic Catheter

American Edwards Laboratories (Santa Ana, Calif.) manufactures a commercially available Toposcopic catheter (previously only a research tool) which is able to bypass fixed narrowings or strictures. The catheter is composed of a thin walled flexible tube passed through a conventional catheter with its end turned inside out and bonded to outside of the conventional catheter (Fig. 10.13A). When pressure is applied to the catheter, the flexible inner tube advances by turning itself inside out (eversion) and creating a frictionless motion forward in order to gain access to the strictured or narrowed lumen of the duct (Fig. 10.13B). Once the "topo" (advancing portion) has turned a corner or negotiated a stricture, the inner catheter can be advanced slowly through the stricture or the narrowing. The internal lumen of the toposcopic catheter collapses as the catheter is advanced. Contrast media can be instilled through the new internal catheter or by releasing the pressure on the "topo" to create a lumen for contrast installation without altering the position of the catheter within the duct (79).

The major role of the toposcopic catheter is gaining access to the obstructed biliary or pancreatic ducts through difficult strictured areas for further therapeutic intervention. Once through the narrowed area, insertion of a guidewire with subsequent insertion of stents or catheters for aspiration of fluids, administration of chemical agents and/or dilatation is feasible. The toposcopic catheter can facilitate access to the gallbladder via the cystic duct by everting the "topo" element into the cystic duct once the cystic duct lumen is entered (79). With the newer methods of gallstone dissolution, the combination of specifically perfusing the gallbladder by this catheter creates new opportunities for the nonsurgical management of gallstone disease.

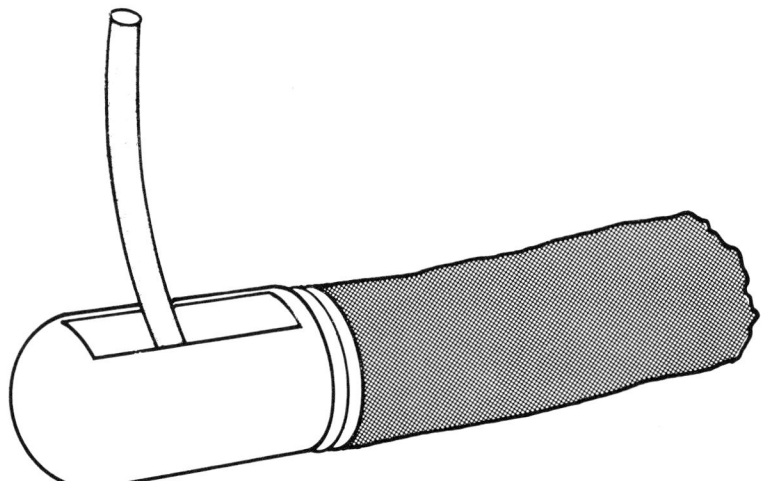

FIGURE 10.12. MOTHER AND BABY ENDOSCOPE

Experimental "mother and baby" endoscope. (Modified from Cotton PB: Research techniques in endoscopic retrograde cholangiopancreatography (ERCP). *Clin Gastroenterol* 7: 681, 1978.)

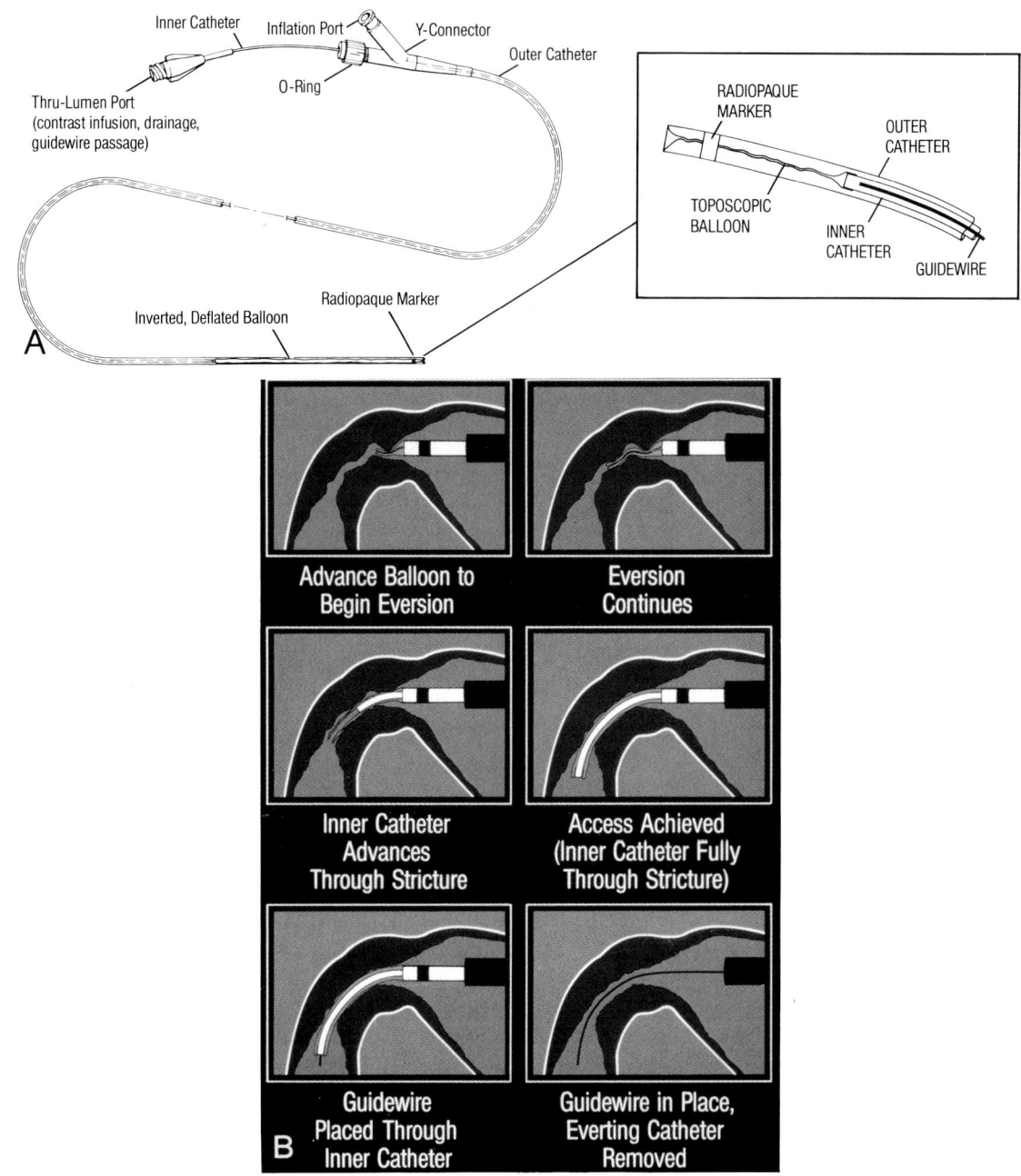

FIGURE 10.13. TOPOSCOPIC CATHETER
Toposcopic catheter. (Courtesy of American Edwards Laboratories, 17221 Red Hill Avenue, Irvine, CA, P.O. Box 11150, Santa Ana, CA 92711.) *A:* Diagram of catheter. *B:* Illustration of its use.

REFERENCES

1. Cotton PB: Research techniques in endoscopic retrograde cholangiopancreatography (ERCP). *Clin Gastroenterol* 7:667–683, 1978.
2. Cotton PB: Progress report: ERCP. *Gut* 18:316–341, 1977.
3. Siegel JH: ERCP update: diagnostic and therapeutic applications. *Gastrointest Radiol* 3:311–318, 1978.
4. Zimmon DS: Endoscopic retrograde cholangiopancreatography in the diagnosis and management of hepatobiliary disease. In Schiff L (ed): *Diseases of the Liver*, Ed 5. Philadelphia. J. B. Lippincott, 1982, pp 1425–1449.
5. Stewart ER, Geenen JE: Endoscopic retrograde cholangiography. In Berk RN, Ferrucci JT Jr, Leopold GR (eds): *Radiology of the Gallbladder and Bile Ducts, Diagnosis and Intervention.* Philadelphia, W. B. Saunders, 1983, pp 367–400.
6. Kasugai T: Endoscopic retrograde cholangiopancreatog-

raphy. In Kasugai T (ed): *Endoscopic Diagnosis in Gastroenterology.* New York, Igaku Shoin, 1982, pp 171–178.
7. Katon RM, Lee TG, Parent JA, Bilbao MK, Smith FW: Endoscopic retrograde cholangiopancreatography (ERCP): experience with 100 cases. *Dig Dis Sci* 19:295–306, 1974.
8. Anacker H, Weiss HD, Kramann B: Indications, contraindications, and complications. In *Endoscopic Retrograde Pancreaticocholangiography ERPC).* New York, Springer-Verlag, 1977, pp 25–30.
9. Goodman MW, Ansel HJ, Vennes JA, Lasser RB, Silvis SE: Is intravenous cholangiography still useful? *Gastroenterology* 79:642–645, 1980.
10. Venu RP, Geenen JE et al: Endoscopic retrograde cholangiopancreatography: diagnosis of cholelithiasis in patients with normal gallbladder x-ray and ultrasound studies. *JAMA* 249:758, 1983.
11. Ruddell WSJ, Ashton MG et al: Endoscopic retrograde cholangiopancreatography and pancreatography in investigation of post cholecystectomy patients. *Lancet* 1:444, 1980.
12. Cooperman M, Ferrara JJ, Carey LC, Thomas FB, Martin EW, Fromkes JJ: Idiopathic acute pancreatitis: the value of endoscopic retrograde cholangiopancreatography. *Surgery* 90:666–670, 1981.
13. Feller ER: Endoscopic retrograde cholangiopancreatography and the diagnosis of unexplained pancreatitis. *Arch Intern Med* 144:797, 1984.
14. Meshkinpour H, Mollot M et al: Bile duct dyskinesia: colon clinical and manometric study. *Gastroenterology* 87:759, 1984.
15. Bilbao MK, Dotter CT, Lee TG, Katon RM: Complications of endoscopic retrograde cholangiopancreatography (ERCP): a study of 10,000 cases. *Gastroenterology* 70:314–320, 1976.
16. Mueller PG: Emergency treatment of anaphylactoid reactions to radiographic contrast materials. *Md State Med J* 34:277–279, 1985.
17. Moss AA, Goldberg HI, Stewart G: Radiographic techniques. In Stewart ET, Vennes JA, Geenen JE (eds): *Atlas of ERCP.* St. Louis, C. V. Mosby, 1977, pp 19–28.
18. Sable RA, Rosenthal WS, Siegel J, Ho R, Janowski RH: Absorption of contrast medium during ERCP. *Dig Dis Sci* 28:801–806, 1983.
19. Goldberg M. Systemic reactions to intravascular contrast media: a guide for the anesthesiologist. *Anesthesiology* 60:46–56, 1984.
20. Holfs JC, Renner IG, Ashcaval M, Redeker AG: Hepatitis B surface antigen in pancreatic and biliary sections. *Gastroenterology* 79:191–194, 1980.
21. Ayoola EA: The risk of type B hepatitis infection in flexible fiberoptic endoscopy. *Gastrointest Endosc* 27:60–62, 1981.
22. Dienstag JL, Ryan DM: Occupational exposure to hepatitis B virus in hospital personnel: infection or immunization? *Am J Epidemiol* 115:26–39, 1982.
23. Geenen JE: ERCP and the problems of sepsis. *Gastrointest Endosc* 28:197–199, 1982.
24. Jendrzejewski JW, McAnally T, Jones SR, Katon RM: Antibiotics and ERCP: in vitro activity of aminoglycosides when added to iodinated contrast agents. *Gastroenterology* 78:745–748, 1980.
25. Collen MJ, Hanan MR, Maker JA, Stubrin SE: Modification of ERCP septic complications by the addition of antibiotic to the contrast media. *Am J Gastroenterol* 74:493–496, 1980.
26. Katon RM, Bilbao MK: Complications. In Stewart ET, Vennes JA, Geenen JE (eds): *Atlas of Endoscopic Retrograde Cholangiopancreatography.* St Louis: C. V. Mosby, 1977, pp 29–32.
27. Roszler MH, Campbell WL: Post-ERCP pancreatitis: association with urographic visualization during ERCP. *Radiology* 157:595–598, 1985.
28. Helm EB: ERCP and biliary infections. *Clin Gastroenterol* 12:115–123, 1983.
29. Shahmir M, Schuman BM: Complications of fiberoptic endoscopy. *Gastrointest Endosc* 26:86–91, 1980.
30. Nebel OT, Silvis SE, Rogers G, Sugawa C, Mandelstam P: Complications associated with endoscopic retrograde cholangiopancreatography: results of the 1974 ASGE survey. *Gastrointest Endosc* 22:34–41, 1975.
31. Silvis SE, Nebel O, Rogers G, Sugawa C, Mandelstam P: Endoscopic complications: results of the 1974 American Society for Gastrointestinal Endoscopy survey. *JAMA* 235:928–930, 1976.
32. Bedogni G, Bestoni G, Contini S, Fabbian F, Pedrazzoli C, Ricci E: Endoscopic sphincterotomy in patients with Billroth II partial gastrectomy: comparison of three different techniques. *Gastrointest Endosc* 30:300–304, 1984.
33. Katon RM, Bilbao MK, Parent JA, Smith FW: Endoscopic retrograde cholangiopancreatography in patients with gastrectomy and gastrojejunostomy Billroth II: a case for the forward look. *Gastrointest Endosc* 21:164–166, 1975.
34. Ariyama J: Direct Cholangiography. In Herlinger H, Lunderquist A, Wallace S (eds): *Clinical Radiology of the Liver.* New York, Marcel Dekker, 1983, pp 471–516.
35. Harbin WP, Mueller PR, Ferrucci JT Jr: Transhepatic cholangiography: complications and use patterns of the fine needle technique. *Radiology* 135:15–22, 1980.
36. Freeny PC, Ball TJ: ERCP and PTC in the evaluation of suspected pancreatic carcinoma. *Cancer* 47:1666–1678, 1981.
37. Burcharth F: Nonsurgical drainage of the biliary tract. *Semin Liver Dis* 2:75–86, 1982.
38. Denning DA, Ellison EC, Carey LC: Preoperative percutaneous transhepatic biliary decompression lowers operative morbidity in patients with obstructive jaundice. *Am J Surg* 141:61–65, 1981.
39. Nakayama T, Ikeda A, Okuda K: Percutaneous transhepatic drainage of the biliary tract: technique and results in 104 cases. *Gastroenterology* 74:554–559, 1978.
40. Hatfield ARW, Terblanche J, Fataar S, Kernoff L, Tobias R, Girdwood AH, Harris Jones R, Marks IN: Preoperative external biliary drainage in obstructive jaundice. *Lancet* 2:896–899, 1982.
41. Norlander A, Kalin B, Sundblad R: Effect of percutaneous transhepatic drainage upon liver function and postoperative mortality. *Surg Gynecol Obstet* 155:161–166, 1982.
42. Yashimoto S, Ohnishi R, Dol S, Kawai K: Endoscopic retrograde pancreatic parenchymography. *Radiology* 141:219–222, 1981.
43. Vennes JA: Endoscopic technique. In Stewart ER, Vennes JA, Geenen JE (eds): *Atlas of Endoscopic Retrograde Cholangiopancreatography (ERCP).* C. V. Mosby, St. Louis, 1977, pp 4–18.
44. Classen M, Leuschner U, Schreiber HW: Stenosis of the papilla vateri and common duct calculi. *Clin Gastroenterol* 12:203–214, 1983.
45. Gregg JA: The intraductal secretin test: an adjunct to ERCP. *Gastrointest Endosc* 28:199–203, 1982.
46. Escourrous J, Frexinous J, Ribet A: Biochemical studies of pancreatic juice collected by duodenal aspiration and endoscopic cannulation of the main pancreatic duct. *Dig Dis* 23:173–177, 1978.

47. Bourgeois MD, Dunham F, Verhest A, Creamer M: Endoscopic biopsies of the papilla of Vater at the time of endoscopic sphincterotomy: difficulties in interpretation. *Gastrointest Endosc* 30:163–166, 1984.
48. Freeny PC, Kidd R, Ball TJ: ERCP guided percutaneous fine needle pancreatic biopsy. *West J Med* 132:283–287, 1980.
49. Geenen JE: Sphincter of Oddi manometry. *Clin Gastroenterol* 12:109–114, 1983.
50. Meshkinpour H, Mollot N, Eckerling GB, Bookman C: Bile duct dyskinesia: clinical and manometric study. *Gastroenterology* 87:759–762, 1984.
51. Stewart ET, Vennes JA, Geenen JE: *Atlas of Endoscopic Retrograde Cholangiopancreatography.* St. Louis, C. V. Mosby, 1977, pp 334–341.
52. Geenen JE, Tooulie J, Hogan WJ, Dodds WJ, Stuart ET, Mavrelis P, Riedel D, Venu R: Endoscopic sphincterotomy: follow-up evaluation on the effects of the sphincter of Oddi. *Gastroenterology* 87:754–758, 1984.
53. Bergdahl L, Holmlund DEW: Retained bile duct stones. *Acta Chir Scand* 142:145–149, 1976.
54. Geenen JE, Vennes JA, Silvis SE: Resume of a seminar on endoscopic retrograde sphincterotomy (ERS). *Gastrointest Endosc* 27:31–38, 1981.
55. Neuhaus B, Safrany L: Complications of endoscopic sphincterotomy and the treatment. *Endoscopy* 13:197–199, 1981.
56. Liguory C, Girault F, Coffin JC: Complications of endoscopic sphincterotomy in the sphincter of Oddi. In *Proceedings of the Third Gastroenterology Symposium, Nice, 1976.* Basel, Karger, 1977, pp 232–239.
57. Friedman CJ: A new complication of endoscopic papillotomy (Letter). *Gastrointest Endosc* 29:62, 1983.
58. Dunham F, Bourgeois N, Gelin M, Jeanmart J, Toussaint J, Cremer M: Retroperitoneal perforations following endoscopic sphincterotomy: clinical course in management. *Endoscopy* 14:92–96, 1982.
59. Nakajima M, Kawai K: Endoscopic sphincterotomy (EST) of the papilla of Vater. In Kasugai T (ed): *Endoscopic Diagnosis in Gastroenterology.* New York, Igaku Shoin, 1982, pp 200–211.
60. Koch H, Rosch W, Schaffner O, Demling L: Endoscopic papillotomy. *Gastroenterology* 73:1393–1396, 1977.
61. Wurbs D: Endoscopic papillotomy. *Scand Gastroenterol* (suppl) 77:107–115, 1982.
62. Siegel JD: Endoscopic papillotomy in the treatment of biliary tract disease: 258 procedures and results. *Dig Dis Sci* 26:1057–1064, 1981.
63. Siegel JH, Yatto RP: ERCP and endoscopic papillotomy in patients with a Billroth II gastrectomy: report of a method. *Gastrointest Endosc* 29:116–118, 1983.
64. Kozarek RA, Sanowski RA: Endoscopic choledochoduodenostomy. *Gastrointest Endosc* 29:119–121, 1983.
65. Siegel JH: Duodenoscopic sphincterotomy in the treatment of the "sump syndrome." *Dig Dis Sci* 26:922–928, 1981.
66. McSherry CK, Fisher MG: Common bile duct stones and biliary intestinal anastomoses. *Surg Gynecol Obstet* 153:669–676, 1981.
67. Safrany L, Cotton PB: A preliminary report: urgent duodenoscopic sphincterotomy for acute gallstone pancreatitis. *Surgery* 89:424–428, 1981.
68. Venu RP, Toouli J, Geenen JE, Stewart ET, Hogan WJ: Migrating common bile duct stones. *Dig Dis Sci* 26:949–953, 1981.
69. Kawai K, Akasaka Y, Murakami K, Tada M, Kohli Y, Nakajima M: Endoscopic sphincterotomy of the ampulla of Vater. *Gastrointest Endosc* 20:148–151, 1974.
70. Startiz M, Poralla T, Dormeyer HH, Mayer zum Bushchenfelde KH: Endoscopic removal of common bile duct stone through the intact papilla after medical sphincter dilation. *Gastroenterology* 88:1807–1811, 1985.
71. Marshall SB, Stassen WN: Multiquadrant precut papillotomy for extraction of large impacted common bile duct stones. *Gastrointest Endosc* 31:336–338, 1985.
72. Siegel JH, Harding GT, Chateau F: Endoscopic decompression and drainage of benign and malignant biliary obstruction. *Gastrointest Endosc* 28:79–82, 1982.
73. Nagai N, Toki F, Oi I, Suzuki H, Kozu T, Takemoto T: Continuous endoscopic pancreatocholedochal catheterization. *Gastrointest Endosc* 23:78–81, 1976.
74. Hagenmuller F, Soehendra N: Non-surgical biliary drainage. *Clin Gastroenterol* 12:297–316, 1983.
75. Leung JWC, DelFavero GD, Cotton PB: Endoscopic biliary prostheses: a comparison of materials. *Gastrointest Endosc* 31:93–95, 1985.
76. Bedogni G, Oselladore D, Ricci E, Rossoni R: Endoscopic papillosphincterotomy. In: *Operative Endoscopy of the Digestive Tract.* Padova (Italy), Piccin Medical Books, 1984, pp 109–163.
77. Toki F, Nakamura M: Transduodenal pancreatocholangioscopy. In Takemoto T, Kasugai T (eds): *Endoscopic Retrograde Cholangiopancreatography.* New York, Igaku-Shoin, 1979, pp 109–122.
78. Bedogni G, Osseladore D, Ricci E, Rossoni R: Cholangioscopy. In *Operative Endoscopy of the Digestive Tract.* Padova, Italy, Piccin Medical Books, 1984, pp 165–203.
79. Goldstein SR, Shook DR, Peterson J, Markle DR, Doppman JL, Patterson RE, Dooley J: The toposcopic catheter and the fiberoptic pH probe-two medical instruments of potential use to gastroenterologists. *Gastrointest Endosc* 29:236–240, 1983.

11

Anomalies and Congenital Disorders

BRUCE M. MARKLE, M.D., ARNOLD C. FRIEDMAN, M.D., AND
LEORA SACHS, M.D.

ANOMALIES OF THE GALLBLADDER AND BILIARY TRACT

Anomalies of the Gallbladder

Conceptually, anomalies of the gallbladder can be subdivided into alterations in form and alterations in position.

Form

The most common abnormality is the Phrygian cap, present in 2-6% of the population (1-3). The name is derived from a similarly shaped hat worn by former slaves in ancient Greece as a sign of their liberation (4). It is of no clinical significance, and is merely a kinking or folding of the fundus on itself. Oral cholecystography is characteristic (Fig. 11.1A–C). Similar folding may occur more proximally, in which case the appearance must be differentiated from the thicker compartmentalization seen at times in adenomyomatosis (Fig. 11.1D and E). A poststimulation examination during oral cholecystography often shows filling of Rokitansky-Aschoff sinuses in the latter condition (3). In either a septated gallbladder in adenomyomatosis or prominent Phrygian cap deformity, CT may spuriously suggest a double gallbladder. Proper use of the infinite scan planes available in real-time sonography will exclude double gallbladder. Quite rarely, multiple thin septations are present in the gallbladder (multiseptate gallbladder) (Fig. 11.1F and G). Bile may stagnate in pockets predisposing to stone formation in this anomaly (2, 3, 5). Both in congenitally septate gallbladder and annular adenomyomatosis, biliary scintigraphy can show delayed filling of one or more of the more distal compartments, correlating well with stasis in these regions (6). Externally, the multiseptate gallbladder is mildly bosselated. Histologically, the walls of the septa have a layer of muscle between two epithelial surfaces (7). The diagnosis can be made by oral cholecystography or sonography.

Agenesis of the gallbladder is a rare condition in humans (but normal in the rat and horse) that is attributed either to failure of development (2, 8) of the gallbladder bud or failure of recanalization. The cystic duct may or may not be present (8). Associated conditions include biliary atresia, left-sided isomerism (polysplenia), rectovaginal fistula, imperforate anus, and absence of one or more bones (1, 9). The patient may, however, be otherwise normal. The condition in the past was diagnosed at surgery undertaken for right upper quadrant symptoms in the face of nonvisualization at oral cholecystography or sometimes intravenous cholangiography. Today, a chance at suspecting a correct diagnosis is afforded by sonography and CT combined with radionuclide scintigraphy. If a gallbladder cannot be found in its usual location with careful sonography and is present nowhere else in the abdomen on CT and biliary scintigraphy, congenital absence must be considered in the absence of surgical scars.

Hypoplastic or rudimentary gallbladder is congenital and of no clinical significance. The gallbladder should function and contain no stones to exclude chronic cholecystitis. Another cause of a small gallbladder to be excluded in children and young adults is cystic fibrosis (10). Gallbladder abnormalities are said to be present in one-third to one-half of patients with cystic fibrosis (3). Typical findings include small size, poor function, marginal irregularities, web-like trabeculations, and usually no calculi. At pathologic examination, the abnormal gallbladders contain thick, colorless bile and mucus accumulates intracellularly and in submucosal cysts (3, 10).

Duplication of the gallbladder is a rare anatomic curiosity (Fig. 11.2). In order to establish the diagnosis, two distinctly separate lumens and cystic ducts must be demonstrated. The latter may join before entering the common duct. The accessory gallbladder may be ectopic, but the two gallbladders are usually about equal in size. Pathogenetic theories include persistence of a developmental outpouching in the cystic, hepatic or common duct that would normally regress or an incomplete recanalization. Triple gallbladder

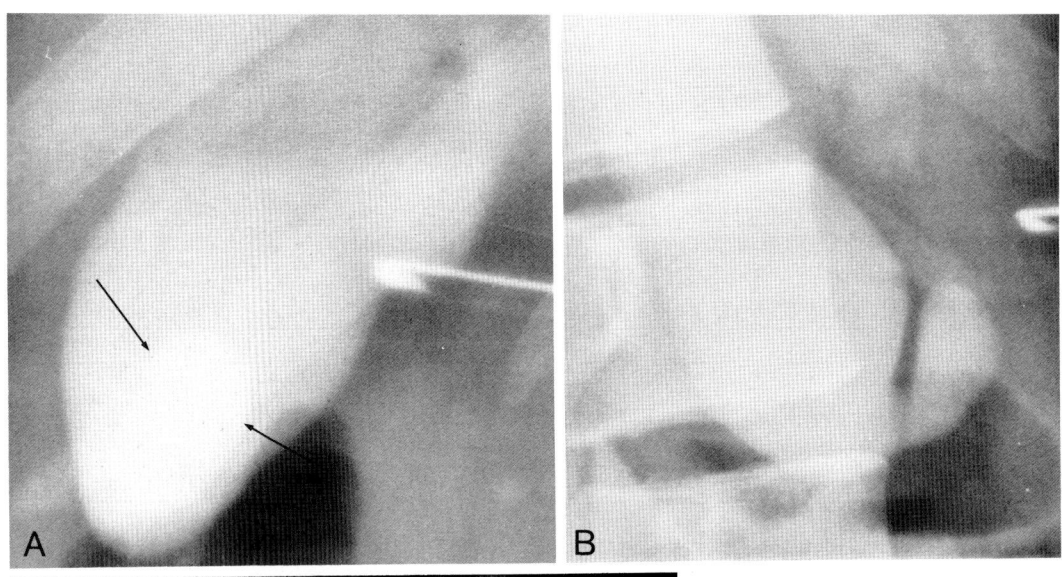
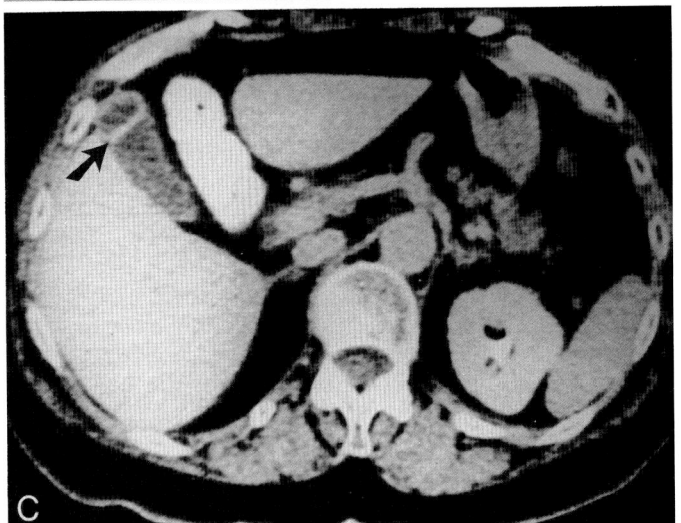

FIGURE 11.1. GALLBLADDER SEPTATIONS AND FOLDS

A and B: Typical phrygian cap deformity on AP and oblique spot from an oral cholecystogram. C: CT of a phrygian cap (arrow). D and E: More proximal folding, both before (C) and after (D) a fatty meal. F and G: Multiseptate gallbladder, post-fat oral cholecystogram (F) and sonogram (G).

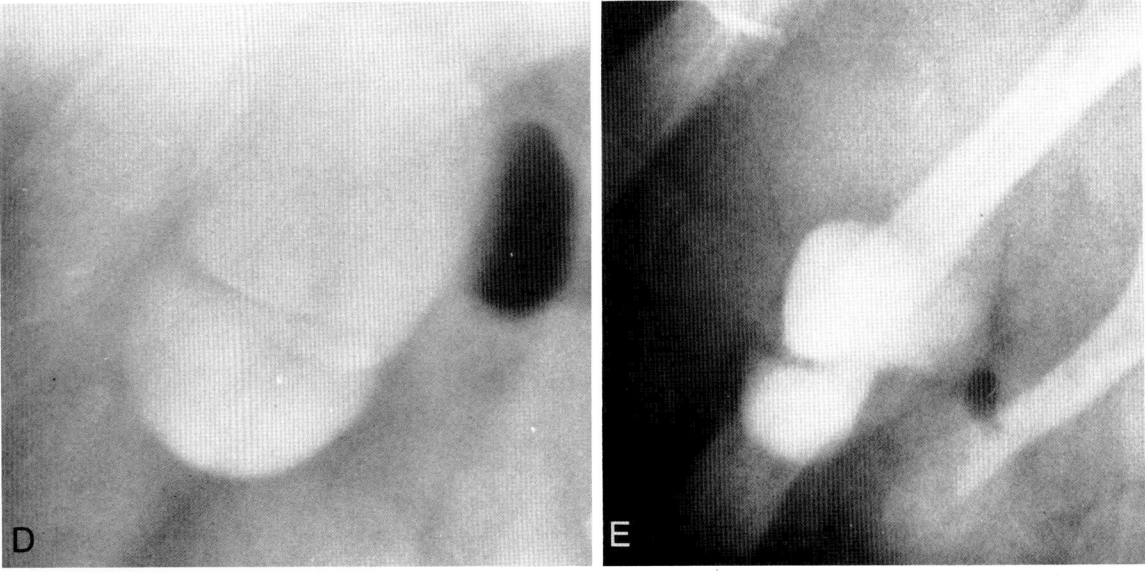

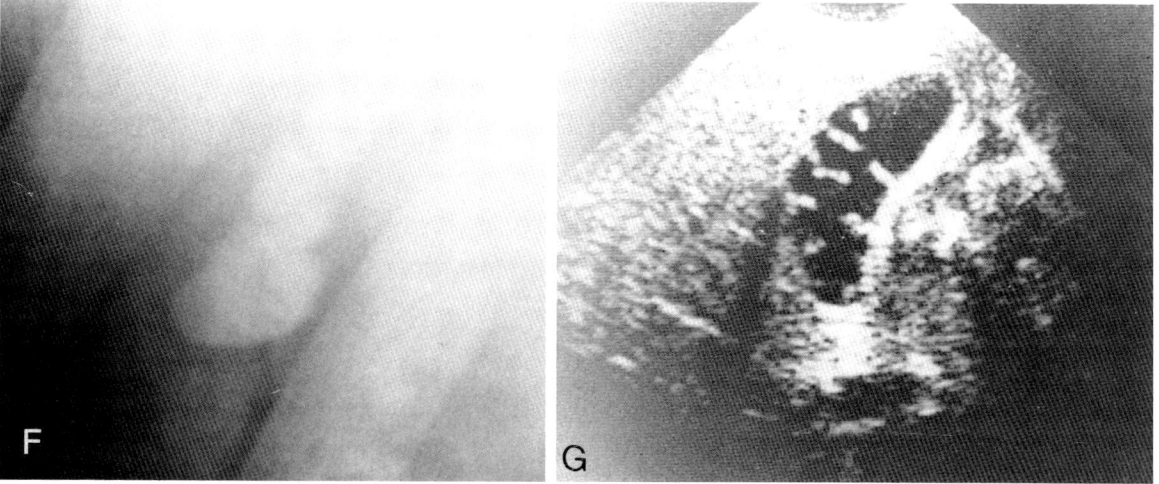

FIGURE 11.1*F* AND *G*

has been reported rarely in humans. A bifid gallbladder has two cavities but one cystic duct (Fig. 11.2). These anomalies of number have little or no clinical significance (2, 3, 5) except that they may predispose somewhat to stones and/or intermittent cystic duct obstruction (11). A congenital gallbladder diverticulum is easily confused with a double or bifid gallbladder (Fig. 11.2). It results from persistence of a cystohepatic duct and may or may not cause stasis and stone formation. Histologically, it contains all the normal wall layers (5).

Position

Left-sided gallbladders occur in association with situs inversus or as an isolated finding (3, 5) (Fig. 11.3). The gallbladder can also be transverse in the midline (situs ambiguus) (1). Intrahepatic gallbladder refers to a gallbladder completely surrounded by hepatic parenchyma. Although partial embedding is not uncommon, complete intrahepatic position is very unusual. Cholecystectomy is more difficult when the gallbladder is intrahepatic (5), and erroneous interpretation of radionuclide liver-spleen scans may result. Radionuclide biliary scintigraphy will avoid potential mistakes if intrahepatic gallbladder is considered a possibility. Errors in sonography or CT could occur but not as often as on sulfur colloid scans. Other rare positional anomalies include the following locations: suprahepatic, near the posterior portion of the spine, along the inferior vena cava, in the falciform ligament or the transverse megacolon or even in the anterior abdominal wall (5, 12) (Fig. 11.3). The above positional anomalies have little or no clinical significance besides the imaging problems they present. The most common positional anomaly, however, the "floating" gallbladder, predisposes to torsion or herniation through the foramen of Winslow. A floating gallbladder is completely surrounded by peritoneum and attached to the liver by a mesentery (2, 5, 13).

Volvulus of a nonherniated gallbladder is more common than herniation. There is a 3:1 female to male ratio and patients are typically thin women in the 6th to 8th decades of life. Presenting signs and symptoms are similar to those of acute cholecystitis. If not treated, progression to gangrene and peritonitis occurs. Imaging characteristics will be those of acalculous cholecystitis.

Herniation through the foramen of Winslow may be intermittent and asymptomatic, cause vague discomfort, or initiate strangulation (3, 14). Conventional radiologic findings (in nonstrangulated cases) include displacement of the opacified gallbladder medial to the duodenal bulb, with the gallbladder draped over the apex of the bulb, best seen on an UGI after an oral cholecystogram (15). CT and sonography may not be specific, only showing a cystic structure in the lesser sac. A correct diagnosis can be suggested if a gallstone is present. Comparison with a biliary scintigram may be helpful if reflux into the stomach can be ruled out on scintigraphy. Percutaneous aspiration was needed to make the diagnosis in a case with strangulation (13).

Biliary Tract Anomalies

Biliary ductal anomalies are found in 2.4% of autopsies, 2.8% of surgical dissections, and 5–13% of operative cholangiograms (5). Aberrant

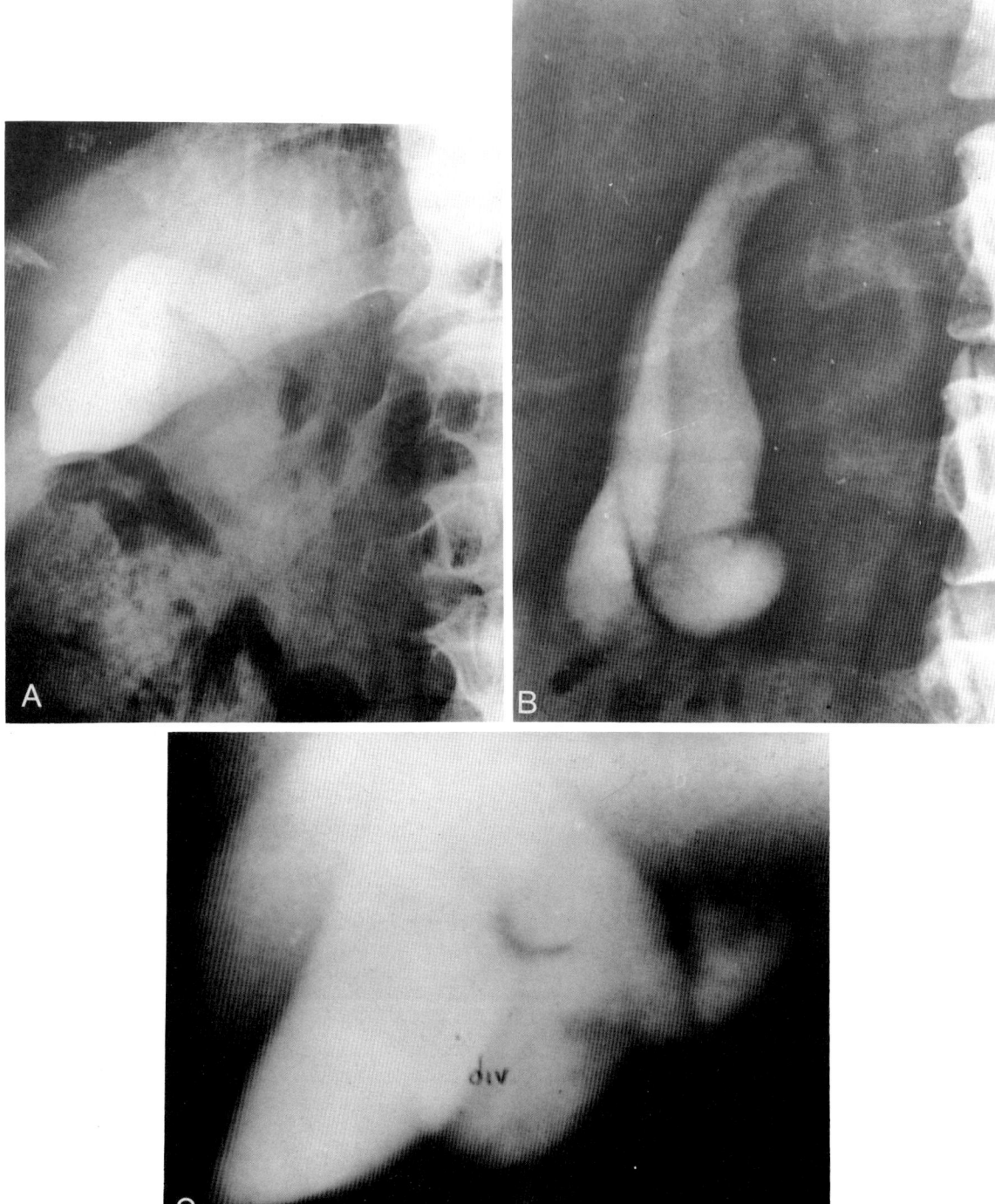

FIGURE 11.2. GALLBLADDER DUPLICATION, BIFID GALLBLADDER, AND GALLBLADDER DIVERTICULUM
These anomalies are difficult if not impossible to differentiate from each other on cholecystography. A: Duplicated gallbladder. B: Bifid gallbladder. C: Gallbladder diverticulum (*div*). (Courtesy of Dr. Caro, Cali, Colombia.)

intrahepatic ducts drain a circumscribed portion of hepatic parenchyma. Most commonly, either an anterior or posterior segment right lobe duct drains into the left main rather than the right main hepatic duct. The aberrant duct may join the common hepatic duct, common bile duct,

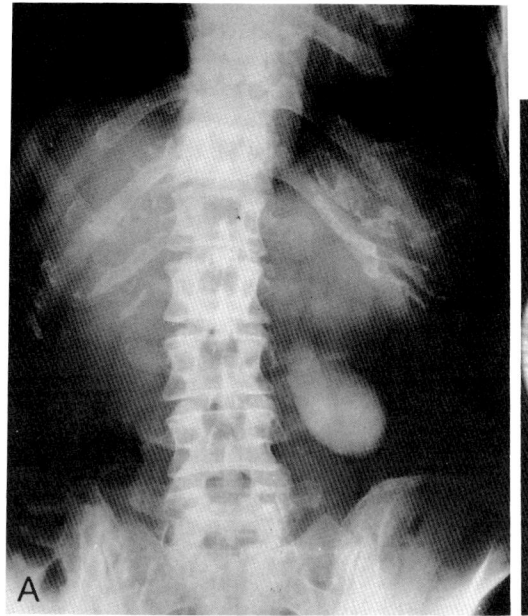
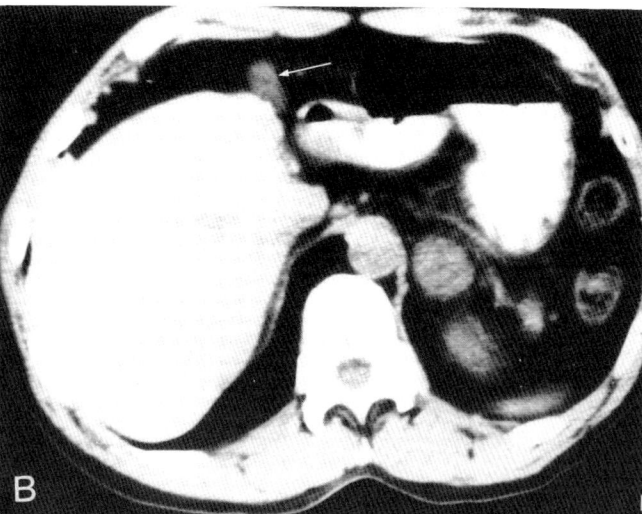

FIGURE 11.3. LEFT-SIDED GALLBLADDER

A: Left-sided gallbladder, isolated anomaly. *B:* Unusual anterior and medial gallbladder (*arrow*) position secondary to congenital absence of the left lobe of the liver. Note placement of stomach where the left lobe would normally be.

cystic duct, or insert low in the right hepatic duct (Fig. 11.4). Rarely, it can run through the gallbladder bed or even enter the gallbladder itself. In the latter instance it is easily torn at cholecystectomy and will then produce a postoperative bile leak if unrecognized. This type of aberrrant duct is >2 mm in diameter and must be distinguished from embryologic remnant cystohepatic duct(s) which are 0.5–1 mm in diameter and of no significance even when torn. Rarely, a significantly sized aberrant left hepatic duct will enter the common bile duct (2, 5, 9).

The hepatic ducts may join either higher or lower than normal (Fig. 11.5). The latter is of clinical significance in gallbladder surgery, especially when the cystic duct enters into the right

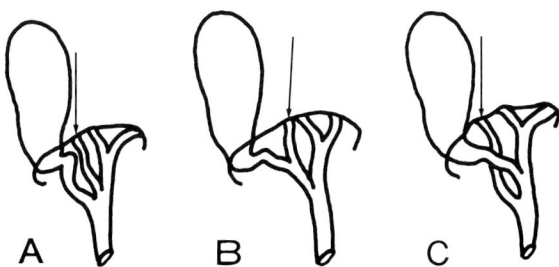
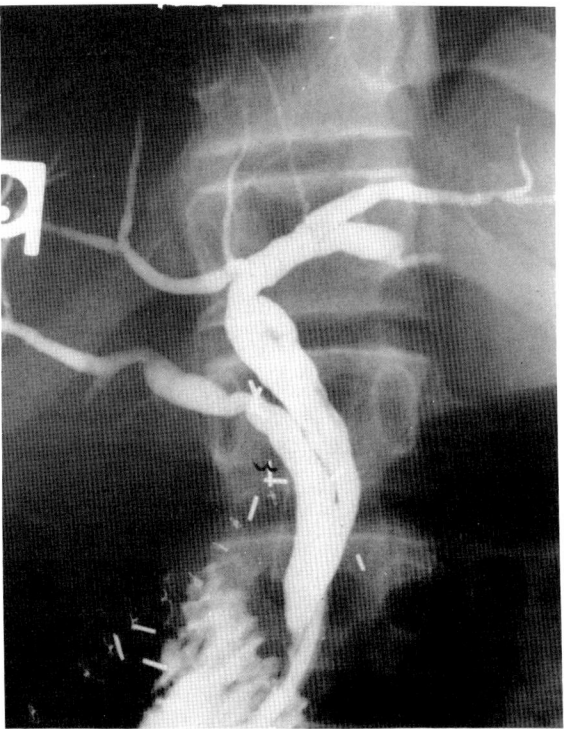

FIGURE 11.4. ABERRANT (ACCESSORY) HEPATIC DUCTS (*ARROW*)

A: Joining common hepatic duct. *B:* Joining cystic duct. *C:* Joining common bile duct.

FIGURE 11.5. ABERRANT DUCTAL ANATOMY

T-tube cholangiogram: low juncture of left and right hepatic ducts. T-tube is in left main hepatic duct. Note drainage of part of the right lobe by a duct which joins the left hepatic duct.

hepatic duct, or the right hepatic duct enters into the cystic duct prior to joining the left hepatic duct. Duplications of the cystic duct or common bile duct are extremely rare. Subvesical ducts are uncommon small anomalous branches in the inferior portion of the right lobe in close proximity to, but not communicating with, the gallbladder (2, 5, 9).

Finally, congenital tracheobiliary fistula is a rare anomaly that presents with respiratory distress and cough productive of bilious sputum. The fistula starts near the carina, traverses the diaphragm and usually communicates with the left hepatic duct. Pneumobilia is usually seen on an abdominal film. In the past, the fistula was demonstrated preoperatively by bronchography (1). Today, radionuclide biliary scintigraphy might suffice for preoperative proof of the diagnosis (16–18).

REFERENCES

1. Singleton EB: Pediatric diseases of the gallbladder and bile ducts. In Berk RN, Ferrucci JT Jr, Leopold GR (eds): *Radiology of the Gallbladder and Bile Ducts, Diagnosis and Intervention.* Philadelphia, W. B. Saunders, 1983, pp 515–159, 544.
2. Netter FH: *The Ciba Collection of Medical Illustrations.* Vol. 3, *The Digestive System, Part III, Liver, Biliary Tract, and Pancreas.* Summit, NJ, Ciba Pharmaceutical Products, 1957, p 123.
3. Berk RN: Oral cholecystography. In Berk RN, Ferrucci JT Jr, Leopold GR (eds): *Radiology of the Gallbladder and Bile Ducts, Diagnosis and Intervention.* Philadelphia, W. B. Saunders, 1983, pp 121–142.
4. Boyden EA: The phrygian cap in cholecystography. *AJR* 33:589, 1935.
5. Pontes JF,: Pinotti WH: Anomalies of the gallbladder and biliary system. In Bockus HL (ed): *Gastroenterology.* Philadelphia, W. B. Saunders, 1976, pp 651–665.
6. Kramer EL, Rumancik WM, Harkavy L, Tiu S, Banner JH, Sanger JJ: Hepatobiliary scintigraphy of the compartmentalized gallbladder. *AJR* 145:1205–1206, 1985.
7. Croce ES: The multiseptate gallbladder. *Arch Surg* 107:104, 1973.
8. Navani SV, Wilde W, Kin R: Agenesis of the gallbladder. *AJR* 101:625–627, 1967.
9. Hatfield PM, Wise RE: Anatomic variation in the gallbladder and bile ducts. *Semin Roentgenol* 11:157–164, 1976.
10. Kramer NR, Karasick D, Karasick S: "Micro-gallbladder"—a clue to cystic fibrosis. *J Can Assoc Radiol* 34:271–272, 1983.
11. Granot E, Deckelbaum RJ, Gordon R, Okon E, Sherman Y, Schiller M: Duplication of the gallbladder associated with childhood obstructive biliary disease and biliary cirrhosis. *Gastroenterology* 85:946–950, 1983.
12. Youngwirth JD, Peters JC, Perry MC: The suprahepatic gallbladder. *Radiology* 149:57–58, 1983.
13. Schoenfield LJ: *Diseases of the Gallbladder and Biliary System* (Clinical Gastroenterology Monographs). New York, John Wiley & Sons, 1977.
14. Bach B, Satin R, Palayew M, Lisbona R, Tessler F: Herniation and strangulation of the gallbladder through the foramen of Winslow. *AJR* 142:541–542, 1984.
15. Vint WA: Herniation of the gallbladder through the epiploic foramen into the lesser sac: radiologic diagnosis. *Radiology* 86:1035–1040, 1966.
16. Savitch I, Kew MC, Levin J: Demonstration of a biliary bronchial fistula using ^{99m}Tc-P-butyl IDA imaging. *Clin Nucl Med* 8:139–140, 1983.
17. Blue PW, Versteg HJ, Cole FN et al: Bronchobiliary fistula-Demonstration with ^{99m}Tc-PIPIDA imaging. *Clin Nucl Med* 8:272–273, 1983.
18. Giulianotti PC, Mazzuca N, Mosca F et al: Demonstration of bronchobiliary fistula with ^{99m}Tc-diethyl IDA cholescintigraphy. *Clin Nucl Med* 9:41–42, 1984.

NEONATAL JAUNDICE, HEPATITIS, EXTRAHEPATIC BILIARY ATRESIA, AND BILE DUCT PAUCITY

Jaundice in the Neonate and Infant

Because of functional immaturity of a normal neonate's hepatobiliary system, jaundice is clinically identifiable in over half the normal neonate population. The neonate and premature infant's limited hepatic metabolic reserve is also easily exceeded by the demands imposed by systemic abnormalities such as hypoxia, acidosis, hemorrhage, infection or nonbiliary gastrointestinal dysfunction. Jaundice is not by itself a cardinal sign of primary hepatobiliary disease. The need for imaging evaluation of the hepatobiliary system is usually reserved for those circumstances where jaundice is abnormally prolonged, or is accompanied by other physical signs such as abdominal distension or a palpable mass; or when the jaundice is not explained by a metabolic, hematologic, nutritional, or infectious cause. Prolonged cholestatic jaundice is the most common abnormality for which imaging consultation is obtained. Mechanical (surgical) obstruction of the biliary tree is a very uncommon cause of jaundice in the neonate or young infant.

Physiologic jaundice is the most common cause of neonatal jaundice. It is due to a variety of enzymatic and other metabolic insufficiencies that affect the conjugation of bilirubin. It has its onset by the third day of life and usually resolves by 8 days of life. The bilirubin levels do not exceed 12 mg/100 ml in full-term infants (15 mg/100 ml in prematures). The chief indicators of *pathologic* jaundice in the neonate are: (*a*) onset of jaundice before 3 days of age, (*b*) bilirubin level above 12 mg/100 ml, (c) persistence of jaundice beyond 8 days of life, and (d) a direct reacting bilirubin component exceeding 1.5 mg/100 ml (1–3).

Breast-fed infants may have noncholestatic jaundice which persists into the second week of life. This is due to factors in the milk which impair conjugation of bilirubin and is readily remedied by supplementing the infants diet with formula. Pathologic causes of noncholestatic jaundice (unconjugated hyperbilirubinemia) include a wide variety of etiologies including sepsis, Rh/ABO incompatibility, red blood cell defects, drug effects, congenital enzyme deficiencies, systemic metabolic disease such as hypothyroidism, and the exaggerated enterohepatic circulation induced by gastrointestinal tract obstruction such as intestinal atresia or Hirschsprung's disease (1–3). Rarely, a massive hemolysis results in plugging of the biliary tree with thick bile, producing a mixed cholestasis picture. Mild, reversible, sonographically detectable common bile duct dilatation has been reported in such a case (4).

When neonatal jaundice is accompanied by a palpable abdominal mass, imaging methods become critical to the diagnosis of possible surgical disease. A palpable right upper quadrant mass in a jaundiced neonate may be due to hepatomegaly, a dilated gallbladder, a biliary or gastrointestinal cyst in the porta hepatis or an adrenal hemorrhage (producing jaundice by an increased bilirubin load). Renal origin masses (e.g., cysts, hydronephrosis) are of doubtful significance in the assessment of the jaundice, except as a possible source of generalized sepsis. Ultrasonography and radionuclide imaging of the hepatic parenchyma and biliary tree are currently the cornerstones of the imaging approach. Ultrasonography clarifies the nature and origin of the mass while 99mTc-IDA scintigraphy documents the patency of the biliary tree and the patent connections, if any, between the biliary tree and any cystic abdominal mass.

Dilatation of the gallbladder may account for a palpable mass in a jaundiced neonate. The gallbladder is normally less than 6 cm in length in the newborn (average length approximately 2.5 cm) (4). However, the overall clinical picture helps determine the importance of the finding of a distended gallbladder. The gallbladder is most frequently dilated in response to generalized sepsis, typically B-streptococcal sepsis, without necessarily representing a surgically important source for the sepsis (5). Nonetheless, should acalculous cholecystitis be present, clinical evaluation of the infant's abdomen will be the most important determinant of the need for surgical diagnosis and treatment (6).

The fasting accompanying intravenous hyperalimentation in sick neonates may also lead to a dilated, "hydropic" gallbladder and clinical jaundice, chiefly due to nonsurgical cholestasis (7). No anatomic ductal dilatation is present by sonography, and a patent biliary tree is demonstrable by hepatobiliary scintigraphy. The gallbladder will return to normal size once the general health of the patient is restored and oral feeding is reestablished. However, its return to normal size lags behind the reinstitution of feedings and clinical resolution of the jaundice, sometimes by weeks.

The presence of gallstones as determined by ultrasonography also has a markedly variable significance, depending on the clinical state of the neonate. In a sick newborn infant with jaundice, cholelithiasis is strongly associated with the presence of life-threatening surgical pathology, including obstructing choledocholithiasis and perforation of the biliary tree (8). Prompt surgical treatment is mandatory for survival.

However, gallstones discovered in an infant of several weeks or months of age, accompanying the cholestasis induced by prolonged fasting or accompanying the subacute disease of neonatal hepatitis are less clearly important surgically. Apparent gallstones, as determined by ultrasound criteria, may be discovered in patients with hemolysis or neonatal hepatitis, and may play no clear cut role in the patient's pathology. They may spontaneously disappear without surgical intervention or apparent morbidity. In this circumstance, the absence of sonographically dilated bile ducts, and scintigraphic demonstration of a patent biliary tree help to allow the conservative approach of watchful waiting (9).

A cystic right upper quadrant mass in the face of neonatal jaundice is likely due to choledochal cyst, gastrointestinal tract duplication cyst or a bile pseudocyst from a spontaneous biliary tract perforation. This latter entity is rare but probably second only to extrahepatic biliary atresia as a surgical cause of jaundice in the neonate (10). Choledochal cyst is quite infrequent as a cause of neonatal jaundice, usually presenting in the older child or adult. It may be differentiated sonographically from intestinal duplication cyst by the cardinal sonographic finding of continuity between the cyst and the extrahepatic bile ducts, typically the common hepatic duct. Anteromedial displacement of the duodenum, as seen on plain film or upper gastrointestinal series, is a classic finding. The biliary origin of choledochal cyst may be confirmed by 99mTc-IDA scintigraphy, showing a photon-deficient mass in the porta hepatis, which gradually accumulates activity as the excreted agent accumulates in the cyst. When obstruction is high grade, no such accumulation occurs and the sonographic findings must stand as the primary noninvasive imaging descriptor of the mass (3).

Neonatal Hepatitis, Extrahepatic Biliary Atresia, and Bile Duct Paucity

Cholestatic jaundice (mixed, predominantly conjugated hyperbilirubinemia) which persists beyond the first weeks of life, or with onset in the first weeks of life may be due to a variety of congenital, metabolic, or inflammatory process. The diagnosis of metabolic disease (e.g. α_1-antitrypsin deficiency), congenital infection (the TORCH infections) or congenital storage diseases depends on clinical and laboratory diagnostic methods. When these known causes of cholestatic hepatobiliary disease have been excluded, a population of patients with idiopathic cholestatic jaundice remain (1, 2, 11, 12).

Unlike older children and adults, discrete extrahepatic biliary obstructions with sonographically recognizable dilatation of proximal bile ducts are extremely rare but reported in this age group (13).

With high frequency transducers, (>7.5 MHz), the common bile duct can be visualized in many, but not all newborns (normal luminal diameter ≤ 1 mm) (4). A normally shaped, dilated duct is a rare, useful finding; failure of visualization is not a reliable indicator of abnormality.

Neonatal Hepatitis

Neonatal hepatitis ("giant cell hepatitis") is a clinicopathologic syndrome characterized by persistent, unexplained cholestatic jaundice and histologic findings of: (a) intracellular and extracellular cholestasis; (b) distortion of the plates of hepatocytes; (c) giant cell transformation of hepatocytes; (d) occasional foci of cell necrosis, extramedullary hematopoiesis and hemosiderin accumulation in some cases; and (e) no significant fibrosis in early stages.

Abnormal elevation in liver enzyme levels are present. Jaundice and hepatosplenomegaly are the chief abnormalities found on physical examination. No mechanical (surgical) bile duct obstruction is present in these patients. In most cases the jaundice fluctuates or remits spontaneously and there is no specific treatment other than general care and support with maintenance of adequate nutrition.

Unfortunately, the initial clinical and laboratory picture overlaps with that of extrahepatic biliary atresia, a progressive sclerosing disease of the extrahepatic biliary ducts which leads ultimately to the complete mechanical obstruction of the extrahepatic biliary tree.

Biliary Atresia

Biliary atresia occurs in association with other anomalies in as many as 15% of cases, chiefly polysplenia and trisomy 18 (14). Nonetheless, the accumulated data suggest that biliary atresia is not a simple developmental defect. Arguments against the notion of a congenital etiology include: (a) It is primarily a disease of 1–3-month-old infants. Patients most frequently are clinically *well* as neonates, and the biliary obstruction is a progressive process (12); (b) it is extremely rare in stillborns (15); and (c) a gross and microscopic inflammatory component is readily evident in 6–8-week-old patients. A lesion resembling biliary atresia can be produced by interruption of the vascular supply of the common bile duct (12), but a vascular etiology does not explain the progressive liver disease which is seen in most patients, even in the face of adequate surgical bile drainage. Chemical injury by certain bile acids and infectious agents (rubella, cytomegalovirus, and recently, Reovirus 3) have also been proposed (16). There is speculation that a vascular pathogenesis might account for the group of patients with biliary atresia and polysplenia syndrome, since many vascular anomalies accompany the syndrome, and the pattern of hepatic parenchymal disease is somewhat different from the nonsyndromic cases.

All, or some portion of the extrahepatic ducts are reduced to a thick fibrous cord. A variable amount of inflammation is present grossly around the extrahepatic duct with little intrahepatic (cellular) inflammation (12). Patent, microscopic duct channels can be identified histologically in the bed of the porta hepatis. (17). In the first month of life, histology of the liver may be indistinguishable from that of neonatal hepatitis and the two diseases may, in fact, be different final processes of a single initial disease state (18, 19).

A small percentage of cases of biliary atresia have obstruction of the distal extrahepatic biliary ducts with a spared, patent proximal common hepatic duct. Such cases were originally classified as "correctable" forms since a choledochoenterostomy or portocholecystostomy could by-pass the point of mechanical obstruction (20). Rarely reported are examples of discrete diaphragms of the distal ducts (21) or discrete obstructions of the distal-most common bile duct in association with complex malformations of the duodenum and pancreas (22). These are probably true congenital obstructions, unrelated to extrahepatic biliary atresia, an inflammatory and fibrosing process. Biliary atresia's similarity to neonatal hepatitis and its progressive liver disease even in the face of adequate post operative bile flow support this concept (23, 24).

If untreated, the vast majority of cases of extrahepatic biliary atresia progress to irreversible biliary cirrhosis and death (25). However, many patients with biliary atresia can now be salvaged by replacement of the sclerosed bile ducts with a surgically created bile drainage pathway. Such a conduit is created by direct anastomosis of a loop of small intestine to the bed of the porta hepatis after resection of the fibrous bile duct remnant: the portoenterostomy procedure pioneered by Dr. Morio Kasai (26, 27). The progressive nature of biliary atresia, and early surgical experience dictate that this procedure be performed by 3 months of life, preferably by 6–8 weeks of life (23, 26). The primarily intrahepatic cholestasis of neonatal hepatitis will not be corrected by such a procedure, and the added trauma of an operative exploration of the porta hepatis imposes a significant added risk to these patients (28). Therefore, a nonoperative differential diagnostic method is extremely important in these infants.

Liver biopsy after the first month of life will help differentiate the two diseases. While the histology of biliary atresia shows many of the same features as neonatal hepatitis, it will demonstrate an additional cardinal feature: proliferation of bile ducts in all portal tracts of a specimen. Percutaneous liver biopsy may correctly separate these two entities in as much as 94% of cases (1). Unfortunately, most laboratory tests show wide ranges of overlapping values for both diseases, (alkaline phosphatase, 5′-nucleotidase, γ-glutamyltranspeptidase, α-fetoprotein, bile acids, and lipoprotein-X) (29). The only proven, noninvasive method of successfully separating neonatal hepatitis (intrahepatic disease) from biliary atresia (progressive extrahepatic obstruction) is hepatobiliary scanning with ^{99m}Tc-labeled iminodiacetic acid compounds ^{99m}Tc-IDA (30).

Early attempts to evaluate neonatal jaundice with ^{131}I-rose bengal suffered from the problems of poor image resolution, and unacceptably high false positive studies. Hypothetically, the short physical half-life of ^{99m}Tc might preclude delayed visualization of excreted, extrahepatic activity. However, Majd et al have shown that the improved rate of bile flow induced by the administration of phenobarbital provides adequate demonstration of excreted agent in those patients with a patent biliary tree but who show delayed excretion because of poor hepatocellular extraction of the agent from the blood stream (31).

The ^{99m}Tc-IDA scan of a patient with neonatal hepatitis is shown in Figure 11.6. Activity is seen in hepatic parenchyma, but the intrahepatic and extrahepatic ducts are not discretely visualized nor is the gallbladder usually visualized. However, delayed images show intestinal activity, indicating the presence of a patent biliary tree. The ^{99m}Tc-IDA scan of a patient with extrahepatic biliary atresia is shown in Figure 11.7.

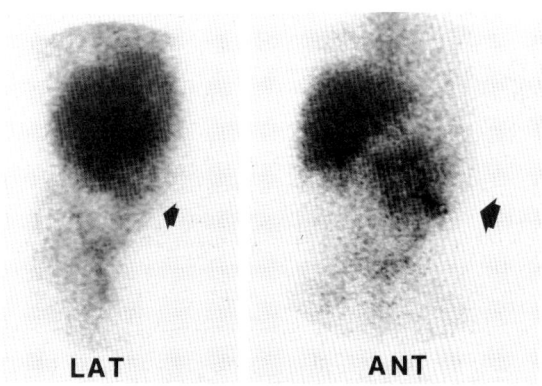

FIGURE 11.6. NEONATAL HEPATITIS
Good hepatic uptake and obvious excretion into the intestine (*arrow*) is apparent.

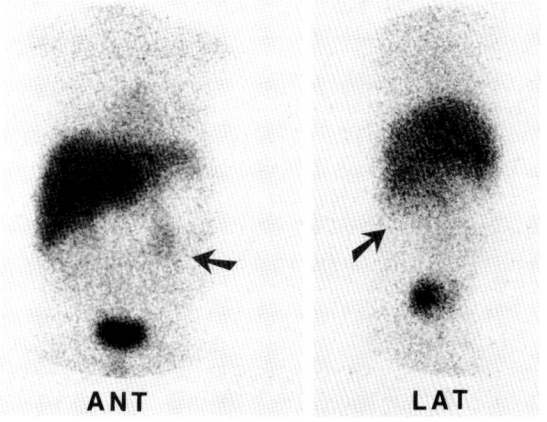

FIGURE 11.7. EXTRAHEPATIC BILIARY ATRESIA
Good hepatic uptake of tracer with no intestinal visualization. Lateral view shows only renal activity outside the liver (*arrow*).

There is good hepatic uptake of the radionuclide on early images, but multiple delayed images (up to 24 hr) fail to demonstrate intestinal activity, indicating complete biliary obstruction. Because of poor hepatobiliary clearance of the agent, renal activity is prominent. Differentiation of renal from intestinal activity is made with lateral view images; renal activity is confined to the posterior portion of the abdominal cavity.

The ^{99m}Tc-IDA scan of a patient with severe neonatal hepatitis is shown in Figure 11.8. The hepatic uptake is very poor. No intestinal activity is present, but this is due primarily to the very weak hepatic extraction of the agent, not due to extrahepatic bile duct obstruction. The scans of biliary atresia patients do not show such weak hepatic activity.

The abnormalities of hepatic uptake and clearance of ^{99m}Tc-IDA compounds in these different disease states may also be detected by computer-generated time-activity curves (32). In patients with hepatitis or hyperalimentation-induced liver disease, comparative hepatic and cardiac curves show hepatic activity which never exceeds cardiac activity, and gradual hepatic clearance parallels cardiac clearance. The observed hepatic activity may represent only hepatic perfusion. Extensive hepatocyte damage is seen on biopsy in such patients. In patients with biliary atresia, an initial phase of *increasing* hepatic activity, reflecting active hepatic uptake, is followed by a curve parallel or divergent from cardiac pool clearance.

When the *combined* criteria of (a) good hepatic uptake and (b) failure of excretion, are applied in a patient who has had an adequate course of phenobarbital therapy, the diagnosis of biliary obstruction, likely biliary atresia, is made and the patient is referred for surgical exploration, intraoperative cholangiography and liver biopsy. If a gallbladder is found at surgery, a cholangiogram is performed. If a small but patent biliary tree is found, no surgical reconstruction is done. If the ducts are completely obstructed, the porta hepatis is dissected and a Kasai procedure is performed. The sensitivity of ^{99m}Tc-IDA scanning for biliary atresia is 100%. The specificity of the scan when the above-mentioned criteria are met is 94% (31). Potential pitfalls in the hepatobiliary diagnosis of biliary atresia include: (a) inadequate phenobarbital therapy (serum level <15 μg/ml) (31), (b) cystic fibrosis (presumably viscid bile causing bile duct obstruction) (see Chapter 2, Cystic Fibrosis), and (c) diarrhea present at the time of the scan, washing out the intestinal activity (33).

The ultrasound evaluation of these patients has proven to be of limited value in our experience. One cannot always clearly identify a common bile duct lumen even in normals; absence of the duct visualization sonographically does not indicate biliary atresia. Biliary atresia may

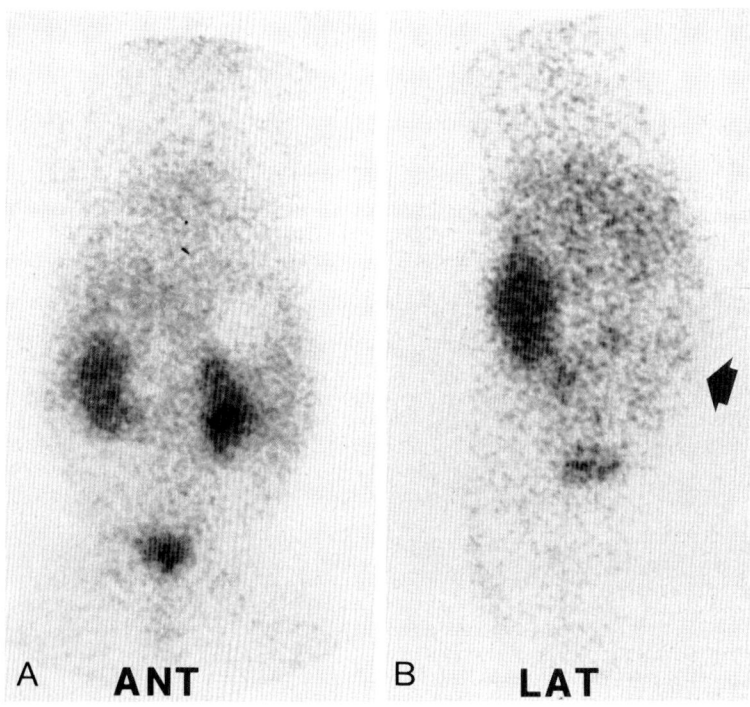

FIGURE 11.8. SEVERE NEONATAL HEPATITIS

Very poor hepatic uptake of tracer with absent intestinal activity (*A*). A very delayed lateral view (*B*) shows some anterior abdominal (intestinal) activity (*arrow*).

involve all or a portion of the extrahepatic tree including the gallbladder; the sonographic presence or absence of the gallbladder is not distinctive. Patients with neonatal hepatitis have small gallbladders from diminished bile flow, so the size of the gallbladder is not distinctive. We have explored the possibility of changes in size of the gallbladder in response to fasting and feeding as a possible differentiating criterion. But we have observed a small gallbladder contract in response to feeding and resume its initial size after fasting in a patient ultimately proven to have biliary atresia. A white mucus and fluid filled gallbladder and distal bile duct were found at surgery, distal to the atretic bile duct segment. And to date, no specific pattern of hepatic parenchymal echogenicity has successfully separated these two entities.

The value of ultrasonography is to (a) demonstrate a dilated bile duct in the very rare cases of discrete distal extra hepatic atresia with patent or dilated proximal ducts (2, 13), or (b) demonstrate the presence of neonatal obstruction from choledochal cyst. However, choledochal cyst may *coexist* with biliary atresia, so the presence or absence of adequate hepatic uptake and excretion of hepatobiliary scanning agent is still of paramount importance to the diagnosis.

Bile Duct Paucity (Alagille's Syndrome)

Bile duct paucity is a histologic description of a pattern of reduced numbers of bile ducts in the interlobular portal tracts. It has been referred to as "intrahepatic biliary atresia" but is not directly related to extrahepatic biliary atresia. This histologic finding may accompany liver disease of known cause (α_1-antitrypsin deficiency, viral hepatitis, cystic fibrosis) or it may be a primary abnormality without any other cause of liver and biliary disease (34).

Bile duct paucity may occur as part of a distinctive syndrome characterized by a typical facies and peripheral pulmonic stenosis with variable presence of ocular abnormalities, vertebral abnormalities, mental retardation and growth failure. This syndromic form is known as "arteriohepatic dysplasia" or Alagille's syndrome and is likely transmitted as an autosomal dominant abnormality (35).

The clinical course of patients with bile duct paucity of whatever cause is extremely variable. An individual's prognosis ranges from early death to a normal life span. Some cases of primary bile duct paucity and Alagille's syndrome present in early infancy and mimic biliary atresia. While most patients with bile duct paucity have patent central hepatic ducts and a patent extrahepatic biliary tree, a few are indistinguishable from extrahepatic biliary atresia even at surgical exploration (Fig. 11.9) (36). Prior to exploration, hepatobiliary scintigraphy will again distinguish most patients with complete biliary obstruction from those with a patent biliary tract. However, in a few cases, operative cholangiography and open liver biopsy will be required to correctly define the pattern of hepatic and bile duct involvement.

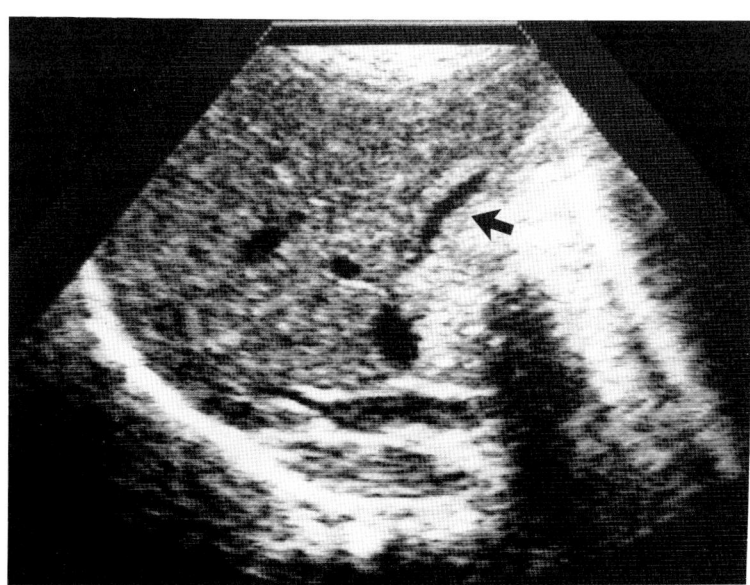

FIGURE 11.9. SONOGRAPHY IN A PATIENT WITH SEVERE JAUNDICE AND OBSTRUCTED APPEARANCE ON HEPATOBILIARY SCAN

There is minimal, if any, inhomogeneity in the hepatic parenchyma. A small gallbladder (*arrow*), but no common bile duct lumen is shown. Operative cholangiography showed a patent 1-mm duct. Biopsy showed severe intrahepatic cholestasis—probable Alagille's syndrome. Sonographic imaging cannot differentiate the liver parenchymal abnormalities of neonatal hepatitis, biliary atresia, and bile duct paucity.

REFERENCES

1. Ferry, GD, Selby ML, Udall J, Finegold M, Nichols B: Guide to early diagnosis of biliary obstruction in infancy. *Clin Pediatr* 24:305–311, 1985.
2. Mathis RK, Andres JM, Walker WA: Liver disease in infants. Part II: Hepatic disease states. *J Pediatr* 90:864–880, 1977.
3. Markle BM, Potter BM, Majd M: The jaundiced infant and child. *Semin Ultrasound* 1:123–133, 1980.
4. Carroll BA, Oppenheimer DA, Muller HH: High-frequency real-time ultrasound of the neonatal biliary system. *Radiology* 145:437–440, 1982.
5. Peevy KJ, Wiseman HJ: Gallbladder distension in septic neonates. *Arch Dis Child* 57:75, 1982.
6. Robinson AE, Erwin JH, Wiseman HJ, Kodroff MB: Cholecystitis in the newborn. *Radiology* 122:749–751, 1977.
7. Barth RA, Brasch RC, Filly RA: Abdominal pseudotumor in childhood: distended gallbladder with parenteral hyperalimentation. *AJR* 136:341, 1981.
8. Brill PW, Winchester P, Rosen MS: Neonatal cholelithiasis. *Pediatr Radiol* 12:285–288, 1982.
9. Keller MS, Markle BM, Laffey PA, Chawla HS, Jacir N, Frank J: Spontaneous resolution of cholelithiasis in infants. *Radiology* 157:345, 1985.
10. Lilly JR, Weinbtraub WH, Altman RP: Spontaneous perforation of the bile ducts and bile peritonitis in infancy. *Surgery* 75:664–673, 1974.
11. Thaler M, Gellis S: Studies in neonatal hepatitis and biliary atresia. *Am J Dis Child* 116:257, 1968.
12. Witzleben C: Extrahepatic biliary atresia: concepts of cause, diagnoses, and management. *Perspect Pediatr Pathol* 5:41–62, 1979.
13. Gates GF: Biliary system. In *Atlas of Abdominal Ultrasonography in Children*. New York, Churchill Livingstone, 1978, pp 79–115.
14. Chandra RS: Biliary atresia and other structural anomalies in the congenital polysplenia syndrome. *J Pediatr* 85:649–655, 1974.
15. Hays DM: Biliary atresia: the current state of confusion. *Surg Clin North Am* 53:1257–1273, 1973.
16. Morecki R, Glaser JH, Horwitz MS: Etiology of biliary atresia: the rode of reo 3 virus. In Daum F and Fisher SE (eds): *Extrahepatic Biliary Atresia*. New York, Marcel Dekker, 1983.
17. Chandra RS: Bile duct and hepatic morphology in biliary atresia: Correlation with bile flow following portoenterostomy. In Daum F and Fisher SE (eds): *Extrahepatic Biliary Atresia*. New York, Marcel Dekker, 1983.
18. Brough A., Bernstein J: Conjugated hyperbilirubinemia early infancy, a reassessment of liver biopsy. *Hum Pathol* 5:507, 1974.
19. Landing B: Considerations on the pathogenesis of neonatal hepatitis, biliary atresia, and choledochal cyst—the concept of infantile obstructive cholangiopathy. *Prog Pediatr Surg*, 6:113, 1974.
20. Koop CE: Biliary obstruction in the newborn. *Surg Clin North Am* 56:373–377.
21. Fisher M, Chen SH, Dekker A: Congenital diaphragm of the common hepatic duct. *Gastroenterology* 54:605, 1968.
22. Fisher M, Chen SH, Dekker A: Congenital diaphragm of the common hepatic duct. *Gastroenterology* 54:605, 1968.
23. Altman RP: The portoenterostomy procedure for biliary atresia: a five year experience. *Ann Surg* 188:351–362, 1978.
24. Kasai M: Results of surgery for biliary atresia. In Javitt NB (ed).: *Neonatal Hepatitis and Biliary Atresia*. DHEW Publication No. (NIH) 79-1296, Bethesda, Md.: National Institutes of Health, 1978, pp 417–429.
25. Hitch DC, Shikes RH, Lilly JR: Determinants of survival after Kasai's operation for biliary atresia using actuarial analysis. *J Pediatr Surg* 14:310–314, 1979.
26. Kasai M, Suzuki H, Ohashi E et al: Technique and results of operative management of biliary atresia. *World J Surg* 2:571–580, 1978.
27. Lilly JR, Altman RP: Hepatic portoenterostomy (the Kasai operation for biliary atresia). *Surgery* 78:76–86, 1975.
28. Lawson E, Boggs J: Long term follow-up of neonatal hepatitis: safety and value of surgical exploration. *Pediatrics* 55:560, 1974.
29. Sunaryo FP, Watkins JB: Evaluation of diagnostic techniques for extrahepatic biliary atresia. In Daum F and Fisher SE (eds): *Extrahepatic Biliary Atresia*. New York, Mercel Dekker, 1983.
30. Majd M, Altman RP, Reba RC: Hepatobiliary scintigraphy with ^{99m}Tc-PIPIDA in infants and children. *J Nucl Med* 20:680, 1979.
31. Majd M: Radionuclide studies in the evaluation of neonatal jaundice. In Daum F and Fisher SE (eds): *Extrahepatic Biliary Atresia*. New York, Marcel Dekker, 1983.
32. Leonard JC, Hitch DC, Manion CV: The use of diethyl-IDA ^{99m}Tc clearance curves in the differentiation of biliary atresia from other forms of neonatal jaundice. *Radiology* 142:773–776, 1982.
33. Altman RP: Personal communication.
34. Witzleben CL: Bile duct paucity ("intrahepatic atresia"), *Perspect Pediatr Pathol* 7:185–200, 1982.
35. Alagille D: Intrahepatic biliary atresia (hepatic ductular hypoplasia). In Berenberg SR (ed): *Liver Disease in Infancy and Childhood*. Baltimore, Williams & Wilkins, 1976, p 129.
36. Kahn EI, Daum F: Arteriohepatic dysplasia: evaluation of the extrahepatic biliary tract, porta hepatis and hepatic parenchyma. In Daum F, Fisher, SE (eds): *Extrahepatic Biliary Atresia*. New York, Marcel Dekker, 1983.

HEPATOBILIARY CYSTIC MALFORMATIONS (POLYCYSTIC LIVER DISEASE, CONGENITAL HEPATIC FIBROSIS, CAROLI'S DISEASE, CHOLEDOCHAL CYST)

The pathogenesis of congenital biliary ductal malformations is unclear. Malformations arising from interference with first trimester development can be indistinguishable from acquired deformities resulting from inflammatory diseases occurring later in life. Clinical manifestations depend on anatomic location and degree of disturbance of bile flow. Dilatation of extrahepatic ducts (choledochal cyst) or major intrahepatic ducts (Caroli's disease) may lead to stasis, cholangitis, and progressive biliary disease. Lesions affecting terminal interlobular bile ducts (congenital hepatic fibrosis) or resulting in noncommunicating cysts (polycystic disease) cause little or no disturbance in bile flow. Differences in anatomic appearance and clinical effects should not obscure the probability that all of the above malformations are etiologically related as they occur in combinations with each other and cystic kidney disease. The relative clinical importance of the hepatic and renal diseases is variable.

Polycystic Liver Disease

Clinical Findings

Polycystic disease of the liver is an autosomal dominant embryologic malformation associated with adult polycystic kidney disease in 50% of cases (1, 2). Multiple hepatic cysts have been reported in children with tuberous sclerosis (3). It is thought to be caused by defective development of intrahepatic bile ducts in the portal tracts (1) Females are affected about twice as often as males, with age of presentation usually in the fifth through the eighth decades of life (1). Only about 15% are symptomatic; signs and symptoms include pain, dyspepsia, abdominal mass, and hepatomegaly without hepatic dysfunction (1, 2, 4). Surgery is usually unwarranted, and prognosis is dependent on presence or absence of kidney disease (1, 2).

Pathology

Depending on the number and size of the cysts, the liver can be either normal in size or greatly enlarged, with or without deformity of the outer surface (1). The number of cysts varies from 2 or 3 to too numerous to count (1). Cysts may be diffusely scattered or restricted to one lobe, usually the left (1). Although average diameter is 1.2 cm, size varies from entirely microscopic to huge (2, 4). Hepatic parenchyma between the cysts is normal (1, 2, 4). Cyst fluid is usually clear or yellow but may be brown due to the presence of old blood (1). Histologically, the cystic regions are related to bile ducts in the portal areas. The cysts are surrounded by a fibrous tissue capsule and lined by a columnar epithelium which may be flattened or absent in larger cysts (1).

Radiology

Plain films often show hepatomegaly. Curvilinear or amorphous dystrophic calcification in the cyst wall is an unusual finding (1), occurring after intracystic hemorrhage (5). Excretory urography may demonstrate multiple intrahepatic radiolucencies, and radionuclide scans will show cold areas corresponding to the larger cysts (Fig. 11.10). Sonography and CT will demonstrate clearly those cysts larger than 1–2 cm in diameter (Fig. 11.10). Aggregates of smaller cysts may appear echogenic on a sonogram because of the multiple acoustic interfaces of closely spaced walls. On the other hand, CT of such a region may show a homogeneous water density because of inability to resolve the walls. On both cholangiography and hepatic angiography polycystic disease has an appearance similar to avascular metastases: splaying and draping of bile ducts and vessels, respectively. Lack of any encasement suggests the correct diagnosis.

Congenital Hepatic Fibrosis

The autosomal recessive type of polycystic kidney disease has a spectrum of clinical presentation but all clinical forms have both hepatic and renal disease (6). In the infantile form, the renal disease is fatal and there is incidental portal fibrosis and bile duct hyperplasia. In the juvenile form there is congenital hepatic fibrosis and renal tubular ectasia and the hepatic disease predominates clinically (6). The underlying disorder may be maldistribution of connective tissue which is interposed between parenchyma and interlobular bile ducts in embryonic liver and surrounds collecting tubules in embryonic kidney causing cystic malformation of these structures (7).

Clinical Findings

Although most often presenting in early childhood, congenital hepatic fibrosis can present in infancy or early adulthood (2, 6–8). Clinical features include hepatosplenomegaly, portal hypertension and bleeding varices. Longevity is greater than with most other causes of portal hypertension because of relatively normal liver function (7, 8). Serum protein, bilirubin and transaminases are usually normal. Alkaline phosphatase is sometimes elevated (1). Misdiagnosis initially as cirrhosis is not uncommon (1). Both hepatocellular and cholangiocellular carcinoma may occur as complications (1). Renal function in these patients is either normal or somewhat impaired (6).

Pathology

Liver biopsy shows bands of fibrous tissue coursing through an otherwise undistorted hepatic parenchyma (2, 8). Embedded in these bands are excess numbers of distorted terminal interlobular bile ducts which form multiple microscopic and tiny macroscopic cysts (7). Rarely, these cysts communicate with bile ductules to

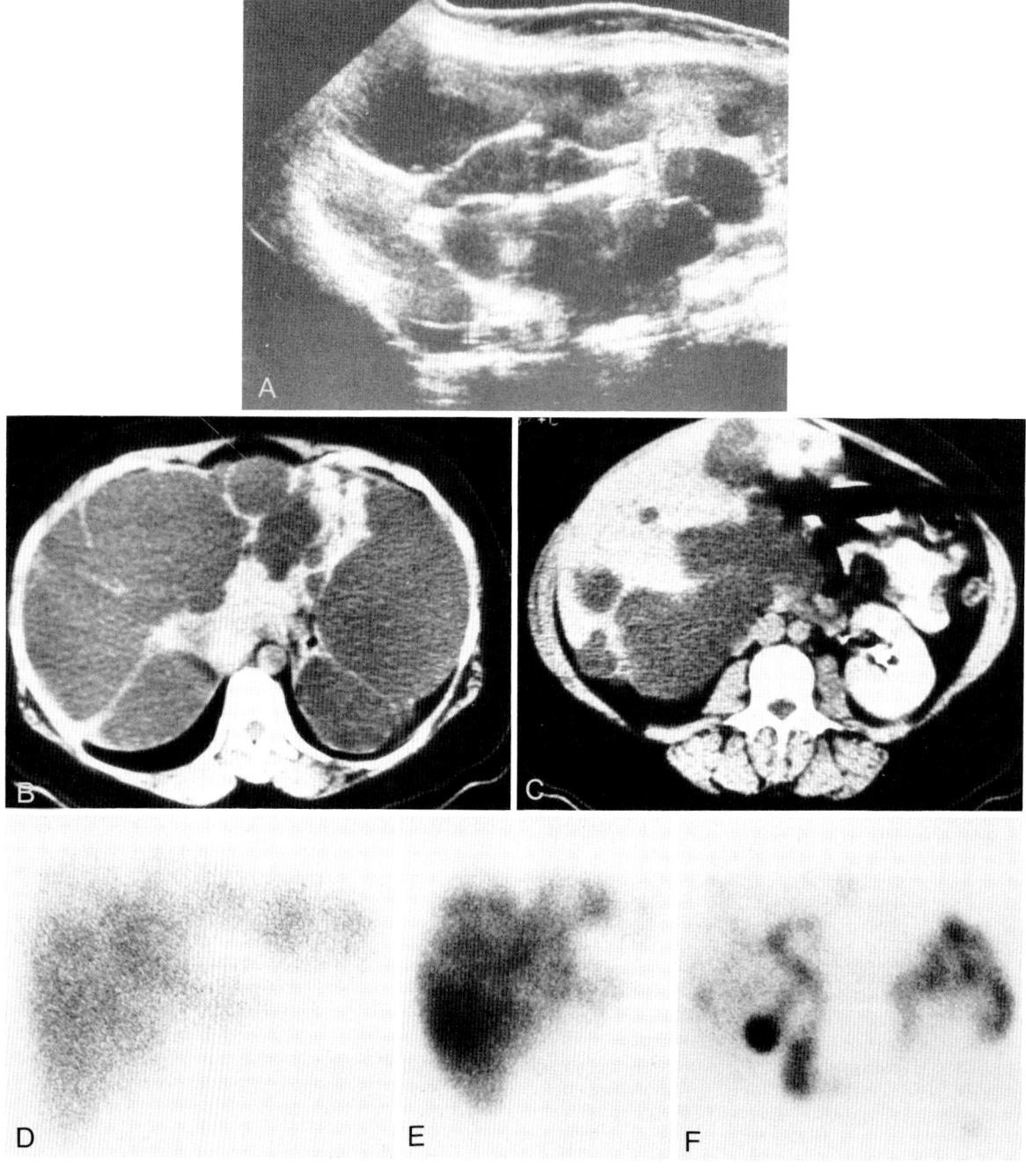

FIGURE 11.10. POLYCYSTIC LIVER DISEASE

A: Parasagittal sonogram through the right lobe shows multiple cystic regions in an enlarged liver. B and C: CT scans in the same patient demonstrate the multiple liver cysts more clearly. The kidneys were normal. D–F: Scintigraphic findings in polycystic liver in a different patient. Sulfur colloid scan (D) shows multiple space-occupying masses that do not communicate with the biliary tree on early (E) or delayed (F) images from a hepatobiliary scintigram.

the extent of interfering with bile flow and intrahepatic ducts dilate giving the appearance of Caroli's disease (7). Further blurring the distinction between congenital hepatic fibrosis and Caroli's disease is the frequent presence of histologic findings compatible with congenital hepatic fibrosis in patients with Caroli's disease (1, 7). Hypoplasia or compression of portal vein branches occurs in the fibrous bands with occasional defects in main portal veins (1). Renal cysts and tubular ectasia are usually present in congenital hepatic fibrosis, and choledochal cyst may be present (1).

Radiology

Plain films demonstrate hepatosplenomegaly and sometimes renal enlargement (2). Varices can be shown by barium meal. Excretory urography shows nephromegaly and some degree of tubular ectasia in conjunction with cortical and medullary cysts which deform the contour and distort the collecting system (Fig. 11.11A and D). Sonography or CT can demonstrate renal cysts and tubular ectasia (Fig. 11.11B and C), in addition to ascites, varices, splenomegaly and an abnormal liver, suggesting the correct cause of the liver disease in the appropriate clinical context (9). Often the only liver abnormalities depicted will be an increased echogenicity on ultrasound (Fig. 11.11E and F), and a normal or slightly enlarged liver of normal density on CT consistent with cirrhosis (9, 10). Large linear regions of low density have been seen on CT that may correspond to the fibrotic bands (3). At times, cystic dilatation of intrahepatic ducts as in Caroli's disease is demonstrable (Fig. 11.11E and F). In addition to varices, portography has demonstrated duplication of the intraheptic portal veins in some children with congenital hepatic fibrosis and portal hypertension (11). This appearance of dual portal branches of unequal caliber following parallel courses often into the periphery is not seen in other causes of portal hypertension (11). Both the major and minor portal vein branches may be affected.

Caroli's Disease (Congenital Dilatation of Intrahepatic Bile Ducts)

Caroli's disease is intermediate between congenital hepatic fibrosis and choledochal cyst and is associated in reports with both, but most cases of Caroli's disease are distinct enough in clinical course and treatment to justify separate classification (6). Most cases are nonfamilial (1). As hepatic artery occlusion and liver infarction can lead to communicating bile cysts, there is speculation that perinatal hepatic artery occlusion might be a causative factor in Caroli's disease (12).

Clinical Findings

Presentation is usually in childhood or early adulthood although it may occur at any time (1, 7). Abdominal pain, fever, and gram-negative sepsis may be presenting features (1). Jaundice is usually absent or minimal but increases during episodes of cholangitis. Malabsorption is frequent but liver function is fairly normal and portal hypertension is absent (1). Cholelithiasis, choledocholithiasis, liver abscesses, and cholangiocarcinoma are complications (1, 7). Symptoms subside temporarily with infection control and/or calculus passage but invariably recur. Palliative treatment includes antibiotics, biliary drainage, and stone removal. Ultimate prognosis is poor but the course is usually extended with sepsis eventually being fatal (7).

Pathology

Caroli's disease is characterized by cystic dilatation of the major intrahepatic bile ducts. The "cysts" are lined with cuboidal epithelium and are in continuity with branches of the main intrahepatic bile ducts (1, 7). Liver biopsy may reveal associated congenital hepatic fibrosis (1, 7). Both renal cystic disease and tubular ectasia may be present although not usually clinically significant (1, 6, 7, 9, 10, 12, 13).

Radiology

Plain films occasionally show small intrahepatic calculi or medullary nephrocalcinosis (Fig. 11.12A). Excretory urography can demonstrate the renal tubular ectasia and cortical or medullary cysts which are often associated (13). Oral cholecystography or intravenous cholangiography may show calculi, and the latter occasionally has shown faint, irregular, patchy collections of contrast throughout the liver (1, 13). Sulfur colloid liver scans can show branching areas of diminished uptake corresponding to dilated ducts (Fig. 11.13A). Although rose bengal hepatobiliary imaging usually showed only delayed bowel visualization, ^{99m}Tc-HIDA and its analogs can successfully depict saccular dilatation of the intrahepatic bile ducts (Fig. 11.13B–D) (10). Sonography demonstrates sonolucent intrahepatic tubular structures converging towards the porta hepatis representing grossly dilated ducts (Fig. 11.12B) (10). Cystic areas can be shown to communicate with ducts by careful angulation of the transducer. Clumps of echogenic sludge and occasionally shadowing calculi are sometimes demonstrated in continuity with dilated ducts. CT shows branching low density tubular structures which extend to the periphery of the liver and communicate with localized ectatic areas (Fig. 11.12C–E) (9). Sometimes higher density

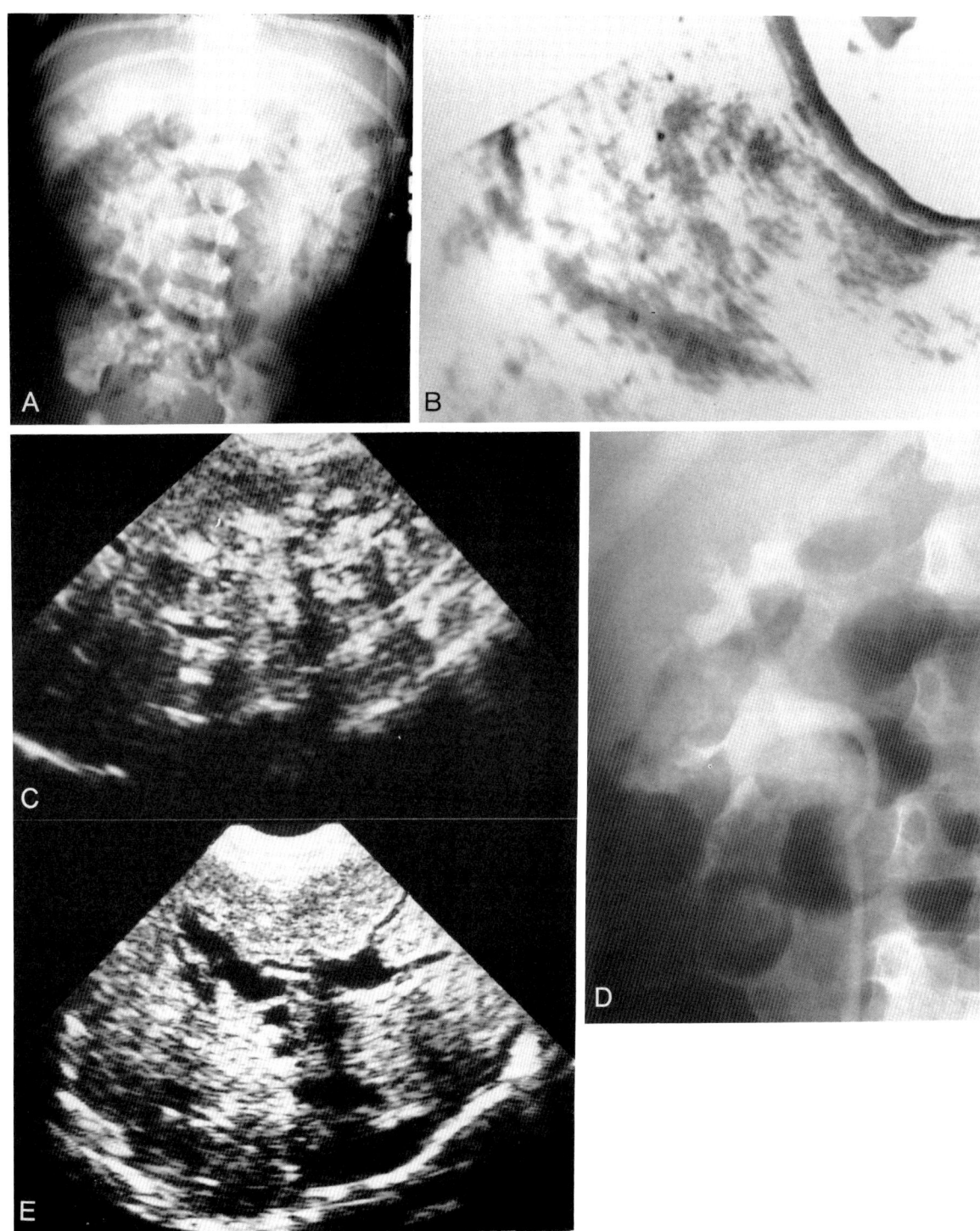

FIGURE 11.11. CONGENITAL HEPATIC FIBROSIS

A: Delayed film from an IVP in a neonate with poor renal function demonstrating striations typical of infantile polycystic kidney. *B:* Prone parasagittal sonogram of the left kidney at the same time shows an enlarged, echogenic kidney compatible with infantile polycystic disease. The right kidney looked similar. *C:* Parasagittal sonogram of the right kidney six years later revealed milder nephromegaly, increased medullary echogenicity, and shadowing from the regions of the papillae, suggesting evolution to juvenile polycystic disease. Renal function was near normal. *D:* IVP at the same time as (*C*) shows tubular ectasia, consistent with juvenile polycystic disease or medullary sponge kidney. *E:* Transverse sonogram of the liver also at age 6 shows dilated deformed bile ducts and an abnormally echogenic liver. The portal veins appear to have abnormally thick, bright walls. *F:* More cephalad view demonstrates cystic regions that did not appear to communicate with the biliary tree and an abnormally increased echo texture. The patient was well with only minimal liver function abnormalities. (Case courtesy of Kathleen Eggli, M.D., Walter Reed Army Medical Center, Washington, D.C.)

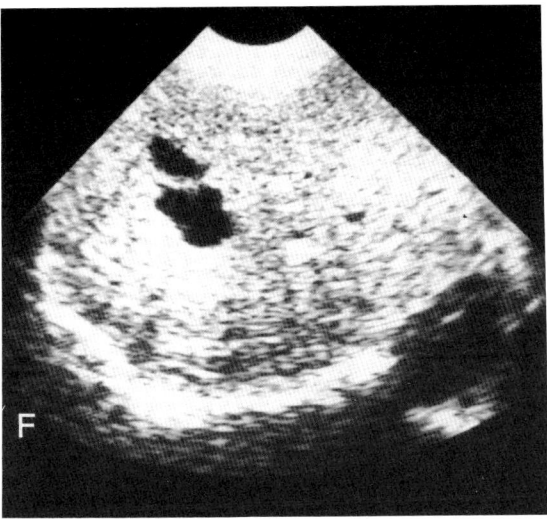

FIGURE 11.11*F*

material within the ducts representing debris or non-calcified stones is seen (9). Intrahepatic calcifications seen on plain films can be proven to be within ducts. If cystic areas predominate, their communication with the biliary tree can be proven with a repeat scan after intravenous infusion of Cholografin. Direct cholangiography by any route demonstrates saccular dilatation of the intrahepatic biliary tree with communicating cystic spaces, almost always involving both lobes (Fig. 11.12*F, G*) (12). The common bile duct is dilated as well in most illustrated cases, although there is no obstruction to the flow of contrast material into the duodenum (14, 15). Differential diagnosis includes multiple intrahepatic abscesses communicating with the biliary tree (Fig. 11.14) (2). Angiography will show displacement of vessels around the larger saccular dilatations (13).

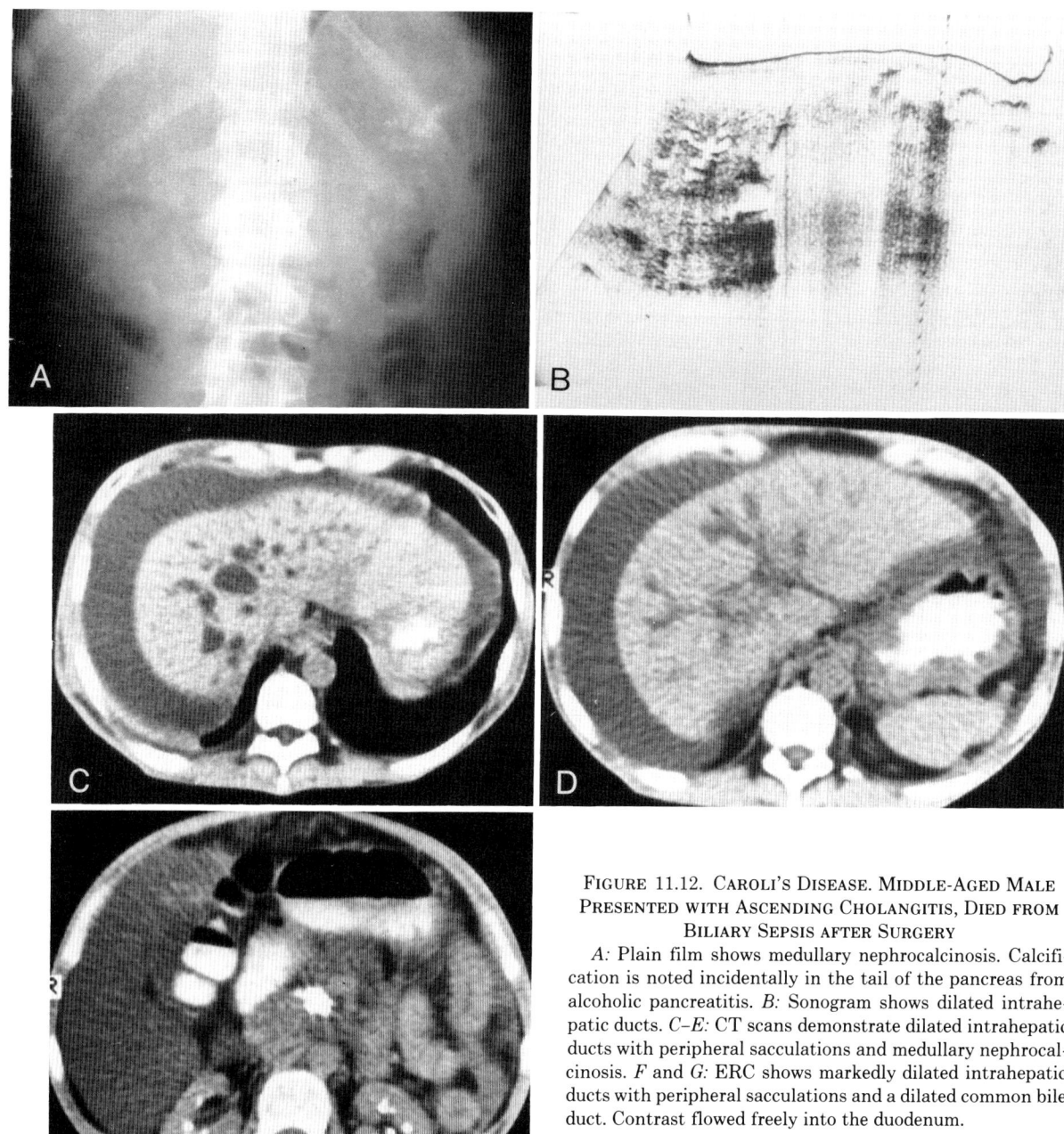

FIGURE 11.12. CAROLI'S DISEASE. MIDDLE-AGED MALE PRESENTED WITH ASCENDING CHOLANGITIS, DIED FROM BILIARY SEPSIS AFTER SURGERY

A: Plain film shows medullary nephrocalcinosis. Calcification is noted incidentally in the tail of the pancreas from alcoholic pancreatitis. *B:* Sonogram shows dilated intrahepatic ducts. *C–E:* CT scans demonstrate dilated intrahepatic ducts with peripheral sacculations and medullary nephrocalcinosis. *F* and *G:* ERC shows markedly dilated intrahepatic ducts with peripheral sacculations and a dilated common bile duct. Contrast flowed freely into the duodenum.

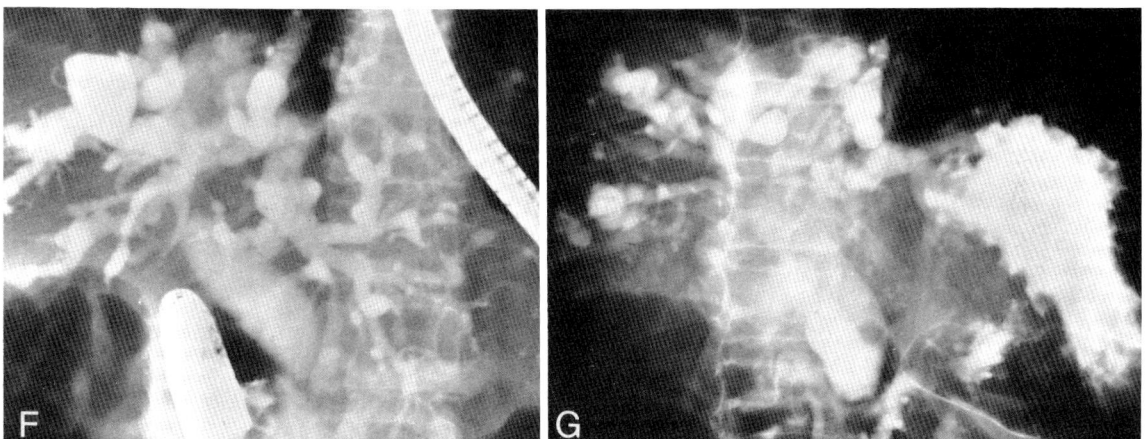

FIGURE 11.12*F* AND *G*

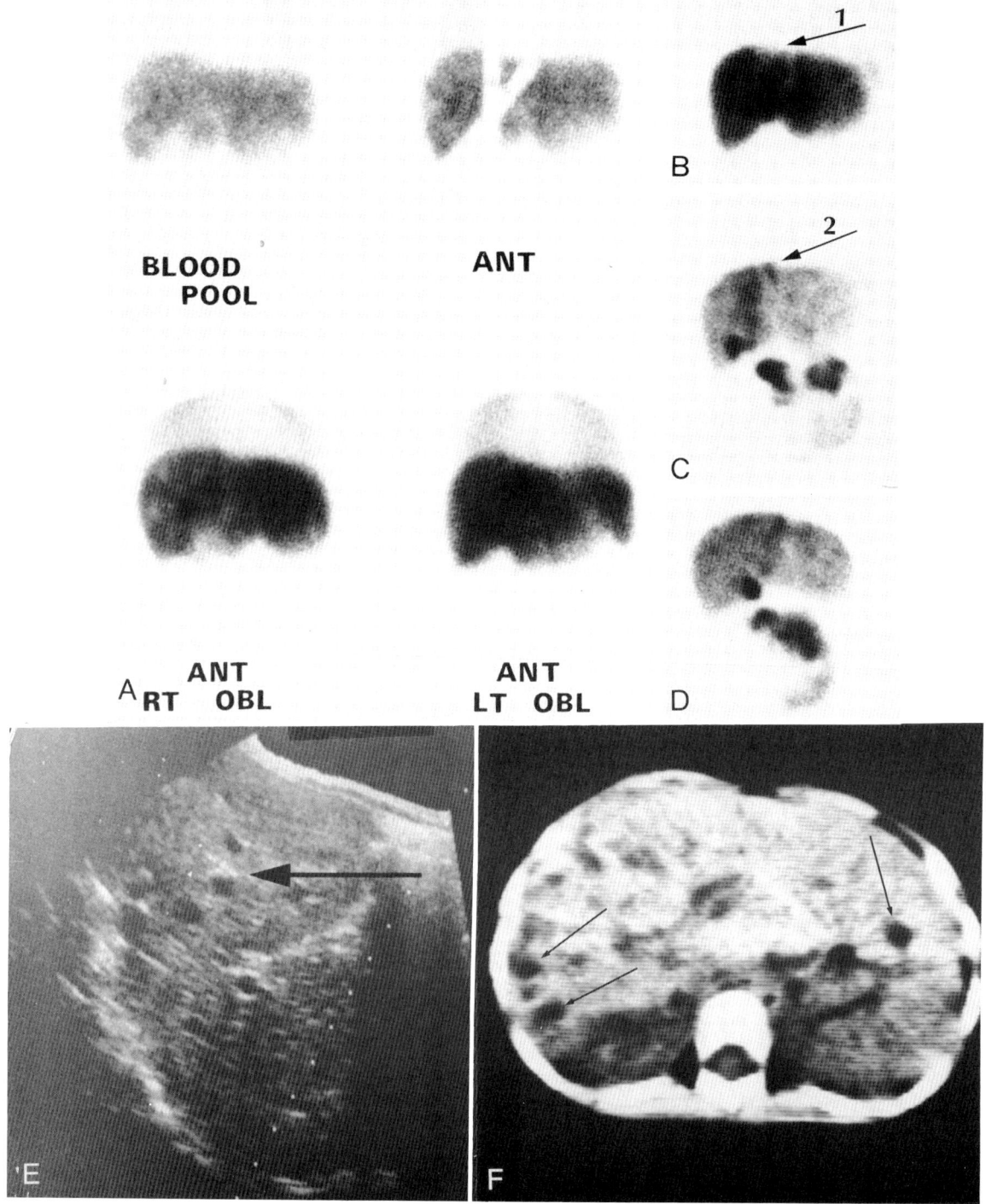

FIGURE 11.13. CAROLI'S DISEASE IN A CHILD

A: Blood pool (top row) and sulfur colloid (bottom row) scans show multiple small masses. B: A 15-min hepatobiliary scan shows a peripheral defect (arrow) that becomes hot on a 60-min image (C). C and D: Scans of 60-min images (AP and RAO) show multiple intrahepatic hot spots due to activity within dilated ducts. Compare (D) to the RAO colloid scan in (A). E and F: Correlative parasagittal sonogram and CT showing dilated intrahepatic ducts, some of which look cystic (arrows). (A–D are from Sty JR, Babbitt DP, Boedecker RA, Thompson N: ^{99m}Tc-PIPIDA biliary imaging in children. Clin Nucl Med 4:315–324, 1979.)

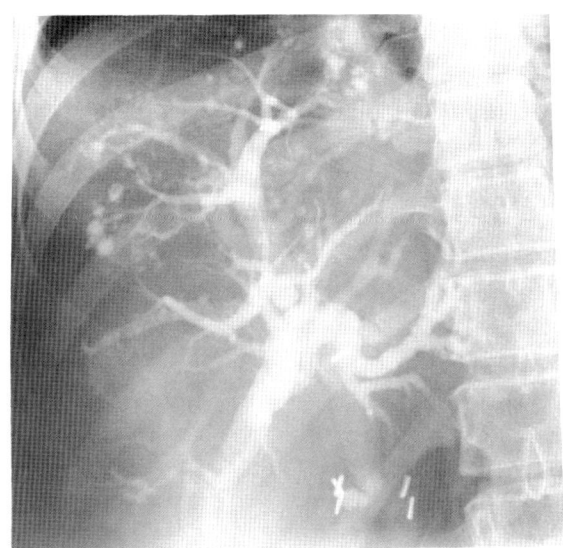

FIGURE 11.14. CAROLI'S DISEASE WITH PERIPHERAL SACCULES AS THE STRIKING FEATURE
Intrahepatic ducts are less markedly dilated compared to Figure 11.12. Differentiation from small intrahepatic abscesses requires clinical correlation.

Choledochal Cyst (Congenital Cystic Dilatation of the Common Bile Duct)

Type I choledochal cyst refers to aneurysmal dilatation of the common bile duct often accompanied by distal narrowing. Types II and III refer to choledochal diverticulum and choledochocele, respectively, and are discussed under those headings. Several theories of pathogenesis exist. Choledochal cyst presenting in childhood or adult life may be caused by anomalous union of the common bile duct and the main pancreatic duct. The normal common pancreaticobiliary channel is less than or equal to 5 mm in length. The anomaly is an elongated channel, usually 2–4 cm in length. The angle of the pancreaticobiliary junction is about 90° in the majority, and less than 90° in some. Most of the latter present relatively later in life. The anomaly leads to reflux of pancreatic secretions into the common bile duct (pancreatic secretory pressure is higher than that in the biliary tract). This is thought to lead to cholangitis, scarring, partial obstruction, wall weakening, and obstructive dilatation (3, 16–18). Choledochal cyst in neonates is frequently associated with dilatation, stenosis or atresia of other portions of the biliary tree and/or polycystic disease of the liver (1, 3). A recently advanced theory to explain this association is that choledochal cyst is part of the spectrum of infantile obstructive cholangiopathy (viral cholangitis) (19). Other theories are deficient embryologic development of the common bile duct wall leading to dilatation, and obstruction from an angulation caused by an anomalous course through the duodenal wall (18).

Clinical Findings

Choledochal cysts may present at any age from the neonate to the elderly. It usually presents in females less than ten years old (1). There is a preponderance among Japanese and other orientals (1, 7, 20). Presentation varies from nearly asymptomatic to fatal bile peritonitis from rupture (18). The classic clinical triad of intermittent jaundice, pain, and abdominal mass is only seen in about 30% (1, 3, 7, 18–22). In recent series using newer diagnostic techniques, fewer patients have the triad than in older series, reflecting earlier diagnosis (18). Infants usually present with persistent jaundice with or without a palpable mass in the right upper quadrant (3). The palpable mass may vary between examinations in size and tenseness. In older children and adults colicky right upper quadrant pain is often associated with intermittent jaundice and fever (cholangitis) (1, 20). Complications of choledochal cyst that at times are presenting features include recurrent pancreatitis, cholangitis, biliary stones, compression of adjacent organs and cholangiocarcinoma (1, 5, 7, 18, 20). Portal hypertension may be caused by portal vein compression by the cyst (1).

Preferred treatment is total removal of the dilated segment of common bile duct with Roux-en-Y choledochojejunostomy at the liver hilum to eliminate the possibility of subsequent development of malignancy in a residual cyst (20). Long term complications occur in 65% of operated patients including ascending cholangitis, anastomotic stricture, cirrhosis, residual intrahepatic biliary disease, steatorrhea, and intestinal obstruction from adhesions (3).

Pathology

Choledochal cysts are often 2–3 cm in diameter but may be much larger with a fluid capacity of up to 10 liters and a transverse diameter of 15 cm (1, 18, 19). The usual morphology is globular or fusiform dilatation of the common bile duct just below the site of entry of the cystic duct (18). There is dilatation of the left and right main intrahepatic ducts in continuity with the dilated common bile duct in up to 45% of patients (20, 22). The cystic duct is often dilated as well but the gall bladder is usually of normal size (18). Choledochal cysts are partially retroperitoneal and contain a thin, dark brown fluid that may be high in amylase (1, 18). Histologically there is fibrosis and chronic inflammation in the cyst wall (2–10 mm thick) with little or no recognizable epithelial or smooth muscle elements (1, 18).

Radiology

Most often, choledochal cysts produce mass effects on the intraperitoneal portions of the gastrointestinal tract. Retroperitoneal displacements are caused by secondary effects in the pancreatic head or unusually large cysts.

Plain films and barium contrast studies can demonstrate a subhepatic soft tissue mass in the right upper quadrant displacing the first and second portions of the duodenum and the antrum anteriorly and to the left accompanied by downward displacement of the anterior segment of the hepatic flexure (Fig. 11.15) (18). Large choledochal cysts extending into the head of the pancreas (usually seen in infants) or comitant pancreatitis can cause cephalad displacement of the antrum and widening of the duodenal sweep (Fig. 11.16) (18, 21). Esophageal varices may be present if there is biliary cirrhosis or portal vein compression (18). Calcification in the cyst wall is unusual, but opaque calculi may be present (18). Excretory urography rarely demonstrates a right upper quadrant lucency displacing the right kidney downward (Fig. 11.16C). Right-sided hydronephrosis is rare (Fig. 11.17) (18). Oral cholecystography and intravenous cholangiography may opacify the cyst if performed between attacks of hepatic dysfunction (Figs. 11.18A and B, and 11.19A) (18, 22). ^{99m}Tc IDA derivatives can usually identify choledochal cysts even in the presence of jaundice (Fig. 11.19B). Findings include normal uptake by the liver followed by accumulation and stasis in centrally dilated bile ducts and the cyst (22). Sulfur colloid scans will show only nonspecific defects in the porta hepatis (21) Sonography is usually diagnostic showing a fluid-filled mass in the porta hepatis separate from the gallbladder (Figs. 11.16D and E, 11.20A). Demonstrating a dilated cystic duct or dilated hepatic ducts entering the mass supports the diagnosis further and is more easily done with real time than static B-mode (22). Sometimes CT is helpful in delineating relationships to surrounding structures and showing the distal duct which is often obscured by gas in the duodenum on sonography (Fig. 11.16 F and G). Unless there are superimposed calculi or sludge (Fig. 11.21), choledochal cysts are sonolucent and have CT numbers similar to bile (Fig. 11.16F and G). Differential diagnosis of sonolucent, low

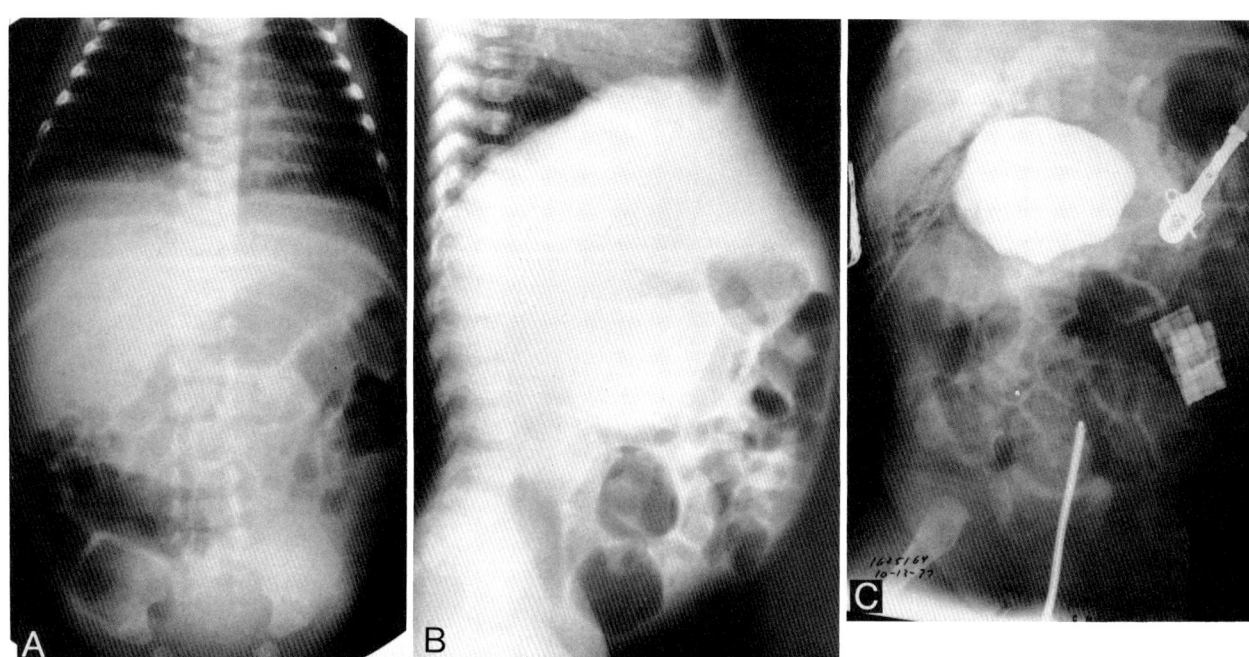

FIGURE 11.15. CHOLEDOCHAL CYST

A and B: Large, supramesocolic soft tissue mass displacing duodenum and antrum anteriorly and to the left, and displacing colon caudally. C: OR cholangiogram of the large choledochal cyst.

density masses in the porta hepatis on sonography and CT would include hepatic cyst, pancreatic pseudocyst, enteric duplication, hepatic artery aneurysm, and perforation of the extrahepatic bile duct (22). CT scanning after oral calcium ipodate or low doses of intravenous Cholografin can prove that the low density mass is biliary (Fig. 11.18C) (3, 23). Direct cholangiography, either percutaneous, retrograde or operative is sometimes needed for fine anatomic detail (Figs. 11.15C, 11.16H, 11.18D, 11.19C) and demonstration of calculi (Figs. 11.22 and 11.23) (18). ERCP or operative cholangiography sometimes demonstrates an anomalous relationship of the biliary and pancreatic ducts (Fig. 11.20B) (18, 20). Angiography, although rarely necessary, can show an avascular mass, sometimes with a rim around it, along with displacement of the gastroduodenal artery (18, 21). The cholangitis which is frequently associated can cause hypervascularity and tortuosity of the arterial branches in the cyst wall (18).

Using any imaging modality the critical point is differentiating choledochal cyst from acquired obstruction. This is only difficult when the cyst is not disproportionately larger than the rest of the biliary tree. Choledochal cyst has an abrupt change in caliber at its junction with normal biliary ducts and absence of duct dilatation in the hepatic periphery, although the left and right main hepatic ducts may be dilated (20). Acquired obstruction shows gradual tapering towards the hepatic periphery (20). Uncomplicated choledochal cyst does not cause dilatation of peripheral intrahepatic ducts even when there is obstructive jaundice. If choledochal cyst is suspected by reason of disproportionate common bile duct dilatation and dilated peripheral ducts are present, an additional obstructing lesion such as cholangiocarcinoma must be suspected (20).

REFERENCES

1. Sherlock S: *Cysts and Congenital Biliary Abnormalities in Diseases of the Liver and Biliary System*. Oxford, Blackwell Scientific Publications, 1981, pp 406–412.
2. McNulty JG: *Radiology of the Liver*. Philadelphia, W. B. Saunders, 1977, pp 167–172.
3. Berger PE, Kuhn JP: Computed tomography of the hepatobiliary system in infancy and childhood. *Radiol Clin North Am* 19:431–441, 1981.
4. San Felippo PM, Beahrs OH, Weiland LH: Cystic disease of the liver. *Ann Surg* 179:922–925, 1974.
5. Kutcher R, Schneider M, Gordon DH: Calcification in polycystic disease. *Radiology* 122:77–80, 1977.
6. Rabinowitz JG: Abnormalities of the liver and other organs. *Radiol Clin North Am* 18:286–293, 1980.
7. Thaler MM: Biliary Disease in Infancy and Childhood. In Sleisenger MH, Fordtran JS (eds): *Gastrointestinal Disease, Pathophysiology Diagnosis Management*. Philadelphia, W. B. Saunders, 1983, pp 1337–1344.
8. Franken EA Jr., Smith WL, Siddigui A: Liver disease in pediatrics. *Radiol Clin North Am* 18:248–251, 1980.
9. Kaiser JA, Mall JC, Salmen BJ, Parker JJ: Diagnosis of Caroli disease by computed tomography: report of two cases. *Radiology* 132:661–664, 1979.
10. Mittelstaedt CA, Volberg FM, Fischer GJ, McCartney WH: Caroli's disease: sonographic findings. *AJR* 134:585–587, 1980.
11. Odievre M, Chaumont P, Montagne JP, Alagille D: Anomalies of the intrahepatic portal venous system in congenital hepatic fibrosis. *Radiology* 122:247–430, 1977.
12. Doppman JL, Dunnick NR, Girton M, Fauci AS, Popvsk MA: Bile duct cysts secondary to liver infarcts: report of a case and experimental production by small vessel hepatic artery occlusion. *Radiology* 130:1–5, 1979.
13. Mujahed Z, Glenn F, Evans JA: Communicating cavernous ectasia of the intraphepatic ducts (Caroli's disease). *AJR* 113:21–26, 1971.
14. Sty JR, Sullivan P, Wagner R, Starshak, RJ: Hepatic scintigraphy in Caroli's disease. *Radiology* 127:732, 1978.
15. Lucaga J, Gomez JL, Molino C, Atienza JG: Congenital dilation of the intrahepatic bile ducts (Caroli's disease). *Radiology* 127:746–778, 1978.
16. Babbitt DP, Starshak RJ, Clemett AR: Choledochal cyst: a concept of etiology. *AJR* 119:57–62, 1973.
17. Kimura K, Ohto M, Ono T, Tsuchiya Y, Saisho H, Kawamura K, Yogi Y, Karasawa E, Okuda K: Congenital cystic dilatation of the common bile duct: relationship to anomalous pancreaticobiliary ductal union. *AJR* 128:571–577, 1977.
18. Ghahremani GG, Lu CT, Woodlief RM, Chuang VP: Choledochal cyst in adults. A clinical and radiological study in ten cases. *Gastrointest Radiol* 1:305–313, 1977.
19. Landing BH: Consideration of the pathogenesis of neonatal hepatitis, biliary atresia and choledochal cyst—the concept of infantile obstructive cholangiopathy. *Progr Pediatr Surg* 6:113, 1974.
20. Araki T, Itai Y, Tasaka A: CT of choledochal cyst. *AJR* 135:729–734, 1980.
21. Singleton EB: Pediatric Diseases of the Gallbladder and Bile Ducts. In Berk RN, Ferrucci JT, Leopold GR (eds): *Radiology of the Gallbladder and Bile Ducts*. Philadelphia, W. B. Saunders, 1983, pp 524–529.
22. Han BK, Babock DS, Gelfand MH: Choledochal cyst with bile duct dilatation: sonography and Tc^{99m}-IDA cholescintigraphy. *AJR* 136:1075–1079, 1981.
23. Pretorius DH, Gosink BB, Olson LK: CT of the opacified biliary tract: use of calcium ipodate. *AJR* 138:1073–1075, 1982.

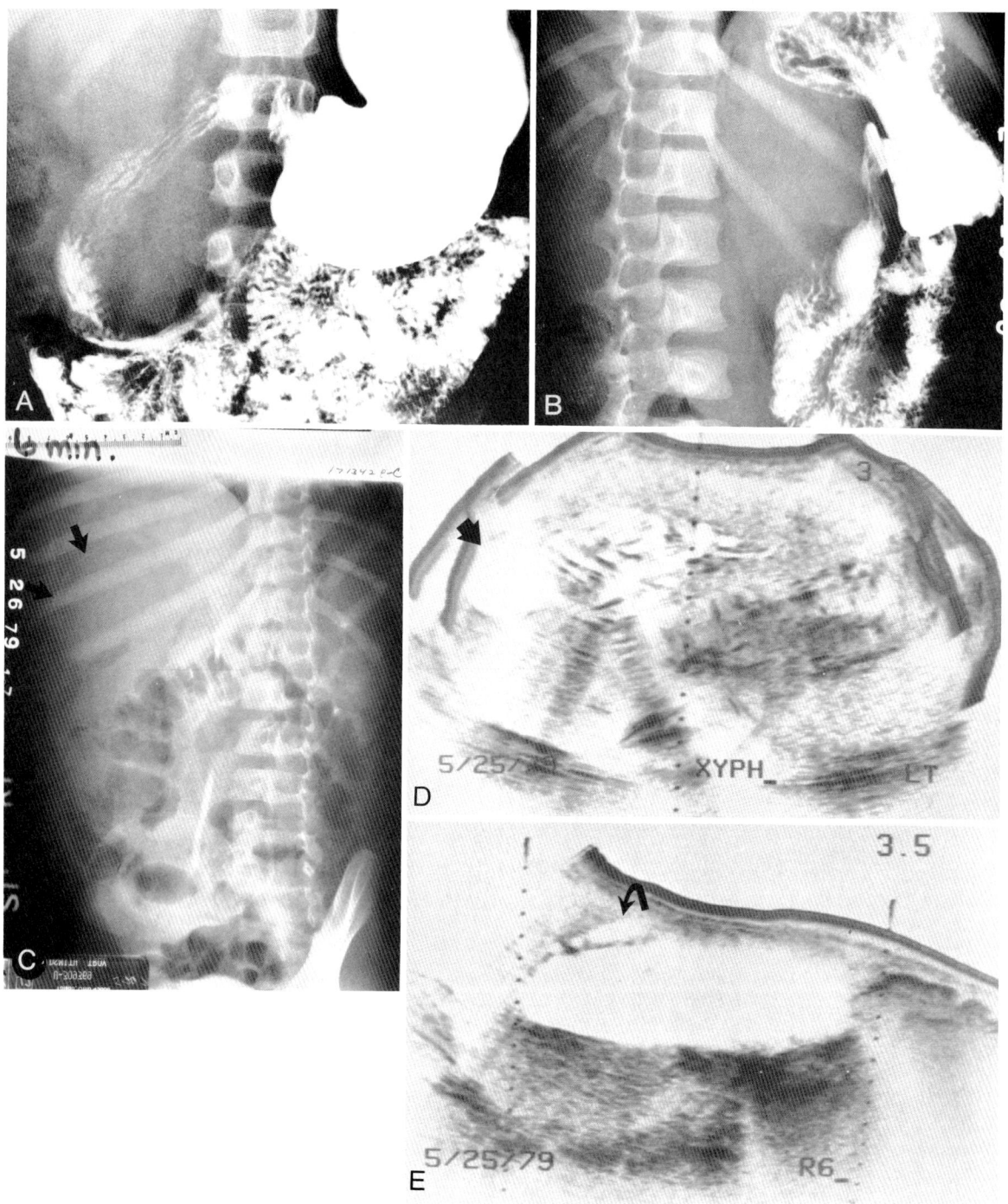

FIGURE 11.16. CHOLEDOCHAL CYST

A, B: UGI series shows displacement of the proximal duodenum and antrum anteriorly and to the left. The sweep is widened also because of the huge size of this cyst. *C:* IVP reveals a radiolucent right upper quadrant mass with a pencil thin wall (*arrows*). *D:* Transverse sonogram shows dilated distal intrahepatic ducts and the large cyst (*arrow*). *E:* Parasagittal sonogram showing the normal gallbladder (*curved arrow*) on top of the cyst. *F* and *G:* CT demonstrating the cyst (*arrows*), some dilated distal intrahepatic ducts and the normal gallbladder (*curved arrow*). *H:* Correlative OR cholangiogram.

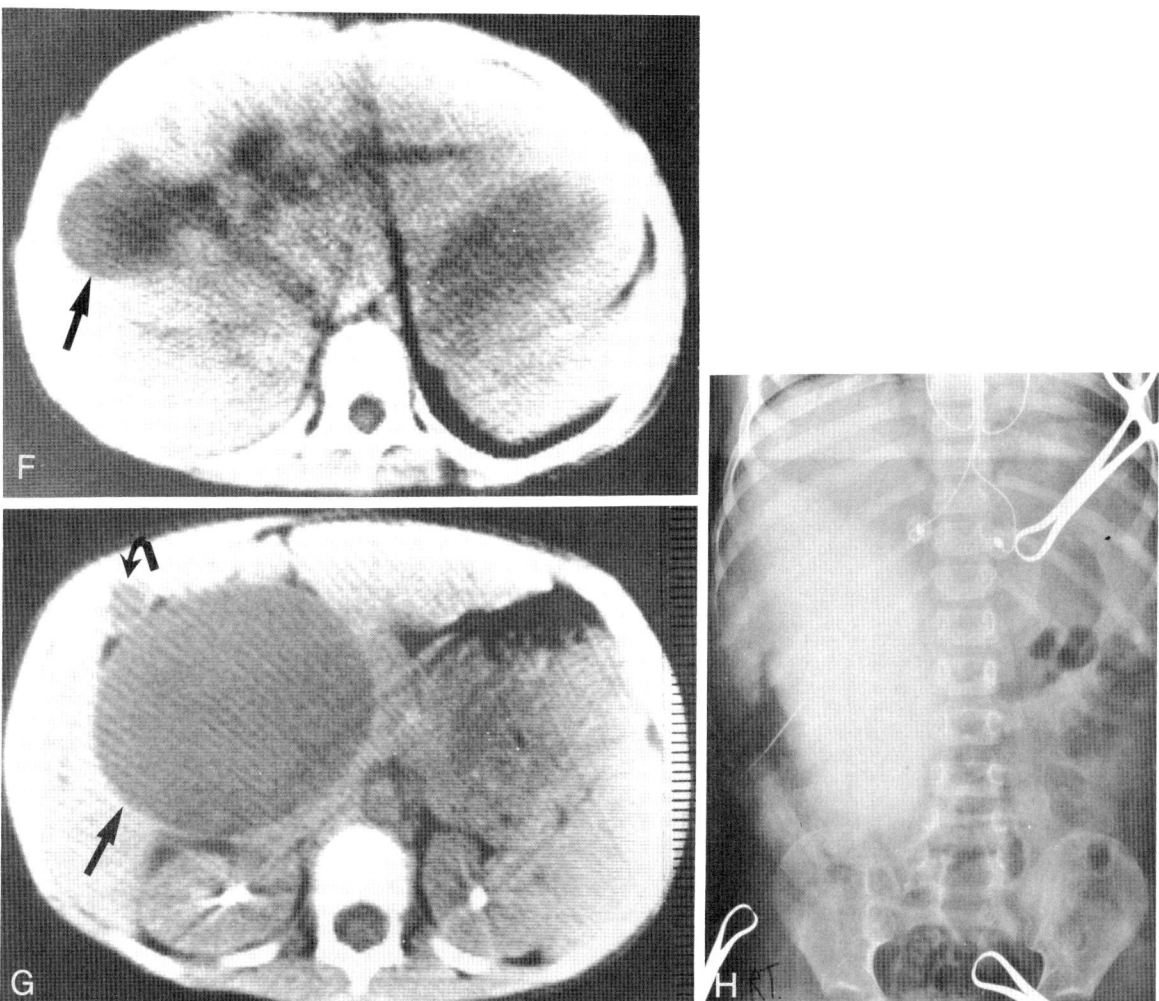

FIGURE 11.16*F–H*

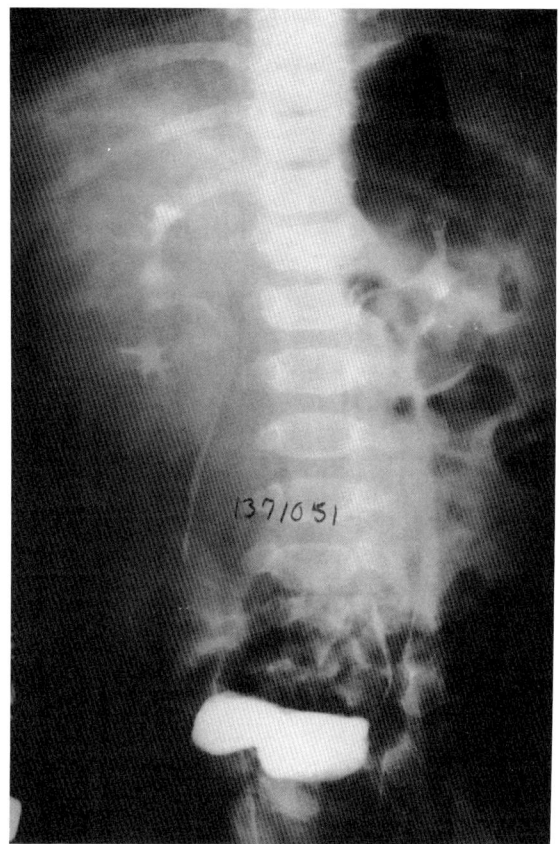

FIGURE 11.17. PANCAKING OF THE RIGHT KIDNEY AND DISPLACEMENT OF THE RIGHT URETER BY A HUGE CHOLEDOCHAL CYST
Right upper quadrant lucency is present, but subtle.

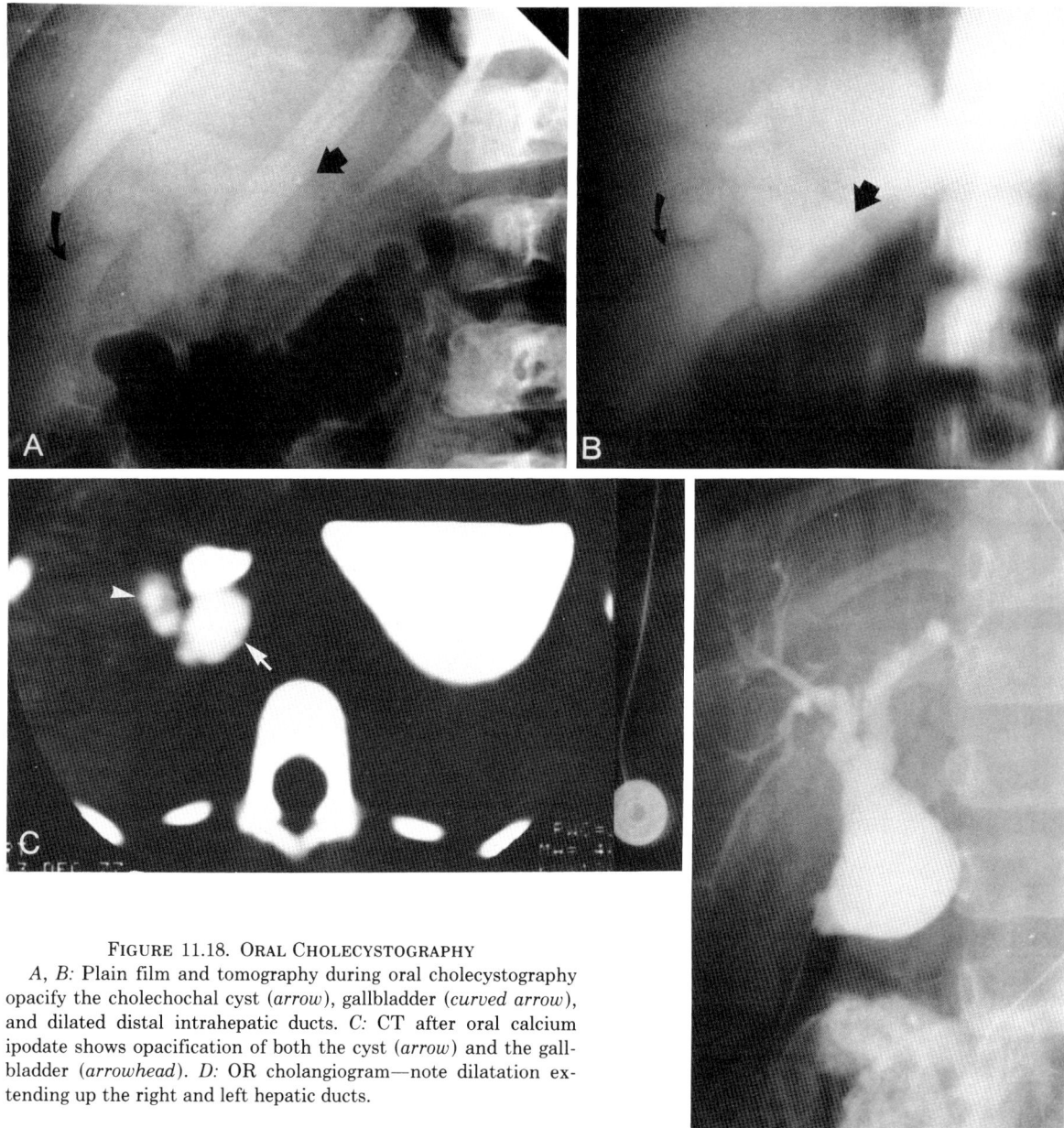

FIGURE 11.18. ORAL CHOLECYSTOGRAPHY

A, B: Plain film and tomography during oral cholecystography opacify the cholechochal cyst (*arrow*), gallbladder (*curved arrow*), and dilated distal intrahepatic ducts. *C:* CT after oral calcium ipodate shows opacification of both the cyst (*arrow*) and the gallbladder (*arrowhead*). *D:* OR cholangiogram—note dilatation extending up the right and left hepatic ducts.

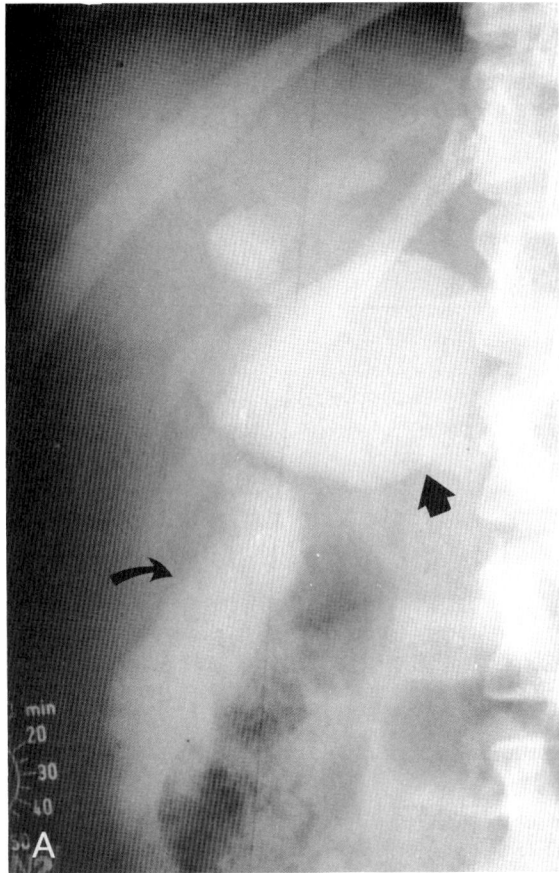
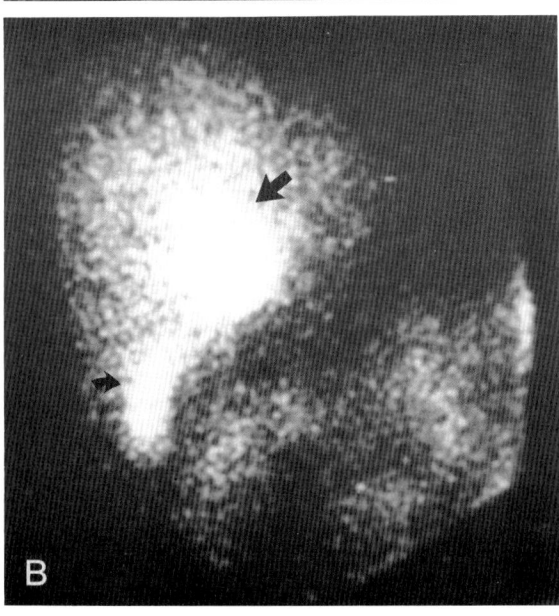
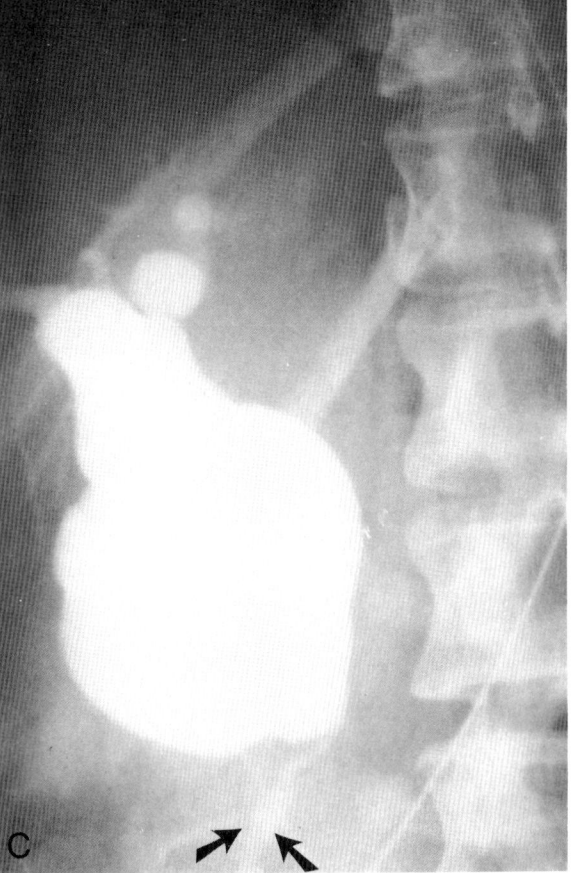

FIGURE 11.19. INTRAVENOUS CHOLANGIOGRAM
A: Intravenous cholangiogram opacifies choledochal cyst (*arrow*), gallbladder (*curved arrow*), and dilated distal hepatic ducts. *B:* Radionuclide cholescintigram with activity in the choledochal cyst (*arrow*) and gallbladder (*curved arrow*). *C:* OR cholangiogram shows the cyst and the dilated distal hepatic ducts. Note flow of contrast into the duodenum (*arrows*).

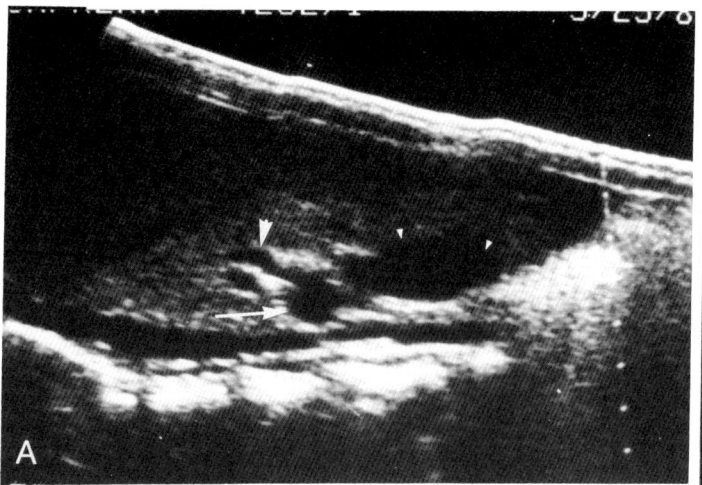
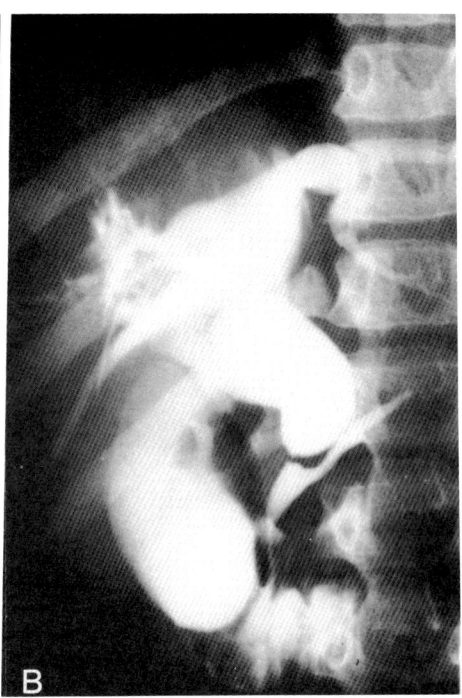

FIGURE 11.20. CHOLEDOCHAL CYST
A: Parasagittal sonogram demonstrates a choledochal cyst (*arrow*) connected to the dilated common duct (*large arrowhead*) and separate from the gallbladder (*small arrowheads*). *B:* PTC reveals the anomalous pancreaticobiliary connection.

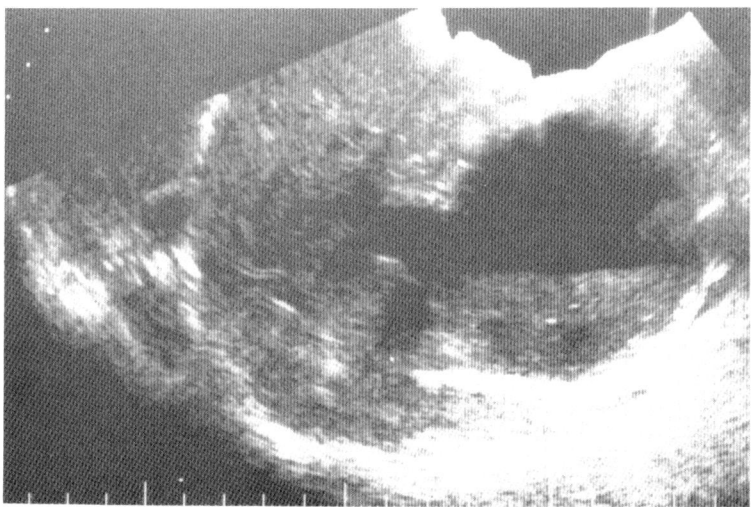

FIGURE 11.21. FLUID-SLUDGE LEVEL IN A HUGE CHOLEDOCHAL CYST

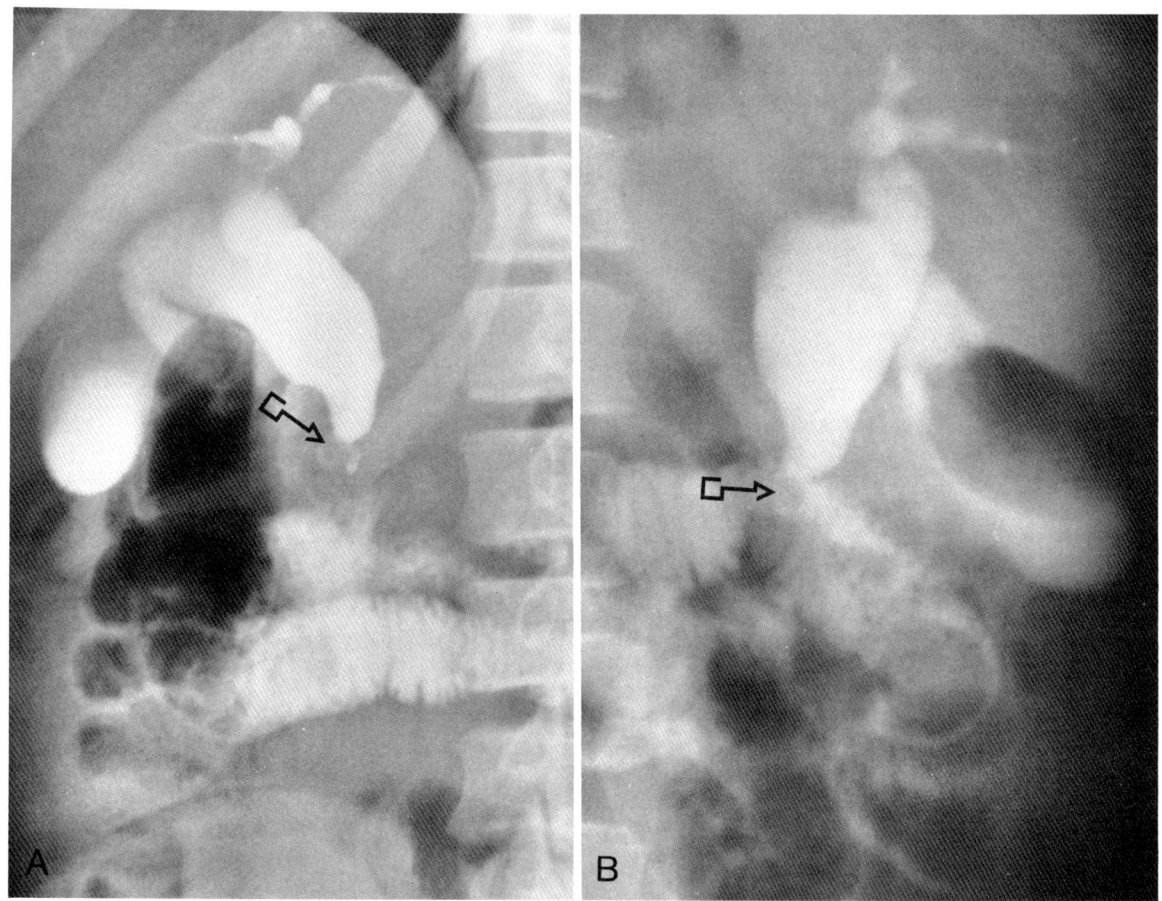

FIGURE 11.22. STONE IMPACTED IN DISTAL ASPECT OF CHOLEDOCHAL CYST
A, B: Stone impacted in distal aspect of a choledochal cyst (*arrows*) on ERCP. Note dilated distal hepatic ducts without dilated proximal intraheptic ducts.

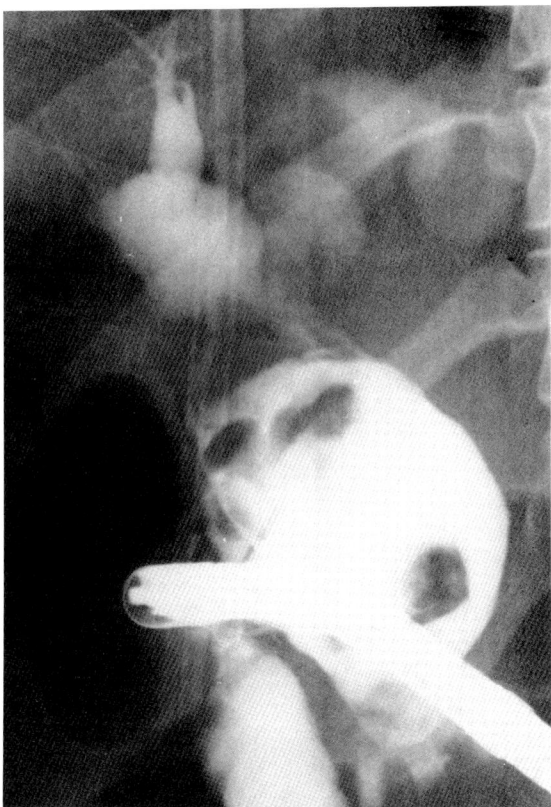

FIGURE 11.23. ERCP
ERCP shows many stones filling a large choledochal cyst, and dilated distal hepatic ducts tapering to normal caliber proximal intrahepatic ducts.

COMMON BILE DUCT DIVERTICULUM (TYPE II CHOLEDOCHAL CYST)

Type II choledochal cyst is a congenital diverticulum of the common bile duct usually protruding from its lateral wall (1, 2). It is a rare anomaly that can be diagnosed in children or adults. Similar diverticula may occur off the lateral margin of the right main hepatic duct (3, 4).

Presentation varies from pain with a palpable mass to asymptomatic. As with type I choledochal cyst, portal hypertension and varices may be produced by portal vein compression. Liver enzymes may be elevated, but jaundice is unusual. Surgical excision is the usual treatment. The diverticula have a fibrous wall lined by flattened and atrophic bile duct epithelium (2).

Sonography will detect bile duct diverticula as sonolucent masses contiguous to the common bile duct or right hepatic duct (Fig. 11.24A). The actual neck connecting the cyst to the duct is difficult to depict (1, 2). Stones or sludge may be present within the diverticulum (3, 4). Cholangiography and radionuclide hepatobiliary scintigraphy may or may not fill the diverticulum since its neck may not be patent (1, 2). When not opacified, a diverticulum may produce a rounded, smooth, extrinsic compression of the adjacent duct of unclear etiology on cholangiography (Fig. 11.24B) (2). Differentiating bile duct diverticula from hepatic cysts or the gallbladder should be difficult on CT because of the limitations of scanning in the axial plane only.

The rare infected choledochal diverticulum can present clinically and radiologically like a neoplasm (Fig. 11.25). The low grade chronic infection causes an inflammatory mass that mimics a carcinoma of the common duct even at surgery.

REFERENCES

1. Morgan CL, Trought WS, Oddson TA, Thompson WM: Type II choledochal cyst: ultrasonographic appearance.

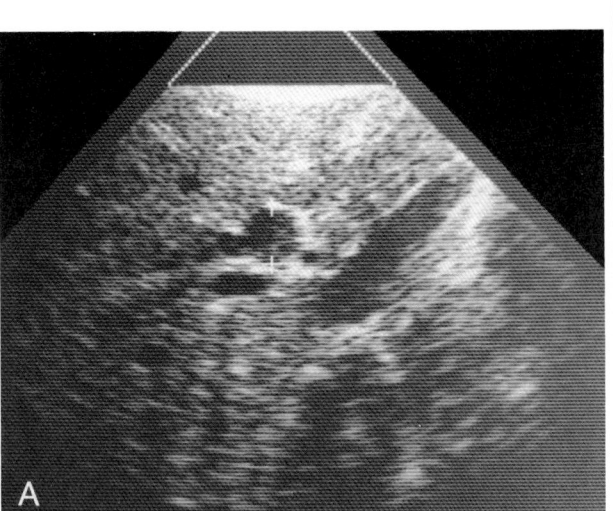
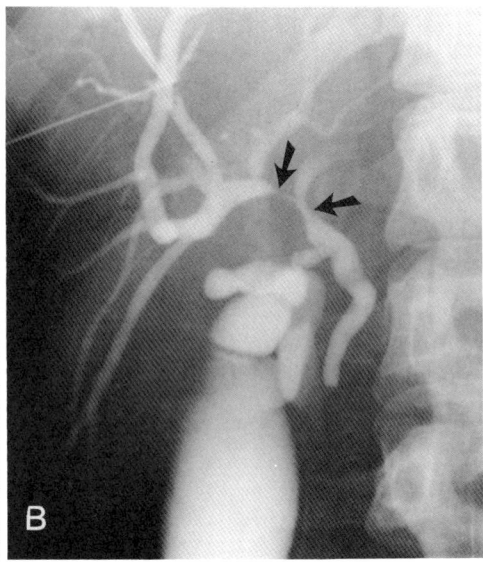

FIGURE 11.24. BILE DUCT DIVERTICULUM
A: Parasagittal real-time sonogram depicting a common bile duct diverticulum (*cursors*) as a round sonolucency intimately related to the biliary tract in the porta hepatis. B: Ensuing transhepatic cholangiogram: non-opacification of the diverticulum. High-grade smooth stenosis at the bifurcation (*arrows*) caused by the diverticulum. (From Richardson JD et al: Type II choledochal cyst: diagnosis using real-time sonography. *J Ultrasound Med* 3:37–39, 1984.)

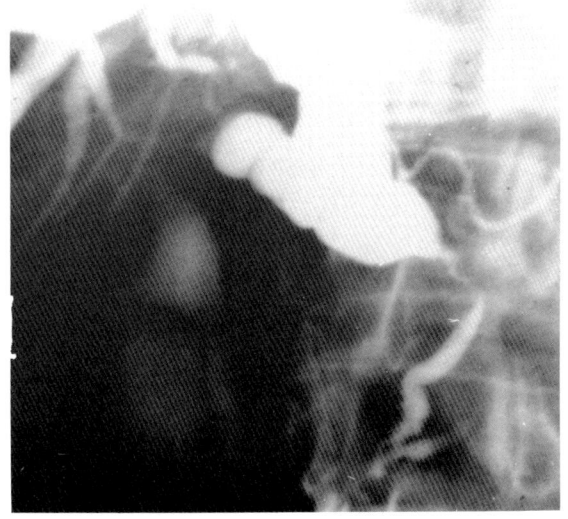

FIGURE 11.25. INFECTED COMMON BILE DUCT
PTC: irregular stenosis of the common bile duct causing a high grade obstruction. Diagnosis of infected common bile duct diverticulum was not made until autopsy. Diagnosis at exploratory laparotomy was unresectable carcinoma of the common duct.

Radiology 132:130, 1979.
2. Richardson JD, Grant EG, Barth KH, Arnstein N, Jacobs N, DeRosa R, Chun BK: Type II choledochal cyst: diagnosis using real-time sonography. *J Ultrasound Med* 3:37–39, 1984.
3. Meyers C, Reynes CJ, Freeark RJ: Diverticulum of the hepatic duct: a rare anomaly. *Radiology* 119:38, 1976.
4. Schey WL, Pinsky SM, Lipschutz HS, Dragomer AS: Hepatic duct diverticulum simulating a choledochal cyst. *AJR* 128:318–320, 1977.

CHOLEDOCHOCELE (TYPE III CHOLEDOCHAL CYST)

Choledochocele is a rare and easily overlooked anomaly of unknown etiology. It has been reported under the names diverticulum of the common bile duct, cyst of the intraduodenal bile duct, cyst of the papilla of Vater, enterogenous cyst of the duodenum and duplication cyst of the duodenum in addition to type III choledochal cyst (1). Analogous to a ureterocele, it is a protrusion of a dilated intramural common duct into the duodenum. Pathogenetic theories include inflammatory reaction at the papilla with obstructive ballooning of the intramural duct, congenital duodenal duplication cyst receiving the common duct, choledochal cyst of the intramural common duct, and congenital common bile duct diverticulum (1, 2).

Clinical Findings

Choledochocele can present in childhood or adulthood. Long-standing episodic abdominal pain, nausea, and vomiting are the most common complaints (2). Biliary colic, episodic jaundice, and pancreatitis are frequent (1, 2). The anomaly may be an incidental finding (2). Treatment is duodenotomy with marsupialization or endoscopic electrosurgical incision (1).

Pathology

Choledochoceles are bile-filled and attached to the posterior or posteromedial wall of the duodenum in the region of the ampulla. Stones or sludge are frequently present. There are two anatomic types which are often not differentiated surgically or radiographically (2). In the first, the common bile duct terminates into the choledochocele which drains into the duodenum via an aperture in its wall. The main pancreatic duct may also empty into the choledochocele. The second type occurs when the choledochocele fills and empties via the common bile duct and the latter drains into the duodenum via a normal papilla. The main pancreatic duct usually inserts into the bile duct proximal to the choledochocele in this variant.

Histologically, the external surface of the choledochocele is covered by duodenal mucosa. The internal surface is lined by duodenal, biliary, or nonspecific enteric epithelium (1).

Radiology

Duodenography will demonstrate a well-defined, smooth filling defect projecting into the

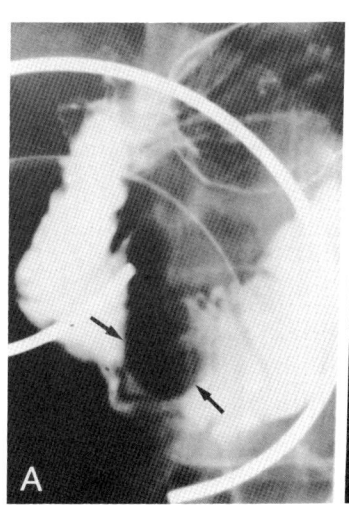
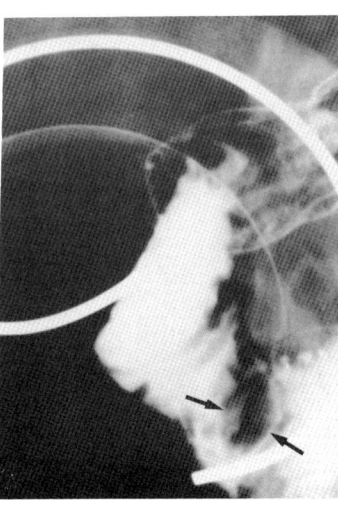
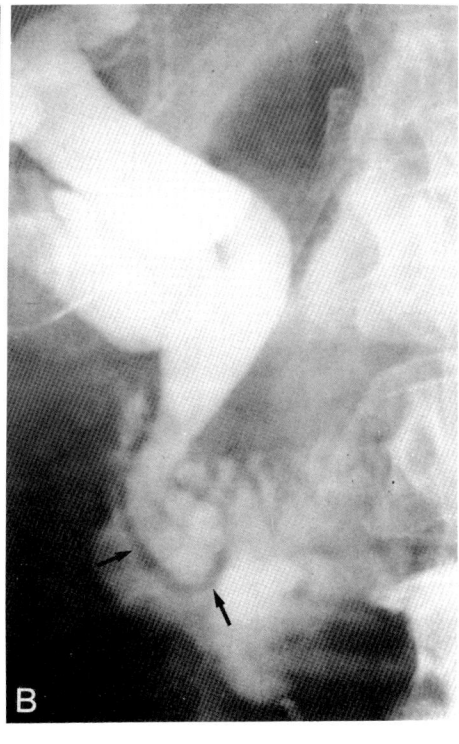

FIGURE 11.26. DUODENOGRAPHY
A: Duodenogram with graded compression: smooth, compressible submucosal mass decreases in size from left to right as compression is increased (arrows). B: Transhepatic cholangiogram: dilated ducts proximal to the choledochocele. Note its thin wall (arrows).

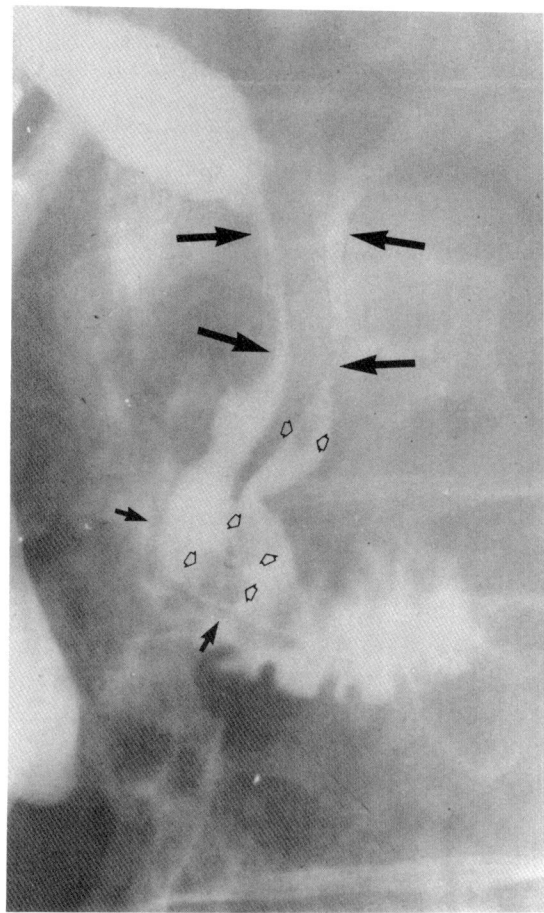

FIGURE 11.27. CHOLEDOCHOCELE
Choledochocele causing pancreatitis; T-tube cholangiogram: choledochocele with thin wall (*small arrows*) containing calculi (*open arrows*). Calculus in pancreatic duct as well (*open arrows*). Adjacent narrowing of common bile and pancreatic ducts (*large arrows*) caused by pancreatitis. Dilated proximal bile ducts.

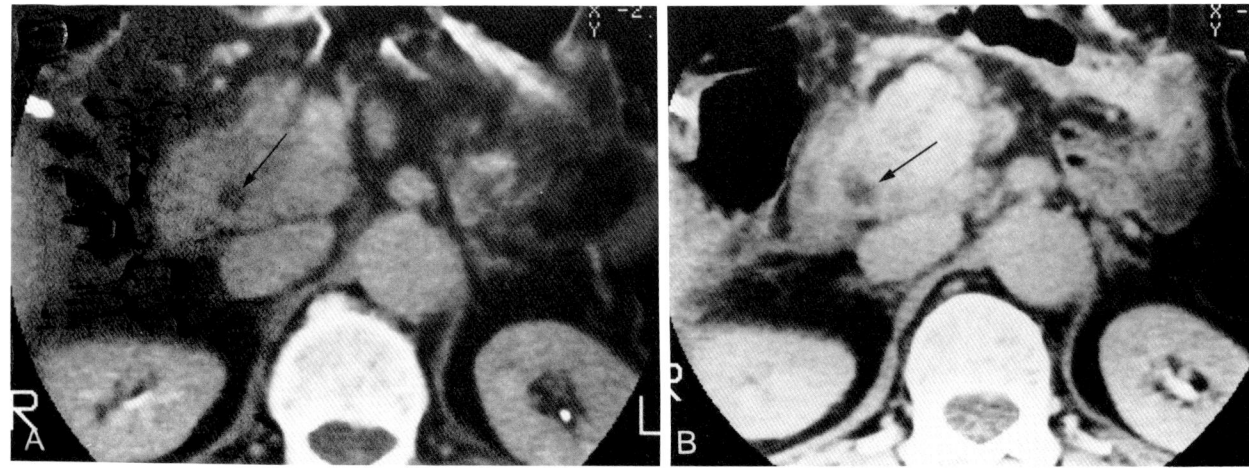

FIGURE 11.28. CT OF CHOLEDOCHOCELE
CT of choledochocele: slightly prominent common bile duct in the head of the pancreas (A, *arrow*) widens into the choledochocele (B, *arrow*, 10 mm caudad to A). Findings are suggestive but not specific.

lumen, either broad-based or narrow and pedunculated (Fig. 1.26A) (2). A change in shape with compression and/or peristalsis is typical. In contradistinction to intraluminal diverticula, choledochoceles will not fill with barium.

Most choledochoceles fill with contrast during intravenous cholangiography, however findings may be nonspecific, ie, dilatation of the common bile duct with delayed excretion or even normal (2). Direct cholangiography best demonstrates the choledochocele as a saccular dilatation of the intramural common bile duct (Figs. 11.26B, and 11.27). Simultaneous opacification of the duodenum is important to show a thin wall and exclude tumor as the cause of obstruction. Choledochocele should be difficult to diagnose by ultrasound, CT (Fig. 11.28), or biliary scintigraphy.

REFERENCES

1. Zimmon DS, Falkenstein DB, Mannon BV, Clemett AR: Choledochocoele: radiographic diagnosis and endoscopic management. *Gastrointest Radiol* 3:349–351, 1978.
2. Scholz FJ, Carrera GF, Larsen CR: The choledochocoele: correlation of radiological, clinical and pathological findings. *Radiology* 118:25–28, 1976.

12

Cholelithiasis and Cholecystitis

LEORA SACHS, M.D., JOEL E. LICHTENSTEIN, M.D., ARNOLD C. FRIEDMAN, M.D., MARK T. BIRNS, M.D., AND JAMES G. SMIRNIOTOPOULOS, M.D.

CHOLELITHIASIS

Gallstones are known to have afflicted humans since earliest recorded history, being found in mummies from 1500 BC (1). Today, gallbladder disease is the most common indication for abdominal surgery in the United States, leading to some 500,000 cholecystectomies per year. Associated expenses approach one billion dollars (2). Calculi are responsible for approximately 95% of this morbidity. About 15–20 million Americans have gallstones, the majority of which are asymptomatic or "silent" (3–5). An additional one million cases are discovered each year. In most series, women outnumber men by about three or four to one. Obesity remains as a possible risk factor (6), but, in other respects the common aphorism of "female, forty, fair, fat, fertile, and flatulent" appears to be invalid. Diabetes, use of oral contraceptives, disturbance of absorption from the distal ileum, and prior truncal vagotomy are, however, associated with increased incidence of gallstones (7–9). The incidence of stones increases with age in both sexes, with peak clinical presentation in the fifties and sixties. The female predominance is less marked in the elderly. Gallstones are rare in childhood when hemolytic anemia is a classic association, though actually seen in only a minority of cases (10). In the dark skinned Pima Indians, 70% of women have gallstones by age 30 and men approach the same prevalence later in life (11).

Pathophysiology

Bile is produced in the liver by the hepatocytes and excreted into the ductal system. In addition to water, the major constituents of bile (over 90% dry weight) are conjugated bile salts, phospholipids (principally lecithin), and cholesterol (12, 13). Bile salts are water-soluble, have detergent properties, and form tiny aggregates in water called micelles. Lecithin and cholesterol are insoluble in water, and are maintained in solution only by being incorporated into the micelles.

The normal gallbladder functions as a reservoir for bile which it concentrates by removing water. Concentration of any of the constituents beyond relatively narrow ranges results in supersaturation with precipitation into solid crystals. Supersaturation of cholesterol may sometimes be caused by enhanced absorption of bile salts and lecithin by the inflamed gallbladder wall during bouts of acute cholecystitis. Bacteria, foreign material, abnormal bile pigments, and mucoproteins have been postulated to form the necessary nidus for initiation of crystallization. Continued growth of the crystals results in macroscopic stones. Aggregation of crystalline cholesterol around a nidus tends to occur in concentric layers forming light-colored, yellowish, soft, rounded, low density, laminated stones. When multiple their impingement upon one another leads to flattened interfaces or large facets. Cholesterol is the constituent most commonly present in excess and forms the main component of most calculi (about 80% in the United States). Pure cholesterol stones are yellowish, soft, and low density. Radiographically, these tend to be lucent and may float in opacified gallbladder bile. However, only about 10% of all cholesterol stones are pure cholesterol. The remainder are mixtures of cholesterol with calcium carbonate and calcium bilirubinate. The calcium content in bile is variable, some of it being bound in the micelles. Inorganic ions such as calcium are incorporated into the growing crystals in amounts depending upon their varying concentration in the bile (14). This produces the laminated appearance frequently seen radiographically as well as grossly. The calcium content of gallstones accounts for the 10–20% which are radioopaque. When calcium carbonate precipitates it produces gray-white particles ranging from sand-like up to several centimeters in diameter. Pure calcium carbonate stones are rare, however.

The incidence of cholesterol stones is about three times as great in women than in men and increases with age. Genetic factors and obesity are additional probable predisposing conditions. Crohn's disease in or resection of the terminal ileum predispose to gallstones by interfering with enterohepatic circulation of bile. Gallbladder stasis seen in diabetes and after truncal vagotomy may be responsible for gallstone formation in some patients. Cystic fibrosis, type IV hyperlipidemia, oral contraceptives, and clofibrate also increase cholesterol gallstone incidence (15).

Pigment stones by definition contain less than 25% cholesterol, and account for about 20% of gallstones in the United States. Calcium bilirubinate is the main component with varying amounts of carbonate. Depending upon the relative amount of pigment they may be black or brown. They usually are multiple, tiny, and may be faceted or irregularly spiculated. Pigment stones are formed after β-glucuronidase deconjugates the soluble bilirubin diglucuronide normally present in bile to free bilirubin which then combines with calcium to form the insoluble calcium bilirubinate. Bile normally contains enough glucaric acid (a β-glucuronidase inhibitor) to prevent deconjugation. Pigment stones occur with increased incidence in hemolytic states, chronic liver disease, and congenital or acquired diseases associated with biliary stasis and/or infection. In hemolytic states, the increased biliary excretion of conjugated bilirubin overwhelms inhibitors of deconjugation leading to nearly pure calcium bilirubinate stones. These tend to be tiny, black, multiple, and often irregular. Biliary stagnation also facilitates deconjugation. Some bacteria produce the enzyme beta-glucuronidase, explaining the increased incidence of pigment calculi in disease states associated with chronic biliary infection (15).

Since the composition of bile is not constant, continued crystalline growth under differing conditions successive layers of precipitates. Hence, stones vary in composition and radiographic appearance.

Natural History and Clinical Considerations

Given conditions favoring precipitation of bile, there is tremendous variability in the physical form of the precipitate and in the resulting clinical manifestations. Stasis may produce a thick sludge which settles under the effect of gravity. Its separation from thinner bile is detected by ultrasound, but the material does not cause the shadowing seen with larger particles. Its chemical and physical nature has been debated but it now seems that sludge is composed of calcium bilirubinate granules and cholesterol crystals (16, 17).

Tiny, sand grain-like, particulate precipitates probably can pass through the cystic and common ducts into the bowel without much notice. Larger particles may remain in the gallbladder indefinitely either as "silent" stones without significant inflammation or they may be associated with chronic cholecystitis. If small stones migrate from the gallbladder lumen they cause symptoms in several ways. They are most likely to obstruct the thin, tortuous cystic duct with its valves of Heister, causing hyperemia and edema of the gallbladder wall. If transient, the result is a typical "gallbladder attack" with biliary colic. Biliary pain will develop in initially asymptomatic patients with gallstones at a rate of approximately 2% per year (18). Biliary "colic" is steady, severe aching or pressure usually in the right upper quadrant or epigastrium at times radiating to the scapula. Onset is sudden and duration is usually 1–3 hr. Nausea is common and vomiting occurs occasionally. Pain subsides after the stone falls back into the gallbladder or passes through the cystic duct. Attacks are unpredictable and no evidence exists that fatty meal ingestion specifically produces an attack of colic. Liver enzymes are usually normal.

Obstructing stones may become dislodged and remain in the gallbladder lumen with a return to normal function. Repeated episodes of obstruction and inflammation related to the persistent presence of the stones often eventuates in decreased absorptive function. Persistent obstruction produces acute inflammation (gallstones are present in about 90% of cases of acute cholecystitis). Absorption diminishes and inflammatory exudate is produced resulting in distention or hydrops. (The term "hydrops" is sometimes reserved for the chronic state in which the duct remains obstructed but the inflammation subsides. Bile salts and pigments are slowly absorbed leaving a mucoid material distending the lumen.) Infection becomes increasingly common with time, cultures being positive in 80% at 1 week (19). If a stone passes through the cystic duct, the ampulla of Vater is the next most likely site of obstruction. Persistent blockage at that point is the most common cause of "surgical" jaundice. Cholangitis and pancreatitis may also result.

The serosal surface of an inflamed gallbladder becomes sticky and may adhere to adjacent structures. With continued inflammation, calculi, especially large ones, may erode through the wall to form a fistula and eventually migrate from the gallbladder lumen into that of another hollow viscus. The proximal duodenum is the classic target organ. If the stone obstructs the bowel, gallstone ileus is the term applied. The point of obstruction is determined by the relative size of the stone and bowel lumen. The terminal ileum is the most common site of such obstruction, but large stones may obstruct more proximally and there may be intermittent transient obstruction before the final site is reached. Alternatively the stone may erode into the hepatic flexure of the colon. In that case, it may be eliminated without obstructing, or it may occlude the colon at a point of relative narrowing, usually in the descending or sigmoid segments. Rarely a gallstone will erode into the antrum of the stomach and may cause gastric outlet obstruction (20).

Mirizzi syndrome has a similar pathophysiology except that a stone, usually impacted in the gallbladder neck or cystic duct, does not extrude completely into another viscus. The inflammatory mass surrounding the diseased, stone-containing gallbladder obstructs the common hepatic duct. The diagnosis may be difficult if the causative stone is poorly mineralized. The syndrome sometimes manifests itself clinically as a mere routine cholecystitis (21). Surgery is difficult, sometimes leading to inadvertent disruption of biliary drainage (22, 23), as described by Mirizzi, an Argentine surgeon also credited with development of operative cholangiography.

Treatment

Cholecystectomy is the definitive treatment for gallstones and is generally indicated in the face of symptoms. Cholecystostomy and drainage may be elected in poor risk patients if the common duct is not also obstructed. Since an acute attack frequently resolves spontaneously, there is debate over immediate versus delayed operation if the disease is not becoming more severe. In any case, there is seldom need for emergency surgery in uncomplicated cholecystitis. Facilities for operative cholangiography should be available. Management of asymptomatic patients with gallstones is controversial. Mortality for elective operation is less than 0.5% and no changes in digestion or even in intestinal bile acid concentration can be determined after cholecystectomy (19, 24–26). On the other hand, the incidence of eventual complications from silent stones is debatable but low and current opinion holds that stones do not cause painless dyspepsia or fatty food intolerance. Observation is often advised in those over the age of 50, whereas prophylactic cholecystectomy is usually recommended in younger patients (15, 27, 28). Marked obesity and cirrhosis are relative contraindications and angina pectoris or recent myocardial infarction are contraindications to prophylactic surgery. Diabetes is an indication for prophylactic surgery because of the increased incidence and severity of septic complications in diabetics. Medical therapy with chenodeoxycholic acid can be considered for some patients. A functioning gallbladder on oral cholecystography is a requirement, as is absence of calcification (dissolution therapy is unsuccessful with bile pigment and calcium carbonate stones). Floating stones (essentially pure cholesterol) are most likely to dissolve. Buoyancy is assessed by oral cholecystography or oral cholecystosonography (sonography after administration of an oral cholecystopaque) (29). Problems with oral dissolution therapy include: only a 15–20% success rate, recurrence after drug cessation, diarrhea and mild transaminase elevation, clinically significant but reversible liver disease, and elevation of serum cholesterol. Long-term safety is unproven (30, 31).

REFERENCES

1. Shehadi WH: The biliary system through the ages. *Int Surg* 64:63–78, 1979.
2. Isselbacher KJ: A medical treatment for gallstones? *N Engl J Med* 286:40–42, 1972.
3. Friedman GD, Kannel WB, Dawber TR: The epidermiology of gallbladder disease: observations in the Framinham study. *J Chronic Dis* 19:273–292, 1966.
4. Ingelfinger FJ: Digestive disease as a national problem. V. Gallstones. *Gastroenterology* 55:102–104, 1968.
5. Wilbur RS, Bolt RJ: Incidence of gallbladder disease in "normal" men. *Gastroenterology* 36:251–255, 1959.
6. Bennion LJ, Grundy SM: Risk factors for the development of cholelithiasis in man. *N Engl J Med* 299:1161–1167, 1221–1227, 1978.
7. Small DM: The formation and treatment of gallstones. In Schiff L, Schiff ER (eds): *Diseases of the Liver*. Philadelphia, J. B. Lippincott, 1982, pp 151–166.
8. Tompkins RK, Kraft AR, Zimmerman E, Lichtenstein JE, Zollinger RM: Clinical and biochemical evidence of increased gallstone formation after complete vagotomy. *Surgery* 71:196–200, 1972.
9. Ihasz M, Griffith CA: Gallstones after vagotomy. *Am J Surg* 141:48–50, 1981.
10. Harned RK, Babbitt DP: Cholelithiasis in children. *Radiology* 117:391–393, 1975.
11. Sampliner RE, Bennett PH, Comess LJ, Rose FA, Burch TA: Gallbladder disease in Pima Indians: demonstration of high prevalence and early onset by cholecystography. *N Engl J Med* 283:1358–1364, 1970.
12. Small DM: Gallstones. *N Engl J Med* 279:588–593, 1968.
13. Small DM: The formation of gallstones. *Adv Intern Med* 16:243–264, 1970.
14. Bouchier IAD: Biochemistry of gallstone formation. *Clin Gastroenterol* 12:25–48, 1983.

15. Schoenfield LJ: *Diseases of the Gallbladder and Biliary System.* Clinical Gastroenterology Monographs. New York, John Wiley & Sons, 1977.
16. Allen B, Bernhoft R, Blanckaert N, Svanvik J, Gooding G, Way L: Sludge is calcium bilirubinate associated with bile stasis. *Am J Surg* 141:51–56, 1981.
17. Filly RA, Allen B, Minton MJ, Bernhoft R, Way LW: In vitro investigation of the origin of echoes within biliary sludge. *J Clin Ultrasound* 8:193–200, 1980.
18. Newman HF, Northrup JD, Rosenblum M et al: Complications of cholelithiasis. *Am J Gastroenterol* 50:476–496, 1968.
19. Way LW, Sleisenger MH: Acute cholecystitis and cholelithiasis and chronic cholecystitis. In Sleisenger MH, Fordtran JS (eds): *Gastrointestinal Diseases.* Philadelphia, W. B. Saunders, 1983, pp 1374–1389.
20. Rigler LG, Borman CN, Noble JF: Gallstone obstruction: pathogenesis and roentgen manifestations. *JAMA* 117:1753–1759, 1941.
21. Clemett AR, Lowman RM: The roentgen features of the Mirizzi syndrome. *AJR* 94:480–483, 1965.
22. Mirizzi PL: Sindrome del conducto hepatico. *J Int Chir* 8:731–777, 1948.
23. Mirizzi PL: Operative cholangiography. *Surg Gynecol Obstet* 65:702–710, 1937.
24. Glenn F: Management of gallstones, particularly the silent variety: advantages of an aggressive surgical approach. In Ingelfinger FJ, Ebert RV, Finland M, Relman AS (eds): *Controversies in Internal Medicine,* Vol 2. Philadelphia, W. B. Saunders, 1974, pp 533–544.
25. Gracie WA, Ransohoff DR: The natural history of silent gallstones: the innocent gallstone is not a myth. *N Engl J Med* 307:798–800, 1982.
26. Donaldson RM Jr: Advice for the patient with "silent" gallstones. *N Engl J Med* 307:815–816, 1982.
27. Fitzpatrick G, Neutra R, Gilbert JJ: Cost-effectiveness of cholecystectomy for silent gallstones. In Bunker JP, Barnes BA, Mosteller R (eds): *Cost, Risks and Benefits of Surgery.* New York, Oxford University Press, 1977, pp 246–261.
28. Wenhert A, Robertson B: The natural course of gallstone disease. *Gastroenterology* 50:376–381, 1966.
29. Lebensart PR, Bloom RA, Meretyk S, Landau EK, Shiloni E: Oral cholecystosonography: a method for facilitating the diagnosis of cholesterol gallstones. *Radiology* 153:255–256, 1984.
30. Pearlman BJ, Marks JW, Bonorris GG et al: Gallstone dissolution—a progress report. *Clin Gastroenterol* 8:12–140, 1979.
31. Schoenfield JJ, Lachin JM: Chenodiol (chenodeoxycholic acid) for dissolution of gallstones: The National Cooperative Gallstone Study. A controlled trial of efficacy and safety. *Ann Intern Med* 95:257–282, 1981.

Radiology

Oral cholecystography (OCG), introduced in 1924 by Graham and Cole (1), augmented by plain film findings and intravenous cholangiography (IVC), was unchallenged until recently in diagnosing gallbladder disease. While plain film findings are likely to remain important, the recent revolution in newer imaging modalities, particularly ultrasound and radionuclide hepatobiliary scintigraphy, have called into question the preeminent roles of the traditional techniques. Computed tomography, while valuable, appears to be less dramatic in this area, and new modalities such as MRI are yet to be fully explored (2–6).

Plain Films

A plain film prior to OCG contrast administration might demonstrate pathology that otherwise would be missed in a small percentage of patients. Such a preliminary film is generally felt to be impractical, however, and is not widely employed. Nevertheless, gallbladder pathology may often be detected on plain films obtained in many other settings. Calculi are by far the most common such finding (Fig. 12.1). Even though only 10–20% of gallstones calcify sufficiently to be seen on plain films, gallstones are so common that they are the most frequent cause of discrete, rounded right-upper-quadrant (RUQ) calcifications. Because there remains a significant differential diagnosis for such densities, ultrasound or OCG should be obtained to confirm the gallbladder as the site of origin. Eighty percent of urinary calculi are sufficiently radioopaque to be observable on plain films, and stones in the right renal collecting system are the most common source of confusion. Less often right renal parenchymal calcifications or calcified renal cysts could be confused for gallstones. Calculi or contrast material in hepatic flexure colonic diverticula may resemble gallstones. Vascular calcifications, particularly ring-like densities, in aneurysms of the renal or porta hepatis vessels may be confusing. Calculi in unusually positioned retrocecal appendices and in Meckel's diverticula have been mistaken for gallstones. Other rare causes of RUQ calcifications include hepatic granulomas (as in chronic granulomatous disease of childhood), hepatic cysts, and granulomas in mesenteric nodes. Residual oily contrast injected into renal cysts and calcareous material in calyceal diverticula may resemble milk of calcium bile (7–9).

Internal fissures caused by stress within brittle gallstones may form a partial vacuum drawing gas out of solution and leading to radiating, streak-like lucencies called the "crow-foot" or "Mercedes-Benz" sign (Fig. 12.2) (10). Potentially, one might diagnose nonopaque stones on plain film by this means, but more often the presence of calcification draws attention to the sign instead. Gas-containing stones tend to float even in nonopacified bile and the presence of gas may thus be predicted on ultrasound or other cross-sectional imaging (even if the gas itself is not found) (11).

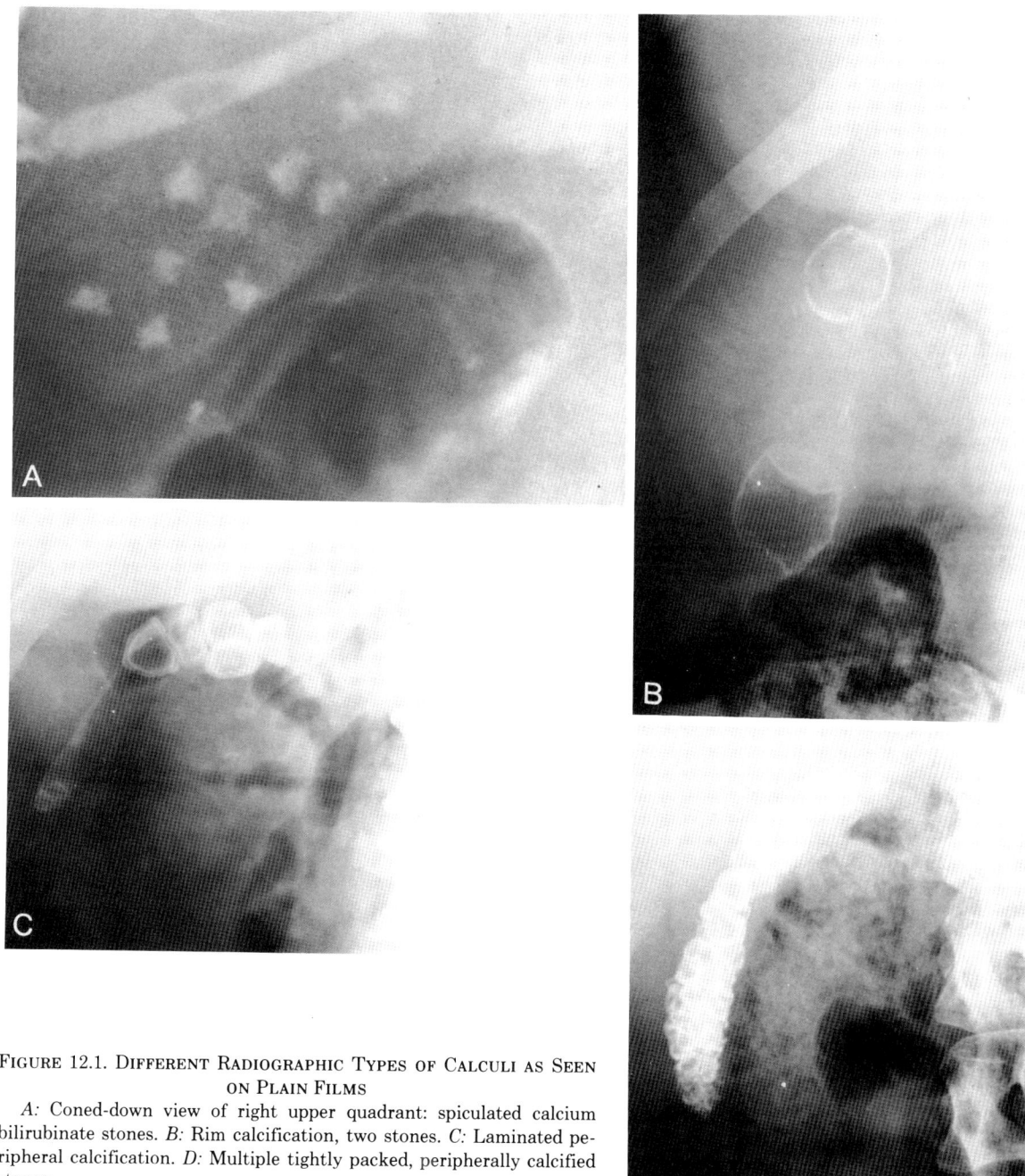

FIGURE 12.1. DIFFERENT RADIOGRAPHIC TYPES OF CALCULI AS SEEN ON PLAIN FILMS

A: Coned-down view of right upper quadrant: spiculated calcium bilirubinate stones. *B:* Rim calcification, two stones. *C:* Laminated peripheral calcification. *D:* Multiple tightly packed, peripherally calcified stones.

Oral Cholecystography

Long considered one of the safest and most accurate of all radiographic studies, OCG remains the primary means of detecting gallbladder disease in many places and is an adjunct to newer modalities in others. The accuracy of OCG was often quoted as 97%; this was based on several circumstances that are now being questioned. Mujahed et al. (12) reported that nonopacification of the gallbladder after two successive doses of oral contrast was a 90% accurate

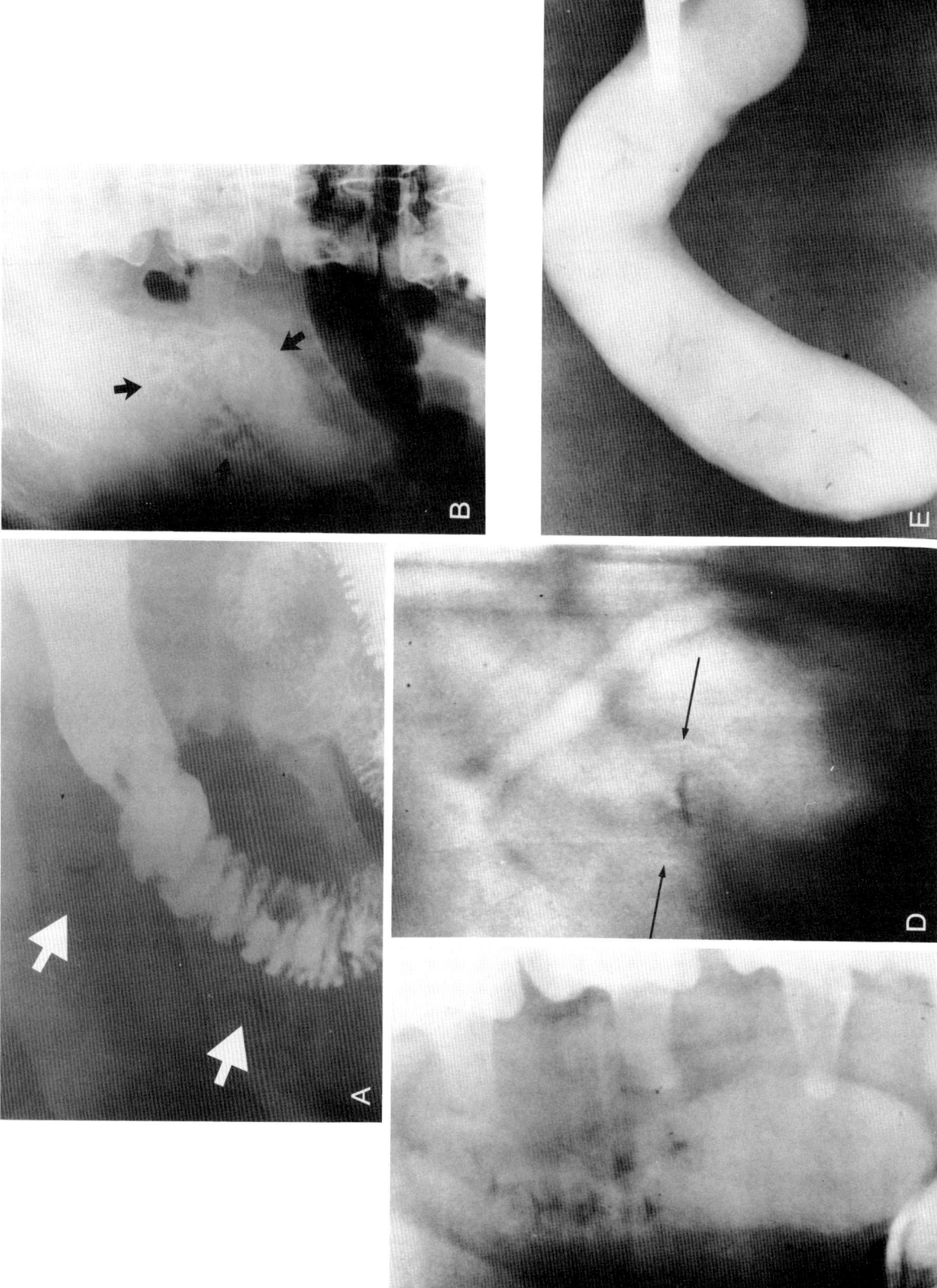

FIGURE 12.2. "Mercedes-Benz" or "Crow's-Foot" Sign

A: Two gallstones (*arrows*) recognized on an UGI primarily on the basis of the central lucency. Faint peripheral calcification was present on close inspection of the original film. *B*: Gallbladder packed with faintly calcified stones with radiolucent centers (*arrows*), plain film. *C*: "Mercedes-Benz" sign on OCG. *D*: Tomogram from an OCG: stone with

indication of disease if extrinsic causes could be excluded. Many of the patients with nonopacification, however, were diagnosed as having chronic acalculous cholecystitis. While this condition undoubtedly occurs, the criteria for its pathological diagnosis are not well defined, making such data subject to question (13, 14).

If the gallbladder is successfully opacified false positives are rare. On the other hand, the possibility of a false negative was not accurately assessed prior to ultrasound availability. Opacification without demonstrated stones was assumed normal and generally no further studies were performed. Stones found on subsequent examination were assumed to have formed in the interim. Recent studies, however, have suggested an OCG false-negative rate as high as 6–8%, with small calculi often overlooked (15–18). Indeed, while the more common problem is obtaining adequate visualization of the gallbladder, early concern that the oral contrast agents would be so dense as to hide small calculi appears to have been well founded.

While the development of oral cholecystography has been relatively stable for many decades, especially since the introduction of iopanoic acid (Telepaque) in 1953, a number of modifications have been suggested. While Telepaque remains the most widely used contrast, other agents have been developed. All are triiodinated aminophenyl compounds, unsubstituted in the number 5 position. When properly employed, there appears to be little difference in their clinical efficacy. All are relatively insoluble in water with Telepaque the most insoluble of all. All agents require glucuronide conjugation in the liver prior to excretion by the hepatocytes. If the contrast reaches the gallbladder via a patent biliary tree and cystic duct, a 6–8-fold concentration by the gallbladder mucosa permits diagnostic opacification. Iopanoic acid depends heavily upon bile salts for absorption across the lipid barrier of the intestine. A fatty meal, prior to contrast administration, will empty the gallbladder, making its bile salt content available for intestinal absorption. Subsequent fasting allows accumulation of new contrast-enhanced bile in the gallbladder. Imaging should be performed at the time of peak opacification, about 14 to 16 hr after ingestion. With other agents, bile salts are less important, and diet and timing somewhat less critical (19).

The usual dose of contrast is 3 g. Inadequate first day visualization averages 15–25% (range 7–53%), but about two-thirds of these cases will have diagnostic visualization after a second dose (12, 20–22). Therefore, some routinely administer two doses on successive days to avoid repeat studies (23, 24). The term "double dose" should be avoided, as it implies administration of twice the usual dose on a single day. Renal toxicity and side effects, such as nausea and diarrhea, are concerns, but even massive overdoses have been relatively well tolerated (25).

Stimulated contraction employing a fatty meal or cholecystokinin (CCK) may be helpful to demonstrate small stones or the findings of hyperplastic cholecystosis. Intravenous CCK has also been suggested to demonstrate functional abnormalities, the so-called dyskinesias, when OCG and ultrasonography fail to demonstrate gallstones in symptomatic patients (26–28). Objective studies have generally not supported its validity, however, for the diagnosis of acalculous cholecystitis or dyskinesia (29, 30).

Tomography may be helpful in otherwise inconclusive oral studies (31). Also, with a nonvisualized gallbladder, it may demonstrate cystic duct obstruction by showing an opacified common duct.

Regardless of the variations employed, attention to careful radiographic technique, including low kilovoltage, horizontal-beam films, optimum grid-film techniques, and careful fluoroscopic positioning with erect compression spot filming is essential (Fig. 12.3A–H).

Radiolucent or mixed calculi are seen as filling defects in a functioning gallbladder (Fig. 12.3I–K). Stones that are calcified on plain films often appear radiolucent on the cholecystogram when compared to the surrounding contrast containing bile. Very rarely, radiolucent gallstones either in the gallbladder or common duct can acquire a peripheral rim radioopacity after administration of an oral cholecystopaque (Fig. 12.4). The phenomenon is limited to pigment-containing stones and is thought to result from a reaction between surface biliverdin in the stone and the contrast material (32).

It may become important to distinguish cholesterol stones from other types radiographically since only cholesterol stones are amenable to chemical dissolution by currently available peroral or percutaneously administered agents. While a spiculated appearance may be typical of bilirubin stones (Fig. 12.1A), calcification alone is not a reliable indicator of other components in the stone's makeup. In a multivariable discriminant analysis of radiographic features, Dolgin et al. (33) found buoyancy to be the only reliable discriminating feature. Apparently only cholesterol stones have sufficiently low specific gravity to float in bile and then only if the bile

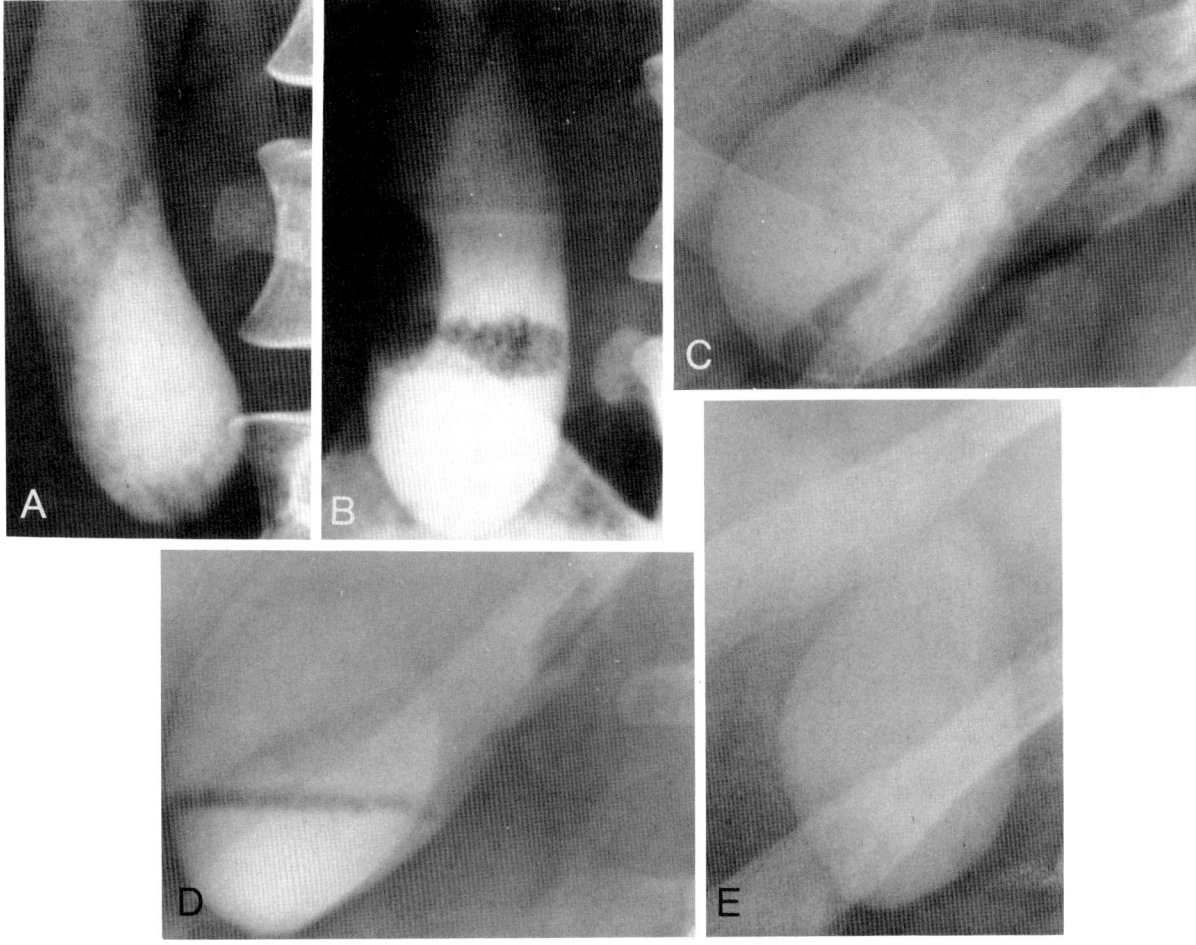

FIGURE 12.3. SOME DIFFERENT APPEARANCES OF CALCULI ON ORAL CHOLECYSTOGRAPHY

A and *B:* Numerous small calculi on the supine film (*A*) layer out on an erect film (*B*). *C* and *D:* Calculi difficult to see on supine film (*C*), but obvious on after layering on erect film (*D*). *E–G:* Calculi are invisible on supine film (*E*), but readily appreciated on erect and decubitus films (*F* and *G*) after layering out (*arrows*). The second apparent layer in (*G*) is an air-fluid level in bowel. *H:* Erect spot film: double layer of stones. The majority of gallstones will sink to a completely dependent position. In this case, the ones that do have central calcification and are probably mixed in composition, whereas the floating stones are radiolucent and probably nearly entirely cholesterol. *I* and *J:* Two examples of centrally calcified stones, small (*I*) and large (*J*). *K:* Multiple lucent faceted stones and large, central partially calcified stone.

specific gravity has been increased by contrast enhancement (34, 35) (Fig. 12.3*A–H*). Buoyancy of stones in noncontrast enhanced bile, as detected by imaging modalities such as ultrasound, is a strong indication of the presence of gas within fissures (equivalent to the radiographic Mercedes-Benz sign) (36).

Intravenous Cholangiography

Primarily a method for demonstrating the duct system, IVC may also be used to examine the gallbladder and assess cystic duct patency (Fig. 12.5*A*). Intravenous injection of a water-soluble contrast which is excreted by the hepatocytes without conjugation permits relatively rapid opacification of the biliary tree. The contrast agents are dimers of the triiodinated benzene rings used in OCG and deliver twice the iodine per molecule, giving faint opacification without need for concentration by the gallbladder. A choleretic effect, however, dilutes the contrast limiting maximum opacification so that tomography is usually required (37, 38). IVC is unsuccessful if liver function is seriously impaired, and delayed films are often required, limiting its utility in acute cases. The contrast has an appreciably higher toxicity than common urographic agents. Also, recent reports suggest a frequency of "adequate visualization" as low as 55% in

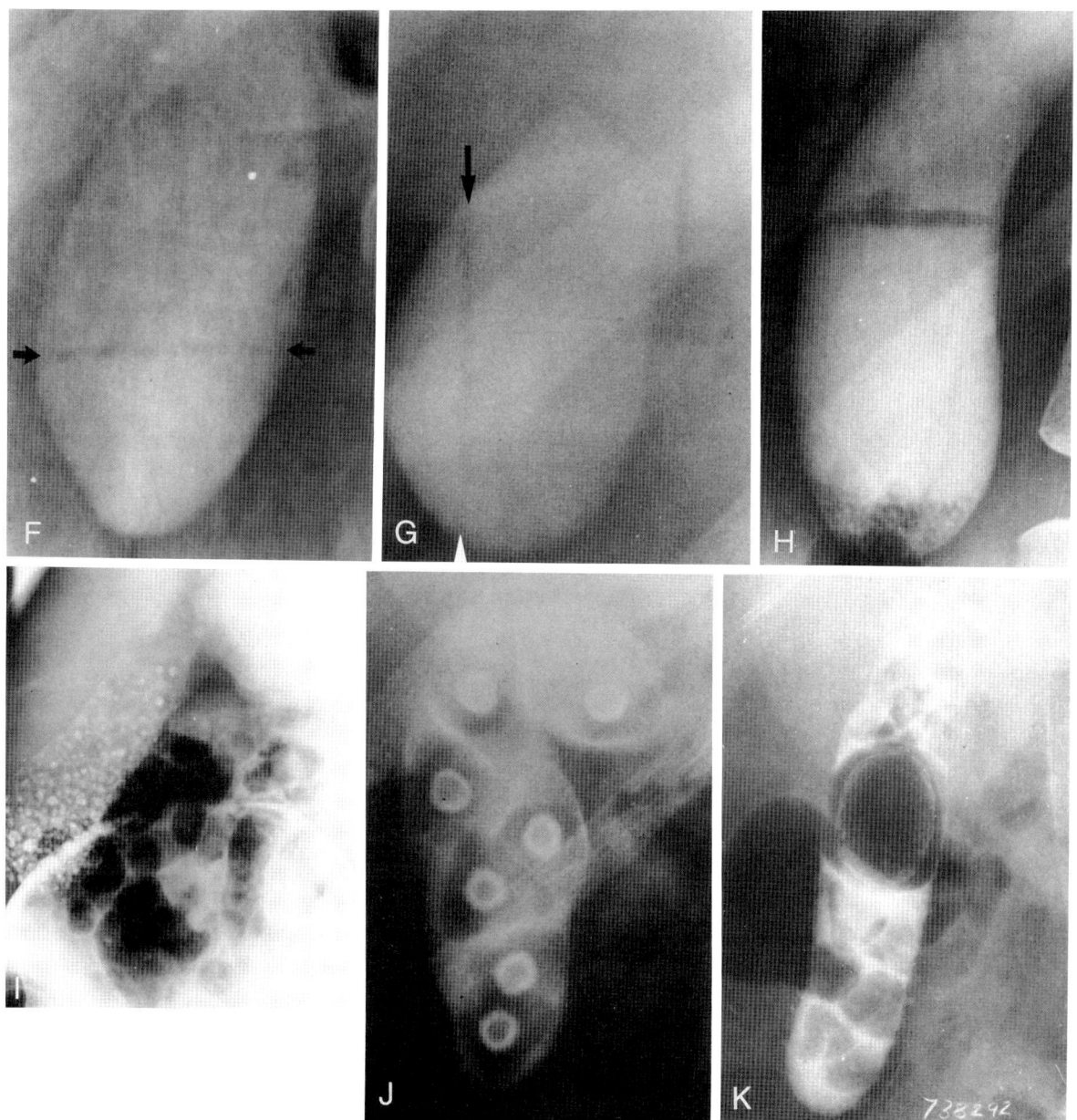

FIGURE 12.3*F–K*

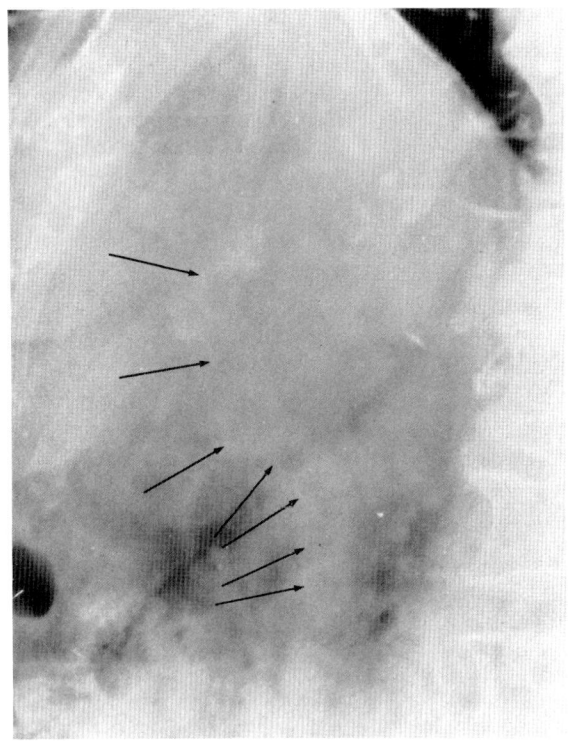

FIGURE 12.4. SECOND-DAY ORAL CHOLECYSTOGRAM
Film from a second day oral cholecystogram: faint coating (*arrows*) of multiple stones in the common duct, which itself is faintly opacified. The film the prior day showed nothing.

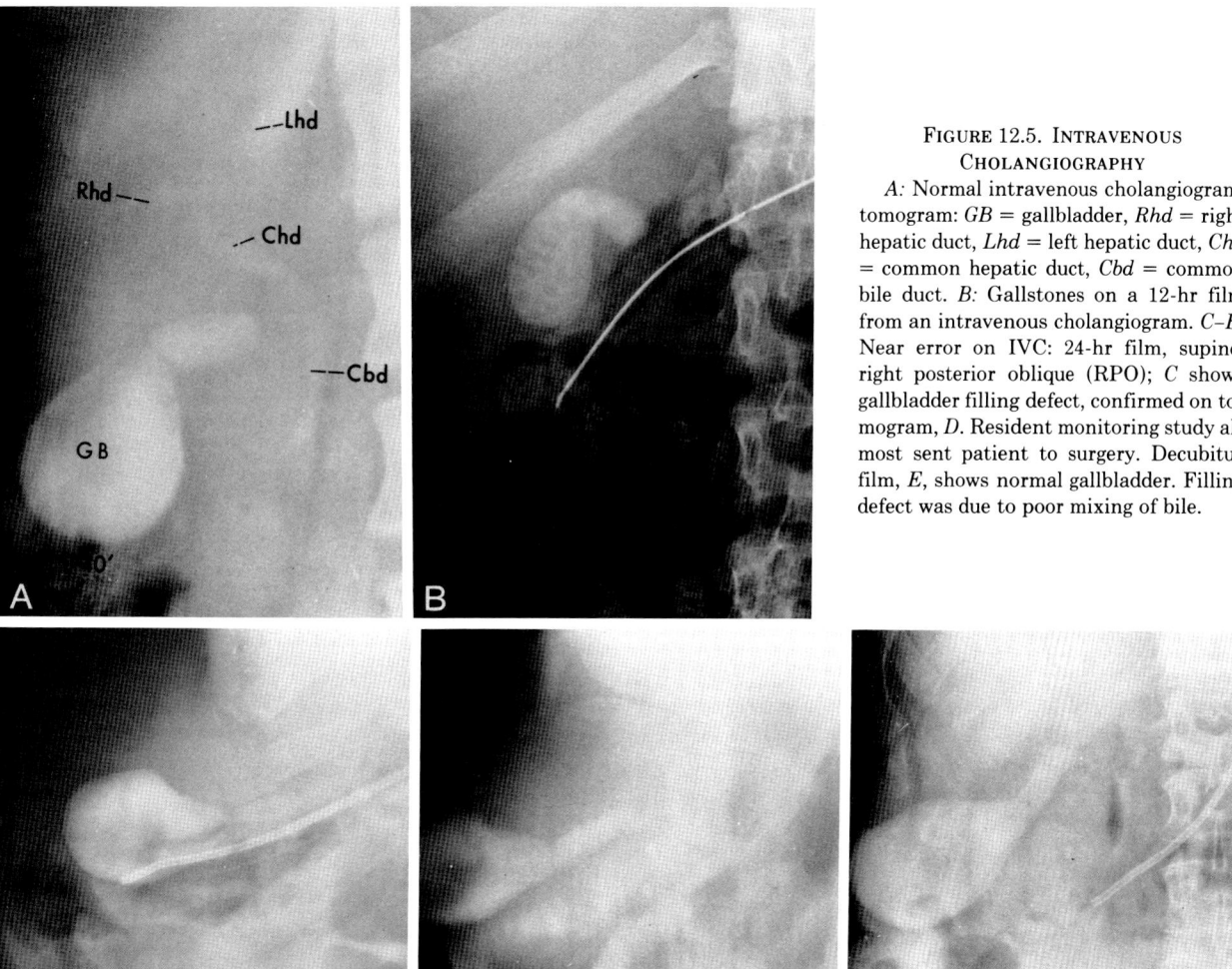

FIGURE 12.5. INTRAVENOUS CHOLANGIOGRAPHY
A: Normal intravenous cholangiogram, tomogram: *GB* = gallbladder, *Rhd* = right hepatic duct, *Lhd* = left hepatic duct, *Chd* = common hepatic duct, *Cbd* = common bile duct. *B:* Gallstones on a 12-hr film from an intravenous cholangiogram. *C–E:* Near error on IVC: 24-hr film, supine, right posterior oblique (RPO); *C* shows gallbladder filling defect, confirmed on tomogram, *D*. Resident monitoring study almost sent patient to surgery. Decubitus film, *E*, shows normal gallbladder. Filling defect was due to poor mixing of bile.

clinical cases and a diagnostic error rate as high as 40% even with visualization (39). The error rate is especially high for stones in the gallbladder (Fig. 12.5*B–E*). These factors, plus the availability of newer, easier, faster and safer modalities, make the IVC obsolete in suspected gallbladder disease.

A thickened gallbladder wall seen on tomography following intravenous injection of urographic contrast has been suggested as a rapid, yet safe, means of diagnosing acute cholecystitis (40). The efficacy of such infusion tomography remains controversial, however, and the technique has never been widely employed (41, 42).

REFERENCES

1. Graham EA, Cole WH: Roentgenologic examination of the gallbladder: preliminary report of a new method utilizing intravenous injection of tetrabromophthalein. *JAMA* 82:613–614, 1924.
2. Havrilla TR, Reich NE, Haaga JR, Seidelmann FE, Cooperman AM, Alfidi RJ: Computed tomography of the gallbladder. *AJR* 130:1059–1067, 1978.
3. Kane RA, Costello P, Duszlak E: Computed tomography in acute cholecystitis: new observations. *AJR* 141:697–701, 1983.
4. Sarva RP, Farivar S, Fromm H, Poller W: Study of the sensitivity and specificity of computerized tomography in the detection of calcified gallstones which appear radiolucent by conventional roentgenography. *Gastrointest Radiol* 6:165–167, 1981.
5. Toombs BD, Sandler CM, Conoley PM: Computed tomography of the nonvisualizing gallbladder. *J Comput Assist Tomogr* 5:164–168, 1981.
6. Hricak H, Filly RA, Margulis AR, Moon KL, Crooks LE, Kaufman L: Work in progress: nuclear magnetic resonance imaging of the gallbladder. *Radiology* 147:481–484, 1983.
7. Berk RN: The plain abdominal radiograph. In Berk RN, Ferrucci JT Jr, Leopold GR (eds): *Radiology of the Gallbladder and Bile Ducts.* Philadelphia, W. B. Saunders, 1983, 2.

8. Darlak JJ, Moskowitz M, Kattan KR: Calcifications in the liver. *Radiol Clin North Am* 18:209–219, 1980.
9. Donner MW, Weiner S: Diagnostic evaluation of abdominal calcifications in acute abdominal disorders. *Radiol Clin North Am* 2:145, 1964.
10. Meyers MA, O'Donahue N: The Mercedes-Benz sign: insight into the dynamics of formation and disappearance of gallstones. *AJR* 119:63–70, 1973.
11. Becker CD, Vock P: Apperance of gas-containing gallstones on sonography and computed tomography. *Gastrointest Radiol* 9:323–328, 1984.
12. Mujahaed Z, Evans JA, Whalen JP: The non-opacified gallbladder on oral cholecystography. *Radiology* 112:1–8, 1974.
13. Berk RN, Ferrucci JT Jr, Fordtran JS, Cooperberg PL, Weissmann HS: The radiological diagnosis of gallbladder disease. *Radiology* 141:49–56, 1981.
14. Howard RJ: Acute acalculous cholecystitis. *Am J Surg* 141:194–198, 1981.
15. Bartrum RJ Jr, Crow HC, Foote SR: Ultrasonic and radiographic cholecystography. *N Engl J Med* 296:538–541, 1977.
16. Cooperberg P, Burhenne HJ: Real time ultrasonography. Diagnostic technique of choice in calculous gallbladder disease. *N Engl J Med* 302:1277–1279, 1980.
17. Crade M, Taylor KJW, Rosenfield AT, Degraff CS, Minihan P: Surgical and pathologic correlation of cholecystography. *AJR* 131:227–229, 1978.
18. Leopold GR, Amberg J, Gosink B, Mittelstaedt C: Gray scale ultrasonic cholecystography: A comparison with conventional radiographic techniques. *Radiology* 121:445–448, 1976.
19. Loeb PM, Berk RN, Janes JO, Perkin L, Moore J: The effect of fasting on gallbladder opacification during oral cholecystography: a controlled study in normal volunteers. *Radiology* 126:395–401, 1978.
20. Berk RN: The consecutive dose phenomenon in oral cholecystography. *AJR* 110:230–233, 1970.
21. Krook PM, Bush WH: Single dose oral cholecystography. *Radiology* 127:643–644, 1978.
22. Stanley RJ, Stanley RJ, Melson GL, Cubillo E, et al: A comparison of three cholecystographic agents: a double blind study with and without prior fatty meal. *Radiology* 112:513–517, 1974.
23. Burhenne HJ, Obata WG: Single visit oral cholecystography. *N Engl J Med* 292:627–632, 1975.
24. Burhenne HJ, Morris DC, Graeb DA: Single visit oral cholecystography for in-patients. *Radiology* 140:505–506, 1981.
25. Gelfand DW, Ott DJ, Klein AA: Massive iopanoic acid (Telepaque) overdose without ill effects. *AJR* 130:1174–1175, 1978.
26. Nathan MH, Newman A, Murray DJ, Camponovo R: Cholecystokinin cholecystography: a four year evaluation. *AJR* 110:240–251, 1970.
27. Sargent EN, Boswell W, Hubsher J: Cholecystokinetic cholecystography: efficacy and tolerance studies of ceruletide. *AJR* 130:1051–1055, 1978.
28. Griffen W, Bivins BA, Rogert EL: Cholecystokinin cholecystography in the diagnosis of gallbladder disease. *Ann Surg* 191:636–640, 1980.
29. Berk RN: Cholecystokinin cholecystography in the diagnosis of chronic acalculous cholecystitis and biliary dyskinesia. *Gastrointest Radiol* 1:325–330, 1977.
30. Dunn EH, Christensen EC, Reynolds J, Fordtran J: Cholecystokinin cholecystography. *JAMA* 228:997–999, 1974.
31. Stephens DH, Gisvold JJ, Carlson HC: Tomography of the gallbladder in oral cholecystography. *Gastrointest Radiol* 1:93–98, 1976.
32. Salzman E: The 4-day cholecystographic test. *Semin Roentgenol* 11:171–173, 1976.
33. Dolgin SM, Schwartz S, Kressel HY et al: Identification of patients with cholesterol or pigment gallstones by discriminant analysis of radiographic features. *N Engl J Med* 304:808–811, 1981.
34. Culp WC: Buoyancy of gallstones in varying concentrations of contrast media. *AJR* 143:79–80, 1984.
35. Scheske GA, Cooperberg PL, Cohen MM, Burhenne HJ: Floating gallstones: the role of contrast material. *J Clin Ultrasound* 8:227–231, 1980.
36. Strijk SP, Boetes C, Rosenbusch G: Floating stones in a nonopacified gallbladder: ultrasonic sign of gas-containing gallstones. *Gastrointest Radiol* 6:261–263, 1981.
37. Eckelberg ME, Carlson HC, McIlrath DC: Intravenous cholangiography with intact gallbladder. *AJR* 110:235–239, 1970.
38. Scholz FJ, Larsen CR, Wise RE: Intravenous cholangiography: recurring concepts. *Semin Roentgenol* 11:197–202, 1976.
39. Goodman MW, Ansel JH, Vennes JA, Lasser RB, Silvis SE: Is intravenous cholangiography still useful? *Gastroenterology* 79:642–645, 1980.
40. Moncada R, Cardoso M, Danley R et al: Acute cholecystitis: 137 patients studied by infusion tomography of the gallbladder. *AJR* 129:583–585, 1977.
41. Morin ME, Baker DA, Marsan RE: Visualization of the gallbladder wall at excretory urography: implication for infusion tomography of the gallbladder. *Radiology* 125:35–38, 1977.
42. Katzberg RW, Glasier CM, Booker JL, Mullins JD, Kopp DT: Infusion tomography and the total body opacification effect: appraisal in the diagnosis of acute cholecystitis. *Radiology* 134:297–302, 1980.

Sonography

Traditionally, only 2% of gallbladders considered normal on technically good oral cholecystograms were thought to have undetected stones. Recent sonographic data suggest a false-negative rate for oral cholecystography of about 7% (1–3).

Initial studies of cholecystosonography between 1974 and 1976 reported a sensitivity for cholelithiasis of 66–84% (4). Between 1976 and 1980 sensitivity increased to 84–97%, and rates of 94–98.9% have been reported since 1980 (2–6). False positives range from 1 to 3% and only 2–3.5% of studies are nondiagnostic (3). One source of false negatives is patients with focal nonshadowing echodensities (3). Real-time sonography is superior to static scanning despite similar resolution (1, 7). A 1981 study of 339 patients found that 97.6% of gallbladders were depicted and 94.5% of gallstones present were detected by real-time, versus 89.5% and 78.8%, respectively, by static scanning. Reasons for these results are as follows: flexible real-time sonography more readily depicts high gallbladders because of better intercostal scanning, shadowing from very small stones is more likely to be shown by real-time because of the infinite number of scan planes possible, and detection of stone motion ("rolling stone" sign) is easier with real-time (4, 7).

Sonography and oral cholecystography both have high sensitivity and specificity. Oral cholecystography may be slightly superior for very small stones (1.0–3.0 mm) and it is superior in determining the number of stones (usually not of any clinical significance). Sonography is faster, without known side effects, more accurate, and more likely to provide a diagnostic study. For these reasons, sonography has rendered oral cholecystography nearly obsolete. The latter is poised for a comeback, however, if oral dissolution therapy becomes feasible on a widespread basis.

Sonographic Findings in Cholelithiasis. At least three typical sonographic patterns occur. The Type I pattern consists of high level intraluminal echoes producing distal acoustic shadowing—the classical gallstone (Fig. 12.6). This appearance is virtually 100% diagnostic. Most often the stone will be freely movable, however, very large stones, stones impacted in the gallbladder neck, and stones adherent to the gallbladder wall will not be mobile (Fig. 12.6C and D). Demonstrating the acoustic shadow is vital since its presence increases diagnostic accuracy from 60% to 100% (8). Theoretically all stones should shadow, however, a multitude of factors influence the formation and perception of an acoustic shadow (9, 10): (a) Particle size: although some in vivo studies report shadowing by stones as small as 2.0 mm (11), others report that no shadow is perceived most of the time when stones are less than 3.0 mm in diameter (12–14). Aggregates of small stones which would not individually cast a perceptible shadow often

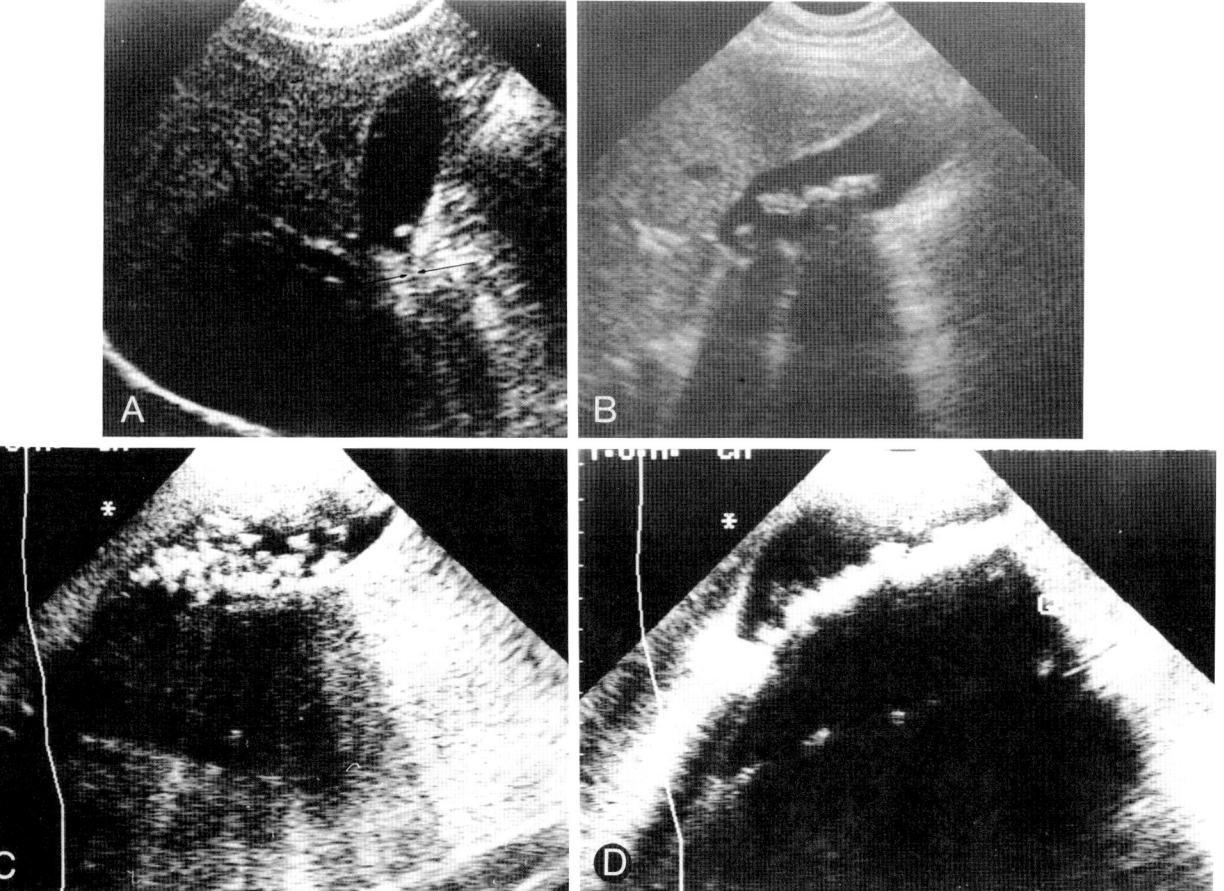

FIGURE 12.6. TYPE I GALLSTONES

A: Pencil-thin shadow (*arrows*) emanating from a tiny gallstone. *B:* High level intraluminal echoes with clean acoustic shadowing. *C* and *D:* Supine and decubitus parasagittal scans respectively showing stone mobility and the importance of patient positioning in demonstrating shadowing, which is seen much better in *D* than *C*.

do so when layered together in the dependent portion of the gallbladder. Scanning in an erect position will regroup the stones, widen the collection, and make the shadow more prominent (11). b) Transducer characteristics: Higher frequency transducers (5 mHz and up) will frequently demonstrate shadowing by smaller stones which cannot be shown using lower frequencies (3.5 mHz and lower). Stones in the focal zone are more likely to shadow than those above or below it. Since the stone must intercept the sonic beam centrally to generate a shadow, its diameter must be relatively large in comparison to beam width and frequency. A stone intercepting the periphery of the beam may be detected as an echogenic focus, yet not cast a shadow. c) Scanning technique: Gain settings used for the liver may obscure acoustic shadows from gallstones; the gain should be lowered to scan the gallbladder. Maximal reflection (echogenicity) and shadowing both occur when the incident beam is perpendicular to the flat surface of a stone (9), so that scanning at different angles may be necessary to demonstrate a shadow. A small stone may cast only a hard to detect pencil-thin shadow (this is just as diagnostic as an obvious shadow, however) (Fig. 12.6A) (15). d) Stone composition: Calcium content, surface characteristics and specific gravity do not affect acoustic shadowing. Stones of the same size do vary in their degree of attenuation in that more highly attenuating stones have a larger average crystal size and more crystalline material (16).

The appearance of acoustic shadowing from a stone differs from that created by gas (17). Acoustic shadowing may be generated in either of two ways: sound absorption or sound reflection. At a tissue-air interface the sonic beam is almost totally reflected leading to reverberation; the beam is reflected from interface to transducer surface repeatedly. Thus the acoustic shadow fills in with regularly spaced horizontal linear echoes and its margins are indistinct. Therefore this type of acoustic shadow is described as "dirty." In contrast, the acoustic shadow cast by a gallstone is primarily due to sound absorption. It is sharply marginated with few if any echoes within it and is described as a "clean" shadow.

Unfortunately, not all gallstone shadows fulfill the criteria for a clean shadow (18). Calcified gallstones (19) and gas-containing fissured stones (20) have been found to generate reverberation artifacts. They are felt to cause reflection as well as sound absorption. In the case of calcified stones, the artifact is primarily a "single" fundamental reverberation echo at twice the transducer-stone distance.

Type II Gallstones: Strong Acoustic Shadowing Originating in the Gallbladder Fossa. Nonvisualization of the gallbladder lumen during cholecystosonography is highly suspicious for pathology with an accuracy of 90% for predicting gallbladder disease (8, 15). Unfortunately, a number of causes for nonvisualization exist that are not clinically significant: postprandial physiologic contraction, obesity, and poor technique. Agenesis and ectopy must be considered. Some patients may have normal, but small gallbladders that are difficult to detect. Carcinoma of the gallbladder may present with nonvisualization at sonography (generally other findings are present, however). When properly coupled with either of two other sonographic signs, nonvisualization of the gallbladder lumen has a high diagnostic accuracy for gallstones (21–23). The first of these is the presence of shadowing echogenic foci in the gallbladder fossa (Fig. 12.7A). The collection of any echoes must be focal and compact, as a broad-based collection of echoes could represent bowel gas (21). The collection must remain in the same position and configuration on longitudinal, transverse, and decubitus views (21). Scanning in the decubitus position will cause gas to rise within a viscus, whereas stones in a contracted gallbladder will remain relatively unchanged. Differentiating between clean and dirty shadowing may be helpful (Fig. 12.7B). Despite all efforts, if large amounts of bowel gas are present the diagnosis will be difficult. Other less common pitfalls (all of which can be excluded by a plain film) include: calcified granulomas, surgical clips, and air in the biliary tree.

The second set of findings which, seen when a normal gallbladder lumen is not confidently identified and indicates cholelithiasis, has been called the "double arc-shadow" sign (Fig. 12.8) (21, 22). This complex of findings consists of two echogenic curvilinear parellel lines, separated by a thin sonolucent rim, with acoustic shadowing distal to the second line. The anterior line corresponds to the gallbladder wall, the sonolucent rim represents the gallbladder lumen and the second (shadowing) line is the stone. This appearance always indicates cholelithiasis and until recently was thought to represent a thickened, contracted stone-filled gallbladder. Pathologic correlation has shown, however, that most patients with this sonographic picture have normal sized thin-walled gallbladders. Two-thirds of patients do have a large number of stones filling the gallbladder (22).

Type III Gallstones: Focal Nonshadowing Opacities. The presence of focal nonshadowing

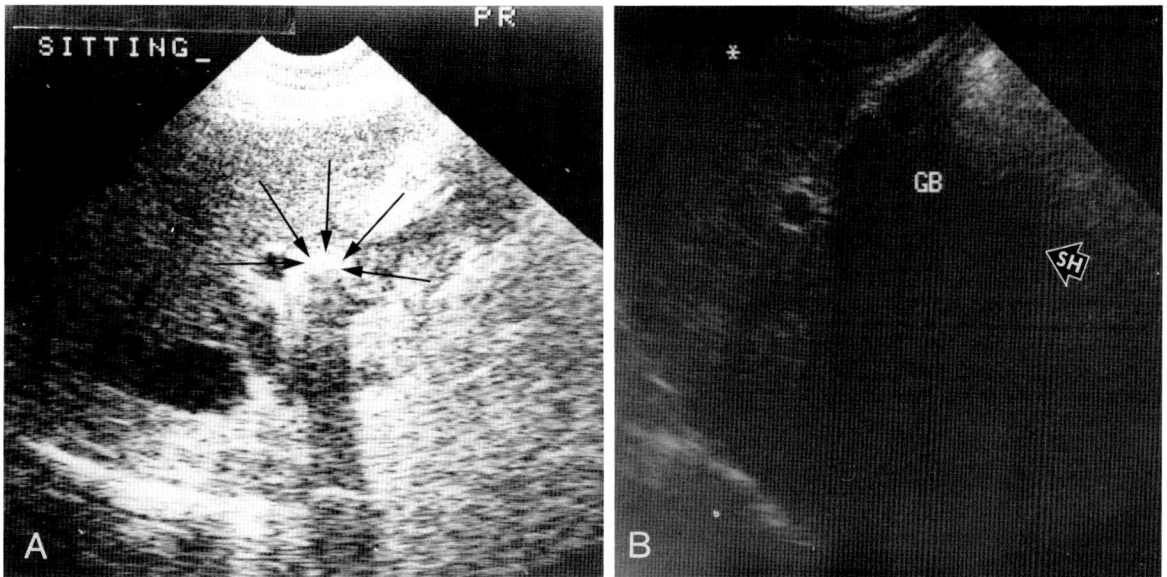

FIGURE 12.7. TYPE II GALLSTONES
A: Compact, shadowing echogenicity (arrows) in the gallbladder fossa region. B: Strong, clean acoustic shadowing (SH, arrow) from the gallbladder fossa (GB).

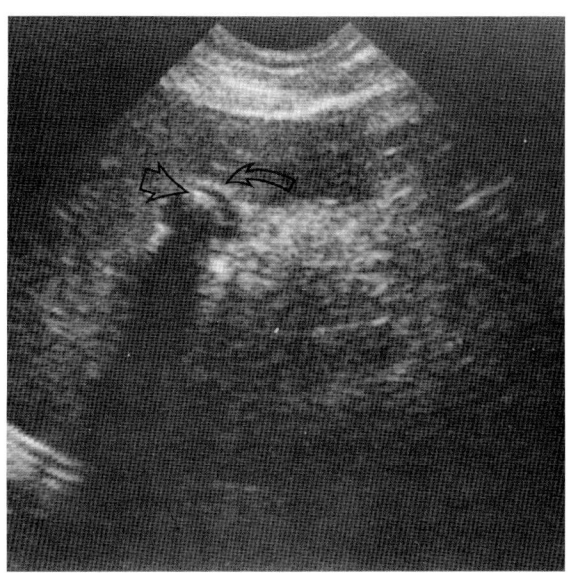

FIGURE 12.8. TYPE II GALLSTONES
"Double arc-shadow": The anterior wall of the gallbladder (curved arrow), the anterior wall of the stone (arrow) and a small amount of intervening bile are depicted.

opacities under 5.0 mm in diameter within the gallbladder lumen is suspicious for, but not a reliable indicator of gallstones (Fig. 12.9). In studies that offer surgical proof, only 60–80% of patients with this sonographic appearance will have gallstones (3, 8, 24). The issue is often clinically resolvable by either a repeat sonogram on a later date or an oral cholecystogram. The former may show disappearance or shadowing while the latter may depict a calculus (Fig. 12.9).

Larger, freely mobile nonshadowing masses are fairly uncommon (17). Most turn out to be hematoma, pus, aggregated sludge, or parasites (e.g., ascaris, fasciola hepaticum, clonorchis sinensis). Some large nonshadowing masses will progress into a classic shadowing gallstone on follow-up examination.

Floating Stones. The phenomenon of floating gallstones is well known to radiologists from oral cholecystography. The specific gravity of bile (1.01–1.04) is generally less than that of gallstones (1.04–1.058), consequently the latter tend to sink. Bile is usually stratified, with lighter layers at the top. Oral cholecystopaques raise the specific gravity of bile (1.03–1.085) often causing stones to float in the bile stratum closest to their own specific gravity (Fig. 12.10) (25). Although most stones will be seen to float sonographically only after a cholecystopaque has been given (if the gallbladder functions), gas-containing stones (20, 26, 27) and relatively pure cholesterol stones (13) may float spontaneously because of a lower specific gravity (1.01–1.035 for gas-containing stones (Fig. 12.11).

Floating stones, when very small, appear as an echogenic, interrupted horizontal line running through the gallbladder lumen. Shadowing may be faint or absent. Rescanning in the erect position will cause realignment and may elicit shadowing since the beam will be parallel instead of perpendicular to the row of stones. When

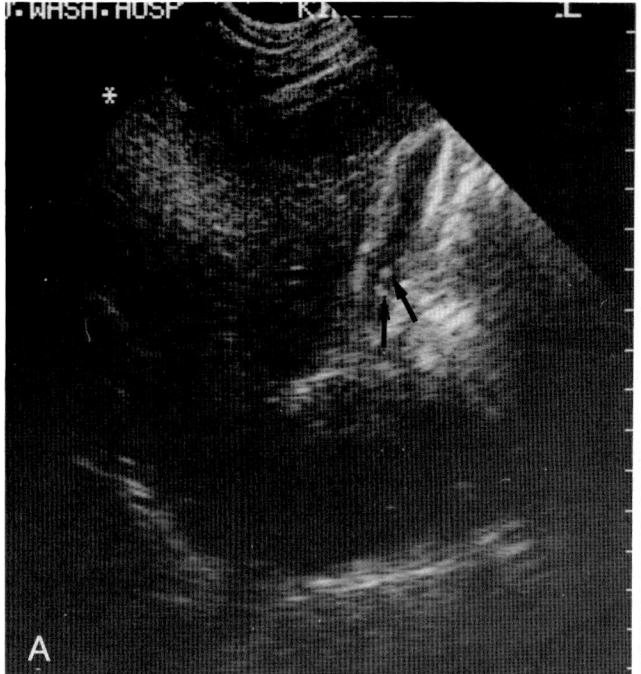
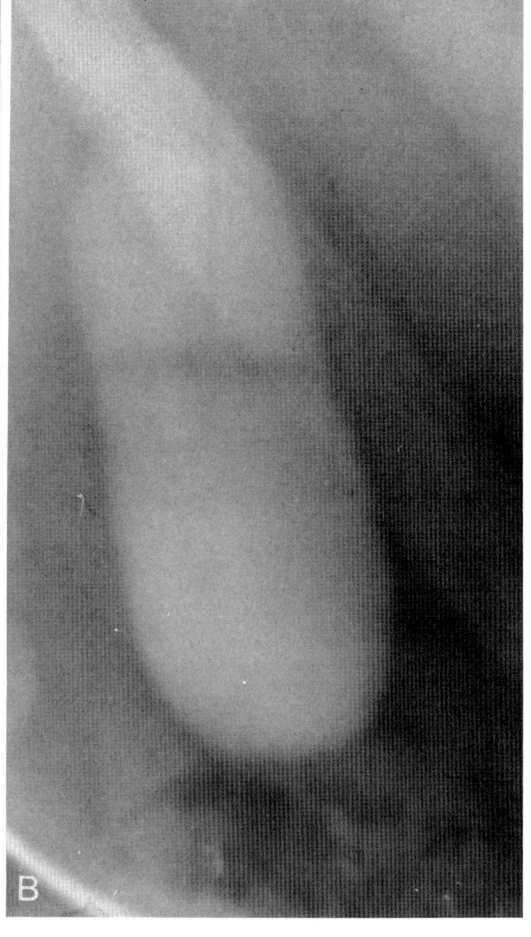

FIGURE 12.9. TYPE III GALLSTONES
A: Small non-shadowing echodensities (arrows) are seen in a contracted gallbladder. B: Oral cholecystogram—small stones layer out on an erect spot film.

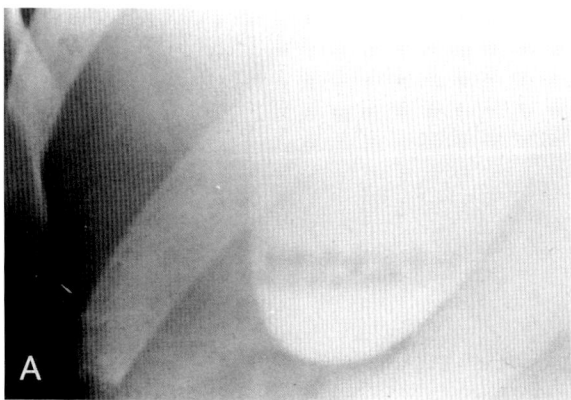
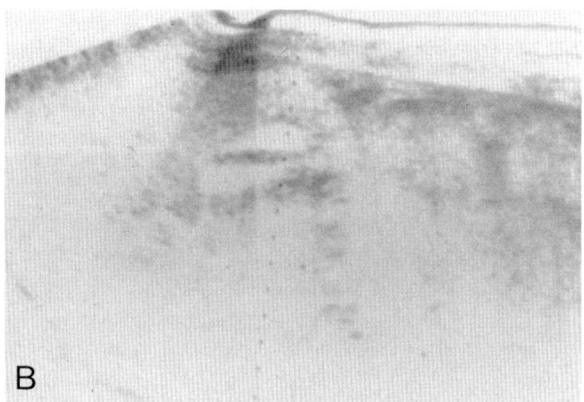

FIGURE 12.10. STONES FLOATING AFTER AN OCG
A: Double layer of floating stones on an upright spot film. B: Same finding on a parasagittal sonogram done immediately afterwards. An erect scan would have shown shadowing to better advantage.

larger, floating stones are depicted as a shadowing echodense line. Very low specific gravity stones can float so close to the anterior wall of the gallbladder that only their shadow will be seen (28). As mentioned in the technique section, sonography after ingestion of an oral cholecystopaque can sometimes resolve an initially equivocal sonogram by inducing layering of small, nonshadowing echodensities. If the "oral cholecystosonogram" is unsuccessful, the patient can proceed directly to oral cholecystography (29).

Sludge. Biliary sludge (echogenic bile) is a

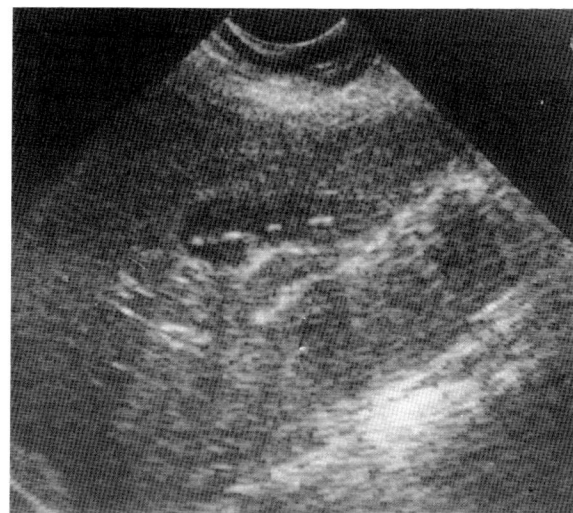

FIGURE 12.11. SPONTANEOUSLY FLOATING STONES
An interrupted echogenic line crosses the gallbladder lumen. Two of the stones faintly shadow.

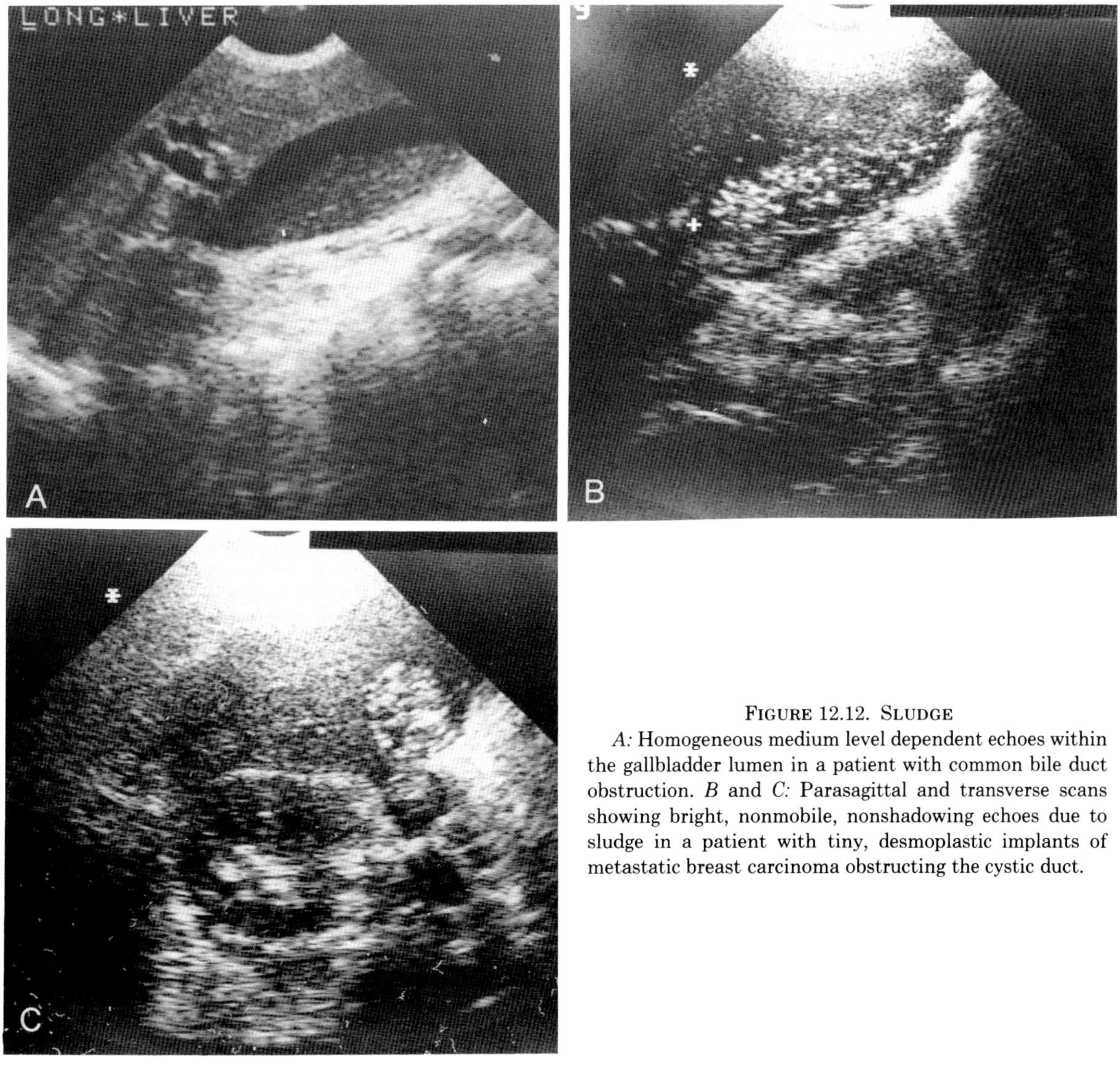

FIGURE 12.12. SLUDGE
A: Homogeneous medium level dependent echoes within the gallbladder lumen in a patient with common bile duct obstruction. B and C: Parasagittal and transverse scans showing bright, nonmobile, nonshadowing echoes due to sludge in a patient with tiny, desmoplastic implants of metastatic breast carcinoma obstructing the cystic duct.

much discussed entity in the sonographic literature. Sludge can be seen in patients with biliary stasis either nonobstructive (prolonged fasting, hyperalimentation, hemolysis (usually sickle cell disease)) or obstructive (any cause of cystic duct or common bile duct obstruction) (Fig. 12.12). Occasionally sludge can also be depicted in the common duct. When the cause is merely fasting, the sludge will disappear after a meal (30, 31).

Biliary sludge, by itself, is not an indication for cholecystectomy.

In vitro investigations have shown that sludge consists of particulate matter, primarily calcium bilirubinate granules with lesser amounts of cholesterol crystals (32). Sludge is depicted as medium to coarse, moderately bright echoes usually dependent in the gallbladder lumen. A fluid-fluid level is sometimes seen and there is no acoustic

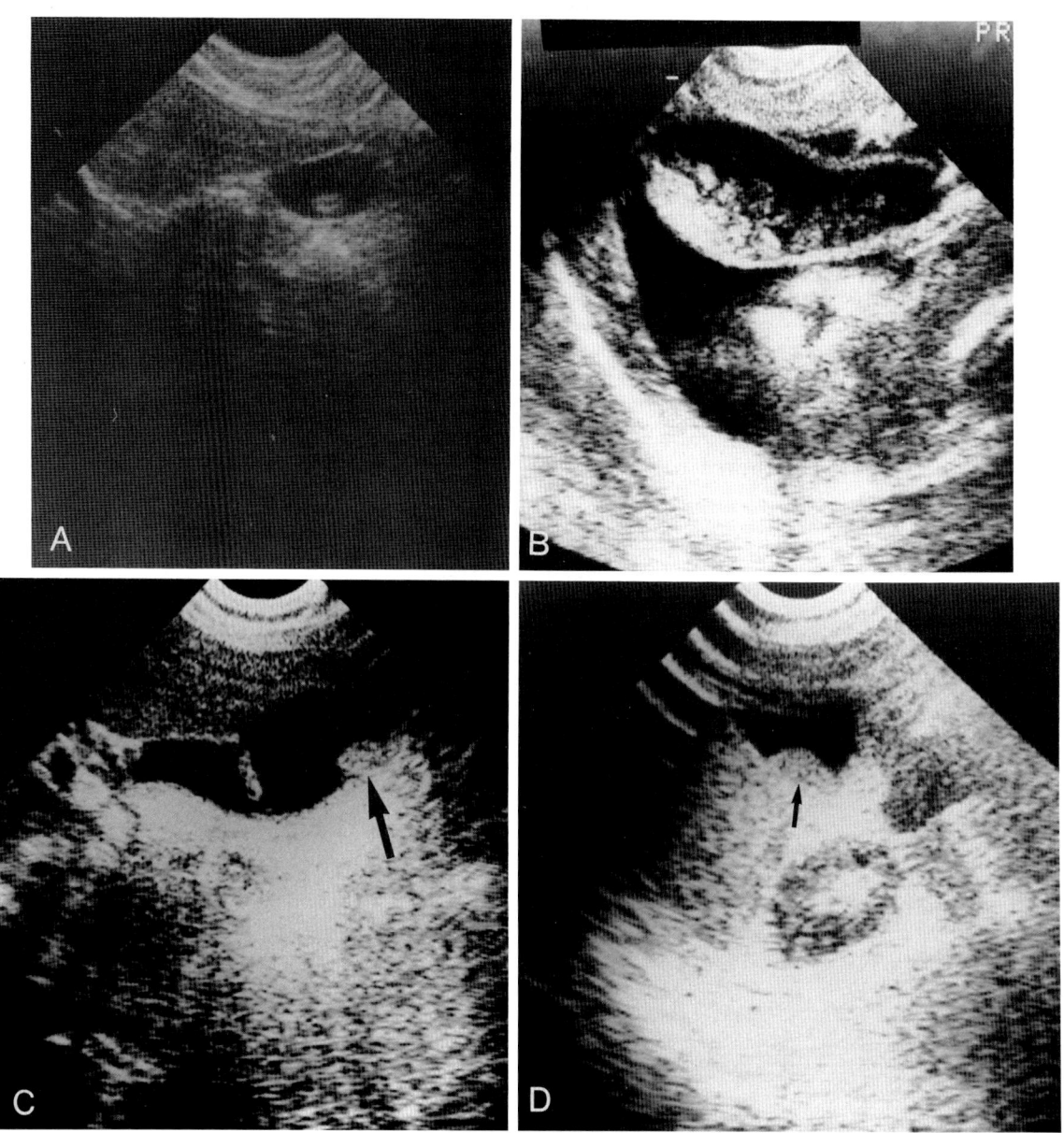

FIGURE 12.13. SLUDGE BALLS

A: This mobile, nonshadowing mass was not seen on a subsequent examination, consistent with tumefactive sludge. *B:* Multiple sludge balls in a patient with ascites. Biliary stasis and gallbladder distention (10.7 cm in length) probably due to parenteral feeding. *C* and *D:* Parasagittal and transverse scans of an echogenic, nonmobile sludge-ball (*arrows*).

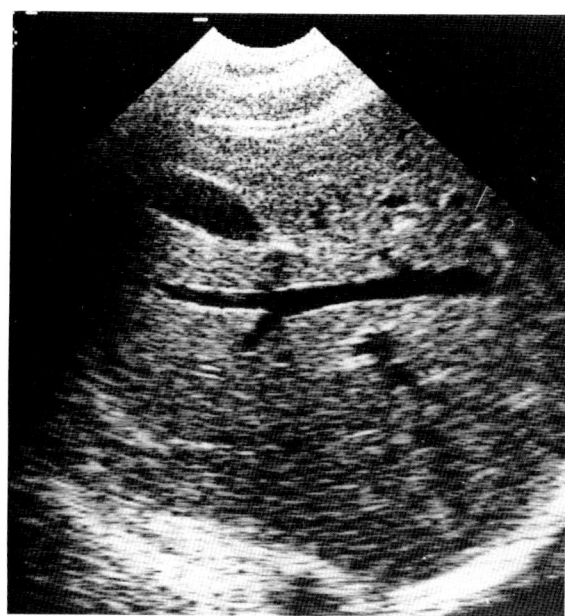

FIGURE 12.14. PSEUDO SLUDGE FROM VOLUME-AVERAGING
Low level artifactual echoes in the gallbladder.

shadowing. Although gravity dependent, sludge shifts position only slowly when the patient is moved (30, 31). The latter feature can sometimes permit differentiation from multiple small calculi, pus, blood, or mucus, which move faster and may otherwise look the same. Sludge is generally fairly homogeneous, and the presence of high level echo(es) within it suggests coexistent small stone(s).

Sludge can form a conglomerate mass or "sludge ball" (Fig. 12.13) (33). These well-defined nonshadowing masses are difficult to differentiate from gallbladder carcinoma (34). Awareness of this entity should prompt a repeat examination after resumption of normal eating habits. Although biliary sludge does not generally seem to predispose to stone formation Britten et al described the formation of three gallstones from sludge balls over the course of two years (35).

Slice thickness artifacts or beam averaging in the diverging portion of the sonic beam gives rise to "pseudo-sludge." These spurious echoes are created by averaging of echoes from adjacent hepatic parenchyma with anechoic bile (Fig. 12.14). This effect is visible in any curved fluid-filled structure, e.g., aorta, urinary bladder, large renal cyst. Changing the patient's position and taking advantage of the infinite scan planes afforded by real-time scanning will determine the true nature of these echoes (36).

REFERENCES

1. Cooperberg PL, Pons MS, Wong P, Stoller JL, Burhenne HJ: Real-time high resolution ultrasound in the detection of biliary calculi. *Radiology* 131:789–790, 1979.
2. Birnholz JC: Population survey: ultrasonic cholecystography. *Gastrointest Radiol* 7:165–167, 1982.
3. McIntosh DM, Penney HF: Gray-scale ultrasonography as a screening procedure in the detection of gallbladder disease. *Radiology* 136:725–727, 1980.
4. Krook PM, Allen FH, Bush WH, Malmer G, MacLean MD: Comparison of real-time cholecystosonography and oral cholecystography. *Radiology* 135:145–148, 1980.
5. Raptopoulos V, Moss L, Reuter K, Kleinman P: Comparison of real-time and gray-scale static ultrasonic cholecystography. *Radiology* 140:153–154, 1981.
6. Hessler PC, Hill DS, Detorie FM, Rocco AF: High accuracy sonographic recognition of gallstones. *AJR* 136:517–520, 1981.
7. Clair MR, Rosenberg ER, Ram PC, Bowie JD: Comparison of real-time and static-mode gray-scale ultrasonography in the diagnosis of cholelithiasis. *J Ultrasound Med* 1:201–203, 1982.
8. Crade M, Taylor KJ, Rosenfield AT, de Graff CS, Minihan P: Surgical and pathological correlation of cholecystosonography and cholecystography. *AJR* 131:227–229, 1978.
9. Gonzalez L, MacIntyre WJ: Acoustic shadow formation by gallstones. *Radiology* 135:217–218, 1980.
10. Taylor KJ, Jacobson P, Jaffe CC: Lack of an acoustic shadow on scans of gallstones: a possible artifact. *Radiology* 131:463–464, 1979.
11. Filly RA, Moss AA, Way LW: In vitro investigation of gallstone shadowing with ultrasound tomography. *J Clin Ultrasound* 7:255–262, 1979.
12. Carroll BA: Gallstones: In vitro comparison of physical, radiographic, and ultrasonic characteristics. *AJR* 131:223–226, 1978.
13. Good LI, Edell SL, Soloway RD, Trotman BW, Mulhern C, Arger PA: Ultrasonic properties of gallstones. *Gastroenterology* 77:258–263, 1979.
14. Grossman M: Cholelithiasis and acoustic shadowing. *J Clin Ultrasound* 6:182–184, 1978.
15. Harbin WP, Ferrucci JT, Wittenberg J, Kirkpatrick RH: Nonvisualized gallbladder by cholecystosonography. *AJR* 132:727–728, 1979.
16. Purdom RC, Thomas SR, Kereiakas JG, Spitz HB, Goldenberg NJ, Krugh KB: Ultrasonic properties of biliary calculi. *Radiology* 136:729–732, 1980.
17. Jeanty P, Ammann W, Cooperberg P et al: Mobile intraluminal masses of the gallbladder. *J Ultrasound Med* 2:65–71, 1983.
18. Sommer FG, Taylor KJ: Differentiation of acoustic shadowing due to calculi and gas collections. *Radiology* 135:399–403, 1980.
19. Parulekar SG: Ultrasonic detection of calcification in gallstones: "the reverberation shadow." *J Ultrasound Med* 3:123–129, 1984.
20. Rubaltelli L, Talenti E, Rizzato G, Bulzacchi A, Angelini F, Zucchi C: Gas-containing gallstones: their influence on ultrasound images. *J Clin Ultrasound* 12:279–282, 1984.
21. Conrad MR, Leonard J, Landay MJ: Left lateral decubitus sonography of gallstones in the contracted gallbladder. *AJR* 134:141–144, 1980.
22. Cunningham JJ, Carswell EL: Strong acoustical shadowing from the gallbladder bed: ultrasonic-pathologic correlation. *Gastrointest Radiol* 7:367–369, 1982.
23. Raptopoulos V, D'Orsi C, Smith E, Reuter K, Moss L,

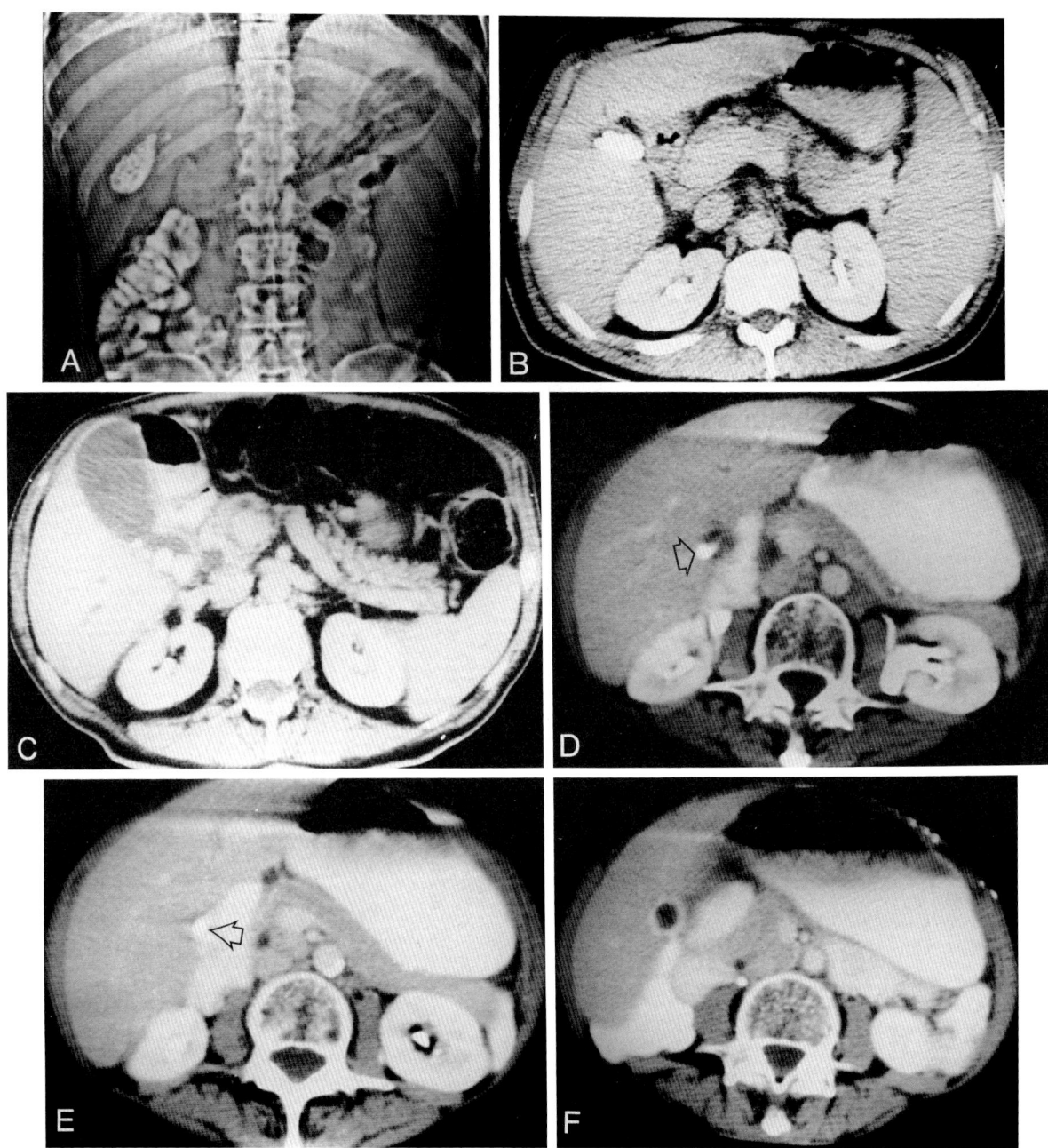

FIGURE 12.15. OPAQUE STONES ON CT

A and *B:* Hemolytic anemia: splenomegaly and very dense gallstones on topogram (*A*) and CT (*B*). Note streak artefacts from the stones. *C:* Four gallstones in the neck of the gallbladder. *D–F:* Cephalocaudad progression of scans showing a stone in the cystic duct (*arrows*) cephalad to a small gallbladder with a slightly thickened, prominently enhanced wall consistent with cholelithiasis and chronic cholecystitis (the patient had no acute symptoms). *G:* Seven small calcified gallstones.

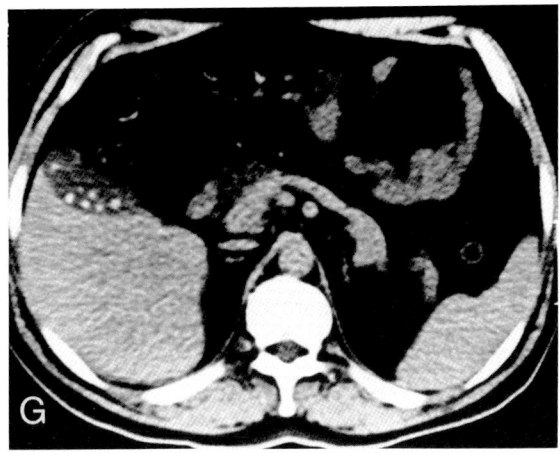

FIGURE 12.15G

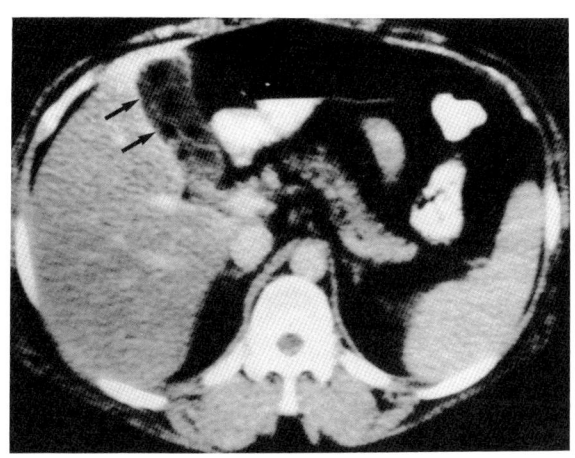

FIGURE 12.16. CHOLESTEROL LUCENT STONES IN THE GALLBLADDER (*arrows*)

23. Kleinman P: Dynamic cholecystosonography of the contracted gallbladder: the double-arc-shadow sign. *AJR* 138:275–278, 1982.
24. Simeone JF, Mueller PR, Ferrucci JT, Harbin WP, Wittenberg J: Significance of nonshadowing focal opacities at cholecystosonography. *Radiology* 137:181–185, 1980.
25. Scheske GA, Cooperberg PL, Cohen MM, Burhenne HJ: Floating gallstones: the role of contrast material. *J Clin Ultrasound* 8:227–231, 1980.
26. Strijk SP, Boetes C, Rosenbusch G: Floating stones in a nonopacified gallbladder: ultrasonographic sign of gas-containing gallstones. *Gastrointest Radiol* 6:261–263, 1981.
27. Dunne MG, Johnson ML: Gas within gallstones on CT. *AJR* 134:1065–1066, 1980.
28. Kane RA: Ultrasonographic evaluation of the gallbladder. *CRC Crit Rev Diagn Imaging* 17:107–159, 1982.
29. Lebensart PR, Bloom RA, Meretyk S, Landau EK, Shiloni E: Oral Cholecystosonography: a method for facilitating the diagnosis of cholesterol gallstones. *Radiology* 153:255–256, 1984.
30. Conrad MR, Janes JO, Dietchy J: Significance of low level echoes within the gallbladder. *AJR* 132:967, 1979.
31. Gosink BB, Leopold GR: Ultrasound and the gallbladder. *Semin Roentgenol* 11:185, 1976.
32. Filly RA, Allen B, Minton MJ, Bernhoft R, Way LW: In vitro investigation of the origin of echoes within biliary sludge. *J Clin Ultrasound* 8:193–200, 1980.
33. Fakhry J: Sonography of tumefactive biliary sludge. *AJR* 139:717–719, 1982.
34. Anastasi B, Sutherland GR: Biliary sludge-ultrasonic appearance simulating neoplasm. *Br J Radiol* 54:679–681, 1981.
35. Britten JS, Golding RH, Cooperberg PL: Sludge balls to gallstones. *J Ultrasound Med* 3:81–83, 1984.
36. Fiske CE, Filly RA: Pseudo-sludge, a spurious ultrasound appearance within the gallbladder. *Radiology* 144:631–632, 1982.

Computed Tomography

Gallstones are frequent incidental findings on CT scans performed for other reasons. Because of partial voluming and/or isodensity, CT may fail to detect calculi that are easily seen by ultrasound or oral cholecystography. On the other hand, using mostly a second generation 18-sec scanner and 13 mm slice thickness, Havrilla and coworkers (1) detected 78% of gallstones prospectively and 94% retrospectively. One proba-

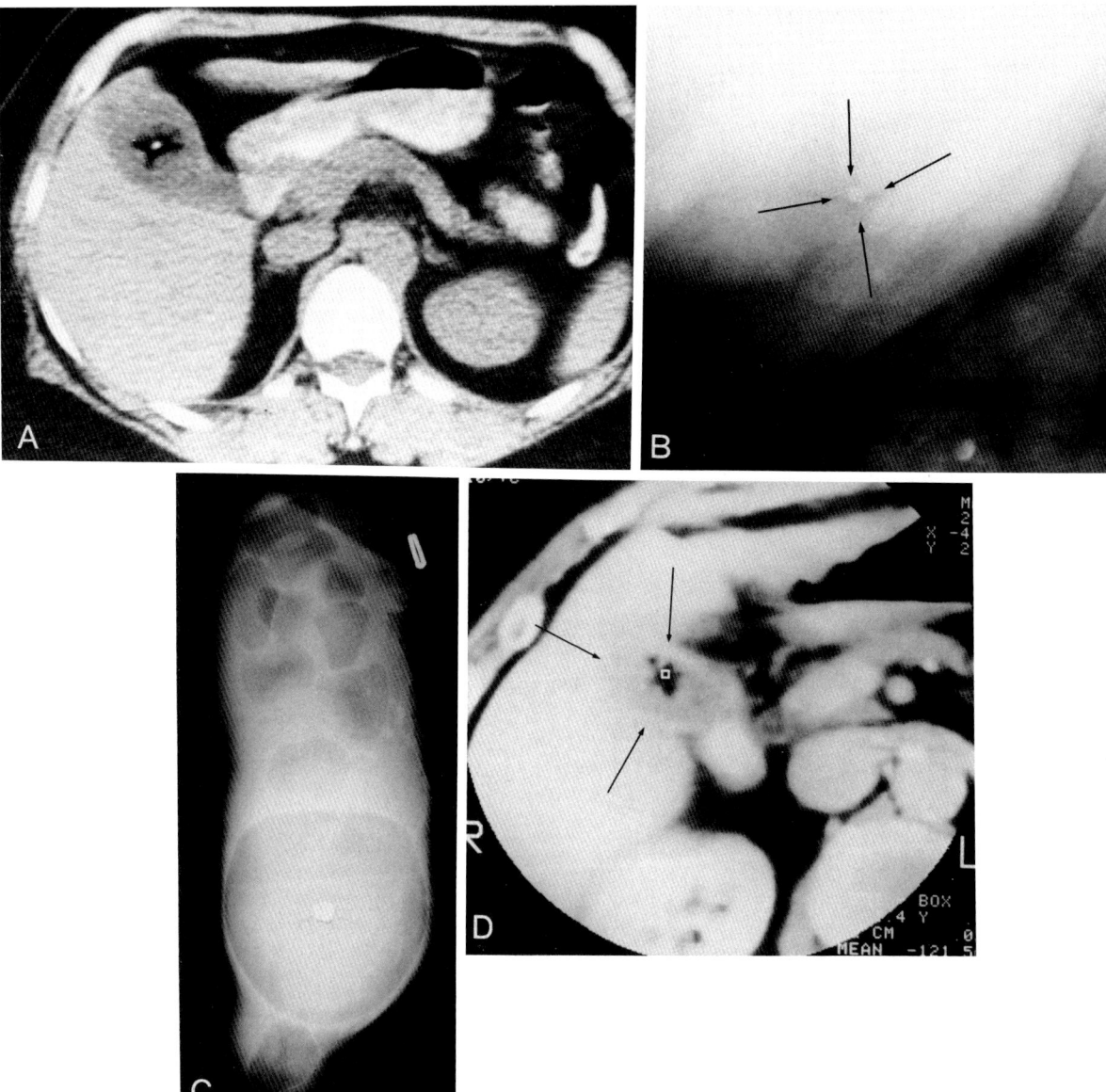

FIGURE 12.17. GAS-CONTAINING STONE WITH CENTRAL CALCIFICATION

A–C: Unusual fissured gas-containing stone with a dot of central calcification (*A*). The cleft was seen in retrospect on the plain film as well (*arrows, B*). The calcification and the fissuring are well seen on the specimen radiograph (*C*). *D:* More typical gas-containing (*cursor*) stone within the gallbladder (*arrows*). Mean CT number was −127 H, higher than air because of partial voluming.

bly could detect nearly all gallstones with current equipment using thin sections and narrow window widths, but sonography is clearly a superior modality. Most gallstones are seen on CT as opacities within the lower attenuation bile (Fig. 12.15). Some are nearly isodense with or less dense than bile and require narrow windows for visualization (Fig. 12.16). Rarely, a stone will be isodense save for a central, triradiate gas-containing cleft, the CT version of the Mercedes-Benz sign (Fig. 12.17) (2). A study of 25 gallstones in vitro (water bath) showed that calcified gallstones sink, gas-containing stones float, and that CT numbers of calculi varied from −188 HU to +178 HU (−500 to +500 scale) (3).

REFERENCES

1. Havrilla TR, Reich NE, Haaga JR, Seidelmann FE, Cooperman AM, Alfidi RJ: Computed tomography of the gallbladder. *AJR* 130:1059–1067, 1978.
2. Dunne MG, Johnson ML: Gas within gallstones on CT. *AJR* 134:1065, 1980.
3. Moss AA, Filly RA, Way LW: In vitro investigation of gallstones with computed tomography. *J Comput Assist Tomogr* 4:827–831, 1980.

ACUTE CHOLECYSTITIS

Clinical Findings

The vast majority (90% or more) of patients with acute cholecystitis have cystic duct obstruction by a gallstone (1). As opposed to biliary colic, the obstruction is persistent. The inflammation is multifactorial: increased intraluminal pressure, ischemia, enzymes and bile acids, and bacteria. Up to 30% of patients admitted for acute cholecystitis will not give a history suggestive of cholelithiasis. Their pain is right upper quadrant or epigastric and increases with motion. Nausea is frequent and vomiting may occur. The accompanying fever is usually low grade. Local guarding may hinder palpation. Murphy's sign (commonly misinterpreted in the radiologic literature as merely local tenderness) is inspiratory arrest and increased tenderness upon palpation of the right upper quadrant during deep inspiration. It is fairly specific although not that frequently elicited as defined above (1–3).

Leukocytosis is frequent. One-third to one-half of these patients will have elevations in alkaline phosphatase, transaminases, and/or bilirubin (3).

In about 75% symptoms will resolve within 3 days of onset with conservative treatment, presumably after the stone passes or falls back. Unless cholecystectomy (or cholecystostomy) is done, the remaining 25% will develop complications such as necrosis, perforation, and/or empyema (1, 2). On the other hand, as many as half of the patients suspected of having acute cholecystitis will have no gallbladder pathology. Common diseases that may mimic acute cholecystitis include right-sided pneumonia, pyelonephritis, or pyonephrosis, pancreatitis and peptic ulcer disease. Less commonly, liver disease such as hepatocellular carcinoma or metastases, pelvic inflammatory disease, ovarian or enteric pathology, and coronary artery disease may present with acute right upper quadrant pain. Therefore a need exists for early and rapid confirmation of a clinical diagnosis of acute cholecystitis both to prevent unnecessary emergency surgery in those patients who have another disease and to operate promptly when indicated in those patients who do indeed have acute cholecystitis to forestall complications.

REFERENCES

1. Schein CJ: *Acute Cholecystitis.* New York, Harper & Row, 1972.
2. Schoenfield LJ: *Diseases of the Gallbladder and Biliary System* (Clinical Gastroenterology Monographs). New York, John Wiley & Sons, 1977.
3. Gagic N, Frey CF, Gaines R: Acute cholecystitis. *Surg Gynecol Obstet* 140:868–874, 1975.

Radiology

Plain Films

The abdominal plain film is usually normal in acute cholecystitis, but it may reveal calcified gallstones. In severe cases, small bowel ileus in the form of dilated loops with air-fluid levels usually localized to the right upper quadrant may be seen (1, 2). Sometimes concomitant dilatation of the colon will be present. Very uncommonly in uncomplicated acute cholecystitis, the gallbladder is enlarged enough to be visible as a mass by virtue of adjacent bowel displacement.

Contrast Gastrointestinal Examination

Acute cholecystitis is almost never encountered on a barium examination in a modern radiology department. Historically, duodenography demonstrated, at times, luminal narrowing, fold thickening, spasm, and irritability involving the postbulbar duodenum. The superolateral aspect characteristically is preferentially affected (3). Occasionally, barium enema can show a smooth, extrinsic impression along the superior margin at or near the hepatic flexure. Sometimes luminal narrowing is present from edema or spasm (4, 5).

REFERENCES

1. Weens HS, Walker LA: The radiologic diagnosis of acute cholecystitis and pancreatitis. *Radiol Clin North Am* 2:89, 1964.
2. Frimann-Dahl J: *Roentgen Examinations in Acute Abdominal Diseases.* Springfield, Ill., Charles C Thomas, 1960, p 34.
3. Berk RN: Radiology of the gallbladder and bile ducts. *Surg Clin North Am* 53:973, 1973.
4. Ghahremani GG, Meyers MA: The cholecysto-colic relationships: a roentgen-anatomic study of the colonic manifestations of gallbladder disorders. *AJR* 125:21, 1975.
5. Crawford A: An irregularity in transverse colon diagnosis. *Aust NZ J Surg* 41:50, 1971.

Oral Cholecystography and Intravenous Cholangiography

Oral cholecystography was of limited usefulness in the diagnosis of acute cholecystitis even before the development of newer imaging modalities, because of both the inherent delay after ingestion of contrast and lack of specificity. If performed, the usual finding was nonvisualization. If the common duct could be seen and/or conjugated contrast detected in the bowel in the presence of nonvisualization, cystic duct obstruction was highly likely. Gallbladder opacification and stone detection was highly unusual in the acute setting because of the cystic duct obstruction (Fig. 12.18). Intravenous cholangiography could diagnose cystic duct obstruction by virtue of common duct visualization and no gallbladder opacification at 24 hr, but again a substantial delay was necessary. Therefore these tests have been completely discarded in favor of sonography

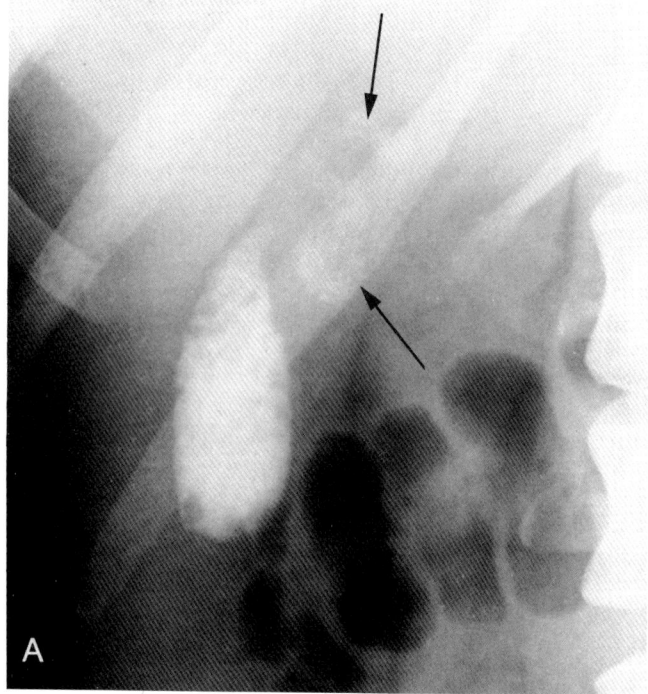

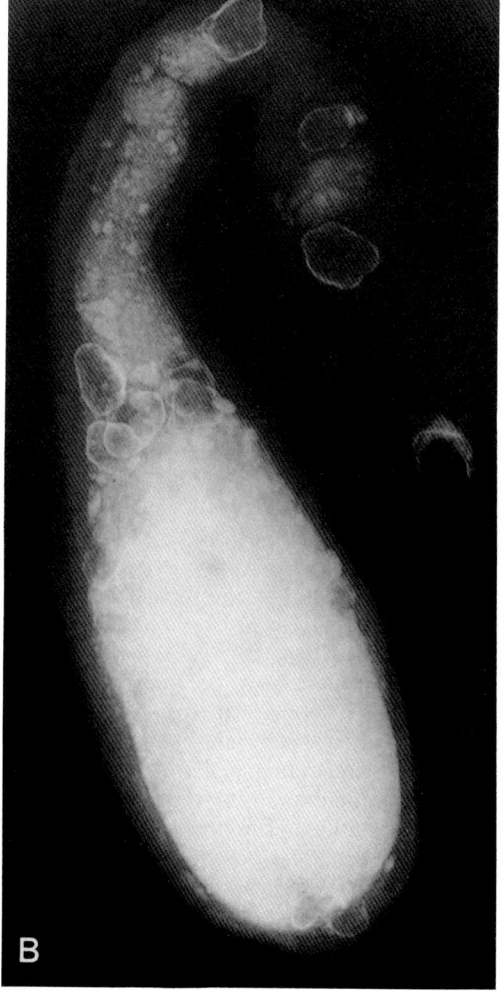

FIGURE 12.18. ORAL CHOLECYSTOGRAM IN ACUTE CHOLECYSTITIS

A: Oral cholecystogram in acute cholecystitis showing many gallstones and stones in the cystic duct (*arrows*). An unusual case. *B:* Specimen radiograph confirming the cholecystographic findings.

and radionuclide biliary scintigraphy for diagnosis of acute cholecystitis.

Ultrasound

Both ultrasound and hepatobiliary scintigraphy have been advocated as the test of choice for "emergency" diagnosis of acute cholecystitis. Both methods are excellent, but conflicting sensitivities and specificities have been reported. In part, this is due to the application of different pathological criteria for determining the presence or absence of acute changes in gallbladder specimens, different patient populations, and variable inclusion of nondiagnostic studies when calculating data. The current trend seems to be toward using cholescintigraphy for the diagnosis of acute cholecystitis and sonography for the detection of cholelithiasis and other chronic gallbladder problems in a more elective fashion. Certainly, the skills available in a given health care setting must be taken into account before choosing which test to order when acute cholecystitis is suspected. However, in many institutions clinicians are currently obtaining both examinations to "rule out" acute cholecystitis, which is usually a wasteful duplication of effort (1).

High sensitivities in the range of 85–95% have been reported for both sonography and cholescintigraphy in the diagnosis of acute cholecystitis, but specificities are somewhat lower (64–100% for sonography and 74–94% for cholescintigraphy) (2–7). Variations in the diagnostic criteria applied can alter the number of false positives by sonography. For example, use of a relatively low number for normal gallbladder wall thickness will increase the number of false positives and use of the sonographic Murphy's sign may decrease the number of false positives.

False positive or equivocal cholescintigrams can occur in the following settings: chronic cholecystitis, alcoholism, pancreatitis, total parenteral nutrition, narcotic use, and severe jaundice.

With respect to cholescintigraphy in the diagnosis of acute cholecystitis, the advantages of ultrasound are: speed (5 min compared to 1–4 hr), more consistent evaluation of adjacent structures, lack of dependence on hepatic excretory function and, usually, less cost (Fig. 12.19). Disadvantages are: relatively nonspecificity of findings with some dependence on secondary subjective signs, and greater operator dependence requiring the presence of more experienced personnel (Fig. 12.20).

Diagnostic Criteria for Acute Cholecystitis. The mere demonstration of gallstones alone by no means implies cystic duct obstruction and acute cholecystitis. Additional findings that suggest this diagnosis include: gallbladder wall thickening, gallbladder wall sonolucency, gallbladder distention and the sonographic Murphy's sign. Signs of complicated cholecystitis include: pericholecystic fluid, coarse nonshadowing nondependent echodensities within the gallbladder, and the presence of a pseudomembrane.

Gallbladder Wall Thickening. The thickness of the nearer subhepatic wall is measured to avoid artifact from underlying bowel gas and mesentery. The true thickness of the wall is measured sonographically as determined by pathologic correlates (8, 9) and it is less than 3.0–3.5 mm in 98% of the population (8–12). A thickened gallbladder wall in acute cholecystitis (Fig. 12.21) has been reported by many, usually with a sensitivity under 50% (8, 10), but sensitivity of about 70% was reported in two series (11, 13). Naturally these measurements must be obtained on distended gallbladders.

Unfortunately, gallbladder wall thickening can be seen in several other conditions; 10–25% of patients with chronic cholecystitis will have wall thickening (12). The hyperplastic cholecystoses, gallbladder perforation, sepsis, renal failure, cirrhosis, right-sided congestive heart failure, ascites and hepatitis have all been associated with thickened gallbladder walls (14). Less commonly, multiple myeloma, acute myelogenous leukemia, and brucellosis have been reported to cause gallbladder wall thickening (14).

Ascites and viral hepatitis are fairly common well-researched causes of gallbladder wall thickening (14–16). Gallbladder wall thickening is especially common in patients with ascites and hypoalbuminemia from alcoholic liver disease. Correlation with autopsy indicates that the finding is artifactually induced by the ascites (Fig. 12.22). Similar thickening can be seen in the urinary bladder wall when there is ascites in the pelvis (17). A number of scanning techniques such as decentering the beam or angulating the transducer can produce a similar artifact, as can immersing an object in a water bath (17, 18). Patients with viral hepatitis and no gallbladder disease may demonstrate sonographic gallbladder abnormalities (Fig. 12.23) (19). Most commonly there is thickening of the gallbladder wall with or without demonstration of three separate layers (20). Gallbladder volume may be reduced to the point of inability to identify the organ. Intraluminal echoes representing abnormal bile can be seen, at times completely filling the lumen. Up to 80% of hepatitis patients may show these changes (20). The sonographic findings are

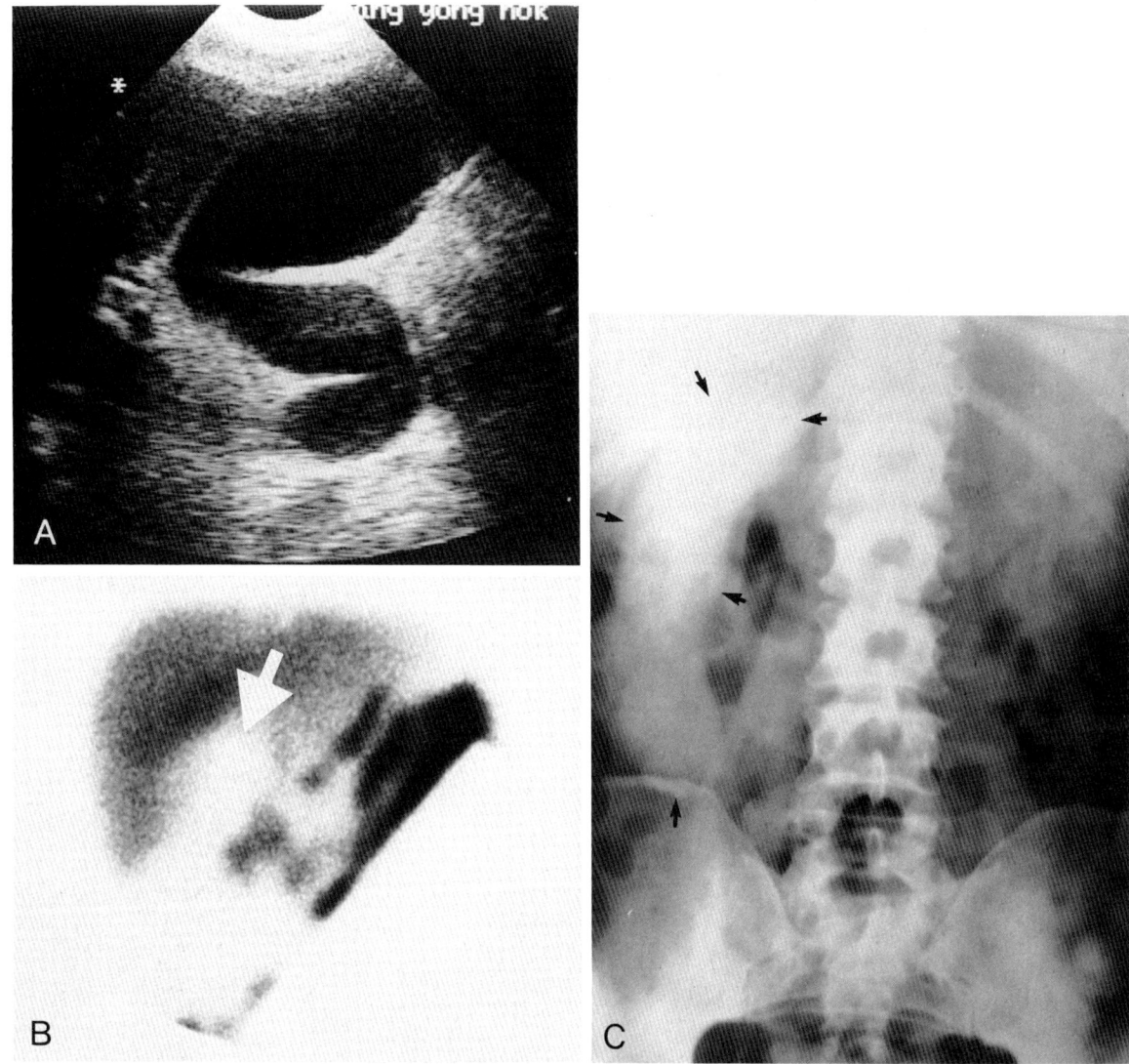

FIGURE 12.19. FALSE-POSITIVE DISIDA SCAN

False-positive DISIDA scan because of a prolonged fast in a patient who developed right upper quadrant pain, fever, and a palpable gallbladder three days after a liver biopsy. He had been NPO during this period. *A:* Markedly distended gallbladder (AP diameter 6.1 mm) but no stones seen on ultrasound. Normal wall thickness. *B:* A 60-min cholescintigram: no gallbladder filling, photopenic gallbladder fossa (*arrow*). A repeat scan 60 min after CCK and reinjection was unchanged. The imaging findings suggest acalculous cholecystitis. The attending physician doubted the diagnosis on clinical grounds, and fed the patient, who improved. His gallbladder became nonpalpable. *C:* Unreliability of distention alone as a criterion for acute cholecystitis is illustrated by this cholecystogram: huge but normally functioning gallbladder (*arrows*) in a diabetic.

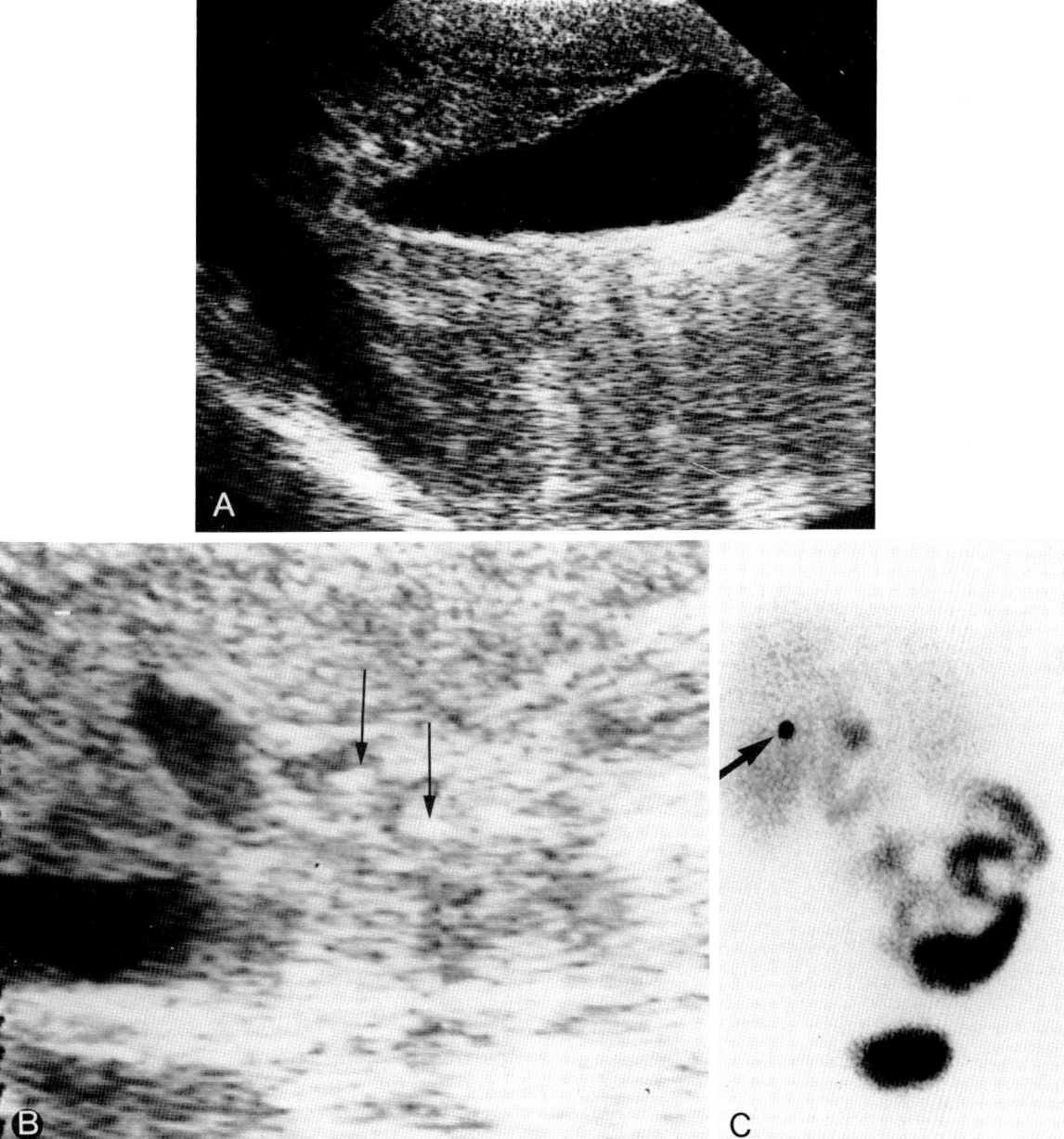

FIGURE 12.20. CYSTIC DUCT STONES AND ACUTE CHOLECYSTITIS
A: Parasagittal scan: tense gallbladder (4.2 mm AP diameter), no obvious stones. *B:* Meticulous scanning through the cystic duct shows two echogenic stones (*arrows*, magnification view). Ultrasound diagnosis is quite difficult. *C:* Confirmatory DISIDA scan: 2 hr—no gallbladder filling (hot cobalt marker over gallbladder, *arrow*). Radionuclide diagnosis is easy.

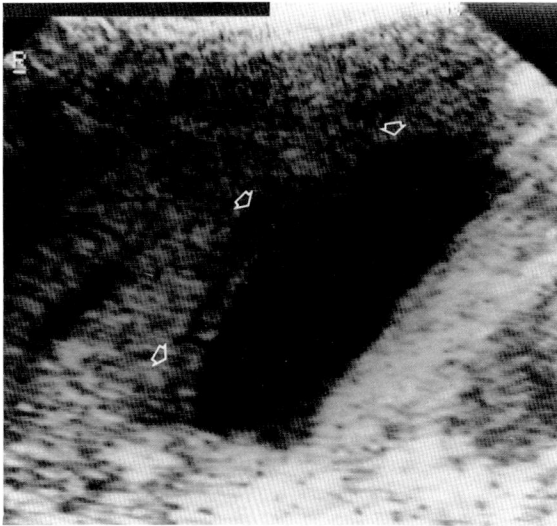

FIGURE 12.21. THICKENED GALLBLADDER WALL IN ACUTE CHOLECYSTITIS
Thickened gallbladder wall (*arrows*) measures 5.4 mm.

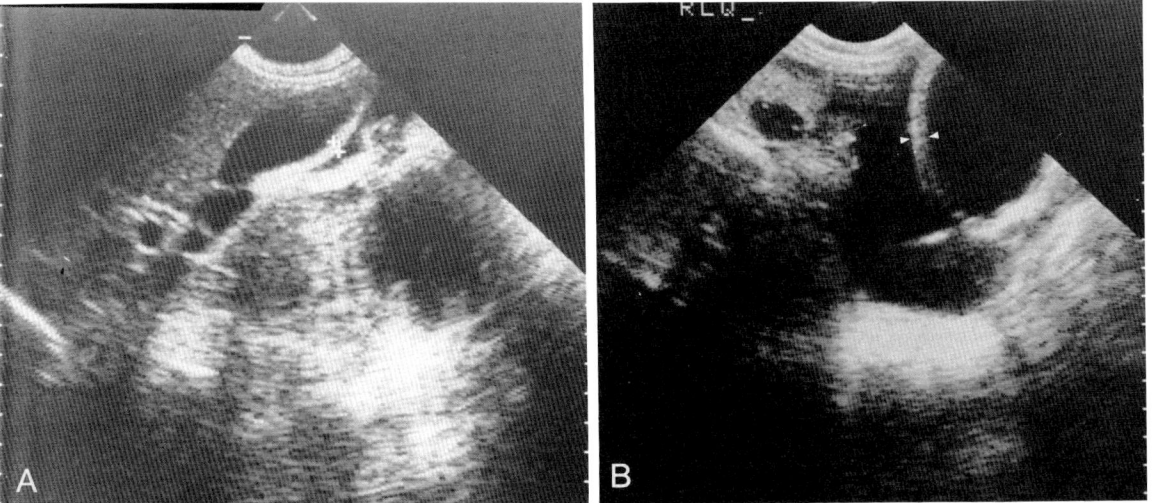

FIGURE 12.22. THICKENED GALLBLADDER WALL DUE TO ASCITES
A: Factitious thickening of the gallbladder wall (*cursors*) due to ascites. *B:* Same phenomenon involving the urinary bladder (*arrowheads*).

completely reversible and should resolve within 20–30 days (20). It is thought that the gallbladder is affected in some way by the inflammation in the adjacent liver.

Gallbladder Wall Sonolucency. More specific than mere wall thickening may be the presence of gallbladder wall sonolucency. Marchal et al. (21) initially described a three-layer configuration consisting of a sonolucent middle layer sandwiched between two outer hyperreflective layers (Fig. 12.24). The sonolucent layer may be either continuous or interrupted (21). Similar observations have been made by Raghavendra who feels that this sonolucent layer is a sensitive indicator of the presence of edema fluid and cellular infiltrate in the gallbladder wall. This finding was present in 70% in his series of 24 patients (11).

Gallbladder Distention. The size of the normal gallbladder is quite variable, but an external AP diameter of more than 4.0–5.0 cm is suspicious for (but certainly not diagnostic of) cystic duct obstruction (Fig. 12.19C). The obstructed gallbladder assumes a globular, tense configuration with loss of its normal pear shape (Fig. 12.20A) (3, 13). Diminished gallbladder emptying from nonobstructive causes may give rise to gallbladder dilatation (Fig. 12.19A). Diabetes mellitus, hyperalimentation, and narcotic analgesia may all cause diminished gallbladder emptying.

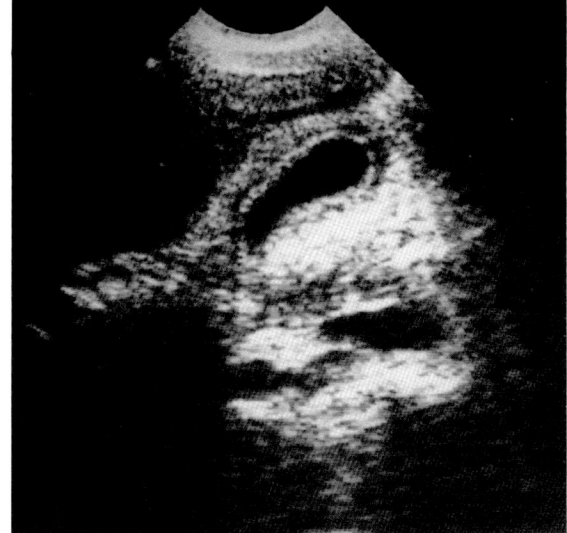

FIGURE 12.23. THICKENED GALLBLADDER WALL DUE TO ACUTE HEPATITIS
Thickened gallbladder wall in a patient with acute hepatitis, not seen on a repeat examination 2 weeks later.

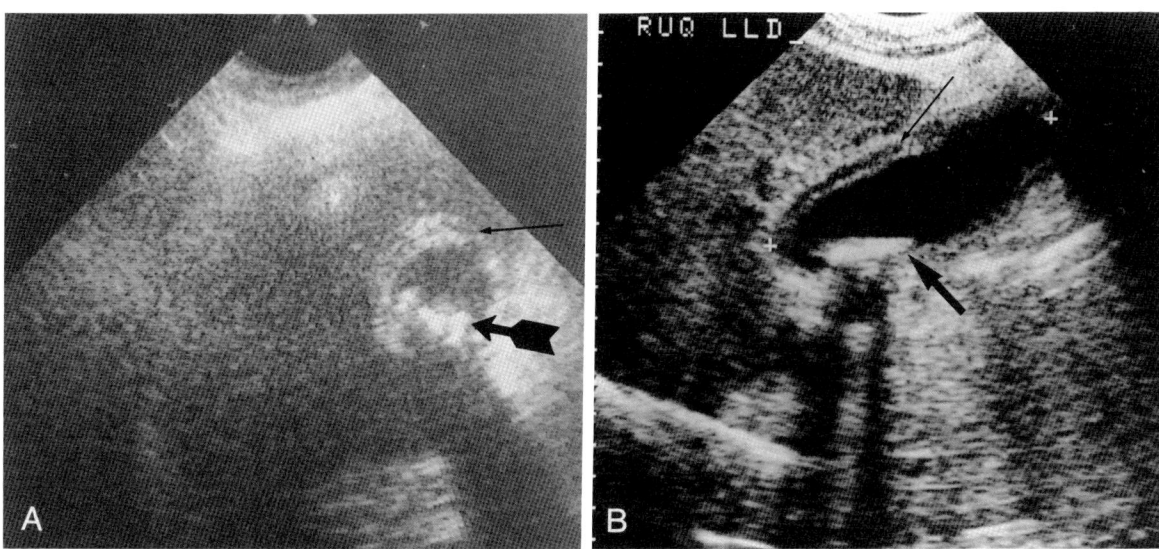

FIGURE 12.24. TRIPLE-LAYERED GALLBLADDER WALL IN ACUTE CHOLECYSTITIS, TWO EXAMPLES
A: Transverse scan: note shadowing stones (*large arrow*) and central lucency within wall (*small arrow*). B: Parasagittal scan: central lucency within wall (*small arrow*) and shadowing stone (*large arrow*).

The WDHA syndrome can lead to gallbladder distention by virtue of the secretin-like effect of vasoactive intestinal polypeptide.

Sonographic Murphy's Sign. The sonographic Murphy's sign (as described in most ultrasound literature) is evaluated by locating the gallbladder in the right upper quadrant and assessing the degree of tenderness by palpation with the transducer. The sign is considered positive if maximal tenderness is elicited over the gallbladder. If the right upper quadrant is diffusely tender, or if no tenderness is elicited, the sign is considered negative. This test is highly subjective and many patients are unable to sense differential pain levels. Nonetheless, many have found it useful (sensitivity of 63% and specificity of 93% in one series, and sensitivity of 94% in another) (13, 22). In clinical practice, patients are referred to "rule out" acute cholecystitis, and the diagnosis will rarely, if ever, be made sonographically when unsuspected clinically. Thus, specificity is far more imporant than sensitivity. Use of a true Murphy's sign during sonography (deep inspiration during pressure over the gallbladder with the transducer producing increased tenderness and inspiratory arrest) is more useful in my opinion. Sensitivity is lower than the more common definition, but specificity is higher in my experience.

REFERENCES

1. Caldwell JH: Ultrasound vs. radionuclide scan in evaluation of acute right upper quadrant abdominal pain: clinician's comments. *J Clin Ultrasound* 11:201–202, 1983.
2. Laing FC, Federle MP, Jeffrey RB, Brown TW: Ultrasonic evaluation of patients with acute right upper quadrant pain. *Radiology* 140:449–455, 1981.
3. Worthen NJ, Uszler JM, Funamura JL: Cholecystitis: prospective evaluation of sonography and ^{99m}Tc-HIDA cholescintigraphy. *AJR* 137:973–978, 1981.
4. Shuman WP, Mack LA, Rudd TG, Rogers JV, Gibbs P: Evaluation of acute right upper quadrant pain: sonography and ^{99m}Tc-PIPIDA cholescintigraphy. *AJR* 139:61–64, 1982.
5. Maturo VG, Zusmer NR, Smoak WM, Stern MH, Gilson AJ, Janowitz WR: The role of biliary scintigraphy and ultrasonography in the diagnosis of cholecystitis. *Rev Interam J Radiol* 6:47–50, 1981.
6. Ralls PW, Coletti PM, Halls JM, Siemsen JK: Prospective evaluation of ^{99m}Tc-IDA cholescintigraphy and grayscale ultrasound in the diagnosis of acute cholecystitis. *Radiology* 144:369–371, 1982.
7. Samuels BI, Freitas JE, Bree RL, Schwab RE, Heller ST: A comparison of radionuclide hepatobiliary imaging and real-time ultrasound for the detection of acute cholecystitis. *Radiology* 147:207–210, 1983.
8. Engel JM, Deitch EA, Sikkema W: Gallbladder wall thickness: sonographic accuracy and relation to disease. *AJR* 134:907–909, 1980.
9. Finberg HJ, Birnholz JC: Ultrasound evaluation of the gallbladder wall. *Radiology* 133:693–698, 1979.
10. Sanders RC: The significance of sonographic gallbladder wall thickening. *J Clin Ultrasound* 8:143–146, 1980.
11. Raghavendra BN, Feiner HD, Subramanyam BR et al: Acute cholecystitis: sonographic-pathologic analysis. *AJR* 137:327–332, 1981.
12. Handler SJ: Ultrasound of gallbladder wall thickening and its relation to cholecystitis. *AJR* 132:581–585, 1979.
13. Laing FC: Diagnostic evaluation of patients with suspected cholecystitis. *Surg Clin North Am* 64:3–22, 1984.
14. Shlaer WJ, Leopold GO, Scheible FW: Sonography of the thickened gallbladder wall: a nonspecific finding. *AJR* 136:337–339, 1981.
15. Fiske CE, Laing FC, Brown TW: Ultrasonographic evidence of gallbladder wall thickening in association with hypoalbuminemia. *Radiology* 135:713–716, 1980.
16. Ralls PW, Quinn MF, Juttner HU, Halls J, Boswell WD: Gallbladder wall thickening: patients without intrinsic gallbladder disease. *AJR* 137:65–68, 1981.
17. Auh YH, Rubinstein WA, Schneider M, Kazam E: Sonographic pseudothickening of the gallbladder with ascites: clinical significance and physical basis. Paper 315. Presented at AIUM, 1981.
18. Lewandowski BJ, Winsberg F: Gallbladder wall thickness distortion by ascites. *AJR* 137:519–521, 1981.
19. Juttner HU, Ralls PW, Quinn MF, Jenney JM: Thickening of the gallbladder wall in acute hepatitis: ultrasound demonstration. *Radiology* 142:465–466, 1982.
20. Maresca G, De Gaetano AM, Mirk P, Cauda R, Federico G, Colagrande C: Sonographic patterns of the gallbladder in acute viral hepatitis. *J Clin Ultrasound* 12:141–146, 1984.
21. Marchal GJ, Casaer M, Baert AL, Goddeeris PG, Kerremans R, Fevery J: Gallbladder wall sonolucency in acute cholecystitis. *Radiology* 133:429–433, 1979.
22. Ralls PW, Halls J, Lapin SA, Quinn MF, Morris UL, Boswell W: Prospective evaluation of the sonographic Murphy sign in suspected acute cholecystitis. *J Clin Ultrasound* 10:113–115, 1982.

Hepatobiliary Scintigraphy

Suspected acute cholecystitis is the most important indication for the use of the ^{99m}Tc-IDA (iminodiacetic acid) agents. The wide clinical use of radionuclide imaging in the workup of patients suspected of having acute cholecystitis began in the late 1970s and early 1980s with the introduction of the ^{99m}Tc-labeled IDA agents. Although there are a number of possible diagnostic strategies for the evaluation of the patient presenting with signs and symptoms suggestive of acute cholecystitis, the radioisotopic study provides the highest overall sensitivity and specificity.

Cholescintigraphic Technique. In the vast majority of instances, there is no need for "patient preparation." However, patients should be fasted for 4–6 hr prior to the study so that the gallbladder is not being stimulated to contract by the endogenous release of CCK. Since most patients suspected to having acute cholecystitis will not have eaten recently, this is rarely a problem. A more important potential problem occurs when a patient is receiving total parenteral nutrition (TPN) and/or has been fasting for a prolonged period, as these clinical situations have been associated with false positive cholescintigrams (1, 2). In cases where the patient has not eaten for more than 24 hr, consideration should be given to pretreating the patient with CCK or its terminal octapeptide analog, sincalide (Kinevac, E. R. Squibb), 30 min prior to the examination. If the patient has not eaten for several days or longer, then it may be helpful to give several doses of CCK simulating a normal feeding pattern and stimulating the gallbladder to contract and empty its viscous bile before beginning the ^{99m}Tc-IDA study. It should be emphasized that this applies to the minority of clinical instances.

The patient is placed supine on the imaging table with the gamma camera positioned so that the superior aspect of the liver is at the uppermost portion of the field of view. This allows for adequate visualization of the liver, biliary tract and small bowel. Five mCi of a ^{99m}Tc-IDA analog (e.g., diisopropylphenylcarbamoyl iminodiacetic acid (Hepatolite), New England Nuclear-Dupont, North Billerica, Mass.) is administered. Imaging is begun at 1 min for the blood pool phase and then at 5-min intervals for the first ½-hr period. This is followed by a scintiphoto at 45 and 60 min. The study may be terminated earlier if labeled bile is definitely seen within the gallbladder and small bowel. Most studies are completed within 20–60 min with normal visualization of the liver, common duct, gallbladder, and duodenum (Fig. 12.25). It is important to monitor the study on the persistence scope to determine if oblique and/or lateral projections are necessary (e.g., to distinguish gallbladder from duodenal sweep) (3). If the gallbladder is not seen in the first hour, obtaining delayed views to 4 hr (e.g., 1½-, 2-, and 4-hr views) improves the specificity of the study and significantly decreases the false positive rate (4). Alternatively, the use of morphine or cholecystokinin has been recommended to improve the specificity while obviating the need for delayed views (5, 6). If the gallbladder fails to visualize in clinical situations known to be associated with biliary stasis (e.g., TPN, prolonged fasting, alcoholism) then delayed images to 24 hr should be considered.

Accuracy. The cholescintigraphic agents have proven to be extremely sensitive and specific in evaluating patients suspected of having acute cholecystitis. When a large number of cases ($N = 736$) from four separate institutions are combined using the criteria of normal biliary-to-bowel-transit (within one hour) and nonvisualization of the gallbladder up to 4 hr (Fig. 12.26), the overall accuracy is 95% with a sensitivity of 97% and a specificity of 94% (7–10). Results from the various articles in the literature will depend on the techniques used to perform the examination, the patient population being studied, the interpretive criteria used, the duration of the study, and the clinical and/or pathological criteria used as the "gold standard." The pathological and/or clinical criteria used will have a major impact on the reported results (Table 12.1)

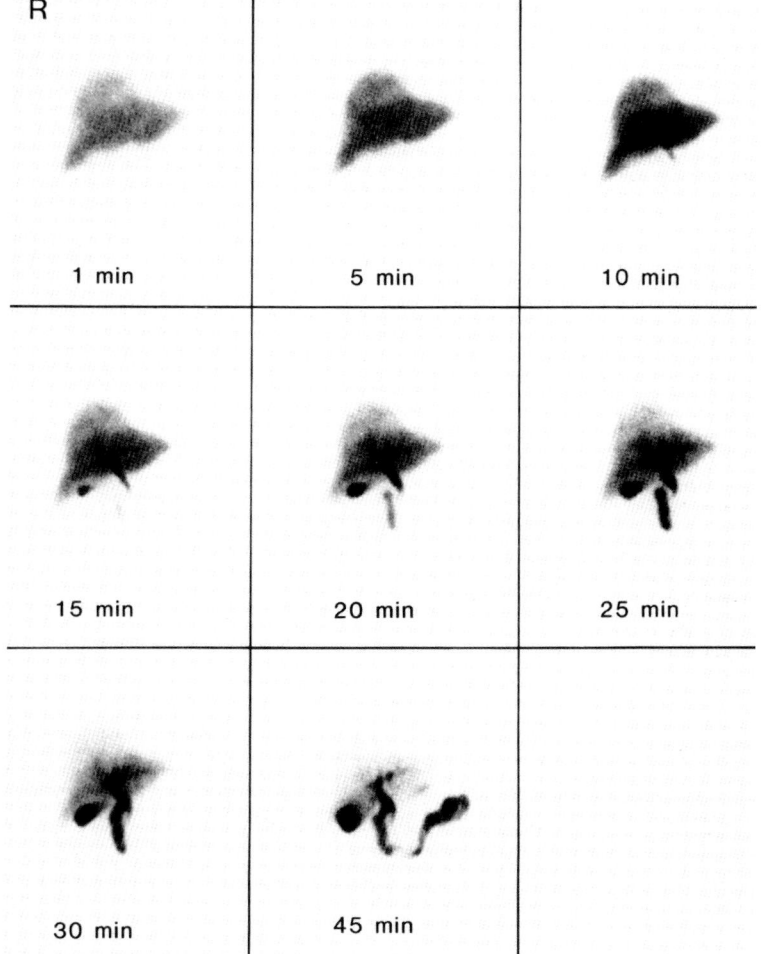

FIGURE 12.25. NORMAL ^{99m}Tc-DISIDA CHOLESCINTIGRAM

Excellent uptake of the radiotracer by the liver is followed by prompt excretion into the common duct, gallbladder, and intestine.

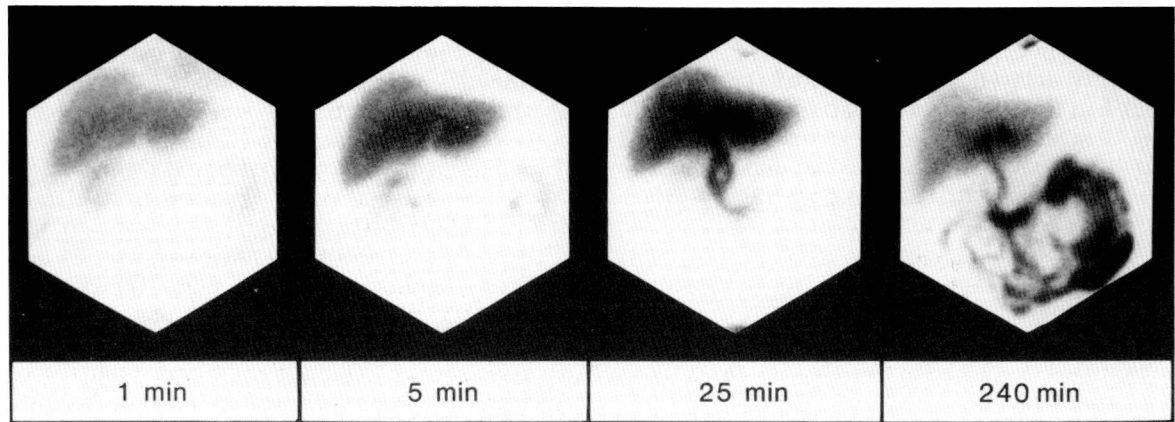

FIGURE 12.26. ACUTE CHOLECYSTITIS WITH CYSTIC DUCT OBSTRUCTION
Excellent uptake of ^{99m}Tc-DISIDA by the liver is followed by prompt excretion into the small bowel. Serial images through four hours failed to visualize the gallbladder.

TABLE 12.1.
EFFECT OF CLINICAL/PATHOLOGIC CRITERIA IN THE RESULTS OF HEPATOBILIARY IMAGING[a]

Criteria	Findings (%)	
	Sensitivity	Specificity
1. Transmural acute inflammatory infiltration	98	91
2. Hemorrhagic necrosis of the gallbladder wall or mucosa	98	94
3. Criteria 2 or complete cystic duct obstruction	98	96
4. Any of the above criteria or relief of pain, fever and leukocytosis following cholecystectomy	95	99

[a] Modified from Freitas JE, Coleman RE, Nagle CE, et al: Influence of scan and pathologic criteria on the specificity of cholescintigraphy. Concise communication. *J Nucl Med* 24:876–879, 1983.

(10). Delayed views up to 4 hr in the setting of normal biliary-to-bowel transit with non-visualization of the gallbladder will improve the specificity of the test with little compromise in the sensitivity and an overall improvement in the accuracy (Table 12.2) (4, 10).

Diagnostic Findings. Weissmann and colleagues (7) described the spectrum of cholescintigraphic findings that can be seen in patients with acute cholecystitis (Table 12.3). In 323 patients studied, there were 143 cases of acute cholecystitis, 96% of whom had nonvisualization of the gallbladder. Less than 1% of patients with acute cholecystitis had normal gallbladder visualization in less than 1 hr. Normal gallbladder visualization in less than 1 hr has repeatedly been confirmed to exclude acute cholecystitis with virtual certainty. In distinction from intravenous cholangiography where the common bile duct must be seen in order to consider the study valid, when there is cholescintigraphic nonvisualization of the gallbladder and common duct with normal transit from the liver to the bowel, a diagnosis of acute cholecystitis can be made. Delayed gallbladder visualization at or later than 1 hr is usually secondary to chronic cholecystitis. However, since 3.5% of patients with acute cholecystitis may exhibit delayed gallbladder visualization, this scintigraphic pattern does not exclude the diagnosis with the same degree of certainty as normal gallbladder visualization in less than 1 hr.

TABLE 12.2.
EFFECT OF DELAYED IMAGING ON THE RESULTS OF HEPATOBILIARY IMAGING IN ACUTE CHOLECYSTITIS[a]

	Findings (%)	
	1 Hour[b]	4 Hours
Sensitivity	100/98	98/95
Specificity	90/88	96/99
Accuracy	93/93	97/98

[a] Data from Choy D, Shi EC, McLean RG, Hoschi R, Murray IP, Ham JM: Cholescintigraphy in acute cholecystitis: Use of intravenous morphine. *Radiology* 151:203–207, 1984, and Freitas JE, Coleman RE, Nagle CE, et al: Influence of scan and pathologic criteria on the specificity of cholescintigraphy. Concise communication. *J Nucl Med* 24:876–879, 1983. Presented as former/latter.

[b] Time of nonvisualization of the gallbladder in patients with normal biliary-bowel transit (1 hr).

When a persistent hepatocyte phase with nonvisualization of the biliary system and absent or markedly delayed visualization of the bowel is identified in an acutely ill patient, common bile duct obstruction should he strongly considered (Fig. 12.27). Although cystic duct patency versus obstruction cannot be assessed with this pattern, a statement regarding the extremely high likelihood of common duct obstruction can be made. Of the 27 patients in the study (7), 22 had obstructing common duct stones, one was felt clinically to have passed a common duct stone, three had neoplastic obstruction of the common duct, and one had acute cholecystitis with ascending cholangitis. Twenty of the 25 patients with irrefutable obstruction also underwent sonography. Significantly, the false negative rate for sonography was 70% (11). This is not surprising when one considers that the sensitivity of sonography for the detection of choledocholithiasis in older series was documented to range from 13 to 30% (12–14). The success of ^{99m}Tc-IDA cholescintigraphy is attributed to its ability to detect functional impedance to bile flow hours to days before anatomic ductal dilatation occurs, and occasionally even before the alkaline phosphatase level and other liver chemistry values suggest the presence of an obstruction. Therefore, when the cholescintigraphic pattern suggests significant common bile duct obstruction in the acute clinical setting, ultrasonography is only helpful if it is positive (15). If it is negative, further evaluation with a more invasive procedure such as an ERCP is indicated. Although intrahepatic cholestasis can yield a similar cholescintigraphic pattern, the differential from acute common duct obstruction is usually readily made clinically.

Identification of diffusely increased activity in the region of the gallbladder fossa in conjunction with gallbladder nonvisualization has been observed to be associated with gangrenous cholecystitis and/or perforation in a high percentage of cases (16–19). Possible mechanisms for this finding include: delayed radiotracer clearance from locally inflamed hepatic tissue due to mechanical obstruction or hepatocyte injury, increased blood flow due to hyperemia from adjacent infection, extravasation of tracer into the gallbladder bed through a gallbladder perforation, and incomplete cystic duct obstruction with faint gallbladder visualization (18). In one report (16) all four cases were associated with acute gangrenous cholecystitis, and in another case report (17) there had been a small perforation of the gallbladder. In 24 patients with pericholecystic increased hepatic activity evaluated by Smith et al. (18), 85% of those who went to surgery during the initial hospitalization had acute cholecystitis, while the remaining 15% had chronic cholecystitis. Of the 9 patients with acute cholecystitis, 4 had acute gangrenous cholecystitis and 5 had gallbladder perforation. (Three of these 9 patients had gangrenous cholecystitis

TABLE 12.3.
CHOLESCINTIGRAPHIC PATTERNS IN ACUTE CHOLECYSTITIS[a]

1. Nonvisualization of the GB	118 (83%)
A. With normal CBD	103 (72%)
B. With medially displaced CBD	9 (6%)
C. With dilated CBD and delayed BBT	3 (2%)
D. With nonvisualized CBD and normal BBT	3 (2%)
2. Nonvisualization of GB and CBD	19 (13%)
A. With no bowel visualization	17 (12%)
B. With delayed BBT	2 (1%)
3. Visualization of GB	6 (4%)
A. <1 hr	1 (0.7%)
B. At 1 hr	2 (1%)
C. >1 hr	3 (2%)

[a] GB = gallbladder, CBD = common bile duct, and BBT = biliary-to-bowel transit. Modified from Weissman HS, Badia J, Surgarman LA, et al: Spectrum of ^{99m}Tc-IDA cholescintigraphic patterns in acute cholecystitis. *Radiology* 138:167–175, 1981.

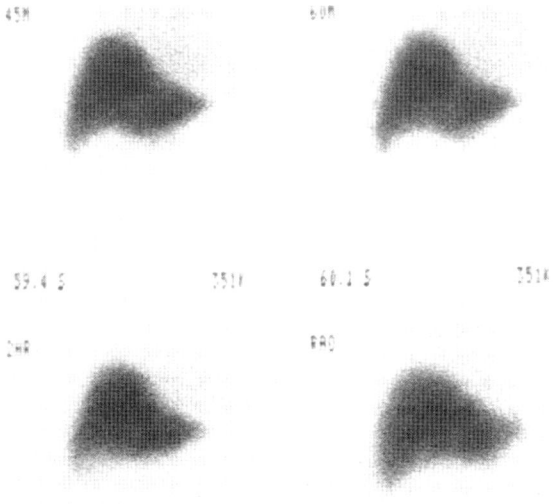

FIGURE 12.27. COMPLETE OBSTRUCTION OF THE COMMON BILE DUCT
The patient presented with acute upper abdominal pain and the suspected clinical diagnosis was acute cholecystitis. Excellent uptake of the ^{99m}Tc-DISIDA was followed by a several hour retention of the radiotracer in the liver. Images at 45 min and 1 and 2 hr are shown. There is no evidence of biliary tract or gallbladder visualization.

and perforation.) Weissmann et al. (19) evaluated 51 consecutive patients with a faint blush of increased activity in the gallbladder fossa and normal visualization of the common duct and intestine. Three patients in this series had incomplete workups. Of the remaining 48 patients, acute cholecystitis was confirmed in 75% (including 27 patients with necrotic changes) and chronic cholecystitis in 25%. The patients were able to be classified into two distinct groups based upon the configuration of abnormal activity. If the activity was bandlike, with linear margins and/or conformed to the contour of the inferior right hepatic lobe, 97% of the patients had acute cholecystitis and 3% had chronic cholecystitis. In those patients where the configuration was rounded suggesting faint gallbladder visualization, 35% had acute cholecystitis while 65% had chronic cholecystitis. Thus, the observation of a faint blush of increased activity in the gallbladder region indicates the presence of significant pathology, and if the activity conforms to the inferior hepatic edge, the likelihood of acute cholecystitis increases significantly to 97% compared with only 35% when the appearance is more suggestive of faint gallbladder visualization. It is also important to note, however, that 27% of patients in the latter group also had gangrenous changes (Fig. 12.30) (19).

False Positives. Though ^{99m}Tc-IDA cholescintigraphy is a simple, safe, noninvasive, accurate diagnostic procedure for suspected acute cholecystitis, other rare causes of gallbladder non-visualization have been identified such as congenital absence of the gallbladder (20) and carcinoma of the gallbladder (21). Chronic cholecystitis, acute pancreatitis, alcoholic liver diseases, hyperalimentation, prolonged and inadequate fasting have been associated with false positive ^{99m}Tc-IDA studies. Each of these need to be evaluated in turn.

Chronic Cholecystitis. There are several possible explanations for reports that indicate a high cholescintigraphic false-positive rate secondary to chronic cholecystitis. As shown by Freitas et al. (10), the most important problem lies in pathologic classification as to what histologically constitutes acute cholecystitis. It is much more appropriate to utilize liberal criteria (cystic duct stone, focal changes, etc.) rather than strict criteria (transmural inflammatory changes). Other problems in the literature include (*a*) differences in statistical criteria used; (*b*) defining the nature of the disorder being studied for example, acute cholecystitis versus "gallbladder disease;" (*c*) symptoms of the patient population selected, for example, acute, subacute, chronic; and (*d*): delayed views (failure to perform, or misinterpretation of significance (3, 4, 10).

Nonetheless, it remains clear that as the prevalence of chronic cholecystitis increases in a patient population, the specificity of real time ultrasound declines markedly while the effect on the ^{99m}Tc-IDA study is minimal. As illustrated by Freitas et al, as the prevalence of chronic cholecystitis increased from 10 to 70%; the positive predictive value for cholescintigraphy decreases from 97 to 81% while that of real time sonography decreases from 75 to 30%. Thus, in the clinical setting of suspected acute cholecystitis, ^{99m}Tc-IDA is the best modality available to the clinician to distinguish acute from chronic gallbladder disease at all prevalence levels. (In actuality, in the acute clinical setting, the prevalence of chronic cholecystitis ranges from 20 to 33% in the literature (22).)

Acute Pancreatitis. Differentiating acute pancreatitis from acute cholecystitis can pose another diagnostic dilemma. This is further complicated by the fact that gallbladder and pancreatic disease can, and do, occur simultaneously. Hepatobiliary scintigraphy has proven to be very reliable in excluding concomitant gallbladder disease in patients with acute pancreatitis. Filling of the gallbladder on ^{99m}Tc-IDA hepatobiliary scans is seen in the majority of patients who do not have concomitant gallbladder diseases. Combining the results reported from three different institutions (23–25), 34 out of 46 patients with acute pancreatitis (79%) demonstrated gallbladder visualization. Of the 12 cases without gallbladder visualization, 10 patients also had acute cholecystitis and two had chronic cholecystitis. Although it was reported by Edlund et al. (26) that five of seven patients with acute pancreatitis failed to show "normal gallbladder visualization," all of those studies were terminated at 1 hr; therefore, the possibility of delayed gallbladder visualization was not evaluated. This is particularly important to assess in this clinical context because of the strong possibility of biliary pancreatitis. The fact that the performance of delayed views may have made an important difference diagnostically is illustrated by the observation that 5 out of 15 patients in one series (23) and 2 out of 16 cases in another series (25) had gallbladders which were not seen by 1 hr but were imaged on delayed views up to 4 hr. In another series (27), the IDA scintigram was a superb means of distinguishing between biliary and nonbiliary causes of pancreatitis; there were normal scans in 95% (19 of 20) of patients with nonbiliary pancreatitis and abnormal scans in 78% (31 of 40) of patients with biliary pancreatitis.

Alcoholic Liver Disease (e.g., Hepatitis and Cirrhosis). Shuman et al. (2) reported nonvisualization or delayed visualization of the gallbladder in 20 of 41 alcoholics. Nine of the 20 presumably had false-positive results. However, 29 alcoholic patients in three other series with nonbiliary acute pancreatitis had normal studies (24, 27, 28). In the series reported by Serafini et al. (27), 6 alcoholic patients with biliary pancreatitis had abnormal cholescintigraphic studies, correctly predicting that biliary disease and not alcohol was the culprit.

Total Parenteral Nutrition. Shuman et al. (2) encountered great difficulty in patients on hyperalimentation. Since this population is definitely more susceptible to acalculous cholecystitis, nonvisualization of the gallbladder may be of prognostic significance even if it does not signify acute cholecystitis. Recognition of this altered physiologic state may identify those patients who would benefit from routine cholecystokinin therapy to keep the gallbladder active, counteract bile stasis, and forestall acalculous cholecystitis.

Prolonged Fasting. Larsen et al. (1) and Kalff et al. (29) have presented case reports suggesting problems in this area, but a well-controlled study of a series of patients is necessary to evaluate the effect of prolonged fasting and to determine if and when optimal fasting (see below) becomes "prolonged" fasting.

Inadequate Fasting. Using normal volunteers, Klingensmith et al. (30) reported that 7 of 11 gallbladders were not visible when studies were commenced 15–30 min after a meal (64% false-positive results). All 11 cases had visualized normally following an overnight fast. Previously, Baker and Marion (31) had shown similar results with ^{99m}Tc-PG (pyridoxylidene glutamate).

False Negatives. It is important that visualization of a dilated cystic duct not be mistaken for gallbladder visualization. Coleman et al. (32) described 9 patients with activity in the dilated patent portion of the cystic duct proximal to the site of cystic duct obstruction that mimicked a small gallbladder. Differentiation between a dilated cystic duct and a "small gallbladder" can be readily accomplished by correlation with sonography. When activity in a dilated, obstructed duct is mimicking a small gallbladder on the scintigram, the sonogram will usually show a normal-sized or a distended gallbladder.

Unexpected Scintigraphic Diagnoses. Weissmann and colleagues (33) described a variety of additional information that can be gleaned from the hepatobiliary study. Nonbiliary pathology was detected in 14% (42 of 294) of patients studied for suspected acute cholecystitis. In describing the findings, the ^{99m}Tc-IDA study was divided into four nonbiliary phases: (*a*) the blood pool phase, which occurs between 1 and 5 min after injection; (*b*) the hepatocyte phase, which occurs between 5 and 20 min after the injection; (*c*) the renal excretion phase (5–15 min); and (*d*) the intestinal phase, which is visualized from 20 to 60 min after injection. The abnormalities identified in each of these phases are summarized in Table 12.4.

TABLE 12.4.
ABNORMALITIES DETECTABLE SERENDIPITOUSLY IN THE VARIOUS PHASES OF THE HEPATOBILIARY SCINTIGRAM

1. Blood Pool Phase
    A. Cardiovascular abnormalities—chamber enlargement, aneurysm, pericardial effusion
    B. Splenic, renal enlargement
    C. Ascites
    D. Hyper or hypovascular lesions, redistribution of flow
2. Hepatocyte Phase
    A. Intrahepatic mass lesions
    B. Contour defects, displacement
3. Renal Excretion Phase
    A. Nonvisualization
    B. Prolonged, enhanced visualization (either primary, e.g., obstruction or secondary, e.g., hepatocellular disease or biliary obstruction)
    C. Intrarenal masses
    D. Changes in size, shape, position, axis
4. Intestinal Phase
    A. Malrotation
    B. Bowel displacement by masses, separation of loops
    C. Nonfilling of loops or persistent activity within loops—obstruction or ischemia, pancreatic or duodenal disorders
    D. Postoperative changes
    E. Gastric reflux

Summary. Clearly, cholescintigraphy with ^{99m}Tc-IDA derivatives is an extremely accurate and efficacious means of evaluating patients suspected of having acute cholecystitis. By careful attention to details, such as proper patient preparation, care in the performance of the examination and an understanding of the potential pitfalls of scan interpretation, the study can add significant additional useful clinical information in the evaluation of the acutely ill patient. Overall, with regard to the controversies that have existed concerning cholescintigraphy and ultrasonography in evaluating patients with acute cholecystitis, it is essential that we keep the proper perspective concerning patient care. As was beautifully summed up by the gastroenterologist, Dr. James Caldwell, in his presentation of the clinician's perspective in the *Journal of Clinical Ultrasound* (34): "We should not labor in a clinical vacuum, and our tests should not be disembodied images unconnected to the total clinical problem. When diagnostic uncertainty exists, consultation among all involved physicians is in order. Understanding by clinicians of differences of techniques, equipment, technical support, imaging agents and experience should resolve conflicts in the patients' interest."

REFERENCES

1. Larsen MJ, Klingensmith WC III, Kuni CC: Radionuclide hepatobiliary imaging: nonvisualization of the gallbladder secondary to prolonged fasting. *J Nucl Med* 23:1003–1005, 1982.
2. Shuman WP, Gibbs P, Rudd TG et al: IDA scintigraphy for cholecystitis: false positives in alcoholism and total parenteral nutrition. *AJR* 138:1–5, 1982.
3. Weissmann HS, Freeman LM: The biliary tract. In Freeman LM (ed): *Freeman and Johnson's Clinical Radionuclide Imaging*, Ed 3. New York, Grune & Stratton, 1984, pp 879–1049.
4. Weissmann HS, Sugarman LA, Badia JD, Freeman LM: Improving the specificity and accuracy of ^{99m}Tc-IDA cholescintigraphy with delayed views. *J Nucl Med* 21:17, 1980.
5. Choy D, Shi EC, McLean RG, Hoschi R, Murray IP, Ham JM: Cholescintigraphy in acute cholecystitis: use of intravenous morphine. *Radiology* 151:203–207, 1984.
6. Freeman LM, Sugarman LA, Weissmann HS: Role of cholecystokinetic agents in ^{99m}Tc-IDA cholescintigraphy. *Semin Nucl Med* 9:186–193, 1981.
7. Weissmann HS, Badia J, Sugarman LA et al: Spectrum of ^{99m}Tc-IDA cholescintigraphic patterns in acute cholecystitis. *Radiology* 138:167–175, 1981.
8. Zeman RK, Burrell MI, Cahow CE et al: Diagnostic utility of cholescintigraphy and ultrasonography in acute cholecystitis. *Am J Surg* 141:446–451, 1981.
9. Mauro MA, McCartney WH, Melmed JR: Hepatobiliary scanning with ^{99m}Tc-PIPIDA in acute cholecystitis. *Radiology* 142:193–197, 1982.
10. Freitas JE, Coleman RE, Nagle CE, et al: Influence of scan and pathologic criteria on the specificity of cholescintigraphy. Concise communication. *J Nucl Med* 24:876–879, 1983.
11. Weissmann HS, Rosenblatt RR, Sugarman LA et al: Early diagnosis of acute common bile duct obstruction by ^{99m}Tc-IDA (iminodiacetic acid) cholescintigraphy (abstr). *J Nucl Med* 21:41, 1980.
12. Laing FC, Jeffrey RB Jr: Choledocholithiasis and cystic duct obstruction: difficult ultrasonographic diagnosis. *Radiology* 146:475, 1983.
13. Gross BH, Harter LP, Gore RM et al: Ultrasonic evaluation of common bile duct stones: prospective comparison with endoscopic retrograde cholangiopancreatography. *Radiology* 146:471, 1983.
14. Cronan JJ, Mueller PR, Simeone JF et al: Prospective diagnosis of choledocholithiasis. *Radiology* 146:467, 1983.
15. Kaplun L, Weissmann HS, Rosenblatt RR, Freeman LM: The early diagnosis of common bile duct obstruction using cholescintigraphy. *JAMA* 245:2431–2434, 1985.
16. Brachman MD, Tanasescu DE, Rammanna L et al: Acute gangrenous cholecystitis: radionuclide diagnosis. *Radiology* 151:209–211, 1984.
17. Cawthon MA, Brown DM, Hartshorne MF et al: Biliary scintigraphy. The "hot rim" sign. *Clin Nucl Med* 9:619–621, 1984.
18. Smith R, Rosen JM, Gallo LN, Alderson PO: Pericholecystic hepatic activity in cholescintigraphy. *Radiology* 156:797–800, 1985.
19. Weissmann HS, Kaplun L, Riley DC, Freeman LM: Clinical significance of faint blush of increased activity in gallbladder fossa region on Tc-99m iminodiacetic acid cholescintigraphy. *Radiology* 157(P):75, 1985.
20. Dickinson CZ, Powers TA, Sandler MP et al: Congenital absence of the gallbladder: another cause of false positive hepatobiliary image. *J Nucl Med* 25:70–71, 1984.
21. Velchik MG, Makler PT, Alavi A: Gallbladder carcinoma. Another cause of distended photon-deficient gallbladder in cholescintigraphy. *Clin Nucl Med* 9:137–138, 1984.
22. Freitas JE: Influence of scan and pathologic criteria on the specificity of cholescintigraphy: concise communication. Reply letter to the editor. *J Nucl Med* 25:728, 1984.
23. Fonseca C, Greenberg D, Rosenthall L et al: ^{99m}Tc-IDA imaging in the differential diagnosis of acute cholecystitis and acute pancreatitis. *Radiology* 130:525–527, 1979.
24. Frank MS, Weissmann HS, Chun KJ et al: Visualization of the biliary tract with ^{99m}Tc-HIDA in acute pancreatitis (abstr). *Gastroenterology* 78:1167, 1980.
25. Ali A, Turner DA, Fordham EW: ^{99m}Tc-IDA cholescintigraphy in acute pancreatitis: concise communication. *J Nucl Med* 23:867–869, 1982.
26. Edlund G, Kemp V, Van der Linden W: Transient nonvisualization of the gallbladder by ^{99m}Tc-HIDA cholescintigraphy in acute pancreatitis: concise communication. *J Nucl Med* 23:117–120, 1982.
27. Serafini NA, Al-Sheikh W, Barkin JS et al: Biliary scintigraphy in acute pancreatitis. *Radiology* 144:591–595, 1982.
28. Glazer G, Murphy F, Clayden GS: Radionuclide biliary scanning in acute pancreatitis. *Br J Surg* 68:766, 1981.
29. Kalff V, Froelich JW, Lloyd R et al: Predictive value of an abnormal hepatobiliary scan in patients with severe intercurrent illness. *Radiology* 146:191, 1983.
30. Klingensmith WC, Spitzer VM, Fritzberg AR et al: The normal fasting and postprandial diisopropyl-IDA ^{99m}Tc-hepatobiliary study. *Radiology* 141:771, 1981.

31. Baker RJ, Marion MA: Scanning with ^{99m}Tc-pyridoxylidene glutamate—the effect of food in normal subjects. *J Nucl Med* 18:793, 1977.
32. Coleman RE, Freitas JE, Fink-Bennett DM et al: The dilated cystic duct sign. A potential cause of false-negative cholescintigraphy. *Clin Nucl Med* 9:134–136, 1984.
33. Weissmann HS, Sugarman LA, Frank MS et al: Serendipity in technetium-99m dimethyl iminodiacetic acid cholescintigraphy. *Radiology* 135:449–454, 1980.
34. Caldwell JH: Ultrasound vs. radionuclide scan in evaluation of acute right upper quadrant abdominal pain: clinician's comments. *J Clin Ultrasound* 11:201, 1983.

Computed Tomography

Although rarely performed with the intention of diagnosing acute cholecystitis, CT is capable of suggesting this diagnosis. Occasionally, the diagnosis will be made on CT when unsuspected clinically (scan obtained for fever of unknown origin (FUO) or other reasons). Other than gallstones, the most common CT finding in acute cholecystitis is wall thickening (1). Although some state that normal wall thickness on CT is 1 mm, we would expect that 2–3 mm is the true upper limit (2, 3). A gallbladder wall thickness of more than 3–5 mm on CT suggests acute cholecystitis (in the proper clinical setting), especially when the gallbladder is not contracted (2, 3). Differential diagnosis of wall thickening on CT would include chiefly chronic cholecystitis, hyperplastic cholecystosis, and carcinoma. Nodularity of the wall and loss of the normal crisp demarcation from the liver may be seen as well. A gallstone in the cystic duct or impacted in the neck of the gallbladder on CT supports a diagnosis of acute cholecystitis, as does an anteroposterior diameter greater than 5 cm. A low density halo around the gallbladder due to edema or early pericholecystic fluid formation is quite suggestive of acute cholecystitis. Fluid collections in the pericholecystic space, subhepatic or subphrenic spaces (21–35 HU) are seen uncommonly and suggest perforation (1, 2). The only specific CT finding for acute cholecystitis is gas in the lumen or wall of the gallbladder or within a pericholecystic abscess. This finding is discussed more fully under emphysematous cholecystitis and is not common. Another uncommon CT manifestation of acute cholecystitis is elevation of the CT numbers of bile within the gallbladder from hemorrhagic cholecystitis (1, 4). On sonography, the intraluminal blood is depicted as echogenic fluid similar to sludge (4). CT differential would include other causes of hemobilia as well as prior contrast administration (intravenous urographic and vicarious excretion or a cholecystopaque) and milk of calcium bile. The former two have to be excluded historically, whereas the latter is usually more opaque, clumpy, and layers dependently. In hemorrhagic cholecystitis, CT is likely to show any stones and/or wall thickening in addition to the high density bile. A finding reported to occur in acute cholecystitis that we feel is not useful is contrast enhancement of the gallbladder wall (2). Visually striking wall enhancement can occur in normals, especially when the gallbladder is not surrounded by enhanced liver. CT gallbladder wall enhancement (to an abnormal degree) has also been reported in acute pancreatitis (along with wall thickening, edematous changes, large volume and high density bile) (5). The theory of the diagnosis of acute cholecystitis on the basis of wall enhancement by urographic contrast due to hyperemia goes back to infusion tomography of the gallbladder, an examination that never gained much credence (6).

REFERENCES

1. Kane RA, Costello P, Duszlak E: Computed tomography in acute cholecystitis: new observations. *AJR* 141:697–701, 1983.
2. Kreel L, Solomon A, Pinto D: Contrast computed tomography in the diagnosis of acute cholecystitis. *J Comput Assist Tomogr* 3:585–588, 1979.
3. Havrilla TR, Reich NR, Haaga JR, Seidelmann FE, Cooperman AM, Alfidi RJ: Computed tomography of the gallbladder. *AJR* 130:1059–1067, 1978.
4. Jenkins M, Golding RH, Cooperberg PL: Sonography and computed tomography of hemorrhagic cholecystitis. *AJR* 140:1197–1198, 1983.
5. Somer K, Kivisaari L, Standertskjold-Nordenstam C-G, Kalima TV: Contrast-enhanced computed tomography of the gallbladder in acute pancreatitis. *Gastrointest Radiol* 9:31–34, 1984.
6. Moncada R, Cardoso M, Danley R, Rodriguez J, Kimura K, Pickelman J, Brandly J: Infusion tomography of the gallbladder: mechanism of gallbladder wall opacification in experimental acute cholecystitis. *AJR* 129:587–590, 1977.

Complications of Acute Cholecystitis

Empyema, gangrene, and perforation of the gallbladder are the major complications of acute cholecystitis and greatly increase the morbidity and mortality of the disease. Unfortunately, there are few signs and symptoms to distinguish the patient with complicated acute cholecystitis from patients with uncomplicated acute cholecystitis. The usual findings of right upper quadrant pain, fever, chills, nausea, and vomiting are generally present. Surprisingly, half of these patients lack a leukocytosis and some are afebrile (1).

Plain Films and Barium Contrast Examinations

Very rarely, the diagnosis of gallbladder perforation secondary to acute cholecystitis can be suggested from the plain film of the abdomen by noting a calcification with the appearance of a gallstone lying free within the peritoneal cavity. Complicated cholecystitis is much more likely than simple acute cholecystitis to produce a mass in the region of the gallbladder fossa as well as all the other findings described on plain films and barium studies in acute cholecystitis.

Sonography

Sonography can be extremely helpful in the preoperative diagnosis of complicated cholecystitis (a recent study correctly diagnosed about 60% of patients with complicated cholecystitis (2). Sonographic findings include wall abnormalities, intraluminal membranes, coarse, nonshadowing, nondependent intraluminal echoes, and localized peritoneal fluid collections. It is not possible to reliably differentiate between empyema and gangrene by ultrasound. Perforation can be suggested and is discussed below.

Wall abnormalities in complicated cholecystitis may be limited to mere thickening, in which case the diagnosis cannot be made. When extremely shaggy, irregular and asymmetric walls with or without focal irregularity or masses are seen, the diagnosis can be suggested (2). These findings are secondary to mucosal ulcers, intraluminal hemorrhage and necrosis. Hyperechoic foci within the wall of the gallbladder have been seen with microabscesses in infected Rokitansky-Aschoff sinuses (3), but these cannot be differentiated from sinuses containing inspissated bile.

Although occasionally seen in uncomplicated acute cholecystitis, intraluminal membranes are more common in gangrenous gallbladders (Fig. 12.28) (2, 4, 5). They correspond to a conglomerate of fibrinous exudate and desquamated mucosa, and are depicted as thin, linear, nonshadowing echoes within the gallbladder lumen.

Another finding in gangrene and empyema of the gallbladder is the presence of multiple medium to coarse, highly reflective intraluminal echoes without shadowing, layering, or gravity dependence. These echoes correspond to purulent exudate and debris within highly viscous bile, and the appearance is not distinguishable from that of blood within the gallbladder (6) or a particularly viscid sludge (Fig. 12.29).

Perforation

Perforation of the gallbladder has greatly decreased in incidence over the past 50 years, but it still occurs in 5–10% of patients admitted emergently for acute cholecystitis and carries a

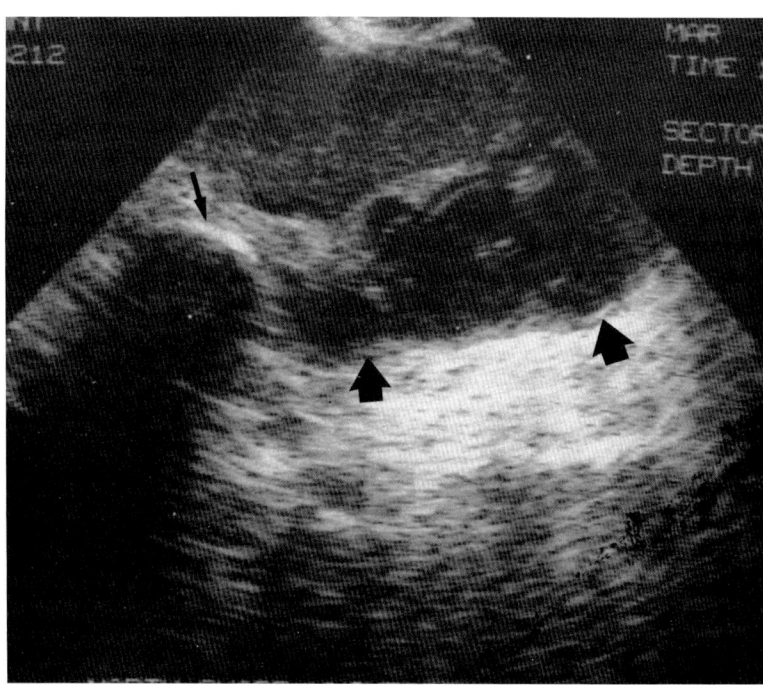

FIGURE 12.28. GANGRENOUS CHOLECYSTITIS
A shadowing calculus is impacted in the neck of the gallbladder (*small arrow*). The lumen (*large arrows*) is filled with membranes and debris.

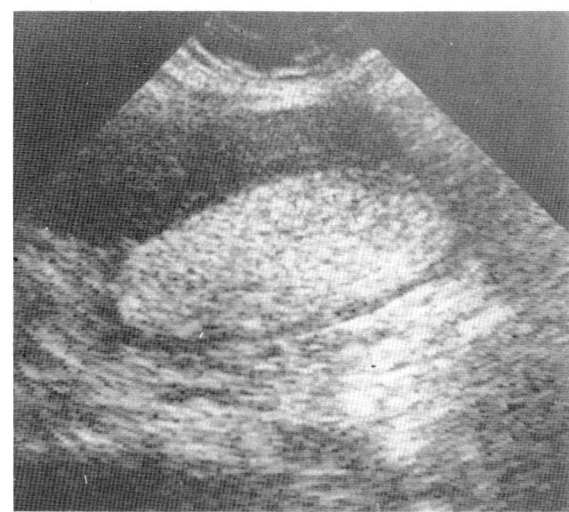

FIGURE 12.29. GALLBLADDER EMPYEMA
Distended gallbladder completely filled with echogenic material that was pus at surgery.

25% mortality (7). Gallbladder perforations are most commonly secondary to acute calculous cholecystitis. Malignancy, infection, trauma, steroid use, and impaired vascularity are contributing factors (7). The usual sequence of events is impaction of a stone in the gallbladder neck, obstruction, distention, impaired vascular supply, necrosis, and perforation. Most perforations occur in the fundus, which has the poorest blood supply. Rokitansky-Aschoff sinuses have been implicated in intrahepatic perforations: they are thought to rupture after becoming infected.

Three types of gallbladder perforations have been described (7). Acute perforations are associated with free spill of bile into the peritoneum with associated peritonitis. Subacute perforations, which are most common, tend to wall off and form pericholecystic abscesses. Chronic perforations are associated with fistulous communication with other organs.

After perforation of the gallbladder, rapid walling off of the inflammation with pericholecystic abscess formation usually occurs. Initially the abscess generally appears as a sonolucent collection surrounding the gallbladder (1, 2, 7, 8), either large or small, with or without other findings (gallstones, even when present, may not be demonstrable). Later in their course (between one and two weeks of age), abscesses are solid, complex pericholecystic masses that are moderately echogenic (highly echogenic foci will be present if there are gas bubbles). A mature abscess (over two weeks in age) will be more anechoic but still sonographically complex. Several entities can simulate pericholecystic abscess sonographically. Small fluid collections adjacent to the gallbladder have been reported in peptic ulcer disease and perforated ulcers (9). Pancreatitis is frequently associated with intra and extraperitoneal fluid collections. Although more commonly left-sided, they may be in the region of the gallbladder. Other causes of intraabdominal inflammatory disease may lead to pooling of fluid in the gallbladder fossa. Demonstrating gallstones and eliciting focal right upper quadrant tenderness is helpful in suggesting pericholecystic abscess.

Gallbladder carcinoma may mimic complicated cholecystitis sonographically. The former is suggested by: a focal mass, proximal biliary tract obstruction (invasion or compression of the common hepatic duct), liver invasion, or regional adenopathy (10). The following signs are nonspecific and are equally likely in either condition: diffuse gallbladder wall thickening, thickening of the hepatoduodenal ligament, and gallstones. A thin smooth, sonolucent halo around the gallbladder suggests cholecystitis (10).

REFERENCES

1. Kane RA: Ultrasonographic diagnosis of gangrenous cholecystitis and empyema of the gallbladder. *Radiology* 134:191–194, 1980.
2. Jeffrey RB, Laing FA, Wong W, Callen PW: Gangrenous cholecystitis: diagnosis by ultrasound. *Radiology* 148:219–221, 1983.
3. Graif M, Horovitz A, Itzchak Y, Strauss S: Hyperechoic foci in the gallbladder wall as a sign of microabscess formation or diverticula. *Radiology* 152:781–782, 1984.
4. Wales LR: Desquamated gallbladder mucosa: unusual sign of cholecystitis. *AJR* 139:810–811, 1982.
5. Farmer DW, Jones TB, Brogdon BG, Daniel SJ: Mucosal fold enlargement: a sonographic finding of gangrenous cholecystitis. *South Med J* 77:659–660, 1984.
6. Jenkins M, Golding RH, Cooperberg PL: Sonography and computed tomography of hemorrhagic cholecystitis. *AJR* 140:1197–1198, 1983.
7. Madrazo BL, Francis I, Hricak H, Sandler MA, Hudak S, Gitschlag K: Sonographic findings in perforation of the gallbladder. *AJR* 139:491–496, 1982.
8. Bergman AB, Neiman HL, Kraut B: Ultrasonographic evaluation of pericholecystic abscesses. *AJR* 132:201–203, 1979.
9. Nyberg DA, Laing FC: Ultrasonographic findings in peptic ulcer disease and pancreatitis that simulate primary gallbladder disease. *J Ultrasound Med* 2:303–307, 1983.
10. Smathers RL, Lee JK, Heiken JP: Differentiation of complicated cholecystitis from gallbladder carcinoma by computed tomography. *AJR* 143:255–259, 1984.

Hepatobiliary Scintigraphy

When gallbladder perforation is a complication of acute cholecystitis with cystic duct obstruction and secondary distension, inflammation, and ischemia, the ^{99m}Tc-IDA study will exhibit gallbladder nonvisualization, indicating the presence of acute cholecystitis. It will not demonstrate biliary leakage into the peritoneum. However, gallbladder perforation can and does occur without cystic duct obstruction (1–3). The main pathogenetic mechanisms include hypoperfusion leading to ischemic necrosis and overwhelming infection (1). Perforation of the gallbladder is the most common cause of bile peritonitis (4). Patients with an acute, free perforation have bile in the peritoneal cavity. Those with a subacute perforation tend to have a pericholecystic or right upper quadrant abscess, while those with chronic perforation form cholecystoenteric or cholecystocutaneous fistulae (1).

Scintigraphic Findings. Several reports have illustrated preoperative detection of gallbladder perforation by ^{99m}Tc-IDA cholescintigraphy (4–7). Possible scintigraphic findings in gallbladder perforation include a blush of activity in the gallbladder region with the inferior margin conforming to the liver contour. This finding may also be seen in gangrenous and uncomplicated cholecystitis (Fig. 12.30). A more complete discussion of pericholecystic increased hepatic activity is given above under Acute Cholecystitis, Hepatobiliary Scintigraphy, Diagnostic Findings. Less commonly observed but more specific is faint gallbladder visualization with later appearance of activity within various peritoneal spaces (subphrenic, subhepatic, paracolic) (7). (See illustration of paracolic IDA in traumatic perforation in Chapter 16.)

REFERENCES

1. Roslyn J, Busuttil RW: Perforation of the gallbladder: a frequently mismanaged condition. *Am J Surg* 137:307, 1979.
2. Williams NG, Socbie IK: Perforation of the gallbladder: analysis of 19 cases. *Can Med Assoc J* 115:1223, 1976.
3. Abdu-Dalu J, Urca I: Acute cholecystitis with perforation into the peritoneal cavity. *Arch Surg* 102:108, 1971.
4. Brunetti JC, Van Heertum RL: Preoperative detection of gallbladder perforation. *Clin Nucl Med* 5:347, 1980.
5. Powers TA, Melton RE: Diagnosis of gallbladder perforation by ^{99m}Tc-disofenin cholescintigraphy. *Clin Nucl Med* 7.201, 1982.
6. Selby JB, Glassman AB: Cholescintigraphic diagnosis of gallbladder rupture. *Clin Nucl Med* 8:64, 1983.
7. Kaplun L, Weissmann HS, Freeman LM: Cholescintigraphic diagnosis of gallbladder perforation (abstr). *Radiology* 153:174, 1984.

Computed Tomography

CT can detect complications of acute cholecystitis although sonography is usually the study of choice. The latter is superior in its depiction of the gallbladder itself, but CT is better at diagnosing perforations. This is because CT can depict small pericholecystic gas collections (Fig.

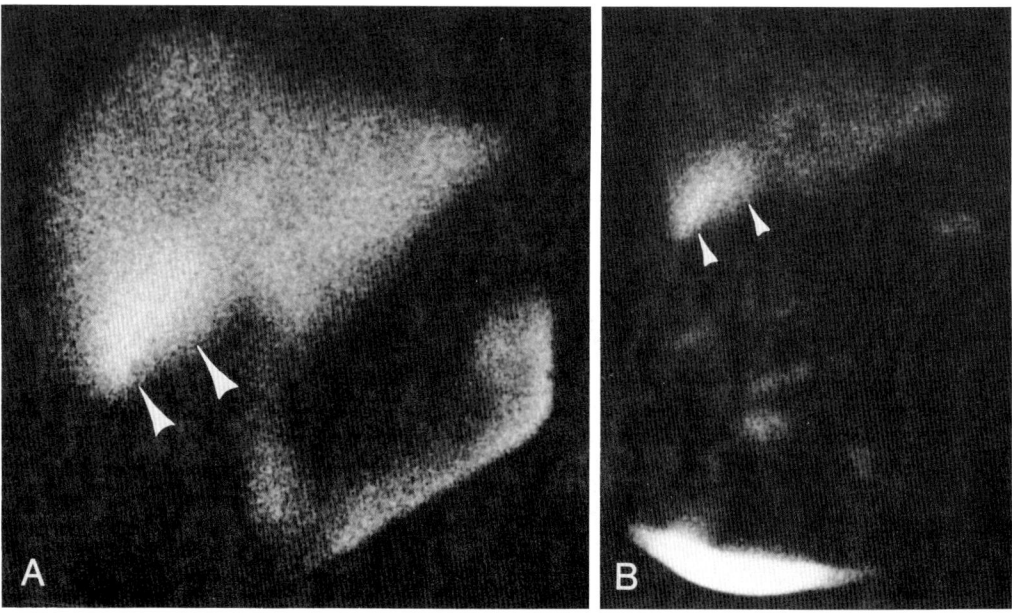

FIGURE 12.30. GANGRENOUS CHOLECYSTITIS
A and *B:* 60-min (*A*) and 3-hr (*B*) delayed scans reveal pericholecystic increased hepatic activity (*arrowheads*) and nonvisualization of the gallbladder in a case of gangrenous cholecystitis.

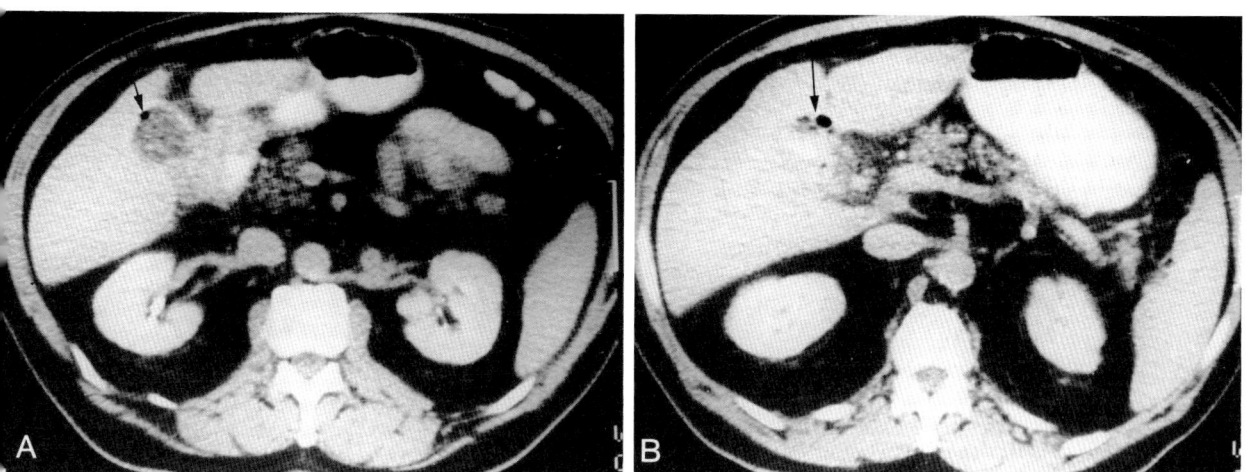

FIGURE 12.31. PERICHOLECYSTIC ABSCESS FROM CONFINED PERFORATION DUE TO ACUTE CHOLECYSTITIS
A: Scan through the gallbladder. *B:* A 10-cm cephalad scan. CT shows pericholecystic gas (*arrows*) and higher than normal density, inhomogeneous gallbladder contents.

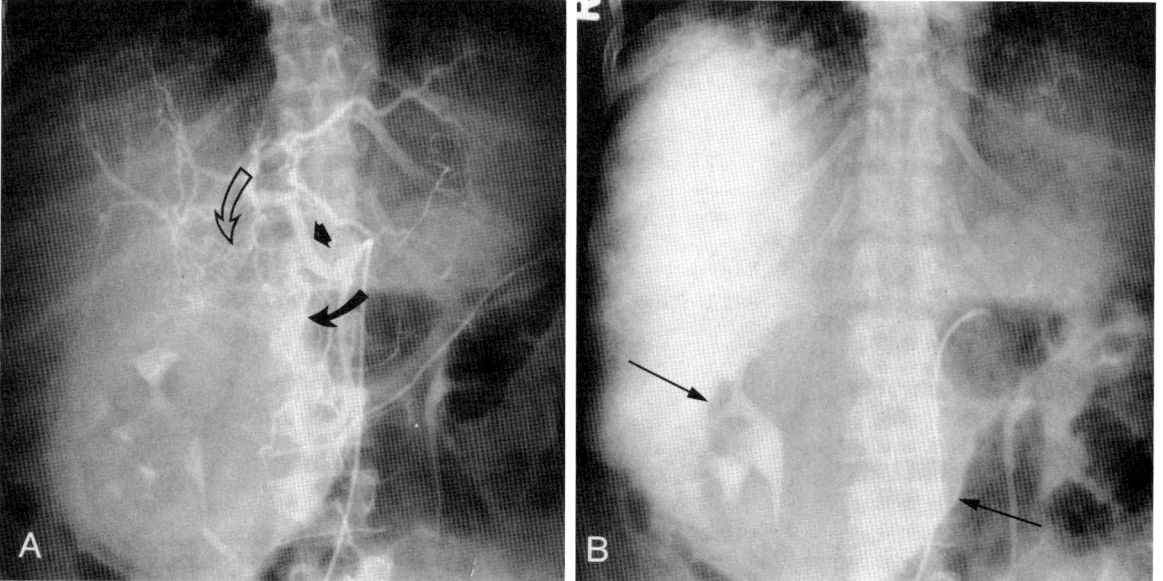

FIGURE 12.32. ANGIOGRAPHY OF COMPLICATED ACUTE CHOLECYSTITIS

Angiography performed to rule out hepatocellular carcinoma in a 51-year-old woman with alcoholism and tender "hepatomegaly." *A:* Arterial phase: right hepatic artery (*closed arrow*) rising from the superior mesenteric artery. The cystic artery (*curved arrow*) is markedly enlarged and its branches splayed, indicating gallbladder enlargement. An intrahepatic branch of the right hepatic artery appears to be slightly enlarged and feeding the gallbladder as well (*curved open arrow*). *B:* Hepatogram phase: mass (*arrows*) is radiolucent and represents a massively dilated gallbladder. At surgery an empyema of the gallbladder was found.

12.31) and differentiate them from bowel gas more easily than ultrasound. CT is also better at detecting a gallstone outside the gallbladder.

As with sonography, empyema and gangrene are hard to differentiate from each other and difficult to distinguish from gallbladder cancer. CT findings in empyema and gangrene include diffuse and sometimes nodular and irregular wall thickening, thickening of the hepatoduodenal ligament, calcified gallstones, streaky soft tissue densities in the pericholecystic fat, and mass effect on the colon in the region of the hepatic flexure. All of the above can be seen in gallbladder cancer (1). Visualization of a well-defined curvilinear low density halo surrounding the gallbladder, corresponding to mural edema or early pericholecystic fluid formation, favors acute cholecystitis over carcinoma. Any soft tissue masses favor carcinoma as do low density intrahepatic masses, which are usually metastases. However, the latter could be hepatic abscesses forming as a complication of cholecystitis (1).

REFERENCE

1. Smathers RL, Lee JKT, Heiken JP: Differentiation of complicated cholecystitis from gallbladder carcinoma by computed tomography. *AJR* 143:255–259, 1984.

Angiography

Although formerly occasionally employed in the evaluation of benign gallbladder disease (1), angiography will only be done today in complicated acute cholecystits if some other disease process is suspected. Gallbladder enlargement due to empyema (or hydrops) can be detected (Fig. 12.32).

REFERENCE

1. Redman HC, Reuter SR: The angiographic evaluation of gallbladder dilatation. *Radiology* 97:367, 1970.

ACALCULOUS CHOLECYSTITIS

Approximately 5–10% of cholecystitis patients have no stones and are diagnosed as having acalculous cholecystitis. Because inflammatory cellular infiltrates can be found in the gallbladders of many asymptomatic adults, the diagnosis of chronic acalculous cholecystitis lacks objective criteria and is sometimes in question (1). This is not a problem when the gallbladder is grossly inflamed or gangrenous (as is generally seen in acute disease). Acute acalculous inflammation is most often seen in situations of altered gallbladder filling and emptying, as occur with sudden immobility or starvation. A combination of concentrated bile, cystic duct obstruction, and vascular compromise are thought to be important in pathogenesis. Acalculous cholecystitis can occur in any patient suffering a major illness. Reported settings include: trauma, burns, surgery, total parenteral nutrition, blood transfusion reactions, anesthesia, mechanical ventilation, and drugs altering sphincter of Oddi function such as narcotics (2–5). Obstruction of the cystic duct by extrinsic inflammation, lymphadenopathy, or metastases are other causes. Infection is usually held to be secondary, but salmonella and cholera may have a special disposition to involve the gallbladder. Symptomatic acalculous inflammation of the gallbladder occurs rarely with typhoid fever, tuberculosis, syphilis, actinomycosis, streptococcal disease, and leptospirosis. In other countries, parasites are a major cause of cholecystitis.

Signs and symptoms are no different from those in stone related acute cholecystitis, but the course is often more fulminant with a higher probability of gangrene and perforation.

Acalculous cholecystitis is especially common relative to the calculous variety in children. Lymphadenopathy obstructing the cystic duct is thought to be the usual cause, but the precise mechanism is not always established. Acute infectious diseases are often precursors. The Kawasaki, or mucocutaneous lymph node, syndrome is particularly associated with acute hydrops in children and may also occasionally occur in adults. Acute acalculous cholecystitis due to lymphadenitis usually resolves spontaneously without need for surgery (6–8).

Radiology

Plain Films and Barium Contrast Examinations

Findings on these examinations are the same as in calculous acute cholecystitis, save for the absence of stones.

Sonography

Sonographic findings are nonspecific by themselves but, when evaluated in conjunction with clinical history may be diagnostic (Figs. 12.33–12.35). The gallbladder is frequently enlarged with a thickened wall which may have a halo around it (3, 9). Sludge or coarse echoes sugges-

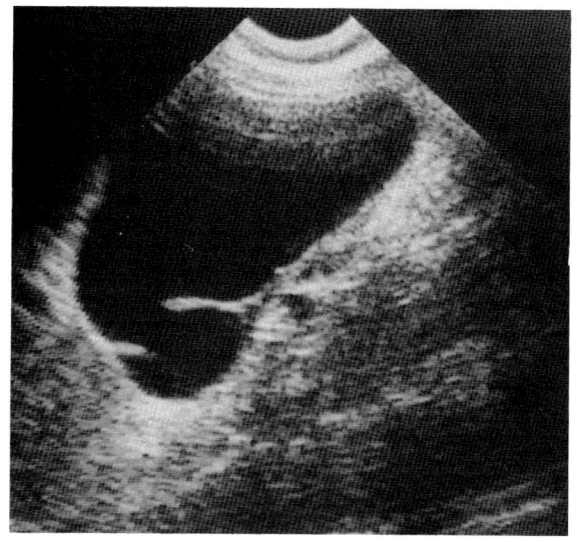

FIGURE 12.33. ACALCULOUS CHOLECYSTITIS
Sonography shows a distended, tense gallbladder with rounding of its contour. No stone was seen, even at surgery.

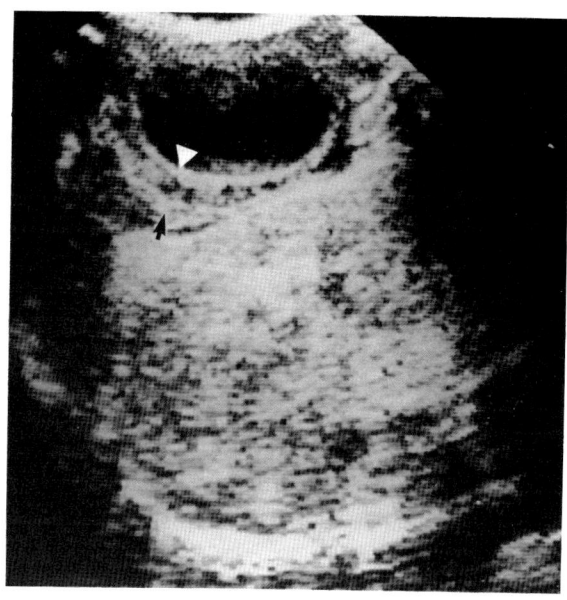

FIGURE 12.34. WALL THICKENING
Marked heterogeneous wall thickening (*arrows*) and no calculi in acalculous cholecystitis.

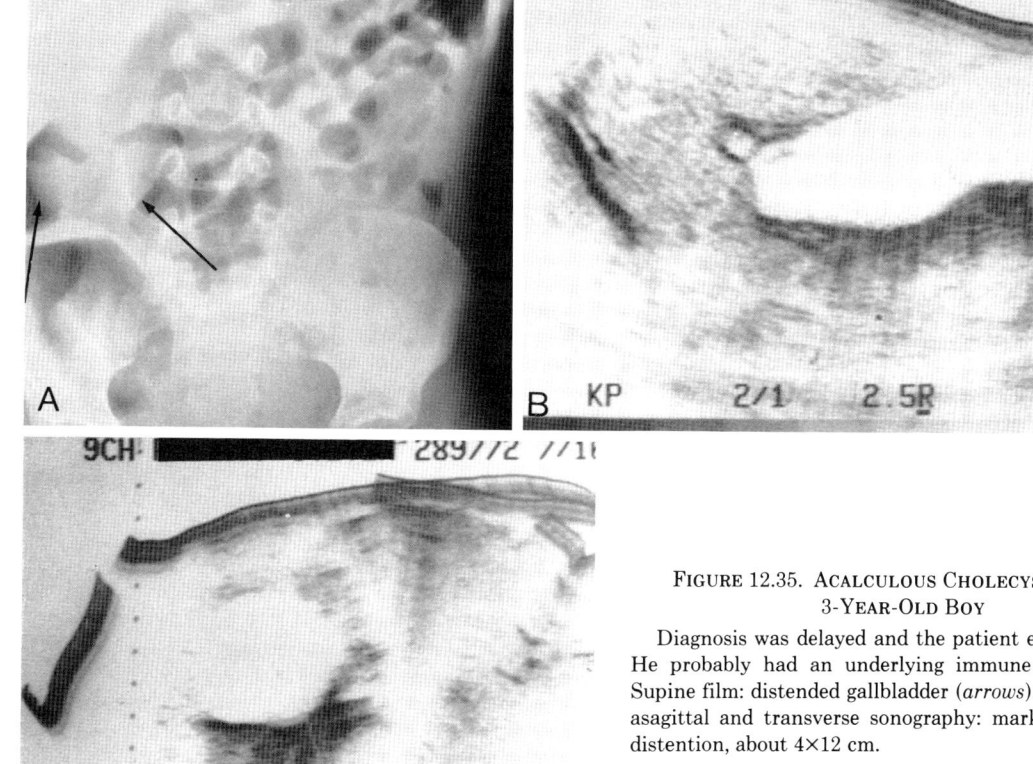

FIGURE 12.35. ACALCULOUS CHOLECYSTITIS IN A 3-YEAR-OLD BOY
Diagnosis was delayed and the patient eventually died. He probably had an underlying immune deficiency. *A:* Supine film: distended gallbladder (*arrows*). *B* and *C:* Parasagittal and transverse sonography: marked gallbladder distention, about 4×12 cm.

tive of pus may be seen within the gallbladder lumen (10). As some of the above findings can be seen in normal patients, it may be useful to perform serial sonography. Progressive enlargement of the gallbladder and thickening of its wall may establish the diagnosis (11). A recent review of 33 patients with documented acalculous cholecystitis yielded a sensitivity of 67% using these sonographic criteria (10). A normal gallbladder sonogram cannot be used to exclude the diagnosis of acute acalculous cholecystitis.

Chronic Acalculous Cholecystitis. A subgroup of patients with chronic acalculous cholecystitis may exist who are difficult to diagnose in that no reliable diagnostic criteria exist using sonography or oral cholecystography. Symptoms in these patients are those commonly associated with cholelithiasis. Cholecystokinin studies have been tried with mixed results. Some patients will respond well to cholecystectomy and many have evidence of inflammatory changes at pathologic examination. Unfortunately, pathologic criteria to make a diagnosis of chronic acalculous cholecystitis are not universally agreed upon, making comparison between series at different institutions difficult.

REFERENCES

1. Berk RN, Ferrucci JT, Jr, Fordtran JS, Cooperberg PL, Weissmann HS: The radiological diagnosis of gallbladder disease. *Radiology* 141:49–56, 1981.
2. Howard RJ: Acute acalculous cholecystitis. *Am J Surg* 141:194–198, 1981.
3. Chen PS, Aliapoulios MA: Acute acalculous cholecystitis, ultrasonic appearance. *Arch Surg* 113:1461–1462, 1978.
4. Davis GB, Berk RN, Scheible WF et al: Cholecystokinin cholecystography, sonography and scintigraphy: detection of chronic acalculous cholecystitis. *AJR* 139:1117–1121, 1982.
5. DuPriest RW Jr, Khaneja SC, Cowley RA: Acute cholecystitis complicating trauma. *Ann Surg* 189:84–89, 1979.
6. Chamberlain JW, Hight DW: Acute hydrops of the gallbladder in children. *Surgery* 68:899–905, 1970.
7. Koss JC, Coleman BG, Mulhern CB Jr, Arger PH, Tuchman DN: Mucocutaneous lymph node syndrome with hydrops of the gallbladder diagnosed by ultrasound. *J Clin Ultrasound* 9:477–479, 1981.
8. Morens DM, Anderson LJ, Hurwitz ES: National surveillance of Kawasaki disease. *Pediatrics* 65:21–25, 1979.
9. Deitch EA, Engel JM: Acute acalculous cholecystitis ultrasonic diagnosis. *Am J Surg* 142:290–292, 1981.
10. Shuman WP, Rogers JV, Rudd TG, Mack LA, Plumley T, Larson EB: Low sensitivity of sonography and cholescintigraphy in acalculous cholecystitis. *AJR* 142:531–534, 1984.
11. Blaquiere RM, Dewbury KC: The ultrasound diagnosis of emphysematous cholecystitis. *Br J Radiol* 55:114–116, 1982.

Hepatobiliary Scintigraphy

Acute acalculous cholecystitis can be difficult to assess clinically as well as sonographically. It often occurs in individuals who have other serious prolonged medical conditions or in postoperative or posttraumatic patients. Most patients with acute acalculous cholecystitis do have a functionally obstructed cystic duct, presumably on the basis of edema. Therefore, cholescintigraphy has proven to be highly accurate in this patient population as well as patients with acute calculous cholecystitis. A total of 43 patients with acute acalculous cholecystitis who were studied preoperatively with ^{99m}Tc IDA have been reported from five institutions (1–5). Thirty-nine of these patients exhibited hepatic uptake and excretion into the intestine: 36 (92%) were true positive cases with gallbladder nonvisualization, and 3 (8%) were falsely negative. In one of the false negative cases (5), duodenal activity was misinterpreted as the gallbladder, so that the accuracy of the study is really somewhat higher, as this error is easily avoidable (6). In four patients, the possibility of acute cholecystitis could not be assessed because they exhibited a persistent hepatocyte phase with no excretion. Since some of the patients with the persistent hepatocyte phase pattern, which suggests common duct obstruction, also had sonograms which demonstrated the presence of gallstones which were not confirmed to be present at the time of surgery, it is possible that these individuals passed their stones prior to surgery and did have common duct obstruction at the time of the ^{99m}Tc IDA study. However, this will always remain an unresolved question. There is evidence in the literature to suggest that it is likely that many patients with a final diagnosis of acute acalculous cholecystitis actually have passed stones prior to surgery (7). Although the overall accuracy of cholescintigraphy in acute acalculous cholecystitis is slightly lower and the false negative rate is slightly higher than in acute calculous cholecystitis, and the persistent hepatocyte phase pattern can pose a diagnostic problem, the fact that the majority of patients do have cystic duct obstruction and scintigraphy is 93% accurate makes it the best diagnostic procedure available.

REFERENCES

1. Zeman RK, Burrell MI, Cahow CE et al: Diagnostic utility of cholescintigraphy and ultrasonography in acute cholecystitis. *Am J Surg* 141:446–451, 1981.
2. Mauro MA, McCartney WH, Melmed JR: Hepatobiliary scanning with ^{99m}Tc-PIPIDA in acute cholecystitis. *Radiology* 142:193–197, 1982.
3. Ramanna L, Salimpour P, Brachman et al: Evaluation of Tc-99m PIPIDA scintigraphy in acalculous cholecystitis (abstr). *J Nucl Med* 23:P90, 1982.
4. Weissmann HS, Berkowitz D, Fox MS et al: The role of technetium-99m iminodiacetic acid (IDA) cholescintig-

5. Shuman WP, Rogers JV, Rudd TG et al: Low sensitivity of sonography in acalculous cholecystitis. *AJR* 142:531–534, 1984.
6. Keller IA, Weissmann HS, Kaplun LL, Freeman LM: The use of water ingestion to distinguish the gallbladder and duodenum on cholescintigrams. *Radiology* 152:811–813, 1984.
7. Anderson AKE, Bergdahl L, Bopvist L: Acalculous cholecystitis. *Am J Surg* 122:3–7, 1971.

Computed Tomography

As cholescintigraphy and sonography are the first line examinations in suspected acalculous cholecystitis, CT is rarely performed. It has been reported that CT findings in acalculous cholecystis are similar to those seen in garden variety acute cholecystitis, but the sensitivity and specificity of CT in this clinical situation have not been studied (1).

REFERENCES

1. Havrilla TR, Reich NR, Haaga JR, Seidelmann FE, Cooperman AM, Alfidi RJ: Computed tomography of the gallbladder. *AJR* 130:1059–1067, 1978.

EMPHYSEMATOUS CHOLECYSTITIS

Emphysematous cholecystitis is a rare clinical entity, distinctly different from acute cholecystitis. Unlike acute cholecystitis, it affects a predominantly male population with a male:female ratio of 2–3:1 and is more common in diabetics. Cholelithiasis is not a major pathogenetic factor, occurring in only half of patients. Prognosis is graver than acute calculous cholecystitis with gangrene occurring in 75% of patients and perforation in 20%. Mortality is close to 15% compared to about 4% in acute calculous cholecystitis (1).

Etiology is uncertain; however, ischemia secondary to small vessel disease or distention may be the precipitating factor. The hallmark is the subsequent bacterial invasion by gas-forming enteric organisms. Common offenders are *Clostridium perfringens* and *Clostridium welchii*, *Escherichia coli*, and less commonly, *Staphylococcus* and *Streptococcus* species.

The majority of patients with emphysematous cholecystitis present with symptoms and signs neither more or less severe than their counterparts with ordinary acute cholecystitis. Most consider the diagnosis a surgical emergency, but others advocate intensive medical therapy (1). We feel that clinical judgment should be exercised individually in each case. We have seen one patient with vague right upper quadrant pain whose abdominal films showed emphysematous cholecystitis for 2 weeks before the finding was recognized and surgery performed with a successful outcome, so that emergency surgery cannot always be necessary.

Radiology

Plain Films

Plain film findings usually become visible only 24–48 hr after the onset of symptoms (Fig. 12.36) (1–3). Gas is seen first in the gallbladder lumen as a round or pear-shaped lucency in the right upper quadrant. An erect film at this time may or may not show an air-fluid level. Occasionally, Rokitansky-Aschoff sinuses will become distended and visible. Subsequently intramural gas forms and is usually seen as a thin curvilinear lucency in the gallbladder wall. Less often gas in the gallbladder wall is bubbly. Intramural gas can be either diffuse or localized. In some patients perforation occurs and mottled pericholecystic lucencies are visible representing pericholecystic abscess formation. Until 1978 it was felt that pneumobilia was not a feature of emphysematous cholecystitis, but three cases were then reported with air in the biliary tree in addition to air in the gallbladder lumen ± air in the gallbladder wall (4). In medically managed patients, the gas may not clear for months even if the treatment is successful (1).

Ultrasound

Sonographic diagnosis of emphysematous cholecystitis depends on the recognition of gas either in the gallbladder wall or lumen (Fig. 12.37). The sudden change of acoustic impedance at a soft tissue-gas interface produces high amplitude echoes (5–7). These bright echoes are distributed throughout the gallbladder wall and/or lumen, and are associated with "dirty" distal acoustic shadowing and reverberation echoes. The presence of reverberations or comet tail artifacts suggest gas rather than calcification. Although a thin rim of gas in the gallbladder wall may not generate reverberations and thus be indistinguishable from calcification, many patients with emphysematous cholecystitis will have abundant intraluminal gas which will cause reverberation (6, 7). Gas within the gallbladder wall may produce focal or diffuse echogenicity without acous-

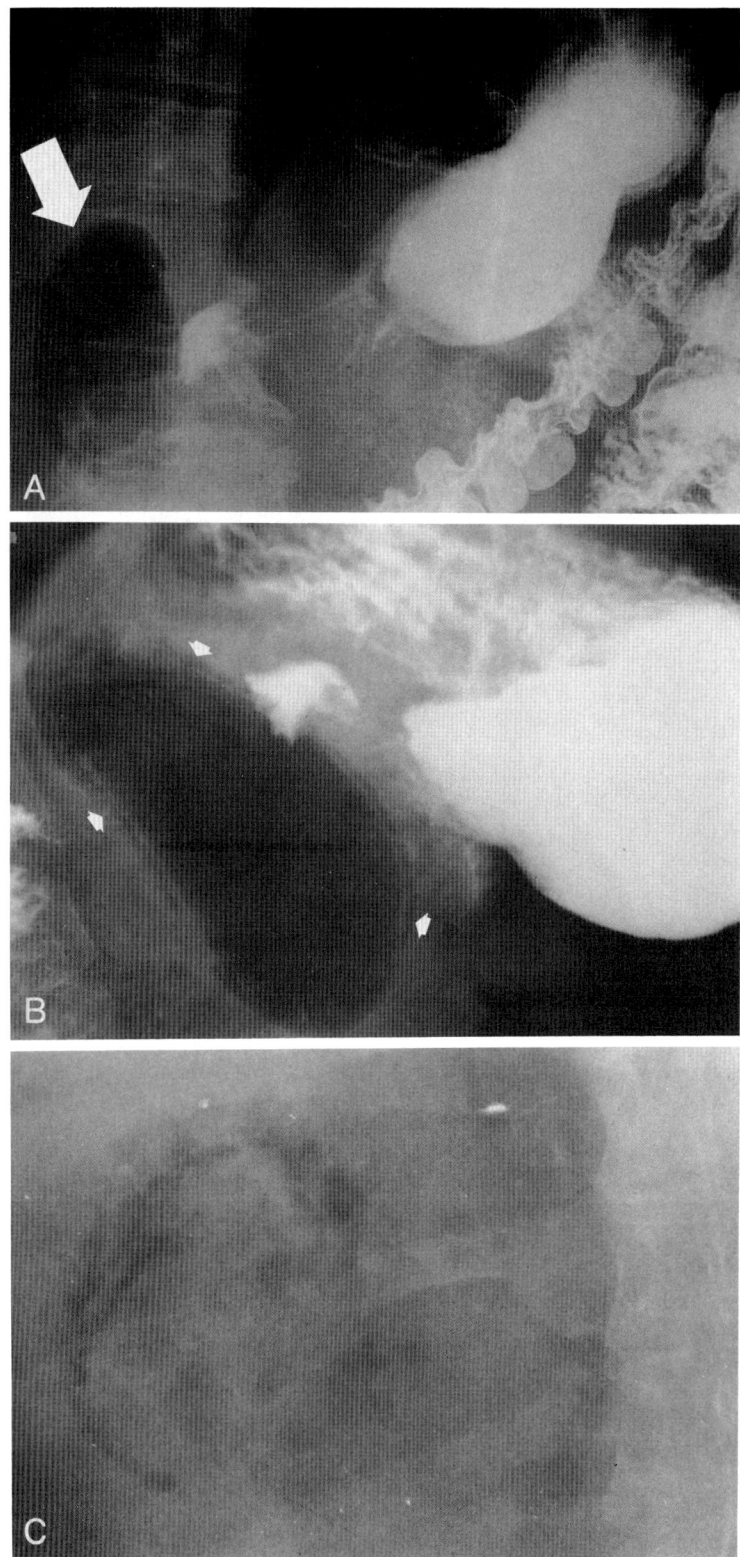

FIGURE 12.36. PLAIN FILM FINDINGS IN EMPHYSEMATOUS CHOLECYSTITIS

A: Gas in lumen only (*arrow*). *B:* Gas in wall, linear and slightly bubbly (*arrows*) and lumen. *C:* Gas in wall only, mostly bubbly. *D* and *E:* Supine and erect films, respectively, showing linear gas in the wall (*arrows*) and intraluminal gas (*open arrows*). Note absence of air-fluid level in the gallbladder. *F* and *G:* Supine and erect films: gas and fluid filled gallbladder (*arrow*) with an air-fluid level. *H* and *I:* Supine film (*H*) shows only bubbly pericholecystic air, but lateral decubitus film (*I*) demonstrates an air-fluid level within the gallbladder (*arrow*).

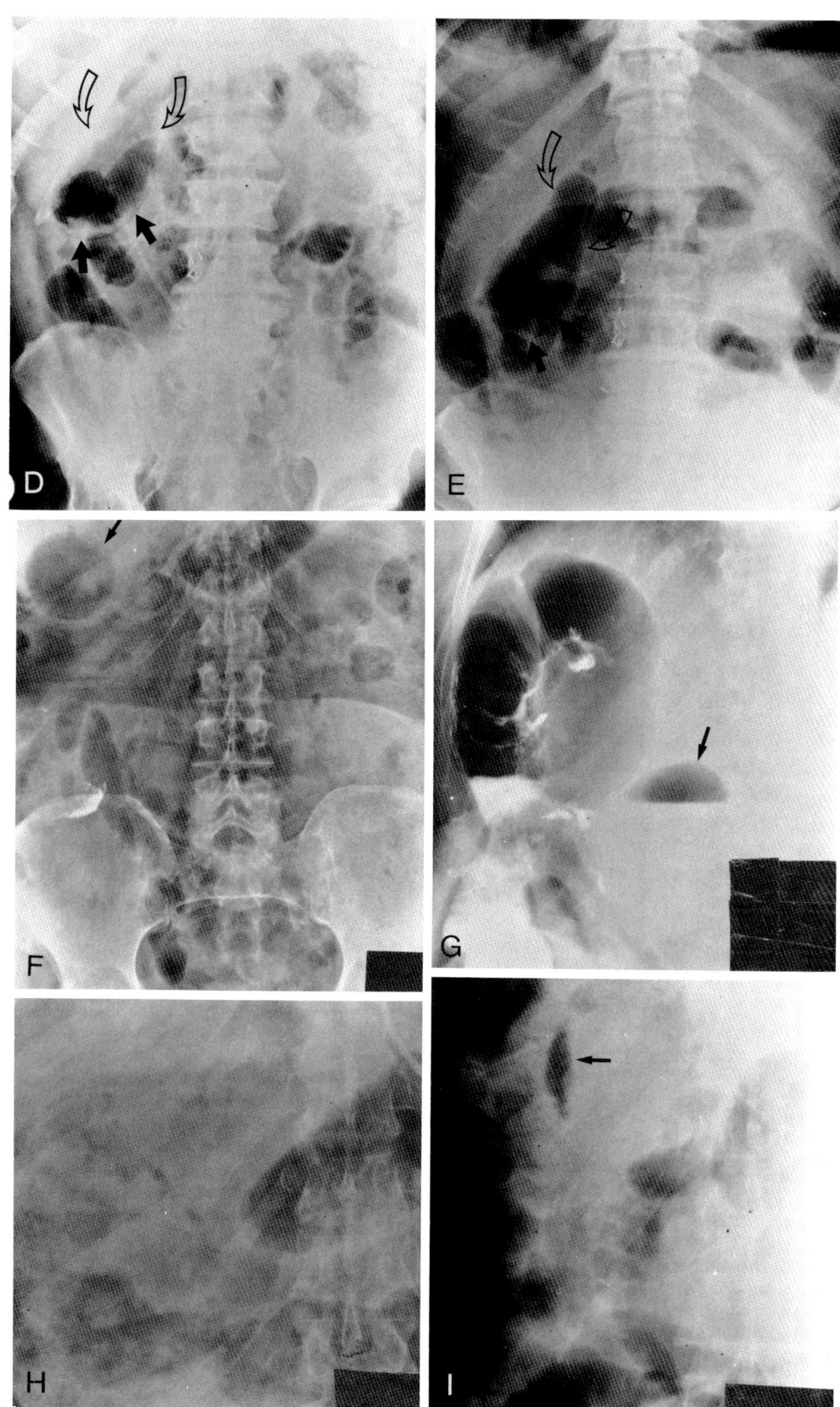

FIGURE 12.36*D–I*

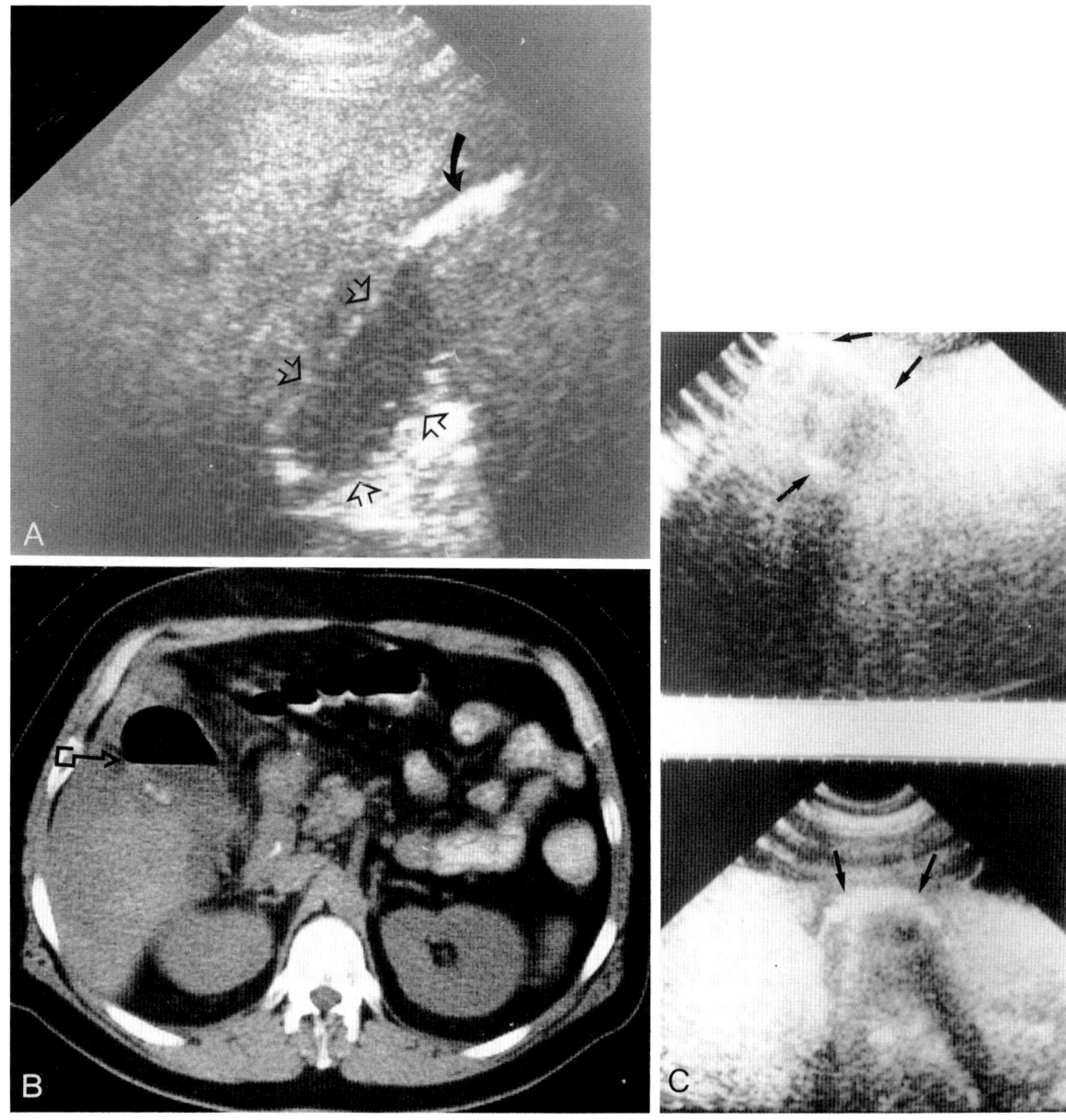

FIGURE 12.37. SONOGRAPHY AND CT OF EMPHYSEMATOUS CHOLECYSTITIS
A: Parasagittal sonogram demonstrates a bright, linear shadowing echo in the fundus (*arrow*). Note that the shadowing is dirty. The remainder of the gallbladder lumen (*open arrows*) shows scattered bright air bubbles. *B:* Corresponding CT: air-fluid level (*arrow*) in fundus. *C:* Different patient: sagittal (*top*) and transverse (*bottom*) sonograms showing bright curvilinear echoes in the gallbladder walls (*arrows*) and dirty shadowing diagnostic of emphysematous cholecystitis.

tic shadowing if it is in the form of microbubbles smaller than the beam width of the transducer (8). If stones are present, they can be obscured by the gas within the gallbladder wall or lumen. The posterior wall of the gallbladder may not be imaged for the same reason. The intraluminal gas will shift to the most superior portion of the gallbladder as the patient is placed in different positions (9).

Emphysematous cholecystitis can be confused sonographically with other entities. A porcelain gallbladder or a large calcified stone may produce a similar appearance, but the shadowing will usually be clean. Large stones may occasionally generate reverberation echoes. Acute or chronic cholecystitis may be associated with a hyperreflective thickened gallbladder wall. Gas-filled loops of bowel in the right upper quadrant may be difficult to differentiate from emphysematous cholecystitis. Prominent Rokitansky-Aschoff sinuses in adenomyomatosis will produce focal echogenicities in the gallbladder wall. Therefore when the diagnosis of emphysematous cholecystitis is suspected sonographically, an abdominal x-ray should be obtained to either confirm the diagnosis or exclude it.

Computed Tomography

CT is almost never necessary for making a diagnosis of emphysematous cholecystitis if plain films and sonograms are properly correlated. Nevertheless, CT may be obtained either as the initial examination or to follow-up an unclear sonogram (10). Intraluminal gas and gas-fluid levels (Fig. 12.37B) will be shown as well as with plain films, pericholecystic gas bubbles, if present, will be shown more convincingly by CT than by plain films, but air in the wall when localized may be demonstrated better by a radiograph because of partial voluming.

REFERENCES

1. Schein CJ: *Acute Cholecystitis.* New York, Harper & Row, 1971, pp 218–222.
2. Nelson SW: Extraluminal gas collections due to diseases of the gastrointestinal tract. *AJR* 115:225–247, 1972.
3. Blum L, Stagg A: Emphysematous cholecystitis. *AJR* 89:840–845, 1963.
4. Harley WD, Kirkpatrick RH, Ferrucci JT: Gas in the bile ducts (pneumobilia) in emphysematous cholecystitis. *AJR* 131:661–663, 1978.
5. Blaquiere RM, Dewbury KC: The ultrasound diagnosis of emphysematous cholecystitis. *Br J Radiol.* 55:114–116, 1982.
6. Parulekar SG: Sonographic findings in acute emphysematous cholecystitis. *Radiology* 145:117–119, 1982.
7. Hunter ND, Macintosh PK: Acute emphysematous cholecystitis: an ultrasonic diagnosis. *AJR* 134:592–593, 1980.
8. Kutcher R, Rosenblatt R, Weissman H: Sonographic appearance of emphysematous cholecystitis. *NY State J Med* 81:1192–1194, 1981.
9. Bloom RA, Fisher A, Pode D, Asaf Y: Shifting intramural gas—a new ultrasound sign of emphysematous cholecystitis. *J Clin Ultrasound* 12:40–42, 1984.
10. Kane RA, Costello P, Duszlak E: Computed tomography in acute cholecystitis: new observations. *AJR* 141:697–701, 1983.

CHRONIC CHOLECYSTITIS

In patients with cholelithiasis the gallbladder will almost always show morphologic findings characteristic of chronic inflammation whether or not the patient has had biliary symptoms. Eventually the gallbladder will become fibrotic, shrunken, thickened, and adherent to surrounding organs and/or omentum. If there are no complications (such as fistula from stone erosion) there are no symptoms per se from chronic cholecystitis. Heartburn, belching, and vague epigastric discomfort which are often attributed to fatty food intolerance occur just as often in patients without gallstones. Clinical diagnosis depends on the recognition of symptoms characteristic of cystic or common duct obstruction. Gallstones are often discovered serendipitously on plain films of the abdomen, sonograms or CT scans performed for reasons unrelated to the gallbladder (1).

REFERENCES

1. Schoenfield LJ: *Diseases of the Gallbladder and Biliary System* (Clinical Gastroenterology Monographs). New York, John Wiley & Sons, 1977.

Radiology

Plain Films and Barium Contrast Examination

Other than the presence of gallstones or porcelain gallbladder, chronic cholecystitis is far less likely than acute cholecystitis to produce any abnormalities on plain films of the abdomen or barium studies. Adhesions from chronic cholecystitis may occasionally angulate and kink the duodenal wall (1).

REFERENCES

1. Berk RN, Ferrucci JT Jr, Leopold GR: *Radiology of the Gallbladder and Bile Ducts, Diagnosis and Intervention.* Philadelphia, W. B. Saunders, 1983, p 30.

Sonography

Sonographic findings in uncomplicated chronic cholecystitis include gallstones and gallbladder wall thickening (Fig. 12.38). The wall thickening is usually smooth, but it may be quite irregular, making carcinoma difficult to exclude (Fig. 12.39). Cholescintigraphic delayed gallblad-

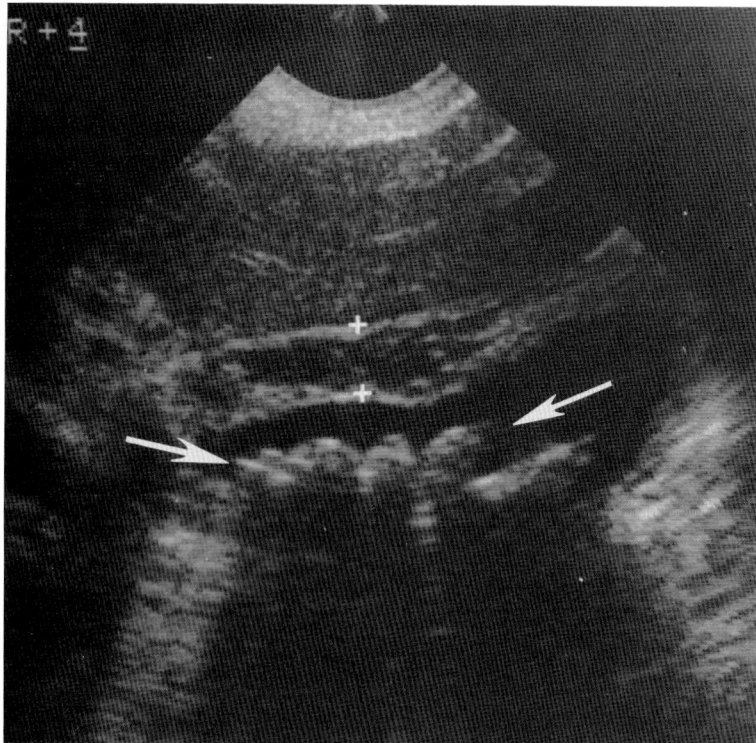

FIGURE 12.38. CHRONIC CHOLECYSTITIS: SONOGRAPHY
Massive gallbladder wall thickening (*cursors*) and multiple shadowing gallstones (*arrows*) in a patient with chronic cholecystitis. The relative lack of symptoms in this case suggested chronic rather than acute cholecystitis. Smoothness of the thickened wall is against a diagnosis of gallbladder carcinoma, although the latter should be considered.

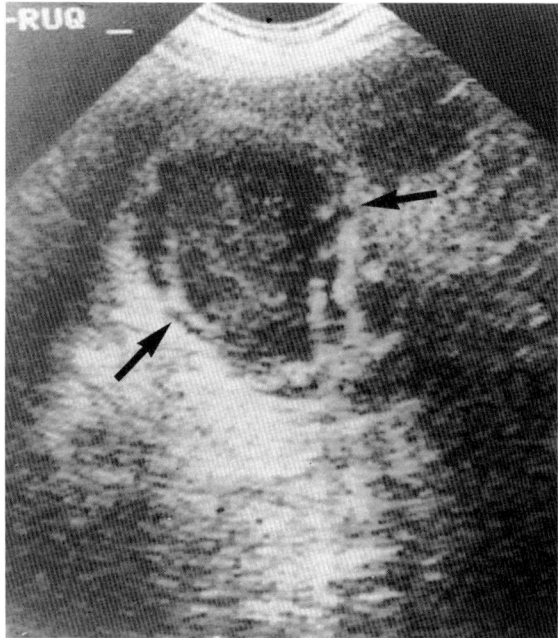

FIGURE 12.39. CHRONIC CHOLECYSTITIS: SONOGRAPHY
Marked irregular gallbladder wall thickening (*arrows*) and sludge within the lumen in a patient with chronic cholecystitis whose sonogram suggests the possibility of carcinoma.

der visualization (1–4 hr) in the face of sonographic cholelithiasis implies chronic cholecystitis.

Cholescintigraphic Evaluation

Chronic cholecystitis is diagnosed by history and ultrasonography and/or oral cholecystography to identify cholelithiasis and/or abnormal gallbladder function. Hepatobiliary scanning plays a very limited role in the workup of patients with chronic cholecystitis, helping to identify the occasional false negative sonogram or OCG. Patients with chronic cholecystitis have a wide spectrum of findings during hepatobiliary scanning: the scan may be completely normal or show delayed (Fig. 12.40) or absent visualization of the gallbladder. (Although false-positive scans for acute cholecystitis are rare, when it does occur, it is usually secondary to chronic cholecystitis) (1, 2). Weissmann et al. reported that delayed visualization of the gallbladder was strongly suggestive of chronic cholecystitis. However, since it is not pathognomonic, sonography should be performed for further evaluation (1). Al-Sheikh et al. (3) reviewed their experience with normal hepatobiliary studies (gallbladder and bowel activity seen by one hour), and noted that if the bowel is visualized before the gallbladder, the likelihood that chronic cholecystitis is present is increased (Fig. 12.41). Although the sensitivity of the finding was poor (45%), its specificity was high (90%). There have been case reports (4, 5) of large gallstones being visualized

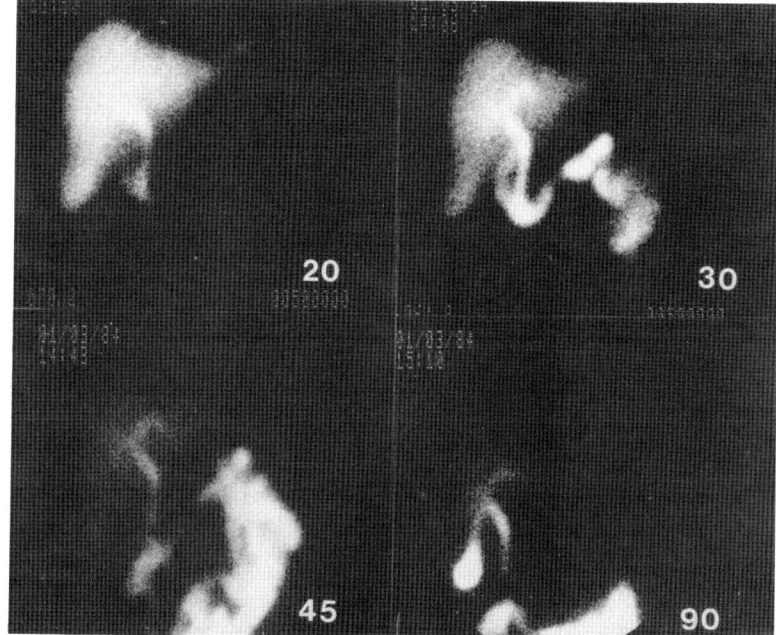

FIGURE 12.40. DELAYED GALLBLADDER VISUALIZATION CONSISTENT WITH CHRONIC CHOLECYSTITIS
There is prompt hepatic uptake, visualization of the common duct and duodenum within the first 20 min. However, the gallbladder is visualized disparately late at 90 min.

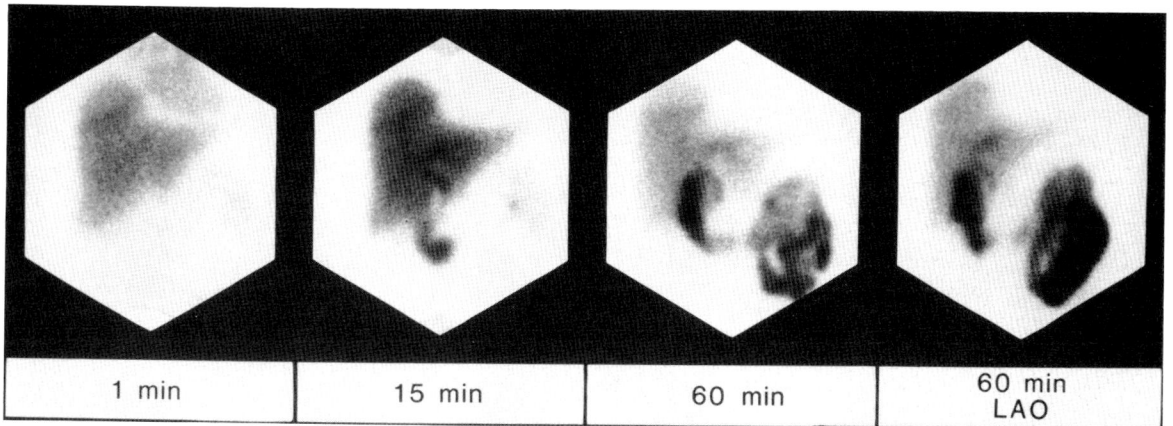

FIGURE 12.41. CHRONIC CHOLECYSTITIS WITH INTESTINAL VISUALIZATION PRECEDING GALLBLADDER VISUALIZATION
There is prompt hepatic uptake with visualization of the common duct and duodenum at 15 min. The gallbladder is visualized at 60 min and is more clearly separated from duodenal activity on the oblique view.

as photopenic regions during hepatobiliary scanning; however, this is a rare occurrence. One complication of cholecystitis can be gallstone ileus, and hepatobiliary scanning may suggest the diagnosis if there is nonvisualization of the gallbladder, and activity in the small bowel does not progress beyond the point of obstruction (6, 7).

Extensive research is currently being conducted with regard to the potential role of cholescintigraphy in the diagnosis of "functional biliary disease" (chronic acalculous cholecystitis—biliary dyskinesia—cystic duct syndrome). Preliminary indications are encouraging; however, further investigations in these traditionally problematic areas are continuing (8, 9).

REFERENCES

1. Weissmann HS, Badia J, Surgarman LA et al: Spectrum of ^{99m}Tc-IDA cholescintigraphic patterns in acute cholecystitis. *Radiology* 138:167–175, 1981.
2. Freitas JE: Influence of scan and pathologic criteria on the specificity of cholescintigraphy: concise communication. Reply letter to the editor. *J Nucl Med* 25:728, 1984.
3. Al-Sheikh W, Hourani M, Barkin JS et al: A sign of symptomatic chronic cholecystitis on biliary scintigraphy. *AJR* 140:283–285, 1983.

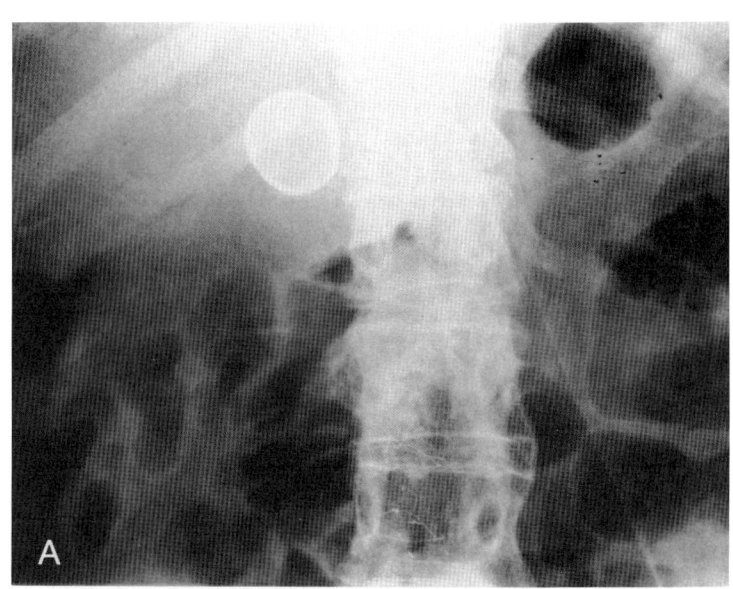

FIGURE 12.42. CT OF CHRONIC CHOLECYSTITIS
A and *B:* Plain film (*A*) shows a large gallstone and CT (*B*) demonstrates a markedly thickened wall (*arrows*) surrounding the stone. *C:* CT of a different patient: slightly thickened, slightly irregular gallbladder wall (*arrow*). Scan was taken during a rapid infusion of 60% contrast. A stone was demonstrated at a different level. Compare to normal gallbladder wall in CT gallbladder anatomy section.

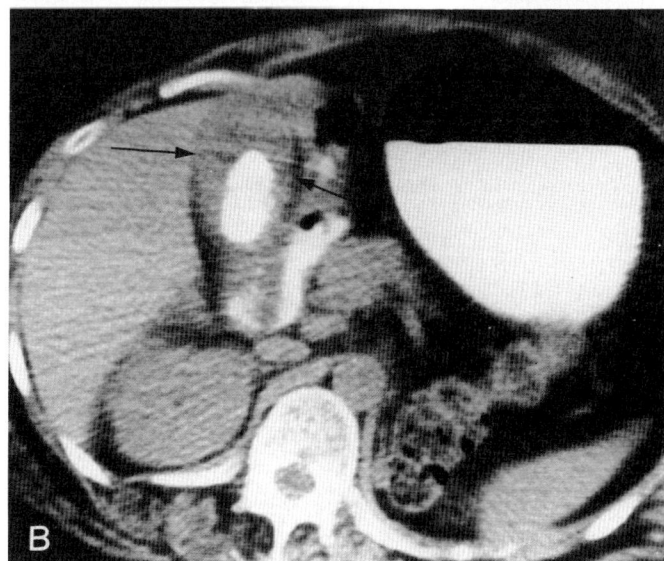

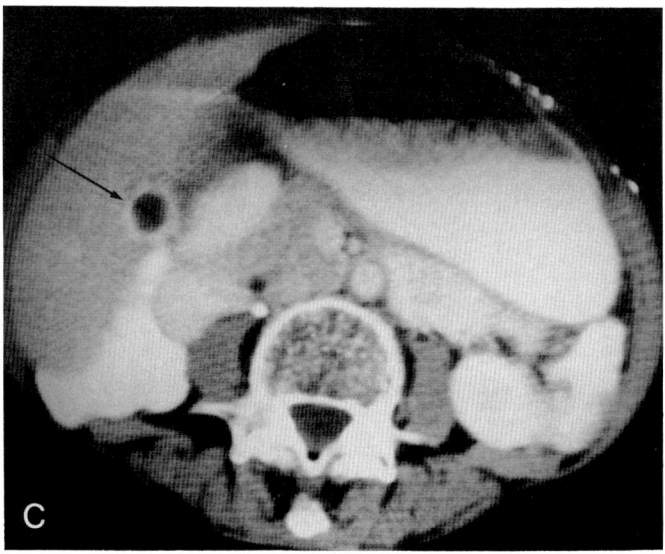

4. Garty I: Visualization of gallstones by hepatobiliary scintigraphy. Two case reports. *Clin Nucl Med* 9:193–195, 1984.
5. Moreno AJ, Yedinak MA, Turnbull GL et al: Cholelithiasis demonstrated on hepatobiliary scintigraphy as a photopenic defect within the inferior portion of the liver. *Clin Nucl Med* 9:655–656, 1984.
6. Bocobo GR, Slavin JD, Rao H, et al: Hepatobiliary imaging in gallstone ileus. *Clin Nucl Med* 9:4–5, 1984.
7. Elkin CM, Weissmann HS, Freeman LM: Gallstone ileus diagnosed by technetium-99m dimethyliminodiacetic acid cholescintigraphy. A case report. *Clin Nucl Med* 9:79–80, 1984.
8. Fink-Bennett D, DeRidder P, Kolozsi W, Gordon R, Rapp J: Cholecystokinin cholescintigraphic findings in the cystic duct syndrome. *J Nucl Med* 26:1123–1128, 1985.
9. Jaros RH: Cholecystokinin (CCK) cholescintigraphy in patients suspected of having acalculous biliary disease. *Radiology* 157:315, 1985.

Computed Tomography

CT is not usually rewarding in chronic cholecystitis; occasionally one can see a thickened gallbladder wall usually accompanied by calculi (Fig. 12.42). One study of patients with nonvisualization on oral cholecystography demonstrated the ability of CT to document a lack of contrast enhancement in gallbladder bile compared to bile in the common duct, diagnostic of cystic duct obstruction (1).

REFERENCE

1. Toombs BD, Sandler CM, Conoley PM: Computed tomography of the non-visualizing gallbladder. *J Comput Assist Tomogr* 5:164–168, 1980.

PORCELAIN GALLBLADDER

Fairly uncommon, porcelain gallbladder occurs in less than 1% of cholecystectomy specimens. Although most patients have had recurrent acute cholecystitis, porcelain gallbladder itself rarely causes symptoms (1). The incidence of associated carcinoma of the gallbladder is probably 10–20% (although figures as high as 60% are quoted), thus prophylactic cholecystectomy is recommended if the patient is a surgical candidate (2). Cholelithiasis is frequently associated.

Pathophysiology

Some speculate that cystic duct obstruction leads to precipitation of calcium carbonate salts in the mucosa. Others feel that the mural calcification is dystrophic and that it occurs in a wall scarred by chronic low grade infection and compromised circulation caused by cystic duct obstruction. A third possibility is irritation of the wall by a stone or other foreign body (3). Histologically, two types of calcification may be seen: flakes of dystrophic calcification within a chronically inflamed and fibrotic muscular wall or numerous microliths scattered diffusely throughout mucosa, submucosa, glandular spaces, and Rokitansky-Aschoff sinuses (4).

Radiology

The radiographic appearance is usually diagnostic: curvilinear (profile) and/or granular (en face) calcification is seen in the gallbladder wall (4). The entire circumference (with a break in the neck) or just a segment of the wall may be calcified (Fig. 12.43). At times it will be unclear from a plain film whether one is dealing with a porcelain gallbladder or a large calcified gallstone (Fig. 12.44); oral cholecystography is then helpful. A porcelain gallbladder is nearly always nonfunctional, whereas a gallbladder containing calculi usually will function. Coexisting gallstones within a porcelain gallbladder will not be seen unless calcified.

Sonography

Three sonographic patterns have been described (3). The first is a highly echogenic shadowing curvilinear structure in the gallbladder fossa, indistinguishable from a contracted gallbladder filled with many calculi or a single large stone. A thin anechoic rim of bile above a calculus can exclude porcelain gallbladder, but a plain film and/or an oral cholecystogram may be needed if the distinction needs to be made. The second pattern consists of visualization of echogenic near and far gallbladder walls with some degree of acoustic shadowing from one or both walls. Emphysematous cholecystitis cannot be distinguished for certain by sonography and a plain film is necessary (Fig. 12.45).

Finally one may see irregular clumps of echoes with posterior acoustic shadowing scattered throughout the gallbladder wall, highly suggestive of porcelain gallbladder; a plain film is merely confirmatory of the sonographic findings in this case.

When scanning a patient with porcelain gallbladder, it is important to search carefully for findings such as intraluminal masses, wall irregularity, or pericholecystic mass that would indicate gallbladder carcinoma.

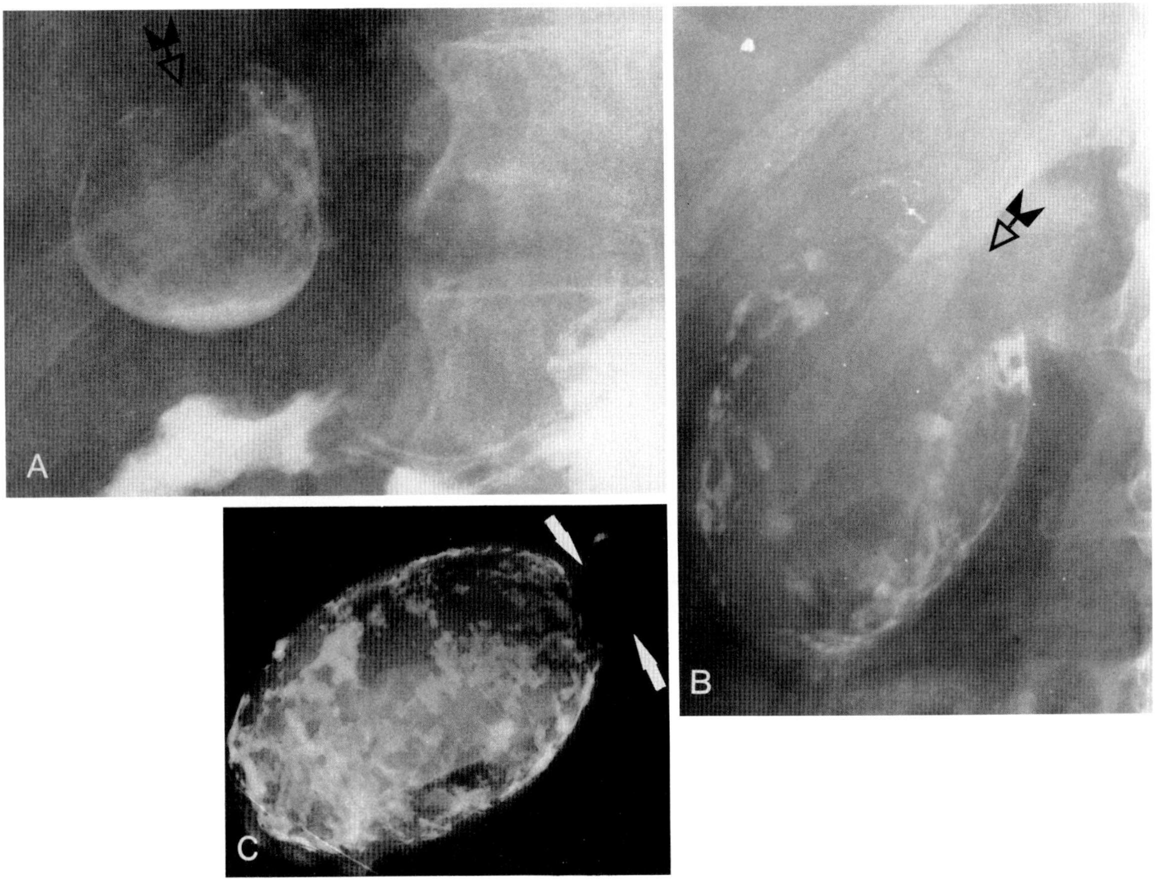

FIGURE 12.43. PORCELAIN GALLBLADDER
A and *B:* Porcelain gallbladders with mostly profile calcification (*A*) and both en face and profile calcification (*B*). Note breaks in calcification in the neck region (*arrows*). *C:* Bivalved specimen x-ray: note absence of calcification in neck (*arrows*).

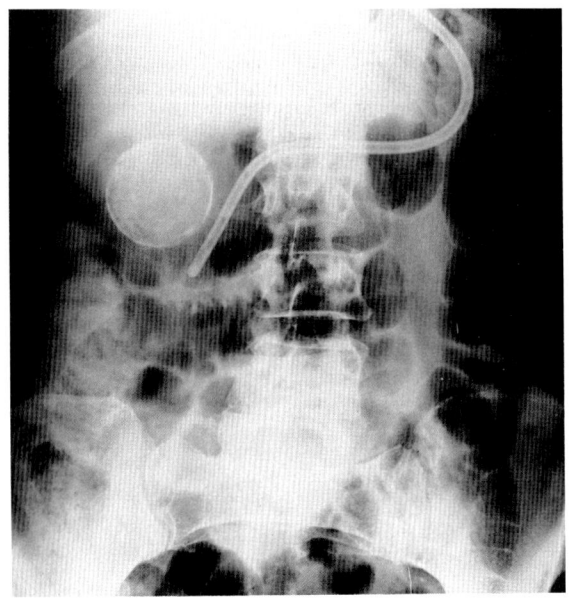

FIGURE 12.44. PORCELAIN GALLBLADDER OR LARGE GALLSTONE?
Complete ring of calcification and circular shape suggest the correct diagnosis of gallstone.

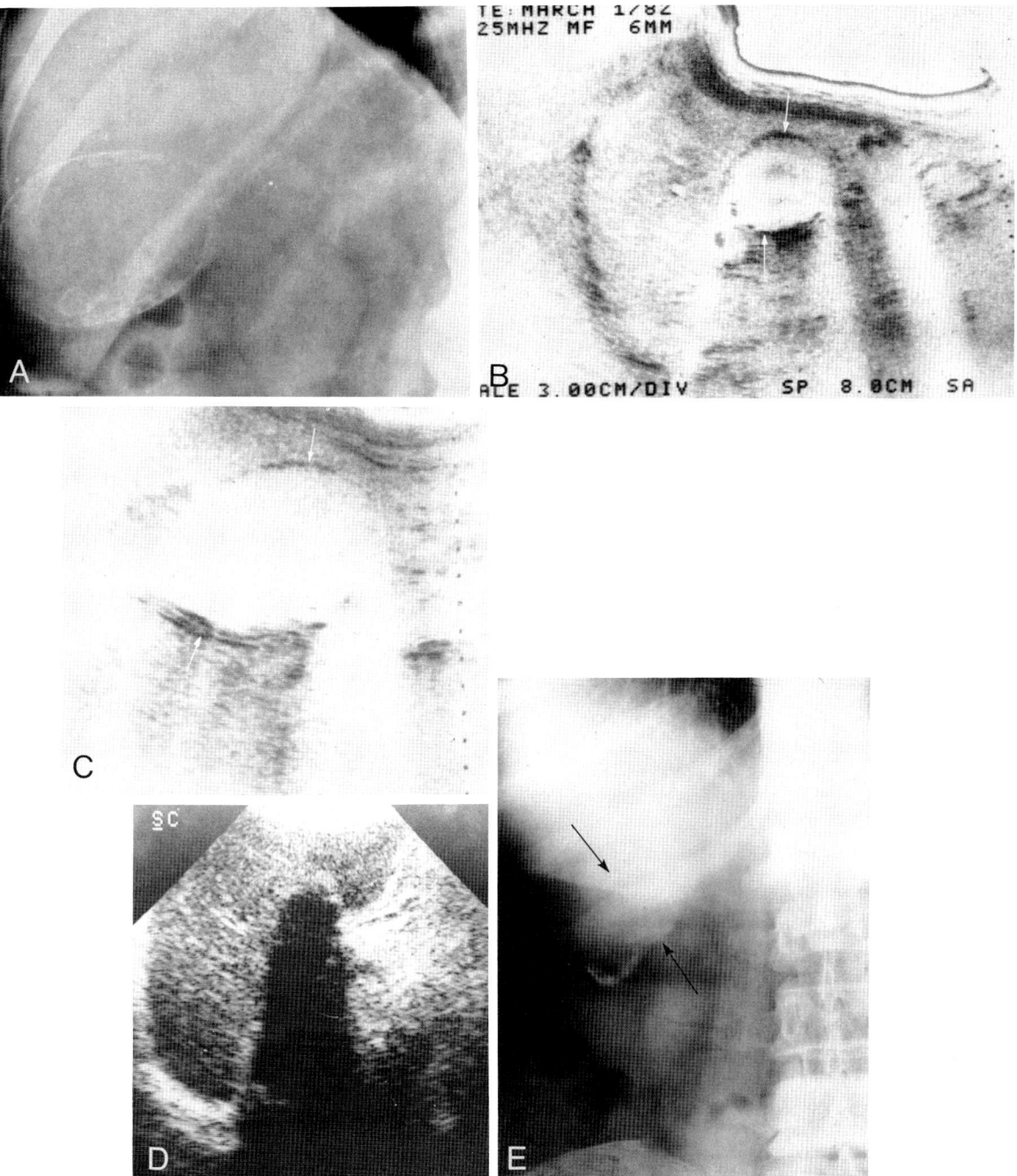

FIGURE 12.45. PLAIN FILM AND SONOGRAPHY OF PORCELAIN GALLBLADDER

A: Plain film calcification. *B* and *C:* Sonography shows echogenic gallbladder walls (*arrows*) consistent with calcification. *D* and *E* (different case): Shadowing from near wall of porcelain gallbladder is so complete that differentiation from a large stone is impossible. Cleanness of shadowing is against a diagnosis of emphysematous cholecystitis. Ovoid plain film calcification (*E, arrows*) suggests porcelain gallbladder rather than stone.

Computed Tomography

CT may be the first study after an abnormal sonogram and can demonstrate the wall calcification of porcelain gallbladder quite exquisitely (Fig. 12.46) (3). Porcelain gallbladder can also be diagnosed on a CT of the abdomen obtained for unrelated complaints. The scans should be scru-

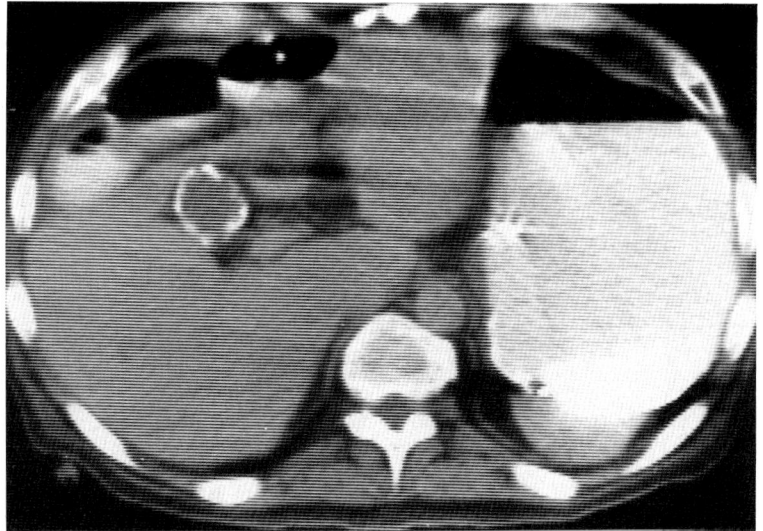

FIGURE 12.46. CT OF PORCELAIN GALLBLADDER
CT: incidental porcelain gallbladder with interrupted wall calcification. A gallstone would generally have continuous calcification and some bile between it and the gallbladder wall.

tinized for evidence of superimposed gallbladder carcinoma.

REFERENCES

1. Schoenfield LJ: *Diseases of the Gallbladder and Biliary System* (Clinical Gastroenterology Monographs). New York, John Wiley & Sons, 1977.
2. Berk RN, Armbuster TG, Saltzstein SL: Carcinoma in the porcelain gallbladder. *Radiology* 106:29–31, 1973.
3. Kane RA, Jacobs R, Katz J, Costello P: Porcelain gallbladder: ultrasound and CT appearance. *Radiology* 152:137–141, 1984.
4. Ochsner SF, Carrera GM: Calcification of the gallbladder ("porcelain gallbladder"). *AJR* 88:847–853, 1963.

MILK OF CALCIUM BILE

Milk of calcium bile or limy bile is formed by the precipitation of particulate material (calcium carbonate, calcium phosphate, and calcium bilirubinate) in the gallbladder giving rise to semifluid or putty-like material. Limy bile is an unusual condition associated in most cases with gallstone obstruction of the cystic duct and chronic cholecystitis. Cholecystectomy is usually indicated, although rarely limy bile disappears spontaneously.

Radiology

A plain film will show diffuse opacification of the gallbladder, at times with a slightly granular appearance (Figs. 12.47–12.49). The appearance of a normal functioning gallbladder can be closely mimicked. A horizontal beam film will show dependent layering of the milk of calcium and will be diagnostic. Affected gallbladders are usually functionless on oral cholecystography (they may opacify slightly), and the danger exists that if a preliminary film prior to contrast administration is not taken, the examination will be considered normal (1).

Sonography

Findings on sonography may be very similar to calculous disease with echodense, shadowing material collecting in the dependent portions of the gallbladder. Features may also be intermediate between sludge and gallstones: highly echogenic shadowing material accumulated in a dependent portion of the lumen forming a fluid-fluid level with lighter bile above it (2, 3). A plain film should always be obtained whenever the condition is suspected on a sonogram.

Computed Tomography

Although rarely performed for this condition, CT is diagnostic, as a bile-calcium level will be seen unless the gallbladder is entirely filled with the milk of calcium (which is not usually the case). The only differential considerations are hemorrhagic cholecystitis, hemobilia, and contrast administration with poor mixing. Milk of calcium will be more attenuating than blood, and contrast material can be excluded by history.

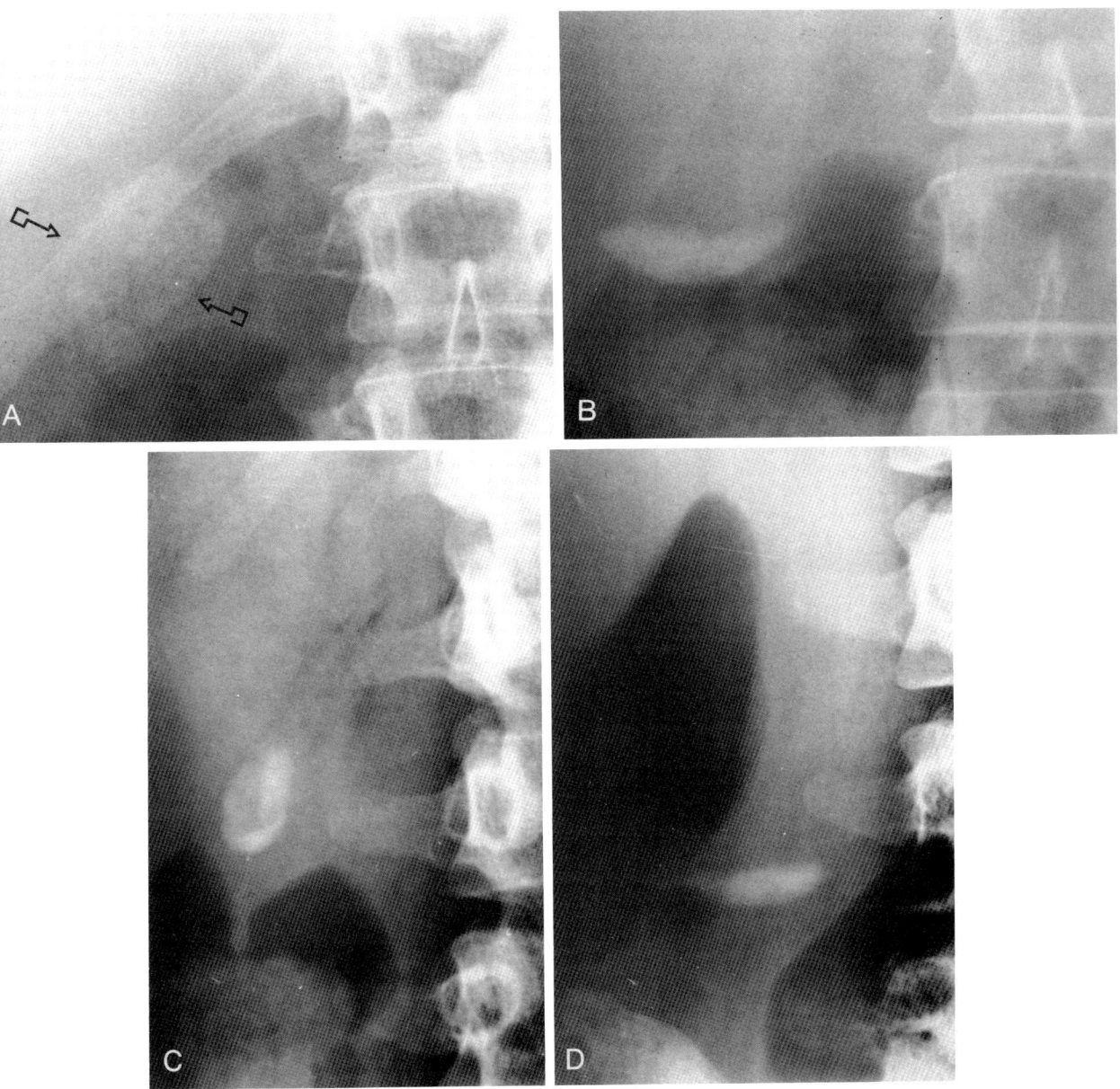

FIGURE 12.47. MILK OF CALCIUM BILE

A: Supine, *B:* erect plain films: en face milk of calcium (*arrows*) and bile-calcium level, respectively. *C* and *D:* A second case with similar findings (supine and erect). *E* and *F:* Specimen radiographs of this case reproduce radiographic findings in erect and decubitus projections.

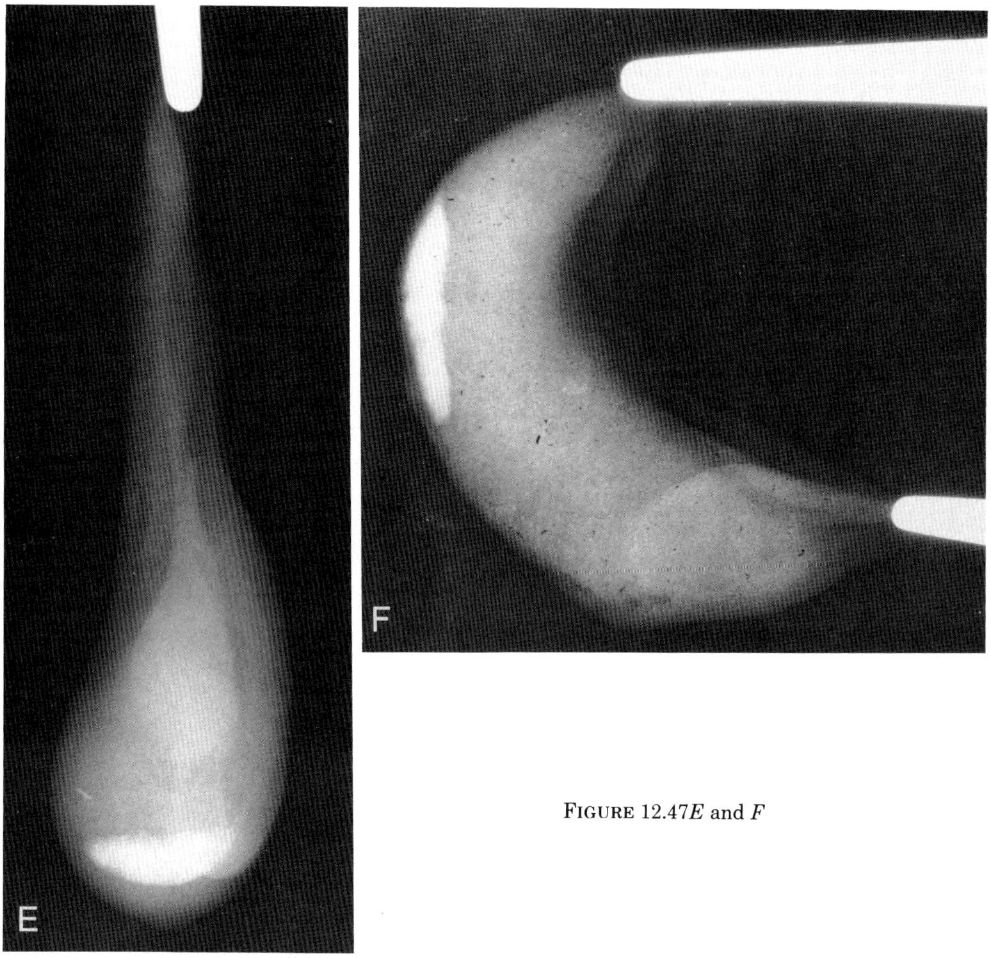

FIGURE 12.47E and F

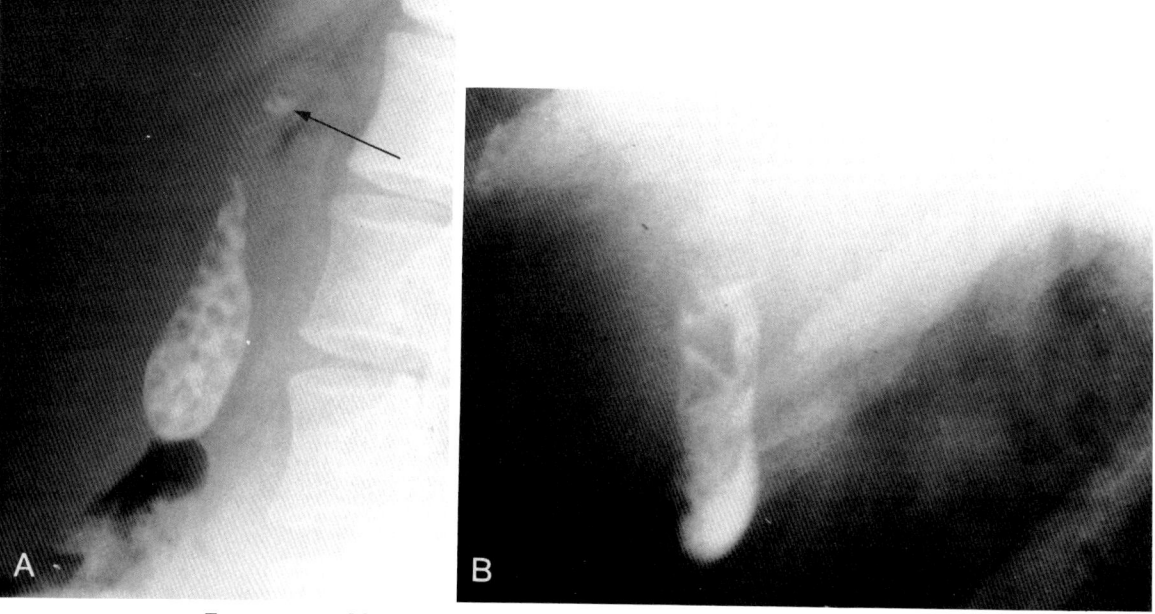

FIGURE 12.48. MILK OF CALCIUM AND LUCENT CALCULI MIMICKING STONES
A and *B:* Plain film (supine): two examples of milk of calcium and lucent calculi mimicking stones in a functioning gallbladder on OCG. Note cystic duct stone in A (*arrow*).

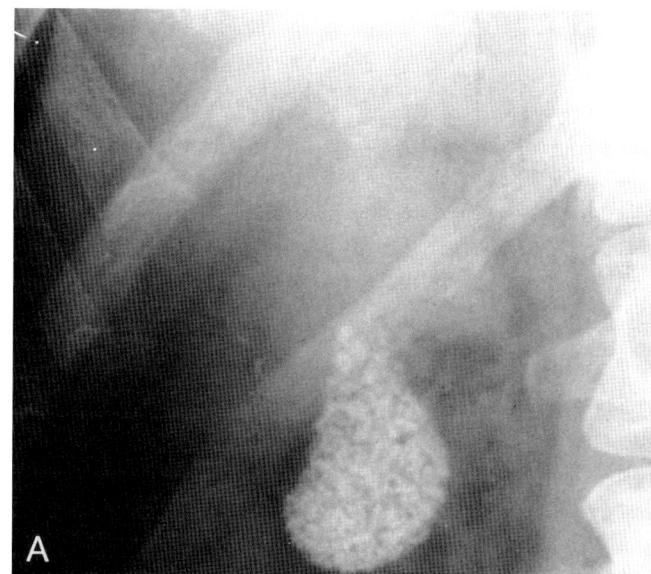
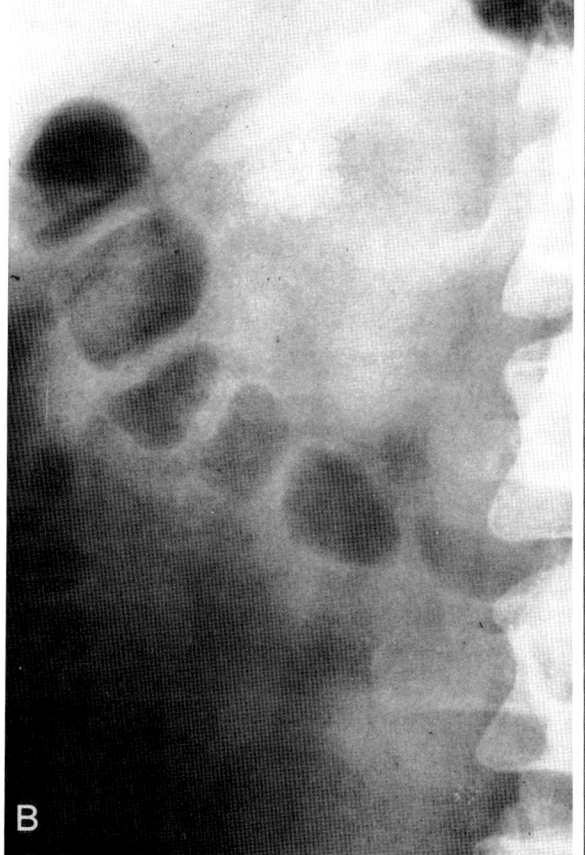
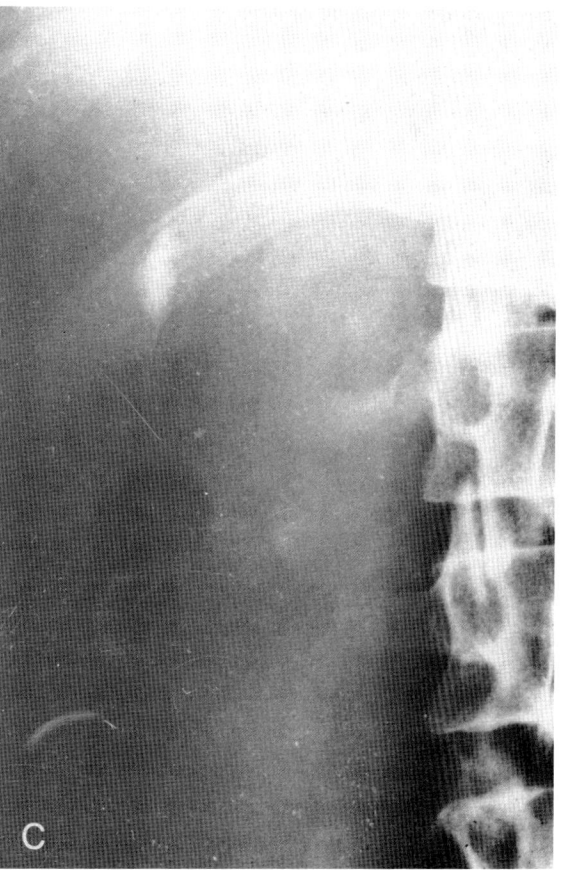

FIGURE 12.49. MILK OF CALCIUM IN TINY CONCRETIONS
A: Plain film (supine): milk of calcium in the form of tiny concretions. *B* and *C:* Supine and decubitus films of tiny concretions showing change in appearance with different positioning.

REFERENCES

1. Besic LR, Krawzoff G, Tiesenga MF: Limey bile syndrome. *JAMA* 193:245–246, 1965.
2. Chun GH, Deutsch AL, Scheible W: Sonographic findings in milk of calcium bile. *Gastrointest Radiol* 7:371–373, 1982.
3. Love MB: Sonographic features of milk of calcium bile. *J Ultrasound Med* 1:325–327, 1982.

HYDROPS OF GALLBLADDER

Hydrops of the gallbladder refers to gallbladder distention by clear, sterile mucus (white bile) (Fig. 12.50). The underlying cause is usually a chronic complete cystic duct obstruction. A nontender mass is visible or palpable in the right upper quadrant in patients with chronic hydrops. Often there are no symptoms, but the patient may have chronic discomfort in the region of the mass. Empyema, gangrene, or perforation rarely supervenes, and cholecystectomy is usually indicated (1).

Radiology

A hydropic gallbladder will sometimes be detected on a plain film or a barium study as a right upper quadrant soft tissue mass displacing and indenting the duodenum inferomedially or indenting the superior aspect of the hepatic flexure (Fig. 12.51). It will not function on oral cholecystography. Sonography will demonstrate an enlarged fluid-filled gallbladder and possibly the cause of the cystic duct obstruction. Sometimes the "white bile" will have low level echoes within it, presumably due to protein aggregates. The appearance of hydrops is not specific and causes of atony and sludge will have to be considered in the differential diagnosis. The diagnosis of hydrops on CT is even less specific (Fig. 12.52). Generally, the only finding is enlargement of the gallbladder beyond an anteroposterior diameter of 4–5 cm (2).

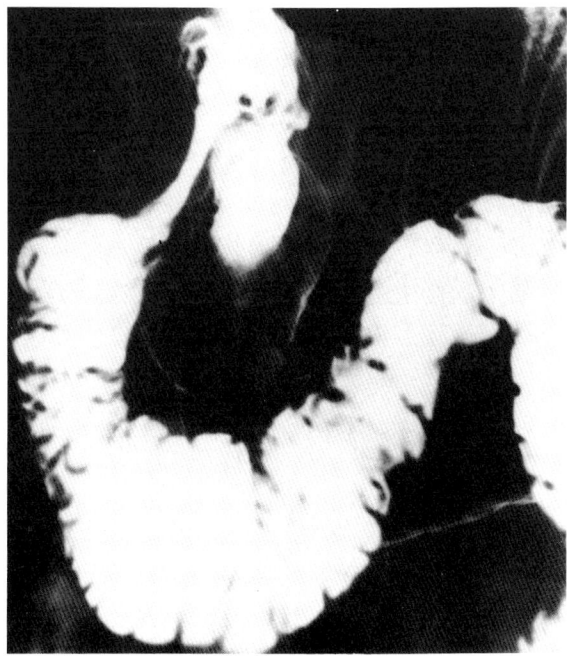

FIGURE 12.51. ENLARGED GALLBLADDER INDENTING THE IMMEDIATELY POST-BULBAR DUODENUM

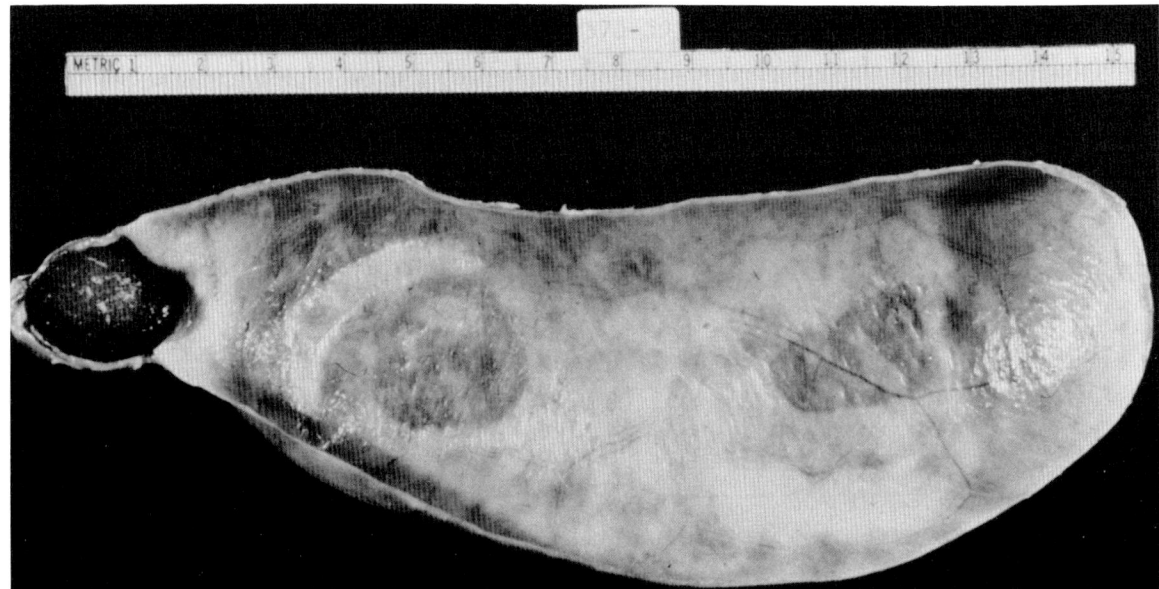

FIGURE 12.50. HYDROPS OF THE GALLBLADDER
Gross specimen of a hydropic gallbladder. Note blue-white coloration (see color plate).

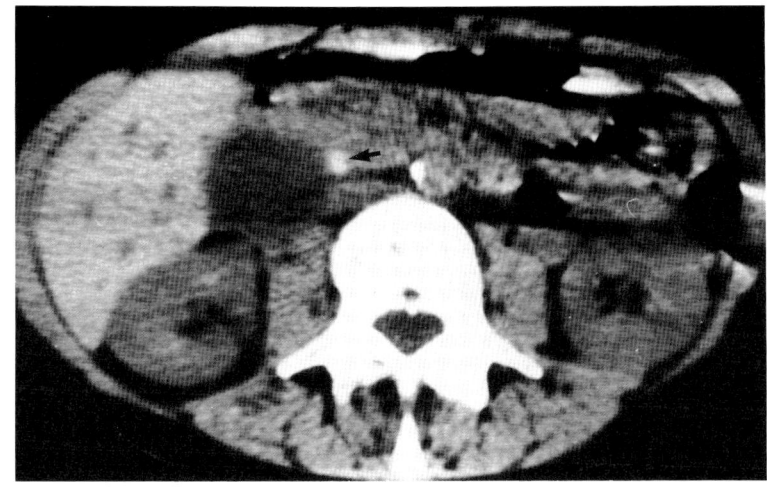

FIGURE 12.52. LARGE HYDROPIC GALLBLADDER
CT immediately after nonfunction on OCG performed for palpable RUQ mass. Large hydropic gallbladder seen as water-density mass between the liver and the opacified common bile duct (*arrow*).

REFERENCES

1. Schoenfield LJ: *Diseases of the Gallbladder and Biliary System* (Clinical Gasteroenterology Monographs). New York, John Wiley & Sons, 1977.
2. Havrilla TR, Reich NR, Haaga JR, Seidelmann FE, Cooperman AM, Alfidi RJ: Computed tomography of the gallbladder. *AJR* 130:1059–1067, 1978.

BILIARY FISTULA

Clinical Findings

Biliary fistulas are incidental findings at cholecystectomy in about 5% of patients, therefore most patients with an internal biliary fistula are asymptomatic. Fistulas to the abdominal wall are exceedingly rare. Over 90% of internal biliary fistulas come about as a result of cholelithiasis and acute or chronic cholecystitis. During repeated episodes of inflammation, adhesions form between the gallbladder and adjacent structures, and eventually any stones erode into adjacent viscera. Fistulas to the duodenum account for 70% of gallstone-related internal fistulas, and most of the remainder are to the stomach or colon. While fistulas not associated with stones more often involve the common bile duct rather than the gallbladder, the gallbladder may be affected. Etiologies include gallbladder and biliary tract carcinoma, other regional invasive neoplasms, diverticulitis, inflammatory bowel disease, trauma, congenital and echinococcal cyst. Additional but rare sites of biliary fistula termination include: jejunum and ileum, hepatic artery, bronchial tree, pericardium, portal vein, renal pelvis, ureter, vagina, ovary, and urinary bladder (1, 2).

Patients may experience clinical improvement after fistula formation, but they are frequently unaware of the event. Cholangitis, gastrointestinal bleeding, diarrhea, and malabsorption may supervene, so that surgery is felt to be indicated even in asymptomatic patients.

Radiology

Plain Films

Gas in the biliary tree is visible on plain films in most patients with a biliary fistula. The usual finding is branching tubular radiolucencies more prominent centrally than peripherally (Figs. 12.53A, 12.54B, 12.55). If only a small amount of gas is present, it may be visible only as bubbles on a supine film so that an erect film helps determine that it is intrabiliary. Portal venous gas is more prominent peripherally, and periportal fat is not as radiolucent as gas. In addition to spontaneous biliary fistula, previous surgery (choledochoduodenostomy, cholecystojejunostomy, sphincterotomy), patulous sphincter of Oddi, and ascending cholangitis with a gas-forming organism should be considered in the differential diagnosis.

Barium Contrast Examination

A barium meal and/or barium enema are frequently useful in detecting and evaluating the cause of a biliary-enteric fistula when the diagnosis is unclear after clinical examination and a plain film (Fig. 12.53B). Gallstone ileus is dis-

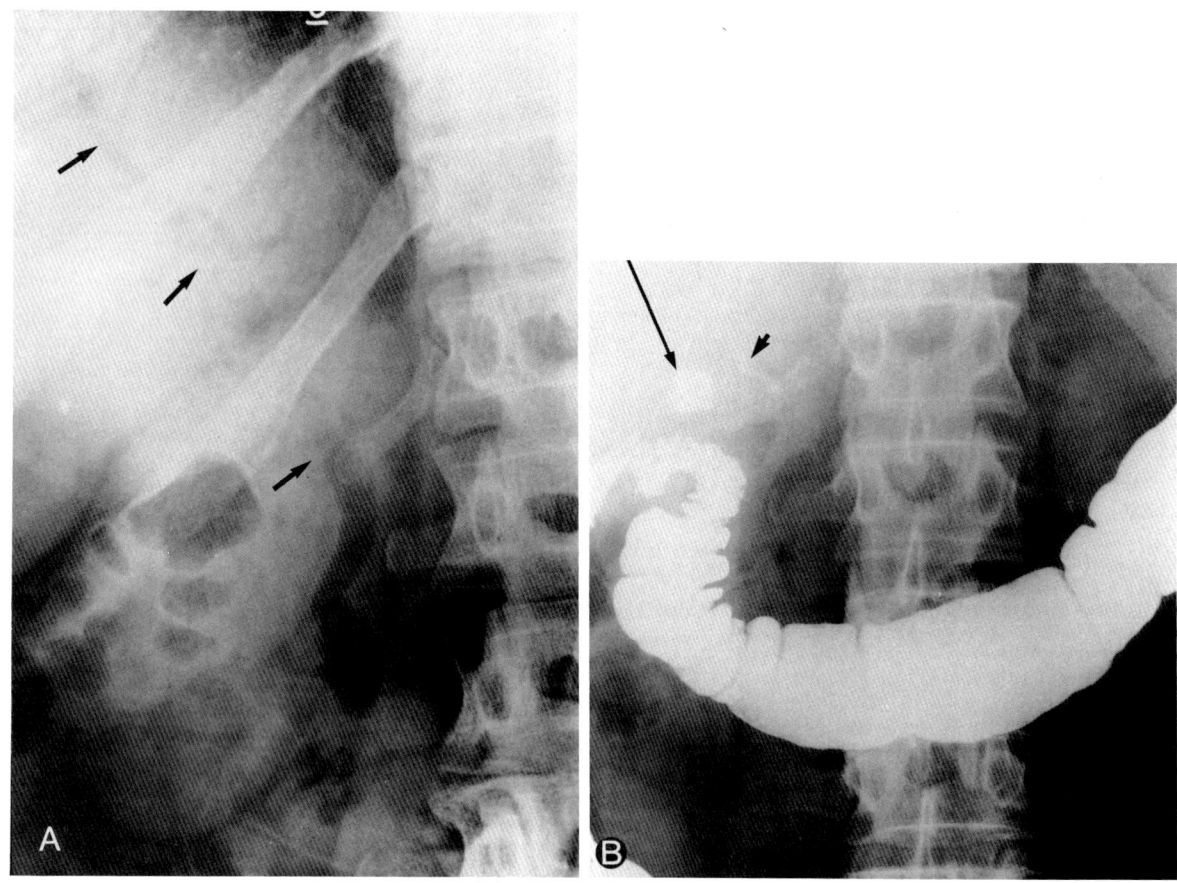

FIGURE 12.53. BILIARY FISTULA

Biliary-colic fistula, from chronic cholecystitis and probably previous gallstone erosion into the hepatic flexure. *A:* Pneumobilia (*arrows*). *B:* Barium enema: gallbladder (*long arrow*) and common duct (*short arrow*) are opacified.

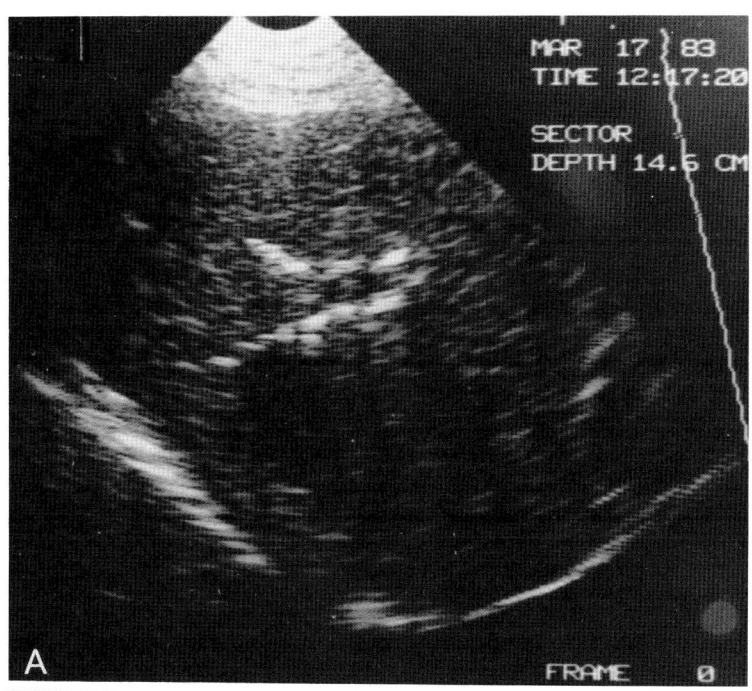
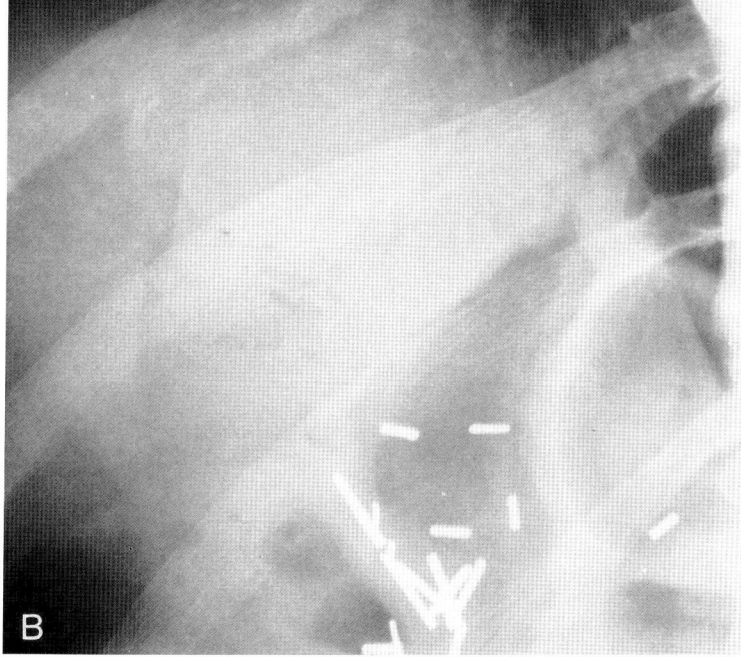

FIGURE 12.54. BILIARY AIR IN A PATIENT S/P WHIPPLE'S PROCEDURE
A: Sonogram shows linear, bright central branching echoes consistent with air in the biliary tree. *B:* Corresponding supine plain film documenting pneumobilia: discontinuous branching lucencies.

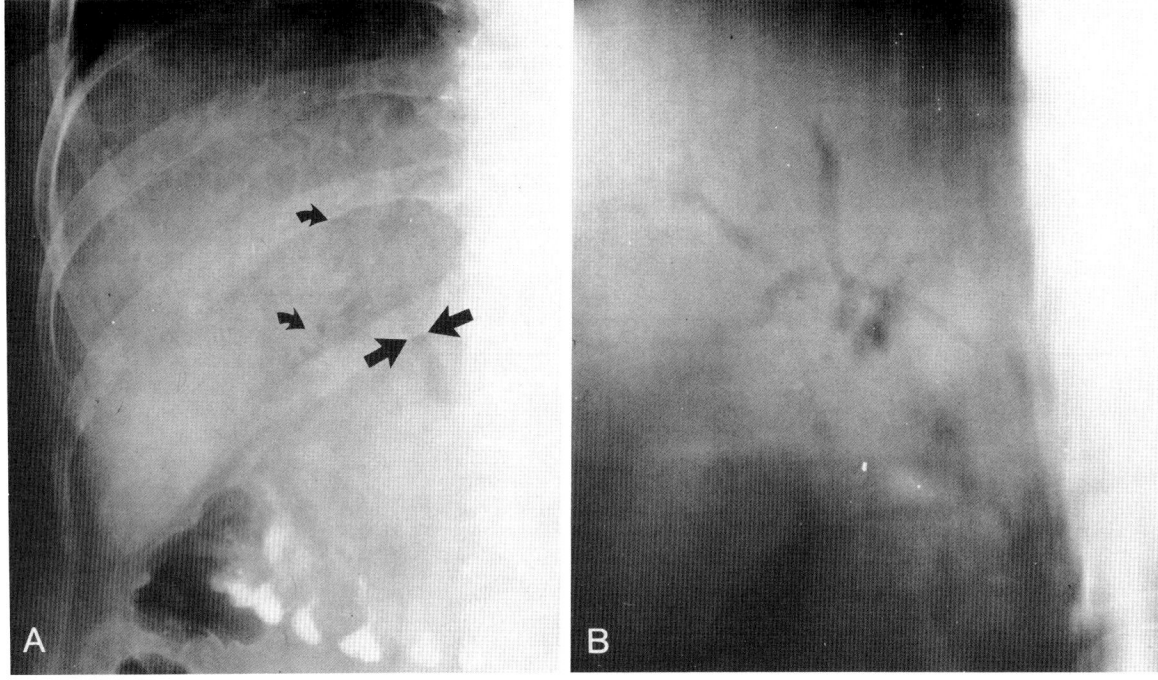

FIGURE 12.55. BILIARY GAS

A: Supine plain film: linear central biliary gas (*large arrows*) and some scattered intrabiliary bubbles (*small arrows*). *B:* Tomography confirms extensive intrabiliary gas.

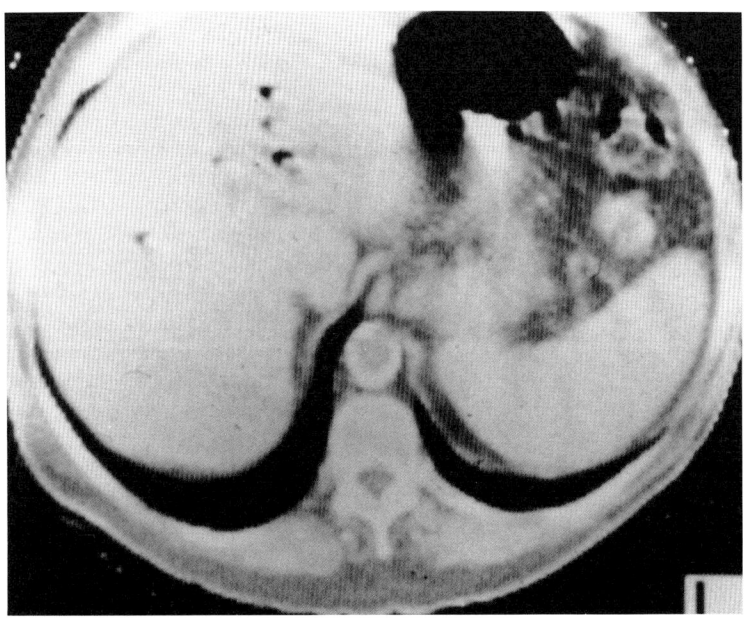

FIGURE 12.56. BILIARY-ENTERIC FISTULA

CT of a biliary-enteric fistula: air and barium in the biliary tree and resultant artefacts.

cussed separately below. Barium examination may be crucial in establishing a diagnosis in the less common causes of biliary enteric fistula such as peptic ulcer disease, carcinoma, diverticulitis or Crohn's disease. Often, however, findings are limited to barium filling the biliary tree and not distinguishable from fistula due to cholelithiasis (2).

Sonography

The role of sonography is limited since the fistula is often too small to be imaged. Air in the biliary tree can be diagnosed when multiple hyperechoic foci are present with dirty shadowing (Fig. 12.54A). Chronic inflammatory changes in the gallbladder may be seen (3). The disappearance of previously documented gallstones in the appropriate clinical context may be suggestive of a fistula, but passage via the common duct is more likely (4).

Computed Tomography

CT can demonstrate gas in the biliary tree with exquisite sensitivity. As most patients will be examined after oral contrast has been given, contrast material may be seen in the biliary tree as well. The resultant multiple air-contrast levels may cause streak artifacts degrading the image (Fig. 12.56). CT will be clinically helpful in a minority of cases when the diagnosis of pneumobilia is unclear from the plain film or neoplastic disease is suspected as the etiology.

Nuclear Medicine

Hepatobiliary scintigraphy is of limited or no value is most biliary fistulae since most etiologies of biliary fistula are associated with cystic duct obstruction (e.g., gallstone ileus). ^{99m}Tc-IDA scintigraphy is most useful in delineating bronchobiliary fistulas (either congenital or traumatic) (5–7), traumatic or postoperative fistulas, and biliary-enteric anastomotic leaks, usually obviating direct cholangiography in these situations.

REFERENCES

1. Scott MG, Pygott F, Murphy L: Significance of gas or barium in the biliary tract. *Br J Radiol* 27:253, 1954.
2. Berk RN, Ferrucci JT Jr, Leopold GR: *Radiology of the Gallbladder and Bile Ducts. Diagnosis and Intervention.* Philadelphia, W. B. Saunders, 1983, pp 46–54.
3. White M, Simeone JF, Muller PR: Imaging of cholecystocolic fistulas. *J Ultrasound Med* 2:181–185, 1983.
4. Caride VJ, Gibson DW: Noninvasive evaluation of bile leakage. *Surg Gynecol Obstet* 154:517–520, 1982.
5. Savitch I, Kew MC, Levin J: Demonstration of a biliary bronchial fistula using ^{99m}Tc- p-butyl IDA imaging. *Clin Nucl Med* 8:139–140, 1983.
6. Blue PW, Versteg HJ, Cole FN et al: Bronchobiliary fistula—demonstration with ^{99m}Tc-PIPIDA imaging. *Clin Nucl Med* 8:272–273, 1983.
7. Giulianotti PC, Mazzuca N, Mosca F et al: Demonstration of bronchobiliary fistula with TC-99m diethyl IDA cholescintigraphy. *Clin Nucl Med* 9:41–42, 1984.

GALLSTONE ILEUS

Clinical Findings

Gallstone ileus (first reported by Bartholin in 1654) is a mechanical intestinal obstruction caused by impaction of one or more gallstones within the intestinal lumen. Although overall it accounts for about 2% of intestinal obstructions, it is considered the etiology of about 20% of intestinal obstructions in patients over the age of 65 (this figure, however, is probably too high) (1). Affected patients are usually in the sixth or seventh decade of life or older, and female preponderance is somewhere between 3 and 16:1. The rate of mortality is high, mostly because of serious concomitant disease. Most often the gallstone passes into the intestinal tract from the gallbladder to the duodenum, although occasionally it will erode into the stomach or the hepatic flexure. Once within the gastrointestinal tract, most stones pass uneventfully per rectum. Occasionally they will be vomited up. Most stones smaller than 2.5 cm pass spontaneously, although ones as large as 5 cm can pass and smaller ones can obstruct. The usual site of obstruction is the terminal ileum (60–70%) somewhat proximal to the ileocecal valve, the first point of critical narrowing generally encountered. Other sites of obstruction include proximal ileum (~25%), distal jejunum (~10), stomach (pylorus), colon (sigmoid), or duodenum (Bouveret's syndrome), all less than 5%. When the sigmoid colon is the point of obstruction, there is usually underlying diverticular disease (1).

The clinical picture of gallstone ileus is similar to that of any mechanical small bowel obstruction, except that symptoms may be intermittent as the stone impacts temporarily at various levels before finally coming to rest permanently. Only half of patients will give a history suggestive of biliary tract disease prior to the obstruction. Enterolithotomy, fistula excision, and cholecystecomy is usually done in one stage unless the patient is too ill, in which case only the intestinal obstruction is treated at the initial operation (1).

REFERENCE

1. Day EA, Marks C: Gallstone ileus. Review of the literature and presentation of 34 new cases. *Am J Surg* 129:552–558, 1975.

Radiology

Plain Films

Rigler's triad describes the classic radiographic findings in gallstone ileus. It is usually expressed as (*a*) distal mechanical small bowel obstruction,

452   LIVER, BILIARY TRACT, PANCREAS, SPLEEN

(b) air in the biliary tree; and (c) calcified stone in the right lower quadrant (1). In practice, gallstone ileus does not always present all of the classic findings and further qualification may be helpful. Any two of the three are highly suggestive but not so completely specific (Fig. 12.57). As indicated above, the site of obstruction is most commonly, but by no means always, in the terminal ileum. Thus, the stone, if visualized, need not necessarily be in the right lower quadrant (Fig. 12.58). Since approximately 85% of gallstones are radiolucent, the condition can exist without being able to see the stone on plain film. In practice, however, gallstone ileus usually follows chronic cholecystitis and involves large stones which frequently contain some calcium. Even so, they may be extremely difficult to find prospectively, especially if overlying the spine or dilated loops of bowel. Rigler included indirect visualization of the offending stone by intestinal contrast in his criteria (Fig. 12.59). The air or contrast in the biliary tract is often not in the ducts as might be expected by the "biliary tree" description. Usually the cystic duct will be chronically obstructed and the fistula will result only in gas in the badly distorted gallbladder which may be difficult to recognize. Also inflammation may seal off the fistula preventing entrance of intestinal air or contrast. Demonstration of a diverticulum-like structure or fistula adjacent to the first duodenal segment on contrast studies in the face of small bowel obstruction is highly reliable for the diagnosis of gallstone ileus (Fig. 12.60) (2). Rigler also included a fourth criterion: a change in the position of a calcification previ-

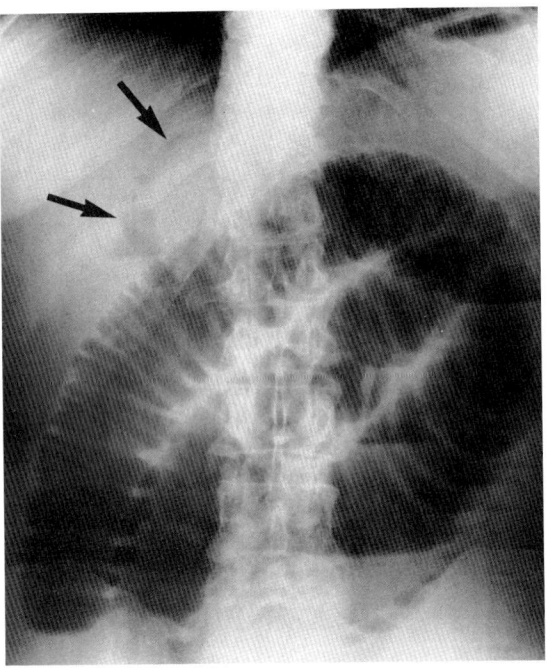

FIGURE 12.57. GALLSTONE ILEUS
Gallstone ileus: small bowel obstruction and air in the biliary tree (*arrows*).

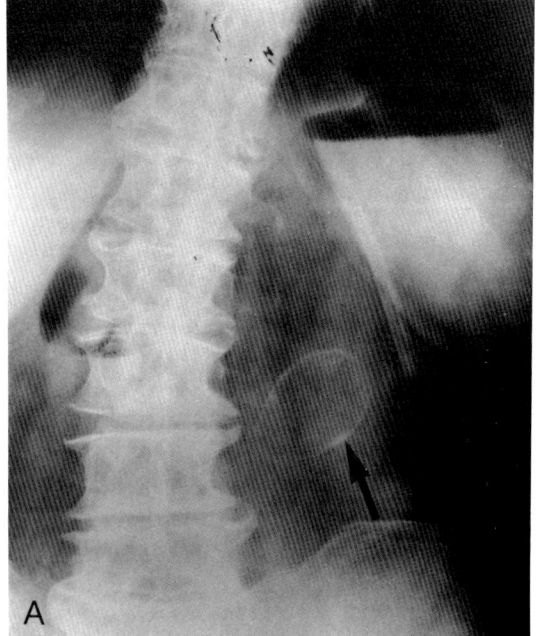
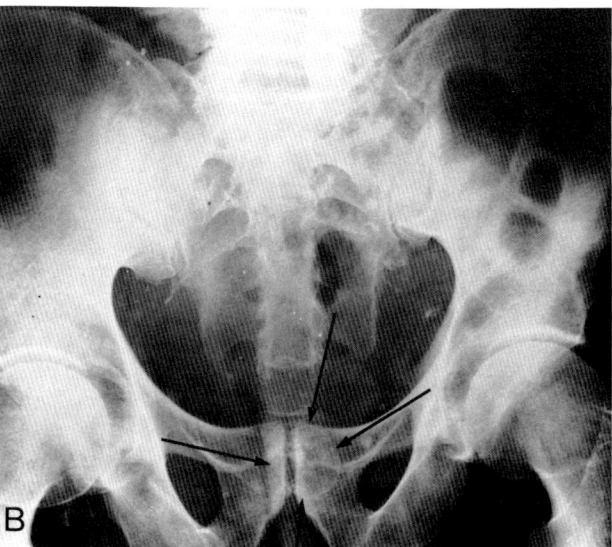

FIGURE 12.58. CALCIFIED ECTOPIC GALLSTONES
A: In jejunum (*arrow*) causing a high small bowel obstruction. *B:* In rectum (*arrow*). This stone passed uneventfully.

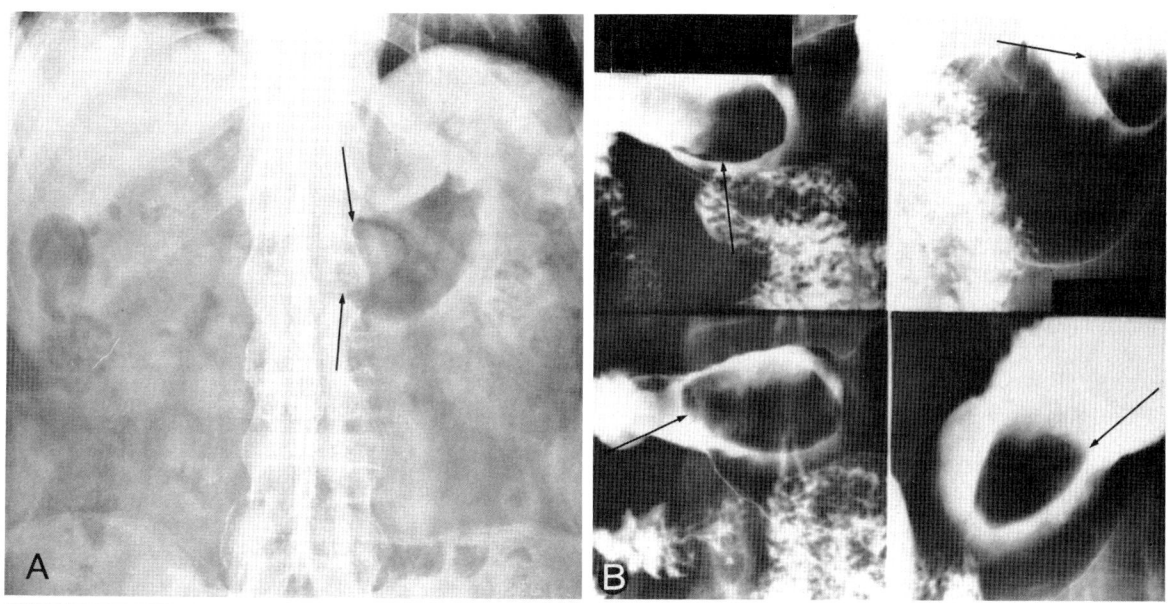

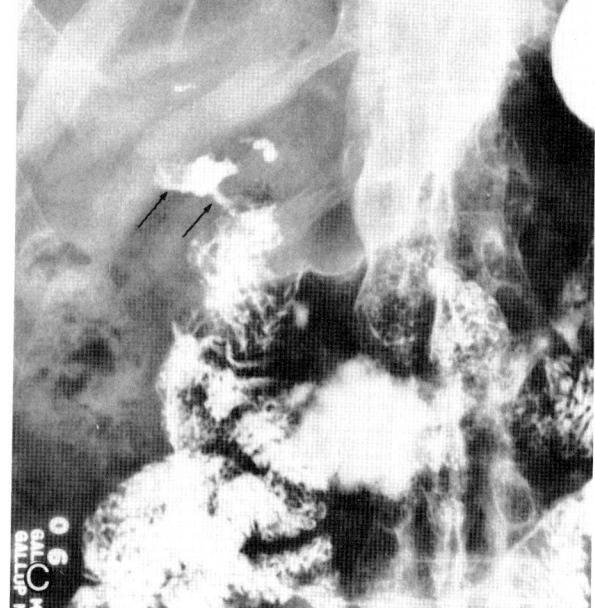

FIGURE 12.59. GALLSTONE BEZOAR
Gallstone bezoar in the stomach, which later passed through the pylorus and transiently obstructed the small bowel. (Case courtesy of Ernest Szechenyi, M.D., Gallup Indian Medical Center.) *A:* Scout film: stone outlined by gas in the stomach (*arrows*). *B:* UGI spot films: mobile intragastric gallstone (*arrows*). *C:* Fistulous tract to the gallbladder (*arrows*).

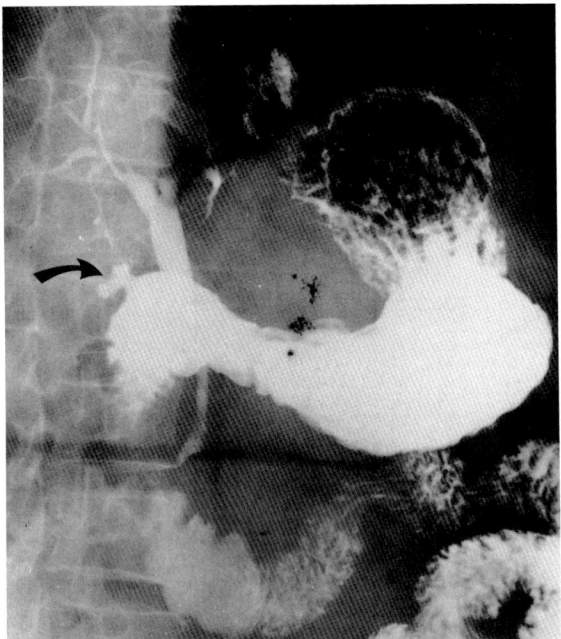

FIGURE 12.60. FILLING OF A DIVERTICULUM-LIKE COLLECTION IN GALLSTONE ILEUS
Filling of a diverticulum-like collection (*arrow*) off the duodenal bulb in addition to the biliary tree in a patient who passed a large gallstone per rectum prior to the study.

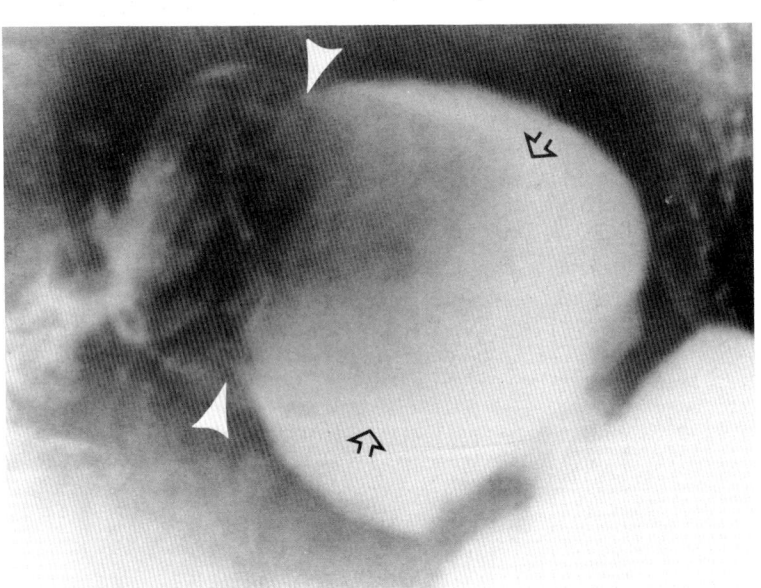

FIGURE 12.61. BOUVERET'S SYNDROME
Gallstone in the duodenal bulb (*arrows*) causing partial obstruction.

ously observed to reside in the gallbladder. An additional special case is the observation of a single large faceted stone in the gallbladder implying that a sister stone that accounted for the facets has moved elsewhere (1, 2).

Contrast Examinations

Oral and intravenous cholecystography are worthless, and barium meal is the procedure of choice in the vast majority of cases. In addition to filling the biliary tree with barium, findings include depiction of a well-contained, localized barium collection lateral to the first portion of the duodenum (Fig. 12.60). Although penetrating ulcer is hard to rule out, absence of duodenal deformity or spasticity mitigates against it (2). A follow-through into the small bowel shows dilatation and dilution, and, eventually, a large smooth intraluminal filling defect corresponding to the stone. A barium meal will also make the correct diagnosis in cases of erosion into the stomach or duodenum (Figs. 12.59 and 12.61).

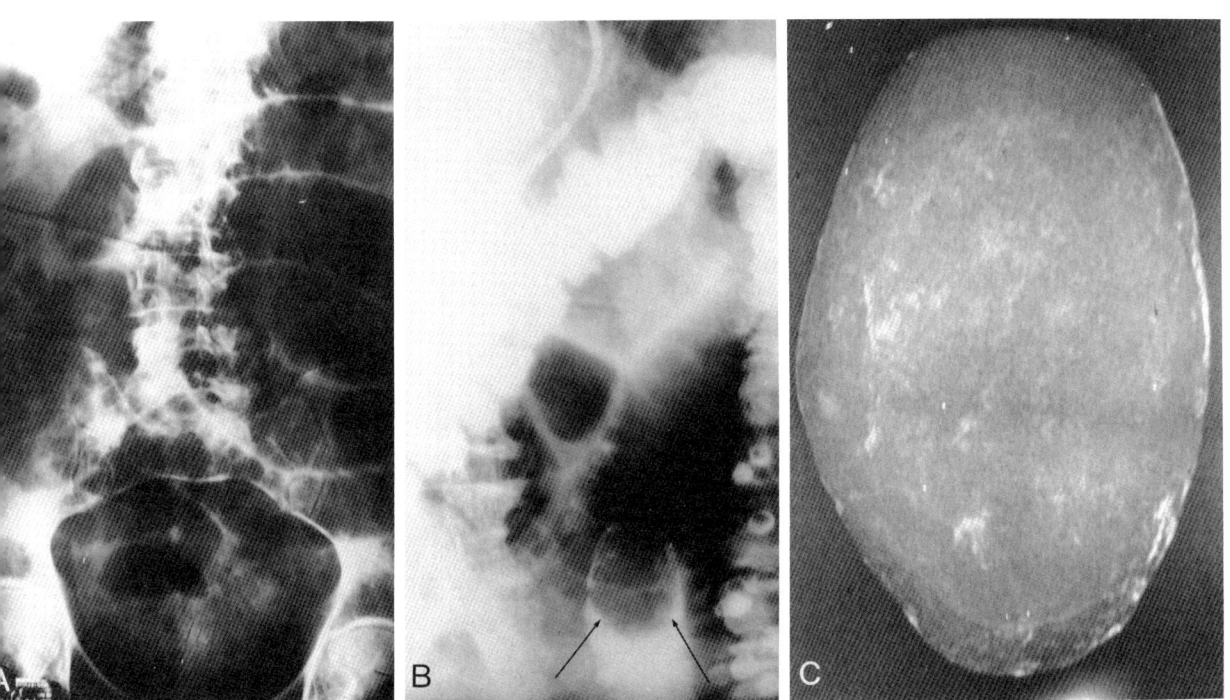

FIGURE 12.62. GALLSTONE ILEUS
A: Plain film shows small bowel obstruction only. *B:* Barium enema with reflux: gallstone obstructing the distal ileum (*arrows*). *C:* Specimen radiograph: poorly mineralized stone. Most gallstones that cause small bowel obstruction are at least partially calcified; they may still be invisible on plain films but might be obvious on CT.

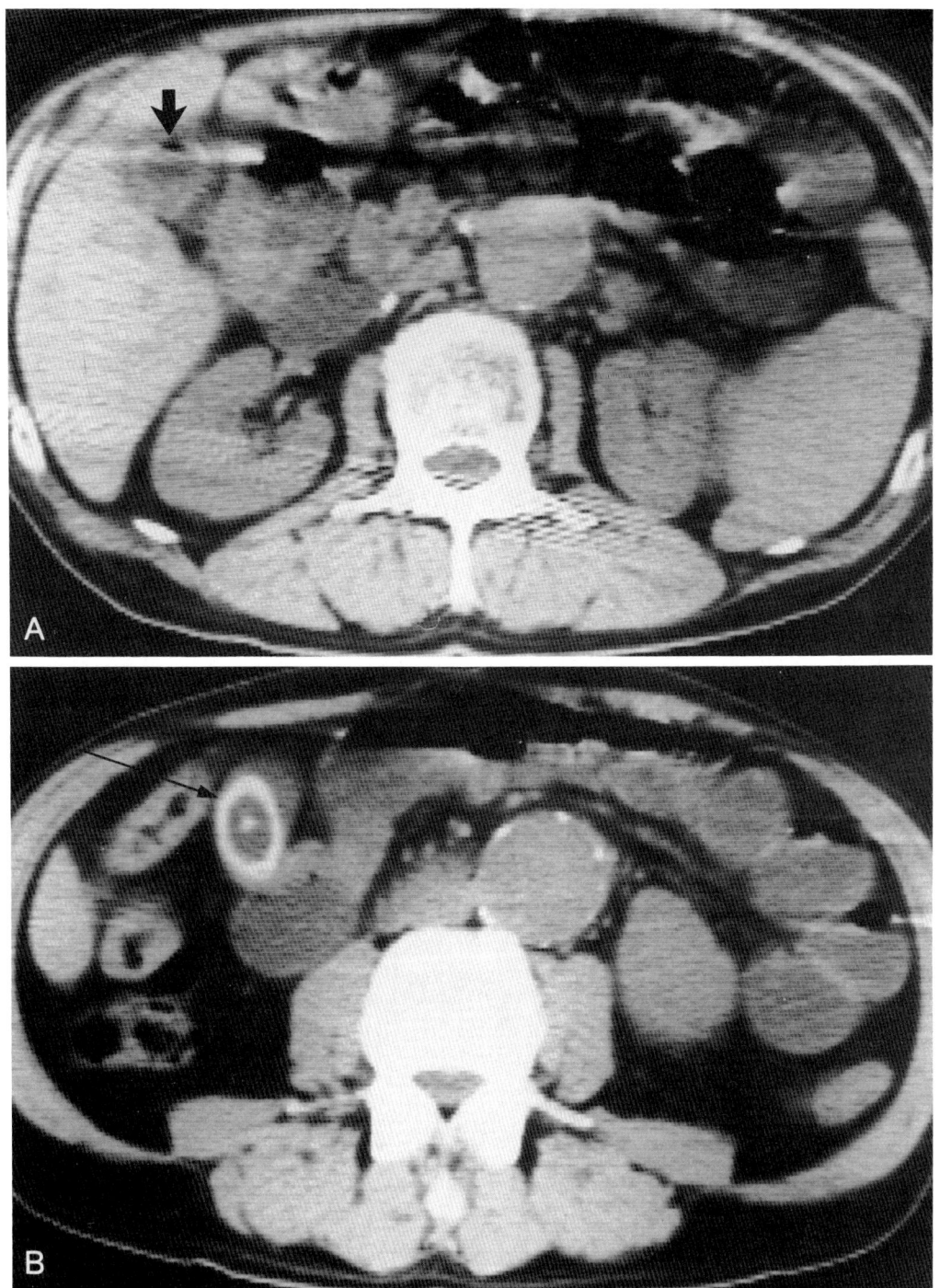

FIGURE 12.63. GALLSTONE ILEUS: CT
CT diagnosis of gallstone ileus. Plain film showed only small bowel obstruction. (Case courtesy of Marc S. Levine, M.D., and Kathryn Grumbach, M.D., Department of Radiology, Hospital of the University of Pennsylvania.) *A:* Small amount of air (*arrow*) in a thick-walled gallbladder. *B:* The obstructing gallstone (*arrow*) is shown within dilated small bowel.

When colonic obstruction is suggested clinically or by the plain film, a barium enema should be the initial procedure. When the gallstone is impacted in the sigmoid, it will be shown as an obturating filling defect generally among diverticula and luminal narrowing. Administration of glucagon may be helpful in relieving spasm. When the obstruction is in the ileum and is mimicking colonic obstruction, an aggressive reflux retrograde small bowel enema can demonstrate the obstructing gallstone (Fig. 12.62). Whether the study is a barium meal or enema, single contrast technique is the method of choice.

Computed Tomography

CT will rarely be done in this clinical situation nor should it be, although theoretically it can make the diagnosis of gallstone ileus, especially if the stone happens not to be obscured by oral contrast material (Fig. 12.63).

REFERENCES

1. Rigler LG, Bormen CN, Noble JF: Gallstone obstruction: pathogenesis and roentgen manifestations. *JAMA* 77:1753, 1941.
2. Galthazar EJ, Schecter LS: Gallstone ileus. The importance of contrast examination in roentgen diagnosis. *AJR* 125:374–379, 1975.

MIRIZZI SYNDROME

The Mirizzi syndrome is an uncommon complication of chronic cholecystitis (named after its discoverer, the Argentine surgeon who pioneered operative cholangiography) in which common hepatic duct obstruction is produced by a stone impacted in the cystic duct, gallbladder neck, or cystic duct remnant (1, 2). The obstruction is not simply a mechanical effect of the calculus; the surrounding chronic inflammatory reaction is contributory. Mirizzi syndrome is thought to occur more frequently in patients with an anomalous or low insertion of the cystic duct. This arrangement requires a rather long cystic duct sharing a common sheath with the common hepatic duct. Most cystic ducts insert into the lateral aspect of the common hepatic duct and a predisposing factor could be a more medial insertion or a spiral course about the common duct (2). Sequelae of unrecognized Mirizzi syndrome include: stricturing of the common duct secondary to inflammatory reaction in the gallbladder and hepatoduodenal ligament and cholecystobiliary fistula after erosion of the impacted stone into the common hepatic duct with a common cavity surrounded by an inflammatory mass (3). Jaundice, ascending cholangitis, or symptoms suggesting merely cholecystitis are the usual presenting features. Recurrent cholangitis and biliary cirrhosis can develop if the patient is untreated.

Correct preoperative diagnosis is vital. During retrograde dissection from the fundus to the neck to free the gallbladder for cholecystectomy, the surgeon normally ligates the first small caliber bile-containing duct he encounters, which is normally the cystic duct. In Mirizzi syndrome it will be the common bile duct, since this structure is relatively small from proximal obstruction and the cystic duct is not readily identified as such because of the gallstone and surrounding inflammation. The above scenario unfolds after an incorrect preoperative diagnosis of cholecystitis and/or choledocholithiasis. An incorrect preoperative diagnosis of carcinoma may be "confirmed" at surgery with the extensive inflammatory adhesions around the gallbladder and hepatoduodenal ligament mimicking an unresectable neoplasm. Inappropriate surgery may then ensue. Unidentified fistulas may leak postoperatively, and an impacted stone can be missed entirely during surgery (3).

Radiology

Noted on a plain film, a large single calcified stone located close to the porta hepatis in the appropriate clinical setting can suggest the diagnosis. Oral cholecystography is quite unlikely to be useful. Intravenous cholangiography has successfully made the diagnosis by showing a large stone immediately adjacent to and deviating the common hepatic duct, but this technique is rarely applied today.

Sonography or CT is now usually the initial imaging examination. Unfortunately, findings are not specific, and the diagnosis is difficult (Figs. 12.64, 12.65). The triad of a stone impacted in the gallbladder neck with dilatation of intrahepatic and common hepatic ducts and a normal common bile duct is quite suggestive if seen (4, 5). At times deviation of the common hepatic duct can be shown. An irregular cavity adjacent to the gallbladder with or without depiction of an extruded stone has been described by two authors (4, 6). Sonographic demonstration of two parallel tubular channels in the position of the common duct led to the successful diagnosis in one case of Mirizzi syndrome due to a stone in a cystic duct remnant (1). An inflammatory mass

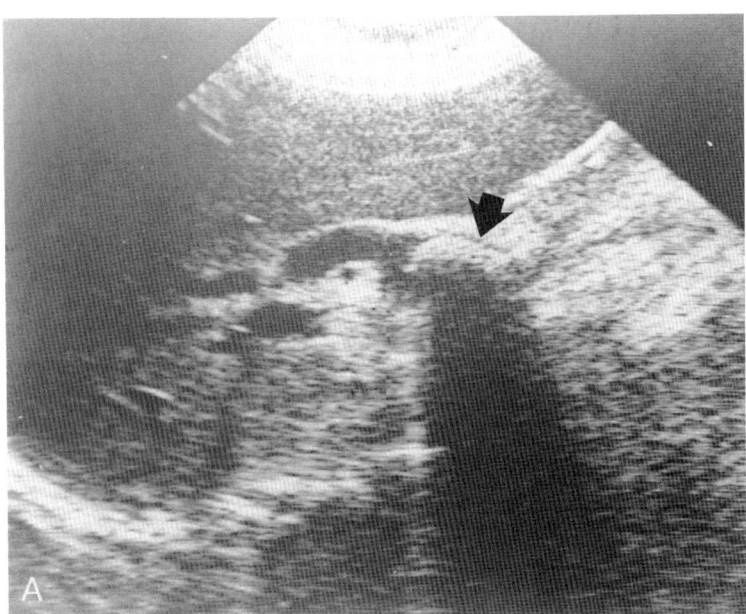
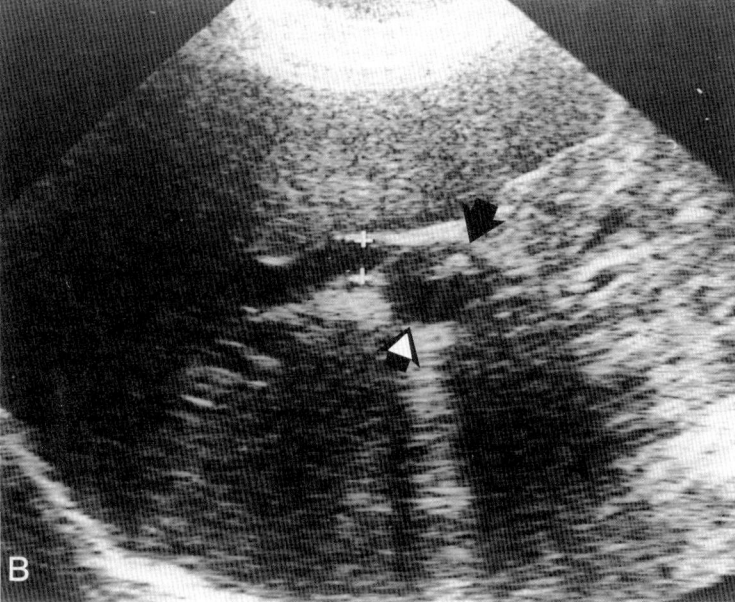

FIGURE 12.64. DIAGNOSIS OF MIRIZZI SYNDROME BY SONOGRAPHY

A: Parasagittal scan of the common duct: apparent intraductal large stone (*arrow*) causing proximal ductal dilatation. *B:* Slightly different angulation: the stone is the echogenic structure within the gallbladder neck (*arrows*). The common duct (*cursors*) measured about 1 cm.

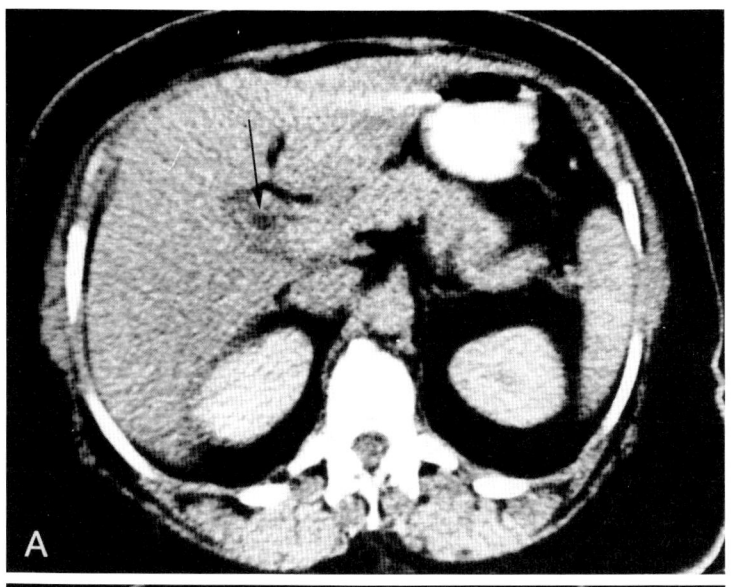
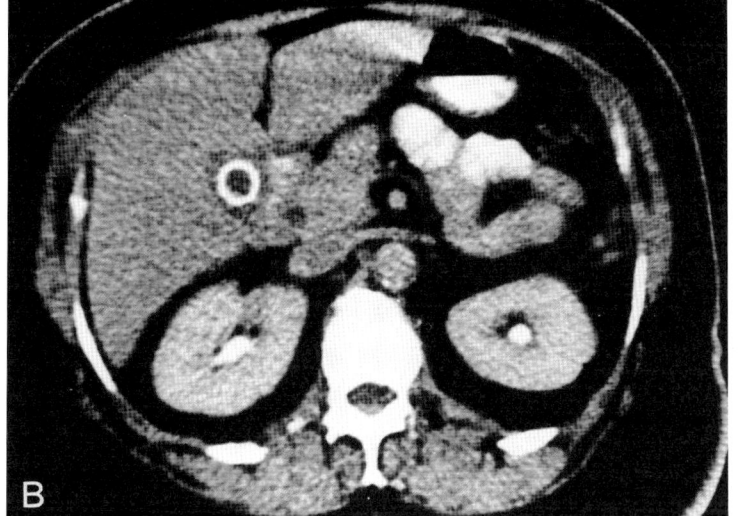
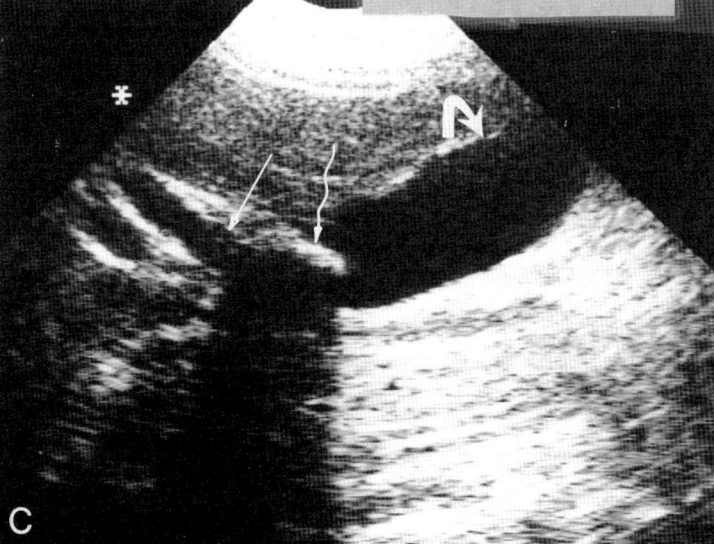

FIGURE 12.65. DIAGNOSIS OF MIRIZZI SYNDROME BY CT
A and *B:* Dilated common hepatic duct (*arrow, A*) just cephalad to a large stone in the neck of the gallbladder (*B*). *C:* Corresponding parasagittal sonogram: shadowing stone (*undulating arrow*) in the neck of the gallbladder (*curved arrow*) obstructing the common hepatic duct (*arrow*).

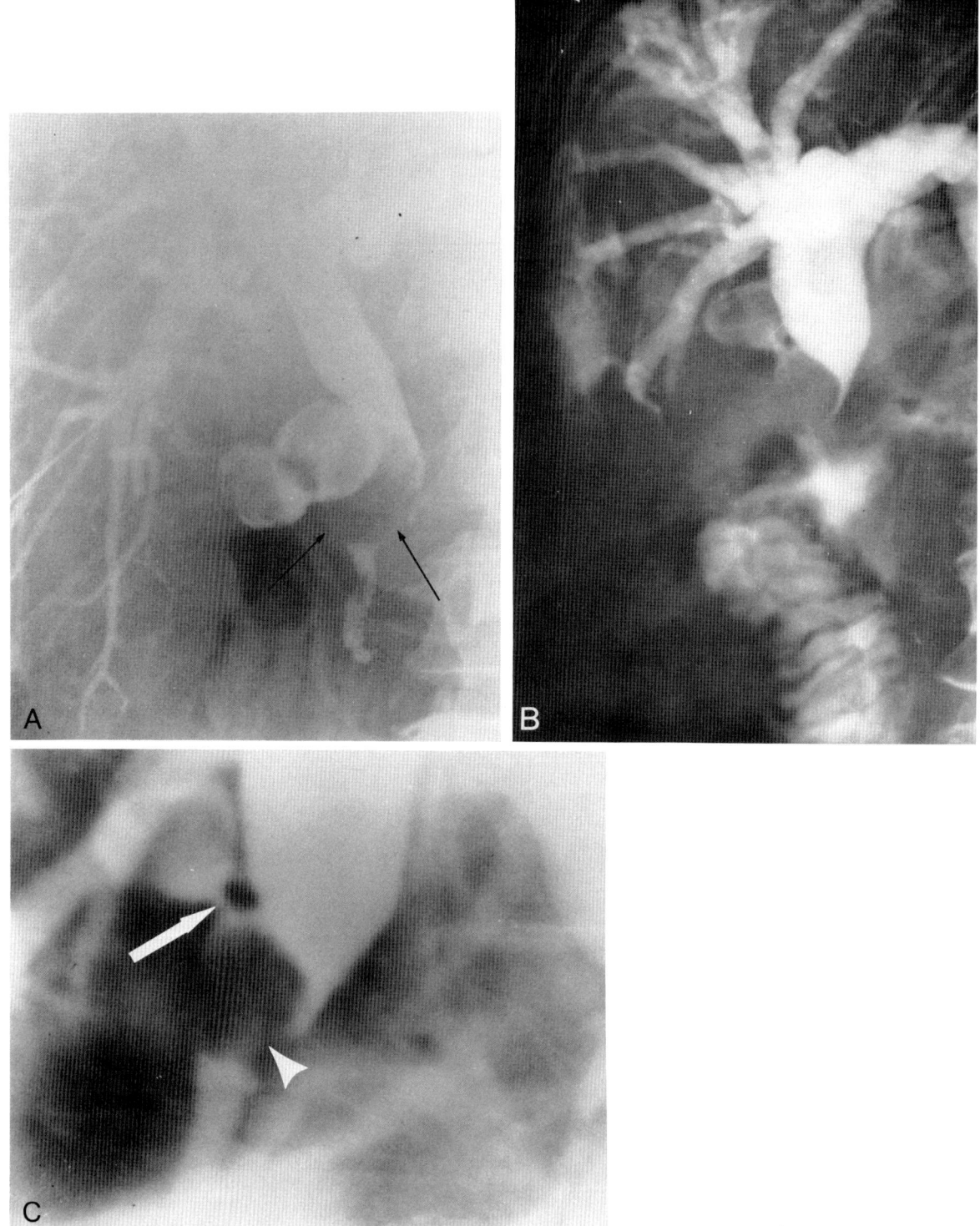

FIGURE 12.66. DIAGNOSIS OF MIRIZZI SYNDROME BY PTC

A: Large gallstone (*arrows*) deviating and obstructing the common hepatic duct. Two additional gallstones are outlined. *B* and *C:* A different case with similar findings of common hepatic duct deviation and obstruction by a gallstone (*arrowhead*). In this case, the fistulous tract whereby the remainder of the gallbladder is filled is demonstrated (*arrow*).

can dominate the sonographic or CT picture to the extent that carcinoma of the gallbladder, cholangiocarcinoma, or even pancreatic carcinoma is suggested.

If the correct diagnosis is suspected confirmation can be obtained by direct cholangiography by either the retrograde or percutaneous route (7, 8). Even if malignancy is thought to be present on the basis of sonography or CT, a cholangiogram is frequently obtained for a preoperative road map or as part of a biliary drainage procedure and presents a second opportunity to make the correct preoperative diagnosis. The primary finding is a smooth, curved segmental stenosis of or lateral extrinsic impression upon the common hepatic duct in the region of the expected insertion of the cystic duct. Unfortunately, a differential diagnosis of periportal adenopathy, enlarged gallbladder from carcinoma or chronic cholecystitis, hepatic or pancreatic neoplasm, and pseudocyst must be entertained if the stone is not calcified and the above is all that is demonstrated. As a result of a high index of suspicion, patience, and delayed filming, any offending stones may be outlined at the point of obstruction via either a cholecystobiliary fistula or the incompletely obstructed cystic duct, clinching the diagnosis (Fig. 12.66A–E). Additionally, cholangiography is useful to delineate the extent and severity of any stricture of the common hepatic duct. If an angiogram is done because of a suspicion of malignancy, a curved lateral impression upon the hepatic artery may be seen, which is not surprising since it is adjacent to the common hepatic duct.

REFERENCES

1. Clemett AR, Lowman RM: The roentgen features of the Mirizzi syndrome. *AJR* 94:480–483, 1965.
2. Koehler RE, Melson GL, Lee JK, Long J: Common hepatic duct obstruction by cystic duct stone: Mirizzi syndrome. *AJR* 132:1007–1009, 1979.
3. Htoo MM: Surgical implications of stone impaction in the gallbladder neck with compression of the common hepatic duct (Mirizzi's syndrome). *Clin Radiol* 34:651–655, 1983.
4. Becker CD, Hassler H, Terrier F: Preoperative diagnosis of the Mirizzi syndrome: limitations of sonography and computed tomography. *AJR* 143:591–596, 1984.
5. Jackson VP, Lappas JC: Sonography of the Mirizzi syndrome. *J Ultrasound Med* 3:281–283, 1984.
6. Pedrosa CS, Casanova R, De La Torre S, et al: CT findings in Mirizzi syndrome. *J Comput Assist Tomogr* 7:419, 1983.
7. Cruz FO, Barriga P, Tocornal J, Burhenne HJ: Radiology of the Mirizzi syndrome: diagnostic importance of the transhepatic cholangiogram. *Gastrointest Radiol* 8:249–253, 1983.
8. Cornud F, Grenier P, Belghiti J, Breil P, Nahum H: Mirizzi syndrome and biliobiliary fistulas: roentgenologic appearance. *Gastrointest Radiol* 6:265–268, 1981.

13
Hyperplastic Cholecystoses and Benign and Malignant Gallbladder Tumors

JOEL E. LICHTENSTEIN, M.D., LEORA SACHS, M.D.,
ARNOLD C. FRIEDMAN, M.D., AND JAMES G. SMIRNIOTOPOULOS, M.D.

THE HYPERPLASTIC CHOLECYSTOSES

Jutras, in 1960, proposed the concept of the hyperplastic cholecystoses to encompass a diverse group of benign, nonneoplastic, proliferative and degenerative gallbladder conditions (1). He believed these to occur in overlapping combinations and to be unified by proliferation of autonomous neural elements or "neuromatosis." Proliferation of the epithelial surface producing greater absorptive area was said to increase contrast density. Muscular dysplasia supposedly increased strength and completeness of gallbladder emptying, referred to as "hyperexcretion." The neuromatosis was invoked to explain unusually rapid onset and speed of contraction or "hyperexcitability." The combination constituted a triad of hyperconcentration, hyperexcitability, and hyperevacuation on fat-stimulated oral cholecystography (OCG), and was thought to be the origin of a variety of biliary dyskinetic symptoms.

Jutras work was a masterpiece of pathological correlation and little can be added to his descriptions of the morphology of cholesterolosis and adenomyomatosis, the two major clinical entities (1, 2). Neuromatosis, requiring vital stains of nonautolysed tissue, however, has not been reproduceably demonstrated, nor have contraction rates and clinical symptoms been reliably correlated with pathology or distinguished from normal. Thus, it is now felt that Jutras classification was unnecessarily complex (3, 4). While details of the etiologies are in doubt and there is debate over clinical significance, cholesterolosis and adenomyomatosis are apparently unrelated to each other pathologically and are distinctive entities without any malignant potential.

The female to male ratio of the hyperplastic cholecystoses is 4–8:1. The actual incidence of these diseases in cholecystectomy specimens is 30–50%, but only 5–10% of oral cholecystograms at most demonstrate any evidence of either cholecystosis (5).

Pathology and Oral Cholecystography

In adenomyomatosis the gallbladder wall is markedly thickened by a hyperplasia of both the epithelial and muscular elements. The gallbladder, in contrast to the rest of the gastrointestinal tract, has no muscularis mucosae separating mucosa from submucosa. The expanding columnar epithelium becomes redundant and appears to grow into, or become enmeshed in, the basket-weave-like structure of the proliferating muscle. This results in the formation of invaginated, epithelial-lined, cystic spaces resembling glands or intramural diverticula (3, 4). These are the Rokitansky-Aschoff sinuses (Fig. 13.1). Increased luminal pressure causing mucosal herniation through points of least resistance is sometimes postulated, but it is doubtful that pressure effects are significant, at least in the early stages (6). The sinuses may protrude through the wall to appear beneath the serosa, but more often they are completely enveloped in the muscle wall which may be up to five or more times normal thickness. If they fill on OCG, the sinuses appear as tiny extraluminal extensions of contrast. Because they often fill with sludge and debris, fat-, or CCK-stimulated contraction may facilitate their demonstration (Figs. 13.2 and 13.3) (7).

Adenomyomatosis may be generalized involving the entire gallbladder. More often, the process is segmental, the thickened region imparting a narrowed, "hourglass" configuration. The segmental, or annular, form is sometimes associated with a relatively thick septum (Fig. 13.4). A

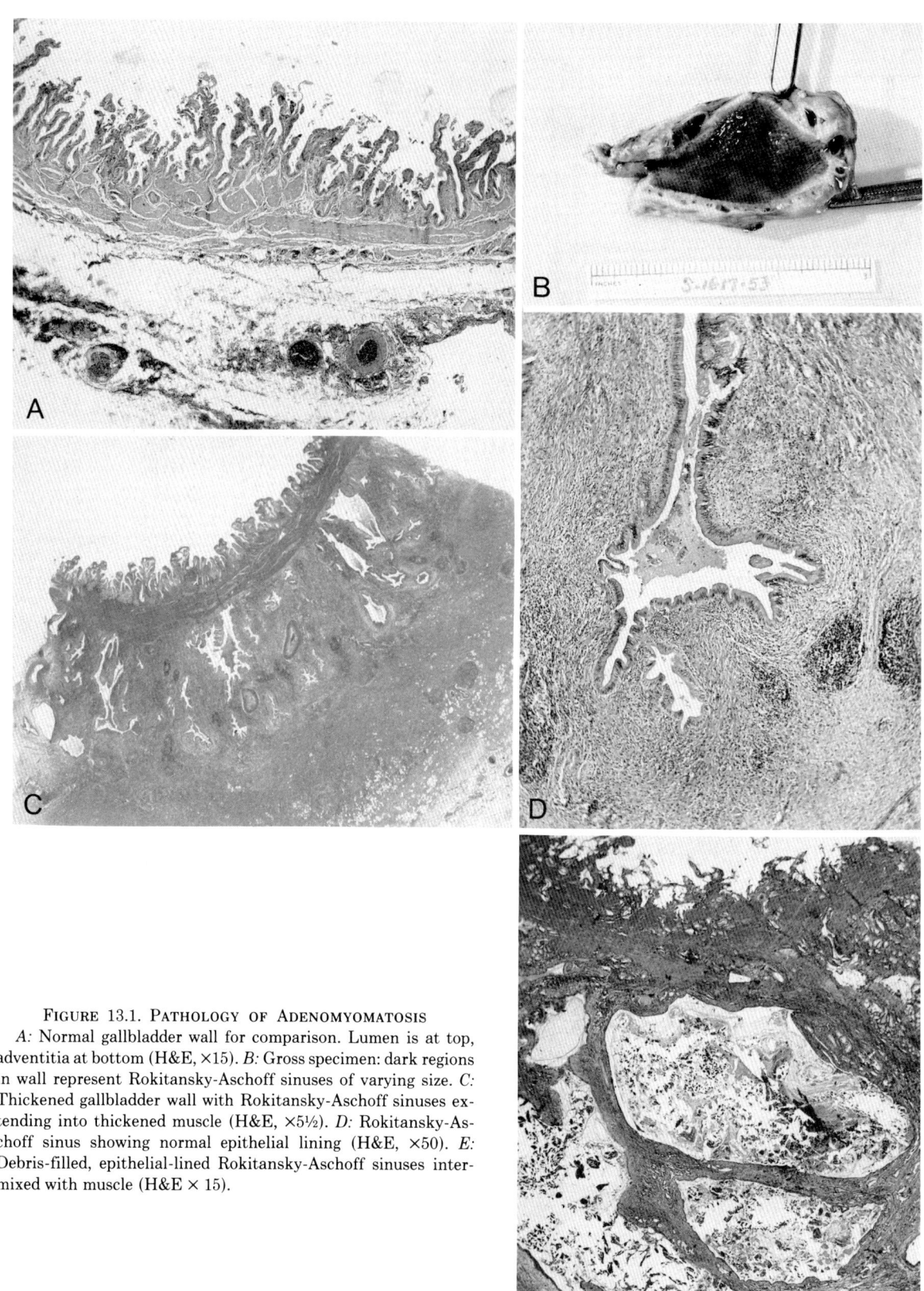

FIGURE 13.1. PATHOLOGY OF ADENOMYOMATOSIS
A: Normal gallbladder wall for comparison. Lumen is at top, adventitia at bottom (H&E, ×15). *B:* Gross specimen: dark regions in wall represent Rokitansky-Aschoff sinuses of varying size. *C:* Thickened gallbladder wall with Rokitansky-Aschoff sinuses extending into thickened muscle (H&E, ×5½). *D:* Rokitansky-Aschoff sinus showing normal epithelial lining (H&E, ×50). *E:* Debris-filled, epithelial-lined Rokitansky-Aschoff sinuses intermixed with muscle (H&E × 15).

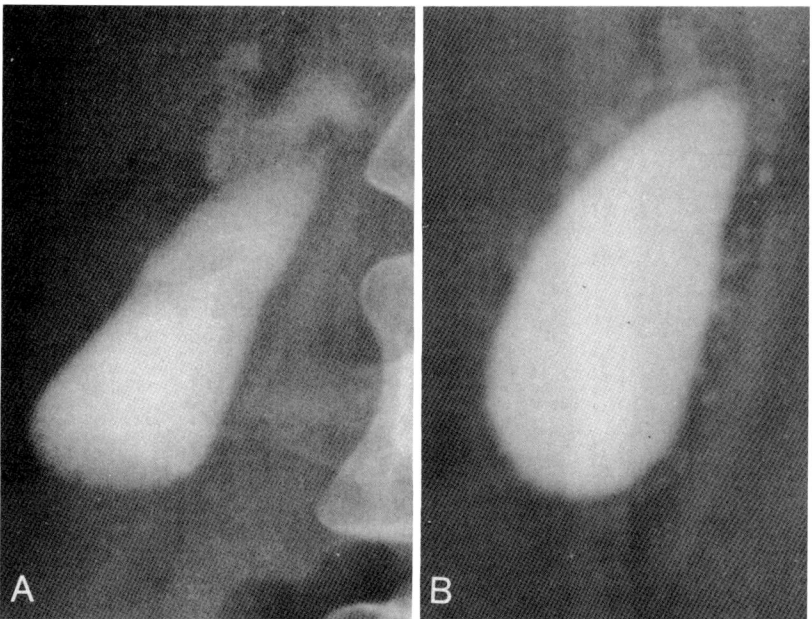

FIGURE 13.2. DIFFUSE ADENOMYOMATOSIS
A and *B:* Diffuse adenomyomatosis before (*A*) and after (*B*) a fatty meal. The prefat film is unremarkable.

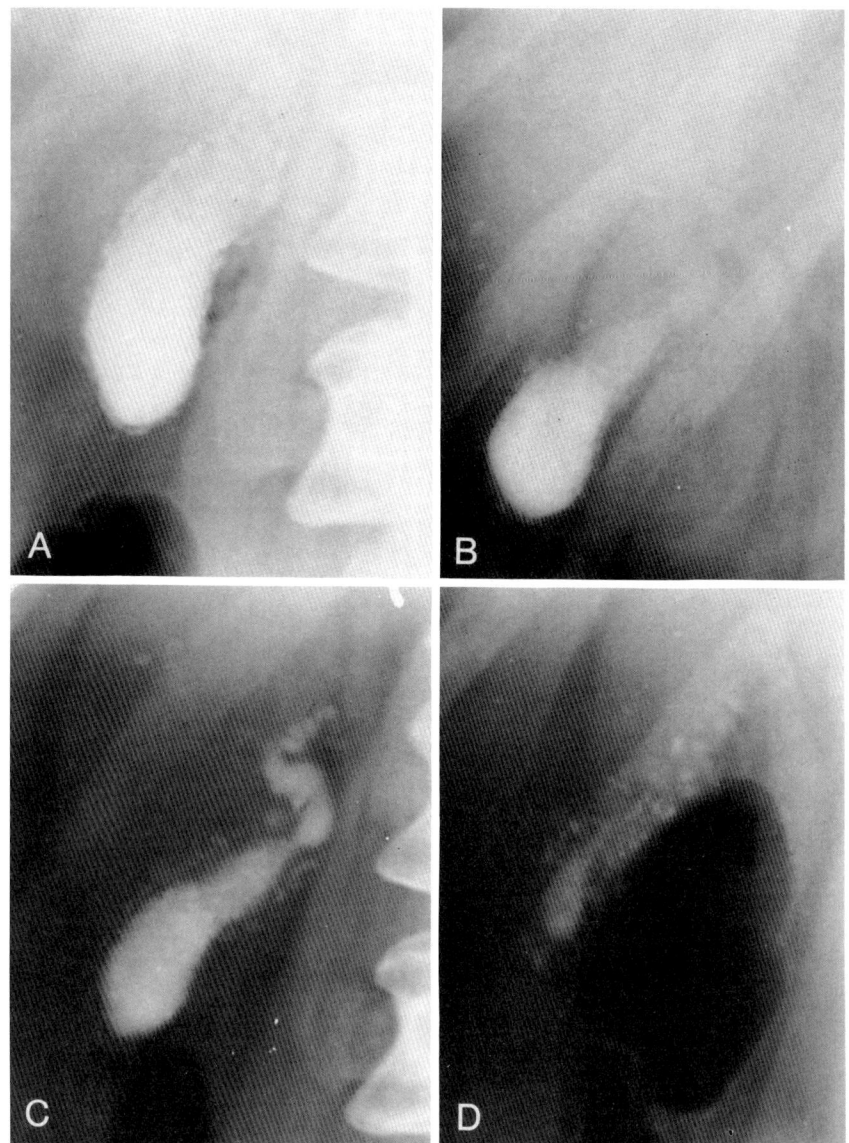

FIGURE 13.3. DIFFUSE ADENOMYOMATOSIS

A–D: Diffuse adenomyomatosis with progressive contraction after a fatty meal. (Case courtesy of Albert Jutras, M.D., who contributed it to the AFIP.)

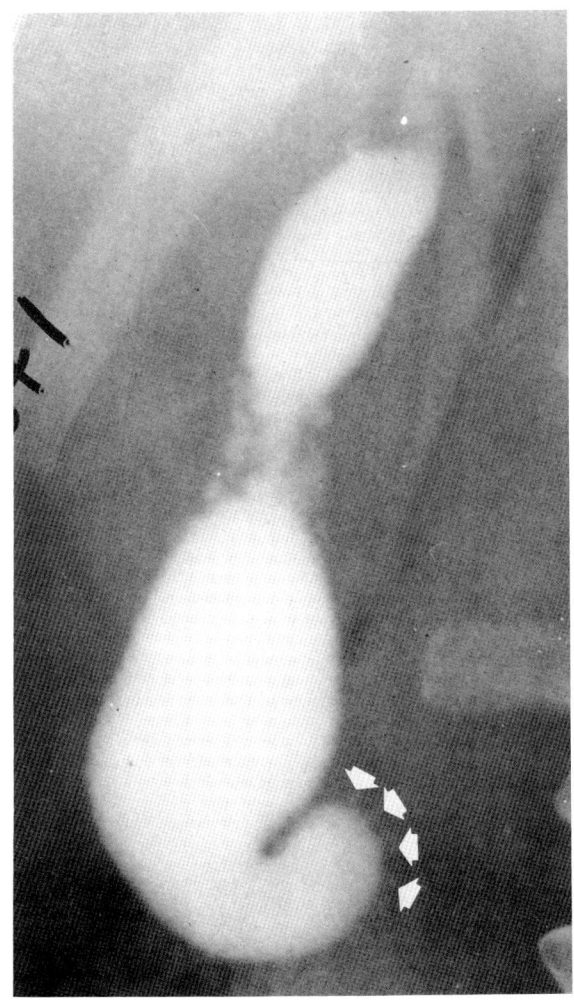

FIGURE 13.4. SEGMENTAL ADENOMYOMATOSIS
Narrowing in the mid-gallbladder with Rokitansky-Aschoff sinus filling there and at the fundus (*arrows*, difficult to appreciate).

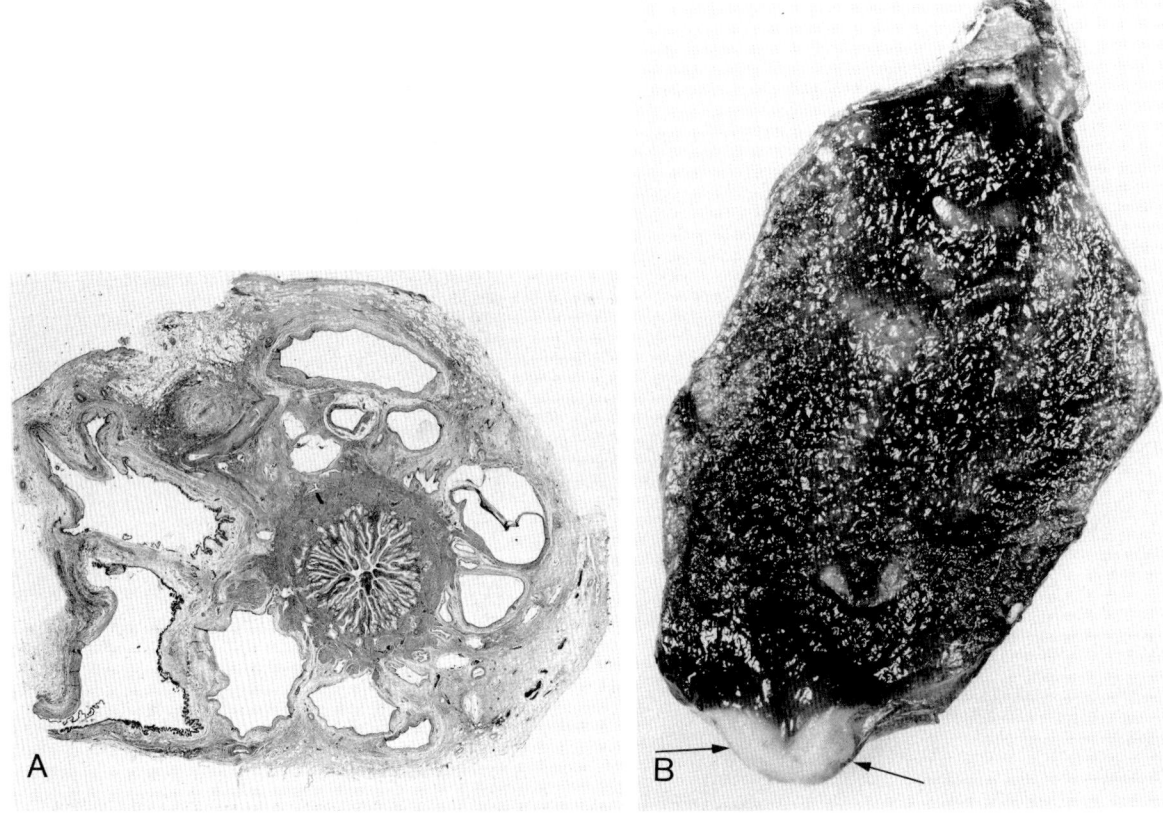

FIGURE 13.5. LOCALIZED FUNDAL ADENOMYOMATOSIS
A: Histology: fundal adenomyoma surrounded by intramural Rokitansky-Aschoff sinuses. *B:* Gross specimen of a fundal adenomyoma (*arrows*).

causal relationship to a transverse congenital septum (sometimes called a "Phrygian cap," although the term originally referred to a simple folding of the fundus suggesting a septum radiographically) has been suggested, but remains doubtful (7, 8). The most common form is a localized lesion in the fundus which has been reported in up to five percent of gallbladders by those with a special interest in the subject (9). Adenomyoma is a separate term commonly applied to the fundal lesion although the histology is essentially the same as that seen in other forms of adenomyomatosis (Fig. 13.5A). Grossly it is a 1–2 cm diameter thickening usually appearing as a smooth sessile filling defect in the fundus of a relaxed, moderately distended gallbladder (Fig. 13.5B). The Rokitansky-Aschoff sinuses are situated in a ring communicating with the lumen through a central umbilicated depression. The radiographic appearance is highly variable depending upon whether the central depression and/or the sinuses fill and whether the lesion is protruding into the lumen or is evaginated as tends to occur with stimulated contraction (Figs. 13.6–13.8).

In cholesterolosis the subepithelial tissue of the gallbladder becomes filled with foamy, cholesterol-laden cells (Fig. 13.9) (10). The etiology and the alleged hyperplastic nature of this process also remain in doubt (11, 12). No relationship to serum or bile cholesterol nor to cholesterol gallstones has been demonstrated. Excess hepatic production of cholesterol precursors, increased absorption of bile cholesterol by the gallbladder mucosa, or impaired transport of cholesterol out of the mucosa have been postulated as etiologies.

Two morphologic forms of cholesterolosis are seen. In the planar form cholesterol-filled cells cause a patchy or diffuse thickening of the usually fine, villous surface pattern of the gallbladder lining. The resulting yellowish excrescences resemble tiny seeds and, when seen against the reddish background of an incidentally inflamed surface, are the source of the term "strawberry gallbladder" (Fig. 13.10A). The size of the ex-

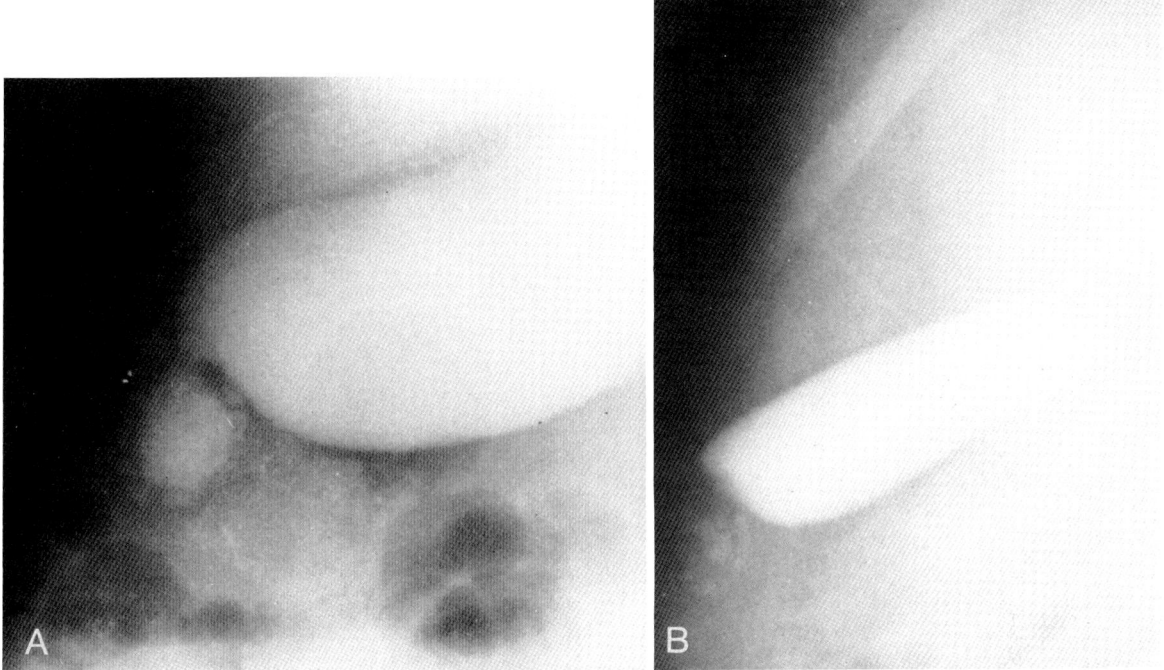

FIGURE 13.6. FUNDAL ADENOMYOMA IN PROFILE

A and B: Waist-like narrowing with distal Rokitansky-Aschoff sinuses involving the fundus before (A) and after (B) a fatty meal.

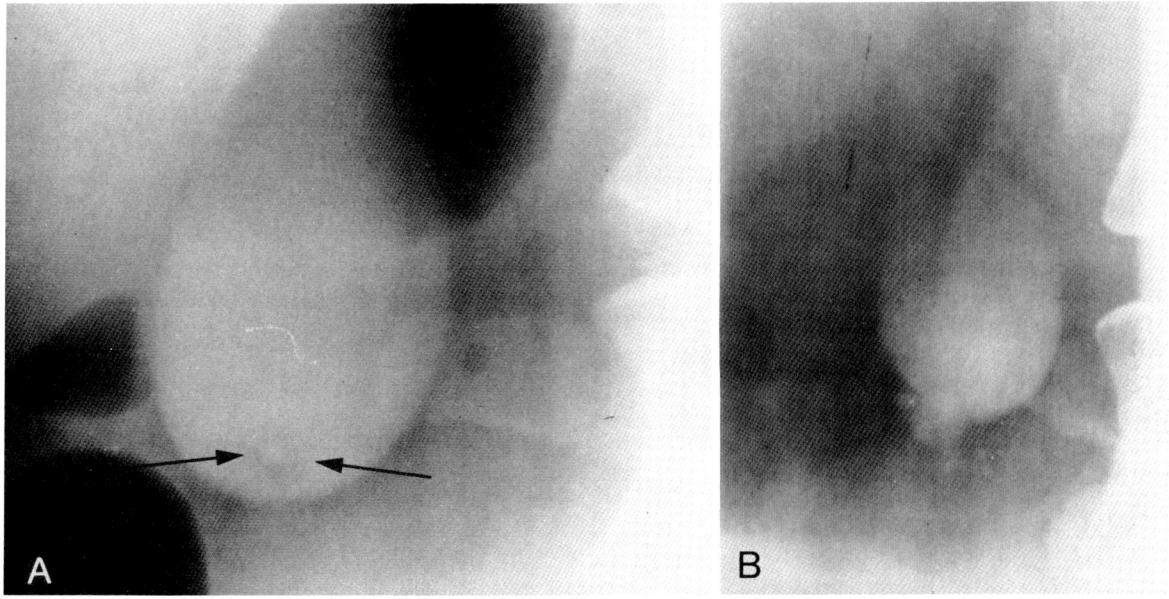

FIGURE 13.7. FUNDAL ADENOMYOMA EN FACE

A and B: Round lucency (*arrows*) with a central dot of contrast (A). More prominent filling of Rokitansky-Aschoff sinuses after a fatty meal (B).

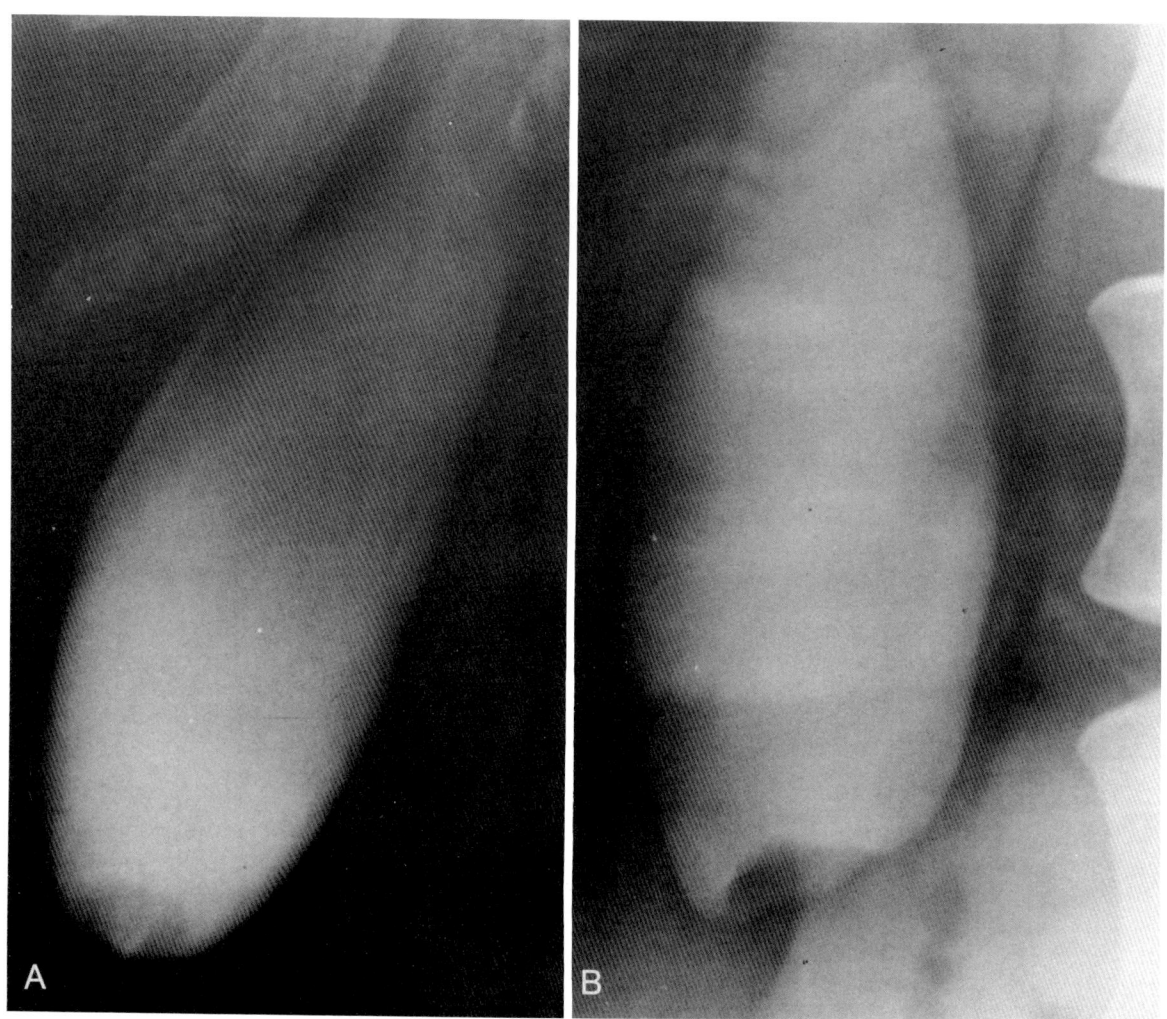

FIGURE 13.8. INVAGINATED FUNDAL ADENOMYOMAS IN PROFILE
A and *B:* Profile invaginated fundal adenomyomas with (*A*) and without (*B*) sinus filling.

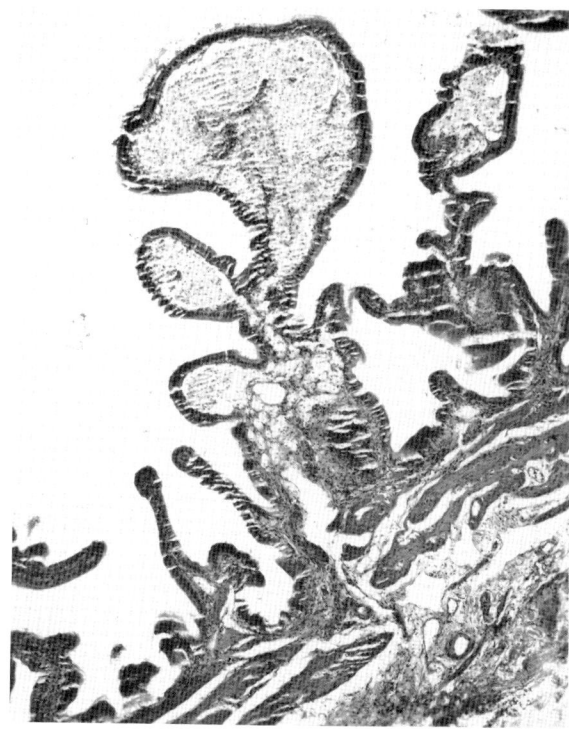

FIGURE 13.9. CHOLESTEROLOSIS
Cholesterolosis: subepithelial, foamy lipid-laden cells (H&E, ×60).

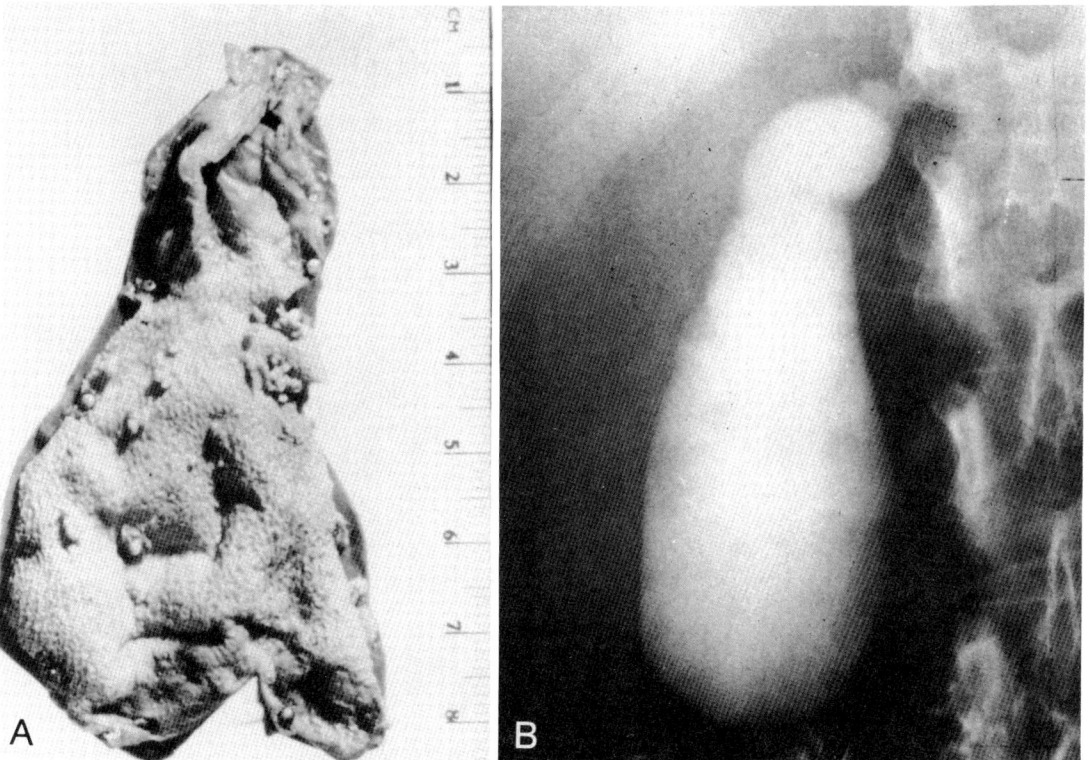

FIGURE 13.10. CHOLESTEROLOSIS
A: Gross specimen of cholesterolosis shows multiple cholesterol polyps against a strawberry mucosal pattern background.
B: The corresponding oral cholecystogram depicts multiple, slightly irregular, difficult to discern nonmobile filling defects. (Case for 13.10A contributed by Albert Jutras, M.D., who contributed it to the AFIP.)

panded villi is barely at the limit of resolution of ordinary oral cholecystography and thus produces little radiographic effect. Occasionally the exaggerated mucosal texture and increased absorption and may produce an unusually well visualized gallbladder with a slightly fuzzy margin permitting a prospective suggestion of the entity especially when associated with multiple cholesterol polyps (Fig. 13.10B). As with adenomyomatosis, the postulated hyperexcitability has been difficult to quantitate for use as a radiographic sign.

The second, or polypoid, form of cholesterolosis is essentially a very localized manifestation of the planar condition. The excrescences become larger but rarely over one centimeter in diameter. Thin, fragile stalks composed only of the cholesterol filled cells covered by single layers of epithelium are sometimes formed. These small polyps may be either solitary or multiple and are, by far, the most common fixed filling defects seen in the gallbladder (Fig. 13.11). It has been suggested that the polyps might break off to form the nidus for gallstones, but this has never been established and no association with stones has been demonstrated.

Clinical Findings

The clinical significance of the hyperplastic cholecystoses remains controversial. The associated neuronal hyperplasia described by Jutras is alleged to cause symptoms based upon increased speed and vigor of contraction. These effects are difficult to quantitate, however. Inflammatory cells are sometimes found in the wall in adenomyomatosis, but are also seen in normal gallbladders. Inflammation may play some role in initiating the hyperplasia, but no consistent association has been shown. The condition is often seen in the presence of stones but, again, no etiologic association has been shown. Some patients appear to suffer biliary colic and are helped by cholecystectomy but any cholelithiasis or cholecystitis present is usually coincidental (Fig. 13.12). Other patients will still have pain after surgery. Management depends to some extent on whether the patient is in the hands of an internist or a surgeon.

Diagnosis of hyperplastic cholecystosis is probably more accurate by oral cholecystography than sonography, but no large comparative series exist.

Sonography

Cholesterolosis

The planar form of cholesterolosis is not readily depicted sonographically. Sometimes a nonspecific wall thickening can be seen. Focal cholesterol polyps are well detected with careful technique as small, echogenic masses that adhere to the wall (Fig. 13.13). Usually nonshadowing, on occasion they exhibit weak shadowing that is less prominent than that seen with a stone of similar size (13). Cholesterol polyps are single or multiple, variable in size but usually small, stationary, and located anywhere in the gallbladder. Gallstones move freely about the gallbladder with changes in patient positioning or merely pumping the gallbladder with the transducer. Most nonshadowing, nonmobile small masses in the gallbladder will be cholesterol polyps, some will be adenomas, and the remainder will be less common entities such as papillomas, carcinoids, or metastases (5).

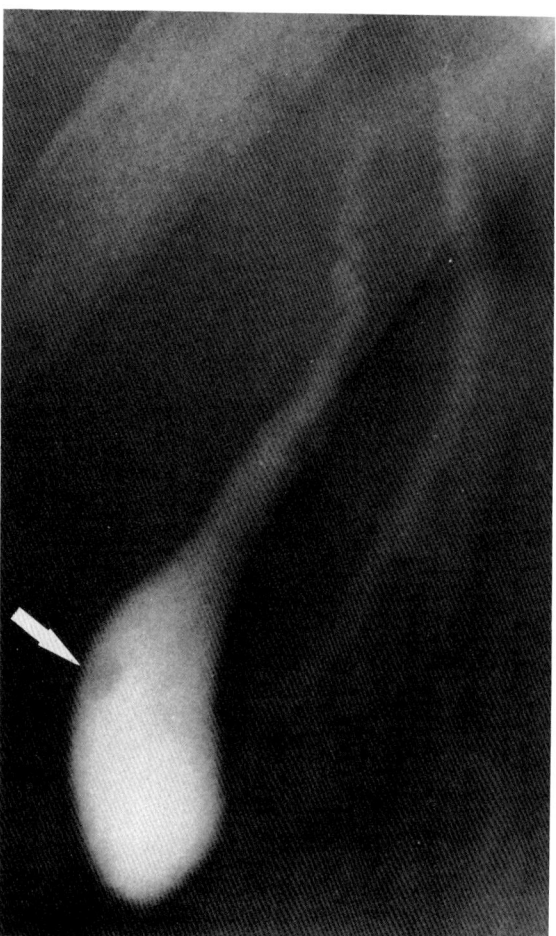

FIGURE 13.11. CHOLESTEROL POLYP
Cholesterol polyp (*arrow*). It was immobile with positional maneuvers.

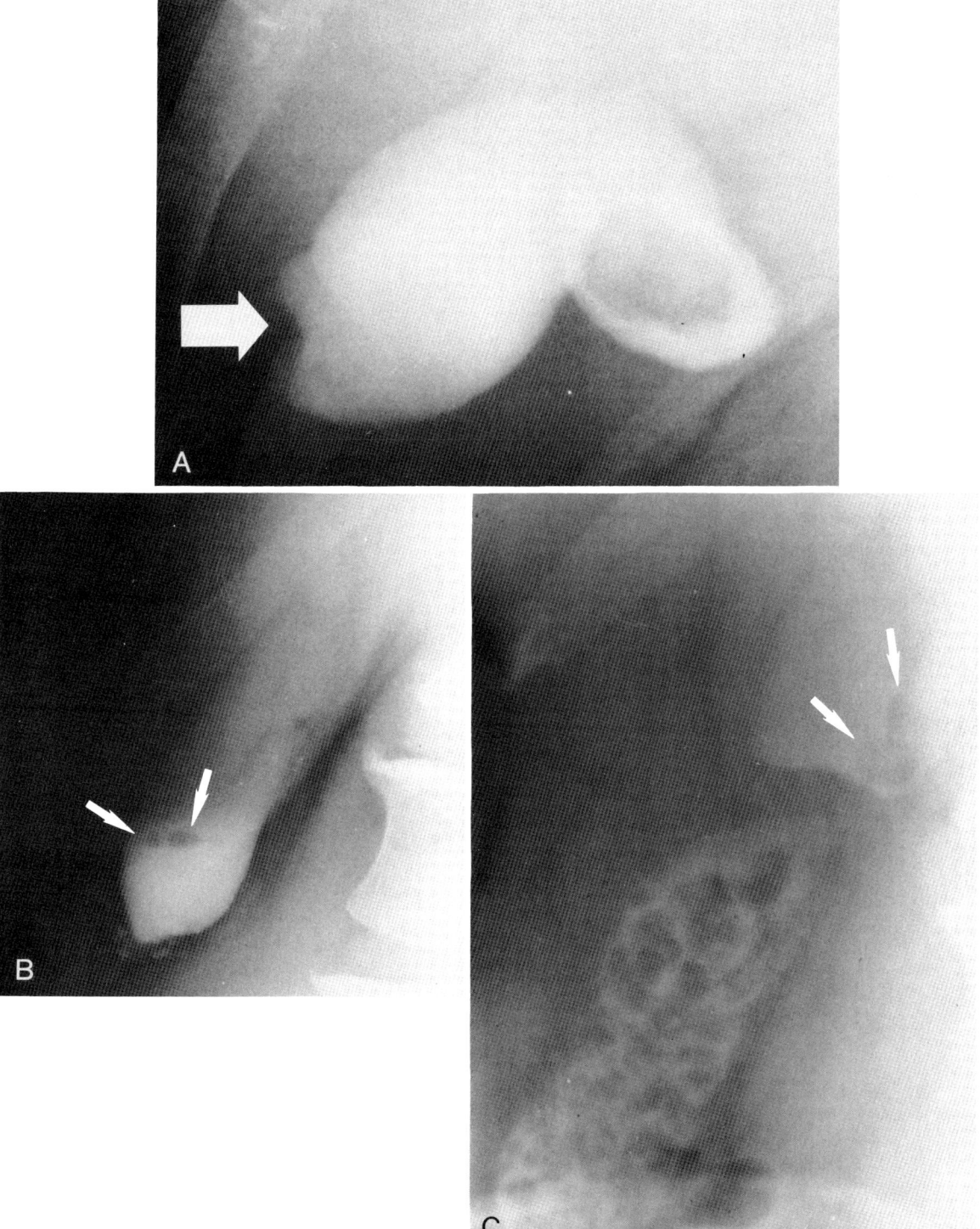

FIGURE 13.12. COEXISTING ADENOMYOMATOSIS AND GALLSTONES

A: Invaginated fundal adenomyoma (*arrow*) and large gallstone in the gallbladder neck. *B:* Floating calculi (*arrows*) and fundal adenomyoma. *C:* Thick septum dividing the gallbladder into two compartments. Two calculi in upper compartment (*arrows*). The lower compartment is packed with stones. Its outline is ragged, due to barely visible opacified Rokitansky-Aschoff sinuses. (Case for 13.12*B* courtesy of Albert Jutras, M.D., who contributed it to the AFIP.)

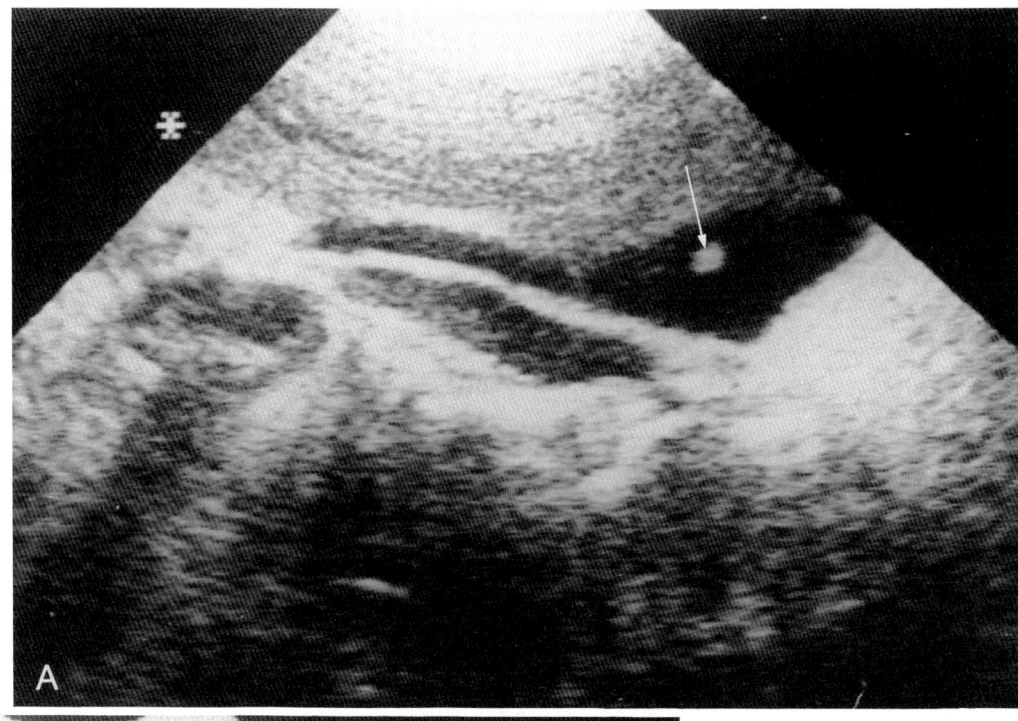

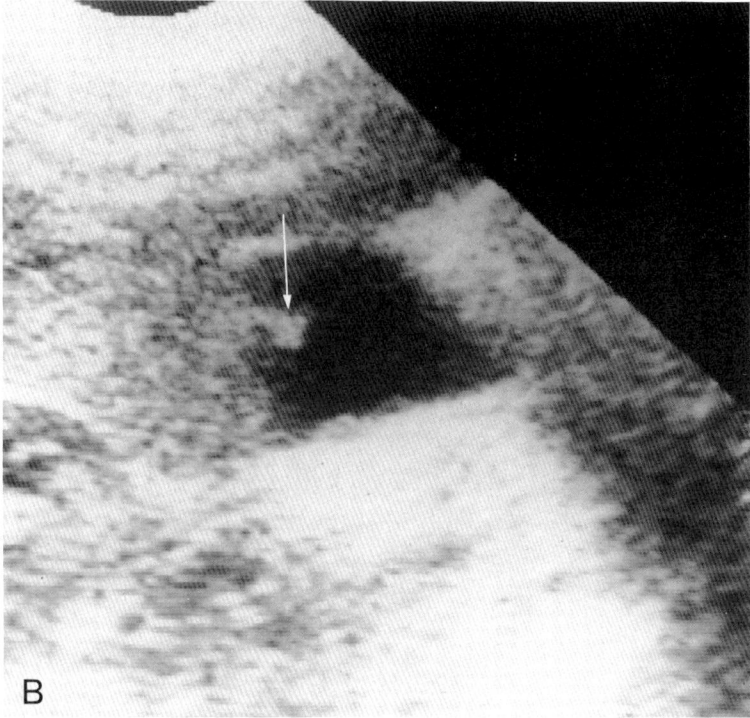

FIGURE 13.13. CHOLESTEROL POLYP
A and *B:* Sagittal (*A*) and transverse (*B*) sonograms of a cholesterol polyp (*arrows*) showing its wall attachment in (*B*).

Adenomyomatosis

Diffuse adenomyomatosis is depicted as diffuse wall thickening with or without Rokitansky-Aschoff sinuses (3). Since the former is so nonspecific, it is necessary to demonstrate the latter to make a diagnosis (Figs. 13.14 and 13.15). These intramural diverticula are anechoic, fluid-filled small spaces within a usually thickened gallbladder wall (5, 10, 14–16). Sinuses may be filled with sludge, debris, or tiny calculi, in which case they will be echogenic or even shadowing

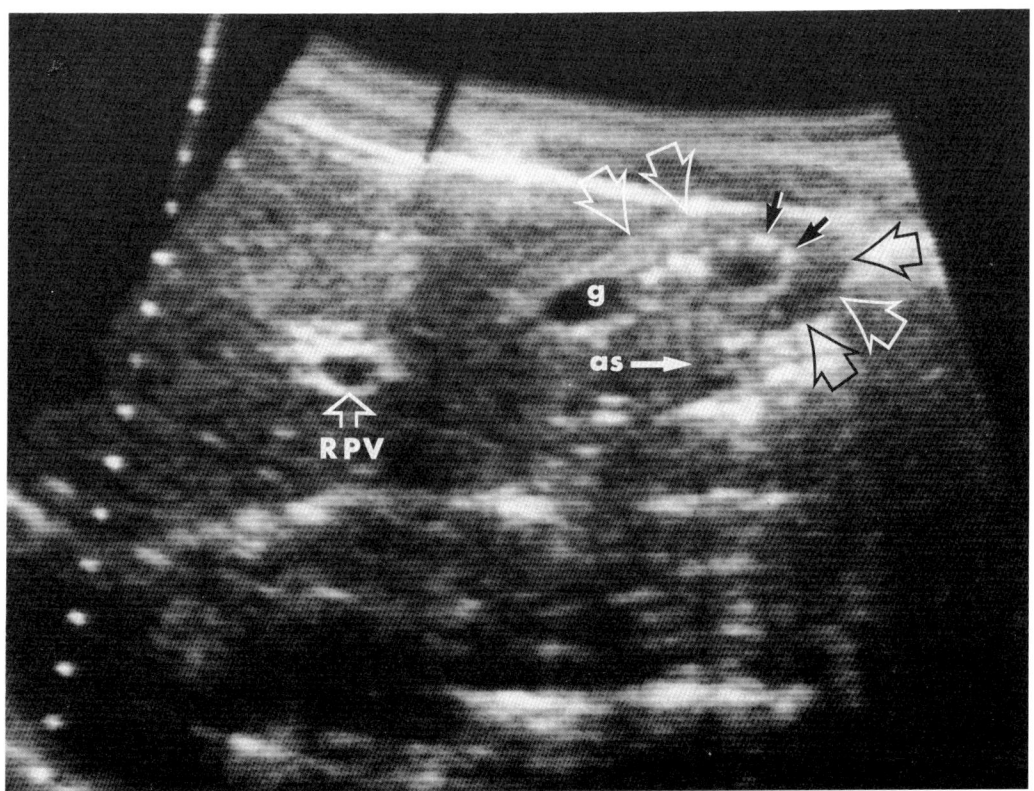

FIGURE 13.14. ADENOMYOMATOSIS

A 35-year-old man with nonvisualized gallbladder on OCG. Sagittal sonogram of the gallbladder (g) shows wall thickening (open arrows) confined to body and fundus of the gallbladder. Note echogenic dots (closed arrows) paralleling the luminal surface in the fundus. as, acoustic shadow from a gallstone; RPV, right portal vein. (From Raghavendra BN, Subramanyam BR, Balthazar EG, Horii SC, Megibow AJ, Hilton S: Sonography of adenomyomatosis of the gallbladder: radiologic-pathologic correlation. Radiology 146:747–752, 1983.)

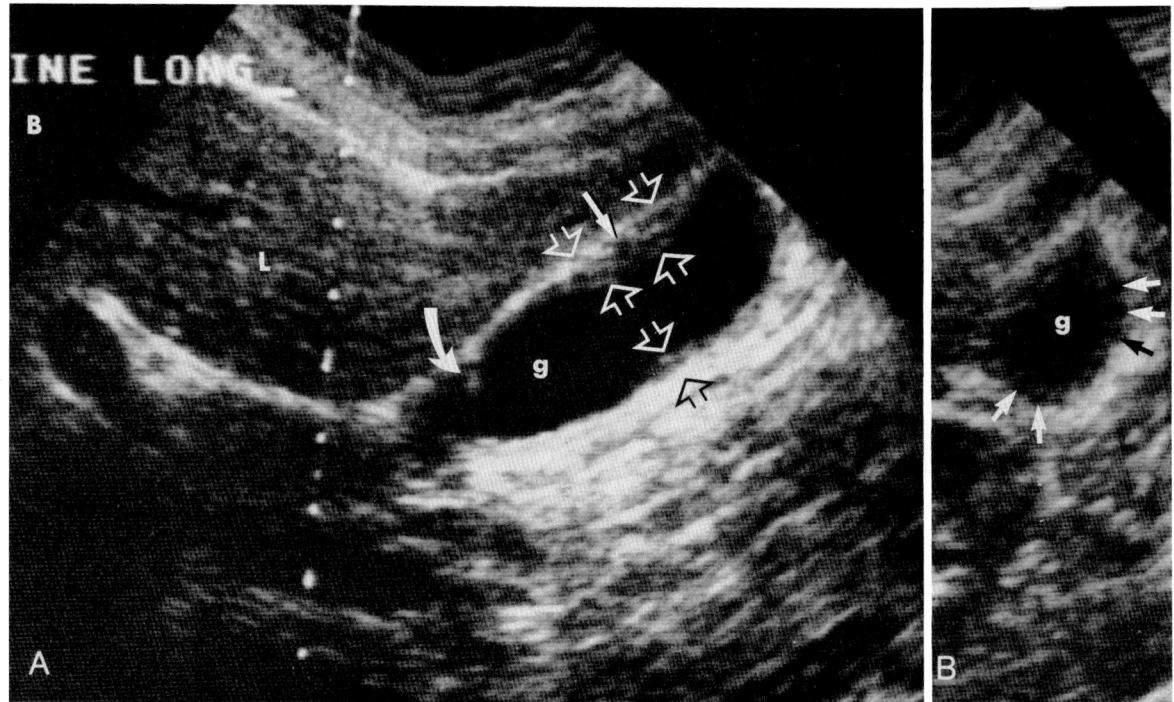

FIGURE 13.15. ADENOMYOMATOSIS

A and B: Sagittal and transverse scans of the gallbladder (g) (L, liver). *Open arrows* point to segmental wall thickening. Note small, rounded anechoic spaces within the wall (*closed, straight arrows*), representing intramural diverticulae. (From Raghavendra BN, Subramanyam BR, Balthazar EG, Horii SC, Megibow AJ, Hilton S: Sonography of adenomyomatosis of the gallbladder: radiologic-pathologic correlation. *Radiology* 146:747–752, 1983.)

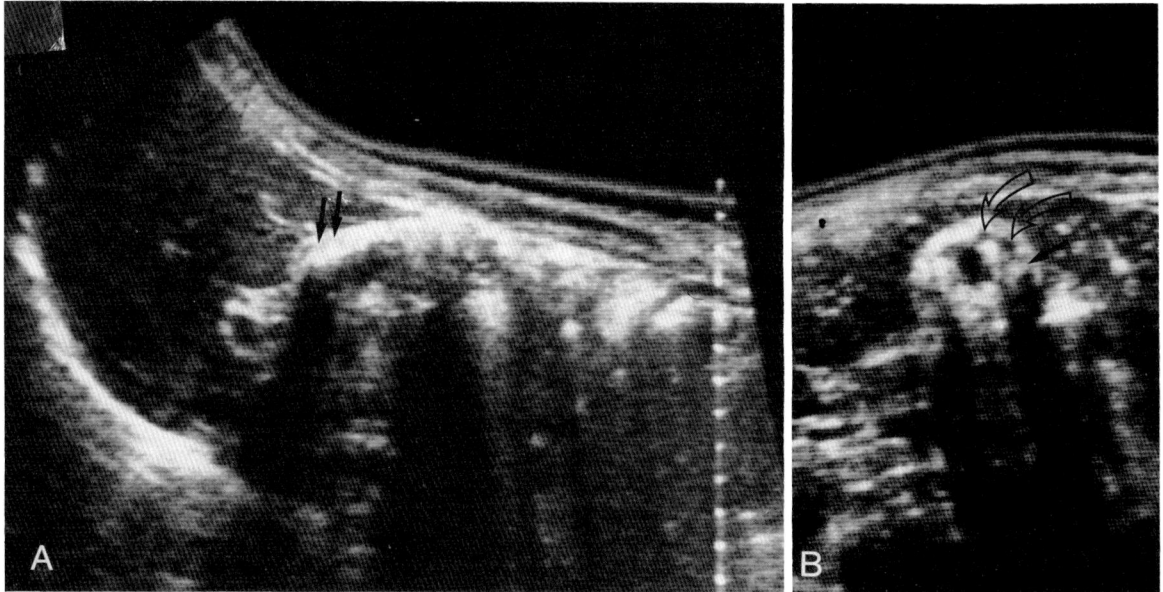

FIGURE 13.16. ADENOMYOMATOSIS

Sagittal and transverse sonograms of the gallbladder. Note intramurally located gallstone (within a Rokitansky-Aschoff sinus) (*arrows*) and fluid-filled Rokitansky-Aschoff sinuses (*curved arrows*). (From Raghavendra BN, Subramanyam BR, Balthazar EG, Horii SC, Megibow AJ, Hilton S: Sonography of adenomyomatosis of the gallbladder: radiologic-pathologic correlation. *Radiology* 146:747–752, 1983.)

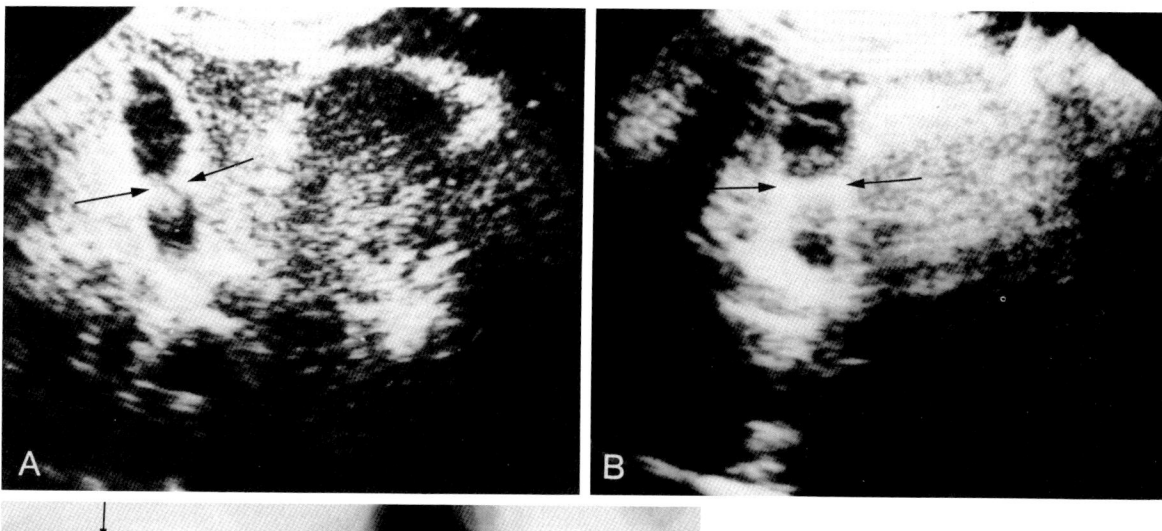

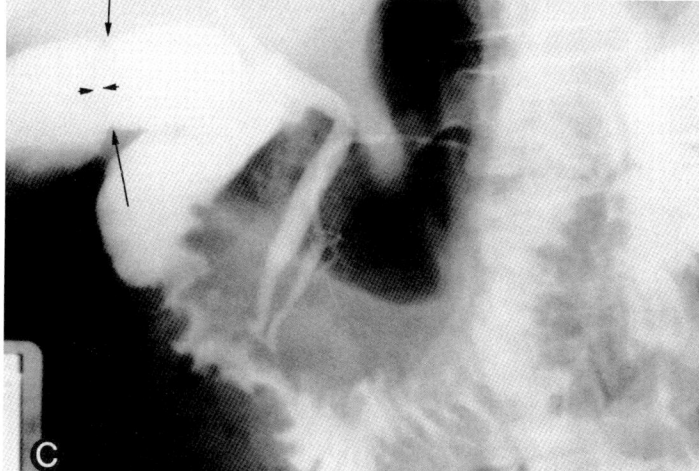

FIGURE 13.17. SEGMENTAL ADENOMYOMATOSIS VS. CONGENITAL SEPTUM
A and *B:* Transverse sonograms: thickly septated gallbladder (*arrows*) confirmed by ERCP (*C, arrows*).

(Fig. 13.16). Post-fatty meal sonography may improve the demonstration of sinuses.

The sonographic appearance of segmental adenomyomatosis ranges from focal wall thickening to a band-like constriction of the gallbladder, separating it into compartments (Fig. 13.17) (15). It may be difficult to decide whether the latter appearance is caused by a congenital septum or adenomyomatosis, although the former are usually thinner than constrictions caused by the latter. Post-fat sonograms can be useful in bringing out otherwise unseen Rokitansky-Aschoff sinuses.

Focal adenomyomatosis, the most common form, usually involves the fundus and is depicted sonographically as a focal wall thickening or mass. Since the abnormality is often mostly extra-luminal, it can be difficult to depict by ultrasound since the fundus of the gallbladder is often surrounded by bowel.

Computed Tomography

Although there is little accumulated experience with CT in either cholecystosis, one would not expect CT to be very contributory. Findings should include diffuse or focal wall thickening, and occasionally small intraluminal masses. Calculi would not be seen except by coincidence, and their absence would mitigate somewhat against the alternative diagnoses of chronic cholecystitis and gallbladder carcinoma.

Hepatobiliary Scintigraphy

^{99m}Tc-IDA scintigraphy may be of value in certain cases of segmental adenomyomatosis by demonstrating delayed filling of the compartment distal to the septum. This scan finding may correlate with stasis and increased incidence of stone formation (17).

REFERENCES

1. Jutras JA, Longtin JM, Levesque MD: Hyperplastic cholecystoses. *AJR* 83:795–826, 1960.
2. Jutras JA, Levesque HP: Adenomyoma and adenomyomatosis of the gallbladder: radiologic and pathologic correlations. *Radiol Clin North Am* 4:483–500, 1966.
3. Berk RN, van derVegt JH, Lichtenstein JE: The hyperplastic cholecystoses: cholesterolosis and adenomyomatosis. *Radiology* 146:593–601, 1983.
4. Berk RN, Lichtenstein JE: Cholecystoses. In Bockus HL et al (eds): *Gastroenterology*. Philadelphia, W.B. Saunders, 1985 (in press).
5. Price RJ, Stewart ET, Foley WD, Dodds WJ: Sonography of polypoid cholesterolosis. *AJR* 139:1197–1198, 1982.
6. Culver GJ, Berens DL, Bean BC: The relationship of stenosis to Rokitansky Aschoff sinuses of the gallbladder. *AJR* 77:47–54, 1957.
7. Colosimo C Jr, Vecchiloli A, Colagrande C: Hyperplastic cholecystosis: study by ceruletide-assisted cholecystography. *Gastrointest Radiol* 8:255–259, 1983.
8. Aguirre JR, Boher RO, Guraieb S: Hyperplastic cholecystoses: a new contribution to the unitarian theory. *AJR* 107:1–13, 1969.
9. Fotopoulos JP, Crampton AR: Adenomyomatosis of the gallbladder. *Med Clin North Am* 48:9–36, 1964.
10. Sagar G, Naik DR: Ultrasound diagnosis of adenomyomatosis of the gallbladder. *Br J Radiol* 57:432–435, 1984.
11. Salmenkivi K: Cholesterolosis of the gallbladder: a clinical study based on 269 cholecystectomies. *Acta Chir Scandinav* (Suppl) 324:1–93, 1964.
12. Tilvis RS, Aro J, Strandberg TE, et al: Lipid composition of bile and gallbladder mucosa in patients with acalculus cholesterolosis. *Gastroenterology* 82:607–615, 1982.
13. Ruhe AH, Zachman JP, Mulder BD, Rime AE: Cholesterol polyps of the gallbladder: ultrasound demonstration. *J Clin Ultrasound* 7:386–387, 1979.
14. Raghavendra BN, Subramanyam BR, Balthazar EG, Horii SC, Megibow AJ, Hilton S: Sonography of adenomyomatosis of the gallbladder: radiologic-pathologic correlation. *Radiology* 146:747–752, 1983.
15. Detweiler DG, Biddinger P, Staab EV, Delany DJ, Shirkoda A, Mittelstaedt CA: The appearance of adenomyomatosis with the newer imaging modalities: a case with pathologic correlation. *J Ultrasound Med* 1:295–298, 1982.
16. Rice J, Sauerbrei EE, Semogas P, Cooperberg PL, Burhenne HJ: Sonographic appearance of adenomyomatosis of the gallbladder. *J Clin Ultrasound* 9:336–337, 1981.
17. Kramer EL, Rumancik WM, Harkavy L, Tiu S, Banner HJ, Sanger JJ: Hepatobiliary scintigraphy of the compartmentalized gallbladder. *AJR* 145:1205–1206, 1985.

BENIGN TUMORS

Benign gallbladder polyps and tumors are a diverse group of lesions, many quite rare, which are often the subject of overlapping and confusing nomenclature and classification. Most current classifications are modifications of that proposed by Christensen and Ishak (1) based on the largest series in the literature, 180 cases collected at the Armed Forces Institute of Pathology. There has been a unfortunate tendency, particularly among radiologists, to refer to any fixed filling defect in the gallbladder as a "papilloma," a vague term not included in the World Health Organization nomenclature for the gallbladder. "Polyp" is a generic term referring to any protrusion from a surface. It should not be used to imply specific pathology.

The most common small polyps are produced by several forms of hyperplasia or heterotopia and are not neoplastic in the true sense. Many are found incidentally in gallbladders removed for cholelithiasis and cholecystitis so that their role in symptom production is problematic. Frequently they are not a primary cause of symptoms. The reported incidence of gallbladder polyps varies widely with the material included and the classification used. It generally ranges from less than 1% to 10%, with the best data suggesting their presence in about 4–5% of surgically removed gallbladders and less than 0.5% of gallbladders seen radiologically (2–6).

Radiographically the various benign gallbladder polyps tend to resemble one another. They generally present as fixed intraluminal filling defects usually between 0.2 and 1.5 cm in diameter. They are best seen on oral cholecystograms following stimulated contraction. Calculi, the far more common filling defects, can usually be distinguished by their dependent position and mobility with changes in body position. Stones sometimes become fixed to the gallbladder wall whence they might be confused with polyps. There is debate as to how often this happens, the consensus being that it is infrequent. In any case, stones are usually more echogenic than soft tissue tumors and much more likely to cause shadowing on ultrasound examination which has emerged as the method of choice for primary evaluation of the gallbladder. Differentiation from carcinoma may be a concern, but carcinoma is unlikely if the lesion can be detected by oral cholecystography since carcinoma is almost always associated with chronic cholecystitis and, hence, nonfunction and nonvisualization on OCG (3).

Cholesterol polyps account for over 90% of benign gallbladder polyps (7, 8), and were discussed previously in the hyperplastic cholecystosis section, as were adenomyomas, the other common benign gallbladder "tumor." What follows is a discussion of the remaining causes of benign gallbladder polyps or tumors.

Hyperplasia

Elfving has described an adenomatous hyperplasia differing from adenomyomatosis in that it involves only the epithelial elements of the mucosa (9). Two types, one a villous form with tall papillary mucosal projections, and the other a spongy type with ramifying, sometimes cystically dilated, glands are seen. Such lesions comprised 10% of the AFIP series, some cases being focal, but most being diffuse (1). Cholelithiasis and cholecystitis were commonly associated with the hyperplasia in these cases so that the role of the hyperplasia in symptom production was unclear especially as some patients were asymptomatic. Mucosal hyperplasia is found in cholesterolosis but a causal relationship is not clear. The hyperplastic mucosa shows no cellular atypia and no relationship to carcinoma has been documented. No radiographic manifestations have been described.

A different form of adenomatous mucosal hyperplasia, or dysplasia, with atypical mitoses, loss of cellular polarity, nuclear hyperchromatism and disorganization of mucosal architecture has also been described (10, 11). The separation from carcinoma in situ is somewhat arbitrary and indeed such changes are often found adjacent to areas of invasive carcinoma. Most cases of carcinoma in situ have been in adenomatous polyps (see below) and only recently found separately (12). In the absence of polyps, radiographic manifestations would not be expected.

Adenomas

Although infrequent in the general population, and far less common than cholesterol polyps and localized fundal adenomyomatosis, adenomas are the most common benign true neoplasms of the gallbladder. They may be stalked or sessile, and either papillary or smooth. Mixed forms also occur (Figs. 13.18 and 13.19). Smooth adenomas are composed of vascularized stroma and proliferating glands, some of which become cystically dilated. The papillary tumors have delicate branching projections covered with columnar or cuboidal epithelium. The papillary adenoma is undoubtedly the origin of the term "papilloma" which should probably be discarded since it has been used so indiscriminately for almost any gallbladder filling defect. Size varies up to several centimeters, but most are less than 2 cm (1, 4, 5). They may arise in any part of the gallbladder and are multiple in about one third of cases. When multiple they are generally few in number, but a recent case of diffuse "papillomatosis" has been reported associated with ulceractive colitis and sclerosing cholangitis (13). They have been reported in both Gardner syndrome and in Peutz-Jeghers syndrome (14, 15).

Radiographically they appear as small fixed

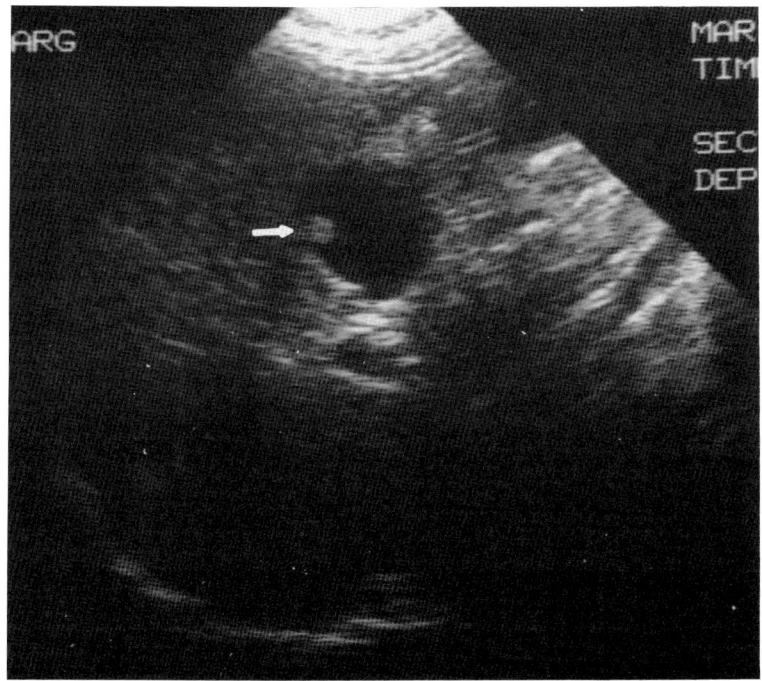

FIGURE 13.18. ADENOMATOUS POLYP Small, nonshadowing mass (*arrow*) adherent to the gallbladder wall consistent with an adenomatous polyp. Cholesterol polyps sometimes are slightly more echogenic and shadow slightly, although the distinction cannot be reliably made.

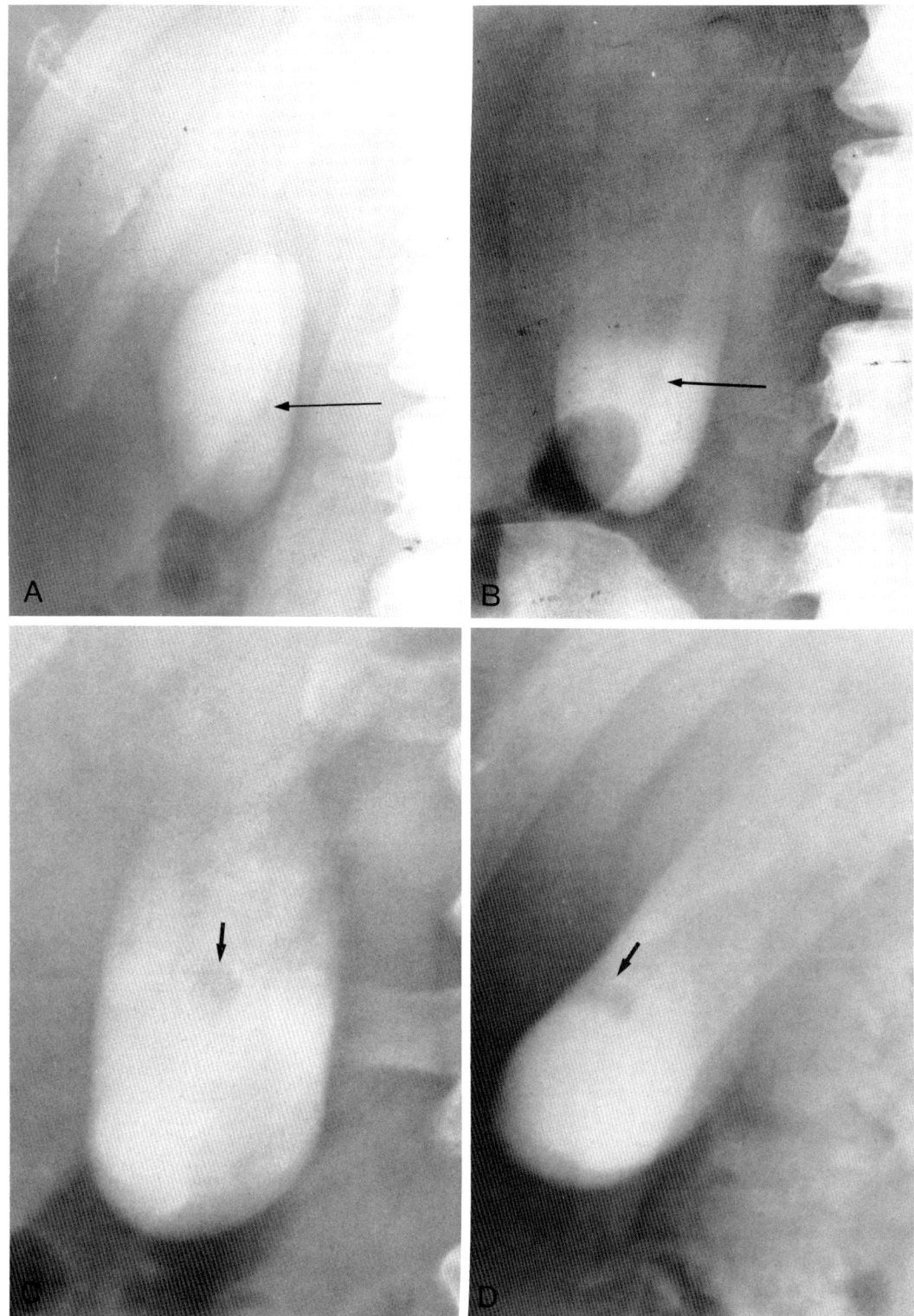

FIGURE 13.19. ADENOMATOUS POLYP

A and *B:* Supine and erect spot films of a small, nonmobile filling defect (*arrow*) that proved to be an adenomatous polyp.
C and *D:* Erect AP and oblique spots demonstrate wall attachment of an adenomatous polyp (*arrow*).

filling defects with nothing to definitively distinguish them from the more common cholesterol polyps by OCG or ultrasound, especially when they are multiple. Perhaps high resolution CT or MRI may eventually be able to distinguish between the two on the basis of tissue characteristics.

Carcinoma in situ has been found within the adenoma in a number of cases, but usually also in association with gallstones. Nevertheless, the premalignant potential of adenomas remains in debate. It is generally believed that adenomas have a very low malignant potential in the absence of stones (1, 2). Most carcinomas have been felt to arise de novo independent of adenomas, although a recent study disputes this, reporting transition from adenoma to carcinoma and finding adenomatous residues in 19% of invasive carcinomas (16). All benign adenomas were less than 12 mm and all containing malignancy were greater than that leading to the suggestion that polyps greater than one centimeter be removed.

Heterotopias

Gallbladder tumors composed of a variety of heterotopic tissues have been described but are very uncommon (1, 17). These tend to appear as submucosal nodules of 1.0–2.5 cm diameter causing the overlying mucosa to bulge smoothly toward the lumen. Such lesions might be confused for the more common focal form of adenomyomatosis especially when they happen to occur in the fundus, but the majority of lesions have been found in the gallbladder neck. Lack of Rokitansky-Aschoff sinuses is a helpful differential point. Gastric tissue appears to be the most common type followed by pancreatic (18, 19). Several types of gastric epithelial cells have been found, and both acinar and islet cell tissue have been found in the pancreatic ectopias. Gastric ulcer and pancreatitis have been reported in such lesions but are very rare (20). It should be noted that goblet cells and mucosa resembling that of the gastric antrum are normally found in the neck of the gallbladder (11). Thyroid and adrenal heterotopias have also been described (17, 21). Heterotopias have generally been assumed to be congenital developmental anomalies arising from common foregut endodermal anlage, although metaplasia is another possibility, especially where foci of relatively flat intestinal tissue is found pathologically. The latter would not be expected to be evident radiologically.

Tumors of Supporting Tissue

There have been occasional reports of tumors arising from a wide variety of the mesenchymal supporting tissues of the gallbladder. Included are examples of leiomyoma, lipoma, hemangioma, lymphangioma, fibroma, neurofibroma, paraganglioma, and several cases of granular cell tumor ("myoblastoma") (11, 22–28). The tissue of origin of the latter is in debate, many authorities doubting it arises from myoblasts, and some suggesting a neural origin. The extrahepatic bile ducts appear to be a more common site for granular cell tumors than the gallbladder. The radiographic features of some of the supporting tissue tumors have yet to be described, and there have been few distinctive features of the rest. Variably sized, submucosal-appearing tumors would be expected in most cases.

Inflammatory and Miscellaneous Polyps

Local inflammatory reaction consisting of fibrous connective tissue stroma densely infiltrated with chronic inflammatory cells and covered with proliferating epithelium is sometimes manifested as polypoid lesions in the gallbladder (Fig. 13.20) 1). The lesions may be large enough to detect sonographically, but they are associated with cholecystitis so that visualization on OCG would be unusual.

Christensen and Ishak (1) originally described seven cases of fibroxanthogranulomatous inflammation presenting pathologically with tumor-like nodules. Goodman and Ishak (29) later

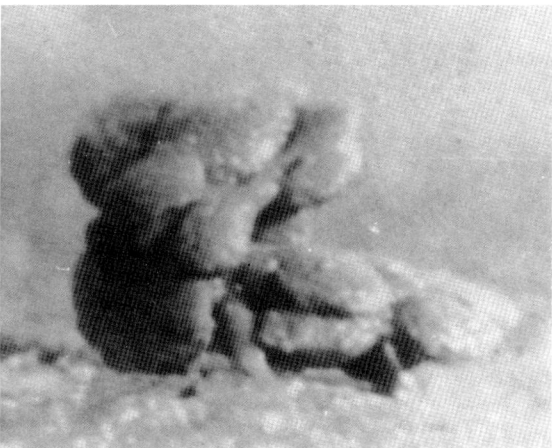

FIGURE 13.20. GROSS SPECIMEN OF AN INFLAMMATORY GALLBLADDER POLYP
(Courtesy of Dr. Albert Jutras, who contributed this case to the AFIP.)

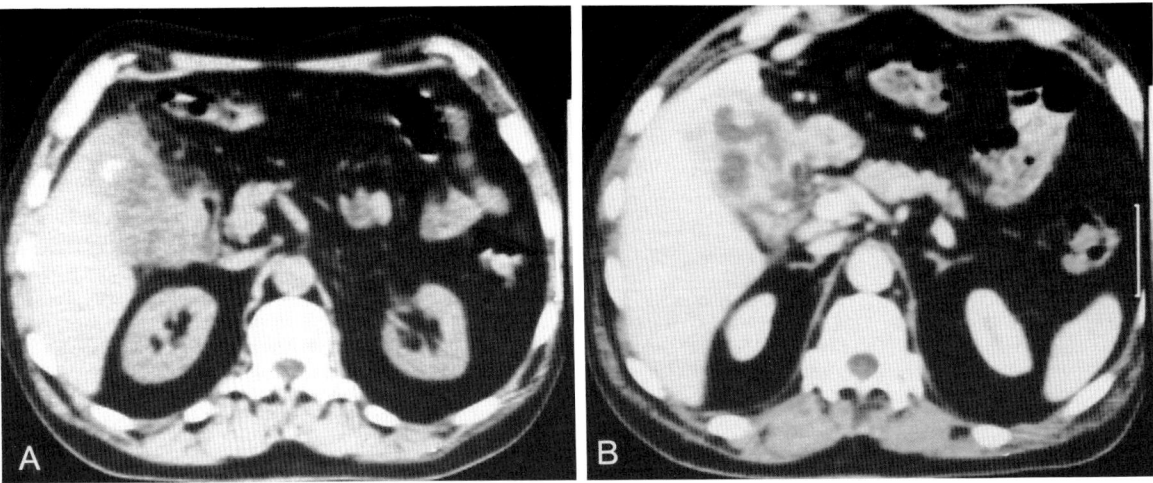

FIGURE 13.21. XANTHOGRANULOMATOUS CHOLECYSTITIS
A and *B:* CT scans of the gallbladder before and after contrast administration: large mass replacing the gallbladder with calcification, irregular wall thickening, and apparent necrosis. The mass has a poorly defined interface with the liver and is inseparable from the duodenum. Diagnosis: xanthogranulomatous cholecystitis. (From Duber C, Storkel S, Wagner PK, et al: Xanthogranulomatous cholecystitis mimicking carcinoma of the gallbladder. CT findings. *J Comput Assist Tomogr* 8:1195, 1984.)

reported an additional 40 cases, modifying the name to xanthogranulomatous cholecystitis. The nodules contained foamy histiocytes mixed with acute and chronic inflammatory cells indicating the reactive nature of the lesions. This entity differs from cholesterolosis and cholesterol polyps in the intramural location of the histiocytes and in the associated inflammatory and granulomatous response. Lesions appear to result from inspissation of bile and sometimes mucin in Rokitansky-Aschoff sinuses with subsequent rupture and inflammation. Extravasation of bile is thought to cause accumulation of histiocytes which phagocytize the insoluble cholesterol and bile lipids. Grossly the lesions form soft yellowish-brown nodules up to 2.5 cm. No specific radiologic manifestations have been reported, and differentiation from carcinoma in cases with larger nodules is probably impossible (Fig. 13.21) (30).

Nodular granulomatous lesions may occur in response to foreign matter such as suture material or, more often, parasite eggs. *Ascaris lumbricoides* is a common cause of the latter, but other parasites including *Paragonimus westermani*, *Schistosoma*, liver flukes such as *Fasciola*, *Clonorchis*, *Opisthorchis*, and even *Filariasis* have all been implicated (1, 11).

A group of hereditary disorders are characterized by abnormal accumulation of sphingolipids. In metachromatic leukodystrophy, a deficiency of the enzyme arylsulfatase-A leads to accumu-

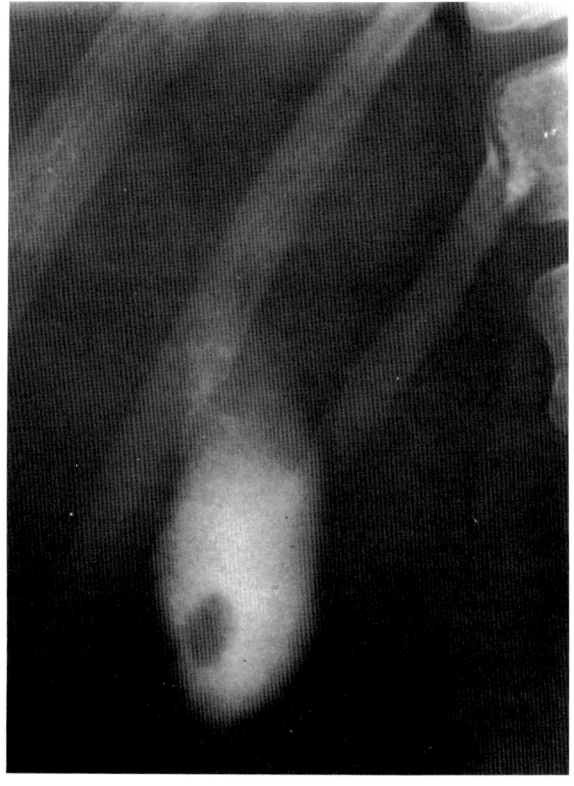

FIGURE 13.22. SULFATIDE CHOLECYSTOSIS
Sulfatide cholecystosis: polypoid mass in the gallbladder in a patient with metachromatic leukodystrophy. (From Kleinman PK, Winchester P, Volberg F: Sulfatide cholecystosis. *Gastrointest Radiol* 1:99–100, 1976.)

lation of metachromatic sulfatides. Neurologic disease secondary to white matter degeneration is the most important problem, but the metachromatic sulfatide also accumulates in nonneural tissue including the gallbladder wall where polypoid growths may result (Fig. 13.22) (31, 32).

REFERENCES

1. Christensen AH, Ishak KG: Benign tumors and pseudotumors of the gallbladder. *Arch Pathol.* 90:423–432, 1970.
2. Eelkema HH, Hodgson JR, Stauffer MH: Fifteen year follow-up of polypoid lesions of the gallbladder diagnosed by cholecystography. *Gastroenterology* 42:144–147, 1962.
3. Grieco VR, Bartone NG, Vasilas A: A study of fixed filling defects in the well opacified gallbladder and their evolution. *AJR* 90:844–853, 1963.
4. Melson GL, Reiter F, Evens RG: Tumorous conditions of the gallbladder. *Semin Roentgenol* 11:269–282, 1976.
5. Ochsner SF, Ochsner A: Benign neoplasms of the gallbladder: diagnosis and surgical implications. *Ann Surg* 151:630–637, 1960.
6. Orloff MJ, Robinson GT: Tumors of the gallbladder. In Bockus HL et al (eds): *Gastroenterology*, Ed 4. Philadelphia, W.B. Saunders, 1985, pp 3677–3692.
7. Jutras JA: Hyperplastic cholecystoses. *AJR* 83:795–827, 1960.
8. Tinsley AR, Mulkerin LE, Van de Linde JM, Todd DW: Polypoid lesions of the acalculous gallbladder. *South Med J* 68:958–962, 1975.
9. Elfving G, Lehtonen T, Teir H: Clinical significance of primary hyperplasia of gallbladder mucosa. *Ann Surg* 165:61–67, 1967.
10. Albores-Saavedra J, Alcantra-Vasquez A, Cruz-Ortiz H, Herrera-Goepfert R: The precursor lesions of invasive gallbladder carcinoma. Hyperplasia, atypical hyperplasia, and carcinoma in situ. *Cancer* 45:919–927, 1980.
11. Weedon D: *Pathology of the Gallbladder.* New York, Masson Publishing USA Inc., 1984, pp 23:136–146, 161–169, 205–211, 213.
12. Bivens BA, Meeker WR Jr, Weiss DL, Griffen WO Jr: Carcinoma in situ of the gallbladder. A dilemma. *South Med J* 68:297–300, 1975.
13. Almagro UA: Diffuse papillomatosis of the gallbladder. *Am J Gastroenterol* 80:274–278, 1985.
14. Tantachamrun T, Borvonaombat S, Theetranot C: Gardner's syndrome associated with adenomatous polyp of the gallbladder: report of a case. *J Med Assoc Thai* 62:441–447, 1979.
15. Foster DR, Foster DBE: Gallbladder polyps in Peutz-Jeghers syndrome. *Postgrad Med J* 56:373–376, 1980.
16. Kozuka S, Tsubone M, Yasui A, Hachisuka K: Relation of adenoma to carcinoma in the gallbladder. *Cancer* 50:2226–2234, 1982.
17. Curtis LE, Sheahan DG: Heterotopic tissues in the gallbladder. *Arch Pathol* 88:677–683, 1969.
18. Keramidas DC, Skondras C, Anagnoston D, Douglas N: Gastric heterotopia in the gallbladder. *J Pediatr Surg* 12:759–762, 1977.
19. Martinez LO, Gregg M: Aberrant pancreas in the gallbladder. *J Can Assoc Radiol* 24:235–238, 1973.
20. Quizilbach AH: Acute pancreatitis occurring in heterotopic pancreas tissue in the gallbladder. *Can J Surg* 19:413–414, 1976.
21. Busuttil A: Ectopic adrenal within the gallbladder wall. *Am J Pathol* 113:231–233, 1974.
22. Shepard VD, Walters W, Dockerty MB: Benign tumors of the gallbladder. *Arch Surg* 45:1–18, 1942.
23. Arbab AA, Brasfield R: Benign tumors of the gallbladder. *Surgery* 61:535–540, 1967.
24. Sewell JH, Miron MA: Benign cavernous hemangioma of the gallbladder. *Arch Pathol* 88:30–31, 1969.
25. Eggleston JR, Goldman RL: Neurofibroma and elastosis of the gallbladder: report of an unusual case. *Am J Gastroenterol* 77:335–337, 1982.
26. Wolf M: Paraganglioma of the gallbladder. *Arch Surg* 107:493, 1973.
27. Aisner SC, Khaneja S, Ramirez O: Multiple granular cell tumors of the gallbladder and biliary tree. *Arch Pathol Lab Med* 106:470–471, 1982.
28. Ishii T, Iri H, Yamamoto S, Shinozawa Y, Sudoh M: Granular cell myoblastoma of the gallbladder. *Am J Gastroenterol* 68:38–44, 1977.
29. Goodman ZD, Ishak KG: Xanthogranulomatous cholecystitis. *Am J Surg Pathol* 5:653–659, 1981.
30. Duber C, Storkel S, Wagner PK et al: Xanthogranulomatous cholecystitis mimicking carcinoma of the gallbladder. CT findings. *J Comput Assist Tomogr* 8:1195, 1984.
31. Dische RM: Metachromatic leucodystrophic polyposis of the gallbladder. *J Pathol* 97:388–390, 1969.
32. Kleinman PK, Winchester P, Volberg F: Sulfatide cholecystosis. *Gastrointest Radiol* 1:99–100, 1976.

GALLBLADDER CARCINOMA

Primary carcinoma of the gallbladder is not common, representing only 1–3% of malignancies at autopsy. However, it is the fifth most common gastrointestinal tract malignancy as well as the most common primary biliary tract malignancy. It is seen in 1% of patients with gallstones and generally occurs in the 6th and 7th decades of life with a female preponderance of 4:1 (1). Gallstones are found in 65–95% of carcinomatous gallbladders (2), and carcinoma of the gallbladder is frequently associated with cholecystitis, suggesting chronic irritation as an inciting factor. An increased incidence is present in automotive, rubber, textile, and metal workers (3).

Clinical Findings

Onset is usually insidious with upper abdominal mass, right upper quadrant pain, jaundice, and weight loss as common presenting signs and symptoms. About 25% have symptoms suggesting acute cholecystitis, and 50% have a past history suggestive of gallbladder disease (1). Prognosis is poor since the disease is usually far advanced at the time of diagnosis. Average survival is only 6 months after the first symptoms appear, and almost all patients die from biliary obstruction and/or liver failure within a year of diagnosis. Carcinoma in situ, found incidentally at cholecystectomy for stones, may occasionally be cured by resection. Radiation and chemotherapy are generally ineffective.

Pathology

The overwhelming majority of gallbladder cancers are adenocarcinomas (85%), with the remainder divided among anaplastic carcinoma, squamous cell carcinoma, adenosquamous carcinoma, carcinoid, melanoma, and rare sarcomas. The scirrhous form invades and infiltrates the gallbladder wall and ultimately obliterates the organ in a mass of tumor. The papillary form tends to grow into and fill the lumen. Spread is by direct extension into the liver, other adjacent organs and the hepatoduodenal ligament. Metastasis occurs to regional nodes via lymphatics, distantly via the hepatic and portal veins, and down the biliary tree (4). Patterns of spread and dismal prognosis are basically the same for all histologic varieties of gallbladder cancer.

Radiology

Oral Cholecystography

The gallbladder fails to opacify in at least two-thirds of patients with carcinoma of the gallbladder usually due to cystic duct obstruction. An abnormal soft tissue mass or contour irregularity suggestive of malignancy was only seen in 10% in a series of 330 cases (Fig. 13.23) (5).

Plain Films and Barium Studies

A right upper quadrant mass can be seen on a plain film of the abdomen in advanced gallbladder carcinoma (Fig. 13.24A). Barium studies are useful in selected cases to demonstrate direct extension to the duodenum, anterior limb of the hepatic flexure, and cholecystoenteric fistulas (Fig. 13.24).

Sonography

Three major sonographic patterns of gallbladder carcinoma have been recognized. The most common (Type I) is replacement of the gallbladder by a complex mass, seen in 40–50% of patients (Figs. 13.25A and B, 13.26A). In 20% of patients there is diffuse or focal irregular thickening of the gallbladder wall (Type II (Fig. 13.25D). Least commonly seen is an irregular,

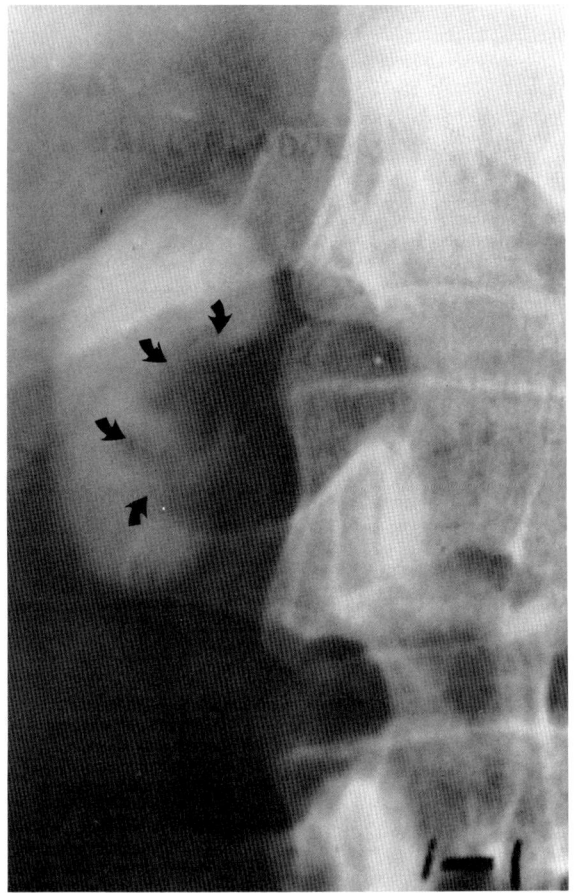

FIGURE 13.23. ORAL CHOLECYSTOGRAM OF GALLBLADDER CANCER
Irregular mass representing a gallbladder carcinoma (*arrows*).

polypoid mass within the lumen (Type III) (Fig. 13.25E). Of course, some cases exhibit combinations of the above three patterns (6). In various series, ultrasound has a prospective accuracy of 50–88% in the diagnosis of gallbladder cancer. Many of the false positives that occur are due to misinterpretation of inflammatory changes as malignancies (7).

Type I. The gallbladder is either replaced or surrounded by soft tissue mass, and may vary in size from normal to markedly enlarged. Its shape can be normal, nodular, or markedly irregular (8). The texture of the mass is frequently inhomogeneously hypoechoic, with any anechoic regions present representing either necrosis or residual bile (9, 10). Gallstones trapped within the mass are depicted as shadowing echodensities. The lack of a clear demarcation between the liver and the gallbladder mass supports a diagnosis of gallbladder carcinoma. The Type I pat-

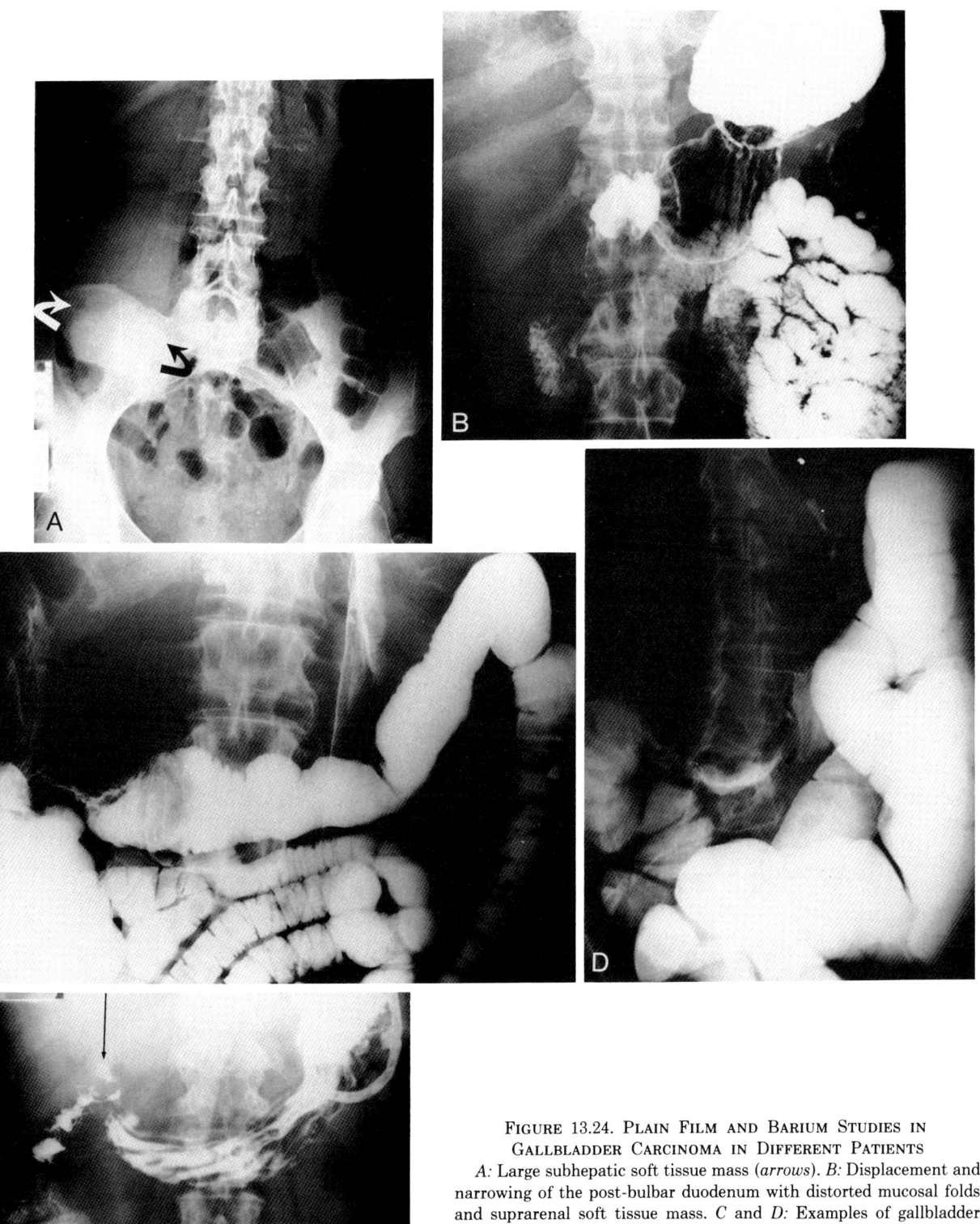

FIGURE 13.24. PLAIN FILM AND BARIUM STUDIES IN GALLBLADDER CARCINOMA IN DIFFERENT PATIENTS

A: Large subhepatic soft tissue mass (*arrows*). *B:* Displacement and narrowing of the post-bulbar duodenum with distorted mucosal folds and suprarenal soft tissue mass. *C* and *D:* Examples of gallbladder carcinoma partially obstructing the hepatic flexure. Concentric narrowing in *C* and eccentric in *D*. *E:* UGI: filling of gallbladder lumen (*arrow*) and colon via an irregular fistula.

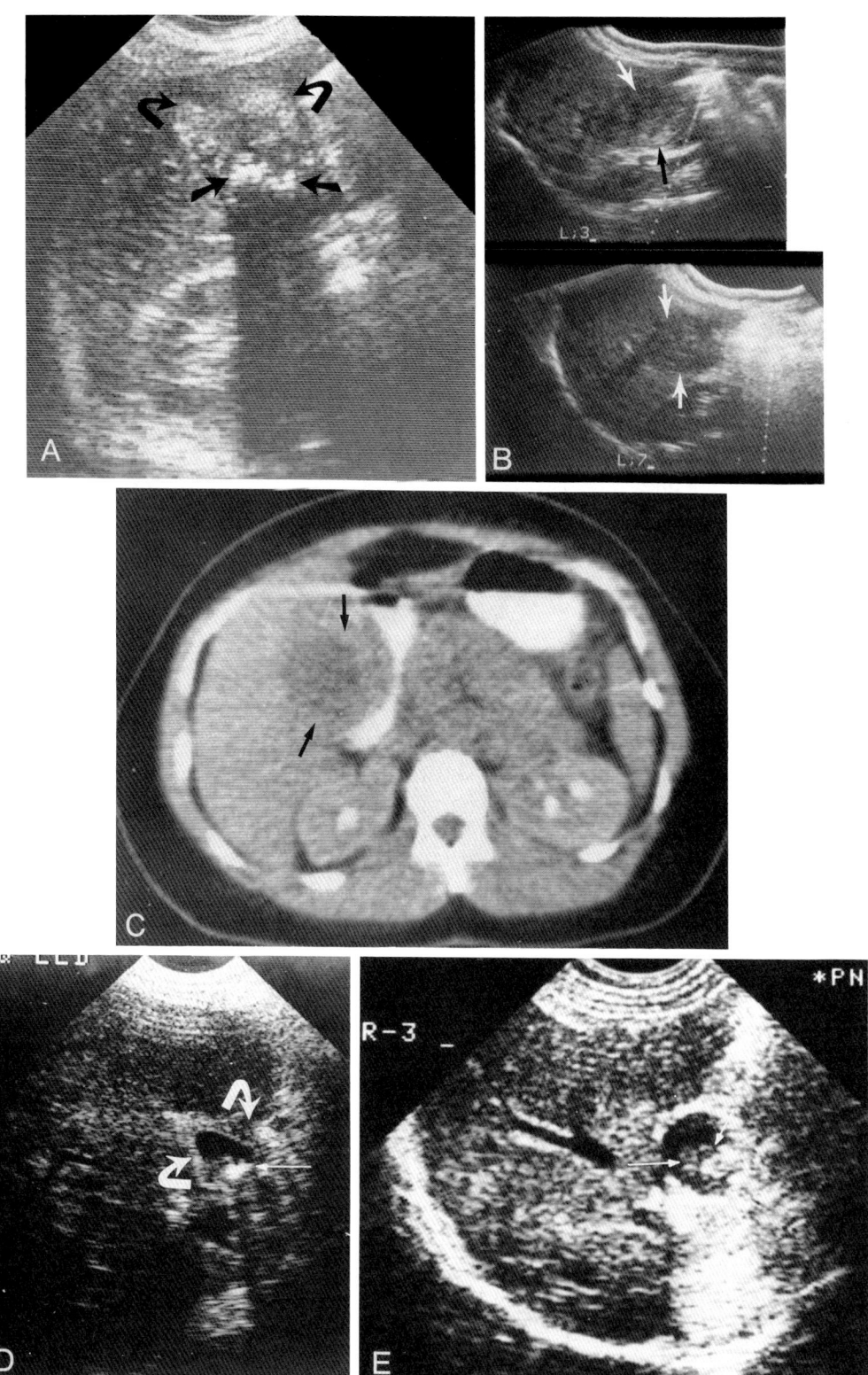

FIGURE 13.25. A SPECTRUM OF SONOGRAPHIC FINDINGS IN CARCINOMA OF THE GALLBLADDER
A: Carcinoma of the gallbladder and cholelithiasis: shadowing calculi (*arrows*) surrounded by a massively thickened wall not clearly demarcated from liver parenchyma (*curved arrows*). *B:* Parasagittal sonogram in a different patient: gallbladder replaced by a large mass (arrows) inseparable from the liver. *C:* CT of the same patient as *B:* similar findings (*arrows*) with medial displacement of the duodenum. *D:* Sagittal scan, left lateral decubitus position, different patient: markedly thickened gallbladder wall (*curved arrows*) and shadowing calculus (*arrow*) embedded in a mass. *E:* Fungating intraluminal mass (*arrows*) in a different patient.

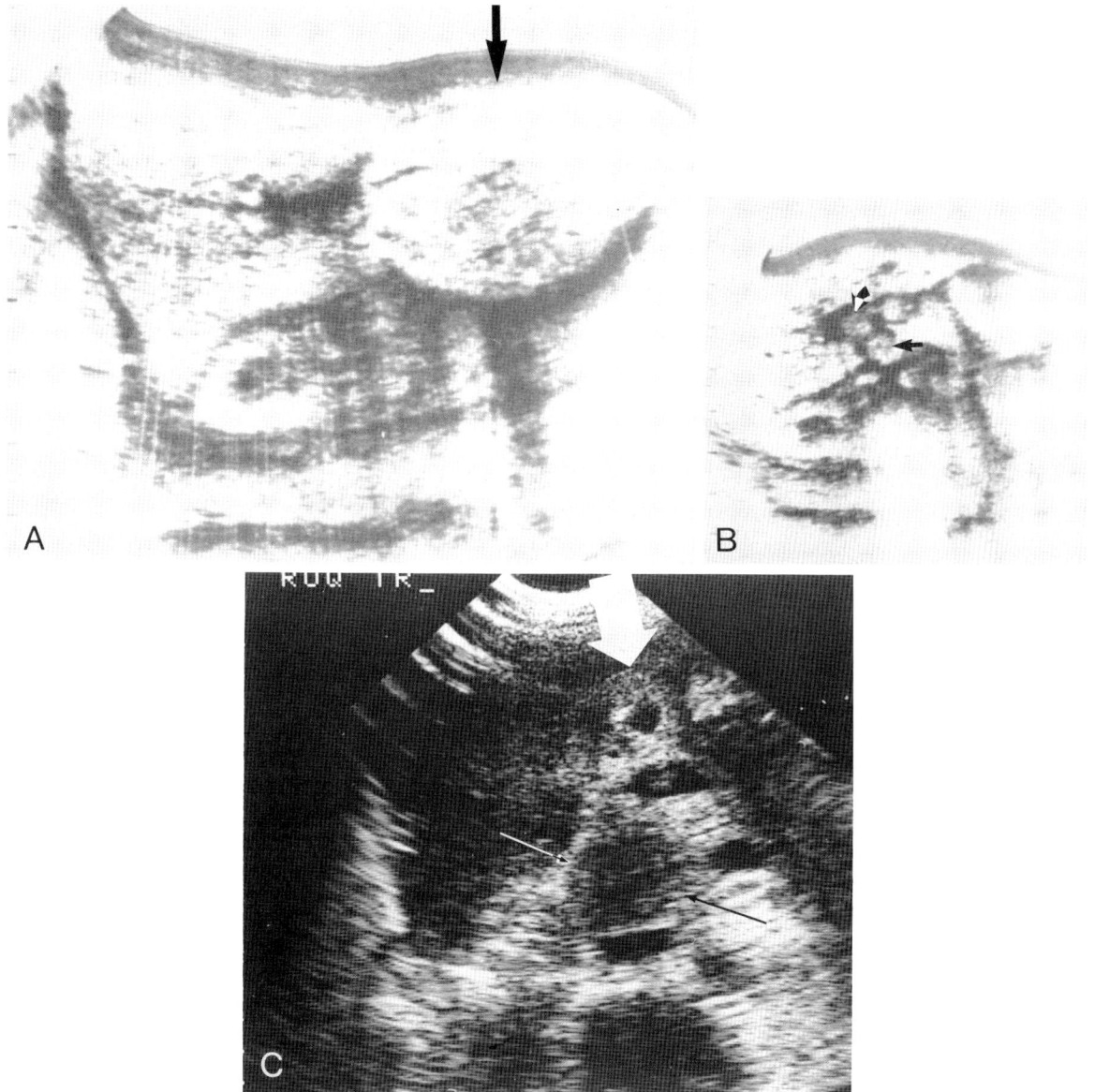

FIGURE 13.26. SONOGRAPHY SHOWING ADENOPATHY FROM GALLBLADDER CARCINOMA METASTASES
A: Parasagittal scan through right lobe: large, subhepatic mass (*arrow*). *B:* Adenopathy in the hepatoduodenal ligament (*arrows*). *C:* Transverse scan: large, hyoechoic mass in the region of the head of the pancreas (*thin arrows*), just anterior to the inferior vena cava, representing peripancreatic adenopathy from carcinoma of the gallbladder. A thick-walled gallbladder representing the primary is also seen (*large arrow*).

tern of gallbladder carcinoma may be confused with intra or extrahepatic tumors or abscesses, or hydatid disease.

Type II. Thickening of the gallbladder wall is relatively nonspecific and can be seen in acute or chronic cholecystitis and the hyperplastic cholecystoses. Wall thickening is usually asymmetric and irregular in gallbladder carcinoma. A correct diagnosis with this pattern is strongly dependent on demonstrating ancillary findings such as mass, adenopathy, or invasion of the liver or other adjacent structures. Occasionally, sludge may layer out and give an erroneous impression of posterior wall thickening and mimic an infiltrating carcinoma. Sludge is usually brighter than the hypoechoic thickened wall of a carcinomatous gallbladder, however (11).

Type III. A fungating intraluminal mass without shadowing or movement after positional changes suggests gallbladder carcinoma. These lesions usually have a wide base as opposed to a narrow stalk (11). Acoustic shadowing from adjacent stones is a frequent finding. Polypoid intraluminal gallbladder carcinomas are usually in the infundibulum or fundus rather than in the body. Distortion of the gallbladder contour is a useful additional sign suggesting carcinoma. Differential diagnostic considerations of this type of carcinoma include cholesterol polyps, mucosal hyperplasia, blood clot, adenoma, and other unusual benign masses. While the above may simulate carcinoma sonographically, they are not likely to prevent opacification of the gallbladder on an oral cholecystogram.

Ancillary Sonographic Findings in Gallbladder Carcinoma. Ancillary findings are: (a) cholelithiasis: although most patients have associated cholelithiasis, only 60% of these are depicted sonographically (Fig. 13.25A and D), (b) liver masses: the liver may become involved either by direct neoplastic extension or hematogenous spread. Lack of a distinct margin between the gallbladder mass and the liver suggests invasion, whereas a clear cleavage plane suggests the opposite (Fig. 13.27A); (c) biliary ductal dilatation: extension to the porta hepatis via the hepatoduodenal ligament causes biliary obstruction and dilatation of the intrahepatic ducts

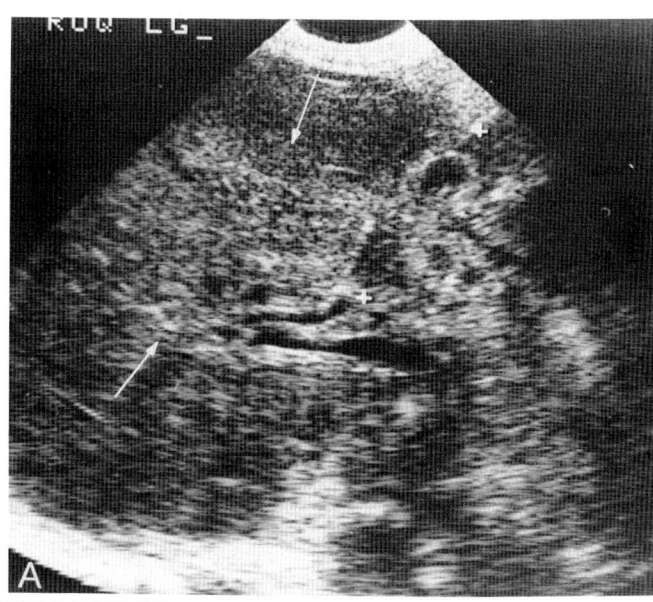

FIGURE 13.27. SONOGRAPHY OF LOCAL EXTENSION

A: Parasagittal scan: large mass in gallbladder bed (*cursors*) extending directly into the liver (*arrows*). *B:* Parasagittal scan in another patient: solid mass (*arrows*) represents extension of gallbladder carcinoma up the hepatoduodenal ligament anterior to the portal vein. *C:* Transverse scan of same patient as *B:* dilated ducts (*arrows*) in the left lobe of the liver.

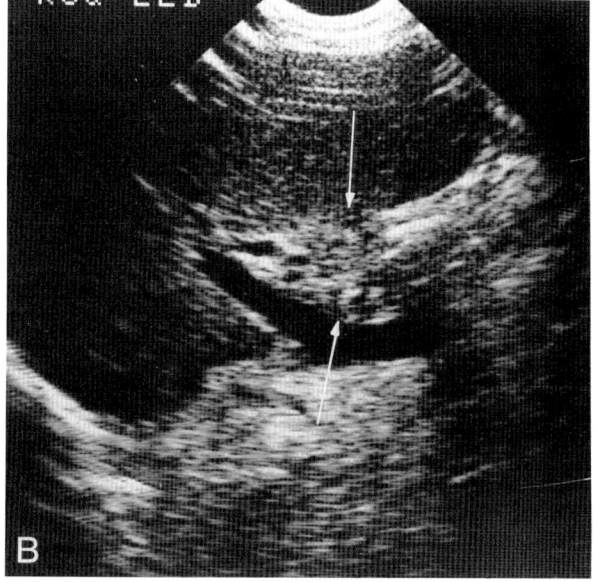
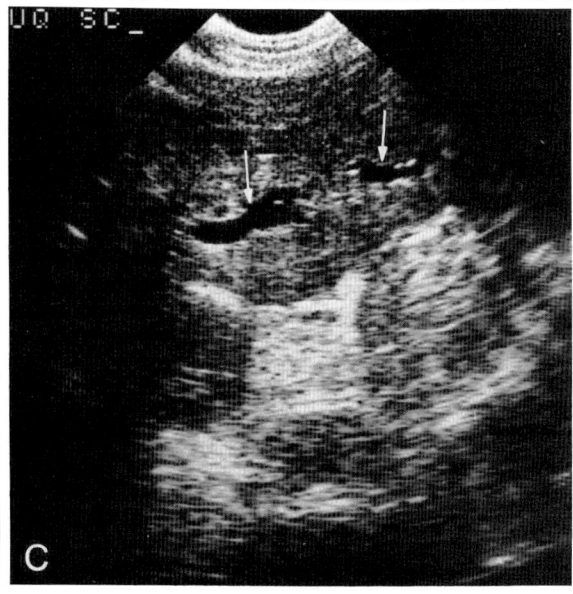

(Figs. 13.27A and C). The common duct may be dilated if the cause of obstruction is peripancreatic nodes or direct duct invasion; and (d) adenopathy: the typical sites for nodes to be seen sonographically is the peripancreatic region and the porta hepatis (Fig. 13.26) (8, 10).

Sonographic False Negatives. The diagnosis of carcinoma of the gallbladder may be missed for a number of reasons. In some series at least 10% of the gallbladders were not depicted (8–11). Reverberation artifacts can obscure the anterior wall of the gallbladder and conceal a mass (10). Diffusely infiltrating tumors often are not distinguishable from complicated cholecystitis or xanthogranulomatous cholecystitis. The latter is a xanthogranulomatous reaction to intramural extravasation of bile caused by rupture of a Rokitansky-Aschoff sinus. Adenopathy in either the peripancreatic region or the porta hepatis may be so prominent that a misdiagnosis of carcinoma of the pancreas or cholangiocarcinoma is made, respectively.

Computed Tomography

The most common CT finding in carcinoma of the gallbladder is a slightly enhancing mass in

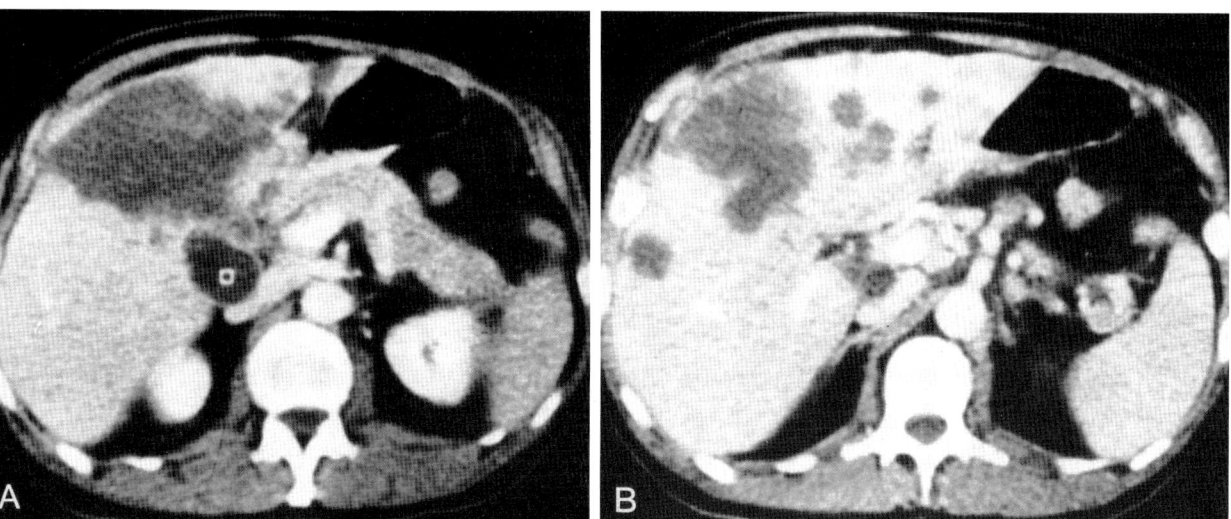

FIGURE 13.28. CT SCAN OF GALLBLADDER CARCINOMA SHOWING MASSIVE LIVER INVASION
A: Residual gallbladder lumen (cursor) and large intrahepatic mass. B: Multiple liver metastases.

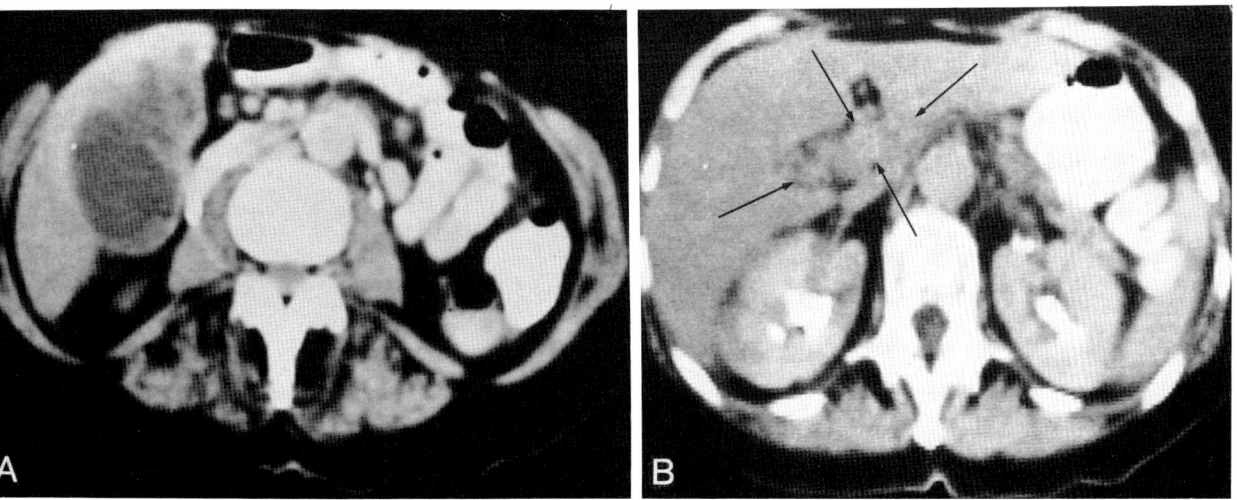

FIGURE 13.29. SONOGRAPHY OF ADENOPATHY DUE TO GALLBLADDER CARCINOMA
A: Irregularly thick-walled, massively enlarged gallbladder with some intraluminal mass caused by gallbladder carcinoma.
B: More cephalad scan in the same patient: peribiliary nodes extending up into the porta hepatis (*arrows*).

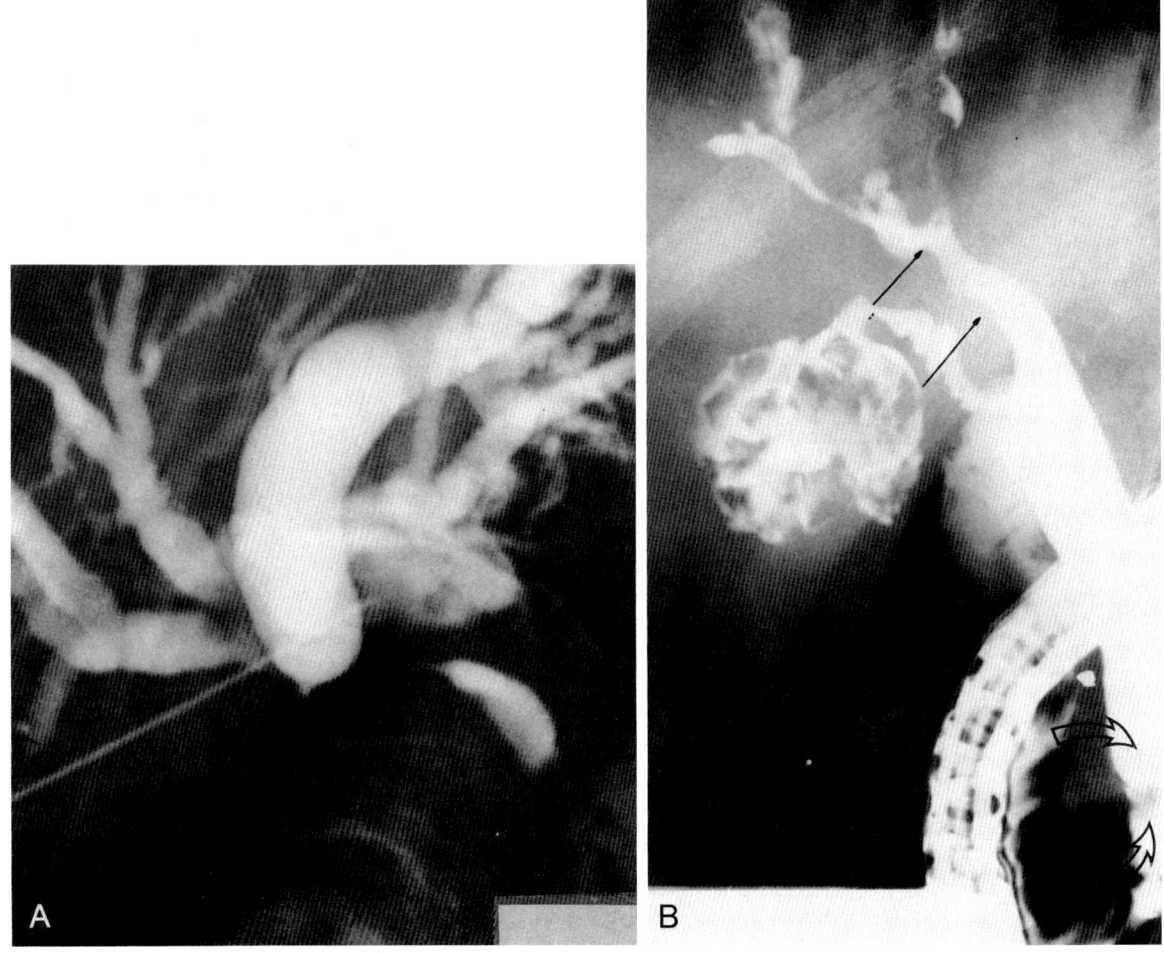

FIGURE 13.30. DIRECT CHOLANGIOGRAPHY OF GALLBLADDER CARCINOMA, TWO DIFFERENT CASES
A: PTC: obstruction high in the porta hepatis, direct extension of gallbladder carcinoma. *B:* ERCP: encasement of the bifurcation and mass effect on the common hepatic duct (*arrows*). Note gallstones and the incidental common duct stones (*curves arrows*).

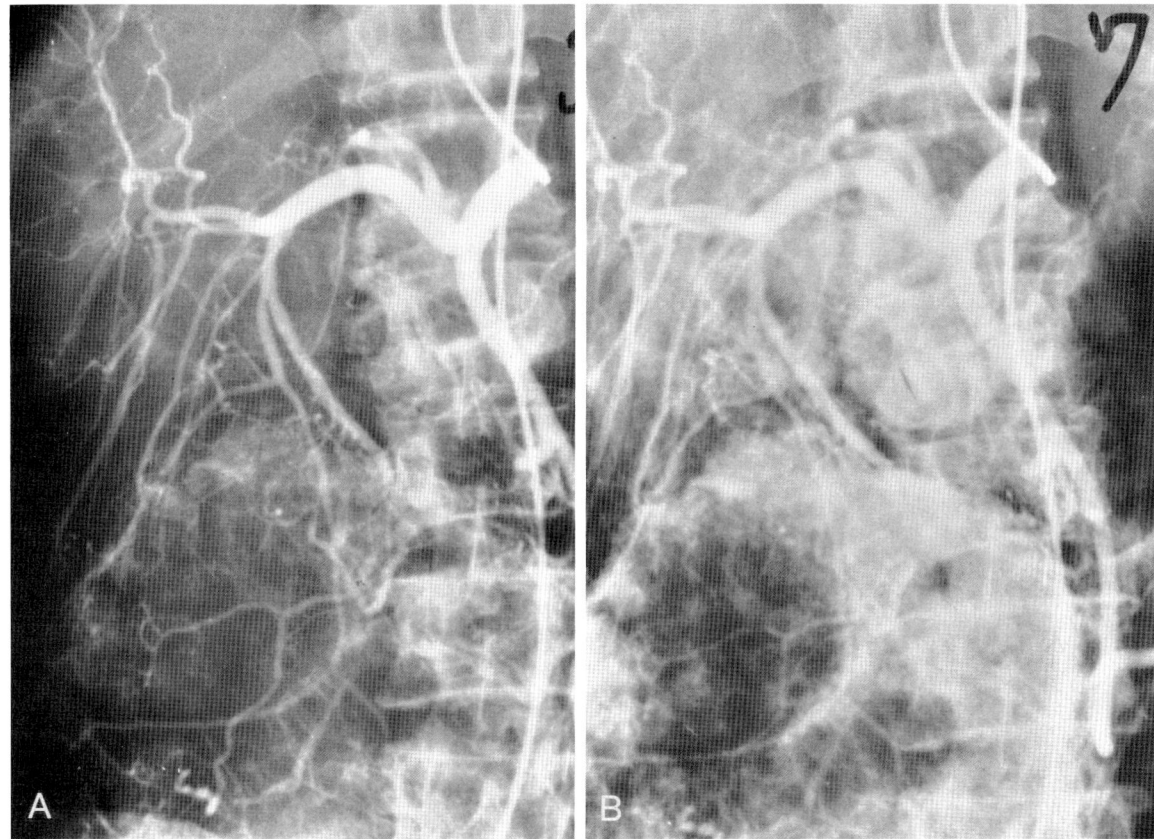

FIGURE 13.31. ANGIOGRAPHY OF GALLBLADDER CARCINOMA
A: Hepatic arteriogram, early. *B:* Late arterial phase. Arteriograms show enlarged cystic artery branches, neovascularity, and tumor blush caused by a large gallbladder carcinoma.

the region of the gallbladder that replaces most or all of the gallbladder (Fig. 13.25C). Direct extension into the adjacent liver is quite frequent, and manifests itself first as an ill-defined border and then as a low density region of hepatic parenchyma (Fig. 13.28) (11–13).

Less common configurations are irregular (or smooth) wall thickening and intraluminal masses (Fig. 13.29A). Both types exhibit mild to moderate contrast enhancement, and are difficult to distinguish from complicated cholecystitis unless ancillary findings of malignancy are present. Liver invasion is less commonly seen than with the massive configuration described above (11–13). Interestingly, while contrast enhancement improves depiction of wall thickening and intraluminal mass in gallbladder carcinoma, it may raise the attenuation of any extraluminal mass present to that of hepatic parenchyma, thereby obscuring it. Thus, optimal depiction may require plain and enhanced scans.

Ancillary findings in descending order of frequency include: gallstones, wall calcification, dilated intra or extra hepatic bile ducts, lymphadenopathy (peripancreatic, pericholedochal (Fig. 13.29B), paraaortic) ascites, hepatic metastases, coexisting empyema with intraluminal gas, and extension into stomach or duodenum. All except gallstones and intraluminal gas are helpful in staging and differentiation from complicated cholecystitis. Biliary obstruction at the level of the porta is due to direct extension up the hepatoduodenal ligament or adenopathy, while obstruction of the common bile duct is from peripancreatic adenopathy or intraductal tumor spread (13, 14).

Cholangiography

In general, patients with gallbladder carcinoma who come to cholangiography will have fairly advanced disease. Infiltration, encasement, and obstruction of the common duct in the region of the cystic duct with nonfilling of the gallbladder are characteristic but not pathognomonic. Obstruction by nodes in the region of the pancreas or porta hepatis can be the major findings

(Fig. 13.30). Rarely, the common duct will be normal and an irregular obstruction of the cystic duct to carcinoma of the gallbladder can be shown by retrograde filling (15). Even more rarely, the gallbladder will fill and the carcinoma can be demonstrated as an irregular filling defect within the lumen.

Angiography

Prior to the advent of ultrasound and CT, angiography was used in both the diagnosis and staging of gallbladder cancer (16–19). Findings include enlargement of the cystic artery, irregular and interrupted arteries in the gallbladder wall, uneven wall thickness, minimal neovascularity, and mild tumor blush (Fig. 13.31). Liver involvement is manifested by neovascularity off the right hepatic artery, early filling of hepatic veins, tumor blush and defects in the hepatogram. Lymph node metastases cause arterial and/or venous displacement or encasement.

REFERENCES

1. Schoenfeld LJ: *Diseases of the Gallbladder and Biliary System* (Clinical Gastroenterology Monographs). New York, John Wiley & Sons, 1977.
2. Harolds JA, Dennehy DC: Preoperative diagnosis of gallbladder carcinoma by ultrasonography. *South Med J* 74:1024–1025, 1981.
3. Carter SJ, Rutledge J, Hirsch JH, Vracko R, Chikos PM: Papillary adenoma of the gallbladder: ultrasonic demonstration. *J Clin Ultrasound* 6:433–435, 1978.
4. Vaittenen E: Carcinoma of the gallbladder. A study of 390 cases diagnosed in Finland from 1953–1967. *Ann Chir Gynaecol Fenn (Suppl)* 59:168, 1970.
5. Vaittenen E: Carcinoma of the gallbladder. *Ann Chir Gynaecol Fenn* 59:47, 1970.
6. Raghavendra BN: Ultrasonographic features of primary carcinoma of the gallbladder: report of five cases. *Gastrointest Radiol* 5:239–244, 1980.
7. Bondestam S: Sonographic diagnosis of primary carcinoma of the gallbladder. *Diagn Imaging* 50:197–200, 1981.
8. Yeh HC: Ultrasonography and computed tomography of carcinoma of the gallbladder. *Radiology* 133:167–173, 1979.
9. Dalla Palma L, Rizzatto G, Pozzi-Mucelli RS, Bazzocchi M: Grey-scale ultrasonography in the evaluation of carcinoma of the gallbladder. *Br J Radiol* 53:662–667, 1980.
10. Weiner SN, Koenigsberg M, Morehouse H, Hoffman J: Sonography and computed tomography in the diagnosis of carcinoma of the gallbladder. *AJR* 142:735–739, 1984.
11. Ruiz R, Teyssou H, Fernandez et al: Ultrasonic diagnosis of primary carcinoma of the gallbladder: a review of 16 cases. *J Clin Ultrasound* 8:489–495, 1980.
12. Itai Y, Araki T, Yoshikawa K, Furui S, Yashiro N, Tasaka A: Computed tomography of gallbladder carcinoma. *Radiology* 137:713–718, 1980.
13. Weiner SN, Koenigsberg M, Morehouse H, Hoffman J: Sonography and computed tomography in the diagnosis of carcinoma of the gallbladder. *AJR* 142:735–739, 1984.
14. Thorsen MK, Quiroz F, Lawson TL, Smith DF, Foley WD, Stewart ET: Primary biliary carcinoma: CT evaluation. *Radiology* 152:479–483, 1984.
15. McNulty JG: Preoperative diagnosis of carcinoma of the gallbladder by percutaneous transhepatic cholangiography. *AJR* 101:605–607, 1967.
16. Abrams RM, Meng C-H, Firooznia H et al: Angiographic demonstration of carcinoma of the gallbladder. *Radiology* 94:277–282, 1970.
17. Kido C, Hibino K, Kaneko M et al: Angiography of gallbladder cancer. *Nippon Acta Radiol* 34:1–11, 1974.
18. Gothlin J, Petterson H: Angiography in malignant and chronic inflammatory lesions of the gallbladder. *Acta Radiol Diagn* 17:343–352, 1976.
19. Sprayregen SS, Messinger NH: Carcinoma of the gallbladder: diagnosis and evaluation of regional spread by angiography. *AJR* 116:382–392, 1972.

Other Gallbladder Malignancies

As noted above, 85% or more of gallbladder cancer is identifiable as adenocarcinoma. It is almost impossible to quantify the remaining cases because of controversy and overlap in grouping and nomenclature (1). The most common of these unusual tumors is spindle cell sarcoma, but even these have been extensively subdivided into various and overlapping types (2, 3). Malignancies of most of the common mesenchymal tissue types have been described. There is reason to believe that many of those described as anaplastic or undifferentiated sarcomas may actually be anaplastic variants of epithelial carcinomas upon closer examination (4). Occasional biphasic tumors appear to have extensively intermixed foci of malignant elements of both epithelial (carcinoma) and mesenchymal (sarcoma) elements and are referred to as carcinosarcomas (5).

Clinically and radiologically there is little to separate any of these tumors from the more common adenocarcinoma. The age range, female predominance, and association with stones is similar as is the mode of spread and prognosis.

Carcinoid and oat cell carcinomas may occur in the gallbladder and may deserve separate mention because of unique clinical features (6, 7). These arise in Kulschitsky (argentaffin) cells thought to be derived from neural crest tissue. Such tissue is part of the APUD (amine precursor uptake and decarboxylase) system. While carcinoid syndrome has apparently not been seen, the possibility of endocrine function remains. The oat cell tumors have been similar to those in other sites in that they tend to be large at presentation with extensive central necrosis, and are highly lethal. They tend to grow submucosally. Carcinoembryonic antigen (CEA) reactivity has been limited or absent and response to chemotherapy has been better than in adenocarcinoma. Association with stones has not been obvious with carcinoids.

Melanocytes have been shown to occur naturally in the gallbladder and are thought to be derived from neural crest ectoderm. Although metastatic melanoma is much more common, rare isolated melanomas of the gallbladder are considered to be primary (8, 9). The tumors have tended to be large, intraluminal polyps occurring in the absence of other potential primary lesions even on follow-up. Junctional activity indicating transition from adjacent benign melanocytes as seen in primary melanoma in other sites has been demonstrated.

REFERENCES

1. Weedon D: *Pathology of the Gallbladder.* New York: Masson Publishing USA Inc., 1984, pp 240–254.
2. Willen R, Willen H: Primary sarcoma of the gallbladder. A light and electromicroscopical study. *Virchows Arch Pathol Anat* 396:91–102, 1982.
3. Carpentier Y, Lambilliotte JP: Primary sarcoma of gallbladder. *Cancer* 32:493–497, 1973.
4. Appelman HD, Coopersmith N: Pleomorphic spindle-cell carcinoma of the gallbladder. *Cancer* 25:535–541, 1970.
5. Born MW, Ramey WG, Ryan SF, Gordon PE: Carcinosarcoma and carcinoma of the gallbladder. *Cancer* 53:2171–2177, 1984.
6. Bosl GL, Yagoda A, Camara-Lopes LH: Malignant carcinoids of the gallbladder: third reported case and review of the literature. *J Surg Oncol* 13:215–222, 1980.
7. Albores-Saavedra J, Soriano J, Larraza-Hernandez O, Aguirre J, Henson DE: Oat cell carcinoma of the gallbladder. *Hum Pathol* 15:639–646, 1984.
8. Carle G, Lessels AM, Best PV: Malignant melanoma of the gallbladder. *Cancer* 48:2318–2322, 1981.
9. Peison B, Rabin L: Malignant melanoma of the gallbladder. *Cancer* 37:2448–2454, 1976.

Secondary Gallbladder Tumors

Metastatic involvement of the gallbladder may be considered in four forms (1, 2). Systemic, presumably blood-borne, metastases tend to appear as small, flat, subepithelial nodules. With continued growth the nodules progress to intraluminal polyps which may be pedunculated. In 1000 autopsies in cancer patients, 5.8% had gallbladder metastases excluding direct extension (3). Melanoma was the cause of gallbladder metastasis in nearly two thirds in a large series (1). Systemic metastases may also cause subserosal nodules. In a large series of melanoma cases from Memorial Hospital in New York, 15% involved the gallbladder, the majority being subserosal (4).

Direct extension of tumor into the gallbladder occurs from malignancies of adjacent tissues and from metastatic deposits in the porta hepatis. Gastric and pancreatic primaries are the most likely sources.

The serosal surface is commonly involved with implants in cases of diffuse intraperitoneal spread with stomach, colon and ovary the most common sources.

Extensive lymphatic permeation with metastatic tumor has also been described (1).

Radiology

Metastases, especially from melanoma, may appear as small nodules on the luminal surface or as larger irregular filling defects on cholecystograms and cholangiograms (Fig. 13.32) (5–7). Central erosion to form "target" or "bull's eye" lesions common in the rest of the gastrointestinal tract is apparently uncommon in the gall-

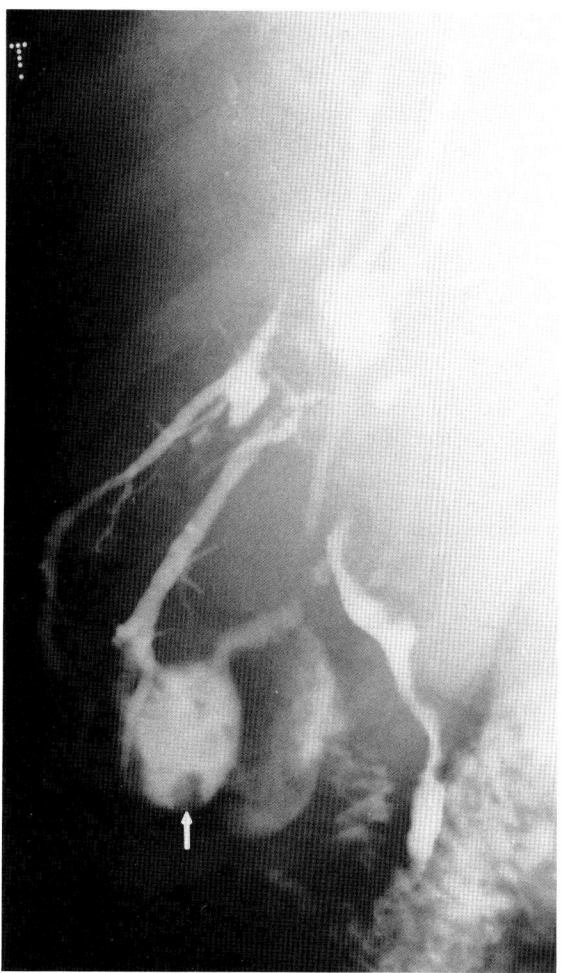

FIGURE 13.32. GALLBLADDER METASTASES
PTC: gallbladder metastases from colon carcinoma appearing as nodular masses. Arrow points to the largest. Peribiliary metastases deform common duct.

LIVER, BILIARY TRACT, PANCREAS, SPLEEN

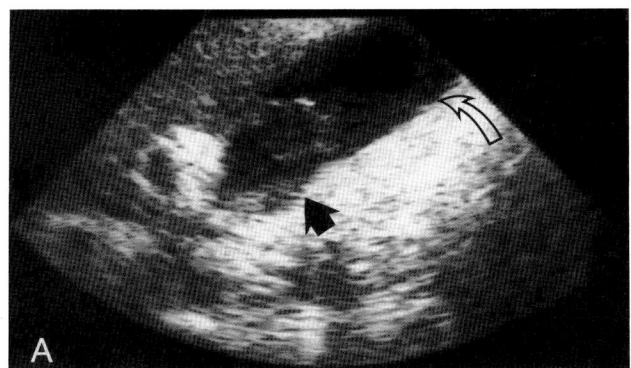

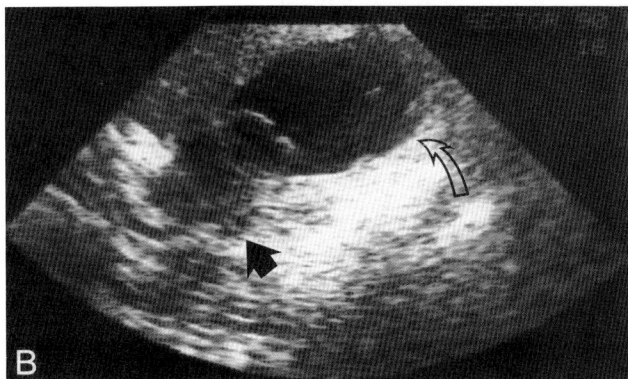
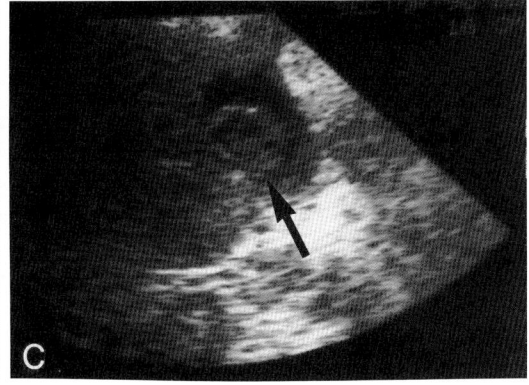

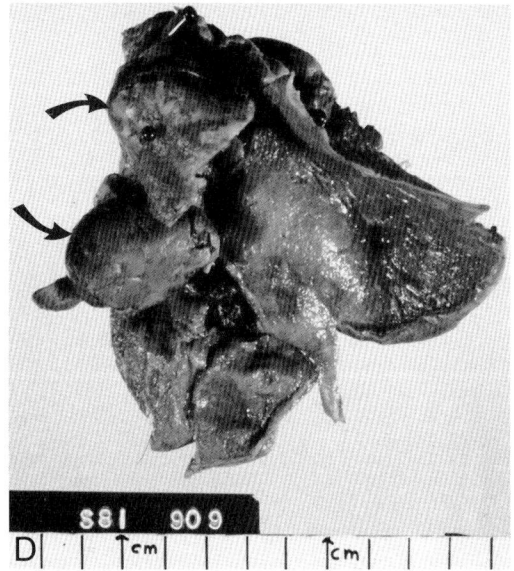

FIGURE 13.33. METASTATIC MELANOMA PRESENTING CLINICALLY AS ACUTE CHOLECYSTITIS

A: Supine, long axis view of the gallbladder: apparent debris (*open arrow*) lying dependent in the gallbladder. A mass is suspected (*closed arrow*) because of the abnormal configuration of the gallbladder neck. *B:* Erect long axis view: lobulated mass (*closed arrow*) in the neck of the gallbladder; debris (*open arrow*) layers out dependently. *C:* Erect transverse view of the gallbladder neck: lobulated sessile mass (*arrow*) partially fills the lumen of the gallbadder. *D:* Resected specimen, opened: metastatic melanoma nodules (*arrows*) attached to the wall in the region of the neck of the gallbladder. (From Bundy AL, Ritchie WG: Ultrasonic diagnosis of metastatic melanoma in the gallbladder presenting as acute cholecystitis. *J Clin Ultrasound* 10:285–287, 1982.)

bladder. As calculi are associated with approximately 90% of primary carcinoma of the gallbladder and are seen only coincidentally with metastases, their absence may provide a differential diagnostic clue (8). Several appearances of metastases to the gallbladder have been seen with ultrasound and would presumably apply to other cross sectional imaging modalities as well (9). Focal thickening of the gallbladder wall, particularly with fixed, nonshadowing, intraluminal soft tissue masses is suggestive. More advanced disease is associated with more diffuse wall thickening and more extensive intraluminal filling defects, often with evidence of central necrosis. Gallbladder metastases can mimic acute cholecystitis clinically and sonography can sometimes suggest the correct diagnosis in this situation (Fig. 13.33) (10).

REFERENCES

1. Willis RA: *The Spread of Tumors in the Human Body*, Ed 2. London, Butterworths, 1952, pp 218–219.
2. Weedon D: *Pathology of the Gallbladder.* New York. Masson Publishing USA Inc., 1984, pp 259–302.
3. Abrams HL, Spiro R, Goldstein N: Metastases in carcinoma. Analysis of 1000 autopsied cases. *Cancer* 3:74–85, 1950.
4. Das Gupta T, Brasfield R: Metastatic melanoma: a clinicopathological study. *Cancer* 17:1323–1339, 1964.
5. Balthazar EJ, Javors B: Malignant melanoma of the gallbladder. *Am J Gastroenterol* 64:332–335, 1975.
6. Goldstein HM, Beydoun MT, Dodd GD: Radiologic spectrum of melanoma metastatic to the gastrointestinal tract. *AJR* 129:605–612, 1977.
7. Shimkin PM, Soloway MS, Jaffe E: Metastatic melanoma of the gallbladder. *AJR* 116:393–395, 1972.
8. Daunt N, King DM: Metastatic melanoma in the biliary tree. *Br J Radiol* 55:873–874, 1982.
9. Phillips G, Pochaczevsky R, Goodman J, Kumari S: Ultrasound patterns of metastatic tumors in the gallbladder. *J Clin Ultrasound* 10:379–383, 1982.
10. Bundy AL, Ritchie WG: Ultrasonic diagnosis of metastatic melanoma in the gallbladder presenting as acute cholecystitis. *J Clin Ultrasound* 10:285–287, 1982.

14

Radiology of Jaundice Including Choledocholithiasis and Biliary Neoplasms

ARNOLD C. FRIEDMAN, M.D., LEORA SACHS, M.D., AND
MARK T. BIRNS, M.D.

JAUNDICE

Diagnostic imaging of the jaundiced patient has advanced dramatically in the last 10 years. It was not uncommon as recently as the early 1970s for a jaundiced patient to have to undergo exploratory laparotomy to rule out biliary obstruction. The rapid evolution in diagnostic ultrasound has rendered obsolete screening tests for biliary obstruction such as infusion hepatotomography and sulfur colloid liver spleen scanning that were touted in the literature as recently as 1979 (1, 2) (Fig. 14.1). Ultrasound plays the pivotal role in evaluating the jaundiced patient by differentiating obstructive from nonobstructive jaundice. However, when positive for obstruction, ultrasound rarely stands alone and usually at least one additional test, generally PTC, ERCP, or CT, is required. When no obstruction is seen, nonobstructive jaundice is usually considered to be the correct diagnosis. If clinical suspicion of obstruction is sufficiently high, however, direct cholangiography should still be performed. Hepatobiliary scintigraphy is extremely useful also in selected cases. Clinicians will find the radiologist who is well versed in interpretation of all these studies to be the most valuable consultant. As in all aspects of diagnostic radiology, clinical correlation is often vital. For example, afferent loop obstruction is not likely to be considered by the radiologist in the differential diagnosis of jaundice unless he knows of the prior surgery (Fig. 14.2).

The fact that laparotomy is rarely needed for differential diagnosis of jaundice and often not required for therapy since percutaneous and endoscopic biopsy and drainage techniques are now widely available should be a source of satisfaction for the medical community.

REFERENCES

1. Cynn WS, Levin BL, Gureghian PA, Chait A: Infusion hepatotomography for evaluation of obstructive jaundice. *AJR* 1323:187–190, 1979.
2. Morin ME, Baker DA, Marsan RE: Demonstration of dilated biliary ducts by total-body opacification. Differentiation of surgical from non-surgical jaundice. *Radiology* 121:307–309, 1976.

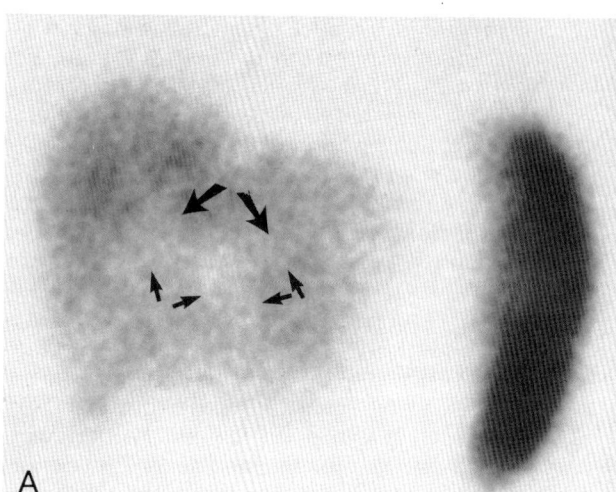
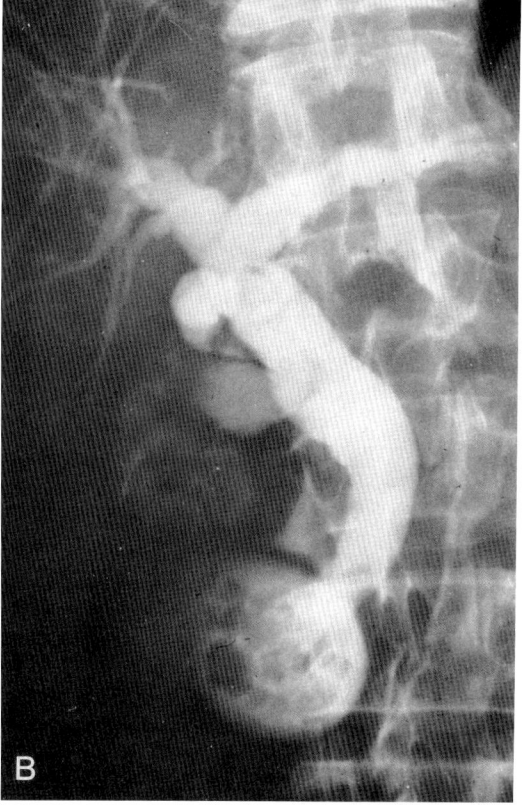

FIGURE 14.1. OBSTRUCTIVE JAUNDICE

Obstructive jaundice differentiated from hepatocellular disease by sulfur-colloid liver spleen scan, a test neither sensitive or specific enough to be used today for this purpose. *A:* Central, linear branching region of decreased activity (*arrows*) representing dilated ducts. Note colloid shift to the spleen. *B:* Corresponding PTC (frontal film) opacifies the dilated biliary tree and shows gallstone. An oblique film (not shown) demonstrated an impacted calculus in the distal common bile duct. Bilirubin was 18, unusually high for benign disease.

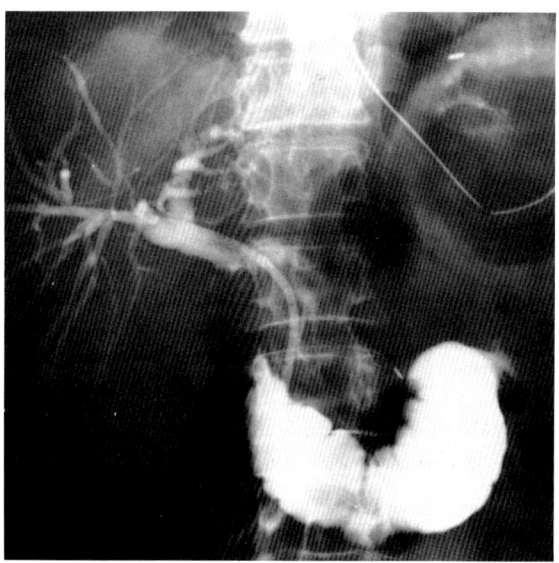

FIGURE 14.2. AFFERENT LOOP OBSTRUCTION FROM CARCINOMA

Biliary drainage demonstrating afferent loop obstruction from recurrent gastric carcinoma post surgical Billroth II gastroenterostomy. Had the clinical history been known, the correct diagnosis could have been sought by sonography or CT.

Sonography

Accuracy

Sonography is almost as accurate as CT or direct cholangiography in distinguishing obstructive from nonobstructive jaundice. However, it is not nearly as good as these other modalities in pinpointing the exact level or cause of obstruction. Nevertheless, it is the preferred screening procedure because of its rapidity, noninvasiveness, and relatively low cost. Early studies reported accuracies of 82–94% (1–4). More recent studies report less favorable results. Baron et al. (5) compared CT and sonography in the evaluation of jaundice. The latter defined the level of obstruction in 60% and the cause in 38%, whereas the former correctly localized the site in 88% and the cause in 70%. Another study (6) determined the site in only 27% and the etiology in 30% using ultrasound. These low percentages can be attributed to several factors. There can be a high rate of technical failure in depicting the entire course of the common duct due to overlying bowel gas or obesity. The most common problem is the failure to detect calculi in nondilated common ducts. Small ampullary tumors are not seen. Metastatic pancreatic carcinoma can be hard to differentiate from lymphoma and pancreatic neoplasms may be hard to distinguish from inflammatory masses. Infiltrative cholangiocarcinoma may mimic an inflammatory or traumatic stricture, although abrupt termination of the common duct usually indicates malignancy or a calculus whereas smooth tapering is associated with a benign stricture (7).

The most common causes of biliary obstruction are pancreatic carcinoma (26–47%) and choledocholithiasis (19–42%) (8). Less common etiologies include intra and extrahepatic neoplasms, pancreatitis, parasitic diseases such as ascariasis, and recurrent pyogenic cholangitis. Liver cysts, especially in polycystic liver disease, may cause common duct obstruction (9–11). A gallstone impacted in the cystic duct may cause common hepatic duct obstruction (Mirizzi syndrome). Aortic aneurysm is another unusual cause of common duct obstruction (12).

Discrepancies between the Degree of Jaundice and Duct Size

The size of the biliary tree does not always correspond to the clinical degree of jaundice. Patients may have duct dilatation without obstruction, obstruction with normal enzymes, and obstruction without dilatation.

Biliary dilatation has been reported in nonjaundiced patients (13–15). Although the serum bilirubin is not elevated, the alkaline phosphatase is elevated in 75–80%, and serum GGTP is even more sensitive. This clinical situation is usually found with early or partial obstruction. Patients with choledocholithiasis often have intermittent obstruction with a ball-valve effect. About half of patients with common duct stones are not jaundiced (15). Slowly enlarging tumors may produce biliary dilatation prior to clinically demonstrable jaundice. Patients who have obstruction of only one of the two major intrahepatic ducts (or segmental ductal obstruction) leading to segmental intrahepatic biliary dilatation will not be jaundiced although they will usually have chemical abnormalities. For this reason, it is vital to scan the entire biliary tree (13, 16). Conversely, there are patients with obvious jaundice due to obstruction who have nondilated biliary systems. Beinart et al. (17) reported 9% nondilated but obstructed systems in a series of 150 percutaneous cholangiograms. Muhletaler et al. (18) reported nine similar patients. These cases included patients with both partial and complete obstructions. Explanations for this phenomenon include acute obstruction without time to dilate, ball-valve effect, and periductal tumor growth or scarring preventing dilatation.

A time lag is known to exist between the onset of obstruction and the demonstration of ductal dilatation, although the precise time is unknown (19–21). The gallbladder can function as a reservoir, decompressing the biliary tree during the first 24 hours of obstruction. Additional observations indicate that the distal common duct alone may dilate while the proximal common duct remains normal. Extrahepatic ducts are thought to dilate prior to intrahepatic ducts, according to LaPlace's law, although some investigators think that peripheral biliary dilatation is a sensitive indicator of obstruction. Assessment of early peripheral biliary dilatation may be quite subjective: a 1–2 mm separation of the walls of peripheral ductules and the demonstration of parallel channels (duct anterior to portal venule) are useful indicators of peripheral dilatation (Fig. 14.3) (22, 23). In cases of relatively short periods of obstruction, biliary ducts will return to normal, particularly with benign disease. This has been observed to occur as rapidly as within 43 hr, and as slowly as 1 week (19, 24). With repetitive episodes or longstanding obstruction, the elastic fibers in the biliary tree are damaged leading to a "floppy" duct (19). The floppy duct is normal in size in its undisturbed

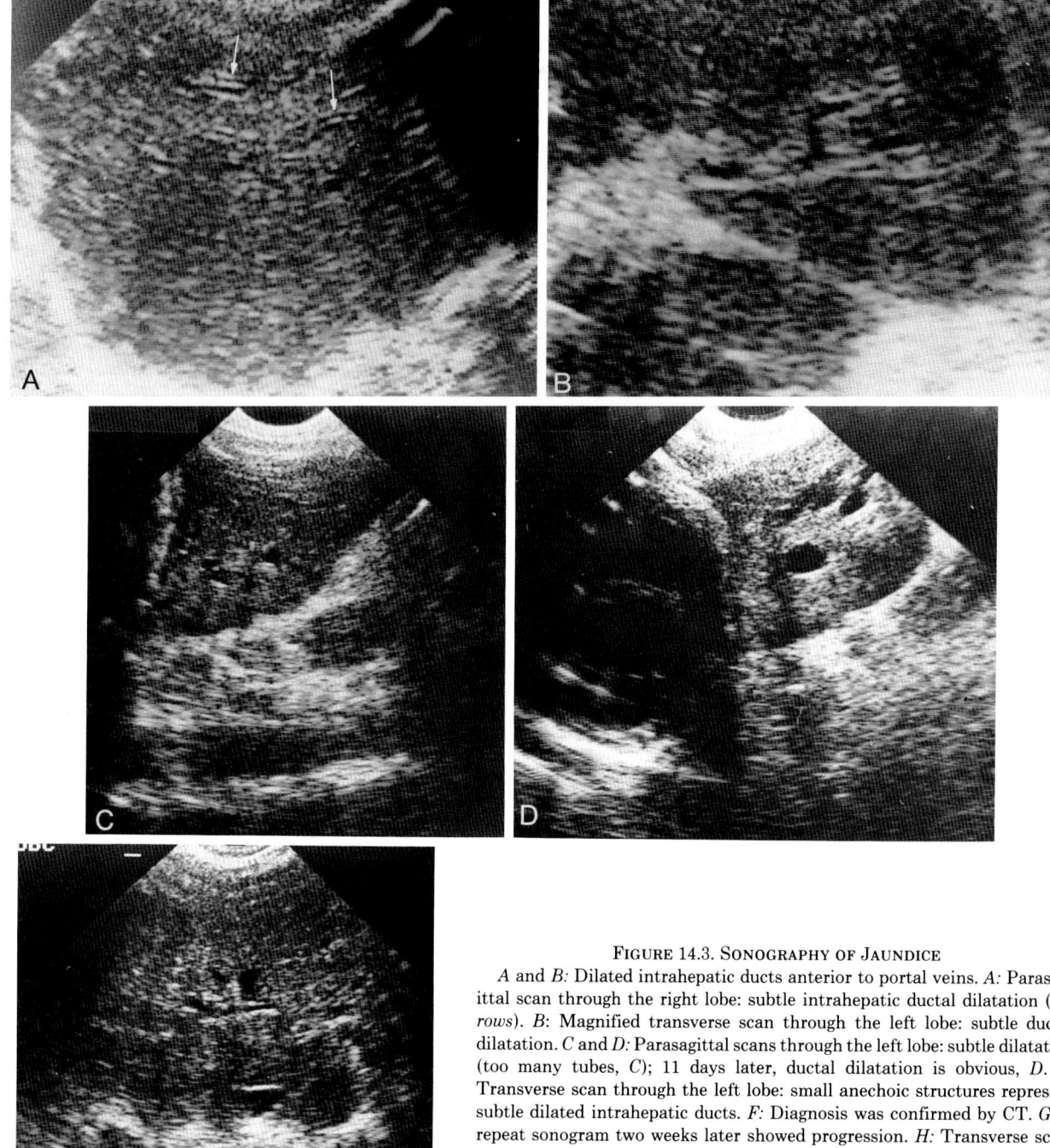

FIGURE 14.3. SONOGRAPHY OF JAUNDICE

A and *B:* Dilated intrahepatic ducts anterior to portal veins. *A:* Parasagittal scan through the right lobe: subtle intrahepatic ductal dilatation (*arrows*). *B*: Magnified transverse scan through the left lobe: subtle duct dilatation. *C* and *D:* Parasagittal scans through the left lobe: subtle dilatation (too many tubes, *C*); 11 days later, ductal dilatation is obvious, *D*. Transverse scan through the left lobe: small anechoic structures represent subtle dilated intrahepatic ducts. *F:* Diagnosis was confirmed by CT. *G:* repeat sonogram two weeks later showed progression. *H:* Transverse scan gross intrahepatic ductal dilatation. *I:* Transverse scan: dilated left and right main hepatic ducts (*arrows*) anterior to portal vein.

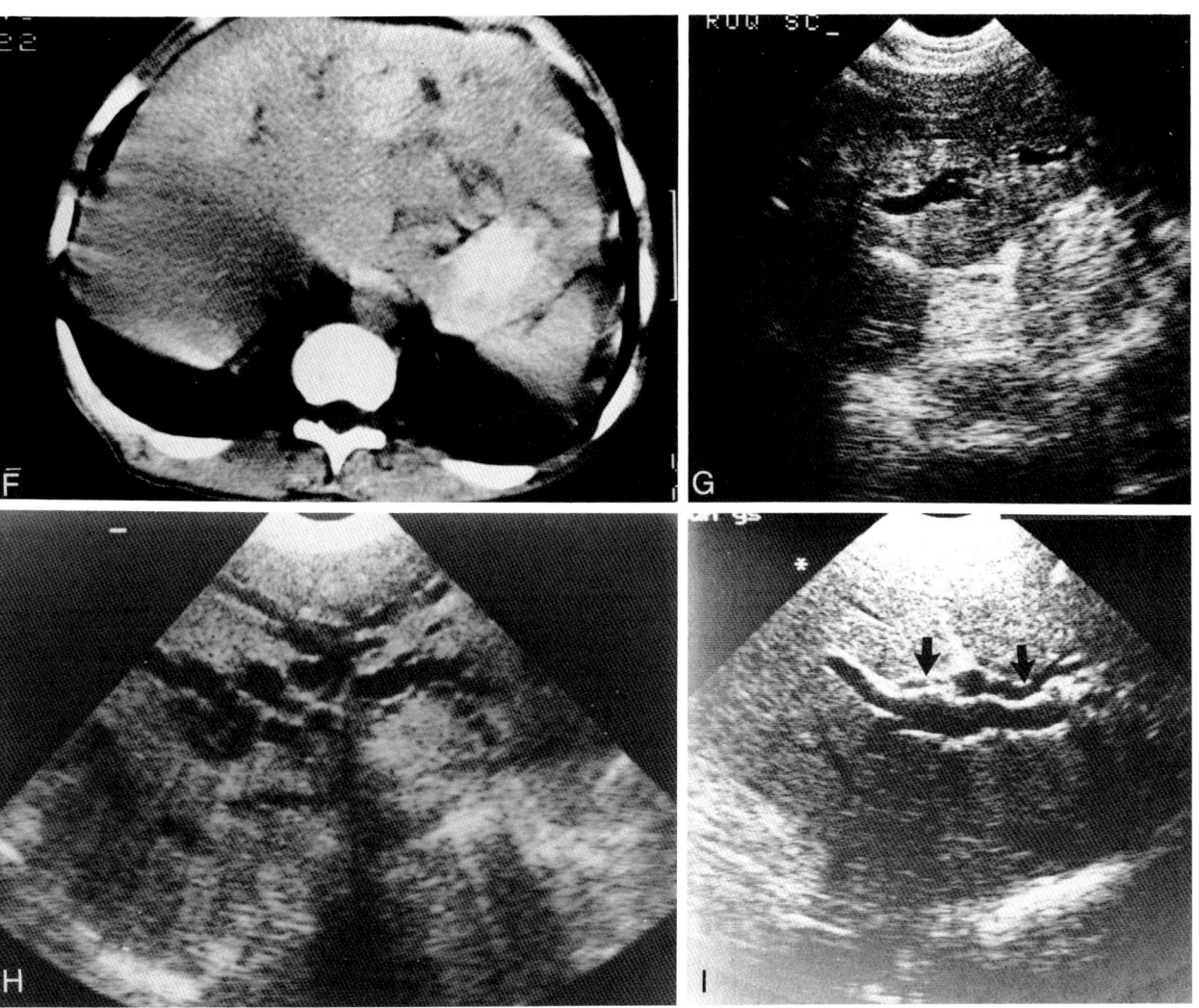

FIGURE 14.3*F–I*

state (i.e., during sonography). However, under the pressure of an injection during cholangiography, it will dilate to an abnormal size. The duration and magnitude of obstruction required to product irreversible ductal dilatation is not known.

Sequential scanning of the biliary tree in monkeys with surgical common bile duct ligation has confirmed clinical observations (25). Dilatation of the gallbladder and distal common duct occurs at about 24 hr. Dilatation progresses proximally with intrahepatic ducts affected at about 1 week. Bilirubin elevation was first detected within 48–72 hr. After release of the obstruction, dilatation resolved in reverse order with the distal common duct returning to normal last, at 30–50 days.

REFERENCES

1. Klingensmith WC, Johnson ML, Kuni CC, Dunne MG, Fitzberg AR: Complementary role of ^{99m}Tc diethyl-IDA and ultrasound in large and small duct biliary tract obstruction. *Radiology* 138:177–184, 1981.
2. Vas W, Salem S: Accuracy of sonography and transhepatic cholangiography in obstructive jaundice. *J Can Assoc Radiol* 32:111–113, 1981.
3. Haubek A, Pederson JH, Burcharth F, Gammelgaard J, Hancke S, Willumsen L: Dynamic sonography in the evaluation of jaundice. *AJP* 136:1071–1074, 1981.
4. Koenigsberg M, Wiener SN, Walzer A: The accuracy of sonography in the differential diagnosis of obstructive jaundice: a comparison with cholangiography. *Radiology* 133:157–165, 1979.
5. Baron RL, Stanley RJ, Lee JT et al: A prospective comparison of the evaluation of biliary obstruction using computed tomography and ultrasonography. *Radiology* 145:91–98, 1982.

6. Honickman SP, Mueller PR, Wittenberg J et al: Ultrasound in obstructive jaundice: prospective evaluation of site and cause. *Radiology* 147:511–515, 1983.
7. Jones TB, Dubuisson RL, Hughes JJ, Robinson AE: Abrupt termination of the common bile duct: a sign of malignancy identified by high-resolution real-time sonography. *J Ultrasound Med* 2:345–348, 1983.
8. Sauerbrei EE: Ultrasound of the common bile duct. *Ultrasound Annu.* 1–45, 1983.
9. Hollinsworth AB: Letter to the editor. *JAMA* 247:462, 1981.
10. Clinkscales NB, Trigg LP, Poklepovic J: Obstructive jaundice secondary to benign hepatic cyst. *Radiology* 154:643, 1985.
11. Ergun H, Wolf BH, Hissong SL: Obstructive jaundice caused by polycystic liver disease. *Radiology* 136:435–436, 1980.
12. Spinelli GD, Kleinclaus DH, Wenger JJ, Christman DL, Matter DF, Warter PC: Obstructive jaundice and abdominal aortic aneurysm: an ultrasonographic study. *Radiology* 144:872, 1982.
13. Zeman R, Taylor KJ, Burrell MI, Gold J: Ultrasound demonstration of anicteric dilatation of the biliary tree. *Radiology* 134:689–692, 1980.
14. Weinstein DP, Weinstein BJ, Brodmerkel GJ: Ultrasonography of biliary tract dilatation without jaundice. *AJR* 132:729–734, 1979.
15. Weinstein BJ, Weinstein DP: Biliary tract dilatation in the nonjaundiced patient. *AJR* 134:899–906, 1980.
16. Myracle MR, Stadalnik RC, Blaisdell FW, Farkas JP, Matin P: Segmental biliary obstruction: diagnostic significance of bile duct crowding. *AJR* 137:169–171, 1981.
17. Beinart C, Efremidis S, Cohen B, Mitty HA: Obstruction without dilatation importance in evaluating jaundice. *JAMA* 245:353–356, 1981.
18. Muhletaler CA, Gerlock AJ, Fleischer AC, James AE: Diagnosis of obstructive jaundice with nondilated bile ducts. *AJR* 134:1149–1152, 1980.
19. Mueller PR, Ferrucci JT, Simeone JF, vanSonnenberg E, Hall DA, Wittenberg J: Observation on the distensibility of the common duct. *Radiology* 142:467–472, 1982.
20. Floyd JL, Collins TL: Discordance of sonography and cholescintigraphy in acute biliary obstruction. *AJR* 140:501–502, 1983.
21. Scheske GA, Cooperberg PL, Cohen MM, Burhenne HJ: Dynamic changes in the caliber of the major bile ducts, related to obstruction. *Radiology* 135:215–216, 1980.
22. Conrad MR, Landay MJ, Janes JO: Sonographic "parallel channel" sign of biliary tree enlargement in mild to moderate obstructive jaundice. *AJR* 130:279–286, 1978.
23. Weill F, Eisenchar A, Zeitner F: Ultrasonic study of the normal and dilated biliary tree. *Radiology* 127:221–224, 1978.
24. Gooding GA: Acute bile duct dilation with resolution in 43 hours: an ultrasonic demonstration. *J Clin Ultrasound* 9:201–202, 1981.
25. Shawker TH, Jones BL, Girton ME: Distal common bile duct obstruction: an experimental study in monkeys. *J Clin Ultrasound* 9:77–82, 1981.

Computed Tomography

Current third and fourth generation CT is accurate in detecting dilated bile ducts (thus differentiating obstructive from nonobstructive jaundice) in over 95% of patients (1, 2). Second generation equipment had only a 75% success rate (3, 4). False negatives occur in that some patients truly have obstruction without measurable biliary dilatation, and false positives occur in patients with dilated ducts but no obstruction. Relative frequency of false negatives and false positives depends on where one wishes to be on a receiver operating curve. Intermittently obstructing calculi or subtle strictures/ampullary stenosis may be missed (5), and some form of direct cholangiography should be resorted to when clinical data are suggestive of intermittent or low grade obstruction despite negative CT and sonography. Similarly, some patients with dilated ducts and no other pathology will need direct cholangiography to prove absence of obstruction.

CT is also quite reliable in demonstrating the level of obstruction and its etiology. In one large series, the level of obstruction was shown in 97% and its etiology (using clinical data such as presence or absence of a primary as well as CT appearance) correctly determined in 94% (4).

As with sonography, it is not uncommon to see dilated extrahepatic ducts on CT in the absence of dilated intrahepatic ducts in patients with obstructive jaundice. Better visualization of the extrahepatic duct accounts for most of the improvement going from second generation scanners to more advanced equipment (3). Slight peripheral ductal dilatation seen on sonography may still be missed on CT because of partial voluming and other artifacts (6).

Dilated intrahepatic bile ducts are depicted as linear, branching or circular structures of near water density, which enlarge and become confluent as they approach the porta hepatis (Fig. 14.4A and B). Visualization of any portion of the intrahepatic biliary tree (in the absence of biliary air or cholangiographic contrast material) implies dilated ducts (7). On noncontrast scans or when levels of urographic contrast material are low, the biliary tree can usually be differentiated from portal veins by comparison to the inferior vena cava. The former will be less dense than the cava, whereas the latter will be isodense (8). As one scans down through the pancreas from the porta hepatis, dilated extrahepatic ducts appear as a series of low density rings (Fig. 14.4C–F). If the level of obstruction is in the porta at the bifurcation, no rings will be seen. If it is suprapancreatic, one to two rings will be seen. Pancreatic obstructions result in three to six rings and ampullary obstruction in seven to eight rings (the above assumes 10 mm slices at 10 mm intervals) (1). Most physicians do not count rings but determine the level of obstruction by com-

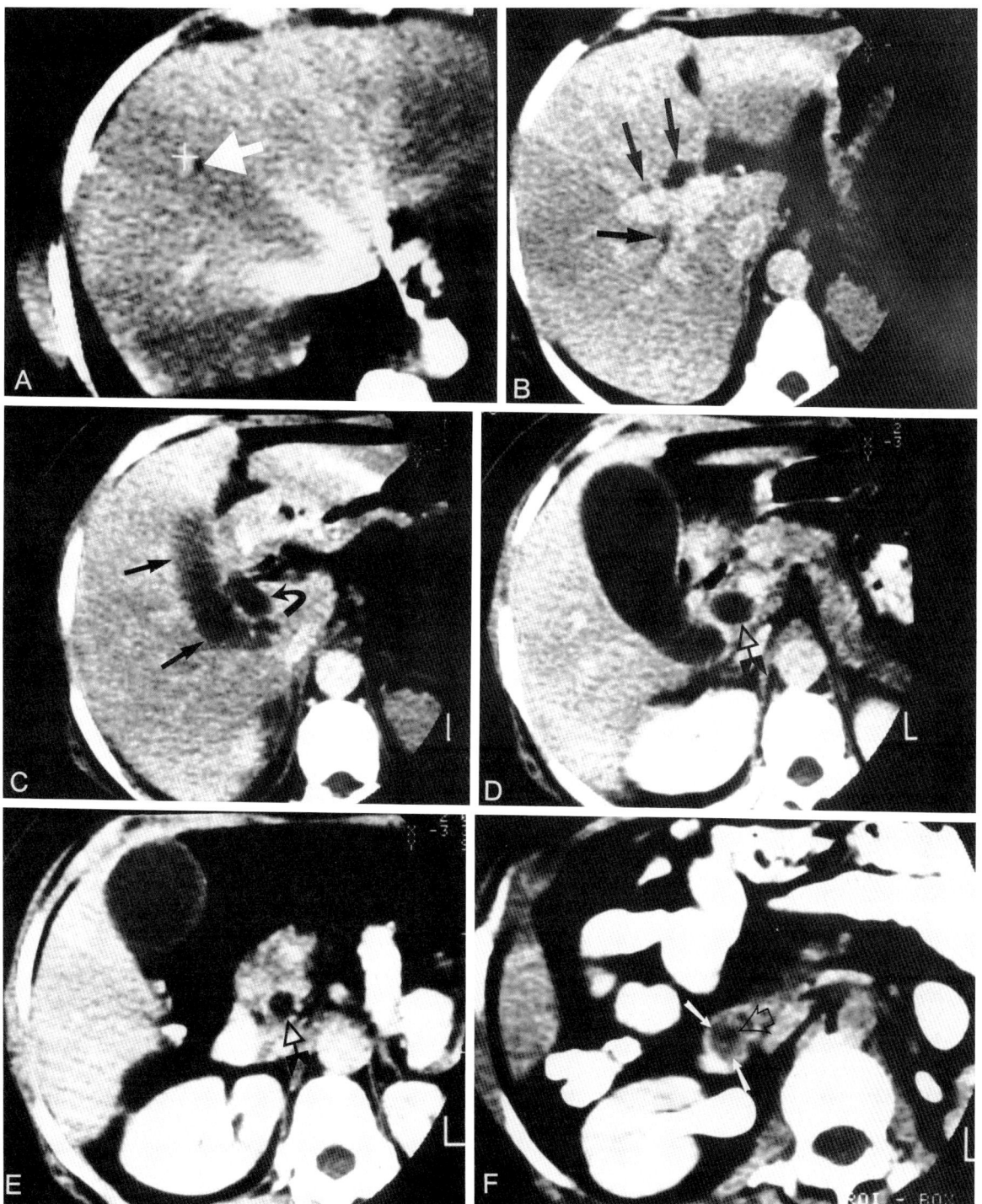

FIGURE 14.4. CT OF JAUNDICE

CT scan of ampullary carcinoma with high-dose contrast enhancement showing excellent delineation of dilated ducts. *A:* Dilated peripheral duct (*arrow*) adjacent to a portal vein branch (*cross*). *B:* Dilated ducts approaching the porta hepatis (*arrows*). *C:* Dilated, slightly transverse common duct (*curved arrow*) just above the pancreas medial to the gallbladder (*arrows*). *D* and *E:* Dilated common bile duct in the head of the pancreas (*arrow*). *F:* Stellate configuration (*open arrow*) of the abrupt termination within a soft tissue mass (*arrows*) at the ampulla.

paring the last dilated ductal segment to the adjacent anatomy. Absolute diameter measurements are less useful and less accurate than in sonography (see discussion of CT of the normal biliary tree in Chapter 9). It is important to visualize a normal duct below the level of obstruction to be certain of the correct level and avoid being fooled when the duct is horizontal or tortuous. The size of the gallbladder is not reliable in determining a level of obstruction (1). When the left hepatic duct is more dilated than the right, it may or may not indicate a local problem. Sometimes the left is more dilated than the right by virtue of its longer extrahepatic course. The converse is rarely the case without a localized abnormality being present (1).

In attempting to differentiate malignant from benign obstruction, many factors need to be analyzed. The degree of intrahepatic or extrahepatic dilatation is not absolutely reliable, although very large intrahepatic ducts do suggest malignancy. Isolated extrahepatic dilatation is frequently benign (stone). A long dilated horizontal segment of extrahepatic duct can be seen in either benign or malignant disease. Abrupt termination over 1.5 cm or less in the absence of a calculus with or without mass suggests malignancy, and gradual tapering over 2 cm or more suggests benignity (2, 4). The configuration of the last ring of the dilated ductal system has been analyzed: irregularity (triangular, stellate, or nodular) suggests malignancy (Fig. 14.4F), as does a nipple (one or two tiny rings below the last large ring) or a rounded configuration (last ring is followed by nonvisualization). Multiple rings gradually decreasing in size correlate with a tapered, long-segment stenosis consistent with benignity (4). The above analysis is subject to the same caveats as an analysis of the configuration of a stricture or an obstruction on a cholangiogram. Finally, a soft tissue mass surrounding a biliary obstruction suggests malignancy quite strongly, with the exceptions of a focal pancreatitis, the occasional benign neoplasm, and rarely, inflammatory adenopathy.

Localized, segmental intrahepatic biliary dilatation is well demonstrated by CT. These patients are often not jaundiced, and may have only an elevated alkaline phosphatase. Differential diagnosis includes intrahepatic calculi, recurrent pyogenic cholangitis, sclerosing cholangitis, congenital fibropolycystic diseases, and intrahepatic metastases (5, 9). The etiology can usually be worked out from the CT. When segmental obstruction is chronic, the affected ducts will be crowded together, the parenchyma that they drain will be atrophic and the remainder of the liver may undergo compensatory hypertrophy (10).

REFERENCES

1. Pedrosa CS, Casanova R, Rodriquez R: Computed tomography in obstructive jaundice. *Radiology* 139:627–634, 1981.
2. Baron RL, Stanley RJ, Lee JKT, Koehler RE, Levitt RG: Computed tomographic features of biliary obstruction. *AJR* 140:1173–1178, 1983.
3. Shimizu H, Ida M, Takayama S, Seki T, Yoneda M, Nakaya S, Yanagi T, Bando B, Sato S, Uchiyama M, Okumura T, Miura S, Fujisawa M: The diagnostic accuracy of computed tomography in obstructive biliary disease: a comparative evaluation with direct cholangiography. *Radiology* 138:411–416, 1981.
4. Pedrosa CS, Casanova R, Lezana AH, Fernandez MC: Computed tomography in obstructive jaundice. *Radiology* 139:635–645, 1981.
5. Ferrucci JT, Adson MA, Mueller PR, Stanley RJ, Stewart ET: Advances in the radiology of jaundice: a symposium and review. *AJR* 141:1–20, 1983.
6. Zeman RK, Dorfman GS, Burrell MI, Stein S, Berg GR, Gold JA: Disparate dilatation of the intrahepatic and extrahepatic bile ducts in surgical jaundice. *Radiology* 138:129–136, 1981.
7. Koehler RE, Stanley RJ: Computed tomography of the gallbladder and bile ducts. In Berk RN, Ferrucci JT Jr, Leopold GR (eds): *Radiology of the Gallbladder and Bile Ducts, Diagnosis and Intervention.* Philadelphia, W. B. Saunders, 1983, pp 245–252.
8. Haaga JR, Alfidi RJ, Ament A: The biliary system. In Haaga JR, Alfidi RJ eds): *Computed Tomography of the Whole Body.* St. Louis, C. V. Mosby, 1983, pp 628–635.
9. Araki T, Itai Y, Tasaka A: Computed tomography of localized dilatation of the intrahepatic bile ducts. *Radiology* 141:733–736, 1981.
10. Myracle MR, Stadalnik RC, Blaisdell FW, Farkas JP, Matin P: Segmental biliary obstruction: diagnostic significance of bile duct crowding. *AJR* 137:169–171, 1981.

Hepatobiliary Scintigraphy

Radiology has made great strides in the evaluation and treatment of the jaundiced patient. When subacute or chronic obstruction must be differentiated from parenchymal liver disease as the cause of jaundice, ultrasonography remains an excellent noninvasive method for evaluation of the biliary tree. CT, transhepatic cholangiography, and endoscopic retrograde cholangiography can be applied as necessary in the further workup of these patients (1). Currently, as a primary modality, hepatobiliary scintigraphy is of more limited utility, although historically it had played a major role (2–7). When ultrasound or CT is not available, hepatobiliary imaging may provide useful information which will aid in the workup of the jaundiced patient (8–11). Patients with obstructive jaundice typically may demonstrate hepatic uptake and excretion with visualization of the larger biliary radicles to the level of the obstruction (Fig. 14.5) or simply show hepatic uptake with delayed or absent excretion of the tracer into the intestine and nonvisualization of the biliary system (Fig. 14.6). Patients with hepatocellular disease may exhibit decreased hepatic uptake with commensurately diminished excretion and visualization of nondilated common duct and intestine (Fig. 14.7) or depressed hepatic uptake with biliary nonvisualization and delayed or absent bowel visualization (Fig. 14.8). It has been demonstrated in humans (12–15) and in dogs (16) that ^{99m}Tc-IDA studies are highly sensitive in detecting early acute obstruction prior to the development of dilated ducts or jaundice. When early or low-grade obstruction is suspected in patients with mildly abnormal liver function, hepatobiliary scanning should be considered when the ultrasound examination is normal (12, 14, 15). Segmental bile duct obstruction from carcinoma (10, 17) or stones (18, 19) can be evaluated with the cholescintigraphic agents. These findings can vary from uniformly decreased activity in the affected regions (19), dilated ducts proximal to the obstruction (11), a photon-deficient area at the site of the stone(s), photon-deficient branching structures due to the dilated obstructed ducts (17), or even prolonged retention of tracer in the area drained by the obstructed system (20).

The postoperative patient presenting with pain or jaundice presents a different diagnostic problem. Ultrasound examinations may show ductal dilatation from the past obstruction, such as due to the passage of stones, or to previous biliary tract surgery, while the hepatobiliary examination will demonstrate whether the system is functionally patent (14, 21). A spectrum of cholescintigraphic patterns have been observed in patients with postcholecystectomy syndrome (Table 14.1) (21). Of the patients with ductal dilatation and intestinal visualization in less than 1 hr, 85% simply had residual dilatation. The remaining 15% had retained common duct stones (21). Since a small amount of labeled bile

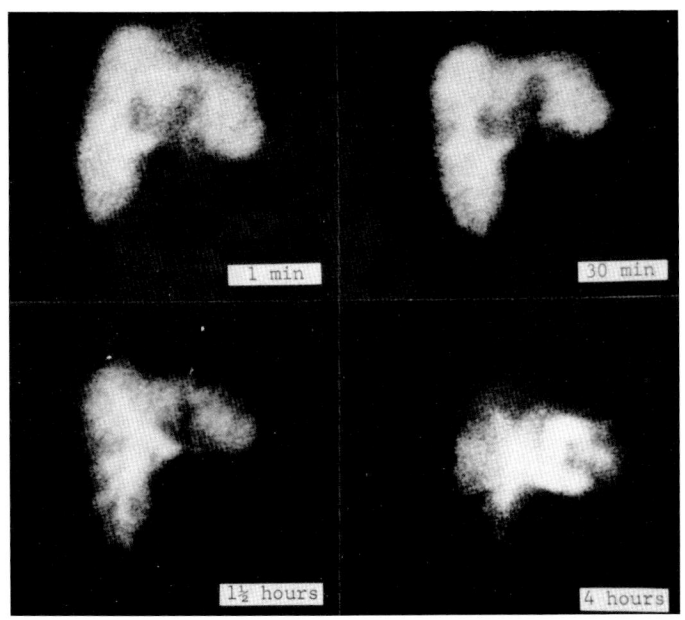

FIGURE 14.5. HEPATOBILIARY SCAN DEPICTING OBSTRUCTED DUCTS

Different degrees of right and left hepatic duct obstruction. The dilated ducts are clearly visualized as branching photon-deficient areas on the 1- and 30-min studies. The right-sided ducts fill in at 1½ hr while the left-sided ducts do not fill until 4 hr. This indicates that the left side is more obstructed at the time of this study. Multiple common and intrahepatic duct stones were found at laparotomy. (From Weissmann HS, Freeman LM: The Biliary Tract. In *Freeman and Johnson's Clinical Radionuclide Imaging*, Orlando, FL, Grune & Stratton, 1984, pp 879–1049.)

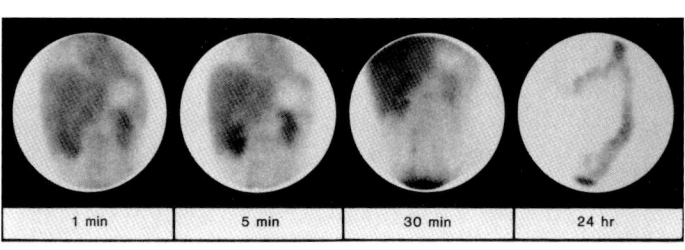

FIGURE 14.6. NON-SPECIFIC HEPATOBILIARY STUDY IN A PATIENT WITH COMMON BILE DUCT OBSTRUCTION

Bilirubin was 12. Note the relatively slow clearance of the hepatobiliary tracer from the blood pool and extensive excretion by the kidneys. By 30 min there is no bowel activity seen. Bowel activity was not present on the one hour and four hour images (which are not included). Activity is seen in the colon on the 24-hr image.

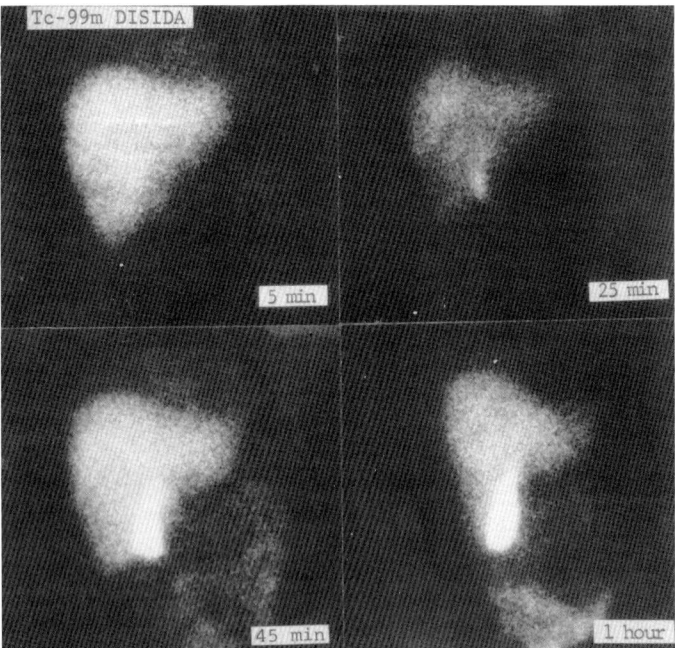

FIGURE 14.7. NONOBSTRUCTIVE JAUNDICE
Normal Tc-99m DISIDA cholescintigram documenting a patent biliary system in a patient whose bilirubin level was 18.5 mg/100 ml. Prompt hepatic uptake is identified within the first 5 min, followed by normal visualization of the common bile duct, gallbladder and intestine within the first 45–60 min. (From Weissmann HS: Cholescintigraphy In Berk, Ferrucci, Leopold: *Radiology of the Gallbladder and Bile Ducts—Diagnosis and Intervention*, Philadelphia, W. B. Saunders, 1983, pp 261–313.)

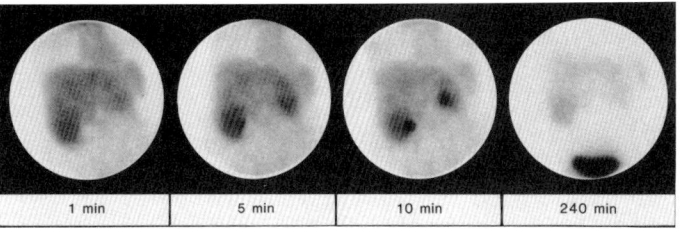

FIGURE 14.8. HEPATOCELLULAR DYSFUNCTION
Hepatobiliary scan on a patient with severe hepatocellular dysfunction. The study shows poor extraction of the tracer from the cardiac blood pool, significant excretion of the material via the kidneys and no activity in the small bowel by 4 hr.

may be able to pass a partially obstructing lesion and result in intestinal visualization in less than 1 hr, the observation of abnormal retention in the common duct is a more significant finding. In the postcholecystectomy patient, an unobstructed common duct should decrease in activity between 1 and 2 hr; if it increases or remains constant, then partial obstruction should be considered and further evaluation (e.g., ERCP) is indicated (21, 22). Ninety-four percent of the patients who showed a "complete" ductal obstructive pattern on ^{99m}Tc-IDA scanning (prompt hepatic uptake, nonvisualization of the common bile duct, and absent or delayed intestinal visualization between 2 and 4 hr) had obstructing lesions confirmed by subsequent workup while sonography was falsely negative in 50% of those studied with both techniques. Thus, this is another clinical setting where scintigraphy can be more sensitive than sonography. Therefore, if the ^{99m}Tc-IDA study is positive and the sonogram is negative, further evaluation is indicated such as with an ERCP. The overall accuracy of cholescintigraphy in determining if the recurrent postcholecystectomy symptoms are biliary in origin is high. Thus, the ^{99m}Tc-IDA study can be used effectively as a simple, noninvasive screening procedure in these patients.

Several small studies have shown that intrahepatic cholestasis can be suggested by ^{99m}Tc-IDA findings of disproportionately increased parenchymal transit time (compared to any decreased hepatocyte clearance) in the absence of any evidence of large-duct obstruction on sonography, scintigraphy or CT (23). The same scintigraphic findings are described in Dubin-Johnson syndrome. The above observations require confirmation in larger series of patients. Intrahepatic cholestasis is defined as an obstruction to bile flow distal to the hepatocyte and proximal to the large bile ducts. Conditions associated with canalicular membrane dysfunction are: pregnancy, elevated serum estrogens or some androgens, sepsis, general anesthesia, Hodgkin's disease, phenothiazides, viral and alcoholic hepatitis, and benign recurrent cholestasis. Diffuse

TABLE 14.1.
RELIABILITY OF CHOLESCINTIGRAPHIC FINDINGS IN POSTCHOLECYSTECTOMY PATIENTS ($N = 125$)[a]

Finding	PTS Studied	IDA Study Correct	Percent Correct[b]	Remarks
I. Evaluation of Ductal Patency				
A. Normal cholescintigram	35	34	97	CBD stricture missed
B. Ductal dilatation and functional patency	20	17	85	3 missed cases had retained CBD stones
C. Partial obstructive patterns	5	5	100	—
1. Dilated common bile duct (CBD) with delayed B-BT				
2. Abnormal ductal time activity dynamics				
a. With ductal dilatation and normal B-BT	16	15	93.8	1 missed case had a pancreatic mass. No other abnormality was found
b. With ductal dilatation and abnormal B-BT	3	3	100	—
c. Delayed vis. of dilated CBD and delayed B-BT	5	5	100	—
3. Nonvisibility of CBD with delayed B-BT	1	1	100	—
D. "Complete" ductal obstructive pattern	19	18	94.7	1 case of cholangitis without anatomically obstructing lesion identified
II. Cystic Duct Remnant	12[c]	11	91.7	1 remnant seen on ERCP
III. Biliary Leaks	9	9	100	—

[a] Several patients demonstrated more than one pattern, but they have then classified according to the major findings.
[b] Overall accuracy: 94.4%.
[c] Three additional remnants were surgically identified in patients who had "complete" ductal obstruction pattern.

small bile duct obstruction can cause the same scintigraphic picture and is seen in primary biliary cirrhosis, sclerosing cholangitis, bacterial cholangitis, and some cases of infiltrating cholangiocarcinoma.

In summary, although the cholescintigraphic examination has a very limited role in the evaluation of patients with painless jaundice, ^{99m}Tc-IDA scanning has particular advantage in identifying patients with early or intermittent obstruction and can also detect localized intrahepatic obstruction. Another important role for the radioisotopic test is in evaluation of the functional status of biliary drainage in patients with previous obstruction or biliary surgery (eg, postcholecystectomy (Fig. 14.9), biliary-enteric anastomosis) where the ducts may be permanently ectatic and/or the anatomy is altered. The study is also useful in evaluating liver transplant patients (Fig. 14.10).

Pediatrics

There is occasionally a need to evaluate a child for acute cholecystitis either with or without the association of cholelithiasis. In these situations, as in adult practice, ^{99m}Tc-IDA cholescintigraphy remains the method of choice in the diagnostic workup. Similarly, as in adults, when older children present with cholestatic jaundice, ultrasound or computed tomography should be the first imaging test to be performed with the radioisotopic agent reserved for equivocal cases, acute or intermittent obstruction, or for the evaluation of children following biliary tract surgery where patency of the system can easily be defined and complications such as bile leaks detected. However, nuclear medicine plays a very important role in the evaluation of the newborn infant with clinically significant hyperbilirubinemia.

Jaundiced neonates usually fall into two categories, neonatal hepatitis or biliary atresia, and the differentiation is extremely important in choosing the correct therapeutic modality. Biliary atresia patients need early surgical correction of their congenital defect, while neonates with hepatitis do not require surgery and have a significant surgical risk. Studies in the late 1950s and early 1960s (24–28) showed the value of the ^{131}I-rose bengal excretion test in making the diagnosis of biliary atresia. The method involves

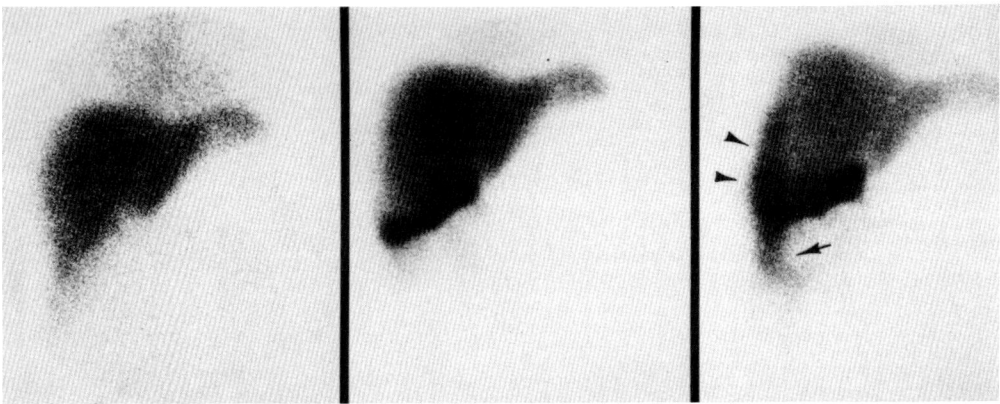

FIGURE 14.9. POSTCHOLECYSTECTOMY BILE LEAK
Postcholecystectomy biliary scan showing activity along the right pericolic gutter (*single arrow*) and up along the lateral margin of the liver (*double arrowhead*).

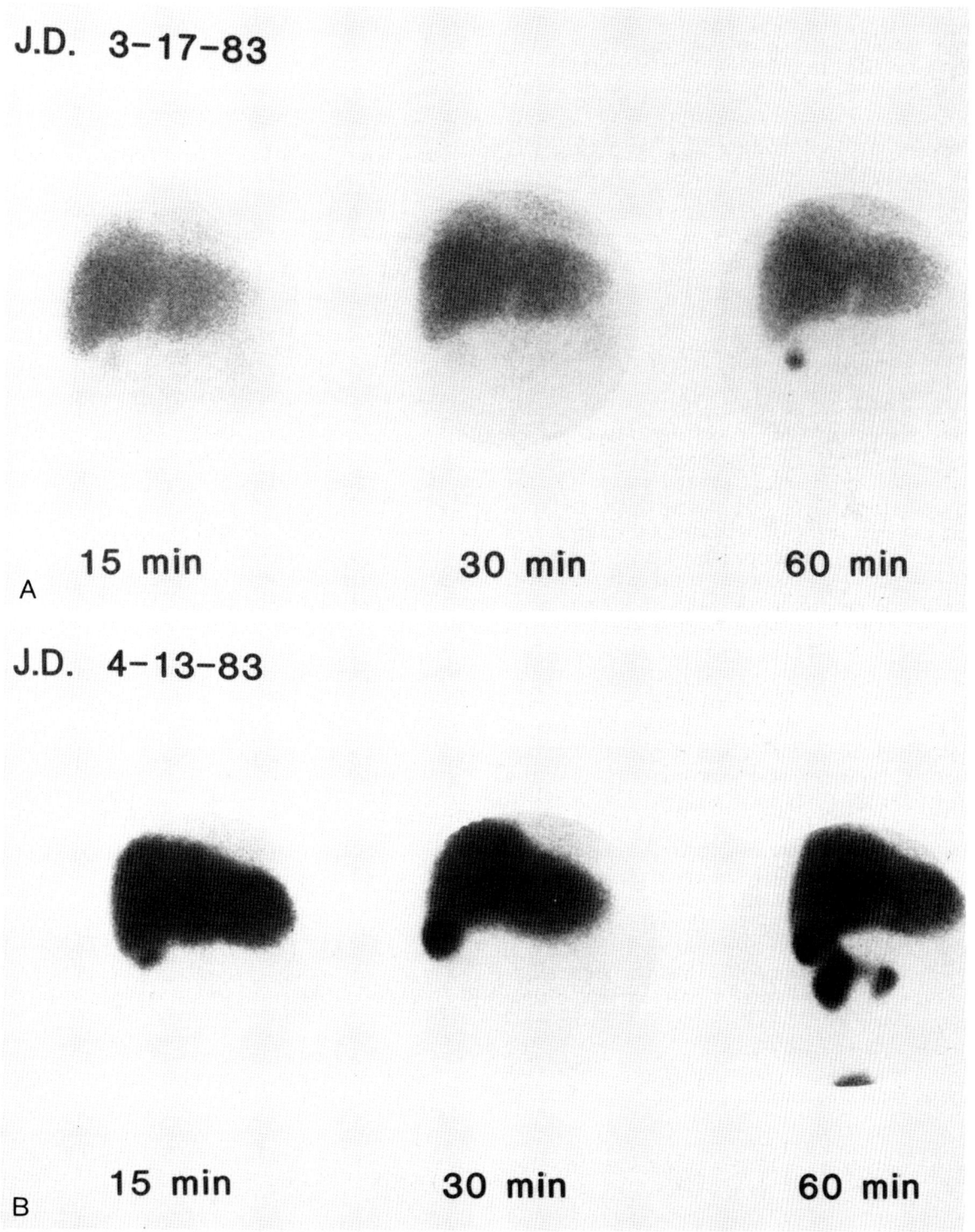

FIGURE 14.10. LIVER TRANSPLANT PATIENT
A: Liver transplant patient showing only minimal clearance of activity into the bowel by 60 min during an episode of acute rejection. *B:* The repeat study following therapy shows significantly better extraction and excretion into the gallbladder by 30 min and into the bowel by 60 min (via the choledochojejunostomy). (The study is courtesy of Dr. Merle Loken.)

the administration of one microcurie of ^{131}I-rose bengal intravenously and collecting all stool for 3 days. The test has been criticized by some as tedious, technically demanding (as urine must be kept separate from the stool) and with a large overlap in results between the two groups (29). Other groups defend the technique (30, 31) as dependable and accurate. Reviewing their experience in 84 patients, the group from the Hospital for Sick Children in Toronto reported an accuracy of 91% and a specificity of 88% using a fecal excretion of less than 7% as the criteria for complete biliary obstruction (31). They do caution regarding the necessity of uncontaminated stool specimens which requires great care, especially for the female patient.

Hepatobiliary scanning with the IDA agents has been a recent addition to the evaluation of the jaundiced infant (29, 30, 32–36). The image pattern varies in patients with neonatal hepatitis from normal to markedly abnormal liver extraction with bowel activity usually seen by 24 hr, except for patients with severe hepatocellular damage and markedly elevated bilirubin levels where intestinal activity may not be identified. In contrast, the child with biliary atresia will show good hepatic uptake with no bowel excretion by 24 hr. Gerhold and colleagues (35), using a combination of hepatic uptake and bowel appearance as diagnostic criteria, report a sensitivity of 97% and a specificity of 82% for biliary atresia. Majd et al. (29) report on the use of phenobarbital pretreatment (5 mg/kg/day) in two divided doses for about 5 days prior to the hepatobiliary study to stimulate the bile excretion of the ^{99m}Tc-IDA agents in children with hepatitis, thereby increasing the accuracy of the test. Additionally, it is recommended that the administered dose should be 1 mCi or greater.

Congenital anomalies in the biliary tract can also be evaluated by the hepatobiliary tracers. Caroli's disease (congenital dilatation of the intrahepatic bile ducts) will be seen as multiple photon-deficient areas during the hepatocyte phase with delayed "filling in" of these ectatic bile ducts (37). Choledochal cysts, which may present with abdominal pain, jaundice and an abdominal mass, can be evaluated well by the combination of ultrasound or CT and radionuclide imaging with the IDA agents (38–40). The appearance consists of a photon-deficient area in the region of the gallbladder/common duct during the hepatocyte phase with delayed and persistent activity filling in this region. Occasionally, an ectopic (intrahepatic) gallbladder may have a similar apearance (41).

REFERENCES

1. Berk RN, Cooperberg PL, Gold RP et al: Radiography of the bile ducts. A symposium on the use of new modalities for diagnosis and treatment. *Radiology* 145:1–9, 1982.
2. Nordyke RA: Biliary tract obstruction and its localization with radioiodinated rose bengal. *Am J Gastroenterol* 33:563–573, 1960.
3. Eyler WR, Schuman BM, Du Sault LA et al: The radioiodinated rose bengal liver scan as an aid in the differential diagnosis of jaundice. *AJR* 94:469–476, 1965.
4. Burke G, Halko A: Dynamic clinical studies with radioisotopes and the scintillation camera. II. Rose bengal ^{131}I liver function studies. *JAMA* 198:140–150, 1966.
5. Neibling HA: Use of ^{131}I-rose bengal scans in diagnosis of biliary obstruction. *Am Surg* 38:328–332, 1972.
6. Davies ER, Morris JN, Read AE et al: ^{131}I-rose bengal scanning and clearance ratios in the investigation of jaundiced patients. *Clin Radiol* 27:227–235, 1976.
7. Winston MA, Blahd WH: ^{131}I-rose bengal imaging techniques in differential diagnosis of jaundiced patients. *Semin Nucl Med* 2:167–175, 1972.
8. Pors-Nielson S, Trap-Jensen J, Lindenberg J et al: Hepatobiliary scintigraphy and hepatography with Tc-99m diethylacetanilido-imino-diacetate in obstructive jaundice. *J Nucl Med* 19:452–457, 1978.
9. Fonseca C, Rosenthall L, Greenberg D et al: Differential diagnosis of jaundice by ^{99m}Tc-IDA hepatobiliary imaging. *Clin Nucl Med* 4:135–142, 1979.
10. Weissmann HS, Rosenblatt R, Sugarman LA et al: The role of nuclear imaging in evaluating cholestasis—an update. *Semin Ultrasound* 1:134–142, 1980.
11. Pauwels S, Piret L, Schoutens A et al: ^{99m}Tc-diethyl-IDA imaging: Clinical evaluation in jaundiced patients. *J Nucl Med* 21:1022–1028, 1980.
12. Weissmann HS, Rosenblatt R, Sugarman LA, Badia JD, Freeman LM: Early diagnosis of acute common bile duct obstruction by ^{99m}Tc-IDA (iminodiacetic acid) cholescintigraphy. *J Nucl Med* 21:41, 1980.
13. Weissmann HS, Sugarman LA, Frank MS, Badia J, Freeman LM: Spectrum of ^{99m}Tc-HIDA cholescintigraphic findings in acute cholecystitis. *Radiology* 138:167–175, 1981.
14. Zeman RK, Lee C, Jaffe MH et al: Hepatobiliary scintigraphy and sonography in early obstruction. *Radiology* 153:793–798, 1984.
15. Kaplun L, Weissmann HS, Rosenblatt RR, Freeman LM: The early diagnosis of common bile duct obstruction using cholescintigraphy. *JAMA* 254:2431–2434, 1985.
16. Zeman RK, Taylor KJW, Rosenfield AT et al: Acute experimental biliary obstruction in the dog: sonographic findings and clinical implications. *AJR* 136:965–967, 1981.
17. Zeman RK, Gold JA, Gluck L et al: ^{99m}Tc-HIDA scintigraphy in segmental biliary obstruction. *J Nucl Med* 22:456–458, 1981.
18. Yeh SH, Liu OK, Huang MJ: Sequential scintiphotography with technetium-99m pyridoxylidene glutamate in the detection of intrahepatic lithiasis: Concise communcations. *J Nucl Med* 21:17–21, 1980.
19. Gupta S, Owshalimpur D, Cohen G et al: Scintigraphic detection of segmental bile-duct obstruction. *J Nucl Med* 23:890–891, 1982.
20. Weissmann HS, Freeman LM: The Biliary Tract. In Freeman LM, Weissmann, HS (eds): *Freeman and Johnson's Clinical Radionuclide Imaging*. Ed 3, Vol 2. New York, Grune & Stratton, 1984.

21. Weissmann HS, Gliedman ML, Wilk PJ et al: Evaluation of the postoperative patient with ^{99m}Tc-IDA cholescintigraphy. Semin Nucl Med 12:27–52, 1982.
22. Badia JD, Weissmann HS, Heller SL, Freeman LM: ^{99m}Tc-IDA cholescintigraphic assessment of common bile duct time activity dynamics in postcholecystectomy patients. Radiology 157:315, 1985.
23. Kuni CC, Klingensmith WC III, Fritzberg AR: Evaluation of intrahepatic cholestasis with radionuclide hepatobiliary imaging. Gastrointest Radiol 9:163–166, 1984.
24. Geppert LJ, Brent RL: Radioactive rose bengal: An aid in the differential diagnosis of the jaundiced infant. Am J Dis Child 94:544, 1957.
25. Brent RL, Geppert LJ: The use of radioactive rose bengal in the evaluation of infantile jaundice. Am J Dis Child 98:720–730, 1959.
26. Ghadimi H, Sass-Kortsak A: Evaluation of the radioactive rose bengal test for the differential diagnosis of obstructed jaundice in infants. N Engl J Med 265:351–358, 1961.
27. White WE, Welch JS, Darrow DC et al: Pediatric appliation of the radioiodine (^{131}I)-rose bengal method in hepatic and biliary system disease. Pediatrics 32:239–250, 1963.
28. Sharp HL, Krivit W, Lowman JT: The diagnosis of complete extrahepatic obstruction by rose bengal ^{131}I. J Pediatr 70:46–53, 1967.
29. Majd M, Reba RC, Altman RP: Effect of phenobarbital on ^{99m}Tc-IDA scintigraphy in the evaluation of neonatal jaundice. Semin Nucl Med 9:194–204, 1981.
30. Collier BD, Treves S, Davis MA et al: Simultaneous ^{99m}Tc-P-butyl-IDA and ^{131}I-rose bengal scintigraphy in neonatal jaundice. Radiology 134:719–722, 1980.
31. Antico VF, Denhartog P, Ash JM et al: The ^{131}I-rose bengal excretion test is not dead. Clin Nucl Med 10:171–172, 1985.
32. Majd M, Reba RC, Altman RP: Hepatobiliary scintigraphy with ^{99m}Tc-PIPIDA in the evaluation of neonatal jaundice. Pediatrics 67:140–145, 1981.
33. Leonard JC, Hitch DC, Manion CV: The use of diethyl-IDA-^{99m}Tc clearance curves in the differentiation of biliary atresia from other forms of neonatal jaundice. Radiology 142:773–776, 1982.
34. Sty JR, Starshak RJ, Thorp SM: Preliminary clinical experience with ^{99m}Tc-disofenin as a biliary imaging agent in pediatrics. Clin Nucl Med 7:210–212, 1982.
35. Gerhold JP, Klingensmith WC, Kuni CC et al: diagnosis of biliary atresia with radionuclide hepatobiliary imaging. Radiology 146:499–504, 1983.
36. Kirks DR, Coleman RE, Filston HC et al: An imaging approach to persistent neonatal jaundice. AJR 142:461–465, 1984.
37. Sty JR, Hubbard AM, Starshak RJ: Radionuclide hepatobiliary imaging in congenital biliary tract ectasia (Caroli's disease). Pediatr Radiol 12:111–114, 1982.
38. Weissmann HS, Gold M, Goldstein RD, Sugarman LA, Freeman LM: Choledochal cyst complicated by acute cholecystitis and bypass obstruction: diagnostic role of ^{99m}Tc-HIDA cholescintigraphy. Clin Nucl Med 6:395–398, 1981.
39. Sugihara M, Suzuki Y, Yokoyama S et al: Radionuclide imaging in the diagnosis of choledochal cysts and intrahepatic duct dilatation. Clin Nucl Med 4:325–326, 1979.
40. Huang M-J, Liaw YF: Intravenous cholescintigraphy using ^{99m}Tc-labeled agents in the diagnosis of choledochal cysts. J Nucl Med 23:113–116, 1982.
41. Dumont M, Danais S: Intrahepatic gallbladder simulating choledochal cysts on DISIDA scintigraphy. Clin Nucl Med 9:657–658, 1984.

Plain Films and Barium Studies

Since the vast majority of stones in the common duct (and intrahepatic biliary tract) are radiolucent, a plain film only occasionally will demonstrate these calculi (Fig. 14.11). Differentiation from pancreatic calculi, gallstones, renal calculi, and hepatic granulomata (depending on location) is often difficult. A stone impacted in the ampulla of Vater may cause a prominent papilla on a barium meal examination (Fig. 14.12).

When a UGI series is performed on a jaundiced patient with biliary obstruction, indirect evidence of dilatation of the gallbladder and common bile duct may be seen. The distended common bile duct produces a tubular impression upon the posterior surface of the duodenum, usually the post-bulbar segment (1) (Fig. 14.13). Mass effects can be produced along the medial aspect of the duodenal sweep as well (2) (Fig. 14.13). Rarely, the duct becomes enlarged enough to indent the antrum as well (Fig. 14.14). A markedly enlarged gallbladder can indent and displace the duodenum and/or the anterior hepatic flexure (1) (Fig. 14.13).

REFERENCES

1. Berk RN: Barium studies of the gastrointestinal tract. In Berk RN, Ferrucci JT Jr, Leopold GR (eds): Radiology of the Gallbladder and Bile Ducts, Diagnosis and Intervention. Philadelphia, W. B. Saunders, 1983, pp 30–46.
2. Gold RP: Medial indentation of the duodenal sweep by common bile duct dilatation. AJR 133:233, 1979.

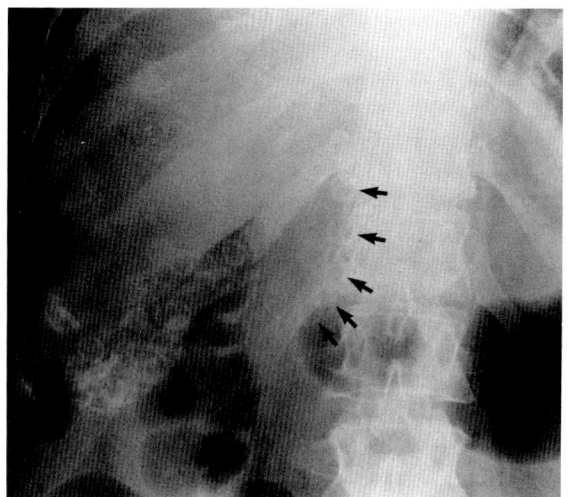

FIGURE 14.11. CALCIFIED COMMON DUCT STONES
Multiple calcified common duct stones (*arrows*) and multiple gallstones in a patient who presented with ascending cholangitis.

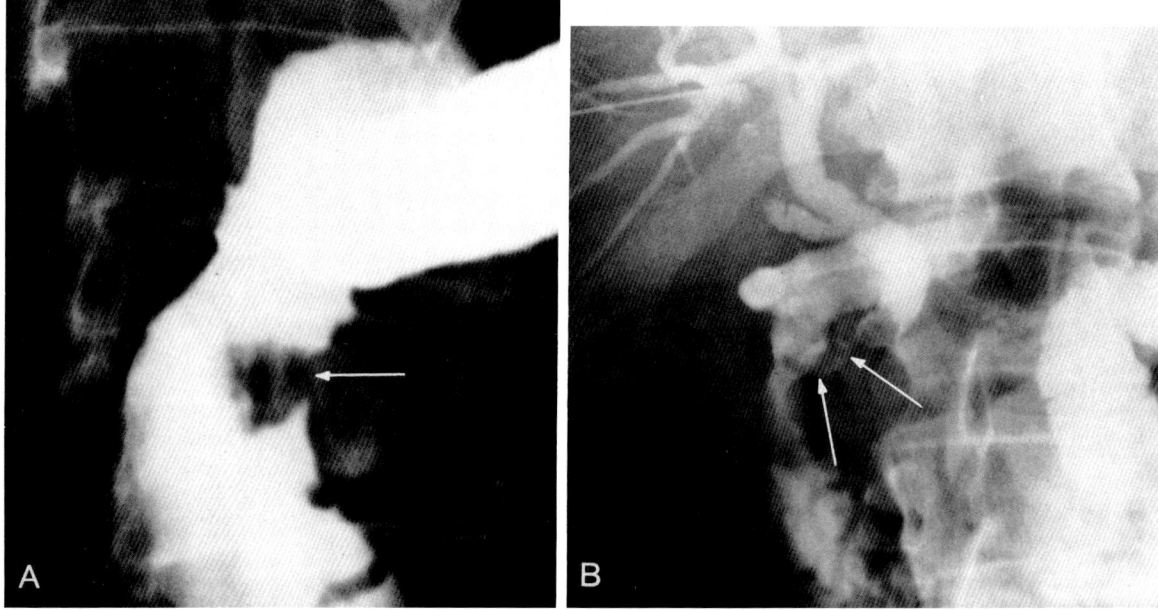

FIGURE 14.12. CALCULUS IMPACTED IN THE AMPULLA PRODUCING A PROMINENT PAPILLA. DIFFERENTIAL DIAGNOSIS INCLUDES PANCREATITIS, AMPULLARY TUMOR AND CHOLEDOCHOCOELE
A: UGI: prominent papilla (*arrow*). Deformed bulb from ulcer disease. *B:* PTC: stone impacted in the ampulla (*arrows*) and a proximal second stone.

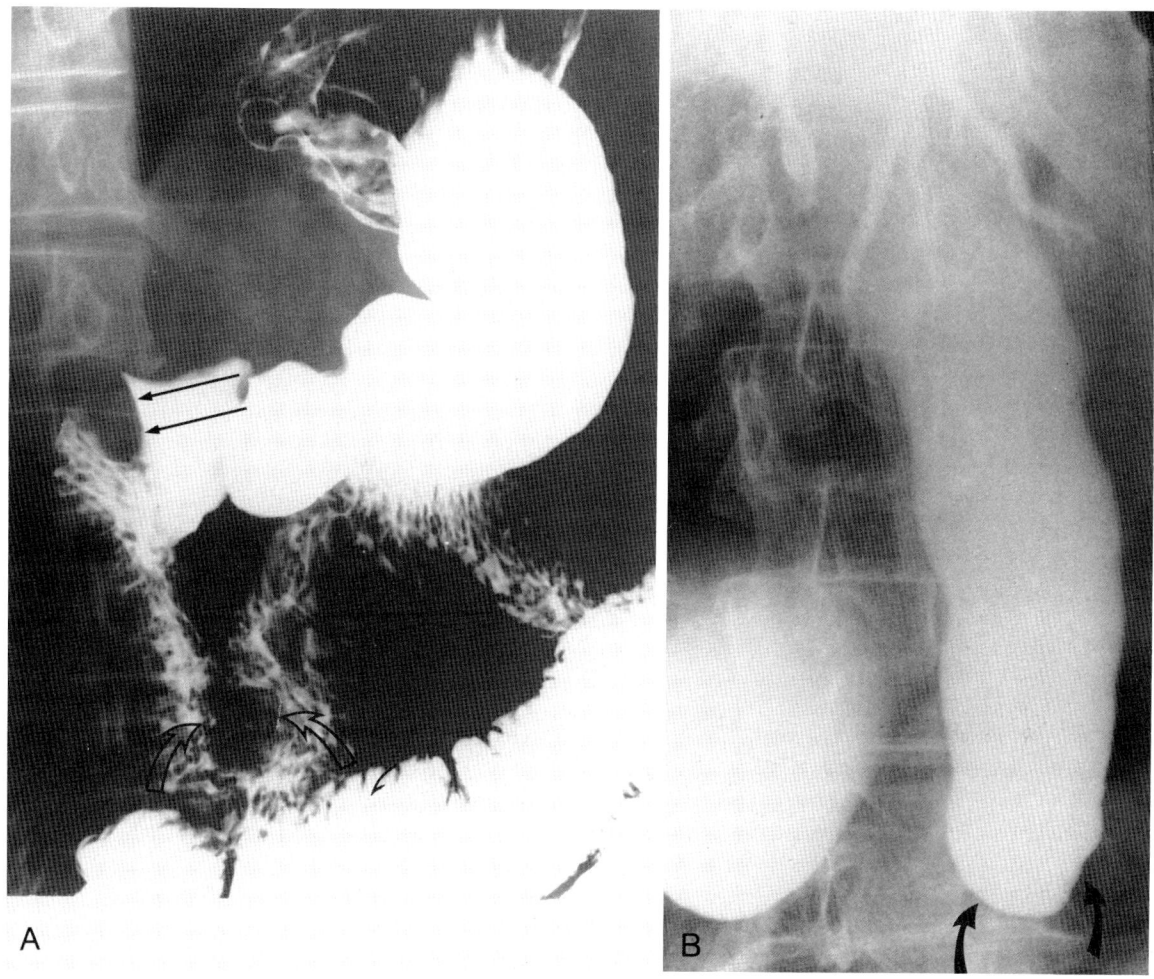

FIGURE 14.13. DILATED COMMON BILE DUCT: UGI
Dilated common bile duct indenting the post-bulbar duodenum; enlarged gallbladder displacing the descending duodenum medially. *A:* UGI shows the tubular impression of the common duct on the duodenum (*arrows*) and the medially displaced duodenum. The ampullary carcinoma causing the obstruction is seen as well (curved arrows). *B:* PTC, massively dilated common duct and gallbladder. Irregularly round abrupt obstruction (*arrows*) suggests malignancy.

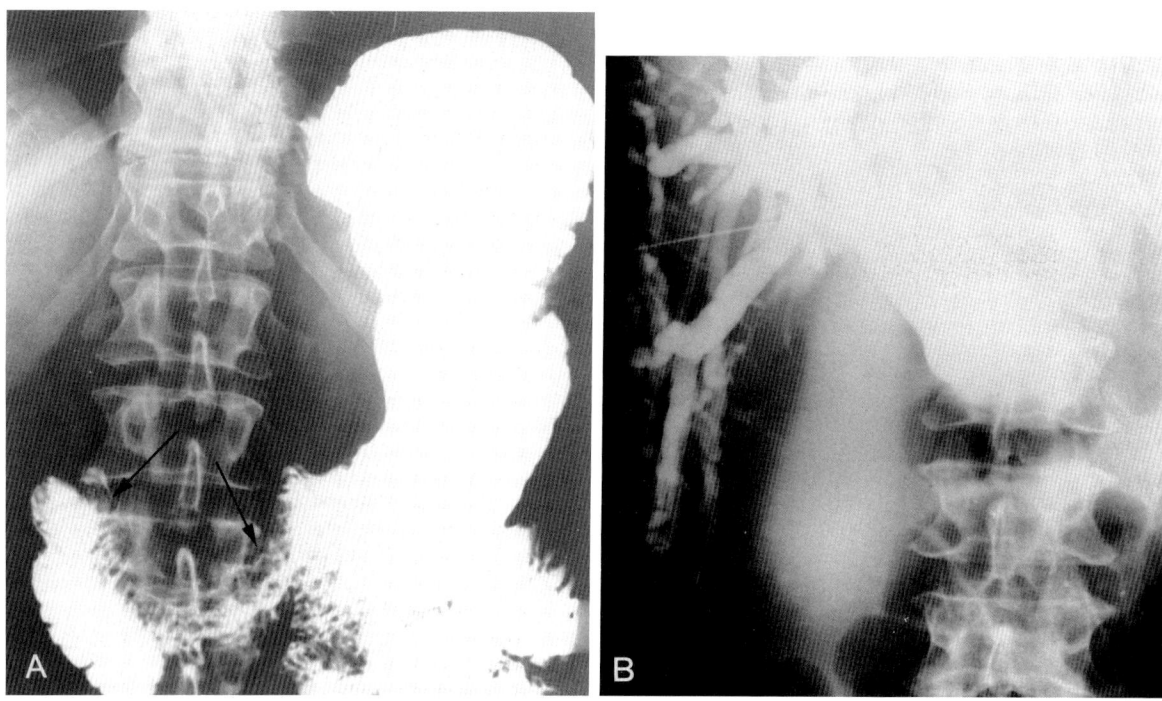

FIGURE 14.14. MASSIVE COMMON BILE DUCT DILATATION: UGI
A: Massive common bile duct dilatation displacing the antrum and proximal duodenum (*arrows*) on UGI. *B:* Confirmatory PTC.

CHOLEDOCHOLITHIASIS

Choledocholithiasis complicates the course of approximately 15% of cholecystectomy patients and 3–4% of post-cholecystectomy patients (1). Common duct stones can originate in the gallbladder and then pass into the common bile duct via the cystic duct or develop primarily in the intrahepatic or extrahepatic ducts. Common duct stones can remain free, or obstruct partially, completely, or intermittently.

Clinical Findings

Although choledocholithiasis may be asymptomatic, biliary colic, cholangitis, jaundice, or pancreatitis generally occur given sufficient time.

Biliary colic from acute impaction of a common duct stone is clinically indistinguishable from the pain caused by acute cystic duct obstruction (2). Acute cholangitis, manifested by fever, chills, and jaundice occurs with common duct obstruction and infection with enteric organisms, often *Escherichia coli*. Usually, response to antibiotics is satisfactory and definitive treatment can be undertaken on a nonurgent basis, but sometimes pus accumulates in the ducts in the face of a complete obstruction and emergency biliary drainage is necessary to prevent septic shock. Emergency palliative drainage can be accomplished via the percutaneous transhepatic route.

Jaundice occurs when the intraductal pressure rises above 25 cm of water, suppressing hepatic bile flow and causing reflux of conjugated bilirubin into the bloodstream via lymphatics. Serum bilirubin rarely rises above 12 mg/100 ml, and serum alkaline phosphatase increases before the bilirubin. Transaminases are elevated in about 75% of patients with acute common bile duct obstruction (2).

Treatment of common duct stones depends to an extent on whether their origin is in the gallbladder or the ductal system. If their origin is in the gallbladder, the latter is removed if still present, and the common duct is explored and all stones are removed. Choledochoduodenostomy or sphincteroplasty is usually unnecessary. However, if the stones are primary within the common duct, ampullary stenosis is often present, and, regardless of ampullary stenosis, primary common duct stones are apt to recur unless a choledochoduodenostomy is done. Cholangitis after choledochoduodenostomy is related to obstruction at the stoma, not reflux of duodenal contents (3). Patients with common duct stones who are poor surgical candidates may be treated by endoscopic sphincterotomy with stone extraction or spontaneous passage. If this technique is unavailable or unfeasible (e.g., prior Billroth II), stone extraction and ampullary dilatation can be performed percutaneously (4).

Pathology

Primary common duct stones are ovoid and single or multiple. They are soft and readily crushed into fragments (biliary mud). On cross-section, two common variations are alternating light and dark brown rings or a dark brown center surrounded by a light yellow periphery (3). Secondary common duct stones that have formed in the gallbladder will have the same varieties as gallstones, with the exception that they must be small enough to have passed through the cystic duct (although they can grow larger once in the common duct).

REFERENCES

1. Coehlo JC, Buffara M, Pozzobon CE, Altenburg FL, Artigas GV: Incidence of common bile duct stones in patients with acute and chronic cholecystitis. *Surg. Gynecol Obstet* 158:76–80, 1984.
2. Schoenfield LJ: *Diseases of the Gallbladder and Biliary System* (Clinical Gastroenterology Monographs). New York, John Wiley & Sons, 1977.
3. Madden JL, Vanderheyden L, Kandalaft S: The nature and significance of common duct stones. *Surg Gynecol Obstet* 126:3–8, 1968.
4. Huggins MJ, Friedman AC, Fenster HA: Transhepatic removal of impacted intrahepatic and common duct stones: case report. *Milit Med* 148:935–937, 1983.

Sonography

Sonography is traditionally considered relatively insensitive to common duct stones (1). Einstein reported a 22% sensitivity in a series of 138 patients with common duct stones, although 77% had dilated ducts demonstrated sonographically (2). Gross found a 25% sensitivity in 90 documented cases (3), whereas Cronan reported a sensitivity of 13% (64% had dilated ducts) (4). However, recent reports by Laing using transverse scanning of the intrapancreatic portion of the common duct and erect or semierect positioning in addition to the traditional parasagittal scans gave an improved sensitivity of 75% for common duct stones (5, 6) (Fig. 14.15). Other helpful maneuvers include longitudinal coronal

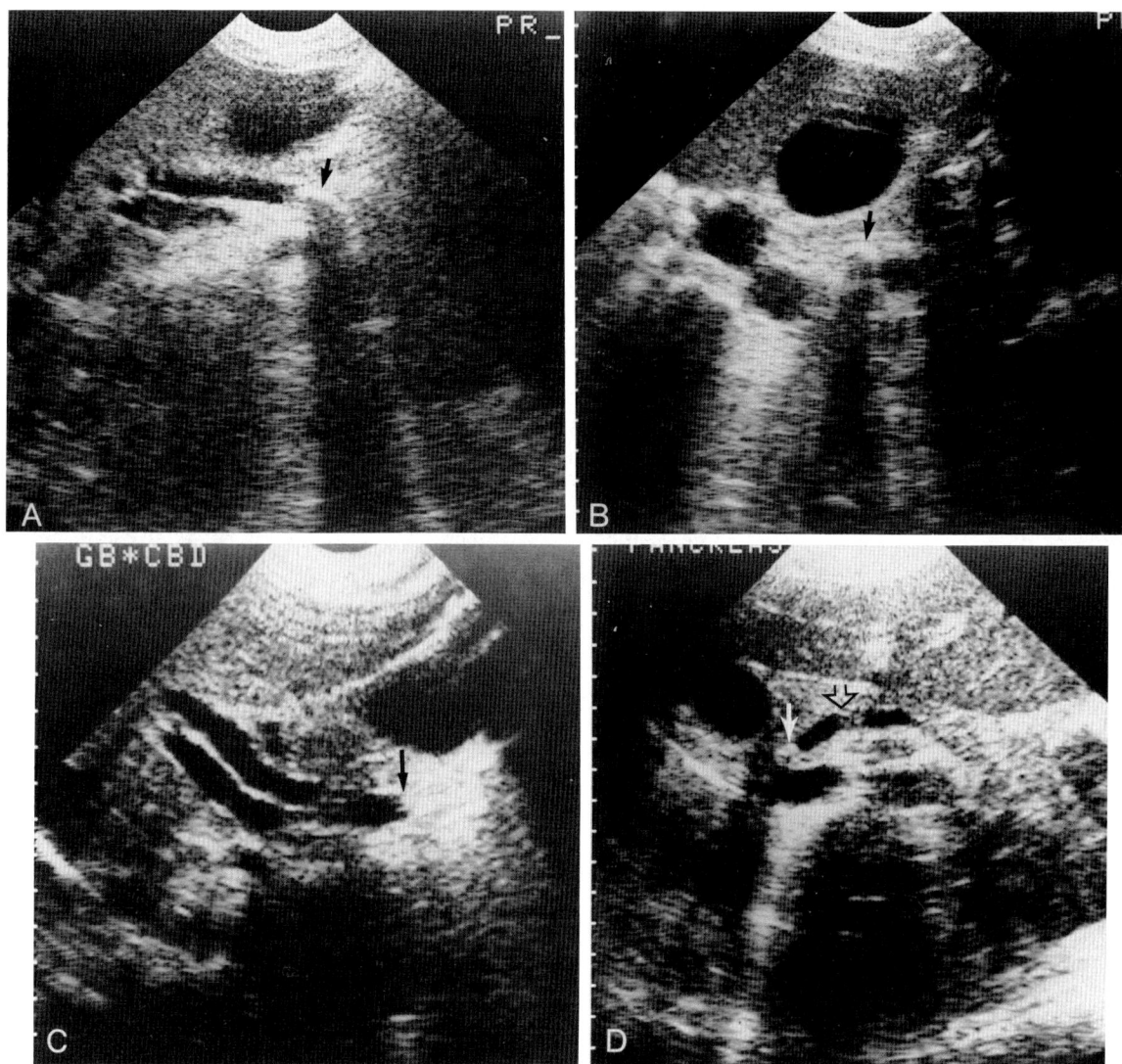

FIGURE 14.15. VALUE OF TRANSVERSE SCANNING

A and *B:* Sagittal (*A*) and obliqued transverse (*B*) scans both show a shadowing calculus in the more distal common duct (*arrows*). Absence of surrounding bile suggests impaction. *C* and *D:* A different patient. The sagittal scan (*C*) shows a dilated common duct with abrupt termination (*arrow*) in the region of the pancreas but no calculus, whereas the transverse scan (*D*) successfully demonstrates the calculus impacted in the ampulla of Vater (*arrow*). Note dilated pancreatic duct (*open arrow*).

views with the patient in various degrees of left posterior obliquity, filling the antrum and duodenum with water, and occasionally Trendelenburg positioning to allow a distal common duct stone to sink to a more accessible proximal position.

Demonstrating dilated ducts is insufficient for a diagnosis of choledocholithiasis. It is necessary to demonstrate a definite echogenic focus within the common duct. In contrast to stones in the gallbladder, only 60–80% of stones in the common duct shadow (Fig. 14.16) (2, 7). Common duct stones frequently lodge in the distal retroduodenal common duct and are often obscured by overlying bowel gas. The surrounding bile pool is small or nonexistent, adding to the difficulty in detection. Even when the diagnosis of choledocholithiasis is successfully made sonographically, more stones are often present at surgery than are shown by sonography (7), and the stone seen on ultrasound is often not the obstructing stone (Fig. 14.17). The larger the duct size the more easily stones are depicted and it is hard to see stones in normal-sized ducts.

Most of the many pitfalls in scanning the common duct for stones result in false positives.

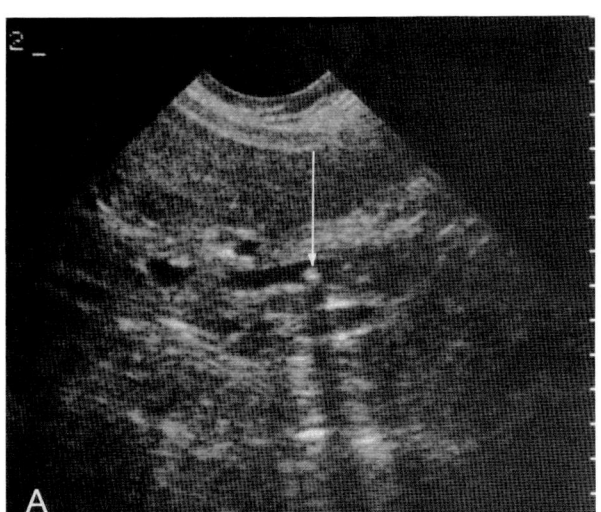
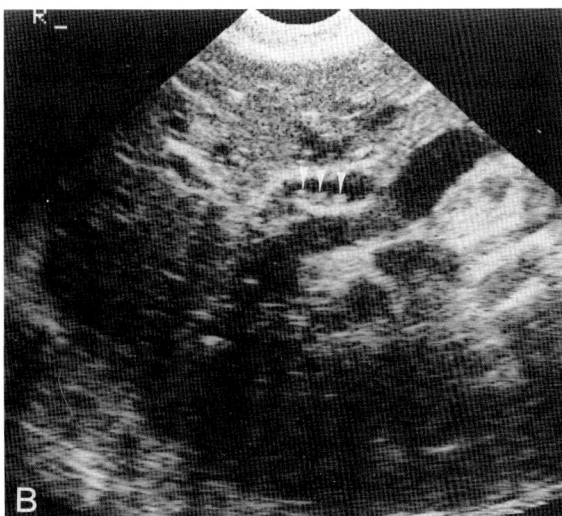
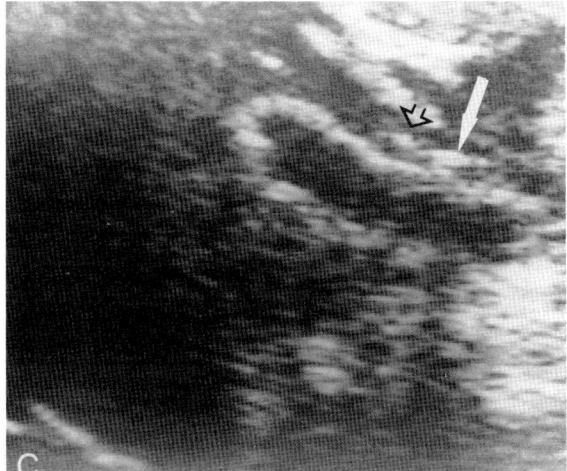

FIGURE 14.16. COMMON DUCT CALCULI MAY OR MAY NOT SHADOW

A: Small shadowing calculus (*arrow*), sagittal scan. *B:* Three small, nonshadowing calculi (*arrowheads*), sagittal scan. *C:* Nonshadowing biliary mud (*open arrow*) proximal to a shadowing calculus (*closed arrow*).

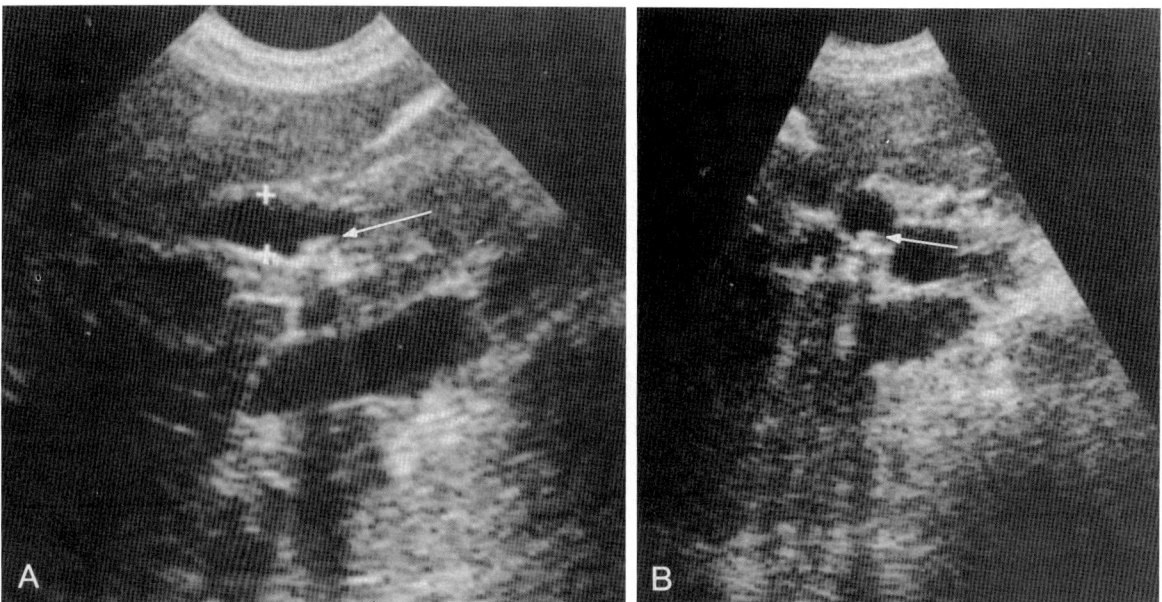

FIGURE 14.17. STONE IN DILATED COMMON DUCT
Stone in dilated common duct (1.2 cm, *cursors*) seen as shadowing echogenicity (*arrow*) on sagittal (A) and transverse (B) scans. The obstructing stone was more distal and not seen.

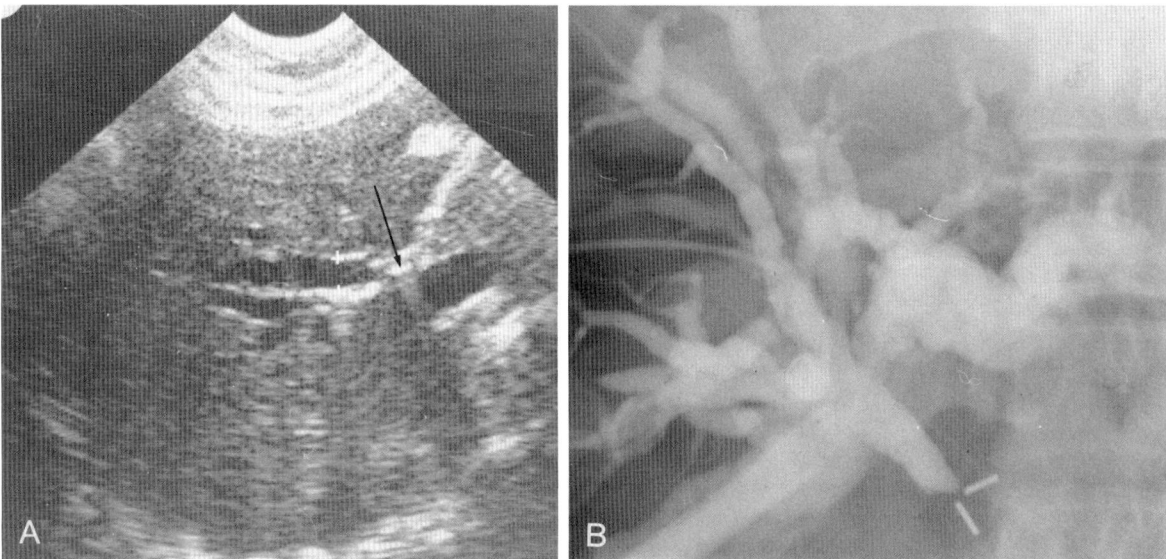

FIGURE 14.18. SURGICAL CLIP MIMICKING COMMON DUCT STONE
A: Parasagittal sonogram shows a dilated common duct (*cursors*) terminating abruptly with an apparent calculus (*arrow*).
B: Percutaneous cholangiogram: surgical clips obstructing the common duct.

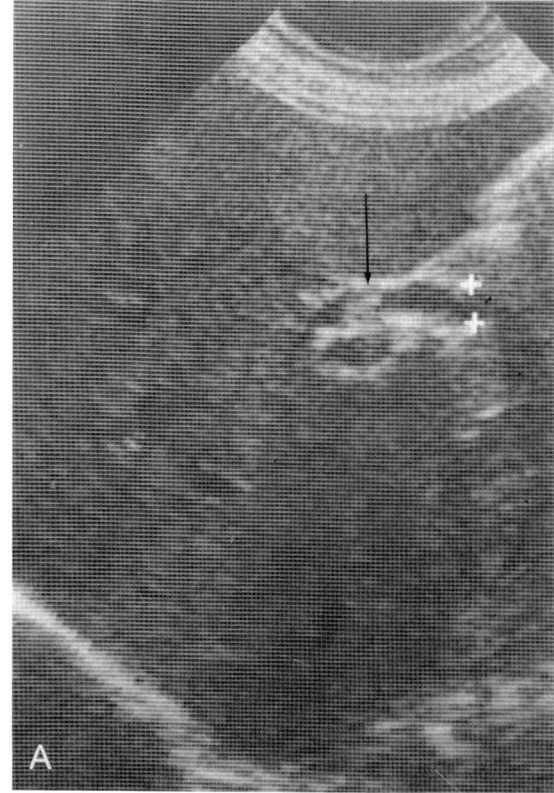
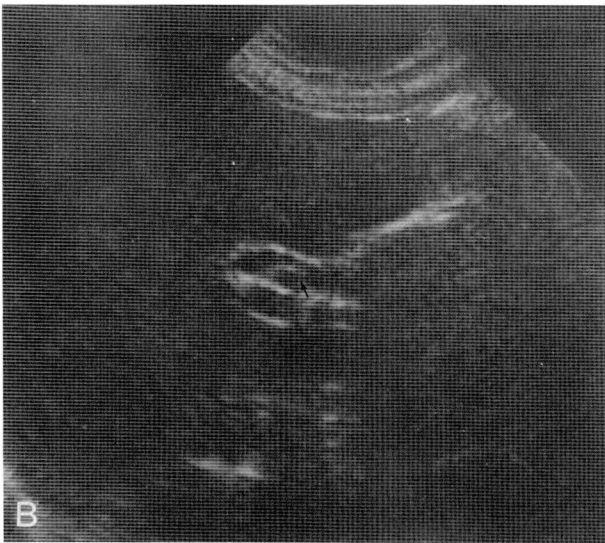

FIGURE 14.19. RIGHT HEPATIC ARTERY SIMULATING COMMON DUCT STONE
A: Echogenic focus (*arrow*) within the common duct (*cursors*). B: Slightly different angulation demonstrating indentation of the common duct by the right hepatic artery (*arrow*) and no intraductal abnormality.

Any highly reflective structure in the porta hepatis can be projected into the common duct. Surgical clips may generate "comet-tail" reverberation echoes, but even with plain film correlation it may be difficult to serparate clip from stone (Fig. 14.18) (7). The right hepatic artery may indent the wall of the common duct and cause an intraluminal echodensity separate from the rest of the artery to appear (7–9) (Fig. 14.19). An endoprosthesis may be mistaken for a calculus (9). Cystic duct remnants or folds in a dilated common duct can be misinterpreted as a stone (7). Finally, intraductal tumors or mucous plugs can be indistinguishable from stones.

In light of the less than perfect detectability of common duct stones, post-cholecystectomy patients with elevated alkaline phosphatase levels should have ERCP despite a normal biliary sonogram.

REFERENCES

1. Coelho JC, Buffara M, Pozzobon CE, Altenburg FL, Artigas GV: Incidence of common bile duct stones in patients with acute and chronic cholecystitis. *Surg Gynecol Obstet* 158:76–80, 1984.
2. Einstein DM, Lapin SA, Ralls PW, Halls JM: The insensitivity of sonography in the detection of choledocholithiasis. *AJR* 142:725–728, 1984.
3. Gross BH, Harter LP, Gore RM et al: Ultrasonic evaluation of common bile duct stones: prospective comparison with endoscopic retrograde cholangiopancreatography. *Radiology* 146:471–474, 1983.
4. Cronan JJ, Mueller PR, Simeone JF: Prospective diagnosis of choledocholithiasis. *Radiology* 146:467–469, 1983.
5. Laing FC, Jeffrey RB: Choledocholithiasis and cystic duct obstruction: difficult ultrasonic diagnosis. *Radiology* 146:475–479, 1983.
6. Laing FC, Jeffrey RB, Wing VW: Improved visualization of choledocholithiasis by sonography. *AJR* 143:949–952, 1984.
7. Parulekar SG, McNamara MP: Ultrasonography of choledocholithiasis. *J Ultrasound Med* 2:395–400, 1983.
8. Mitchell SE, Clark RA: A comparison of tomography and sonography in choledocholithiasis. *AJR* 142:729–733, 1984.
9. Mueller PR, Cronan JJ, Simeone JF, vanSonnenberg E, Hall DA: Choledocholithiasis: ultrasonographic caveats. *J Ultrasound Med* 2:13–16, 1983.

Computed Tomography

CT sensitivity for the detection of common duct stones is quite high: greater than 80% in four to five fairly large series using third or fourth generation equipment with short scanning times (1–5). The series with only a 50% detection rate saw only calcified stones, detecting noncalcified stones only in retrospect (1). Several technical factors will aid sensitivity: 5 mm collimation scans at 5 mm intervals through the extrahepatic ducts, targeting to a small field of view, soft tissue high resolution algorithms, and close physician supervision. These factors aid mostly in detecting stones that are noncalcified and nearly isodense with bile. These stones will account for essentially all the false negatives. Calcified stones are easily detected with almost any technique except for two potential pitfalls: oral contrast material in a duodenal diverticulum mimicking a calcified stone and prior administration of cholecystographic or cholangiographic contrast material, both of which can increase the attenuation in the common bile duct simulating a calcified stone on one or several slices. When scanning specifically for common duct calculi one generally gives intravenous contrast to aid in the detection of dilated intrahepatic ducts but omits oral contrast at least initially.

CT appearances of common duct calculi include: (*a*) radioopaque calcification (Figs. 14.20 and 14.21), (*b*) soft tissue density in the dependent portion of the common duct with an anterior crescent of low density bile (Fig. 14.22), (*c*) intraluminal soft tissue density surrounded by lower density bile, (*d*) a faint rim of increased density along the peripheral margin of an otherwise low density calculus (Fig. 14.22), and (*e*) mottled regions of increased density centrally

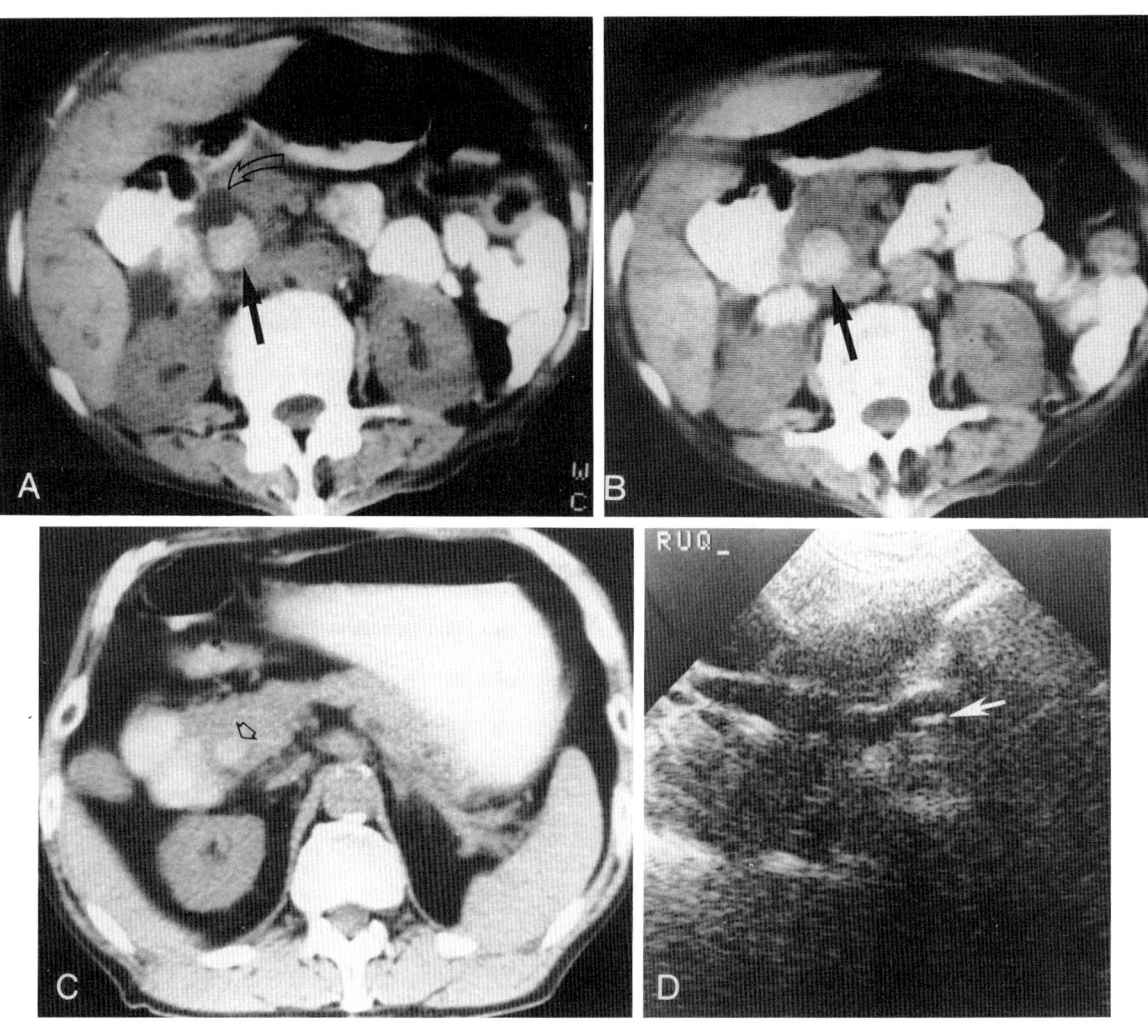

FIGURE 14.20. LARGE COMMON DUCT STONES: CT

A and *B:* Abrupt termination. A dilated common duct at a large stone lodged in the ampulla. *A:* Duct (*curved arrow*) and stone (*arrow*). *B:* 5 mm. caudad to (*A*): impacted stone (*arrow*) and thin lucent crescent of bile anterior to the stone. *C* and *D:* CT with correlative ultrasound of a 1 cm stone. *C:* CT through the head of the pancreas: 1 cm impacted stone (*arrow*). *D:* Sagittal sonogram: nonshadowing calculus is depicted (*arrow*) despite bowel gas interference.

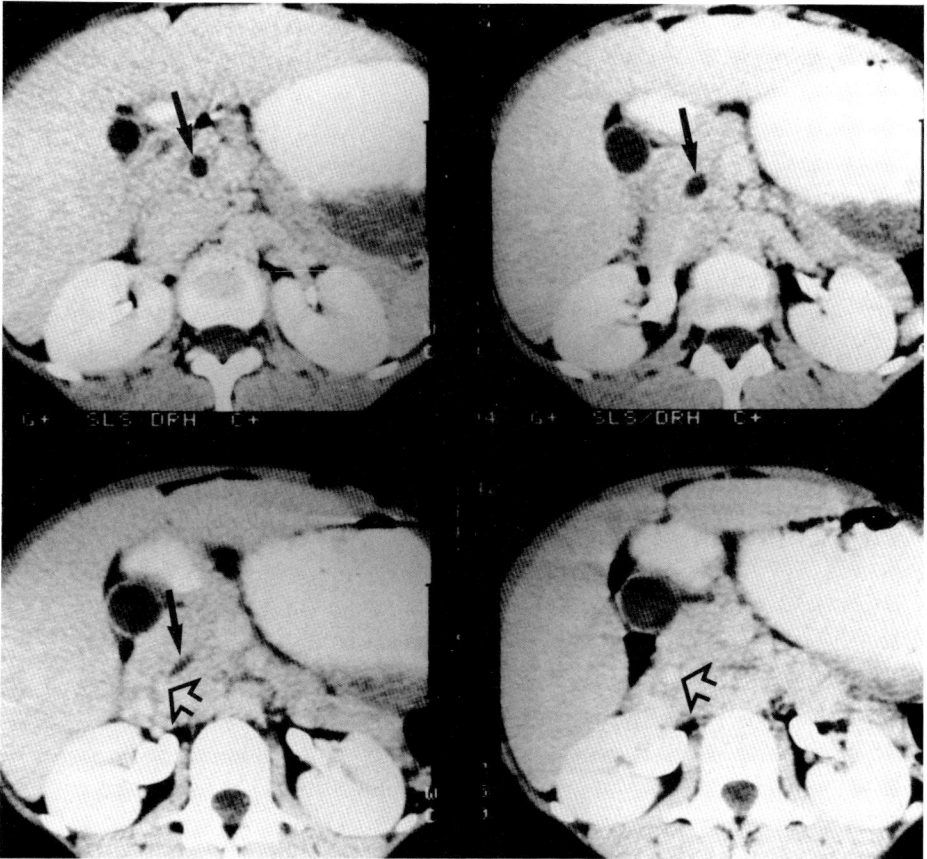

FIGURE 14.21. CALCIFIED CALCULUS IN DISTAL BILE DUCT: CT

Small calcified calculus (*open arrows*) in the most distal common bile duct. Thin sections and high-dose intravenous contrast improve depiction of dilated intrapancreatic common duct (*closed arrows*) which ends abruptly at the stone. Top left most cephalad, then top right, bottom left and bottom right in cephalocaudad progression.

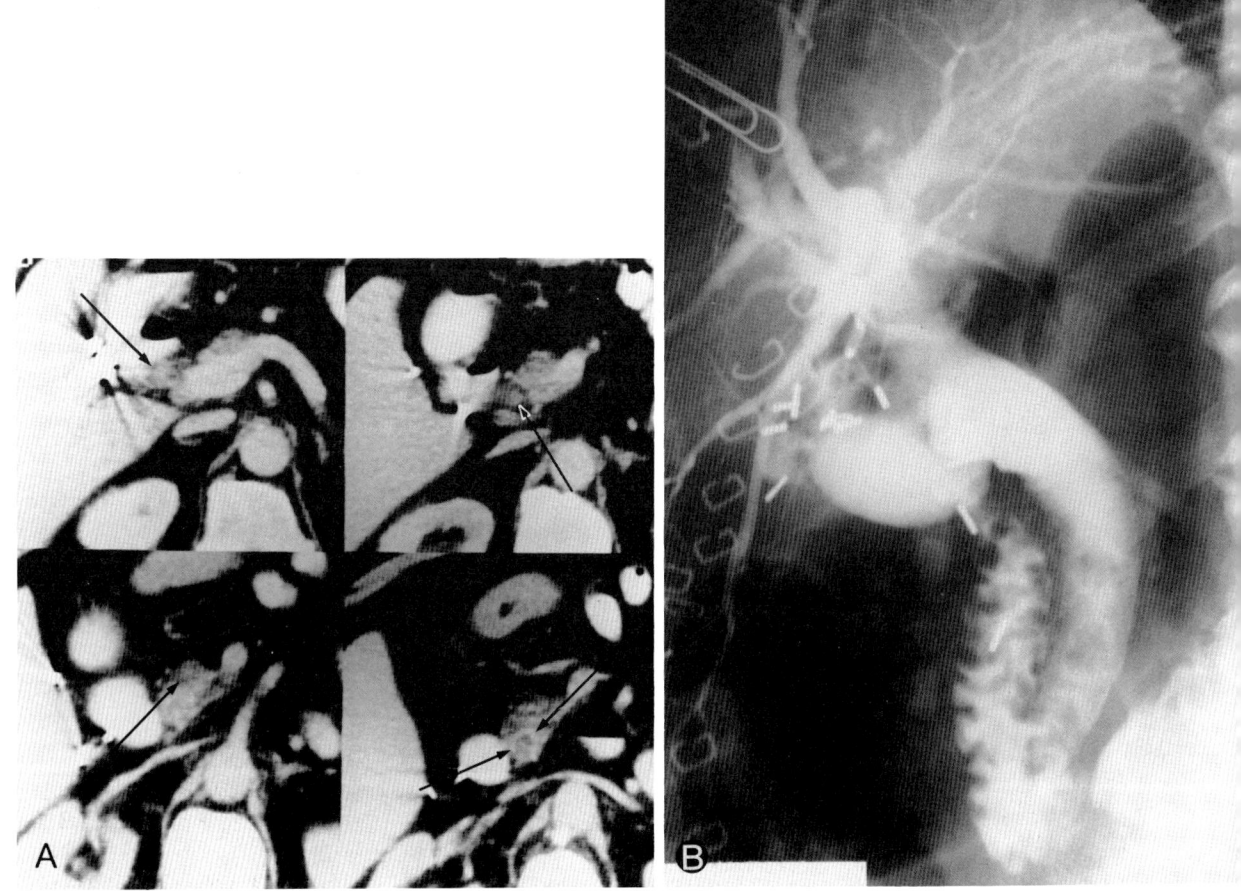

FIGURE 14.22. CT SHOWING MULTIPLE CALCULI IN THE COMMON BILE DUCT

A: The proximal ducts were dilated and water density (not shown). (*Top left*) Common bile duct is filled with soft tissue density material (the calculus) instead of water density bile (*arrow*). (*Top right*) Intraluminal soft tissue density (*arrow*) partially surrounded anteriorly by bile. (*Bottom left*) Mottled regions of increased attenuation within the duct (*arrow*). (*Bottom right*) High density rim surrounding otherwise mostly low density calculus (*arrows*). *B:* Corresponding transhepatic cholangiogram on the same patient: multiple calculi.

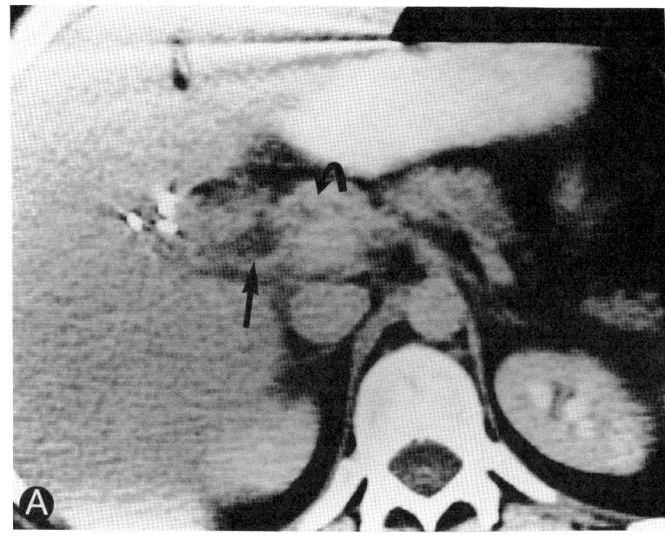
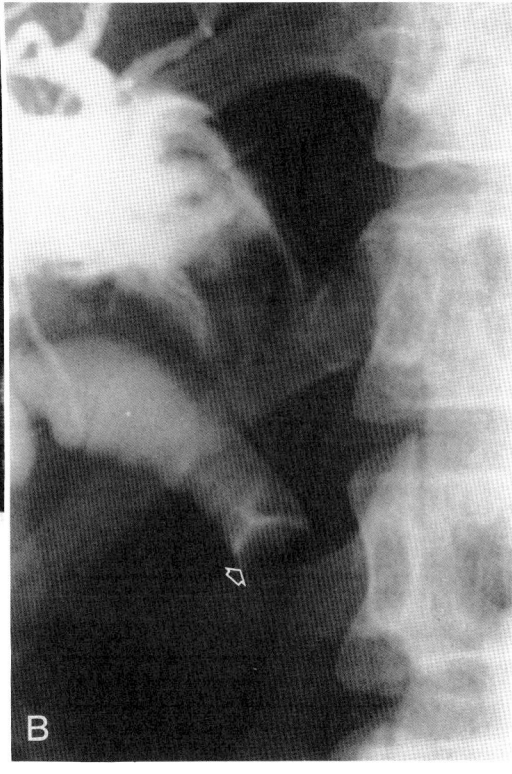

FIGURE 14.23. NONCALCIFIED STONE: CT
A: CT scan interpreted as abrupt obstruction with no mass consistent with stone. In retrospect, a noncalcified stone is demonstrated as higher than normal attenuation within the duct (arrow). B: Corresponding cholangiogram.

within the common duct elevating its attenuation to greater than that of normal bile (Fig. 14.22) (2, 3). When the stone is impacted in the ampulla, bulging into the duodenum can be seen mimicking a choledochocoele or an ampullary tumor (3). Dilated ducts both intra and extrahepatic proximal to the stone are a frequent but not mandatory finding. When dilated, the ducts will usually terminate abruptly at the level of the calculus, although a tapered, gradual obstruction can occur (2–5). An abrupt obstruction accompanied by the absence of a soft tissue mass at the point of obstruction suggests choledocholithiasis even without depiction of the stone (Fig. 14.23). Some primary ductal carcinomas will, however, not have a mass detected by CT. Polypoid ductal carcinomas also must be included in the differential diagnosis when a noncalcified soft tissue density "stone" is seen on CT.

REFERENCES

1. Suzuki M, Takaskima T, Funaki H, Uogoshi M, Isobe T, Matsuda Y, Kanno S, Ushitani K, Fuchuh K: CT diagnosis of common bile duct stone. *Gastrointest Radiol* 8:327–331, 1983.
2. Jeffrey RB, Federle MP, Laing FC, Wall S, Rego J, Moss AA: Computed tomography of choledocholithiasis. *AJR* 140:1179–1183, 1983.
3. Baron RL, Stanley RJ, Lee JKT, Koehler RE, Levitt RG: Computed tomographic features of biliary obstruction. *AJR* 140:1173–1178, 1983.
4. Mitchell SE, Clark RA: A comparison of computed tomography and sonography in choledocholithiasis. *AJR* 142:729–733, 1984.
5. Pedrosa CS, Casanova R, Lezana AH, Fernandez MC: Computed tomography in obstructive jaundice; II. The cause of obstruction. *Radiology* 139:635–645, 1981.

Cholangiography

Despite the fact that only 15% (at most) of common duct or intrahepatic biliary calculi are sufficiently opaque to be recognized on a plain film, one should always obtain a scout film prior to opacification of the biliary tree to search for calcification, air, foreign body, etc., all of which might cause confusion if only post-injection radiographs are obtained (1, 2). The entire biliary tree should be opacified during cholangiography; although calculi are most frequently extrahepatic, as many as 16–25% can be intrahepatic (3). Direct cholangiography is probably the only way to reliably diagnose cystic duct remnant stones (Fig. 14.24).

Although ducts are usually dilated in the presence of calculi (Figs. 14.25–14.27), it is now recognized that stones may be present in normal caliber ducts (3, 4) (Fig. 14.28). Stones rarely

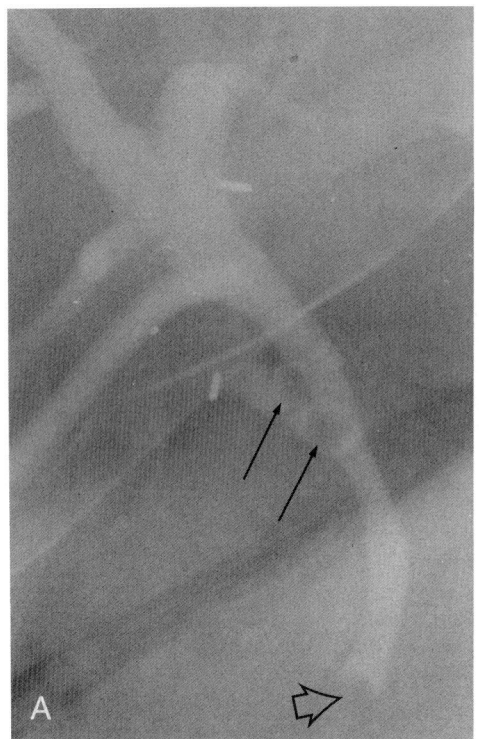
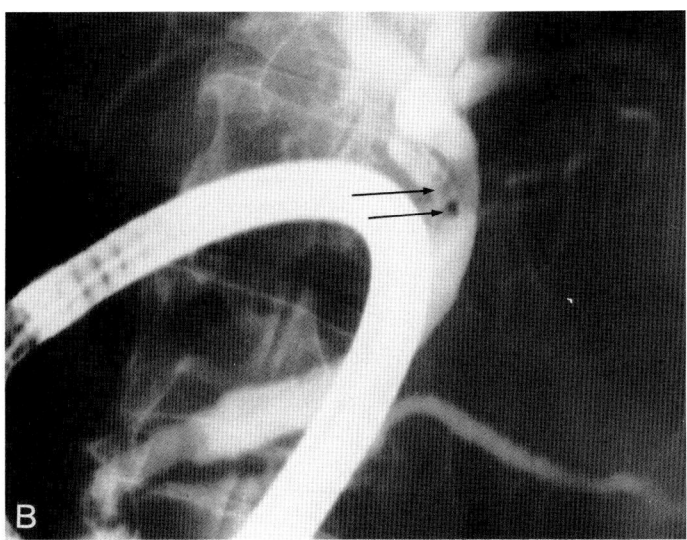

FIGURE 14.24. CYSTIC DUCT REMNANT CALCULI
A and *B:* Cystic duct remnant calculi (*arrows*). *A:* T-tube cholangiogram. *B:* ERCP. The former also shows a stone impacted distally (*open arrow*).

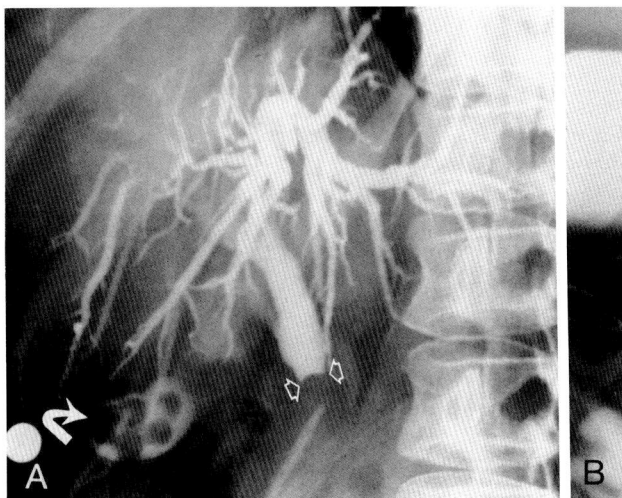
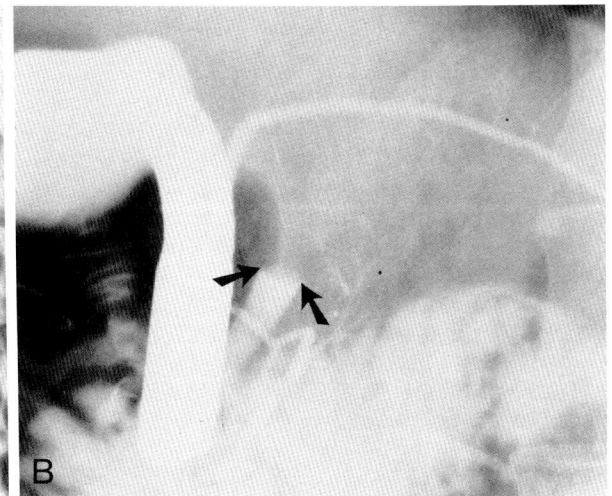

FIGURE 14.25. MENISCUS SIGN, IMPACTED STONES
A: Semierect film, PTC: meniscus above a stone (*arrows*). Gallstones also present (*curved arrow*). Ducts dilated proximally. *B:* ERCP: meniscus from below (*arrows*).

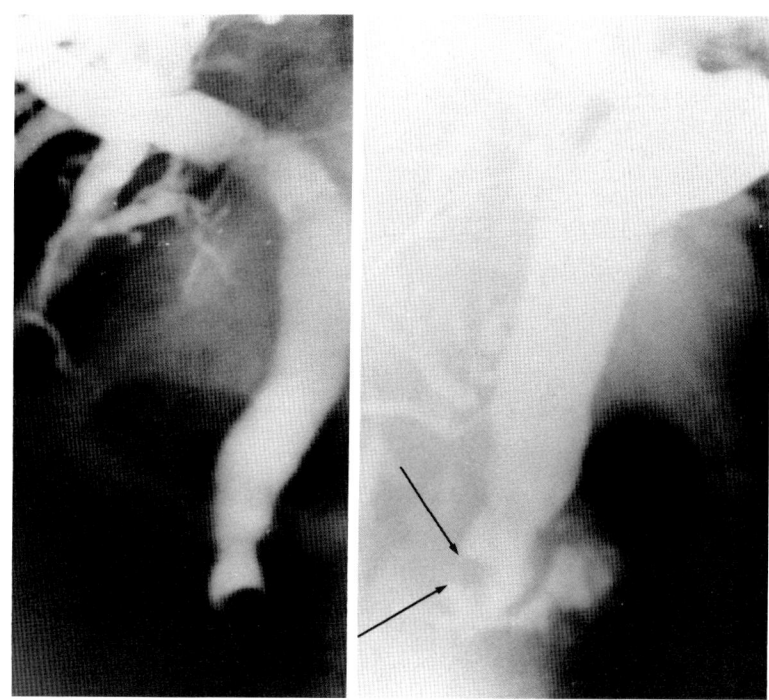

FIGURE 14.26. POLYPOID CARCINOMA
Film on left shows meniscus, but opposite obliquity on right shows attachment to the wall (*arrows*).

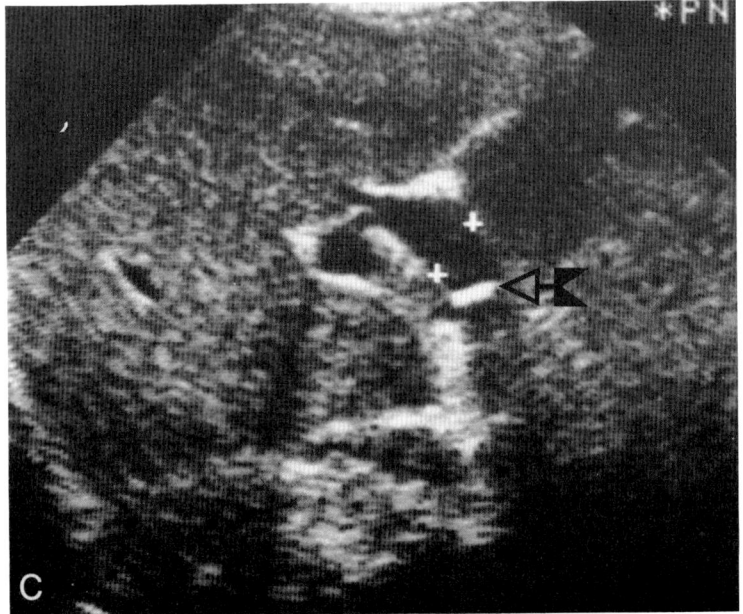

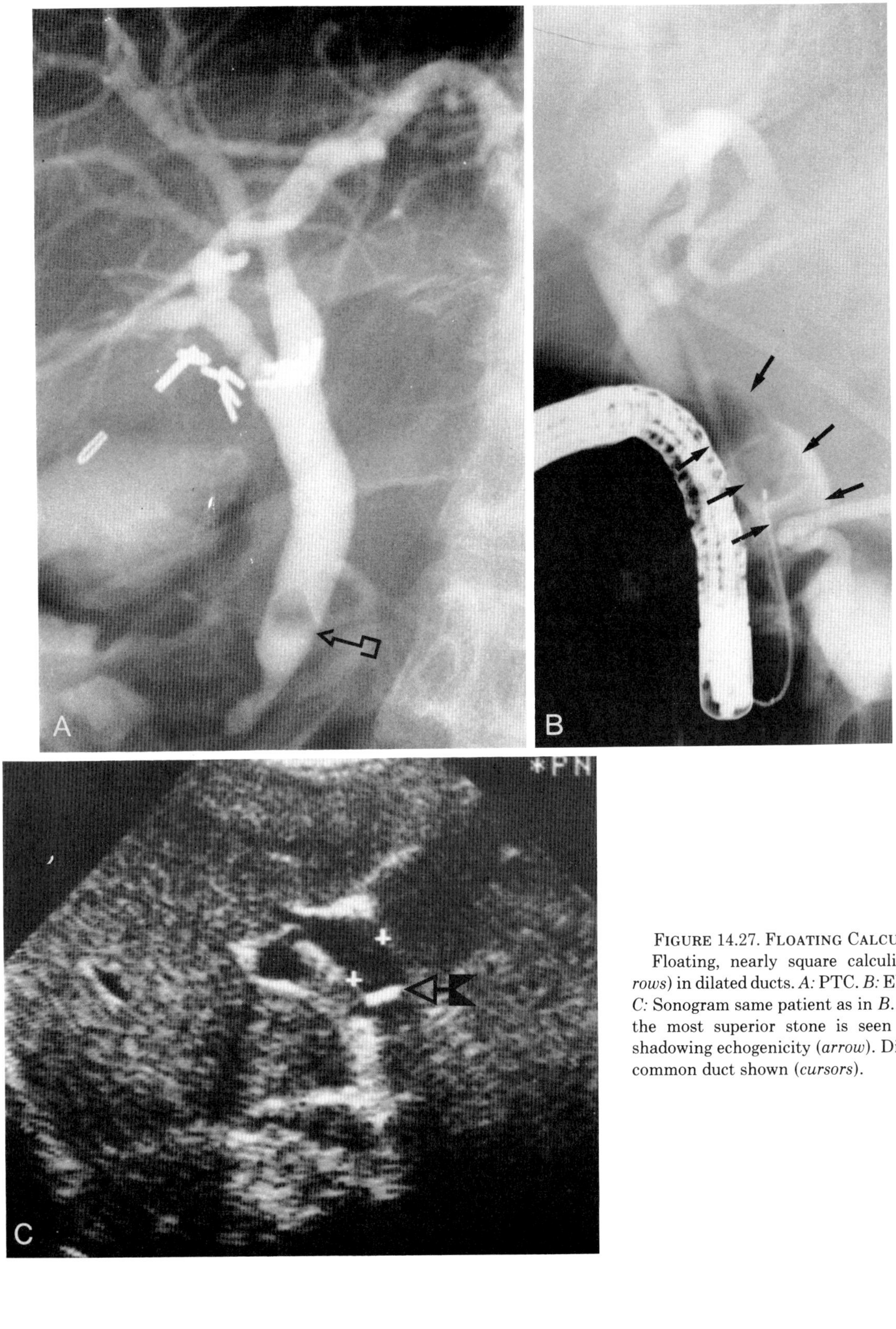

FIGURE 14.27. FLOATING CALCULI
Floating, nearly square calculi (*arrows*) in dilated ducts. *A:* PTC. *B:* ERCP. *C:* Sonogram same patient as in *B*. Only the most superior stone is seen as a shadowing echogenicity (*arrow*). Dilated common duct shown (*cursors*).

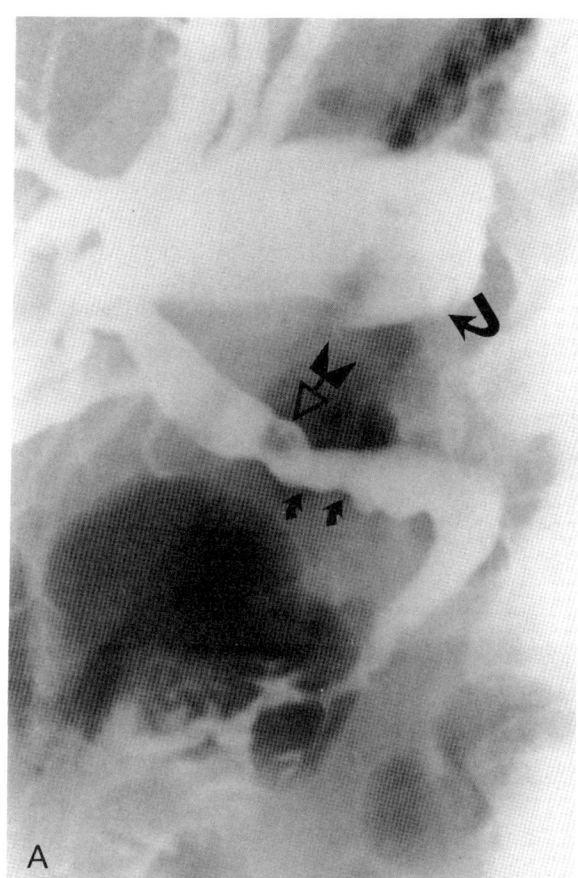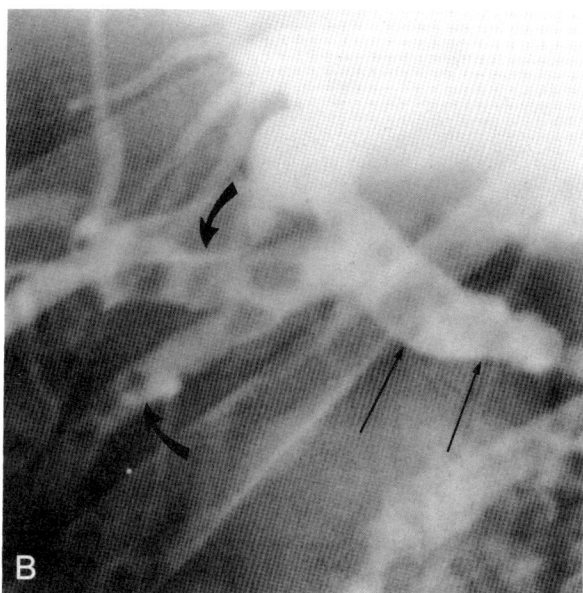

FIGURE 14.28. BILIARY CALCULI IN NONDILATED DUCTS

Biliary calculi in nondilated ducts, post surgery cholecystectomy, no significant abnormality on sonography. *A:* PTC: calculus (*large arrow*) in common duct proximal to mild stricturing (*small arrows*). Free flow of contrast into duodenum on this semierect film. Large contrast collection (*curved arrow*) is subcapsular. *B:* Compression coned down spot film: lucencies are multiple calculi in the proximal common duct (*arrows*) and intrahepatic biliary tree (*curved arrows*).

cause complete obstruction to the flow of cholangiographic contrast unless impacted in the periampullary duct (5). In this circumstance, low grade biliary infection is frequent and it is critical to avoid overinjection which could precipitate septic shock (4). Impacted stones produce a meniscus on either their superior or inferior surface (depending on the route of cholangiography) (Fig. 14.25) (3). Multiple obliquities should be obtained to confirm the presence of the meniscus in all projections to differentiate stone from polypoid tumor. The latter will be adherent to the wall in at least one projection (Fig. 14.26). Of course, a stone adherent to one wall and producing obstruction may cause confusion. Polypoid tumors frequently expand the duct, whereas stones do not (5). Floating biliary stones are filling defects that are generally either ovoid and slightly irregular, faceted, or even nearly square (Fig. 14.27). Sometimes mud-like plugs pack entire radicles and appear as elongated filling defects (4). When multiple stones are present, cholangiography will show them all, whereas noninvasive tests often do not (Fig. 14.27). Differential diagnosis must include polypoid tumor (discussed above), blood clot, admixture defect, and air bubble.

Blood clots are associated with grossly bloody bile, and will clear on reexamination after the cause of the hemobilia is corrected. Admixture defects are caused by poor mixing of contrast with unopacified bile and usually appear as filling defects anteriorly in the contrast column in the suprapancreatic common duct. Rotating the patient and erect filming will abolish the admixture defect. Similarly, a periportal pseudo-obstruction can be produced in the supine position because of contrast material layering in the dependent portions of the intrahepatic biliary tract. Turning the patient to his left and then partially erect will redistribute the contrast material and demonstrate the real site of obstruc-

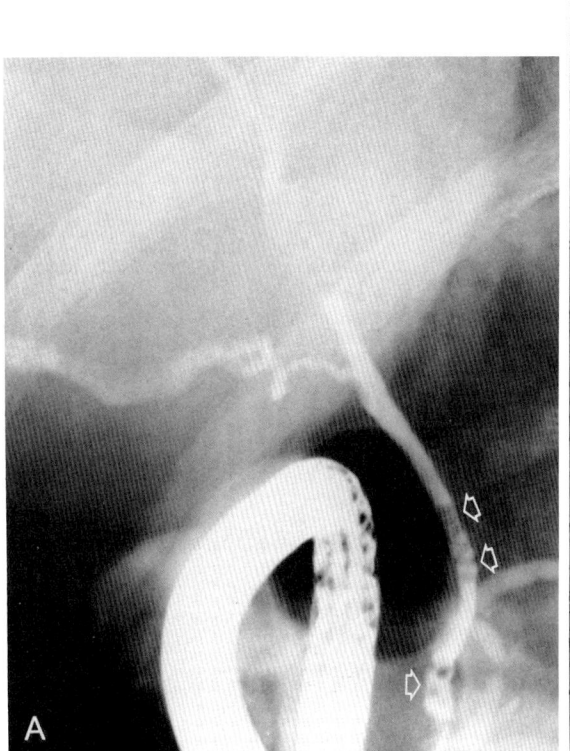
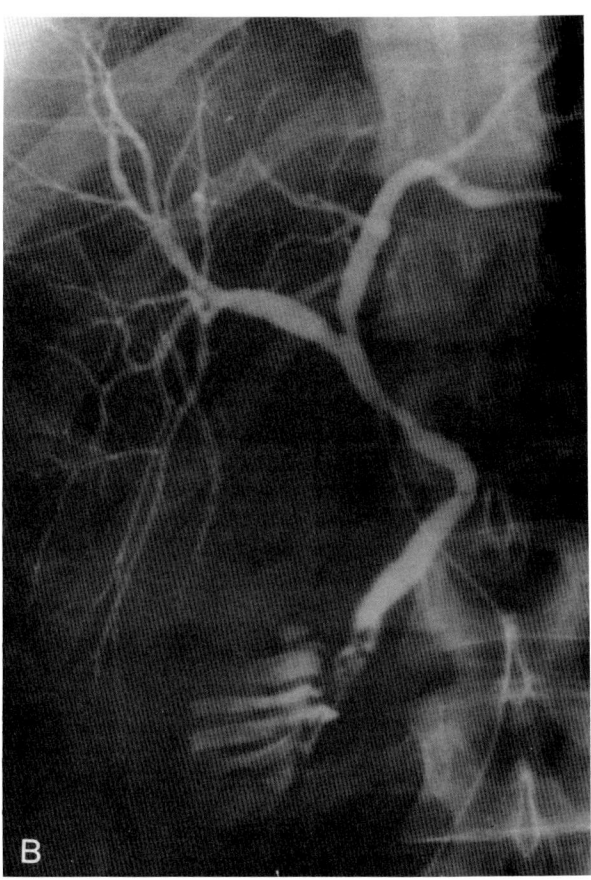

FIGURE 14.29. BUBBLES VERSUS STONES

A: ERCP: multiple tiny air bubbles (*arrows*) mimicking stones in the common duct. Their near perfect roundness suggests the correct diagnosis. Unfortunately, the patient was explored for presumptive stones. *B:* Operative cholangiogram: nonobstructing calculi in the distal common duct not all that different in appearance from the bubbles in *A*. The stones are not quite round on close inspection.

tion, if one is present (4). Air bubbles can be extremely difficult to distinguish from stones (Fig. 14.29). If proper care is taken during ERCP or PTC, air bubbles will rarely be introduced, but this is less easily accomplished during T-tube cholangiography. When pneumobilia is already present (e.g., biliary-enteric anastomosis) air bubbles often form during cholangiography and create difficulty. Air bubbles are usually round and smooth whereas stones are seldom perfectly round and smooth. Air bubbles tend to coalesce. They rise in the erect position while stones usually fall (according to conventional wisdom) (3, 6). It has recently been shown by in vitro experiments (7) that stones also usually float in concentrations of contrast material commonly employed during cholangiography. With currently recommended technique (for operative and T-tube cholangiography) of relatively high iodine concentration and high kilovoltage, almost all stones will float (8). It would appear that the reason the rule of thumb "bubbles rise and stones sink" works is that in vivo, stones are quite often stuck in the distal duct (held down by edema, inflammation and/or scarring) and cannot rise. When all else fails and doubt remains whether one is dealing with air bubbles or stones, the best course is to repeat the examination at a later date. Even this may not help when there is a biliary-enteric anastomosis.

REFERENCES

1. Lahey FH, Swinton NW: Stones in the common and hepatic bile ducts. N Engl J Med 213:1275, 1935.
2. Waugh JM, Johnston EV, Cain JC: Surgical aspects of choledocholithiasis. JAMA 154:734, 1954.
3. Larsen CR, Scholz FJ, Wise RE: Diseases of the biliary ducts. Semin Roentgenol 11:259–267, 1976.
4. Ferrucci JT Jr, Mueller PR, vanSonnenberg E: Transhepatic cholangiography. In Berk RN, Ferrucci JT Jr, Leopold GR (eds): Radiology of the Gallbladder and Bile Ducts. Diagnosis and Intervention. Philadelphia, W. B. Saunders, 1983, pp 328, 350–355.
5. Stewart ET, Geenen JE: Endoscopic retrograde cholangiography. In Berk RN, Ferrucci JT Jr, Leopold GR (eds): Radiology of the Gallbladder and Bile Ducts. Diagnosis and Intervention. Philadelphia, W. B. Saunders, 1983, p 373.
6. Goldberg HI: Operative and postoperative cholecystocholangiography. Semin Roentgenol 11:208, 1976.
7. Culp WC: Buoyancy of gallstones in varying concentrations of contrast media. AJR 143:79–81, 1984.
8. Thompson WM, Halvorsen RA, Gedgaudas RK, Kelvin FM, Rice RP, Woodfield S, Johnson GA: High kvp vs. low kvp for T-tube and operative cholangiography. Radiology 146:635–637, 1983.

BILIARY-ENTERIC ANASTOMOSES

Patients with biliary-enteric anastomoses need radiologic evaluation for functional obstruction and bile duct anatomy when clinical problems such as right upper quadrant pain, abnormal liver function tests, cholangitis, jaundice, or even fever of unknown origin surface. Proper study is most important for those patients whose surgery was for benign disease and who have a long life expectancy. Methods commonly employed include: plain radiography, barium reflux cholangiography, intravenous cholangiography, sonography, radionuclide cholescintigraphy, CT, ERCP, and PTC.

Plain Radiography

Pneumobilia indicates a patent biliary-enteric communication but does not imply lack of obstruction to the flow of bile (Fig. 14.30). Conversely, lack of intrabiliary air does not necessarily imply inadequacy of the anastomosis (1).

Barium Reflux Cholangiography

Although well tolerated by and easily eliminated from the biliary tree, barium cannot always be made to reflux through the surgical anastomosis from the gastrointestinal tract. Even when reflux is easily obtained, adequate demonstration of the anatomy is hampered by the possible obscuration of stones and/or the stoma by the dense barium in the ducts and the overlying gastrointestinal tract, respectively (Figs. 14.31 and 14.32). Calculi are hard to differentiate from discontinuous filling, and fistulas may be missed (2–5). The use of delayed upright films to evaluate emptying of barium from the biliary tree has led to both false positives and false negatives for obstruction in my experience.

Intravenous Cholangiography

Fraught with false positives and false negatives in the intact biliary system, this study becomes essentially uninterpretable in the presence of a biliary-enteric anastomosis (1, 3, 6).

Sonography

Presence or absence of dilatation of intra and extrahepatic ducts can usually be assessed. Refluxed air can be difficult or impossible to differentiate from calculi, however. Unfortunately, the

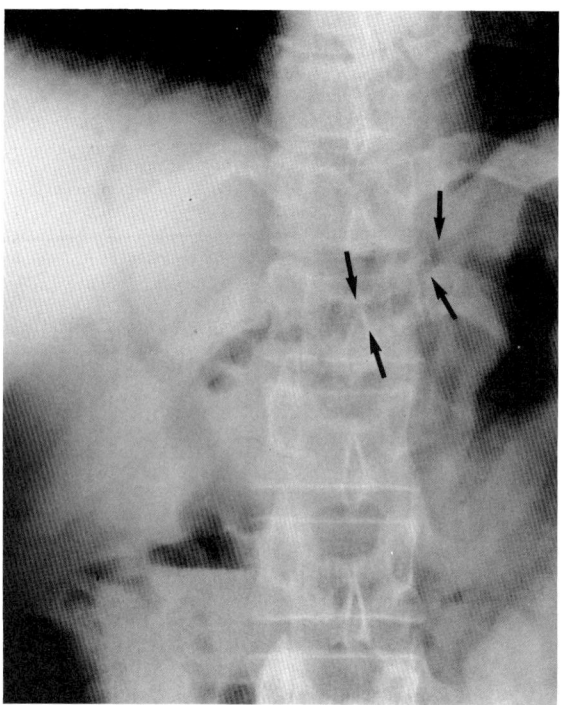

FIGURE 14.30. PNEUMOBILIA
Large amount of gas in the biliary tree after choledochoduodenostomy. Note excellent visualization of the left hepatic duct (arrows). Nevertheless, recurrent (or retained) calculi were present on further evaluation.

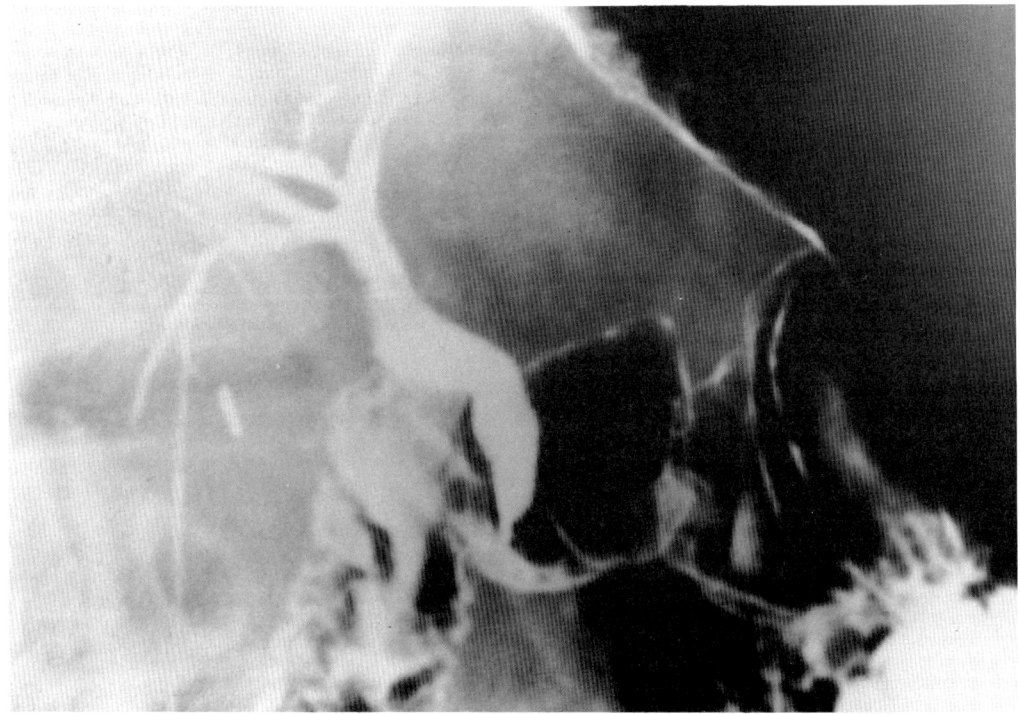

FIGURE 14.31. NORMAL CHOLEDOCHODUODENOSTOMY: DOUBLE CONTRAST UGI

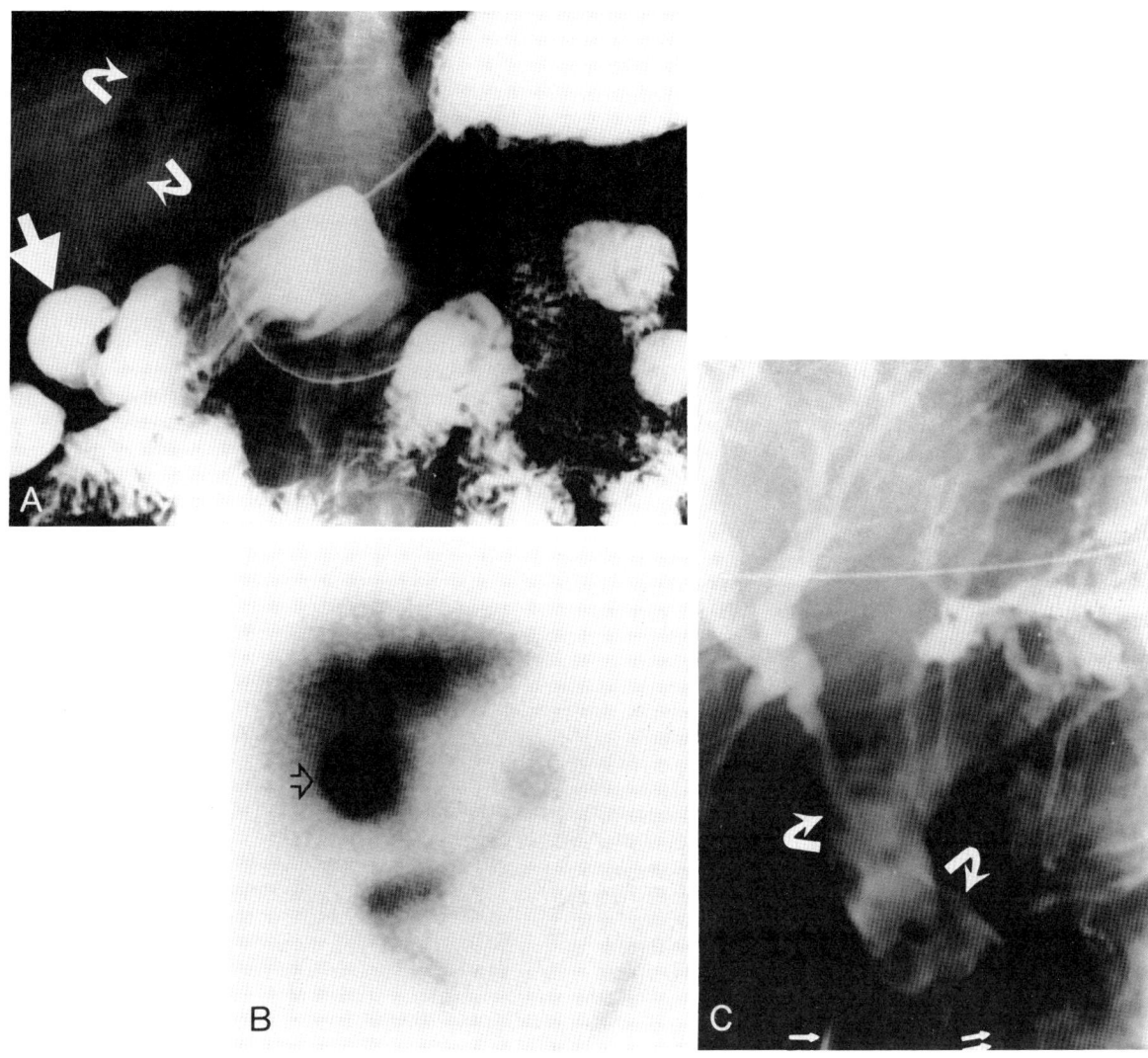

FIGURE 14.32. CBD STONES AFTER CHOLEDOCHOJEJUNOSTOMY

A: Filling of the gallbladder (*arrow*) on UGI and air but no barium in the biliary tree (*curved arrows*). *B:* Radionuclide cholescintigram at ten minutes, performed because of persistently elevated alkaline phosphatase and abdominal pain, shows prompt filling of the gallbladder (*arrow*) and small intestine. *C:* PTC: common duct packed with biliary mud (primary duct calculi: *curved arrows*). Erect film shows contrast dribbling through a high-grade stenosis on its way into jejunum (*double arrows*) and filling cystic duct (*single arrow*). This case illustrates unreliability of noninvasive tests in the face of appropriate clinical data suggesting obstruction.

biliary tree is frequently dilated prior to surgery in this group of patients, and this dilatation can persist even with relief of obstruction. Persistently dilated unobstructed ducts cannot be differentiated from recurrently obstructed ducts by sonography unless a baseline postoperative study is available to show interval increase in duct diameter (7).

Hepatobiliary Scintigraphy

This radionuclide study is useful in deciding whether the biliary tree is functionally obstructed. Delayed washout with prominent retention of activity in hepatic parenchyma and bile ducts at 4 hr postinjection and delayed appearance of intestinal activity (at or beyond 1 hr) suggests obstruction (7). Although advocated as a method of deciding which patients with dilated ducts need cholangiography, false negatives do occur, so that the study cannot replace clinical judgment (Fig. 14.32). As with sonography, a postoperative baseline examination is invaluable; the examination is much more accurate when searching for interval change (7).

Computed Tomography

In my experience, CT is most useful in these patients as an adjunct to cholangiography to help differentiate calculi from air bubbles. Oral contrast is best withheld, at least initially. CT can confirm that sonographically detected calculi are not intrabiliary gas (Fig. 14.33).

Cholangiography

PTC can detect stomal narrowing (usually concentric) anatomically and by delayed drainage of contrast material (Figs. 14.32, 14.34, and 14.35). Stones can usually be differentiated from air bubbles by appropriate positional maneuvers. Cholangiography usually, but not invariably, is the definitive test for the evaluation of biliary-enteric anastomoses (Figs. 14.32 and 14.33). Transhepatic balloon dilatation of anastomotic strictures can be performed as a reasonable alternative to repeat surgery when clinically indicated. Long-term success rates are high (Fig. 14.35). Most recommend stenting for 1–3 months, but some successful balloon dilatations have been reported without stenting (8–11).

ERCP offers the same benefits of direct cholangiography afforded by PTC in these patients but is technically quite difficult because of altered anatomy (Fig. 14.36). If successful, it does

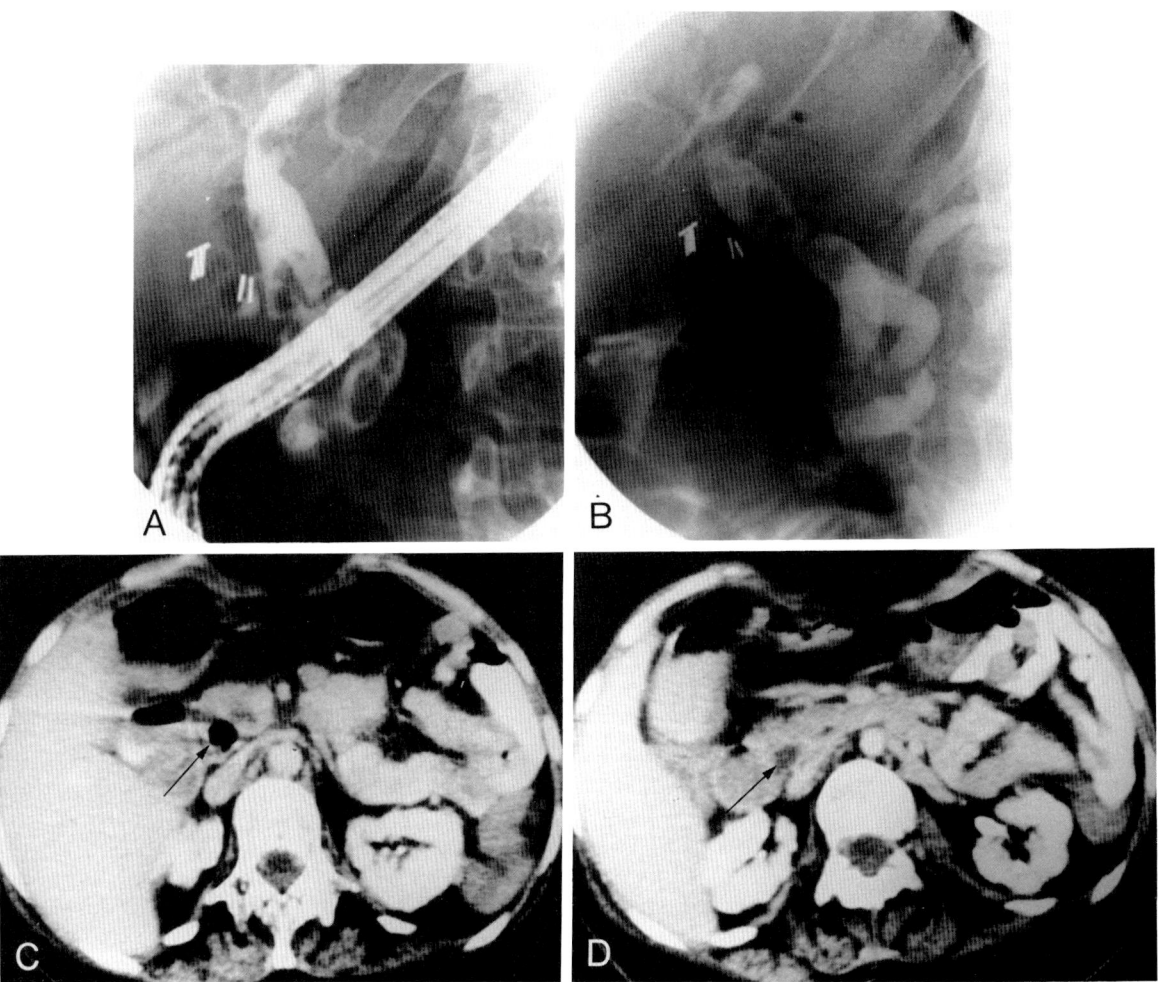

FIGURE 14.33. CASE ILLUSTRATING THE DIFFICULTY THAT MAY BE ENCOUNTERED IN DIFFERENTIATING AIR FROM CALCULI IN A PATIENT POST SURGICAL CHOLEDOCHODUODENOSTOMY

A and *B:* ERCPs 3 months apart both show multiple lucent filling defects (air bubbles) of various shapes mimicking calculi in addition to air in the biliary tree. *C* and *D:* Representative CT scans showed only air (*C, arrow*) and bile (*D, arrow*) in the extrahepatic ducts. At surgery, there were no calculi.

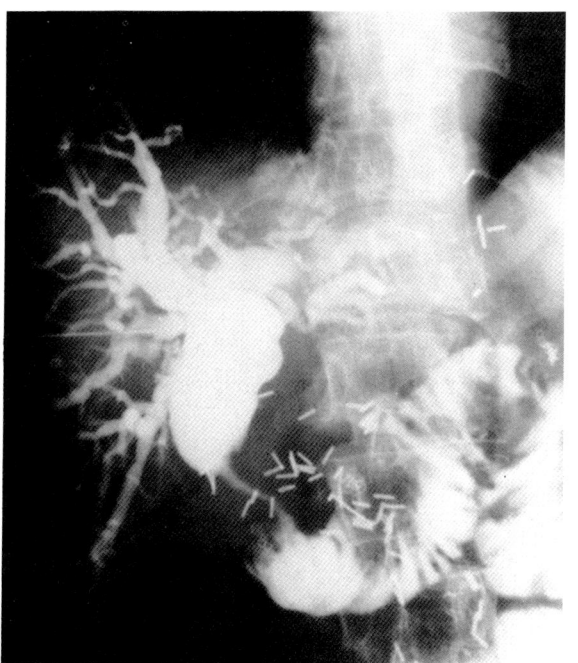

FIGURE 14.34. PTC SHOWING ANASTOMOTIC NARROWING
Clinical history is needed to differentiate benign anastomotic stricture from tumor recurrence. This PTC shows an anastomotic narrowing due to recurrent ampullary carcinoma post surgical Whipple procedure. Some mass effect is present, but clinical information is vital in suggesting the malignant nature of the stricture.

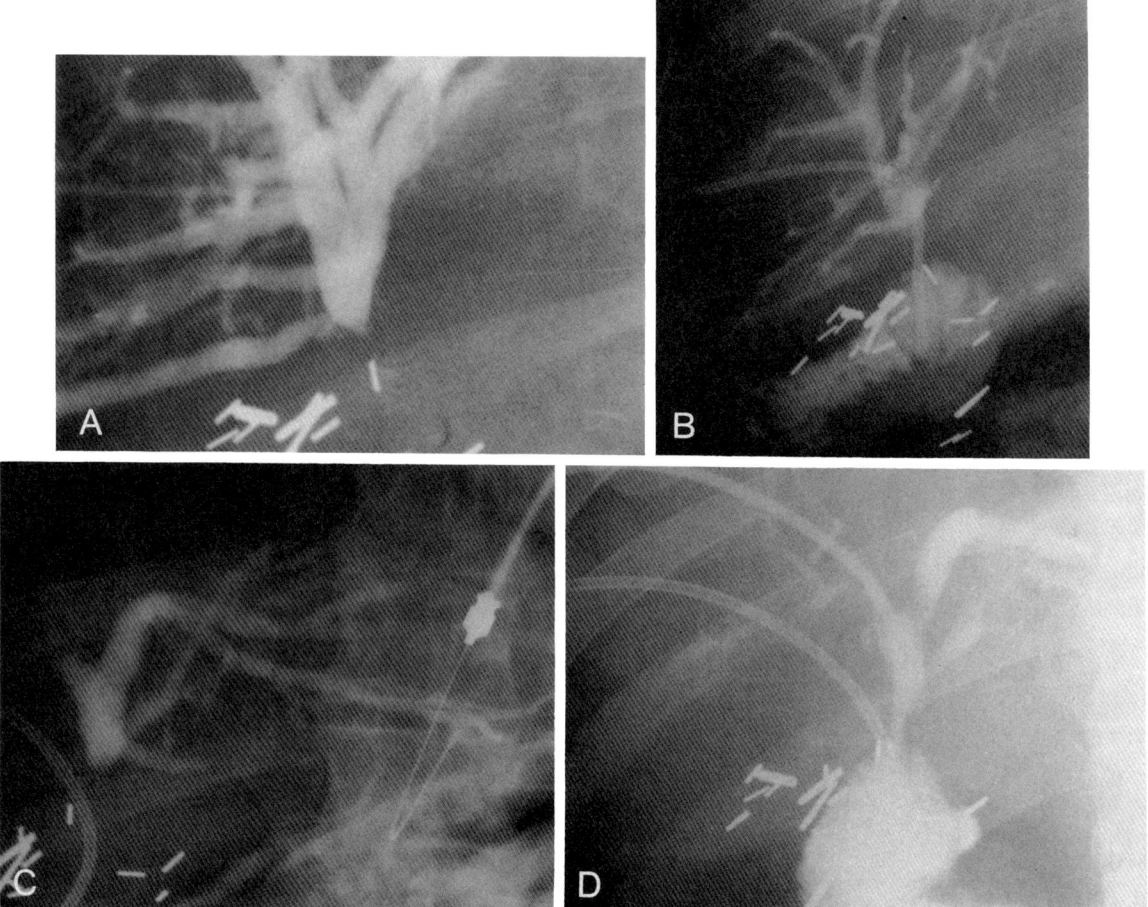

FIGURE 14.35. ANASTOMOTIC STRICTURE POST SURGICAL HIGH CHOLEDOCHOJEJUNOSTOMY FOR IATROGENIC COMMON DUCT INJURY

Patient had elevated enzymes, recurrent bouts of cholangitis and secondary sclerosing cholangitis on liver biopsy, and had been forced into early retirement. He was able to return to work after transhepatic internal drainage. *A:* PTC of right-sided ducts: no flow through anastomosis. *B:* Drainage catheter traversing the stricture. No opacification of left side. *C:* Subxiphoid puncture of the left side: complete obstruction to the flow of contrast and no cross-filling. *D:* Second drainage tube drains the left system from a right-sided approach. Serial transhepatic dilatation of both sides was performed up to 22F and soft catheters were placed. The patient felt so well six months later that he refused to have the catheters removed.

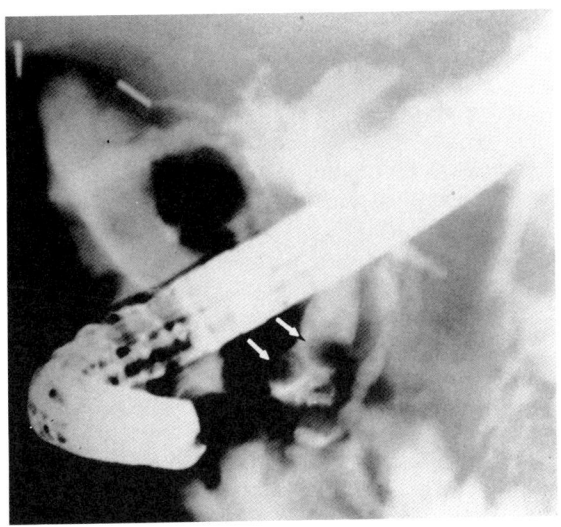

FIGURE 14.36. SUMP SYNDROME
Two retained calculi (*arrows*) in bypassed portion of distal common bile duct post surgical choledochoduodenostomy. PTC would be likely not to opacify this bypassed segment and therefore miss these calculi.

afford the advantages of direct visualization of the anastomosis and pancreatography (1).

REFERENCES

1. Gold RP, Price JB: Thin needle cholangiography as the primary method for the evaluation of the biliary-enteric anastomosis. *Radiology* 136:309–316, 1980.
2. Lucas CE, Read RC: Barium cholangiography. *Radiology* 87:1043–1047, 1966.
3. Wise RE, Keefe JP: Radiologic evaluation of hepaticojejunal anastomoses. *Surg Clin North Am* 48:579–585, 1968.
4. Classen M, Fruhmorgen P, Kozu T et al: Endoscopic-radiologic demonstration of biliodigestive fistulas. *Endoscopy* 3:138–142, 1971.
5. Sorby WA, Ham JM: A new method for roentgenologic assessment of the stoma after choledochoduodenostomy. *Surg Gynecol Obstet* 135:437–439, 1972.
6. Mujahed Z: Non-opacification of the gallbladder and bile ducts. *Radiology* 112:297–298, 1974.
7. Zeman RK, Lee C, Stahl RS, Cahow CE, Viscomi GN, Neumann RD, Gold JA, Burrell MI: Ultrasonography and hepatobiliary scintigraphy in the assessment of biliary-enteric anastomoses. *Radiology* 145:109–115, 1982.
8. Moore PT, Clark RA: An update of interventional biliary radiology. *Semin Ultrasound CT MR* 5:349–368, 1984.
9. Tegtmeyer CJ: The interventionalists's role in biliary tract drainage. *Diagn Imaging* 44–51, Dec. 1984.
10. Martin EC, Fankuchen EI, Laffey KJ, Sibley RE: Percutaneous management of benign biliary disease. *Gastrointest Radiol* 9:207–212, 1984.
11. Molnar W, Stockum AE: Transhepatic dilatation of choledochoenterostomy strictures. *Radiology* 129:59–64, 1978.

CHOLANGIOCARCINOMA

Cholangiocarcinoma is an uncommon tumor, with an autopsy incidence of 0.3–0.5% (1, 2). The tumor is two to three times more common in males than females, with a peak incidence in the sixth and seventh decades. A higher incidence of cholangiocarcinoma is associated with inflammatory bowel disease, sclerosing cholangitis, and gallstones (2, 3). Cholangiocarcinomas have been reported to arise within the walls of congenital bile duct cysts (4).

Clinical Findings

The most common presenting sign is jaundice, frequently accompanied by weight loss, pruritus, and anorexia. Additional possible complaints include abdominal pain, acholic stools, weakness, and diarrhea. Obstruction of a segmental duct alone may produce elevated alkaline phosphatase and sometimes fever without jaundice. Tumors originating below the cystic duct often cause gallbladder distention.

Laboratory studies usually reveal elevations in alkaline phosphatase and bilirubin frequently with slight aminotransferase elevation as well.

Cholangiocarcinomas are slow growing tumors that, due to their critical location, produce obstructive symptoms early. They generally are small (2 cm or less) at the time of diagnosis. Despite this, prognosis is poor in general with the five-year survival rate of bile duct cancer being 5% in the Lahey Clinic experience (5). Patients succumb eventually to the complications of biliary obstruction rather than metastatic disease. These include: cholangitis, biliary cirrhosis, liver abscess, suppurative pylephlebitis, portal hypertension and periportal fibrosis. Prognosis is best for polypoid carcinomas and worst for diffuse sclerosing carcinomas with focal stenotic lesions intermediate. Carcinomas limited to the more distal duct have a longer average survival and higher probability of surgical cure (2). Decision regarding surgical palliation versus attempted excision versus percutaneous or endoscopic drainage requires consideration of many factors including the systemic effects of invasion or disseminated cancer, potential relief of obstructive symptoms, potential life extension, and total cost of the effort. Lesions without a proven diagnosis should be approached surgically if possible.

Pathology

Cholangiocarcinomas originate most frequently in the larger bile ducts (1, 6, 7). Rates in large series are as follows: 8–13% intrahepatic ducts, 10–26% at the confluence of the hepatic ducts (Klatskin tumor (3)), 15–30% proximal common duct and 30–36% distal common duct. In a smaller series of 63 patients from the Mayo Clinic, distribution of common duct carcinoma was proximal third, 54%, middle and distal third, 21% each, and 5% involved most or all of the common duct (5). Most are adenocarcinomas and a minority are other histologies such as squamous cell and anaplastic. Growth patterns are either infiltrating and scirrhous, nodular, or papillary. The former is the most common (3, 7) and characteristically presents as a focal biliary stricture, often without evidence of mass (8), at times producing longer strictures or even infiltrating a large part of the biliary tree mimicking sclerosing cholangitis. Differentiation from benign causes of stricturing is made more difficult by the fact that malignant cells may be hard or impossible to detect in the midst of the extensive desmoplastic reaction that these neoplasms may incite. Only about 5% of cholangiocarcinomas are of the papillary type, which present as intraluminal masses (8).

Radiology

The foregoing discussion excludes cholangiocarcinomas arising in the peripheral biliary tree, since these are radiologically hepatic masses and are discussed in the section on the liver in this book.

Ultrasound

Sonography will demonstrate biliary dilatation proximal to the tumor in the vast majority of cases. Proximal cholangiocarcinomas are more readily imaged by ultrasound than distal ones which are often obscured by bowel gas. Key to successful differentiation from choledocholithiasis or benign stricture is demonstration of a mass either within or surrounding the ducts at the point of obstruction. This is usually not possible. Wall thickening at the point of obstruction can be seen with benign strictures. Cholangiocarcinoma should be suspected when abrupt obstruction is seen and no stone or mass is demonstrable. When masses have been seen, they have been described as persistent intraluminal echoes without shadowing by most authors (6–9), although Dillon describes irregularly defined coarse acoustic shadows arising from the mass as being specific for cholangiocarcinoma (10). Subramanyan (7) describes some tumors as echogenic bands crossing the bile ducts. The sonographic differential diagnosis of an intraluminal nonshadowing mass includes nonshadowing calculi and uncommon benign tumors such as adenoma, papilloma or a polyp, as well as gallbladder or hepatocellular carcinoma extending into the duct, blood clot, or sludge (the latter is usually accompanied by sludge in the gallbladder).

In patients with cholangiocarcinoma the gallbladder may be either small or distended. The biliary tract proximal to the obstruction is either mildly or markedly dilated (7). At the level of the tumor, the bile ducts will be narowed if the process is primarily desmoplastic and widened if there is an obturating intraluminal mass. "Cystic" appearing dilatation of the biliary tree has been reported in a patient with sclerosing cholangitis who developed cholangiocarcinoma. This is suggestive of superimposed neoplasm in patients with known sclerosing cholangitis since the latter does not usually cause that marked a biliary dilatation on sonography (11). Sonographic demonstration of dilatation of intrahepatic ducts without any evidence of extrahepatic dilatation is suspicious for a Klatskin tumor, with or without the demonstration of small tumor masses in the porta hepatis (3, 7). A key finding is failure to demonstrate the confluence of the right and left hepatic ducts in the portal region. Invasion of the liver is suggested by lack of margination of the hepatic parenchyma. The left and right sides may or may not be equally dilated. It is not possible to reliably differentiate between Klatskin tumor and adenopathy in the porta hepatis, although adenopathy is more likely to produce a sonographically visible mass (Fig. 14.37). Metastatic carcinoma is less likely if there is no known primary. Lymphoma is usually associated with adenopathy elsewhere in the abdomen, whereas cholangiocarcinoma generally is not until far advanced. When abrupt common bile duct obstruction is seen without evidence of stone or mass, cholangiocarcinoma is a consideration, especially if a normal pancreas is well-depicted. If a mass is seen, carcinoma of the pancreas is far more likely (Fig. 14.38).

Computed Tomography

Published experience with CT in extrahepatic cholangiocarcinoma has been limited. Klatskin tumors more often than not have produced visible soft tissue masses in the region of the com-

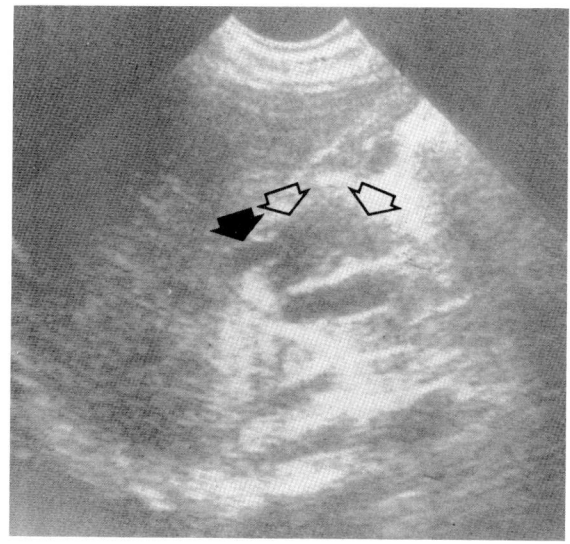

FIGURE 14.37. LYMPHOMA
Parasagittal scan: abrupt obstruction of the very proximal common hepatic duct (*closed arrow*) with a large soft tissue mass (*open arrows*). The latter argues against cholangiocarcinoma. Diagnosis: lymphoma.

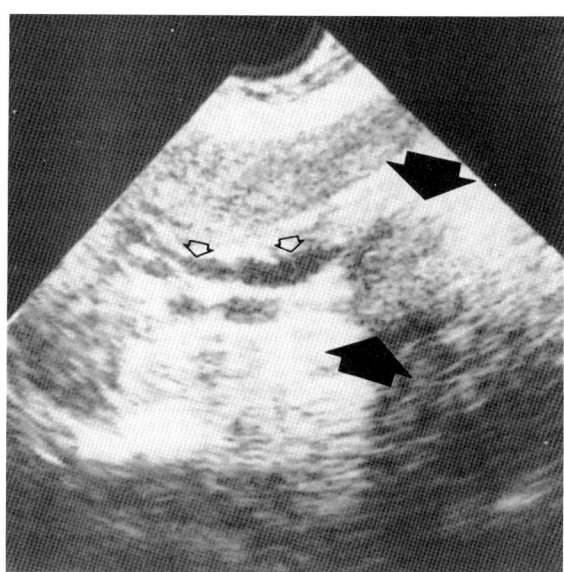

FIGURE 14.38. CARCINOMA OF THE PANCREAS
Parasagittal scan: suprapancreatic abrupt common bile duct obstruction (*open arrows*). Large mass (*closed arrows*) favors the correct diagnosis of carcinoma of the pancreas.

mon hepatic duct in the porta hepatis at the level of obstruction in addition to marked proximal ductal dilatation (12–14) (Fig. 14.39). Usually these masses are small and sometimes fairly low density. Lymphoma and metastatic nodes tend to produce larger masses. When there is a large mass invading the liver (often contrast-enhanc-ing) the lesion is better classified as an intrahepatic cholangiocarcinoma. Bile duct cancers originating in the distal common hepatic duct or the proximal common bile duct usually have no associated mass, and the diagnosis may be suggested by abrupt biliary obstruction at the appropriate level without a visualized mass or calculus. Distal common duct cancers may or may not have an associated mass. If a mass is present, it could be neoplasm or secondary pancreatitis, and the two are usually indistinguishable. Pancreatic carcinoma is far more likely a diagnosis in the presence of a mass. Again, abrupt obstruction in the absence of a mass or calculus (or the presence of a very small mass) suggests the diagnosis of primary bile duct cancer (or, when very distal, ampullary carcinoma). Finally, a diffuse sclerosing cholangiocarcinoma, as is the case with sclerosing cholangitis, is apt to cause a minimal, irregular biliary dilatation even in the face of markedly high laboratory values for obstructive jaundice (13).

Cholangiography

Percutaneous transhepatic cholangiography (PTC) and endoscopic retrograde cholangiopancreatography (ERCP) are still the best modalities available for depicting bile duct neoplasms. From a diagnostic standpoint, it is important to know whether or not previous biliary surgery has been performed. Iatrogenic postoperative strictures are typically long and smooth as opposed to bile duct carcinoma which is shorter with an irregular margin. The classic Klatskin tumor at the bifurcation is an irregular stricture with prestenotic dilatation (Fig. 14.40). One or both of the left and right main ducts may be affected in addition to the proximal common hepatic duct. With high-grade obstruction, contrast may not fill either or both main intrahepatic ducts during ERCP even after deep selective cannulation of the common duct. After excluding technical difficulties as the cause of underfilling, this appearance is quite suggestive of cholangiocarcinoma (Fig. 14.40B). PTC has the advantage of being able to delineate the intrahepatic ductal anatomy in this situation. Other entities that may produce a similar cholangiographic appearance to Klatskin tumor are: metastatic adenopathy (Fig. 14.40C), lymphoma, hepatocellular carcinoma (Fig. 14.40D), or, less likely, cirrhotic nodules (12, 15, 16).

Bile duct carcinoma has been classified cholangiographically as either obstructive, stenotic, or protuberant (polypoid and intraluminal) (15) (Fig. 14.41). The obstructive type is the most

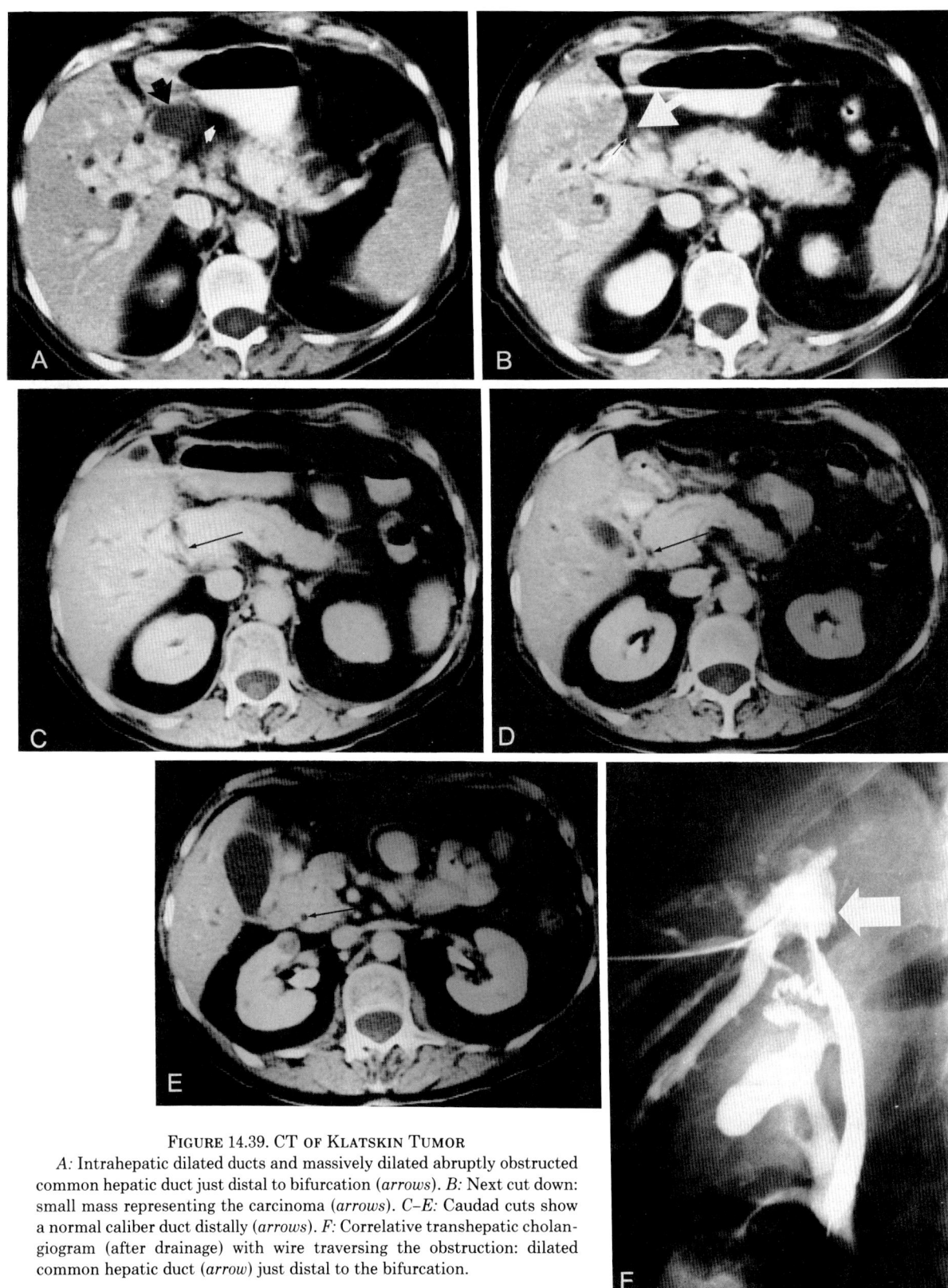

FIGURE 14.39. CT OF KLATSKIN TUMOR

A: Intrahepatic dilated ducts and massively dilated abruptly obstructed common hepatic duct just distal to bifurcation (*arrows*). *B:* Next cut down: small mass representing the carcinoma (*arrows*). *C–E:* Caudad cuts show a normal caliber duct distally (*arrows*). *F:* Correlative transhepatic cholangiogram (after drainage) with wire traversing the obstruction: dilated common hepatic duct (*arrow*) just distal to the bifurcation.

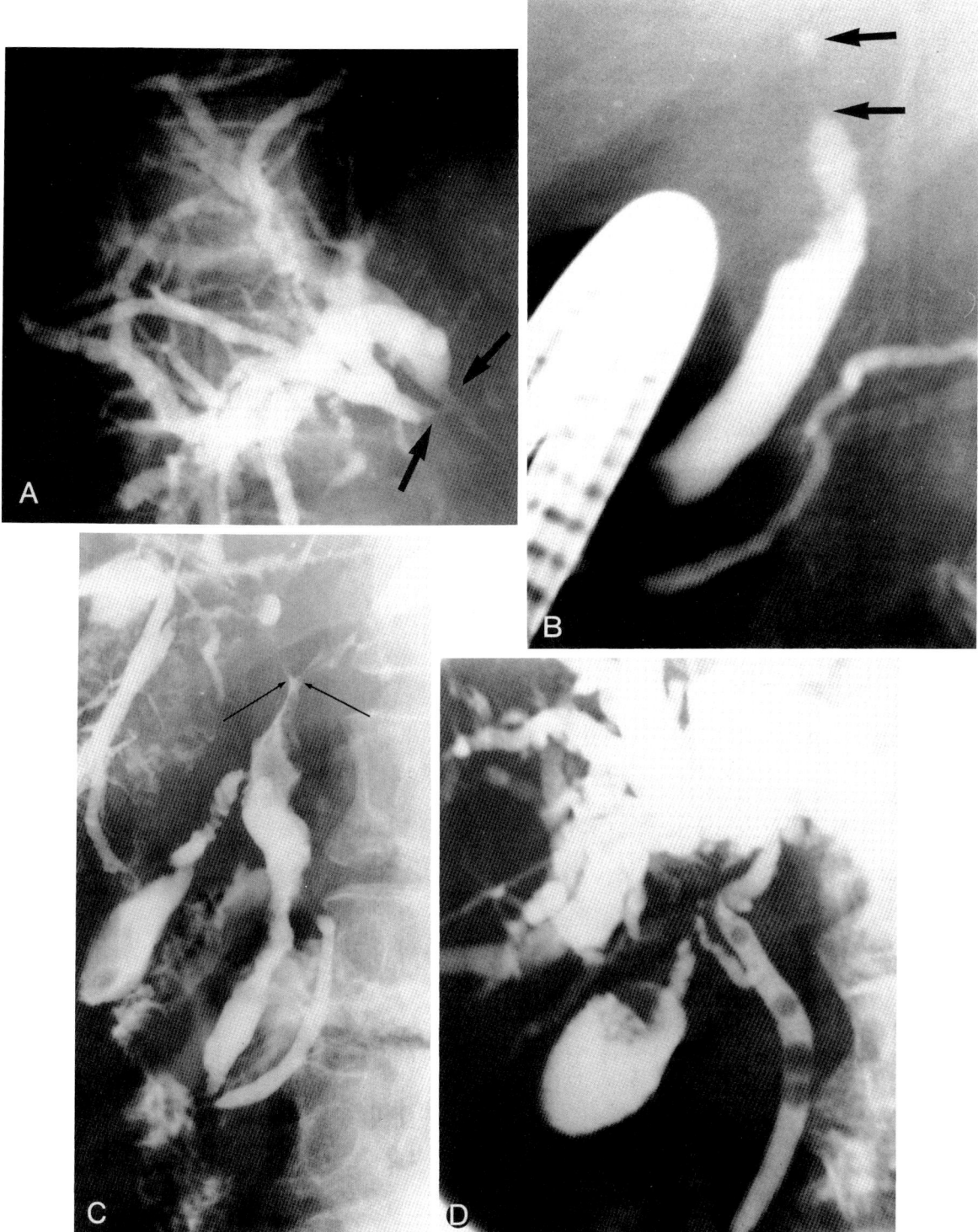

FIGURE 14.40. KLATSKIN TUMOR OR METASTATIC DISEASE?
A and *B:* Klatskin tumor. *A:* PTC, LPO projection: slightly tapered abrupt obstruction at the bifurcation (*arrows*). *B:* ERCP: complete obstruction of the common bile duct (*arrows*) above the pancreas. *C:* Metastatic colon carcinoma: marked stenosis at the bifurcation (*arrows*), with irregular contour abnormalities involving nearly the entire common duct, indistinguishable from advanced cholangiocarcinoma. *D:* Intrahepatic primary hepatocellular carcinoma invading the porta hepatis and producing a high grade obstruction on PTC. Filling defects in common duct are air bubbles.

frequent, occurring in about 70% of cholangiograms and appearing as a U- or V-shaped obstruction with a nipple, rat-tail, smooth, or irregular termination (7, 8) (Fig. 14.42). PTC rather than ERCP is necessary to evaluate the intrahepatic biliary tree, although if this lesion is encountered at ERCP, some success at proximal filling has been reported using a balloon catheter (15–18). Most apparent obstructions can be traversed with a guidewire (Fig. 14.39F). The stenotic type is depicted as a strictured, rigid lumen with irregular margins and prestenotic dilatation (Fig. 14.43). The length of the stenosis may be long or short. Diffuse sclerosing cholangiocarcinoma causes widespread stricturing throughout the biliary tree, (both intra- and extra-hepatic) resembling sclerosing cholangitis (Fig. 14.44).

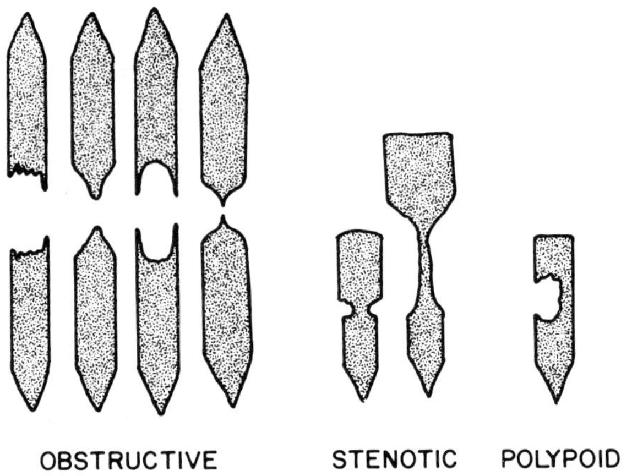

FIGURE 14.41. COMMON TYPES OF BILE DUCT CARCINOMA
Diagrammatic representation of types of common bile duct carcinoma. (Modified from Ligoury C, Canard JM: Tumors of the biliary system. *Clin Gastroenterol* 12:274, 1983.).

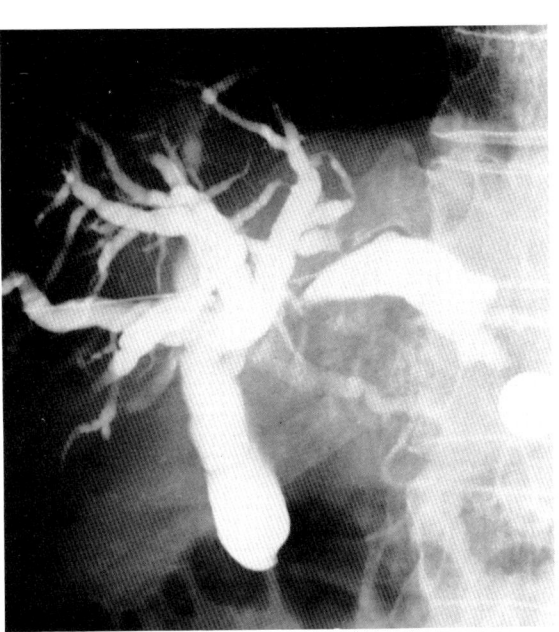

FIGURE 14.42. OBSTRUCTION FROM CHOLANGIOCARCINOMA
PTC: irregular U-shaped obstruction from cholangiocarcinoma.

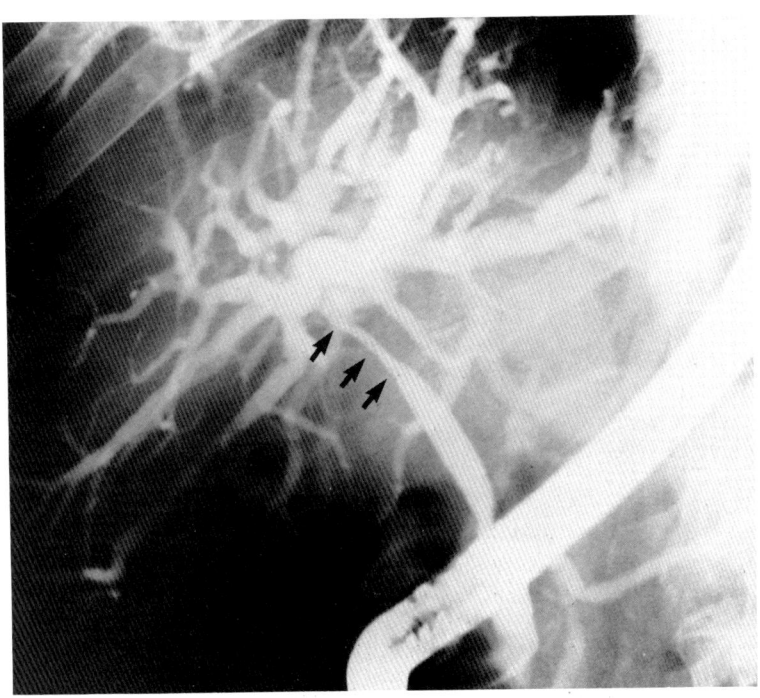

FIGURE 14.43. STENOTIC CHOLANGIOCARCINOMA
Long segment stricture (*arrows*).

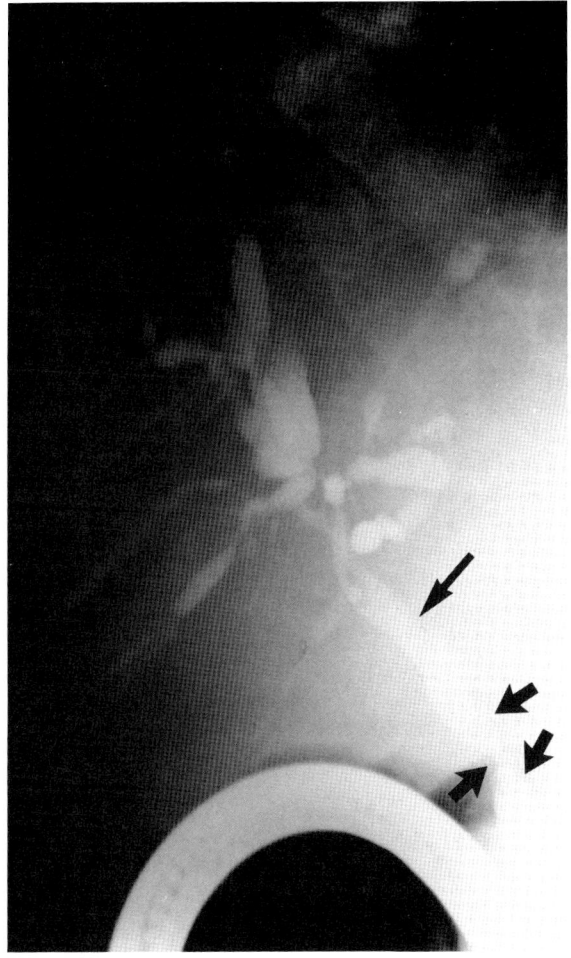

FIGURE 14.44. DIFFUSE SCLEROSING CHOLANGIOCARCINOMA
ERCP: diffuse sclerosing cholangiocarcinoma involving intra and extrahapatic ducts. Nodular lesion (*long arrow*) and irregular long stricture in the common duct (*arrows*) suggest the correct diagnosis rather than sclerosing cholangitis.

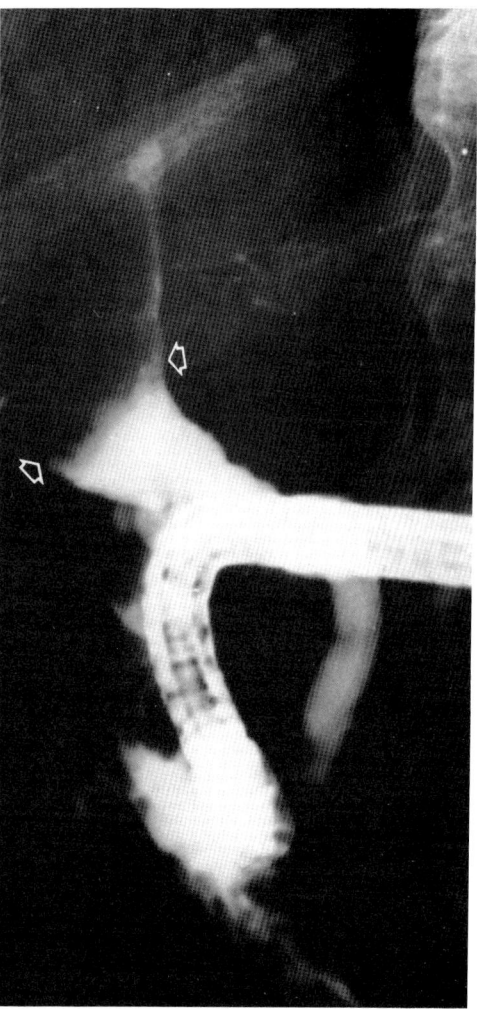

FIGURE 14.45. PAPILLARY CARCINOMA
ERCP: Large intraluminal filling defect with irregular margins (*arrows*). Papillary carcinoma of the common hepatic duct. Note widening of the duct by the mass.

Clues to the correct diagnosis include absence of diverticula in the extrahepatic biliary tree, more severe disease in the extrahepatic biliary tree, and prominent dilatation of ducts. The differentiation really rests on positive biopsy or cytology for malignancy, and malignant cells are often difficult to find because of the extensive desmoplastic reaction induced by the tumor. The protuberant type (about 5%) (Fig. 14.45) appears as an intraluminal filling defect usually with irregular margins attached at one point to the wall (filming in several obliquities may be needed to demonstrate the attachment). The duct is often widened in the region of the mass (15).

Using either PTC or ERCP, brush biopsy, bile juice cytology, and percutaneous aspiration biopsy can be performed. Although technically difficult, forceps biopsy can be done during ERCP. False positivies for atypia may occur in forceps biopsies after endoscopic sphincterotomy for stent placement (19).

Nuclear Medicine

Hilar cholangiocarcinomas manifest themselves as a prominent porta hepatis sometimes with centrifugally radiating linear regions of decreased activity (flare pattern) on sulfur-colloid scans (Fig. 14.46). Hepatobiliary scintigraphy can demonstrate the level and degree of biliary obstruction present. Avidity for gallium is usually not present.

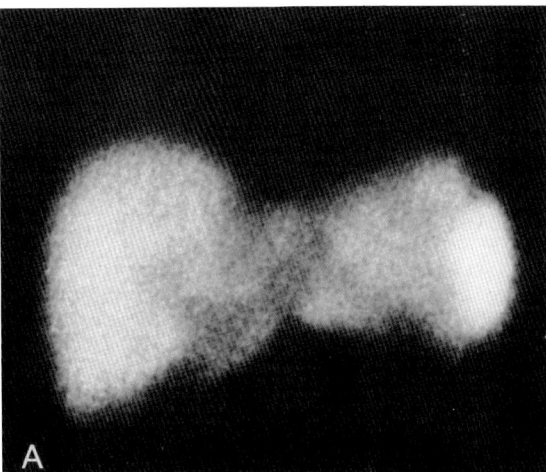
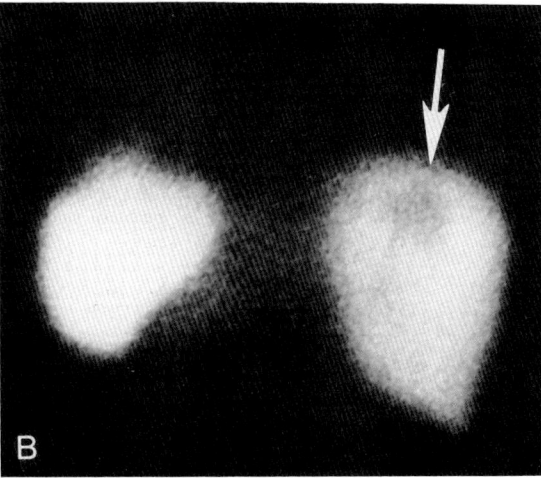

FIGURE 14.46. HILAR CHOLANGIOCARCINOMA
Hilar cholangiocarcinoma, flare sign. Anterior sulfur colloid scan. *A:* A central region of photon deficiency radiating towards the periphery. *B:* The posterior view shows an intrahepatic metastasis (*arrow*).

Angiography

Angiography is rarely employed in the evaluation of bile duct carcinoma. However, as palliation of biliary obstruction improves and survival is lengthened, vascular complications such as portal hypertension from portal venous invasion may be seen more frequently (1). Angiographic findings in bile duct carcinomas include: vascular encasement and/or occlusion with or without fine neovascularity in the region of the liver hilum, tubular lucencies in the hepatogram representing dilated ducts, focal encasement of the portal vein near its bifurcation, and arterioarterial collaterals in the region of the liver hilum (20).

Interventional Aspects

Treatment alternatives include: external biliary drainage, internal biliary drainage (either with capping of the external portion of the catheter or with internal stenting), and radical biliary-enteric anastomosis. Percutaneous transhepatic drainage is useful preoperatively to lower the bilirubin to below 10 mg/dl as several studies have shown a decrease in perioperative mortality with a lower bilirubin (21-24). Having a drainage catheter in place allows rapid identification of the anatomy at surgery since the surgeon can palpate the catheter (22, 23). Permanent palliative decompression with either internal or external drainage can be accomplished percutaneously in nonsurgical candidates (22-24). Although purely internal stents can be placed percutaneously, the endoscopic route, if available, is preferable for internal stenting since trauma to the liver is minimized. A combined percutaneous/endoscopic approach can be useful, giving one the ability to pull rather than have to push an endoscopically placed stent across the obstruction (25).

Temporary decompression can be performed during ERCP for obstruction (or cholangitis). Permanent placement of a nasobiliary catheter or an internal biliary stent may be performed following endoscopic sphincterotomy at the time of the diagnostic procedure (23, 26-28). A straight Amsterdam type of stent prosthesis offers the best flow rate; pigtails reduce the flow rate (16). Larger stents up to 12 F have been advocated (27).

In a recent review, external drainage or internal drainage with or without endoprosthesis insertion were able to reduce bilirubin markedly in 63% and moderately in 17%. Little or no reduction occurred in 20%. Complications occurred in 18% of transhepatic procedures with acute pancreatitis and cholangitis the most frequent. Bile leakage and hemobilia were seen in 1-3%. Complication rates were somewhat lower with endoscopic procedures (21, 23, 29, 30). These figures are a rough guideline at best, as in any given institution complication and success rates will depend primarily on the skill and judgment of the operator rather than on the technique used. Finally, common duct cancers that are at or near the bifurcation, in which the left and right main hepatic ducts either do not communicate or have impending noncommunication, require drainage of each side to avoid sepsis (colonization of the drained side will lead to sepsis in the obstructed side if only one side is drained, despite the fact that bilirubin can be nearly normalized if only one of the two major ducts is opened up).

Surgical Considerations

Preoperative assessment of bile duct cancers will facilitate intraoperative evaluation. Surgical exploration and assessment will offer resectability in as many as 40% in the best (or most aggressive) hands (25). The surgical approach must be individualized.

Resectability is rare and surgical palliation is difficult for proximal bile duct cancers. Silastic catheters inserted into both hepatic ducts and bilateral hepatojejunostomies allow for permanent drainage and improved long-term results in Klatskin tumors (31, 32). Alternatively, standard choledochoenterostomy or hepatico-enterostomy can be performed if feasible (21, 33). Tumors that are not resectable require operative dilatation and stent placement. However, this can be accomplished transhepatically (or, with somewhat more difficulty, endoscopically). Partial hepatectomy has not substantially improved overall survival except in lesions sufficiently proximal to the hilum of the liver to be considered intrahepatic cholangiocarcinomas (15, 21, 34).

Middle segment lesions require prophylactic cholecystectomy (to preclude cystic duct obstruction) with biliary bypass via an anastomosis between the jejunum and the hepatic bifurcation (21, 35).

Resection via pancreaticoduodenectomy for distal common bile duct cancers can be performed with a 5-yr survival rate approaching 30%, but an operative mortality of 5–10%. In nonresectable cases, palliation by choledocho- or cholecysto-jejunostomy is usually feasible (35).

Radiotherapy with Iridium-192 wires placed across proximal bile duct carcinomas either percutaneously or surgically has had some success. Chemotherapy has been disappointing (15, 36).

Summary

Bile duct carcinoma generally carries a poor prognosis, but a better one than carcinoma of the pancreas. Preoperative diagnostic studies are required to define anatomic location and extent of the lesion and to make a pathologic diagnosis if possible. Surgical resection should always be considered, but it is possible in only some instances. Percutaneous and endoscopic nonsurgical methods of palliation are widely available and often preferable to surgery when all factors are considered.

REFERENCES

1. Gold JA, Sostman HD, Burrell MI: Cholangiocarcinoma with portal vein obstruction. *Radiology* 130:15–20, 1979.
2. Nichols DA, MacCarty RL, Gaffey TA: Cholangiographic evaluation of bile duct carcinoma. *AJR* 141:1291–1294, 1983.
3. Meyer DG, Weinstein BJ: Klatskin tumors of the bile ducts: sonographic appearance. *Radiology* 148:803–804, 1983.
4. Todani T, Tabuchi K, Watanabe Y, Kobayashi T: Carcinoma arising in the wall of congenital bile duct cysts. *Cancer* 44:1134–1141, 1979.
5. Warren KW, Tan EGC: Disease of the gallbladder and bile ducts. In Schiff L (ed): *Diseases of the Liver*. Philadelphia, J. B. Lippincott, 1975, pp 1278–1335.
6. Levine E, Maklad NF, Wright CH, Lee KR: Computed tomographic and ultrasonic appearances of primary carcinoma of the common bile duct. *Gastrointest Radiol* 4:147–151, 1979.
7. Subramanyam BR, Raghavendra BN, Balthazar EJ, Horil SC, Lefleur RS, Rosen RJ: Ultrasonic features of cholangiocarcinoma. *J Ultrasound Med* 3:405–408, 1984.
8. Schnur MJ, Hoffman JC, Koenigsberg M: Ultrasonic demonstration of intraductal biliary neoplasms. *J Clin Ultrasound* 10:246–248, 1982.
9. Bondestam S, Kivilaakso EO, Standertskjold-Nordemstam CM, Holmstrom T, Hastbacka J: Sonographic diagnosis of a bile duct polyp. *AJR* 135:610–611, 1980.
10. Dillon E, Peel AL, Perkin GJ: The diagnosis of primary bile duct carcinoma (cholangiocarcinoma) in the jaundiced patient. *Clin Radiol* 32:311, 1981.
11. Gluskin LE, Payne JA: Cystic dilatation as a radiographic sign of cholangiocarcinoma complicating sclerosing cholangitis. *Am J Gastroenterol* 78:661–664, 1983.
12. Kuno N: Carcinoma of the biliary tract. In Takemoto T, Kasugai T (eds): *Endoscopic Retrograde Cholangiopancreatography*. New York, Igaku-Shoin, 1979, pp 229–258.
13. Thorsen MK, Quiroz F, Lawson TL, Smith DF, Foley WD, Stewart ET: Primary biliary carcinoma: CT evaluation. *Radiology* 152:479–483, 1984.
14. Haaga JR, Alfidi RJ, Ament A: The biliary system. In Haaga JR, Alfidi RJ (eds): *Computed Tomography of the Whole Body*. St. Louis, C. V. Mosby, 1983, p 637.
15. Ligoury C, Canard JM: Tumors of the biliary system. *Clin Gastroenterol* 12:269–285, 1983.
16. Silverstein FE, Rohrmann CA, Templeton FE: Extrahepatic conditions of the biliary tree. In Stewart ET, Vennes JA, Geenen JE (eds): *Atlas of Endoscopic Retrograde Cholangiopancreatography*. St. Louis, C. V. Mosby, 1977, pp 272–333.
17. Anacker H, Weiss HD, Kramann B: ERCP in diseases of the biliary tract. In *Endoscopic Retrograde Pancreaticocholangiography (ERPC)*. New York, Springer-Verlag, 1977, pp 97–104.
18. Ikeda S, Shimoto H, Tanaka M, Matsumoto S, Itoh H: Cholangiography of intrahepatic bile ducts in hepatolithiasis by endoscopic placement of an indwelling balloon catheter. *Gastrointest Endosc* 31:181–187, 1985.
19. Bourgeois N, Dunham F, Verhest A, Cremer M: Endoscopic biopsies of papilla of Vater at the time of endoscopic spincterotomy: difficulties and interpretations. *Gastrointest Endosc* 30:163–166, 1984.
20. Walter JF, Bookstein JJ, Bouffard EV: Newer angiographic observations in cholangiocarcinoma. *Radiology* 118:19–23, 1976.
21. Adson MA, Farnell MB: Hepatobiliary cancer—surgical considerations. *Mayo Clin Proc* 55:686–699, 1981.

22. Ring EG: Percutaneous intubation of malignant biliary strictures. In Moody FG (ed): *Advances in Diagnosis and Surgical Treatment of Biliary Tract Disease.* New York, Masson Publishing U.S.A. Inc., 1983, pp 119-128.
23. Hagenmuller F, Soehendra N: Non-surgical biliary drainage. *Clin Gastroenterol* 12:297-316, 1983.
24. Denning DA, Ellison EC, Carey CC: Preoperative percutaneous transhepatic biliary decompression lowers operative morbidity in patients with obstructive jaundice. *Am J Surg* 141:61-65, 1981.
25. Brasch KW: Malignant disease of the distal bile duct. In Moody FG (ed): *Advances and Diagnosis of Surgical Treatment of Biliary Tract Disease.* New York, Masson Publishing U.S.A. Inc., 1983, pp 109-118.
26. Burcharth F, Jansen LI, Oleson K: Endoprosthesis for internal drainage of the biliary tract. *Gastroenterology* 77:133-137, 1979.
27. Siegel JH: Improved biliary decompression using large caliber endoscopic prostheses. *Gastrointest Endosc* 30:21-23, 1984.
28. Siegel JH, Harding GT, Chakau F: Endoscopic decompression and drainage of benign and malignant biliary obstruction. *Gastrointest Endosc* 28:79-82, 1982.
29. Leung JWC, Favero GD, Cotton PB: Endoscopic biliary prostheses. A comparison of material. *Gastrointest Endosc* 31:93-95, 1985.
30. Burcharth F: Non-surgical drainage of the biliary tract. *Semin Liver Dis* 2:75-86, 1982.
31. Cameron JL, Gayler BW, Zuidema GD: The use of silastic transhepatic stents in benign and malignant biliary strictures. *Ann Surg* 188:552-560, 1978.
32. Longmire WP: Malignant disease of the proximal bile ducts. In Moody FG (ed): *Advances in Diagnosis and Surgical Treatment of Biliary Tract Disease.* New York, Masson Publishing U.S.A. Inc., 1983, pp 103-108.
33. Vierling JM: Hepatobiliary complications of ulcerative colitis and Crohn's disease. In Zakim D, Boyer TD (eds): *Hepatology: A Textbook of Liver Disease.* Philadelphia, W. B. Saunders, 1982, pp 821-822.
34. Longmire WP, McArthur MS, Bastunis EA, Hiatt J: Carcinoma of the extrahepatic biliary tree. *Ann Surg* 178:333-345, 1973.
35. Warren KW, Tan EGC: Diseases of the gallbladder and bile ducts. In Schiff L (ed): *Diseases of the Liver.* Philadelphia, J. B. Lippincott, 1975, pp 1278-1335.
36. Tsuzuki T, Ogata Y, Iida S, Nakanishi I, Takenaka Y, Yoshii H: Carcinoma of the bifurcation of the hepatic ducts. *Arch Surg* 118:1147-1151, 1983.

MISCELLANEOUS BILE DUCT TUMORS

Benign

Benign bile duct tumors are most frequently found in the periampullary region or the common bile duct, and are quite unusual in the common hepatic duct or the intrahepatic ducts. Papillomas and adenomas are most common, other possibilities include: lipoma, fibroma, cystadenoma, and granular cell myoblastoma. Biliary cystadenoma is discussed in the liver section of this book, as it is usually intrahepatic. It may, however, present as a filling defect in the extrahepatic ducts (1).

Papilloma and Adenoma

Papillomas are usually sessile tumors with a broad base, consisting of a framework of vascular connective tissue covered by a single layer of columnar epithelium. They can be multifocal, but even then are usually confined to a small segment of the common duct. Frequently atypia are present, and papillomas may recur if not widely excised. A case of "ascending papillomatosis" has been reported consisting of multiple small filling defects in the ducts after resection of an ampullary papilloma (1, 2).

Adenomas are usually single, smooth, well-circumscribed tumors arising in the bile duct wall. They consist of epithelial glandular structures surrounded by a fibrous tissue stroma (2).

Clinically, biliary adenomas or papillomas usually present with obstructive jaundice. Other signs and symptoms include biliary colic, dyspepsia, weight loss, chills, fever, or hemobilia causing heme positive stools. Cholangiographically, they present usually as solitary (occasionally multiple) filling defects or obstructions, whose margins may be round, closely resembling stones. Demonstration of wall attachment by the proper obliquity is suggestive of tumor, although adherent stone is a possibility (2). Sonographically, they are moderately echogenic nonshadowing filling defects. The lack of shadowing suggests a tumor rather than a stone. On CT, they are soft tissue masses indistinguishable from non-calcified stones. Fibromas have the same imaging characteristics as adenomas, but lipomas can be specifically diagnosed by CT as fat density masses.

Treatment is wide excision and bilioenteric anastomosis (2).

Granular Cell Myoblastoma

These are benign neurogenic tumors, about twenty of which have been reported in the biliary tree. The vast majority occur in young (ages 14-45) black females who present with either obstructive jaundice or biliary colic. They are usually single, although about 10% are multifocal. Half occur in the common bile duct and 40% occur in the cystic duct, with the remainder in the common hepatic duct. Granular cell myoblastoma of the cystic duct may present with acute cholecystitis due to cystic duct obstruction.

Cholangiography of granular cell myoblastoma of the common duct will demonstrate a subepithelial smooth mass with eccentric duct narrowing and partial obstruction (3).

Prognosis is good after wide excision.

Malignant

Biliary cystadenocarcinomas are not distinguishable from cystadenomas roentgenologically. Hepatocellular carcinoma involving the bile ducts is discussed in the section on the liver in this book, and ampullary carcinoma is discussed in the pancreatic adenocarcinoma section. Discussed below are villous tumors, carcinoids, metastases, and rhabdomyosarcoma, a tumor of childhood.

Villous tumors can arise in the ampulla or distal common bile duct, or grow up into the biliary tree from the duodenum. Almost all villous tumors of the upper GI tract are malignant. They present with obstructive jaundice, weight loss, pain, nausea, and/or anemia. The cholangiographic appearance is distinctive when fronds, feathery margins or interstices are demonstrated (Fig. 14.47) (3). Prognosis is good if complete resection is possible before metastases have occurred.

Carcinoids are APUD cell neural crest derivative tumors that can arise in the extrahepatic bile ducts or ampulla. They present most commonly with obstructive jaundice. Those of biliary origin are polypoid filling defects on cholangiography. Ampullary carcinoids have the same imaging characteristics as ampullary carcinomas. Prognosis is excellent if the carcinoid is resectable (3).

Metastases affecting intrahepatic ducts are associated with hepatic parenchymal changes that dominate the imaging picture and are therefore discussed in the liver section on metastatic disease. With regard to the extrahepatic ducts, intraductal metastasis is unusual; smooth extraluminal obstruction by nodes is more common. Primary malignancies of the lung, breast, colon, testicle, prostate, pancreas, gallbladder and melanoma can cause intraductal metastasis. These present cholangiographically as single or multiple filling defects attached to the wall (Fig. 14.48A). Mucosal destruction and/or luminal obliteration can occur (3). CT and sonography can show extrinsic discrete nodal masses when metastases or lymphomatous nodes are extraluminal and, less commonly, intraductal soft tissue masses corresponding to intraluminal metastases (Fig. 14.48B).

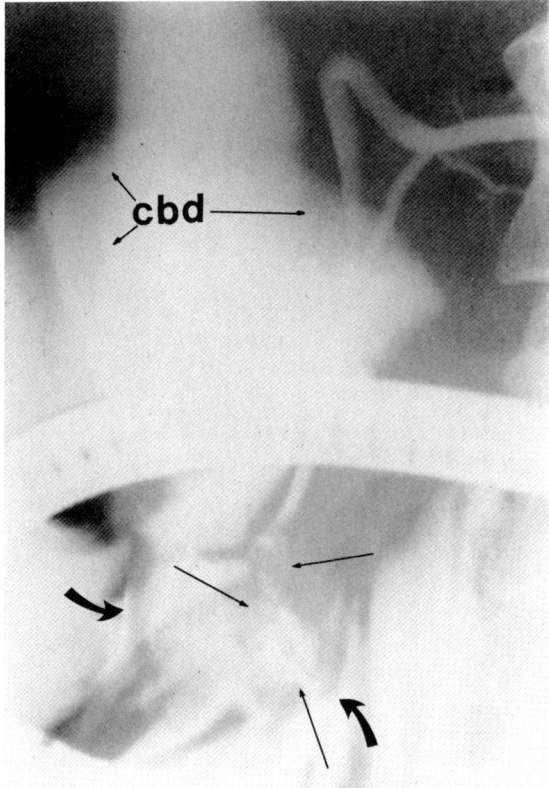

FIGURE 14.47. VILLOUS TUMOR OF THE AMPULLA
ERCP of a villous tumor of the ampulla in a patient with Gardner's syndrome (increased incidence of periampullary tumors): polypoid mass (*curved arrows*) with contrast-filled interstices (*straight arrows*). The common duct (*cbd*) is dilated.

Embryonal Rhabdomyosarcoma (Sarcoma Botryoides) of the Biliary Tree

Sarcoma botryoides is a variant of embryonal rhabdomyosarcoma that arises in close proximity to the mucosal surface of a hollow viscus or body cavity. After choledochal cyst, sarcoma botryoides is probably the most common cause of obstructive jaundice in children past infancy (2, 4).

Clinical Findings. Age range is 16 months to 11 yr with an average age at onset of 4 yr and a female preponderance of almost 2:1 (2, 4). Children present with malaise, fever, and jaundice that is often initially attributed to viral hepatitis. The average survival after onset of symptoms is 5.3 months, with a range of less than 1 month to over 16 months. Although late metastases occurs, death is usually from local invasion of contiguous structures (4). Wide surgical resection, radiation and chemotherapy yield

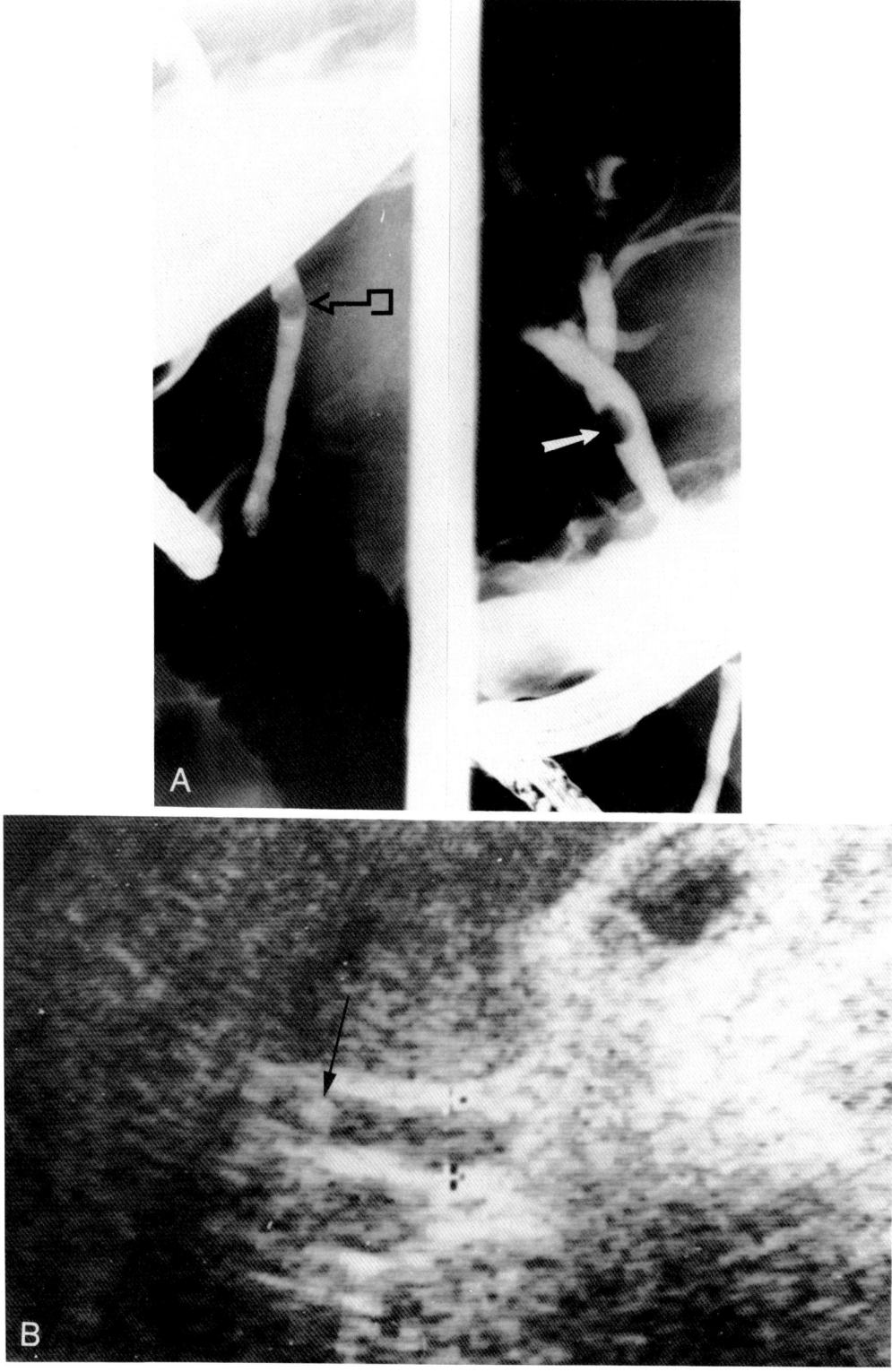

FIGURE 14.48. BILIARY METASTASES FROM CARCINOMA OF THE PANCREAS
A: ERCP: two intrabiliary metastases (*arrows*). Both are attached to the wall, although one is seen in profile and the other en face. *B:* Sonography demonstrated only the more proximal mass as a nonshadowing echogenicity (*arrow*) in the nondilated common duct (*cursors*, 4.2 mm).

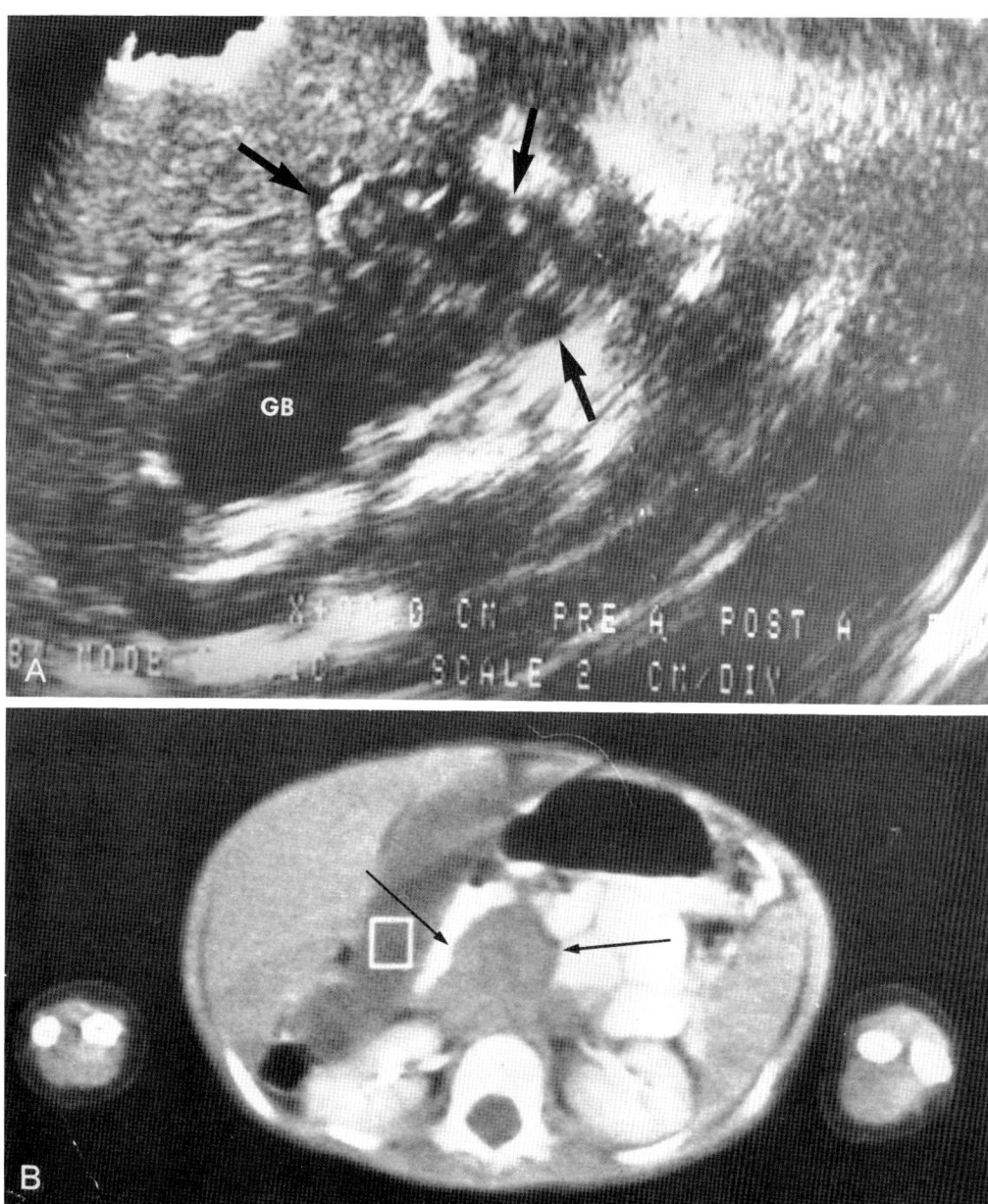

FIGURE 14.49. BILIARY SARCOMA BOTRYOIDES
Sonography and CT in a child with biliary sarcoma botryoides. *A:* Oblique transverse sonogram: complex mass filling a dilated common duct (*arrows*) medial to the gallbladder (*GB*). *B:* Corresponding CT: soft-tissue mass medial to the duodenum in the region of the common bile duct (*arrows*). *Cursor* is over the dilated gallbladder.

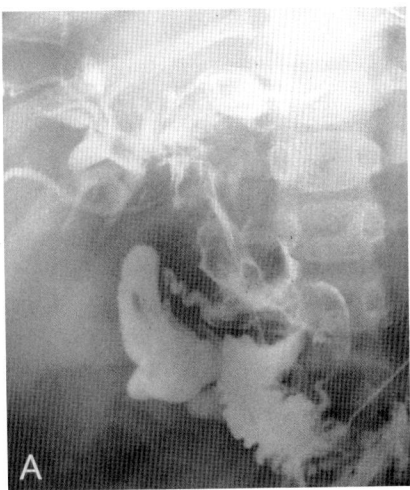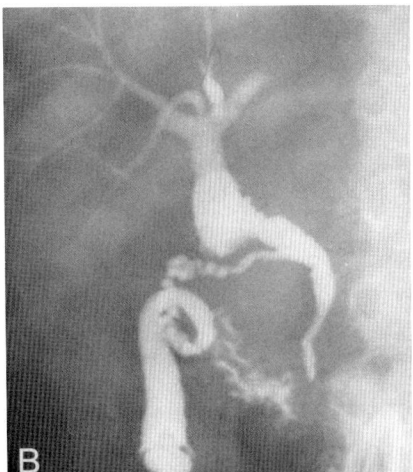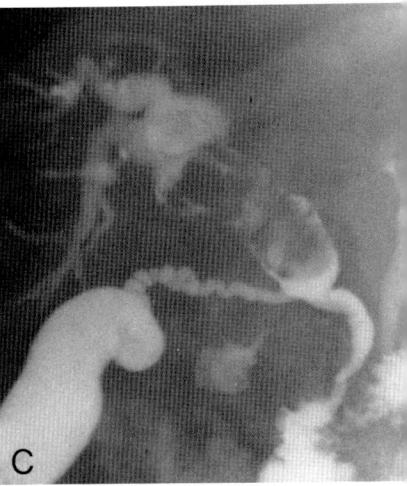

FIGURE 14.50. SARCOMA BOTRYOIDES IN AN 8-YEAR-OLD GIRL
A: PTC: grape-like projections from a large, bulky intraluminal mass involving intra and extrahepatic ducts. *B:* Tumor regression after radiation therapy. *C:* Recurrence of the tumor four months after initial examination. (From Janes JO, Laughlin CL, Goldberger LE, Berk RN: Differential features of some unusual biliary tumors. *Gastrointest Radiol* 7:341–348, 1982.)

significant prolongation of life and palliation but not cure (2, 4).

Pathology. Biliary sarcoma botryoides usually grows from or along the wall of the common bile duct beneath the lining mucosa with projections into the lumen. It has a yellow, shiny, gelatinous appearance. The projecting polyps often undergo hemorrhage and necrosis, and the tumor may slough and fill the lumen with debris. When it originates intrahepatically, sarcoma botryoides grows from the major ducts in the hilum along and into the extrahepatic biliary tree as a yellow, soft, lobulated mass with large cystic spaces into which protrude polypoid projections (4).

The polypoid projections are covered by biliary epithelium overlying a dense zone of neoplastic cells (cambium layer) resembling rhabdomyoblasts. Cells with cross-striations are hard to find, but racket-shaped cells and elongated cells with eosinophilic cytoplasm are typically present. There are no PAS-positive globules. The pattern of tumor growing about small biliary radicals with intraluminal projection is present at a microscopic level in intrahepatic regions of solid tumor (4).

Radiology. Duodenography may demonstrate an extraluminal mass effect medially, along the second portion of the duodenum. Sonography and CT will show intrahepatic duct dilatation and a soft tissue mass in the region of the common bile duct and/or porta hepatis (Fig. 14.49). Sonolucent or low density regions representing necrosis may be present. Direct cholangiography is suggestive of the histologic diagnosis (Fig. 14.50). There are grape-like intraluminal filling defects usually in extrahepatic ducts that obstruct the duct only after the tumor has reached a considerable size. Ducts proximal to the obstruction are usually not as dilated as ducts containing the tumor (2).

REFERENCES

1. Larsen CR, Scholz FJ, Wise RE: Diseases of the biliary ducts. *Semin Roentgenol* 11:259–267, 1976.
2. Orloff MJ, Charters AC: Tumors of the gallbladder and bile ducts. In Bockus HL (ed): *Gastroenterology*. Philadelphia, W. B. Saunders, 1976, pp 837–838.
3. Janes JO, Laughlin CL, Goldberger LE, Berk RN: Differential features of some unusual biliary tumors. *Gastrointest Radiol* 7:341–348, 1982.
4. Davis GL, Kissane JM, Ishak KG: Embryonal rhabdomyosarcoma (sarcoma botryoides) of the biliary tree. Report of five cases and review of the literature. *Cancer* 24:333–342, 1969.

15

Inflammatory Cholangitis, Parasitic Diseases, Primary Biliary Cirrhosis, and Papillary (Ampullary) Stenosis

MARK T. BIRNS, M.D., ARNOLD C. FRIEDMAN, M.D., and LEORA SACHS, M.D.

ACUTE (ASCENDING) CHOLANGITIS

Acute cholangitis is an inflammatory condition of the biliary ductal system usually associated with bacterial infection and characterized by fever, abdominal pain, and jaundice. The entire major ductal system and even the gallbladder is generally involved. Infection is more evident in the contents of the biliary tract than in the duct walls themselves. Often there is no grossly purulent material present and the bile remains clear despite heavy bacterial contamination. Although the etiology is nearly always related to biliary obstruction with ductal dilation, acute cholangitis is seen more frequently with some causes of obstruction than others. Acute cholangitis is seen frequently with choledocholithiasis, ampullary carcinoma, ampullary stenosis, and bilioenteric anastomotic strictures but relatively seldom with cholangiocarcinoma, pancreatic carcinoma, and biliary obstruction from nodal metastases. *Escherichia coli* is the most common offender (1).

Acute cholangitis usually subsides in 1–3 days, either after appropriate antibiotic therapy or because the obstruction has spontaneously remitted. Persistent complete obstruction leads to the accumulation of purulent material under pressure (suppurative cholangitis) with potential complications such as septicemia, shock, and miliary hepatic abscess formation (2).

Radiology

Most often, the role of radiology is to define the etiology of the obstruction, and no other additional findings are present. In cases of suppurative cholangitis, intrabiliary pus can be depicted in several ways (Fig. 15.1). Sonography will show echogenic material within dilated ducts, and CT can demonstrate the pus as relatively high density material within dilated ducts. On cholangiography, pus appears as intrabiliary irregular filling defects. Abscesses, if present, can be shown by CT and ultrasound, but their connection to the biliary tree is most likely to be appreciated at cholangiography as round to oval amorphous collections of intraparenchymal contrast filling from one or more dilated biliary radicles (Fig. 15.2) (3–6). Percutaneous or endoscopic biliary drainage may be necessary as an emergency lifesaving procedure, especially in the suppurative variety of acute cholangitis (7). Choice of route depends on the exact clinical circumstances and the expertise available.

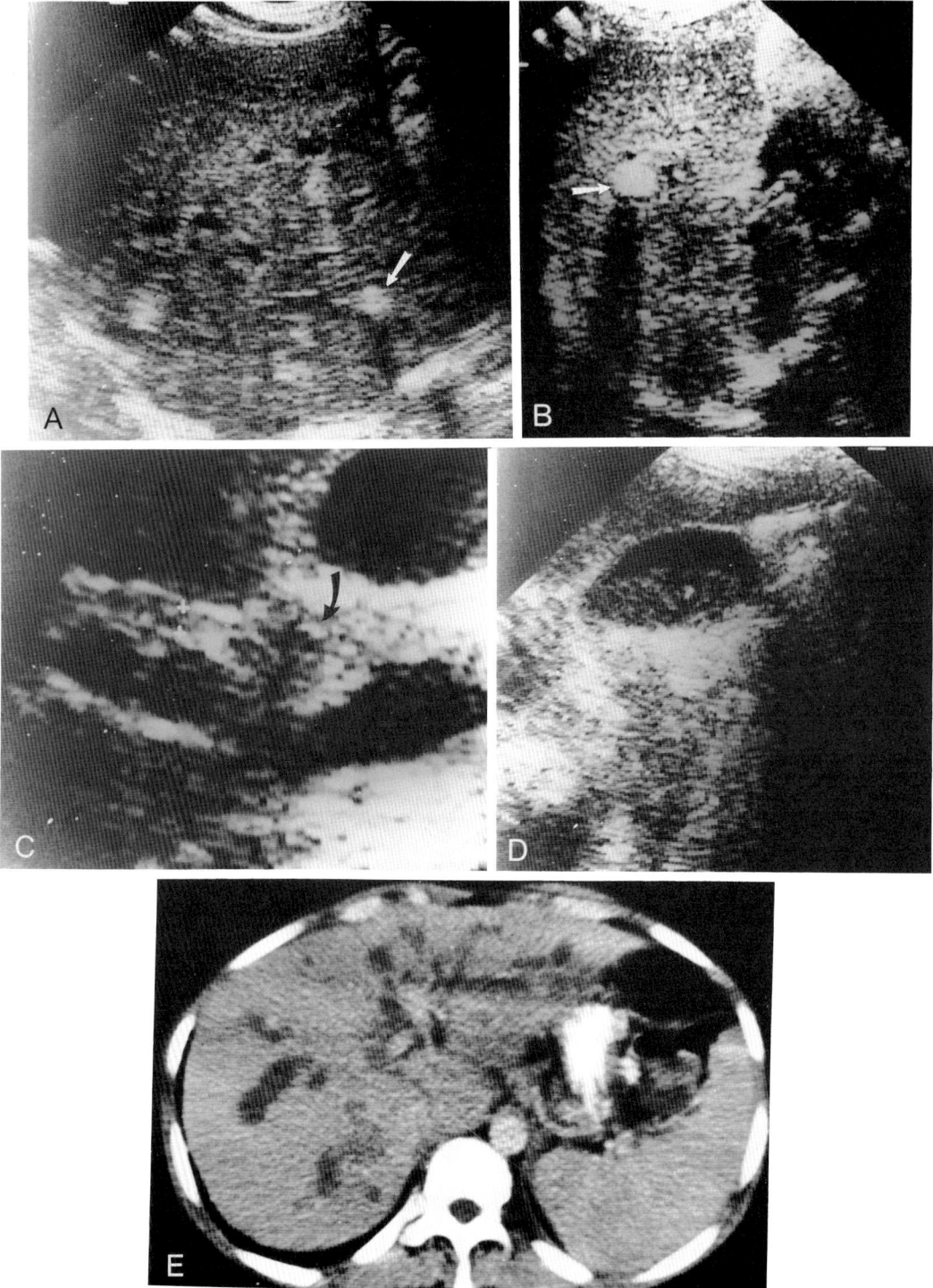

FIGURE 15.1. ACUTE SUPPURATIVE CHOLANGITIS

A and B: Longitudinal sonograms: in addition to dilated ducts, there are several echogenic foci, some of which shadow (arrows), which correspond to pus-filled ducts. C: Normal caliber common duct (0.43 cm, cursors) filled with echogenic pus. Note enlarged lymph node (arrow). D: Purulent material within the gallbladder. E and F: CT: dilated ducts, some of which contain high density material. A right posterior duct has quite high attentuation material within it (arrow), corresponding to the collection on sonography that cast the best defined shadow. G: operative cholangiogram: dilated ducts with ragged margins due to contrast intermingling with purulent bile.

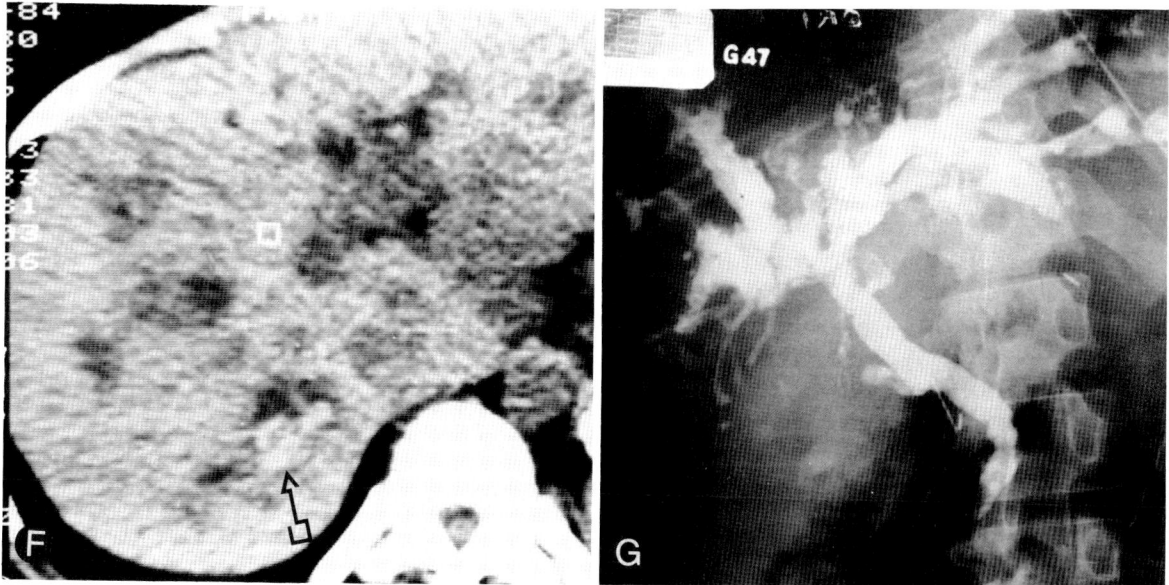

FIGURE 15.1*F* and *G*

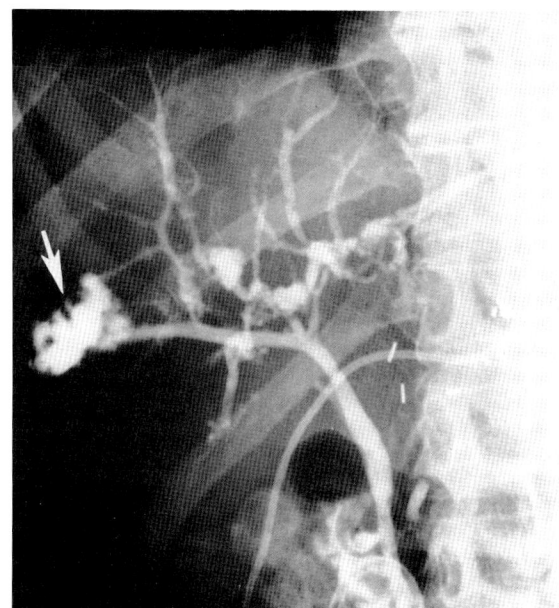

FIGURE 15.2. ACUTE SUPPURATIVE CHOLANGITIS WITH ABSCESSES

Intrahepatic abscesses due to biliary drainage catheter malfunction. Note largest abscess cavity (*arrow*) and duct contour irregularity with some filling defects due to pus.

REFERENCES

1. Caroli J, Rosner D: Acute cholangitis. In Bockus HL et al. (eds): *Gastroenterology*, Philadelphia, W. B. Saunders, 1976, pp 865–867.
2. Schoenfield LJ: *Diseases of the Gallbladder and Biliary System*. Clinical Gastroenterology Monographs. New York, John Wiley & Sons, 1977.
3. Ferrucci JT Jr, Mueller PR, vanSonnenberg E: Transhepatic cholangiography. In Berk RN, Ferrucci JT Jr, Leopold GR (eds): *Radiology of the Gallbladder and Bile Ducts Diagnosis and Intervention*. Philadelphia, W. B. Saunders, 1983, pp 360–361.
4. Stewart ET, Geenen JE: Endoscopic retrograde cholangiography. In Berk RN, Ferrucci JT Jr, Leopold GR (eds): *Radiology of the Gallbladder and Bile Ducts. Diagnosis and Intervention*. Philadelphia, W. B. Saunders, 1983, p 381.
5. Haaga JR, Alfidi RJ, Ament A: The biliary system. In Haaga JR, Alfidi RJ (eds): *Computed Tomography of the Whole Body*. St. Louis, C. V. Mosby, 1983.
6. Grossman RI, Ring EG, Oleaga JA et al: Diagnosis of pyogenic hepatic abscesses by percutaneous transhepatic cholangiography. *AJR* 132:919–920, 1979.
7. Kadir S, Bassiri A, Barth KH, Kaufman SL, Cameron JL, White RI Jr: Percutaneous biliary drainage in the management of biliary sepsis. *AJR* 138:25–30, 1982.

RECURRENT PYOGENIC CHOLANGITIS

(Oriental Cholangiohepatitis, Intraphepatic Pigment Stone Disease, Biliary Obstruction Syndrome of the Chinese)

Recurrent pyogenic cholangitis (RPC) is a disease of uncertain etiology endemic to Indochina, South China, Taiwan, Japan, and Korea (1, 2). It is most prevalent in the low socioeconomic status rural population (3). Sporadic cases occurring in other parts of the world are usually in Asian immigrants. The distribution of *Clonorchis sinensis* is identical that of RPC, suggesting that *Clonorchis* is an etiologic agent. However, the frequency of *Clonorchis* infestation in RPC patients is not much higher than that in Asians without RPC (2). Other parasites implicated include *Opisthorchis viverrini*, *Fasciola hepatica*, *Ascaris*, and *Entamoeba coli* (3). Parasites could cause RPC by acting as a nidus for stone formation and causing stasis, predisposing to secondary bacterial infection. The second theory of pathogenesis implicates recurrent portal sepsis from gastroenteritis. Infection with beta glucuronidase-producing *E. coli* then leads to bilirubin deconjugation and pigment stone formation (3).

Clinical Findings

RPC is characterized by recurrent attacks of right upper quadrant pain, fever, chills, and jaundice (4). Each episode lasts several days and usually gradually subsides. Males and females are equally affected and the peak age range is 20–50 yr (2). The initial or subsequent attacks can lead to severe sepsis and obstructive jaundice necessitating decompression (4). RPC is the third most common cause of an acute abdomen in Hong Kong after appendicitis and perforated ulcer (2).

Physical examination usually reveals right upper quadrant tenderness and hepatomegaly (3, 4). Splenomegaly may be present and the gallbladder may be palpably enlarged (4). Routine laboratory tests generally show leukocytosis, elevated alkaline phosphatase, and often an elevated bilirubin. Bile cultures usually grow *E. coli* (3, 4).

The natural history of the disease is exacerbation and remission of cholangitis leading to progressive destruction of biliary radicals and cirrhosis. Antibiotics are helpful in treating acute attacks. Surgical treatment can entail emergency decompression, lobectomy, and/or stone removal. Although surgery is almost always palliative only, lobectomy can be curative if the disease is confined to the left lobe (1, 3).

Pathology

Intra- and extrahepatic ducts are markedly dilated (often on the order of 3–4 cm) proximal to multiple strictures (1, 2). The ducts frequently contain soft bile pigment stones which are variably calcified, biliary mud, and/or pus. Calculi are more prominent in the intrahepatic ducts than in the extrahepatic ducts (3). Cholelithiasis is present in only 15–20% (3, 4). Usually multiple ducts are affected, although isolated involvement of the left hepatic duct does occur occasionally (2).

Histologically there is pericholangitis, periportal fibrosis, and polymorphonuclear cell infiltration along duct walls and portal tracts (3).

Radiology

Plain films of the abdomen are reported to show pneumobilia in 3% of cases either due to gas-producing organisms or patulousness of the sphincter of Oddi (1). Intrahepatic calcifications representing stones are occasionally seen (Fig. 15.3C and 15.4 G), but the majority of stones are not calcified sufficiently for radiographic detection. Oral cholecystography and intravenous cholangiography are rarely useful because of impaired hepatic function.

Sonography

Ultrasound is capable of depicting most dilated ducts and some of the calculi in RPC (2). However, some difficulties exist (Fig. 15.4A and B). Highly reflective echoes with shadowing could be either calculi or air. Calculi can be missed altogether if tightly packed within a duct or if small. Dilated ducts can be overlooked if they are packed with stones and/or mud (3).

Computed Tomography

CT is capable of easily differentiating biliary air from calculi. The latter are usually radiodense in RPC because of the calcium within the bilirubinate stones (3). Biliary mud and/or pus-filled ducts are depicted as tubular or sausage-

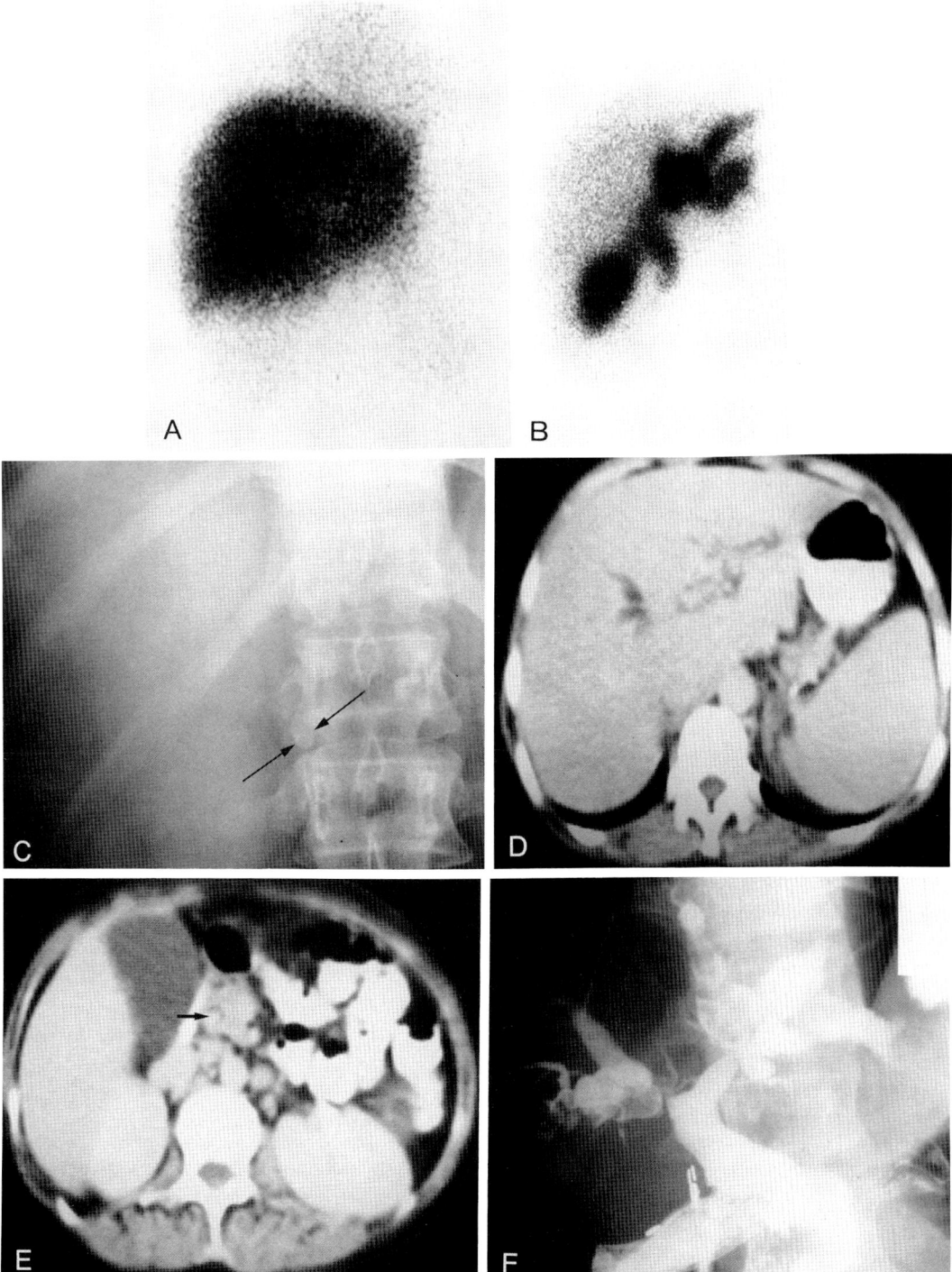

FIGURE 15.3. RECURRENT PYOGENIC CHOLANGITIS

Forty-year-old male Vietnamese refugee with acute right upper quadrant pain and elevated alkaline phosphatase from recurrent pyogenic cholangitis. *A* and *B:* HIDA scan showing good hepatic uptake and excretion into a dilated biliary tree with delayed transit to bowel but a patent cystic duct. *C:* Plain film shows a calculus in the common duct (*arrows*). *D* and *E:* CT scans showing dilated intrahepatic ducts filled with noncalcified stones and a calcified stone in the distal common duct (*E, arrow*). *F:* T-tube cholangiogram demonstrating dilated intra- and extrahepatic ducts and calculi proximal to strictures.

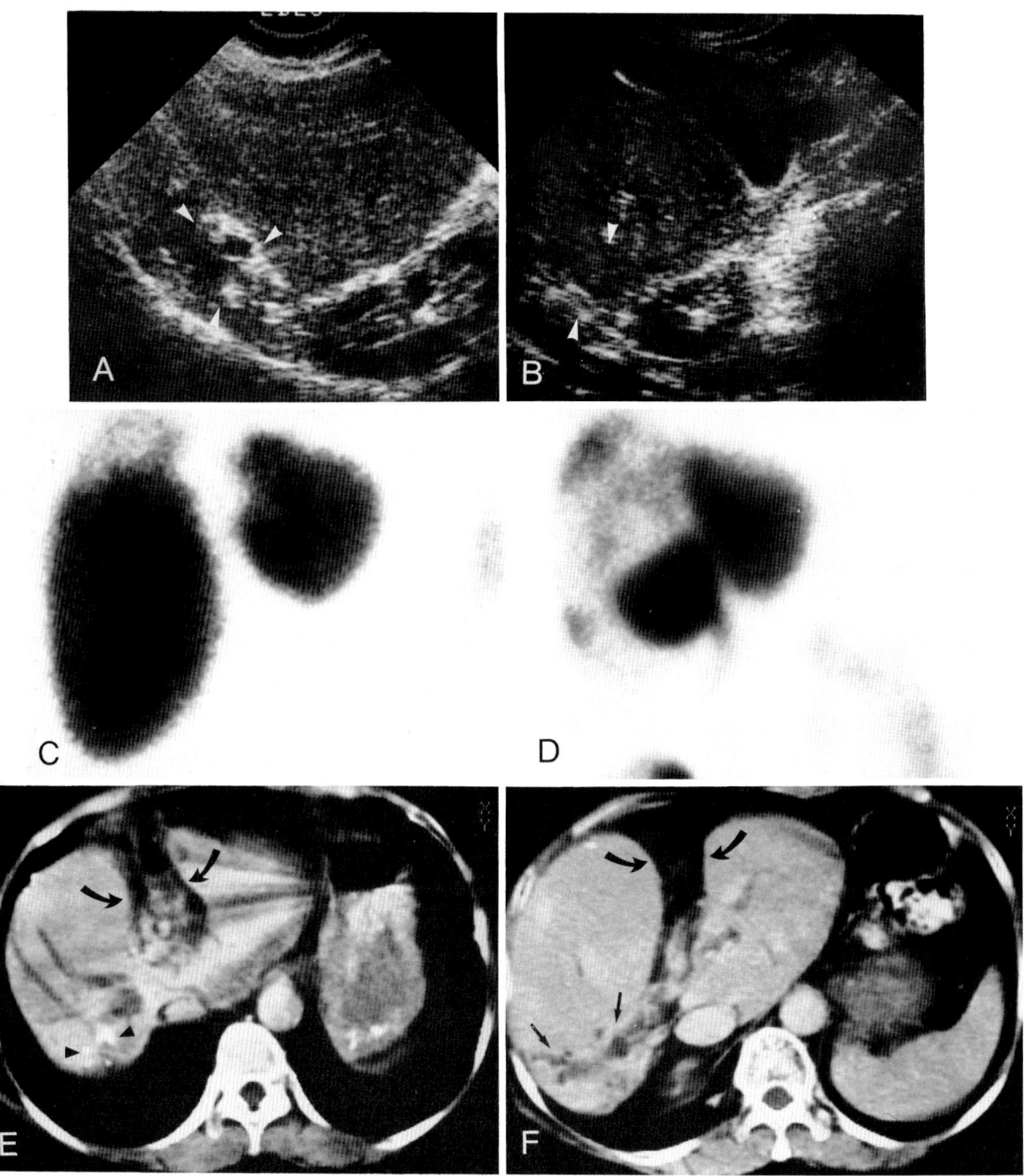

FIGURE 15.4. RECURRENT PYOGENIC CHOLANGITIS

Fifty-two-year-old Filipino woman with recurrent attacks of right upper quadrant pain, low grade fever, and mild jaundice. *A* and *B:* Parasagittal and transverse sonograms of the liver showing a large inferior right lobe, a complex posterior right lobe mass (*arrowheads*), and a large sonolucency with low level echoes initially interpreted as gallbladder. *C:* Ten-minute HIDA scan demonstrates enlargement of right and left hepatic lobes, diminished uptake superiorly on the right, and a void between right and left lobes corresponding to the sonolucency. *D:* A 2-hr delayed scan shows persistent activity within the liver in multiple regions suggesting multifocal obstructions. The cold regions at ten minutes are now warm. Excretion into the small bowel has occurred. *E* and *F:* CT slices through the liver demonstrate nonuniform intrahepatic duct dilatation. The predominant duct dilatation was in the regions of the liver that had prolonged HIDA retention, and these regions were diminished in size, whereas those portions of the liver with minimal duct dilation had parenchymal hypertrophy. The complex mass on sonography was atrophic liver with dilated ducts (*arrows*). The sonolucency and isotopic void was destroyed medial segment of left lobe (*curved arrows*). Intraductal calcifications were also depicted (*arrowheads*). *G* and *H:* PTC using right lateral approach showing dilated intra and extrahepatic ducts and nonopacification of the left lobe. Intraductal calcifications (*arrows*) are seen as on CT. The gallbladder is faintly opacified (*arrowhead*) and the duodenum is displaced medially by the hypertrophied portion of the right lobe. *I:* Direct subxiphoid puncture of the destroyed medial segment of the left lobe shows a cavity packed with soft stones and debris that probably resulted from a massively dilated duct (*arrows*). Most of the other contrast is subcapsular and some is residual from the previous right-sided injection.

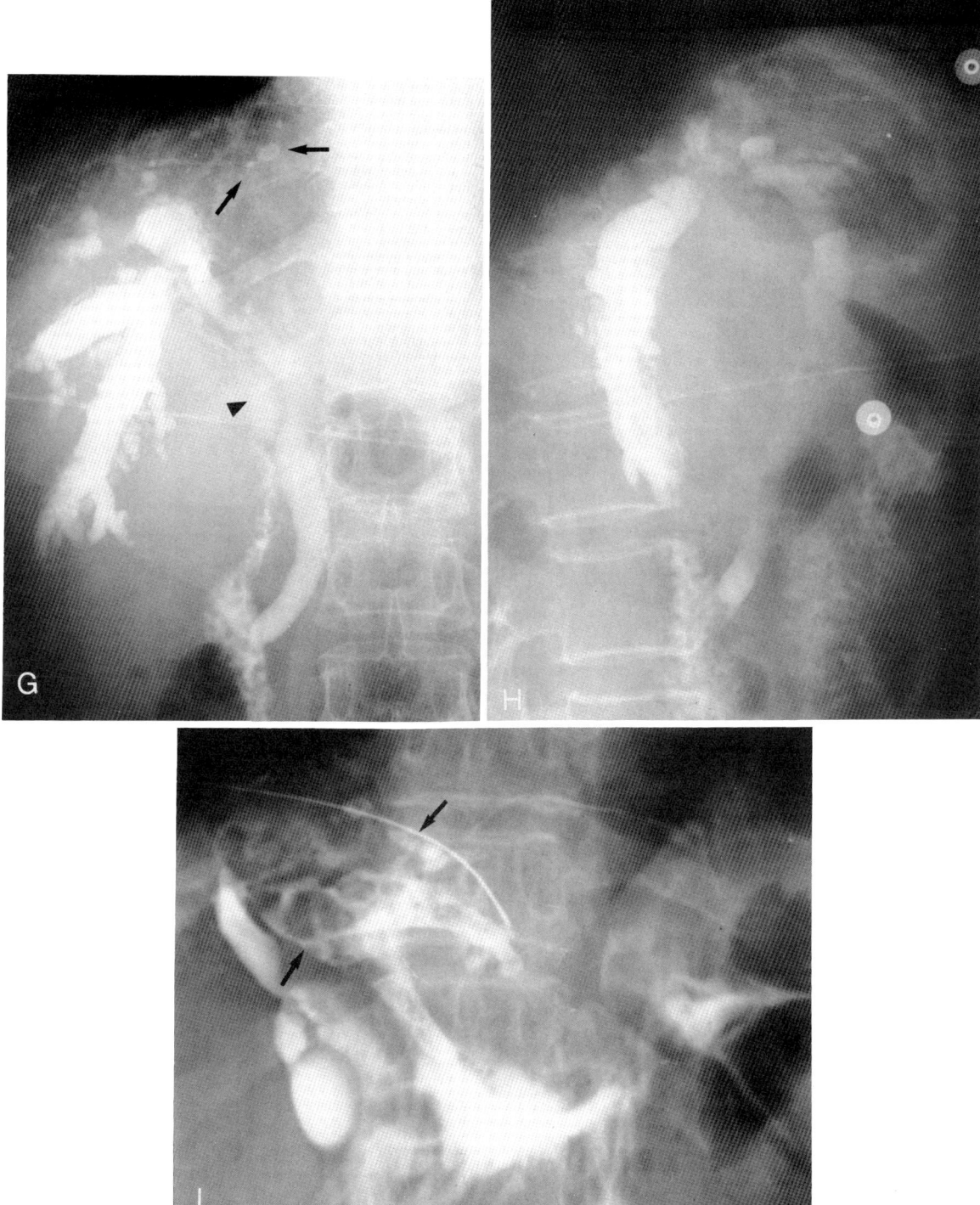

FIGURE 15.4G–I

shaped low density structures compared to the contrast enhanced hepatic parenchyma (Figs. 15.3D and E and 15.4E and F).

Cholangiography

Direct cholangiography in RPC will demonstrate decreased arborization of intrahepatic radicals, distorted branching angles with stretching of branches, dilated ducts proximal to smooth strictures, and filling defects from stones and debris (4). The common duct is usually involved. Some regions may be unopacified because of tight packing of stones and mud, necessitating multiple punctures for complete evaluation (Figs. 15.3F and 15.4G–I). Endoscopic retrograde cholangiopancreatography (ERCP) and percutaneous transhepatic cholangiography (PTC) carry the risk of exacerbating cholangitis and sepsis in these patients and antibiotic prophylaxis is mandatory.

RPC can be extremely difficult to distinguish from Caroli's disease complicated by cholangitis and stone formation. Features favoring Caroli's disease are small extrahepatic ducts compared to the size of the intrahepatic ducts, renal cystic disease, and a disease onset in adolescence or childhood. The saccular, cystic changes in the intrahepatic ducts seen in Caroli's disease can be mimicked by abscesses in RPC.

REFERENCES

1. Wastie, ML, Cunningham IGE: Roentgenologic findings in recurrent pyogenic cholangitis. *AJR* 119:71–77, 1973
2. Ralls, PW, Colletti PM, Quinn MF, Lapin SA, Morris UL, Halls J: Sonography in recurrent oriental pyogenic cholangitis. *AJR* 136:1010–1012, 1981.
3. Federle MP, Cello JP, Laing FC: Recurrent pyogenic cholangitis in Asian immigrants. Use of ultrasonography, computed tomography, and cholangiography. *Radiology* 143:151–156, 1982.
4. Ho CS, Wesson DE: Recurrent pyogenic cholangitis in Chinese immigrants. *AJR* 122:368–374, 1974.

BILIARY ASCARIASIS AND OTHER MISCELLANEOUS PARASITES

Infestation by *Ascaris lumbricoides* is a worldwide problem, estimated to affect one-fourth of the population. The southeastern United States is among the endemic regions (1). Adult worms are several inches in length and reside in the jejunum. Common clinical presentations include vomiting of worms, passage of worms per rectum, and small bowel obstruction secondary to the formation of a large worm bolus. Adult worms have a propensity to migrate from the small intestine through the ampulla of Vater to lodge in the gallbladder and biliary tree. The pancreatic duct may also be affected (2). In some endemic areas ascariasis is second only to gallstones as a cause of biliary symptoms, and second only to appendicitis as a cause of acute abdomen in children. Parasitic infestation has been implicated in the pathogenesis of recurrent pyogenic cholangitis.

Clinical Findings

Clinical manifestations are usually seen in children. Most present with uncomplicated biliary colic. Nausea, vomiting, and fever may be associated. Although jaundice is rare, liver enzyme abnormalities are common and serum bilirubin is occasionally slightly elevated. Patients may present with acute cholecystitis and/or acute biliary obstruction, but complications such as ascending cholangitis and worm-containing liver abscess are rare.

Ultrasound

Sonography is reliable for diagnosis, evaluation of degree of biliary dilation, and following response to therapy. Five different signs have been described in characterizing the worms' sonographic appearance (3–5) (Figs. 15.5–15.8). The "strip sign" occurs when a worm is depicted as a long, thin linear, echogenic strip within the lumen of either the intra- or extra-hepatic ducts or within the gallbladder. Demonstration is dependent on good visualization of the portal structures and variant anatomy may lead to interpretive errors. When the worm-containing duct is viewed in cross-section a "bull's-eye" appearance of a central specular echo within the duct is obtained. On occasion, a central anechoic tube is seen within the worm (the "inner tube" sign), probably representing the worm's digestive tract. With heavier infestations and many biliary worms, multiple overlapping longitudinal interfaces may be present within a duct(s), the "spaghetti" sign. The worms may also coil up within the gallbladder or ducts, assuming a spiral configuration. Real-time examination is useful in demonstrating worm motility (6). Biliary ascariasis has been diagnosed sonographically in patients both with and without biliary dilatation and with or without symptoms. Worms can be shown to move in and out of the biliary tree without causing dilatation. Although usually only a few worms are present within the biliary

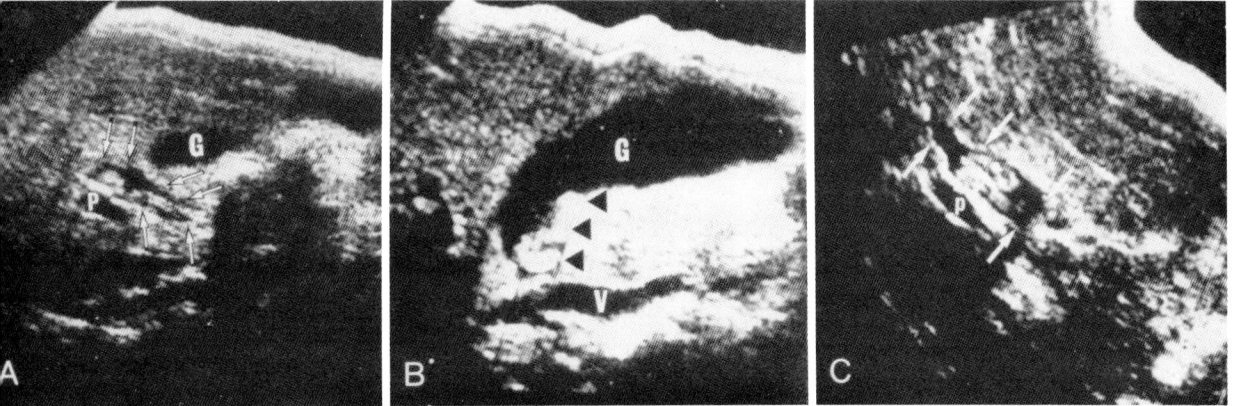

FIGURE 15.5. BILIARY ASCARIASIS

A: Innertube appearance of common duct worm. Distended common duct (*arrows*) containing a thick, echogenic strip representing the worm. The anechoic sliver within the worm is probably its digestive tract. P = portal vein, G = gallbladder. *B:* Coiled worm (*arrowheads*) within the neck of the gallbladder (G) in the same patient. V = inferior vena cava. *C:* The worm is coiled within the common duct (*arrows*) 7 days later. P = portal vein. (From Schulman A, Loxton AJ, Heydenrych JJ, Abdurahman KE: Sonographic diagnosis of biliary ascariasis. *AJR* 139:485–489, 1982.)

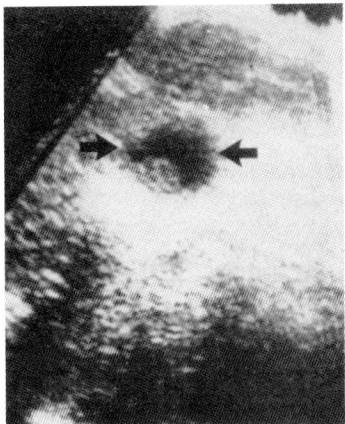

FIGURE 15.6. BILIARY ASCARIASIS

Coiled worm seen in the gallbladder (*arrows*) on a transverse scan, indistinguishable from a sludge ball. (From Schulman A, Loxton AJ, Heydenrych JJ, Abdurahman KE: Sonographic diagnosis of biliary ascariasis. *AJR* 139:485–489, 1982.)

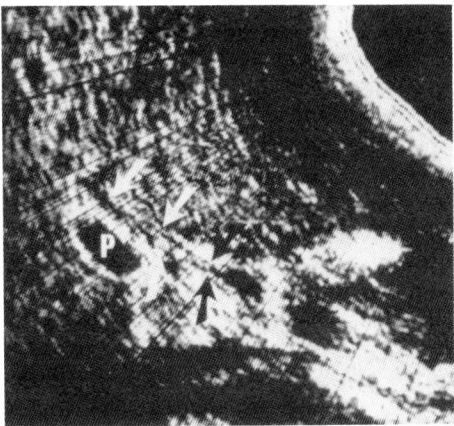

FIGURE 15.7. BILIARY ASCARIASIS

Echogenic strip running longitudinally in the common duct (*arrows*) representing an ascarid. P = portal vein. (From Schulman A, Loxton AJ, Heydenrych JJ, Abdurahman KE: Sonographic diagnosis of biliary ascariasis. *AJR* 139:485–489, 1982.)

tract, up to 49 worms were reportedly present in one Chinese patient (3).

Discrepancies between oral cholecystography, intravenous cholangiography, and sonography in biliary ascariasis have been reported (positive sonogram and negative radiographic study). Although this has led to the suggestion that contrast materials may act as a vermifuge, sonography may merely be a more sensitive technique.

Clonorchis sinensis, Fasciola hepatica, and Opisthorchis viverrini are liver flukes endemic in the Far East which also inhabit the biliary tract. They can present as mobile, echogenic, nonshadowing masses within the gallbladder or biliary tree indistinguishable from ascariasis (2).

Cholangiography and Cholecystography

Ascaris worms may be detected in the common bile duct or the biliary radicles as smooth, cylindrical lucencies on direct cholangiography or intravenous cholangiography (Fig. 15.9). Rarely barium will reflux through the sphincter of Oddi during an upper GI series and demonstrate a worm in the common duct. Eggs and other remnants from biliary parasites can act as the nidus for gallstone formation (7), but actual depiction of a worm in the gallbladder by cholangiography or cholecystography is not common (8). *C. sinensis, F. hepatica,* and *O. viverrini* may be directly depicted by cholangiography as curved, crescen-

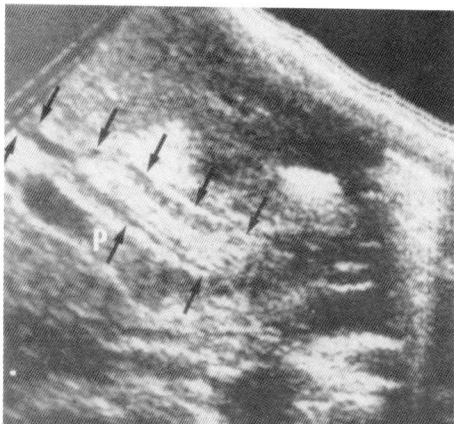

FIGURE 15.8. BILIARY ASCARIASIS
Spaghetti Sign: common duct expanded (*arrows*) around many echogenic worms. P = portal vein. (From Schulman A, Loxton AJ, Heydenrych JJ, Abdurahman KE: Sonographic diagnosis of biliary ascariasis. *AJR* 139:485–489, 1982.)

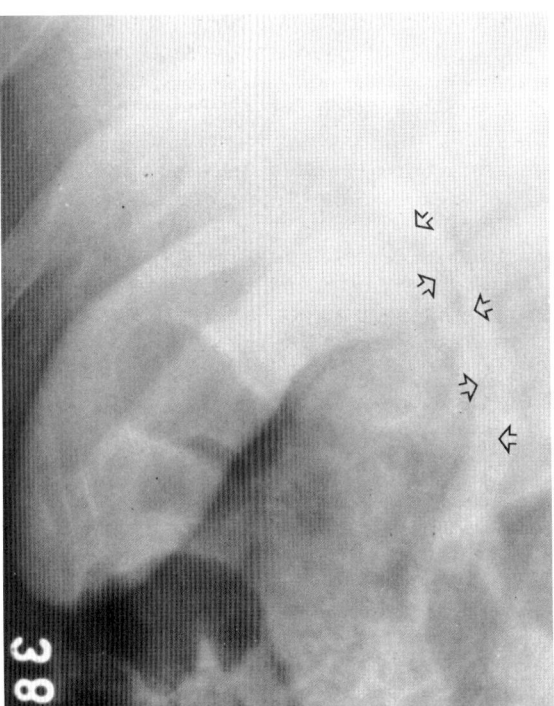

FIGURE 15.9. BILIARY ASCARIASIS
Intravenous cholangiogram: ascarid seen as a long, tubular filling defect (*arrows*).

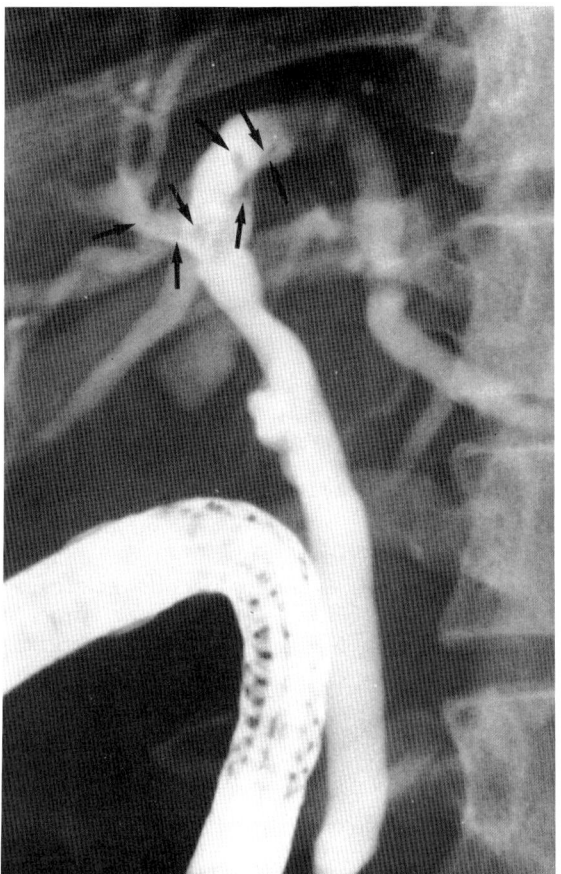

FIGURE 15.10. RECURRENT PYOGENIC CHOLANGITIS
ERCP of a 20-year-old Oriental woman demonstrates persistent rod-shaped filling (*arrows*) defects that represent parasites (*Clonorchis sinensis* and *Fasciola hepatica* were recovered from her bile). She went on to develop intrahepatic calculi consistent with recurrent pyogenic cholangitis.

tic filling defects or semilunar mounds with or without ductal dilatation (7) (Fig. 15.10).

Computed Tomography

Although not commonly used for biliary ascariasis, CT should be able to detect the disease with a fairly high degree of sensitivity if the same technical factors for detecting common duct calculi are adhered to. The worm will be shown as a soft-tissue density within the common duct, which may or may not be dilated. As opposed to a noncalcified stone, which is usually seen on only one or two cuts, the soft-tissue density of a worm will be present on several adjacent slices.

REFERENCES

1. Reeder MM, Palmer PS: *The Radiology of Tropical Diseases.* Baltimore, Williams & Wilkins, 1981, pp 411–438.
2. Itzchak Y, Rubinstein Z, Shilo R: Ultrasound in tropical diseases. In *Ultrasound Annual 1983.* New York, Raven Press, 1983, pp 69–93.
3. Schulman A, Loxton AJ, Heydenrych JJ, Abdurahman KE: Sonographic diagnosis of biliary ascariasis. *AJR* 139:485–489, 1982.
4. Schulman A, Roman T, Dalrymple R, Fataar S, Morton P: Sonography of biliary worms (ascariasis). *J Clin Ultrasound* 10:77–78, 1982.

5. Cremin BJ: Ultrasonic diagnosis of biliary ascariasis: "a bull's eye in the triple O." Br J Radiol 55:683–684, 1982.
6. Cerri GG, Leite GJ, Simoes JB et al: Ultrasonic Evaluation of ascaris in the biliary tract. Radiology 146:753–754, 1983.
7. Reeder MM: Tropical diseases of the liver and bile ducts. Semin Roentgenol 10:229–243, 1975.
8. Cremin BJ, Fisher MB: Biliary ascariasis in children. AJR 126:352, 1976.

PRIMARY SCLEROSING CHOLANGITIS AND PERICHOLANGITIS

Primary sclerosing cholangitis is a disease of unknown etiology, which, because of increasing use of ERCP and PTC and greater clinical awareness, is being diagnosed more frequently and at an earlier stage than in the past (1). Prior to 1980, fewer than 100 cases were reported in the English literature including no large series (1). The hallmark of the disease is involvement of all or some of the biliary tree including the gallbladder by a chronic, fibrosing inflammatory process. In order to exclude secondary sclerosing cholangitis (an identical pathologic process caused by chronic low grade obstruction and/or infection) there must be no stones or previous biliary surgery (ruling out a postoperative stricture). A reasonable period of clinical follow-up is necessary to exclude diffuse sclerosing cholangiocarcinoma (2, 3). Pericholangitis is an entity often associated with ulcerative colitis, occasionally with Crohn's disease, in which cholangiographic abnormalities identical to sclerosing cholangitis are present but confined to the intrahepatic ducts (2, 4). In the past pericholangitis was often confused with primary biliary cirrhosis because of the distribution of cholangiographic abnormalities (3). It is the most common hepatic complication of ulcerative colitis, and it is often asymptomatic with elevation of alkaline phosphatase the only sign in spite of well-developed histologic abnormalities (4). Some consider pericholangitis not as a separate entity, but merely the milder end of the spectrum of primary sclerosing cholangitis, probably with a better prognosis, in which, at least initially, only intrahepatic ducts are involved (2).

Sclerosing Cholangitis

Although the etiology of primary sclerosing cholangitis is unknown, several theories have been advanced. One is portal phlebitis from *E. coli* bacteremia secondary to colonic mucosal disease, leading to pericholangitis, fibrosis and obliteration of bile ducts. Another proposes that absorption of immunogenic substances such as endotoxins in large quantitites through damaged mucosa causes deposition of large immune complexes in the liver. The failure to document increased circulating immune complexes in ulcerative colitis with extraintestinal manifestations compared to uncomplicated ulcerative colitis has not been supportive of this concept (6). The elevation in hepatic copper seen in sclerosing cholangitis is not necessarily pathogenetic since elevated copper levels are seen in chronic large bile duct obstruction of any cause (5).

Clinical Findings

Primary sclerosing cholangitis is a progressive disease without a known cure. It is associated with a variety of disorders, the most common of which is ulcerative colitis (50–75%) (2, 5). Other associated or underlying disorders include: Crohn's disease (colitis or ileocolitis), mediastinal and retroperitoneal fibrosis, pancreatitis, orbital pseudotumor, thyroiditis, hypothyroidism, chronic active hepatitis, immunodeficiency syndromes, and Peyronie's disease (2, 5). In cases associated with inflammatory bowel disease, little correlation exists between the activity of the bowel disorder and the cholangitis. Sclerosing cholangitis occasionally will manifest itself clinically prior to the inflammatory bowel disease (2). Despite anecdotal reports to the contrary, colectomy is not considered beneficial in the treatment of sclerosing cholangitis (6).

Primary sclerosing cholangitis occurs typically in young and middle-aged men with a male-to-female ratio of 2:1. Mode of presentation varies from asymptomatic elevation of alkaline phosphatase or merely pruritus to the signs and symptoms of large bile duct obstruction: fever, jaundice, right upper quadrant pain, nausea and vomiting (5–7). End-stage sequelae (cirrhosis, portal hypertension) can be presenting features in up to 17% (6). Laboratory studies show a nearly universal elevation of alkaline phosphatase which is greater than 3 times normal in 85%. SGOT elevations are found in 85%, and elevated bilirubin in 67%, with serologic and autoimmune markers such as antimitochondrial antibody absent or present only in low titer (5).

With involvement of the extrahepatic biliary tree, prognosis is poor. Therapy is generally unsatisfactory. Treatment is intended to improve biliary drainage, reverse the primary pathologic process, treat underlying disease, and symptomatically treat sequelae such as pruritus, malnutrition, and cholangitis. Surgery must be individualized based on the level and degree of obstruction and is used to relieve obstruction, although it has no positive influence on the progression of the disease. Balloon dilatation via ERCP or PTC is feasible but long-term benefit is unclear (8, 9). Surgical placement of stents across a hepatojejunostomy with subsequent percutaneous toilet has had some long-term palliative success (10).

Medical therapy including steroids, antibiotics, cytotoxic agents, and choleretics alone or in combination has been disappointing (5). Using D-penicillamine in an effort to decrease hepatic copper levels has been initiated and results are pending (5, 8). Cholestyramine to reduce pruritus and fat-soluble vitamin replacement are useful in concert with an obstruction-relieving procedure (7).

Liver transplantation is a new viable option with 1 yr survivals approaching 70%. Since the procedure is made more difficult if there has been prior biliary surgery, palliative procedures in potential transplant candidates should be postponed (11).

Pathology

Pathologically the extrahepatic ducts are thickened with a small lumen and described as cord or rope-like. Intrahepatic ducts are almost always affected; early studies based on surgical findings and underfilled cholangiograms underestimated the frequency and extent of intrahepatic duct involvement (1). Histologically the duct walls are surrounded by an infiltrate of lymphocytes, plasma cells, and sometimes eosinophils with a varying degree of fibrosis and epithelial desquamation (2, 6–8, 11). Four stages are recognized: initially enlargement of portal tracts with an increase in connective tissue, edema, and bile ductular proliferation (Stage 1), then connective tissue extension into the parenchyma (Stage 2), followed by formation of fibrous septa (Stage 3), and finally biliary cirrhosis (Stage 4) (8). Although strictly speaking, hepatic histology is never diagnostic of primary sclerosing cholangitis and must be correlated with cholangiography, the constellation of small bile ducts surrounded by a cuff of fibrous tissue, reduced numbers of bile ducts, ductular proliferation, copper deposition, and piecemeal necrosis is very suggestive.

Radiology

Ultrasound

Sonographic abnormalities that suggest sclerosing cholangitis have been recently reported (12). Extensive thickening of intrahepatic and extrahepatic ducts is depicted as brightly echogenic tissue surrounding the portal venules and the common duct (Fig. 15.11). The wall of the latter was thickened up to 1.4 cm in one case. Intraluminal debris consisting of nonshadowing, mobile echogenic particles can be present, consistent with either pus, biliary sludge, or desquamated bile duct epithelium. Although the above findings are quite suggestive, a sclerosing cholangiocarcinoma cannot be excluded. As described in the CT section below, irregular multisegmental intrahepatic biliary dilatation seen sonographically can suggest sclerosing cholangitis.

Computed Tomography

Multifocal discontinuous areas of minimal intrahepatic biliary dilatation without a mass suggests sclerosing cholangitis on CT (13, 14) (Fig. 15.12). These slightly dilated ducts are characteristically beaded or irregularly contoured. However, smooth dilatation can be seen proximal to a high grade central stenosis. Irregular thickening of the gallbladder wall is an occasional finding.

Cholangiography

ERCP is generally preferable to PTC in sclerosing cholangitis in view of its higher success rate in the absence of dilated intrahepatic ducts (1, 15). PTC may be needed if certain regions of the liver are unopacified by ERCP in order to differentiate underfilling from real obstruction. The most common abnormal finding is diffuse or multifocal strictures involving both intra and extrahepatic ducts (Fig. 15.13) (1, 8, 16, 17). Extrahepatic ducts may be uninvolved, especially when the underlying disease is ulcerative colitis (1, 16–18). It is quite unusual for extrahepatic ducts to be involved without intrahepatic involvement; if this appears to be the case, underfilling or another diagnosis must be suspected (16). Strictures are typically short and annular (1–2 cm) with a predilection for bifurcations. They alternate with normal or minimally dilated segments giving a beaded appearance. Long, confluent strictures, pruning, and diminished arborization are seen in more advanced disease (Fig.

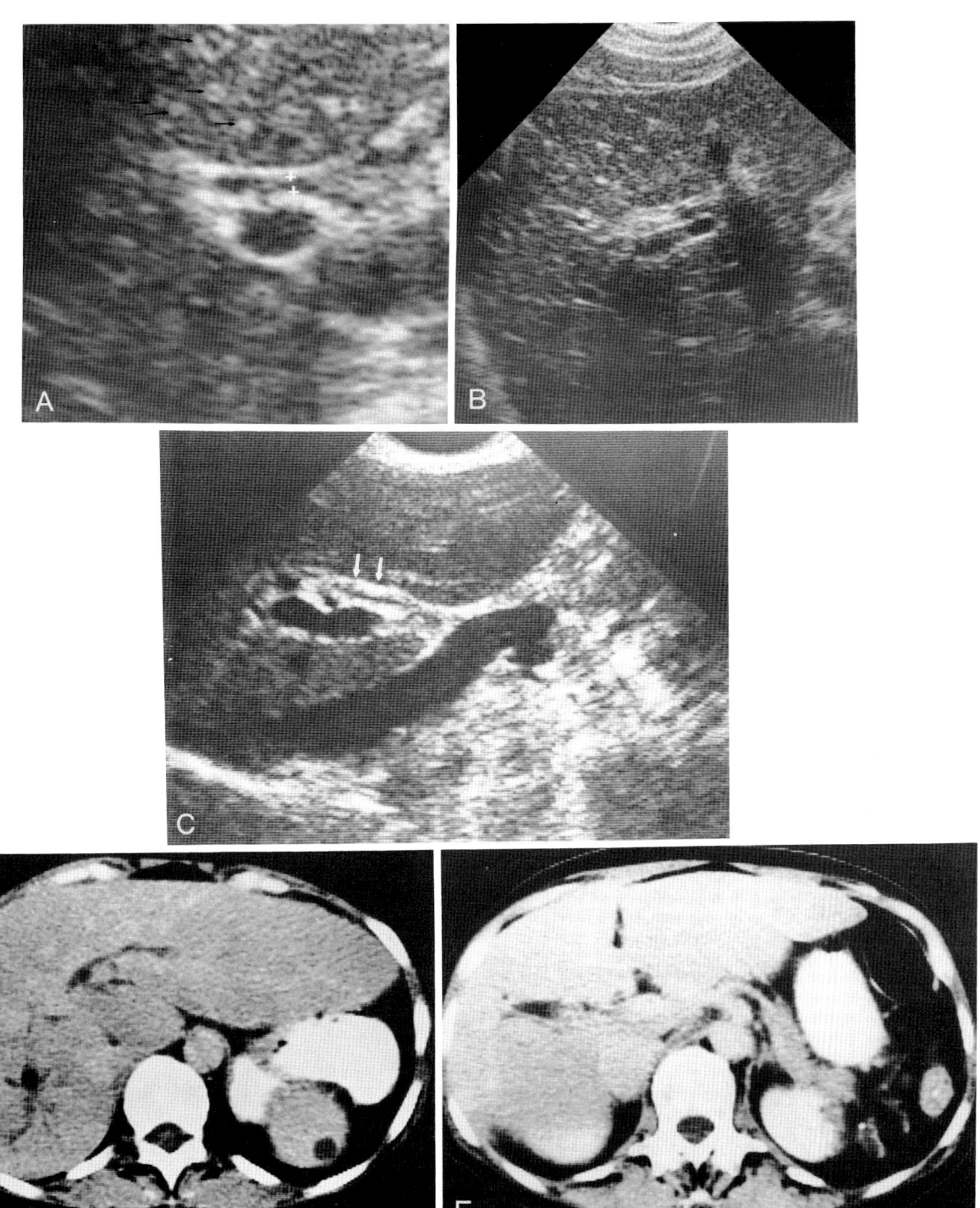

FIGURE 15.11. PRIMARY SCLEROSING CHOLANGITIS

A: Magnified scan of the common duct (*cursors*): brightly echogenic wall thickening with normal luminal caliber. Prominent echogenic thickening of portal venule walls (*arrows*). *B:* Nonmagnified view to give better perspective of portal venules. Cholangiogram (not shown) was typical of sclerosing cholangitis. *C–G:* Different patient with higher grade obstruction from sclerosing cholangitis. *C:* Thickened, bright common duct wall (*arrows*) but normal luminal caliber. *D* and *E:* Continuous but irregularly dilated ducts, level of obstruction at porta hepatis. *F:* Magnified view of level of obstruction: nondilated ducts with enhancing walls but no mass. *G:* PTC: smooth and beaded dilatation proximal to a high grade confluent smooth stricture at the bifurcation. Suboptimal filling distally, but both the common hepatic duct and the cystic duct look shaggy. Intrahepatic ducts involved to a greater degree than extrahepatic ducts.

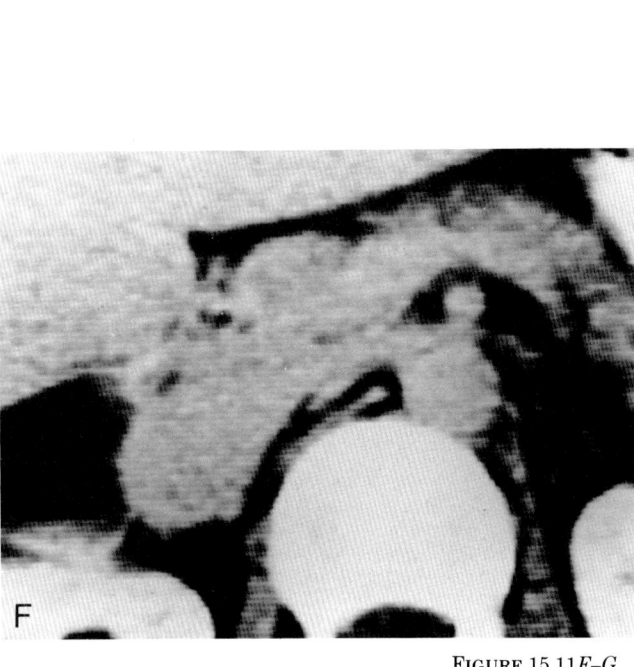
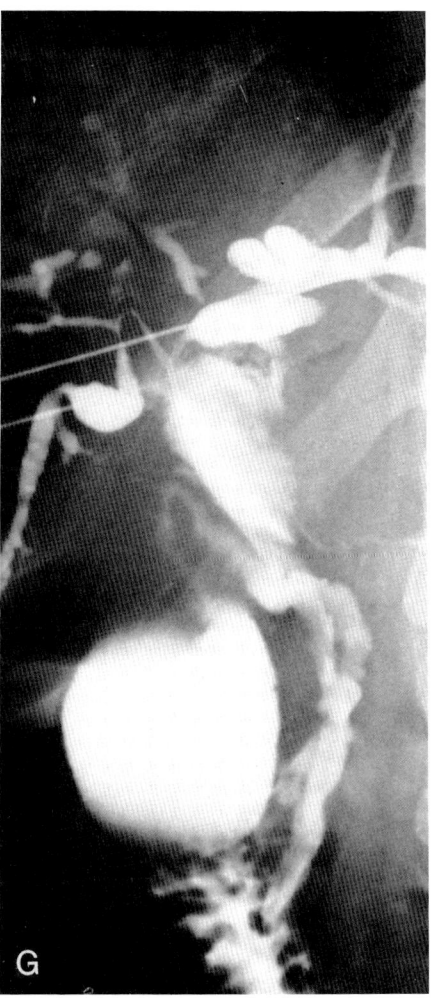

FIGURE 15.11F–G

15.11G). Small outpouchings (diverticula or pseudodiverticula), sometimes associated with 1–2 mm length band-like strictures, are more frequent in the extrahepatic ducts than the intrahepatic ducts and practically are pathognomonic (Figs. 15.13 and 15.14). They occur in primary sclerosing cholangitis associated with any underlying entity, not just inflammatory bowel disease and their pathologic correlate is not known (1). About one-half of patients with primary sclerosing cholangitis will have ductal mural irregularity, ranging from a brush border to shaggy to frankly nodular with coarse filling defects (Fig. 15.14). These irregularities are more common in the extrahepatic ducts. Diffuse ductal dilatation is quite infrequent, although segmental dilatation proximal to a high grade stenosis is not. Cystic duct abnormalities are present in about 20% (Figs. 15.13 and 15.14B), and gallbladder wall irregularities are seen quite uncommonly (1, 17). 8% of patients in one series had pancreatic duct abnormalities, consisting of many short strictures, beading, narrowing with serrations, or smooth strictures with intervening ectasia. Most had no clinical pancreatitis (1). One study evaluated serial cholangiography over time: extrahepatic duct disease was frequently stable and intrahepatic disease often progressed (6).

Differential Diagnosis

Sclerosing cholangiocarcinoma cannot be excluded even by negative histology and cytology (which can be obtained both percutaneously under fluoroscopic guidance and via intraluminal brushings). Diffuse stricturing favors sclerosing cholangitis, as do band-like strictures and diverticula. Carcinoma can be ruled out only by long-term follow-up. Inflammatory bowel disease predisposes to carcinoma as well as sclerosing cho-

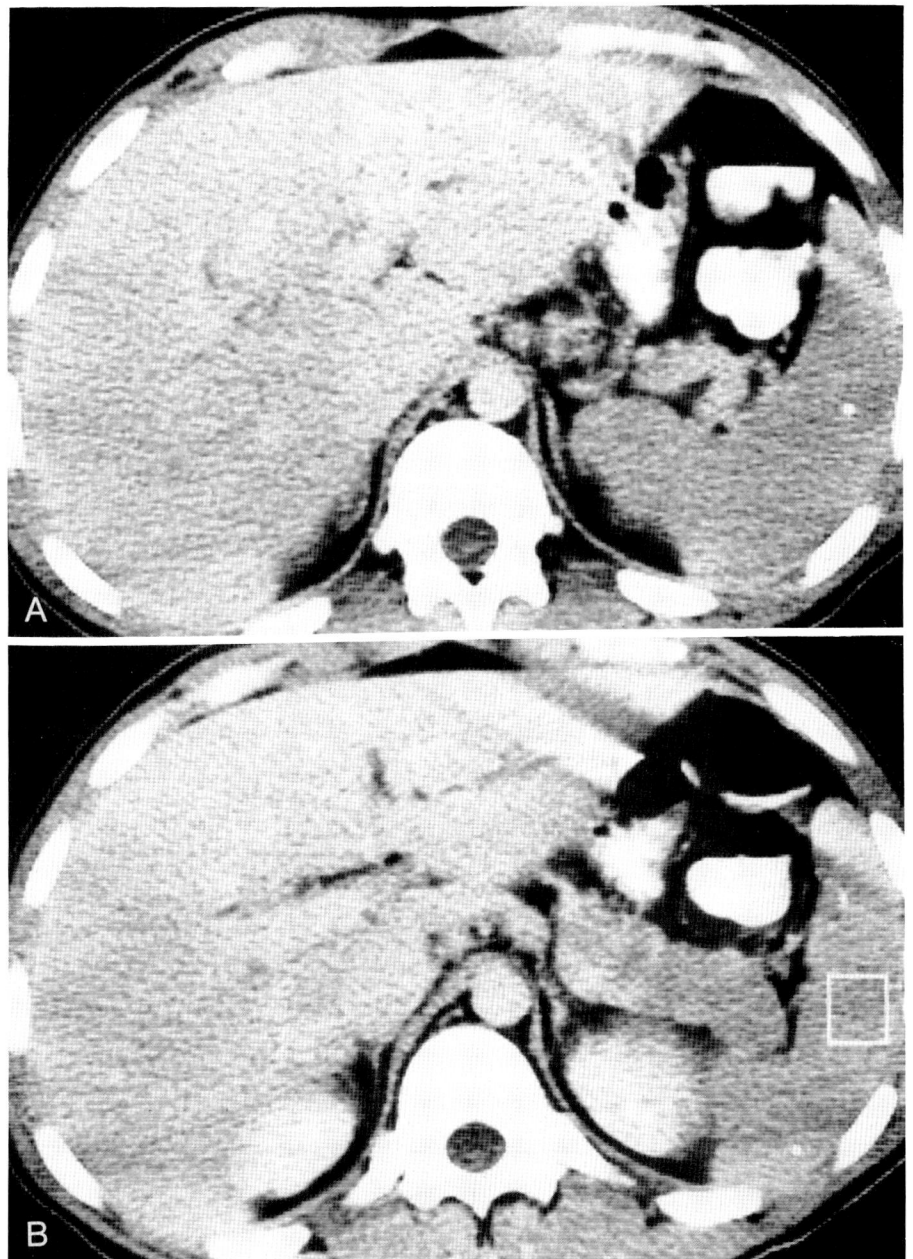

FIGURE 15.12. PRIMARY SCLEROSING CHOLANGITIS
A and *B:* CT scan showing minimally dilated, discontinuous, irregular intrahepatic ducts. Cholangiogram (not shown) correlated.

langitis. In view of the absence of effective therapy for either condition, absolute differentiation is usually only of academic interest. Secondary sclerosing cholangitis looks the same as primary sclerosing cholangitis on liver biopsy, and must be distinguished by cholangiographic demonstration of stones or cholangiography and history compatible with traumatic stricture, ampullary stenosis or anastomotic stricture. Although acute ascending cholangitis is rarely studied cholangiographically, if it is the picture may resemble sclerosing cholangitis. Distinction may be made by clinical history and reexamination documenting resolution after treatment. Differentiation of

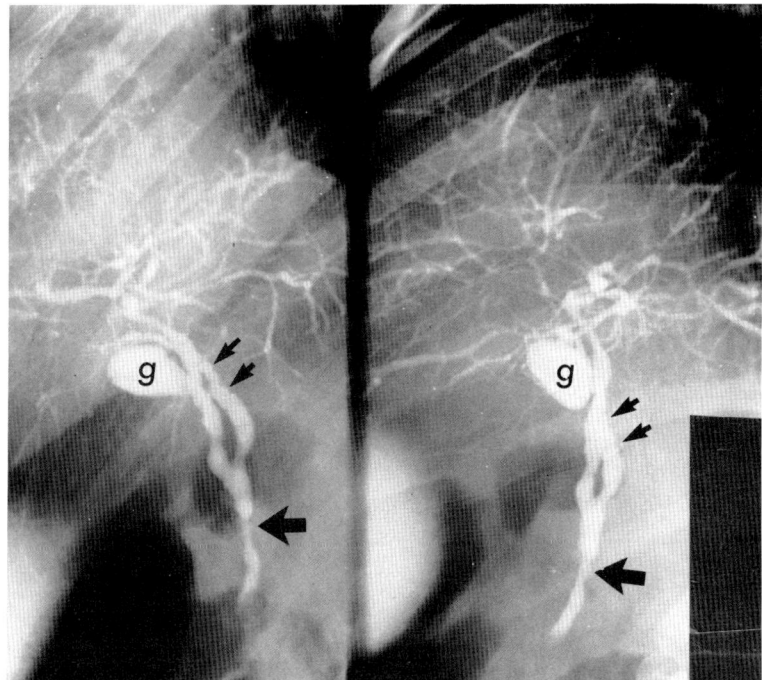

FIGURE 15.13. PRIMARY SCLEROSING CHOLANGITIS
ERCP: diffuse, irregular intrahepatic stricturing with a shaggy cystic duct (*short arrows*), partial gallbladder filling (*g*), and short segment stricture with a diverticulum or ulceration in the common bile duct (*large arrow*).

primary sclerosing cholangitis from primary biliary cirrhosis may be difficult when disease is limited to intrahepatic ducts (Fig. 15.15). The latter disease is characterized less by biliary stricturing than by cirrhotic changes: crowding and tortuosity of ducts within contracted hepatic segments and extrinsic deformity with spreading secondary to compensatory hypertrophy (1). Clinically, titers of antimitochondrial antibodies are high, which is not the case in sclerosing cholangitis.

Interventional Radiology

Stricture dilatation can be performed serially either percutaneously or endoscopically and eventually converted to internal drainage. Because of the nature of the disease, it is preferable to maintain easy access to the biliary tree, and surgical stenting of a choledochojejunostomy or a hepatojejunostomy permits easy percutaneous access via the barium-filled jejunum after stent removal. In this way, biliary toilet can be performed repetitively as an outpatient without having to traverse the liver repetitively (9, 10).

Nuclear Medicine

Hepatobiliary scintigraphy can be a valuable study in this group of patients, both for initial diagnosis and, especially, for noninvasive follow-up. The hepatogram phase will generally show patchy parenchymal activity. The most specific findings consist of multiple focal hot spots appearing as early as 15 min postinjection and persisting for 60 min or longer. These correspond to focally dilated ducts on cholangiography. Another important finding that can be seen is delayed isotope clearance of various segments of liver parenchyma. These segments are drained by severely stenosed ducts that may not be filled at all on cholangiography (19). Further experience with hepatobiliary scintigraphy in sclerosing cholangitis is needed before its clinical efficacy relative to other diagnostic methods can be properly assessed. Sulfur colloid scanning is unrewarding in this disease.

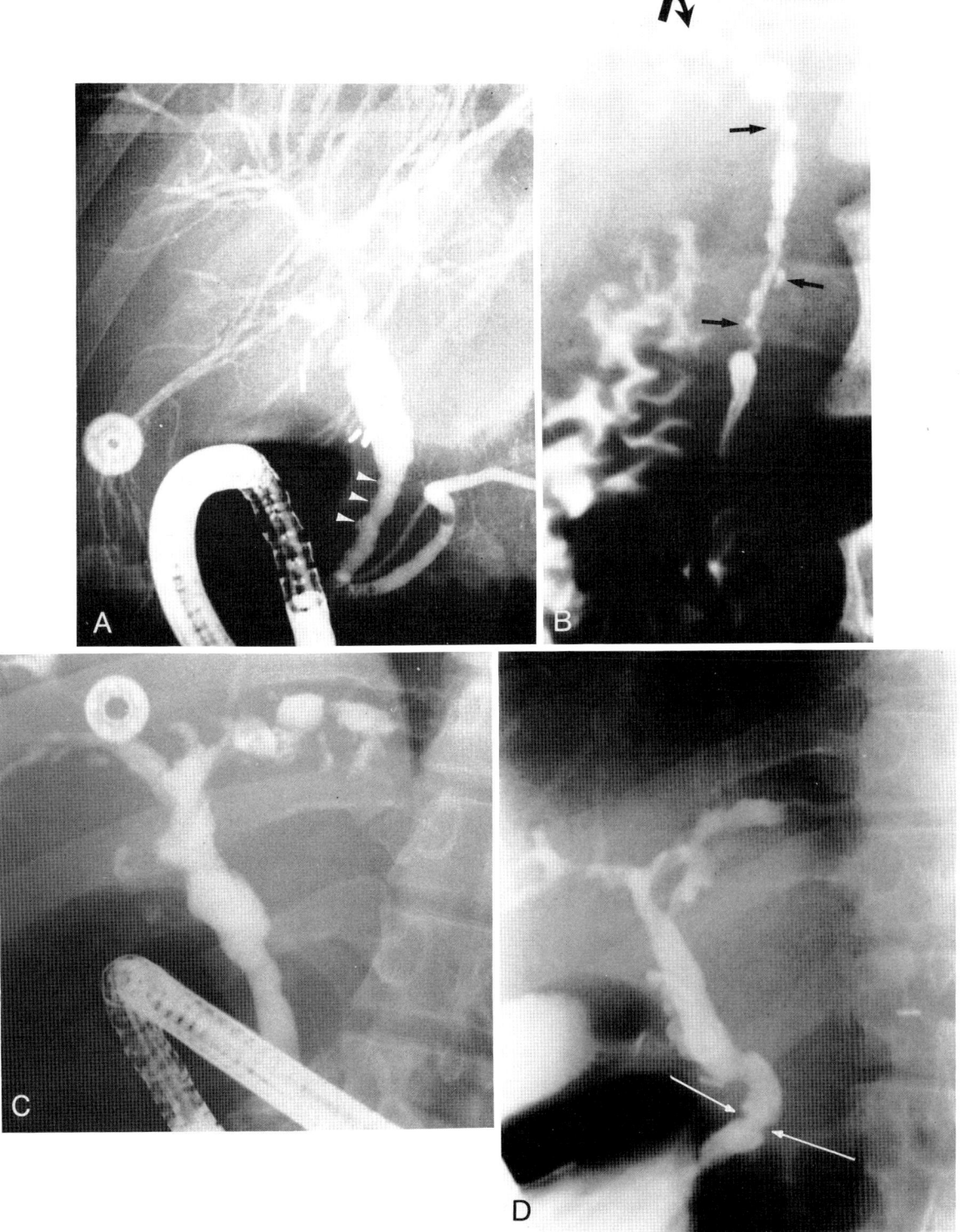

FIGURE 15.14. PRIMARY SCLEROSING CHOLANGITIS

Four cases of sclerosing cholangitis with wall irregularities. *A:* Diffuse irregular intrahepatic stricturing with diverticula in the common bile duct (*arrowheads*), ERCP. *B:* PTC: coned-down view of the common bile duct showing multiple band-like strictures and diverticula (*arrows*). Cystic duct is involved (*curved arrow*). *C:* Nodular irregularity of the common duct wall and intrahepatic strictures. *D:* Band-like stricture in distal common duct (*arrows*) due to sclerosing cholangitis. Intrahepatic disease present as well.

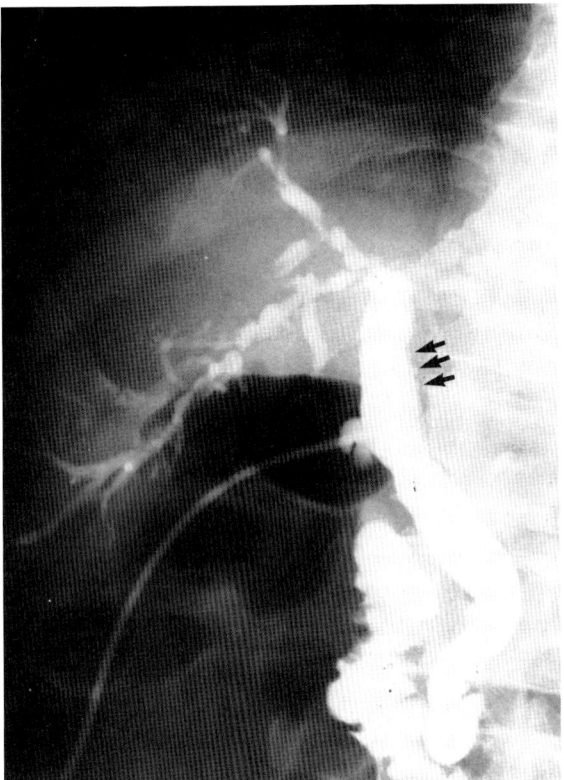

FIGURE 15.15. PRIMARY SCLEROSING CHOLANGITIS
A 57-yr-old man with a 20-yr history of episodic jaundice. Operative cholangiogram: beaded intrahepatic ducts with multiple strictures. Despite overwhelming intrahepatic involvement, the diagnosis is primary sclerosing cholangitis, not biliary cirrhosis. A few diverticula (arrows) are present in the common hepatic duct. The long course is consistent with the hypothesis of better prognosis with predominant intrahepatic disease.

REFERENCES

1. MacCarty RL, La Russo, NF, Weisner RH, Ludwig J: Primary sclerosing cholangitis: findings on cholangiography and pancreatography. Radiology 149:39–44, 1983.
2. Sherlock S: Diseases of the Liver and Biliary System. London, Oxford & Blackwell Scientific, 1981, pp 239–243.
3. Bhathal PS, Powell LW: Primary intrahepatic obliterating cholangitis: a possible variant of "sclerosing cholangitis." Gut 10:886–893, 1969.
4. Mistilis SP: Pericholangitis and ulcerative colitis. Ann Intern Med 63:1–25, 1965.
5. Weisner RH, La Russo NF: Clinicopathologic features of the syndrome of primary sclerosing cholangitis. Gastroenterology 79:200–206, 1980.
6. Warren GH, Kern F: The biliary tract and inflammatory bowel disease. Clin Gastroenterol 12:255–268, 1983.
7. Vierling JM: Hepatobiliary complications of ulcerative colitis and Crohn's disease. In Zakim D, Boyer TD (eds): Hepatology: A Textbook of Liver Disease. Philadelphia, W. B. Saunders, 1982, pp 818–821.
8. La Russo NF, Weisner RH, Ludwig J, MacCarty RL: Current concepts: primary sclerosing cholangitis. N Engl J Med 310:899–903, 1984.
9. Martin EC, Fankuchen EJ, Laffey, KJ, Sibley RE: Percutaneous management of benign biliary disease. Gastrointest Radiol 9:207–212, 1984.
10. Kaufman SL, Cameron JL, Adams PE, Kadir S, Mitchell SE, Chang R, White RI: The management of surgically placed silastic transhepatic biliary stents. AJR 142:347–350, 1984.
11. Schwartz SI: Sclerosing cholangitis. In Moody FG (ed): Advances in Diagnosis and Surgical Treatment of Biliary Tract Disease, New York, Masson, 1983, pp 155–158.
12. Carroll BA, Oppenheimer DA: Sclerosing cholangitis: sonographic demonstration of bile duct wall thickening. AJR 139:1016–1018, 1982.
13. Rahn NH, Koehler RE, Truss CD, Sagel SS, Stanley RJ: CT appearance of sclerosing cholangitis. AJR 141:549–552, 1983.
14. Ament A, Haaga J, Wiedenmann S, Barkmeir J, Morrison S: Primary sclerosing cholangitis: CT findings. J Comput Assist Tomogr 7:795–800, 1983.
15. Longmire WP: When is cholangitis sclerosing? Am J Surg 135:312–320, 1978.
16. Chen L, Goldberg HI: Sclerosing cholangitis: broad spectrum of radiographic features. Gastrointest Radiol 9:39–47, 1984.
17. Rohrmann CA, Ansel HJ, Freeny PC, Silverstein FE, Protell RL, Fenster LF, Ball T, Vennes JA, Silvis SE: Cholangiographic abnormalities in patients with inflammatory bowel disease. Radiology 127:635–641, 1978.
18. Blackstone MO, Nemchausky BA: Cholangiographic abnormalities in ulcerative colitis associated pericholangitis which resemble sclerosing cholangitis. Dig Dis Sci 23:579–585, 1978.
19. Ament AE, Bick RJ, Miraldi FD, Haaga JR, Wiedenmann SD: Sclerosing cholangitis: cholescintigraphy with ^{99m}Tc-labeled DISIDA. Radiology 151:197–201, 1984.

PERICHOLANGITIS ASSOCIATED WITH INFLAMMATORY BOWEL DISEASE

The term "pericholangitis" is poorly descriptive for what has been more aptly referred to as "portal triaditis," usually seen in association with inflammatory bowel disease (1, 2). The term "pericholangitis" focuses attention only on the ductular changes; however, pericholangitis involves the entire portal triad. The incidence of pericholangitis in patients with inflammatory bowel disease ranges from 4% in retrospective studies to 83% in prospective studies of surgical patients undergoing liver biopsy prior to colectomy(3).

Hepatic dysfunction is common in patients with inflammatory bowel disease, but other en-

TABLE 15.1.
HEPATOBILIARY LESIONS ASSOCIATED WITH
INFLAMMATORY BOWEL DISEASE[a]

Frequent	Uncommon	Rare
Pericholangitis	Cirrhosis	Abscess
Fatty liver	Sclerosing cholangitis	Pylephlebitis
	Cholangiocarcinoma	Amyloidosis
	Hepatoportal fibrosis	Granulomatous hepatitis
	Chronic active hepatitis	

[a] Modified from B. Gastel (6), p. 227.

tities besides pericholangitis must be considered. Overall, liver function abnormalities are seen in 15% of patients with ulcerative colitis (4) with histologic abnormalities found in 94% of wedge liver biopsies of ulcerative colitis patients undergoing colectomy. Of those patients with histologic abnormalities, 73% have inflammatory changes, 45% have fatty infiltration, and cirrhosis is seen in 3.8% (5). The most common liver lesions in inflammatory bowel disease are listed in Table 15.1.

Clinical Findings

Pericholangitis manifests itself clinically in three forms which have identical pathologic changes. The first form is asymptomatic biochemical cholestasis. Symptomatic forms are either cholestatic (recurrent or sustained, with jaundice, pruritus, and fever) or cholangitic (with recurrent attacks of fever, abdominal pain, tender hepatomegaly, and leukocytosis) (3, 4, 6–8). A patient may manifest all three forms during the course of his disease.

Pericholangitis usually occurs in patients with extensive bowel disease but may be seen in limited colonic disease and may or may not parallel the severity of the bowel disease. The inflammatory bowel disease is usually moderate to severe, universal in extent, and present for at least one year prior to the discovery of pericholangitis (5). While pericholangitis is usually relatively benign, progression to chronic liver disease and secondary biliary cirrhosis can occur. Pericholangitis and sclerosing cholangitis have been described independently of each other, but they are well known to occur together and may, in fact, represent different parts of the spectrum of the same disease (9). Pericholangitis is not static but rather waxes and wanes.

Pathology

Pericholangitis is a diffuse process with the intensity of the inflammation varying from one portal tract to another. Early on, the inflammatory process is largely limited to the portal regions and it consists of an infiltrate of polymorphonuclear cells, lymphocytes, and plasma cells. Portal zones may be expanded and the inflammatory infiltrate may extend into the interlobular spaces or the periportal liver lobules. Periductal inflammation is conspicuous with ductal epithelium showing degenerative features similar to those seen in primary biliary cirrhosis (7, 8, 10). In more advanced disease, periductal and portal fibrosis occur with ductular proliferation seen as well as development of portal-portal bridging. This may vary from one portal tract to another in the same biopsy specimen (7, 8, 10). Extension into the extrahepatic ducts may be seen, although the process is usually limited to intrahepatic ducts (10). Other histologic changes common to other chronic liver diseases may be seen, such as piecemeal necrosis and fibrosis (3, 8, 10).

Progression of pericholangitis through three stages (acute, subacute, and chronic) has been described (3, 7, 10). Changes characteristic of the acute stage are the portal tract and periductular inflammation described above coupled with occasional parenchymal changes. In the subacute stage, fibroblastic proliferation with an increase in connective tissue and decreased cellular infiltration and edema compared to the acute stage is present. Additionally, accumulation of a hyaline-like material in bile duct walls can be seen. Subacute pericholangitis is probably a transition between acute and chronic disease. In chronic disease concentric fibrosis around the bile ducts and portal tracts may extend into the lobules causing broad fibrous bands (2). Periportal fibrosis spreading between lobules results in a stellate appearance and may involve lymphatic and venous channels. Inflammation may be absent making the etiology of the fibrosis difficult or impossible to ascertain, but acute changes may be present in the same sample, making diagnosis possible.

Acute histologic changes found early in disease may resolve spontaneously or in response to therapy, but extensive fibrosis is irreversible.

Pathogenesis

Theories advanced include portal vein bacteremia (3, 7–11), toxins released from diseased

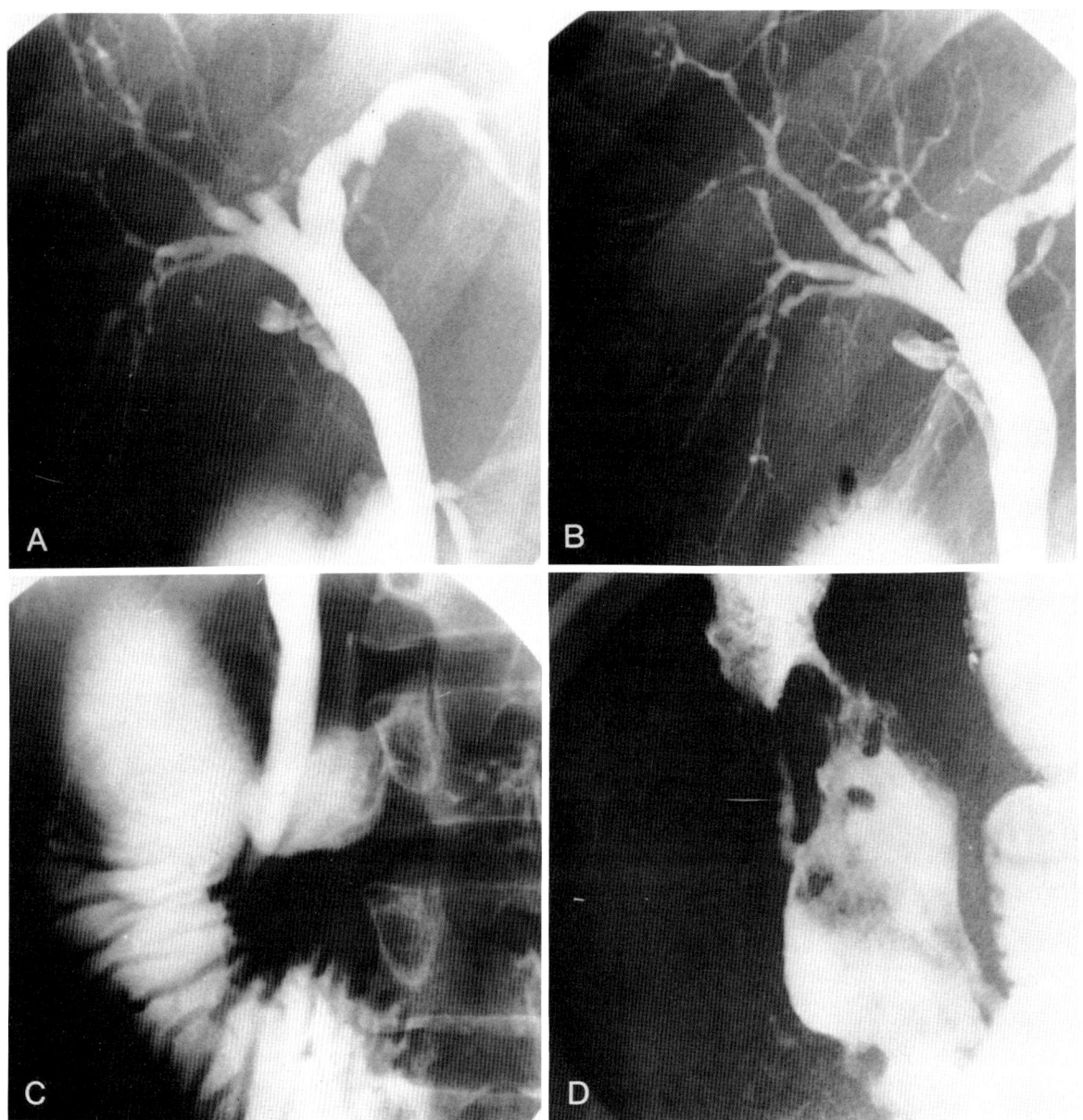

FIGURE 15.16. PERICHOLANGITIS
Pericholangitis with underlying quiescent Crohn's disease: at the time of the cholangiogram the only clinical problem was elevated alkaline phosphatase. *A* and *B:* ERCP: multiple short strictures affecting intrahepatic ducts only. *C:* Normal distal common bile duct. *D:* Barium enema with reflux several years earlier: advanced ileocolitis seen on spot film of terminal ileum.

bowel (3), hepatotoxicity of lithocolic acid (3, 8, 11), and antigen-antibody immune complex deposition (3, 5, 8, 11).

Treatment

Treatment is expectant because of the usual relatively benign course. Serial liver biopsy and clinical observation is mandatory, as what is initially considered pericholangitis may, in fact, turn out to be the more serious chronic active hepatitis or sclerosing cholangitis. Long-term antibiotic or corticosteriod therapy has not been shown to be efficacious. The benefit of colectomy is controversial (3, 10, 12). If colectomy is chosen, the optimal time is after evidence of progressive histologic change accumulates but before irreversible fibrosis develops. Symptomatic medical therapy is the same as that described in this book for sclerosing cholangitis and primary biliary cirrhosis.

Radiology

Cholangiography and other imaging studies show findings identical to primary sclerosing cholangitis, except that abnormalities are generally limited to the intrahepatic biliary tree (3, 9, 13) (Fig. 15.16).

REFERENCES

1. Stauffer MH, Sauer WG, Dearing WH et al: The spectrum of cholestatic hepatic disease. *JAMA* 191:829–837, 1965.
2. Schmid R: Clinical gastroenterology conference: differential diagnosis of jaundice and ulcerative colitis. *Gastroenterology* 73:357–374, 1977.
3. Vierling JM: Hepatobiliary complications of ulcerative colitis and Crohn's disease. In Zakim D, Boyer TD (eds): *Hepatology: A Textbook of Liver Disease.* Philadelphia, W. B. Saunders, 1982, pp 797–824.
4. Scully RE: Case records of the Massachusetts General Hospital. *N. Engl. J Med* 298:445–452, 1978.
5. Eade MN: Liver disease and ulcerative colitis; I. Analysis of operative liver biopsies in 138 consecutive patients having colectomy. *Ann Intern Med* 72:474–487, 1970.
6. Gastel B: Clinical conferences at the Johns Hopkins Hospital. *Johns Hopkins Med J* 141:224–232, 1970.
7. Mistilis SP: Pericholangitis and ulcerative colitis; I. Pathology, etiology and pathogenesis. *Ann Intern Med* 63:1–26, 1965.
8. Warren GH, Kern F: Pericholangitis: the biliary tract and inflammatory bowel disease. *Clin Gastroenterol* 12:255–268, 1983.
9. Blackstone MO, Nemchausky BA: Cholangiographic abnormalities in ulcerative colitis-associated pericholangitis which resemble sclerosing cholangitis. *Dig Dis Sci* 23:579–585, 1978.
10. Mistilis SP: Liver disease and bowel disorders. In Schiff I (ed): *Diseases of the Liver.* Philadelphia, J. B. Lipincott, 1975, pp 1373–1383.
11. Perrett AD, Higgins G, Johnston HH, Massarella GR, Truelove SC, Wright R: The liver and ulcerative colitis. *Q J Med* 158:211–238, 1971.
12. Eade MN, Cooke WT, Brooke BN: Liver disease and ulcerative colitis; II. The long-term effect of colectomy. *Ann Intern Med* 72:489–497, 1970.
13. Rohrmann CA, Ansel HJ, Freeny PC, Silverstein FE, Protell RL, Fenster LF, Ball T, Vennes JA, Silvis SE: Cholangiographic abnormalities in patients with inflammatory bowel disease. *Radiology* 127:635–641, 1978.

PRIMARY BILIARY CIRRHOSIS

Primary biliary cirrhosis is a chronic cholestatic hepatitis of unknown etiology which is relentlessly progressive over decades. It causes a significant fibrotic reaction within the liver and, eventually, cirrhosis. There are four overlapping histologic stages (1). A better name for the disease is chronic nonsuppurative destructive cholangitis; nevertheless, the less cumbersome term primary biliary cirrhosis is commonly used even in the earliest stages of the disorder when cirrhosis is absent. Differential diagnosis usually includes extrahepatic bile duct obstruction, sclerosing cholangitis, chronic active hepatitis, drug-induced cholestatis, and pericholangitis.

Etiology and Pathogenesis

Several theories have been advanced as to the etiology of primary biliary cirrhosis including cell-mediated autoimmunity, humoral autoimmunity, and immune-complex deposition. A genetic predisposition has also been invoked (1–6). Although copper levels well above those seen with mere biliary obstruction and cholestasis (and exceeded only in Wilson's disease and Indian childhood cirrhosis) are found in primary biliary cirrhosis, copper accumulation is secondary since its reduction does not significantly alter th course of the disease (1). Interestingly, elevated copper levels are also present extrahepatically in primary biliary cirrhosis, similar to the pattern seen in Wilson's disease.

Clinical Findings

Primary biliary cirrhosis occurs throughout the world with a point prevalence in England. A 9–10:1 female to male ratio exists with the typical patient being a woman between the ages of 35 and 55. The most common presentation (about 60%) is the insidious onset of pruritus, which precedes jaundice by many months. Pruritus is worse at night and most severe on the hands and feet as well as regions of pressure such as belt lines. Fatigue is a common additional complaint. Simultaneous onset of pruritus and jaundice or onset of jaundice alone are less common presenting features. Other physical findings are hepatomegaly or hyperpigmentation (about 50%) and xanthelasma/xanthoma (about 25%). As the disease progresses, scratch marks occur as the result of unremitting pruritus. Late manifestations include osteomalacia and pathologic fractures, digital clubbing, and signs and symptoms of portal hypertension and hepatic failure. Other associated autoimmune and collagen diseases include: rheumatoid arthritis, scleroderma, Sjögren's syndrome, CRST syndrome, Hashimoto's thyroiditis, renal tubular acidosis, and lupus (1–3, 7, 8). Alkaline phosphatase is almost invariably elevated in both relatively asymptomatic and symptomatic patients, and its elevation (usually 2–3 times normal) is out of proportion to that of any elevation in bilirubin or aminotransferases. Serum bile acids, bilirubin, and cholesterol are raised in about ⅔ (1, 2, 8, 9). The serum bilirubin is an important prognostic factor: when it exceeds 2 mg/dl, the disease is in an accelerated phase, a linear rise in bilirubin may occur, and an inverse relationship of bilirubin level to life expectancy exists (2, 3, 8). IgM is increased as much as 4-fold in 95% of patients, and antimitochondrial antibody is present in 81–100% with a high titer in ½ (1, 2). Antimitochondrial antibodies are non-organ-specific and directed against an antigen of the inner membrane of the mitochondrial cristae. Although they have no role in the pathogenesis of the disease, the presence of antimitochondrial antibodies confirms the diagnosis of primary biliary cirrhosis by virtue of their absence in mechanical bile duct obstruction. Antimitochondrial antibodies are sometimes present in cryptogenic cirrhosis and surface antigen negative lupoid chronic active hepatitis (1–3). Other autoimmune markers which may be present are: antinuclear antibody (30–50%), antismooth muscle antibody (30–40%), rheumatoid factor (25–60%), and antithyroid antibody (15–26%). These markers are more prevalent in chronic hepatitis (1).

Pathology

Initially (Stage 1), liver biopsy shows inflammation of septal and larger interlobular bile ducts. Epithelioid granulomas may be present in the portal tracts, and signs of cholestasis may be absent. Stage 2 disease is charaterized by fibrosis, acute and chronic inflammatory infiltration and ductular proliferation. Ducts are reduced and replaced by ill-defined lymphoid aggregates and cholestasis is present. In Stage 3, the inflammation subsides and relatively acellular septa extend from portal tracts into and around lobules. The appearance is no longer pathognomonic of biliary cirrhosis, but it can be interpreted as compatible.

Stage 4 is end-stage cirrhosis with regenerating nodules. The etiology can be suggested by a dearth of bile ducts or lymphocyte accumulation (1, 3, 4). Overlap between stages is common—Stage 1 lesions are occasionally seen in Stage 4 livers.

Radiology

ERCP is the preferred modality for evaluating the biliary tree in this disease since intrahepatic ducts are not dilated. ERCP is indicated in primary biliary cirrhosis to exclude obstructive biliary disease. In primary biliary cirrhosis, the extrahepatic ducts are normal except occasionally when filling defects are seen due to inspissated bile (10). Gallstones are present in up to 35% of patients (1). The intrahepatic biliary tree may be normal, narrowed, or both narrowed and shortened with decreased branching (Fig. 15.17). Ducts may be tortuous and of mildly varying caliber (10, 11). The decreased branching has been termed the "tree-in-winter" appearance (3). Narrowing alone is hard to call on a single study but is more easily appreciated as an interval

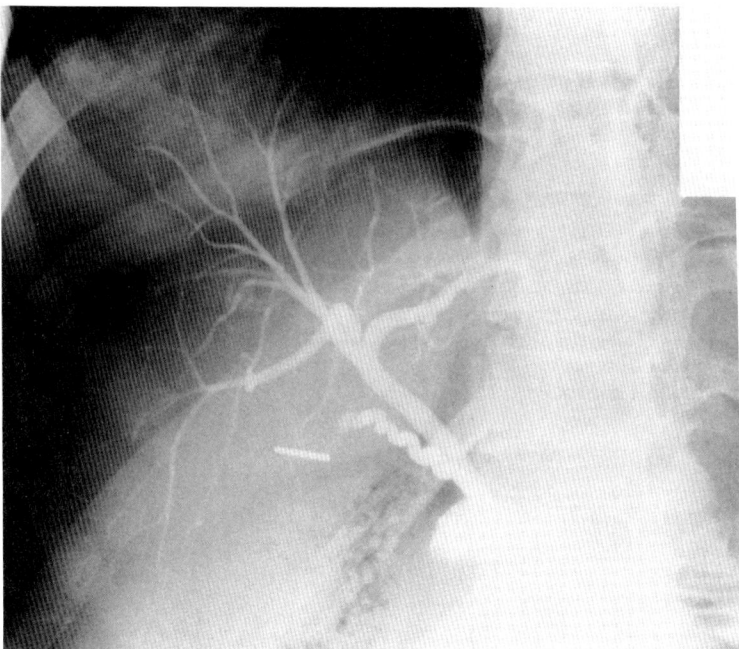

FIGURE 15.17. PRIMARY BILIARY CIRRHOSIS
ERCP: normal extrahepatic ducts. Intrahepatic ducts undulate and are attenuated with diminished branching, consistent with primary biliary cirrhosis.

change on serial examinations. Normal cholangiography does not exclude the disease, and positive findings suggest advanced disease. In fact, the cholangiographic abnormalities just described correlate well with cirrhosis (5, 11). The lack of correlation with bile duct histologic abnormalities should not be surprising since the characteristic pathologic changes are seen in ducts smaller than those examined radiographically.

The major differential diagnosis cholangiographically (besides cirrhosis) is primary sclerosing cholangitis or pericholangitis associated with inflammatory bowel disease. Primary biliary cirrhosis has less stricturing than the latter two diseases and the changes in the intrahepatic biliary tree are more peripheral (12). Normal extrahepatic ducts are not useful in differential diagnosis, but abnormal extrahepatic ducts rule out primary biliary cirrhosis. Prior to the recognition that primary sclerosing cholangitis and pericholangitis need not affect the extrahepatic biliary tree, primary biliary cirrhosis was overdiagnosed cholangiographically in the presence of abnormal intrahepatic ducts and normal extrahepatic ducts (Fig. 15.18).

Course

Though the progression of primary biliary cirrhosis is variable the long-term prognosis is poor. Patients presenting with cholestatic symptoms and jaundice have a mean survival of 5.5–6 yr, with a range of 3–11 yr (1, 3). The survival of "asymptomatic" patients who only manifest deranged liver chemistries can vary from 2 to 20 yr (1, 3, 9). These patients may be free of hepatobiliary symptoms for up to 10 yr following diagnosis; however, once symptoms develop, their prognosis is similar to that seen with initially symptomatic patients. Independent discriminators of a poor prognosis are an elevated serum bilirubin, age, and hepatomegaly upon presentation of the disease (1, 2, 8). Liver biopsies specimens showing bridging fibrosis or cirrhosis also portend a poor prognosis (1, 2, 8). Granulomas and bile destruction without cirrhosis are seen more frequently in asymptomatic patients and imply better prognosis (1, 5). The histologic finding of fibrosis limited to portal areas correlates with longer survival, as does the presence of epithelioid granulomas (1, 2, 8).

Treatment

The conventional treatment of PBC is directed at the symptoms and complications of the disease (Table 15.2).

Experimental Modalities

Current experimental modalities include corticosteroids (may exacerbate metabolic bone dis-

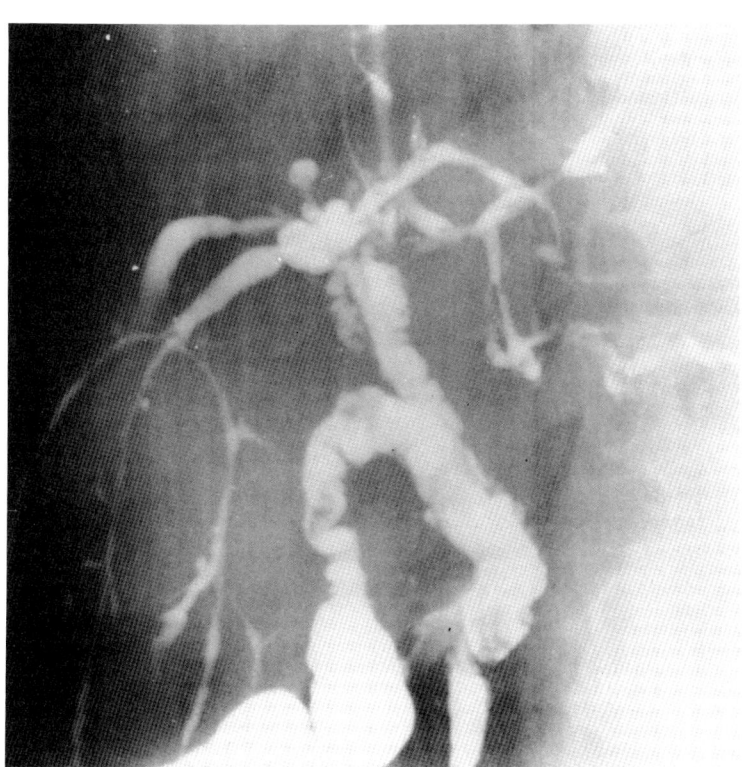

FIGURE 15.18. SCLEROSING CHOLANGITIS
Operative cholangiogram through the gallbladder, called primary biliary cirrhosis in 1959. Almost certainly secondary cirrhosis due to primary sclerosing cholangitis. Intrahepatic ducts are far more diseased than extrahepatic ducts with stricturing and drop out of branches. Linear strictures and diverticula are present in extrahepatic duct. Note splaying of ducts in lower right lobe, probably due to nodular regeneration.

TABLE 15.2.
TREATMENT OF PRIMARY BILIARY CIRRHOSIS

Problem	Treatment
Pruritus	Cholestyramine (concentrate around A.M. meal)
	Phenobarbital
	Atarax or periactin
Steatorrhea and malabsorption	40 g fat restricted diet medium chain triglyceride supplements parenteral vitamins A, D, and K
Bleeding	Parenteral vitamin K
Gallstones	Surgery for symptomatic stones
	Avoid clofibrate
Xanthomas and xanthomatous neuropathy	Plasmapheresis, plasma exchange, cholestyramine
Proximal myopathy	1,25-(OH)-vitamin D or calcium infusions
Jaundice	Phenobarbital
Bone disease osteomalacia/osteoporosis	(Osteomalacia responds to therapy, osteoporosis does not)
	Increase dietary calcium, oral water-soluble vitamin D preparation, parenteral vitamin D, calcium infusions for bone pain, sunlight
Portal hypertension	Treat sequelae according to Child's classification

ease, however); cyclosporin-A (modulated immune function); azathioprine and chlorambucil (early trials reveal no benefit); plasmapheresis to remove immune complexes; and pencillamine which lowers hepatic copper concentration, reduces circulating immune complexes and autoantibodies, and might inhibit events leading to hepatic fibrosis (1, 3–6, 13). Pencillamine therapy has a 40% incidence of side effects, and unfortunately a recent study showed it to be ineffective in arresting the disease process (13).

REFERENCES

1. Vierling JM: Primary biliary cirrhosis. In Zakim G, Boyer TD (eds): *Hepatology: A Textbook of Liver Disease.* Philadelphia, W. B. Saunders, 1982, pp 825–862.
2. Roll J, Boyer JL, Barry D, Klatskin G: Prognostic importance of clinical and histologic features in asymptomatic and symptomatic primary biliary cirrhosis. *N Engl J Med* 308:1–7, 1983.
3. Herlong HF: Primary biliary cirrhosis. In Bayless TM (ed): *Current Therapy in Gastroenterology and Liver Disease, 1984–1985.* St. Louis, C. V. Mosby, 1984, pp 430–435.
4. Foulk WT, Baggenstoss AH: Biliary cirrhosis. In Schiff L (ed): *Diseases of the Liver,* Ed 4. Philadelphia, J. B. Lippincott, 1975, pp 940–970.
5. Sherlock S: Primary biliary cirrhosis. In Wright R, Alberti KGMM, Karran S, Millwood-Sadler GH (eds): *Liver and Biliary Disease.* Philadelphia, W. B. Saunders, 1979, pp 715–734.
6. James SP: Primary biliary cirrhosis (editorial). *N Engl J Med* 312:1055–1056, 1985.
7. Reynold TB, Dennison EK, Frankle HD, Liberman FL, Peters RL: Primary biliary cirrhosis with scleroderma, Raynaud's phenomenon and telangectasia. *Am J Med* 50:302–312, 1971.
8. Christensen E, Crowe J, Doniach D, Popper H, Ranek L, Rodes J, Tygstrup N, Williams R: Clinical pattern and course of disease in primary biliary cirrhosis based on an analysis of 236 patients. *Gastroenterology* 78:236–246, 1980.
9. Long RG, Scheuer PJ, Sherlock S: Presentation and course of asymptomatic primary biliary cirrhosis. *Gastroenterology* 72:1204–1209, 1977.
10. Legge DA, Carlson HC, Dickson ER, Ludwig J: Cholangiographic findings in cholangiolitic hepatitis. *Radiology* 102:16–20, 1971.
11. Summerfield JA, Elias E, Nikapota VLB, Dick R, Sherlock S: The biliary system in primary biliary cirrhosis. *Gastroenterology* 70:240–243, 1976.
12. MacCarty RL, LaRusso NF, Wiesner RH, Ludgwig J: Primary sclerosing cholangitis: findings on cholangiography and pancreatography. *Radiology* 149:39–44, 1983.
13. Dickson ER, Fleming TR, Wiesner RH, Baldus WP, Fleming CR, Ludwig J, McCall JT: Trial of penillamine in advanced primary biliary cirrhosis. *N Engl J Med* 312:1011–1015, 1985.

PAPILLARY (AMPULLARY) STENOSIS

The symptoms caused by disorders of the sphincter of Oddi are similar irrespective of the origin of the obstruction. Whether it is due to fibrosis of the papilla or disturbance of the physiologic function, its clinical presentation is a manifestation of the segment of the sphincter affected (1). Classically, papillary stenosis may be difficult to differentiate from choledocholithiasis since it may be associated with recurrent right upper quadrant or epigastric pain, laboratory evidence of cholestasis or pancreatitis or both, and dilation of the bile and/or pancreatic ducts revealed on radiographic studies (1, 2).

Anatomy and Physiology

The ampulla of Vater, named after the anatomist Abraham Vater (1720), is the choledochoduodenal connection usually found in the middle third of the descending duodenum on the medial wall. The main pancreatic duct usually forms an anastomosis with the common bile duct. The walls of both distal ducts are thickened by the presence of sphincter muscle causing a protrusion into the lumen, the papilla of Vater (3).

The anatomic makeup of the papilla of Vater is similar to other sphincters with longitudinal and transverse muscle fibers running below the lamina epithelialis. The anterior surface of the ampulla is covered by a single layer of epithelium with inlaid mucosal glands and a generous capillary network (1). The sphincter of Oddi, described by Oddi in 1887, is a complex system of annular muscles which are interconnected to those of the common bile duct as well as to those of the duodenum. A vascular plexus is present in the area as is a nerve plexus from both the sympathetic and parasympathetic nervous systems (1). The sphincter discharges bile and pancreatic juice in a timed manner but is a one-way barrier, thereby preventing reflux and infection by isolating the pancreatic and biliary systems from the remainder of the GI tract. The flap-like partition between the pancreatic and bile ducts prevents duodenobiliary reflux as well as duodenopancreatic reflux but still allows synchronous flow (1). The intrinsic pressure in the pancreatic duct is two to three times higher than that within the bile duct which, in turn, is higher than the intraduodenal pressure. The pressure differentials allow for a forward gradient only (4). Manometrically, a 4–6 mm long high pressure zone can be demonstrated at the sphincter of Oddi (1).

Etiology

Primary papillary stenosis may arise as a result of congenital malformations of the papilla. Acute and chronic inflammation of the papilla may also result in stenosis (5). Adenomyosis, similar to that seen with prostatic hypertrophy, can also narrow the outflow tract (1, 6, 7).

Secondary papillary stenosis occurs in association with cholelithiasis in 26% or choledocholithiasis in 64% by direct mechanical trauma to the area of the distal sphincter (stone passage) or continued irritation of the biliary tract inducing reflex spasm of the papilla. Ninety percent of papillary stenoses arise from these causes. Previous surgical manipulation is another less common cause (1). Benign and malignant periampullary neoplasms must be excluded.

Interestingly, there is an association with functional stenosis of the papilla and cases of pancreas divisum. The latter has been found to be present in 3.3% of patients with chronic abdominal pain undergoing ERCP but is more frequent (12%) in patients who have a prior history of pancreatitis.

Clinical Findings

Papillary stenosis may present as RUQ abdominal pain associated with laboratory evidence of cholestasis or pancreatitis or both, depending on the segment of sphincter affected. Isolated stenosis of the biliary sphincter may occur but stenosis only involving the pancreatic sphincter is rare. The common sphincter is most often affected making differentiation from choledocholithiasis difficult (1, 8).

Radiology

Papillary stenosis may cause sonographic bile duct and sometimes pancreatic duct (Fig. 15.19A and B) dilatation. A study of Warshaw et al. (9) using serial sonography of the pancreatic and common hepatic ducts following intravenous injection of secretin demonstrated a measurable increase in the pancreatic duct diameter in 83% of symptomatic patients with papillary stenosis. A positive test result was associated with a 90% success rate (relief of pain) following surgical sphincterotomy (9). The use of hepatobiliary scintigraphy has also been suggested as being a valuable, minimally invasive method of diagnosing papillary stenosis by the observation of a prolonged bile-to-bowel transit time of more than 45 minutes (10). During this study, the diagnosis of papillary stenosis was confirmed by ERCP which paralleled the results of the scintigram. CT is useful (Fig. 15.19E) only in showing no mass lesions (although this does not exclude neoplasm) when sonographic depiction of the anatomy is suboptimal.

The single most valuable study for assessing the diagnosis of papillary stenosis is ERCP. Direct endoscopic inspection of the ampulla is possible. Tumors of the papilla or surrounding duodenum may be identified and forceps or snare biopsy of the papilla may be carried out to support the diagnosis (1). Endoscopic sphincterotomy may be necessary to obtain tissue samples. Additionally, aspiration of secretions, cytology,

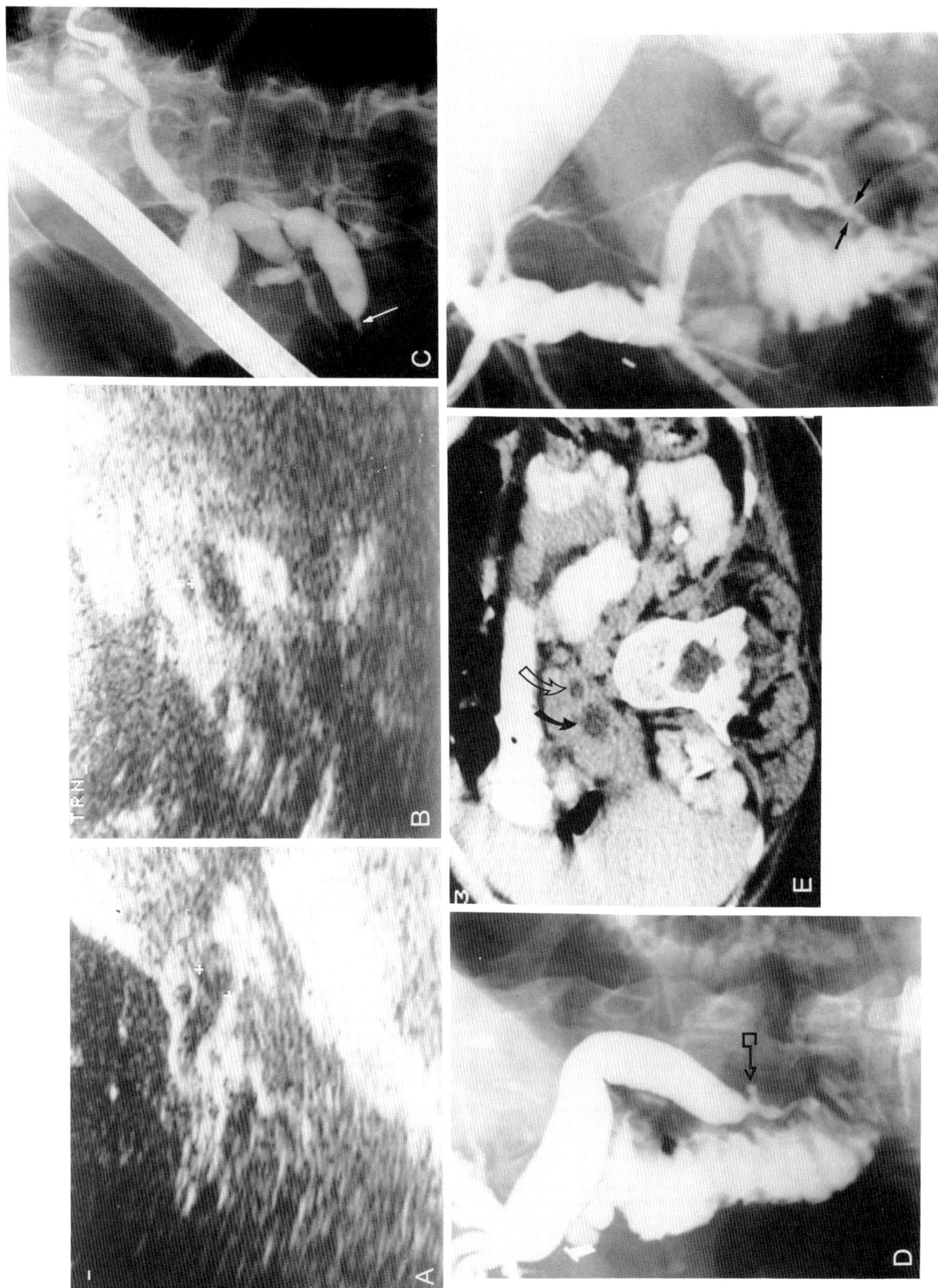

manometry of the spincter of Oddi, and instillation of contrast media for radiographic study is possible all at the same time (1).

Fibrotic Papillary Stenosis

Cholangiography (Fig. 15.19D) usually reveals some degree of biliary tree dilatation associated with a long smooth narrowing or beak at the distal end of the biliary tree. Prestenotic dilatation of the ampulla may be present (7). A delay in drainage of the contrast material also lends support to the diagnosis (the normal post-cholecystectomy biliary tree empties in 45 minutes in the supine position.) The pancreatogram, when obtainable, may demonstrate a mild degree of main duct dilatation (Fig. 15.19C). The differential diagnosis between benign and malignant stenoses is difficult although complete obstruction usually indicates a malignant stricture (1, 7). Glucagon may be required to relax the sphincter of Oddi for cannulation and to differentiate spasm from anatomic stenosis (11) (Fig. 15.19F). The success rate for ERCP with papillary stenosis is only 82%; therefore, PTC may sometimes be required (Fig. 15.19D).

Other authors in the surgical literature have defined papillary stenosis of the papilla of Vater as a narrowing that does not permit easy passage of a No. 3 Bakes Dilator from the common bile duct into the duodenum (12). Encountering this stenosis with the above maneuver at the time of elective cholecystectomy is said to necessitate a transduodenal sphincteroplasty.

Diagnosis of Functional Papillary Stenosis

Endoscopic manometry of the sphincter of Oddi during ERCP may reveal phasic contractions of the sphincter that are abnormally high with retrograde contractions and a paradoxical cholecystokinin octopeptide response (13–15) (Fig. 15.20). Manometric findings may help differentiate purely functional papillary stenosis from other causes of postcholecystectomy pain syndrome (16). Only a small difference in pressure was found in functional versus fibrotic stenosis. Functional stenoses showed a nonlinear pressure-diameter relationship when distended by probes of increasing diameter. Fibrotic stenoses could not be probed or could only be probed minimally (17).

Hepatobiliary Scintigraphy in the Diagnosis of Papillary Stenosis

Recent work suggests that the ^{99m}Tc-IDA hepatobiliary scintigram may have a major role to

FIGURE 15.19. PAPILLARY (AMPULLARY) STENOSIS

Surgically proven papillary stenosis in a 35-yr-old woman with pain and elevated alkaline phosphatase 7 yr after cholecystectomy. The patient underwent choledochoduodenostomy, and multiple biopsies of the stenotic region showed only fibrosis. A: Parasagittal sonogram: dilated common duct (8 mm, cursors). B: Transverse sonogram: dilated main pancreatic duct (3.5 mm, cursors). C: ERCP: markedly dilated main pancreatic duct proximal to a smooth narrowing at the ampulla (arrow). The common bile duct could not be cannulated. D: PTC: dilated intrahepatic and extrahepatic ducts. Irregular narrowing of distal common bile duct compatible with either neoplasm or benign stenosis. Preampullary "diverticulum" (arrow), a finding we have seen in some cases of papillary stenosis, of uncertain significance, possibly a type II choledochal cyst. E: CT: Dilated common bile (closed arrow) and pancreatic (open arrow) ducts. No evidence of a mass. F: Spasm of the distal common duct (arrows) due to recent stone passage in a different patient. Followup examination showed a return to normal.

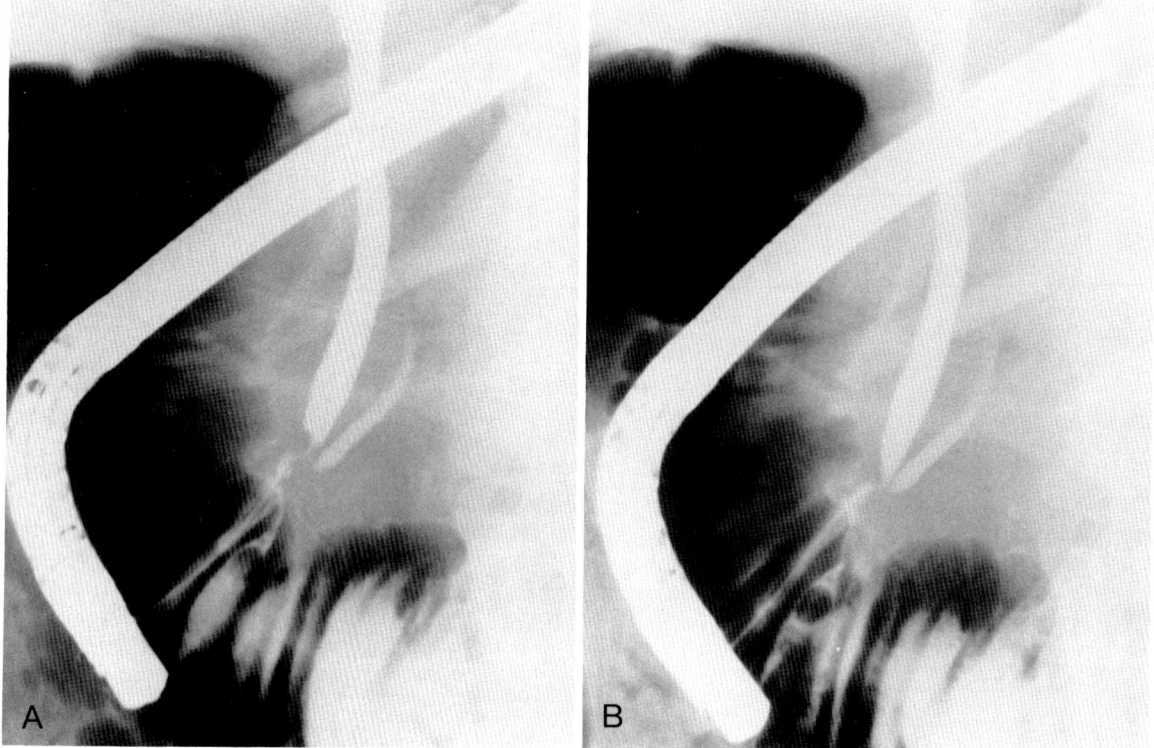

FIGURE 15.20. FUNCTIONAL PAPILLARY STENOSIS

The ampullary segment of the common bile duct is initally tight (A) but eventually relaxes (B). This patient, a young female, had typical biliary pain. Her common duct did not drain well, and her pain was relieved by endoscopic sphincterotomy. Manometry would have been useful.

play in noninvasive screening for papillary stenosis, both functional and anatomic. In one study (18), patients with abnormal scans had a mean basal sphincter pressure of 38.5 mm Hg (compared to a normal of 15 ± 4 mm Hg). Criteria for defining the scan as abnormal included delayed biliary intestinal transit (greater than 1 hr) abnormal time-activity dynamics (ductal activity at 2 hr equal to or greater than that at 1 hr) obstruction (no intestinal activity) and apparent ductal dilatation. The scintigram was also useful as an objective means of assessing therapeutic response. In another study, hepatobiliary scintigraphy detected 9 of 10 cases of papillary stenosis (using ERCP as the gold standard) with retention of activity at 2 hours in visually prominent ducts considered the best sign of abnormal drainage (19).

Treatment

The treatment of papillary stenosis is logically endoscopic sphincterotomy (Fig. 15.21). Endoscopic sphincterotomy can be performed in either fibrotic or functional papillary stenosis, the fibrotic type usually being somewhat more difficult to freely cannulate with the sphincterotome. Use of a catheter which permits application of a high-frequency current in order to pass through a stenosis has been described thereby allowing easier passage for a biliary endoprosthesis (20).

The papillotome is a plastic catheter with a wire snare which leaves the lumen of the catheter 3 cm from the tip and returns to the lumen 3 mm from the tip. This can then be made into a bowstring configuration. Application of an electric current after exact positioning on deep cannulation allows this wire to function as a knife. A cutting needle may also be used to incise the roof of the papilla when the sphincterotome may not be introduced (1). After opening up the ampulla, completion of the sphincterotomy can be performed with a normal papillotome. Other authors advocate constructing a fistula between the duodenum and bile duct, bypassing the distal stenosis (1). The obvious advantage of the sphincterotomy is the ability to remove stones and concretions in the bile duct when present.

Results following endoscopic sphincterotomy are generally good. Complete relief of symptoms or marked improvement of symptoms are seen

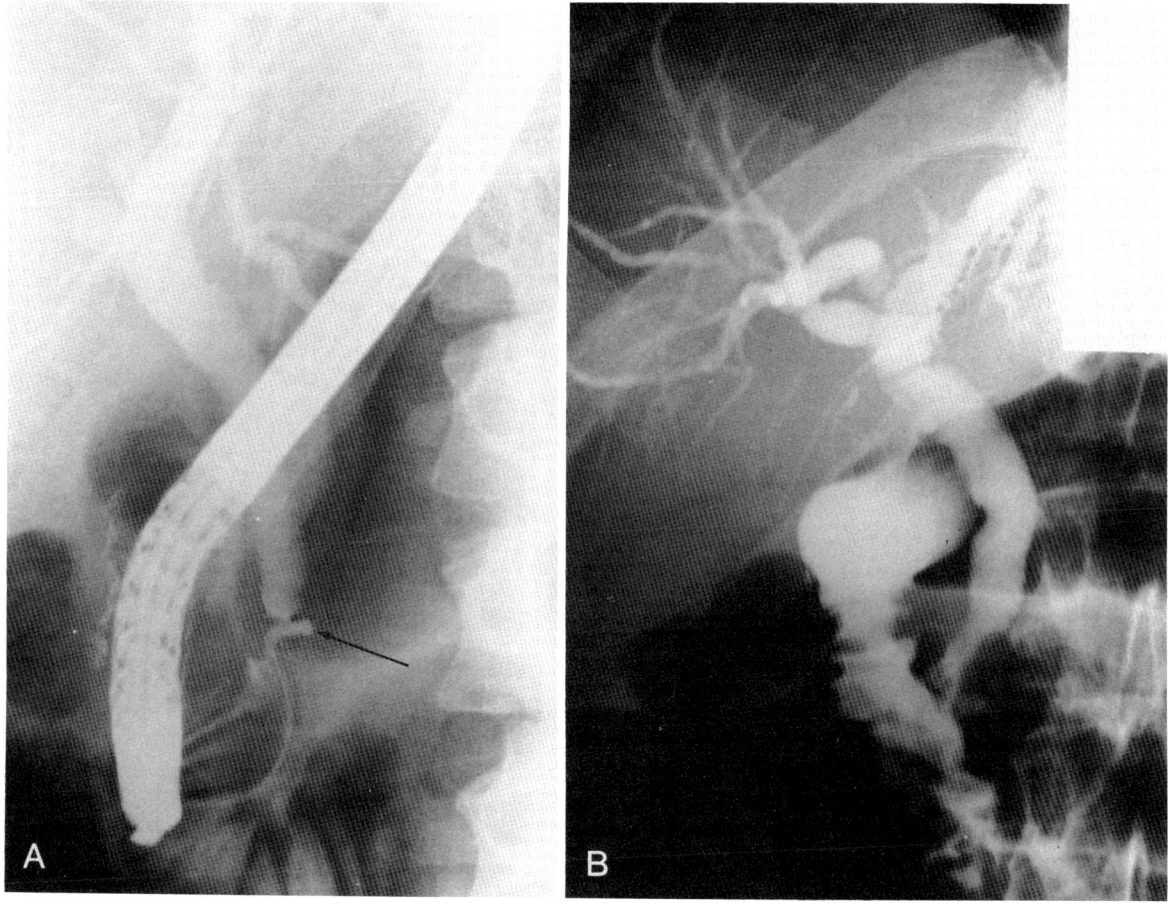

FIGURE 15.21. PAPILLARY (AMPULLARY) STENOSIS
Endoscopic sphincterotomy. A: ERCP: ampullary stenosis. Note periampullary diverticulum (arrow). B: Wide-open ampulla after sphincterotomy.

in over 90 percent of cases (1, 7, 21–24). In contrast, the morbidity rate is generally comparatively low (4.8–7.4%) and mortality negligible (0.7%) for patients undergoing sphincterotomy, although one study reported higher rates of morbidity and mortality in patients undergoing sphincterotomy for papillary stenosis than in patients having the same procedure for choledocholithiasis (1, 25). The adequacy of biliary drainage can be determined by follow-up cholangiography or manometry. Manometric pressure in the bile ducts has been shown to fall from 11.2 mm Hg to 1.1 mm Hg following endoscopic sphincterotomy. Bile duct sphincter activity seen manometrically was present in only 21% of patients following endoscopic sphincterotomy (4). Incision length decreased during the first year following endoscopic sphincterotomy without further reduction in length after 2 yr. Manometric pressures also seem to remain unchanged after the initial decrease for at least 2 yr (26).

Long-term follow-up reveals that restenosis is more common following endoscopic sphincterotomy for papillary stenosis (11.5 percent) then for choledocholithiasis (2.93%) (1, 27, 28). Recurrent stenosis may be treated again by renewed endoscopic papillotomy (28). Endoscopic balloon dilation to 15 mm has been used for benign papillary stenosis (29), but reportedly, the danger of cicatrized recurrent stenosis has been found to be higher with this method (1).

The alternative to endoscopic sphincterotomy is surgical sphincterotomy which can be transduodenal papillotomy, transduodenal partial sphincterotomy, transduodenal total sphincterotomy or sphincteroplasty (1, 30).

Some authors advocate that whenever possible, an attempt to determine whether an associated papillary stenosis is present in patients undergoing elective cholecystectomy should be made. Sphincterotomy would be able to be performed during cholecystectomy in appropriate patients so as to avoid a later procedure that may become necessary because of post-cholecystectomy syndrome. Preoperative use of the morphine-prostigmine test to induce ampullary spasm causing an elevation of the serum amylase or lipase was found to be of value in selecting patients with suspected papillary stenosis. Once suspected, ERCP was used to confirm the diagnosis both in this group and in patients with atypical biliary pain (31).

REFERENCES

1. Classen M, Leuschner U, Schreiber HW: Stenosis of the papilla Vateri and common duct calculi. *Clin Gastroenterol* 12:203–214, 1983.
2. Albot G: Functional disorders of Oddi's sphincter and of the duodenobiliary system. In *The Sphincter of Oddi: Proceedings of the Third Gastroenterological Symposium, Nice, 1976.* Basel, Switzerland, Karger, 1977, pp 123–128.
3. Menuck L, Amberg J: The bile ducts. *Radiol Clin North Am* 14:499, 1976.
4. Gregg JA, Carr-Locke DL: Endoscopic pancreatic and biliary manometry in pancreatic, biliary, and papillary disease and after endoscopic sphincterotomy and surgical spincterotomy. *Gut* 25:1247–1254, 1984.
5. Laurent J, Floquet J, Guibal F, Watrin B, Vosse A: Primary and secondary chronical odditis. In *The Sphincter of Oddi: Proceedings of the Third Gastroenterological Symposium, Nice, 1976.* Basel, Switzerland, Karger, 1977, pp 131–136.
6. Fernandez-Cruz L, Palacin A, Pera C: Benign strictures of the terminal common bile duct. In *The Sphincter of Oddi; Proceedings of the Third Gastroenterological Symposium, Nice, 1976.* Basel, Switzerland, Karger, 1977, pp 137–144.
7. Classen M: Endoscopic approach to papillary stenosis. *Endoscopy* 13:154–156, 1981.
8. Nardi GL: Papillitis and stenosis of the sphincter of Oddi. *Surg Clin North Am* 53:1149–1160, 1973.
9. Warshaw AL, Simeone J, Schapiro RH, Hedberg SE, Mueller PE, Ferruci JT Jr.: Objective evaluation of ampullary stenosis with ultrasonography and pancreatic stimulation. *Am J Surg* 149:65–72, 1985.
10. Pace RF, Chamberlain MJ, Pass RB: Diagnosing papillary stenosis by technetium-99m HIDA scanning. *Can J Surg* 26:191–193, 1983.
11. Setakis N, Vennart W, Gardner AM, Nayak P: A preoperative test of the function of the sphincter of Oddi. *Ann R Col Surg Engl* 66:175–178, 1984.
12. Griffith CA: Diagnosis of papillary stenosis by calibration. Follow-up 15 to 25 years after sphincteroplasty. *Am J Surg* 143:717–720, 1982.
13. Geenen JE: Part two: sphincter of Oddi manometry. *Clin Gastroenterol* 12:108–114, 1983.
14. Toouli J, Roberts-Thompson K, Dent J, Lee J: Manometric disorders in patients with suspected sphincter of Oddi dysfunction. *Gastroenterology* 88:1243–1250, 1985.
15. Geenen JE, Hogan WJ, Dodds WJ, Stewart ET, Arndorfer RC: Intraluminal pressure recording from the human sphincter of Oddi. *Gastroenterology* 78:317–324, 1980.
16. Bortolotti M, Calletti GC, Brocchi E, Bernsani G, Caletti T, Guizzardi G, Labo G: Endoscopic manometry in the diagnosis of the post cholecystectomy pain syndrome. *Digestion* 28:153–157, 1983.
17. Hancke E: Intraoperative mural pressure measurements in the papilla of Vater (author's translation). *Langenbecks Arch Chir* 354:293–298, 1981.
18. Lee RGL, Gregg JA, Koroshetz AM, Hill TC, Clouse ME: Sphincter of Oddi stenosis: diagnosis using hepatobiliary scintigraphy and endoscopic manometry. *Radiology* 156:793–796, 1985.
19. Zeman RK, Burrell MI, Dobbins J, Jaffe MH, Choyke PL: Postcholecystectomy syndrome: evaluation using biliary scintigraphy and endoscopic retrograde cholangipancreatography. *Radiology* 156:787–792, 1985.
20. Sauerbruch T, Pfulgbeli P: Catheter for the electrocoagulation of bile duct stenosis. *Endoscopy* 16:229–230, 1984.
21. Geenen JE, Vennes A, Silvis SE: Resume of a seminar on endoscopic retrograde sphincterotomy (ERS). *Gastrointest Endosc* 27:31–38, 1981.
22. Neese T, Meoptolemos JP, Carr-Locke DL: Successes, failures, early complications and their management following endoscopic sphincterotomy: results in 394 consecutive patients from a single center. *Br J Surg* 72:215–219, 1985.
23. Rosch W, Reimann JF, Lux G, Linder HG: Long-term follow-up after endoscopic sphincterotomy. *Endoscopy* 13:152–153, 1983.
24. Mustard R, MacKenzie R, Jamieson C, Haber GB: Surgical complications of endoscopic sphincterotomy. *Can J Surg* 27:215–217, 1984.
25. Siegel JH: Endoscopic papillotomy and the treatment of biliary tract disease: 258 procedures and results. *Dig Dis Sci* 26:1057–1064, 1981.
26. Geenen JE, Tooulie J, Hogan WJ, Dodds WJ, Stewart ET, Mavrelis P, Riedel D, Venu R: Endoscopic sphincterotomy: follow-up evaluation of the effects on the sphincter of Oddi. *Gastroenterology* 87:754–758, 1984.
27. Richieri JP, Belissier G: Early papillary stenosis following successful endoscopic sphincterotomy for residual common bile duct stones. *Endoscopy* 16:77–78, 1984.
28. Ell CH, Geocze ST, Riemann JF: Successful endoscopic treatment of extensive recurrent papillary stenosis six years after endoscopic papillotomy. *Endoscopy* 16:246–248, 1984.
29. Staritz M, Ewe K, Meyerzumbuchenfelde KH: Endoscopic papillary dilatation (EPD) for the treatment of common bile duct stones and papillary stenosis. *Endoscopy* 15:197–198, 1983.
30. Anderson TM, Pitt HA, Longmire WP: Experience with sphincteroplasty and sphincterotomy in pancreatobiliary surgery. *Ann Surg* 201:399–406, 1985.
31. Gregg JA, Clark G, Barr C, McCartney A, Milano A, Volcjak C: Post-cholecystectomy syndrome and its association with ampullary stenosis. *Am J Surg* 139:374–378, 1980.

16

Trauma to the Gallbladder and Biliary Tract

ARNOLD C. FRIEDMAN, M.D., DAVID S. BALL, D.O., AND LEORA SACHS, M.D.

BILIARY TRACT

Clinically significant biliary tract trauma is rarely the result of a blunt or penetrating injury; instead the etiology is usually surgical, especially cholecystectomy. Surgical biliary tract trauma and its sequelae will be discussed first, followed by blunt and penetrating trauma, and then hemobilia, bilhemia, and, finally, biloma, conditions that usually result from accidental or iatrogenic biliary trauma.

Surgical Trauma

The majority of iatrogenic extrahepatic bile duct injuries happen during routine cholecystectomy. About 20% occur during emergency cholecystectomy with a small percentage resulting from other operations, such as gastric resections. Over 90% of benign biliary strictures are surgically induced (1, 2), and the estimated frequency of iatrogenic injury to the extrahepatic ducts during biliary surgery is about 0.25% (3).

Clinical Findings

When the common hepatic or common bile duct is ligated, the patient will become jaundiced within the first few postoperative days. Transection, on the other hand, results in an initial period of excessive bile drainage followed by spontaneous biliary fistula. The latter will stenose or close and jaundice then ensues. Prior to fistula formation, bile pooling in the subphrenic or subhepatic space can form a biloma with or without superimposed infection (4). Common mechanisms of injury include: (*a*) blind applications of a hemostat or ligature to arrest bleeding of the cystic artery, hepatic artery, or portal vein, either directly injuring the common duct or imparing its vascular supply; (*b*) clamping and tying the common duct in the mistaken belief that it is the cystic duct; and (*c*) excessive traction on the neck of the gallbladder, tenting the common duct (1, 2, 4). Injuries to the extrahepatic biliary tract are more common when the cystic duct is apposed to either the common duct or the right hepatic duct. Transection of anomalous biliary ducts and slippage of the cystic duct ligature must be included in the clinical differential diagnosis of excessive bile drainage postoperatively; the drainage will usually resolve spontaneously in these instances (1).

In general, the earlier the diagnosis is made, the easier the surgical repair. The first repair is crucial, with each failure the next attempt is less likely to succeed because of scarring (1). The most popular form of repair is some type of biliary-enteric anastomosis, usually either choledochojejunostomy or hepatojejunostomy, because excision of the stricture with end-to-end anastomosis has a very high recurrence rate. The biliary-enteric anastomosis is usually stented by a transhepatic tube(s) for several months postoperatively (4). Stricture recurrence or anastomotic narrowing can present after an initial symptom-free period of 5–10 yr (3).

Radiology

If an external fistula is present, a fistulogram with water-soluble contrast should be the first study performed, and it will often demonstrate the biliary obstruction or stenosis. Sonography or CT can demonstrate dilated ducts above a stricture or obstruction, and generally no soft-tissue mass will be seen (5). The obstruction or stenosis will usually be abrupt, an exception to the rule of thumb that abrupt obstructions not due to calculi are malignant. Radionuclide biliary scintigraphy may be useful in selected cases to demonstrate extravasation (Fig. 16.1) or confirm

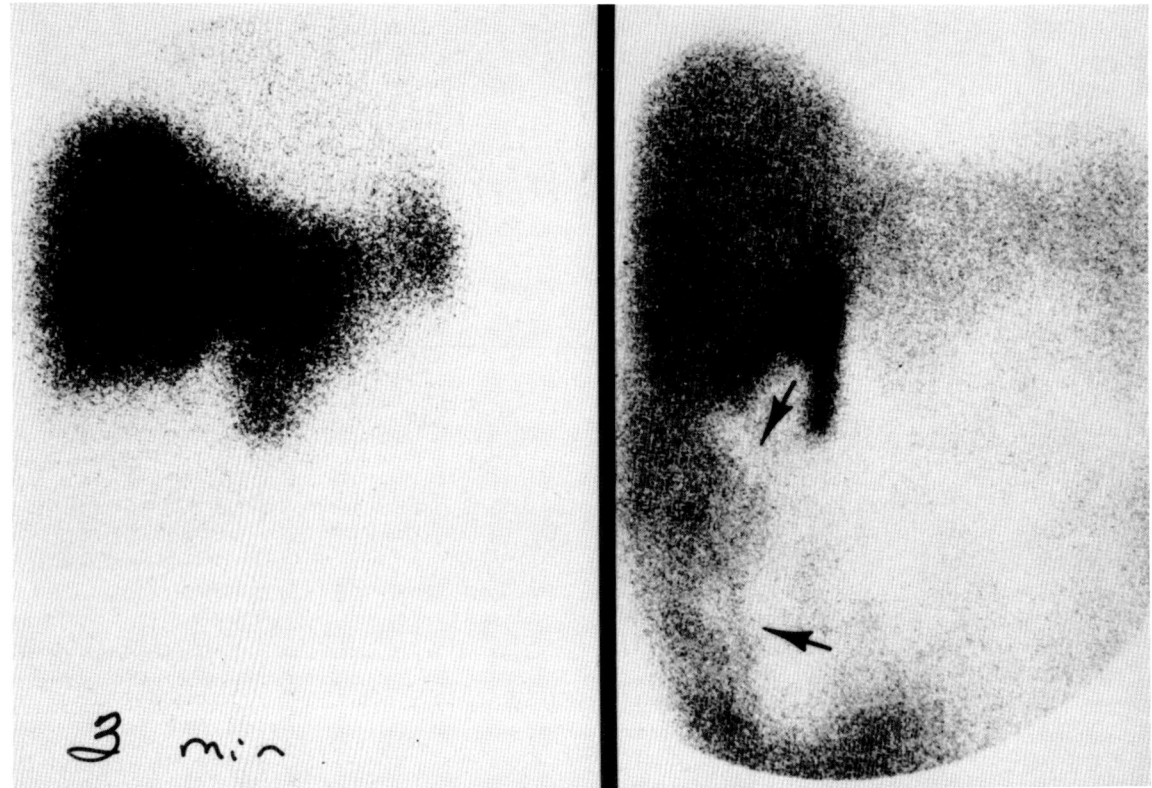

FIGURE 16.1. EXAMPLE OF A POSTCHOLECYSTECTOMY LEAK
Radionuclide hepatobiliary scan. *Arrows* demonstrate activity along the right pericolic gutter. (Scans courtesy of Dr. Scott Swenson.)

obstruction by showing delayed or absent bile-to-bowel transit and prolonged retention of activity in the biliary tract. Definitive diagnosis and preoperative mapping is provided by direct cholangiography via the most convenient route. Iatrogenic strictures are usually in the mid common duct, smooth and concentric and vary in severity from mild narrowing to total obstruction (Fig. 16.2). The obstructed end is funneled or convex distally, as opposed to the meniscus of an impacted calculus. Occasionally postoperative strictures can be elongated, irregularly annular, or even web-like (2, 6). Surgical clips are usually present in the vicinity of the stricture. Extravasation can be demonstrated in cases of transection. Anastomotic strictures complicate biliary-enteric anastomoses in about 30% of attempted reconstructions and are usually circumferential, fairly short segment narrowings often accompanied by proximal primary intrahepatic calculi (6). No matter what its radiologic appearance, any mid-common duct stricture in a patient who has had a cholecystectomy for benign disease is probably iatrogenic. Other benign causes of strictures in the common duct include inflammation (sclerosing cholangitis, infection, pancreatitis), erosion by a gallstone or impaction of a gallstone, external accidental trauma, arterial infusion chemotherapy (Fig. 16.3), and, rarely, congenital stenosis (2) (Fig. 16.4).

Interventional Radiology in Post-Traumatic Stricture

Postoperative biliary strictures are less amenable to percutaneous dilatation than anastomotic strictures, but little is lost by the attempt and some are cured. Most respond to balloon dilatation initially, but some require coaxial dilatation. Postdilatation stenting is necessary; periods as long as 6 months to 1 yr have been advocated, although others have had success with shorter periods. Inflation of a balloon across the stricture for 24 hr has been advocated by some, but size of the balloon, frequency, duration, and number of dilatations, size of the stent, and duration of stenting are parameters whose optimal values have yet to be determined. Despite best efforts, postoperative strictures tend to recur at some time after stent removal (7–10).

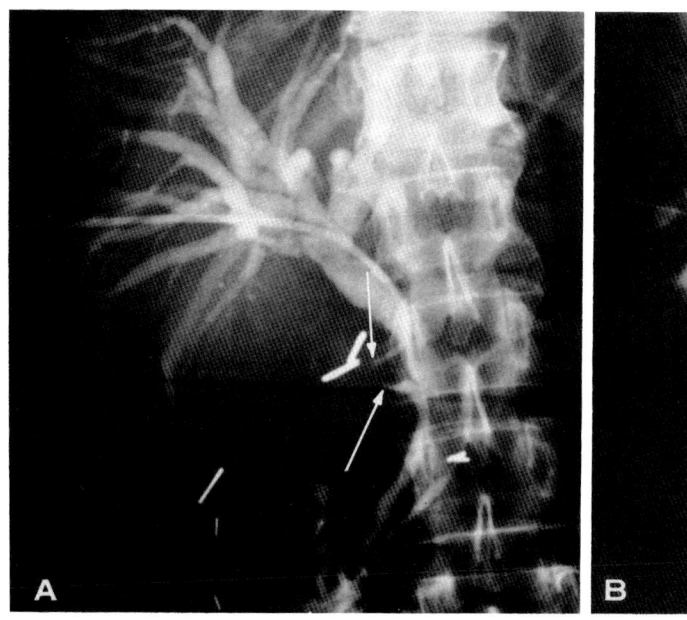
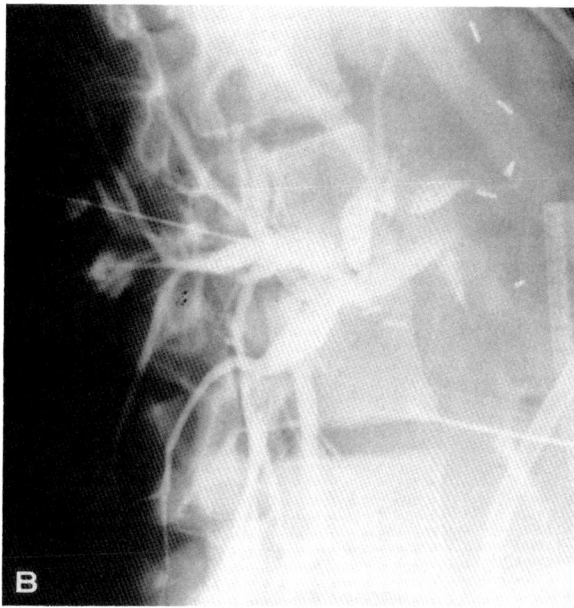

FIGURE 16.2. POSTOPERATIVE STRICTURE

A: Film during biliary drainage: catheter tip and the proximal portion of the common duct distal to the stricture (*arrows*) are tented toward the clips around either the cystic duct or cystic artery which injured the common duct during cholecystectomy. The catheter could not be advanced through the stricture. *B:* Percutaneous transhepatic cholangiography (PTC) in a different case: Postoperative obstruction at the level of the bifurcation. Surgery was for a hepatic adenoma. This is an unusual site for traumatic stricture, and the cholangiographic appearance is not distinguishable from that of a Klatskin tumor except for the clips.

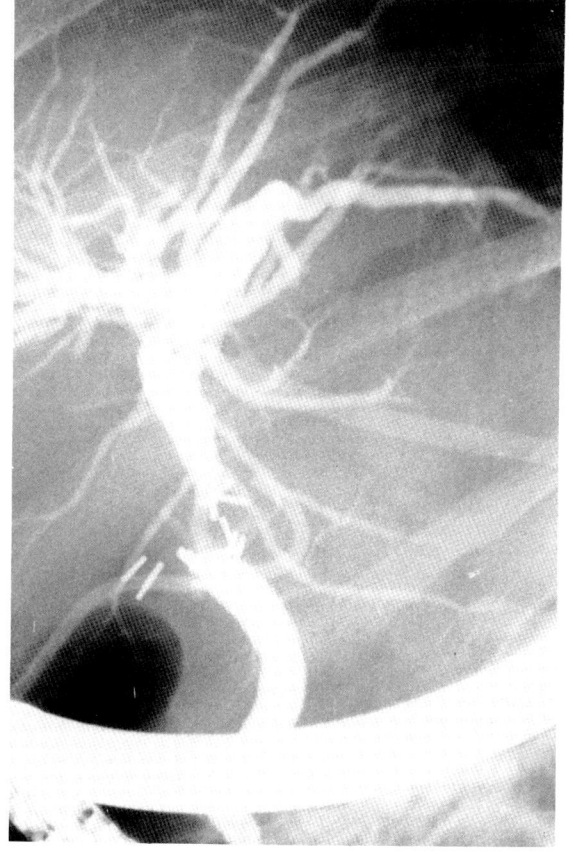

Blunt and Penetrating Biliary Trauma

Tears and partial or complete separation of major extrahepatic bile ducts may occur at any place between the bifurcation of the common hepatic duct and the duodenum as a result of blunt trauma. The majority of distal injuries are associated with pancreatic trauma and often require Whipple procedures. Isolated blunt injury to the common duct is not common (Fig. 16.5). Injuries to the intrahepatic ducts are associated with hepatic trauma and the latter determines the therapy. Penetrating wounds of the extrahepatic biliary tract are relatively easily repaired (11).

Emergency radionuclide hepatobiliary scintigraphy is quite useful in suspected biliary trauma for demonstrating extravasation and any associated liver injury. Vascular integrity can be grossly assessed by a radionuclide angiogram. The liver parenchyma is evaluated 5–15 min. after the injection by multiple projections during the parenchymal phase. Subsequent scintigrams assess the possibility of biliary tract disruption with free or loculated bile collections (12–14).

FIGURE 16.3. IATROGENIC STRICTURE

ERCP: mid-common duct stricture due to arterial infusion chemotherapy (catheter is the arterial line).

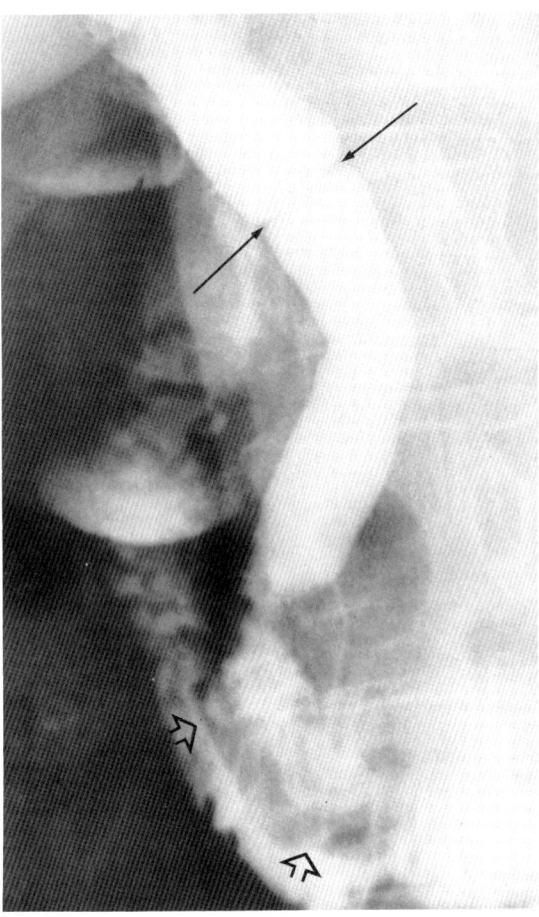

FIGURE 16.4. BILIARY WEB
Congenital web (*arrows*) proximal to an ampullary carcinoma (*open arrows*). Although an incidental finding, the web hindered passage of a guidewire making biliary drainage more difficult.

Delayed views beyond 1 hr are essential in order to detect small or slow leaks. In the Montefiore experience (13), 14 of 23 leaks would have been missed had delayed views not been obtained. For increased sensitivity, lateral and oblique views in addition to frontal projections should be obtained as necessary as the study is actively monitored. A review of both blunt and penetrating noniatrogenic biliary trauma concluded that the parenchymal phase of the hepatobiliary scan was as sensitive as the sulfur-colloid scan for intrahepatic hematomas or other liver lesions and gave the added advantage of assessment of the biliary tract (Fig. 16.6). In their series, 7 of 21 patients did have scintigraphic evidence of biliary disruption (15). Interestingly, nonfilling of the gallbladder in this series usually did not imply cholecystitis or gallbladder perforation (because of intercurrent factors such as hyperalimentation and pancreatitis).

An emergency ERCP can give better anatomic display of any injury to intrahepatic or extrahepatic bile ducts, and CT is the method of choice for evaluating any associated injury to the hepatic or pancreatic parenchyma. Many of these patients will be explored without the benefit of any preoperative imaging because of other associated intraabdominal injuries.

Hemobilia

Differential diagnosis of hemobilia includes trauma, inflammatory disease, cholelithiasis, neoplastic diseases in the pancreaticohepatobiliary region, and vascular abnormalities such as aneurysms, arteriovenous fistulas, and varices in the gallbladder wall in portal hypertension (16, 17). Patients present clinically with intermittent right upper quadrant pain, jaundice, and occult gastrointestinal blood loss.

Radiology

Definitive diagnosis rests with either direct endoscopic observation of blood entering the duodenum from the ampulla of Vater or angiographic demonstration of a bleeding site in the liver, gallbladder, or biliary tract. If no active bleeding is seen, demonstration of an arteriovenous fistula (see Fig. 7.8), hepatic artery aneurysm, or a cholangiographic cavity is strongly supportive evidence (16, 18–23). Intrabiliary blood appears as lucent filling defects that may be elongated or even casts of the biliary tree on direct cholangiography. Cholangiographic diagnosis of hemobilia is made by correlation with clinical history and demonstration of clearing on a subsequent study. Differential includes mainly calculi and polypoid tumors. CT performed after angiography may demonstrate extravasated contrast in the gallbladder or biliary tract that could not be detected angiographically (24).

Sonography

Sonography is a mandatory complement to CT in the diagnosis of hemobilia to exclude mere calculi as the cause of dependent high densities (suspicious for clots) seen on gallbladder CT. Clots are nonshadowing echogenicities on ultrasound, whereas all substantially sized stones will shadow with proper technique. Blood filling the gallbladder may also be depicted as merely low-level echoes indistinguishable from sludge. Over time, echogenicity tends to decrease (16, 17).

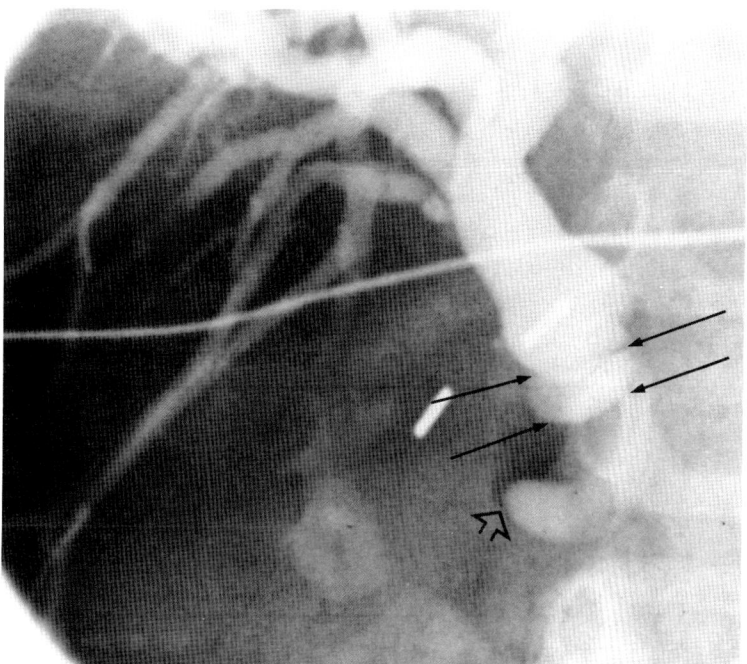

FIGURE 16.5. BILIARY TRAUMA
Post-traumatic common duct stricture in a 3-yr-old boy. A cholecystectomy was done for rupture emergently after an automobile accident. Three months postoperatively he developed jaundice and hepatomegaly. The PTC shows two web-like strictures (*closed arrows*) above a complete obstruction (*open arrow*).

Computerized Tomography

Although the sensitivity of CT in detecting hemobilia is not known, specificity is quite good when combined with ultrasound as described above. Blood can only enter the gallbladder from above if the cystic duct is patent. When the concentration of blood in the bile exceeds 70%, clots form and cause inhomogeneous increased attenuation within the gallbladder lumen. When the bile is completely replaced by blood, there will be homogeneously increased attenuation >50–60 HU on the order of 80 HU. Clots may persist in the gallbladder for up to 2 weeks on CT (16, 17). Milk of calcium bile might cause a problem in CT differential diagnosis of increased intraluminal attenuation in the gallbladder since it does not always shadow on ultrasound, but this is a rare condition and its attenuation is usually considerably higher than blood. It is mandatory that recent administration of biliary or urographic contrast material be excluded before hemobilia is diagnosed on CT on the basis of increased gallbladder attenuation. After a diagnosis of hemobilia is made noninvasively, angiography will usually be necessary for differential diagnosis and treatment.

Nuclear Medicine

Radionuclide studies using labeled red cells are useful in localizing occult gastrointestinal hemorrhage. They are quite sensitive to active gastrointestinal bleeding. It is not clear to what extent background activity in the liver would interfere with detection of hemobilia. CT has the advantage of being able to detect blood in the gallbladder after bleeding has stopped.

Angiography

Selective angiography is necessary to confirm the underlying pathology, locate the vascular lesions precisely, and perform either balloon or embolic occlusion. Angiographic techniques have several advantages over surgery: in some cases the bleeding site cannot be found during surgery, ligation of the main hepatic artery will not prove successful in arresting bleeding if there is a rapidly developing collateral arterial supply or if the bleeding is from a veno-biliary fistula, and partial hepatectomy carries appreciable mortality and is not feasible when multiple abnormalities are present (25).

Bilhemia

Bilhemia, as defined by passage of bile into the blood stream via a fistula between the biliary tract and the venous system is distinctly uncommon. The cause is trauma, often as a result of percutaneous transhepatic interventional procedures, but sometimes blunt trauma. Biliohepatic vein fistula will have a more rapidly rising rate

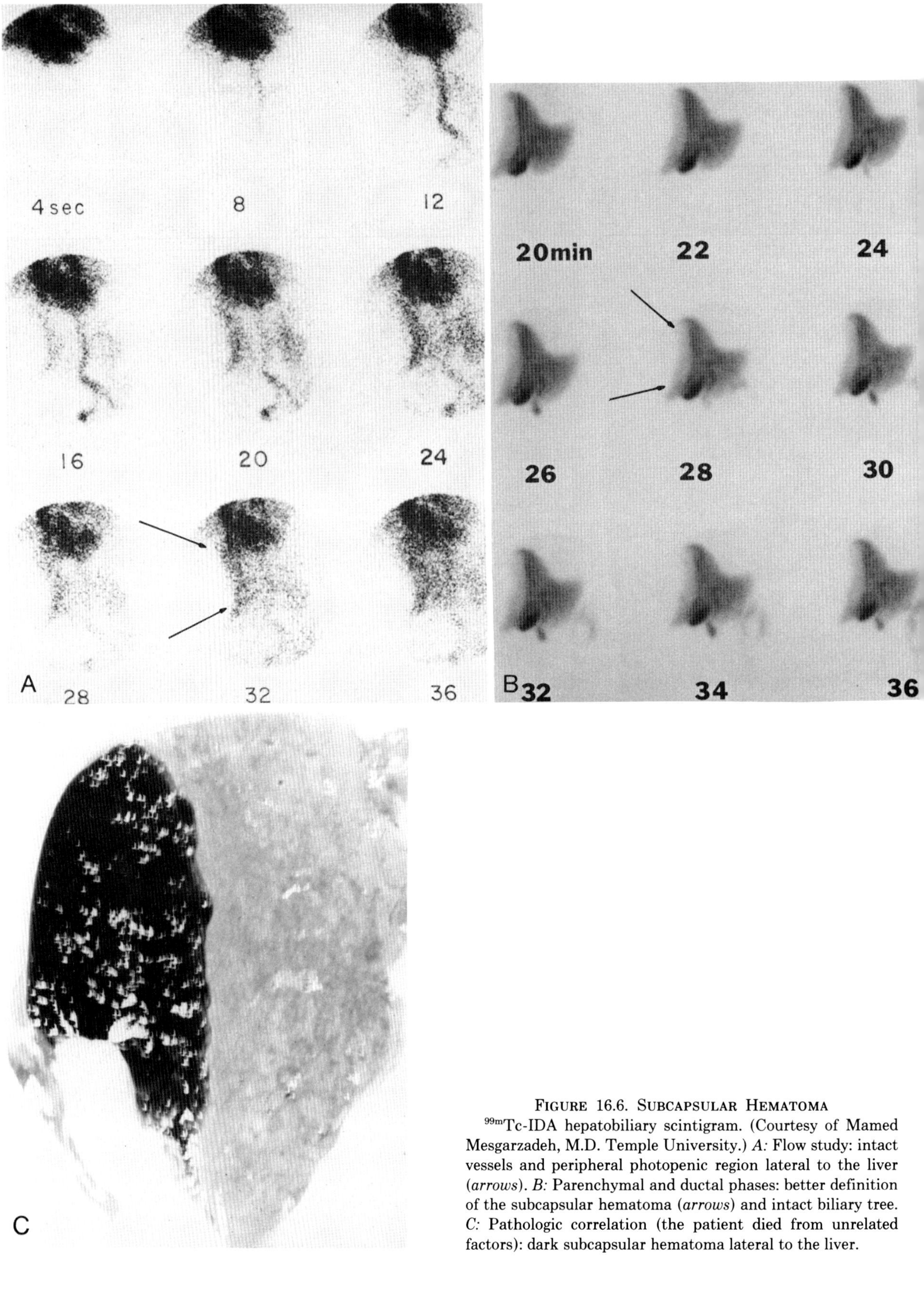

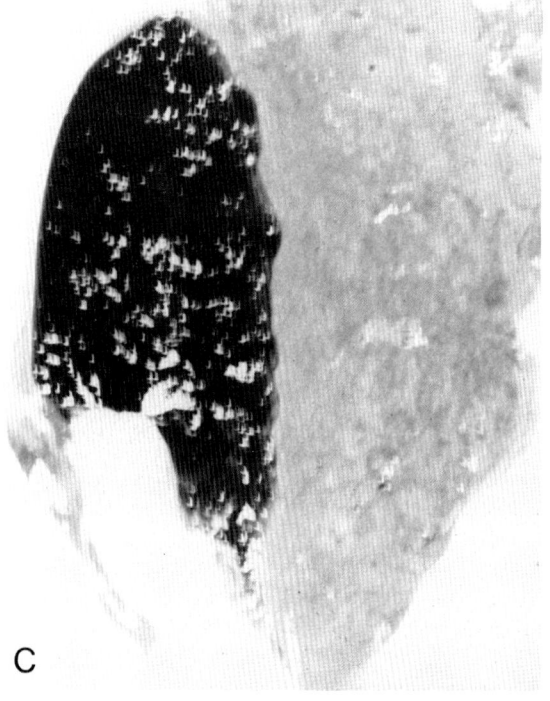

FIGURE 16.6. SUBCAPSULAR HEMATOMA
^{99m}Tc-IDA hepatobiliary scintigram. (Courtesy of Mamed Mesgarzadeh, M.D. Temple University.) *A:* Flow study: intact vessels and peripheral photopenic region lateral to the liver (*arrows*). *B:* Parenchymal and ductal phases: better definition of the subcapsular hematoma (*arrows*) and intact biliary tree. *C:* Pathologic correlation (the patient died from unrelated factors): dark subcapsular hematoma lateral to the liver.

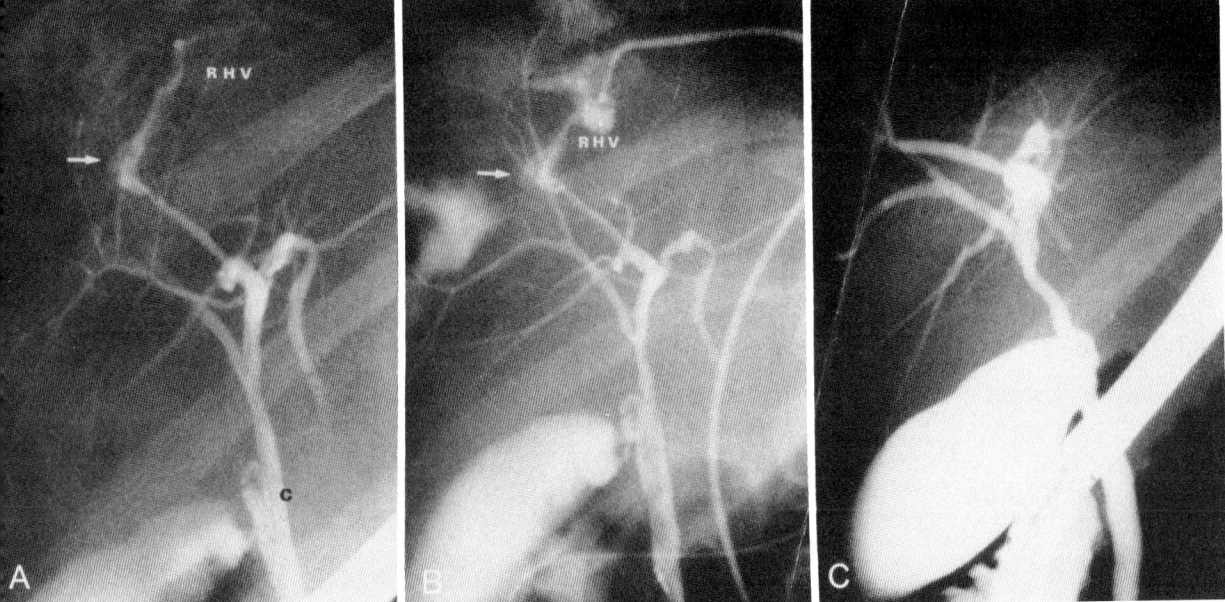

FIGURE 16.7. BILHEMIA

A: Endoscopic retrograde cholangiogram. Bile ducts injected by catheter (c) positioned in common bile duct. Opacification of fistula (arrow) and segmental branch of right hepatic vein (RHV). B: Selective opacification of segmental branch of right hepatic vein, fistula (arrow), and bile ducts. Balloon catheter then positioned at tip to diagnostic catheter. C: Endoscopic retrograde cholangiogram 3½ weeks later. Normal biliary pattern. (From Struyven J, Cremer M, Pirson P, Jeanty P, Jeanmart J: Post-traumatic bilhemia: diagnosis and catheter therapy. AJR 138:746–747, 1982.)

of jaundice than either bilioportal fistula or hemobilia because of the positive pressure gradient between the biliary tract (6–10 cm water) and the hepatic vein (0–6 cm water). Clinical and laboratory findings cannot otherwise differentiate between bilhemia and hemobilia.

Radiology

Direct cholangiography is necessary for proper diagnosis and therapy. ERCP is preferable to PTC because the biliary tree is not dilated (Fig. 16.7). Either a branch of the hepatic or the portal vein will be opacified. Venography of the appropriate vein will opacify the biliary tract. Direct occlusion of the fistula with a detachable balloon via ERCP or venography is the treatment of choice, resulting in faster recovery than drainage of the biliary tract (which lowers biliary pressure below hepatic venous pressure, promoting closure of the fistula) (26).

REFERENCES

1. Netter FH: *The Ciba Collection of Medical Illustrations. Volume 3, Digestive System, Part III, Liver, Biliary Tract and Pancreas.* Ciba Pharmaceutical Products, 1957, p 123.
2. Larsen, CR, Scholz FJ, Wise RE: Diseases of the biliary ducts. *Semin Roentgenol* 11:260–262, 1976.
3. Berci G, Hamlin JA: Operative and postoperative cholangiography. In Beck RN, Ferrucci JT Jr, Leopold GR (eds): *Radiology of the Gallbladder and Bile Ducts, Diagnosis and Intervention.* Philadelphia, W. B. Saunders, 1983, p 401.
4. Smith R: Traumatic strictures of the bile ducts. In Bockus HL (ed): *Gastroenterology.* Philadelphia, W. B. Saunders, 1976, pp 874–881.
5. Love L, Kucharski P, Pickleman J: Radiology of cholecystectomy complications. *Gastrointest Radiol* 4:33–40, 1979.
6. Ferrucci JT Jr, Mueller PR, vanSonnenberg E: Transhepatic cholangiography. In Beck RN, Ferrucci JT Jr, Leopold GR (eds): *Radiology of the Gallbladder and Bile Ducts, Diagnosis and Intervention.* Philadelphia, W. B. Saunders, 1983, p 355.
7. Martin EC, Fankuchen EI, Laffey KJ, Sibley RE: Percutaneous management of benign biliary disease. *Gastrointest Radiol* 9:207–212, 1984.
8. Tegtmeyer CJ: The interventionalist's role in biliary tract drainage. *Diagn Imaging*, Dec. 44–51, 1984.
9. Moore PT, Clark RA: An update of interventional biliary radiology. *Semin Ultrasound CT MR* 5:349–368, 1984.
10. Salomonowitz E, Castaneda-Zuniga WR, Lund G, Cragg AH, Hunter DW, Coleman CC, Amplatz K: Balloon dilatation of benign biliary strictures. *Radiology* 151:613–616, 1984.
11. Glenn F: Trauma, perforation, fistula. In Bockus HL (ed): *Gastroenterology.* Philadelphia, W. B. Saunders, 1976, pp 886–887.
12. Shristensen PB, Oester-Joergensen E, Schoubye J et al: Scintigraphy with ^{99m}Tc-(2,6-diethylacetanilide)-imino-

13. Weissmann HS, Byun KJC, Freeman LM: Rose of ^{99m}-Tc-IDA scintigraphy in the evaluation of hepatobiliary trauma. *Semin Nucl Med* 13:199-222, 1983.
14. Colletti P, Siegel ME, Ralls PW et al: Hepatobiliary scintigraphy scintiangiography in trauma. *J Nucl Med* 24:8, 1983.
15. Zeman RK, Lee CH, Stahl R et al.: Strategy for the use of biliary scintigraphy in non-iatrogenic biliary trauma. *Radiology* 151:771-777, 1984.
16. Krudy AG, Doppman JL, Bissonette MB, Girton M: Hemobilia: computed tomographic diagnosis. *Radiology* 148:785-789, 1983.
17. Daneman A, Matzinger MA, Martin DJ: Posttraumatic hemorrhage into the gallbladder. *J Comput Assist Tomogr* 7:59-61, 1983.
18. Katz MC, Meng CH: Angiographic evaluation of traumatic intrahepatic psuedoaneurysm and hemobilia. *Radiology* 94:95-99, 1970.
19. Ryvicket MJ, Schatz SL, Deutsch AM, Cohen HR: Angiographic demonstration of bleeding into the gallbladder. *Radiology* 136:326, 1980.
20. Atiyeh FF, McSweeney J, Fortner JG: Hemobilia complicating needle liver biopsy: a case report with arteriographic demonstration. *Radiology* 118:559-560, 1976.
21. Druy EM: Hepatic artery-biliary fistula following percutaneous biliary drainage. *Radiology* 141:369-370, 1981.
22. Ranniger K, Menguy R, Kittle CF, Abrams E: Angiographic diagnosis of an intrahepatic aneurysm as a cause of unexplained bleeding. *Radiology* 90:507-509, 1968.
23. Sandblom PH: *Hemobilia*. Springfield, Ill., Charles C Thomas, 1972, pp 5-117.
24. Vujic I, Stanley JH, Tyminski L, Cunningham JT, Adams K: Computed tomographic demonstration of hemobilia. *CT* 7:219-222, 1983.
25. Hirsch M, Avinoach I, Keynan A, Khodadadi J: Angiographic diagnosis and treatment of hemobilia. *Radiology* 144:771-772, 1982.
26. Struyven J, Cremer M, Pirson P, Jeanty P, Jeanmart J: Post-traumatic bilhemia: diagnosis and catheter therapy. *AJR* 138:746-747, 1982.

BILOMA (BILIARY CYST)

First described by Whipple in 1898 as a biliary cyst in a patient who had been kicked by a horse, an abnormal collection of bile is now commonly called a biloma since the term was coined in 1979 by Gould and Patel (1, 2). Bilomas are either extrahepatic or intrahepatic walled off bile collections that form secondary to duct disruption or hepatic tissue necrosis with bile leakage. They may be caused by trauma or spontaneous perforation of the biliary tree. Actual bile leakage may or may not be present at the time of diagnosis. Traumatic etiologies include both penetrating and blunt trauma, cholecystectomy, and percutaneous transhepatic procedure (1, 3). Spontaneous perforation of the biliary tree usually occurs for unknown reasons in the anterior common bile duct near the cystic duct junction in infants younger than 5 months of age (4).

Clinical Findings

Bilomas tend to develop 2-6 weeks after trauma but may present as late as several years. Symptoms and signs include fullness, tightness, and/or pain in the region of the collection. Symptoms occur as the biloma slowly accumulates bile and grows. Fever and leukocytosis are generally present when the biloma is infected (3, 5). Hemobilia may occur. Bilomas also may be asymptomatic fortuitous findings (3). Infants with spontaneous bile duct perforation and bilomas present with jaundice and abdominal mass(es) (4).

Treatment of bilomas consists of percutaneous aspiration and catheter drainage. The catheter should be removed when sonography or CT shows resolution and drainage has ceased, usually in 10-24 days (1, 5). Infected bilomas require antibiotics in addition. Surgery is required in those cases with persistent leakage. When an active leak is present at the time of aspiration, the catheter tip should be placed as close as possible to the site of the leak (5).

Pathology

Bilomas can be either unilocular or multilocular and are well-encapsulated. Although most are either right subphrenic or right subhepatic, they can be left-sided as well (5). The aspirated fluid is either yellow, clear yellow-brown or bilious. When infected, the fluid is purulent initially and becomes yellow or bilious after 1-2 days of catheter drainage (5). Although an initial Multistix test is positive for bilirubin in only about 50%, a chemical analysis is always positive (5).

Radiology

Nuclear Medicine

Cholescintigraphy confirms the diagnosis of biloma when a cystic mass accumulates radionuclide on delayed images. Occasionally the early hepatocyte phase will show a photopenic region corresponding to the biloma (3). The precise location of the leak is often demonstrated and unsuspected additional biliary-enteric fistulas may be demonstrated (11). Useful information is also garnered when cholescintigraphy shows no leak in a patient with a proven biloma. After percutaneous catheter drainage of a biloma, the hepatobiliary scan can document the presence or absence of persistent leakage (5). Direct cholangiography is rarely necessary since the advent of current ^{99m}Tc-IDA agents.

Ultrasound

Uncomplicated bilomas are either anechoic or hypoechoic with fine internal echoes (1, 3, 5). Occasionally they have a few internal septations and/or a small amount of debris (Fig. 16.8). They are well-circumscribed with good through transmission and a smooth back wall (Fig. 16.9) (1, 3). When infected they tend to have more numerous and coarser internal echoes (1). Bilomas can be subphrenic, subhepatic, subcapsular, or intrahepatic.

Computed Tomography

Uncomplicated bilomas are unenhancing water density sharply defined collections in or around the liver (Figs. 16.8 and 16.9). Infection can be suggested when rim enhancement or gas is present. As is true with sonography, specific diagnosis of biloma requires cholescintigraphy and/or aspiration (6).

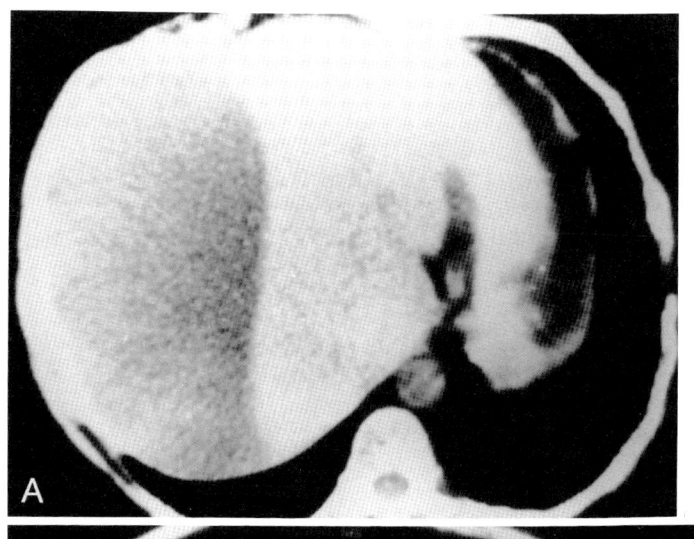
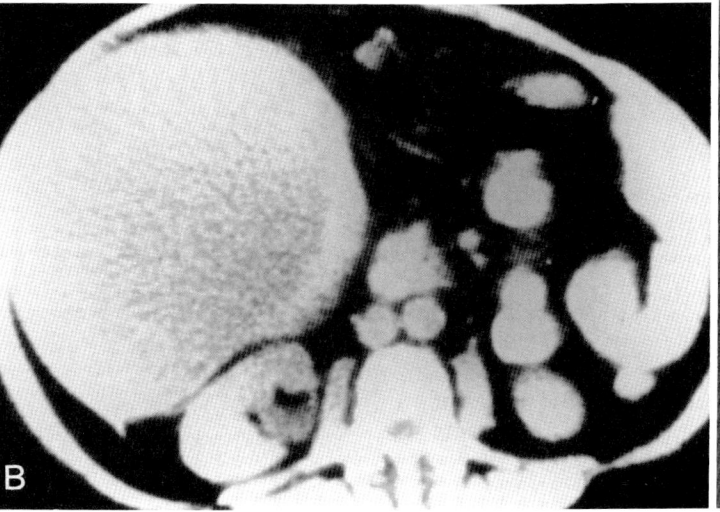
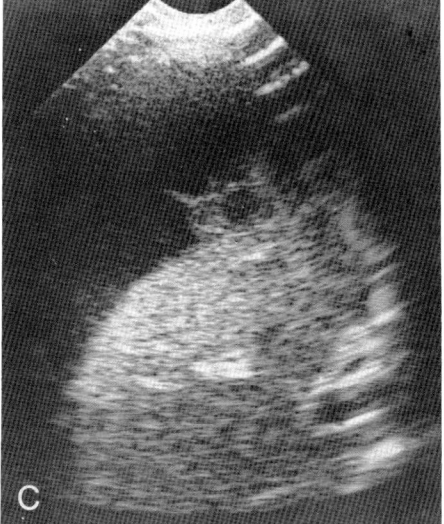

FIGURE 16.8. BILOMA
A and B: Unenhanced CT: large, subcapsular low density biloma. C: Sonogram: mostly anechoic biloma with a small amount of echoes representing debris.

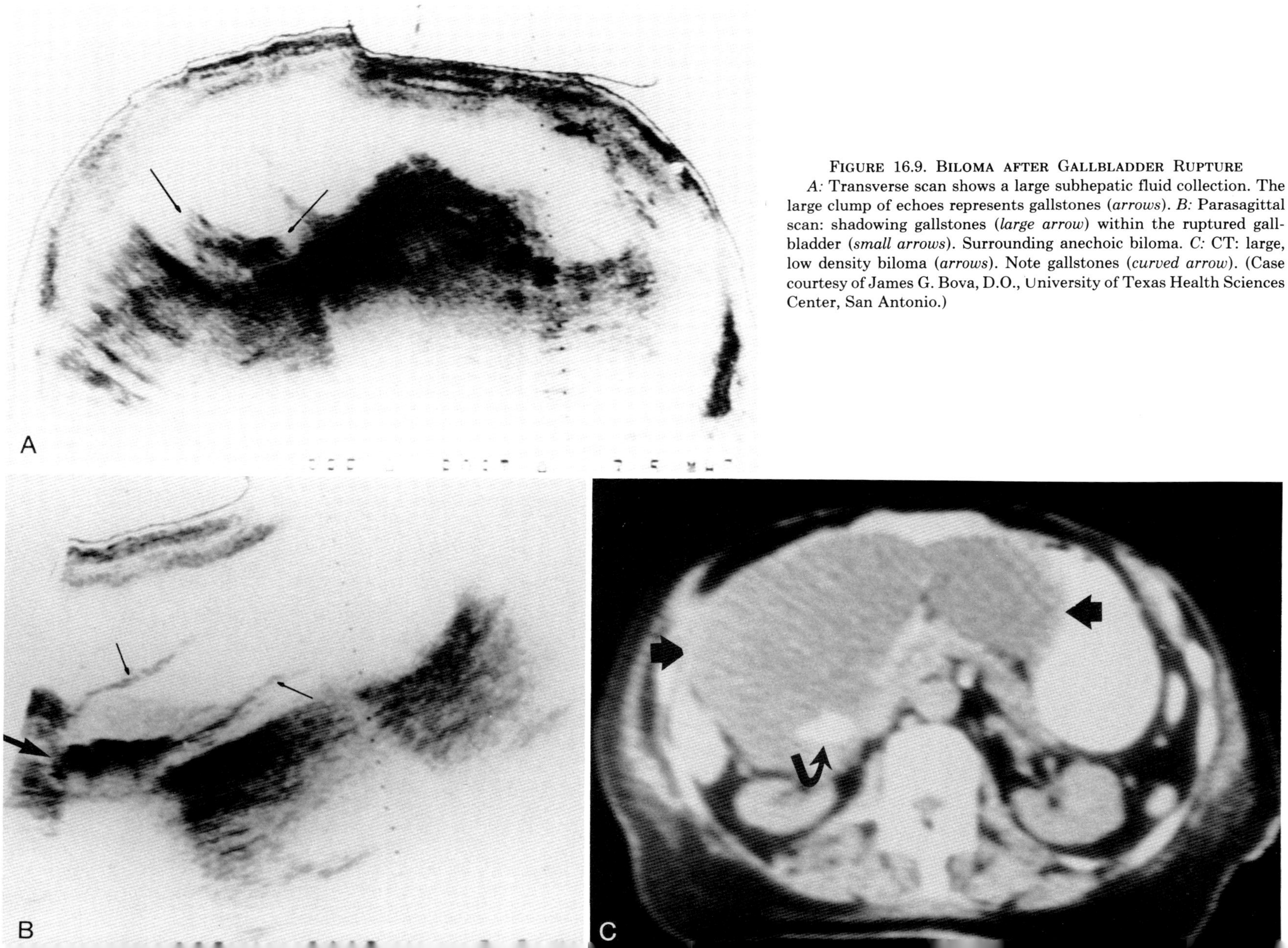

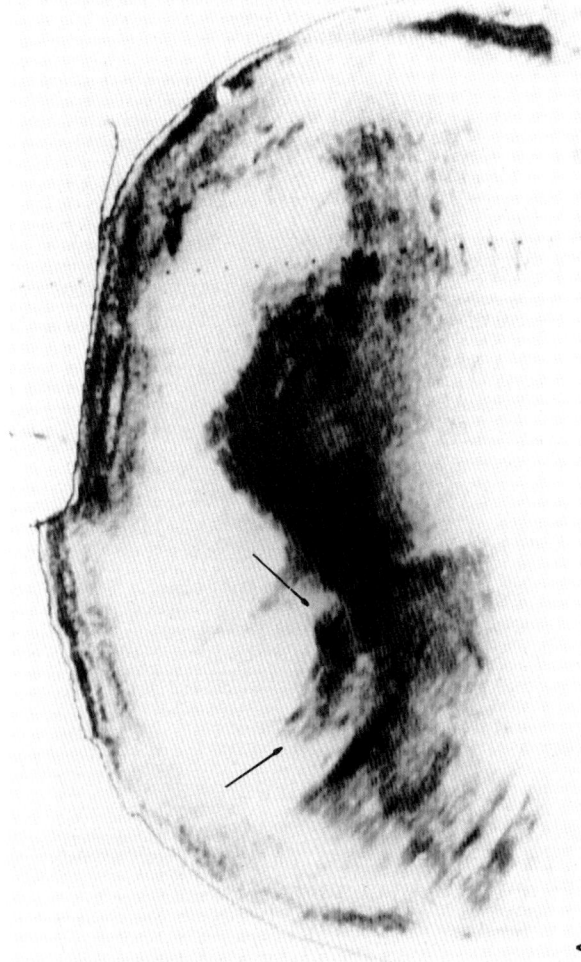

FIGURE 16.9. BILOMA AFTER GALLBLADDER RUPTURE
A: Transverse scan shows a large subhepatic fluid collection. The large clump of echoes represents gallstones (*arrows*). *B*: Parasagittal scan: shadowing gallstones (*large arrow*) within the ruptured gallbladder (*small arrows*). Surrounding anechoic biloma. *C*: CT: large, low density biloma (*arrows*). Note gallstones (*curved arrow*). (Case courtesy of James G. Bova, D.O., University of Texas Health Sciences Center, San Antonio.)

REFERENCES

1. Kuligowska E, Schlesinger A, Miller KB, Lee VW, Grosso D: Bilomas: a new approach to the diagnosis and treatment. *Gastrointest Radiol* 8:237–243, 1983.
2. Gould L, Patel A: Ultrasound detection of extrahepatic encapsulated bile: "biloma." *AJR* 132:1014–1015, 1979.
3. Esensten M, Ralls PW, Coletti P, Halls J: Posttraumatic intrahepatic biloma: sonographic diagnosis. *AJR* 140:303–305, 1983.
4. Hoffman AD: Spontaneous perforation of the common bile duct in infancy (pediatric case of the day). *AJR* 142:1070–1072, 1984.
5. Mueller PR, Ferrucci JT Jr, Simeone JF, Cronan JJ, Wittenberg J, Neff CC, van Sonnenberg E: Detection and drainage of bilomas: special considerations. *AJR* 140:715–720, 1983.
6. Lorenz R, Beyer D, Peters PE: Detection of intraperitoneal bile accumulations: significance of ultrasonography, CT, and cholescintigraphy. *Gastrointest Radiol* 9:213–217, 1984.

GALLBLADDER

Gallbladder injuries are uncommon with only 278 incidents (3.7%) in major series of 7600 abdominal injuries in the English literature (1, 2). The gallbladder is well shielded and cushioned by the rib cage, liver, right kidney, and vertebral bodies. The exact mechanism by which blunt trauma causes injury to this protected organ and/or the common bile duct are unknown, although three methods have been postulated: compression against the vertebral column (3), sudden increase of intracholecystic pressure (4), and shearing force producing avulsion of the common duct near its fixed junction with the pancreatic duct (5). The gallbladder is injured more frequently than the portal vein or hepatic artery, possibly due to the relatively greater fixation of the common bile duct, leaving the gallbladder more susceptible to avulsion (6).

Penn's review of gallbladder trauma in 1962 classified gallbladder injuries into four types, using the divisions of Smith and Hastings (7) as a guide.

1. *Contusion*—following blunt trauma this probably occurs more frequently than is recognized. Proof of injury is virtually impossible, however vague right upper quadrant pain which is transient would be characteristic. Rarely a contused area may become necrotic and perforate secondary to ischemia.

2. *Avulsion*—the gallbladder is torn from its bed and hangs by its neck or is free in the abdominal cavity except for attachment to the common bile duct and hepatic artery (traumatic cholecystectomy). This may occur with minor trauma to an acutely inflamed gallbladder such as retching (8), or horseback riding (9). More commonly this occurs with a crushing deceleration injury to the driver of a motor vehicle by the steering wheel (10, 11).

3. *Laceration*—usually follows penetrating trauma but may also be seen with blunt trauma, or on an iatrogenic basis (liver biopsy). It is possible that distension occurs secondary to alcohol ingestion, making the gallbladder more prone to rupture (2). This type of injury is not seen with chronic cholecystitis as the fibrotic thickened wall and local inflammatory reaction are thought to provide better than normal resistance to tearing (12). Occasionally delayed rupture of the gallbladder may follow development of an intramural hematoma with subsequent necrosis.

4. *Traumatic cholecystitis*—follows direct trauma to the gallbladder, or bleeding from the intrahepatic biliary tree into the gallbladder. The retained blood may occlude the cystic duct, precipitate infection and progress to gangrene of the gallbladder. Patients present with jaundice, hematemesis and melena. Alternatively injury to the cystic artery causing thrombosis may cause infarction of the gallbladder.

A fifth classification was added by Solheim (13), biliary peritonitis without perforation. A mucosal tear allows bile to seep through the remainder of the intact gallbladder wall. A rare complication of blunt trauma is cholecystocutaneous fistula secondary to a gallstone becoming embedded in the abdominal wall from rupture of the gallbladder (14).

Bile peritonitis need not be devastating if leakage is noninfected; a self limited mild chemical irritation is characteristic, although prolonged leakage may predispose to secondary infection.

Diagnosis

Physical examination, laboratory studies, and peritoneal lavage can all be misleading. In Soderstrom's series, peritoneal lavage was performed in 28 of 31 cases; all samples were positive for blood and negative for bile. The correct diagnosis is usually not suspected preoperatively (2).

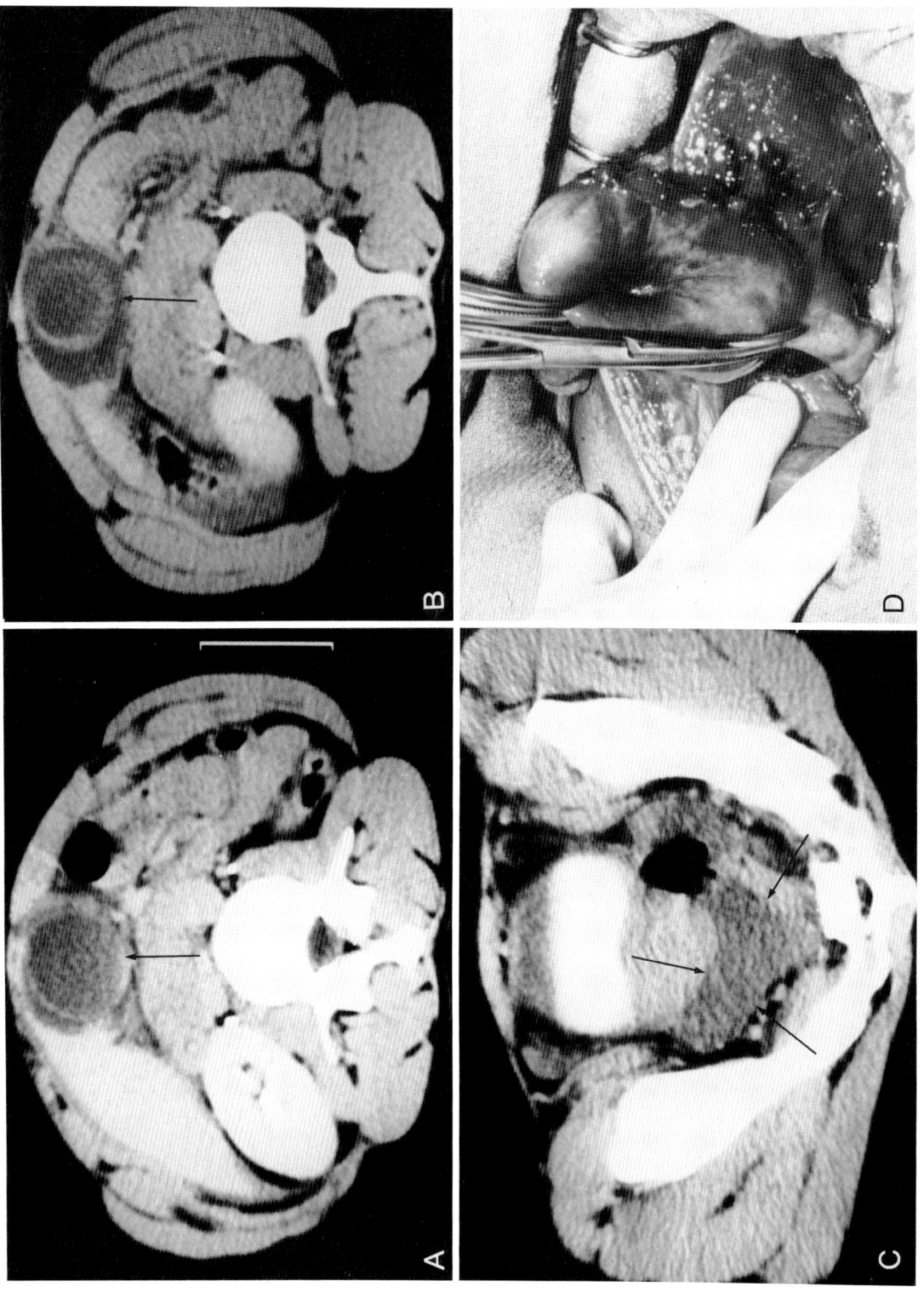

FIGURE 16.10. GALLBLADDER TRAUMA

Avulsion of the gallbladder as the only injury during an automobile accident. *A* and *B*: CT shows a large amount of fluid surrounding a distended gallbladder (*arrow*). A small amount of free intraperitoneal fluid is seen at the liver tip and in the right flank. *C*: A large collection of fluid is present in the cul-de-sac (*arrows*). *D*: At surgery, the gallbladder and its veins were completely avulsed from the liver save for the intact cystic artery and duct. The fluid seen on CT was nonclotted blood. The gallbladder was probably predisposed to trauma because of its unusually midline position, which was caused by hepatomegaly (the patient is an alcoholic).

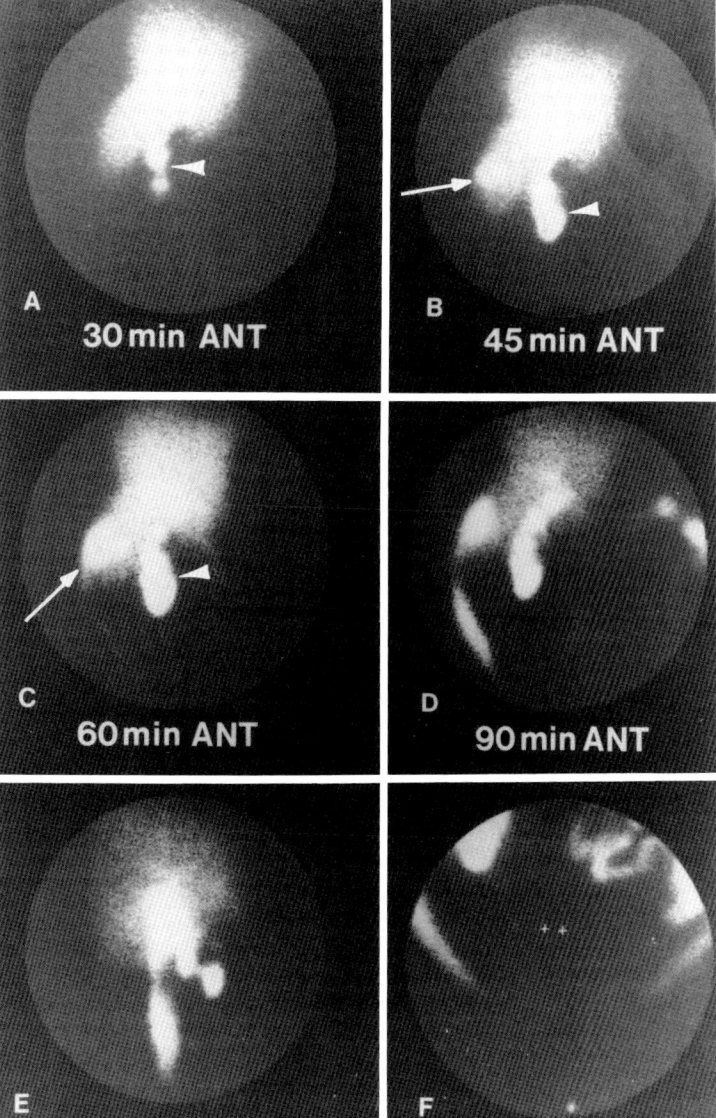

FIGURE 16.11. RUPTURED GALLBLADDER
Courtesy of Mamed Mesgarzadeh, M.D., Temple University. Early ^{99m}Tc-IDA imaging shows liver and gallbladder (arrowheads) and perihepatic pooling of activity (arrows) (A–C). Radioactivity appears in both gutters simultaneously at 90 min (D). Right lateral (E) and low anterior (F) images show activity moving along in both gutters (++ indicates umbilicus).

Radiology

Plain Film

Although nonspecific, plain films may show a mass impression on the hepatic flexure or signs of free fluid (15). Free intraperitoneal cholelithiasis is a more specific but undoubtedly rare sign of rupture (16). As gallbladder trauma is rarely an isolated finding, right anterior lower rib fractures or free air could suggest trauma severe enough to cause gallbladder injury.

Ultrasound

The associated injuries of blunt or penetrating trauma may preclude sonography, but pericholecystic fluid collections, hepatic or splenic lacerations and hematomas are usually readily detected (17, 18). The presence of a blood/bile fluid/fluid level is suggestive of gallbladder/ductal injury (18). The absence of a gallbladder within the gallbladder fossa in a patient with trauma who has not had prior cholecystectomy might suggest avulsion.

Computerized Tomography

CT can depict gallbladder location, intracholecystic blood bile levels, pericholecystic fluid collections, hepatic lacerations, and other associated trauma to the viscera (17, 18) (Fig. 16.10). Several cases of isolated blunt gallbladder trauma are presented in the literature, but as this is rarely the only injury, the finding of multiple regions of injury may increase the suspicion of gallbladder/ductal injury (1, 2). Contrast administration usually shows enhancement of the gallbladder wall if the arterial supply is intact.

Nuclear Medicine

Hepatobiliary scintigraphy studies may show leakage of the agent throughout the peritoneal cavity with or without visualization of the gallbladder in patients with gallbladder trauma (Fig. 16.11) (19–23). Absence of gallbladder visualization as an isolated finding in the setting of trauma does not necessarily imply gallbladder trauma. Other reasons for nonfilling include: prior cholecystectomy, hyperalimentation, and pancreatitis or other severe intercurrent illness (24).

Treatment

Contusions and minor lacerations may be managed expectantly with serial noninvasive studies, large lacerations may be oversewn. True rupture of the gallbladder or avulsion is treated with emergency cholecystectomy.

REFERENCES

1. Penn I: Injuries of the gallbladder. *Br J Surg* 49:636–641, 1962.
2. Soderstrom CA, Maekawa K, DuPriest RW, Cowley RA: Gallbladder injuries resulting from blunt abdominal trauma. *Ann Surg* 193:60–65, 1981.
3. Lee D, Sacher J, Vogel TT: Primary repair in transection of duodenum with avulsion of the common duct. *Arch Surg* 111:592, 1976.
4. Fletcher WS: Non-penetrating trauma in the gallbladder and extrahepatic bile ducts. *Surg Clin North Am* 52:711–717, 1972.
5. Maier WP, Lightfoot WP, Rosemond GP: Extrahepatic biliary ductal injury in closed trauma. *Am J Surg* 116:103, 1968.
6. Wiener I, Watson LC, Wolna FJ: Perforation of the gallbladder due to blunt abdominal trauma. *Arch Surg* 117:805–807, 1982.
7. Smith SW, Hastings TN: Traumatic rupture of the gallbladder. *Ann Surg* 139:517–520, 1954.
8. Shannon J: Avulsion of the gallbladder from the liver bed. Report of a case with hydrops and massive hemoperitoneum. *N Engl J Med* 253:521, 1955.
9. Campos E, Errandonea J: Case cited in Penn (1), p 639.
10. Khodadadi S, Mihich M, Finally R, Milleritzky M: Avulsion of the common bile duct after blunt abdominal injury (literature review). *Injury* 14:447–450, 1983.
11. Kaehr D, Jones LM, Miller SF, Finley RK: Traumatic cholecystectomy. *J Trauma* 24:655, 1984.
12. Brickley HD, Kapan A, Freeark et al: Immediate and delayed rupture of the extrahepatic biliary tree following blunt abdominal trauma. *AJR* 100:107, 1960.
13. Solheim K: Blunt gallbladder injury. *Injury* 3:246, 1972.
14. Grimes OF, Steinbach HL: Case cited in Penn (1), p 639.
15. Fielding JWL, Strachan CJL: Jaundice as a sign of delayed gallbladder perforation following blunt abdominal trauma. *Injury* 6:66, 1975.
16. Wolfson RH, Moore EE, Murr PC: Free intraperitoneal cholelithiasis: a sign of traumatic performation of the gallbladder. *J Emerg Med* 1:223–225, 1984.
17. Daneman A, Matzinger MA, Martin DJ: Post-traumatic hemorrhage into the gallbladder. *J Comput Assist Tomogr* 7:59–61, 1983.
18. Gohesman L, et al: Diagnosis of isolated perforation of the gallbladder following blunt trauma using sonography and CT scan. *J Trauma* 24:280–281, 1984.
19. Weissman HS, Byun JC, Freeman LM: Role of ^{99m}Tc scintigraphy in the evaluation of hepatobiliary trauma. *Semin Nucl Med* 3:199–222, 1983.
20. Powers TA, Melton RE: Diagnosis of gallbladder perforation by ^{99m}Tc disofenin cholescintigraphy. *Clin Nucl Med* 7:201–202, 1982.
21. Selby JB, Glassman AB: Cholescintigraphic diagnosis of gallbladder rupture. *Clin Nucl Med* 8:64–65, 1983.
22. Wilson DG, Lieberman LM: Perforation of the gallbladder diagnosed preoperatively. *Eur J Nucl Med* 8:145–147, 1983.
23. Kaplun L, Weissmann HS, Freeman LM: Cholescintigraphic diagnosis of gallbladder perforation. *Radiology* 153(P):174, 1984.
24. Zeman RK, Lee CH, Stahl R et al: Strategy for the use of biliary scintigraphy in non-iatrogenic biliary trauma. *Radiology* 151:771–777, 1984.

17

MRI of the Gallbladder and Biliary Tract

ARNOLD C. FRIEDMAN, M.D.

NORMAL ANATOMY

The appearance of the normal gallbladder is highly dependent on when the MRI is done in relation to meals (Fig. 17.1A–C). Hepatic bile (nonconcentrated) is low intensity on T1-weighted spin echo images with a long average T1 of 2324 ms (range 917–3152 ms, 0.35T) (1). After a meal the gallbladder contracts and refills with fresh hepatic bile. Therefore it has low intensity on T1-weighted images and higher intensity (exceeding that of liver) on T2-weighted sequences (average T2 = 122 ms range 98–171 ms) (1) (Fig. 17.1D and E). On the other hand, concentrated bile has a shorter T1 (average T1 = 584 ms, range 302–914 ms, 0.35T) and a slightly shorter T2 (average 100 ms, range 57–119 ms) (1). Therefore, the normal fasting gallbladder containing concentrated bile has a high intensity on both T1-weighted and T2-weighted images due to a relatively short T1 and a still prolonged T2. Differences between concentrated and dilute (hepatic) bile are probable due to higher water content of the latter (lengthens T1 and T2) and the higher lipid concentration of the former (shortens T1) (1). If imaging is performed after the administration of a cholecystogogue, dilute low intensity bile can be seen floating on top of concentrated high intensity bile in normal patients (1) (Fig. 17.1F and G).

Intrahepatic bile ducts are not seen on MR in normal individuals. The extrahepatic common duct can be seen as a low intensity structure anterior to the portal vein when sufficient fat is present in the porta hepatis and hepatoduodenal ligament (Fig. 17.2). The common bile duct is readily depicted on axial projections in its intrapancreatic portion as it is of lower intensity than normal pancreas. The intrapancreatic common bile duct is more often depicted by MRI than ultrasound or routine CT (CT performance can be improved by high contrast doses and thin sections).

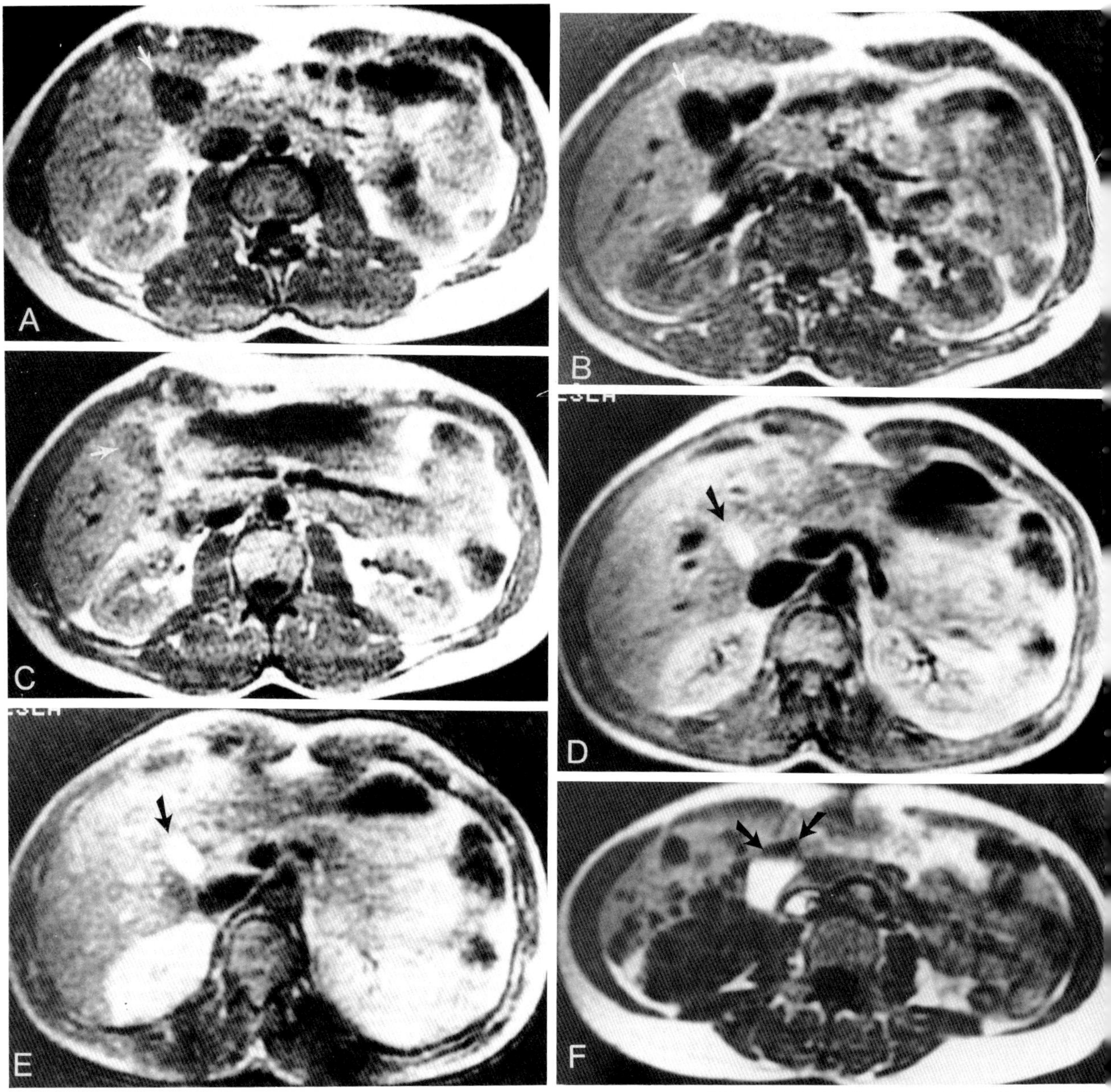

FIGURE 17.1. MRI GALLBLADDER AND BILIARY TRACT
A and B: Normal, nonfasting gallbladder (arrow), very low intensity on T1-weighted images. SE 28/500 and IR 310/1500, respectively. C: Fasting gallbladder (arrow)—SE 28/500—higher intensity than (A), same subject. D and E: Nonfasting gallbladder (arrows): more T2-weighted images, SE 28/2000 and 56/2000, respectively, show high intensity. F and G: Postprandial gallbladder, IR 310TI/1500TR: dilute low intensity bile (arrows) floating on top of high intensity, concentrated bile (F). A coronal scan (G) shows only the high intensity bile, missing the fluid level, SE 28/500. This patient has polycystic disease of the kidneys and liver (note multiple low intensity cysts best seen on F. The gallbladder was more easily identified on MRI than ultrasound.

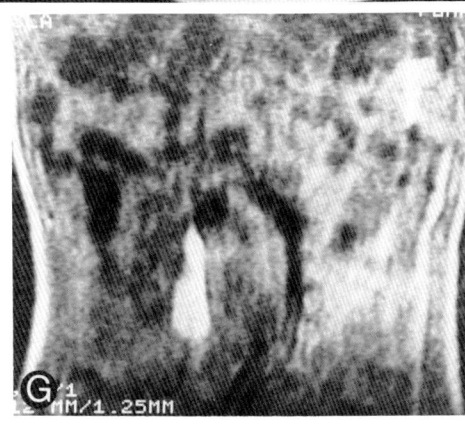

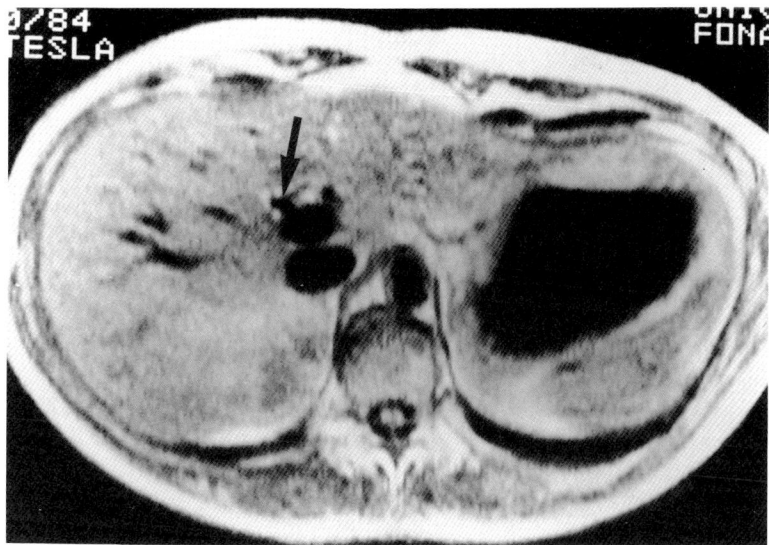

FIGURE 17.2. MRI OF GALLBLADDER AND BILIARY TRACT
Normal common duct (*arrow*) anterior to the portal vein and to the right of the hepatic artery.

GALLBLADDER DISEASE

Regardless of their chemical composition, gallstones are depicted as low intensity filling defects (1, 2). Their lack of signal can be attributed to a lack of mobile protons. Chronic cholecystitis manifests itself as a low intensity gallbladder after appropriate dietary manipulation due to the inability of the diseased gallbladder to concentrate bile (1). Acute cholecystitis can be suggested when an irregular low intensity rind surrounds the gallbladder (increased T1 due to edema and inflammation) (2). No MRI experience with cholecystoses or carcinoma of the gallbladder has been reported. We have studied two cases of gallbladder carcinoma with MRI in which the extent of the neoplasm was depicted by MRI about as well as by sonography, both of which were better than CT (Fig. 17.3).

In view of the speed, accuracy, sensitivity, and relatively low cost of ultrasound and despite claims to the contrary (1), I find it hard to believe that MRI will ever replace ultrasound as a first line test for gallbladder disease.

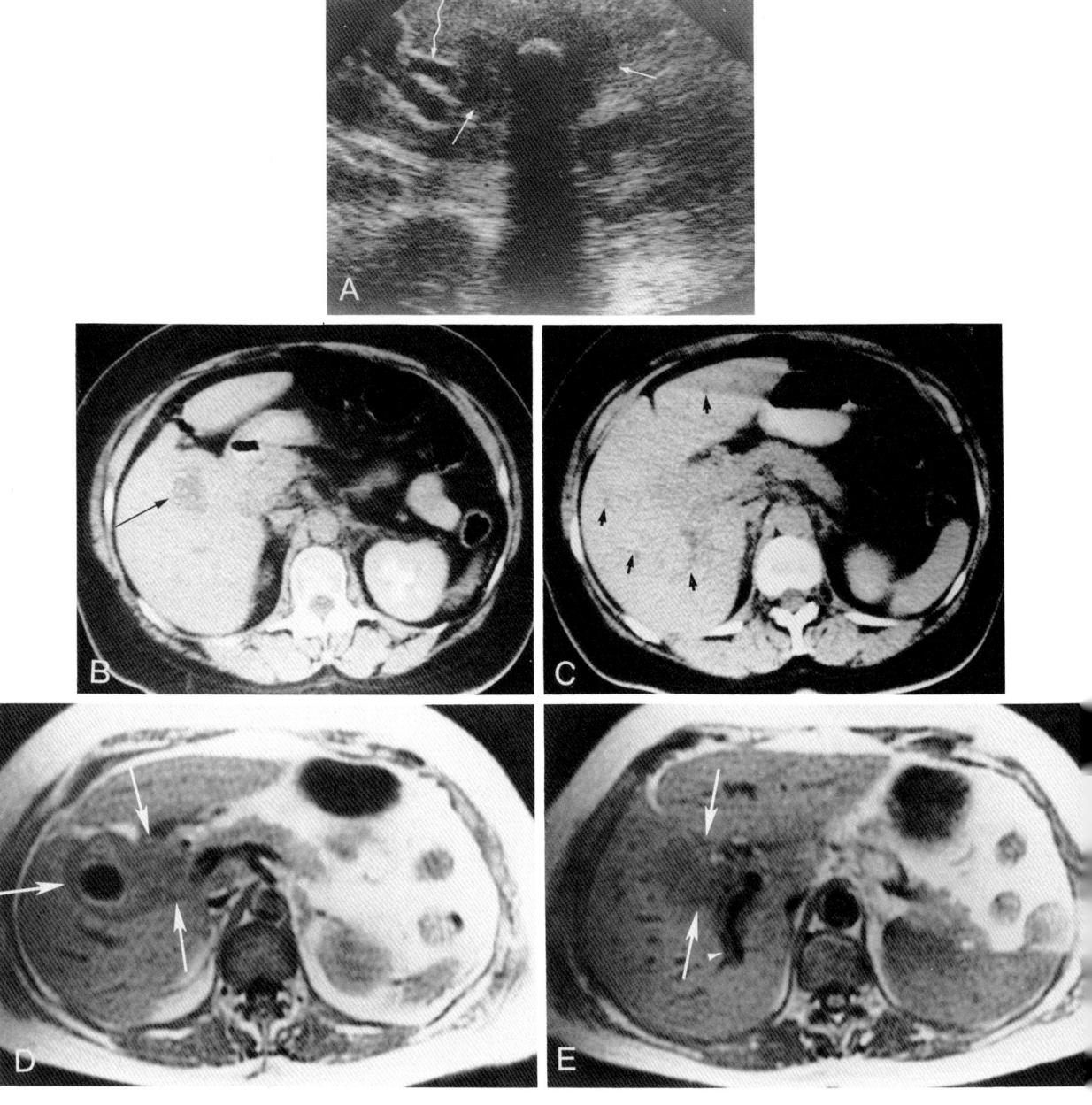

FIGURE 17.3. CARCINOMA OF THE GALLBLADDER—MRI SUPERIOR TO CT

A: Parasagittal sonogram: hypoechoic mass (*arrows*) surrounding a shadowing gallstone and obstructing the common duct (*undulating arrow*). Note poor demarcation between the mass and the liver, suggesting invasion. *B* and *C:* Contrast-enhanced CT: faintly calcified gallstone surrounded by a small amount of bile is seen (*large arrow*). Mass in porta hepatis/head of pancreas region poorly defined. Dilated intrahepatic ducts (*small arrows*). *D* and *E:* SE 28/1000 MRI at comparable levels. Hypointense mass surrounding gallbladder invading the head of the pancreas and liver (*arrows*). Large round region of nearly absent signal is gallstone, surrounded by thin rim of high signal representing bile. Dilated bile duct (*arrowhead*). *F* and *G:* SE 28/2000 MRI: mass is now hyperintense (*arrows*). Note intensity difference between head of pancreas (*curved arrow*) where tumor has spread versus the remainder of the gland. *H* and *I:* PTC: gallstone surrounded by small amount of contrast (*large arrow*) and long segment encasement of common duct (*arrows*).

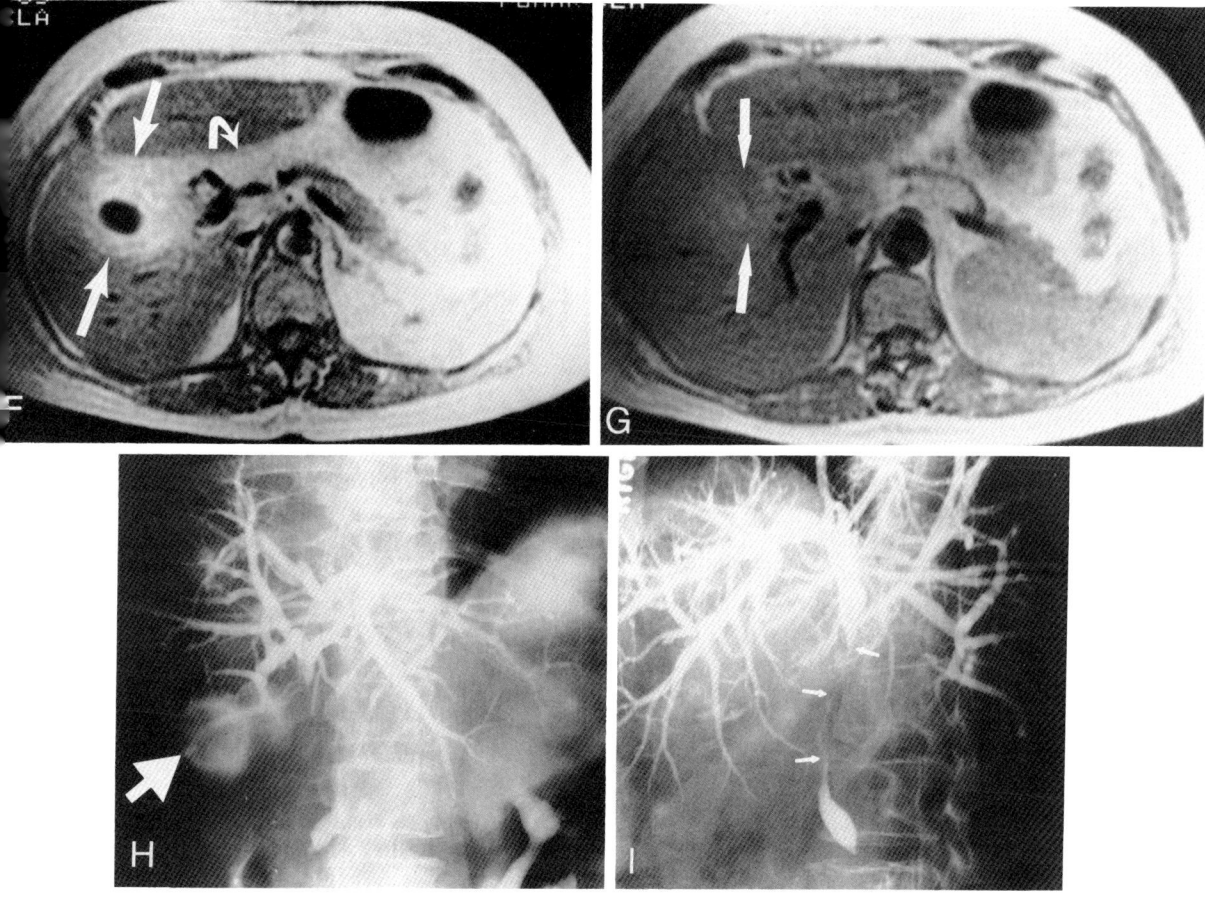

FIGURE 17.3F–I

BILIARY OBSTRUCTION

The dilated biliary tree in obstructive jaundice can be demonstrated by MRI (2, 3), but not, in our experience, as well as by CT and ultrasound (Fig. 17.4). Dilated intrahepatic bile ducts will be seen adjacent to portal vein radicles, and the common duct will be larger than normal. Bile in dilated biliary ducts has a T1 of 300–400 ms at 0.04T (3), and 550–980 ms at 0.15T (4, 5). Since both dilated ducts and portal vein radicles have about the same signal intensity on spin echo sequences, a method of increasing contrast between them would be useful. At 0.15T, saturation recovery imaging with a short TR accomplishes this goal because of paradoxical enhancement in portal veins from flowing blood (4). Intravenous MR contrast agents can increase venous signal intensity and delineate dilated ducts analogous to urographic contrast material in CT.

Preliminary work has shown that MRI may be useful in patients with sclerosing cholangiocarcinoma of the biliary tree (6). If born out, this would be an advance, since noninvasive studies are often noncontributory in this condition. Abnormalities depicted in descending order of frequency include: diffuse increase in signal in the peripheral hepatic parenchyma and/or focal regions(s) of decreased signal (presumably due to metabolic changes secondary to obstruction), segmental biliary dilatation, distorted portal vein radicles, and discrete mass (6).

In view of the current availability of both sensitive and accurate noninvasive functional and anatomic studies (sonography, CT and scintigraphy) and the exquisite anatomic detail and relative safety afforded by invasive direct cholangiography (either endoscopic or transhepatic) it is hard to envision a major role for MRI in the biliary tree unless significant advances in equipment are achieved.

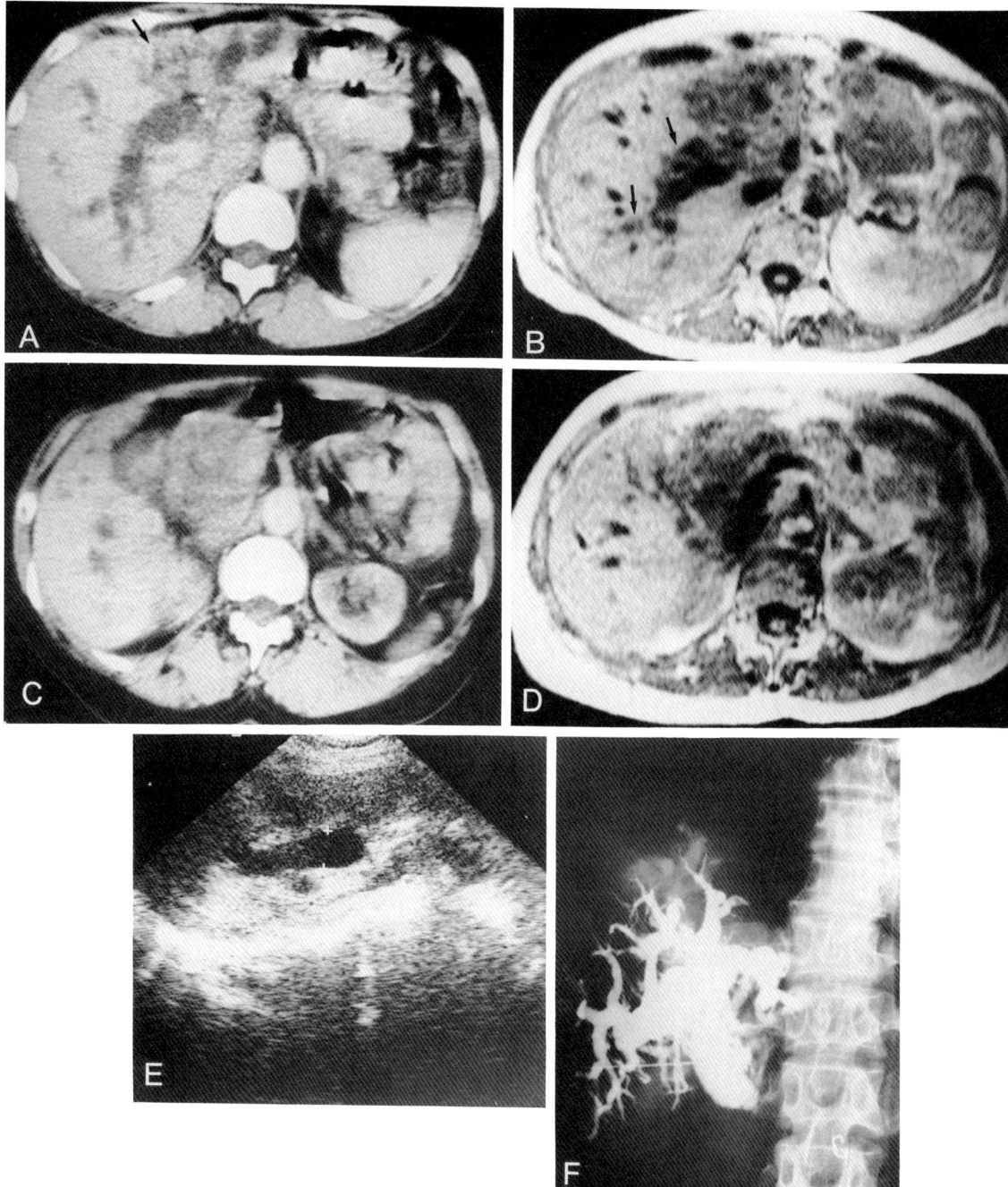

FIGURE 17.4. MRI OF GALLBLADDER AND BILIARY TRACT
Superiority of contrast-enhanced CT and sonography in showing dilated bile ducts in a case of carcinoma of the pancreas. *A:* CT: obvious dilated ducts in homogeneous low attenuation in left lobe (*arrow*). Probable direct extension of tumor. *B:* SE 28/500 MRI at slightly lower level. Obvious hypointense tumor. Dilated ducts (*arrows*) not as obvious. *C:* CT: large mass in head and neck of pancreas. Obvious dilated ducts. *D:* SE 28/500 MRI at comparable level: obvious hypointense mass in head of pancreas, but dilated ducts not seen. *E:* Parasagittal sonogram: large abruptly obstructed common duct (*cursors*). *F:* Percutaneous transhepatic cholangiography: huge, obstructed intra and extrahepatic ducts.

REFERENCES

1. Hricak H., Filly RA, Margulis AR, Moon KL, Crooks LE, Kaufman L: Work in progress: nuclear magnetic resonance imaging of the gallbladder. *Radiology* 147:481-484, 1983.
2. Moon KL, Hricak H, Margulis AR, Bernhoft R, Way LW, Filly RA, Crooks LE: Nuclear magnetic resonance imaging characteristics of gallstones in vitro. *Radiology* 148:753-756, 1983.
3. Smith FW, Mallard JR, Reid A, Hutchison JMS: Nuclear magnetic resonance tomographic imaging in liver disease. *Lancet* 1:963-966, 1981.
4. Doyle FH, Pennock JM, Banks LM, McDonnell MJ, Bydder GM, Steiner RE, Young IR, Clarke GJ, Pasmore T, Gilderdale DJ: Nuclear magnetic resonance imaging of the liver: initial experience. *AJR* 138:193-200, 1982.
5. Buonocore E, Borkowski GP, Pavlicek W, Ngo F: NMR imaging of the abdomen: technical considerations. *AJR* 141:1171-1178, 1983.
6. Kerlan RK, Wall SD, Margulis AR, Hricak H, Goldberg HI: MR imaging in the detection of cholangiocarcinoma. Presented at the 70th Scientific Assembly and Annual Meeting of the RSNA, Washington, D.C., Nov. 25-30, 1984.

18

Interventional Biliary Radiology

DOUGLAS M. COLDWELL, M.D., PH.D.

Pancreatic and biliary diseases are among the most common causes of hospital admissions. Noninvasive imaging modalities rely on differences in x-ray attenuation, acoustic impedance or relaxation time to depict the biliary ductal system, rather than installation of contrast. Consequently, fine anatomic details are not well seen. Percutaneous transhepatic cholangiography (PTC) enables one to visualize the biliary ducts directly. While it is an invasive procedure, it provides the most accurate information concerning biliary pathology. It also achieves access to the biliary tract for various interventional procedures. An overview of biliary pathology will first be given in this chapter followed by a description of the technical aspects of PTC and subsequent interventions. The diagnostic radiology and interventional aspects of specific disease entities are also discussed elsewhere in this book under their own heading.

BENIGN STRICTURES

The two major categories of benign strictures seen in the bile ducts are those arising from either iatrogenic causes or sclerosing cholangitis. Such a stricture most commonly arises in the common bile duct months to years after a patient has had a cholecystectomy with subsequent T-tube placement. On PTC, these appear as smoothly contoured strictures at the site of the previous surgical exploration (Fig. 18.1). A malignant stricture must be excluded as neoplasm may occur in the post operative patient. In practice, a stricture in the mid common bile duct in a patient who is post cholecystectomy is most likely of iatrogenic origin while a similar appearing stricture in a patient whose gallbladder has not been removed is most likely a malignancy.

Primary sclerosing cholangitis is a rare and idiopathic disease resulting in focal or diffuse fibrosis of the bile ducts. It is most common in males over 40 years of age and can be an isolated disease or associated with inflammatory bowel disease or multifocal fibrosclerosis (e.g., retroperitoneal fibrosis, fibrosing mediastinitis). Secondary sclerosing cholangitis may be caused by choledocholithiasis, tumor, postoperative trauma, intra-arterial infusion chemotherapy, or persistent/recurrent infection (1, 2). Both the focal and the diffuse forms may involve either the intra- or extrahepatic ducts. On PTC, the ducts are narrow and beaded. These patients present with jaundice, pruritus, right upper quadrant abdominal pain, and cholangitis. Biliary cirrhosis, portal hypertension, and hepatic failure will eventually develop. The mean survival of these patients after diagnosis is 10 yr. The treatment of choice is drainage of the bile ducts either externally or preferably internally. Balloon dilatation of strictures has had some success. It is unclear whether these methods of treatment actually extend the patient's survival (3).

Other causes of biliary stenosis include chronic pancreatitis and ampullary (papillary) stenosis. Chronic relapsing pancreatitis may cause stricturing of the intrapancreatic portion of the common bile duct. The chronic inflammation results in fibrosis and a smooth stricturing of the common bile duct, usually without complete obstruction. Calcification in the head of the pancreas suggests this diagnosis. An indentation on the common bile duct may also be present caused by a pseudocyst which should be well delineated by CT and sonography. Postoperative strictures of the ampulla of Vater are usually benign, but when there is irregular tapering of the distal common bile duct into the ampulla it is difficult to exclude an ampullary carcinoma.

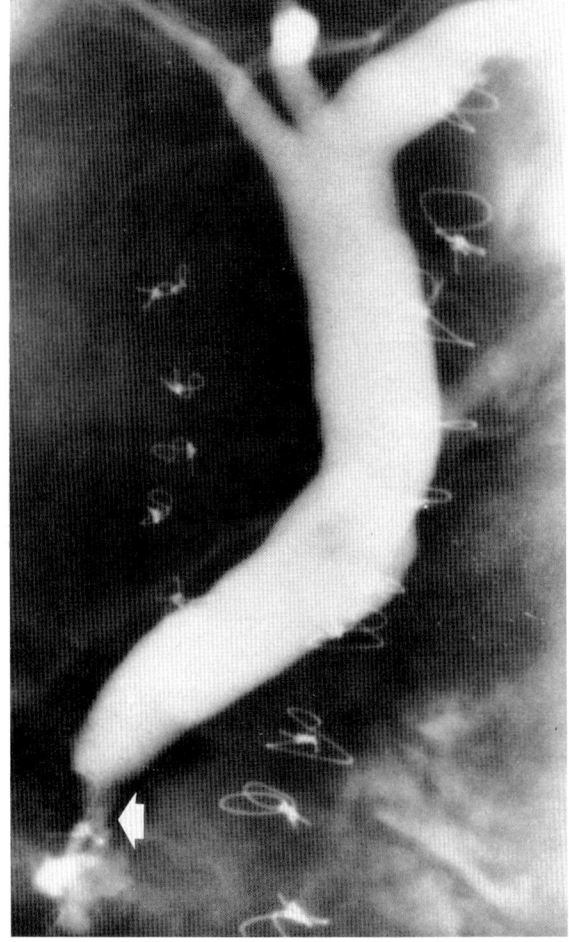

FIGURE 18.1. POSTOPERATIVE STRICTURE AFTER A CHOLECYSTECTOMY AND COMMON DUCT EXPLORATION (*arrow*)

MALIGNANT STRICTURES

The primary causes for malignant strictures in the biliary system are cholangiocarcinoma, metastatic disease to the periportal nodes, carcinoma of the pancreas, ampullary carcinoma, and lymphoma. Less commonly, carcinoma of the gallbladder and hepatocellular carcinoma invade the biliary tree also causing stricturing. Biopsy of the stricture is necessary to confirm the diagnosis.

Cholangiocarcinoma may be found in either the extra- or intrahepatic biliary system. Predisposing factors to the formation of a cholangiocarcinoma include ulcerative colitis (0.4% of these patients), choledochal cyst, parasitic infestation, and sclerosing cholangitis. Cholangiocarcinoma associated with sclerosing cholangitis is usually a diffuse fibrosing form of adenocarcinoma. Presenting symptoms usually are weight loss, jaundice, and pruritus. A form of cholangiocarcinoma occurring at the confluence of the hepatic ducts is known as a Klatskin tumor which refers only to its position and not a particular histology (Fig. 18.2). Cholangiocarcinomas usually spread contiguously along the biliary tree (4, 5). Radiographic findings of biliary ductal carcinoma include complete obstruction of the biliary system with either a blunt termination, or a "rat tail" appearance. The latter is an irregular tapering of the contrast column in its distal end as shown in Figure 18.2. Cholangiocarcinoma arising from the intrahepatic biliary ductal system may infiltrate into the parenchyma of the liver causing solitary or multiple stenoses of the bile ducts (6). Pathologically, this is the same type as the carcinoma of the extrahepatic bile duct with similar progression and prognosis.

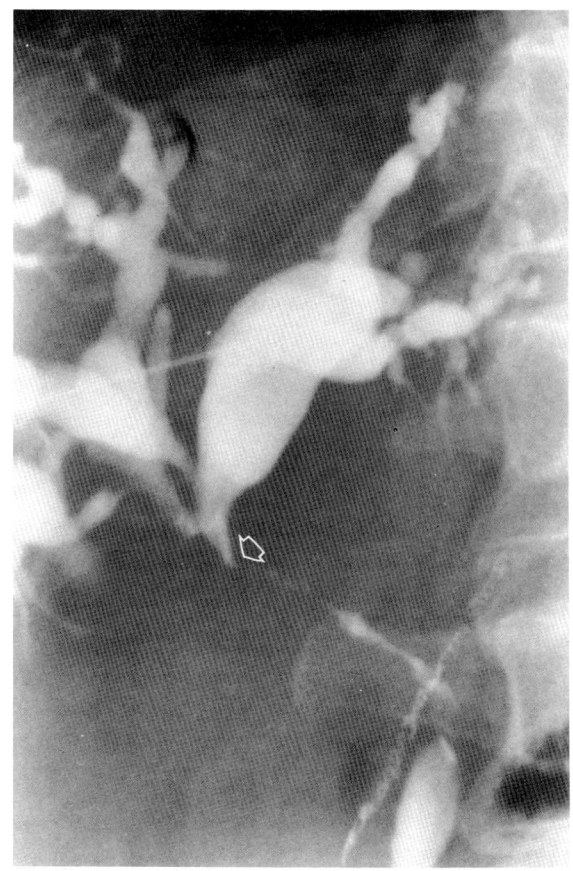

FIGURE 18.2. CHOLANGIOCARCINOMA
Occurrence at the confluence of the right and left intrahepatic ducts (Klatskin tumor) showing the typical "rat tail" appearance (*arrow*).

original diagnosis to death approximately 5 months. Patients usually present with pain, weight loss, and jaundice. Most patients with carcinoma in the head of the pancreas will be icteric at diagnosis. Sonography and CT demonstrate the actual mass in the head of the pancreas as well as enlarged bile ducts. PTC will show tapering of the common bile duct in its mid to distal one third (Fig. 18.4). The common bile duct is usually obstructed and the contrast column will end either abruptly or in the expected "rat-tail" appearance (8).

Carcinoma of the ampulla of Vater is a form of extrahepatic biliary ductal carcinoma with a prognosis somewhat better than other forms of this disease. It is usually well demarcated and localized at the time of its presentation with jaundice. The cholangiographic appearance is either that of a stricture or a polypoid mass (Fig. 18.5). If the tumor is resected with "clean" margins, long-term survival is possible. Stenting the biliary-enteric anastomosis may be helpful (9).

Carcinoma of the gallbladder or hepatocellular carcinoma, with their tendency to infiltrate the liver parenchyma, may not only encroach upon but grow into the biliary tree (Fig. 18.6) and produce intraluminal defects within the bile ducts on cholangiography.

Enlargement of the lymph nodes in the periportal region may obstruct the common hepatic or common bile duct. This lymphadenopathy may be due to metastatic disease commonly from gastrointestinal, breast, or lung primaries. These nodes may also be involved with lymphoma or even benign processes such as tuberculosis or sarcoid. The cholangiographic pattern is one of a smooth obstruction which can be tapered at both ends (Fig. 18.3). Regional radiation therapy can produce dramatic results. Direct infiltration of gallbladder carcinoma or hepatocellular carcinoma into this region may also occur (7).

Pancreatic duct cell adenocarcinoma is an extremely aggressive malignancy. It occurs more often in men than women in the population aged 65–85. It is associated with diabetes mellitus but apparently antecedent diabetes mellitus may be merely an early sign of the malignancy. The prognosis is grave with the average time from

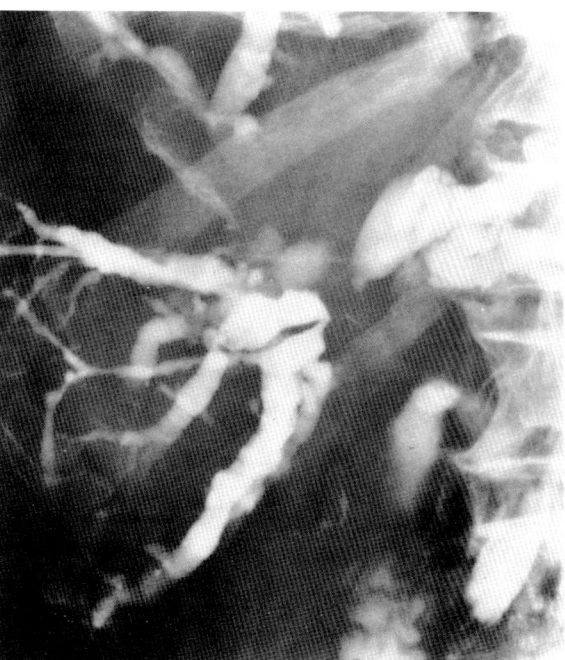

FIGURE 18.3. PERIPORTAL ADENOPATHY
Metastatic colon carcinoma obstructing the left and right hepatic ducts at the bifurcation.

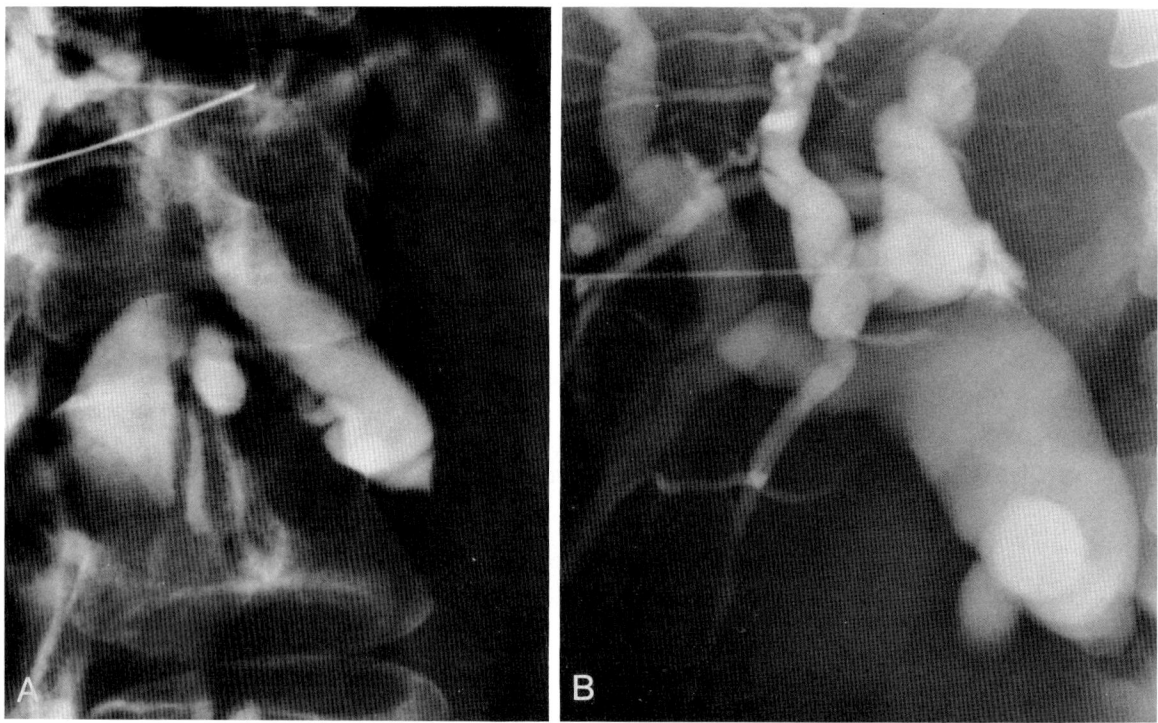

FIGURE 18.4. PANCREATIC CARCINOMA
A: Carcinoma occluding the distal common bile duct (oblique view, abrupt tapered obstruction). *B:* This pancreatic carcinoma obstructed the distal common bile duct producing marked ductal dilatation and a blunt obstruction.

FIGURE 18.5. POLYPOID PERIAMPULLARY CARCINOMA
Lesion was proved to be adenocarcinoma on resection (*closed arrow*). Reflux is present into the pancreatic duct (*open arrow*).

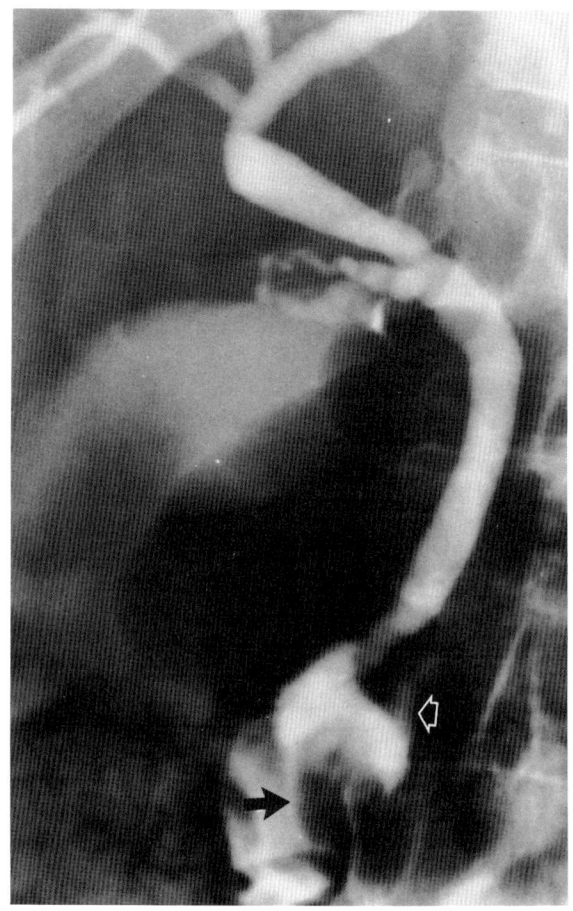

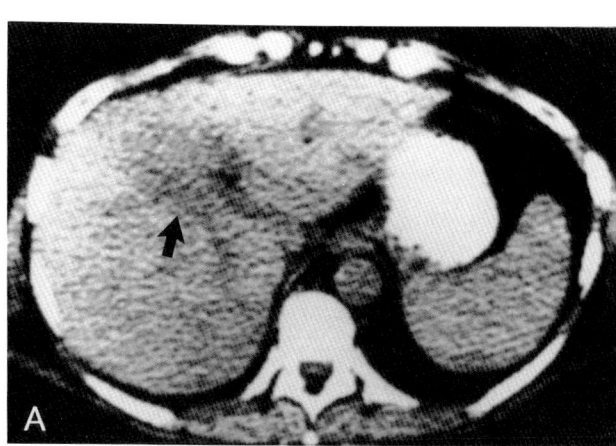
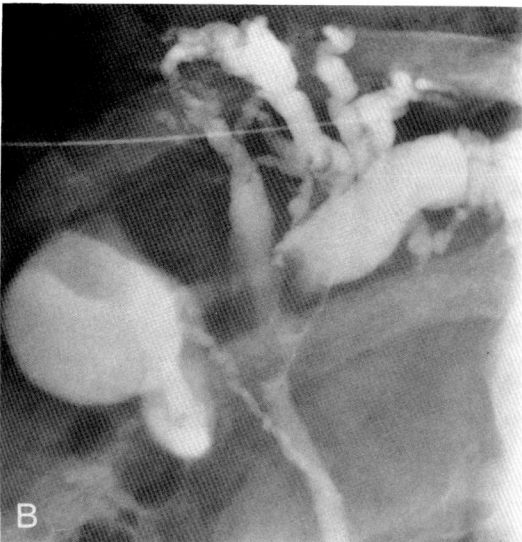

FIGURE 18.6. HEPATOCELLULAR CARCINOMA
A: CT scan showing low attenuation region near porta hepatis (*arrow*) which, on biopsy, was proven to be a hepatocellular carcinoma. *B:* The PTC demonstrates a filling defect at the confluence of the intrahepatic ducts representing invasion of the hepatoma into the biliary system.

OTHER BILIARY CONDITIONS

Choledocholithiasis

Stones within the intra- or extrahepatic biliary ducts are readily identifiable on transhepatic cholangiography but are often seen first on ultrasound and less commonly CT. It is not unusual for more calculi to be shown by PTC than the noninvasive techniques. Calculi may completely obstruct the biliary system when they impact at the ampulla. Partial or even no obstruction is generally the case with more proximal calculi. Low grade infection is common and care should be taken not to overinject during PTC otherwise septic shock may ensue. It is important to distinguish actual calculi in the bile ducts from admixture defects due to inspissated bile. Bile calculi are most commonly angular but may be rounded. Biliary calculi can be removed with a basket either percutaneously or endoscopically. Calculi may also be dissolved using monooctanoin infused through a catheter in the common bile duct (10). The differential diagnosis of choledocholithiasis includes blood clot, admixture defect, polypoid tumor (ampullary carcinoma or hepatocellular carcinoma), and extraductal mass impression.

Cirrhosis

Cirrhosis of the liver from any cause may produce tortuous corkscrewing of the bile ducts as a result of fatty infiltration and shrinkage of the liver parenchyma. The ducts are usually small but will enlarge if obstruction from a superimposed hepatocellular carcinoma occurs.

Congenital Anomalies

Primary congenital abnormalities of the biliary tree include choledochal cyst and Caroli's disease. The first, choledochal cyst, is a congenital cystic dilatation of the common bile duct. One etiology postulated is anomalous insertion of the common bile duct into the pancreatic duct proximal to the ampulla of Vater allowing reflux of pancreatic enzymes into the biliary tree leading to inflammation and fibrosis. The subsequent obstruction of the extrahepatic biliary system causes dilatation of the common bile duct. Another theory is that these cysts are the result of an infantile viral cholangitis. Three major types occur. Type I is a cystic dilatation of most of the common bile duct. Type II (choledochal diverticulum) is a saccular dilatation extending off of the common bile duct (Fig. 18.7). Type III (choledochocele) is cystic dilatation of the distal common bile duct extending into the duodenum at the ampulla of Vater (11).

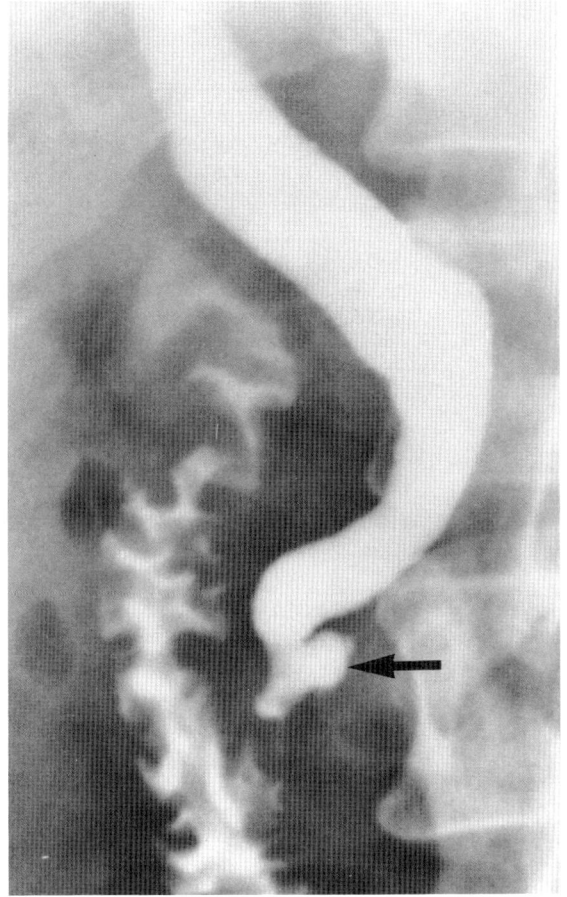

FIGURE 18.7. TYPE II CHOLEDOCHAL CYST (*arrow*)

Caroli's disase is a saccular dilatation of the intrahepatic bile ducts. These saccular dilatations communicate with one another and predispose toward intrahepatic biliary calculi and cholangitis. Portal hypertension and cirrhosis are not usually seen (12).

TECHNIQUE OF PERCUTANEOUS TRANSHEPATIC CHOLANGIOGRAPHY

Patient Preparation

Since this is an invasive procedure, adequate patient preparation is essential. Many patients undergoing PTC will have significant liver disease and alterations in clotting parameters; preliminary laboratory results including prothrombin time, activated partial thromboplastin time, bleeding time, and complete blood count should be known before the procedure is begun. Prophylactic antibiotics should be administered when the ducts are dilated. The antibiotics found most useful in this setting have been ampicillin (2 g per 24 hr IV or 1 g IV within 1 hr before the procedure) and gentamicin (80 mg per 24 hr IM). These antibiotics should be continued for a minimum of 48 hr after the last biliary manipulation. Premedication with valium may be useful. Adequate analgesia during the procedure may be obtained with intravenous Demerol (25 mg bolus) or Fentanyl (50 μg bolus). Fentanyl provides a more profound anesthesia and its dosage can be titrated more exactly than Demerol. As is the case with Demerol, Fentanyl is reversible with Narcan. Other patient preparations include intravenous access and cardiac monitoring.

Placement of the Thin-Walled 22-Gauge Needle

The puncture site is chosen from the lateral approach in the mid axillary line at a position one intercostal space below the most caudad level of excursion of the right hemidiaphragm (several centimeters below the right costophrenic angle). The site is adequately cleaned with iodine-containing soap and the skin anesthesized with lidocaine (1% without epinephrine). Deep anesthesia through the liver capsule can then be obtained with either lidocaine or Marcaine. Marcaine provides a more profound anesthesia locally and is excellent for deadening the liver capsule. A small skin incision is made with a scalpel and the needle is placed in a direction aiming toward the xyphoid while the patient suspends respiration. The needle thrust should be performed under continuous fluoroscopic monitoring.

If an anterior approach is employed for placement of the needle in the left hepatic ducts the entry site is chosen adjacent to the left costal margin immediately below the level of the xyphoid process. Sterilization of the skin and local anesthesia is then performed and the thin-walled needle inserted perpendicularly to the skin surface to a depth of 4–6 cm. A 22-gauge spinal needle may be adequate for a left-sided puncture. The puncture is made with the patient inspiring and then suspending respiration. Sonographic guidance may be helpful in selected cases, especially with left duct punctures.

From either puncture site the needle is then slowly withdrawn as tiny puffs of contrast (significantly less than 1 ml) are injected. If vascular structures are opacified the contrast will flow away from the needle tip toward the heart or toward the periphery of the liver. The needle tract itself and occasionally lymphatic structures will be opacified. When contrast enters a biliary duct, it assumes a stationary linear configuration and does not become diluted. After the ducts are seen, further contrast is injected and the patient maneuvered so that the contrast will flow down and identify the site of obstruction. This may entail rolling the patient from side to side, adopting the prone position or placing the patient in an almost erect position. The entire ductal system, including both right and left branches, should be examined during the cholangiogram. It must be emphasized that over-distention of the ductal system should be avoided as this may precipitate septic shock because of cholangiovenous reflux of infected bile (13) (Fig. 18.8).

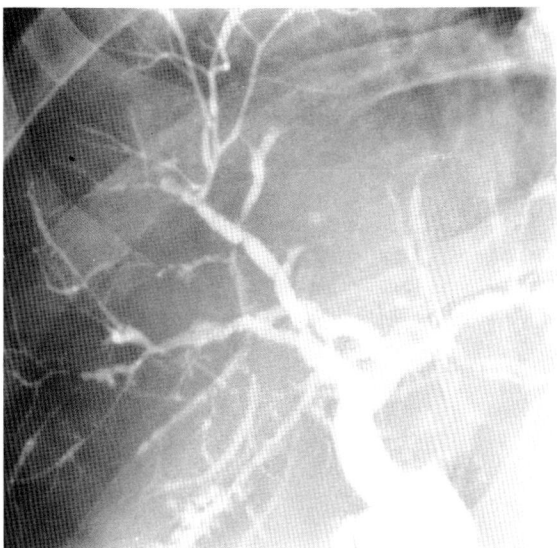

FIGURE 18.8. OVERINJECTION, T-TUBE CHOLANGIOGRAM
Note multiple ill-defined regions of parenchymal staining, especially in the lower right lobe. The patient went into septic shock after the injection.

Dilated ducts are nearly always opacified and nondilated ducts are visualized 70–90% of the time depending on the numbers of passes attempted.

Biliary Drainage

If drainage of an obstructed system has been elected, a guide wire must be placed and a catheter advanced into the biliary ducts. Proper needle placement is important in initiating the biliary drainage procedure. This, more often than not, necessitates repuncturing the patient. A horizontal beam lateral film with the bile ducts opacified is compared with the overhead frontal views of the biliary system to select a duct that leads directly to the common hepatic duct with only a gentle curve and no acute angulation. The 22-gauge needle used in the original puncture should be left in place as a marker. A new puncture is then made with a 21-gauge Chiba needle or a 19-gauge sheathed needle. The latter is a 5-French sheath over a 19-gauge needle which then allows passage of a 0.038-inch guide wire. If possible, it is desirable to puncture below the 9th intercostal interspace, thereby avoiding traversing the pleural space. A low puncture may create too much of an angle for the drainage catheter, however (14). If a 21-gauge Chiba needle is used, a 0.018-inch wire is then advanced into the ducts followed by a 7.5 French dilator. This catheter should have a side hole in it which is large enough to pass the 0.038-inch guide wire for further manipulations.

It is unusual for the wire to pass straightaway into the common hepatic duct without further active direction. This may be accomplished with the use of a short (30 cm) 6.5 French cobra catheter (Cook, Inc.) which makes it possible to direct a 3 mm J wire down to the common duct. A Benson wire can be directed down the common duct even if its initial direction is peripheral. It can be "bounced" off a distal bile duct and curve on itself and thereby end up in the common hepatic duct. A limited attempt is made to cross the point of obstruction during the initial procedure. Excessive manipulations at this time can lead to complications. If the obstruction is not readily traversed, external drainage is performed and 24–48 hr later, after the system has decompressed, the obstruction may then be crossed. When the drainage procedure is for acute suppurative cholangitis external drainage and minimal manipulation is recommended until the infection is under control.

To cross the obstruction, the short cobra catheter is advanced to the level of the obstruction and, using a Benson wire, gentle probing motions can be made until a tract is found. After the tract is identified the catheter can then be advanced through the tract into the duodenum. A stiffer wire is then placed through the cobra catheter. This wire may be a Lunderquist exchange wire or a THG wire (0.038-inch) (Cook Inc.). Advancing this well into the duodenum provides great stability and ease of placement for a biliary drainage catheter.

The most commonly used biliary drainage catheter is a Cope catheter (Cook, Inc.) which is made of a soft pliable material and has side holes present in both the rounded tip and proximally along the shaft of the catheter itself. This allows bridging of the obstruction with holes in the catheter within the biliary tree above the obstruction tree and below the obstruction in the duodenum. The Cope catheter may be either a 10 or 12 French size. The 8 French size is usually too small to drain the viscous bile. After consecutive dilatations have been made with fascial dilators, the Cope catheter is advanced over the wire with its stiffener to a point where it can easily make a gentle curve into the common duct and duodenum. The stiffener is then held at this point and the catheter advanced over the wire into the duodenum. The stiffener and wire are removed and contrast gently instilled through the catheter. Gentle puffing of the contrast will identify the side holes. One must insure that the side holes are within the biliary system and not intraparenchymal, subcapsular, or extrahepatic. There is a string on the outside end of the Cope catheter which extends through it to coil the distal end to prevent the catheter from migrating. When placing the wire or the stiffener through the Cope catheter, place slight tension on the string in order to keep the string from coiling in the lumen of the catheter causing obstruction of the catheter. Coiling or kinking of the catheter in the peritoneal cavity outside the liver or subcapsularly causes the patient great pain. A firm wire will help keep the catheter from bending but alternatively a stiffer Ring catheter can be used. The Teflon Ring catheter may be advanced over the wire and left in the duodeunum to be replaced with a Cope catheter when the soft tissue tract matures (Fig. 18.9). At a convenient point during the procedure, bile should be aspirated for culture and cytology as clinically indicated.

Post Procedure

If only a cholangiogram is performed without complication, a hemoglobin and hematocrit are obtained approximately 4 hours after the procedure is completed. This will provide information concerning the presence of a subcapsular hematoma or, more important, active bleeding.

If a catheter is placed to drain the biliary system, meticulous records should be kept of the catheter output. The catheter is initially left on external drainage and can be converted into internal drainage by merely closing the stopcock after a period of 2–4 days. Post procedural injection of contrast into the biliary system can be made to insure that the catheter remains well-positioned and is draining adequately. The catheter itself may be flushed with sterile saline 2–4 times per day to ensure continued patency. This is particularly important in the first few days after a tube has been placed as the bile which is initially drained is very viscous and can easily obstruct the catheter (15, 16).

Complications

Other than the pain during the procedure, the most significant complication seen is hemobilia. This usually clears within 48 hr but occasionally a vasobiliary fistula will form causing persistent hemobilia (Fig. 18.10). Embolization of the fistula can be performed with a stainless steel coil or Gelfoam pledgets. This of course, requires identification of the fistula, which can sometimes be accomplished by a catheter cholangiogram (biliovenous fistula) but may require arteriogra-

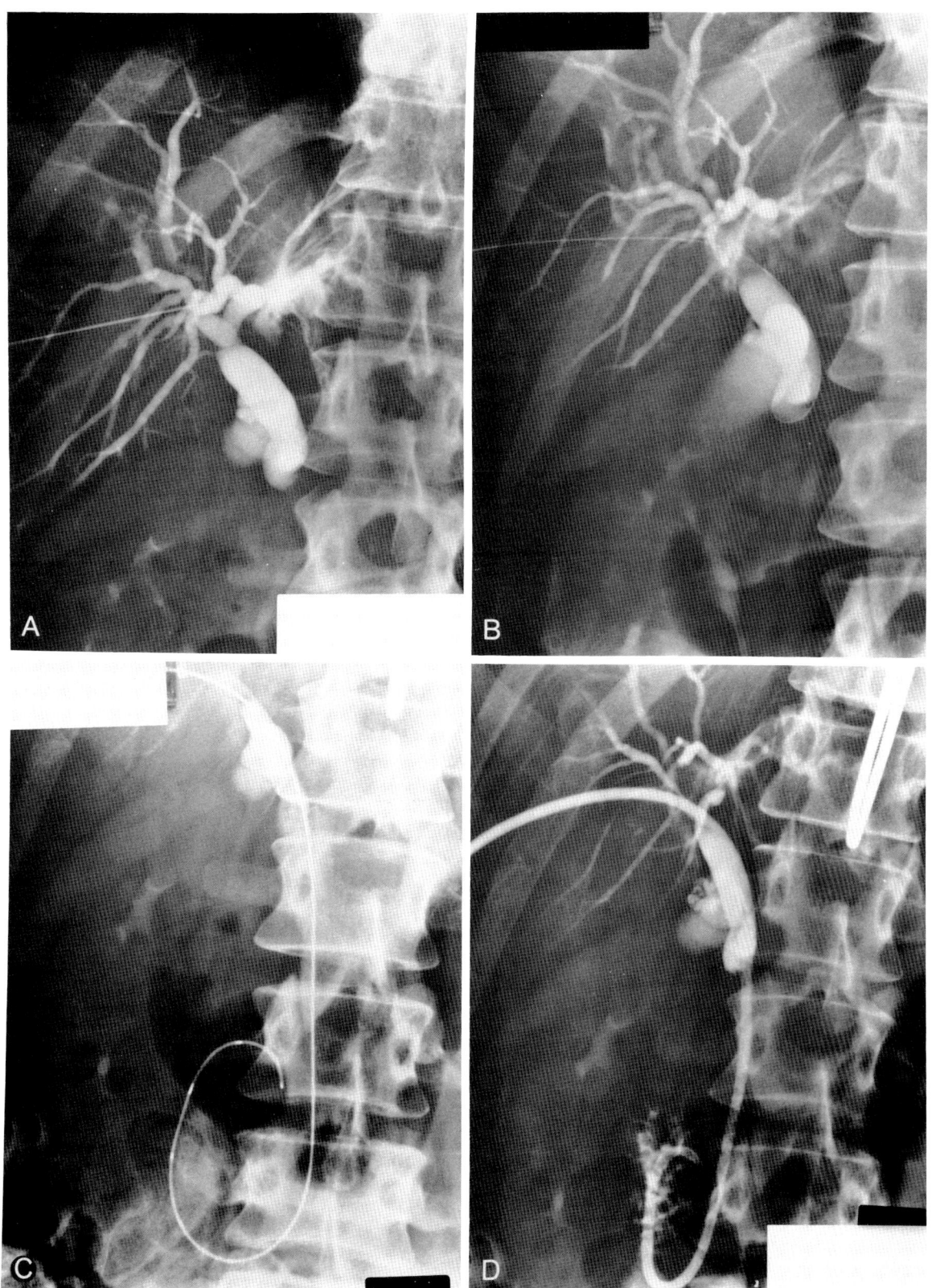

FIGURE 18.9. PERCUTANEOUS TRANSHEPATIC BILIARY DRAINAGE
A: The PTC shows obstruction by a pancreatic carcinoma in the distal common bile duct. *B:* An 0.018-inch guide wire is advanced through the 21-gauge Chiba needle. *C:* A catheter is placed through the obstruction and a heavy 0.038-inch wire secured in the duodenum. *D:* A 10 French Cope catheter is advanced beyond the obstruction into the duodenum.

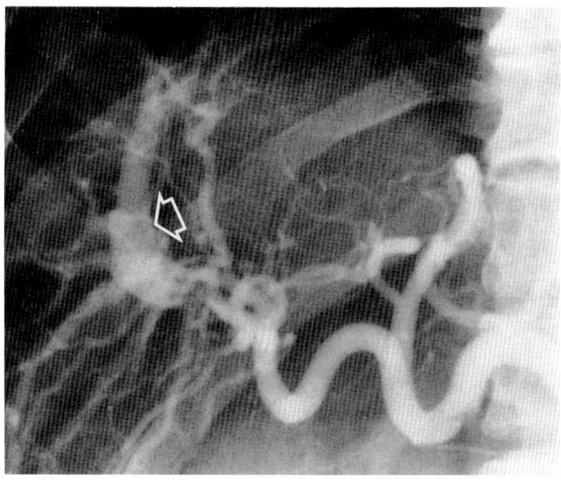

FIGURE 18.10. HEMOBILIA POST-PTC
Hepatic arteriography shows an arterioportal fistula with early filling of the portal vein (arrow). Feeding vessels were occluded successfully with stainless steel coils.

phy (arterioportal fistula) or even hepatic venography.

The other major complication is infection. This may occur acutely as septic shock or insidiously. Fully 50% of tumor patients who remain on internal drainage become infected (17). The most common organisms are, as expected, colonic bacteria. When the left side and right side are both obstructed and do not communicate with each other, each must be drained even though decompression of only 30% of the liver is sufficient for palliation. This is because an isolated, undrained left system is likely to become infected (18).

After the drainage catheter has been in place for a week or more and converted to internal drainage, it may become occluded with inspissated bile. This will cause bile to leak around the tube. The catheter should then be replaced with a larger bore catheter and left on external drainage until the bile becomes less viscous.

OTHER BILIARY SPECIAL PROCEDURES

Tumor Biopsy

Biopsy of either a primary biliary carcinoma or carcinoma in the head of the pancreas may be achieved via the biliary drainage tract. A relatively stiff guide wire (THG or Lunderquist exchange guide wire) is first placed through the existing biliary drainage tube. The catheter is removed leaving the guide wire in the duodenum. A 9 French thin-walled sheath through which both the biopsy instrument and guide wire may pass is then placed over the wire and positioned with its opening at the level of the stenosis. A small brush is first passed through the stenosis to obtain a cytologic specimen. If an adequate specimen is not obtained with this instrument, a 22-gauge Chiba needle is then placed through the sheath and an aspiration biopsy is taken at the stenosis. It may be necessary to slightly bend the distal portion of the needle to facilitate entry into the tumor mass. The sheath then can be removed and a new drainage catheter placed in the duodenum. Transient hemobilia is common post procedure but actual vasobiliary fistulas are uncommon. A percutaneous approach from the ventral aspect of the abdomen can also be used as the stenosis can be easily seen by injecting contrast into the sheath. Depth of the lesion can be determined from a prior CT or sonogram (19, 20).

Placement of Biliary Endoprostheses

Biliary drainage catheters extending from the intrahepatic ducts into the duodenum can be converted to permanent endoprostheses. A wire is passed through the catheter into the duodenum (usually a stiff THG or Lunderquist wire). Over this wire a stent is placed and pushed so that it both bridges the obstruction and enters the duodenum. An angioplasty balloon catheter is usually used to push the endoprosthesis. A loop of sutures extends from the proximal end of the stent to a polyethylene button which is placed subcutaneously, thus the prosthesis can be pulled. The combination of balloon catheter and suture control of the prosthesis allows the stent to be moved until optimal placement is achieved. A straight catheter is left in the ductal system peripheral to the stent for access and drainage.

It is important that the patient be drained externally for a period of time until the bile is less viscous to decrease the likelihood of obstruction of the stent. After 2–4 days, the external catheter is removed if a cholangiogram demonstrates that the stent remains in proper position. The complication rate has been reported to be 13% and includes migration and perforation of the duodenum and portal biliary fistula. If the stents become either obstructed or migrate, they may be replaced either percutaneously or endoscopically (21, 22). Recently the use of very large endoprostheses inserted via a peroral endoscopic-transhepatic push-pull method has been described (23).

Biliary Stenosis Dilatation

Dilatation of a benign biliary tract stenosis can be an attractive alternative to surgery. These strictures are usually postoperative and successful dilatation is more likely within two months of the surgery. A balloon catheter is placed over a wire bridging the stenosis and inflated. It is important that the catheter be made of polyethylene or wire reinforced polyvinyl as a simple polyvinyl balloon will not tolerate the stress of the stenosis dilatation. A biliary drainage catheter is then placed through the stenosis as a stent. A cholangiogram is then performed within several days to weeks after the procedure to assess its success. Although choledochoenterostomy strictures may not require stenting after dilatation, intrinsic biliary strictures probably do. The optimal duration of stenting is unclear, as is the long-term success rate (20, 24).

Drainage of an Obstructed Left Hepatic System

If only the left hepatic system is obstructed, a left hepatic puncture may be made and a catheter advanced into the duodenum as described previously. If both sides are obstructed and do not communicate, a catheter may be advanced through the obstruction into the left intrahepatic system via the right tract. This is achieved by placing a wire through the existing catheter from the right system into the duodenum to maintain access into the duodenum. Over this wire a 9 French sheath is advanced and a second wire placed. The first wire should be set aside so that access to the tract beyond the obstruction into the duodenum is not lost. The second wire is the working wire and over this wire a 6.5 French RIM (Cook, Inc.) catheter is advanced. This catheter has a sharp curve in it and can be used to seek out the orifice of the left ducts. When the orifice is found, a Benson wire is gently passed through the obstruction into the left ducts and is followed by the catheter. A stiff wire (usually a THG wire) is then placed through the catheter instead of the probing wire. The catheter is removed and several dilators passed over this wire into the left ducts. An 8 to 10 French feeding tube with multiple sideholes or an APD Drain (Medi-tech, Inc.) can then be passed along the wire into the left ducts. The right drainage system is then replaced and the patient left on external drainage until any hemobilia clears. The tubes then can be joined at their proximal ends with a male-male connector. This will allow internal drainage of bile and little external paraphernalia. Two endoprostheses can also be placed although it is usually difficult if not impossible to get an endoprosthesis into the left ducts via the right tract. A right endoprosthesis may be placed in addition to a feeding tube in the left allowing continued access but with only one external catheter (Fig. 18.11).

Biliary Stone Removal

Percutaneous biliary stone extraction usually is performed through a T-tube tract that has been allowed to mature for 4–6 weeks. A catheter and wire may be placed along the T-tube tract so that the catheter tip is immediately proximal to the calculus. A steerable basket is then placed through this 9 French catheter and the stone ensnared. The stone and catheter can then be removed together. As this occurs via a mature T-tube tract it may be unnecessary to keep a wire through the tract to the duodenum, however, leaving a wire as a safety guide can be helpful to speed the procedure. Manipulation of the stone with an angiographic catheter passed over a wire may be useful to place the stone in a position that is closer to the T-tube tract and

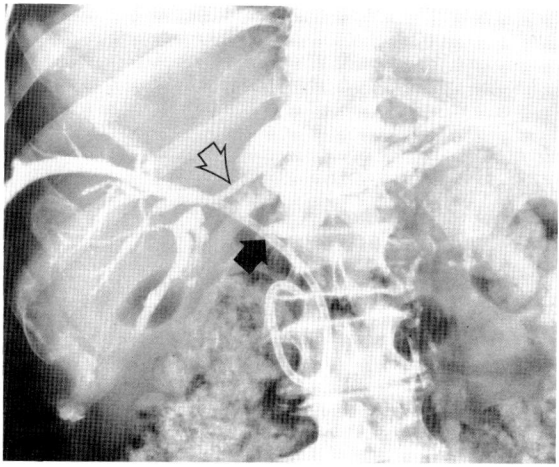

FIGURE 18.11. DRAINAGE OF AN OBSTRUCTED, ISOLATED LEFT SYSTEM

The drain decompressing the left duct (*open arrow*) is present and attached to the right drain (*closed arrow*) to allow the entire biliary tree to drain internally.

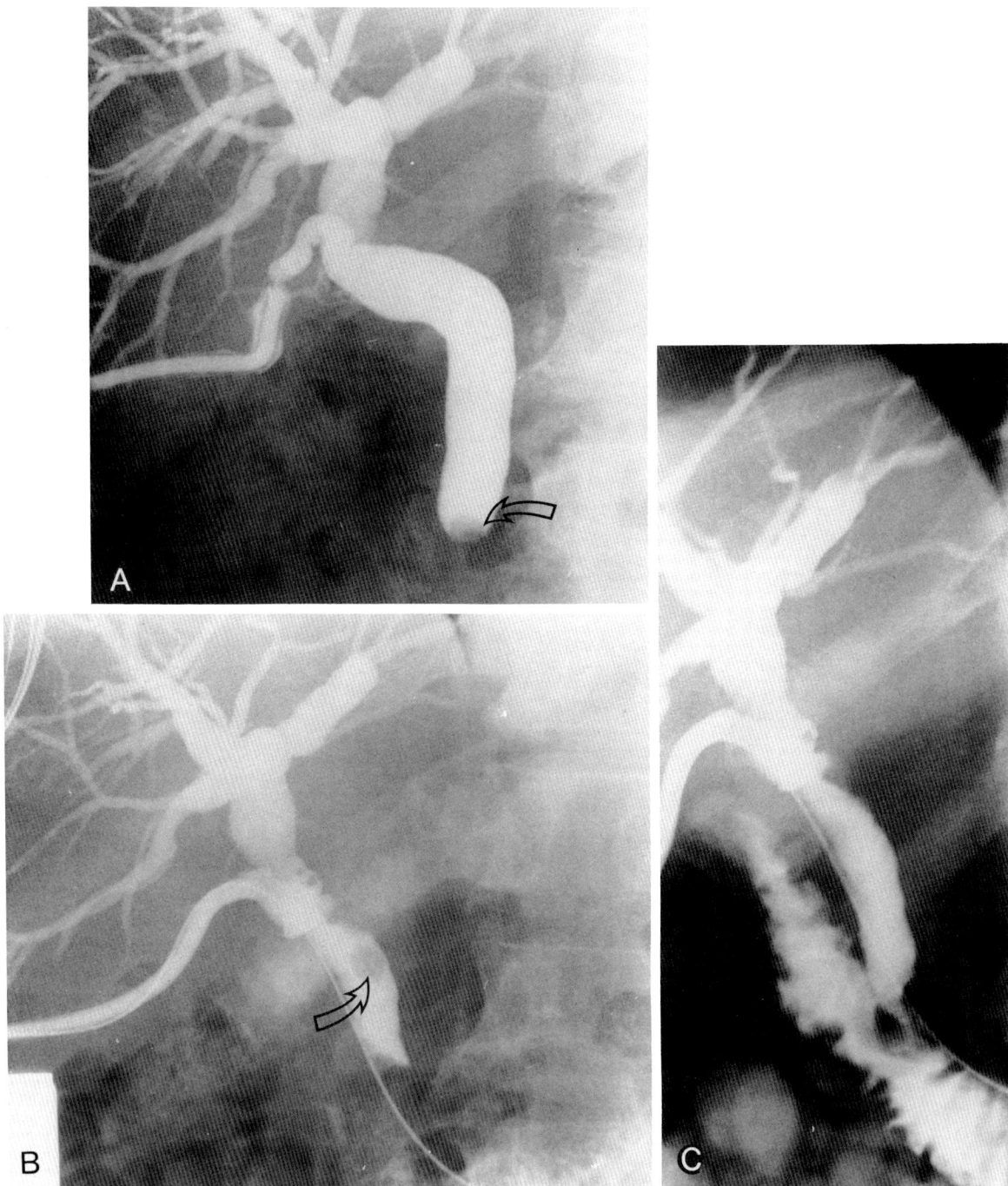

FIGURE 18.12. T-TUBE TRACT STONE EXTRACTION USING GUIDEWIRE, BALLOON, AND FRAGMENTATION
A: Cholangiogram through steerable catheter: stone (*arrow*) impacted at ampulla which could not be snared. *B:* Guidewire advanced into duodenum, Gruntzig balloon passed into duodenum, inflated and stone (*arrow*) pulled back into common bile duct, where it was snared. The stone was then pulled against the T-tube tract and fragmented. The fragments were then snared and extracted. *C:* Completion cholangiogram: no calculi. Note edema at the ampulla.

therefore more accessible to the stone basket (Fig. 18.12). Retained stones in the intrahepatic ducts may be flushed into the common bile duct with injections of contrast or saline or manipulation with either a wire or angiographic catheter (25, 26). Large stones may require fragmentation

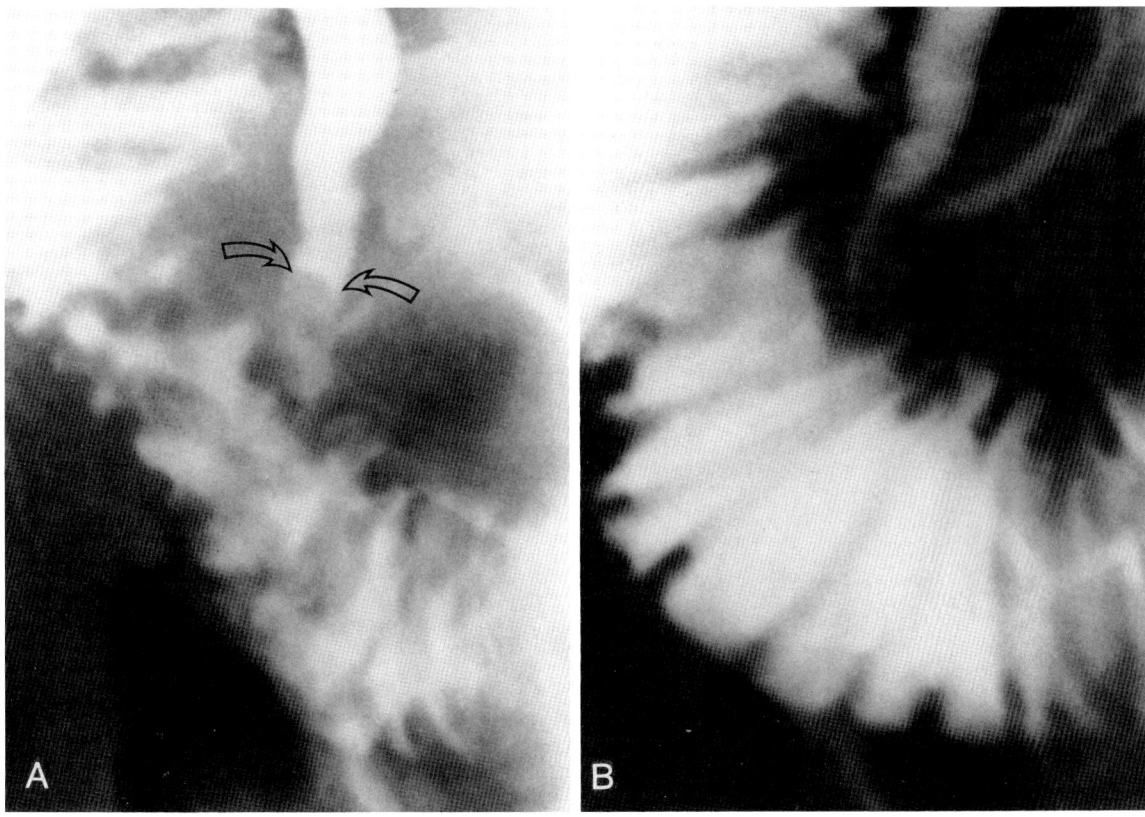

FIGURE 18.13. T-TUBE TRANSAMPULLARY STONE DELIVERY

Stone (*arrows, A*) impacted at ampulla which could not be snared. Completion cholangiogram shows absence of stone (*B*) after intravenous glucagon administration and pushing of the stone into the duodenum with the steerable catheter.

by the basket or even lithotripsy before they can be removed. Infusion of monooctanoin may be helpful to reduce size of cholesterol stones, or occasionally, completely dissolve them (27, 28). If stones cannot be removed via the T-tube tract they can sometimes be pushed through the ampulla into the duodenum (Fig. 18.13). Overall, percutaneous stone removal via the T-tube tract is successful in about 95% of cases (29). Although endoscopic sphincterotomy with or without stone extraction is the preferred nonsurgical therapy for common duct calculi when no T-tube tract is present, percutaneous transhepatic stone extraction is a feasible alternative when the endoscopic technique is unsuccessful or the required expertise is unavailable. Rather large stones can be safely extracted through the liver, although pushing them through the ampulla seems preferable (30) (Fig. 18.14). When necessary, balloon dilatation of the ampulla can be performed to permit stone passage (31).

Percutaneous Transhepatic Portography

A variation on the transhepatic cholangiography theme is the percutaneous transhepatic portal venogram (Fig. 18.15). The procedure is that of a transhepatic cholangiogram except one injects contrast searching for portal venous flow rather than stasis in a duct. Portal veins can be recognized by characteristic flow to the lateral portion of the liver or centrally and inferiorly if there is hepatofugal flow in portal hypertension. A catheter is then advanced into the portal vein and an injection of contrast can then be made. Sequential filming will reveal hepatofugal or hepatopetal flow of contrast and permit evaluation of the portal venous system. Recanalization of the umbilical vein can be seen as well as esophageal or gastric varices. Occlusion of the portal vein due to tumor or thrombus is easily noted (32).

Selective catheterization of the coronary vein may be performed for sclerosis of bleeding esophageal varices. Occlusive agents which have been used include stainless steel coils, Gelfoam, and alcohol. Unfortunately, this treatment has not resulted in long-term cures and is most useful as a temporizing measure (33–38). It has been supplanted to a large extent by endoscopic sclero-

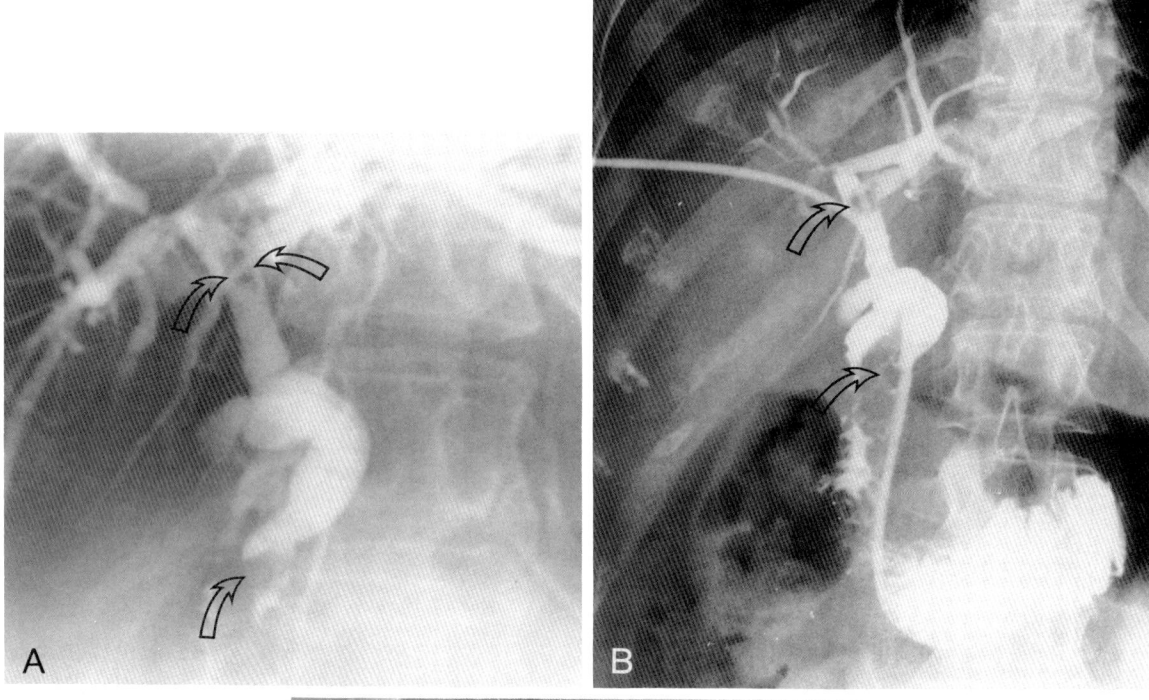
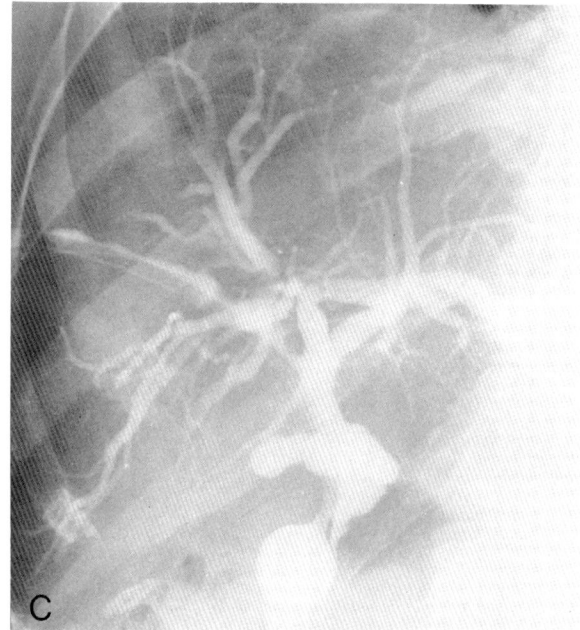

FIGURE 18.14. PERCUTANEOUS TRANSHEPATIC STONE REMOVAL

Elderly woman with metastatic breast cancer and two known retained calculi (these were impacted to the extent that they could not be removed at surgery). Postoperatively, the T-tube fell out and the tract could not be recannulated. The patient had had a sphincteroplasty for ampullary stenosis and ERCP was unsuccessful. *A:* Transhepatic cholangiogram: two retained stones (*arrows*). *B:* Ring catheter in duodenum bypassing the calculi. A tract was allowed to form and dilated up to 14 F. The stones were dislodged by inflating a Gruntzig balloon catheter distal to them and forcibly pulling back on the catheter. The distal calculus was pushed into the duodenum, but the proximal stone had to be extracted through the liver. This was done without complication, despite the stone's size of 8–10 mm. *C:* Completion cholangiogram: no calculi. A Foley catheter had to be inflated to retain the contrast in the biliary tree because of the sphincteroplasty. It was left in the biliary tree and slowly withdrawn over the course of a week as one would do with a T-tube.

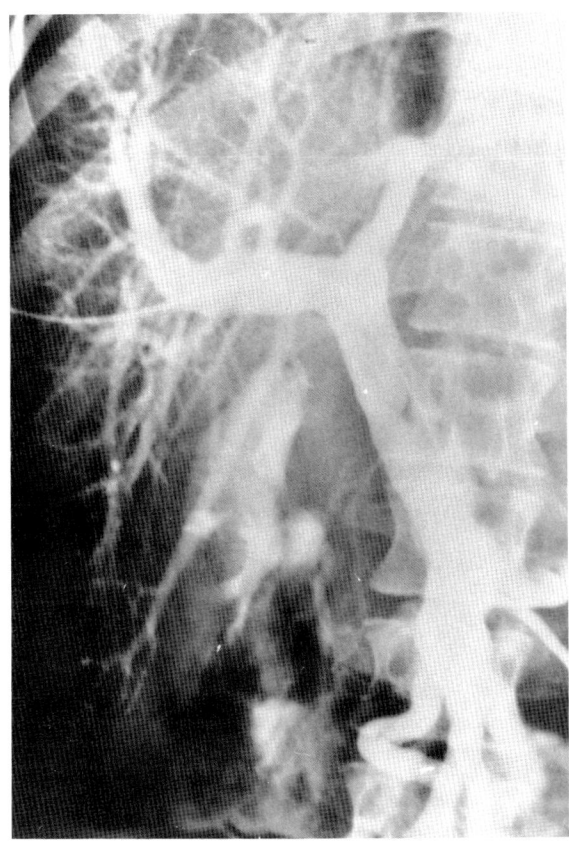

FIGURE 18.15. TRANSHEPATIC PORTOGRAM
Filling of superior mesenteric vein but not splenic vein—splenic vein occlusion.

therapy. Transhepatic portal venography is also employed for pancreatic venous sampling to evaluate islet cell tumors.

When the transhepatic portal venography is terminated a small 2 × 4 mm plug of Gelfoam is placed through the catheter into the liver parenchyma as the catheter is withdrawn. This stanches any hemorrhage into the liver parenchyma. Complications of this procedure are unusual and certainly are no greater than the usual angiographic risks.

Percutaneous Cholecystostomy

When PTC is not possible for technical or other reasons, percutaneous cholecystostomy offers an alternative for biliary interventions or cholangiography. It offers a therapeutic alternative to surgical cholecystostomy in patients with acute cholecystitis. The gallbladder is generally localized sonographically, and the actual puncture is made either using fluoroscopic or sonographic guidance. An anterior transhepatic approach is favored to minimize the risk of intraperitoneal bile leakage. The remainder of the procedure is carried out fluoroscopically. As vasovagal reactions have been reported after gallbladder puncture, atropine and other life-support equipment should be at hand (39, 40).

Radiation Therapy

Internal radiation therapy via radium or iridium seeds and/or wires implanted into indwelling biliary catheters has had effectiveness in palliation of extrahepatic bile duct cancers and metastatic or lymphomatous periportal adenopathy. Combined interstitial and external radiation has resulted in long-term survival of some patients with cholangiocarcinoma (40–42).

REFERENCES

1. Warren KW, Athanassiades S, Monge J: Primary sclerosing cholangitis. *Am J Surg* 111:23, 1965.
2. Pien EH, Zeman RK, Benjamin SB, Barth KH, Jaffe MH, Choyke PL, Clark LR, Paushter DM: Iatrogenic sclerosing cholangitis following hepatic arterial chemotherapy infusion. *Radiology* 156:329, 1985.
3. Martin EC, Fankuchen EI, Laffey KJ, Sibley RE: Percutaneous management of benign biliary disease. *Gastrointest Radiol* 9:207–212, 1984.
4. Ross AP, Braasch JW: Ulcerative colitis and carcinoma of the proximal bile duct. *Gut* 14:94, 1973.
5. Warren KW, Mountain JD, Lloyd-Jones W: Malignant tumors of the bile ducts. *Br J Surg* 59:501, 1972.
6. Bismuth H, Malt RA: Carcinoma of the biliary tract. *N Engl J Med* 301:704, 1979.
7. Arnaud JP, Graf P, Graanfort JL et al: Primary carcinoma of the gallbladder: review of 25 cases. *Am J Surg* 138:403, 1979.
8. Ferrucci JT, Wittenberg J, Sarno RA, Dreyfuss JR: Fine needle transhepatic cholangiography: a new approach to obstructive jaundice. *AJR* 127:403, 1976.
9. Cady B, Macdonald JS, Gunderson LL: Cancer of the hepatobiliary system. In DeVita VT, Hellman S, Rosenberg SA (ed): *Cancer: Principles and Practice of Oncology*. Philadelphia, J. B. Lippincott, 1985, pp 741–770.
10. Hoffman AF, Schmack B, Thistle JL et al: Clinical experience with monooctanoin for dissolution of bile duct stones: An uncontrolled multicenter trial. *Dig Dis Sci* 26:954–955, 1981.
11. Babbitt DP, Starshak RK, Clemett AR: Choledochal cyst: a concept of etiology. *AJR* 119:57, 1973.
12. Makuuchi M, Bandai Y, Ito T et al: Ultrasonically guided percutaneous transhepatic bile drainage. *Radiology* 136:165–169, 1980.
13. Oleaga JA, McLean GK, Frieman DB, King EJ: Interventional biliary radiology. In King EJ, McLean GK (eds): *Interventional Radiology Principles and Techniques*. Boston, Little, Brown, Company, 1981, pp 245–378.
14. Neff CC, Mueller PR, Ferrucci JT Jr et al: Serious complications following transgression of the pleural

space in drainage procedures. *Radiology* 152:335–341, 1984.
15. Ferrucci JT Jr, Mueller PR, Harbin WP: Percutaneous transhepatic biliary drainage: technique, results and applications. *Radiology* 135:1, 1980.
16. Cope C: Improved anchoring of nephrostomy catheters: loop technique. *AJR* 135:402, 1980.
17. Carrasco, HC: Personal communication.
18. Mueller PR, Ferrucci JT Jr, Van Sonnenberg E et al: Obstruction of the left hepatic duct: diagnosis and treatment by selective fine-needle cholangiography and percutaneous biliary drainage. *Radiology* 145:534–536, 1982.
19. Walker AN, Feldman PS, Covell JL, Tegtmeyer C: Fine needle aspiration under percutaneous transhepatic cholangiographic guidance. *Acta Cytol* 26:767–771, Nov-Dec, 1982.
20. Moore PT, Clark RA: An update of interventional biliary radiology. *Semin Utrasound CT MR* 5:349–368, 1984.
21. Jonsson K, Hellekant C: Percutaneous insertion of an endoprosthesis in obstructive jaundice. *Radiology* 139:749, 1981.
22. Coons HG, Carey PH: Biliary endoprosthesis: yes or no? *AJR* 145:429, 1985.
23. Kerlan RK, Ring EJ, Pogany AC et al: Biliary endoprosthesis insertion using a combined per oral transhepatic method. *Radiology* 150:828–830, 1984.
24. Burhenne HJ, Morris DC: Biliary stricture dilatation: Use of the Gruntzig balloon catheter. *J Can Assoc Radiol* 31:196–197, 1980.
25. Ellman BA, Berman HL: Treatment of common duct stones via transhepatic approach. *Gastrointest Radiol* 6:357, 1981.
26. Perez MR, Oleaga JA, Freiman DB, McLean GK, Ring EJ: Removal of a distal common bile duct stone through percutaneous transhepatic catheterization. *Arch Surg* 114:107, 1979.
27. Teplick SK, Haskin PH: Monooctanoin perfusion for in vivo dissolution of biliary stones: a series of 11 patients. *Radiology* 153:379, 1984.
28. Butch RJ, MacCarty RL, Mueller PR, Ferrucci JT Jr, Simeone JF, Teplick SK, Haskin PH: Monooctanoin perfusion treatment of intrahepatic calculi. *Radiology* 153:375, 1984.
29. Burhenne HJ: Percutaneous extraction of retained biliary tract stones: 661 patients. *AJR* 134:888–890, 1980.
30. Huggins MJ, Friedman AC, Fenster HA: Transhepatic removal of impacted intrahepatic and common duct stones: case report. *Milit Med* 148:935–937, 1983.
31. Centola CAP, Jander HP, Stauffer A et al: Balloon dilatation of the papilla of Vater to allow biliary stone passage. *AJR* 136:613–614, 1981.
32. Lunderquist A, Vang J: Transhepatic catheterization and obliteration of the coronary vein in patients with portal hypertension and esophageal varices. *N Engl J Med* 291:646, 1974.
33. Yune HY, Klatte EC, Richmond BD et al: Absolute ethanol in thrombotherapy of bleeding esophageal varices. *AJR* 138:1137, 1982.
34. Keller FS, Rosch J, Dotter CT et al: Embolization in the treatment of bleeding gastroesophageal varices. *Semin Roentgenol* 16:103, 1981.
35. Witt WS, Goncharenko V, O'Leary JP et al: Interruption of esophageal varices. Steel coil technique. *AJR* 135:829, 1980.
36. Uflacker R: Percutaneous transhepatic obliteration of gastroesophageal varices using absolute alcohol. *Radiology* 146:621, 1983.
37. Keller FS, Rosch J, Dotter CT: Transhepatic obliteration of gastroesophageal varices with absolute ethanol. *Radiology* 146:615, 1983.
38. Sos TA: Transhepatic portal venous embolization of varices: pros and cons (opinion). *Radiology* 148:569, 1983.
39. Pearse DM, Hawkins IF Jr., Shaver R, Vagel S: Percutaneous cholecystostomy in acute cholecystitis and common duct obstruction. *Radiology* 152:365–367, 1984.
40. VanSonnenberg E, Wing VW, Pollard JW, Casola G: Life threatening reactions associated with percutaneous cholecystostomy. *Radiology* 151:377, 1984.
41. Hershkovic A, Heaston D, Engler MJ et al: Irradiation of biliary carcinoma. *Radiology* 139:219–222, 1981.
42. Conroy RM, Shahbazian AA, Edwards KC et al: A new method for treating carcinomatous biliary obstruction with intracatheter radium. *Cancer* 49:1321–1327, 1982.
43. Hishikawa Y, Shimada T, Miura T et al: Radiation therapy of carcinoma of the extrahepatic bile ducts. *Radiology* 146:787–789, 1983.

SECTION III
The Pancreas

19

Embryology, Anatomy, Histology, and Physiology

ARNOLD C. FRIEDMAN, M.D., AND MARK T. BIRNS, M.D.

EMBRYOLOGY

The pancreas arises as two diverticula off the foregut. Together with the common bile duct, the ventral diverticulum rotates backward behind the duodenum to fuse with the dorsal diverticulum. The ventral diverticulum becomes most of the head of the pancreas as well as the uncinate process (Fig. 19.1A–D).

The main pancreatic duct is a combination of the fusion of the ducts of the dorsal and ventral pancreas at approximately 6 weeks in the developing fetus. The proximal end of the duct of the ventral pancreas fuses to the duct of the dorsal pancreas between the middle and the distal third of the latter duct (1). Thus, the main pancreatic duct beginning in the head of the pancreas is derived from the ventral portion and the proximal pancreatic duct from the dorsal portion of the gland. The accessory pancreatic duct, the duct of Santorini, is the remaining distal portion of the dorsal pancreatic duct and empties into the duodenum via the minor papilla. The main pancreatic duct, or duct of Wirsung, is the main excretory pathway in approximately 91% of adults (1, 2), variations are common. To parallel the nomenclature of the biliary tree, the pancreatic duct in the tail is referred to as "proximal" and that in the head as "distal" in this book.

Tubules bud off the main ducts and give rise laterally and at blind ends to the vesicles which differentiate into acini. Both acinar cells (exocrine) and islet cells (endocrine) are derived from duct epithelium, which retains its multipotential nature into adulthood. Solid nests of cells along the embryonal ducts detach from the lumen and become the islets of Langerhans. Some acinar cells retain their ductal character and connect acini to the ducts (Fig. 19.2).

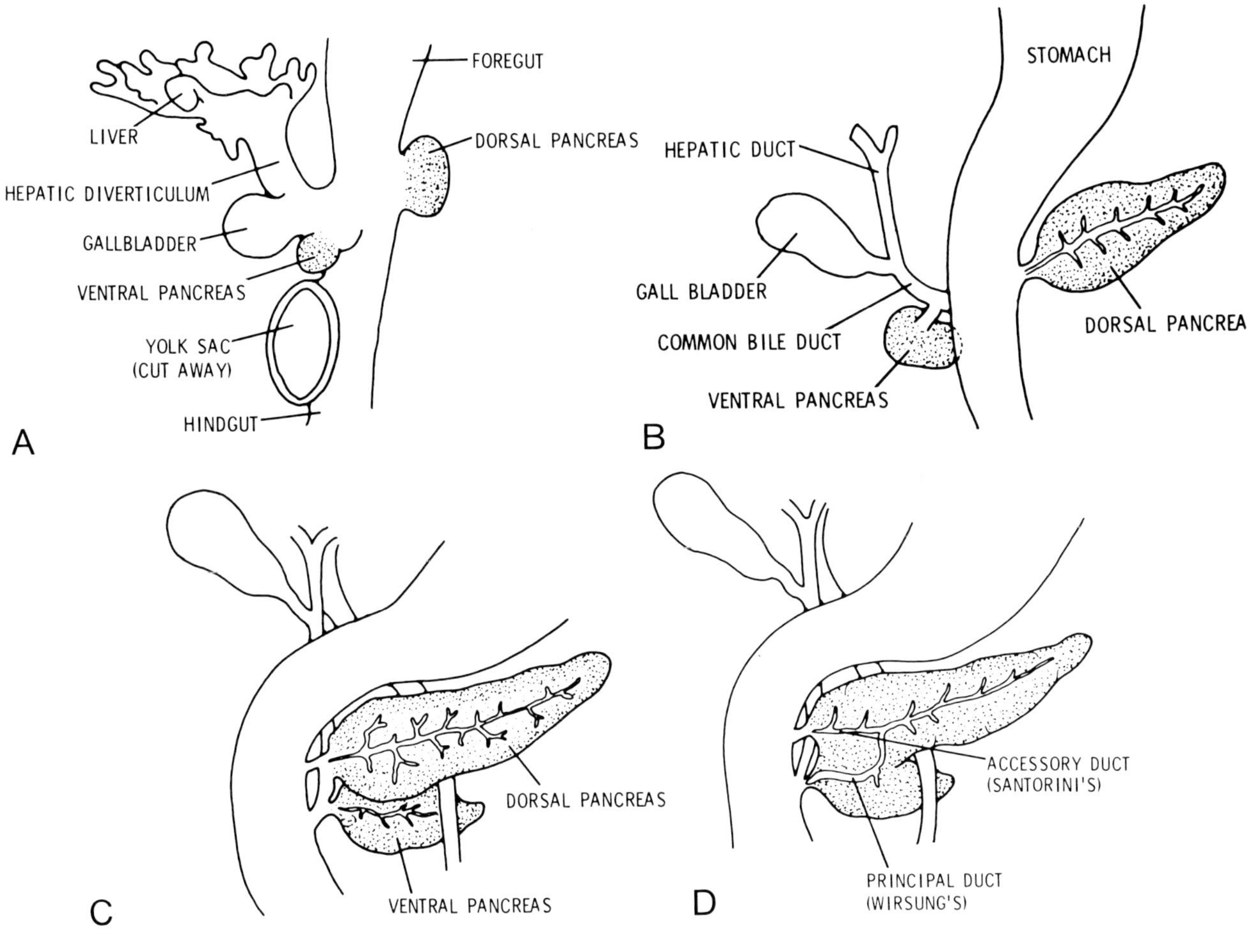

FIGURE 19.1. SUCCESSIVE STAGES OF DEVELOPMENT OF THE PANCREAS

ANATOMY

The adult pancreas is approximately 15 cm in length, 3–5 cm in width, and 2–3 cm in thickness with an average weight of 80 g. Its surface is pale yellow-tan, finely nodular, and firm to palpation (3).

The posterior surface of the gland is devoid of peritoneum except for the tail—thus, the head and body are retroperitoneal and the tail is intraperitoneal since it is ensheathed within the splenorenal ligament. It is connected to the splenic flexure via the splenorenal and phrenicocolic ligaments (Fig. 19.3) (4). The pancreas extends from the duodenal loop to the splenic hilum diagonally across the body at about the L1–L2 level (Fig. 19.4). The head is globular and gives rise to the uncinate process which projects like a hook to the left behind the superior mesenteric vein. The neck narrows, goes behind the pylorus and in front of the portal vein and widens as it becomes the body, which bulges up almost to the level of the celiac axis. The transverse mesocolon attaches to the anterior surface of the head and the inferior aspect of the body and tail (Fig. 19.5). The root of the small bowel mesentery attaches near the inferior border of the

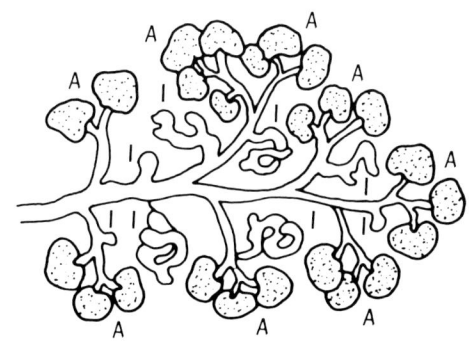

FIGURE 19.2. DEVELOPMENT OF ACINI (*A*) AND ISLETS (*I*)

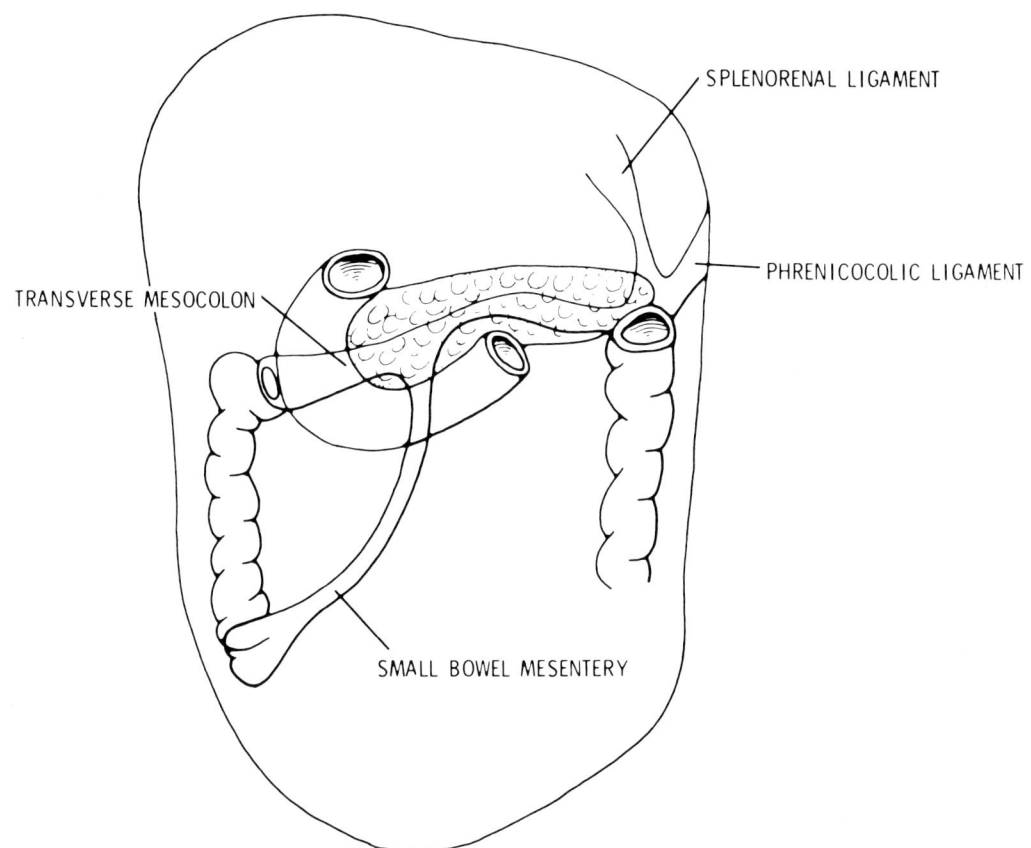

FIGURE 19.3. PERITONEAL ATTACHMENTS IN THE REGION OF THE PANCREAS

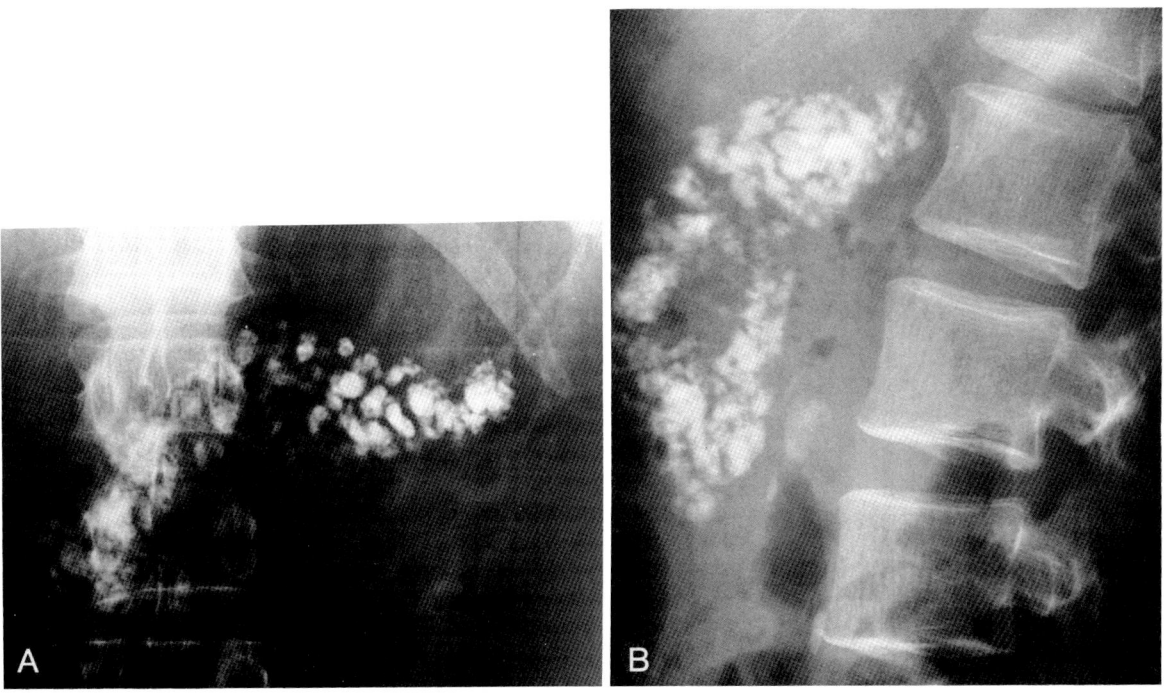

FIGURE 19.4. PANCREATIC IDIOPATHIC CALCIFICATION
AP and lateral films in a patient with idiopathic pancreatic calcification illustrating the normal position of the pancreas. The pancreas is, of course, normally invisible on plain radiography.

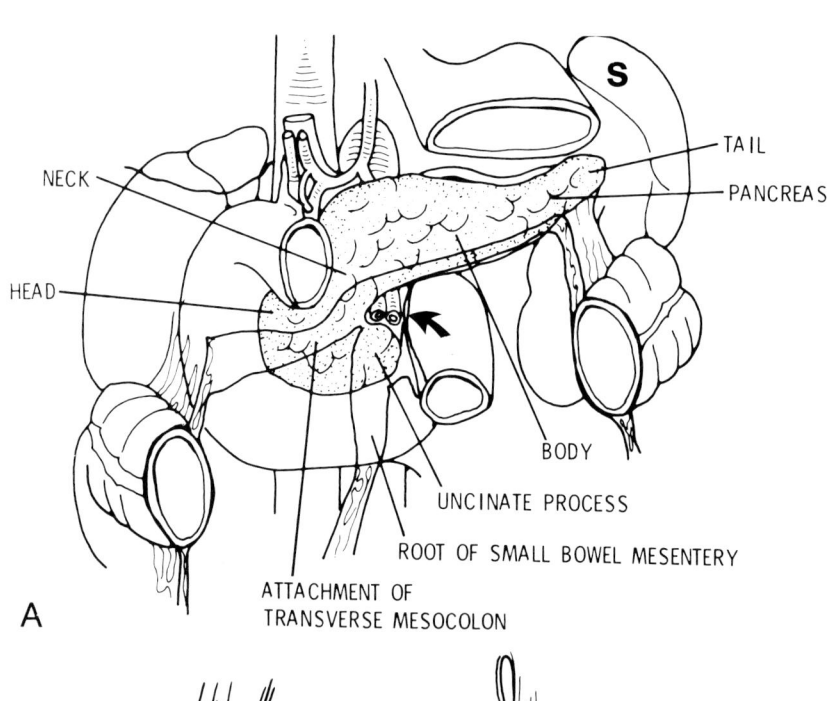
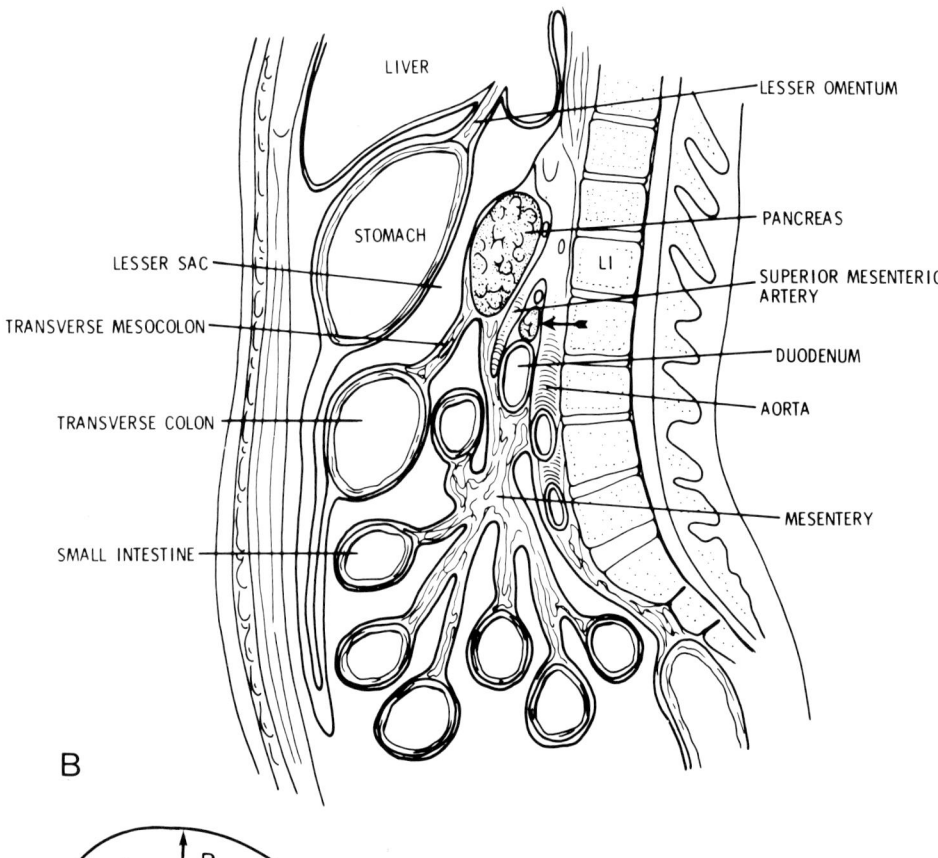
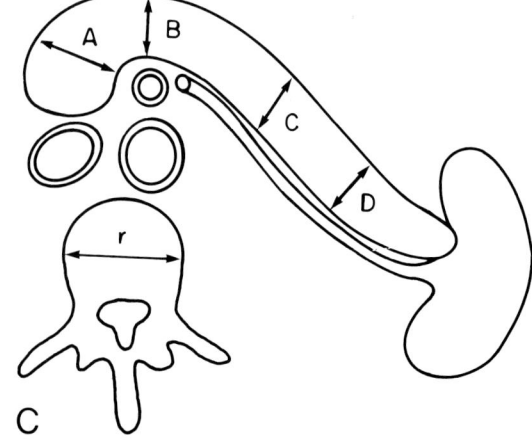

FIGURE 19.5. PANCREATIC ANATOMY
A: Anterior frontal view of the pancreas showing its relationships to the duodenum, superior mesenteric vessels (*arrow*), and mesenteric attachments, and spleen (*S*). *B:* Sagittal midline view through the head of the pancreas and uncinate process (*arrow*). *C:* Although absolute measurements cannot be relied upon, the following are offered as a guide: $A = 2.5$ cm, $B = 1.9$ cm, $C = 2.0$ cm, $D = 1.5$ cm, all ± 0.3 cm. Also the diameter of the head (*A*) should not exceed the transverse diameter of the vertebral body (*r*), and the diameter of the proximal body (*C*) should not exceed $2/3 r$.

pancreas (Fig. 19.5). The duodenojejunal junction at the ligament of Treitz just anterior and inferior to the pancreas demarcates the body and tail (4). The tail tapers as it curves posteriorly to cross the upper portion of the left kidney to enter the splenic hilum. Pancreatic size can be estimated from its transverse diameter (Fig. 19.5C).

RADIOLOGIC ANATOMY

Normal Sonographic Anatomy

The pancreas lies in the upper retroperitoneum in the anterior pararenal space draped across the aorta and inferior vena cava. It is divided anatomically into a head, neck, body and tail (5). The neck lies anterior to the superior mesenteric vein and proximal portion of the main portal vein which is formed by the junction of the superior mesenteric and splenic veins (Fig. 19.6). The head of the pancreas lies lateral to the neck, nestled in the C-loop of the duodenum (Fig. 19.7A). In this area it lies anterior to the inferior vena cava and right crus of the diaphragm. The inferior medial portion of the head is called the uncinate process which varies greatly in size. It lies posterior to the superior mesenteric vein and, in about 5% of patients,

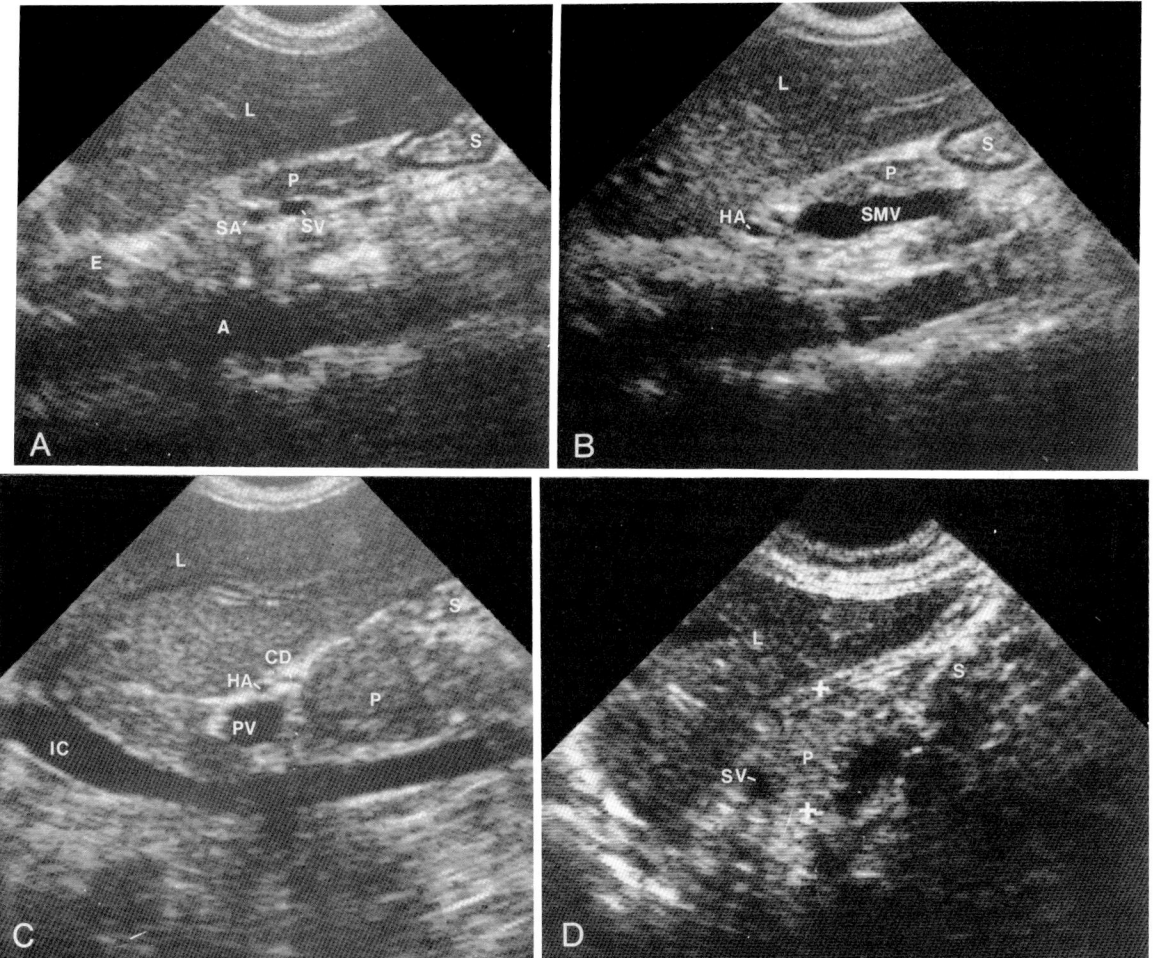

FIGURE 19.6. SONOGRAPHIC ANATOMY OF PANCREAS
Longitudinal scans of the normal pancreas through the area of the body (A), neck (B), head (C), and tail (D). See text. Aorta (A), pancreas (P), stomach (S), liver (L), hepatic artery (HA), splenic artery (SA), splenic vein (SV), and esophageal gastric junction (E).

posterior to the proximal superior mesenteric artery. Below the uncinate process, both these vessels cross the third portion of the duodenum to enter the small bowel mesentery. The actual position of the pancreatic head can vary and may be more to the left of the midline lying directly anterior to the abdominal aorta, or it may be more inferior and even lie as low as the sacral promontory (6, 7). Even with these variations in position, the pancreatic head still maintains its relationship to the duodenum and surrounding vascular structures, including the portal and superior mesenteric veins and the hepatic, splenic, and gastroduodenal arteries and common bile duct.

The body of the pancreas lies anterior to the abdominal aorta below the origin of the celiac axis and anterior to the origin of the superior mesenteric artery (Fig. 19.6). Connective tissue, small lymph nodes and a variable amount of fat are present between the anterior wall of the aorta and the posterior margin of the pancreas. The body is delineated on its right side by the neck of the pancreas and on its left by a line drawn alongside the lateral margin of the adjacent lumbar vertebral body (Fig. 19.7). To the left of this line lies the tail of the pancreas. It is related posteriorly to the left crus of the diaphragm, left adrenal gland and left kidney from which it is separated by the anterior portion of Gerota's fascia. The tail is usually at a more superior level (41%) or at the same level (51%) as the body, however, it can be at a lower level (2%) and its tip usually abuts the spleen just inferior to its hilus (8). When the left kidney has been removed, the tail assumes a more medial and dorsal

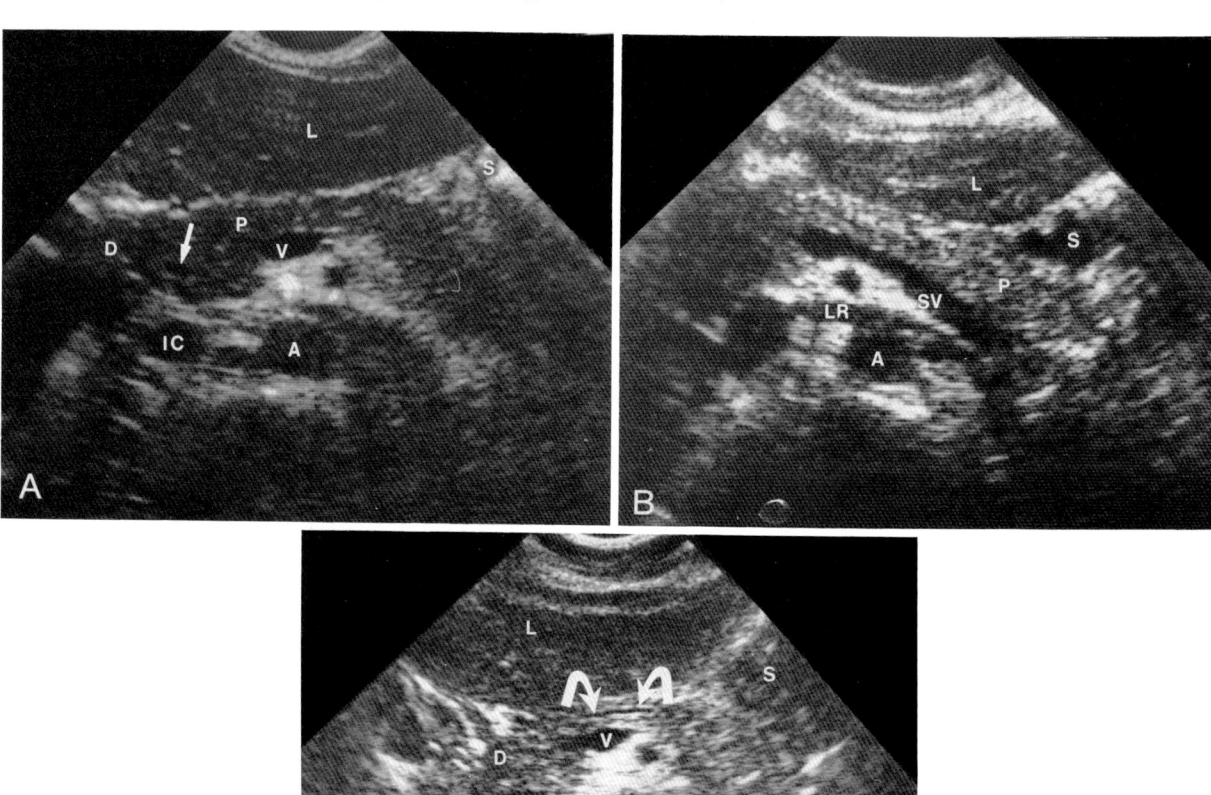

FIGURE 19.7. SONOGRAPHIC ANATOMY OF PANCREAS

Transverse scans of the normal pancreas. *A:* In scan the pancreatic tail is poorly seen. *B:* Following the ingestion of water it is better defined. *C:* Scan shows the normal pancreatic duct in the body of the pancreas. See text. Aorta (*A*), inferior vena cava (*IC*), pancreas (*P*), pancreatic duct (*curved arrows*), splenic vein-portal vein confluence (*V*), splenic vein (*SV*), common bile duct (*arrow*), duodenum (*D*), liver (*L*), stomach (*S*), and left renal vein (*LR*).

position. The anterior aspect of the neck, body, and tail including the upper anterior portion of the pancreatic head are related to the lesser sac which is a potential space that separates the pancreas from the stomach (Fig. 19.8). As mentioned previously, the relationship of the pancreas to the surrounding vascular anatomy is fairly constant (7). The splenic vein runs from the splenic hilus along the posterosuperior aspect of the pancreatic tail and body, slightly posterior and inferior to the splenic artery (Figs. 19.7 and 19.8). The splenic artery near the splenic hilus can lie anterior to the pancreatic tail depending upon the position of the tail and the tortuosity of the artery. The common hepatic artery can be seen arising from the celiac axis in most patients (92%) (9). It can be traced along the superior margin of the first portion of the duodenum where it divides into the proper hepatic artery and gastroduodenal artery (Fig. 19.6). The latter runs an inferior course onto the anterior surface of the pancreas near the junction of the neck and body where it divides into the superior pancreaticoduodenal artery and right gastroepiploic artery (Fig. 19.9). The proper hepatic artery courses superiorly along the anterior aspect of the portal vein medial to the common bile duct and in the porta hepatis divides into the right and left hepatic arteries. In about 15% of patients, the right hepatic artery arises from the proximal superior mesenteric artery in which case it (replaced right hepatic artery) runs along the posterior aspect of the portal vein to the porta hepatis where it enters the right lobe of the liver (10).

The normal common bile duct runs along the anterior margin of the main portal vein in the free edge of the lesser omentum with the proper hepatic artery along its medial aspect. The duct enters the pancreatic parenchyma where the portal vein crosses anterior to the inferior vena cava and can be identified running somewhat posteriorly and inferiorly in the pancreatic parenchyma to enter the second portion of the duodenum at the level of the ampulla of Vater (Figs. 19.7, 19.9–19.11). It is usually joined by the pan-

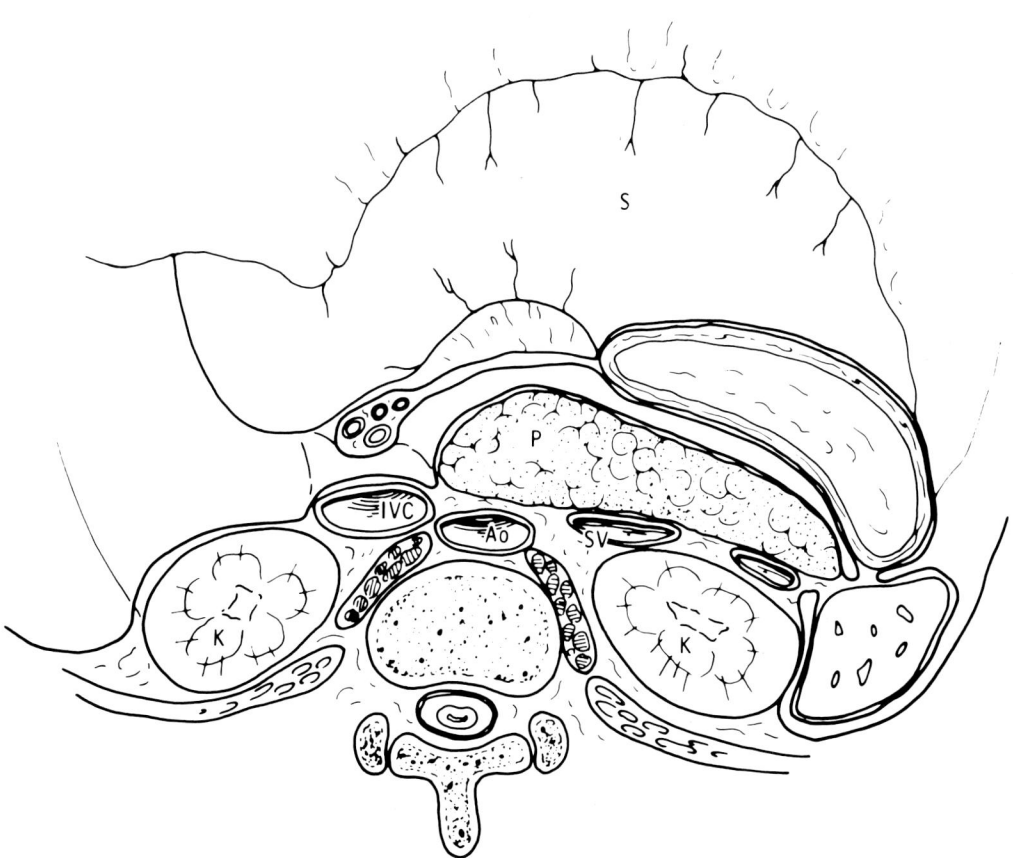

FIGURE 19.8. PANCREATIC ANATOMY

Axial view of the pancreas (*P*) showing its relationship to the stomach (*S*), kidneys (*K*), inferior vena cava (*IVC*), aorta (*Ao*) and spleen. The lesser sac is the potential space between the stomach and the pancreas.

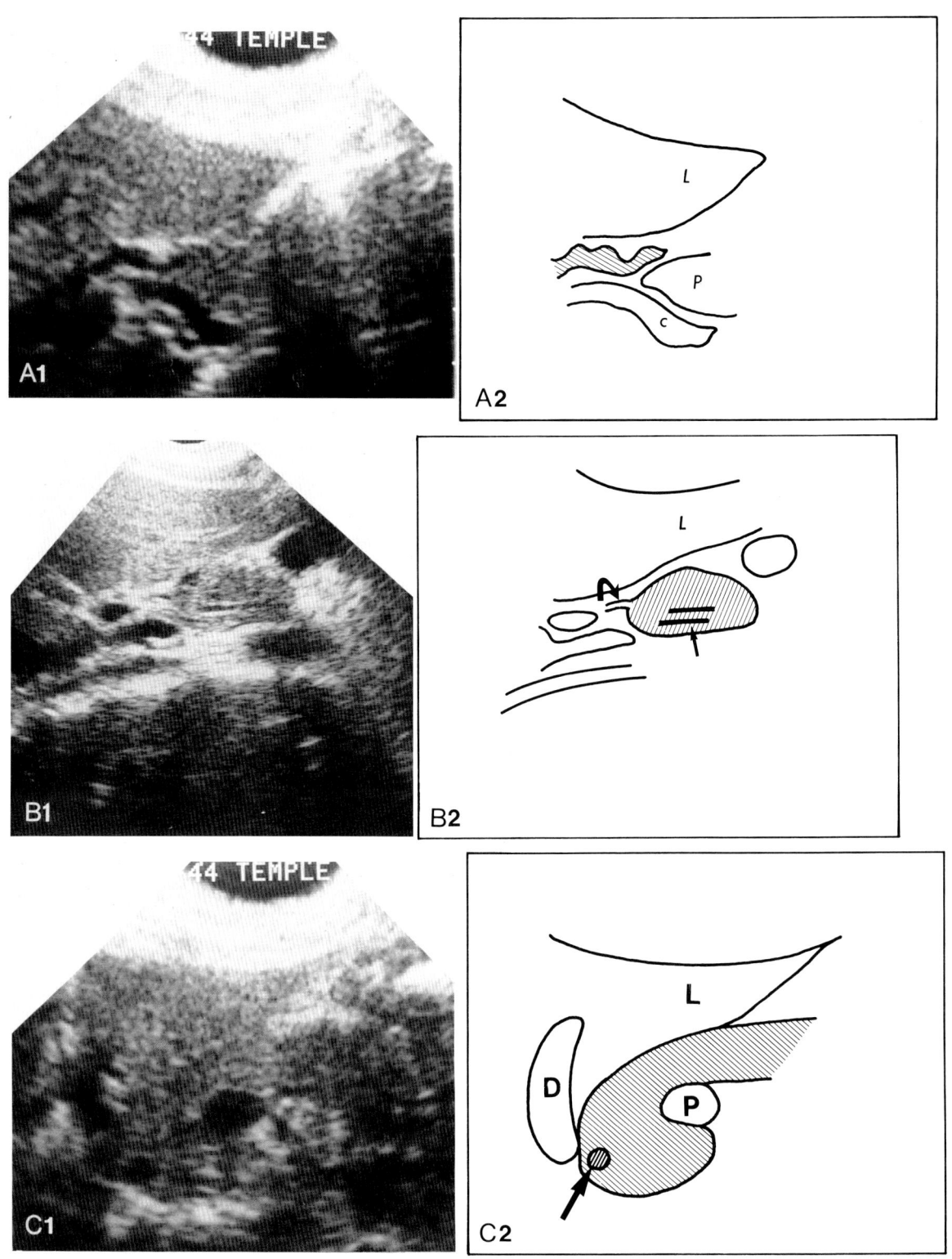

FIGURE 19.9. PANCREATIC ANATOMY

A: Sagittal sonogram through the neck of the pancreas showing the gastroduodenal artery (*shaded*), common duct (*C*), pancreas (*P*), and liver (*L*). *B:* Sagittal scan through the head of the pancreas (*shaded*). Intrapancreatic common bile duct is seen (*arrow*) as is gastroduodenal artery (*curved arrow*). *L* = liver. *C:* Transverse scan through head and body (*shaded*) shows pancreatic parenchyma nearly isoechoic to liver (*L*). The normal distal common duct is seen as a sonolucent circle (*arrow*). *D* = duodenum, *P* = confluence of superior mesenteric and splenic veins.

creatic duct just prior to where it enters the duodenum.

A thin layer of connective tissue surrounds the pancreas as it has no distinct capsule. Thin septa arise from this connective tissue layer and enter into the gland substance dividing it up into lobules. Each lobule is drained by a small branch of the pancreatic duct. Richly innervated peripancreatic areolar tissue dips in between lobules. The normal echogenicity of the pancreatic parenchyma is homogeneous and its echogenicity is at least equal to (48%) and in most cases is greater (52%) than that of the adjacent liver (Figs. 19.6 and 19.12) (11). The amount of fat present between the lobules of the gland and to a lesser extent the interlobular fibrous tissue determines the degree of echogenicity of the gland (12). The degree of fatty infiltration increases with age, however, it can also occur with marked obesity, diabetes mellitus, and steroid therapy (13, 14). Fatty replacement may be so marked that the echogenicity of the gland blends in with that of the surrounding retroperitoneal fat making the pancreatic outline impossible to identify (Fig. 19.13) (6, 11, 13, 14). In such patients, the gland can be assessed only by examining the normal anatomic landmarks of the gland and the homogeneity of its echogenicity. It is only by doing this that small focal processes in the gland will be detected (15). In comparing pancreatic echogenicity to that of the liver, one has to be certain that diffuse liver disease is not present and that a portion of liver at the same depth from the skin as the pancreas is used for comparison. This area should be within the focal zone of the transducer being used (16). If the fluid-filled stomach is used for visualization of the pancreas, the pancreas will appear more echogenic than liver at the same depth because of good through transmission through the fluid.

Normal intrapancreatic structures that can be identified include the common bile duct, pancreatic duct, and some small arterial and venous branches. The common bile duct in the head of the pancreas should measure no more than 4 mm in its internal diameter (Figs. 19.7 and 19.9). The main pancreatic duct (duct of Wirsung) can be seen in approximately 80% of patients in the central portion of the body of the pancreas (Figs. 19.7 and 19.14) (17–19). It is less frequently seen in the head (32%) or tail (12%). It may be seen as a fluid-filled tube with well-defined echogenic walls and should not have an internal diameter of greater than 2–3 mm (20, 21). It has been shown to increase slightly in size with age (22). When no fluid is present, it can be seen as a linear echogenic line. One should make sure not to mistake the hypoechoic posterior wall of the stomach or a vascular variant such as doublesplenic vein or a low-lying splenic artery as a dilated pancreatic duct (23). The accessory pancreatic duct (duct of Santorini) which runs transversely in the upper anterior portion of the pancreatic head is usually not seen sonographically (24). It drains into the duodenum superior and slightly anterior to the ampulla of Vater (5, 21). The anterior and posterior arcades of the superior and inferior pancreaticoduodenal arteries can sometimes be seen in the parenchyma of the pancreatic head just medial to the duodenum.

The size of the normal pancreas varies greatly and depends upon the age and size of the patient (25–27). Top normal measurements for the anteroposterior measurements for adults is given

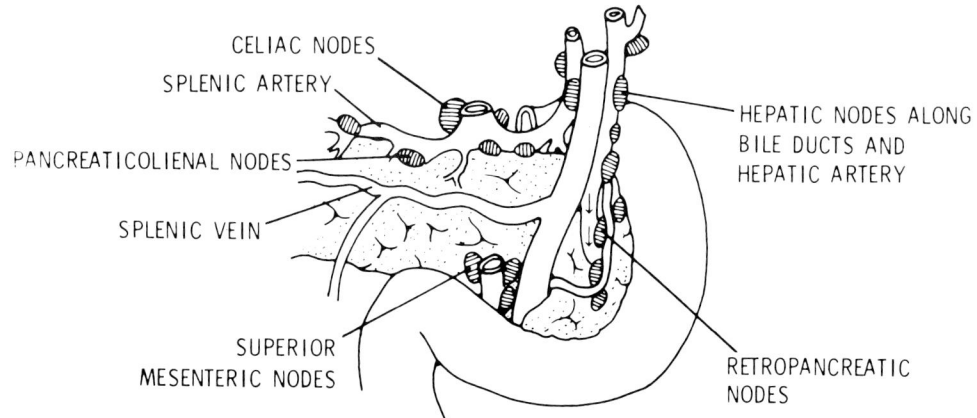

FIGURE 19.10. PANCREATIC ANATOMY

Posterior view of regional nodes also showing common bile duct (*arrows*) going through the pancreatic head before entering the duodenum.

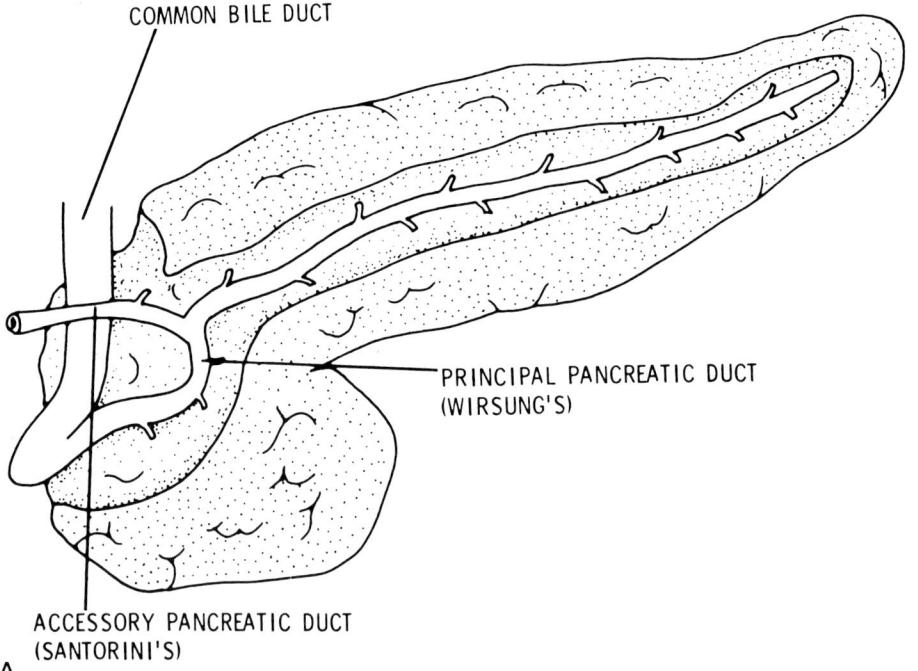
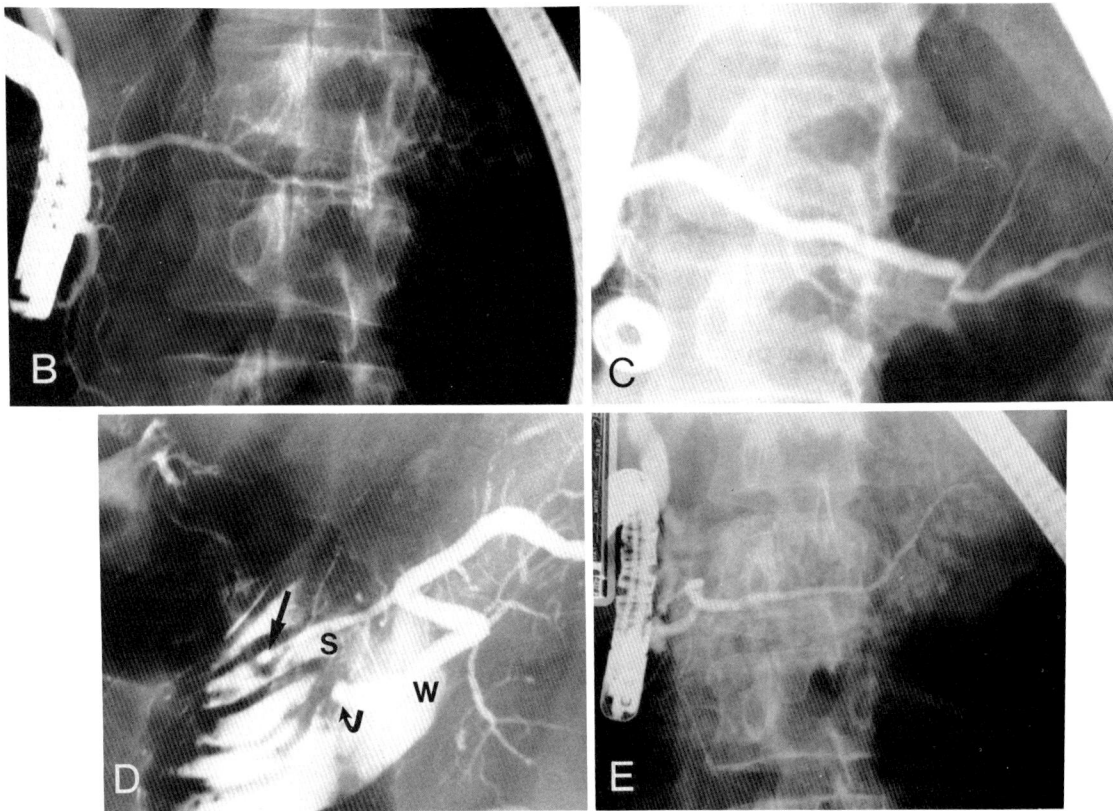

FIGURE 19.11. PANCREATIC ANATOMY

A: Anterior frontal view of the pancreas showing pancreaticobiliary ductal anatomy. *B:* Normal endoscopic retrograde pancreatogram in a young patient. Note good opacification of branches to the uncinate process inferiorly. Slight RPO projection. *C:* Slightly dilated main pancreatic duct which is normal for age in this 55-yr-old. *D:* Major (*curved arrow*) and minor (*straight arrow*) papillae and Santorini's duct (S) and the duct of Wirsung (W). *E:* Normal pancreatogram with acinarization due to overinjection.

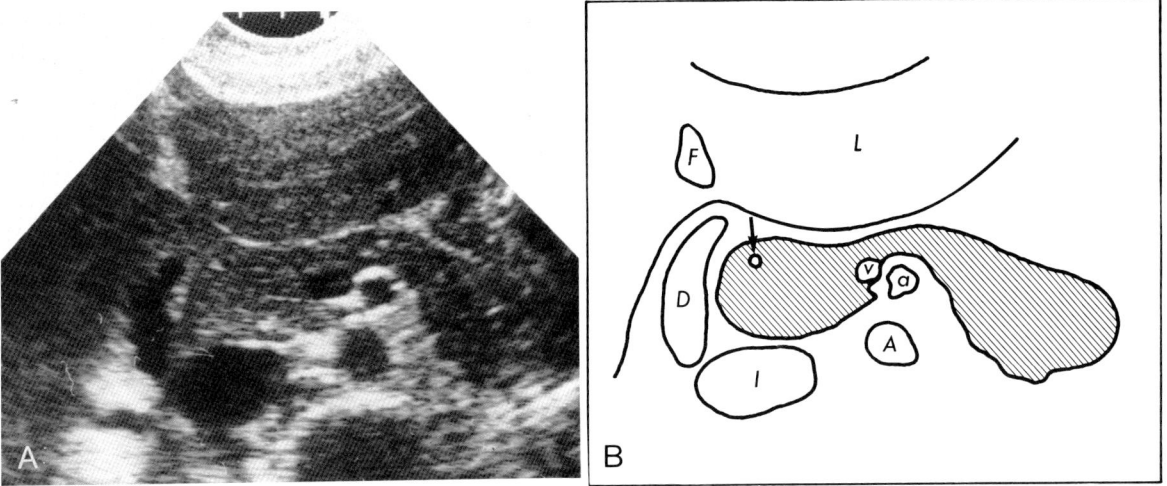

FIGURE 19.12. PANCREATIC ANATOMY

A and *B:* Normal transverse scan of the pancreas (*shaded*) with echo texture slightly greater than liver. *D* = duodenum, *L* = liver, *F* = fat in falciform ligament, *I* = inferior vena cava, *A* = aorta, *a* = superior mesenteric artery, *v* = superior mesenteric vein; *arrow* points to gastroduodenal artery.

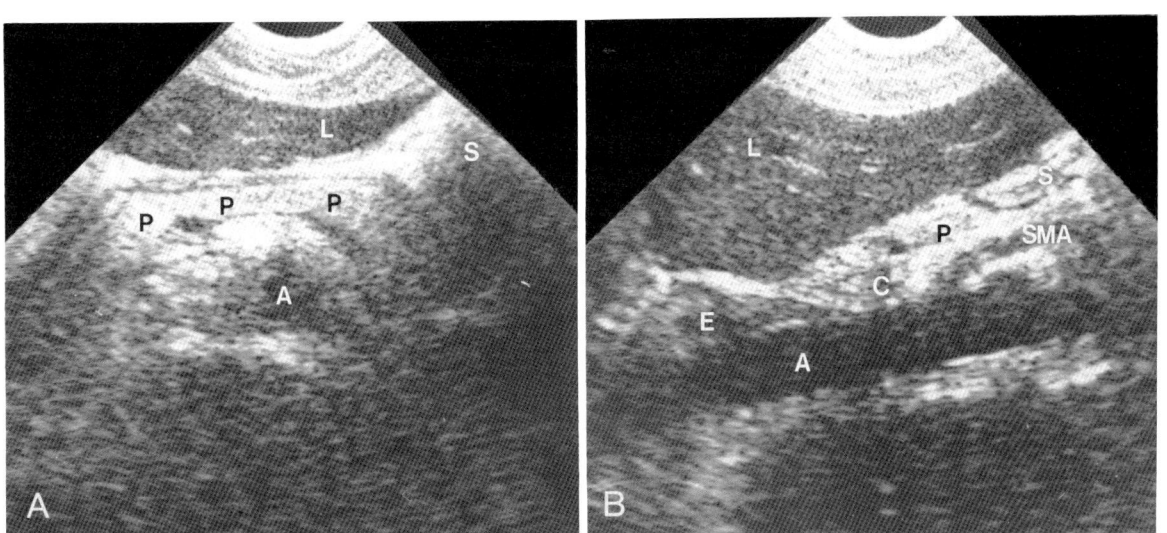

FIGURE 19.13. PANCREAS OBSCURED BY FAT

A and *B:* Transverse and longitudinal scans of the normal pancreas (*P*). The pancreatic outline is difficult to see as it blends with the surrounding retroperitoneal fat. See text. Aorta (*A*), celiac axis (*C*), superior mesenteric artery (*SMA*), Liver (*L*), esophageal gastric junction (*E*), and stomach (*S*).

as follows: 3 cm for the head, 1 cm for the neck, 2.2 cm for the body, and 2.8 cm for the tail. These measurements should be obtained from front-to-back at right angles to the long axis of the gland in the area being measured, since the pancreas is a curved organ draped across the spine and great vessels. The measurement of the gland can change as much as 8 mm depending upon the phase of respiration, being thicker in inspiration (28). The maximum craniocaudal dimensions for the gland are 6 cm for the head, 3.6 cm for the body, and 2.5 cm for the tail. One should be cautious about using absolute numbers in diagnosing pancreatic enlargement. The symmetry and contour of the gland have to be taken into account as the neck and body of the pancreas including the tail are smaller in their front-to-back dimensions than the head (29).

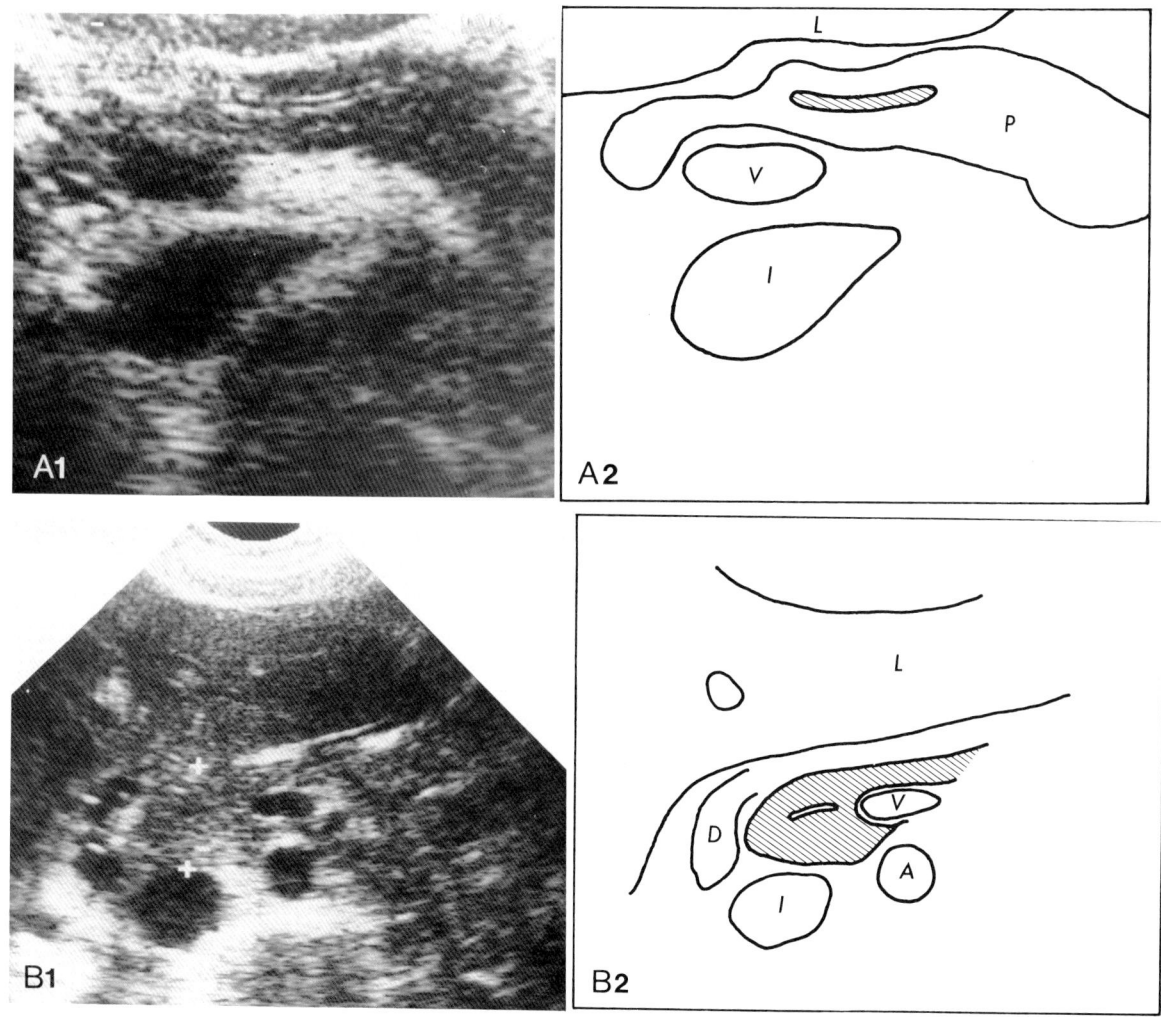

FIGURE 19.14. PANCREATIC DUCT
A: Normal pancreatic duct (*shaded*) on a transverse scan. Note echogenic walls. P = pancreas, I = inferior vena cava, V = confluence of superior mesenteric and splenic veins, L = liver. *B:* Normal pancreatic duct in transverse section of the head of the pancreas (*shaded*). Note pointed uncinate process behind venous confluence (V). L = liver, D = duodenum, I = inferior vena cava, A = aorta. *C:* Normal pancreatic duct (*shaded*) in the tail of the pancreas). Transverse scan. L = liver, V = confluence of superior mesenteric and splenic veins. *D:* Angled transverse scan of the normal pancreatic duct (*shaded*) in the neck and head. L = liver.

Sonography of the Pancreas

Technique of Examination

If a sonographic examination of the pancreas is to be performed, it is best done prior to any contemplated barium studies of the gastrointestinal tract. The dilute barium mixture used for CT scanning generally does not interfere with a pancreatic sonogram. Patients are kept fasting for 4–6 h prior to the examination but are allowed clear liquids up to 1 hr before the examination to prevent dehydration. We have not found degassing agents such as simethicone (80 mg 4 times a day for 2 days) to be clinically useful in providing better visualization of the pancreas.

The study is best performed with a real-time unit which allows more rapid evaluation of the gland. The highest frequency transducer (3.5–7.0 mHz) with an appropriate focal length should be used (16). If the patient is to be scanned in the upright position, the skin to pancreas distance is greater than in the supine position and might warrant a change in transducer to one that has a deeper focal zone (30). Scanning should be

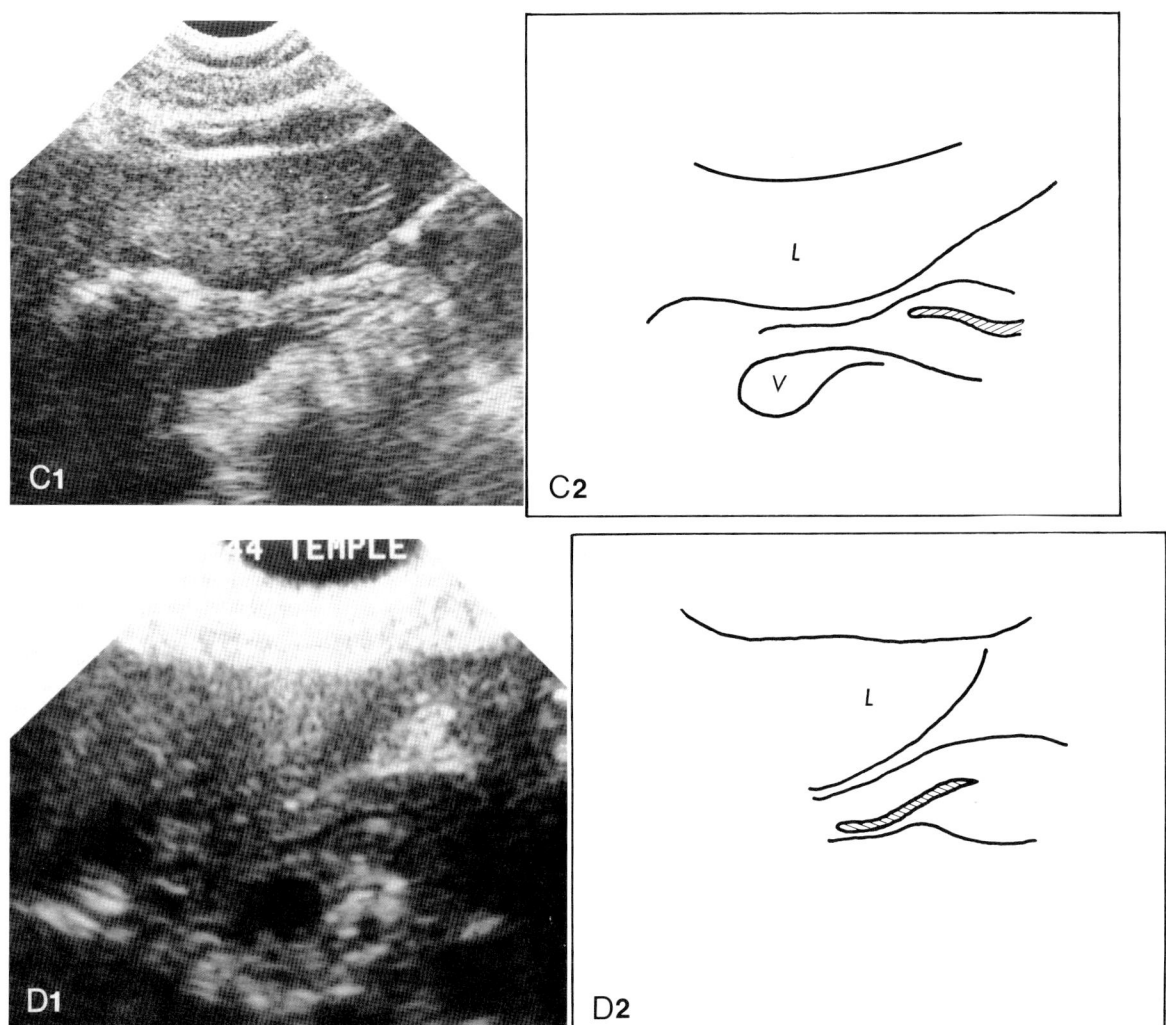

FIGURE 19.14C and D

started longitudinally in the midline. The aorta should be identified with the body of the pancreas situated between the celiac axis and superior mesenteric artery. The pancreatic duct may be identified in the central portion of the gland with the splenic vein along its posterosuperior aspect and the splenic artery along its superior aspect (Fig. 19.6). Following the splenic vein to the right, it will join with the superior mesenteric vein and the neck of the pancreas can be seen anterior to this area. Continuing to the right, we are now in the head of the pancreas. The pancreatic head is often best seen by angling the transducer to the right rather than moving laterally, since air in the distal stomach or proximal duodenum may preclude visualization. By angling to the right in this fashion, the portal vein can be identified anterior to the inferior vena cava and the common bile duct will be seen running from the anterior aspect of the portal vein into the parenchyma of the pancreatic head (Fig. 19.6). Moving further to the right, the superior portion of the common bile duct and area of the porta hepatis should be evaluated along with the gallbladder and remaining liver.

The pancreatic tail may not be visualized as one moves to the left of midline due to the presence of gas in the stomach. This can sometimes be overcome by keeping the transducer in the midline and by angling to the left along the long axis of the pancreatic tail (Fig. 19.6). In such instances, the left lobe of the liver, depending on its size, can be used as a soft tissue window. The area of the pancreatic tail can also be evaluated by scanning intercostally and using the spleen as an acoustic window with the patient in the right decubitus position.

Transverse scanning should be started just

below the xiphisternum in the midline (Fig. 19.7). The superior portion of the liver is examined in deep suspended inspiration while the remaining liver and porta hepatis may be evaluated in quiet respiration if technically possible. The size of the common bile duct and the presence or absence of stones in the gallbladder is noted. The portal vein is followed inferiorly to the area of the pancreas. At this point, by changing the angulation of the transducer appropriately, the splenic vein can be displayed along most of its length with the superior portion of the pancreatic body and tail along its anterior aspect (Fig. 19.7). Moving inferiorly, the common bile duct can be identified in the lateral portion of the head of the pancreas (Figs. 19.7 and 19.9). The gas and/or fluid-filled duodenum will demarcate the lateral aspect of the head while the uncinate process will be seen posterior to the superior mesenteric vein (Fig. 19.14B). The pancreatic body is usually easily seen anterior to the aorta and proximal superior mesenteric artery. One may have to change the angulation of the transducer to adequately visualize the entire pancreatic tail (Fig. 19.7). The sonographic image of the pancreatic tail differs from the CT image as the former underestimates its size and extent and makes its tip appear more dorsal in position (31).

The sonographic appearance of the stomach and duodenum varies depending upon whether they are empty or contain a varying amount of fluid, food, or air (Fig. 19.7). The antral area of the stomach, when empty, is seen as a thin echogenic line which represents the mucosa surrounded by a hypoechoic area due to the muscular layer of the stomach (Fig. 19.6). It has a varying complex pattern when filled with fluid and food and is highly reflective when air is present as it abuts the anterior wall with the patient in the supine position. This varying sonographic pattern can also be seen in the duodenum.

Using a skillful scanning technique and attention to detail, a diagnostic examination of the pancreas can be obtained in up to 90% of patients using the above technique (25, 32). Adequate visualization of the pancreatic tail is less than that of the head and body due to presence of gas in the stomach. By giving the patient four cups of de-gassed water, the ingested water in the stomach can be used as a sonic window to provide adequate visualization of the tail (Fig. 19.7). Since the axis of the stomach varies in different patients, the scanning position may have to be altered to provide adequate visualization and in some instances, erect scanning may be necessary (33). Due to the good-through transmission through the stomach, the gain curve and output setting will have to be adjusted. Despite an adequate scanning technique, the pancreatic tail is better evaluated by computed tomography and, in fact, the anterior pararenal fat can be sonographically mistaken for the tip of the pancreatic tail (31).

This water technique may also be used to evaluate the head and body of the pancreas by appropriate positioning of the patient (33). It can also help resolve the problem with pseudomasses of the pancreas produced by the fluid-filled stomach, duodenum or proximal small bowel. Using real-time ultrasound, such pseudomasses can be shown to change in appearance with time due to the presence of peristalsis. Real-time evaluation also helps resolve pseudo-masses produced by duodenal diverticula, a feces-filled splenic flexure and a dilated afferent loop following a Billroth II operation. Pseudo-masses due to ectatic or aneurysmal vessels can be confirmed using doppler ultrasound.

If the above technique fails to provide a diagnostic examination of the pancreas, then a CT scan should be performed.

Computed Tomography of the Normal Pancreas

Normal Anatomy

The basic normal anatomy of the pancreas has been described previously under the normal sonographic anatomy portion of this chapter. This section will deal primarily with the anatomy that is best depicted by the axial computed tomographic image.

The normal pancreas is quite variable in size, shape, and orientation (Fig. 19.15). The number of contiguous 1 cm slices needed to encompass the gland depends upon the obliquity of the tail and varies from 6 to 10 slices. In the adult patient, the outline of the pancreas may be smooth or lobulated depending on the amount of fat in the retroperitoneum and between the pancreatic lobules. The size of the pancreatic head, neck, body, and tail usually agree with those obtained sonographically except in those cases where the true pancreatic outline is lost due to its echo texture blending with that of the surrounding retroperitoneal fat. This can make the pancreatic tail or the entire pancreas appear homogeneously enlarged on the sonogram, however, this problem can be resolved by CT. Abso-

 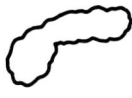 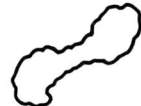 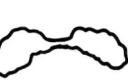

FIGURE 19.15. SOME COMMON VARIATIONS IN PANCREATIC CONFIGURATION
(Modified from Partain CL, Staab EV, McCarthey WH: Multiple imaging modalities for the study of pancreatic disease. *Semin Nucl Med* 9:36–42, 1979.)

lute numbers for pancreatic size should not be used alone in diagnosing pancreatic enlargement as they vary depending on the age and body habitus of the patient. What is important in judging pancreatic size is the symmetry of the gland with the head (3 cm) being slightly larger in its anteroposterior diameter than the body (2.2 cm) and the tail (2.8 cm). In a couple of percent of normal individuals, the pancreatic tail can appear somewhat bulbous and measure larger than the head. A small intrapancreatic mass may produce a bulge along only one border of the pancreas; and if this occurs in the uncinate process, its normally tapered medial margin may become rounded.

The previously described normal vascular landmarks of the pancreas are best identified by the use of intravenous iodinated contrast. Its use may not be necessary, however, in those patients with abundant retroperitoneal fat. Oral contrast (a dilute barium suspension) is used in every patient to outline the stomach, duodenum, remaining small bowel and adjacent portions of colon.

On the most superior CT slice one will usually see the base of both lungs, the liver, stomach and spleen and the crus of the diaphragm (Fig. 19.16). Proceeding inferiorly, the tail and body of the pancreas will come into view along with the branches of the celiac axis, the splenic vein, adrenal glands, kidneys and area of the porta hepatis (Fig. 19.17A and B). The junction of the splenic and superior mesenteric veins to form the portal vein will be seen behind the neck of the pancreas (Figs. 19.16 and 19.17C). On the ensuing slices, the head of the pancreas will be seen nestled in the duodenal C-loop with the low density common bile duct (3–6 mm) in its lateral portion. The pancreatic duct can be identified in the parenchyma of the body as it is here that the duct runs in a horizontal fashion along the axis of the transverse x-ray beam of the CT scan (Fig. 19.17E and F). The uncinate portion of the head varies in size; however, it always has a nice tapered medial margin (Figs. 19.16 and 19.17D). It lies behind the superior mesenteric vein and in about 5% behind the superior mesenteric artery as well. The gallbladder is identified along the under surface of the liver lateral and anterior to the portal vein, common bile duct and hepatic artery as they run in the free edge of the lesser omentum. It is usually identified on the images through the head of the pancreas. The area of the lesser sac is a potential space between the stomach anteriorly and the superior portion of the head and the body and tail of the pancreas posteriorly (Fig. 19.8). The inferior recess of the lesser sac is obliterated due to fusion of the layers of peritoneum of the greater omentum and transverse mesocolon. On the slices below the stomach, the transverse colon will come into view while the hepatic and splenic flexure vary in position with the latter being at a higher level then the former. When abundant fat is present in the retroperitoneum, the anterior and posterior pararenal fascia (Gerota's fascia) and the lateroconal fascia can be seen (Fig. 19.17).

Technique of Examination

The patient is given 2–3 cups (250–700 ml) of a dilute (2%) barium sulfate suspension by mouth 30–45 min prior to the examination. This will ensure adequate opacification of the stomach, duodenum, and remaining small bowel. If a nasogastric tube is in place, the barium suspension may be injected slowly through the tube and the tube withdrawn into the esophagus. With the patient on the CT table, a further half-cup may be given to ensure adequate opacification of the stomach and duodenum. If a CT scanner with a slow scan time (i.e., 18 sec) is being used, intravenous glucagon (1.0 mg) should be administered immediately before the start of the examination to eliminate motion artifacts from bowel peristalsis.

For routine scanning we use an air-charged rapid drip of 150 ml of 60% contrast running through at least a 19-gauge butterfly needle during the scan. Supplemental bolus injections can be done to resolve questions that might arise on initial review of the scans. Dynamic scanning with automatic table incrementation during bolus injection is needed for optimal detection of small islet cell tumors. Multiple small bolus (one prior to each slice) is an alternate technique that

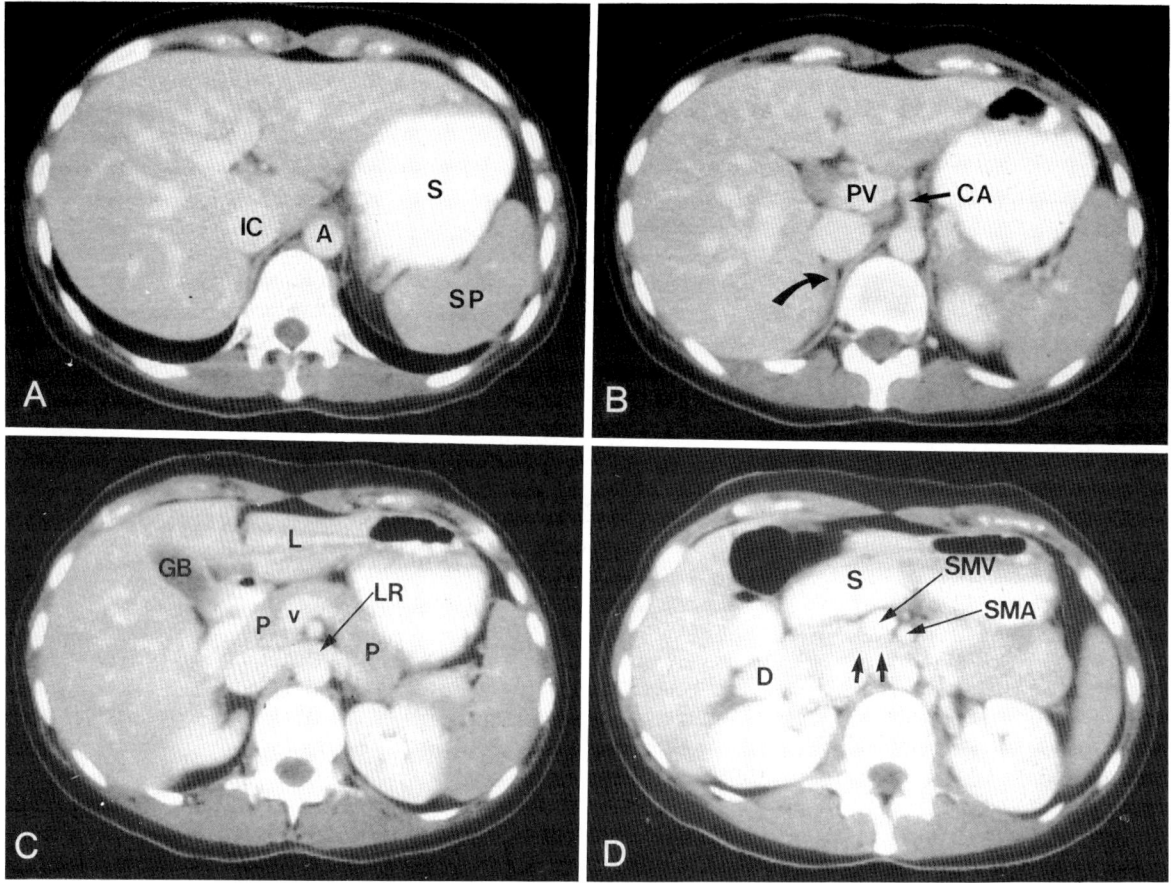

FIGURE 19.16. PANCREATIC ANATOMY ON CT: SPARSE RETROPERITONEAL FAT
Normal CT scan of the pancreas from superior (A) to inferior (D). See text. Aorta (A), inferior vena cava (IC), spleen (SP), stomach (S), liver (L), portal vein (PV), pancreas (P), portal vein, splenic vein confluence (V), left renal vein (LR), superier mesenteric artery (SMA), duodenum (D), gallbladder (GB), celiac axis (CA), right adrenal gland (*large arrow*), superior mesenteric vein (SMV), and uncinate process (*small arrows*).

may be useful (34). If pancreatic hemorrhage is suspected, a noncontrast examination should be performed initially to avoid masking the high density area of hemorrhage.

Proper attention to technique and the administration of contrast (oral/intravenous) is necessary so as to avoid misdiagnosing pseudotumors due to underfilled loops of bowel or duodenal diverticula or due to ectatic or aneurysmal vessels (35). Clinical history is also important as oral contrast will not always opacify the afferent loop following a Billroth II operation and this can simulate a pancreatic head mass.

Although recommended by Foley, we have not found sagittal reconstruction of the images to be of clinical value in neoplastic or inflammatory diseases of the pancreas (36). Others have performed pancreatic CT immediately following ERCP (37, 38). This technique can determine whether intrapancreatic gas is all within the pancreatic ductal system and in the post-operative patient who is being considered for further surgery, it can determine the amount of remaining pancreas and the location of a bowel anastomosis if present (38). It may also be useful in outlining the entire extent of pancreatic fistulas.

The CT scan is routinely performed using 1-cm thick slices spaced at 1-cm intervals to include all the liver and pancreas. The patient is instructed to hold his or her breath in expiration while each CT slice is being obtained. The study can then be extended if necessary and/or 0.5-cm slices can be performed through suspicious areas if necessary, i.e., question of a small mass or dilated pancreatic duct or small calculus in the common bile duct (39, 40). The technique used includes an mA of 320 and a kVP of 120 unless the patient is extremely large in which case the mA is increased to 400. The exact window level and window width at which a CT scan is photo-

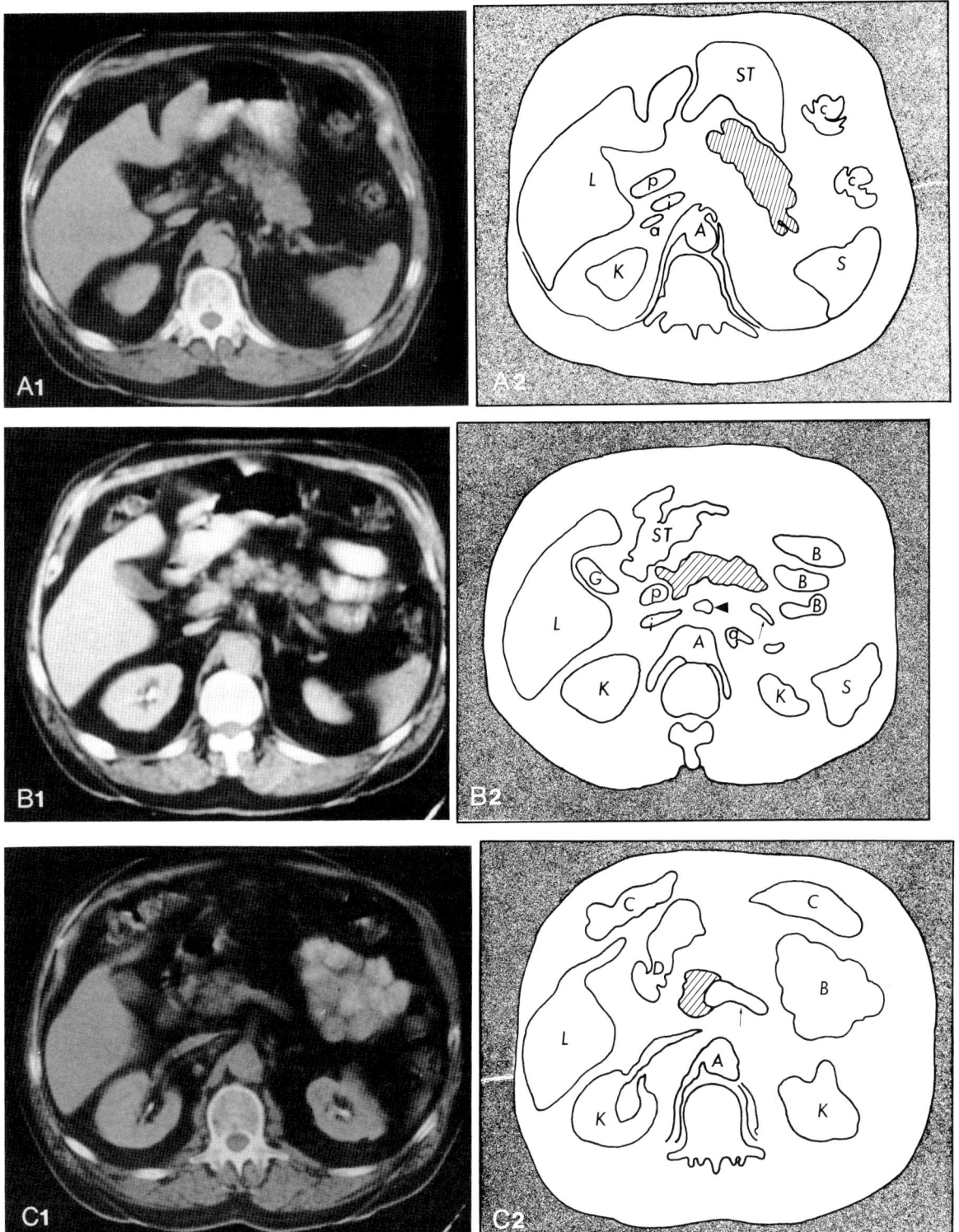

FIGURE 19.17. PANCREATIC ANATOMY ON CT: ABUNDANT RETROPERITONEAL FAT

A: Normal tail and body of pancreas (*shaded*). *B:* Normal neck and body of pancreas (*shaded*). *C:* Normal head of pancreas (*shaded*). *D:* Normal uncinate process (*shaded*). S = spleen, C = colon, ST = stomach, L = liver, P = portal vein, i = inferior vena cava, a = adrenal, K = kidney, A = aorta, G = gallbladder, *arrowhead* = superior mesenteric artery, *arrow* = splenic vein, D = duodenum, *feathered arrow* = superior mesenteric vein. *E:* Normal pancreatic duct in the body of the pancreas (*arrows*). Normal common bile duct in the head of the pancreas (*larger arrow*). *F:* Normal pancreatic duct in the neck of the pancreas (*arrows*).

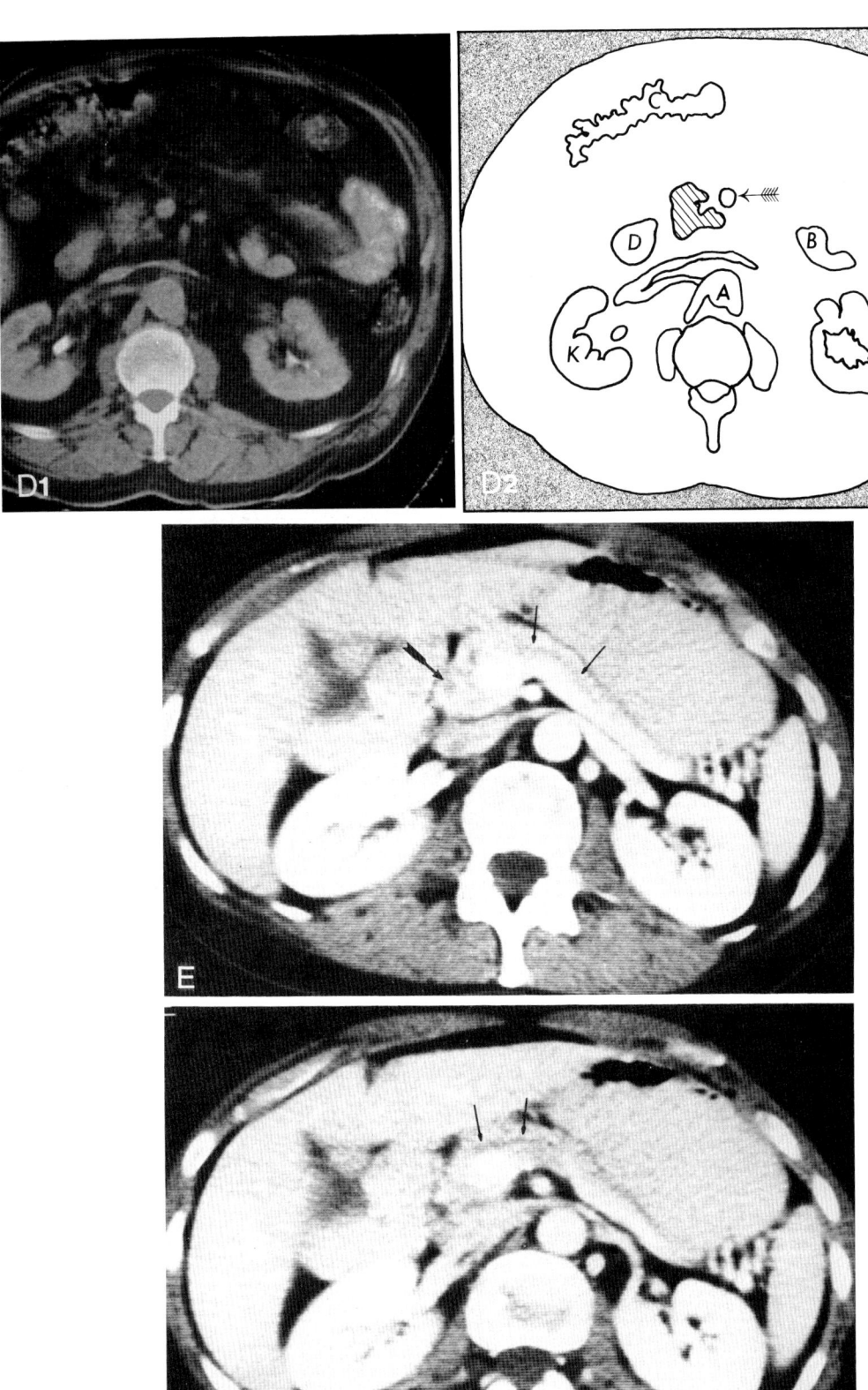

FIGURE 19.17D–F

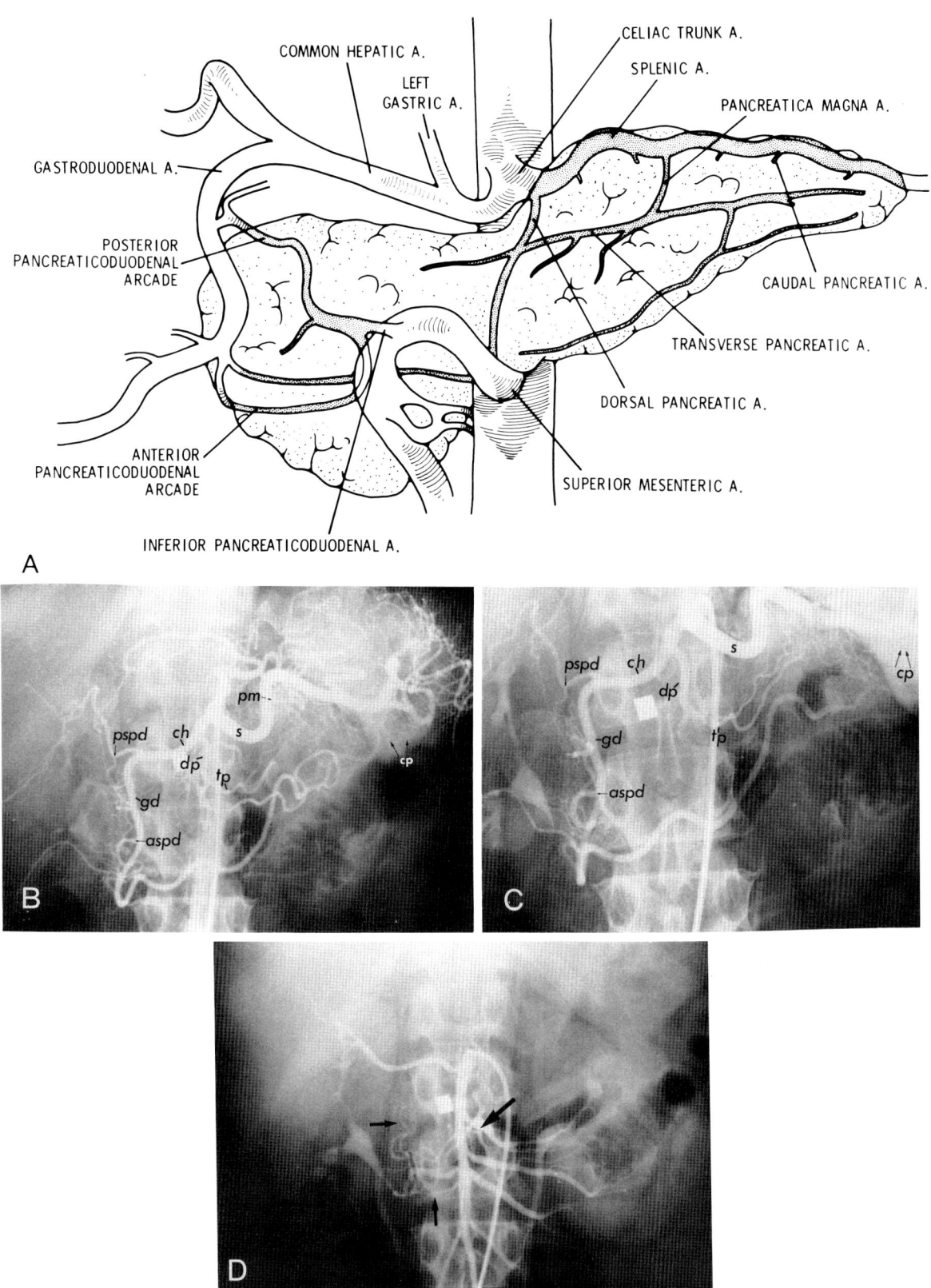

FIGURE 19.18. PANCREATIC ARTERIAL ANATOMY

A: Arteries of pancreas. *B* and *C:* Celiac arteriogram, conventional and magnification views, respectively. s = splenic artery, ch = common hepatic artery, gd = gastroduodenal artery, pm = pancreatica magna artery, dp = dorsal pancreatic artery, $pspd$ = posterior superior pancreaticoduodenal artery, $aspd$ = anterior superior pancreaticoduodenal artery, tp = transverse pancreatic artery, and cp = caudal pancreatic artery. *D:* Inferior pancreaticoduodenal arcade, superior mesenteric artery injection (*arrow*).

graphed depends on the body habitus (fat, thin) of the patient and the personal choice of the reviewing physician, but it is usually at a level of 50–80 HU and a window width of 300–500 HU.

Arterial, Venous, and Lymphatic Anatomy

The arterial supply to the pancreas arises from the celiac and superior mesenteric arteries. The relationships of the pancreatic arteries are extremely variable and their distribution differs on an individual patient basis (Fig. 19.18) (41). With some exceptions, pancreatic veins are similar in size and course to corresponding arteries (Fig. 19.19) (42). The veins draining the pancreas enter either the portal or the superior mesenteric vein. Lymph nodes are distributed along the vascular pathways (Figs. 19.10 and 19.20). The body and tail are drained by pancreaticolienal nodes adjacent to the splenic artery and vein.

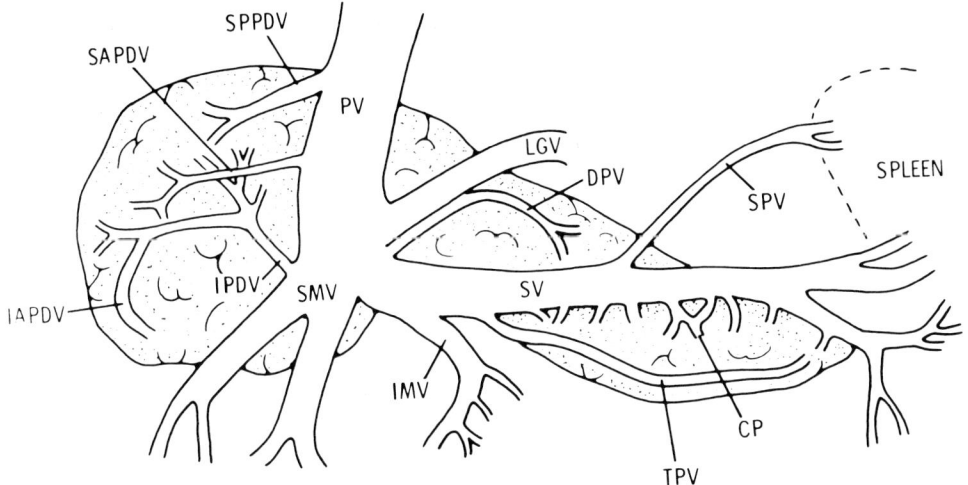

FIGURE 19.19. PANCREATIC VENOUS ANATOMY
PV = portal vein, *SV* = splenic vein, *SMV* = superior mesenteric vein, *IMV* = inferior mesenteric vein, *SPV* = splenic polar vein, *LGV* = left gastric vein, *DPV* = dorsal pancreatic vein, *TPV* = transverse pancreatic vein, *CP* = caudal pancreatic vein, *SPPDV* = superior posterior pancreaticoduodenal vein, *SAPDV* = superior anterior pancreaticoduodenal vein, *IPDV* = inferior pancreaticoduodenal vein, *IAPDV* = inferior anterior pancreaticoduodenal vein.

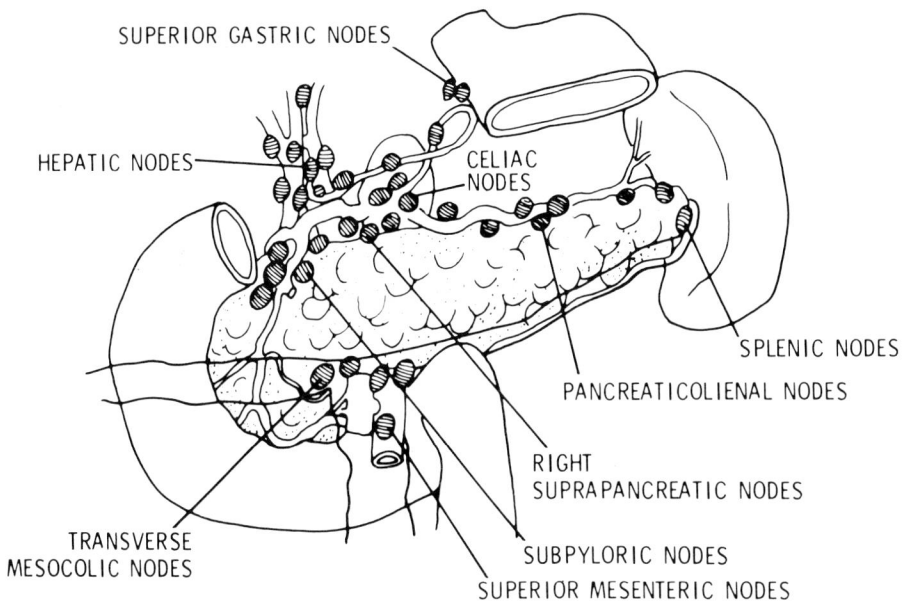

FIGURE 19.20. ANTERIOR FRONTAL VIEW OF REGIONAL LYMPH NODES

The head of the pancreas is drained by superior and inferior head nodes and anterior and posterior pancreaticoduodenal nodes. Some drainage from the head and proximal body is upward toward nodes in the porta hepatis and inferiorly towards superior mesenteric, mesocolic and para-aortic nodal chains (43).

Ductal Anatomy

The main pancreatic duct is centrally located in the body and tail of the pancreas and is oriented nearly transverse in the abdomen in most patients. In one series of 111 cases, the course of the main pancreatic duct from the tail to the neck was ascending in 49.6% of cases, horizontal in 35.8%, sigmoid in 10.3%, and descending in 4.3% (4). Upon reaching the neck of the pancreas, it descends toward the ampulla, paralleling the course of the common bile duct. The length of pancreatic duct may vary, however mean length is approximately 205 mm with a range of 107–270 mm (4, 44, 45). The width of the normal pancreatic duct is often larger in the head and smaller in the tail (3–4 mm in the head of the pancreas, 2–3 mm in the body, and 1–2 mm in the tail). There is some dilatation of the duct normally with age (4). Two areas of narrowing may be seen normally in the main pancreatic duct—at the orifice and in the neck of the gland where embryologic fusion occurred. Pathologic strictures may occur in these same areas but usually should be obvious because of the resulting prestenotic ductal dilatation (46). Average maximum diameter of the main pancreatic duct as measured in autopsy series was 2.9 mm in patients up to age 50 and an average of 3.5 mm in patients over that age (47, 48).

HISTOLOGY

The exocrine portion of the pancreas consists of acini bound into lobules by connective tissue interlobular septa. The ductal epithelium is cuboidal in main ducts, columnar in interlobar ducts, and flat in the terminal ducts. The latter flat epithelium can be confused with endothelium. Some ductal epithelial cells are ciliated while others are mucin secreting. Acinar cells are arranged in a single layer around a lumen and are pyramidal (Fig. 19.21). During the resting phase, the lumen is small and the cell cytoplasm is filled with zymogen granules which are emptied into the lumen during active enzyme secretion. The endocrine portion of the pancreas is composed of rounded masses of cells irregularly dispersed throughout the entire organ parenchyma, usually most numerous in the tail. Islets may lie in connective tissue septa and occasionally in peripancreatic areolar tissue. They have a ribbon-like arrangement of cells between which there are capillaries whose endothelial lining is apposed to the secreting cells. This ribbon pattern is exaggerated in islet cell hyperplasia and occasionally in neoplasms. The islets contain beta (β), alpha (α), delta (δ), and pancreatic polypeptide cells in descending order of frequency. β Cells secrete insulin, α cells glucagon, δ cells vasoactive intestinal polypeptide and somatostatin, and pancreatic polypeptide cells a polypeptide of unknown activity. On routine staining, the islet cells look alike. They can be differentiated with special immunoperoxidase stains by light microscopy and by analysis of their enzyme granules by electron microscopy (1, 2).

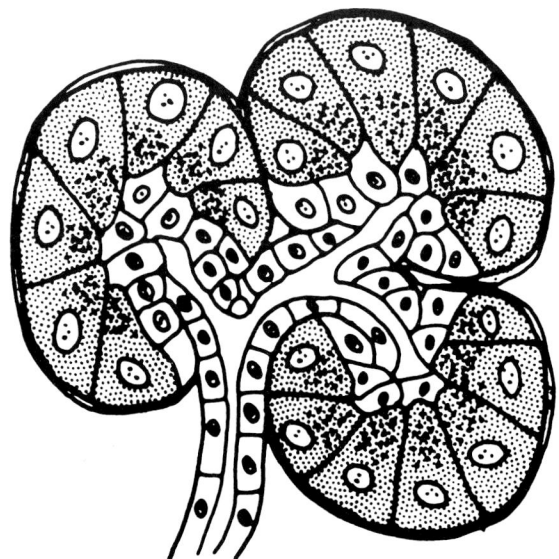

FIGURE 19.21. PANCREATIC HISTOLOGY
Drawing of acinus and terminal duct shows acinar cells (*stippled*) and ductular epithelium (*clear*).

PANCREATIC EXOCRINE FUNCTION

Pancreatic Secretion

The pancreas, despite its important contributions to digestion, has remained inaccessible to both direct diagnostic and functional testing by virtue of its anatomic location. Recent advances in medical technology have enabled us to better "image" the pancreas to define suspect lesions as well as quantitate secretory output. Since the pancreas shares many anatomic and physiologic features with the salivary glands, particularly the parotid, it has been referred to "the salivary gland of the abdomen" (49). It is capable of performing both exocrine and endocrine functions and through a series of negative feedback loops, its output is autoregulated.

Pancreatic Anatomy and Physiology

The macroanatomy of the pancreas previously described connects to the ultrastructure of the gland by means of progressively decreasing diameter excretory ducts progressing from the main pancreatic duct to extralobular ducts which drain interlobular and finally interlobular systems connecting with the acinus. These ducts are lined by epithelial cells which contain carbonic anhydrase and secrete water and electrolytes; they do not contain zymogen granules. Additionally, the walls of these ducts contain elastic fibers which control pancreatic fluid secretion into the duodenum (49).

At the glandular end of the duct, the secretory acinus lined by enzyme-secreting cells containing zymogen granules resemble truncated pyramids. The entire array of digestive enzymes is secreted by the acinar cells. Ductular cells may protrude into the acinus and are then known as centroacinar cells and share the same secretory capacity as the cells lining the ducts (50).

The pancreas can be broken down physiologically into the exocrine pancreas which compromises about 90% of the mass of the pancreas and the endocrine pancreas which secretes hormones making up about 4% (the remainder comprised by supportive structures). The exocrine pancreas consists of two parts—the ductal epithelium which secretes water and electrolytes and acinar cells which secrete digestive enzymes.

Water and Electrolyte Secretion

Water, bicarbonate, and electrolytes are secreted into pancreatic juice by the centroacinar and the ductal cells of the pancreas. This output is dependent upon stimulation by secretin. The pancreas produces 1–4 liters of an isotonic pancreatic juice daily containing sodium at 140 mEq per liter, potassium at 6 mEq per liter, calcium, and magnesium with bicarbonate and chloride comprising the major anions. These vary reciprocally and together total 150 mEq per liter. At high flow rates, the bicarbonate concentration is high, approaching 150 mEq per liter, and the chloride concentration is low. At low flow rates, this concentration is reversed (51). As flow rates increase, less time is available for bicarbonate to exchange with chloride. The pH varies directly with bicarbonate concentration and may vary over a range of 7.5–8.5.

From micropuncture studies, juice from the intralobular ducts draining the acini exhibit a high secretion of the chloride component with a progressive increase in bicarbonate secretion as the pancreatic juice passes into the larger interlobular ducts. Most water in volume is added by the extralobular ducts (52).

Carbon dioxide in pancreatic capillaries diffusing into the cells eventually becomes the source of bicarbonate in pancreatic juice. Bicarbonate is accompanied by sodium via an active transport mechanism into the pancreatic lumen, since the concentration of bicarbonate in the pancreatic lumen is in excess of that found in either extracellular or intracellular fluid (50, 51). Bicarbonate is easily generated by the reactions of ubiquitous carbon dioxide with a hydroxyl molecule from water and catalyzed by carbonic anhydrase to bicarbonate. Bicarbonate is then extruded across the luminal border. Interference with the secretion of this bicarbonate containing juice is possible with the use of carbonic anhydrase inhibitors. For this reason, bicarbonate output rather than the absolute bicarbonate concentration is the more sensitive indicator of pancreatic disease.

Enzyme Secretion

Enzymes are secreted by acinar cells into the acinar lumen by a process similar to reverse pinocytosis. Secretory proteins are synthesized on membrane-bound ribosomes and are transported through the endoplasmic reticulum to the Golgi complex. Condensing vacuoles are created by "packing" secretory proteins with secretory granules which subsequently mature into zymogen granules during fasting. Since no secretory stimulus is present, these granules increase in size and number at the apical region of the cell. Discharge of these enzymes into the lumen occurs by merging the membrane of the zymogen granule with the cell membrane at the apical portion of the cell (53).

Pancreatic juice contains three major enzyme groups: amylolytic, lipolytic, and proteolytic (50).

Amylase is secreted in pancreatic juice in the active state. Its substrate is starch.

The lipolytic enzymes are forms of lipase which hydrolyze insoluble esters of glycerol at an oil-water interface. Pancreatic juice also contains phospholipase.

Proteolytic enzymes come from trypsinogen and chymotrypsinogen, the former which is activated by gut enterokinase and trypsin and the latter by trypsin. These enzymes act on proteins and peptide chains to break them into short chain peptides and amino acids. Other proteolytic enzymes includes procarboxypeptidase, elastase, ribonuclease, deoxyribonuclease.

Clinically, measurement of serum amylase and lipase are only useful in assessing pancreatic inflammation.

Control of Pancreatic Secretion

Pancreatic secretion is finally controlled by hormonal and neural mechanisms. Major stimulation results from the presence of fat, amino acid, and acid into the duodenum. Secretin is released from cells in the duodenal mucosa in response to an acid load, increasing the output of water and bicarbonate (50). It also acts through a feedback loop to shut off gastrin simulated acid production. The release of cholecystokinin (pancreozymin) is stimulated by amino acids and peptones in the duodenum. Cholecystokinin is a trophic hormone for the pancreas and acts to increase the output of pancreatic enzymes (50). Since the terminal sequence of gastrin is similar to cholecystokinin, it can compete for the parietal cell receptor site thereby inhibiting gastric acid secretion and gastric motility. Conversely, gastrin may stimulate pancreatic enzyme release and gallbladder contraction because of its similarity to cholecystokinin, although it is less potent then cholecystokinin (51). Pancreatic growth can be stimulated by continued administration of cholecystokinin or gastrin whereas secretin decreases the weight of the pancreas (54).

Electrical stimulation of the vagus nerve causes output of an increased volume of juice rich in enzymes from the pancreas. Parasympathomimetic drugs produce the same response as does insulin-induced hypoglycemia. Surgical transection of the vagus nerve reduces stimulated pancreatic secretion but does not result in clinical impairment of digestion.

Since man is an intermittent feeder, pancreatic secretion is greatest during the digestion phase (49).

REFERENCES

1. Robbins SL, Cotran SR: *Pathologic Basis of Disease*. Philadelphia, W. B. Saunders, 1979, pp 1092-1093.
2. Netter FH: In Oppenheimer E (ed): *Ciba Collection of Medical Illustrations—The Digestive System. Part III—Liver, Biliary Tract, and Pancreas*. New York, Ciba, 1957, pp 25-27.
3. Frantz VK: Tumors of the pancreas. In *Atlas of Tumor Pathology*, Sect. 7, Fasc. 27-28. Washington, D.C., Armed Forces Institute of Pathology, 1959, pp 7-10, 36-75.
4. Meyers MA: *Dynamic Radiology of the Abdomen*. New York, Springer-Verlag, 1976, p 24.
5. Williams P, Warwick R: The pancreas. In *Gray's Anatomy*, Ed. 36. Philadelphia, W. B. Saunders, 1980, pp 1368-1374.
6. Kreel L, Sandin B, Slavin G: Pancreatic morphology: a combined radiological and pathological study. *Clin Radiol* 24:154-161, 1973.
7. Sample WF: Techniques for improved delineation of normal anatomy of the upper abdomen and high retroperitoneum with Gray-scale ultrasound. *Radiology* 124:197-202, 1977.
8. Neumann CH, Hessel SJ: CT of the pancreatic tail. *AJR* 135:741-745, 1980.
9. Ralls PW, Quinn MF, Rogers W, Halls J: Sonographic anatomy of the hepatic artery. *AJR* 136:1059-1063, 1981.
10. Marchel G, Kint E, Nijssens M, Baert A: Variability of the hepatic arterial anatomy: a sonographic demonstration. *J Clin Ultrasound* 9:377-381, 1981.
11. Filly RA, London SS: The normal pancreas: acoustic characteristics and frequency of imaging. *J Clin Ultrasound* 7:121-124, 1979.
12. Marks D, Spinelli G, Warter P: Ultrasonically guided percutaneous pancreatography. *J Clin Ultrasound* 11:401-404, 1983.
13. Patel S, Bellon EM, Haaga J, Park CH: Fat replacement of the exocrine pancreas. *AJR* 135:843-845, 1980.
14. Walters MN: Adipose atrophy of the exocrine pancreas. *J Pathol Bacteriol* 92:547-557, 1966.
15. Taylor KJW, Buchin PJ, Viscomi GN, Rosenfield AT: Ultrasonographic scanning of the pancreas: prospective study of clinical results. *Radiology* 138:211-213, 1981.
16. Jaffe CC, Harris DJ: Sonographic tissue texture: influence of transducer focusing pattern. *AJR* 135:343-347, 1980.
17. Hadidi A: Pancreatic duct diameter: sonographic measurement in normal subjects. *J Clin Ultrasound* 11:17-22, 1983.
18. Lawson TL, Berland LL, Foley WD, Stewart ET, Geenan JE, Hogan WJ: Ultrasonic visualization of the pancreatic duct. *Radiology* 144:865-871, 1982.
19. Ohto M, Saotome N, Saisho H, Tsuchiya Y, Ono T, Okuda K, Karasawa E: Real-time sonography of the

pancreatic duct: application to percutaneous pancreatic ductography. *AJR* 134:647–752, 1980.
20. Bryan PJ: Appearance of normal pancreatic duct: a study using real-time ultrasound. *J Clin Ultrasound* 10:63–66, 1982.
21. Parulekar SG: Ultrasonic evaluation of the pancreatic duct. *J Clin Ultrasound* 8:457–463, 1980.
22. Kreel L, Sandin B: Changes in pancreatic morphology associated with aging. *Gut* 14:962–970, 1973.
23. Sanders RC, Chang R: A variant position of the splenic artery mimicking the pancreatic duct. *J Clin Ultrasound* 10:391–393, 1982.
24. Eisenscher A, Weill F: Ultrasonic visualization of Wirsung's duct: dream or reality? *J Clin Ultrasound* 7:41–44, 1979.
25. Arger PH, Mulhern CB, Bonavita JA, Stauffer DM, Hale J: An analysis of pancreatic sonography in suspected pancreatic disease. *J Clin Ultrasound* 7:91–97, 1979.
26. DeGraaff CS, Taylor KJW, Simmonds BD, Rosenfield AJ: Grayscale echography of the pancreas. *Radiology* 129:157–161, 1978.
27. Niederau C, Sonnenberg A, Muller JE, Erckenbrecht JF, Scholten T, Fritsch WP: Sonographic measurements of the normal liver, spleen, pancreas and portal vein. *Radiology* 149:537–540, 1983.
28. Higashi Y, Sakazaki T, Hirata, Murakami K, Matsuura K: Pancreatic thickening during ultrasonography—variations with respiration and scanning planes. Presented (Paper 304) at the American Institute of Ultrasound in Medicine Meeting, San Francisco, August 1981.
29. Johnson ML, Mack LA: Ultrasonic evaluation of the pancreas. *Gastrointest Radiol* 3:257–266, 1978.
30. Kwa A, Bowie JD: Transducer selection for pancreatic ultrasound based on skin to pancreas distance in the supine and upright position. *Radiology* 134:541–542, 1980.
31. Suramo J, Lobela P, Labde S, Myllyla V, Pannilo M: The "ghost tail" of the pancreas in ultrasonography. *Eur J Radiol* 2:139–140, 1982.
32. Lawson TL: Sensitivity of pancreatic ultrasonography in the detection of pancreatic disease. *Radiology* 128:733–736, 1978.
33. Bowie JD, MacMahon H: Improved techniques in pancreatic sonography. *Semin Ultrasound* 1:170–177, 1980.
34. Rossi P, Baert A, Marchal W, Tipaldi L, Wilms W, Pavone P: Multiple bolus technique vs. single bolus or infusion of contrast medium to obtain prolonged contrast enhancement of the pancreas. *Radiology* 144:929–931, 1982.
35. Churchill RJ, Reynes CJ, Love L: Pancreatic pseudotumors: computed tomography. *Gastrointest Radiol* 3:251–256, 1978.
36. Foley WD, Lawson TL, Berland LL, Chintapalli K, Berninger WH, Reddington RW: Reformatted coronal display of upper abdominal computed tomography: comparison with ultrasonography. *J Comput Assist Tomogr* 5:946–502, 1981.
37. Frick MP, O'Leary JF, Salomonowitz E, Stoltenberg P, Hutton S, Gedgaudas E: Pancreas imaging by computed tomography after endoscopic retrograde pancreatography. *Radiology* 150:191–194, 1984.
38. Jaffe MH, Glazer GM, Amendola MA, Nostrant T, Wilson JAP: Endoscopic retrograde computed tomography of the pancreas. *J Comput Assist Tomogr* 8:63–366, 1984.
39. Berland LL, LawsoN TL, Foley WD, Greenen JE, Stewart ET: Computed tomography of the normal and abnormal pancreatic duct: correlation with pancreatic ductography. *Radiology* 141:715–724, 1981.
40. Callen PW, London SS, Moss AA: Computed tomographic evaluation of the dilated pancreatic duct: the value of thin section collimation. *Radiology* 134:253–255, 1980.
41. Reuter SR, Redman HC: *Gastrointestinal Angiography*. Philadelphia, W. B. Saunders, 1977, pp 31–64.
42. Keller FS, Niles NR, Rosch J, Dotter CT, Stenzel-Poore M: Retrograde pancreatic venography: autopsy study. *Radiology* 135:285–293, 1980.
43. Eaton SB Jr, Ferrucci JT Jr: *Radiology of the Pancreas and Duodenum*. Philadelphia, W. B. Saunders, 1973, pp 1–17.
44. Anacker H: Radiological anatomy of the Pancreas. In Anacher H (ed): *Efficiency and Limits of Radiologic Examination of the Pancreas*. Stuttgart, George Thieme Verlag, 1975, pp 29–42.
45. Ansel HJ: Normal pancreatic duct (ch 6). In Vennes JA, Geenen JE (eds): *Atlas of Endoscopic Retrograde Cholangiopancreatography*. Stewart ET, St. Louis, C. V. Mosby, 1977, p 43.
46. Short WF: Pancreatography. In Eaton SB, Ferrucci JT Jr (eds): *Radiology of the Pancreas and Duodenum*. Philadelphia, W. B. Saunders, 1973, p 261.
47. Kizu M: Normal endoscopic cholangiopancreatogram (chapter 12). In Takemoto T, Kasugai T (eds): *Endoscopic Retrograde Cholangiopancreatography*. New York: Igaku-Shoin 141, 1979.
48. Salmon PR: Re-evaluation of ERCP as a diagnostic method. *Clin Gastroenterol* 7:651, 1978.
49. Davenport HW: Pancreatic secretion. In *Physiology of the Digestive Tract*. Chicago, Yearbook, 1982.
50. Rudick J: Physiology of pancreatic secretion. *Surg Clin North Am* 61:47, 1981.
51. Meyer JH: Pancreatic physiology. In *Gastrointestinal Disease*. Sleisenger and Fordtran, eds. Philadelphia, W. B. Saunders, 1978.
52. Lightwoord R, Reber HA: Micropuncture study of pancreatic secretion in the cat. *Gastroenterology* 72:61, 1977.
53. Scheele GA: The secretory product in the pancreatic exocrine cell. *Mayo Clin Proc* 54:420, 1979.
54. Brooks FP: Applied physiology of the exocrine pancreas. *Prac Gastroenterol* 2:4, 1978.

20

Anomalies and Congenital Disorders

BRUCE M. MARKLE, M.D., ARNOLD C. FRIEDMAN, M.D.,
AND MARK T. BIRNS, M.D.

PANCREATIC ARTERIOVENOUS FISTULA

Pancreatic arteriovenous fistulas are very rare, and are either isolated or part of the spectrum of hereditary hemorrhagic telangiectasia (Osler-Weber-Rendu disease) (1, 2). Angiographic diagnostic criteria are dilated feeding arteries, a focal group of racemose arterioles and venules, and shunting into dilated draining veins. Upper gastrointestinal tract endoscopy and barium studies are unlikely to show any abnormalities. Treatment has been surgical, although transcatheter embolotherapy is an alternative.

REFERENCES

1. Brinley JL, Palubinskas AJ: Congenital arteriovenous malformation of the pancreas. Br J Radiol 50:219–222, 1977.
2. Chuang VP, Pulmano CM, Walter JF et al: Angiography of pancreatic arteriovenous malformation. AJR 129: 1015–1018, 1977.

PANCREAS DIVISUM

Pancreas divisum is a congenital anomaly caused by failure of fusion of the ducts of Wirsung and Santorini. Consequently, the duct of Santorini drains the superior head and the body and tail, whereas the duct of Wirsung is small and drains only the inferior head and uncinate process (1). Autopsy studies suggest that this anomaly is present in 4–11% of the population (1).

Clinical Findings

Although pancreas divisum can be an incidental finding, it appears to predispose toward pancreatitis. The incidence of divisum in the general population is 3–6.7%, while 12–26% of patients with idiopathic recurrent pancreatitis have this anomaly (1–3). The clinical disease pattern is recurrent acute pancreatitis. It is felt that the duct of Santorini and its accessory ampulla are too small in some patients to transmit the necessary volume of secretions when the duct of Wirsung does not join (1). Surgical sphincteroplasty of the minor papilla may afford relief in those patients with pancreas divisum and recurrent acute pancreatitis (1). The concept that pancreas divisum predisposes to pancreatitis has been disputed by Delhaye and coworkers, who consider it an incidental anatomic variant present in 10% of the population (4).

One of the tests advocated to make the diagnosis of pancreas divisum is the intravenous injection of secretin (1 mg per kg body weight) which according to Simeone produces dilatation of the sonographically monitored duct 30–60 sec after injection (Fig. 20.1) (5). Morphine and prostigmine elicited a similar response. There was good correlation between a positive response and relief of symptoms following surgical sphincterotomy. These results are disputed by Bolondi et al. (6), who have shown that intravenous secretin can product dilatation of the pancreatic duct in normal human volunteers.

Radiology

Pancreatography is the only reliable method for achieving the diagnosis of pancreas divisum. The duct of Wirsung is short and tapered and will show early acinarization because of its shortness (Fig. 20.1A). Radiographic changes of pancreatitis will not be seen in the duct of Wirsung, but may be seen if the duct of Santorini is opacified either by cannulation at ERCP (often not technically possible) or at surgery (Fig. 20.1B) (1). In 3% of unselected autopsy patients, there is no duct of Wirsung (1).

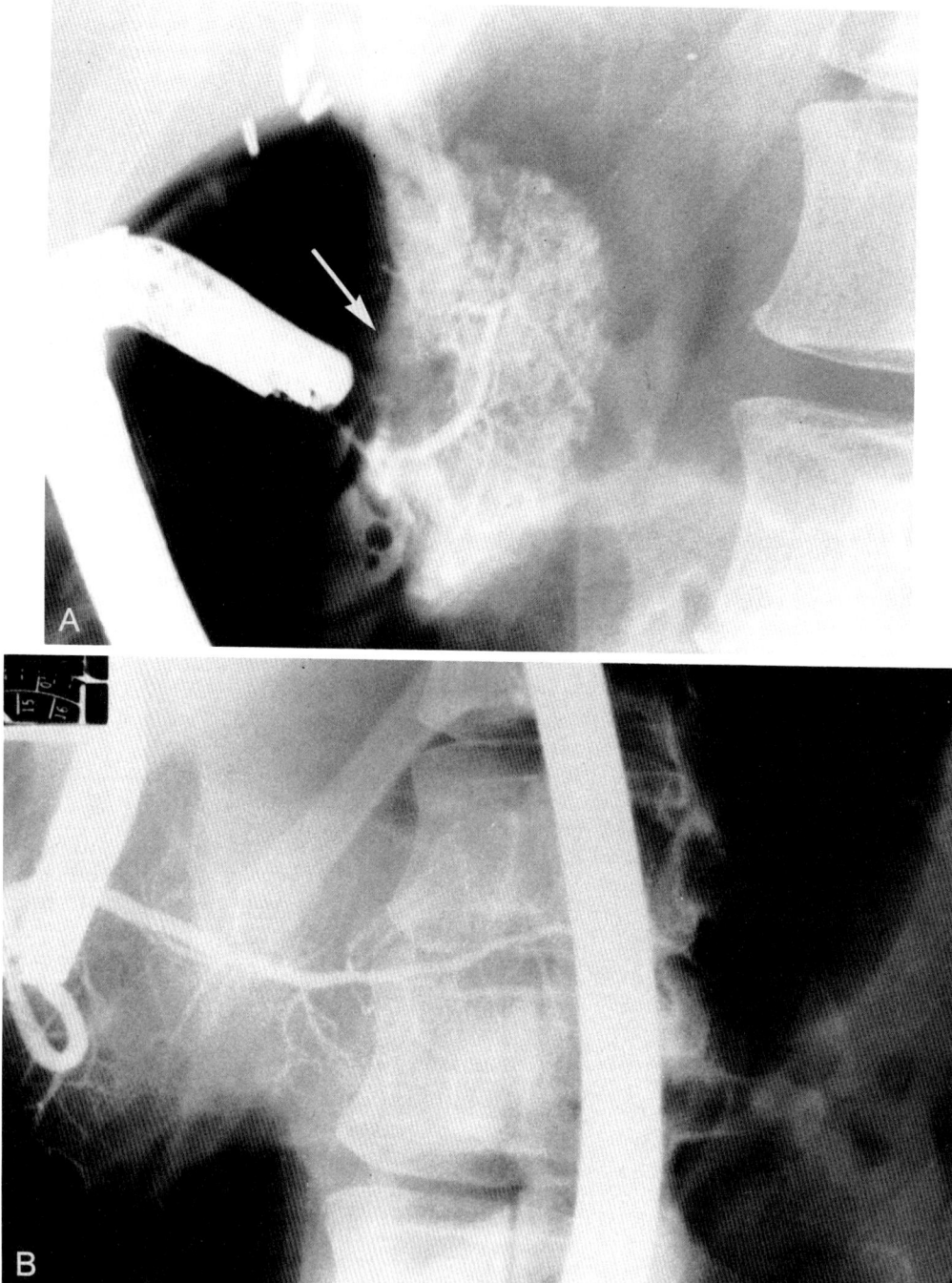

FIGURE 20.1. PANCREAS DIVISUM

A: Injection of the duct of Wirsung at the major papilla (note residual contrast in common bile duct, *arrow*). The duct of Wirsung is small and there was early acinization with normal injection pressure. Note normal parenchyma distal to the duct termination, a differentiating feature from ductal obstruction. *B:* Cannulation of the minor papilla reveals the duct of Santorini to be draining the majority of the pancreas. No evidence of pancreatitis.

REFERENCES

1. Richter JM, Schapiro RM, Mulley AG, Warshaw AL: Association of pancreas divisum and pancreatitis and its treatment by sphincteroplasty of the accessory ampulla. *Gastroenterology* 81:1104–1110, 1981.
2. Gold RP, Berman H, Fakhry J, Heier S, Rosenthal W, DelGuercio L: Pancreas divisum with pancreatitis and pseudocyst. *AJR* 143:1343–1344, 1984.

3. Warshaw AL, Richter JM, Schapiro RH: The cause and treatment of pancreatitis associated with pancreas divisum. *Ann Surg* 198:443–462, 1983.
4. Delhaye M, Engelholm L, Cremer M: Pancreas divisum: congenital anatomic variant or anomaly? *Gastroenterology* 89:951–958, 1985.
5. Simeone JF, Mueller PR, Butch RJ, Ferrucci JT, Wittenberg J, White M: Ultrasound evaluation of the pancreatic and common duct following pharmacologic stimulation with morphine/prostigmine and secretin. *Radiology* 153:108, 1984.
6. Bolondi L, Gaiani S, Gullo L, Labo G: Secretin administration induces a dilatation of main pancreatic duct. *Dig Dis Sci* 29:802–808, 1984.

ANNULAR PANCREAS

Annular pancreas is an uncommon congenital anomaly wherein a ring of normal pancreatic tissue encircles the second portion of the duodenum. Because of varying degrees of associated duodenal obstruction, this anomaly may manifest in the immediate neonatal period, may first manifest in adulthood, or may very rarely be discovered incidentally at autopsy (1). Roughly one-half of cases are seen in childhood, one-half in later life (2). Annular pancreas is the most common congenital anomaly of the pancreas, comprising 62% of one large surgical series in children, all other congenital lesions being much more rare (pancreatic duct atresia, intrapancreatic gastric duplication, pancreatic hypoplasia, partial or complete pancreatic agenesis) (2).

As many as 75% of cases of annular pancreas are associated with other congenital anomalies. Intrinsic duodenal obstruction is a major feature of neonatal cases, and may take the form of duodenal atresia, stenosis or duodenal diaphragm; the pancreatic ring is usually inseparable from the duodenal wall. Additional extrinsic duodenal obstruction may be present due to Ladd's bands from concomitant intestinal malrotation. Coexisting common congenital anomalies include Down's syndrome (trisomy-21), esophageal atresia, tracheoesophageal fistula and imperforate anus. Table 20.1 lists reported associated abnormalities (1, 3–11).

Embryology

Theories about the origin of annular pancreas center on abnormal migration and rotation of the anlagen of the pancreatic head. At approximately 4 weeks of gestation, two pancreatic anlagen arise from the ventral surface of the primitive gastrointestinal tube as branches of the hepatic bud. The left ventral anlage atrophies, while the right ventral anlage rotates posteriorly, then toward the left to fuse with the dorsal anlage (the precursor of the pancreatic neck, body, and tail) (9). The most widely accepted theory is that of Lecco (12) which proposes that the tip of the right ventral anlage remains attached to the surface of the duodenum and that this pancreatic primordium is then stretched around the duodenum during its normal rotation process to leave a ring of normal pancreatic tissue surrounding the second portion of the duodenum. Histological and immunohistochemical studies on tissue from a case of resected annular pancreas show that the tissue is very similar to normal pancreatic head tissue (suggesting ventral anlage origin) (13). Microdissection studies (14, 15) and cholangiographic studies (2, 6) of the ductal patterns of annular pancreas support Lecco's theory by showing a duct which encircles the duodenum and directly joins the main pancreatic duct of Wirsung (a ventral anlage structure). Other pathologic specimens and cholangiograms show the duct of the annular segment draining separately from the duct of Wirsung, suggesting that failure of atrophy of the left ventral anlage may be responsible for such cases (16).

Pathology

Pathological specimens of annular pancreas show histologically normal pancreatic tissue which intermingles with the smooth muscle bundles of the duodenal muscularis. In some cases

TABLE 20.1.
ANOMALIES ASSOCIATED WITH ANNULAR PANCREAS[a]

* Down's syndrome (Trisomy 21)
* Duodenal atresia
* Duodenal stenosis
* Duodenal diaphragm
* Malrotation; Ladd's bands
* Esophageal atresia
  Preduodenal portal vein
* Tracheoesophageal fistula
* Imperforate anus
  Hirschsprung's disease
  Situs inversus viscerum
  Congenital absence of the pancreatic neck and tail

Other reported concurrences
  Hemivertebra
  Lung agenesis
  Microcephaly
* Congenital heart disease (Down's syndrome)
  Absent radius
  Cornelia de Lange syndrome

[a] Asterisk connotes common associations.

the pancreatic tissue extends very close to the mucosa (8). The annulus may be from 2–5 cm in length. Intrinsic duodenal atresia, stenosis, or diaphragm frequently coexists. Approximately 85% of annular pancreas are in the second portion of the duodenum; 15% are found in the first or third portions. The relationship of the obstructing ring to the papilla of Vater is variable. The duodenum proximal to the annulus typically shows wall hypertrophy (9).

Clinical Presentation

The clinical manifestations of annular pancreas are chiefly due to duodenal obstruction. Neonates display persistent vomiting following birth. Frequently a history of polyhydramnios in the mother is elicited, a manifestation of intrauterine fetal GI tract obstruction (2, 9). When annular pancreas is present in association with esophageal atresia, tracheoesophageal fistula, or imperforate anus, the signs and symptoms of these latter anomalies may easily obscure the manifestations of the annular pancreas. Such infants have enigmatic feeding difficulties following surgical repair of their other anomalies, and the diagnosis of annular pancreas is delayed, usually discovered only after barium studies are initiated. While one half of neonates with annular pancreas may have jaundice, multiple, nonsurgical factors are the source of the jaundice (1, 10).

In older children and adults, the degree of duodenal obstruction is not significant until inflammatory changes in the annulus narrow the duodenum, or symptoms of pancreatitis or ulcer disease bring the patient to medical attention (6, 9, 16). In a large review of symptomatic and surgically treated cases, 60% of adults complained of nausea and vomiting; 70%, abdominal pain and 10%, hematemesis (17). It is not clear whether duodenal obstruction from the annulus precedes and precipitates the above conditions or vice versa. Occasionally kinking of a dilated, redundant duodenum proximal to the annulus produces a sudden obstruction (13, 19). Rare clinical features are hemorrhage, jaundice, and hypoglycemia (13, 19).

Imaging Studies

The imaging diagnosis of annular pancreas is based on demonstration of high grade duodenal obstruction in neonates. A dilated air-and-fluid filled duodenum and stomach, with little or no gas in more distal bowel, give the "double bubble" appearance on plain radiographs (Fig. 20.2). In this situation one can only diagnose high grade congenital duodenal obstruction. The surgeon will diagnose the exact cause of the obstruction, be it intrinsic duodenal obstruction, annular pancreas, or both. Concomitant intestinal malrotation with Ladd's bands and volvulus are also surgical diagnoses in such cases. Positive contrast study is not necessary. Ultrasonography may show a dilated, fluid-filled duodenum, whether performed on a neonate, or performed on a fetus as part of a maternal obstetrical study (Fig. 20.3). In this latter situation, polyhydramnios will frequently be apparent (20).

In older children and adults, the first portion of the duodenum may show mild or no dilatation on plain radiographs.

Duodenographic findings depend on the degree of obstruction present (Figs. 20.4A and B and 20.5). If complete obstruction is present one may only see a dilated duodenum proximal to the lesion (16). With lesser degrees of obstruction there is eccentric narrowing with lateral notching and medial retraction of the duodenal sweep at the level of the annulus (16, 18). The mucosa is intact unless there is superimposed ulcer disease or pancreatitis (16). Associated signs that may be present include reverse peristalsis, a dilated bulb, pyloric incompetency, and gastric dilatation (18). These findings are extremely difficult to differentiate from postbulbar ulcer, pancreatitis or pancreatic carcinoma, especially considering the frequency with which the former two coexist with annular pancreas in adults (2). Although 85% of annular defects are in the second portion of the sweep, other locations in the duodenum are possible (16). Single contrast upper gastrointestinal study may occasionally miss the findings (21). Double contrast study, with gaseous distension of the duodenum, is superior.

Sonography typically shows only apparent enlargement of the pancreatic head (6). Computed tomography may also show only pancreatic head enlargement, but may also show a central density of high attenuation value which represents contrast material in the narrowed duodenal segment (22). CT may also show a peninsular protrusion of tissue into the duodenal lumen (23). Other cases show circumferential thickening of the apparent duodenal wall in conjunction with an enlarged pancreatic head (24) (Fig. 20.4C and D).

ERCP can be expected to be diagnostic in the 85% of cases in which the annular duct opens into the main pancreatic duct (6), and nondiagnostic if it drains separately into the duodenum. When depicted, the duct of the annulus

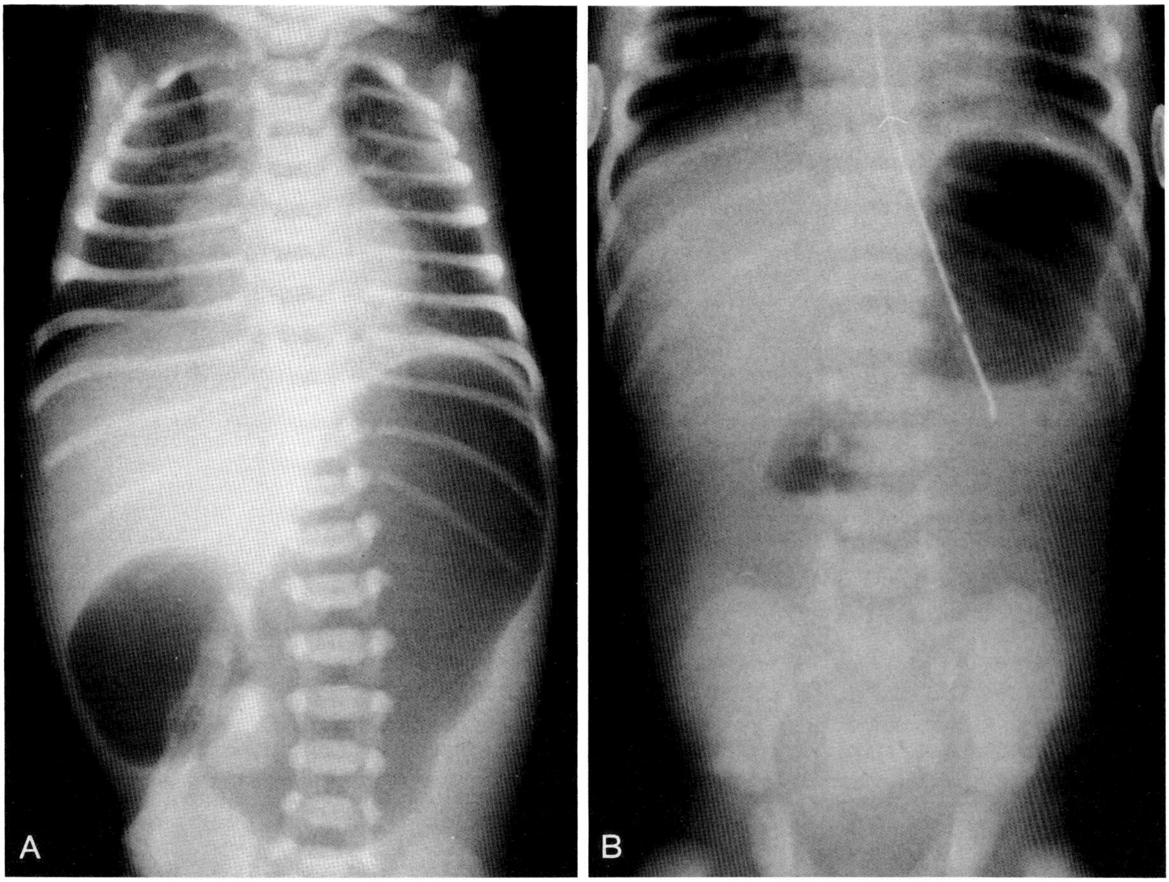

FIGURE 20.2. ANNULAR PANCREAS
The radiographic "double bubble" sign: (A) in a neonate with spontaneous gaseous distension, and (B) in a neonate with partial decompression of the stomach and obstructed duodenum.

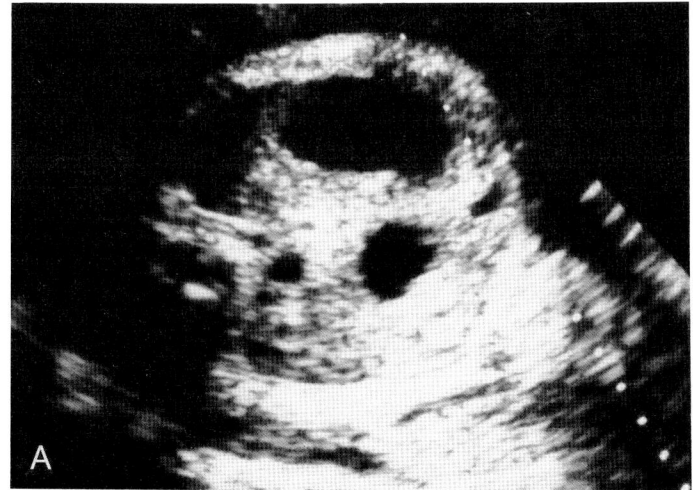
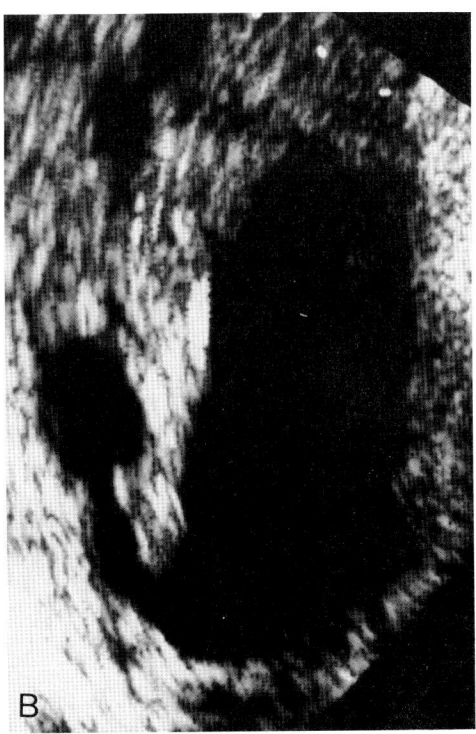

FIGURE 20.3. ANNULAR PANCREAS
The sonographic "double bubble" sign in a fetus: (A) Transverse fetal abdomen section, shows two fluid-filled structures which prove to be distended stomach and duodenum on coronal view. (B). (Courtesy of Jon Meilstrup, M.D., Department of Radiology Walter Reed Army Medical Center.)

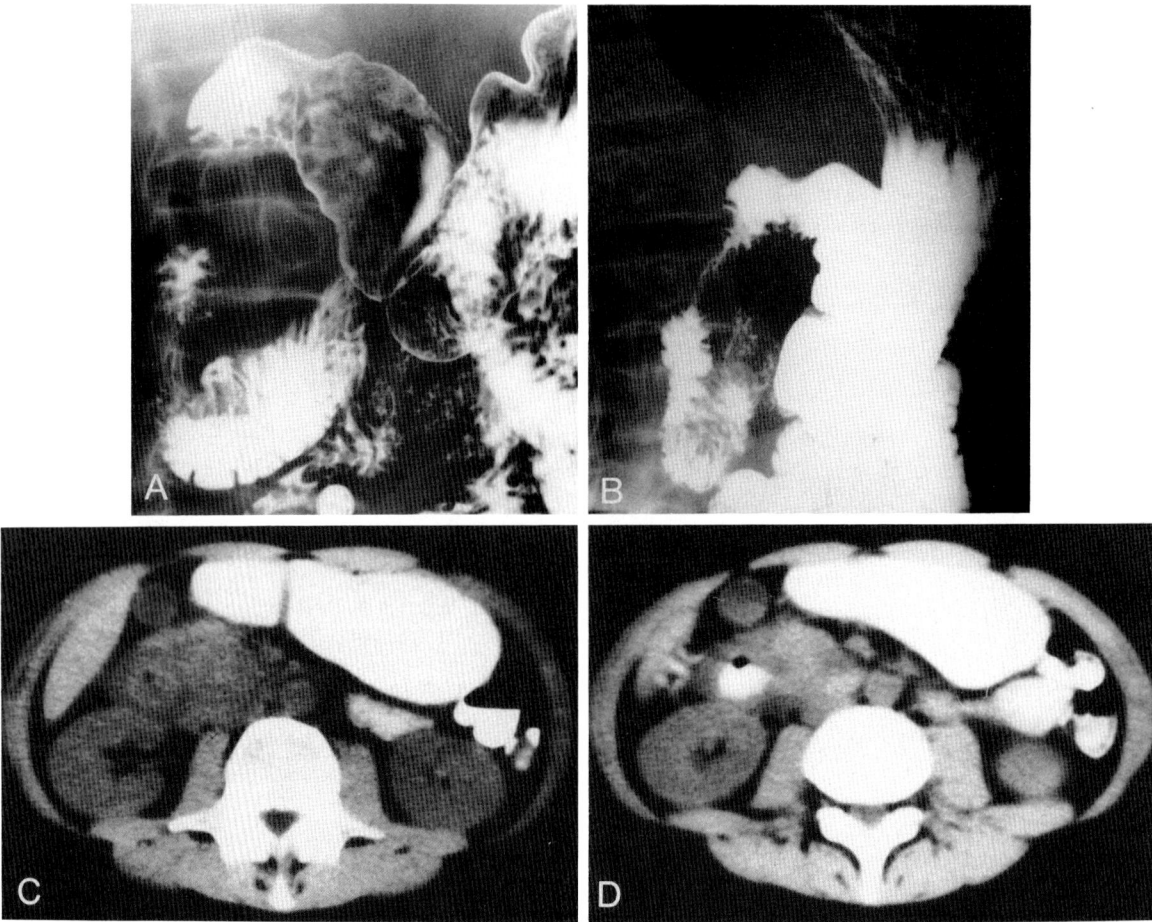

FIGURE 20.4. ANNULAR PANCREAS
Alcoholic with recurrent acute pancreatitis and annular pancreas. *A* and *B:* Two films from an UGI demonstrate narrowing of the proximal descending duodenum with slightly thickened but intact folds and moderate dilatation of the bulb. *C* and *D:* CT scans of the same patient with and without contrast in the duodenum showing thickening of the anterior, lateral and posterior aspects of the descending duodenum suggesting annular pancreas. The head of the pancreas is mildly enlarged from pancreatitis. (Case courtesy of Dr. Kam F. Chan.)

will be seen originating on the left anterior surface of the duodenum passing posteriorly around the duodenum and opening into the main pancreatic duct or common bile duct near the ampulla (6, 15). Occasionally, concomitant biliary obstruction will be present (6) (Fig. 20.6).

Celiac angiography may show an anomalous branch from the posterior superior pancreaticoduodenal artery, which courses in a right and caudal direction to supply the annular segment (23).

Treatment

The goal of surgery for annular pancreas is to bypass the obstructed duodenal segment. Since the anomalous pancreatic tissue is intimately entwined with the muscle fibers of the duodenal wall, it is usually firmly attached to the duodenum and is extricated only with difficulty. In addition, since the pancreatic ring contains a normal pancreatic duct, surgical division of the ring is often complicated by pancreatitis, pancreatic fistula, or such severe local fibrosis that re-obstruction of the duodenum occurs (2, 9). Duodenoduodenostomy or duodenojejunostomy is the recommended procedure to avoid the marginal ulcerations that occur with gastroenterostomy. In the past, mortality rates have ranged from 11 to 34% (2, 8), deaths being primarily in neonates who succumb to other anomalies or to pneumonitis (1).

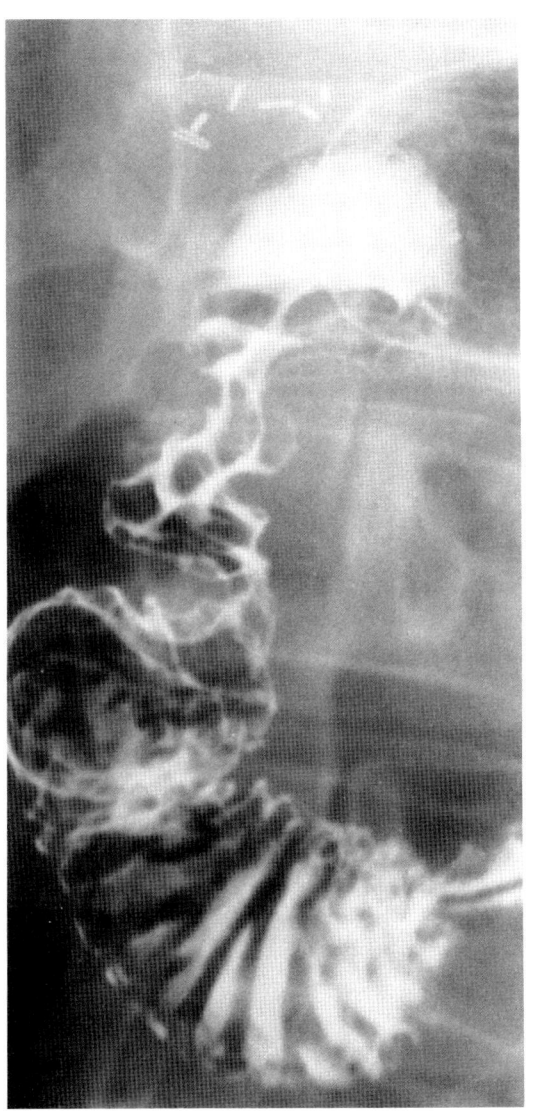

FIGURE 20.5. ANNULAR PANCREAS
A spot film of the duodenum shows marked narrowing of the proximal descending duodenum with contour distortion and thickened and distorted folds. The patient was a 40-yr-old moderate alcohol abuser.

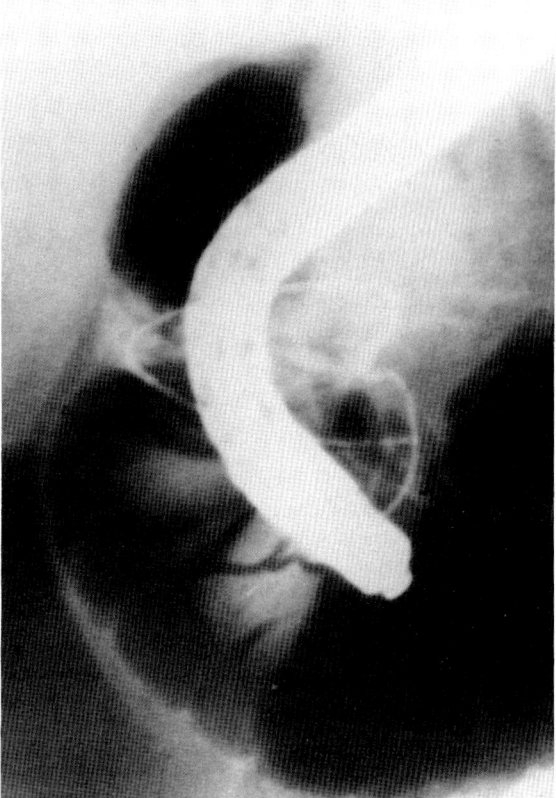

FIGURE 20.6. ANNULAR PANCREAS
ERCP showing a ring around the duodenum formed by the pancreatic duct in annular pancreas. (Courtesy of American Society of Gastrointestinal Endoscopy.)

REFERENCES

1. Merrill JR, Raffensberger JG: Pediatric annular pancreas. *J Pediatr Surg* 11:921–925, 1976.
2. Kiernan PD, Remine SG, Kiernan PC, Remine WH: Annular pancreas. Mayo Clinic experience from 1957 to 1976 with review of the literature. *Arch Surg* 115:46–50, 1980.
3. Welch KJ: The pancreas. In: Ravitch MM, Welch KJ, Benson CD, Aberdeen E, Randolph JG (eds): *Pediatric Surgery*. Chicago: Year Book, 1979, pp 902–912.
4. Ermak TH, Grendell JH, Brandborg LL: The pancreas, anatomy, embryology, and developmental anomalies. In: Sleisenger MH and Fordtran JS (eds): *Gastrointestinal Disease*. Philadelphia, W. B. Saunders, 1983, pp. 1415–1425.
5. Ruben GD, Templeton JM Jr, Ziegler MM: Situs inversus: the complex inducing neonatal intestinal obstruction. *J Pediatr Surg* 18:751–756, 1983.
6. Dharmsathaphorn K, Burell M, Dobbins J: Diagnosis of annular pancreas with endoscopic retrograde cholangiopancreatography. *Gastroenterology* 77:1109–1114, 1979.
7. Free EA, Gerald B: Duodenal obstruction in the newborn due to annular pancreas. *AJR* 103:321–325, 1965.
8. Salonen I: Congenital duodenal obstruction. *Acta Peadiatr Scand (Suppl)* 272:1–87, 1978.
9. Ravitch MM: The pancreas in infants and children. *Surg Clin North Am* 55:377–385, 1975.
10. Andrassy RJ, Mahour H: Gastrointestinal anomalies associated with esophageal atresia or tracheoesophageal fistula. *Arch Surg* 114:1125–1128, 1979.
11. Wick MR, Simmons PS, Ludwig J, Kleinberg F: Duodenal obstruction, annular pancreas, and horseshoe kidney in an infant with Cornelia de Lange syndrome. *Minn Med* 65:539–541, 1982.
12. Lecco TM: Zur Morphologie des pankreas annulare. *Sitzungsb Akad Wissench* 119:391–406, 1910.
13. Sessa F, Fiocca R, Tenti P, Solcia E, Tavani E, Pliteri S: Pancreatic polypeptide rich tissue in the annular pancreas. A distinctive feature of ventral primordium derivatives. *Virchows Arch (Pathol Anat)* 399:227–233, 1983.
14. Baldwin WM: A specimen of annular pancreas. *Anat Rec* 4:299–304, 1910.
15. Ikeda Y, Irving IM: Annular pancreas in a fetus and its three-dimensional reconstruction. *J Pediatr Surg* 19:160–164, 1984.
16. Glazer G, Margulis A: Annular pancreas: etiology and diagnosis using endoscopic retrograde cholangiopancreatography. *Radiology* 133:303–306, 1979.
17. Gilroy JA, Adams AB: Annular pancreas. *Radiology* 75:568–571, 1960.
18. Dodd GD, Nafis WA: Annular pancreas in the adult. *AJR* 75:333–342, 1956.
19. Faegenburg D, Bosniak M: Duodenal anomalies in the adult. *AJR* 88:642–657, 1962.
20. Clark JFJ, Hales E, Ma P, Rosser S: Duodenal atresia in utero in association with Down's syndrome and annular pancreas. *J Natl Med Assoc* 76:190–192, 1984.
21. MacGregor AMC, Green BJ, Stern MA: Symptomatic annular pancreas in the adult. *Br J Surg* 56:713–715, 1969.
22. Novetsky GJ, Berlin L, Smith C, Epstein AJ: CT diagnosis of annular pancreas. *J Comput Assist Tomogr* 8:1031–1032, 1984.
23. Inamoto K, Ischikawa Y, Itoh N: CT demonstration of annular pancreas: case report. *Gastrointest Radiol* 8:143–144, 1983.
24. Afzal A, Chan KF, Song IS: Annular pancreas. *J Comput Assist Tomogr* 6:409–410, 1982.

SCHWACHMAN-DIAMOND SYNDROME

First reported by Schwachman and Diamond in 1964, this is a congenital disease that has a familial tendency but uncertain genetics (1). In addition to pancreatic insufficiency, there are major hematologic and skeletal disturbances.

Clinical Findings

Patients present in infancy with failure to thrive, diarrhea with or without steatorrhea, growth retardation, normal sweat electrolytes, and normal glucose tolerance (1). Recurrent respiratory and skin infections may lead to septicemia, pneumonia, and disseminated hemorrhage (2). The above are caused by bone marrow hypoplasia which results in neutropenia or pancytopenia (1). Although the prognosis for normal growth is poor and morbidity can be serious, this disease should be separated from cystic fibrosis which carries a worse prognosis (1).

Pathology

Autopsy has shown absence of pancreatic exocrine tissue and replacement by mature adipose tissue with well-preserved islets (1).

Radiology

Skeletal

Bony abnormalities include dwarfism with or without metaphyseal chondrodysplasia (2, 3), abnormal tubulation of bone, focal absence of normal metaphyseal calcification, hypoplasia of the fifth middle phalanges, bilateral clinodactyly, narrowing of the sacrosciatic notches, and retarded bone age (2).

Computerized Tomography

The pancreas is replaced by fat and the main pancreatic duct is depicted as a relative radiodensity (Fig. 20.7).

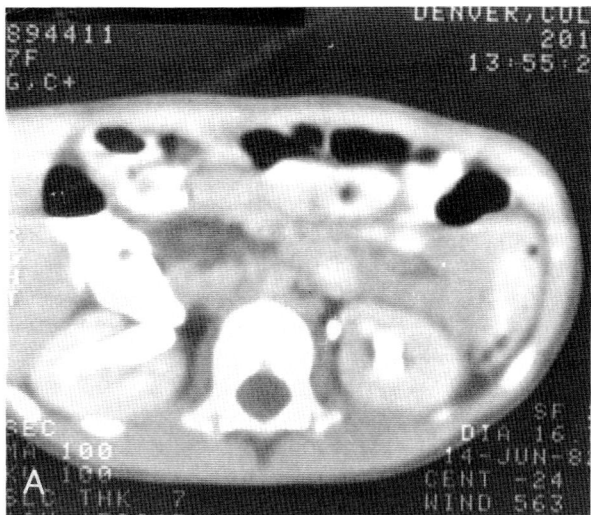 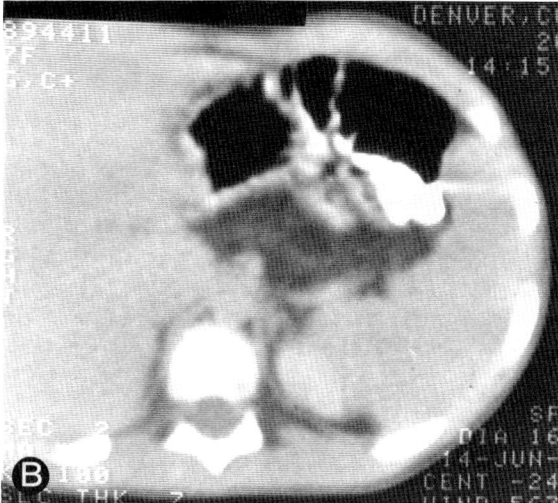

FIGURE 20.7. SCHWACHMAN'S SYNDROME
A and *B:* CT scans of a child with Schwachman's syndrome showing complete fat replacement of the pancreas. The thin relative radiodensity coursing through the fat is the pancreatic duct.

REFERENCES

1. Schwachman H, Diamond LK, Oski FA, Khaw K: The syndrome of pancreatic insufficiency and bone marrow dysfunction. *J Pediatr* 5:645–663, 1964.
2. McLennan TW, Steinbach HL: Schwachman's syndrome: the broad spectrum of bony abnormalities. *Radiology* 112:167–173, 1974.
3. Taybi H, Mitchell AD, Friedman GD: Metaphyseal dystostosis and the associated syndrome of pancreatic insufficiency and blood disorders. *Radiology* 95:563–571, 1969.

CYSTIC FIBROSIS

Cystic fibrosis is a multisystem disorder characterized by widespread abnormalities of mucus secreting glands and abnormal loss of electrolytes in sweat. The major common clinical manifestations of cystic fibrosis are chronic infection with obstructive disease of the lungs, and malabsorption due to pancreatic insufficiency. The original description of the disease comes from a pathologic summary of "celiac" disease wherein an entity with striking fibrosis, fatty replacement, and cyst formation in the pancreas was noted to cause characteristic patterns of clinical disease: (*a*) neonatal death from intestinal obstruction, (*b*) death before 6 months of age from malabsorption, and (*c*) malabsorption and respiratory disease in older infants and children (1).

Cystic fibrosis occurs in 1 in 1,500 live births in Caucasians; it is much less common in blacks and Orientals. It is the single most common cause of exocrine pancreatic insufficiency in childhood (2). The basic defect in cystic fibrosis is unknown. Patients may rarely escape diagnosis until adulthood, yet the pathologic changes of cystic fibrosis have been demonstrated in a fetus (3). Although there is a general positive correlation between the age of the patient and the severity of his disease, degree of impairment is variable at any age. Ten percent of patients will have no pancreatic dysfunction (2, 4).

The long-term goals of therapy are to maximize nutrition and growth, chiefly by providing a low fat, high protein, high calorie diet in combination with pancreatic enzyme replacement.

Pathology

In the very young, the pancreas may appear normal. With increasing degrees of involvement the pancreas shows initially increased lobulation, then variable degrees of fibrosis and replacement by fat. Small macroscopic cysts may be seen in longstanding cases (2, 5, 6).

Histology shows focal inspissation of eosinophilic material in acini and ductules as the earliest change. With increasing disease, there is progressive dilatation of acini and ductules, and atrophy of the parenchyma, such that islands of parenchyma are surrounded by collagen and fat;

cysts are the only remnants of the pancreatic ducts. In the most advanced cases, there is a mass of adipose tissue in which scattered groups of islets of Langerhans and scattered foci of parenchyma remain (Fig. 20.8) (2).

Clinical Findings

In the majority of cases, steatorrhea and creatorrhea are the major clinical problems directly referable to the pancreatic insufficiency (7). The steatorrhea is markedly exacerbated by failure to take adequate pancreatic enzyme replacement or by intake of a high fat diet. Some patients, usually those older patients with more normal pancreatic function, present with acute pancreatitis, usually exacerbated by diet, alcohol intake or tetracycline administration (8, 9). While hyperglycemia and glycosuria can be demonstrated in many patients, clinical diabetes mellitus is apparent in only 1–2% of patients. Patients may occasionally be misdiagnosed as having celiac disease if the pulmonary symptoms are not yet apparent. Other gastrointestinal tract symptoms may be the first recognizable symptoms of cystic fibrosis: growth failure, idiopathic hypoproteinemia; cirrhosis and portal hypertension; recurrent abdominal pain and fecal impaction; rectal prolapse (4).

Radiology

Any of the chronic changes described below may be absent in those few patients who lack significant pancreatic dysfunction. However, the typical imaging patterns of acute pancreatitis may be recognized in this group of patients (8).

Plain film radiography plays little role in the assessment of pancreatic disease in cystic fibrosis. Pancreatic calcifications may be present (10), but only rarely are dense concretions (11) (see section on plain films in chronic pancreatitis). Fatty infiltration of the liver is a rare finding with untreated severe malabsorption (Fig. 20.9).

Gastrointestinal Tract Barium Examinations

The radiologic findings and treatment of me-

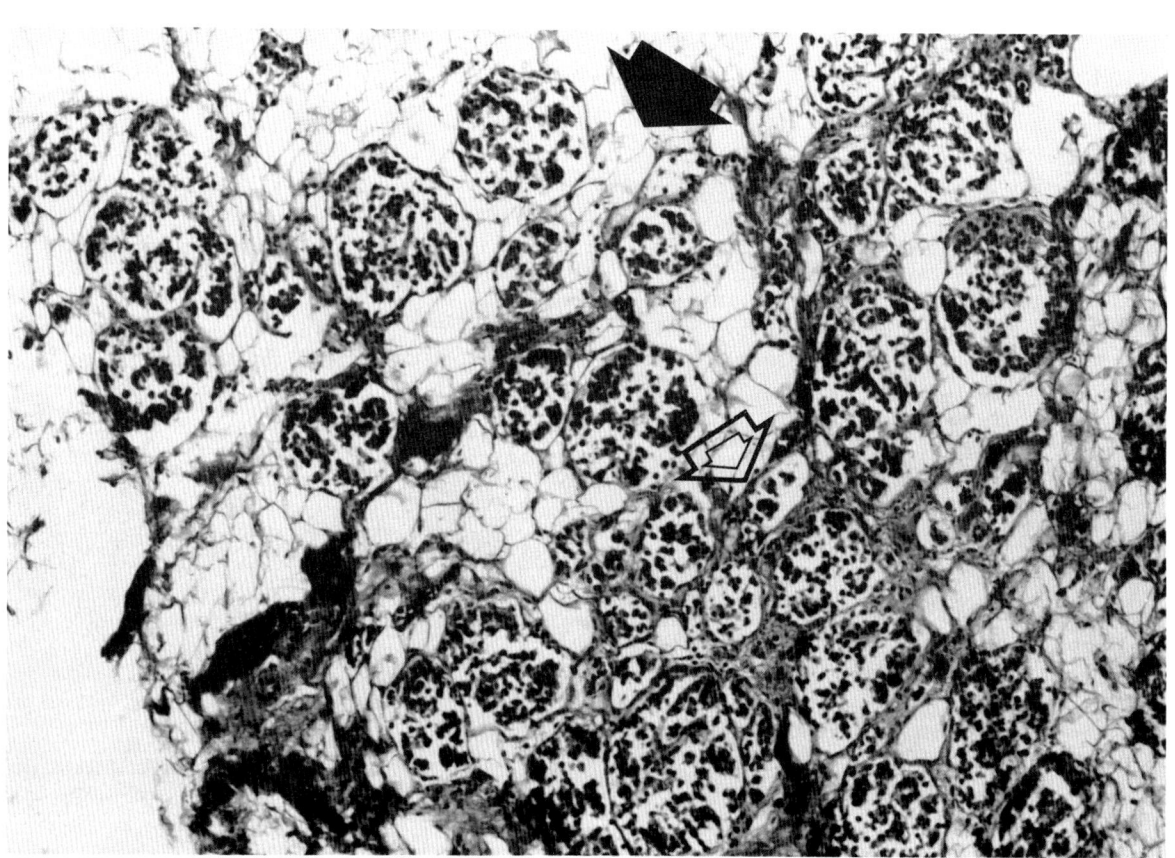

FIGURE 20.8. CYSTIC FIBROSIS
Advanced cystic fibrosis of the pancreas. Islets of Langerhans are the only remaining pancreatic tissue, separated by fat (*arrow*) and fibrosis (*open arrows*).

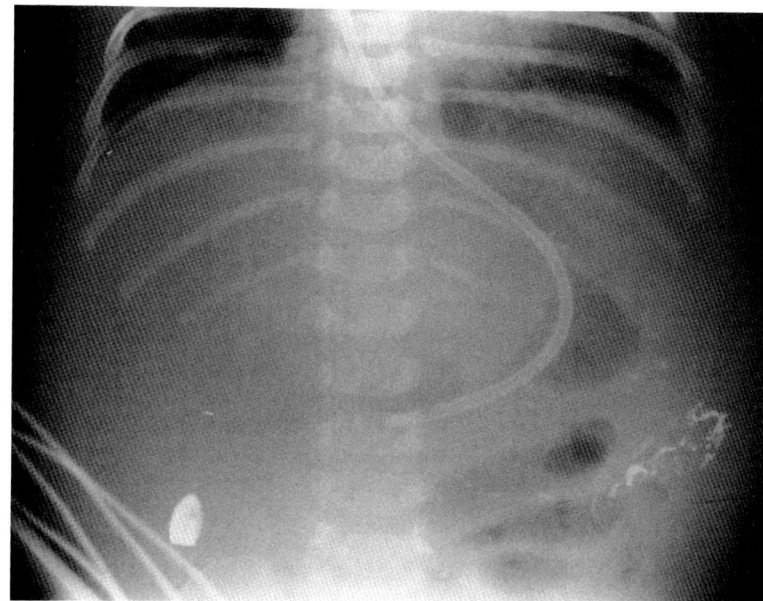

FIGURE 20.9. CYSTIC FIBROSIS
Right upper quadrant lucency due to fatty infiltration of the liver in an infant with cystic fibrosis who is starving because of lack of pancreatic enzyme replacement. (Courtesy of Marie Capitanio, M.D., St. Christopher's Hospital for Children, Philadelphia.)

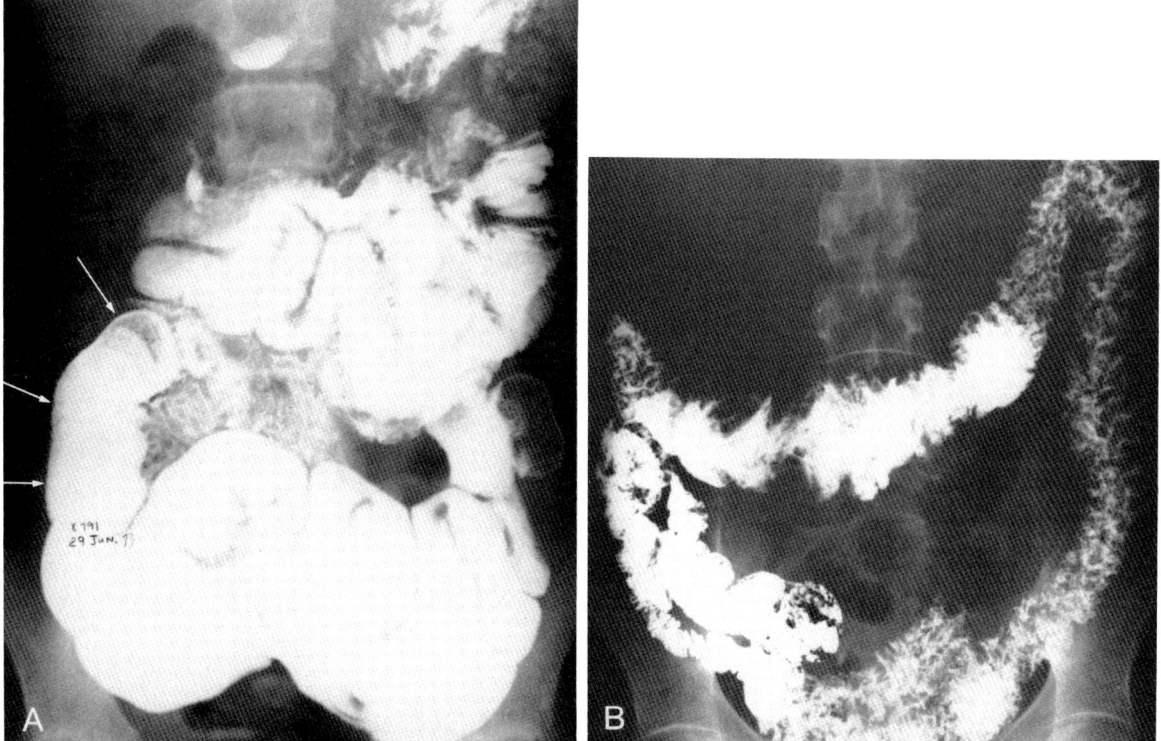

FIGURE 20.10. CYSTIC FIBROSIS
A: Small bowel series: granular mucosal pattern due to abnormal intestinal secretions (*arrows*) and thickened jejunal folds in the left upper quadrant. Note large amount of stool in colon. Cystic fibrosis, child. *B:* Evacuation film from a barium enema: incomplete evacuation and jejunization of mucosa. Cystic fibrosis, adolescent.

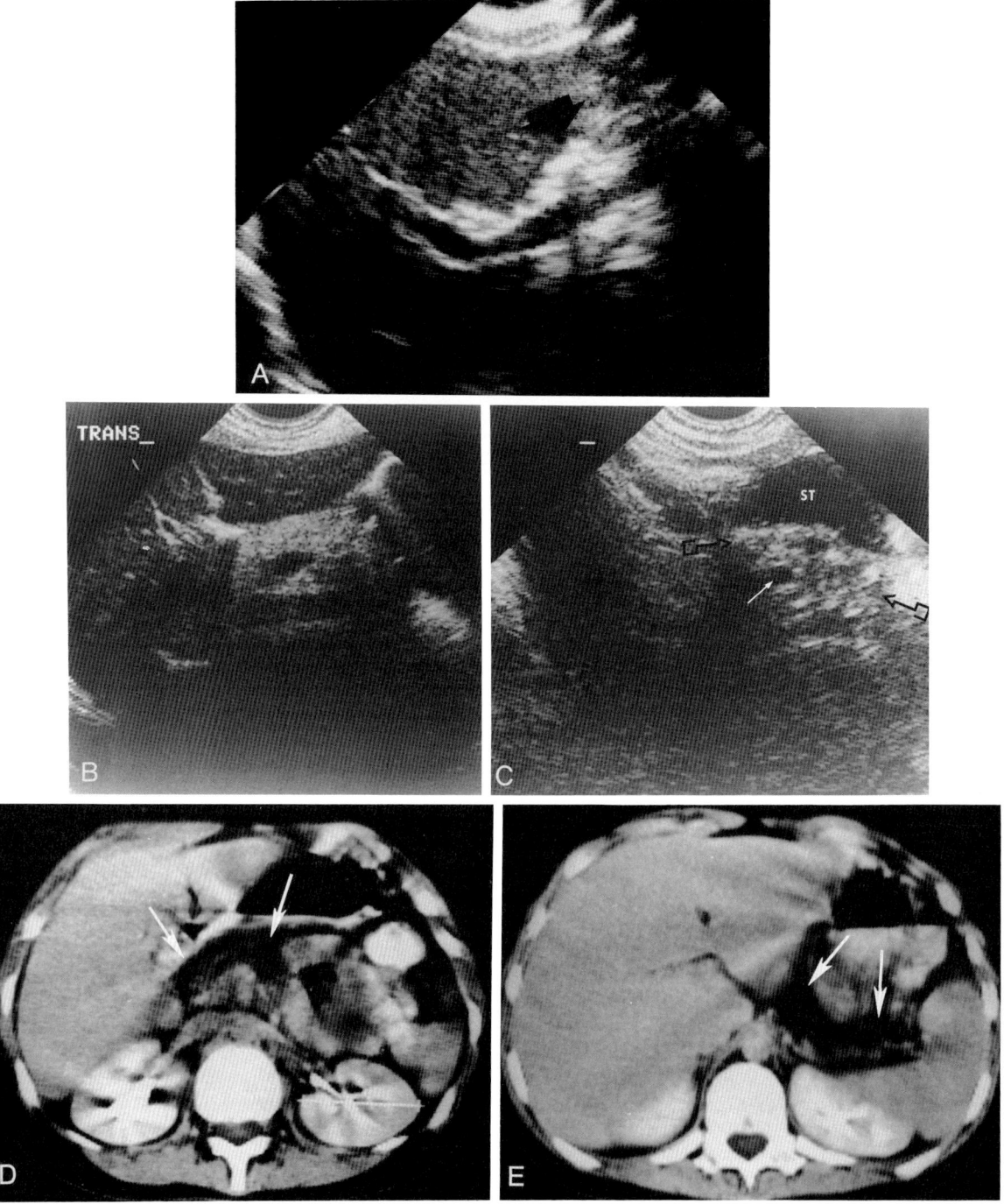

FIGURE 20.11. ULTRASONOGRAPHY AND CT OF ADVANCED CYSTIC FIBROSIS

A: Transverse section through the splenoportal venous junction shows a densely echoic pancreatic head (*arrow*). (This patient's histology shown in Fig. 20.8.) *B:* Transverse scan through the head and body of the pancreas: uniform, hyperechoic texture. Cystic fibrosis, adolescent. *C:* Transverse scan through the tail (*arrows*) in the same patient via a water-filled stomach (*ST*): coarse, heterogeneous echo texture with one small cyst (*white arrow*). *D* and *E:* CT of same patient as in *B* and *C:* fatty replacement of the pancreas (*arrows*).

conium ileus are well known and beyond the scope of this textbook. Less well known are duodenographic changes in cystic fibrosis consisting of thickened folds, nodular filling defects, mucosal smudging, dilatation and redundancy (11). The etiology is thought to be related to irritation by unbuffered gastric acid.

Small bowel abnormalities can also occur, consisting of thick or course folds in the proximal jejunum, and occasionally jejunal dilatation (Fig. 20.10A). Histologic correlation with the duodenal and small bowel abnormalities has revealed shortening and clubbing of villi with distention of crypts and dilatation of Brunner's glands and a thick mucosal coat of adherent mucus (12).

A distinctive picture in the colon can be seen on barium enema (Fig. 20.10B). The postevacuation film can show coarse redundant and hyperplastic mucosa, reminiscent of the normal jejunum, termed "jejunization" of the colon (13). Marginal defects can be produced by tenacious fecal material. Histologically, colonic mucosa shows dilated and gaping crypts with goblet cell hyperplasia. The surface is covered by adherent mucus (12).

Ultrasonograms are markedly affected by the pathologic changes of fibrosis, fatty replacement, calcification, and cyst formation in the pancreatic ductules. All of these changes increase the echogenicity of the pancreas (6, 14–16). Occasionally the cysts are macroscopic and can be discerned as discrete cysts (Fig. 20.11) (5, 6). Assessment of pancreatic echogenicity may be hampered by concomitant liver disease causing increased hepatic echogenicity. However, a quantitative assessment of pancreatic echo amplitude has shown a clear increase in pancreatic echogenicity (17). Often, the changes are striking (Fig. 20.11).

Computed tomography of the pancreas has a variable appearance. Small calcifications may give the pancreas a diffuse or focal increase in attenuation value, whereas extensive fatty replacement is depicted as a normal pancreatic contour with attenuation values in the range of fat (−90 to −120 HU). The latter pattern is usually present in older adolescents and young adults (6).

REFERENCES

1. Anderson DH: Cystic fibrosis of the pancreas and its relation to celiac disease. Am J Dis Child 56:344–399, 1938.
2. Oppenheimer EH, Esterly JR: Pathology of cystic fibrosis. Review of the literature and comparison with 146 cases. Perspect Pediatr Pathol 2:241–278, 1975.
3. Matsuo T, Ikeda T, Mori Y, Nonaka M, Fujiwara H, Yun K: Cystic fibrosis of the pancreas in a human fetus. Acta Pathol Jpn 28:77–82, 1978.
4. Schwachman H: Gastrointestinal manifestations of cystic fibrosis. Pediatr Clin North Am 22:787–805, 1975.
5. Churchill RJ, Cunningham DG, Henkin RE, Reynes CJ: Macroscopic cysts of the pancreas in cystic fibrosis demonstrated by multiple radiologic modalities. JAMA 245:72–74, 1981.
6. Daneman A, Gaskin K, Martin DJ, Cutz E: Pancreatic changes in cystic fibrosis: CT and sonographic appearances. AJR 141:653–655, 1983.
7. Park RW, Grand RJ: Gastrointestinal manifestations of cystic fibrosis: a review. Gastroenterology 81:1143–1161, 1981.
8. Schwachman H, Lebenthal E, Khaw KT: Recurrent acute pancreatitis in patients with cystic fibrosis with normal pancreatic enzymes. Pediatrics 55:86–95, 1975.
9. Doershuk CF, Boat TF: Cystic fibrosis. In Berman RE, Vaughn VC, Nelson WE (eds): Textbook of Pediatrics. Philadelphia, W. B. Saunders, 1983, pp 1086–1099.
10. Iannaccone G, Antonelli M: Calcification of the pancreas in cystic fibrosis. Pediatr Radiol 9:85–89, 1980.
11. Taussig LM, Saldino RM, DiSant'Agnese PA: Radiographic abnormalities of the duodenum and small bowel in cystic fibrosis of the pancreas. Radiology 106:369–376, 1973.
12. Berk RN, Lee FA: The late manifestations of cystic fibrosis of the pancreas. Radiology 106:377–381, 1973.
13. Haller JO, Heffer ET, Kassner EG, Pinck RL: Unusual radiographic manifestations of cystic fibrosis. Rev Interam Radiol 2:41–42, 1977.
14. Willi UV, Reddish JM, Teele RL: Cystic fibrosis: its characteristic appearance on abdominal sonography. AJR 134:1005–1010, 1980.
15. Phillips HE, Cox KL, Reid MH, McGahan JP: Pancreatic sonography in cystic fibrosis. AJR 137:69–72, 1981.
16. Wilson-Sharp RC, Irving HC, Brown RC, Chalmers DM, Littlewood JM: Ultrasonography of the pancreas, liver, and biliary system in cystic fibrosis. Arch Dis Child 59:923–926, 1984.
17. Shawker TH, Linzer M, Hubbard VS: Chronic pancreatitis: the diagnostic significance of pancreatic size and echo amplitude. J Ultrasound Med 3:267–272, 1984.

ized clinically into acute
21

Pancreatitis

MICHAEL C. HILL, M.D., MARK T. BIRNS, M.D.,
ARNOLD C. FRIEDMAN, M.D., DONALD G. MITCHELL, M.D.,
LEONARD BODNER, M.D., AND SEYMOUR S. SPRAYREGEN, M.D.

Pancreatitis is separated clinically into acute and chronic forms. Acute pancreatitis is characterized by single or repeated episodes (acute relapsing pancreatitis) of pancreatic inflammation and pain. Following resolution, normal anatomy and function are restored. By definition, chronic pancreatitis is characterized by permanent damage, either functional or anatomic (1). It may be initiated by a severe attack of abdominal pain, but it usually begins insidiously with mild recurrent bouts of pain (2). In some patients pain is almost constant, whereas in a small percentage exocrine and endocrine insufficiency develop without pain (2). Thus, a long period of observation may be necessary to differentiate acute relapsing pancreatitis from chronic pancreatitis.

ACUTE PANCREATITIS

Etiology and Pathogenesis

Alcoholism and biliary tract disease account for the vast majority of cases of acute pancreatitis in adults in the United States (2–4). Other causes include hypercalcemia (especially hyperparathyroidism) (2, 5, 6); hyperlipidemia (Types I and V) (2, 4, 7); viral infection (mumps (8), hepatitis (9)); mononucleosis (10); drugs (6) (azathioprine, thiazide, sulfonamides, furosemide, tetracycline, estrogens, L-asparaginase, chlorthalidone, steroids, ethracrynic acid, phenformin and procainamide); surgery and blunt or penetrating trauma (2); renal transplantation (11); penetrating ulcer (2); pancreatic neoplasms or tumor lysis; parasites (12) (ascariasis, clonorchis sinensis); vasculitis, (especially polyarteritis nodosa) (2); and structural abnormalities of the biliary and pancreatic ducts (choledochocele, pancreas divisum) (13). In children the most common causes of acute pancreatitis are trauma, systemic diseases, and drugs (14, 15). Approximately 20% of patients with acute pancreatitis have no apparent underlying or predisposing cause (2).

Acute pancreatitis is caused by the destructive effects of pancreatic enzymes: proteolysis, lipolysis and hemorrhage. Trypsin is likely to play a key role as it is capable of activating proenzymes and is itself a protease (2, 3). Lipase and elastase (which digest the elastic tissue in vessels) are also important (2, 3). At present, only theories exist as to what triggers these enzymes; these include bile reflux, hypersecretion, obstruction, alcohol-induced change, and duodenal reflux (3). Biliary reflux has been considered an important mechanism of activation of pancreatic enzymes since Opie noted a gallstone impacted in the ampulla blocking the outflow of both pancreatic and common bile ducts at the autopsy of a patient with acute pancreatitis (2, 3). A common channel exists at the termination of the biliary and pancreatic ducts in the majority of adults (2). However, fatal pancreatitis has been seen in patients whose pancreatic and bile ducts enter the duodenum separately (2). Pancreatic secretory pressure normally exceeds that in the biliary tree (2). Despite this conflicting evidence, there is unquestionably an increased incidence of acute pancreatitis in patients with gallstones even without choledocholithiasis, and cholecystectomy is often curative (2).

The hypersecretion-obstructive theory proposes that pancreatic ducts rupture from hypersecretion in the presence of partial ductal obstruction. However, pancreatic duct obstructive lesions are not common in acute pancreatitis (3). The mechanism of the production of acute pancreatitis in chronic alcoholics is unclear—occasional heavy ingestion in a healthy individual rarely causes pancreatitis (2). Acute pancreatitis in alcoholics is usually superimposed on chronic pancreatitis in which ducts are obstructed by stones, protein plugs and fibrosis (2). Alcohol stimulates pancreatic secretion by increasing gastric acid output and secretin release (2). The combination of hypersecretion and partial duct obstruction then causes acute pancreatitis. Hyperlipidemia (Type IV) in alcoholics may be a factor (7).

Duodenal contents can reflux into the pancreatic duct and activate pancreatic enzymes if the sphincter of Oddi is damaged by biliary stones or rendered lax by alcohol (3).

Acute pancreatitis develops not uncommonly in patients with hyperparathyroidism and other hypercalcemic states (3, 5). Pancreatitis complicates hyperparathyroidism as often as 7–12% (3, 5). Hypercalcemia may both activate trypsinogen and increase pancreatic secretion (2, 3, 5).

Unless hypertriglyceridemia is controlled in patients with Types I or V hyperlipidemia, recurrent acute pancreatitis is common (3). A proposed mechanism is lipolysis by peripancreatic lipase resulting in high concentrations of toxic free fatty acids causing hypercoagulability and ischemia (3).

Renal transplant patients may develop pancreatitis months to years after the operation (11, 14, 15). Precipitating factors include steroids and other immunosuppressive agents, hyperparathyroidism, and opportunistic infection (14, 15).

Trauma, either blunt, penetrating, or surgical, may cause acute pancreatitis, probably disrupting or temporarily obstructing small and/or large ducts (2, 16, 17).

Pancreatic carcinoma uncommonly presents clinically with acute pancreatitis. In one series of 255 patients with proven carcinoma of the pancreas, 3% had acute pancreatitis (18). Conversely, carcinoma is found in only 1–2% of patients with acute pancreatitis (18). Mechanisms include both duct obstruction and activation of trypsinogen by the tumor (18). Similarly, metastases and lymphoma can cause acute pancreatitis (19).

Tumor lysis pancreatitis, a complication of chemotherapy, is thought to occur because of the direct inflammatory effect on the pancreas of local tumor cell necrosis (20).

Pathology

In the milder acute edematous pancreatitis, the gland is swollen and edematous but otherwise well-preserved (3, 4). Microscopically, edema, congestion, and leukocytic infiltration predominate, and there is a return to normal structure and function after resolution (3, 4). Acute hemorrhagic pancreatitis is characterized by proteolytic destruction of pancreatic parenchyma, hemorrhage from blood vessel wall necrosis, fat necrosis, and accompanying inflammation (3). Grossly, there are areas of blue-black hemorrhage and gray-white necrotic softening with foci of yellow-white fat necrosis in and about the pancreas (3). Fat necrosis is often found in peripancreatic and other intraabdominal fat depots and occasionally in distant sites as a result of enzymatic dissemination via the blood stream (3). Free intraperitoneal fluid with floating oil droplets is frequently present (3). Areas of fat necrosis become infiltrated first by neutrophils and then later by histiocytes and lymphocytes and extensive calcification may eventually occur (4).

Secondary bacterial infection may complicate hemorrhagic pancreatitis after 3 to 4 days resulting in suppurative necrosis or abscess formation (3). If the patient survives acute hemorrhagic pancreatitis, the end result often is pancreatic fibrosis, calcification and duct dilatation (3).

Clinical Findings

Severe upper abdominal pain in a band-like distribution sometimes radiating to the back is the outstanding symptom, often accompanied by nausea, vomiting, abdominal distention, and constipation (2). Patients rarely may present without abdominal pain (21). Physical findings of abdominal tenderness are often unimpressive compared to the intense pain (2). Three days to a week after the onset of symptoms, hemorrhagic changes (blue to yellow-brown discoloration) may be apparent in the flanks or the periumbilical region. The former (Grey Turner's sign) and the latter (Cullen's sign) are due to extravasation of blood from the anterior pararenal space to the properitoneal fat plane via the posterior pararenal space (2, 22). Systemic manifestations of metastatic fat necrosis include erythematous tender subcutaneous nodules, polyarthralgia, eosinophilia, aseptic necrosis, osteolysis and bone infarcts (2, 21).

Elevation of serum amylase and lipase are the most helpful laboratory findings, although not completely specific (2). Blood calcium and magnesium levels may be depressed in patients with extensive fat necrosis indicating poor prognosis (2). Liver enzymes may be elevated either by partial common duct obstruction from pancreatic edema or underlying disease (2).

REFERENCES

1. Perrier CV: Symposium on the etiology and pathologic anatomy of chronic pancreatitis, Marseilles 1963. *Dig Dis Sci* 9:371–376, 1964.
2. Snodgrass PJ: Diseases of the pancreas. In Wintrobe, MM et al (eds): *Harrison's Principles of Internal Medicine*. New York, McGraw-Hill, 1974, pp 1571–1577.
3. Robbins SL, Cotran SR: *Pathologic Basis of Disease*. Philadelphia, W. B. Saunders, 1979, pp 1096–1102.
4. Rosai J: *Ackerman's Surgical Pathology*. St. Louis, C. V. Mosby, 1981, pp 664–668.
5. Mixter CG, Keynes WM, Cope O: Further experience with pancreatitis as a diagnostic clue to hyperparathyroidism. *N Engl J Med* 266:265–271, 1962.
6. Mallory A, Kern F Jr: Drug-induced pancreatitis: a critical review. *Gastroenterology* 78:813–820, 1980.
7. Cameron JL, Capuzzi DM, Zuidema GD: Acute pancreatitis with hyperlipemia. *Am J Med* 56:482–487, 1974.
8. Feldstein JD, Johnson FR, Kallick CA: Acute hemorrhagic pancreatitis and pseudocyst due to mumps. *Ann Surg* 180:85–88, 1974.
9. Achord JL: Acute pancreatitis with infectious hepatitis. *JAMA* 205:129–132, 1968.
10. Wislocki LC: Acute pancreatitis in infectious mononucleosis. *N Engl J Med* 275:322–323, 1966.
11. Schnyder PA, Brasch RC, Salvatierra O: Gastrointestinal complications of renal transplantation in children. *Radiology* 130:361–366, 1979.
12. Reeder MM, Palmer PES: *Radiology of Tropical Diseases*. Baltimore, Williams & Wilkins, 1981, pp 414–470.
13. Richter JM, Schapiro RH, Mulley AG, Warshaw AL: Association of pancreas divisum and pancreatitis, and its treatment by sphincteroplasty of the accessory ampulla. *Gastroenterology* 81:1104–1110, 1981.
14. Fernandez JA, Rosenberg JC: Post-transplantation pancreatitis. *Surg Gynecol Obstet* 143:795–798, 1976.
15. Robinson DO, Alp MH, Grant AK et al: Pancreatitis and renal disease. *Scand J Gastroenterol* 12:17–20, 1977.
16. White TT, Morgan A, Hopton D: Postoperative pancreatitis. *Am J Surg* 120:132–137, 1970.
17. Bardenheier JA III, Kaminski DL, William VL: Pancreatitis after biliary tract surgery. *Am J Surg* 116:773–776, 1968.
18. Levine E: Carcinoma of the pancreas presenting as acute pancreatitis: CT diagnosis. *Gastrointest Radiol* 6:29–33, 1981.
19. Niccolini DG, Grahm JH, Banks PA: Tumor-induced acute pancreatitis. *Gastroenterology* 71:142–145, 1976.
20. Spiegel RJ, Magrath IT: Tumor lysis pancreatitis. *Med Pediatr Oncol* 7:169–172, 1979.
21. Boswell SH, Baylin CJ: Metastatic fat necrosis and lytic bone lesions in a patient with painless acute pancreatitis. *Radiology* 106:85–86, 1973.
22. Meyers MA: *Dynamic Radiology of the Abdomen. Normal and Pathologic Anatomy*. New York, Springer-Verlag, 1976, pp 265–277.

Radiology

Although the diagnosis of acute pancreatitis is primarily clinical and based on history, physical findings, and blood tests, radiology is often important. At times the clinical diagnosis is difficult and corroborating radiologic evidence is helpful (Fig. 21.1). Surgically correctible lesions need to be identified radiologically and complications often can be diagnosed only by radiologic techniques.

Chest Film

Pleuropulmonary abnormalities have been reported in 14–71% of patients with acute pancreatitis (1). Findings include diaphragmatic elevation, atelectasis, infiltrates, and effusions—abnormalities almost always affecting the lung bases (1). Except for pleural effusions, these abnormalities are equally frequent on either side and are commonly bilateral (1). Pleural effusion is usually unilateral and left-sided and occurs in about 5% of patients with acute pancreatitis (Fig. 21.2C) (1, 2). Pleural fluid amylase is elevated to levels higher than those in the serum in 85% of effusions from pancreatitis, and this elevation in a unilateral left-sided effusion is considered almost pathognomonic for pancreatitis (1, 2). The pathogenesis of these pleuropulmonary changes in acute pancreatitis is incompletely understood. Possible pathways for spread to the chest of enzymes and inflammation include fenestrations in the diaphragm, the hiatal openings, and transdiaphragmatic lymphatics. Diffuse alveolar infiltrates (noncardiac pulmonary edema) may be seen in patients with acute pancreatitis as part of the adult respiratory distress syndrome (3). Free fatty acids in the circulation and elevated triglycerides can damage the alveolar lining, causing alveolar filling with fluid (4).

Skeletal Films

Polyarthralgia, tender erythematous subcutaneous nodules, osteolytic bone lesions, bone infarcts, and aseptic necrosis are well-documented manifestations of metastatic fat necrosis in acute pancreatitis (1, 5). Fever and eosinophilia are usually also present (5). These symptoms may occur during or shortly after an attack of pancreatitis (5). The true incidence of bone changes in pancreatitis is unknown since most patients are not subjected to skeletal survey, however, estimates of 6% have been made (1). Osteolysis generally affects the long bones and the tubular bones of the hands and feet (5). Radiographs demonstrate punched out and permeative destruction of cancellous bone and endosteal erosion which may destroy the cortex and result in periosteal reaction (Fig. 21.1) (5).

Although unproven, it is felt that these lesions result from high levels of lipase in the circulation which lead to lipolysis and fat necrosis within

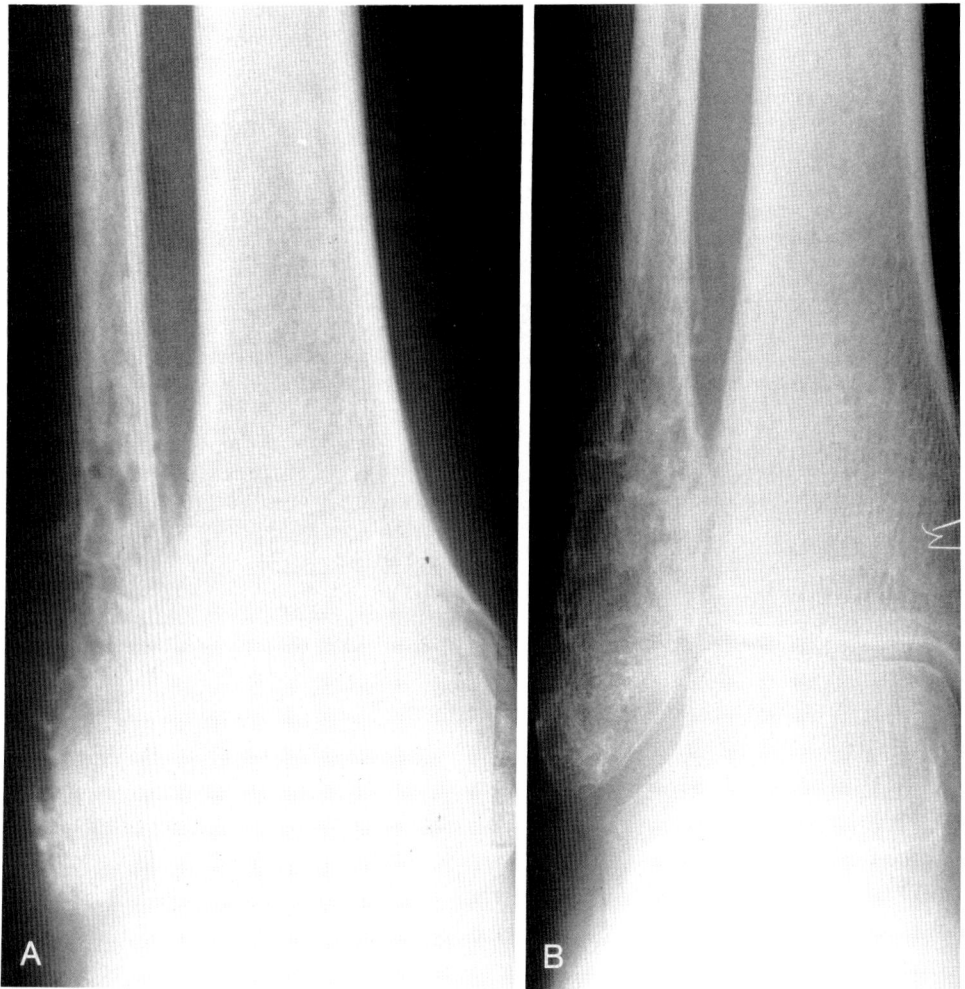

FIGURE 21.1. ACUTE PANCREATITIS

A: Patient with acute pancreatitis without abdominal pain and a red, swollen, painful ankle. There is soft tissue swelling, permeative and moth-eaten lytic changes and periosteal reaction in the distal fibula. Noted also is periosteal reaction in the distal tibia. *B:* Seven weeks later without specific therapy. There is a healing of the distal fibula. Seven months later a radiograph was normal. (Case courtesy of Dr. Angus Robertson.)

bones and in the subcutaneous tissues (5). The inflammatory response to liberated free fatty acids may cause a hyperemia in turn leading to osseous resorption. The osteolytic lesions heal spontaneously over weeks to months, and rarely calcification develops in the areas of subcutaneous fat necrosis (1, 5).

Two additional bone lesions can be seen as a result of acute pancreatitis, although they are more common in chronic pancreatitis—aseptic necrosis and metaphyseal infarcts (1, 5). The former tend to occur in the femoral and humeral heads and are radiographically identical to the subarticular abnormalities seen in other causes of aseptic necrosis (1, 5). Metaphyseal infarcts tend to occur in the distal femur and proximal tibia and are indistinguishable from bone infarcts seen in other diseases (1, 5). There are several reasons for bone ischemia to develop in pancreatitis: edema and increased pressure in the marrow cavity from fat necrosis, direct enzyme damage to vascular endothelium, and circulating vasoactive substances (1, 5).

The bone and soft tissue lesions of pancreatitis have been seen in duct cell adenocarcinoma (1, 5) and acinar cell carcinoma of the pancreas (6), so that, while they are suggestive of pancreatitis, they are not pathognomonic.

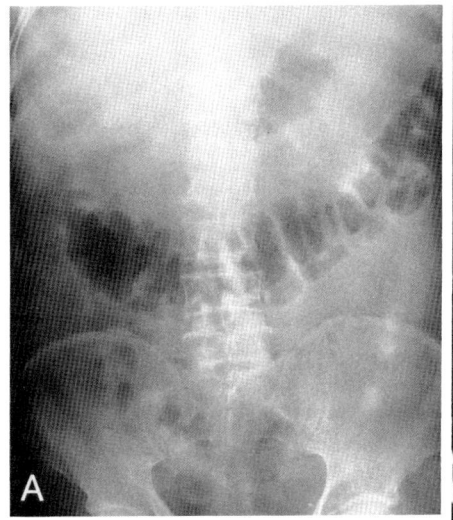
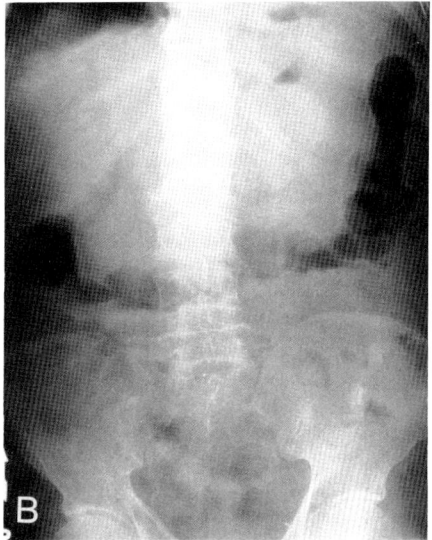
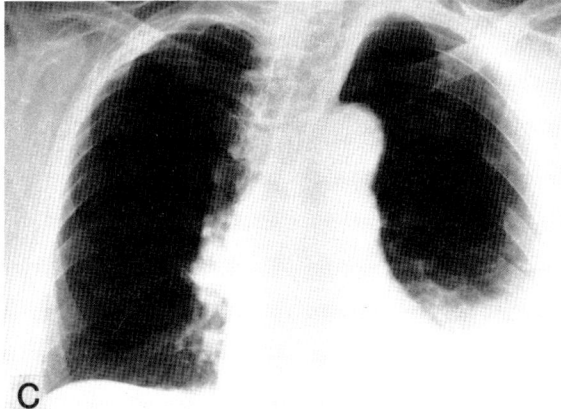

FIGURE 21.2. ACUTE PANCREATITIS

A and *B:* Supine and erect films of the abdomen demonstrate the colon cut-off sign in acute pancreatitis. Note separation of the stomach and transverse colon probably by phlegmon. *C:* Large left-sided pleural effusion in same patient. *D* and *E:* Bilateral large pleural effusions in a different patient apparently permeating through the diaphragm—the effusions could be connected to a lesser sac fluid collection (*arrow*) which, in turn, could be traced back to the acutely inflamed pancreas (not shown).

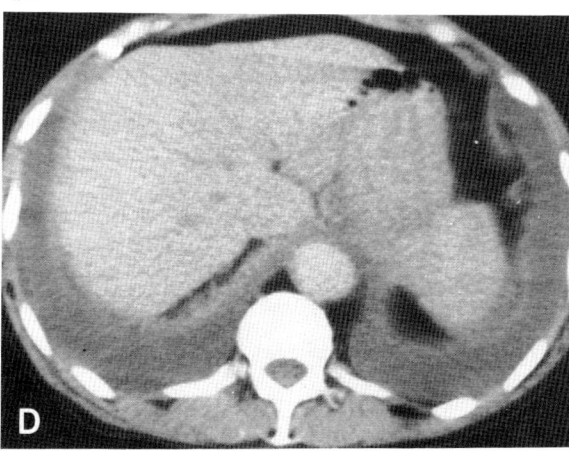
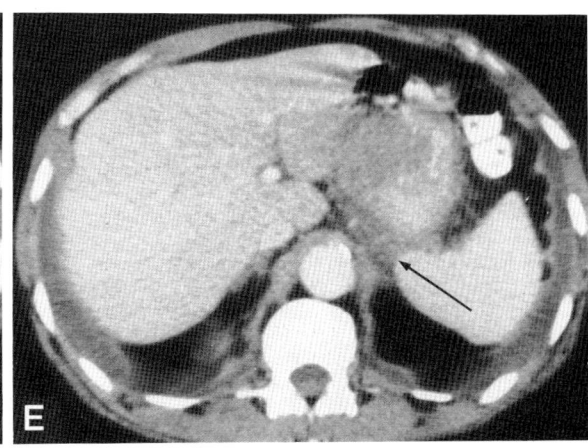

Abdominal Films

There have been many radiographic findings on plain abdominal films described in the literature. Some are reliable in the proper clinical context, and almost always indicative of pathology, others are not.

The colon cut-off sign, defined by Brascho, is infrequently encountered but reliable (1, 7). It refers to a dilated transverse colon with abrupt

662   LIVER, BILIARY TRACT, PANCREAS, SPLEEN

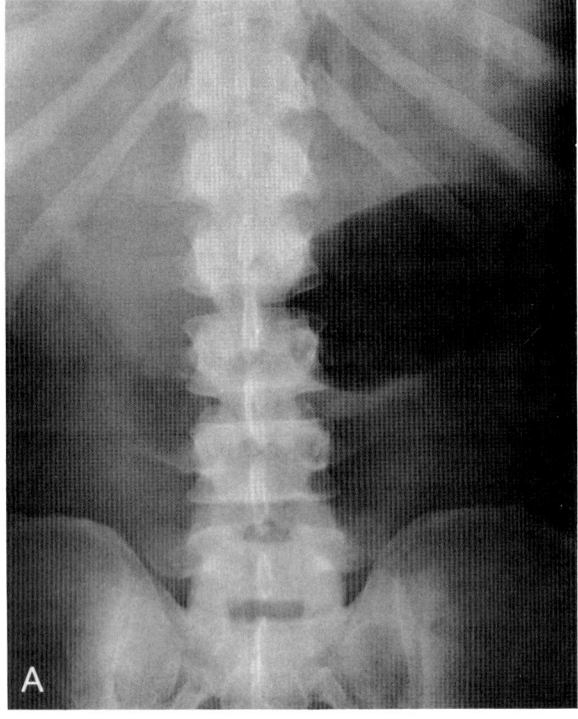

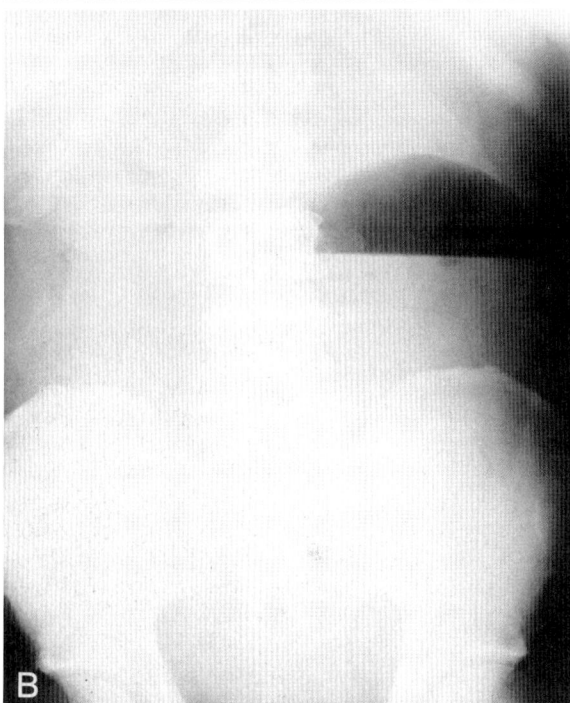

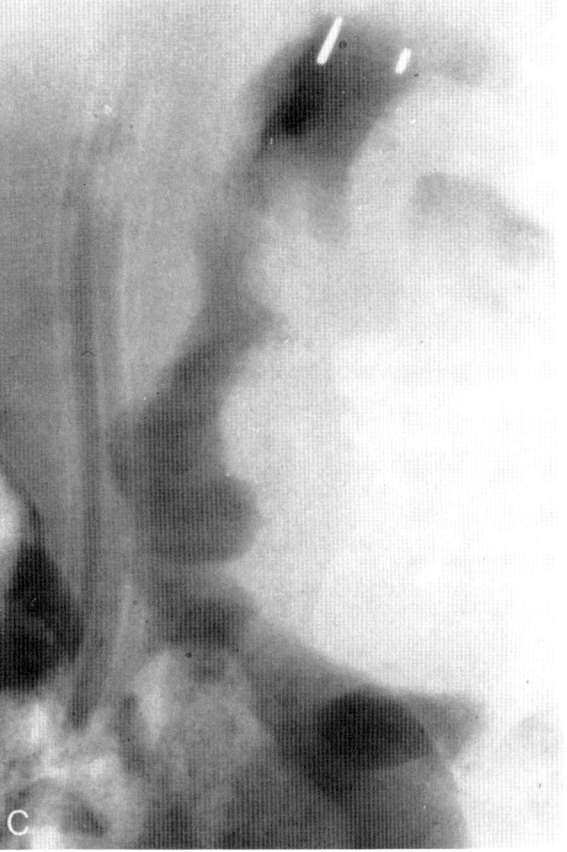

FIGURE 21.3. ACUTE PANCREATITIS
A and *B:* Supine and erect films of the abdomen showing a sentinel loop in acute pancreatitis. *C:* Duodenal ileus and Frostberg 3 sign in an acute exacerbation of chronic pancreatitis. Coned-down AP view of duodenum.

change to a relatively gasless descending colon (Fig. 21.2) (1, 7–9). The point of transition is often at the anatomic splenic flexure (1, 7, 9). Distention of the transverse colon can be caused by a paralytic ileus from enzymes in the transverse mesocolon (8). Extension of the inflammatory process into the phrenicocolic ligament can result in spasm and obstruction at the anatomic splenic flexure (8). Less commonly, there is predominant extension to the region of the hepatic flexure via the mesocolon, or to the ascending colon through the duodenum, producing more proximal obstruction (8).

A sentinel loop (localized segment of gas-containing dilated small bowel) is frequently (10–55%) seen in acute pancreatitis, although it is a nonspecific finding (1, 7–9). Dilation to 3 cm or more with an air-fluid level help differentiate a true sentinel loop from a chance finding in a normal patient (Fig. 21.3A and B) (9). Duodenal ileus is present and manifested by air in the duodenum with or without dilatation in 20–45% of patients and is more specific (Fig. 21.3C) (1, 7, 9). Gaseous distention may be localized to the terminal ileum and cecum (9). Spread of pancreatic enzymes down the small bowel mesentery is responsible for spasm of some small bowel segments and dilatation of others (8). Induration of the root of the mesentery can compress the third portion of the duodenum leading to proximal dilatation (8).

The renal halo sign has been recently described in acute pancreatitis (10). The lateral margin of the perirenal fat is usually not seen on plain films because it blends imperceptibly with the pararenal fat (10). When there is inflammation in the anterior pararenal space, the resultant water density contrasts with the perirenal fat to produce a radiolucent halo around the kidney (9). The sign will be produced by anterior pararenal exudate of any etiology, but in pancreatitis the left side is more commonly involved (9).

A characteristic but rare plain film finding in acute pancreatitis is an indistinct mottling in the peripancreatic area or throughout the abdomen from intra-abdominal fat necrosis (1, 7–9, 11). Small, irregularly rounded relatively radiodense water density areas are intermingled with lucent fat in normal fat-containing areas such as the pancreatic bed, small and large bowel mesentery, and the omentum (1, 7–9, 11). The major factor responsible for the densities is hydrolysis of fat, not calcium deposition (1, 11). The radiologic finding is rare and associated with hypocalcemia, metastatic fat necrosis and a high mortality (9). Another characteristic but rare plain film finding in the initial stage of acute pancreatitis is intrapancreatic gas (9). This is due to acute gangrenous or acute suppurative pancreatitis and has a poor prognosis (7). Later in the clinical course, gas can be seen in the pancreatic region due to either abscess, enteric fistula, or rarely, necrotic tissue alone. Plain film findings consist of small gas bubbles throughout the region of the pancreas (7, 12–14), or less commonly a large gas pocket or a long air-fluid level (Fig. 21.4) (1, 12–14).

Less valuable radiologic signs reported to occur in acute pancreatitis are the "gasless abdomen," pancreatic enlargement, and obliteration of the left psoas margin (1, 9). The "gasless abdomen" correlates best with vomiting and is also seen in high intestinal obstructions, intestinal infarction and ileus as well as in normals (1, 9). Pancreatic enlargement, detected by indentation of the duodenal sweep and separation of the stomach and colon is difficult to evaluate reliably on plain films (Fig. 21.2) (9). Obliteration or poor definition of the left psoas shadow, although occurring in pancreatitis, occurs too often in normals to have any value by itself in an individual case (9). There is a low incidence

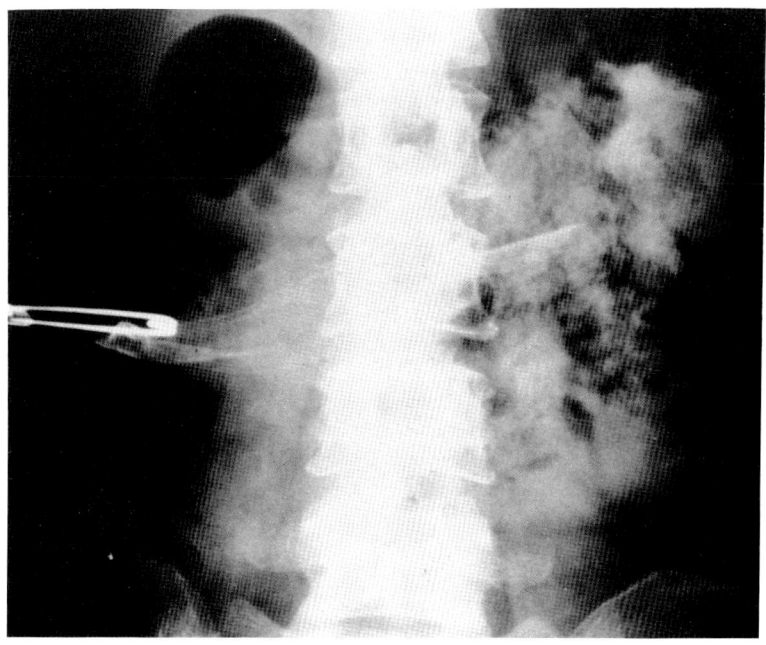

FIGURE 21.4. ACUTE PANCREATITIS
Acute gangrenous pancreatitis with gas bubbles in the region of the body and and tail of the pancreas and the lesser sac.

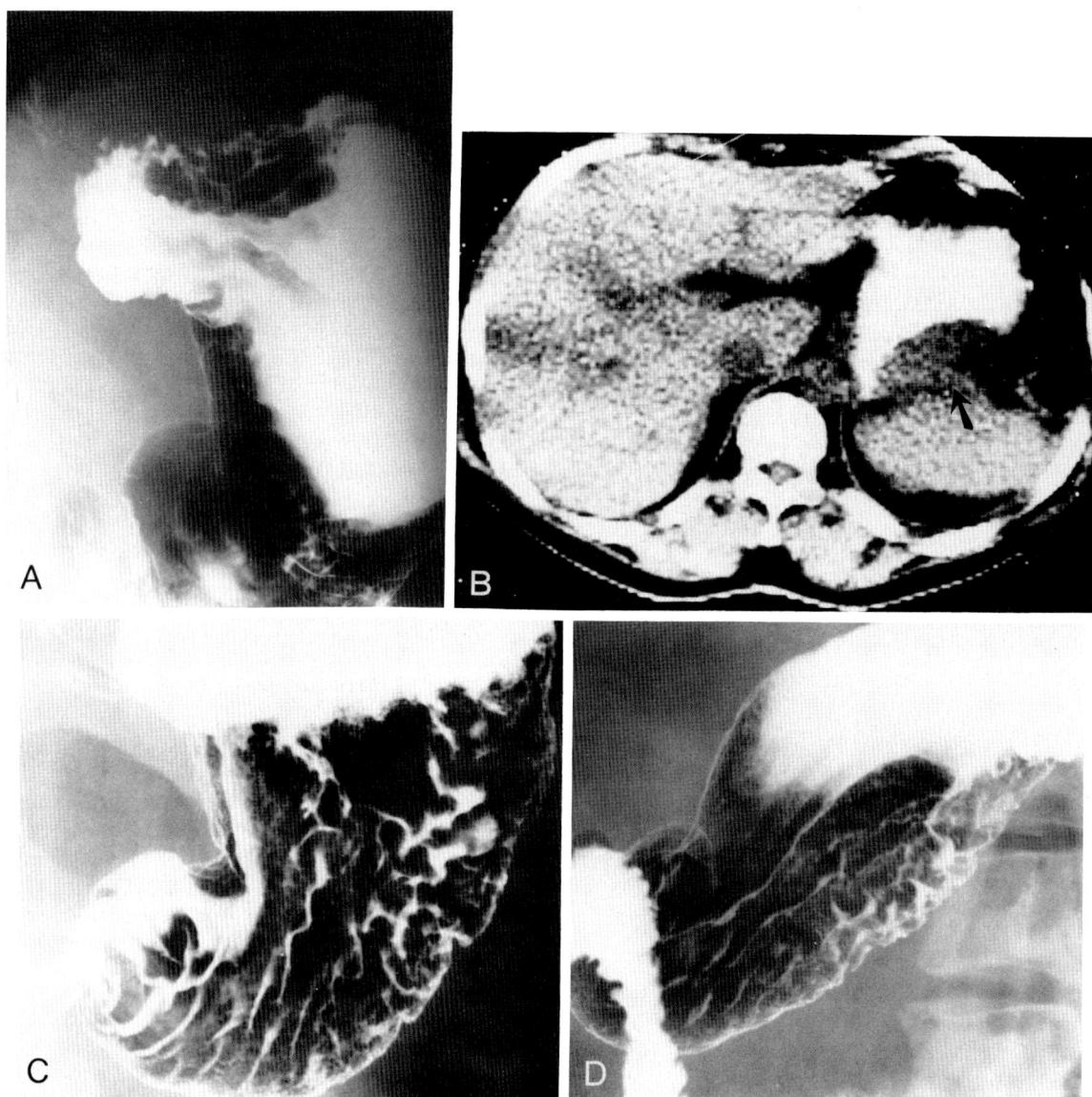

FIGURE 21.5. ACUTE PANCREATITIS THICKENING AND DISTORTING GASTRIC FOLDS
A: Nondistensible region of thick folds in the fundus. *B:* CT scan showing superior extension of a phlegmon (*arrow*) producing the changes in (*A*). Lower cuts showed a phlegmon anterior to an enlarged pancreas. *C* and *D:* Anteroposterior and oblique films showing thickened and distorted gastric folds. Note selective posterior wall involvement.

of pancreatic calcification in acute pancreatitis, as calcification is associated more with chronic pancreatitis (9).

Ascites is often present in early acute pancreatitis and disappears with clinical improvement. If it persists, a pancreaticoperitoneal fistula or a leaking pseudocyst should be suspected.

Barium Contrast Examinations

Esophagus. Acute pancreatitis can cause splenic vein obstruction leading to splenomegaly with gastric varices alone or esophagogastric varices (1).

Stomach. Gastric abnormalities observed during or immediately after episodes of acute pancreatitis include nonspecific, functional changes such as spasticity, irregular contractility or dilatation with atony (1, 15). Enlarged, tortuous edematous rugal folds may be seen diffusely throughout the stomach or predominantly posteriorly in the antrum and along the greater curvature (Fig. 21.5) (1, 15). Widening of the retrogastric space from pancreatic enlargement and/or inflammation in the lesser sac is common (Fig. 21.6). In 20% of cases there are localized contour irregularities in the posterior wall and/or lesser curvature (15). These changes develop after a delay of a few days to a week and correlate in degree with the severity of pancreatitis (15).

The radiographic changes affecting the stomach result from the effects of activated enzymes and the subsequent inflammatory response. All of the above findings usually resolve completely in weeks to months following the acute attack (1, 15).

Duodenum. The most common abnormality seen in acute pancreatitis is diminished peristalsis which is often associated with edematous folds (1, 8). Widening of the duodenal sweep with mass effect on the inner border and downward displacement at the ligament of Treitz may be seen as a result of pancreatic enlargement (Fig. 21.7) (1, 8). Edematous swelling of the papilla (Poppel's sign) may also be present (1, 8). Occasionally, acute pancreatitis can cause segmental narrowing and fold thickening in the duodenum (Fig. 21.8).

Although a normal barium meal examination cannot exclude acute pancreatitis, abnormalities in the stomach or duodenum are present in greater than 80% of cases (16).

Small Bowel. Fold thickening can be seen in the jejunum and ileum in acute pancreatitis from enzyme spread down the mesentery (Fig. 21.9) (1, 8). Microaneurysms, pseudoaneurysms, stenosis and occlusion can occur in mesenteric vessels in severe acute pancreatitis. Mucosal atrophy and strictures or frank infarction may occur as a result in the small bowel (8).

Colon. Abnormalities in the colon are caused

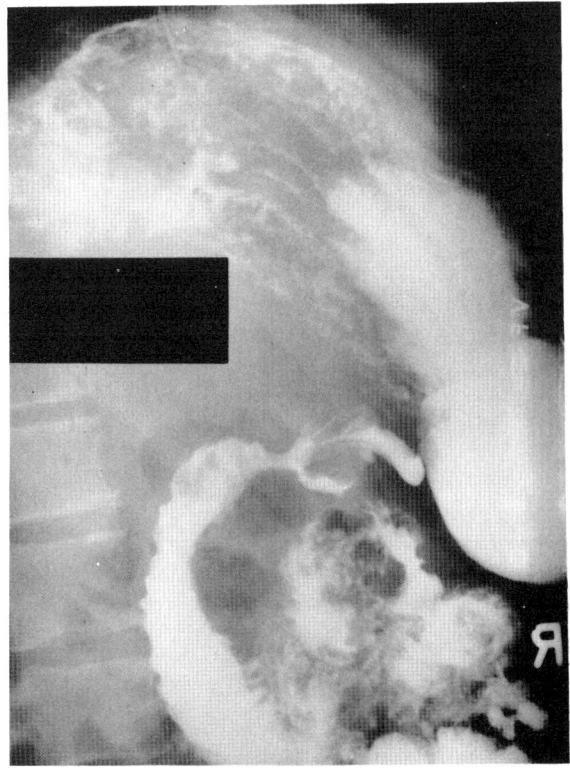

FIGURE 21.6. ACUTE PANCREATITIS
Retrogastric mass from acute pancreatitis. Note also distortion of duodenal bulb and widening of the sweep with mass effect along its anteromedial border.

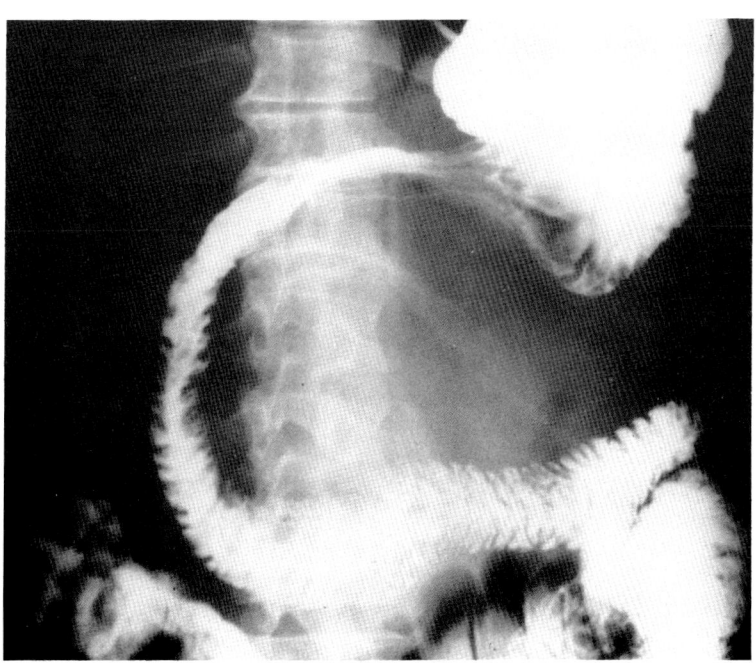

FIGURE 21.7. ACUTE PANCREATITIS
Widening of the C-loop, superior antral displacement and inferior displacement of the duodenojejunal junction by acute pancreatitis.

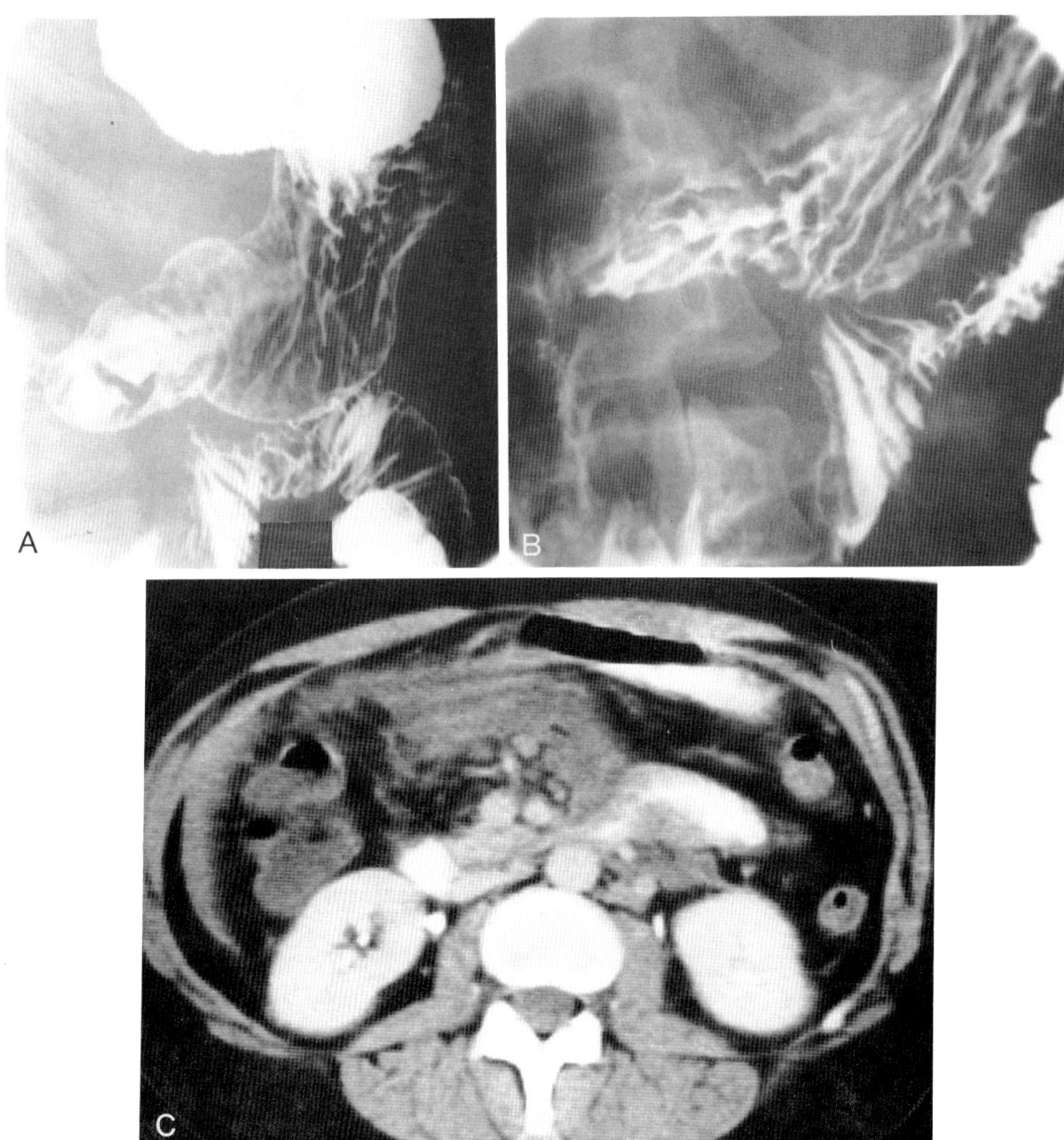

FIGURE 21.8. ACUTE PANCREATITIS

A and *B:* Thickening and distortion of folds and segmental narrowing at the duodenojejunal junction in acute pancreatitis. *C:* CT of the same patient showing encasement of the duodenojejunal junction by a pancreatic phlegmon. This patient has Type IV hyperlipidemia and her acute pancreatitis was precipitated by alcohol abuse.

by spread of inflammatory fluid across the transverse mesocolon and phrenicocolic ligament to the splenic flexure (8, 17). Thus, the region of the anatomic splenic flexure is the portion of the colon most often involved in acute pancreatitis (17, 18). The transverse colon, hepatic flexure and descending colon are less commonly affected in descending order of frequency (1, 8, 17, 18). The inferior haustral row tends to be involved earlier and to a greater extent than the superior row (8) (see Chapter 22, radiology of duct cell adenocarcinoma). Spread inferiorly through the anterior pararenal space is the cause of changes in the descending colon (17). Barium enema will reveal narrowing, irregular nodular margins and distorted but intact mucosal folds in the affected

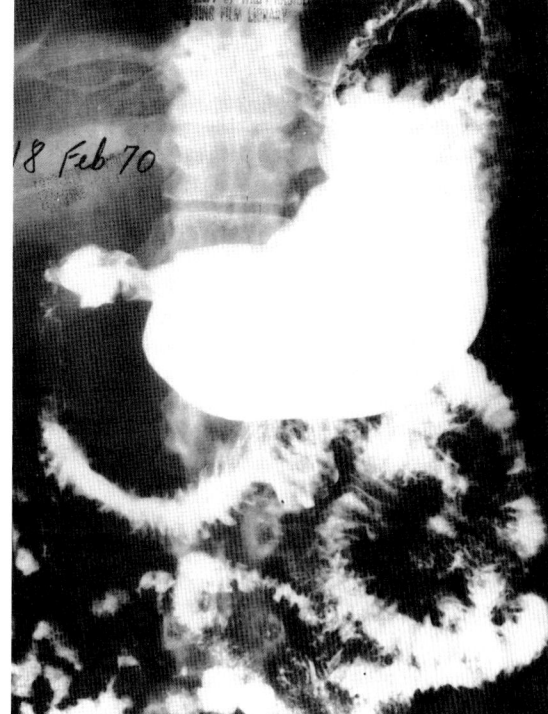

FIGURE 21.9. ACUTE PANCREATITIS
Diffuse fold thickening, segmental narrowing and separation of loops in the small bowel in acute pancreatitis. Hemorrhage, edema, and/or fat necrosis in the mesentery are probably responsible for the separation of loops. Note the mass effect in the head of the pancreas.

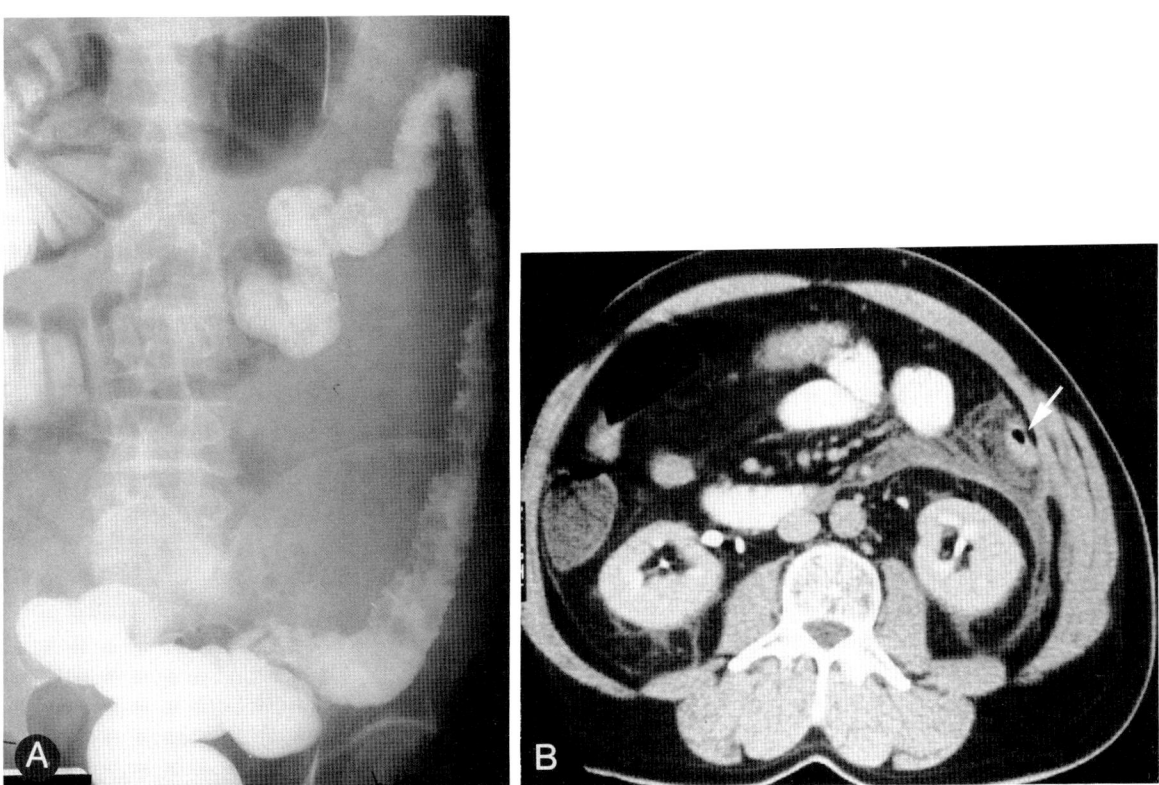

FIGURE 21.10. ACUTE PANCREATITIS
A: Crampy abdominal pain and left lower quadrant fullness in a patient with acute pancreatitis. Barium enema shows narrowing, nodularity, and fold distortion in the descending colon and splenic flexure. *B:* A CT scan one day before the enema showed a pancreatic fluid collection in the left anterior pararenal space surrounding the descending colon (*arrow*). (Case courtesy Dr. Richard Strax.)

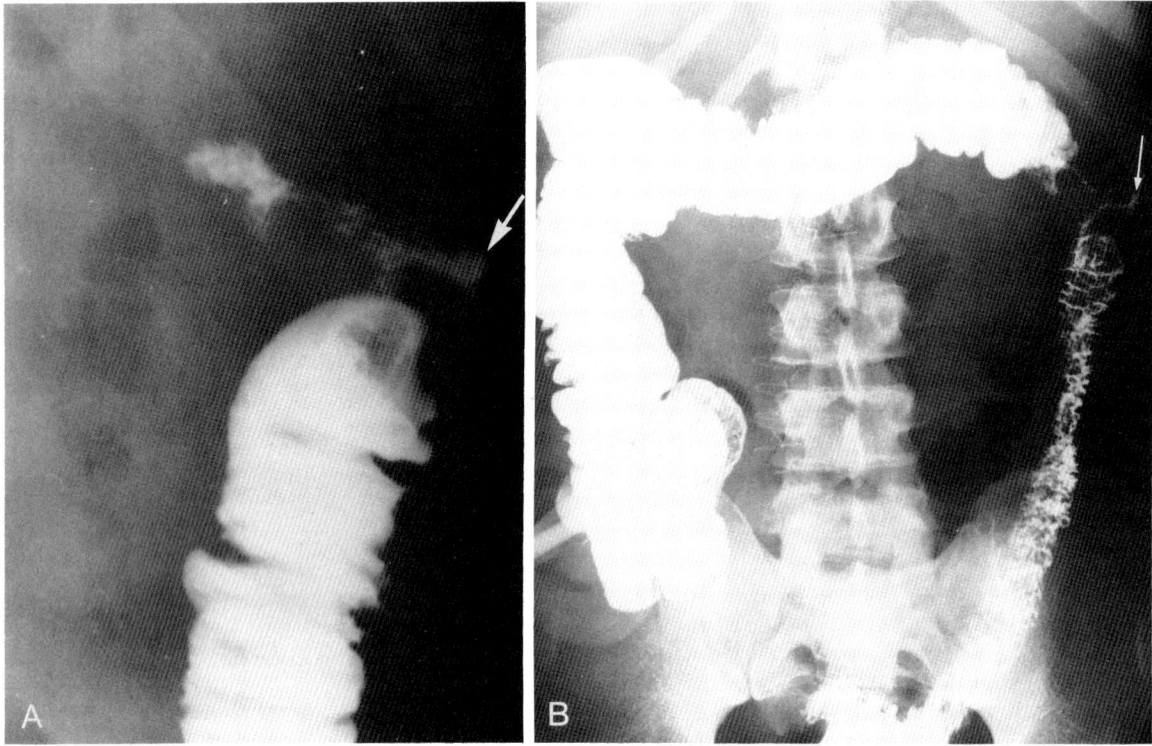

FIGURE 21.11. ACUTE PANCREATITIS

A patient with acute pancreatitis after an alcoholic binge developed large bowel obstruction. An emergency cecostomy was performed. A: Barium enema demonstrating high grade obstruction at the anatomic splenic flexure and a beginning sinus tract (arrow). B: Retrograde enema via the cecostomy tube outlining the obstruction and sinus tract (arrow) from above.

portion of colon (Fig. 21.10) (1, 8, 17, 18). If the disease process is severe, there can be retrograde obstruction and/or erosion through the bowel wall with fistulas and sinus tracts (Fig. 21.11) (8, 18).

A rare complication is colonic ischemia or necrosis due to mesenteric vascular stenosis or occlusion (18). With resolution of pancreatitis, the colon usually reverts to normal but a smooth stricture can be the end result (8, 18).

REFERENCES

1. Eaton SB, Ferrucci JT: *Radiology of the Pancreas and Duodenum*. Philadelphia, W. B. Saunders, 1973, pp 20–22, 24–47, 359–368.
2. Razzaque MA, Hussain SA, Hossain Z, Kumar CK: Pleural effusion with pancreatico-pleural fistula. *Am J Gastroenterol* 68:84–87, 1977.
3. McKenna JM, Chandrasekhar AJ, Skorton D et al: The pleuropulmonary complications of pancreatitis. *Chest* 71:197–204, 1977.
4. Warshaw AL, Lesser PB, Rie M et al: The pathogenesis of pulmonary edema in acute pancreatitis. *Ann Surg* 182:505–510, 1975.
5. Boswell SH, Baylin CJ: Metastatic fat necrosis and lytic bone lesions in a patient with painless acute pancreatitis. *Radiology* 106:85–86, 1973.
6. Cubilla AL, Fitzgerald PJ: Cancer (non-endocrine) of the pancreas. A suggested classification. *Mongr Pathol* 21:99–100, 1980.
7. Brascho DJ, Reynolds RN, Zanca P: The radiographic "colon cut-off sign" in acute pancreatitis. *Radiology* 79:763–768, 1962.
8. Meyers MA: *Dynamic Radiology of the Abdomen. Normal and Pathologic Anatomy*. New York, Springer-Verlag, 1976, pp 265–277.
9. Davis S, Parbhoo SP, Gibson MJ: The plain abdominal radiograph in acute pancreatitis. *Clin Radiol* 31:87–93, 1980.
10. Sussman N, Hammerman AM, Cohen E. The renal halo sign in pancreatitis. *Radiology* 142:323–327, 1982.
11. Berenson JE, Spitz HB, Felson B: The abdominal fat necrosis sign. *Radiology* 100:567–571, 1971.
12. Alexander ES, Clark RA, Federle MP: Pancreatic gas: indication of pancreatic fistula. *AJR* 139:1089–1094, 1982.
13. Woodward S, Kelvin FM, Rice RP, Thompson WM: Pancreatic abscess: importance of conventional radiology. *AJR* 136:871–878, 1981.
14. Torres WE, Clements JL, Sones PJ, Knopf DR: Gas in the pancreatic bed without abscess. *AJR* 137:1131–1133, 1981.
15. Balthazar EJ: Effects of acute and chronic pancreatitis

Nuclear Medicine

Although no longer used in clinical practice, ^{75}Se-selenomethionine scanning of the pancreas was usually positive (75–90%) in patients with pancreatitis (1). Gallium scanning is probably sensitive in acute pancreatitis but of limited usefulness because of nonspecificity. Tanaka and colleagues (2) reported that 7 out of 7 patients with acute pancreatitis had localized increased uptake of gallium-67 in the epigastric area. There have been case reports of gallium-67 localization in infected pseudocysts (3) and diffuse peritoneal uptake of gallium-67 in two patients who died from pancreatitis with widespread inflammation (4). In contrast to acute pancreatitis, in Tanaka's series (2), only 1 of 4 patients with chronic pancreatitis showed any gallium uptake.

Recently indium-111-labeled leukocytes have been shown to localize in infectious and inflammatory processes. Fawcett and coworkers (5) reported two patients with acute pancreatitis who had leukocyte scans, both of which were positive. In the first case, there was diffuse and homogeneous uptake in the region of the pancreas but no focal intense uptake to suggest an abscess. Surgery in this patient revealed only an enlarged, inflamed pancreas. In their second case, the indium white cell scan showed diffuse pancreatic uptake with superimposed areas of more intense uptake suggestive of abscess formation which was subsequently proven at laparotomy. Laird and colleagues (6) studied white blood scanning in 16 cases of acute pancreatitis. Seven scans were positive and all showed evidence of severe pancreatitis or pseudocyst formation, whereas the nine patients with negative scans had mild disease and no complications. Although these are only preliminary reports, it appears that indium-111 white blood cell localization in acute pancreatitis may play a useful role and indicate severe disease or complications such as pseudocyst or abscess formation.

REFERENCES

1. Miale A, Rodriguez-Antunez A, Gill W: Pancreas scanning after 10 years. *Semin Nucl Med* 2:201–219, 1972.
2. Tanaka T, Mishkin FS, Buozas DJ et al: Pancreatic uptake of gallium-67 citrate in acute pancreatitis. *Appl Radiol/NM* 7:163–164, 1978.
3. Kennedy KD, Martin NL, Robinson RG et al: Identification of an infected pseudocyst of the pancreas with ^{67}Ga-citrate: case report. *J Nucl Med* 16:1132–1134, 1975.
4. Myerson PJ, Myerson DA, Spencer RP: Diffuse peritoneal uptake of ^{67}Ga in pancreatic disease: a possible prognostic indicator. *J Nucl Med* 19:1266–1267, 1978.
5. Fawcett HD, Lin MS, Goodwin DA: Indium-111-labeled leukocyte imaging in acute pancreatitis with suspected complicating abscess. *Dig Dis Sci* 24:872–875, 1979.
6. Laird JD, Ferguson WR, Anderson JR: The use of indium-111 labeled white blood cells in the investigation of acute pancreatitis. *J Nucl Med* 24:79, 1983.

Endoscopic Retrograde Pancreatography

During an acute episode of pancreatitis, endoscopic retrograde cholangiopancreatography (ERCP) is relatively contraindicated since injection of contrast material into the inflamed and permeable pancreatic duct may exacerbate the disease (1, 2). The information obtained from the study is also of limited usefulness. In acute or acute-relapsing pancreatitis, there are usually no pancreatographic abnormalities, either in the acute phase or after clinical recovery (2, 3). However, straightening of the pancreatic radicles with minor irregularities in their caliber (Fig. 21.12) may be seen due to edema as well as mild main pancreatic duct dilatation and a nonspecific, hazy parenchymal stain thought to be caused by increased permeability of ductal epithelium. The parenchymal stain is similar to that seen in normal glands after overinjection (2). Tiny pseudocysts may rarely be seen but are again difficult to distinguish from appearances in overinjection (2). One episode of acute hemorrhagic pancreatitis may lead to permanent histologic and functional abnormalities, thus pancreatography in this condition can disclose diffuse or focal changes indistinguishable from chronic pancreatitis (3). ERCP and sphincterotomy is indicated in some patients with acute pancreatitis from a stone impacted in the ampulla of Vater.

Cholangiography

Uncommonly, acute pancreatitis causes biliary obstruction leading to cholangiography. The inflamed, enlarged head of the pancreas can cause medial or lateral displacement of the common bile duct and rigidity of the duct. Long segment narrowing can occur (Fig. 21.13) but obstruction is quite unusual. Since the changes are due to inflammation, they are generally transient. Of

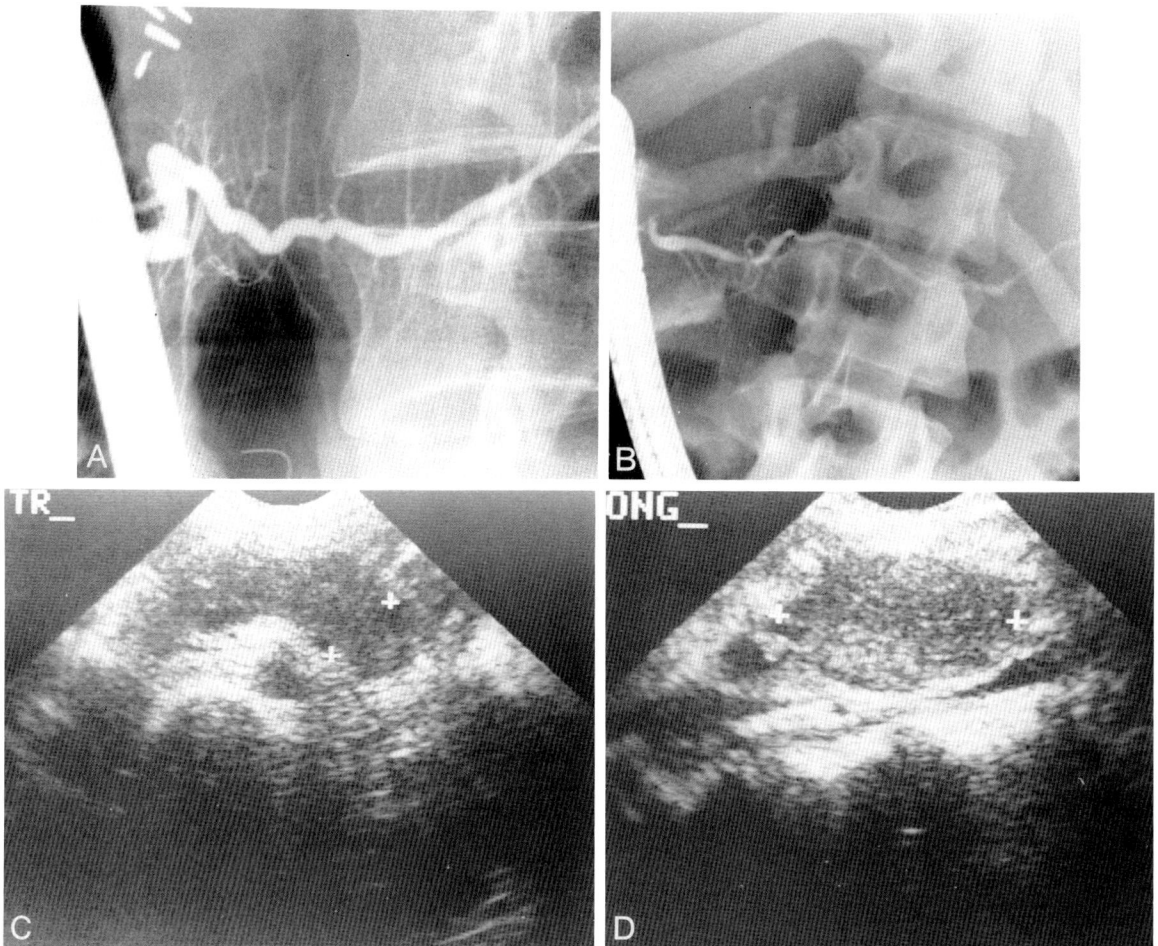

FIGURE 21.12. ACUTE PANCREATITIS

A: ERP in a patient recovering from acute pancreatitis. Elongation and straightening of the superior row of side branches in the body of the pancreas. *B:* ERP in acute viral pancreatitis: multiple tapered long segment narrowings of the main pancreatic duct with poor side branch filling. *C* and *D:* Correlative sonograms, same patient as in *B*, transverse and sagittal, respectively: markedly enlarged, hypoechoic pancreas (*cursors*).

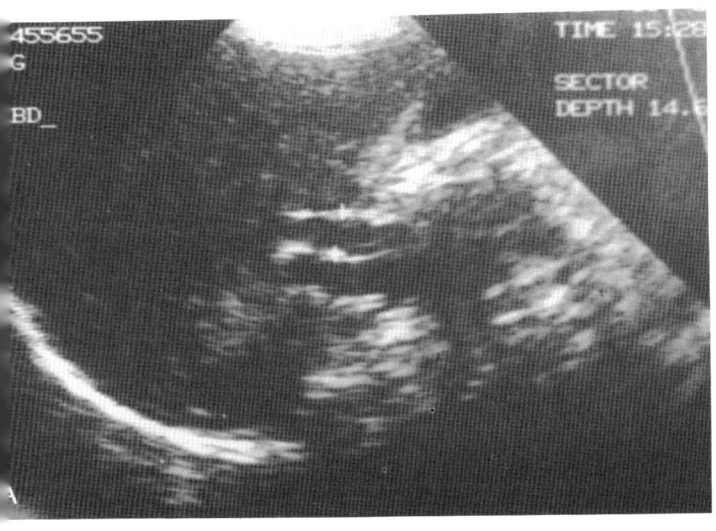
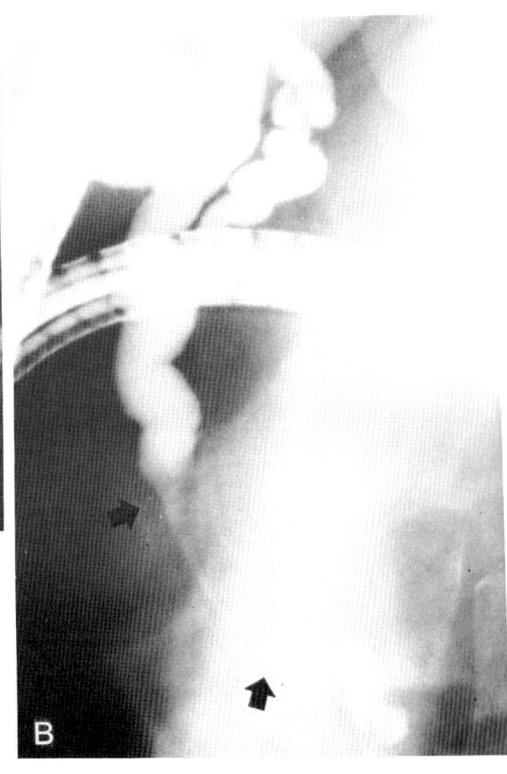

FIGURE 21.13. ACUTE PANCREATITIS
A: Sagittal sonogram shows a dilated, partially obstructed common bile
ct (cursors) just cephalad to an enlarged, hypoechoic pancreas due to
ute pancreatitis. B: ERC in a different patient showing a long, smooth
rrowing of the common bile duct in acute pancreatitis. The identical
pearance can be seen in chronic pancreatitis.

course, in those cases of acute pancreatitis caused by biliary tract pathology, cholangiography will often be crucial in disclosing the etiology of the disease (e.g., stone, choledochocoele, choldedochal cyst).

REFERENCES

1. Kasugai T: Pancreatitis. In Takemoto T, Kasugai T (eds): *Endoscopic Retrograde Cholangiopancreatography.* New York, Igaku-Shoin, 1979, pp 176–202.
2. Short WF: Pancreatography. In Eaton SB, Ferrucci JT Jr (eds): *Radiology of the Pancreas and Duodenum.* Philadelphia, W. B. Saunders, 1973, pp 261–275.
3. Freeny PC, Lawson TL: *Radiology of the Pancreas.* New York, Springer-Verlag, 1982, pp 205–212.

Sonography

The severity of acute pancreatitis varies from being a mild, self-limiting disorder to one with shock and rapid death. It is composed of two separate somewhat overlapping clinical disorders. The milder form, acute edematous pancreatitis, is signaled by the presence of nausea, vomiting, and epigastric pain associated with elevation of the serum and/or urinary amylase (1). Acute necrotizing (hemorrhagic, suppurative) pancreatitis is the severest form of the disease and is accompanied by a drop in hematocrit and serum calcium associated with hypotension despite volume replacement, metabolic acidosis and the adult respiratory distress syndrome (1).

The sonographic appearance of the pancreas is normal in about 29% of patients with the clinical diagnosis of acute pancreatitis (2–4). When pancreatic involvement is sonographically present, it may be diffuse (52%) or focal (48%) and when focal usually involves the head (60%) or the tail (40%) (Fig. 21.14) (4). The involved area is usually but not always hypoechoic due to the presence of edema (2, 3, 5). There may be pancreatic ductal dilatation associated with focal enlargement of the head of the pancreas (Fig. 21.15). In mild pancreatitis (acute interstitial pancreatitis) the swelling of the gland and dilatation of the pancreatic duct usually subside within days to weeks and the echogenicity of the parenchyma returns to normal (2). One should be careful not to mistake fluid-filled bowel, peripancreatic lymphadenopathy, or direct invasion of the pancreas by gastric carcinoma as a focal pancreatic mass (6). It should also be remembered that focal enlargement of the body alone does not occur with inflammatory disease of the pancreas (4). The main complications of acute pancreatitis include the formation of a phlegmon (18%), pseudocyst formation (10%), hemorrhage

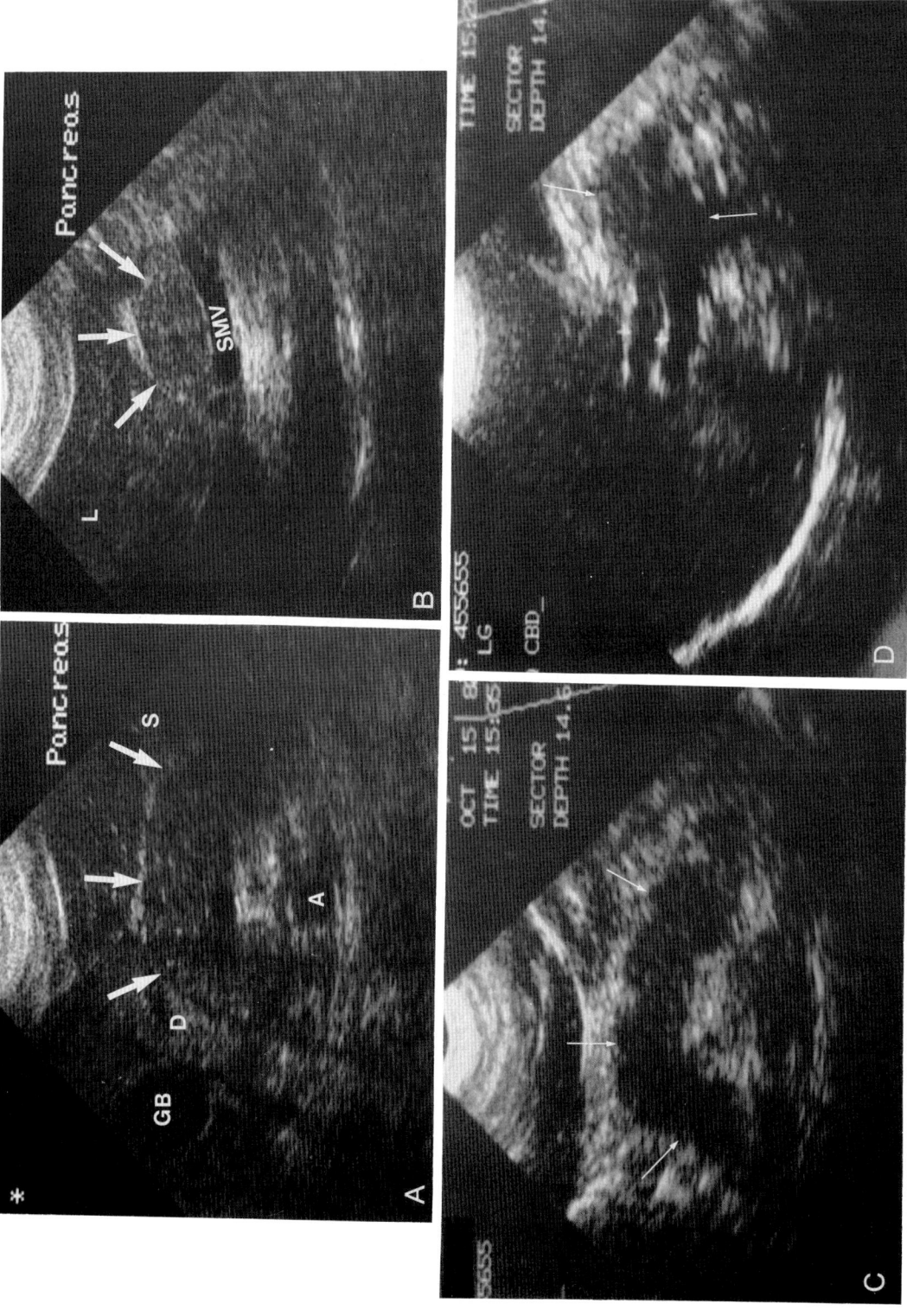

FIGURE 21.14. ACUTE PANCREATITIS

A and *B*: Acute pancreatitis, transverse and longitudinal, respectively. Sonography of a diffusely enlarged pancreas (*arrows*), isoechoic to liver. A = aorta, SMV = superior mesenteric vein, D = duodenum, GB = gallbladder, L = liver, S = stomach. *C* and *D*: Transverse and longitudinal sonograms, respectively, of a case of acute pancreatitis with an enlarged, very hypoechoic gland (*arrows*). Note biliary ductal dilatation (*cursors*).

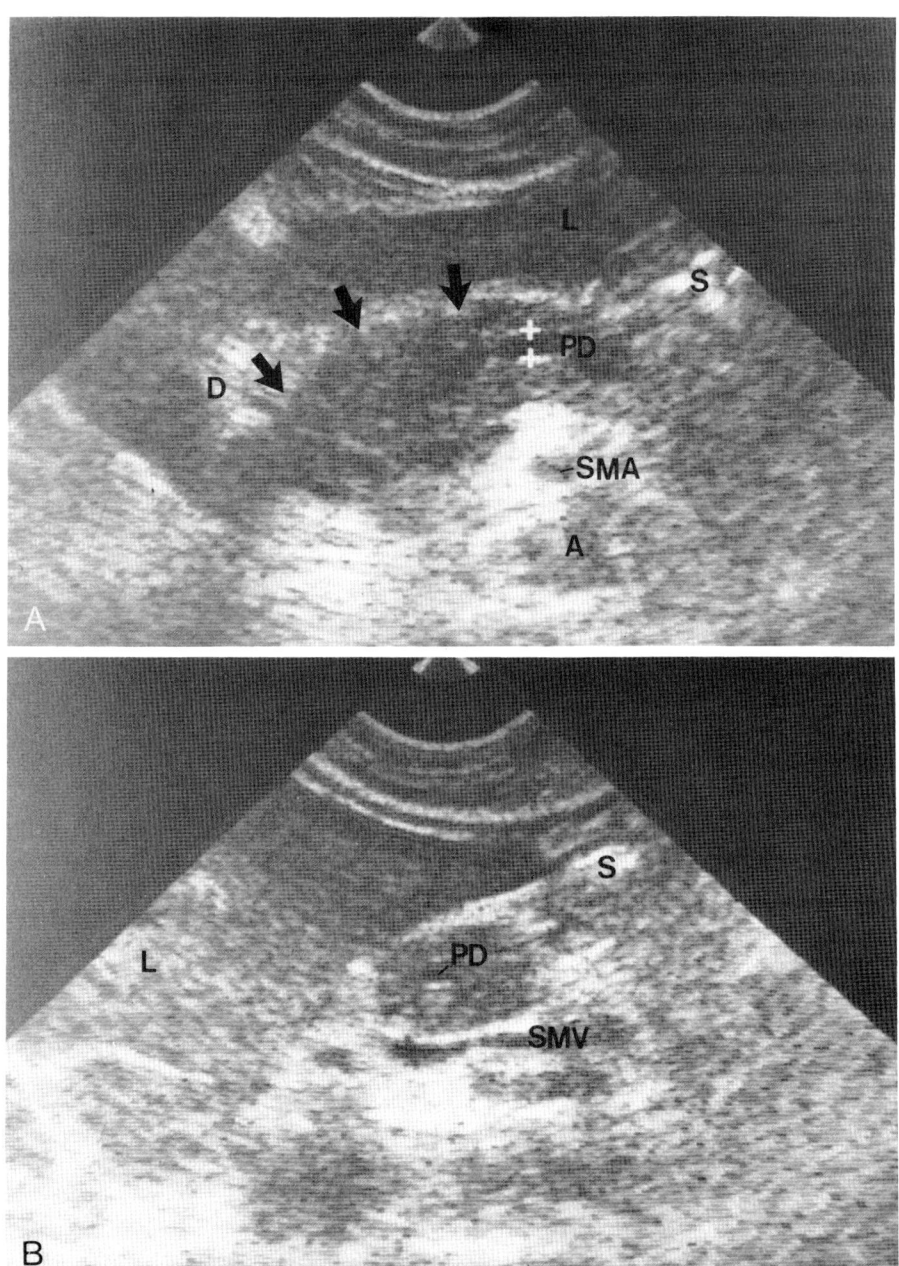

FIGURE 21.15. ACUTE PANCREATITIS (FOCAL)
Transverse (A) and longitudinal (B) scans of the pancreas showing enlargement of the pancreatic head (*arrows*) with a dilated pancreatic duct (PD). Aorta (A), superior mesenteric artery (SMA), stomach (S), liver (L), duodenum (D), and superior mesenteric vein (SMV).

(5%), or development of an abscess (3%) (1, 4, 7, 8).

Pathologically, a *phlegmon* is described as a spreading diffuse inflammatory edema of soft tissues that may be complicated by necrosis and even suppuration (9, 10). As mentioned previously, since the pancreas lacks a capsule, the inflammatory process within the gland can spread easily into the surrounding retroperitoneal soft tissues. Spread of this inflammation occurs in an anterior direction into the area of the lesser sac and anterior pararenal spaces since

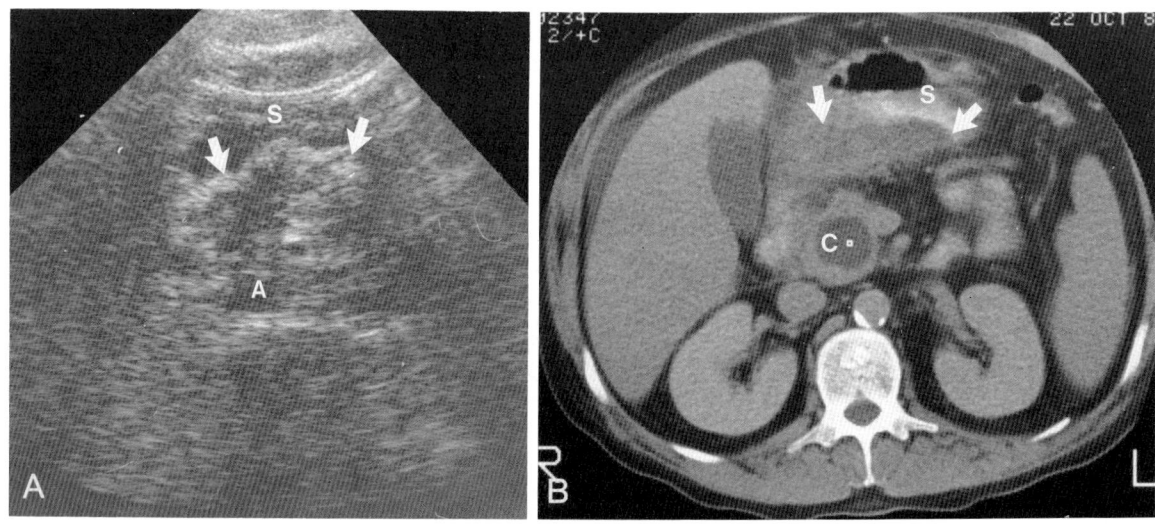

FIGURE 21.16. PHLEGMONOUS PANCREATITIS
A: Transverse sonogram of pancreas showing extension of a phlegmon (arrows) to involve the stomach (S). The pancreatic outline is poorly defined. B: CT scan of the same area reveals similar findings along with a small pseudocyst (C) in the pancreatic head. Aorta (A).

posterior extension is usually prevented by the anterior pararenal fascia (Gerota's fascia) (Fig. 21.16) (10). Medially, this fascia blends with the connective tissue around the aorta and inferior vena cava thus preventing spread of the phlegmon into this area. The phlegmon may involve the right anterior pararenal space and may simulate gallbladder disease by producing thickening of the gallbladder wall and a pericholecystic fluid collection (11). Extension may also occur into the transverse mesocolon and small bowel mesentery and inferiorly into the retroperitoneum and pelvis.

Patients with phlegmonous pancreatitis usually have an associated adynamic ileus which prevents adequate visualization of the retroperitoneum with the patient in the supine position. If this is the case, the patient should be examined in both decubitus views by scanning through the flank. It is only in this fashion that extensive phlegmonous changes in the retroperitoneum may be detected. Although a phlegmonous mass is hypoechoic and has good through transmission, it should not be mistaken for a peripancreatic fluid collection and this can be proven by percutaneous aspiration which will yield no fluid (4). At surgery, such phlegmons are found to represent a boggy edematous mass and possibly necrotic retroperitoneal tissues.

Total necrosis of the pancreas can occur in which the central necrotic portion of the gland is filled with necrotic debris (12). The gland may appear sonographically to be diffusely enlarged and hypoechoic or the entire center may appear cystic with a fluid debris level. The presence of this entity can be proven by ERCP in which the cystic necrotic portion of the gland communicates with the ductal system and will fill with contrast.

Pancreatic Hemorrhage. Hemorrhage occurs in 5% of patients with acute pancreatitis (4). Although such patients are usually extremely ill and have a drop in hematocrit and serum calcium, hemorrhage can occur in the absence of clinical manifestations (1, 8, 13). The sonographic appearance of pancreatic hemorrhage varies depending on the frequency of the transducer used and the age of the hemorrhage (14). In the first 24 hr if a high frequency transducer is used (5–7.5 MHz) the hemorrhage can appear totally echogenic. The degree of echogenicity decreases with time as the red cells undergo lysis and so the mass assumes a complex appearance with less and less echogenicity as time goes by until finally by 96 hr the area of hemorrhage is sonolucent (Fig. 21.17). During its evolution it can also develop a fluid debris level (14). Hemorrhage can occur in the pancreatic phlegmon or in a pseudocyst and these two entities are sonographically indistinguishable. The wall of the hemorrhage in the acute phase is usually irregular, however, with time it becomes more well-defined and finally has the appearance of an uncomplicated pseudocyst (Fig. 21.17) (13).

Aneurysms. Aneurysms can occur secondary to acute pancreatitis and when these rupture a

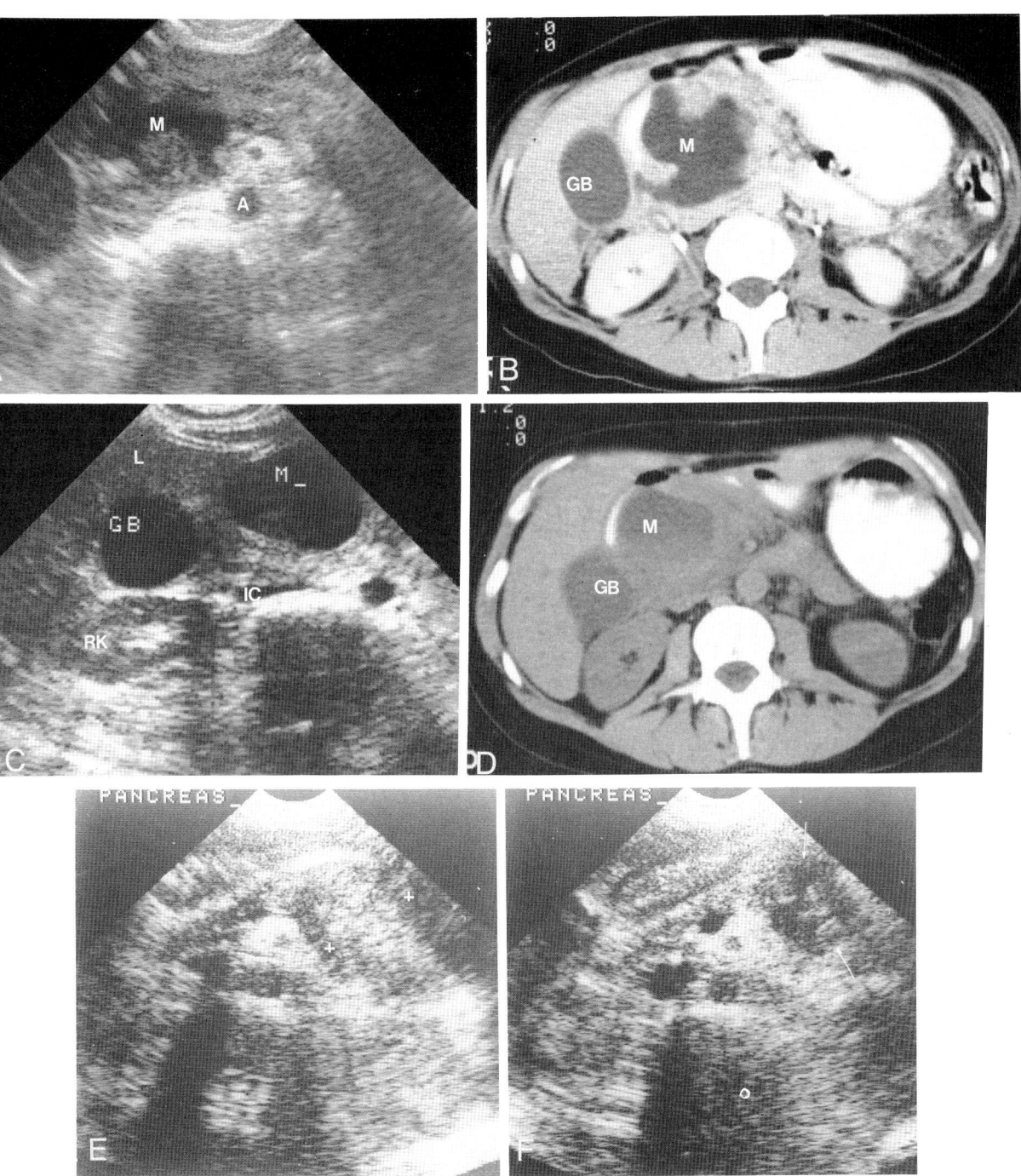

FIGURE 21.17. HEMORRHAGIC PANCREATITIS

A–D Transverse sonogram (*A*) reveals an irregular cystic mass (*M*) in the pancreatic head with echogenic internal contents. A CT through the same area (*B*) shows a fluid containing mass (*M*). A follow up sonogram (*C*) and CT scan (*D*) 10 days after shows the mass (*M*) has been become better defined and resembles a pseudocyst. Aorta (*A*), inferior vena cava (*IC*), gallbladder (*G*), liver (*L*), and right kidney (*RK*). *E–I:* Hemorrhagic pancreatitis evolving into pseudocyst. *E:* Transverse scan: marked enlargement of the tail (*cursors*) from acute hemorrhagic pancreatitis, initially hyperechoic. *F:* Transverse scan 1 week later: smaller, hypoechoic mass as hemorrhage evolves into pseudocyst (*arrows*). *G:* Noncontrast CT scan corresponding to (*E*): high attenuation region in the tail corresponding to hemorrhagic pancreatitis. *H:* Enhanced scan at the same time as (*G*): hemorrhage is less obvious. *I:* CT corresponding to (*F*): evolving pseudocyst in the tail (*arrows*).

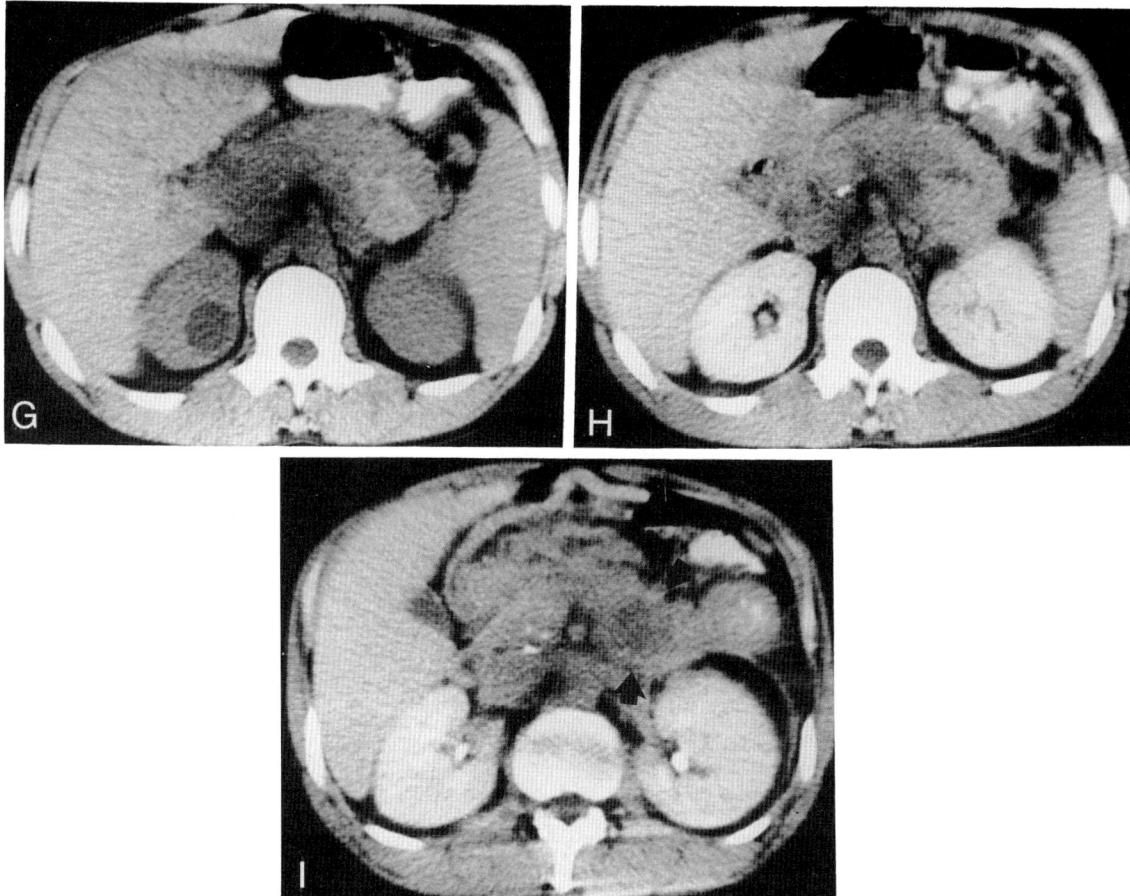

FIGURE 21.17G–I

catastrophic gastrointestinal or intraperitoneal hemorrhage can occur (15). Such aneurysms most commonly involve the splenic artery but can involve other branches of the celiac axis, the superior mesenteric artery and the intrapancreatic arteries (15, 16). Sonographically the aneurysm can be mistaken for a pseudocyst. If doubt exists, a doppler examination or a dynamic CT scan through the "cyst" should be performed.

Since a large percentage of patients with an inflamed pancreas have their disease due to alcohol abuse, the presence of alcoholic liver disease and cirrhosis should be looked for. If cirrhosis is present then the portal venous system should be sonographically assessed looking for gastroesophageal varices and gastrorenal, splenorenal and periportal collateral veins along with a recanalized umbilical vein (17).

Computed Tomography

The CT findings in acute pancreatitis vary in severity. In approximately 29% of patients with this clinical diagnosis, the CT scan of the pancreas will be normal (4, 18). In the remaining patients, findings of varying severity are present. The gland may be focally (48%) or diffusely (52%) enlarged and the involved portion may have a well-defined outline or its interface with the peripancreatic fat may be ill-defined. The attenuation number of the involved pancreas is reduced, presumably secondary to the presence of edema and it is the spread of this edema into the surrounding fat that gives the pancreatic outline its indistinct appearance (see Fig. 21.19). When focal enlargement of the pancreas is present, it most frequently involves the pancreatic head (60%), followed by the tail (40%). One does not see focal enlargement of the true body of the pancreas alone in acute pancreatitis, if this is present then an underlying neoplasm should be suspected (4). Focal enlargement of the head and tail due to inflammation cannot be distinguished from a neoplasm on CT alone. The clinical presentation of acute pancreatitis vs. a pancreatic carcinoma is quite distinct and it is only in a few percent of patients that this distinction is difficult on clinical grounds (4). A follow-up CT is helpful in cases where there is doubt as focal swelling secondary to acute pancreatitis usually subsides within a couple of weeks while a neoplasm would persist (2). Other factors that would help differentiate inflammatory enlargement from a neoplasm include (a) finding adenopathy in the para-aortic and peripancreatic areas, around the base of the superior mesenteric artery and in the porta hepatis as such adenopathy should not present in pancreatitis and (b) the presence of liver metastases (19). Focal swelling of the head of the pancreas can occur with a posterior penetrating peptic ulcer. In such cases, the ulcer crater, if large enough, may be seen on CT. A linear low density band extending from the ulcer crater into the head of the pancreas representing the sinus tract may also be present (20). Acute pancreatitis has also been described secondary to carcinoma of the ampulla of vater (21).

When the inflammatory process in the gland is severe it may spread into the surrounding tissues due to the absence of a pancreatic capsule. This spreading cellulitis or phlegmon (*phlegmonous pancreatitis*) most commonly originates from the body and tail of the pancreas. It has been shown that the density measurements of the most severely affected portion of the pancreas following a rapid intravenous injection of contrast enhances to a lesser degree in patients with acute necrotizing pancreatitis then in those with the milder form of acute pancreatitis (22). The phlegmon usually first spreads anteriorly into the area of the lesser sac and left anterior pararenal space (Figs. 21.16 and 21.18) (23, 24). Posterior extension is usually prevented by the anterior pararenal fascia (Gerota's fascia), however, extension into the posterior pararenal space rarely occurs through the lateroconal fascia. Phlegmon extension from the pancreatic head involves the right anterior pararenal space. In cases with minimal phlegmonous changes there may be only slight thickening of the anterior pararenal fascia (25). Containment of the inflammatory process outside of Gerota's fascia makes the perinephric fat stand out on a plain abdominal radiograph giving rise to the so-called "renal halo" sign (26). Spread can also occur along the transverse mesocolon to involve the transverse colon, into the mesentery of the small bowel (Fig. 21.19) and down the retroperitoneum into the pelvis (27). Intestinal obstruction can result from phlegmonous involvement of the bowel wall (28).

The CT number of the phlegmonous mass can be very low (5-20 HU) and can simulate fluid. It is not a true fluid collection however as percutaneous aspiration will yield no fluid and surgery reveals that the phlegmon is in fact boggy edematous tissue. When a fluid collection occurs within the phlegmon it represents areas of necrosis, hemorrhage and/or abscess formation or focal extrapancreatic accumulations of leaking pancreatic juice. Phlegmonous changes can persist long after the patient has made a full clinical recovery (29). Bilateral pararenal calcifications due to fat necrosis can occur secondary to phlegmonous involvement of these areas (30).

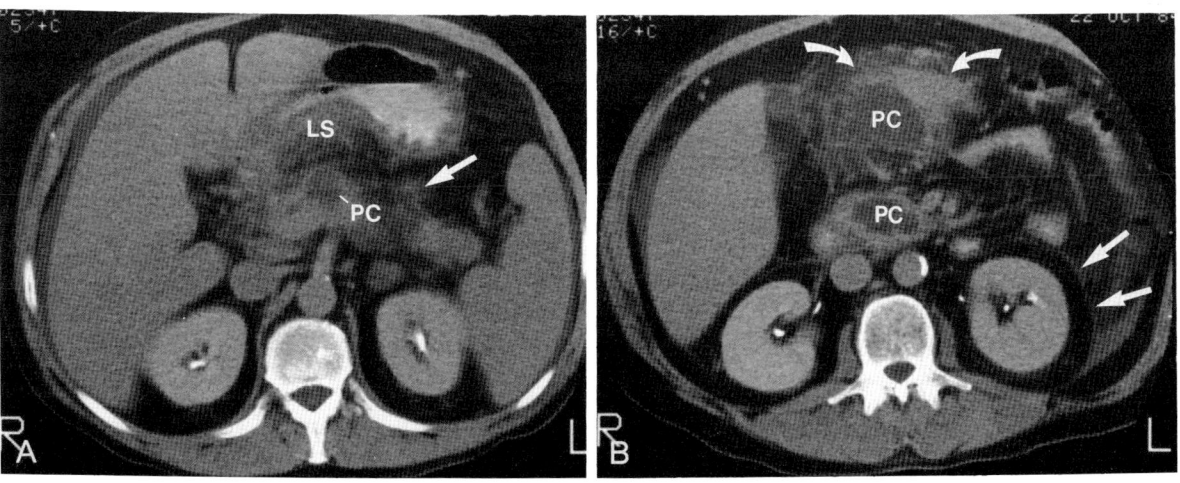

FIGURE 21.18. PHLEGMONOUS PANCREATITIS
CT scan of the pancreas from superior (*A*) to inferior (*B*) reveals a phlegmonous extension involving the lesser sac (*LS*) and the left anterior perirenal space. Two small pseudocysts (*PC*) are seen, one in the head-body and the other in the lower portion of the head and adjoining uncinate process.

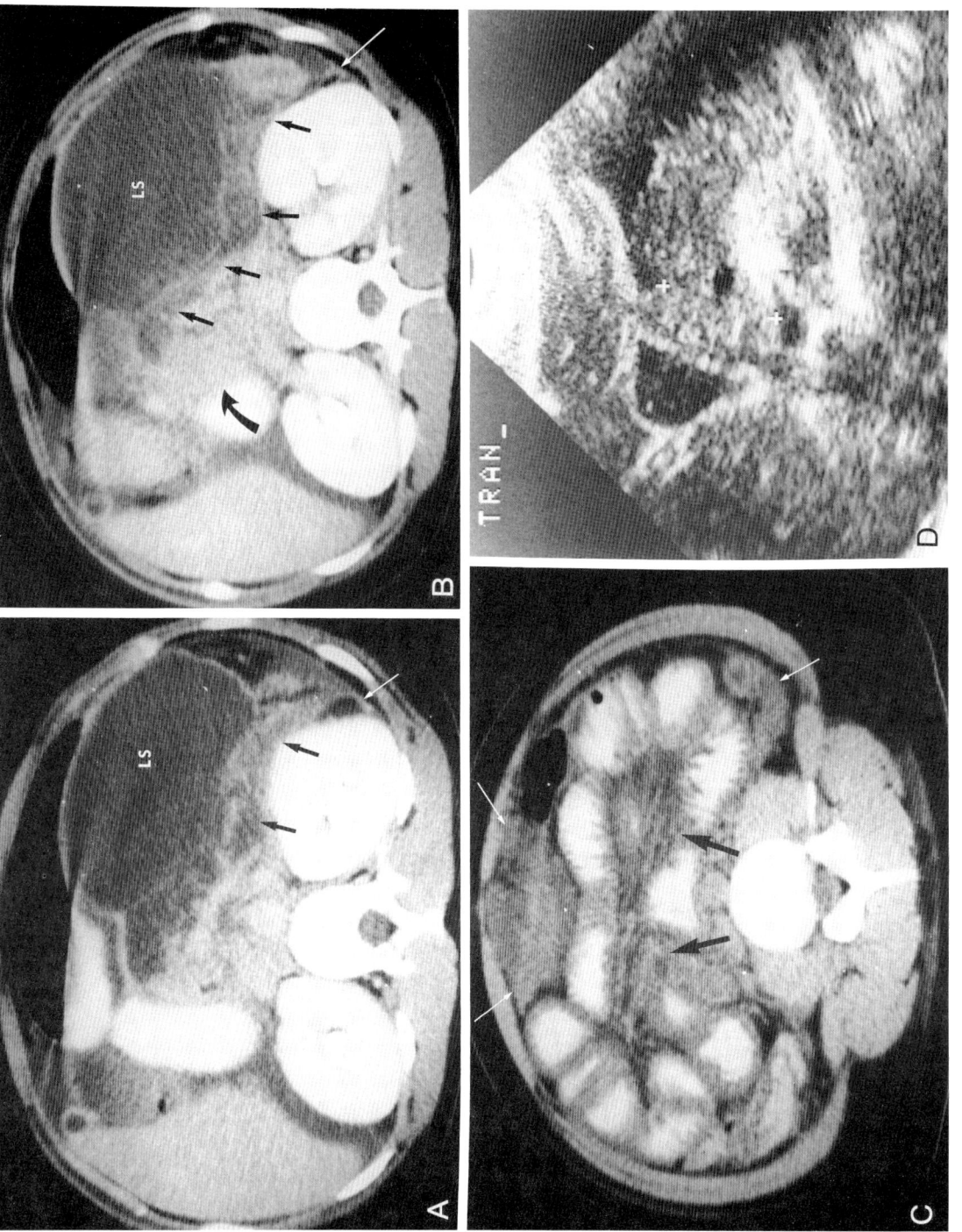

FIGURE 21.19. ACUTE PANCREATITIS

Acute pancreatitis with large fluid collections, ascites, and inflammatory changes in the small and large bowel mesenteries. *A* and *B*: Large lesser sac collection (*LS*), inflammatory changes in the anterior pararenal space with thickening of Gerota's fascia (*white arrow*), ascites, and marked low density in the body and tail of the pancreas (*black arrows*) from inflammation. Head is enlarged (*curved arrow*). *C*: Inflammatory masses in the colonic mesentery (*white arrows*) and small bowel mesentery (*black arrows*) with thickening of the bowel walls. *D*: Transverse pancreatic sonography, same patient: enlarged pancreas (*cursors*) with an abnormal, coarse echo texture.

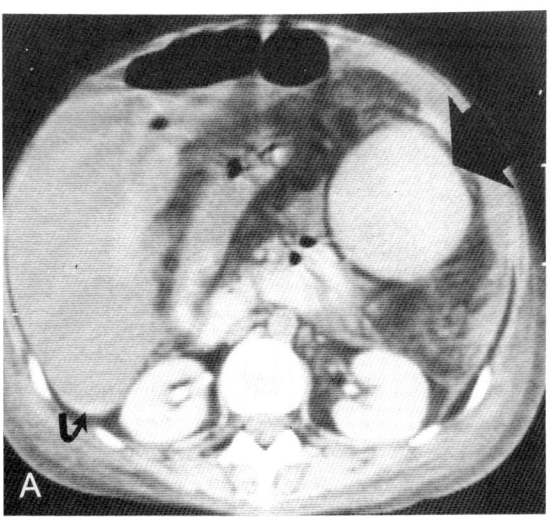
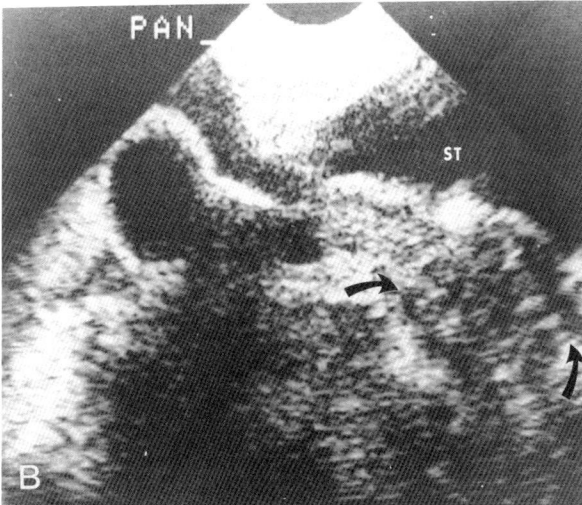

FIGURE 21.20. ACUTE HEMORRHAGIC PANCREATITIS

A: CT: massive hematoma in the tail of the pancreas (*arrow*), inflammatory changes in the left anterior pararenal space and massive hemorrhagic ascites. Note blood in the peritoneal cavity (*curved arrow*). *B:* Corresponding angled transverse sonogram through a water-filled stomach (*ST*): complex mass in the tail of the pancreas (*arrows*) due to resolving hemorrhage three days after the CT.

CT can make the specific diagnosis of *hemorrhagic pancreatitis* when high attenuation values are present in the phlegmon. Such areas of hemorrhage are generally visible to the observers eye as they stand out against the normal low density (5–20 HU) of the surrounding phlegmon (Figs. 21.17 and 21.20). The density of the area of hemorrhage is usually 50–70 HU, however, these high density numbers will only persist for 24–48 hr after the initial event (13). Because of this, when hemorrhagic pancreatitis is suspected, a CT should be performed immediately. As previously mentioned, intravenous iodinated contrast should not be used initially. Clinically unsuspected pancreatic hemorrhage can occur (13). The reverse is also true in that a patient with this clinical diagnosis and a drop in hematocrit and serum calcium may have no CT evidence of hemorrhage. Hemorrhage may not only occur in phlegmonous area but also into pancreatic-peripancreatic fluid collections. Again, its presence is detected by high attenuation values within what should be low density fluid. If followed by CT, phlegmonous areas with hemorrhage can after weeks or months end up having an appearance similar to a pseudocyst (13). One word of caution in diagnosing pancreatic hemorrhage. A pseudocyst can decompress itself into the adjacent stomach or small bowel and so become filled with the orally administered barium suspension. This can then simulate an area of hemorrhage, however, to the trained eye the density of this area is just too high to represent extravasated blood. If doubt exists, an upper GI series could be performed to demonstrate the communication between the bowel and pseudocyst.

Pancreatic or Extrapancreatic Fluid Collections. Fluid collections occur due to rupture of an obstructed pancreatic duct. The collection of fluid may remain in the pancreas itself; however, it may escape beyond the gland because of the absence of a capsule (Fig. 21.19; see also Fig. 21.20). The fluid dissects along tissue planes and can assume an unusual outline but is usually round to oval in shape. The commonest location for such fluid collections is in the lesser sac as only a thin layer of connective tissue and peritoneum separate this space from the gland (see Fig. 21.71). The fluid does not usually escape into the greater peritoneal space as the foramen of Winslow becomes blocked by the surrounding inflammatory process. With the passage of time, such fluid collections if they persist develop a fibrous wall and so become a true *pseudocyst*. From the point of view of surgical management of these fluid collections, it is desirable to wait 6 weeks before operating so that a fibrous wall can develop that can be marsuprialized to the adjacent stomach, duodenum or small bowel. From the CT image alone, the age of a fluid collection cannot be ascertained and so serial studies may have to be performed.

Sonography vs. CT in Pancreatitis: Clinical Considerations

CT has been shown to be better overall (sensitivity/specificity) then sonography in evaluating patients with a pancreatic problem (31). This is especially true of CT units with a fast scanning time (3 sec vs. 18 sec) as they have been shown to reduce the number of both technically unsuccessful and false negative examinations (32).

In acute pancreatitis, diagnostic visualization of the gland will be present sonographically in 62% vs. 98% for CT (4). The decision regarding which modality to use to evaluate the pancreas depends on the body habitus of the patient and on the diagnostic information which is being sought. If the patient is thin and emaciated then sonography is the procedure of choice while CT is appropriate for the big and/or obese patient. Most individuals lie between these two extremes so ones choice has to be made on an individual basis. In the mild form of pancreatitis (acute edematous pancreatitis), both the sonogram and CT will be normal in about 28%. In the severe form of pancreatitis (acute necrotizing), there is often an associated ileus which prevents adequate sonographic evaluation of the gland. Since there may be superimposed hemorrhage or abscess formation, CT is the modality of choice in this clinical setting (27). The pancreas should not appear normal in a patient with this diagnosis and if it does, then the clinical diagnosis has to be reconsidered (27, 29). If biliary pancreatitis is suspected, sonography should be used as the initial examination as gallbladder calculi are best detected by sonography rather than by CT (12). Sonography can detect pseudocysts in the head and body of the pancreas, however, it tends to miss those present in the tail. In a study by Williford et al. (33), CT correctly identified 23 of 24 patients with pseudocysts in a group of 54 patients with this suspected diagnosis. Sonography on the other hand only detected 18 and in 10 of these, the information was incomplete (33). When percutaneous aspiration of a pancreatic/peripancreatic fluid collection is clinically indicated, this is best achieved using sonographic guidance. CT guidance should be reserved for those fluid collections that cannot be identified sonographically or when they are small and deep in location (34).

The CT and sonographic findings of acute pancreatitis, especially phlegmonous changes, can persist following full clinical recovery of the patient and so follow up examinations should not be used unless a complication is suspected (2, 29).

REFERENCES

1. Ranson, JHC: Acute pancreatitis. *Curr Probl Surg* 16:5–83, 1979.
2. Cox KL, Ament ME, Sample WF, Sarti DA, O'Donnell M, Byrne WJ: The ultrasonic and biochemical diagnosis of pancreatitis in children. *J Pediatr* 96:407–411, 1980.
3. Fleischer AC, Parker P, Kirchner SG, James AE: Sonographic findings of pancreatitis in children. *Radiology* 146:151–155, 1983.
4. Silverstein W, Isikoff MB, Hill MC, Barkin J: Diagnostic imaging of acute pancreatitis: prospective study using CT and sonography. *AJR* 137:497–502, 1981.
5. Arger PH, Mulhern CB, Bonavita JA, Stauffer DM, Hale J: An analysis of pancreatic sonography in suspected pancreatic disease. *J Clin Ultrasound* 7:91–97, 1979.
6. Simeone JF, Dembner AG, Mueller PR: Invasion of the pancreas by gastric carcinoma: ultrasonic appearance. *J Clin Ultrasound* 8:501–503, 1980.
7. Coleman BG, Arger PH, Rosenberg HK, Mulhern CB, Ortega W, Stauffer D: Gray-scale sonographic assessment of pancreatitis in children. *Radiology* 146:145–150, 1983.
8. Warshaw AL: Inflammatory masses following acute pancreatitis: Phlegmon, pseudocyst and abscess. *Surg Clin North Am* 54:621–635, 1974.
9. Robbins SL, Cotran RS: The pancreas. In *Pathological Basis of Disease*, Ed. 2. Philadelphia, W. B. Saunders, 1979, pp 1092–1114.
10. Williams P, Warwick R: The pancreas. In *Gray's Anatomy*, Ed. 36. Philadelphia, W. B. Saunders, 1980, pp 1368–1374.
11. Nyberg DA, Laing FC: Ultrasonographic findings in peptic ulcer disease and pancreatitis that simulate primary gallbladder disease. *J Ultrasound Med* 2:303–307, 1983.
12. Burrell M, Gold JA, Simeone J, Taylor K, Dobbins J: Liquefactive necrosis of the pancreas. *Radiology* 135:157–160, 1980.
13. Isikoff MB, Hill MC, Barkin J: The clinical significance of acute pancreatic hemorrhage. *AJR* 136:679–684, 1981.
14. Hill MC, Saunders RC: Gray scale B scan characteristics of intraabdominal cystic masses. *J Clin Ultrasound* 6:217–222, 1978.
15. Stabile BE, Wilson SE, Debas HT: Reduced mortality from bleeding pseudocysts and pseudoaneurysms caused by pancreatitis. *Arch Surg* 118:45–51, 1983.
16. Gooding GAW: Ultrasound of a superior mesenteric artery aneurysm secondary to pancreatitis: a plea for real-time ultrasound of sonolucent masses in pancreatitis. *J Clin Ultrasound* 9:255–256, 1981.
17. Dach JL, Hill MC, Pelaez JC, LePage JR, Russell E: Sonography of hypertensive portal venous system: correlation with arterial portography. *AJR* 137:511–517, 1981.
18. Moss AA, Federle M, Shapiro HA, Ohto M, Goldberg H, Korobkin M, Clemett A: The combined use of computed tomography and endoscopic retrograde cholangiopancreatography in the assessment of suspected pancreatic neoplasm: a blind clinical evaluation. *Radiology* 134:159–163, 1980.
19. Megibow AJ, Bosniak MA, Ambos MA, Beranbaum ER: Thickening of the celiac axis and/or superior mesenteric artery: a sign of pancreatic carcinoma on computed tomography. *Radiology* 141:449–453, 1981.
20. Madrazo BL, Halpert RD, Sandler MA, Pearlberg JL: Computed tomographic findings in penetrating peptic ulcer. *Radiology* 153:751–754, 1984.
21. Wise RH, Stanley RJ: Case report. Carcinoma of the

ampulla of vater presenting as acute pancreatitis. *J Comput Assist Tomogr* 8:158–161, 1984.
22. Kivisaari L, Somer K, Standertskjold-Nordenstam CG, Schroeder T, Kivilaakso E, Lempinen M: A new method for the diagnosis of acute hemorrhagic necrotizing pancreatitis using contrast enhanced CT. *Gastrointest Radiol* 9:27–30, 1984.
23. Dembner AG, Jaffee CC, Simeone J, Walsh J: A new computed tomographic sign of pancreatitis. *AJR* 133:477–479, 1979.
24. Mendez G, Isikoff MB, Hill MC: CT of acute pancreatitis: interim assessment. *AJR* 135:463–469, 1980.
25. Chintapalli K, Lawson TL, Foley WD, Berland LL: Renal fascial thickening in pancreatitis. *J Comput Assist Tomogr* 6:983–986, 1982.
26. Susman N, Hammerman AM, Cohen E: The renal halo sign in pancreatitis. *Radiology* 142:323–327, 1982.
27. Jeffrey RB, Federle MP, Cello JP, Cross RA: Early computed tomographic scanning in acute severe pancreatitis. *Surg Gynecol Obstet* 154:170–174, 1982.
28. Macerollo P, Segal I, Epstein B, Essop R, Elliseos C: Total obstruction of the ascending colon complicating acute pancreatitis. *Am J Gastroenterol* 5:173–175, 1978.
29. Hill MC, Barkin J, Isikoff MB, Silverstein W, Kalser MH: Acute pancreatitis: clinical versus CT findings. *AJR* 139:263–269, 1982.
30. Baker DE, Glazer GM: Bilateral pararenal calcifications resulting from pancreatitis. *AJR* 143:51–52, 1984.
31. Hessel SJ, Siegelman SS, McNeil BJ et al: A prospective evaluation of computed tomography and ultrasound of the pancreas. *Radiology* 143:129–133, 1982.
32. Levitt RG, Stanley RJ, Sagel SS, Lee JKT, Weyman PJ: Computed tomography of the pancreas: three second scanning versus 18 second scanning. *J Comput Assist Tomogr* 6:259–267, 1982.
33. Williford ME, Foster WL, Halvorsen RA, Thompson WM: Pancreatic pseudocyst: comparative evaluation by sonography and computed tomography. *AJR* 140:53–57, 1983.
34. Pelaez JC, Hill MC, Dach JL, Isikoff MB, Morse B: Abdominal aspiration biopsies: sonographic vs. computed tomography guidance. *JAMA* 250:2663–2666, 1983.

CHRONIC PANCREATITIS

Etiology and Pathogenesis

A close correlation exists in the Western Hemisphere, Europe, and Japan between daily alcohol consumption and the risk of developing chronic calcifying pancreatitis (1, 2). A high protein high fat diet is believed to add to the risk. A preponderance of blood group O and an increased frequency of HLA A1 and BW40 suggests a congenital factor in pancreatic intolerance to alcohol (1). Other etiologies are relatively uncommon: biliary tract disease, hyperparathyroidism, hereditary pancreatitis, cystic fibrosis, trauma, tropical pancreatitis, and hyperlipidemia (1). Patients with biliary tract disease usually develop acute rather than chronic pancreatitis (and when they do develop chronic disease they have a morphologically different chronic obstructive pancreatitis) (1–3). In up to 40% there is no recognizable predisposing cause (3). No matter what the etiology, a constant increase in concentration of a peculiar protein, lactoferrin, is present in pancreatic juice (1). Lactoferrin is normally present in zymogen granules but is not found in calculi (1).

The pathogenesis of chronic calcific pancreatitis can be explained by protein hyperconcentration in pancreatic juice (more often from protein hypersecretion than diminished water and bicarbonate secretion), resultant protein precipitates in the ducts (which include a "stone protein" with a high affinity for calcium) and consequently precipitation of calcium carbonate resulting in calculi (1). Precipitations in the ducts cause duct epithelial abnormalities and ductal stenosis. Strictures and/or precipitates cause partial or complete obstruction which lead to lobular atrophy and/or fibrosis and cyst formation (1). Protein hypersecretion and inspissation is responsible for acute pancreatitis after scorpion bites and probably for acute pancreatitis caused by steroids (1). Thus, protein hypersecretion and precipitation could be responsible for exacerbations as well as chronic lesions (1).

Chronic alcohol feeding causes an increase in protein secretion and a slight decrease in bicarbonate secretion (1). Hypercalcemia increases protein secretion as well as facilitating calcification (1). In the initial stages of cystic fibrosis protein secretion is normal, but bicarbonate and water secretion are diminished (1). In tropical pancreatitis there is a good correlation between pancreatitis and protein malnutrition (kwashiorkor) (1). Prussic acid, present in manioc which is a tropical dietary staple, has been implicated as a toxic factor (1).

Clinical Findings

Chronic pancreatitis can be manifested by mild recurrent bouts of pain, constant abdominal or back pain, or in a small number of patients, painless exocrine and endocrine deficiency (2). Alcoholism is usually present for 5–10 yr prior to the development of clinical pancreatitis (2). Initially, exocrine function is minimally impaired, but as insufficiency develops, fat and protein malabsorption occurs with weight loss (2, 3). Diabetes occurs in 10% of cases and impaired glucose tolerance in 14–90% (2, 3). Duodenal obstruction and/or jaundice may occur in

45% of patients with moderate or advanced chronic pancreatitis (3, 4).

Before the acinar cells are greatly diminished in number, confirmation of the diagnosis may be obtained by serum or urine amylase determinations within 8–12 hr of episodes of pain or by serum amylase and lipase response to secretin stimulation (2). The secretin test may also reveal a decrease in the volume and bicarbonate content of pancreatic secretion. A reduction of steatorrhea and weight gain in response to enzyme replacement is a useful therapeutic trial (2).

Hereditary Pancreatitis

Hereditary pancreatitis is an autosomal dominant disorder occurring only in Caucasians, characterized by recurrent bouts of abdominal pain that begin in childhood and chronic pancreatitis which is refractory to therapy (5–7). It is the most common cause of pancreatic calcification in childhood (5). A constant finding is dilatation of the pancreatic ductal system (5). Pseudocysts occurred in 50% in one series (5) and 20% of deaths in patients with this disease have been from carcinoma of the pancreas (6).

Cystic Fibrosis

This autosomal recessive disorder affects many organ systems and usually manifests itself in infancy or childhood, however, because of increased survival of moderately severe cases and failure to recognize mild cases in childhood, more adults with this disease are being encountered (2). Some young adults with "idiopathic" pancreatitis, COPD, or cirrhosis may in fact have cystic fibrosis (2). Pancreatic acini are replaced by fibrotic tissue, multiple cysts, inspissated mucous and eventually fat. The result is exocrine insufficiency which is severe in 80%, mild in 10%, and inapparent in 10% (2). Patients with radiographically visible pancreatic calcification usually have clinically advanced pancreatic disease (6).

Tropical Pancreatitis (Kwashiorkor)

Chronic pancreatitis in underdeveloped countries is frequently associated with a high carbohydrate diet with insufficient protein (6, 8). Abdominal pain is less prominent than in alcoholic pancreatitis but diabetes and steatorrhea are more common (8). Clinical symptoms, histologic changes in acini, and pancreatic lithiasis develop in childhood (8). Ninety-seven percent of affected patients have dilated pancreatic ducts and 50% have intraductal calculi (6).

Treatment

Control of pain is often poor, and patients may become dependent on narcotics. Surgery, when indicated, provides relief of pain in about 60% of cases. It is most effective when a correctible biliary abnormality is present. If there are dilated ducts, a longitudinal pancreaticojejunostomy (Puestow procedure) can divide strictures, remove calculi, and promote drainage (2, 9). A proximal (tail) pancreaticojejunostomy can provide drainage when there is localized proximal obstruction. If there are no dilated ducts, there is no surgical alternative to major resection or total pancreatectomy (2, 9).

REFERENCES

1. Sarles H, Figarella C, Tiscornia O, Colomb E, Guy O, Venrine H, DeCaro A, Multigner L, Lechene P: Chronic calcifying pancreatitis, *Monogr Pathol* 21:48–66, 1980.
2. Snodgrass PJ: Diseases of the pancreas. In Wintrobe, MM et al (eds): *Harrison's Principles of Internal Medicine.* New York, McGraw-Hill, 1974, pp 1571–1577.
3. Robbins SL, Cotran SR. *Pathologic Basis of Disease.* Philadelphia, W. B. Saunders, 1979, pp 1096–1102.
4. Rosai J: *Ackerman's Surgical Pathology.* St. Louis, C. V. Mosby, 1981, pp 664–668.
5. Fried AM, Selke AC: Pseudocyst formation in hereditary pancreatitis. *J Pediatr* 93:950–953, 1978.
6. Ring EJ, Eaton SB, Ferrucci JT, Short WF: Differential diagnosis of pancreatic calcification. *Radiology* 117:446–452, 1973.
7. Buntain W, Wood JB, Woolley MM: Pancreatitis in childhood. *J Pediatr Surg* 13:143–149, 1978.
8. Reeder MM, Palmer PES: *Radiology of Tropical Diseases.* Baltimore, Williams & Wilkins, 1981, pp 414–470.
9. Turner FW: Surgery in chronic pancreatitis. *Can J Surg* 21:63–67, 1978.

Pathology

Chronic pancreatitis has two morphologic patterns: chronic calcifying pancreatitis and chronic obstructive pancreatitis (1–3). Chronic calcifying pancreatitis, by far the more common, is manifested by a nodular, misshapen, hard gland that can be enlarged or shrunken (2, 3). Calculi are present and are almost always within the ductal system. They vary in size from microscopic concretions, to stones, one to several cm in diameter (2). Eosinophilic protein precipitates are also present within the ducts (1). Duct epithelium is often atrophic or absent (1), and may show squamous metaplasia (3). Regions of obstruction and poststenotic dilatation in intralobular or intercalated ducts are common (1). Parenchymal lesions are patchy and irregular (1). Fairly well preserved lobules are present in the midst of fibrotic scars and half-destroyed lobules (1). Aci-

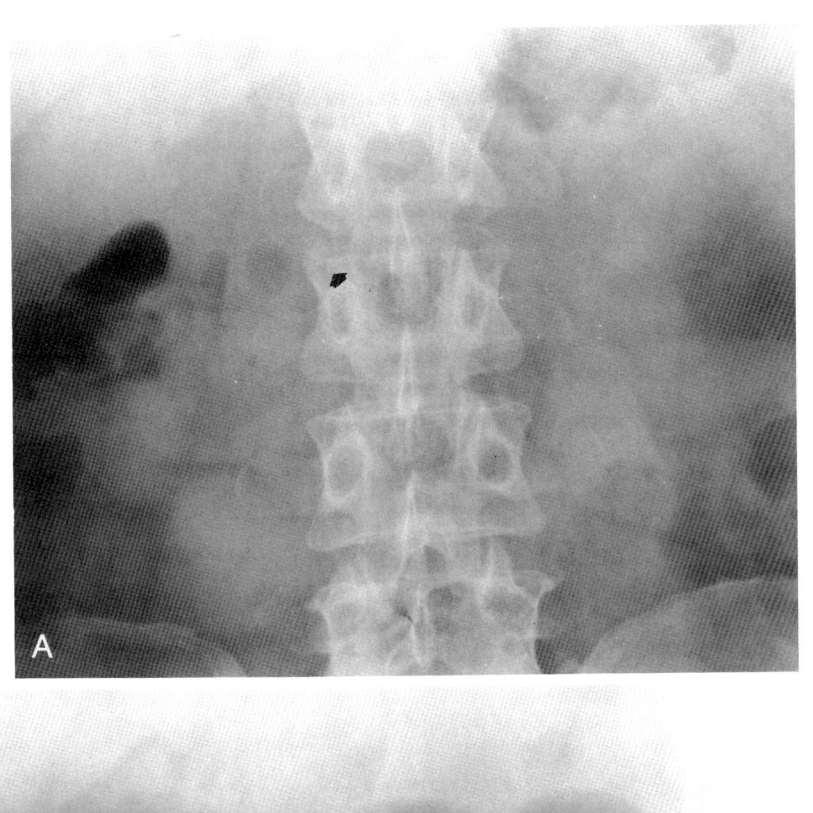
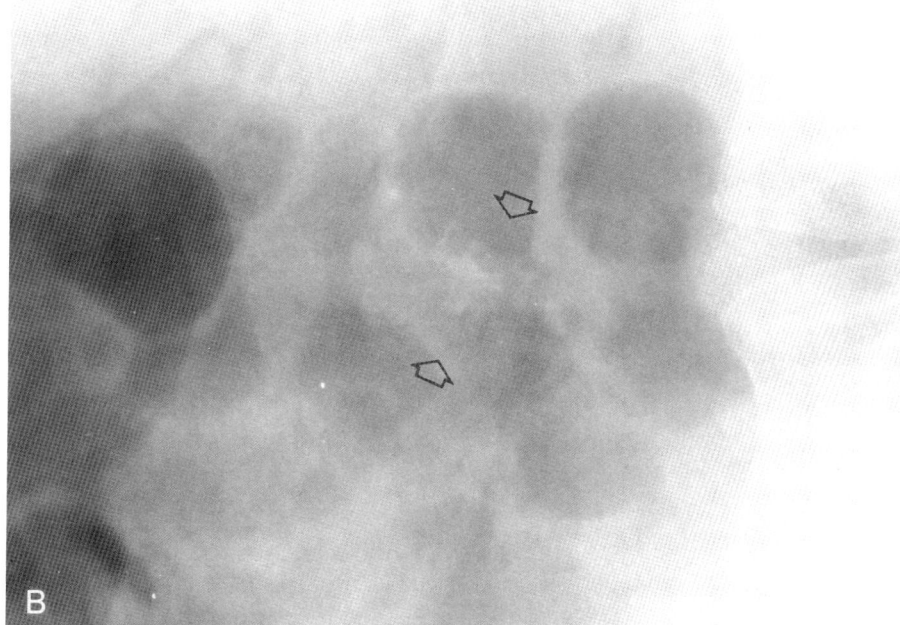

FIGURE 21.21. CHRONIC PANCREATITIS
A: Calcification in the head of the pancreas obscured by spine (*arrow*). Film was read as negative. *B:* Right posterior oblique film of same patient showing calcification limited to the head of the pancreas (*arrows*).

nar atrophy is present but the islets are relatively preserved (2). Cyst formation, in addition to atrophy, may be present because of complete isolation of lobules from the ductal system (1).

Chronic obstructive pancreatitis is caused by slow growing tumors, ampullary stenosis from biliary disease, or surgical duct ligation (1–3). Lesions are regularly distributed in that part of the pancreas proximal to the obstruction (1). Protein plugs and calculi are exceptional (1–3).

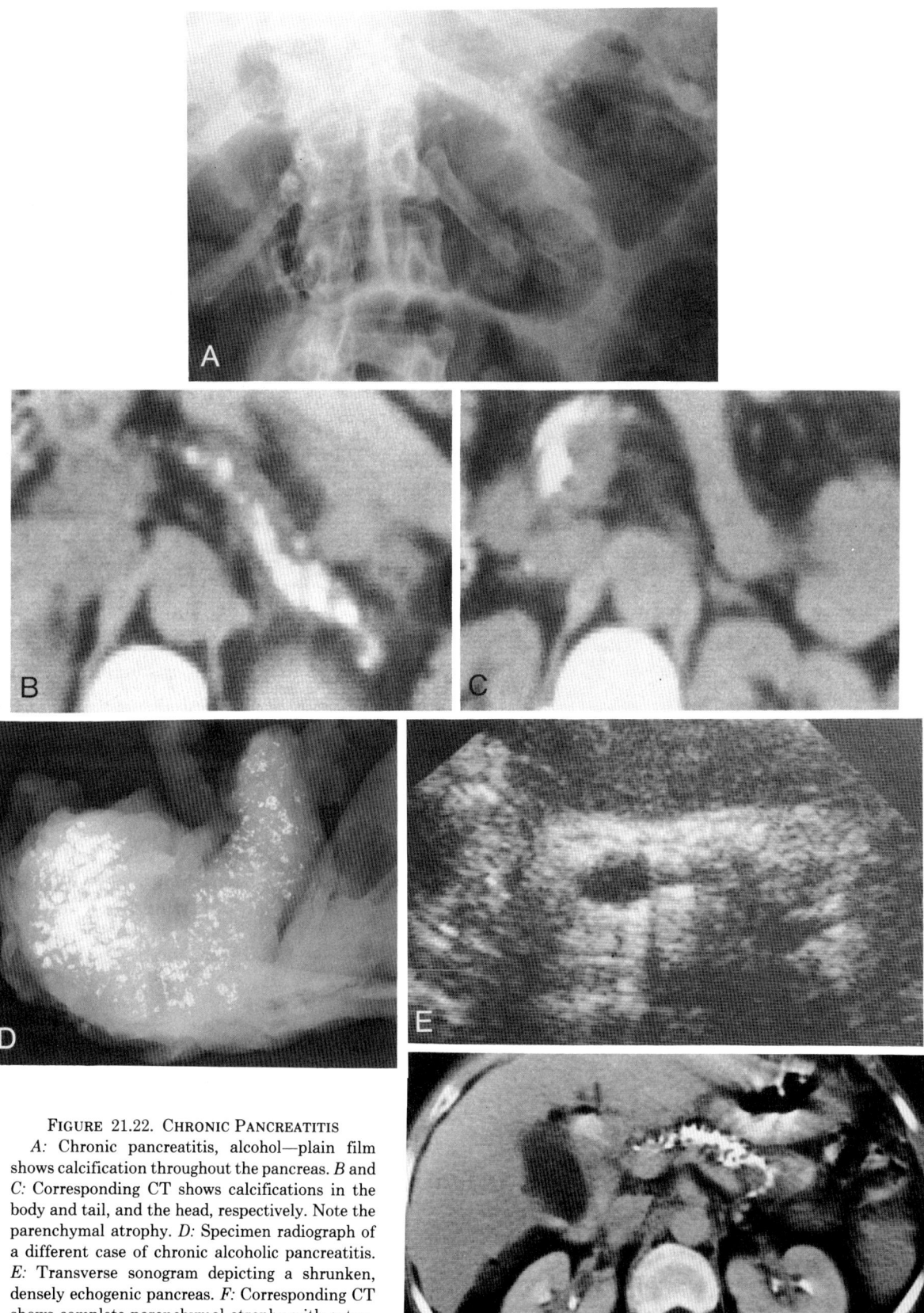

FIGURE 21.22. CHRONIC PANCREATITIS
A: Chronic pancreatitis, alcohol—plain film shows calcification throughout the pancreas. *B* and *C:* Corresponding CT shows calcifications in the body and tail, and the head, respectively. Note the parenchymal atrophy. *D:* Specimen radiograph of a different case of chronic alcoholic pancreatitis. *E:* Transverse sonogram depicting a shrunken, densely echogenic pancreas. *F:* Corresponding CT shows complete parenchymal atrophy with extensive diffuse ductal calcification in alcoholic chronic pancreatitis.

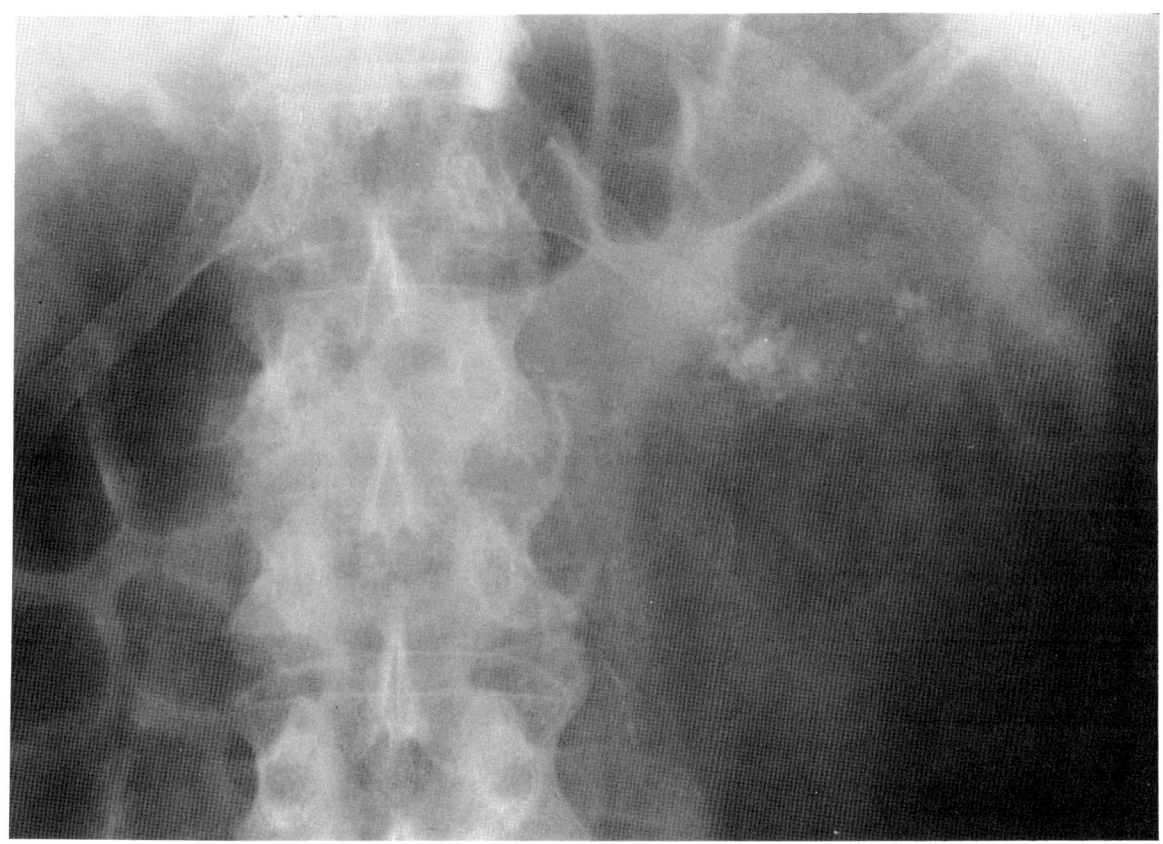

FIGURE 21.23. CHRONIC PANCREATITIS
Solitary left upper quadrant calcifications proven to be in the pancreatic tail by CT. Alcoholic pancreatitis.

Radiology

Plain Films

Demonstration of pancreatic lithiasis on plain films is a fast and inexpensive means of confirming a clinical diagnosis of chronic pancreatitis and effectively excluding carcinoma (1, 4). As calcifications in the head of the pancreas can be rendered nearly invisible by the lumbar spine, shallow oblique films are often helpful (Fig. 21.21). In various series the frequency of plain film calcification has varied from 20 to 50% in alcoholic chronic pancreatitis (2, 4). In one series, a 2-yr follow-up of noncalcified cases showed development of calcifications in nearly all patients (2). By contrast, only 2% or less of patients with chronic pancreatitis from biliary disease develop pancreatic calculi (4).

The calculi of chronic pancreatitis are nearly always intraductal (3, 4). Plain films show numerous, irregular calcifications of varying but usually small size deposited throughout the gland (Fig. 21.22) (4). In alcoholic disease calcifications are limited to the head or tail in 25% and are rarely solitary (Fig. 21.21B, 21.23, and 21.24) (4). True parenchymal calcification is unusual and probably occurs after hemorrhage from trauma or tissue necrosis (4).

Hereditary Pancreatitis. In hereditary pancreatitis plain film calcification occurs in 35–60% (4, 5). Calcifications are rounded and seen throughout the gland. They are often larger than those in cystic fibrosis, the chief differential consideration in children (4).

Hyperparathyroidism. Almost one-half of patients whose hyperparathyroidism causes pancreatitis have plain film calcification indistinguishable from alcoholic pancreatitis (4, 6). However, a high percentage of these patients will have concomitant radiographically detectable nephrocalcinosis (4).

Cystic Fibrosis. Pancreatic calcification is a frequent finding at autopsy in patients with cystic fibrosis but is found only occasionally on plain films, in association with advanced disease (4). The calcifications are finely granular and smaller

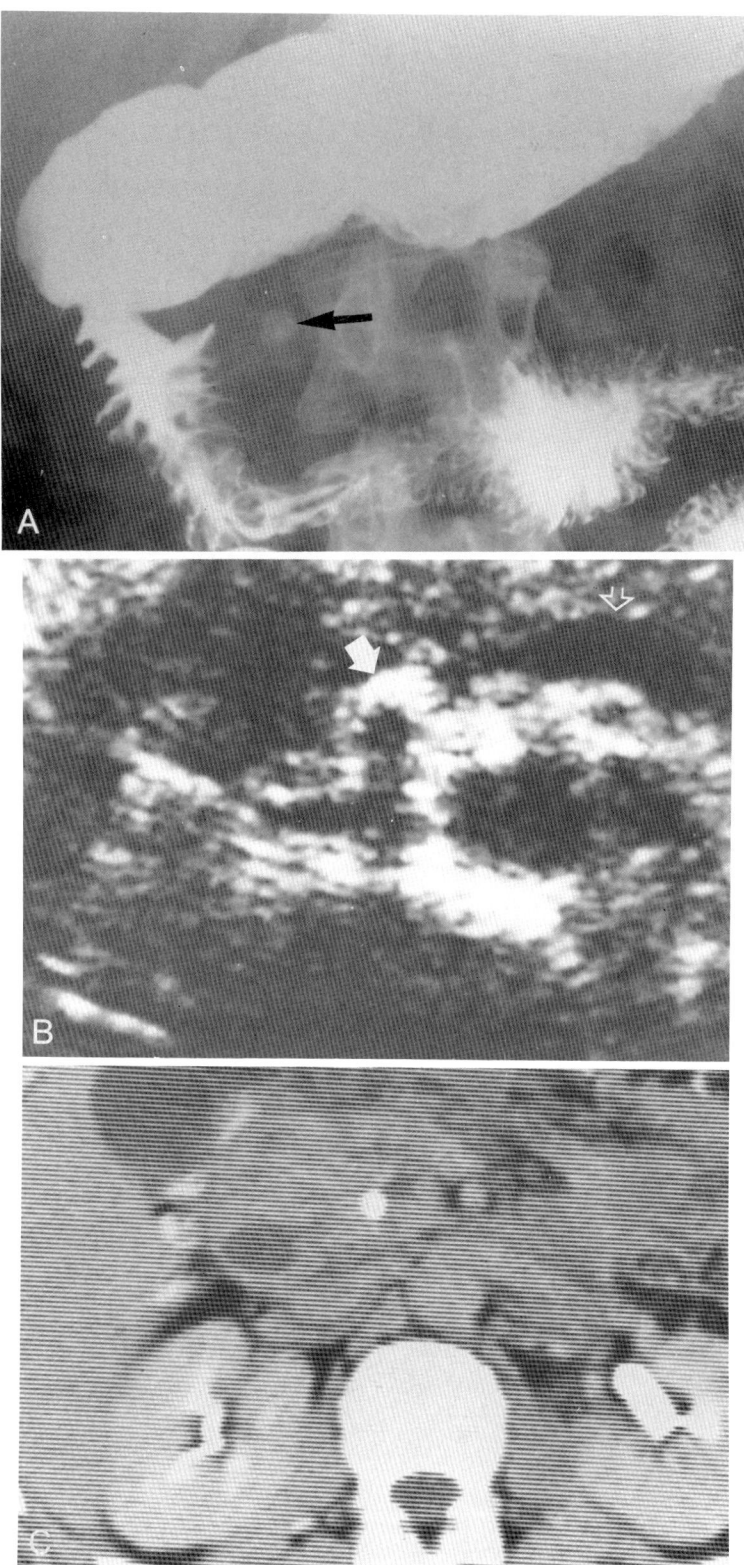

FIGURE 21.24. CHRONIC PANCREATITIS

Solitary intraductal calcification in the pancreatic head in alcoholic chronic pancreatitis. *A:* GI series—note stenotic, distorted duodenum and greater curvature of antrum in addition to pancreatic calcification (*arrow*). *B:* Sonogram—note shadowing from calculus (*arrow*) and dilated pancreatic duct (*open arrow*). *C:* CT—note enlarged head and small pseudocyst in addition to intraductal calculus.

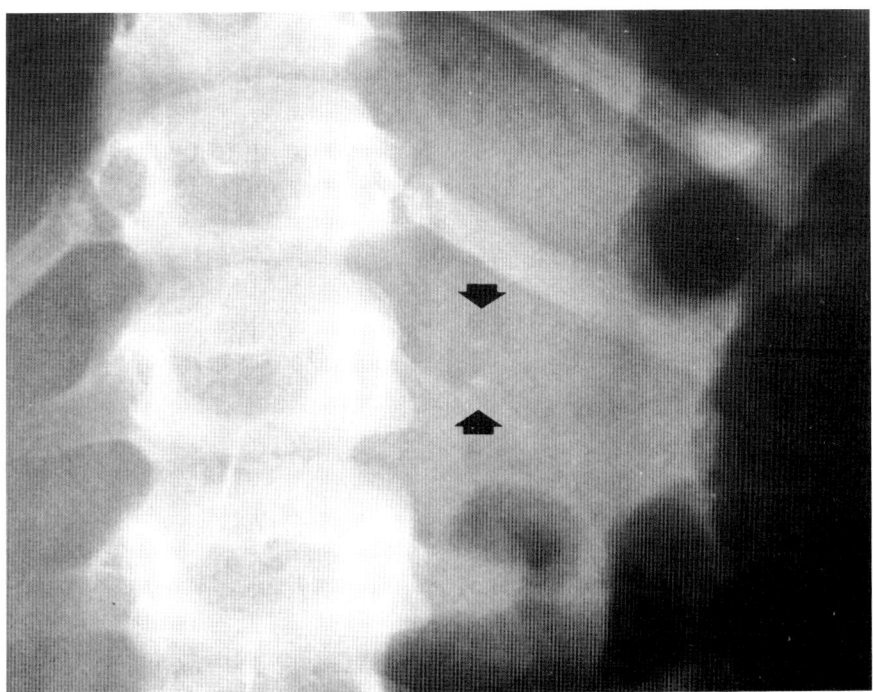

FIGURE 21.25. CHRONIC PANCREATITIS
Tiny pancreatic calcifications to the left of the L1 vertebral body in a patient with cystic fibrosis.

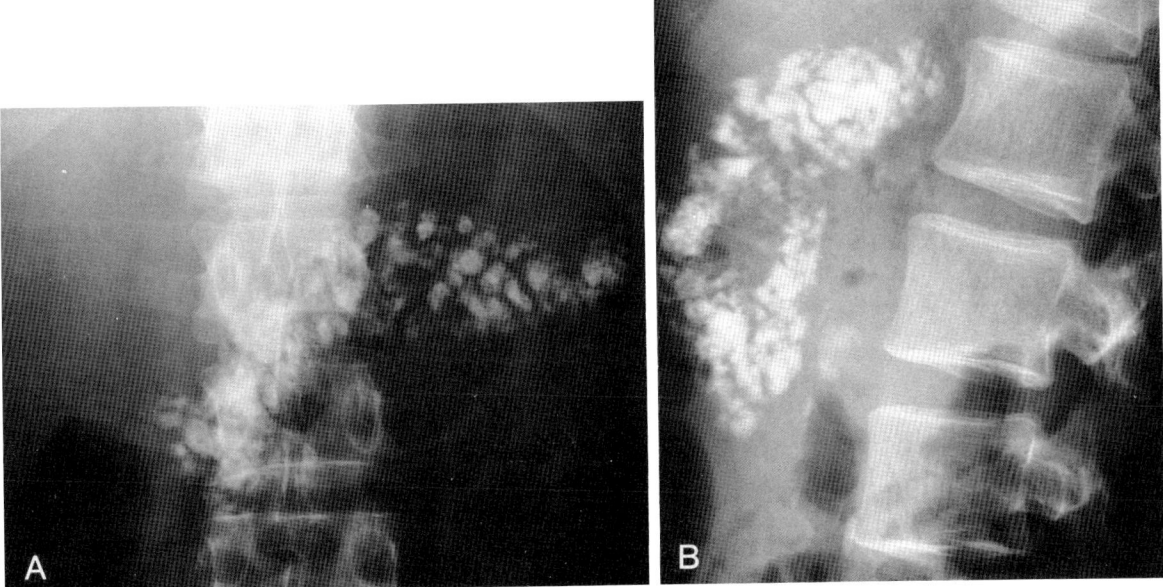

FIGURE 21.26. CHRONIC PANCREATITIS
AP (*A*) and lateral (*B*) abdominal films of a patient with idiopathic pancreatic lithiasis. He was entirely asymptomatic with regard to his pancreas and was not alcoholic. The calcifications were discovered on a skeletal survey for lung cancer metastases.

than those in hereditary pancreatitis (Fig. 21.25) (4).

Idiopathic. There is a set of patients with intraductal pancreatic lithiasis who are not alcoholic and have no pain or any other clinical evidence of pancreatitis (Fig. 21.26) (4). Calculi have been found proximal to regions of nonspecific ductal obstruction in some of these patients, along with ductal dilatation, periductal fibrosis, parenchymal atrophy and fatty replacement.

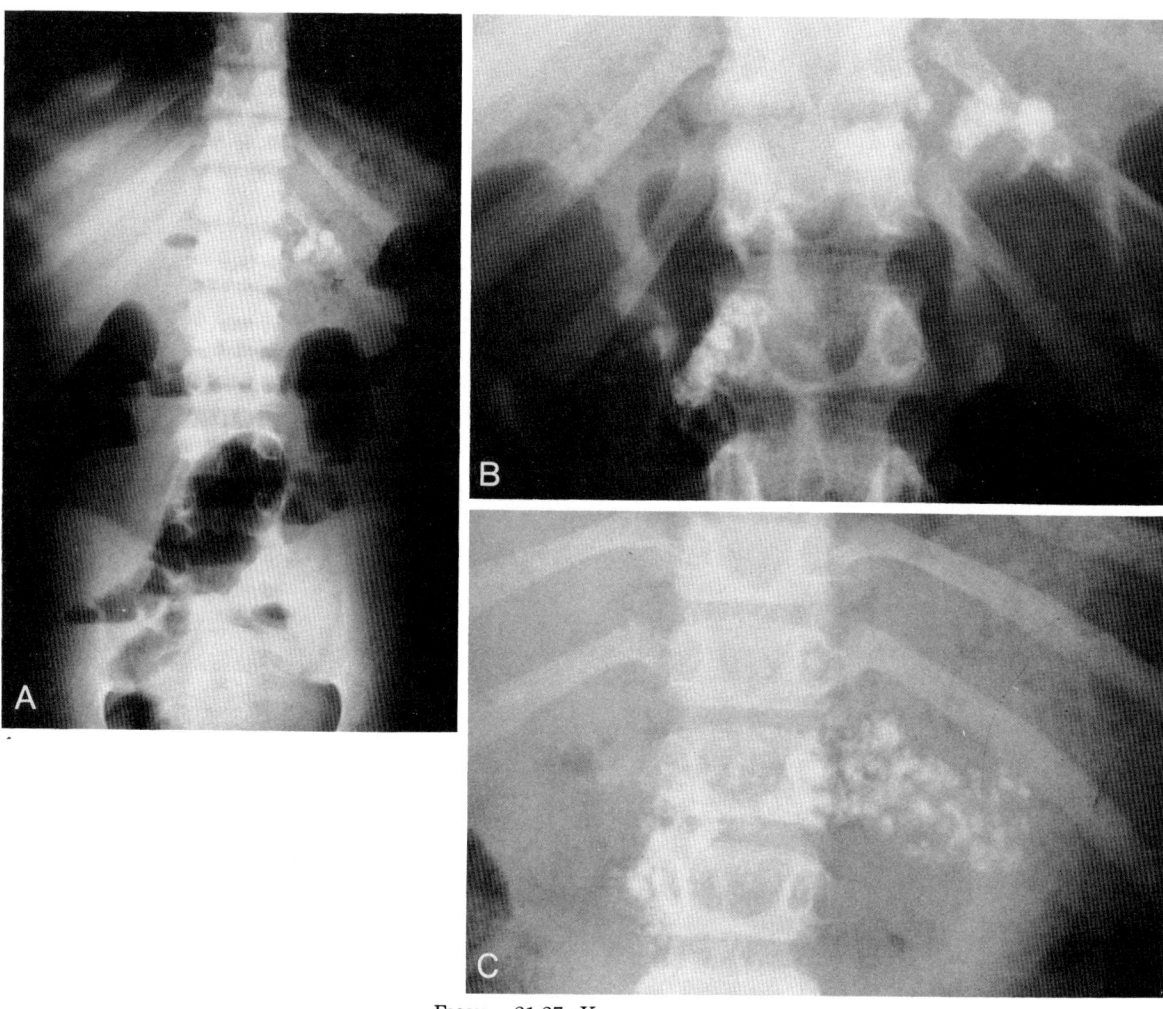

FIGURE 21.27. KWASHIORKOR

A and *B*: A 15-yr-old Haitian girl suffering from Kwashiorkor. Erect film (*A*) shows an ileus and pancreatic calculi. The latter are seen better on the close-up (*B*). Plain film findings are indistinguishable from familial pancreatitis. *C*: Pancreatic calcification in a young refugee from Southeast Asia with kwashiorkor.

These findings are consistent with post obstructive atrophy (7).

Kwashiorkor (Tropical Pancreatitis). Intraductal calculi are seen often in this condition and are indistinguishable from chronic alcoholic pancreatitis (Fig. 21.27) (8).

Barium Contrast Examinations

Stomach and Duodenum. Displacement of the stomach may be caused by focal or diffuse pancreatic enlargement but is often due to a pseudocyst (1, 9). Abnormalities of the gastric folds are present in about 20% of patients with chronic pancreatitis (9). Enlarged, nodular folds are usually localized to areas contiguous to the inflammatory process and are more common in the posterior wall, and proximal half of the stomach (9). Patients with severe pancreatitis occasionally develop profound gastric abnormalities including shrinkage with fold induration mimicking linitis plastica and marked contour abnormalities mimicking primary carcinoma of the stomach (Figs. 21.28 and 21.29). These severe changes are probably caused by a combination of intrinsic mucosal inflammation and perigastric fibrosis and adhesions (9). Surgical biopsy has shown serosal and muscular inflammation and necrosis with submucosal edema and normal mucosa (9), thus, endoscopic biopsy may be negative.

Duodenum. Abnormalities of the duodenum are found in only 10% of patients with chronic pancreatitis using conventional single-contrast

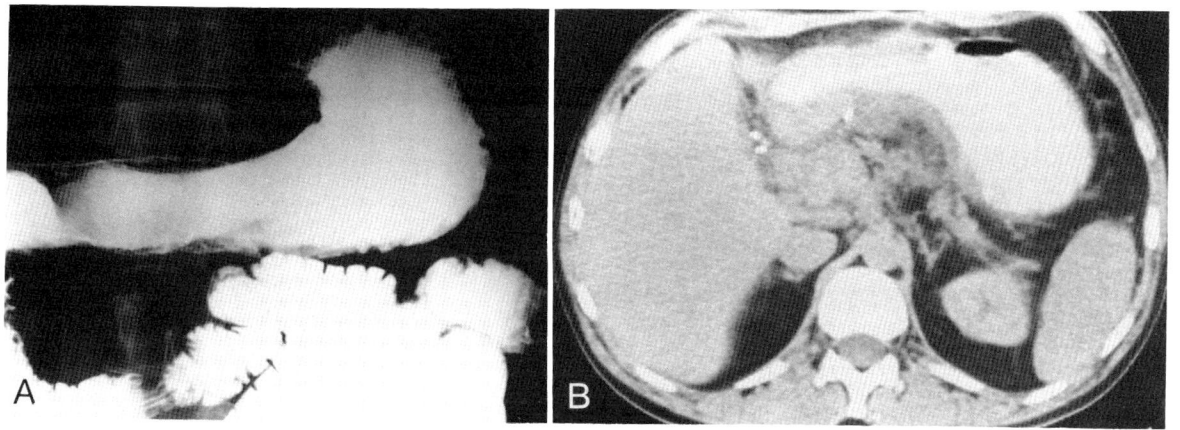

FIGURE 21.28. CHRONIC PANCREATITIS
A: Straightened, rigid antrum with fold thickening from chronic pancreatitis. *B:* Corresponding CT showing thickening of the posterior gastric wall.

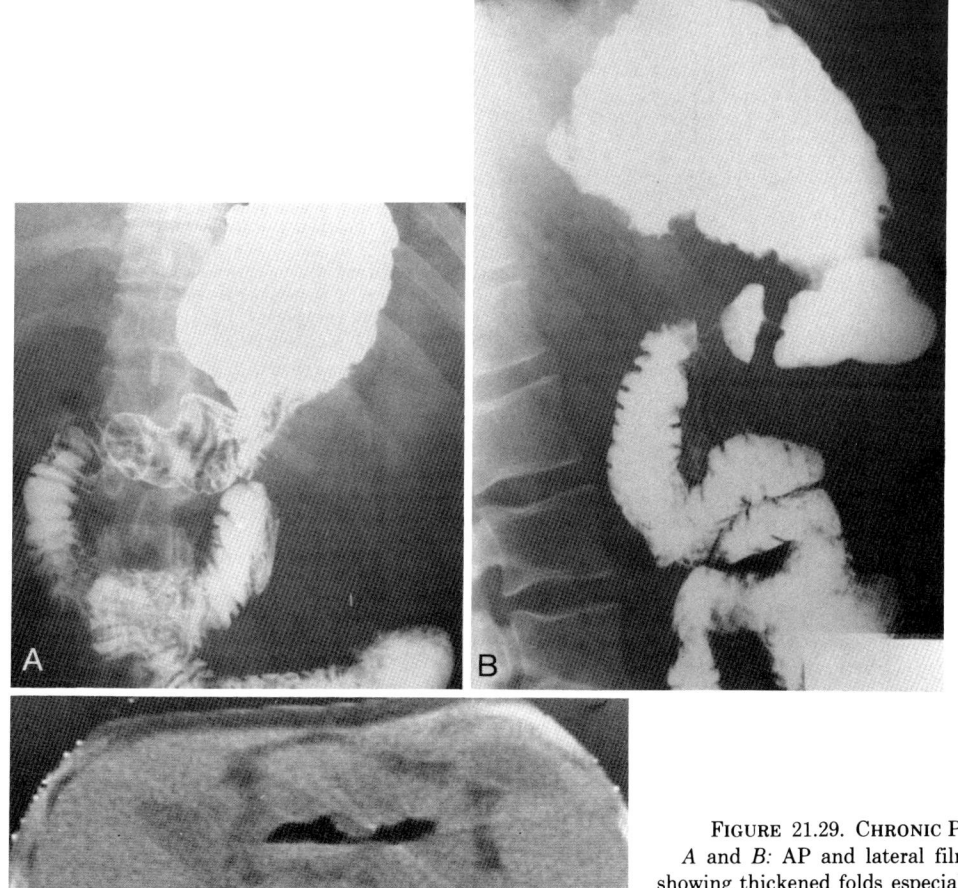

FIGURE 21.29. CHRONIC PANCREATITIS
A and *B:* AP and lateral films of the stomach showing thickened folds especially in the posterior wall and marked gastric distortion with rigidity most marked in the antrum and distal body. The splenomegaly is probably from splenic vein thrombosis. *C:* Corresponding CT showing gross thickening of the wall of the antrum mimicking carcinoma or lymphoma.

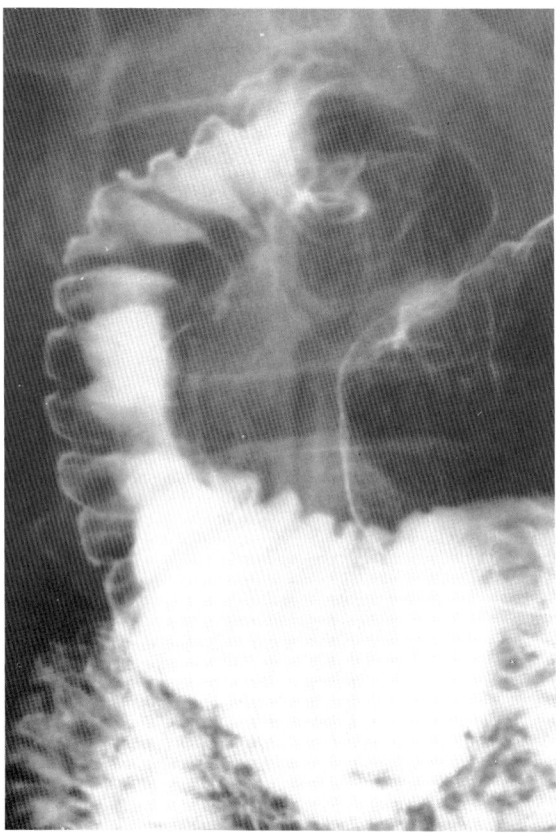

FIGURE 21.30. CHRONIC PANCREATITIS
Mass effect and padding along the medial border of the duodenal sweep with adjacent fold thickening from chronic alcoholic pancreatitis.

examinations but are seen in 64–80% using hypotonic techniques (1). The most common finding is extrinsic mass effect along the inner border of the descending duodenum (Fig. 21.30) (1). Smooth effacement of the folds in the same region may be seen (1). Occasionally spiculation of folds and enlargement of the papilla may occur (1). In severe cases, strictures may be produced causing obstruction (Fig. 21.24A). Depending on the findings, carcinoma of the pancreas and post-bulbar peptic disease are the usual differential diagnosis.

Small Bowel. Chronic pancreatitis patients with steatorrhea from exocrine pancreatic insufficiency generally have a normal small bowel series (1). In fact, a normal radiologic examination in the face of documented steatorrhea might suggest chronic pancreatitis (8). Occasionally, nonspecific small bowel abnormalities such as segmentation, flocculation, dilatation, and prolonged transit time can be seen in pancreatic exocrine insufficiency from chronic pancreatitis (1).

Colon. Most colonic abnormalities occur as complications of acute pancreatitis or pseudocysts. However, the colon may be affected in the same manner by acute exacerbations of chronic pancreatitis.

Skeletal. Approximately 5% of patients with established chronic pancreatitis will have medullary bone infarcts and/or aseptic necrosis of the femoral or humeral heads (1).

REFERENCES

1. Eaton SB, Ferrucci JT: *Radiology of the Pancreas and Duodenum.* Philadelphia, W. B. Saunders, 1973, pp 20–22, 24–47, 359–368.
2. Sarles H, Figarella C, Tiscornia O, Colomb E, Guy O, Venrine H, DeCaro A, Multigner L, Lechene P: Chronic calcifying pancreatitis, *Monogr Pathol* 21:48–66, 1980.
3. Robbins SL, Cotran SR: *Pathologic Basis of Disease.* Philadelphia, W. B. Saunders, 1979, pp 1096–1102.
4. Ring EJ, Eaton SB, Ferrucci JT, Short WF: Differential diagnosis of pancreatic calcification. *Radiology* 117:446–452, 1973.
5. Fried AM, Selke AC: Pseudocyst formation in hereditary pancreatitis. *J Pediatr* 93:950–953, 1978.
6. Mixter CG, Keynes WM, Cope O: Further experience with pancreatitis as a diagnostic clue to hyperparathyroidism. *N Engl J Med* 266:265–211, 1962.
7. Stobbe KC, ReMine WH, Bagestoss AH: Pancreatic lithiasis. *Surg Gynecol Obstet* 131:1090–1099, 1970.
8. Marshak RH, Lindner AE: Malabsorption syndrome. *Semin Roentgenol* 1:138–177, 1966.
9. Balthazar EJ: Effects of acute and chronic pancreatitis on the stomach. Patterns of radiographic involvement. *Am J Gastroenterol* 72:568–580, 1979.

Pancreatography

Indications

The diagnosis of chronic pancreatitis is usually suspected on clinical grounds alone. It may be confirmed by pancreatic secretory studies or the bentiromide test (1, 2). Further support may be obtained by the radiologic findings previously described. ERCP is needed in some cases to confirm the diagnosis, but more often is used to identify the extent of the disease or exclude an underlying biliary tract etiology, an underlying neoplasm, or a pseudocyst. It offers the precise anatomic display of the pancreatic ducts needed prior to surgical treatment of refractory disease (3). ERCP in one large series altered the clinical diagnosis in 54% with a surgical lesion found in 33% (4).

TABLE 21.1.
PANCREATITIS[a]

Morphology	Changes		
	Minimal	Moderate	Marked
PANCREAS			
Main Pancreatic Duct			
Rigidity	±	+	2+
Tortuosity	±	+	2+
Irregular caliber	2−	+	2+
Obstruction	2−	2−	+
Cyst formation	2−	2−	+
Calculi	2−	2−	+
Branch Ducts			
Rigidity	+	2+	2+
Irregular distribution	+	2+	2+
Dilatation	+	2+	3+
Irregular caliber	+	2+	3+
Cystic dilatation	2−	+	2+
Calculi	2−	2−	+
Parenchyma			
Coarse opacification	2−	2−	+
Size of Pancreas			
Diminished	2−	2−	+
BILIARY SYSTEM			
Lower Common Bile Duct			
Rigidity	2−	+	2+
Dilatation	2−	+	2+
Stenosis	2−	+	2+
Irregularity	2−	2−	+

[a] After Kasugai et al. (21).

Radiographic Findings

Many classifications of pancreatitis describing the appearance of the main pancreatic duct have been described. Kasugai and his colleagues combined the results of ERCPs with postmortem pancreatograms and microscopic examination in 245 cases of chronic pancreatitis (5). These ERCPs were divided into groups with minimal changes of chronic pancreatitis (156 cases), moderate chronic pancreatitis (67 cases), and advanced chronic pancreatitis (22 cases) (Fig. 21.31). Recent series have used this classification to describe ductal morphology in relation to pancreatic function (6–8). (Table 21.1). One study supported ERCP as a more sensitive diagnostic technique than pancreatic function testing in that normal secretory function was present in two patients with grossly abnormal pancreatograms (6).

In minimal chronic pancreatitis, the earliest radiographic finding is slight ectasia or clubbing of the side branches of the pancreatic duct (5, 9, 10). The junctions of the side branches with the main pancreatic duct can be minimally narrowed, and side branch filling may be impaired by protein precipitates (9). The main pancreatic duct is often normal, although minimal dilatation with some wall rigidity and irregularity may be present (5, 9, 10) (Fig. 21.32). No abnormalities are seen in the common bile duct.

Moderate chronic pancreatitis is characterized

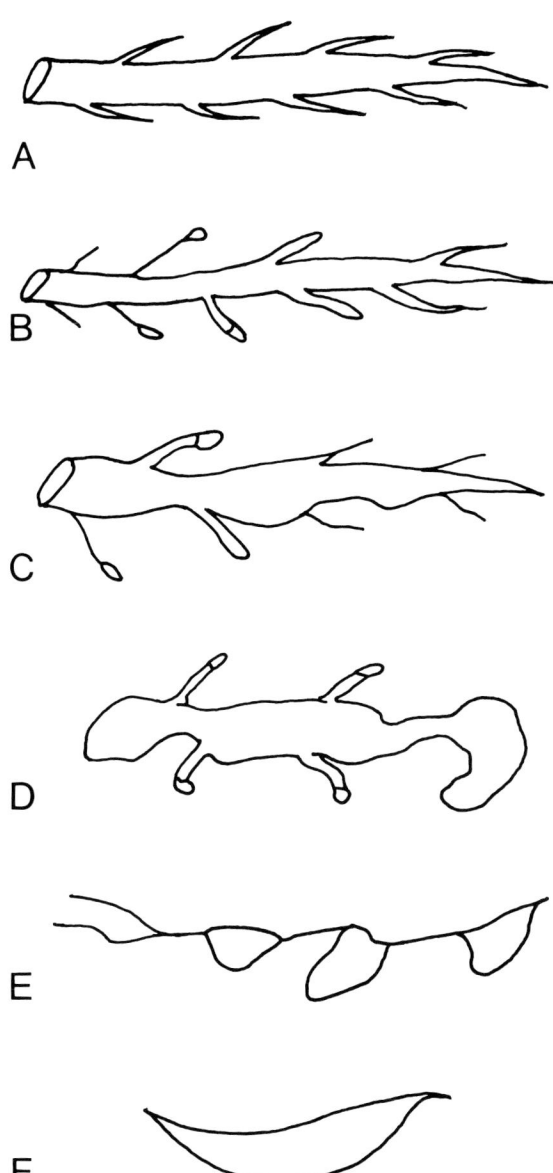

FIGURE 21.31. ARTIST'S VERSION OF PANCREATOGRAPHIC CLASSIFICATION OF CHRONIC PANCREATITIS

A: Normal. *B:* Minimal—ectasia of side branches. *C:* Moderate—dilatation and wall rigidity in main duct, side branch dilatation. *D:* Advanced—severe dilatation and some stenosis of main duct, very dilated side branches and diminished number of branches fill. *E:* Advanced—chain of lakes. *F:* Advanced—tapered, smooth duct obstruction.

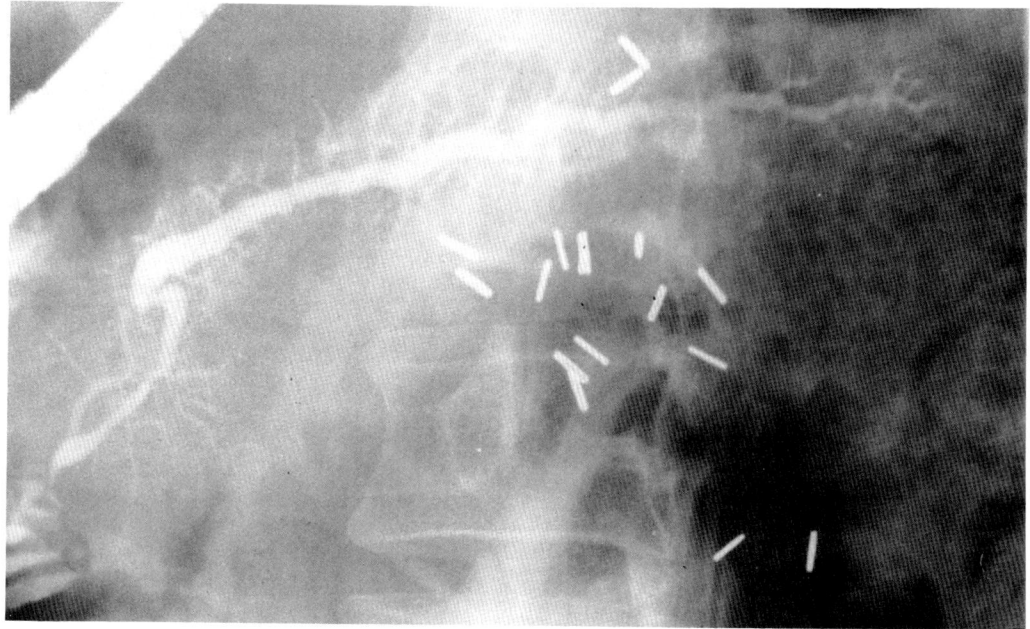

FIGURE 21.32. CHRONIC PANCREATITIS
Mild chronic pancreatitis: mild dilatation with some irregularity of the main pancreatic duct and mild ectasia of the side branches.

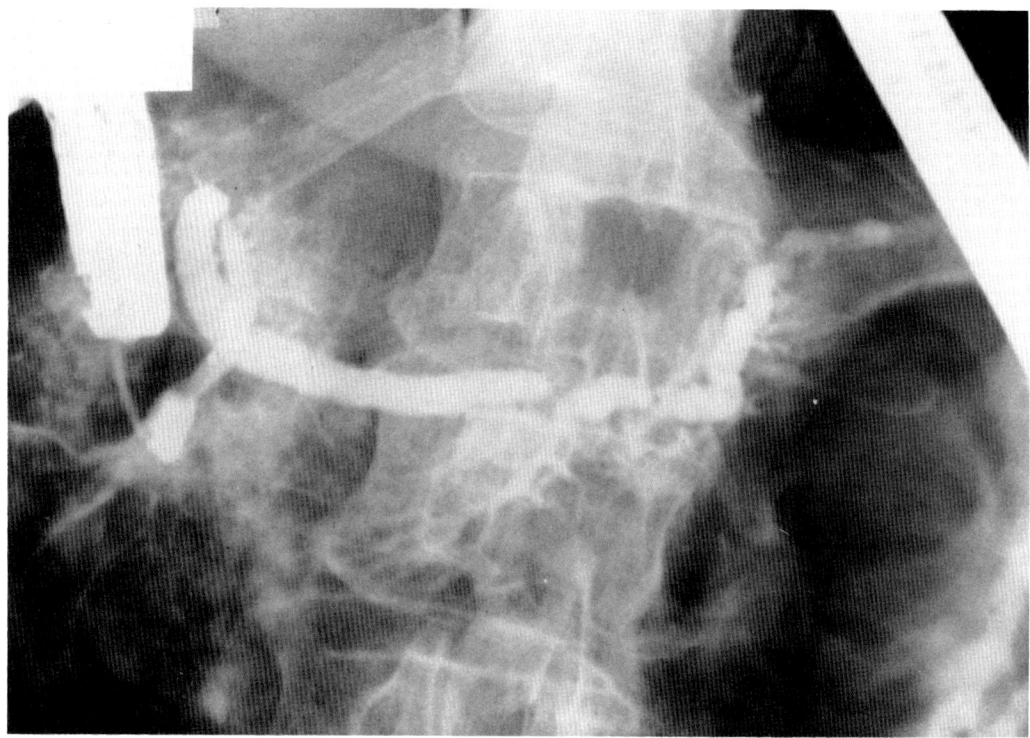

FIGURE 21.33. CHRONIC PANCREATITIS
Moderate chronic pancreatitis: multiple stenoses of the main pancreatic duct, dilated side branches in the proximal body and tail, and regions of absent branch opacification in the head and distal body. There is a coarse acinar pattern.

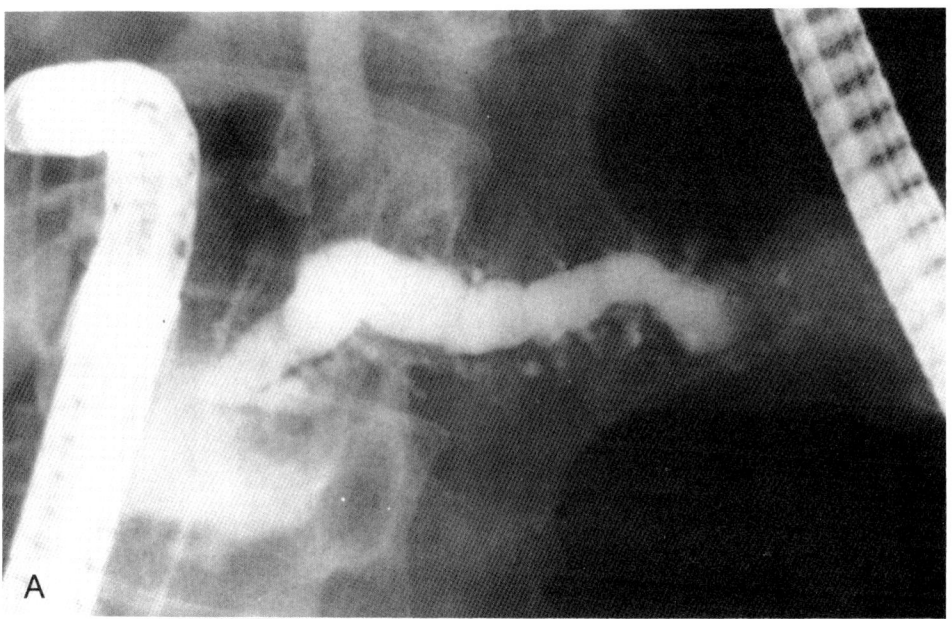

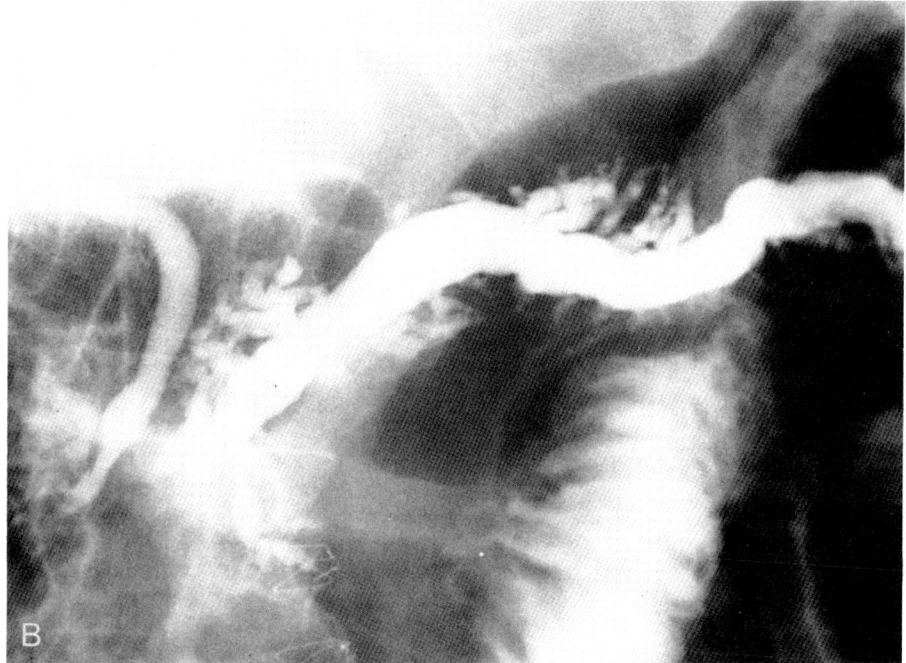

FIGURE 21.34. CHRONIC PANCREATITIS
Advanced chronic pancreatitis. *A:* Markedly dilated, slightly beaded main pancreatic duct. Side branches are dilated but narrowed at their junctions with the main duct. *B:* Markedly dilated main pancreatic duct, and the branches that fill are markedly dilated as well.

by dilatation, tortuosity, wall rigidity and region(s) of stenosis of the main pancreatic duct. Branch ducts show irregular distribution, cystic dilatation, partial stenosis or obstruction, and wall rigidity (5) (Fig. 21.33). A coarse, acinar pattern is an ancillary finding hard at times to differentiate from overfilling (9). The common bile duct may be mildly rigid with associated mild or moderate stenosis (5, 11, 12).

Usually the main duct dilatation is obvious, but when smooth and borderline it may be hard to diagnose especially in the elderly. Uniform tapering is maintained in the normal patient but lost in chronic pancreatitis. Main ductal dilata-

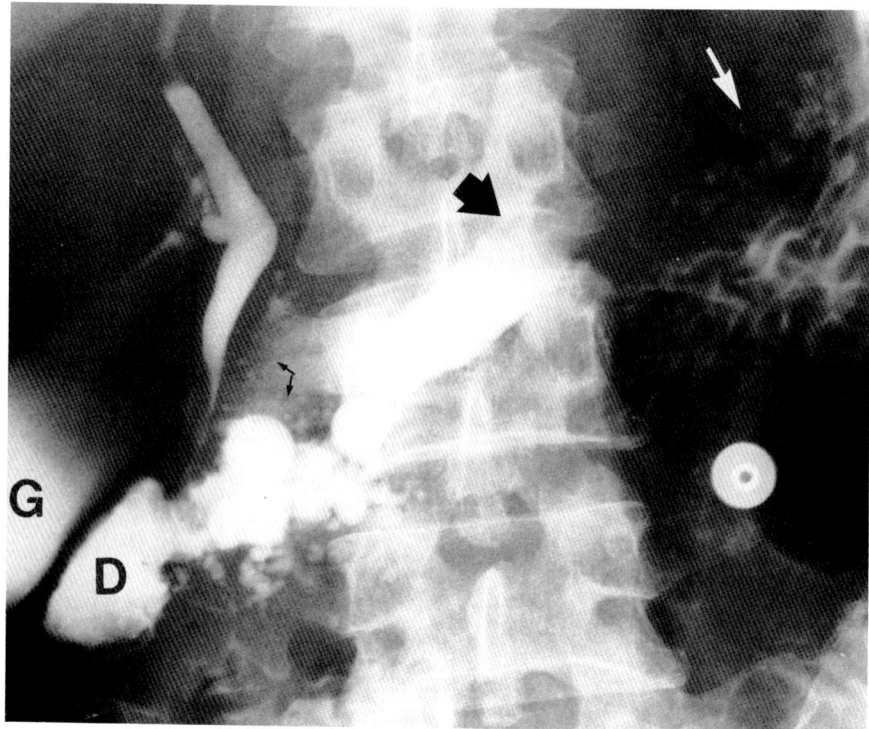

FIGURE 21.35. CHRONIC PANCREATITIS
Chain of lakes in the pancreatic head. Calculi are present in unpacified branches in the head (*small arrows*). The main duct appears obstructed (*large arrow*) but the fading margin indicates underfilling. Calculi are also present in the tail (*white arrow*). Note smoothly narrowed common duct. D = duodenum, G = gallbladder.

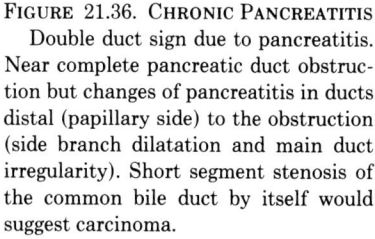

FIGURE 21.36. CHRONIC PANCREATITIS
Double duct sign due to pancreatitis. Near complete pancreatic duct obstruction but changes of pancreatitis in ducts distal (papillary side) to the obstruction (side branch dilatation and main duct irregularity). Short segment stenosis of the common bile duct by itself would suggest carcinoma.

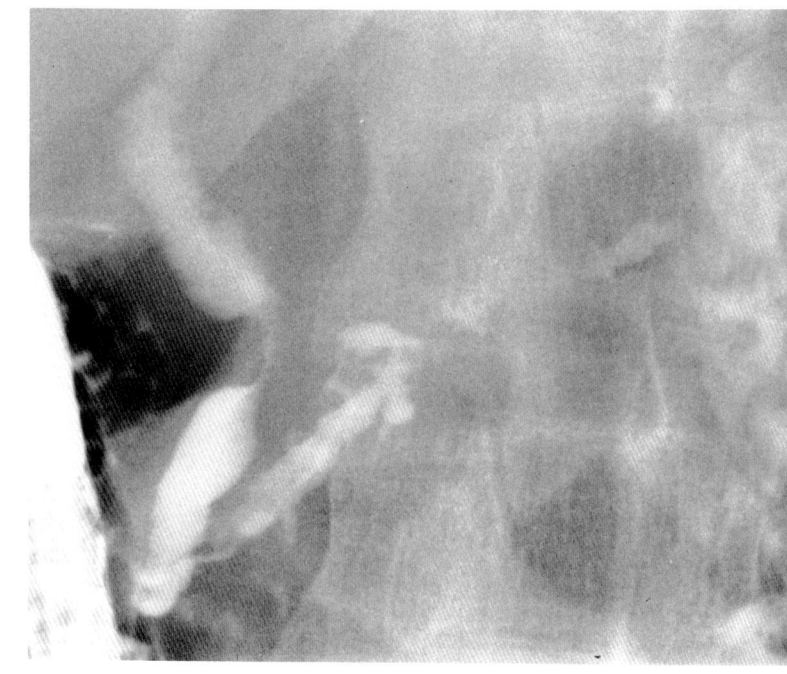

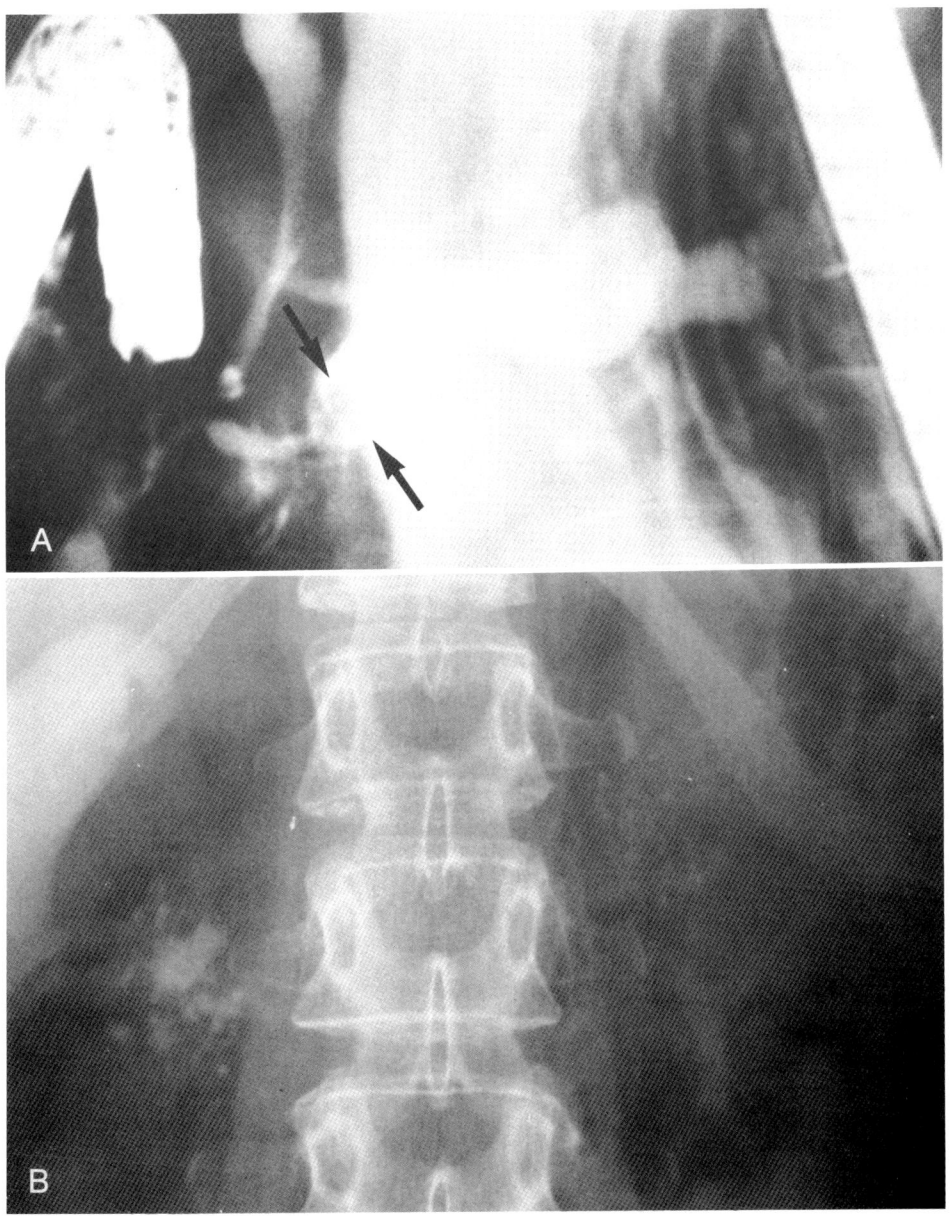

FIGURE 21.37. CHRONIC PANCREATITIS

A: Markedly dilated main pancreatic duct with filling defect (*arrows*) consistent with stone proximal to a high grade stenosis. Dilated side branches distal to stenosis suggest the correct diagnosis of chronic pancreatitis as well. Note smoothly narrowed common bile duct. *B:* Plain film shows the large calculus that was the filling defect and many additional calculi. Contrast in gallbladder from oral cholecystogram.

tion also has associated ectasia of side branches and sometimes calculi, and is never isolated (9).

Advanced chronic pancreatitis is diagnosed when both the main pancreatic duct and side branches are severely involved by dilatation, stenosis, and/or obstruction. The predominant sign is ectasia of the main duct, found in more than 50% of cases (13). The enlarged main duct may be smooth but is more often beaded (10) (Fig. 21.34A). In most instances the entire duct is involved but rarely, with proximal obstruction, the head and body are spared (10).

When advanced disease is not accompanied by obstruction, the main pancreatic duct is tortuous and receives scattered, deformed branches. Better filling than usual of the numerically diminished peripheral branches occurs presumably due to rigidity (10) (Fig. 21.34B). Parenchymal fibrosis prevents acinarization, unless there is overinjection (14). Emptying of the contrast material is prolonged, and can take as long as 26.5 min (15, 16). Stenosis of the main pancreatic duct is very common in advanced pancreatitis and is usually short segment. If longer than 1 cm, carcinoma is suggested (9). Multifocal stenoses and their associated dilatations give the characteristic chain of lakes or string of pearls appearance to the main pancreatic duct (Fig. 21.35). The periampullary main duct is a frequent site of stenosis in chronic pancreatitis (9). Complete obstruction of the main pancreatic duct is an uncommon finding in chronic pancreatitis. It can be due to fibrosis, calculi, abscess, or pseudocyst (14). Except in post-traumatic pancreatitis, the ducts distal to an obstruction in chronic pancreatitis show inflammatory changes (ectasia, beading, multifocal stenosis, marginal irregularity, calculi) (Fig. 21.36), whereas they are normal in obstruction due to carcinoma (9, 14). The configuration of the obstruction is smooth or round in pancreatitis and usually irregular or eccentric in carcinoma. Correlation with plain films, sonography and CT is important in identifying intraductal calculi, which may otherwise be obscured by the contrast injection (Fig. 21.37). Obstructing calculi generally cause a meniscus at the point of obstruction. Non-obstructing calculi are usually shown as filling defects (Fig. 21.37). Calculi seen on plain films may appear to be extraductal on pancreatography but are, in fact, located in unopacified terminal branches (Fig. 21.35) (5). Occasionally focal pancreatitis causes relatively short segment and focal ductal changes and differentiation from neoplasm can be quite difficult (Fig. 21.38) (14, 17).

Parenchymal fibrosis and shrinkage accompanies main pancreatic ductal dilatation. The intrapancreatic common bile duct may therefore be affected in advanced chronic pancreatitis with smooth, concentric narrowing seen in about 15% (Fig. 21.35) (11, 12, 18–21).

The above-described arbitrary grades of pancreatitis are most accurate in cases with the most severe anatomic changes in the main pancreatic duct (6, 7, 17, 22) (Table 21.1). Correlation between structural and functional abnormalities was good in 33% of patients with minimal chronic pancreatitis, 60% and 92.3% respectively in moderate and severe chronic pancreatitis (23–25). Early exocrine dysfunction is therefore not predictable based on radiographic changes of early chronic pancreatitis but severe functional derangement can be predicted from pancreatographic changes of advanced chronic pancreatitis (6, 25).

REFERENCES

1. Orlando RC: Secretin test. In Drossman DA (ed): *Manual of Gastroenterology Procedures*. New York, Raven Press, 1982, pp 65–69.
2. Toskes PP: Bentiromide as a test of exocrine pancreatic function in adult patients with pancreatic exocrine insufficiency. *Gastroenterology* 85:565, 1983.
3. Wong DH, Schuman DM, Grodsinsky C: The value of endoscopic retrograde cholangiopancreatography in the surgical management of chronic pancreatitis. *Am J Gastroenterol* 73:353–356, 1980.
4. Zimmon DS, Falkenstein DB, Abrams RM: Endoscopic retrograde cholangiopancreatography in the diagnosis of pancreatic inflammatory disease. *Radiology* 113:287–292, 1974.
5. Kasugai T: Pancreatitis. In Takemoto T and Kasugai T (eds): *Endoscopic Retrograde Cholangiopancreatography*. New York, Igaku-Shoin, 1979, pp 176–202.
6. Girdwood AH, Hatfield ARW, Bornman PC: Structure and function in non-calcific pancreatitis. *Dig Dis Sci* 29:721–726, 1984.
7. Braganza JM, Hunt JP, Warwick F: Relationship between pancreatic exocrine function and ductal morphology in chronic pancreatitis. *Gastroenterology* 82:1341–1347, 1982.
8. Stern I, Roberts-Thompson IC, Hansky J: Correlation between pancreatic polypeptide response to secretin and ERCP findings in chronic pancreatitis. *Gut* 23:235, 1982.
9. Short WF: Pancreatography. In Eaton SB, Ferrucci JT, Jr (eds): *Radiology of the Pancreas and Duodenum*. Philadelphia, W. B. Saunders, 1973, pp 261–275.
10. Freeny PC, Lawson TL: *Radiology of the Pancreas*. New York, Springer-Verlag, 1982, pp 205–212.
11. Wisloff F, Jacobsen J, Osnes M: Stenosis of the common bile duct in chronic pancreatitis. *Br J Surg* 69:52–54, 1982.
12. Gregg JA, Carr-Locke DL, Gallagher MM: Importance of common bile duct strictures associated with chronic pancreatitis: diagnosis by endoscopic retrograde cholangiopancreatography. *Am J Surg* 141:199, 1981.
13. Anacker H, Weiss HD, Kramann B: The ERPC in lesions of the pancreas and papilla duodeni. In *Endoscopic Retrograde Cholangiopancreatography (ERCP)*. New York, Springer-Verlag, 1977, pp 57–66.
14. Freeny PC, Ball TJ: Evaluation of endoscopic retrograde cholangiopancreatography and angiography in the diagnosis of pancreatic carcinoma. *AJR* 130:683–691, 1978.
15. Ralls PW, Halls J, Renner I, Juttner H: Endoscopic retrograde cholangiopancreatography (ERCP) and pancreatic disease. *Radiology* 134:347–352, 1980.
16. Okuda K, Someya N, Goto A et al: Endoscopic retrograde cholangiopancreatography. *AJR* 117:437, 1973.
17. Salmon PR: Re-evaluation of ERCP as a diagnostic method. *Clin Gastroenterol* 7:651, 1978.
18. Cotton PB: Progress report: ERCP. *Gut* 18:316, 1977.
19. Warshaw AL, Schapiro RH, Ferucci JT, Galdabin JJ: Persistent obstructive jaundice, cholangitis, and biliary cirrhosis due to common bile duct stenosis in chronic pancreatitis. *Gastroenterology* 70:562–567, 1976.
20. Snape WJ, Long WB, Trotman BW: Marked alkaline phosphatase elevation with partial common bile duct obstruction due to calcific pancreatitis. *Gastroenterology* 70:70–73, 1976.
21. Kasugai T, Kino N, Kizu M: Endoscopic pancreatography. II. The pathological endoscopic pancreatocholangiogram. *Gastroenterology* 63:227–234, 1972.
22. DeMagno FP, Malagelada JR, Go VLW: Relationships between pancreatic ductal obstruction and pancreatic secretion in man. *Mayo Clin Proc* 54:157, 1979.

23. Dreiling DA, Janowitz HD: The measurement of pancreatic secretory function. In *CIBA Foundation Symposium on the Exocrine Pancreas*. London, Churchill, 1962, p 225.
24. Gooddale RL, Condie RM, Gajl-Pezalskak et al: Clinical and secretory differences in pancreatic cancer and chronic pancreatitis. *Ann Surg* 194:193–198, 1981.
25. Nagata A, Homma T, Tamai K et al: A study of chronic pancreatitis by serial endoscopic pancreatography. *Gastroenterology* 81:884, 1981.

Cholangiography

Patients with chronic pancreatitis may have transient and recurring mild bouts of jaundice due to common bile duct involvement. The etiology is probably underlying fibrosis and superimposed edema during exacerbations (1). The typical cholangiographic findings are smooth, undulating, long segment, tapered narrowing of the distal common bile duct with possibly some proximal dilatation but almost never complete obstruction (Figs. 21.35, 21.37, 21.39) (1–4). Short segment, smooth, hourglass-shaped narrowing can occur, but is less common (Fig. 21.36). Additional findings that may be present are compression of the distal common bile duct and either medial or lateral displacement, or an angulation at the junction of the middle and distal thirds of the common bile duct (3).

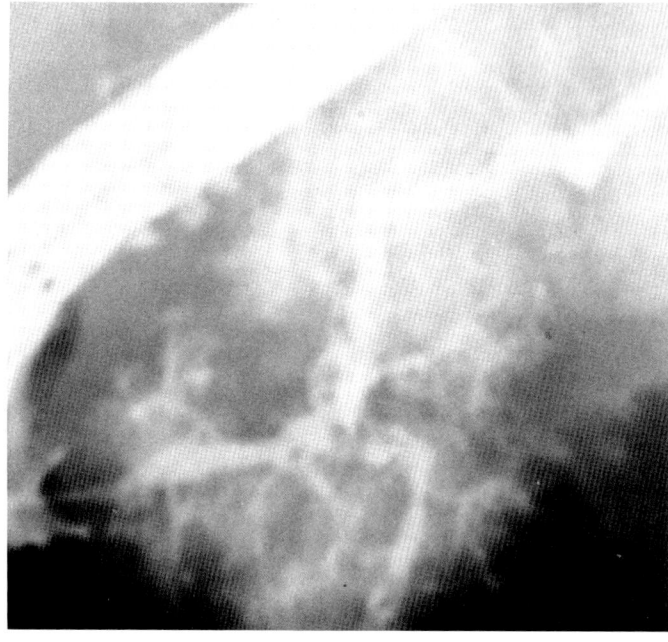

FIGURE 21.38. CHRONIC PANCREATITIS
Field defect (focal lack of acinarization and branch filling, arrows) due to chronic pancreatitis. Correct diagnosis is suggested by irregularities in the main duct and side branches. Field defects are also seen in neoplasms.

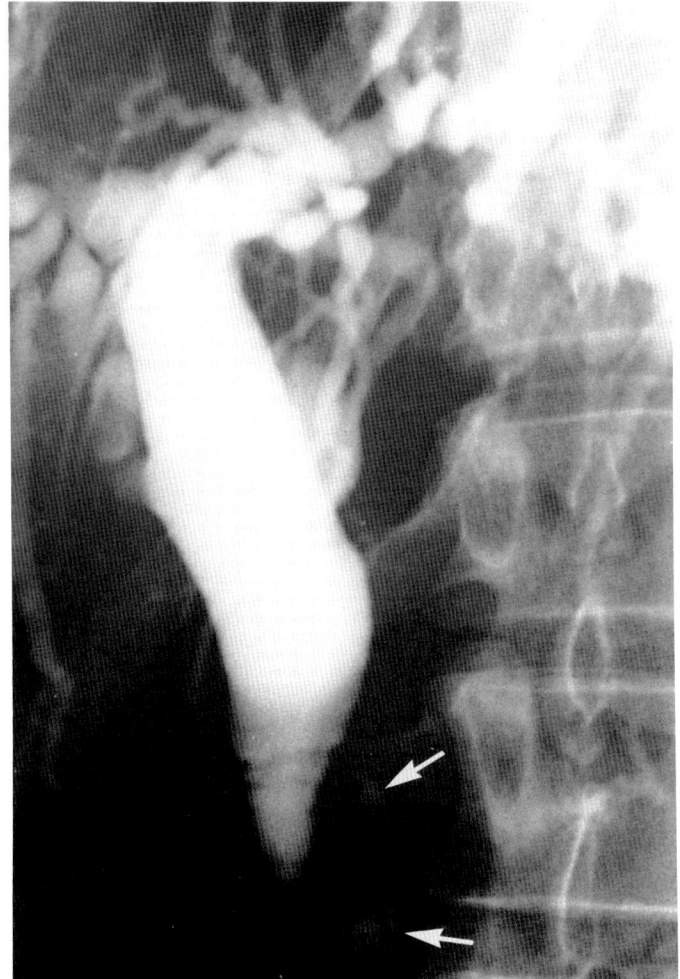

FIGURE 21.39. CHRONIC PANCREATITIS
Transhepatic cholangiogram-tapered obstruction of intrapancreatic common bile duct. Adjacent calcifications (*arrows*) enable the correct diagnosis of chronic pancreatitis.

REFERENCES

1. Wisloff F, Jakobsen J, Osnes M: Stenosis of the common bile duct in chronic pancreatitis. *Br J Surg* 69:52–54, 1982.
2. Ferrucci JT Jr, Mueller PR, vanSonnenberg E: Transhepatic cholangiography. In Berk RN, Ferrucci JT Jr, Leopold GR (eds): *Radiology of the Gallbladder and Bile Ducts, Intervention and Diagnosis.* Philadelphia, W. B. Saunders, 1983, p 357.
3. Eaton SB Jr, Ferrucci JT Jr: *Radiology of the Pancreas and Duodenum.* Philadelphia, W. B. Saunders, 1973, pp 358–359.
4. Lang EK: Percutaneous transhepatic cholangiography. *Radiology* 112:283–290, 1974.

Sonography

Due to the presence of fibrosis within the gland, there is sonographic evidence of increased parenchymal echoes which may be inhomogeneous (62%) (1). The inhomogeneous echo pattern of the pancreas is most marked when calcifications are present (Fig. 21.40). These calcifications are in the ductal system and their distribution may be focal or diffuse and if large enough are associated with acoustical shadowing (2). In the absence of calcifications, the subtle change of the echo pattern of the pancreatic parenchyma can be missed (3, 4). This usually occurs when the gland is not enlarged or has atrophied and has been reported in up to 50% of patients with chronic pancreatitis (4, 5). In such instances, the size and outline of the gland can be difficult to determine as its echogenicity blends with that of the retroperitoneal fat (6). Be that as it may, Lees in one report detected 91% of patients with chronic pancreatitis based upon the echo texture of the gland (7).

The gland is usually irregular in outline (45–60%) and there may be focal (12%) or diffuse enlargement (27–45%) (1, 7). Pancreatic ductal dilatation may be present (41–67%); however, the duct may be difficult to see due to distortion of the gland by a pseudocyst or by pancreatic calcifications (Fig. 21.40) (7–9). Ductal dilatation may not only occur due to obstructing stones but may also be due to a stricture. Stones in a dilated pancreatic duct are more easily identified sonographically than with CT. This is best done in the area of the body of the pancreas as the duct is more difficult to identify in the head and tail of the pancreas. A percutaneous pancreatic ductogram can be performed on a dilated duct using ultrasound guidance if an ERCP fails. Percutaneous drainage of the pancreatic duct has been reported in the treatment of acute or chronic pancreatitis in surgically high risk patients (10–12). Ductal dilatation can be so marked that it can simulate a number of small pancreatic pseudocysts (Fig. 21.41) (13). True pseudocysts are present in approximately 20% of patients with chronic pancreatitis and unlike those associated with acute pancreatitis, these pseudocysts tend not to resolve spontaneously (14).

Patients with chronic pancreatitis can have all the symptoms and signs of pancreatic carcinoma (upper abdominal pain radiating to the back associated with weight loss). If a noncalcified focal mass is found in the pancreas of such a patient, then pancreatic carcinoma has to be

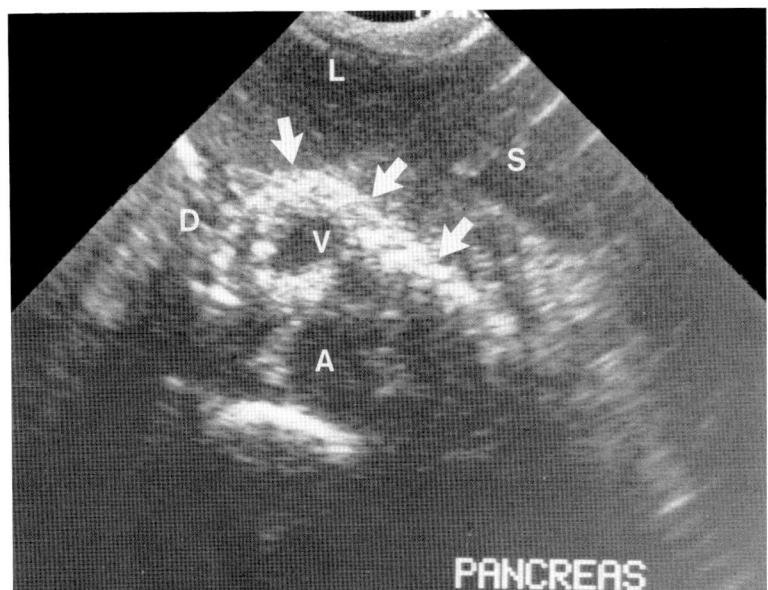

FIGURE 21.40. CHRONIC CALCIFIC PANCREATITIS
Transverse sonogram of the pancreas reveals that it is densely echogenic (*arrows*) due to multiple small calcifications. Aorta (*A*), portal vein, splenic vein confluence (*B*), liver (*L*), stomach (*S*), and duodenum (*D*).

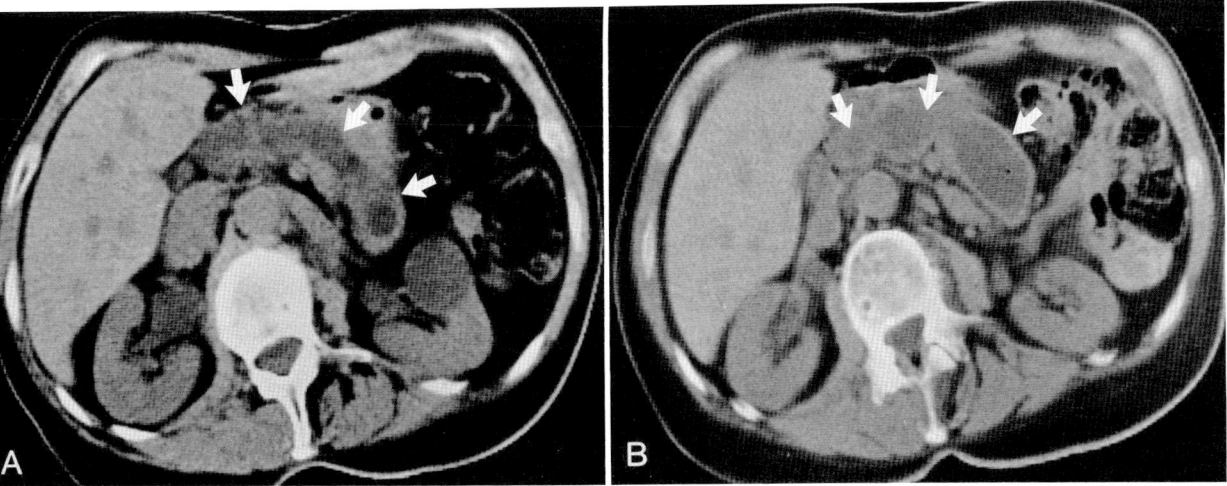

FIGURE 21.41. CHRONIC PANCREATITIS
A and *B*: CT scans of the pancreas show a markedly dilated beaded pancreatic duct (*arrows*).

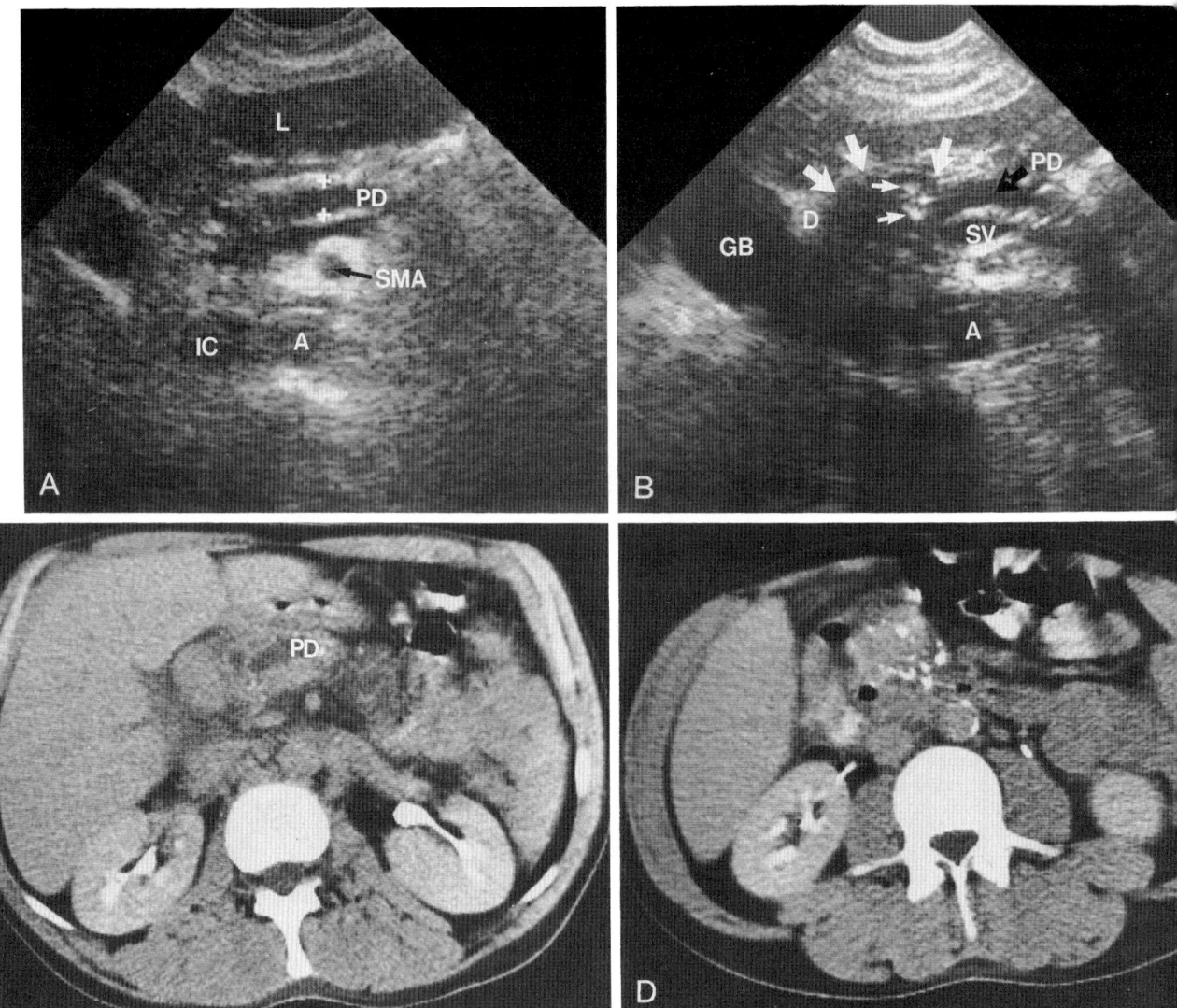

FIGURE 21.42. CHRONIC CALCIFIC PANCREATITIS
Chronic calcific pancreatitis with focal mass in the head. A and B: Transverse sonography reveals a mass (*large arrows*) in the head of the pancreas with foci of high level echoes (*small arrows*) corresponding to calcifications and a dilated pancreatic duct (*PD*). C and D: Corresponding CT: calcifications within the focal mass and dilated pancreatic duct. A = aorta, IC = inferior vena cava, SMA = superior mesenteric artery, SV = splenic vein, L = liver, D = duodenum, and GB = gallbladder.

considered. This diagnosis can be confirmed if adjacent lymphadenopathy is present or liver metastases are found. The presence of the characteristic dense calcifications of chronic pancreatitis within a mass makes it unlikely that it represents a pancreatic cancer (Fig. 21.42). If a diagnostic dilemma exists, then a percutaneous needle aspiration should be considered (15).

Chronic pancreatitis with or without a coexistent carcinoma can be associated with thrombosis of the portal venous system. This usually involves the splenic vein; however, extension to involve the main portal vein can also occur. Echogenic thrombus may be identified within the involved portion of the vein and collateral channels may develop to shunt blood around the area of obstruction. In some instances, the obstructed vein cannot be sonographically identified.

Computed Tomography

The gland in chronic pancreatitis can be normal in size or enlarged or it may be small,

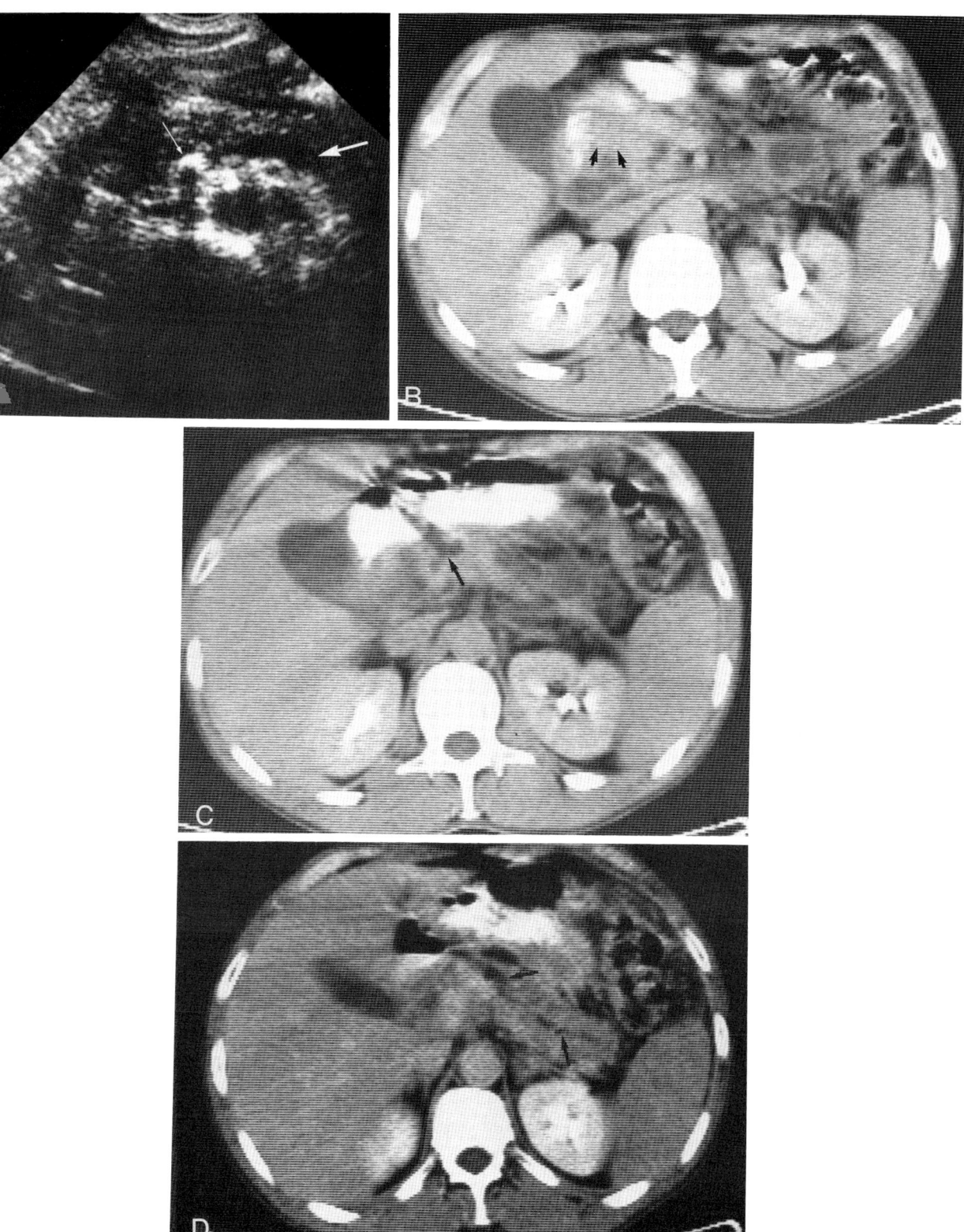

FIGURE 21.43. CHRONIC PANCREATITIS
Patient referred for treatment of "surgically proven malignant desmoid of the pancreas." Review of pathology showed only chronic pancreatitis. *A:* Transverse sonogram nicely shows shadowing calculus (*small arrow*) obstructing the dilated pancreatic duct (*large arrow*). *B–D:* CT from left renal vein cephalad: enlarged head of pancreas with subtle calcifications (*small arrows*), dilated pancreatic duct (*large arrows*), and extensive peripancreatic inflammatory changes. Note relative sparing of the fat around the superior mesenteric artery.

atrophic and replaced by fat (16). When the gland is enlarged, this enlargement may be focal or diffuse (Figs. 21.42 and 21.43). Focal enlargement due to chronic pancreatitis is hard to distinguish on CT grounds alone from carcinoma unless punctate calcifications are present as these are almost never found in carcinoma (except sometimes following chemotherapy) (Figs. 21.42 and 21.43) (17, 18). The incidence of pancreatic carcinoma is low (except for familial pancreatitis) in patients with chronic pancreatitis (16, 17, 19). The calcifications present in chronic pancreatitis (36%) are easily seen on CT and are usually multiple. They may occur in only one part of the gland or may be present throughout. One should not confuse a tortuous calcified splenic artery as pancreatic calcifications and, if any doubt exists, this should be resolved with a bolus injection of intravenous iodinated contrast.

Pancreatic ductal dilatation (greater than 3 mm) is often present (58%) especially when a focal mass with calcification involves the head (Figs. 21.42 and 21.43) (16, 20, 21). The ductal dilatation may be irregular (73%), smooth (15%), or beaded (12%) (21). Associated dilatation of the common bile duct may be present. If pancreatic ductal dilatation is present in the absence of a mass, then a small obstructing carcinoma has to be considered. In such cases, one should look for upper abdominal lymphadenopathy and liver metastases. On occasion, all that is found in chronic pancreatitis is a markedly dilated beaded pancreatic duct which can simulate a number of small intrapancreatic pseudocysts (Fig. 21.41). The incidence of true pseudocyst is more common in chronic (20%) than in acute (10%) pancreatitis and, in the former, the pseudocyst may not be contiguous to the pancreas. Pseudocysts have been previously described under the CT of acute pancreatitis portion of this chapter. Chronic pancreatitis can lead to duodenal stenosis (22).

There may be associated portal venous system thrombosis with chronic pancreatitis. The thrombosis usually involves the splenic vein and may spread to involve the main portal vein and adjacent superior mesenteric vein. The presence of thrombus can be inferred when the normal vein fails to opacify following the use of intravenous iodinated contrast along with the presence of collateral channels. In obstruction of the splenic vein, there may be associated splenomegaly (40%) and collaterals develop via the short gastrics which anastomose with the tributaries of the coronary vein in the fundus of the stomach and via the left gastroepiploic vein which anastomoses with its fellow from the right side and drains into the superior mesenteric vein. If there is complete obstruction of the main portal vein, numerous periportal collaterals develop (cavernous transformation) and similar collaterals develop around the duodenum when there is obstruction of the superior mesenteric vein.

It should be remembered that the diagnosis of chronic pancreatitis can often be made on plain radiographs of the abdomen due to the presence of pancreatic calcifications. This would obviate the need for a sonogram or a CT scan unless some complication of chronic pancreatitis was suspected, i.e., pseudocyst, obstruction of the common bile duct. CT is, however, more sensitive in diagnosing chronic pancreatitis than sonography (3). As a final point, it should be said that in this age of cost containment, CT has been shown to reduce the need for more invasive and expensive studies such as ERCP and angiography (23).

REFERENCES

1. Cotton PB, Lees WR, Vallon AG, Cottone M, Croker JR, Chapman M: Gray-scale ultrasonography and endoscopic pancreatography in pancreatic diagnosis. *Radiology* 134:453–459, 1980.
2. Isikoff MB, Hill MC: Ultrasonic demonstration of intraductal pancreatic calculi: a report of two cases. *J Clin Ultrasound* 8:449–452, 1980.
3. Foley WD, Stewart ET, Lawson TL, Geenan J, Loguidice J, Mather L, Unger GF: Computed tomography, ultrasonography, and endoscopic retrograde cholangiopancreatography in the diagnosis of pancreatic disease: A comparative study. *Gastrointest Radiol* 5:29–35, 1980.
4. Lawson TL: Sensitivity of pancreatic ultrasonography in the detection of pancreatic disease. *Radiology* 128:733–736, 1978.
5. Patel S, Bellon EM, Haaga J, Park CH: Fat replacement of the exocrine pancreas. *AJR* 135:843–845, 1980.
6. Shawker TH, Linzer M, Hubbard VS: Chronic pancreatitis: the diagnostic significance of pancreatic size and echo amplitude. *J Ultrasound Med* 3:267–272, 1984.
7. Lees WR, Vallon AG, Denyer ME, Vahl SP, Cotton PB: Prospective study of ultrasonography in chronic pancreatic disease. *Br Med J* 1:162–164, 1979.
8. Lawson TL, Berland LL, Foley WD, Stewart ET, Geenan JE, Hogan WJ: Ultrasonic visualization of the pancreatic duct. *Radiology* 144:865–871, 1982.
9. Weinstein DP, Weinstein BJ: Ultrasonic demonstration of the pancreatic duct: an analysis of 41 cases. *Radiology* 130:729–734, 1979.
10. Ohto M, Saotome N, Saisho H, Tsuchiya Y, Ono T, Okuda K, Karasawa E: Real-time sonography of the pancreatic duct: application to percutaneous pancreatic ductography. *AJR* 134:647–652, 1980.
11. Matter D, Spinelli G, Warter P: Ultrasonically guided percutaneous pancreatography. *J Clin Ultrasound* 11:401–404, 1983.
12. Gobien RP, Stanley JH, Anderson MC, Vujic I: Percutaneous drainage of pancreatic duct for treating acute pancreatitis. *AJR* 141:795–796, 1983.

13. Kuligowska E, Miller K, Birkett D, Burakoff R: Cystic dilatation of the pancreatic duct simulating pseudocysts on sonography. *AJR* 136:409–410, 1981.
14. Aranha GV, Prinz RA, Esguerra AC, Greenlee HB: The nature and course of cystic pancreatic lesions diagnosed by ultrasound. *Arch Surg* 118:486–488, 1983.
15. Pelaez, JC, Hill MC, Dach JL, Isikoff MB, Morse B: Abdominal aspiration biopsies: sonographic vs. computed tomography guidance. *JAMA* 250:2663–2666, 1983.
16. Ferrucci JT, Wittenberg J, Black EB, Kirkpatrick RH, Hall DA: Computed body tomography in chronic pancreatitis. *Radiology* 130:175–182, 1979.
17. Paulino-Netto A, Dreiling DA, Baronofsky ID: The relationship between pancreatic calcification and cancer of the pancreas. *Ann Surg* 151:530–537, 1960.
18. Dastur KJ, Lewin JR: Computed tomography demonstration of tumor calcification after chemotherapy in a case of pancreatic carcinoma. *Comput Tomogr* 5:351–354, 1981.
19. Robinson A, Scott J, Rosenfeld DD: The occurence of carcinoma of the pancreas in chronic pancreatitis. *Radiology* 94:289–290, 1970.
20. Fishman A, Isikoff MB, Barkin JS, Friedland JT: Significance of a dilated pancreatic duct on CT examination. *AJR* 133:225–227, 1979.
21. Karasawa E, Goldberg HI, Moss AA, Federle MP, London SS: CT pancreatogram in carcinoma of the pancreas and chronic pancreatitis. *Radiology* 148:489–493, 1983.
22. Makrauer FL, Antonioli DA, Banks PA: Duodenal stenosis in chronic pancreatitis. Clinicopathological correlations. *Dig Dis Sci* 27:525–532, 1981.
23. Freeny PC, Marks WM, Ball TJ: Impact of high-resolution computed tomography of the pancreas on utilization of endoscopic retrograde cholangiopancreatography and angiography. *Radiology* 142:35–39, 1982.

Angiography

With the advent of ultrasound and CT, angiography is no longer a primary diagnostic modality for evaluating pancreatitis, and is no longer indicated to detect a suspected pseudocyst. The potential exists, however, for possibly lethal sequelae such as pseudoaneurysms and splenic vein obstruction to go undiscovered if non-invasive modalities are relied upon exclusively (1). If operative intervention becomes necessary because of fulminating course and/or hemorrhage, surgery is especially hazardous since normal tissue planes frequently become obliterated due to severe inflammatory changes (2). The risk of severe operative and perioperative bleeding is high, especially without the benefit of preoperative angiography (3, 4). In isolated cases, pancreatic angiography may be helpful regarding differential diagnosis. Far more important, however, is its role in preoperative planning.

Arteriographic changes associated with pancreatitis depend upon the clinical course of the disease. Comparison between different series is difficult, since only those patients suspected of having complications are studied and the index of suspicion regarding complications varies according to the institution, referring physician and radiologist.

Acute Pancreatitis

In uncomplicated acute pancreatitis, pancreatic angiography may be entirely normal (3, 5), or mild stretching and displacement may be seen indicative of diffuse glandular enlargement by edema (3, 6). Hypervascularity and increased parenchymal stain is common (3, 6–8). Rarely, markedly increased vascularity with arteriovenous shunting may be seen (3, 9). While arterial caliber and contour are typically normal (3), some series report arterial stenosis in more than half (6). Much of this arterial narrowing may be due to superimposed chronic pancreatitis or atherosclerosis. Venous compression secondary to edema may also be seen during the acute phase (3). If recovery is uneventful, arteriographic changes usually revert to normal (3). Acute, hemorrhagic pancreatitis may show an irregular, mottled parenchymal phase and result in focal fibrosis and permanent intrapancreatic or peripancreatic arterial or venous abnormalities (3). (Aneurysms in acute pancreatitis are discussed later under the heading "Aneurysms.")

Chronic Pancreatitis

Arterial Changes. The arteriogram may be normal or indistinguishable from carcinoma (Fig. 21.44) (and see Figs. 22.74 and 22.75). The most common arteriographic finding in some series is increased tortuosity and angulation of pancreatic arcades and intrapancreatic arteries, seen in as many as 88% of cases (6, 10). Tortuosity and angulation without associated narrowing are indicative of pancreatitis, rather than carcinoma (8). Luminal irregularities are seen in between 25 and 75% of cases (5, 6, 9, 11, 12). Nearly half of these consist of a nonspecific "sleeve-like" mild narrowing and straightening of large extrapancreatic arteries unassociated with occlusions or abrupt change in course (5, 10, 12, 13). This finding is indistinguishable from atherosclerosis, and may represent superimposed atherosclerosis (5). Sleeve-like narrowing is thus not a useful diagnostic feature. Atherosclerosis involves primarily large and medium size arteries, while pancreatitis will exhibit prominent involvement of small intrapancreatic arteries.

More specific is a smooth, beaded appearance consisting of alternating areas of dilatation and constriction not unlike fibromuscular dysplasia

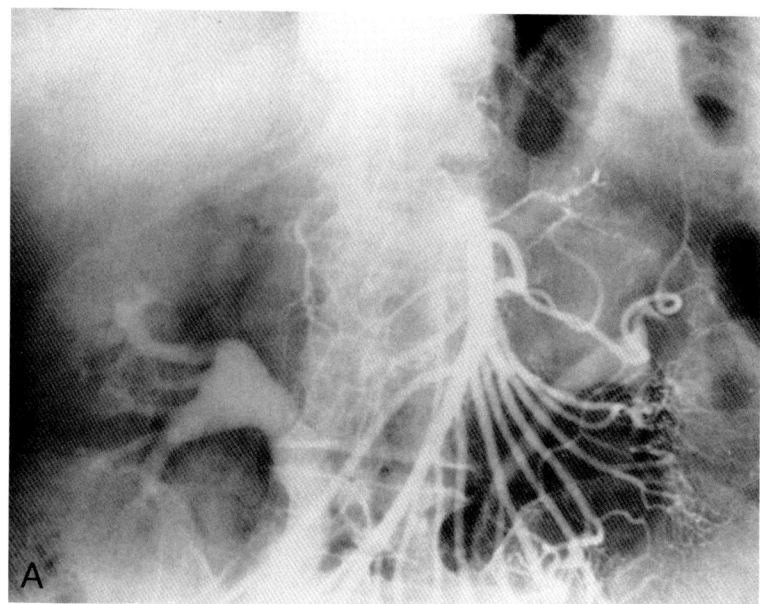
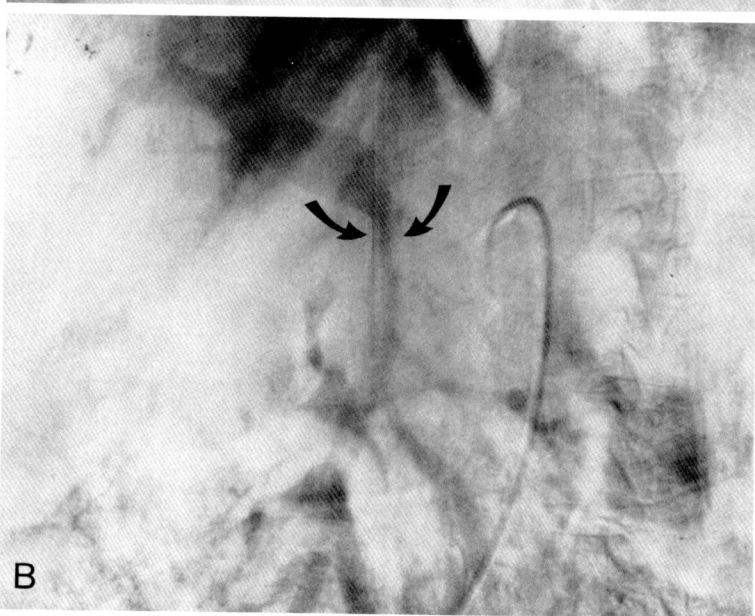

FIGURE 21.44. CHRONIC PANCREATITIS INDISTINGUISHABLE FROM CARCINOMA
Superior mesenteric arteriogram. *A:* Normal arterial phase. *B:* Smooth encasement of the superior mesenteric vein (*arrows*).

(5, 10, 13). Diagnostic criteria may differ, however, and there are reports of arterial beading occuring almost as often in carcinoma (12). Histological specimens reveal medial hypertrophy associated with luminal irregularities, with thickened hyalinized walls and subintimal fibrosis present in advanced cases (14). Arterial irregularities may be most severe in those with chronic calcific pancreatitis (Fig. 21.45). Proximal stenosis of the celiac axis and superior mesenteric artery in association with pancreatitis have been reported, but these appear to represent catheter-induced spasm, which may, in fact, be more frequent in patients with pancreatitis (6, 13). These "stenoses" may be accentuated by the use of vasoconstrictors (6). Actual occlusions of arteries are unusual, present far more often in carcinoma (12). Occasionally, severe scarring of retroperitoneal tissues may cause marked displacement of the pancreas, shifting with the gastroduodenal artery and pancreatic arcades to the left (6).

Venous Changes. Venous compression or occlusion, while not as common as in carcinoma, is present in between 20 and 50% of patients with pancreatitis studied by arteriography (6, 8,

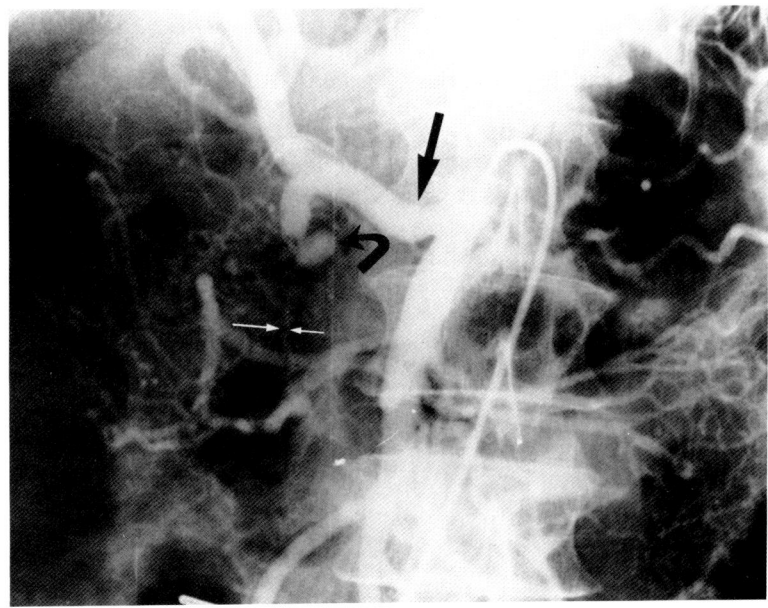

FIGURE 21.45. CHRONIC PANCREATITIS
Encasement of the gastroduodenal artery (*small arrows*) and pseudoaneurysm (*curved arrow*) caused by chronic pancreatitis. Superior mesenteric arteriogram with replaced right hepatic artery (*large arrow*).

9, 12). Most common is splenic vein occlusion or narrowing, which comprised approximately half of vascular complications noted in one series (see Fig. 22.74) (15). Splenic vein occlusion may occur in acute pancreatitis, but is more common with chronic disease (5, 6). The vein may be narrowed due to compression by edema or pseudocysts, or may thrombose. Involvement of the superior mesenteric or portal veins (Fig. 21.44B) (6, 15), is less common and unlikely unless the patient has been ill for several years. A splenic vein which appears occluded radiographically may in fact, however, be patent if the abnormality is caused by kinking or compression (16).

Isolated obstruction of the splenic vein leads to enlargement of collateral vessels and portoportal shunting. Typically, gastroepiploic and short gastric varices develop, draining blood into the portal vein via the coronary vein. Esophageal varices are usually not present unless portal hypertension from cirrhosis is also present since a portosystemic shunt is not needed to decompress the portal system (2, 17). The presence of gastric varices without esophageal varices is thought to be specific for splenic vein occlusion (17). The etiology of splenic vein occlusion is almost always pancreatic, whether from inflammatory or neoplastic disease (17). If normal collateral pathways have been disrupted, such as by prior gastric surgery, colonic varices may develop as a consequence of shunting to the inferior mesenteric system (18). Bleeding from varices, as well as from pseudoaneurysms, is a significant cause of morbidity and mortality associated with pancreatitis (16, 17, 19). Splenic vein obstruction is especially common in patients with pseudocysts (15, 17). The majority of these patients will not have palpable splenomegaly (17).

Parenchymal Changes. Hypervascularity may be seen in any phase of pancreatitis, providing there is active inflammation present. Between 12 and 45% have areas of hypervascularity, depending upon patient population (5, 6, 8, 11, 12). Hypovascular areas are also seen frequently, from 15 to 56% (6, 11). An irregular parenchymal phase may be seen in approximately 25% of cases, usually in patients with chronic pancreatitis of longer than 2 yr duration (5), and should be interpreted as evidence of chronic pancreatitis. Acute hemorrhagic pancreatitis may also, however, show an irregular, mottled parenchymal phase (3). Chronic calcific pancreatitis in particular is characterized by irregularly decreased vascularity, with regions of fibrosis and/or calcification being seen as paucity of vessels and decreased blush (5, 11).

Aneurysms. An uncommon but important arterial finding associated with pancreatitis is aneurysm formation. Although the majority of patients with pancreatitis do not develop this complication, of those with disease severe enough to warrant arteriography, approximately 10% have aneurysms (6, 13, 15, 20, 21). This proportion may, in fact, increase with the decreasing utilization of arteriography for detecting pseudocysts. Aneurysms are extremely uncommon but do occur in pancreatitis patients without either abscess or pseudocyst (4, 22).

Since aneurysms do not occur with pancreatic cancer, when present they are an important differential feature (10, 21) although atherosclerotic aneurysms are found in from 0.16 to 1% of autopsies (23, 24) and could be an incidental finding in a patient with pancreatic carcinoma. Aneurysms may be present in either acute or chronic disease, and appear unrelated to the duration of disease (6), although they do enlarge with time (4, 13, 23). Aneurysms appear uncommon in patients with calcific pancreatitis, even those with pronounced vascular changes. These patients are also less likely to have abscesses since these patients have a less necrotic inflammatory process (6).

The pathogenesis of these aneurysms is poorly understood. There are probably two basic types of aneurysms associated with pancreatitis, although they cannot be differentiated. If the inflammatory process causes partial digestion of the artery wall with loss of elastic tissue, focal dilatation may ensue with development of a true aneurysm (21). "False" aneurysms are thought to result from incorporation of an artery within the wall of an enlarging pseudocyst (Fig. 21.46). With digestion of the artery wall, the vessel ruptures into the pseudocyst converting it into a pseudoaneurysm (4, 10, 23). Alternatively, these pseudoaneurysms may be created as hemorrhage is contained by surrounding inflammatory reaction (2). The distinction between these types of aneurysms is probably not clinically important, since the risk of bleeding and mortality from any aneurysms associated with pancreatitis is high.

The most frequent artery affected by pseudoaneurysm formation in pancreatitis is the splenic artery, which is also the visceral artery most likely to have atherosclerotic aneurysms. Approximately half of pseudoaneurysms will involve the splenic artery (4, 6, 21, 25–28). Next in frequency are gastroduodenal (Fig. 21.45) and pancreaticoduodenal artery aneurysms, the latter even more uncommon (4, 6, 25–27). Any other vessel in proximity to the pancreas may rarely be affected (26, 27).

Gastrointestinal Bleeding and Other Vascular Complications of Pancreatitis. Although vascular complications such as varices and pseudoaneurysms affect only a minority of patients, they are a major cause of mortality in these patients (2, 16, 17, 19, 25). In one series of 14 patients studied preoperatively, 3 had pseudoaneurysms and 6 had splenic or portal vein occlusion (15). The incidence of gastrointestinal bleeding among patients with pancreatitis is low, approximately 2% (27). Among patients with pseudocysts or abscess, the incidence of spontaneous gastrointestinal bleeding is considerably higher (16). Occasionally, however, visceral vessel erosion may occur in the absence of pseudocyst (22). The mortality rate of patients operated on for hemorrhage is near 50%, and even higher in those in whom arteriography was not performed (4). Frequently, the bleeding is of sufficient severity that preoperative angiography is not possible (4). In these cases, the patients might have benefited from elective arteriography earlier in their course, if suspicion regarding

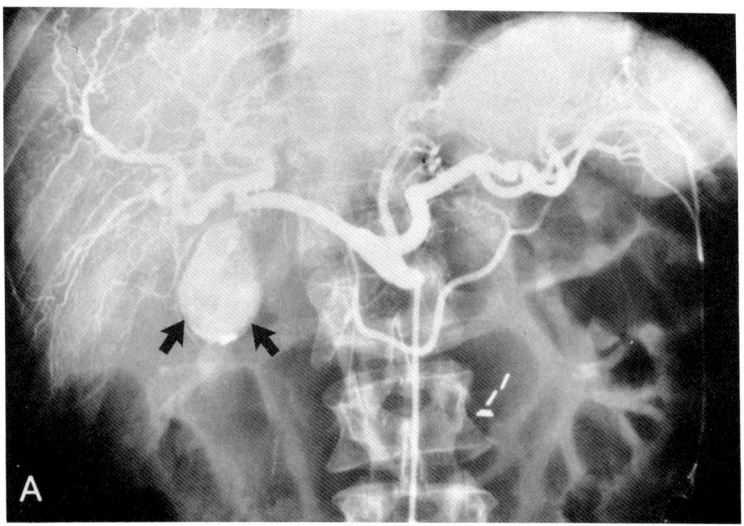
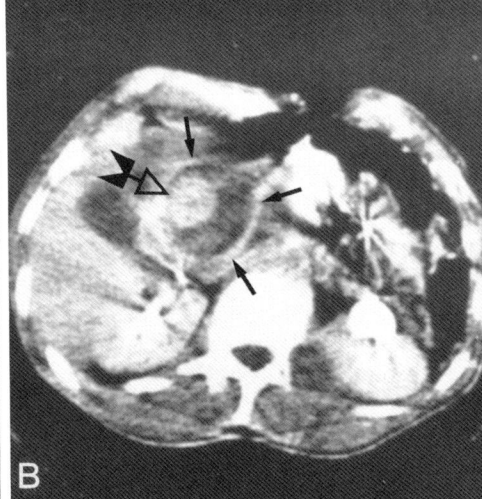

FIGURE 21.46. CHRONIC PANCREATITIS
Pseudoaneurysm within a pseudocyst. A: Large gastroduodenal artery pseudoaneurysm (*arrows*), celiac arteriogram. B: Contrast-enhanced CT shows the pseudoaneurysm (*large arrow*) within a pseudocyst with enhancing walls (*small arrows*).

possible vascular complications had been raised. Thus, arteriography is advocated by some in all patients with pseudocysts detected by ultrasound or CT, although this is not practiced in most institutions (1). Criteria for emergency arteriography include a new or enlarging mass, decrease in size of a preexisting mass (suggestive of rupture of a pseudocyst or pseudoaneurysm), pulsatile mass, decreasing hematocrit, gastrointestinal bleeding, or a pseudocyst with high CT numbers (2, 27). If a pseudoaneurysm is identified, prompt treatment with embolization, balloon occlusion, or surgery is indicated (28). When a visceral artery aneurysm ruptures, the mortality in some series is approximately 75% (23). In a Mayo Clinic autopsy series, the mortality associated with occult splenic artery aneurysms was 6% (19), but is considerably higher if aneurysms secondary to pancreatitis, which are more likely to bleed, are considered separately (29). The most common causes of bleeding associated with pancreatitis are gastritis, ulcer, and varices (27). Bleeding due to pseudoaneurysm is less common, but may be catastrophic, especially into the bowel as is most commonly reported (26–28). Bleeding into the peritoneal cavity (26), pancreatic duct (12, 30) or biliary tree is less common (12, 25). Branches of the splenic artery are the most common sources of hemorrhage when a site is identified angiographically (2, 4, 26, 27, 31). Bleeding may also occur from the gastroduodenal or pancreatoduodenal arteries and rarely from other peripancreatic arteries (2, 4, 26, 27, 31). The bleeding from pseudoaneurysms is usually acute and massive, but rarely may be of a chronic nature (4). Aneurysms of the gastroduodenal artery tend to bleed into the pseudocyst lumen, pancreatic duct, or gastrointestinal tract, while pancreaticoduodenal artery aneurysms tend to bleed into the peritoneal cavity or retroperitoneum (4). The risk of rupture of small vessel visceral aneurysm appears to be as high as 50% (32).

Angiographically, definite diagnosis of a bleeding artery involves demonstrating extravasation, indicative of active bleeding during the injection. Other signs of bleeding aneurysm include delayed emptying and irregularity in the wall of the aneurysm (31). The "flashing artery" sign, consisting of alternate opacification and emptying on sequential films, is thought to be indicative of bleeding of an end artery into a closed space (28). Actual extravasation is seen in a minority of cases, and there may be no sign of bleeding demonstrated angiographically in spite of clinical signs of massive hemorrhage (4, 25, 28, 33). Bleeding into the biliary tree or pancreatic duct, due to intermittent obstruction with clots and subsequent lysis, is especially likely to be episodic, and actual extravasation will only rarely be seen (12, 30). Even if no signs of active bleeding are demonstrated angiographically, depiction of an aneurysm can be considered to constitute indirect evidence of the site of bleeding (27). Rarely, hemorrhage directly into the pancreatic duct may occur in the absence of pseudoaneurysm (34). Frequently, even at surgery, no specific arterial bleeding site will be found. Diffuse hemorrhage from the pseudocyst wall is said to be the most common surgical finding (31, 33). Bleeding which is first encountered at surgery is usually massive and difficult to control (22). This may occur if a pseudocyst is opened at laparotomy without prior angiographic evaluation, and needle aspiration at surgery is thus advocated prior to open drainage (22).

Since bleeding may be intermittent, venous, or from a diffuse surface, or from multiple small arterial bleeding sites, a bleeding site may not be demonstrated even in life-threatening situations. Attempted treatment with vasoconstrictor agents is often unsuccessful, since vessels encased by reactive inflammatory tissue tend to respond suboptimally (35). In such cases, even if a bleeding site cannot be demonstrated, empiric embolization with resorbable materials (e.g., Gelfoam) of encased vessels and aneurysms has been advocated, with promising initial results (33). Gelfoam occludes for approximately 2–3 weeks and allows conservative treatment of pancreatitis, rather than subjecting these high risk patients to surgery. Gelfoam is thought to act in these cases not by creating total ischemia, but by converting pulsatile to nonpulsatile blood flow (33). Massive bleeding which may prove fatal may also result from ruptured gastric varices secondary to splenic vein occlusion. If splenic vein occlusion and gastric varices are seen, treatment by splenectomy is advocated (2, 17, 36, 37) although if generalized portal hypertension is present from portal vein involvement or cirrhosis, a portosystemic shunting procedure may be needed (2). Splenectomy may also be indicated if the splenic artery is eroded or incorporated into a pseudocyst, or if the spleen is extensively involved by the inflammatory process (36).

Other less frequent vascular complications include superior mesenteric artery or vein thrombosis, which may cause infarction of the transverse colon and proximal small bowel (2). In most cases, however, bowel ischemia secondary to pancreatitis is caused by small vessel thrombosis in the bowel wall caused by mesenteric fat necrosis (2, 37).

Differential Diagnosis. The diagnosis of acute pancreatitis is based primarily on clinical data, and angiography is rarely indicated other than to evaluate potential surgical complications. Detection and evaluation of fluid collections is best accomplished by ultrasound and CT. Differential problems include mucinous cystic neoplasm, which may be mistaken for pseudocyst (38). Secondary pancreatitis with or without pseudocysts may be due to occult carcinoma. New onset of pancreatitis in an elderly patient without choledocholithiasis should be viewed as suspicious for underlying carcinoma. In these patients, arteriography may reveal irregularities suggestive of carcinoma, thus aiding in the differential diagnosis (20).

Angiographically, chronic pancreatitis may be difficult to distinguish from carcinoma or atherosclerosis. A normal angiographic examination is unusual in carcinoma, but is not uncommon with pancreatitis (20, 39). Arterial changes due to carcinoma are characterized by serrated or saw-toothed encasement and abrupt angulation, while those due to chronic pancreatitis typically involve alternating areas of constriction and dilatation resulting in a beaded appearance not unlike fibromuscular dysplasia (12). Smooth, arc-shaped arterial displacement by fluid collections is suggestive of pancreatitis. Arterial occlusion is frequent in carcinoma, but is unusual in pancreatitis (12). These findings are highly reliable, but are not pathognomonic (5, 12). Arterial irregularities present in chronic pancreatitis may be difficult to distinguish from those due to atherosclerosis or fibromuscular dysplasia. Smooth, mild, arterial narrowing is nonspecific, seen in both atherosclerosis and pancreatitis and fibromuscular dysplasia. Primary vascular diseases are rarely restricted to the peripancreatic region, however (5, 10). Prominent involvement of small intrapancreatic arteries is typical of pancreatitis, but unusual for atherosclerosis and fibromuscular dysplasia, which tend to affect larger arteries. Venous involvement, if present, cannot be accounted for by atherosclerosis or fibromuscular dysplasia.

Finding aneurysms or pseudoaneurysms is extremely indicative of pancreatitis (21), although an incidental atherosclerotic aneurysm can be present in a patient with carcinoma. Calcification within the wall of the aneurysm is suggestive of atherosclerotic etiology. Atherosclerosis is probably the most common etiology of visceral artery aneurysm, although pancreatitis is almost as common (23, 32). Atherosclerotic aneurysms appear somewhat more common in patients with portal hypertension (29). Splenic artery aneurysms are also seen more frequently in pregnant women, and are subject to rupture in this clinical context as in pancreatitis (23). Whatever the etiology, angiographically demonstrated visceral artery aneurysms should be treated, whether by embolization, balloon occlusion or surgery, providing the patient's clinical condition permits (16).

Hypervascular areas may be seen in pancreatitis with variable frequency, but are rare in carcinoma (12). Inhomogeneous parenchymal staining is also suggestive of chronic pancreatitis (5, 10).

Venous involvement is almost universal in carcinoma (40), but is absent in approximately 60% of cases of pancreatitis (12). Although involvement of both arteries and veins is suggestive of carcinoma, it has been seen in as many as 35% of cases of chronic pancreatitis in some series (6).

Other differential possibilities include duodenal or gastric inflammatory disease involving the pancreas, although diffuse intrapancreatic abnormalities seen with superselective injection support the diagnosis of pancreatitis (10). Retroperitoneal tumors may cause displacement and peripancreatic vascular stenosis, but would not result in prominent intrapancreatic arterial changes (6). In most cases, correlation with other radiographic modalities will establish the diagnosis. Rarely, pancreatitis may be caused by primary vascular diseases, such as drug-induced vasculitis, periarteritis nodosa, malignant hypertension, or severe atherosclerotic occlusive disease (3). In these cases, angiography may be valuable in evaluating the underlying disease process.

Accuracy. Angiography is not a sensitive method for diagnosing pancreatitis, especially in acute cases. The percentage of normal exams will vary greatly according to patient population, and may be below 5% if only superselective techniques are used and only patients with severe and/or chronic disease are studied (11, 12, 15). If superselective techniques are used, most abnormalities detected will involve intrapancreatic arteries only (12). Nearly half the abnormal exams will consist of only nonspecific changes such as smooth narrowing or displacement (5, 12). Control patients studied for other abnormal diseases will frequently have similar nonspecific intrapancreatic abnormalities, greater than 50% in one series (12).

Summary—Role of Angiography in Evaluation of Pancreatitis

The diagnosis of pancreatitis, both acute and chronic, is usually made via clinical, laboratory, and noninvasive radiologic data. Thus, questions regarding the angiographic differential diagnosis of pancreatitis are primarily academic. The true role of angiography in pancreatitis is usually to detect protentially life-threatening complications, and provide a guide for transcatheter or surgical treatment.

In uncomplicated acute pancreatitis or acute exacerbation of known chronic pancreatitis, radiologic examination is often necessary. If symptoms fail to respond to conservative treatment within 5-7 days, evaluation with ultrasonography or computed tomography to detect pancreatic or peripancreatic fluid collections may be indicated. If these fluid collections are detected, and do not respond to treatment or if unexplained blood loss occurs, a case can be made for arteriography to detect pseudoaneurysms or splenic vein obstruction, or to provide a "road map" should a sudden decline in clinical status necessitate emergency surgery. Pseudoaneurysm or splenic vein obstruction are both indications for definitive treatment if the patient's clinical condition permits.

REFERENCES

1. Levin DC, Wilson R, Abrams HL: The changing role of pancreatic arteriography in the era of computed tomography. *Radiology* 136:245-249, 1980.
2. Freeny PC, Lawson TL: *Radiology of the Pancreas.* New York, Springer-Verlag, 1982, pp 364-370.
3. Freeny PC, Lawson TL: *Radiology of the Pancreas.* New York, 1982, pp 364-370.
4. Eckhauser FE, Stanley JC, Zelenock GB, Borlaza GS, Freier DT, Lindenauer SM: Gastroduodenal and pancreaticoduodenal artery aneurysms: a complication of pancreatitis causing spontaneous gastrointestinal hemorrhage. *Surgery* 88:325-344, 1980.
5. Reuter SR, Redman HC, Joseph RR: Angiographic findings in pancreatitis. *AJR* 107:56-62, 1964.
6. Tylen U, Arnesjo B: Angiographic diagnosis of inflammatory disease of the pancreas. *Acta Radiol* 14:215-240, 1973.
7. Aakus T, Hofsli M, Vestad E: Angiography in acute pancreatitis. *Acta Radiol* 8:119-128, 1969.
8. Goldstein HM, Neiman HL, Bookstein JJ: Angiographic evaluation of pancreatic disease. *Radiology* 112:275-282, 1974.
9. Roe M, Greenough WG: Marked hypervascularity and arteriovenous shunting in acute pancreatitis. *Radiology* 113:47-48, 1974.
10. Freeny PC, Lawson TL: *Radiology of the Pancreas.* New York, 1982, pp 106-269.
11. Khademi M, Lazaro EJ, Rickert RR: Selective arteriography in the diagnosis of chronic inflammatory pancreatic disease. *AJR* 119: 141-150, 1973.
12. Gortenuti G, Cavallini G, Vantini I, Angelini G, Piubello W, Frasson F, Dobrilla G: Angiography in chronic pancreatitis and pancreatic cancer. *Gastroenterology* 70:620-626, 1978.
13. Boijsen E, Tylen U: Vascular changes in chronic pancreatitis. *Acta Radiol* 12:34-48, 1972.
14. Howard JM, Nedwich A: Correlation of the histologic observations and operative findings in patients with chronic pancreatitis. *Surg Gynecol Obstet* 132:387-395, 1971.
15. Freeny PC, Ball TJ, Ryan J: Impact of new diagnostic imaging methods on pancreatic angiography. *AJR* 133:619-624, 1979.
16. Levin DC, Eisenberg H, Wilson R: Arteriography in the evaluation of pancreatic pseudocyst. *AJR* 129:243-248, 1977.
17. Muhletaler C, Gerlock AJ, Goncharenko V, Avant GR, Flexner JM: Gastric varices secondary to splenic vein occlusion: radiographic diagnosis and clinical significance. *Radiology* 132:593-598, 1979.
18. Burbige EJ, Tarder G, Carson S, Eugene J, Frey CF: Colonic varices. A complication of pancreatitis with splenic vein thrombosis. *Dig Dis Sci* 23:752-755, 1978.
19. Cosgrove H, Legge D, O'Connel FX, Weir D: Angiographic evaluation of gastrointestinal haemorrhage complicating pancreatic disease. *Clin Radiol* 29:289-293, 1978.
20. Boijsen E: Pancreatic Angiography. In Abrams HL (ed): *Angiography: Vascular and Interventional Radiology,* Ed 3. Boston, Little, Brown, 1983, pp 1452-1455.
21. White RF, Baum S, Suranasir S: Aneurysms secondary to pancreatitis. *AJR* 127:393-396, 1976.
22. Schecter LM, Gordon E, Passaro E Jr: Massive hemorrhage from the celiac axis in pancreatitis. *Am J Surg* 128:301-305, 1974.
23. Bowers J, Koehler PR, Hammar SP, Nelson JA, Tolman KG: Rupture of a splenic artery aneurysm into the pancreatic duct. *Gastroenterology* 70:1152-1155, 1976.
24. Koehler PR, Nelson JA, Berenson MM: Massive extraenteric gastrointestinal bleeding: angiographic diagnosis. *Radiology* 119:41-44, 1976.
25. Wolstenholme JT: Major gastrointestinal hemorrhage associated with pancreatic pseudocyst. *Am J Surg* 127:377-381, 1974.
26. Stanley JC, Frey CF, Miller TA, Lindenauer SM, Child CG: Major arterial hemorrhage. *Arch Surg* 111:435-440, 1976.
27. Gaadacz TR, Trunkey D, Kieffer RF: Visceral vessel erosion associated with pancreatitis. *Arch Surg* 113:1438-1440, 1978.
28. Walter JF, Chuang VP, Bookstein JJ, Reuter SR, Cho KJ, Pulmano CM: Angiography of massive hemorrhage secondary to pancreatic disease. *Radiology* 124:337-342, 1977.
29. Boijsen E, Gothlin J, Hallbook T, Sandblom P: Preoperative angiographic diagnosis of bleeding aneurysms of abdominal visceral arteries. *Radiology* 93:781-791, 1969.
30. Bivins BA, Sachatello CR, Chuang VP, Brady P: Hemosuccus pancreaticus (hemoductal pancreatitis). *Arch Surg* 113:751-753, 1978.
31. Greenstein A, DeMaio EF, Nabseth DC: Acute hemorrhage associated with pancreatic pseudocysts. *Surgery* 69:55-62, 1971.
32. Harris RD, Anderson JE, Coel MN: Aneurysms of the small pancreatic arteries: a cause of upper abdominal pain and intestinal bleeding. *Radiology* 115:17-20, 1975.

33. Vujic I, Anderson BL, Stanley JH, Gobien RP: Pancreatic and peripancreatic vessels: embolization for control of bleeding in pancreatitis. Radiology 150:51–55, 1984.
34. Melville GE, Maxwell DD: Massive lower GI hemorrhage in hemoductal pancreatitis. Gastrointest Radiol 8:145–146, 1983.
35. Eisenberg H, Steer ML: The nonoperative treatment of massive pyloroduodenal hemorrhage by retracted autologous clot embolization. Surgery 79:414–420, 1976.
36. Haff RC, Page CP, Andrassy RJ, Buckley CJ: Splenectomy: its place in operations for inflammatory disease of the pancreas. Am J Surg 134:555–557, 1973.
37. Collins JJ, Peterson LM, Wilson RE: Small intestinal infarction as a complication of pancreatitis. Am J Surg 167:433–436, 1968.
38. Tylen U: Angiographic differentiation between inflammatory disease and carcinoma of the pancreas. Acta Radiol 38:257–272, 1973.
39. Mackie CR, Cooper MJ, Lewis MH, Moossa AR: Nonoperative differentiation between pancreatic cancer and chronic pancreatitis. Ann Surg 189:480–487, 1979.
40. Buranasiri S, Baum S: The significance of the venous phase of celiac and superior mesenteric arteriography in evaluating pancreatic carcinoma. Radiology 102:11–20, 1972.

Pancreatic Function Testing

Pancreatic function testing can be split into direct and indirect methods of collection. The usefulness of these tests may be of some controversy because of limitations of interpretation but overall these procedures may: (a) aid in the differential diagnosis of pancreatic disease, (b) confirm the diagnosis of pancreatic disease, and (c) provide a means of assessing and predicting prognosis of pancreatic disease (1–4).

There are several practical problems that make interpretation of pancreatic function by these tests difficult. The tests of pancreatic secretory capacity may not be an accurate measure of the degree of pancreatic glandular damage (4).

Collection of Pure Pancreatic Juice

Experimentally, collection of pure pancreatic juice can be achieved by creating a permanent fistula opposite the pancreatic duct of dogs. A glass cannula can be passed through the fistula into the duct to collect the pancreatic juice while stimultaneously substances can be placed into the duodenum to test their effect on secretion. The fistula is capped when not in use and pancreatic secretions enter the duodenum normally (1).

Clinically, this can be done via ERCP with selective cannulation of the pancreatic duct. The limitations of this method stem from the incomplete collection of pancreatic juice since there is leakage of juice around the intraductal catheter. Additionally, use of the premedications and sedation required in performing the procedure may affect the response to stimulants. The single advantage is that the pancreatic juice can be collected in the zymogen form prior to the action of proteases activated by enterokinases (4). Fresh, uncontaminated pancreatic juice has no proteolytic activity until activated and then forms several proteolytic enzymes (1).

Tests of Exocrine Pancreatic Function

Tests of exocrine pancreatic function are among the most difficult to perform accurately and interpret because of the number of variables involved. The tests can confirm the clinical diagnosis, evaluate progression of pancreatic disease, and provide direction for management in chronic pancreatic insufficiency. The tests, however, are inadequate in mild pancreatic insufficiency in reflecting the degree of pancreatic damage (4). While morphologic and histologic disturbances may be evident, the secretory test result may be normal. An individual may respond to exogenous stimulants erroneously and reveal impaired secretory response (4). Interpretation of these results of pancreatic secretory capacity cannot be made to correlate perfectly with quantitative changes in pancreatic structure. In a study in 60 patients using ERCP, correlation between the clinical appearance of the pancreas and pancreatic exocrine insufficiency secondary to pancreatic carcinoma was made in 73% (3). Exocrine dysfunction often accompanies carcinoma as well as chronic pancreatitis, since the pancreatic tissue surrounding a cancer loses exocrine function.

Using ERCP versus a pancreozymin-secretin test, obstruction and stenosis was seen to correlate with a decrease in exocrine function in 88.3% of patients (2). The more severe the functional impairment, the more likely ductal alterations were to be present. Likewise, significant ductal abnormality seen by ERCP was predictive of severe excretory dysfunction of the pancreas.

Tests of secretory capacity assess these indices—volume of pancreatic juice secreted, bicarbonate secretion, and secretion of pancreatic enzymes. Although decrease in the capacity to secrete enzymes may represent a decrease in pancreatic mass, little is known whether compensatory mechanisms occur in response to loss of pancreatic acinar function (4).

Techniques for collection of pancreatic juice most commonly involve aspiration of duodenal secretions. However, collection of pancreatic juice from the pancreatic duct at the time of ERCP may be useful. Collection of pancreatic components in the feces does not enjoy widespread clinical use.

Collection by ERCP

After cannulation and opacification of the pancreatic duct with 60% Renografin, secretin stimulation μg/kg is given IV and the pancreatic fluid is collected via the catheter, mixed with aprotinin, a pancreatic enzyme inhibitor, and centrifuged (4).

Secretin Test

Duodenal intubation allows for the collection of duodenal fluid including pancreatic secretion. Currently the gold standard of pancreatic analysis for assessing pancreatic secretory capacity is the secretin stimulation test. Secretin increases the volume and bicarbonate content of pancreatic juice. Although response to IV secretin can vary from one investigation to another due to differences in technique, product used, and laboratory determination, the most recent introduction of Secretin-Kabi (Pharmacia Laboratories) has allowed a constant and reliable response with a lower potential for allergic reactions when the test is properly performed (5).

The test is performed by placing a double lumen radiopaque catheter just beyond the ampulla of Vater with its second lumen within the gastric antrum. Constant but interrupted aspiration is performed while IV secretin 1 ml/kg is injected and the duodenal aspirate is collected for 80 min (5). Each fraction of duodenal aspirate is analyzed for volume and bicarbonate. While a diminished pancreatic reserve is seen with aging, interpretation of the test may help differentiate complete obstruction of the duct due to a pancreatic carcinoma from decreased functional capacity seen with chronic pancreatitis (Table 21.2) (6, 7).

As mentioned before, studies correlating quantitative changes in pancreatic structure by ERCP with the secretin test showed a statistically significant functional impairment of pancreatic secretion with advanced ductal alterations (4, 7, 8).

Bentiromide Test

Because the secretin test and Lundh test meal (measuring postcibal trypsin concentration) are cumbersome, time consuming, and often difficult to interpret, an easy and reliable indirect measurement of pancreatic exocrine function of chymotrypsin has been developed by Toskes (9) and

TABLE 21.2.
INTERPRETATION OF SECRETIN TEST OF EXOCRINE PANCREATIC FUNCTION

Test	Diagnosis	
	Chronic Pancreatitis	Pancreatic Cancer
Cytology	Negative	Positive (60% of cases)
HCO_3	<90 meq/L in all samples	≥90 meq/L in one or more samples
Total volume	≥2 ml/kg	<2 ml/kg

is now commercially available from Adria Laboratories.

An orally administered synthetic peptide (Bentiromide, N-benzoyl-L-tyrosyl-p-aminobenzoic acid) is split by chymotrypsin. Free p-aminobenzoic acid (PABA) is absorbed from the bowel, conjugated by the liver and its metabolites are excreted in the urine. Measurement of the PABA in a 6-hr urine collection following a 500 mg dose of bentiromide was 75% of the ingested dose in normal subjects, 40% in patients with chronic pancreatitis, and 50% with pancreatic carcinoma (10). A concomitant D-xylose test was also suggested to increase specificity in the presence of suspected malabsorption (11). A 5% false positive and 20% false negative rate was seen in one series (9).

Pancreatic Enzymes

Serum Amylase

Pancreatic enzymes enter the circulation via lymphatics in states of pancreatic ductal obstruction. Although the significance of the elevation of amylase is limited by its increase in other conditions (Table 21.3), its elevation usually signifies pancreatic disease (12). The serum amylase concentration rises within 24 hr of the onset of an attack of pancreatitis and returns to normal within 3–5 days. There is no correlation between the degree of elevation and the severity of the episode. In chronic pancreatitis there may be only minimal elevation of the amylase, felt to be secondary to the inability of the damaged gland to produce amylase. Therefore, the diagnostic sensitivity and specificity of serum amylase determinations for pancreatitis only approaches 80% (13). Persistent elevation of serum amylase may signal the presence of a pseudocyst; elevated urinary amylase determinations are more accurate in this regard.

TABLE 21.3.
CAUSES OF HYPERAMYLASEMIA AND/OR HYPERAMYLASURIA

A. Pancreatic disease
  1. Pancreatitis
     a. Acute
        1) Common causes (alcoholism, gallbladder disease, etc.)
        2) Uncommon (vasculitis, uremia, etc.)
        3) Drug-induced
        4) Viral
           a) Hepatitis
           b) Other
        5) Postendoscopy
        6) Postoperative
        7) Renal transplantation
     b. Chronic
     c. Complications
        1) Pseudocyst
        2) Ascites
        3) Abscess
  2. Pancreatic carcinoma
  3. Pancreatic trauma
B. Disorders of nonpancreatic origin (mechanism known)
  1. Renal insufficiency
  2. Salivary-type hyperamylasemia
  3. "Tumor" hyperamylasemia
  4. Salivary gland lesions
     a. Mumps
     b. Calculus
     c. Irradiation sialoadenitis
     d. Maxillofacial surgery
     e. Drugs
  5. Macroamylasemia
C. Disorders of complex origin (mechanism unknown or uncertain)
  1. Biliary tract disease
  2. Intra-abdominal diseases other than pancreatitis
     a. Perforated peptic ulcer
     b. Intestinal obstruction
     c. Ruptured ectopic pregnancy
     d. Mesenteric infarction
     e. Afferent loop syndrome
     f. Aortic aneurysm with dissection
     g. Peritonitis
     h. Acute appendicitis
  3. Cerebral trauma
  4. Burns and traumatic shock
  5. Postoperative hyperamylasemia
  6. Diabetic ketoacidosis
  7. Renal transplantation
  8. Pneumonia
  9. Acquired bialbuminemia
  10. Prostatic disease
  11. Pregnancy
  12. Drugs

Isoamylase

Isoenzymes of amylase exist. P-type comprises 40% of the serum amylase and originates in the pancreas. The S-type, comprising 60% of the serum amylase, originates in the salivary gland. Studies confirm the presence of the P-fraction of amylase in urine to be present to a greater extent during an episode of pancreatitis than the S-type (14, 15). The persistence of a P2 isoamylase peak is consistent with the presence of a pseudocyst (16). A recent study showed an appreciable sensitivity advantage of pancreatic isoenzyme and lipase over total amylase measurement during the recovery phase of pancreatitis. Pancreatic isoamylase and lipase are interchangeable markers of the levels of pancreatic enzymes in the blood (17) in intestinal disorders where the mucosal barriers are disrupted (perforation, ischemia, ulceration, and obstruction). Measurement of pancreatic isoenzyme levels will not distinguish acute pancreatitis from acute intraabdominal catastrophe (18, 19).

Urine Amylase

Since the P-type amylase, originating from the pancreas, is filtered more freely and more rapidly than the S-type isoenzyme, measurement of the urinary amylase reflects predominantly the presence of that fraction. While the majority of serum amylase undergoes clearance by an extrarenal mechanism, urinary excretion accounts for 24% of the amylase removed (20). Serum amylase determination is sensitive to changes in renal function and its usefulness may be limited when renal disease is present. The serum amylase would reflect the failure of excretion in this instance and would thus appear elevated. In acute pancreatitis, wide fluctuations in urinary amylase may occur such that multiple 2-hr urinary collections would be more accurate than a 24-hr specimen (21). The elevation of the urinary amylase may last several days longer than the serum amylase in acute pancreatitis, and subsequently fall to normal. Persistence of the elevations may indicate continued pancreatic inflammation or development of a pseudocyst.

Much controversy exists over the mechanism of the elevation in urinary amylase during pancreatitis; studies suggest that glomerular permeability is normal, that clearance of isoamylases is uniform, not dependent on a specific type (indicating a renal abnormality), and protein reabsorbed by the tubule assessed using β_2-microglobulin is markedly reduced (20–22).

Lipase

Serum lipase is more specific than amylase, rises more rapidly, and remains elevated longer than amylase in acute pancreatitis. The sensitivity of lipase together with amylase in predicting clinical pancreatitis is 83% (13). Conversely, 90% of patients with acute pancreatitis can be shown to have elevated lipase levels (23). Lipase elevations may also occur in other situations which give rise to hyperamylasemia except in parotitis and macroamylasemia (24). Lipase itself injected into adipose tissue does not produce fat necrosis; when injected intraperitoneally in combination with bile salts, typical fat necrosis ensues (24).

REFERENCES

1. Davenport HW: Pancreatic secretion. In *Physiology of the Digestive Tract*. Chicago, Yearbook, 1982, ch 10.
2. Rudick J: Physiology of pancreatic secretion. *Surg Clin North Am* 61:47, 1981.
3. Meyer JH: Pancreatic physiology. In Sleisenger MH, Fordtran JS (eds): *Gastrointestinal Disease*. Philadelphia, W. B. Saunders, 1978, ch 20.
4. Goodale RL, Condie RM et al: Clinical and secretory difference in pancreatic cancer and chronic pancreatitis. *Ann Surg* 194:193, 1981.
5. Drossman DA: Secretin test. In *Manual of Gastroenterology Procedures*. New York, Raven Press, 1982, ch 20.
6. Wormsley KG: Pancreatic function test. *Clin Gastroenterol* 7:529, 1978.
7. DiMagno EP, Malagelada JR, Go VL: The relationship between pancreatic ductal obstruction and pancreatic secretion in man. *Mayo Clin Proc* 54:157, 1979.
8. Kozu T: Correlation between pancreatic ductal morphology and exocrine function comparison of endoscopic retrograde cholangiopancreatography and pancreozymin—secretin test. In *Endoscopic Retrograde Cholangopancreatography*. New York, Igaku-Shoin, 1979.
9. Toskes PP: Bentiromide as a test of exocrine pancreatic function in adult patients with pancreatic exocrine insufficiency. *Gastroenterology* 85:565, 1983.
10. Reber HA: Chronic pancreatitis. In *Gastrointestinal Disease*. Philadelphia, W. B. Saunders, 1978, ch 20.
11. Greenberger NJ, ed. The pancreas. In *1984 Yearbook of Medicine*. Chicago, Yearbook, 1984, ch 37, p 474.
12. Salt WB, Schenker S: Amylase—its clinical significance: a review of the literature. *Medicine* 55:269, 1976.
13. Kayasseh L, Gyr K: Diagnosis of pancreatitis. *Surg Dig Dis* 1:26, 1983.
14. Scheele GA: The secretory product in the pancreatic exocrine cell. *Mayo Clin Proc* 54:420, 1979.
15. Legaz ME, Kenny MA: Electrophoretic amylase fractional as an aid in diagnosis of pancreatic disease. *Clin Chem* 22:57, 1976.
16. Warshaw AL, Lee KH: Aging changes of pancreatic isoamylases and the appearance of "old amylase": in the serum of patients with pancreatic pseudocysts (abstract). *Gastroenterology* 76:1266, 1979.
17. Kolars JC, Ellis CJ, Levitt MD: Comparison of serum amylase, pancreatic isoamylase, and lipase in patients with hyperamylasemia. *Dig Dis Sci* 29:289, 1984.
18. Banks PA, Warshaw AL et al: Identification of amylase isoenzymes in intestinal contents. *Dig Dis Sci* 29:297, 1984.
19. Byrne JJ, Boyd TF: Serum amylase levels in experimental intestinal obstruction. *N Engl J Med* 256:1176, 1957.
20. Warshaw AL, Lee KH: The mechanism of increased renal clearance of amylase in acute pancreatitis. *Gastroenterology* 71:388, 1976.
21. Moossa AR: Diagnostic tests and procedures in acute pancreatitis. *N Engl J Med* 311:639, 1984.
22. Johnson SG, Ellis C et al: Mechanism of the elevated renal clearance of amylase: clearance of cretinine (Cam/Ccr) in acute pancreatitis. *Clin Res* 24:433A, 1976.
23. Brandborg LL: Acute pancreatitis. In Sleisenger MH, Fordtran JS (eds): *Gastrointestinal Disease*. Philadelphia, W. B. Saunders, 1978, ch 91, p 1409.
24. Orda R, Orda A, Baron J, Wiznitzer: Lipase turbidometric assay and acute pancreatitis. *Dig Dis Sci* 29:294, 1984.

COMPLICATIONS OF PANCREATITIS

Pancreatic Abscess

Pancreatic abscesses develop as a sequel to severe hemorrhagic pancreatitis or surgery in the pancreatic region or biliary tract (1). They usually manifest themselves clinically 10–14 days after the onset of pancreatitis or on the 4th to 8th postoperative day (1). It is estimated that 2–6% of patients with acute pancreatitis develop a pancreatic abscess (2), although the percentage is higher in those with severe necrotizing pancreatitis.

Abscesses may develop either as a superinfection of an intra- or extrapancreatic fluid collection or directly in a necrotic pancreas. The mechanism of infection is unclear; enteric organisms are usually the cause (1). Left untreated, mortality approaches 100% (1). With surgical drainage, the mortality in alcoholics is 18% and in postoperative abscesses 62% (1). Postoperative abscesses after pancreatic resection tend to be located near drains and are not as serious as those that occur after biliary surgery, peptic ulcer surgery, splenectomy or pancreatic biopsy (1). Pancreatic abscesses can be very extensive, involving the entire retroperitoneum without respect for fascial boundaries (3), and may occur in remote areas of the abdomen in a manner similar to pseudocysts (2). Frequently large chunks of particulate matter are present within the abscess which are not easily removed by catheters or drains (1).

Clinical Findings

Clinical diagnosis rests on persistence of symptoms beyond 7–10 days or relapse in patients with acute pancreatitis or the development

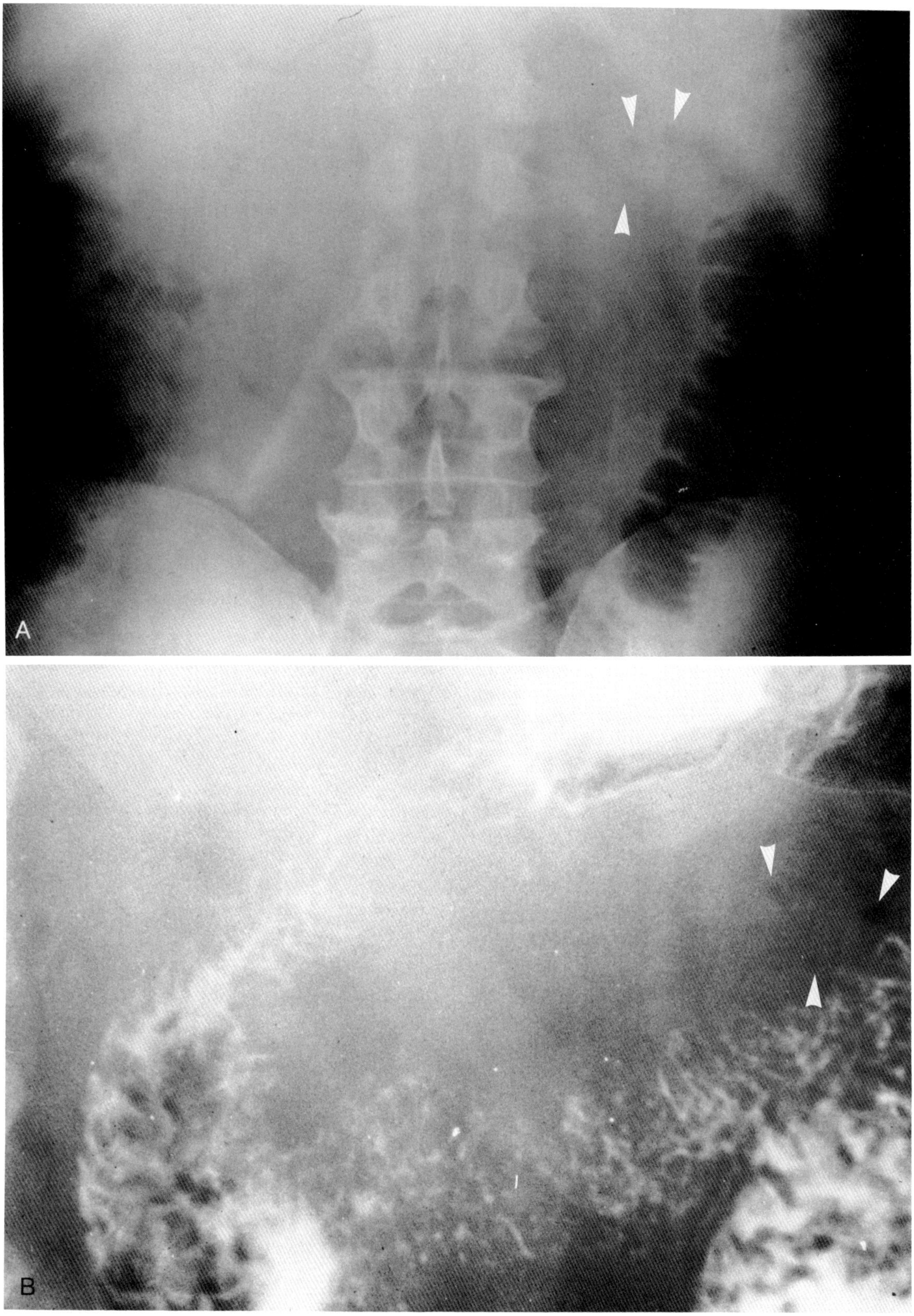

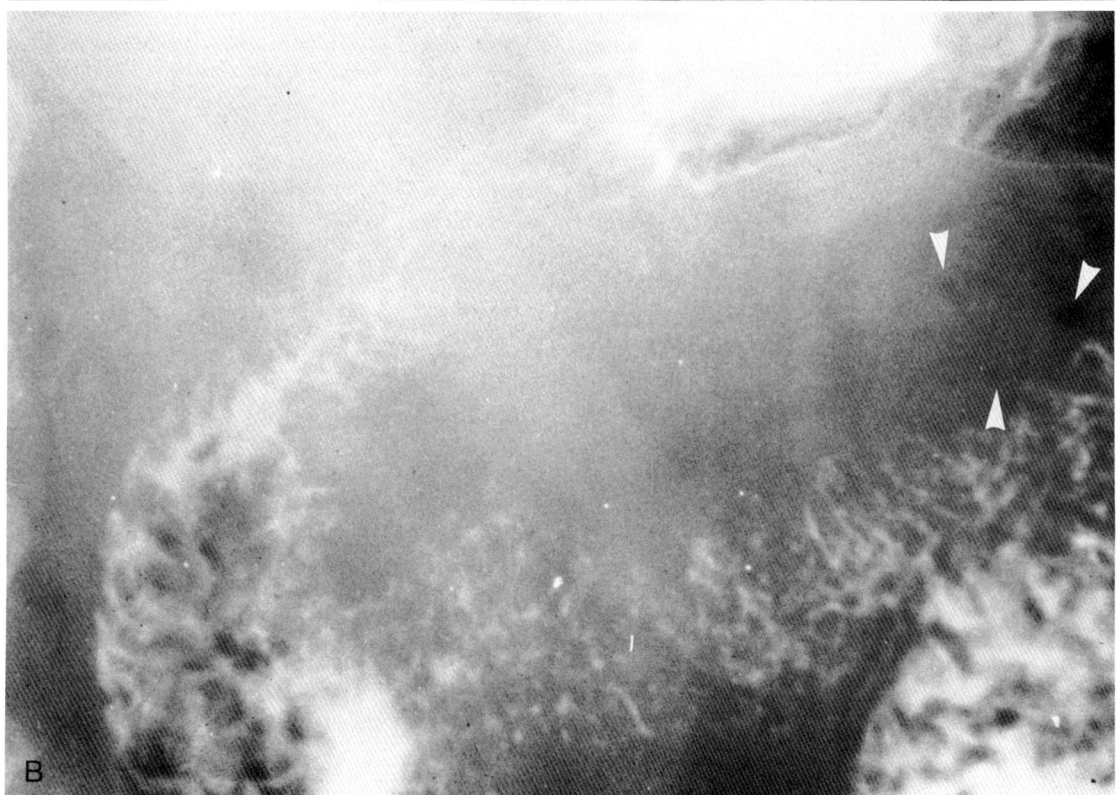

FIGURE 21.47. PANCREATIC ABSCESS
Pancreatic abscess developing 3 weeks after acute alcoholic pancreatitis. *A:* Tiny gas collections (*arrowheads*) noted on plain films with a sentinel loop of jejunum. *B:* UGI demonstrates the gas to be extraluminal (*arrowheads*).

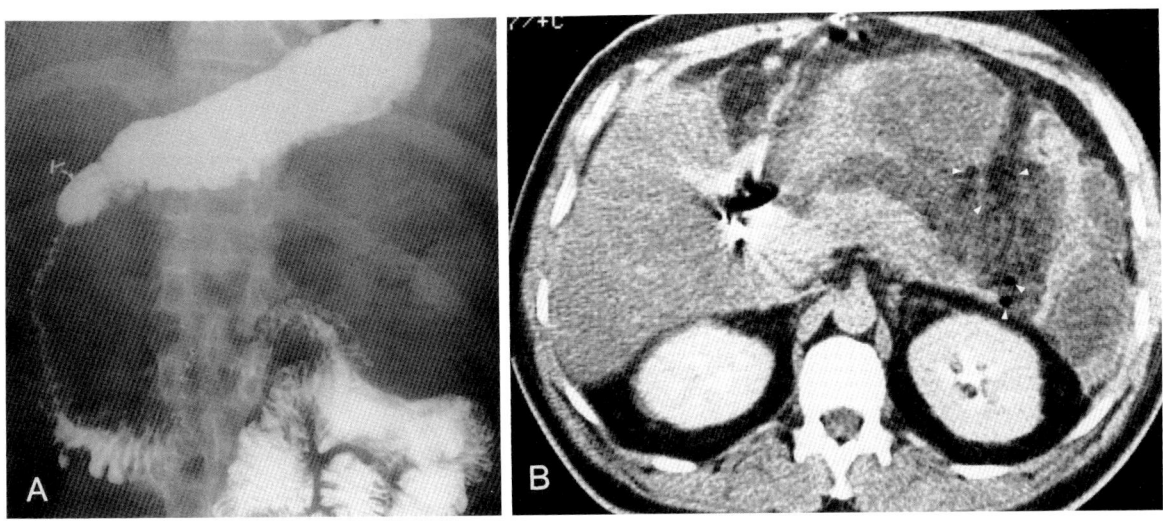

FIGURE 21.48. PANCREATIC ABSCESS

Pancreatic abscess developing 2 weeks after acute postoperative (cholecystectomy) pancreatitis. *A:* Upper gastrointestinal examination shows changes in the stomach and duodenum consistent with acute pancreatitis. There is a soft tissue mass in the left upper quadrant containing small air collections and displacing jejunum. *B:* CT shows air bubbles in a lesser sac abscess (*arrowheads*). The pancreas is nearly normal in size and the mass effects on stomach and duodenum were primarily due to peripancreatic fluid collections.

of fever, prostration and leukocytosis in the postoperative patient. Physical examination may be limited by severe abdominal tenderness and a number of patients will have only minimal findings (2). In up to one-third of patients the diagnosis will not be clinically suspected (2). Laboratory data are similar to pancreatitis and noninfected pseudocyst/phlegmon (2). Findings may include elevated or normal serum amylase, elevated liver function tests, hypoalbuminemia and renal failure.

Radiology

Plain Films. Detection of gas within pancreatic abscesses by plain films occurs in 34–60% of cases (2, 4). The findings range from subtle, small bubbles to large, obvious pockets or air-fluid levels (Figs. 21.47 and 21.48) (1, 2, 4). Mottled gas and fluid may be confused with fecal material (2). The presence of gas may be due to abscess alone, fistula alone, or abscess plus fistula (2, 4). Rarely gas in the pancreatic bed is produced by degenerating tissue after necrotizing pancreatitis without infection or fistula (Fig. 21.49) (5).

Gastrointestinal Contrast Examinations. Contrast examinations of the gastrointestinal tract are helpful both in confirming that the gas collection is extraluminal and demonstrating pancreatic-enteric fistula (Fig. 21.47B) (2, 4). The latter were demonstrated in 20% of abscesses in one recent series (2). Contrast examinations will also demonstrate mass effects and inflammatory changes in regions of the gastrointestinal tract contiguous to the abscess, findings similar to those of pseudocysts (Fig. 21.48A). A combination of plain films and gastrointestinal contrast studies can be expected to suggest the diagnosis of pancreatic abscess nearly 60% of the time (2).

Sonography. The clinical diagnosis of a pancreatic abscess is extremely difficult as patients with acute necrotizing pancreatitis can have all the signs and symptoms of sepsis in the absence of an abscess (6, 7). If there is sonographic evidence of a fluid collection in a patient with acute necrotizing pancreatitis and a persistent fever and leukocytosis then percutaneous aspiration of this fluid collection should be performed as one third will prove to be an abscess (Fig. 21.50) (8). It is extremely important to perform a gram stain on the aspirate as an immediate diagnosis can be made without waiting for a culture provided numerous white cells and bacteria are present. Complications, although unlikely (6%), can occur and include superinfection of a sterile pseudocyst and hemoperitoneum due to puncture of a varix in a patient with associated portal hypertension. The sonographic appearance of the wall and contents of the fluid collection are not of value in determining whether an abscess is present. In abscesses, the wall can vary from

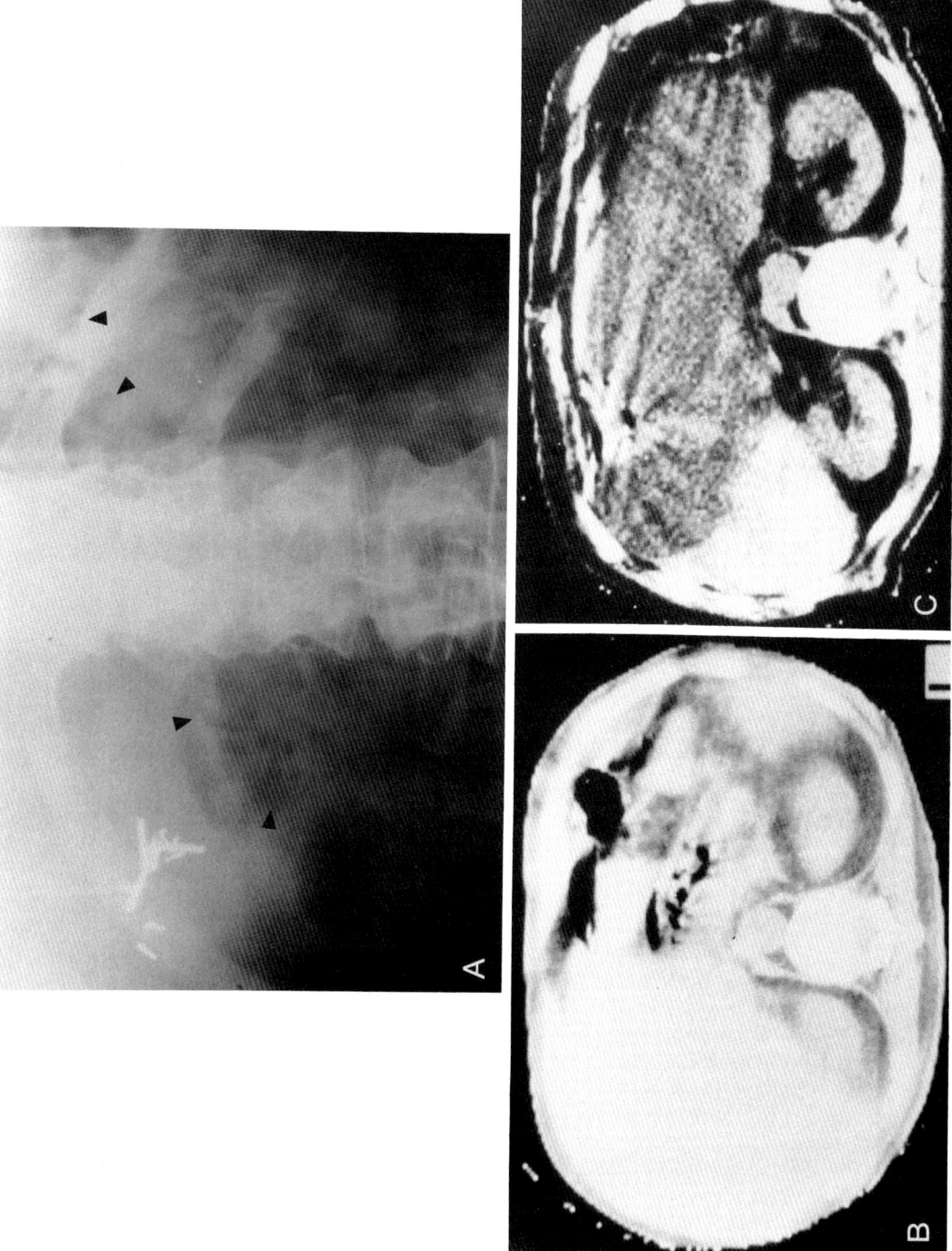

FIGURE 21.49. STERILE NECROSIS

Gas due to tissue necrosis without infection. *A*: Plain film showing gas bubbles throughout the region of the pancreatic bed (*arrowheads*). *B*: Corresponding CT showing pancreatic gas. The patient was asymptomatic at this time and a gallium scan was negative. He continued to recover uneventfully from alcoholic hemorrhagic pancreatitis. *C*: CT scan at the time of presentation with acute hemorrhagic pancreatitis 2 weeks prior to *A* and *B*, showing an enlarged pancreas not separable from hemorrhagic fluid in the lesser sac.

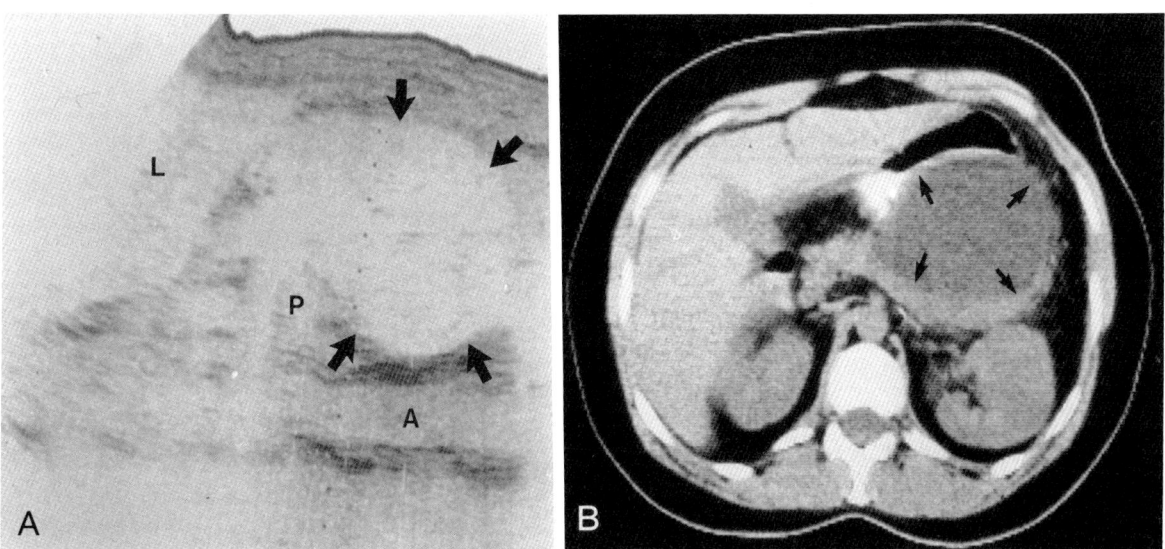

FIGURE 21.50. PANCREATIC ABSCESS

Lesser sac abscess secondary to acute pancreatitis. Proven by percutaneous aspiration using sonographic guidance. *A:* Longitudinal sonogram reveals a large cystic mass with fairly well defined walls (*arrows*) with internal echoes. *B:* CT scan through the abscess. Aorta (*A*), liver (*L*), pancreas (*P*).

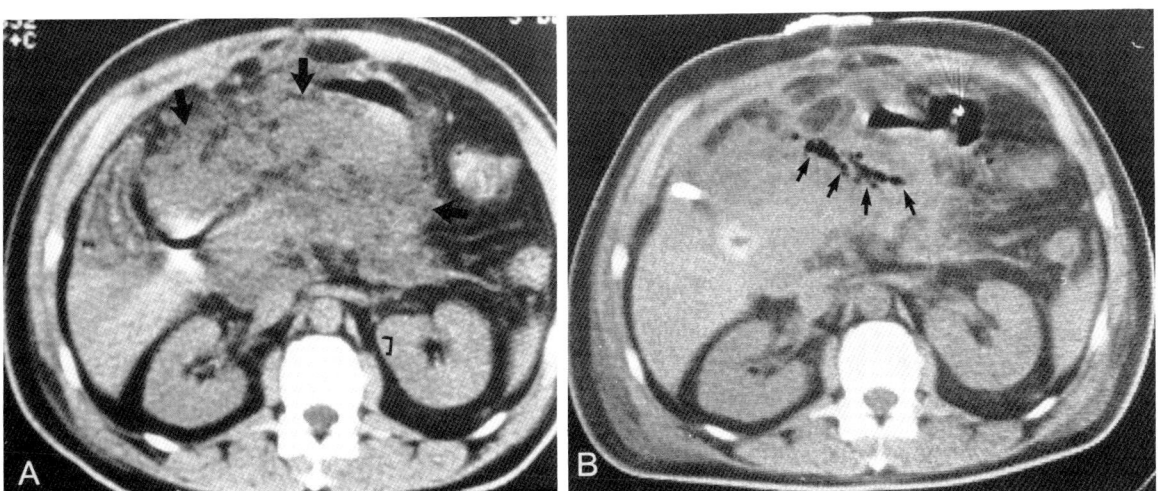

FIGURE 21.51. PANCREATIC ABSCESS

Gas containing abscess secondary to postoperative phlegmonous pancreatitis. *A:* The initial CT scan shows evidence of an extensive phlegmonous pancreatitis (*large arrows*) involving the lesser sac, both anterior pararenal spaces and the transverse mesocolon. *B:* A follow-up CT scan 5 days later reveals bubbles of gas (*small arrows*) in the phlegmon compatible with an abscess. (From Silverstein, W, Isikoff MB, Hill MC, Barkin J: Diagnostic imaging of acute pancreatitis: prospective study using CT and sonography. *AJR* 137:497–502, 1981.)

being thick and irregular to being entirely smooth and well-defined while the contents may be entirely anechoic or be entirely filled with echoes (Fig. 21.50). Thick-walled fluid collections with a lot of internal echoes that are not abscesses usually represent an area of hemorrhage and this can be proven by aspirating sterile nonclotting blood (8, 9).

Sonography can entirely miss a gas-containing pancreatic abscess as it may be mistaken for a gas-filled loop of bowel. Gas-filled abscesses, on occasion may be seen as a densely echogenic mass due to the presence of micro bubbles of air within the abscess (10). If there is any doubt about the presence of a gas-containing pancreatic abscess, plain radiographs of the abdo-

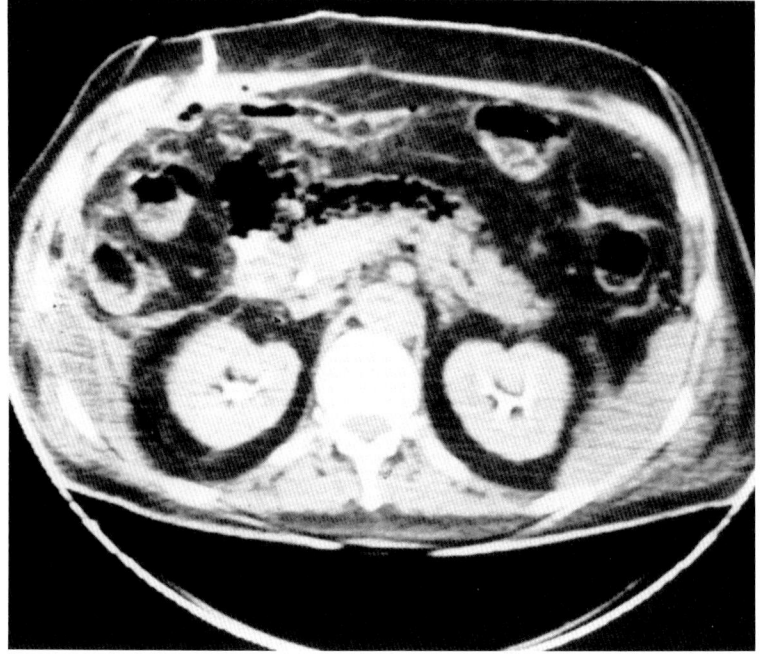

FIGURE 21.52. PANCREATIC ABSCESS
Emphysematous pancreatitis. CT of a patient who was seen 5 days after cholecystectomy and gravely ill, showing gas bubbles anterior to and within the pancreatic parenchyma. The density in head is the lower limb of a T-tube.

men should be obtained as extraluminal gas may be evident in 58% (2). This should be followed by a CT scan if clinically indicated (Fig. 21.51) (2, 11). The presence of a gas collection in the pancreas or associated phlegmon does not always indicate the presence of an abscess. A pancreatic pseudocyst can spontaneously decompress itself into a gas-containing loop of bowel while sterile necrosis of a phlegmon can also occur (5, 12).

Computed Tomography. Pancreatic abscesses are low density fluid collections in the region of the pancreas containing extraluminal gas in about two-thirds of reported cases (Figs. 21.48B, 21.52, and 21.53) (2, 11, 12). When gas is not present, abscesses cannot be distinguished from plegmon or pseudocyst without needle aspiration. When gas is present, the possibilities of fistula or rarely, sterile tissue necrosis have to be considered (Fig. 21.49b). CT may demonstrate extension of pancreatic abscesses via the same intraabdominal pathways described for pancreatitis and pseudocysts, although pancreatic abscesses can obliterate fascial planes (Fig. 21.53) (2, 3).

Intrapancreatic or peripancreatic bubbles of gas in patients with acute necrotizing pancreatitis has to be considered indicative of an abscess which demands surgical draining. If the medical condition of the patient is such that surgery is contraindicated, then confirmation of the abscess by percutaneous aspiration should be considered (8). If the abscess is confirmed then the surgical draining will have to be performed (7). Single large gas collections and those with air-fluid levels may not be abscesses but may represent communications between a pseudocyst and adjacent stomach or intestine (5, 12, 13).

Not all pancreatic abscesses contain gas, as many (36–71%) appear as pancreatic or peripancreatic fluid collections (8, 11). The CT number of the fluid and degree of wall enhancement do not aid in making the diagnosis of an abscess and such a fluid collection could represent uninfected pancreatic juice or an area of old hemorrhage (Fig. 21.53) (11). When such a fluid collection is present in a patient with acute necrotizing pancreatitis, percutaneous aspiration should be considered since 33% of such fluid collections represent abscesses and need surgical drainage (8). The aspirated material should be immediately gram stained and both aerobic and anaerobic cultures should be performed. Although not optimal, percutaneous drainage of an abscess can be performed using ultrasound or CT guidance when the patient's clinical condition is not stable enough for immediate surgery (14). Complications following aspiration are uncommon (6%) but include hemorrhage, superinfection of a previously sterile fluid collection and fatal necrotizing pancreatitis (8, 15, 16).

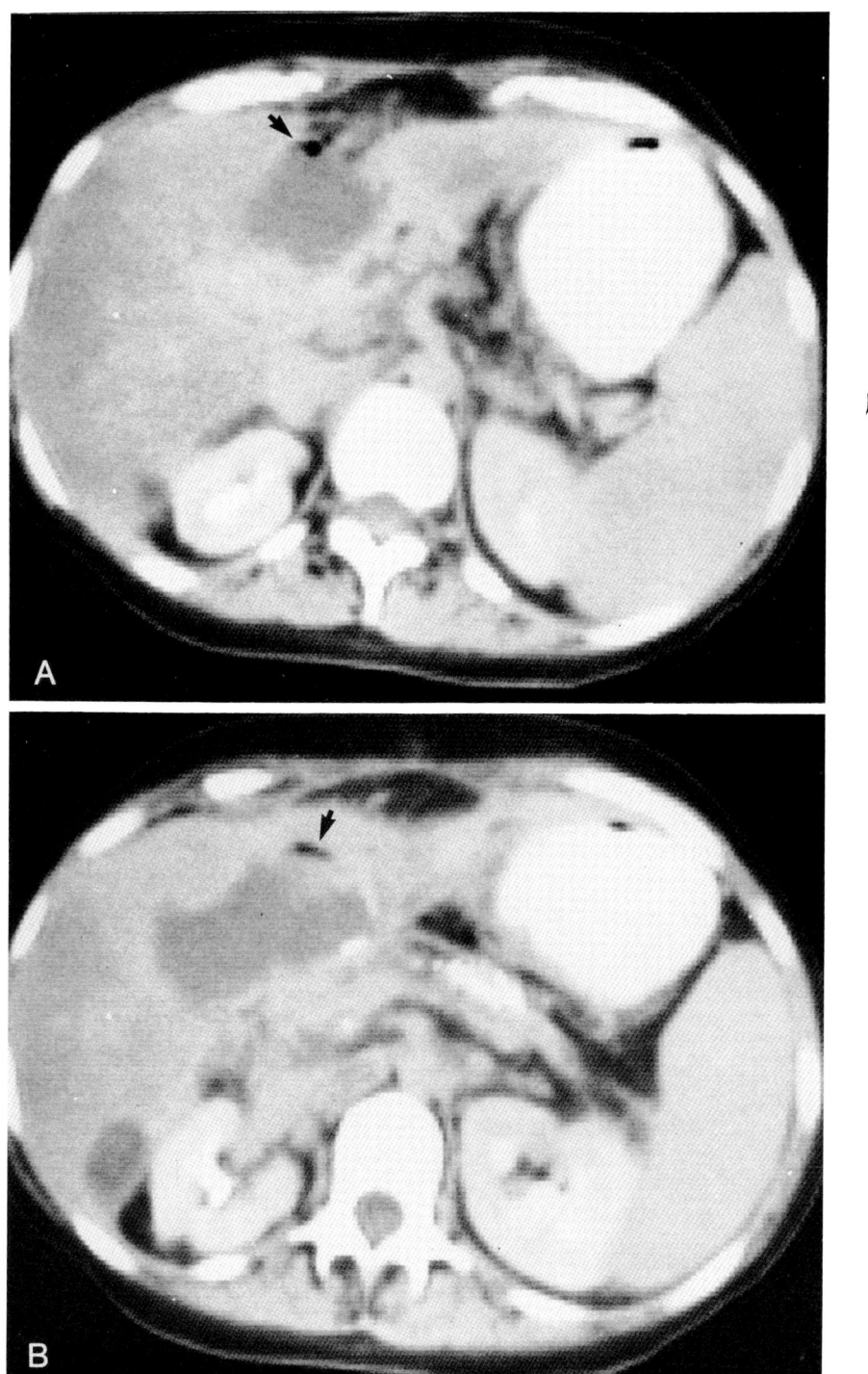

FIGURE 21.53. PANCREATIC ABSCESS
A and *B:* Apparently intrahepatic pancreatic abscess. CT shows an irregular fluid collection containing a small amount of gas (*arrow*). The patient had chronic alcoholic pancreatitis and probably spontaneous infection of a pseudocyst, which had dissected into a recess of the lesser sac. Note splenomegaly from splenic vein thrombosis.

REFERENCES

1. Frey CF, Lindenauer SM, Miller TA: Pancreatic abscess. *Surg Gynecol Obstet* 149:722–726, 1979.
2. Woodard S, Kelvin FM, Rice RP, Thompson WM: Pancreatic abscess: importance of conventional radiology. *AJR* 136:871–878, 1981.
3. Meyers MA: *Dynamic Radiology of the Abdomen. Normal and Pathologic Anatomy.* New York, Springer-Verlag, 1976, pp 265–277.
4. Alexander ES, Clark RA, Federle MP: Pancreatic gas: indication of pancreatic fistula. *AJR* 139:1089–1094, 1982.
5. Torres WE, Clements JL, Sones PJ, Knopf DR: Gas in the pancreatic bed without abscess. *AJR* 137:1131–1133, 1981.
6. Ranson JHC. Acute pancreatitis. *Curr Probl Surg* 16:5–83, 1979.
7. Warshaw AL: Inflammatory masses following acute pancreatitis: phlegmon, pseudocyst and abscess. *Surg Clin North Am* 54:621–635, 1974.
8. Hill MC, Dach JL, Barkin J, Isikoff MB, Morse B: The role of percutaneous aspiration in the diagnosis of pancreatic abscess. *AJR* 141:1035–1038, 1983.
9. Hill MC, Sanders RC: Gray Scale B scan characteristics of intraabdominal cystic masses. *J Clin Ultrasound* 6:217–222, 1978.
10. Kessel HY, Filly RA: Ultrasonographic appearance of gas containing abscesses in the abdomen. *AJR* 130:71–73, 1978.
11. Federle MP, Jeffrey RB, Crass RA, Dalsem VV: Computed tomography of pancreatic abscesses. *AJR* 136:879–881, 1981.
12. Mendez G, Isikoff MB: Significance of intrapancreatic gas demonstrated by CT: a review of nine cases. *AJR* 132:59–62, 1979.
13. Petruschak MJ, Haaga JR, Pardes J: CT demonstration of spontaneous internal drainage of a pancreatic pseudocyst. *Comput Tomogr* 5:534–536, 1981.
14. Karlson KB, Martin EC, Frankuchen EI, Mattern RF, Schultz RW, Casarella WJ: Percutaneous drainage of pancreatic pseudocysts and abscesses. *Radiology* 142:619–624, 1982.
15. Evans WK, Ho CS, McLoughlin MJ, Tao LC: Fatal necrotizing pancreatitis following fine needle aspiration biopsy of the pancreas. *Radiology* 141:61–62, 1981.
16. Pelaez JC, Hill MC, Dach JL, Isikoff MB, Morse B: Abdominal aspiration biopsies: sonographic vs. computed tomography guidance. *JAMA* 250:2663–2666, 1983.

Pancreatic Fistula

Chest

Pancreaticopleural fistulas present with cough, shortness of breath, and chest pain, often without abdominal pain (1–3). This complication should be suspected when pleural effusion persists after other manifestations of pancreatitis have subsided and when the amylase level in the effusion is extremely high. The fistulous track usually is through the aortic or esophageal hiatus into the mediastinum and then into the pleural cavity (1). Pericardial or bronchial involvement can occur. The fistulous track can be opacified by ERCP or contrast injection into the pleural space, but ERCP has failed to demonstrate a fistula in surgically proven cases (1–4). Treatment is usually surgical but low-dose radiotherapy to the pancreatic bed has been successfully employed (1).

Abdomen

Pancreatic-enteric fistulas occur late in the course of pancreatitis either from decompression of a pseudocyst or as a complication of phlegmonous pancreatitis (5). Although patients with spontaneous pseudocyst rupture into bowel may

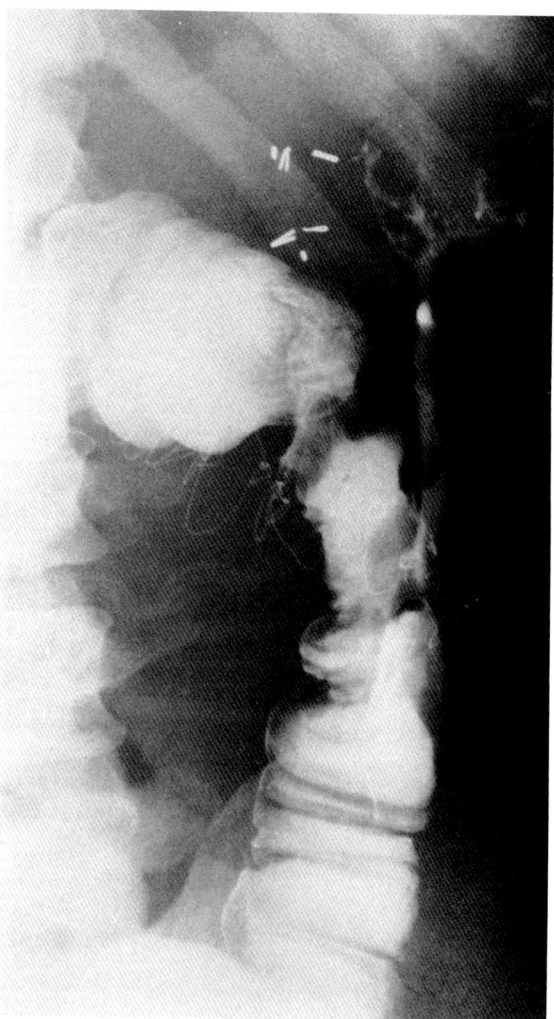

FIGURE 21.54. PANCREATICOCOLONIC FISTULA: BARIUM ENEMA

Pancreaticocolonic fistula developing a month after an attack of acute alcoholic pancreatitis. A left subphrenic abscess resulted. The fistula probably came from drainage of a pancreatic fluid collection into the colon.

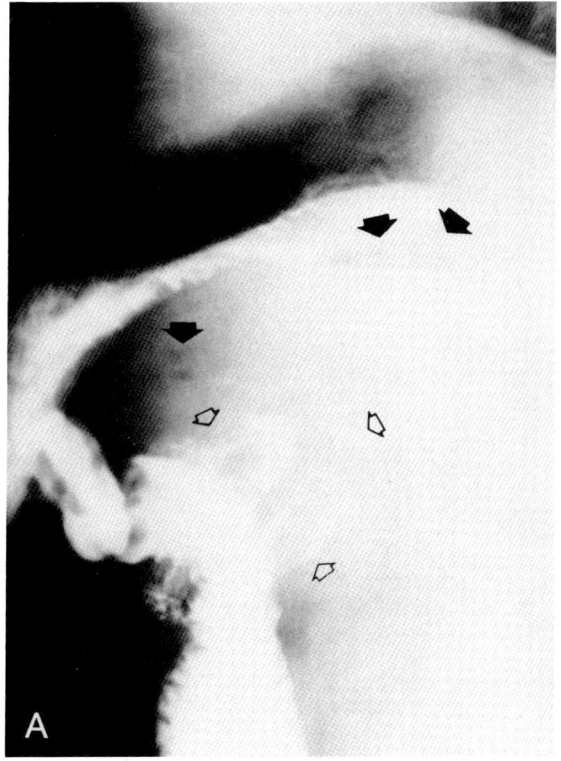
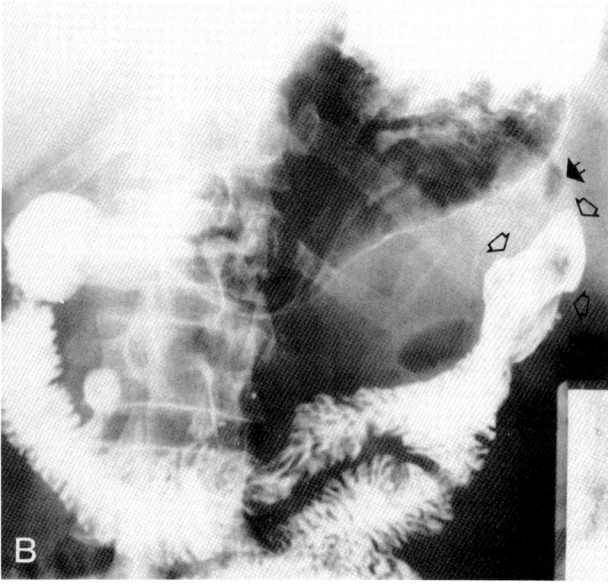

FIGURE 21.55. PANCREATIC FISTULA
A and *B:* Pancreaticoenteric fistula. Frontal and erect lateral films from an UGI demonstrate contrast extravasation from the proximal jejunum (*open arrows*). Communication with the lesser sac abscess (air-fluid level and bubbles, closed arrows) was shown at surgery. Probably spontaneous pseudocyst rupture.

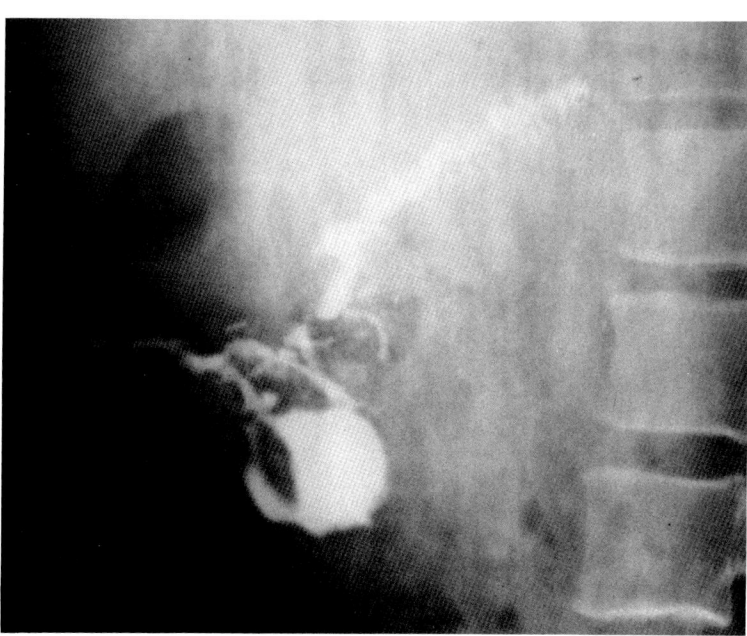

FIGURE 21.56. PANCREATICOCUTANEOUS FISTULA
Fistulogram from anterior abdominal wall demonstrates abscess cavity and pancreatic duct.

actually improve clinically as a result of decompression, the decompression may be incomplete. Signs and symptoms of a fistula may then develop, including diarrhea, fever, and hematochezia (4, 5). Vessels in the bowel wall may be eroded leading to gastrointestinal bleeding which can be exsanguinating (6). The fistula also serves as a pathway for intestinal bacteria and can cause a pancreatic abscess (4). Pancreatic-enteric fistula most often affects the colon in the region of the anatomic splenic flexure (Fig. 21.54). Other areas of the colon, the stomach, esophagus, duodenum, small bowel, skin, and peritoneal cavity are less frequently involved (Figs. 21.55 and 21.56). A pancreatic fistula into the peritoneal cavity results in pancreatic ascites (1, 5).

Radiology

Pancreatic-enteric fistulas must be specifically suspected and sought in order to be radiographically detected. However, in one series, even with appropriate gastrointestinal contrast studies, 20% of fistulas were detected only at surgery (1). ERCP will detect some but probably not all fistulas in patients with pancreatic ascites. A fistula can be recognized on CT by the presence of oral contrast material with or without gas in a peripancreatic phlegmon. Sometimes gas is seen without oral contrast. CT performed without oral contrast after ERCP may give the best delineation of a fistula in selected cases.

Treatment

Fistulas due to pseudocyst rupture into bowel other than colon may be large enough to afford complete decompression (1). If hemorrhage or infection do not develop and the fistula closes, surgery can be avoided. Pancreaticocolonic fistulas are nearly always treated with diverting colostomy because of their great tendency toward hemorrhage and sepsis (1).

REFERENCES

1. Greenwald RA, Deluca RF, Raskin JB: Pancreatic-pleural fistula. Demonstration by ERCP and successful treatment with radiation therapy. *Dig Dis Sci* 24:240–244, 1979.
2. Razzaque MA, Hussain SA, Hossain Z, Kumar CK: Pleural effusion with pancreatico-pleural fistula. *Am J Gastroenterol* 68:84–87, 1977.
3. McKenna JM, Chandrasekhar AJ, Skorton D et al: The pleuropulmonary complications of pancreatitis. *Chest* 71:197–204, 1977.
4. Alsumait AR, Jabbari M, Goresky CA: Pancreaticocolonic fistula: a complication of pancreatitis. *J Can Med Assoc* 119:715–719, 1978.
5. Alexander ES, Clark RA, Federle MP: Pancreatic gas: indication of pancreatic fistula. *AJR* 139:1089–1094, 1982.
6. Dallemand S, Farman J, Stein D, Waxman M, Mitchell W: Colonic necrosis complicating pancreatitis. *Gastrointest Radiol* 2:27–30, 1977.

PANCREATIC PSEUDOCYST

Pancreatic/peripancreatic fluid collections occur due to rupture of an obstructed pancreatic duct. The pancreatic juice that escapes may collect within the pancreas itself; however, due to the absence of a pancreatic capsule, it usually escapes into the adjacent tissues especially into the area of the lesser sac (1–3). This escape of fluid from the gland is probably helpful because if the pancreas had a capsule which retained the fluid, the gland would digest itself. The contents are composed not only of pancreatic juice but also necrotic cellular debris and blood. When the wall of the fluid collection matures, which usually takes about 6 weeks, it is composed of fibrous tissue and is termed a pseudocyst to distinguish it from a true cyst of the pancreas which is lined by epithelium (1). Only 10% of patients with acute pancreatitis develop a pseudocyst which is usually single, round to oval in shape, and can be either small or quite large (4).

Clinical Findings

A pancreatic pseudocyst can appear within a couple of days and can also spontaneously decompress itself by rupturing into either the pancreatic duct, adjacent portion of the gastrointestinal tract usually the stomach or into the common bile duct (5–7). This is believed to occur in approximately 20–30% of cases and usually occurs in 6–8 weeks (5, 8, 9). Factors mitigating against spontaneous resolution include a cyst larger than 5–6 cm, increasing size on serial sonograms, and the presence of multiple cysts (10). If left alone, complications occur (40%) including rupture into the peritoneal space, hemorrhage, and infection (5). Other than the common sites (colon, duodenum, pancreatic duct, stomach, and esophagus) rupture can occur into the pleural cavity, bronchus, neck, aorta, splenic artery, and portal vein (11). Rupture occurs due to the combined effects of enzymatic digestion, pressure necrosis, and vascular ischemia.

A bowel obstruction can occur due to the intramural extension of a pseudocyst between the serosa and muscularis or between the muscularis and mucosa. Sites of involvement can include the stomach, small bowel especially the duodenum, and the colon (5, 12). Pseudocysts can be found anywhere within the abdomen and can dissect up into the mediastinum or into the small bowel mesentery or down the retroperitoneum into the pelvis (see Fig. 21.65) (2, 13). They can also dissect into the parenchyma of the liver, spleen, and kidney and mimic a cyst of these organs (2, 4, 12, 14–17).

The success rate of surgery for pancreatic pseudocysts varies from 16 to 80% (3, 18). They have been treated with a varying degree of success by percutaneous aspiration; however, more than one aspiration may have to be performed (19, 20). To be successful, the pseudocyst should be present for at least 6 weeks prior to aspiration (3). The success rate is greater with percutaneous aspiration if the pseudocyst has a low amylase level and is not contiguous to the pancreas (19). It is less successful in the treatment of pseudocyst of the lesser sac. Another alternative to percutaneous aspiration is percutaneous transgastric drainage with an indwelling catheter that is only removed when drainage has ceased and the fluid collection has disappeared on sonography or CT (21). Another approach that has recently been advocated by Bernardino is percutaneous insertion of a stent between a pseudocyst and the stomach when they abut each other (22). The stent is left in place and is removed endoscopically only when complete drainage of the pseudocyst has occurred as indicated by CT. This technique needs further study to determine its rate of complications before its widespread use can be advocated (22). If a surgical approach is being contemplated, a repeat sonogram should be performed immediately prior to operating to confirm that the pseudocyst is still present and has not spontaneously decompressed itself.

REFERENCES

1. Robbins SL, Cotran RS: The pancreas. In *Pathological Basis of Disease*, Ed. 2, Philadelphia, W. B. Saunders, 1979, pp 1092–1114.
2. Siegelman SS, Copeland BE, Saba GP, Cameron JL, Sanders RC, Zerhouni E: CT of fluid collections associated with pancreatitis. *AJR* 134:1121–1132, 1980.
3. Warshaw AL: Inflammatory masses following acute pancreatitis: phlegmon, pseudocyst and abscess. *Surg Clin North Am* 54:621–635, 1974.
4. Laing FC, Gooding GAW, Brown T, Leopold GR: Atypical pseudocysts of the pancreas: an ultrasonographic evaluation. *Clin Ultrasound* 7:27–33, 1979.
5. Bradley EL, Clements JL: Spontaneous resolution of pancreatic pseudocyst: implications for timing of operative intervention. *Am J Surg* 129:23–28, 1975.
6. DeVanna T, Dunne MG, Haney PJ: Fistulous communication of pseudocyst to the common bile duct: a complication of pancreatitis. *Pediatr Radiol* 13:344–345, 1983.
7. Sarti DA: Rapid development and spontaneous regression of pancreatic pseudocysts documented by ultrasound. *Radiology* 125:789–793, 1977.
8. Bradley EL, Gonzales AC, Clements JL: Acute pancreatic pseudocysts: incidence and implications. *Ann Surg* 184:734;737, 1976.
9. Gonzalez AC, Bradley EL, Clements JL: Pseudocyst formation in acute pancreatitis: ultrasonographic evaluation of 99 cases. *AJR* 127:315–317, 1976.
10. Aranha GV, Prinz RA, Esguerra AC, Greenlee HB: The nature and course of cystic pancreatic lesions diagnosed by ultrasound. *Arch Surg* 118:486–488, 1983.
11. Clements JL Jr, Bradley EL III, Eaton SB Jr: Spontaneous internal drainage of pancreatic pseudocysts. *AJR* 126:985–991, 1976.
12. Bellon EM, George CR, Schreiber H, Marshall JB: Pancreatic pseudocysts of the duodenum. *AJR* 133:827–831, 1979.
13. Gooding GAW: Pseudocyst of the pancreas with mediastinal extension: an ultrasonographic demonstration. *J Clin Ultrasound* 5:121–123, 1977.
14. Baker MK, Kopecky KK, Wass JL: Perirenal pancreatic pseudocysts: diagnostic management. *AJR* 140:729–732, 1983.
15. DeGraaff CS, Taylor KJW, Rosenfield AT, Kinder B: Gray scale ultrasonography in the diagnosis of pseudocysts of the pancreas simulating renal pathology. *J Urol* 120:751–753, 1978.
16. Conrad MR, Landay MJ, Khoury M: Pancreatic pseudocysts: unusual ultrasound features. *AJR* 130:265–268, 1978.
17. Vick CW, Simeone JF, Ferrucci JT, Wittenberg J, Mueller PR: Pancreatitis associated fluid collection involving the spleen: sonographic and computed tomographic appearance. *Gastrointest Radiol* 6:247–250, 1981.
18. Ranson JHC: Acute pancreatitis. *Curr Probl Surg* 16:5–83, 1979.
19. Barkin JS, Smith FR, Pereiras R, Isikoff M, Levi J, Livingston A, Hill MC, Rogers AI: Therapeutic percutaneous aspiration of pancreatic pseudocysts. *Dig Dis Sci* 26:585–586, 1981.
20. MacErlean DP, Bryan PJ, Murphy JJ: Pancreatic pseudocyst: management of ultrasonically guided aspiration. *Gastrointest Radiol* 5:255–257, 1980.
21. Ho CS, Taylor B: Percutaneous transgastric drainage for pancreatic pseudocyst. *AJR* 143:623–635, 1984.
22. Bernardino ME, Amerson JR: Percutaneous gastrocystostomy: a new approach to pancreatic pseudocyst drainage. *AJR* 143:1096–1097, 1984.

Radiology

Plain Films

Abdomen. Pancreatic calcification is present in 10–20% of pseudocysts and almost always represents pancreatic lithiasis. Displacement of calcification may indicate a pseudocyst (Fig. 21.57). Rare cases of cyst wall calcification exist (Fig. 21.58) (1). Soft tissue masses can be detected when pseudocysts are sufficiently large (Fig. 21.59).

Chest. Mediastinal pseudocysts present with chest or abdominal pain and dyspnea (2). Approximately three-fourths occur in the posterior mediastinum and pleural effusion is usually pres-

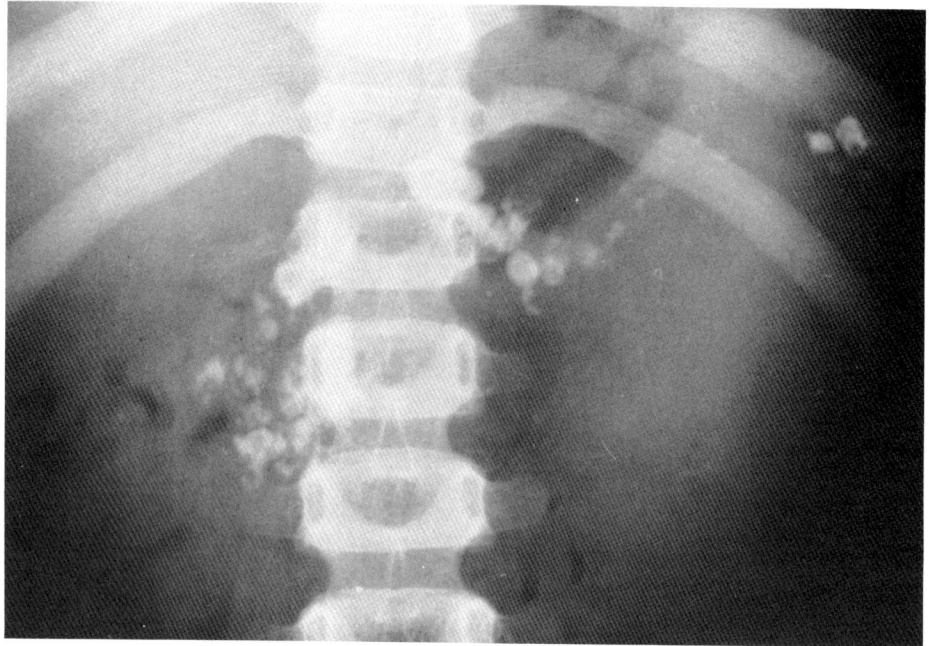

FIGURE 21.57. PANCREATIC PSEUDOCYST
Left upper quadrant soft tissue mass displacing the calculations in the tail of the pancreas.

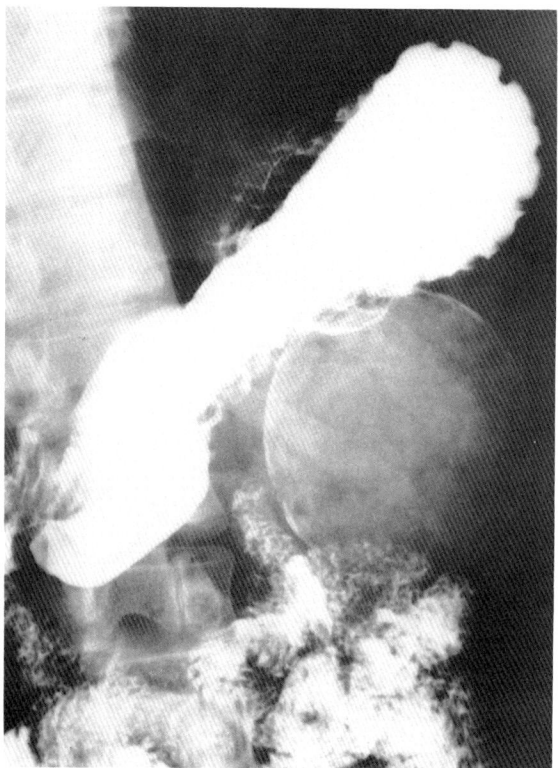

FIGURE 21.58. CALCIFIED PANCREATIC PSEUDOCYST
The calcification is entirely in the wall.

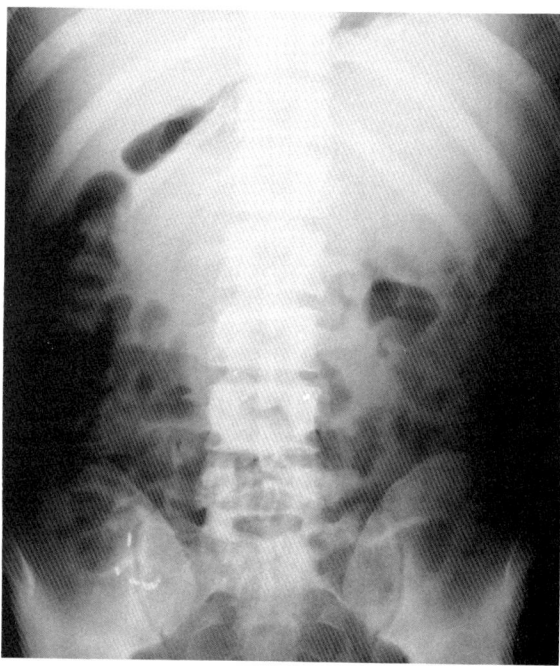

FIGURE 21.59. PANCREATIC PSEUDOCYST
Pseudocysts in the head and tail of the pancreas depicted as soft tissue masses displacing stomach, duodenum, and colon.

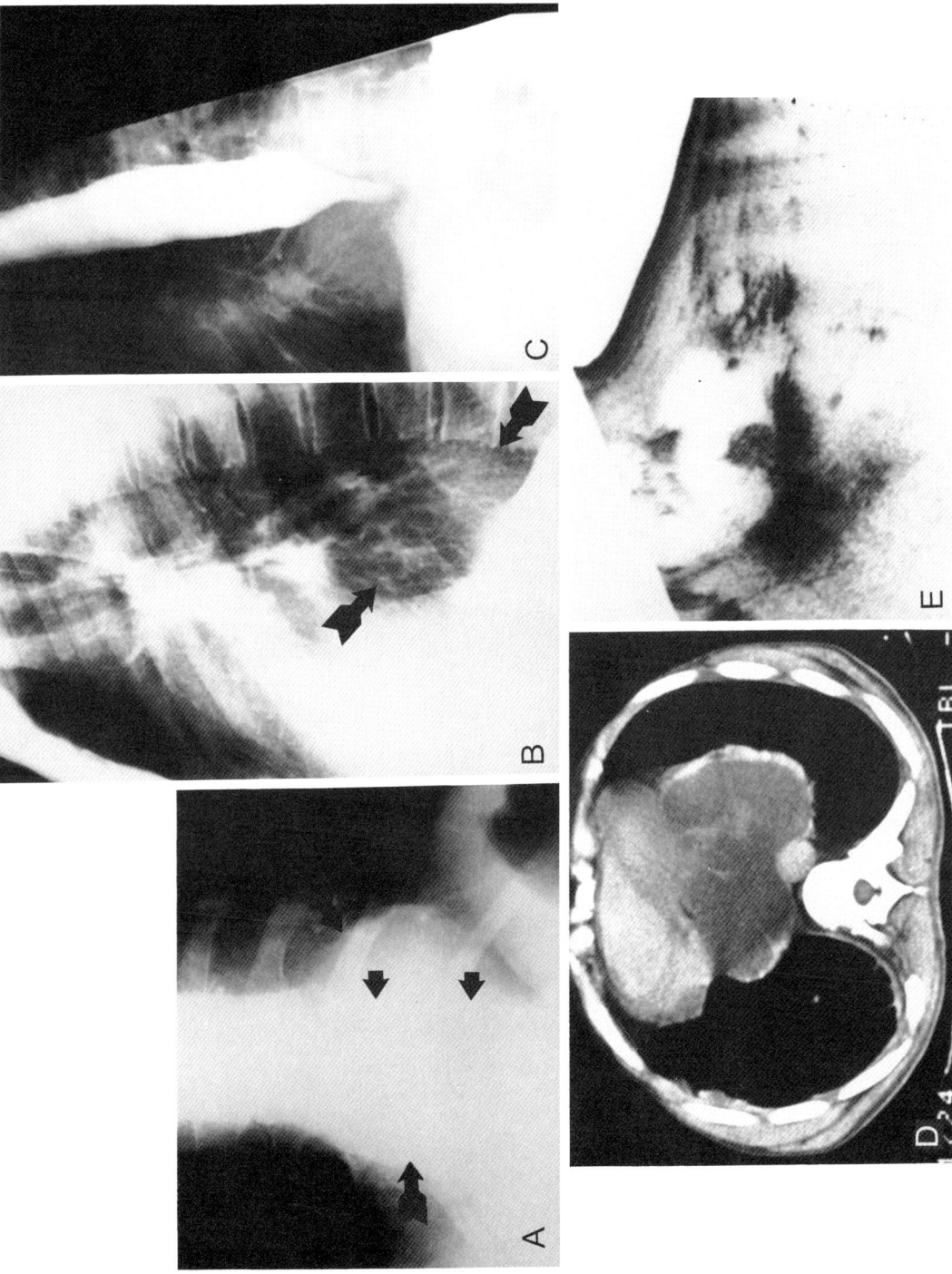

FIGURE 21.60. MEDIASTINAL PSEUDOCYST

A and *B*: Posteroanterior and lateral chest x-rays showing a middle mediastinal mass (*large arrows*) due to a pseudocyst. The left paraspinal line was widened from pleural effusion (*small arrows*, not well shown). *C–E*: Second mediastinal pseudocyst. *C*: Esophagram shows smooth narrowing of the distal esophagus and a surrounding mass. *D*: CT shows the retrocardiac pseudocyst with an enhancing rind and septa. *E*: Septations and nodularity within the pseudocyst are seen on sagittal sonography. (Courtesy of Bruce E. Rubin, M.D., Holy Cross Hospital, Silver Spring, Md.)

FIGURE 21.61. PANCREATIC PSEUDOCYST
Smooth upward displacement of the antrum by a pancreatic pseudocyst.

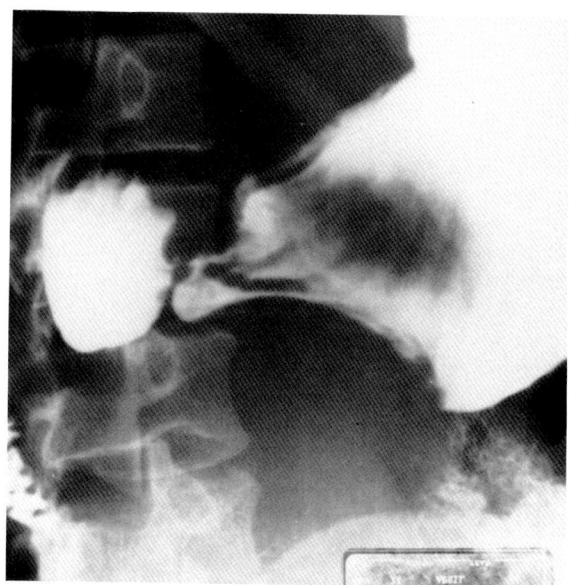

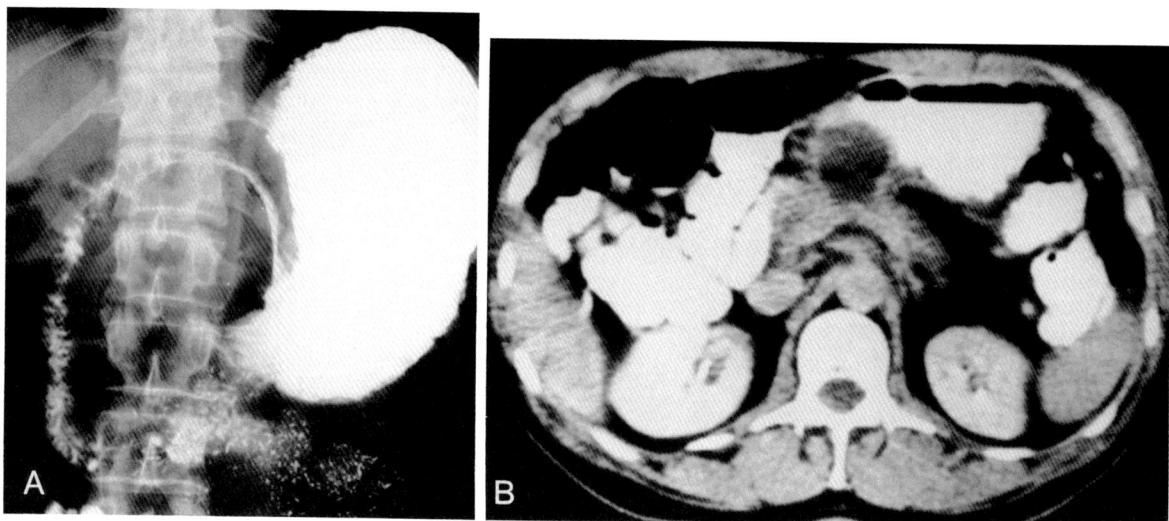

FIGURE 21.62. PANCREATIC PSEUDOCYST
A: Marked elevation and narrowing of the antrum and proximal duodenum by a pseudocyst. Note acute angles suggesting an intragastric mass. *B:* CT of the same patient showing a pseudocyst arising in the body of the pancreas extending into the wall of the stomach.

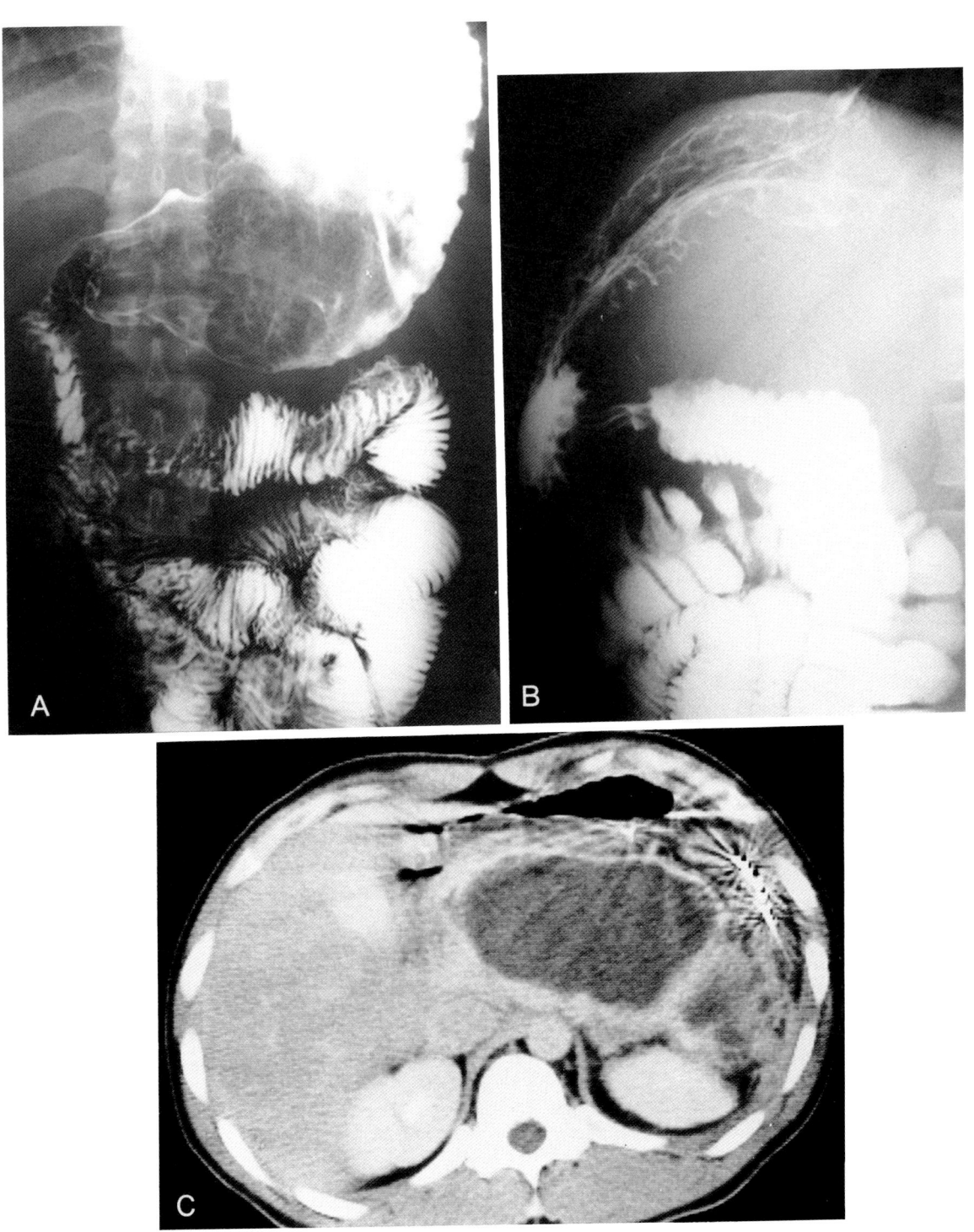

FIGURE 21.63. PANCREATIC PSEUDOCYST
A and *B:* Large pseudocyst. Frontal and lateral films from an UGI showing a large retrogastric space and thickened posterior gastric folds. There is fold thickening in the transverse duodenum and at the duodenojejunal junction, which is displaced inferiorly. *C:* Corresponding CT scan showing a huge pseudocyst flattening the stomach against the anterior abdominal wall. There is mild contrast enhancement of the wall of the pseudocyst.

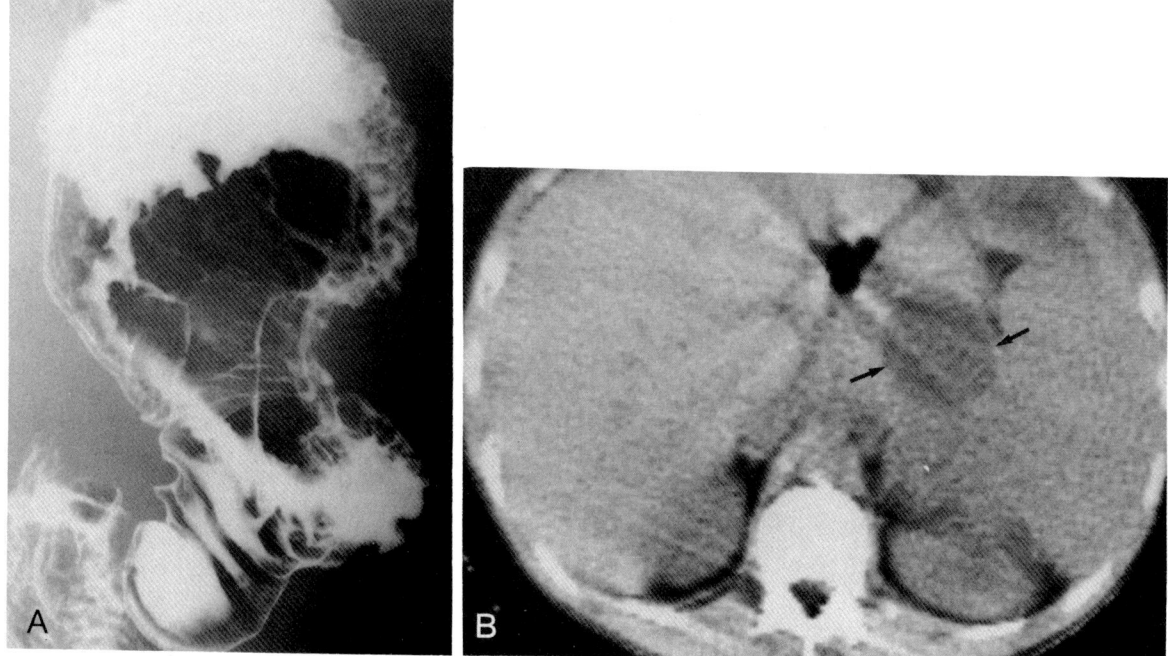

FIGURE 21.64. PANCREATIC PSEUDOCYST
A: Huge gastric folds and marked contour distortion caused by a pancreatic pseudocyst mimicking gastric lymphoma or carcinoma. *B:* Corresponding CT showing a pseudocyst arising from the tail of the pancreas (*arrows*). Note the enlarged spleen, probably from splenic vein obstruction.

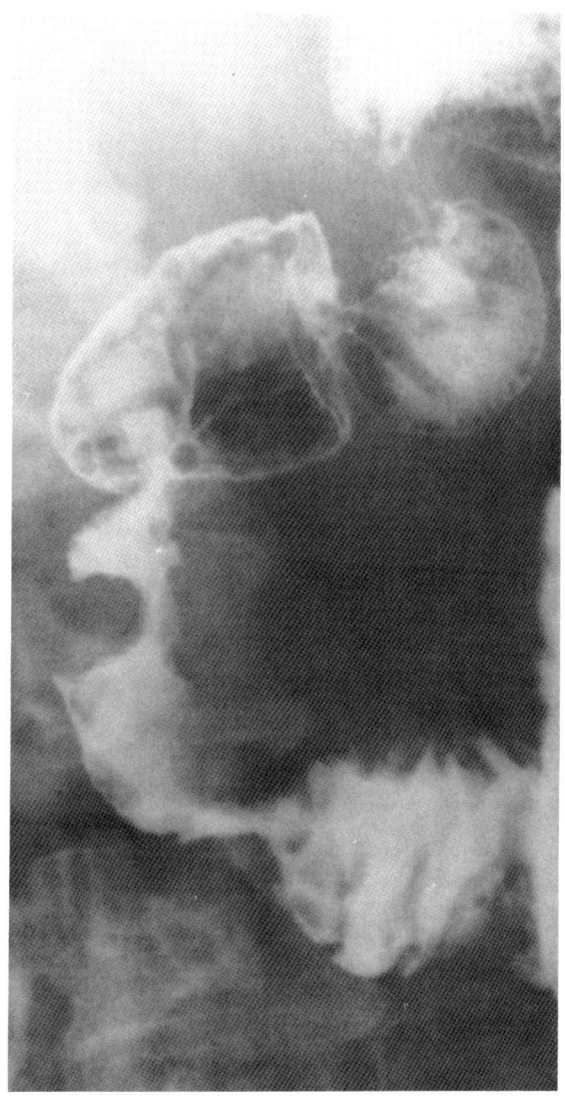

FIGURE 21.65. PANCREATIC PSEUDOCYST
Marked narrowing and distortion with fold effacement in the descending duodenum caused by a pancreatic pseudocyst.

concommitant retrogastric mass (Fig. 21.60) (1, 2).

Stomach and Duodenum. Extrinsic indentation of the posterior stomach or inner duodenal sweep is seen in 80–85% of pancreatic pseudocysts (1). Those in the region of the body of the pancreas indent the body of the stomach and those near the head widen the duodenal sweep (Figs. 21.61–21.65) (1). The duodenojejunal junction is sometimes pushed down by pseudocysts of the tail (Fig. 21.63) (3). Although the mass effect of pseudocysts is often smoothly contoured, mural irregularity and fold thickening is not uncommon (Figs. 21.61–21.65).

Colon. About 40% of pseudocysts indent or displace the splenic flexure or the transverse colon. The mass effect is usually smoothly contoured, but stenosis and/or mucosal irregularity can occur (Fig. 21.66) (1).

ent (Fig. 21.60) (1, 2). Portals of entry into the mediastinum, in descending order of frequency, are the esophageal and aortic hiatuses, the foramen of Morgagni, and erosion through the diaphragm (2).

Barium Contrast Examinations

Esophagus. Mediastinal pseudocysts typically displace the lower esophagus anterolaterally with or without a long, smoothly tapered narrowing (1, 2). There may or may not be a

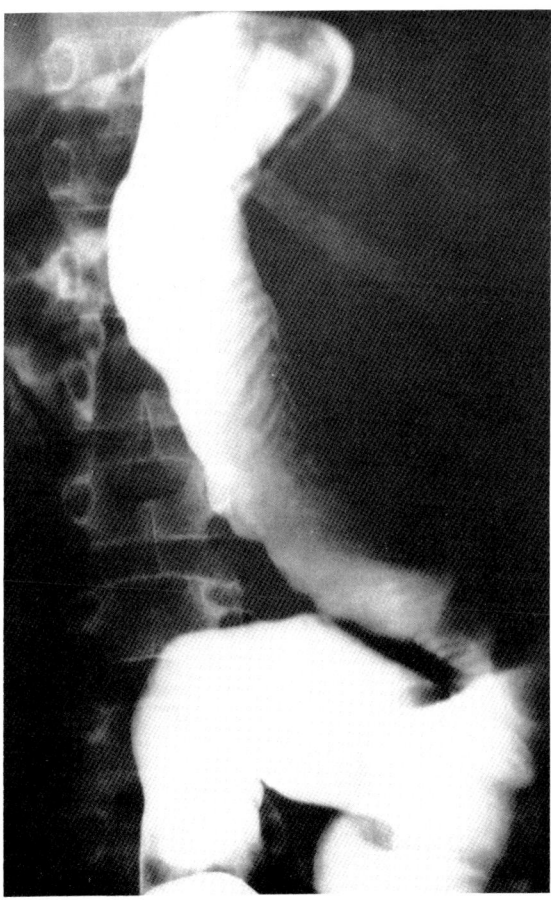

FIGURE 21.66. PANCREATIC PSEUDOCYST
Barium enema showing medial displacement of the splenic flexure and descending colon by a pseudocyst arising in the tail of the pancreas.

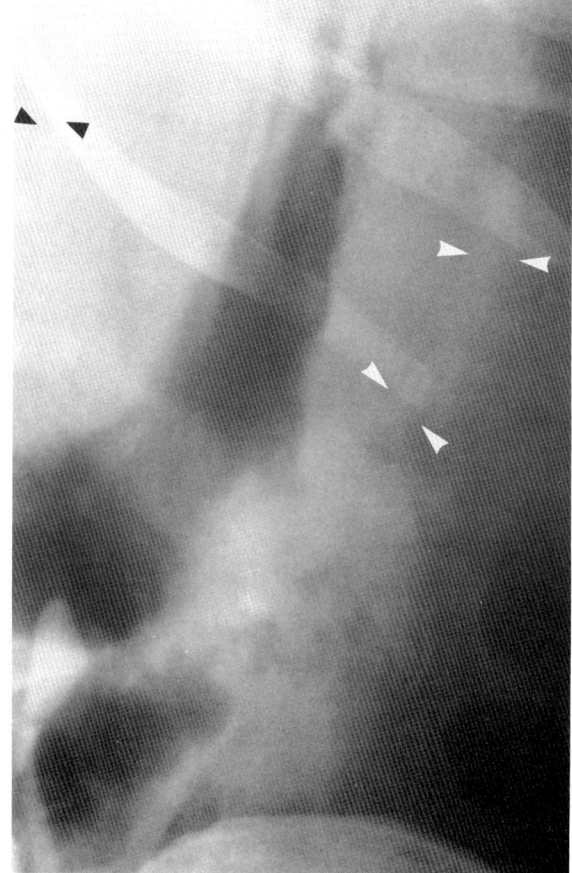

FIGURE 21.67. PANCREATIC PSEUDOCYST
Excretory urogram demonstrating a thick-walled cystic appearing left suprarenal mass (*arrowheads*). Pseudocyst of the tail.

Excretory Urography

Patients with pancreatic pseudocyst can present with back pain and hematuria secondary to involvement of the perirenal space, usually on the left (Figs. 21.67 and 21.68) (4). It is often difficult to discern the extrarenal origin of perirenal pseudocysts because they may become intimately adherent to or even invade the kidney (Fig. 21.68) (1). Their appearance on excretory uroraphy is that of a mass splaying but not invading the collecting system (1). Tomography will demonstrate central lucency and a thick wall by virtue of the total body opacification effect (Fig. 21.67) (5). Differential diagnosis includes necrotic hypernephroma and infected or hemorrhagic cyst (4). Rarely, pseudocysts spread to the pelvis by descending anterior to the spine and they can produce ureteral displacement, compression or hydronephrosis (1), and/or present as a pelvic mass (Fig. 21.69).

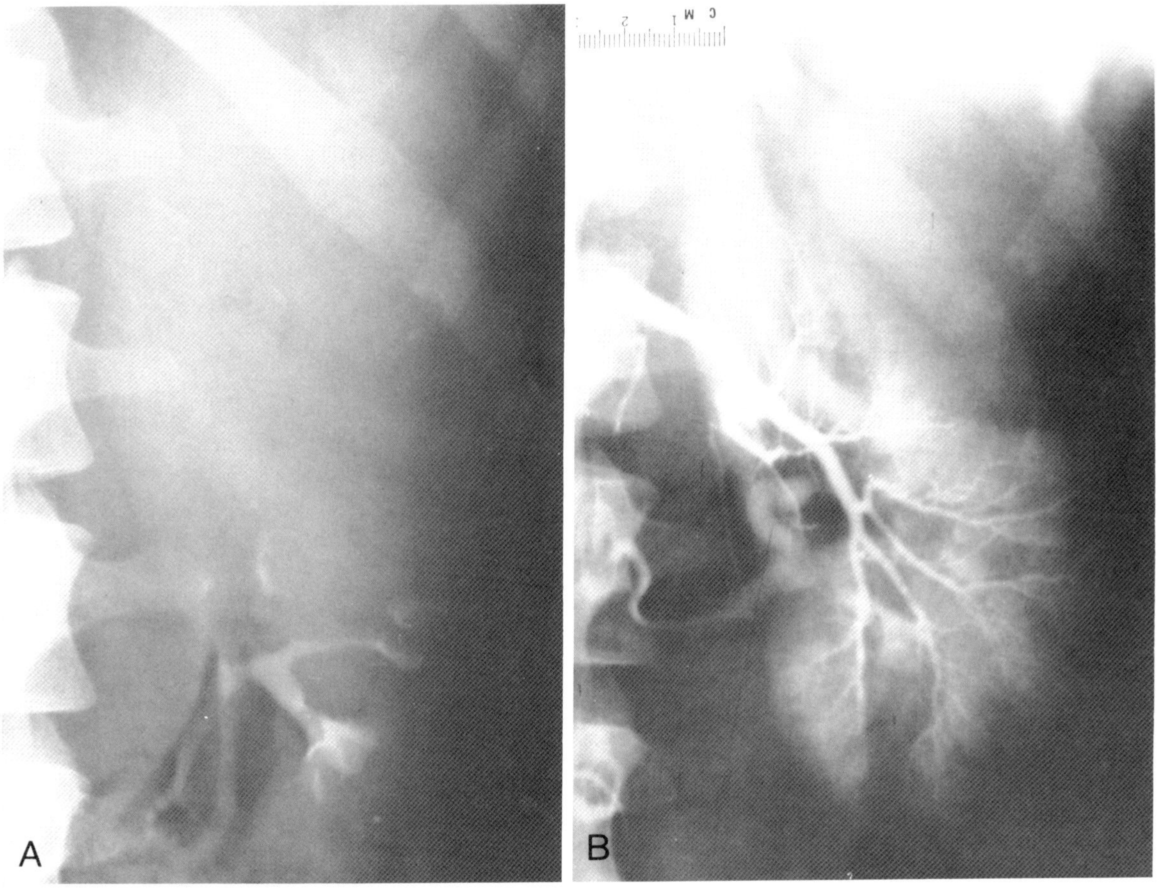

FIGURE 21.68. PANCREATIC PSEUDOCYST
A: Excretory urogram showing a large mass in the upper pole of the left kidney. *B:* Left renal arteriogram demonstrating the mass to be avascular. Surgery revealed an intrarenal pancreatic pseudocyst.

FIGURE 21.69. PANCREATIC PSEUDOCYST
Large pseudocyst obstructing the right ureter.

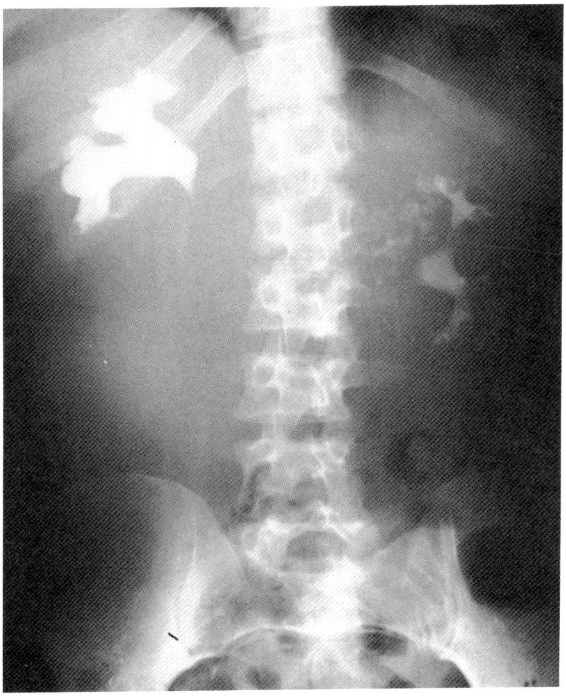

REFERENCES

1. Eaton SB, Ferrucci JT: *Radiology of the Pancreas and Duodenum.* Philadelphia, W. B. Saunders, 1979, pp 20–24, 359–368.
2. Kirchner SG, Heller RM, Smith CW: Pancreatic pseudocyst of the mediastinum. *Radiology* 123:37–42, 1977.
3. Bruna J: A contribution to the roentgenologic diagnostics of pancreatic pseudocysts in children. *Radiol Diagn* 19:723–729, 1978.
4. Davis S, Parbhoo SP, Gibson MJ: The plain abdominal radiograph in acute pancreatitis. *Clin Radiol* 31:87–93, 1980.
5. Morin ME, Marsan RE, Baker DA: Pseudocysts: diagnosis in the adult by total body opacification. *Clin Radiol* 28:229–232, 1977.

Sonography and Computed Tomography

Pseudocysts of the head and body of the pancreas are usually easily seen sonographically and the former, if large enough, can cause not only obstruction of the pancreatic and common bile ducts but also gastric outlet obstruction. When they are located in the tail of the pancreas, they are more difficult to detect, especially when small. The success rate overall in detecting pseudocysts sonographically varies from 50 to 92% (1–3). One has to be careful not to mistake the fluid-filled stomach for a pseudocyst in the tail of the pancreas. If a diagnostic dilemma exists, the patient can be instructed to drink a small amount of water and if the "cystic" structure is the stomach, micro bubbles of air will be seen with real-time sonography. If the patient has a nasogastric tube in place, a small amount of air or fluid can be injected down the tube (4).

The wall of a pancreatic pseudocyst is generally well-defined and smooth, however, it can be irregular especially when hemorrhage is present (3, 5). The contained fluid can be entirely echo-free or have a varying amount of internal echoes or even a fluid-debris level (Figs. 21.70–21.74). As mentioned previously, when the cyst wall is irregular and the contents are very echogenic, the possibility of superimposed hemorrhage (Fig. 21.73) or infection has to be considered although these findings are not diagnostic (5–7). On occasion septations can occur within a pseudocyst, thus mimicking a mucinous cystic neoplasm (Fig. 21.71) (7). This problem can usually be resolved by the clinical history and the presence of other sonographic findings of inflammatory pancreatic disease. Shadowing in a pseudocyst can occur due to air being present or due to calcification within its wall.

The CT number of the fluid in a pseudocyst varies but in uncomplicated cases it usually is close to 0 HU, however, it can be as high as 25–30 HU. The wall is best identified using IV contrast and is usually smooth and thin (3–4 mm). A thick irregular wall may indicate the presence of hemorrhage or an abscess. Overall, CT is better than sonography in detecting pseudocysts, especially those in the area of the tail of the pancreas (8) as compared to the head and body.

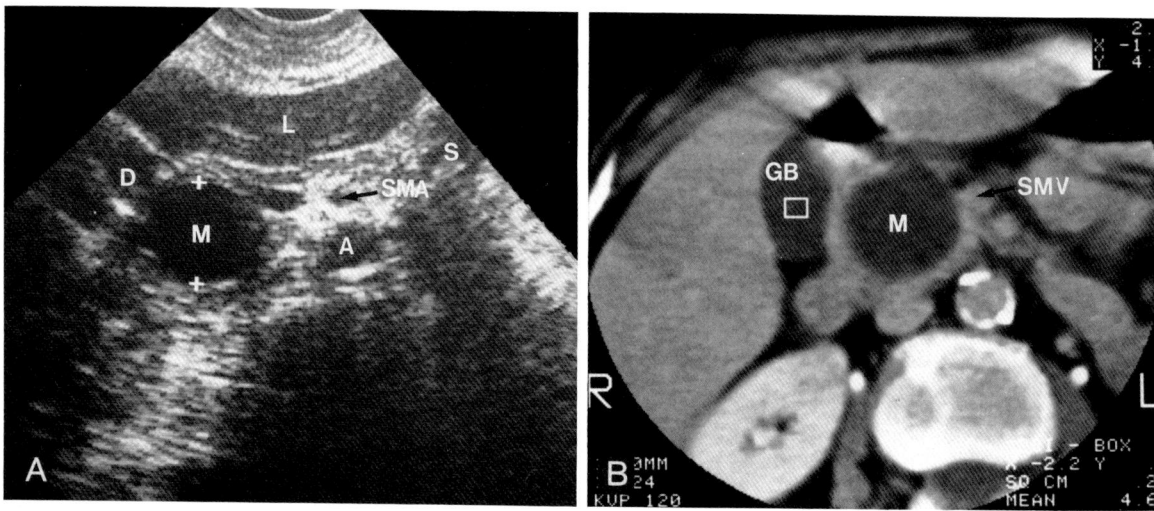

FIGURE 21.70. PANCREATIC PSEUDOCYST
Pseudocyst in the head of the pancreas. *A:* Transverse sonogram reveals a well defined cystic mass in the head of the pancreas. *B:* Corresponding CT scan. Aorta (*A*), superior mesenteric artery (*SMA*), superior mesenteric vein (*SMV*), duodenum (*D*), liver (*L*), stomach (*S*), pseudocyst (*M*), and gallbladder (*GB*).

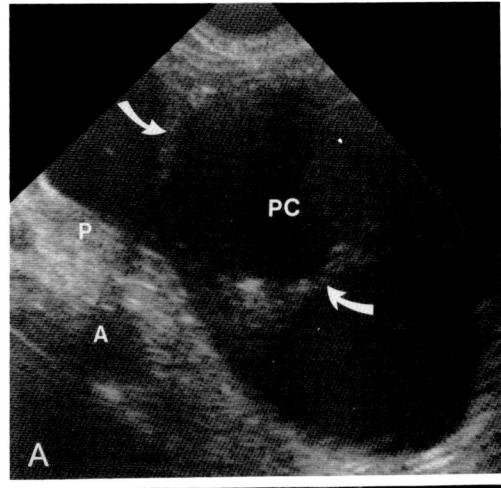
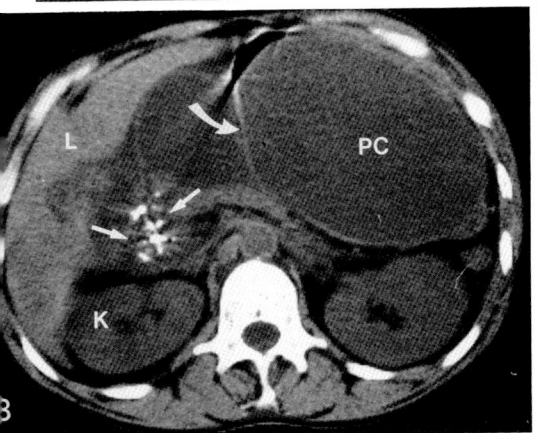
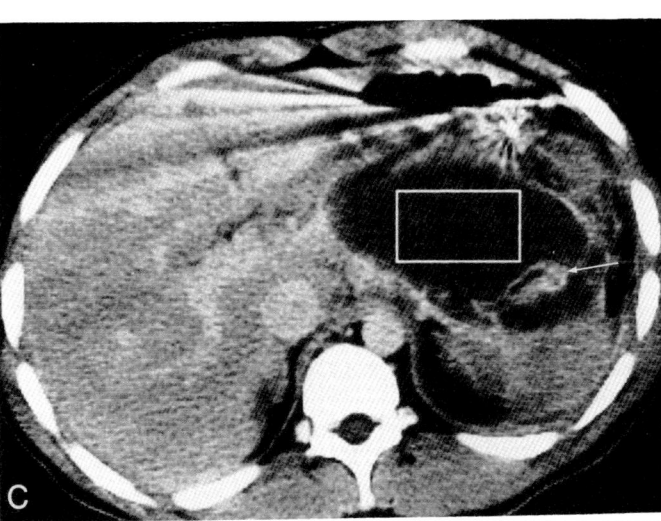
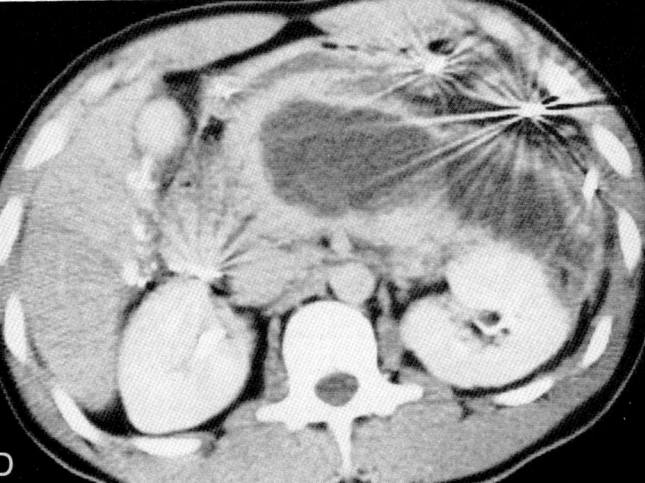
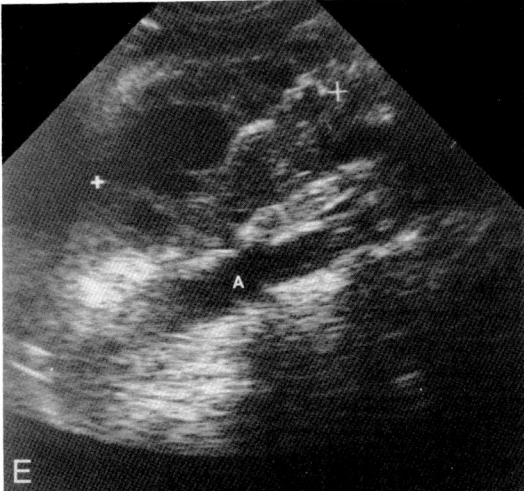

FIGURE 21.71. PANCREATIC PSEUDOCYST

Multiloculated pseudocyst in chronic pancreatitis. *A:* Transverse sonogram of the pancreas demonstrates a large cystic mass (*PC*) with septations (*large arrows*). *B:* Similar findings are present on the CT scan which also reveals irregular punctate calcifications (*small arrows*) in the pancreatic head. Aorta (*A*), pancreas (*P*), liver (*L*), kidney (*K*). *C–E:* Multiloculated, enhancing pseudocyst with internal necrotic debris. *C* and *D:* CT scans showing an enhancing wall and necrotic debris (*arrow*). *E:* Corresponding coronal sonogram shows the complex architecture of this pseudocyst to better advantage (*cursors*). *A* = aorta.

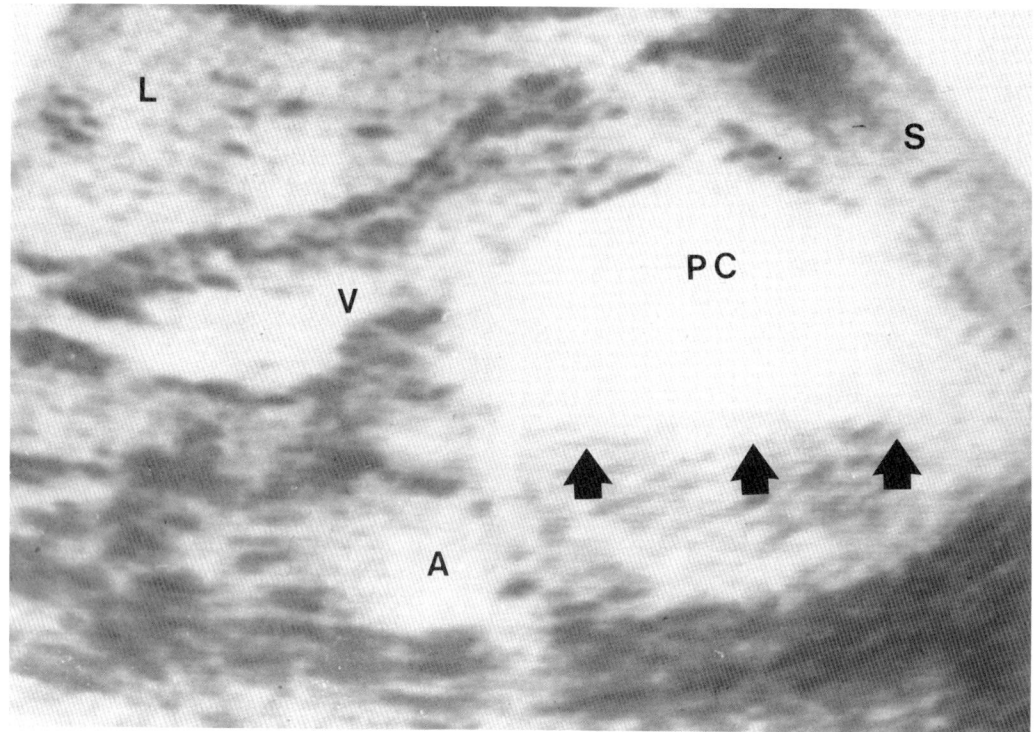

FIGURE 21.72. PANCREATIC PSEUDOCYST
Hemorrhage into a pseudocyst. Proven by percutaneous aspiration using sonographic guidance. Transverse sonogram shown a large, cystic mass (PC) in the tail of the pancreas with a fluid-debris level (arrows). Aorta (A), stomach (S), splenic vein-portal vein confluence (V), and liver (L).

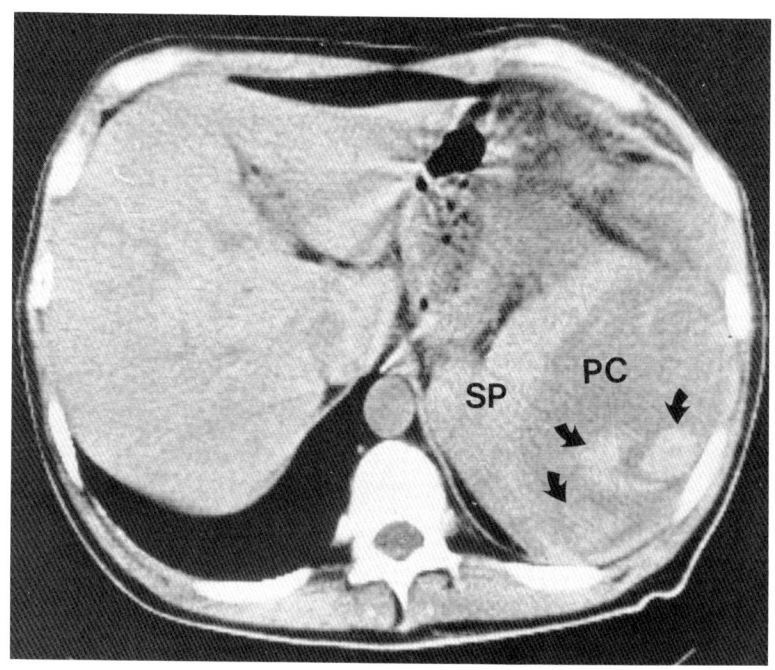

FIGURE 21.73. PANCREATIC PSEUDOCYST
Intrasplenic pseudocyst with hemorrhage. CT scan shows a fluid collection (PC) with high density area (arrows) in the spleen (SP).

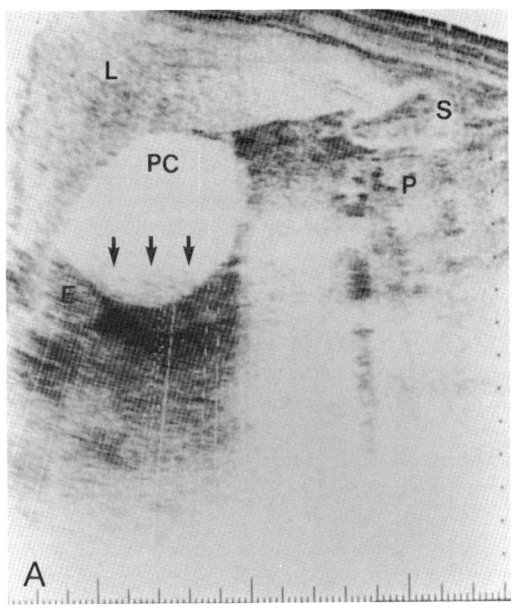 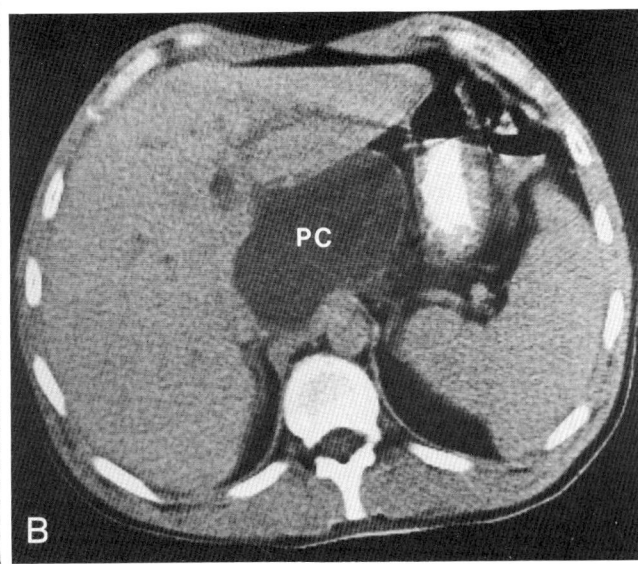

FIGURE 21.74. PANCREATIC PSEUDOCYST

Pseudocyst in chronic pancreatitis. A: Longitudinal sonogram through the left lobe of the liver: well-defined cystic mass with low level dependent echoes (arrows). The calcified body of the pancreas is separate from and inferior to the pseudocyst. B: Corresponding CT through the pseudocyst: sharply marginated thin-walled water density mass. L = liver, S = stomach, E = esophagogastric junction, PC = pseudocyst, P = pancreas.

Pseudocysts usually remain peripancreatic in location but have the ability to dissect to other areas of the abdomen including down the transverse mesocolon to the colon, into the mesentery of the small bowel or sigmoid colon or down the retroperitoneum into the pelvis (Fig. 21.69). They can dissect along the psoas muscle and present as a groin mass. They may also insinuate themselves into the spleen or into the liver especially along the under surface of the left lobe and into the left intersegmental fissure (Fig. 21.53). Dissection may also occur into the chest through the esophageal and the aortic openings of the diaphragm and it can extend up the mediastinum into the neck where it can present as a palpable neck mass. CT is better than sonography in general in evaluating pseudocysts remote from the pancreas (Fig. 21.60).

Pseudocysts are usually single and unilocular but they can be multiple and contain septations and on occasion have calcification in their walls. The presence of septations is not common and when seen, suggests superimposed abscess or hemorrhage. These septations are often better seen sonographically than with CT and if there is any doubt regarding their existence on the CT scan, a sonogram should be performed (Fig. 21.71). When a cystic mass with septation is seen in a patient with no history of alcohol abuse and an otherwise normal-appearing pancreas, then a cystic neoplasm (cystadenoma, cystadenocarcinoma) of the pancreas has to be considered (9, 10). This is especially true if a cyst is present in the area of the pancreatic tail in a young female patient. Other cystic-appearing masses that can simulate a pseudocyst include a fluid-filled loop of bowel or duodenal diverticulum, a choledochocele and an aneurysm of the hepatic or splenic artery. The variant carcinomas of the pancreas can undergo extensive hemorrhage and necrosis and mimic pseudocysts on sonography and CT. This has been reported to occur in ordinary duct cell adenocarcinoma of the pancreas (11), but the reported pathology was not exact.

REFERENCES

1. Gonzalez AC, Bradley EL, Clements JL: Pseudocyst formation in acute pancreatitis: ultrasonographic evaluation of 99 cases. AJR 127:315–317, 1976.
2. Kressel HY, Margulis AR, Gooding GW, Filly RA, Moss AA, Korobkin M: CT scanning and ultrasound in the evaluation of pancreatic pseudocysts: a preliminary comparison. Radiology 126:153–157, 1978.
3. Silverstein W, Isikoff MB, Hill MC, Barkin J: Diagnostic imaging of acute pancreatitis: prospective study using CT and sonography. AJR 137:497–502, 1981.
4. Gooding GAW, Laing FC: Rapid water infusion: a technique in the ultrasonic discrimination of the gas-free

stomach from a mass in the pancreatic tail. *Gastrointest Radiol* 4:139–141, 1979.
5. Hill MC, Sanders RC: Gray scale B scan characteristics of intra-abdominal cystic masses. *J Clin Ultrasound* 6:217–222, 1978.
6. Hill MC, Barkin J, Isikoff MB, Silverstein W, Kalser MH: Acute pancreatitis: clinical versus CT findings. *AJR* 139:263–269, 1982.
7. Laing FC, Gooding GAW, Brown T, Leopold GR: Atypical pseudocysts of the pancreas: an ultrasonographic evaluation. *J Clin Ultrasound* 7:27–33, 1979.
8. Williford ME, Foster WL, Halvorsen RA, Thompson WM: Pancreatic pseudocyst: comparative evaluation by sonography and computed tomography. *AJR* 140:53–57, 1983.
9. Friedman AC, Lichtenstein JE, Dachman AH: Cystic neoplasms of the pancreas. Radiological-pathological correlation. *Radiology* 149:45–50, 1983.
10. Wolfman NT, Ranquist NA, Karstaedt N et al: Cystic neoplasms of the pancreas: CT and sonography. *AJR* 138:37–41, 1982.
11. Kaplan JO, Isikoff MB, Barkin J, Livingston AS: Necrotic carcinoma of the pancreas: "the pseudo-pseudocyst." *J Comput Assist Tomogr* 4:166–167, 1980.

Pancreatography

ERP can be used for the diagnosis of pseudocysts or for preoperative evaluation. Ultrasound and CT are more sensitive in the detection of pseudocysts because roughly one-half of pseudocysts will not be filled by pancreatography (1–4). The risk of infection of a previously sterile pseudocyst during ERP is a relative contraindication. This risk can be diminished by avoiding overfilling and allowing a small amount of contrast material to mix with the cyst contents (5). Pseudocysts usually have a smooth inner wall in contradistinction to the ragged wall of excavated neoplasms or mucinous cystic neoplasms (Figs. 21.75, 21.76, and 21.79), but the occasional case will have a shaggy wall and debris, due to either infection, hemorrhage, or extensive tissue necrosis. Small intrapancreatic pseudocysts are common in chronic pancreatitis and can smoothly displace the pancreatic ducts (Fig. 21.75) (6, 7). If they do not fill, they produce a nonspecific field defect. Pseudocysts can cause main pancreatic duct obstruction (Fig. 21.77), and when they do so without filling, differentiation from neoplasm can be quite difficult (8–10). The terminus is nonspecifically blunt or square in obstruction due to pseudocyst and usually irregular

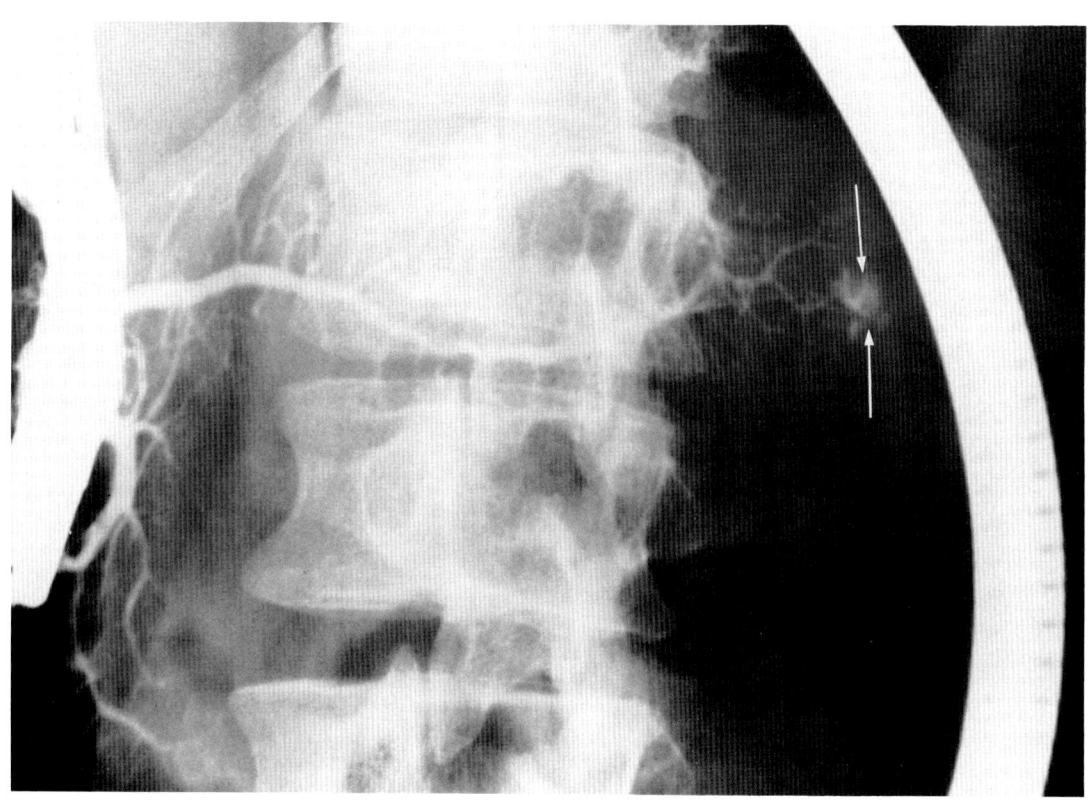

FIGURE 21.75. PANCREATIC PSEUDOCYST
ERP shows a small intrapancreatic pseudocyst in the tail (*arrows*). Only minimal changes of chronic pancreatitis otherwise.

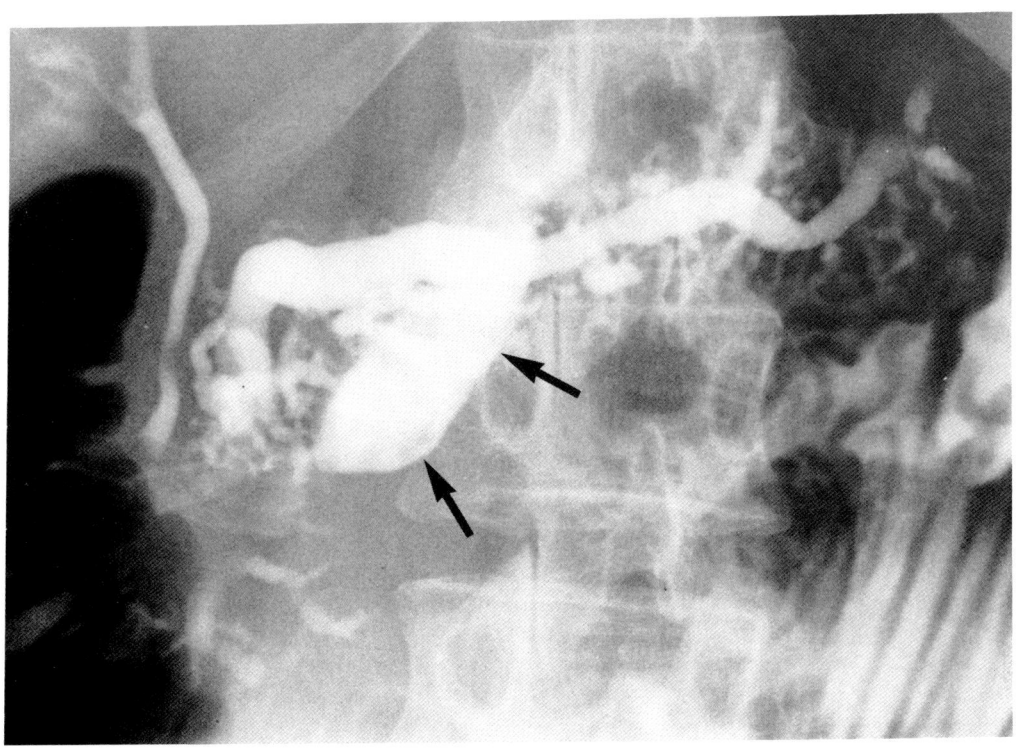

FIGURE 21.76. PANCREATIC PSEUDOCYST
Larger pseudocyst opacified (*arrows*). Advanced chronic pancreatitis.

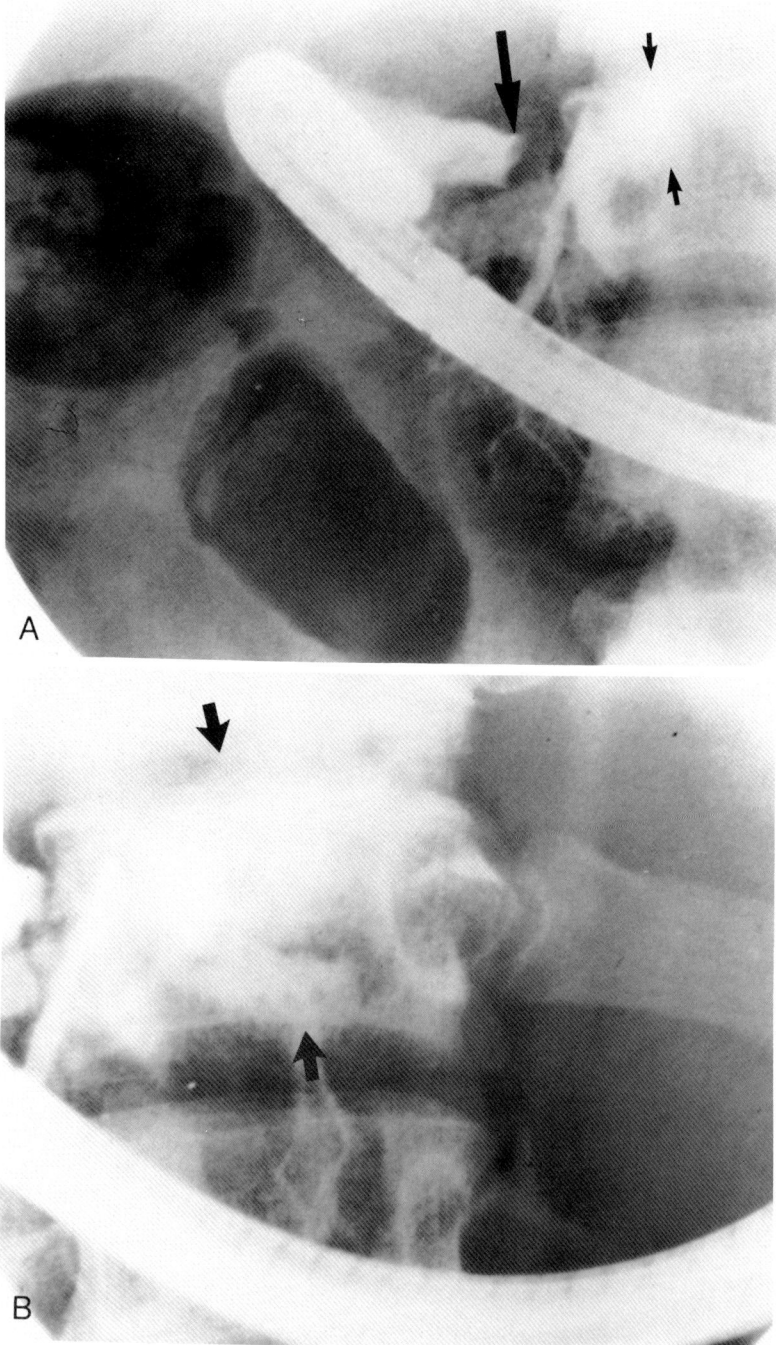

FIGURE 21.77. PANCREATIC PSEUDOCYST
Huge pseudocyst obstructing the pancreatic duct (same case as seen in Figure 21.63 barium studies, pseudocyst). *A:* Distal duct is obstructed (*large arrow*). Branch to uncinate process is filled as is an amorphous contrast collection (*small arrows*). Injection was stopped. *B:* Contrast collection (*arrows*) spreading out into large pseudocyst.

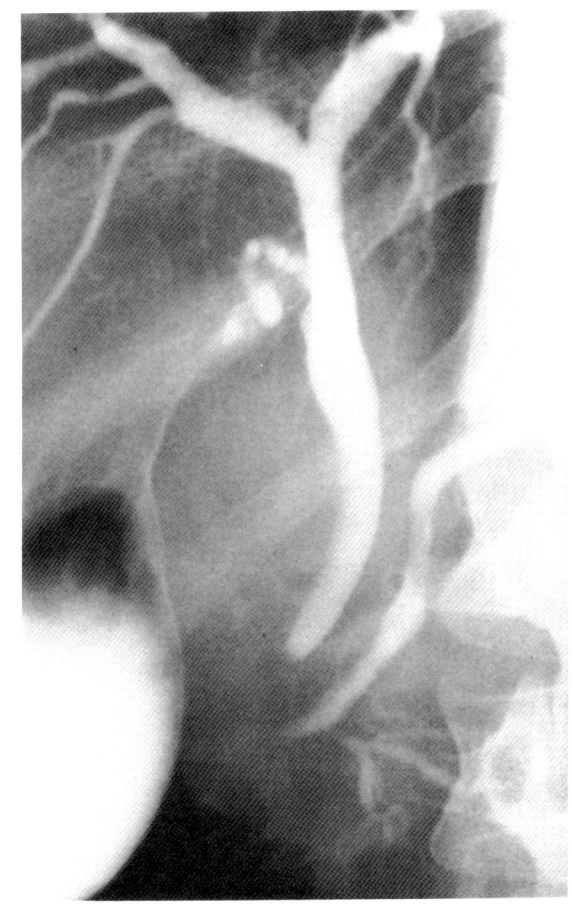

FIGURE 21.78. PANCREATIC PSEUDOCYST
ERCP shows subtle bowing of the common bile duct due to an unopacified pseudocyst just lateral to it.

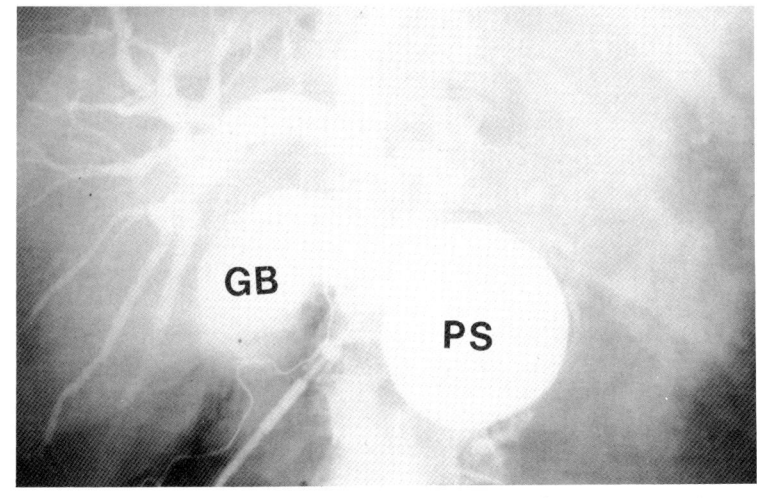

FIGURE 21.79. PANCREATIC PSEUDOCYST
Operative cholangiogram fills a pancreatic pseudocyst (*PS*). *GB* = gallbladder.

and/or eccentric in carcinoma (9), but this distinction is difficult in an individual case. The duct distal to the obstruction often will show changes of pancreatitis when the obstruction is due to pseudocyst (except in trauma) and it will usually be normal in obstructions due to carcinoma.

The pancreatographic appearance of the ductal system distal to the pseudocyst is important preoperative information (11). The presence or absence of loculations can be important, but this information can be obtained more easily with ultrasound.

REFERENCES

1. Anderson BN, Hancke S, Nielsen SAD, Schmidt A: The diagnosis of pancreatic cyst by endoscopic retrograde pancreatography and ultrasonic scanning. *Ann Surg* 185:286–289, 1977.
2. Silvis SE, Vennes JA, Rohrmann CA: Endoscopic pancreatography in the evaluation of patients with suspected pancreatic pseudocysts. *Am J Gastroenterol* 62:452–459, 1974.
3. Rohrmann CA, Silvis SE, Vennes JA: Evaluation of the endoscopic pancreatogram. *Radiology* 113:279–304, 1974.
4. Silvis SE, Schuman DM: Benign conditions of the pancreas. In Stewart ET, Vennes JA, Geenen JE (eds): *Atlas of Endoscopic Retrograde Pancreatography*. St. Louis, C. V. Mosby, 1977, pp 124–128.
5. Bilbao MK, Dotter CT, Lee TG, Katon RM: Complications of endoscopic retrograde cholangiopancreatography (ERCP). A study of 10,000 cases. *Gastroenterology* 70:314–320, 1976.
6. Anacker H, Weiss HD, Kramann B: *Endoscopic Retrograde Pancreaticocholangiography (ERPC)*. New York, Springer Verlag, 1977, pp 67–74.
7. Short WF: Pancreatography. In Eaton SB, Ferruci JT Jr (eds): *Radiology of the Pancreas and Duodenum*. Philadelphia, W. B. Saunders, 1973, pp 261–275.
8. Cotton PB, Beales JSM: Endoscopic pancreatography in the management of relapsing acute pancreatitis. *Br Med J* 1:608–611, 1974.
9. Rohrmann CA, Silvis SE, Vennes JA: The significance of pancreatic ductal obstruction in the differential diagnosis of the abnormal endoscopic retrograde pancreatogram. *Radiology* 121:311–314, 1976.
10. Seifert E, Stender HS, Safrany L, Lesch P, Luska G, Misaki F: X-ray findings of pancreatic cysts diagnosed by endoscopic pancreatocholangiography. *Endoscopy* 6:77–83, 1974.
11. Braasch JW, Gregg JA: Surgical uses of peroral retrograde pancreatography and cholangiography. *Am J Surg* 125:432–436, 1973.

Cholangiography

Pancreatic pseudocysts can cause obstruction of the common bile duct, either by compression or entrapment by inflammation and fibrosis. Mere decompression of the pseudocyst may not be adequate therapy, and a biliary drainage procedure may be necessary to relieve the obstruction (1, 2). The spectrum of cholangiographic findings is similar to that of chronic pancreatitis, with a greater tendency to have curvilinear displacement of the common bile duct (3) (Fig. 21.78). Rarely, pseudocysts can communicate with the biliary tree and cholangiography can demonstrate this finding (Fig. 21.79).

REFERENCES

1. Warshaw AL, Rattner DW: Facts and fallacies of common bile duct obstruction by pancreatic pseudocysts. *Ann Surg* 192:33–37, 1980.
2. Warshaw AL, Schapiro RH, Ferrucci JT Jr, Galdabini JJ: Persistent obstructive jaundice, cholangitis, and biliary cirrhosis due to common bile duct stenosis in chronic pancreatitis. *Gastroenterology* 70:562–567, 1976.
3. Ferrucci JT Jr, Mueller PR, vanSonnenberg E: Transhepatic cholangiography. In Berk RN, Ferrucci JT Jr, Leopold GR (eds): *Radiology of the Gallbladder and Bile Ducts, Intervention and Diagnosis*. Philadelphia, W. B. Saunders, 1983, p 357.

Angiography

The most common complication of pancreatitis is the development of abnormal fluid collections, most frequently referred to by the generic term "pseudocyst." Pseudocyst, phlegmon, fluid collection, and pancreatic abscess are indistinguishable angiographically, and are manifested by smooth, arc-like arterial displacement out of proportion to any luminal irregularities that might be present and avascularity in the capillary phase (1, 2) (Fig. 21.80) (see also Fig. 21.68*B* in discussion on pseudocysts, excretory urography).

In the past, suspected pseudocyst was one of the major indications for arteriography, whereas today sonography and CT are the procedures of choice. If performed in the evaluation of pancreatitis, the purpose of angiography is to create a surgical "road map," or to detect potentially lethal vascular complications. The latter are more common in patients whose pancreatitis is complicated by the development of abnormal fluid collections, indicating extensive inflammation. See section on angiography of pancreatitis for discussion of vascular complications.

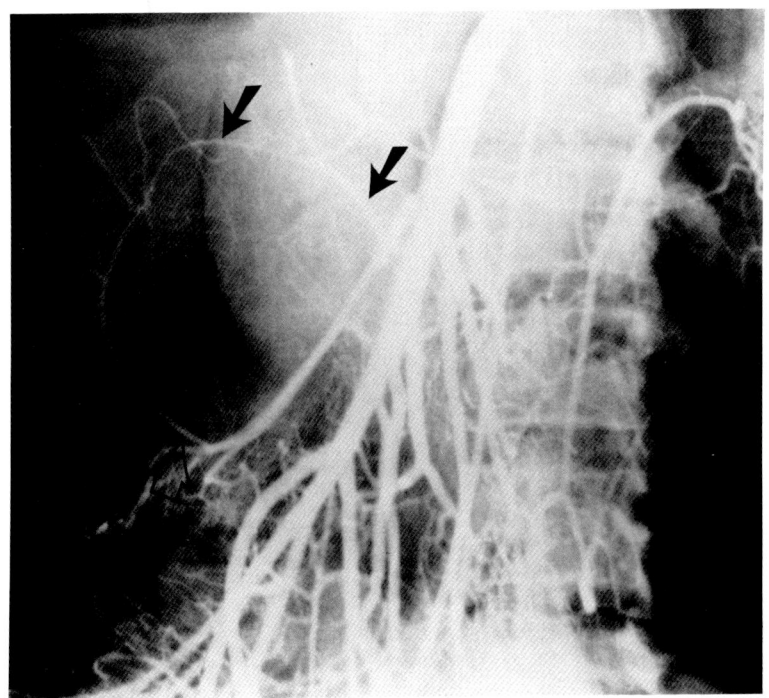

FIGURE 21.80. PANCREATIC PSEUDOCYST
Displacement of the right branch of the middle colic artery (*arrows*) around an avascular mass due to a pancreatic pseudocyst. Superior mesenteric arteriogram.

REFERENCES

1. Levin DC, Eisenberg H, Wilson R: Arteriography in the evaluation of pancreatic pseudocysts. *AJR* 129:243–348, 1977.
2. Tylen U, Arnesjo B: Angiographic diagnosis of inflammatory disease of the pancreas. *Acta Radiol* 14:215–240, 1973.

PANCREATIC TRAUMA

Clinical Findings

The pancreas is relatively protected from abdominal trauma and is involved in only 3–12% of abdominal injuries (1). Most pancreatic injuries occur when the driver is crushed against the steering column in high speed automobile crashes, but some are due to penetrating trauma (2). Mortality was nearly 20% in one series (3) with one-third of survivors having major complications such as pseudocyst, abscess, hemorrhage, or fistula. However, this early mortality is from associated major vascular injury, not the pancreatic injury. Diagnosis is often delayed and hampered by the frequent association with other significant organ or vessel injuries. Penetrating trauma to the upper abdomen that enters the peritoneal cavity usually requires emergency laparotomy and the pancreas should be inspected or injury to it may be overlooked (2). Pancreatic injury may be clinically occult after blunt trauma and a high index of suspicion is important. Elevated levels of serum amylase are suggestive but not specific. Even with complete transection the only clinical evidence of injury may be mild abdominal pain (2).

Treatment

Emergency surgery is indicated in traumatic pancreatitis when there is injury to the main pancreatic duct (3, 4). Some patients with traumatic pancreatitis and a proven intact ductal system probably can be managed conservatively. Simple drainage is adequate for contusions and small lacerations and hematomas (3). Pancreatograms must be obtained as apparent contusions and hematomas can hide a duct transection. Distal pancreatectomy is performed for pancreatic fractures and pancreaticoduodenectomy for extensive damage to the head of the pancreas or combined pancreatic and duodenal injuries (3). Untreated duct injuries lead to strictures, chronic pancreatitis, and pseudocysts.

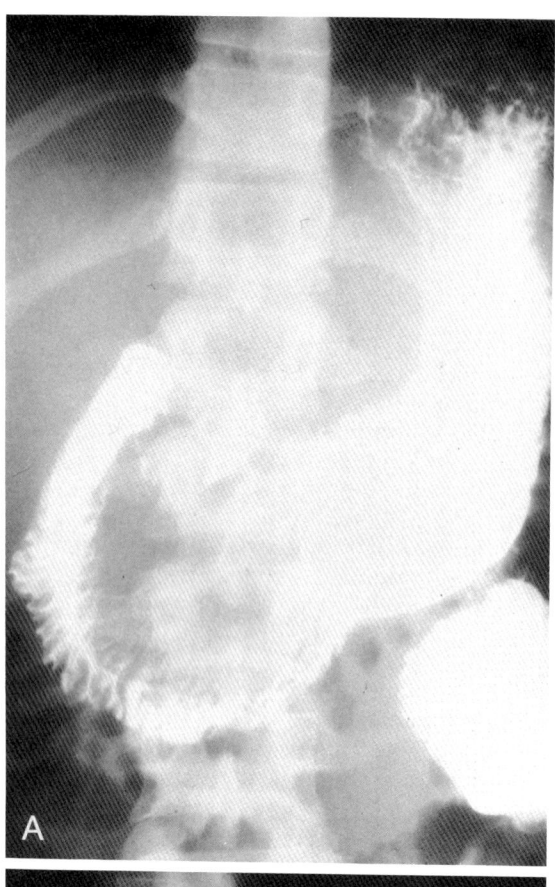
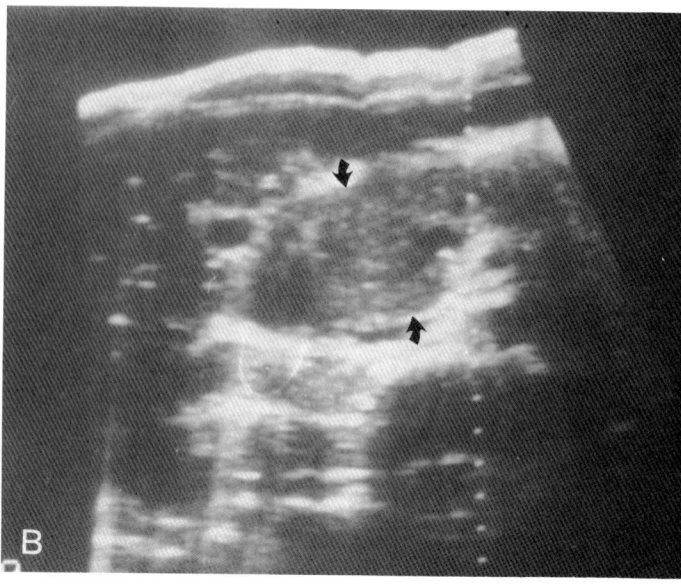
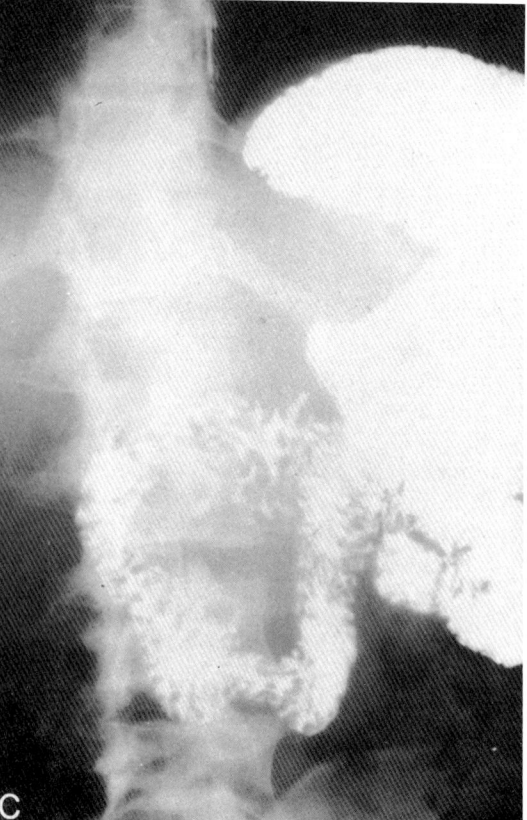
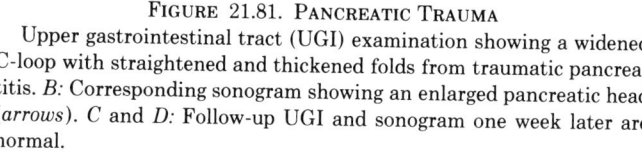
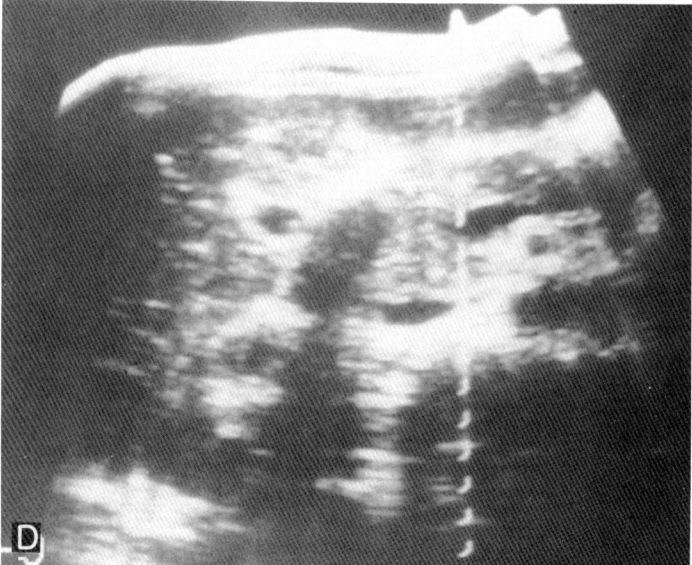

FIGURE 21.81. PANCREATIC TRAUMA
Upper gastrointestinal tract (UGI) examination showing a widened C-loop with straightened and thickened folds from traumatic pancreatitis. *B:* Corresponding sonogram showing an enlarged pancreatic head (*arrows*). *C* and *D:* Follow-up UGI and sonogram one week later are normal.

Pathology

Traumatic lesions include pancreatitis, posttraumatic pseudocyst, contusion, laceration or fracture (complete parenchymal disruption with main pancreatic duct disruption (5). The most common site of transection is the neck or body of the pancreas opposite the vertebral column just to the left of the mesenteric vessels (2). Injuries to the main pancreatic duct cause extravasation of pancreatic juice and/or duct obstruction with proximal pancreatitis and/or pseudocyst formation. Intrapancreatic or peripancreatic hematomas result from associated vascular injury.

Radiology

Contrast Studies

Examination of the upper gastrointestinal tract may disclose evidence of injury to the stomach or duodenum. Mass effects consistent with acute pancreatitis or pseudocyst may be demonstrated (Fig. 21.81).

Ultrasound

Sonography may initially demonstrate evidence of pancreatic enlargement due to pancreatitis or contusion (Fig. 21.81). Later in the patient's course pseudocysts, abscesses, focal pancreatitis, or pseudoaneurysms may be seen (4). These solid or cystic masses are located near the point of ductal stenosis or obstruction (4).

Computed Tomography

Acute traumatic pancreatitis is depicted as diffuse or focal swelling of the gland with or without inflammatory changes in the peripancreatic fat, mesentery, lesser sac or anterior pararenal space (5) (Fig. 21.82).

Pancreatic contusions are nearly isodense masses due to hemorrhage into the gland (1). Fractures are linear sometimes ill-defined low density regions running through the gland (Fig. 21.83). There may be little or no separation of fragments and the density change can be very subtle (1, 2, 5). The neck and body are the most common sites of fracture. The fracture plane may not be seen because of artefact or masking of attenuation difference with parenchyma by hemorrhage and edema, but the diagnosis of pancreatic trauma can be made by CT in most cases of pancreatic fracture. Subtle changes may be the only findings, especially if scans are per-

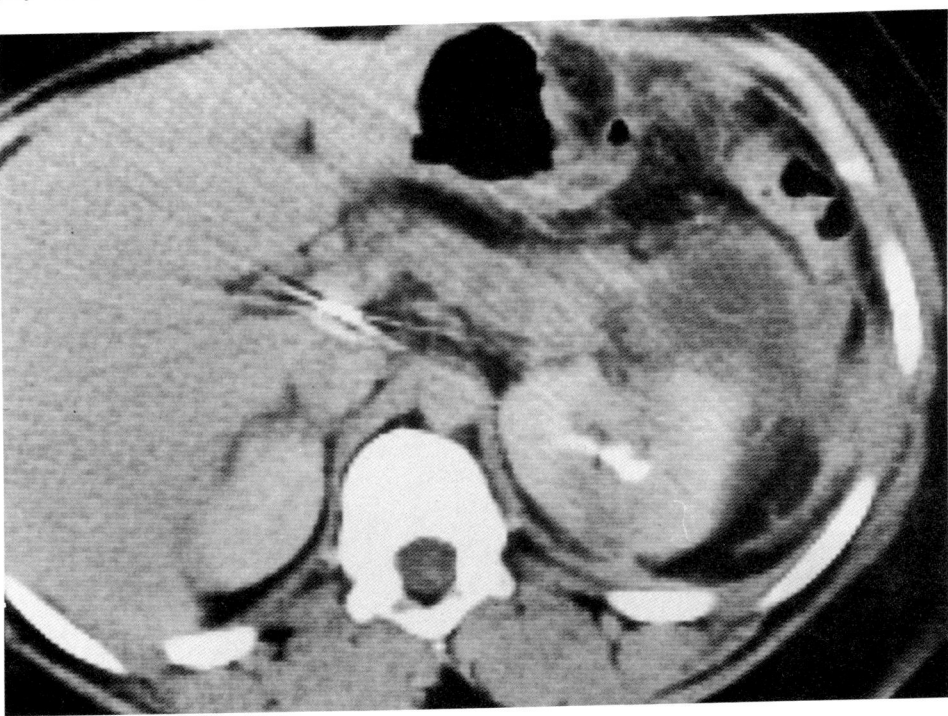

FIGURE 21.82. PANCREATIC TRAUMA
Acute traumatic pancreatitis with inflammatory changes and fluid in the anterior pararenal space. Note the laceration of the left kidney.

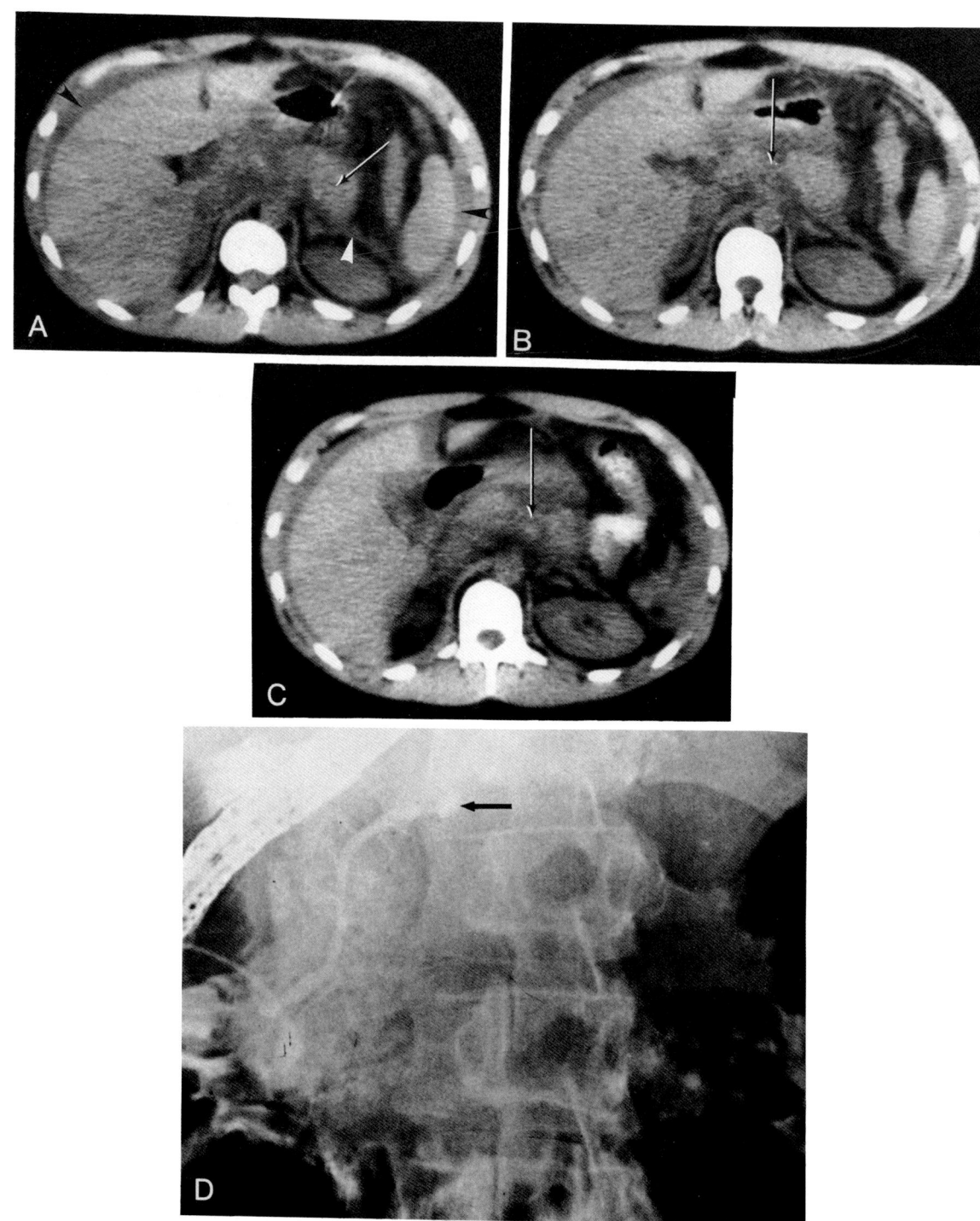

FIGURE 21.83. PANCREATIC TRAUMA

A: CT scan reveals mild enlargement of the body and tail of the pancreas (*arrow*) compatible with traumatic pancreatitis. There is thickening of the anterior pararenal fascia (*white arrowhead*) and ascites (*black arrowheads*) present. *B:* CT scan 1 cm below (*A*) reveals a lucency (*arrow*) separating the body and head of the pancreas, compatible with transection of the pancreas. Again noted is thickening of the anterior pararenal fascia and ascites. *C:* CT scan 2 cm below (*A*) again reveals the lucency (*arrow*) between the body and tail of the pancreas, compatible with transection of the pancreas. *D:* Emergency endoscopic retrograde cholangiopancreatogram reveals transection of pancreatic duct with extravasation of contrast medium (*arrow*). (From Baker LP, Wagner EJ, Brotman S, Whitley NO: Transection of the pancreas. *J Comput Assist Tomogr* 6:411–412, 1982.).

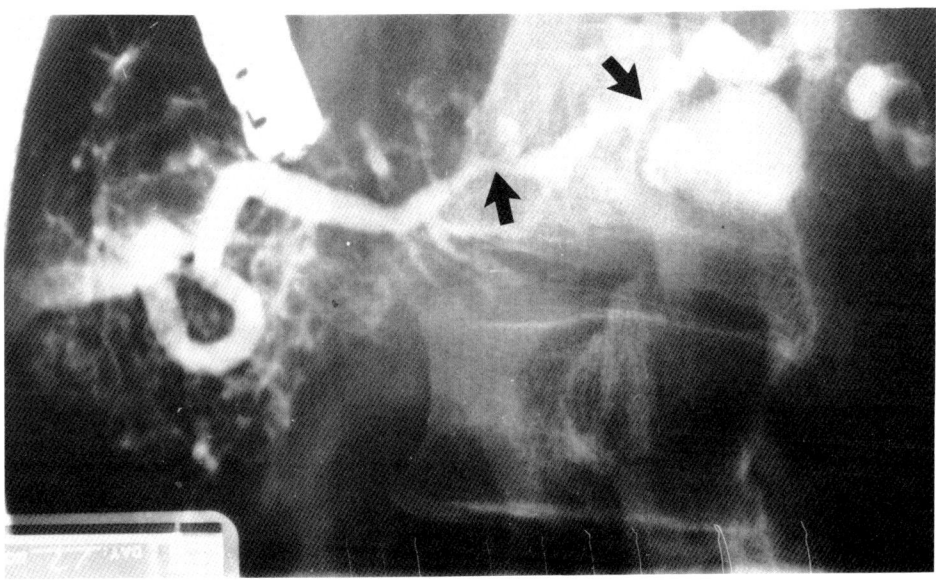

FIGURE 21.84. PANCREATIC TRAUMA

ERCP showing strictures (*arrows*) with duct dilatation and pseudocysts proximally in a patient with chronic post-traumatic pancreatitis.

formed in the first few hours after trauma. These include hemorrhage into and infiltration of the peripancreatic fat, transverse mesocolon, small bowel mesentery, and especially thickening of the perirenal fascia (Fig. 21.83) (1, 5). False negatives occur because parenchymal fractures may be missed or mistaken for streak artifact and false positives occur from artefact or thickening of the perirenal fascia from renal injury (1). Dynamic scanning after bolus contrast injection may facilitate detection of pancreatic fracture by enhancing normal parenchyma (1).

Pseudocysts identical to those of inflammatory origin can be seen within a few days to weeks after an untreated traumatic duct laceration (5). Other complications that can be detected by CT are focal pancreatitis, abscesses, and pseudoaneurysms.

ERCP

Emergency ERCP may be necessary if the results of CT are equivocal or technically adequate scans cannot be obtained and there are no other indications for laparotomy. Traumatic pancreatitis with amylase elevation can occur without disruption, and a normal ductogram can obviate laparotomy in this setting (6). Ductal disruption may be depicted as either duct obstruction or contrast extravasation (Fig. 21.83*D*) (4, 6). Although the classic duct injury is over the vertebral column, disruption may occur at any point (6). ERCP is also useful as a preoperative examination in patients with ductal strictures and pseudocysts that are sequelae of pancreatic trauma (Fig. 21.84).

Although useful in evaluating associated vascular injuries, arteriography has limited use in acute pancreatic injuries (7).

REFERENCES

1. Jeffrey RB Jr., Federle MP, Crass RA: Computed tomography of pancreatic trauma. *Radiology* 147:491–494, 1983.
2. Baker LP, Wagner EJ, Brotman S, Whitley NO: Transection of the pancreas. *J Comput Assist Tomogr* 6:411–412, 1982.
3. Bach RD, Frey, CFL: Diagnosis and treatment of pancreatic trauma. *Am J Surg* 121:20–29, 1971.
4. Vallon AG, Lees WL, Cotton PB: Gray-scale ultrasonography and endoscopic pancreatography after pancreatic trauma. *Br J Surg* 66:169–172, 1979.
5. Federle MP: Trauma. In Wittenberg J (ed): *Syllabus for the Categorical Course on Computed Body Tomography with MRI Correlation.* Presented at the Annual Meeting of the American Roentgen Ray Society, Las Vegas, Nevada, April, 1984, pp 364–367.
6. Taxier M, Sivak MF Jr, Cooperman AM, Sullivan HB Jr: Endoscopic retrograde cholangiopancreatography in the evaluation of trauma to the pancreas. *Surg Gynecol Obstet* 150:65–68, 1980.
7. Soroudi M, Bookstein JJ: Angiography in acute pancreatic transection. *Radiology* 11:309–311, 1975.

FAT REPLACEMENT

A small amount of fat replacement of the pancreas is common and is a normal finding in the obese and elderly (1, 2). In obesity the process is reversible and should be termed fat infiltration (Fig. 21.85) (1) Elderly patients often have associated mild degrees of atrophy of the endocrine and exocrine elements with little or no functional impairment, probably on an atherosclerotic basis (Fig. 21.86) (2). Causes of fat replacement with atrophy include main pancreatic duct obstruction, cystic fibrosis, malnutrition, Schwachman's syndrome, hemochromatosis, and viral infection (1, 2). Cushing's syndrome and steroid therapy are reversible causes of fatty infiltration (Fig. 21.87) (1).

Clinical Findings

In most instances there are no symptoms attributable to pancreatic fat infiltration or replacement. In severe cases associated with atrophy such as complete obstruction, cystic fibrosis and Schwachman's syndrome exocrine function is impaired (1, 2), and patients with hemochromatosis may develop diabetes.

Pathology

Histologic examination reveals fibrofatty replacement of the acini and preservation of islets (1, 2). Ducts are often enlarged (2). The changes are similar to those produced experimentally by ligature of the main pancreatic duct (1, 2).

Radiology

While fatty replacement may be depicted sonographically as increased pancreatic echogenicity, the diagnosis is much more readily appreciated on CT. In milder cases there is a marbling of the pancreatic parenchyma by interspersed fat. Overall size is normal or diminished (Figs. 21.85–21.87). When the process is advanced, the entire parenchyma can be replaced by fat, with the duct seen as a linear density (see discussion in Chapter 20 under Schwachman's syndrome). Rarely the pancreas becomes enlarged by multiple nodular fatty masses (lipomatous pseudohypertrophy (3). In this condition ERCP has shown stretching, draping and thinning of the ducts and angiography has shown stretching and displacement of vessels by avascular masses (3), so that CT is vital to exclude neoplasm.

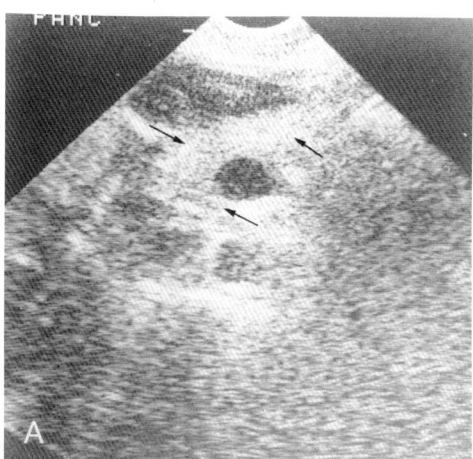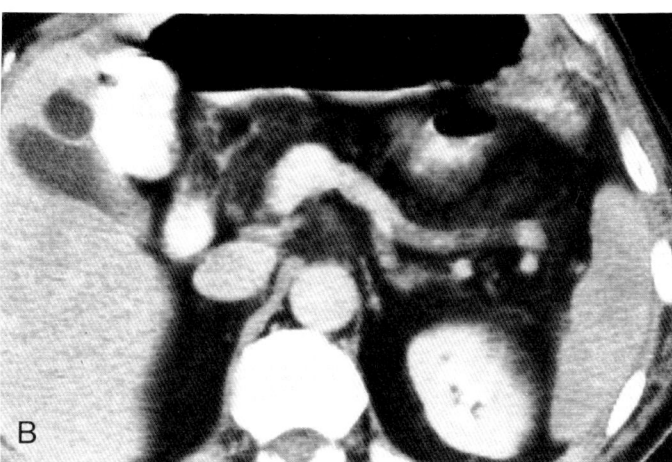

FIGURE 21.85. FAT INFILTRATION

A: Transverse sonogram showing increased echogenicity in the pancreas from fatty infiltration (*arrows*). *B:* A 64-yr-old man with internal obesity. CT shows infiltration of the pancreatic parenchyma by fat giving a marbled appearance. Overall pancreatic size is mildly diminished. No pancreatic symptoms.

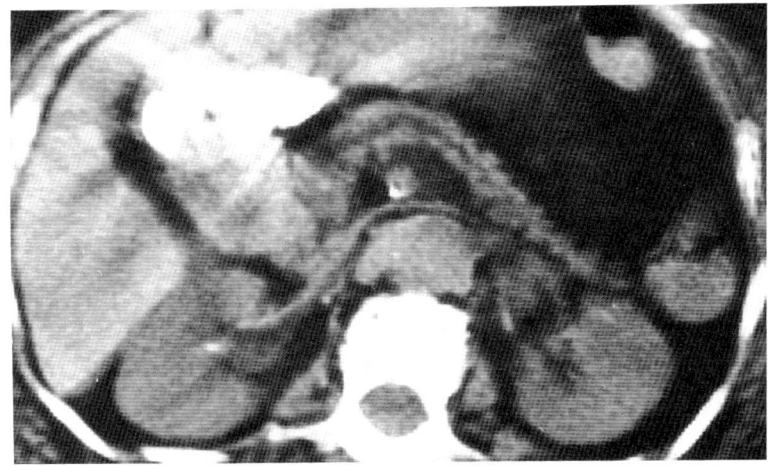

FIGURE 21.86. FAT REPLACEMENT
Marked atrophy of the pancreas in an 85-yr-old woman with no symptoms referable to the pancreas. Fat interdigitates between prominent lobulations. The pancreatic duct is mildly dilated compatible with the patient's age and parenchymal atrophy.

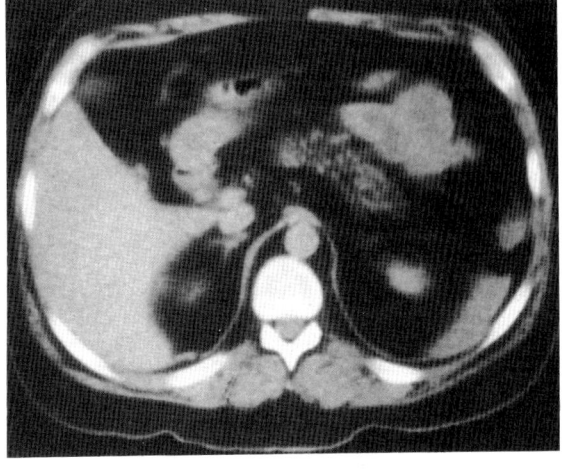

FIGURE 21.87. FAT INFILTRATION
A 35-yr-old woman with Cushing's syndrome has fatty infiltration of a normal-sized pancreas giving a marbled appearance to the gland.

REFERENCES

1. Patel S, Bellon EMN, Haaga J, Park CH: Fat replacement of the exocrine pancreas. *AJR* 135:843–845, 1980.
2. Robbins SJ, Cotran SR: *Pathologic Basis of Disease.* Philadelphia, W. B. Saunders, 1979, pp 1092–1093.
3. Nakamura N, Katada N, Sakakibara A et al: Huge lipomatous pseudohypertrophy of the pancreas. *Am J Gastroenterol* 72:171–174.

22
Pancreatic Neoplasms

ARNOLD C. FRIEDMAN, M.D., ADRIAN G. KRUDY, JR., M.D.,
THOMAS H. SHAWKER, M.D., DONALD G. MITCHELL, M.D.,
MARK T. BIRNS, M.D., LEONARD BODNER, M.D., AND
SEYMOUR S. SPRAYREGEN, M.D.

The various histologic types of cancer may respond differently to treatment regimens. Although most pancreatic neoplasms do not show a significant response to therapy, there are some important exceptions. Underneath the blanket term "cancer of the pancreas" are distinctive morphological types that may prove to have important differences at the molecular level (1). The normal histology of the gland can be used to divide neoplasms into those of the duct(ule) cell, acinar cell, islet cell, and connective tissue cell type (1).

Classification of Pancreatic Neoplasms (1)

I. Duct(ule) cell origin
   A. Cystic
      1. Congenital cyst
      2. Microcystic adenoma
      3. Mucinous cystic neoplasm
   B. Solid
      1. Duct cell adenocarcinoma
      2. Variant carcinomas
         a. Giant cell carcinoma (epulis-osteoid)
         b. Giant cell carcinoma (pleomorphic)
         c. Adenosquamous carcinoma
         d. Mucinous (colloid) carcinoma
         e. Microadenocarcinoma
         f. Anaplastic
      3. Solid and papillary epithelial neoplasm
II. Acinar cell origin
   A. Acinar cell carcinoma
   B. Acinar cell cystadenocarcinoma
III. Indeterminate
   A. Pancreaticoblastoma
   B. Ductuloinsular tumor
IV. Connective Tissue
V. Metastases, lymphoma, leukemia
VI. Islet cell tumors

True Pancreatic Cysts (Congenital)

Epithelial-lined true pancreatic cysts are thought to form by persistence and segmentation of primitive ducts leading to sequestering of nests of ductal secretory cells, fluid production and cyst formation (1). True cysts are usually multiple and associated with cystic disease of other organs, but they can be solitary (1, 2). They are developmental anomalies, not true neoplasms.

Multiple True Cysts

Nine percent of patients with adult polycystic kidney disease have simple pancreatic cysts at autopsy (3); no detection rates are published for ultrasound or CT. There are no symptoms referable to pancreatic cysts in adult polycystic kidney disease. The multiple cysts vary in size from microscopic to 3–5 cm in both adult polycystic kidney disease and von Hippel-Lindau disease (Fig. 22.1A and B).

Seventy-two percent of patients with von Hippel-Lindau disease at autopsy have simple pancreatic cysts, but CT detection rate was only 25% in a recent series (4). Cysts are usually multiple and can be so extensive as to replace the parenchyma and lead to diabetes (4). Pancreatic cysts in von Hippel-Lindau disease appear to be restricted to members of certain families (4). Other pancreatic lesions associated with von Hippel-Lindau disease include duct cell adenocarcinoma, ampullary carcinoma, hemangioblastoma, microcystic adenoma, and nonfunctional islet cell tumor (4).

Solitary True Pancreatic Cyst

Clinical Findings. Solitary true pancreatic cyst is the rarest cystic lesion of the pancreas (5). They usually occur in infants and children, with occasional cases in adults (5). Symptoms and signs are abdominal mass and distension,

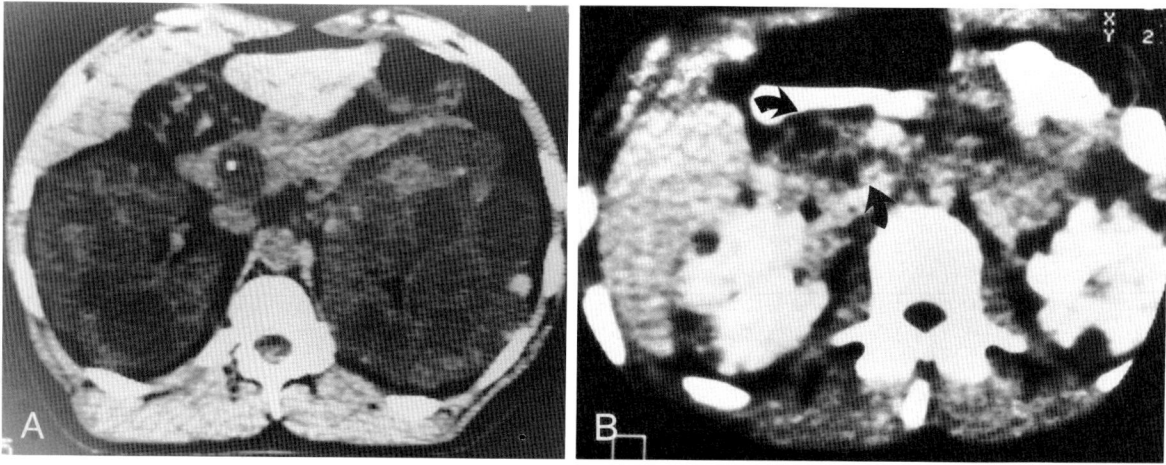

FIGURE 22.1. TRUE PANCREATIC CYSTS, CONGENITAL
A: Polycystic kidney disease with renal and pancreatic (*cursor*) cysts. B: Von Hippel-Lindau disease with multiple renal cysts and cysts throughout the pancreas (*arrows*).

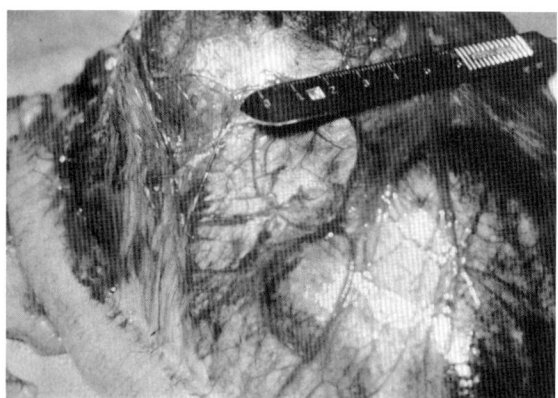

FIGURE 22.2. CONGENITAL PANCREATIC CYST
Gross specimen of a congenital true pancreatic cyst in an infant.

with nausea and vomiting from gastroduodenal compression (5). Treatment has been resection for those cysts in the body or the tail of the pancreas and cystoenterostomy for those in the head (5).

Pathology. True pancreatic cysts can be uni- or multilocular, and they vary in size from 1–2 cm to 13 cm in diameter (Fig. 22.2) (5). The lining can show atrophy of duct epithelial cells, preservation of flattened duct epithelium, or low cuboidal duct epithelium (1). Rarely, there may be heterotopic mucosa in the lining (6). The cysts are delimited by a thin fibrous capsule (1). The cyst fluid is generally easily aspirated and clear yellow, but can be turbid or viscous if there has been hemorrhage or infection (5). Amylase levels are normal (7). Analysis of the lining cells and

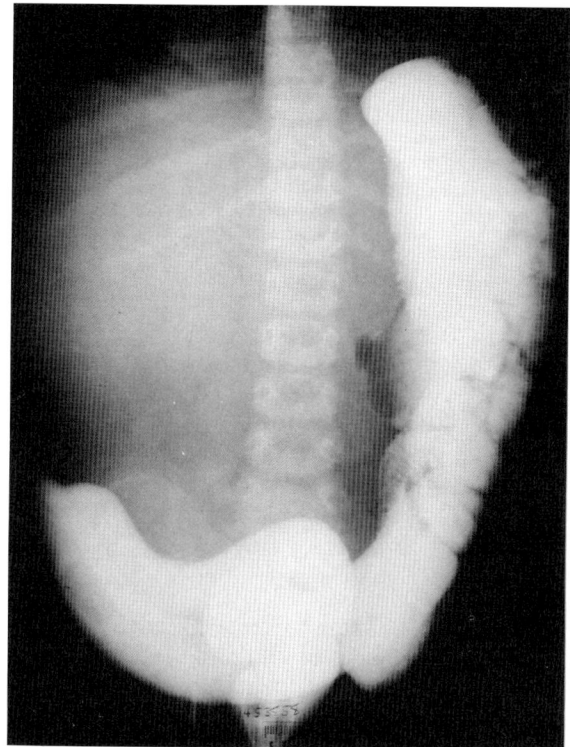

FIGURE 22.3. CONGENITAL PANCREATIC CYST
Barium enema showing colon displacement by a large soft tissue mass which was a congenital pancreatic cyst (same patient as in Fig. 22.2).

cyst fluid will show no significant amounts of glycogen (4), ruling out microcystic adenoma.

Radiology. Plain films and gastrointestinal contrast studies show a nonspecific soft tissue mass (Fig. 22.3). Sonography and CT, although not reported, should show a uni- or multiloculated cyst, without excrescences unless there has been hemorrhage or infection. Angiography will show an avascular mass (5). Cyst puncture is potentially both diagnostic and therapeutic. Contrast injection into the cyst will show non-filling of the pancreatic duct. Conversely, these cysts will not fill on pancreatography. The absence of communication with the duct does not exclude pseudocyst; however, the latter will have markedly elevated levels of amylase in its fluid (7). In the rare instance of an adult with a solitary true pancreatic cyst, mucinous cystic neoplasm probably cannot be excluded by any means short of surgery and pathologic examination of the cyst wall.

REFERENCES

1. Robbins SL, Cotran SR: *Pathologic Basis of Disease.* Philadelphia, W. B. Saunders, 1979, pp 1092–1093.
2. Rosai J: *Ackerman's Surgical Pathology.* St. Louis, C. V. Mosby, 1981, pp 664–696.
3. Shirkhoda A, Mittelstaedt CA. Demonstration of pancreatic cysts in adult polycystic disease by computed tomography and ultrasound. *AJR* 131:1074–1076, 1978.
4. Levine E, Collins DL, Horton WA, Schimke RN: CT screening of the abdomen in von-Hippel-Lindau disease. *AJR* 139:505–510, 1982.
5. Mares AJ, Hirsch M: Congenital cysts of the head of the pancreas. *J Pediatr Surg* 12:547–552, 1977.
6. Frantz VK: Tumors of the pancreas: In: Atlas of Tumor Pathology. Washington, D.C., Armed Forces Institute of Pathology, 1956, pp 7–10.
7. Schwerk WB: Ultrasonically guided percutaneous puncture and analysis of aspirated material of cystic pancreatic lesions. *Digestion* 21:184–192, 1981.

DUCT CELL ORIGIN: CYSTIC NEOPLASMS

Primary cystic neoplasms of the pancreas, which represent 10–15% of pancreatic cysts in surgical series (1, 2), are currently classified as either microcystic adenomas or mucinous cystic neoplasms (3, 4). Prior to the landmark articles by Compagno and Oertel in 1978 (3, 4), the less aggressive mucinous cystic tumors were grouped with the microcystic adenomas under the heading "cystadenoma" and the more aggressive mucinous cystic neoplasms were called "cystadenocarcinoma."

Understandably, radiologists had difficulty separating cystadenoma from cystadenocarcinoma. However, microcystic adenomas and mucinous cystic neoplasms are easily distinguished from each other by their radiologic characteristics which correspond to their differing gross morphology (5).

Microcystic Adenoma

Clinical Findings. Microcystic adenomas occur between the ages of 34–88 with 82% being in patients 60 yr or older. There is a female to male preponderance varying from 3:2 to 9:2 (3, 5–7). Tumors are located in the head, body, and tail with approximately equal frequency; occasionally the entire gland is involved (3, 5–7).

Microcystic adenoma usually presents with nonspecific abdominal symptoms, weight loss, and/or a palpable mass of days to years duration (3, 5–7). Jaundice is not common (3, 5–7). One case presented with an abdominal bruit (4).

Microcystic adenoma may be an incidental finding at laparotomy or postmortem (3). Previously reported asssociation with diabetes, extrapancreatic tumors and other miscellaneous ailments may be chance findings in an elderly population (3). Microcystic adenomas of the pancreas have increased incidence in von Hippel-Lindau syndrome (3, 7).

There has been one case of exsanguination from a ruptured vessel in a microcystic adenoma (3).

Proper radiologic diagnosis of microcystic adenoma is crucial so that asymptomatic and poor risk patients can be spared surgery. It is noteworthy that there were four postoperative deaths out of 24 patients operated for microcystic adenoma in one series (3). Percutaneous aspiration biopsy may be helpful in avoiding surgery by confirming the diagnosis (1, 3, 8). Radiologic confirmation of the pancreas as the organ of origin is necessary for proper interpretation of aspiration biopsies (J. E. Oertel, personal communication).

Pathology. Microcystic adenomas (Fig. 22.4) are usually externally lobulated (Fig. 22.4A) and covered by a thin, incomplete layer of connective tissue (3, 6, 7, 9). They vary in size from 4 to 25 cm in greatest dimension, with a mean of 13 cm (5). They are composed of innumerable small cysts, (Fig. 22.4C), the vast majority of which vary from less than 1 mm to 2 cm in size (3, 5–7, 9). The occasional patient will have a few larger cysts (up to 8 cm) (5). A distinctive feature, when present, is a prominent central stellate fibrotic scar (Fig. 22.4B) which may calcify (3). Hemorrhage into the tumor occurs occasionally, large vessels are present in or adjacent to the tumor, and there is a rich subepithelial capillary network (3).

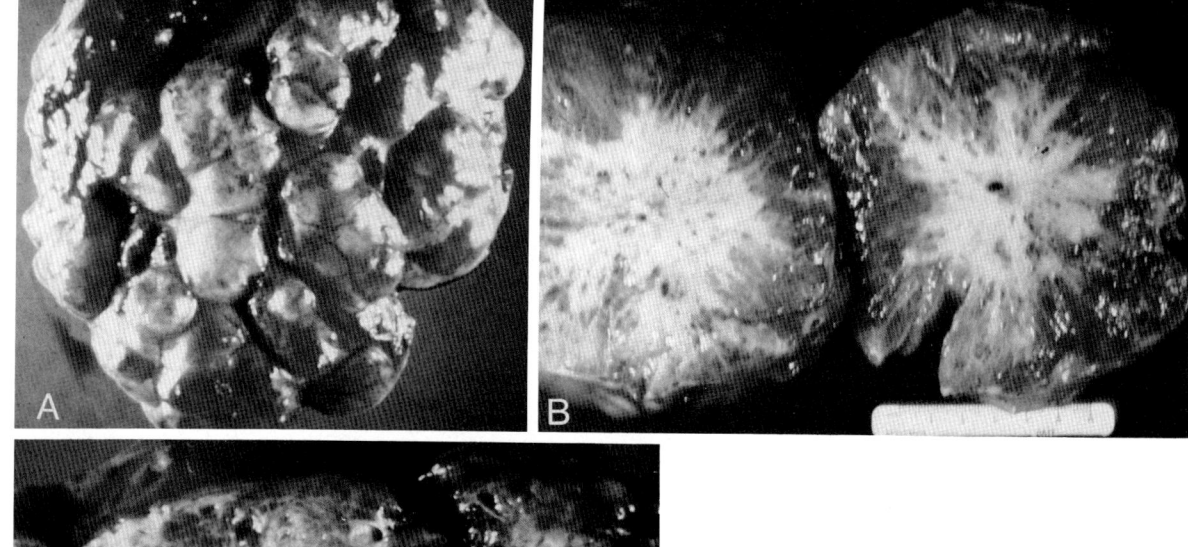
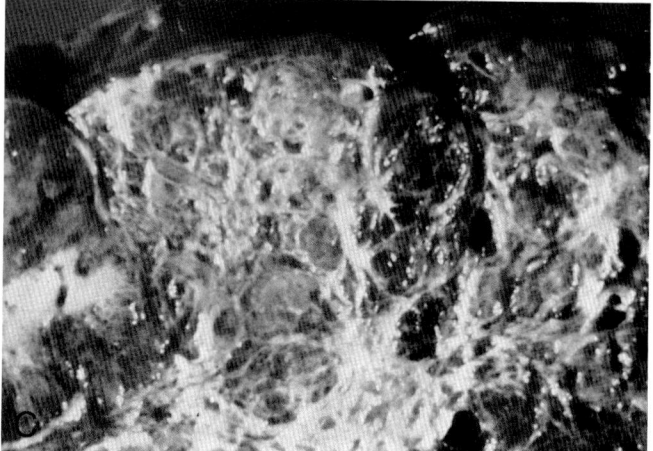

FIGURE 22.4. PRIMARY CYSTIC NEOPLASM
A: Gross specimen of a microcystic adenoma showing the lobulated external surface. *B:* Cut surface of a microcystic adenoma showing the central, stellate, fibrotic scar. *C:* Blow-up of a cut surface of one of the lobules shows that the tumor is composed of tiny cysts.

The tiny cysts (Fig. 22.5) are filled with amorphous, proteinaceous fluid and are at times packed with red blood cells (3). They are separated by a thin, nearly acellular connective tissue network and are evenly lined with cuboidal or flattened epithelial cells. The cells have a clear cytoplasm with a central dense oval nucleus. The cytoplasm, and sometimes the cyst fluid, contains considerable glycogen. Well-formed papillae are rare, nuclear pleomorphism is infrequent and mitoses are almost never seen. Mucin is absent or present in only negligible amounts. The most common misinterpretation is lymphangioma. Electron microscopy shows the cells to be similar to the ductular and centroacinar cells of the fetal pancreas (3).

Radiology. Microcystic adenomas show radiologic calcification (Fig. 22.6) more frequently than any other pancreatic tumor (approximately one-third calcify on plain films) (5). The calcifications can be single or multiple, linear, arcuate or globular, but are always central (5). They represent dystrophic calcification in the central stellate fibrotic scar (3). This is the previously described sunburst calcification (1) said to occur in pancreatic "cystadenomas."

The common sonographic pattern (Fig. 22.7) of microcystic adenomas is a solid mass with mixed hypoechoic and echogenic areas, since almost all of the cysts are less than 2 cm in diameter (3, 5, 6, 9, 10). The uncommon larger cyst can be depicted as such (5). The central stellate fibrotic scar can be depicted as a central radiating echodensity (5). The CT appearance (Fig. 22.8) of the microcystic adenoma is that of a water to muscle density mass, depending on the relative amounts of connective tissue and cyst fluid, as well as the protein content of the cyst fluid (1, 5, 11). Contrast enhancement may occur because of the rich subepithelial capillary network present in these tumors (3, 5). Central calcifications and the central stellate fibrotic scar may be seen (1, 5, 12). Cysts are generally too small to be depicted (1, 5). Due to the absence of a well developed capsule, microcystic adenomas tend to be poorly demarcated on both son-

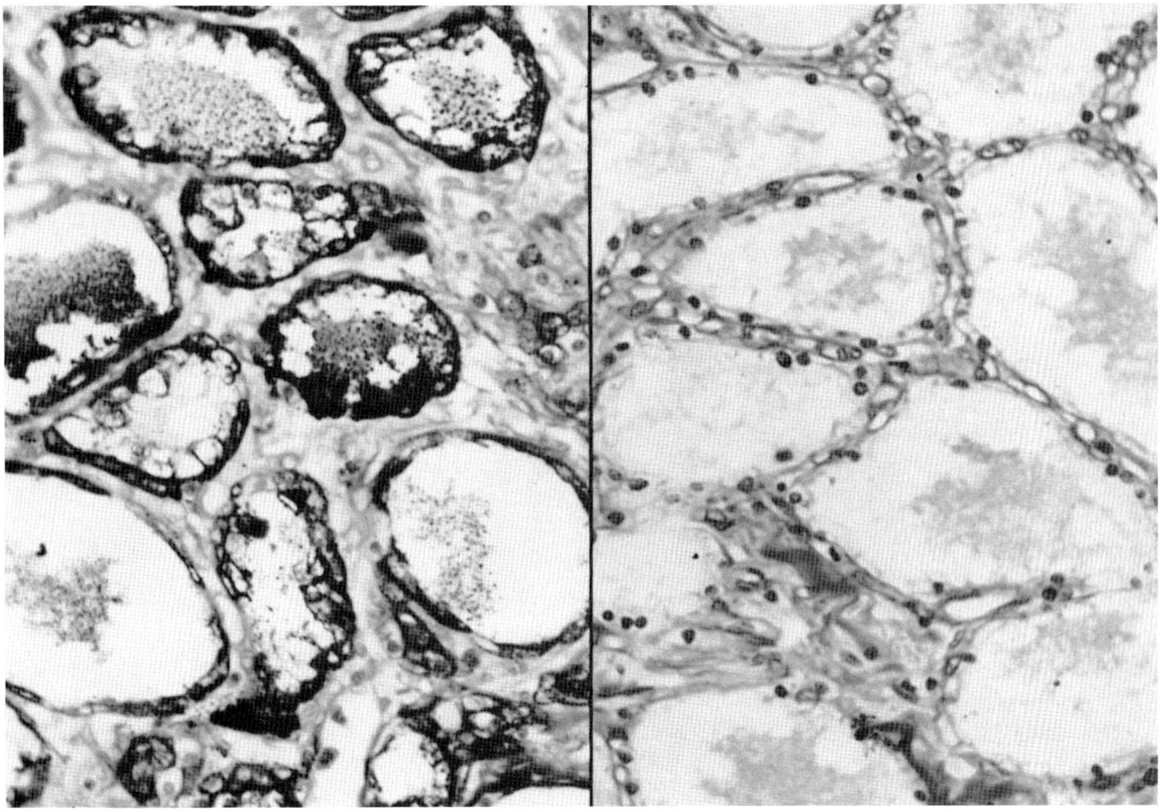

FIGURE 22.5. MICROCYSTIC ADENOMA
Photomicrographs of a microcystic adenoma showing PAS positive intracytoplasmic and intracystic glycogen (*dark areas, left*) that is diastase sensitive (*right*). Note small cysts lined by flattened, benign epithelial cells on right.

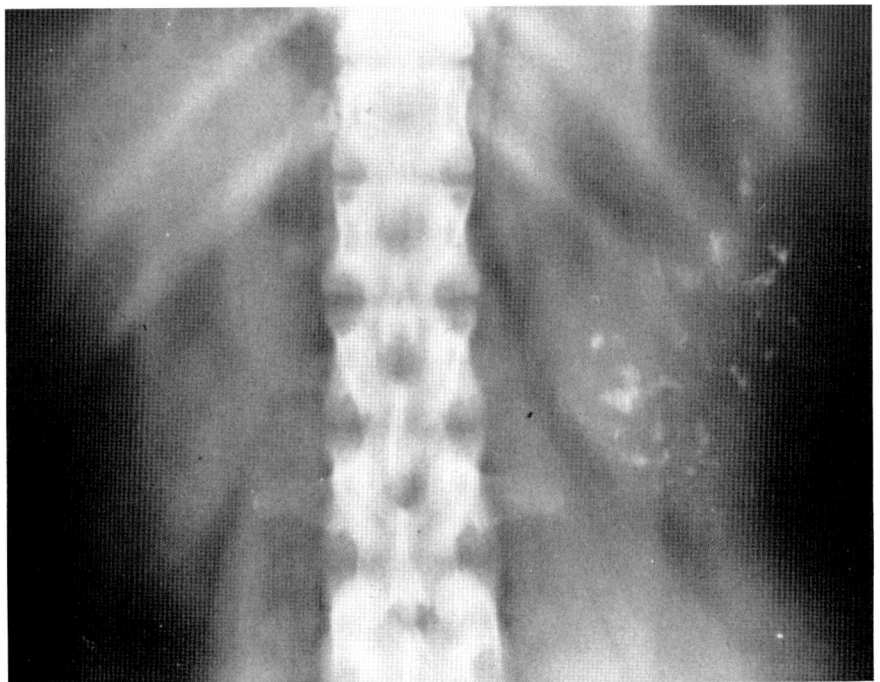

FIGURE 22.6. MICROCYSTIC ADENOMA
Plain film tomogram of a microcystic adenoma showing central calcification.

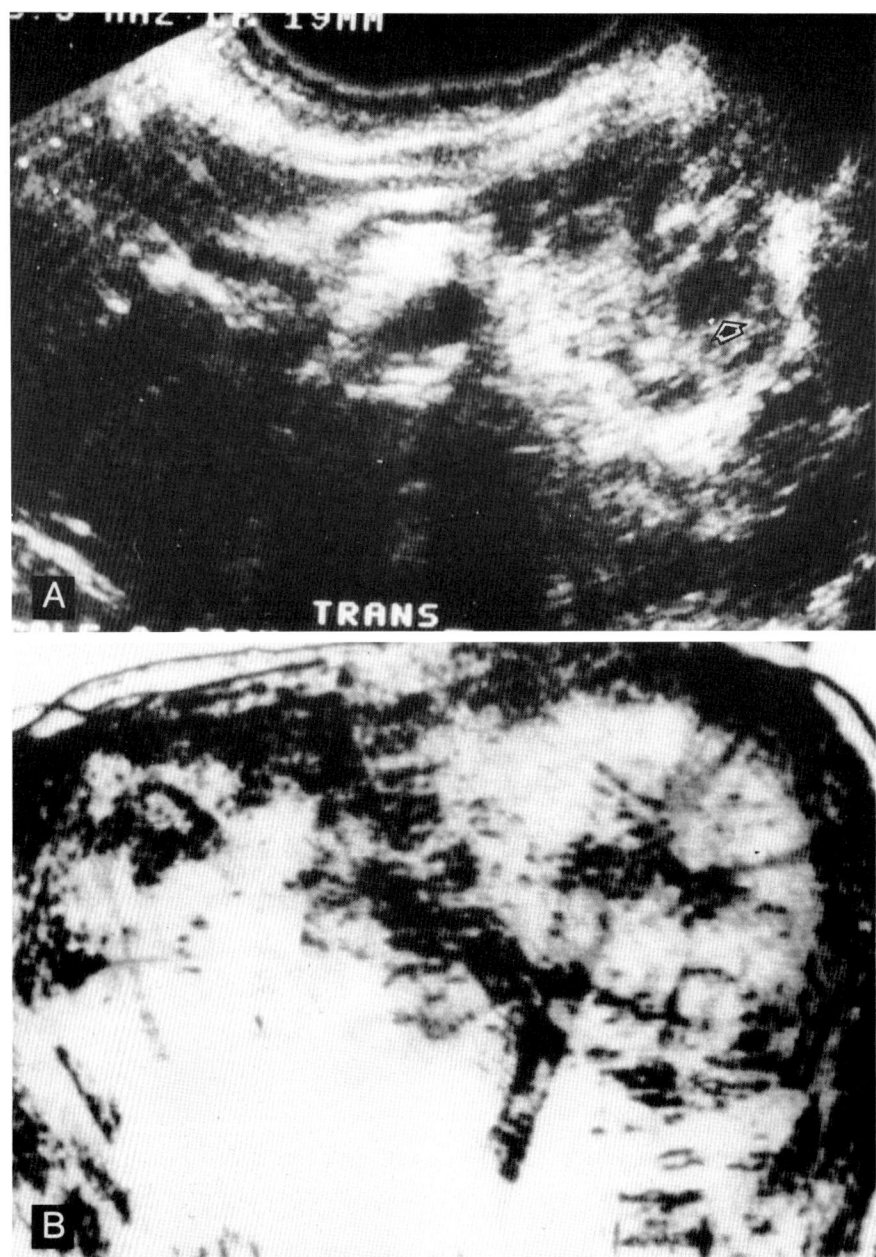

FIGURE 22.7. MICROCYSTIC ADENOMA

A: Transverse sonogram of a microcystic adenoma shows a large, poorly demarcated, mixed echogenicity left upper quadrant mass with one fairly large hypoechoic area which represents an agglomeration of cysts (*arrow*). *B:* Transverse sonogram of a microcystic adenoma shows a mostly hypoechoic mass with an echogenic center, the latter corresponding to the central scar.

ography and CT (5). Demarcation can be shown by CT if there is sufficient contrast enhancement of the tumor relative to surrounding structures (5). Sonography generally is superior in depicting the internal architecture, whereas CT gives a better appreciation of calcification, organ of origin and vascularity (Fig. 22.8*E* and *F*) (5). The gross external lobulations of microcystic adenomas can be shown by either modality (5).

Microcystic adenomas are highly vascular lesions (Fig. 22.9) and demonstrate large feeding arteries, neovascularity and tumor blush, prom-

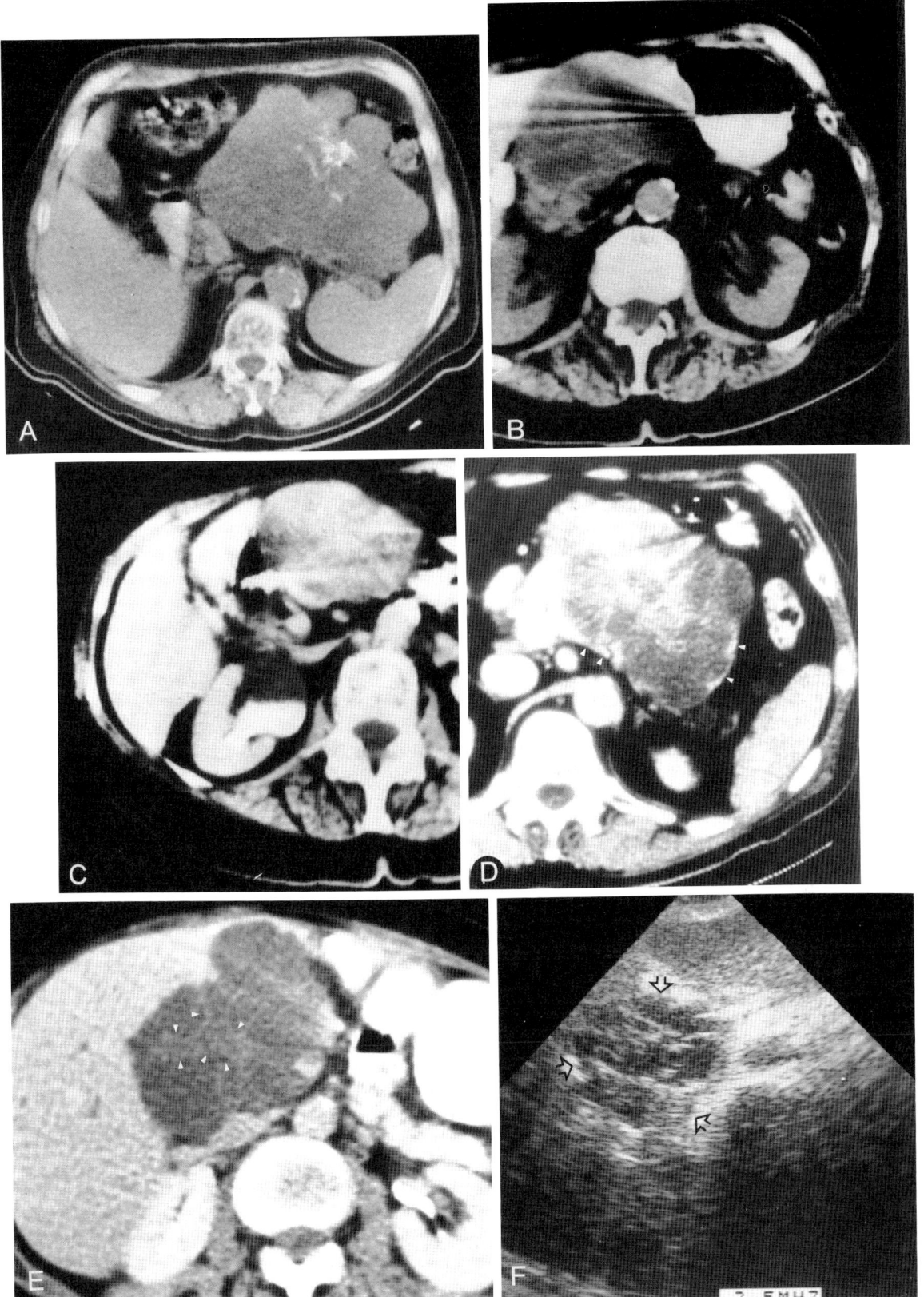

FIGURE 22.8. MICROCYSTIC ADENOMA

A: Unenhanced CT of a microcystic adenoma showing central calcifications in a large, lobulated, near water density mass. *B* and *C:* Unenhanced and enhanced CT scans showing uniform contrast enhancement in a microcystic adenoma. *D:* Bolus infusion dynamic CT scan of a microcystic adenoma showing enhanced peripheral draining veins (*arrowheads*). *E:* Contrast enhanced CT of a microcystic adenoma in the head of the pancreas. It appears to be of uniform low density except for a faintly seen central scar and septations (*arrowheads*). *F:* Sonography of the same case shows a complex, heterogeneous mass (*arrows*).

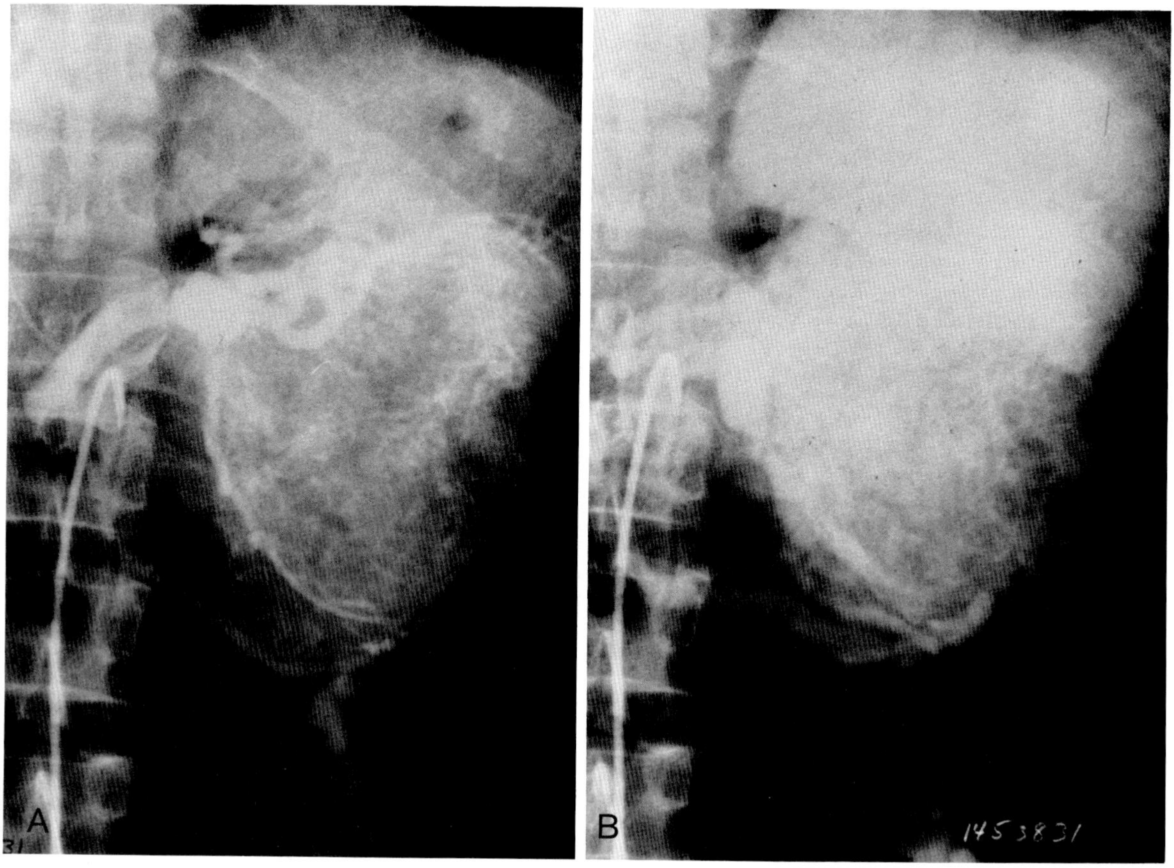

FIGURE 22.9. MICROCYSTIC ADENOMA

A: Arteriogram of a microcystic adenoma shows a hypervascular mass with neovascularity. *B:* Capillary phase from the same study as (*A*) shows early draining veins, tumor blush and small lucencies within the blush most likely corresponding to aggregates of small cysts.

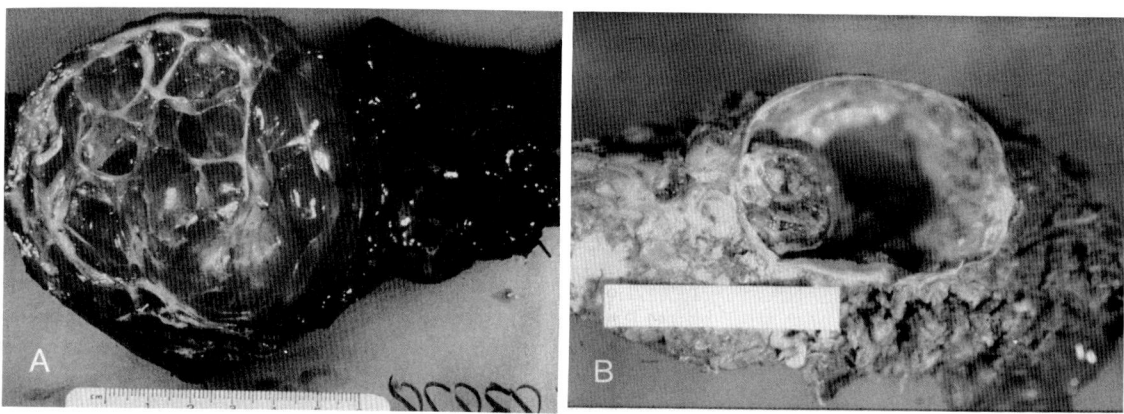

FIGURE 22.10. MUCINOUS CYSTIC NEOPLASM

A: Gross specimen of a mucinous cystic neoplasm that is a thick-walled multiloculated cyst with large cystic spaces. *B:* Gross specimen of a bivalved mucinous cystic neoplasm showing papillary excrescences projecting into the interior. Despite the thick, intact wall this tumor presented with liver metastases and ascites.

inent draining veins and occasional arteriovenous shunting (3, 5–7). These features correlate well with the prominent surface vessels and rich capillary network seen at pathological examination (3, 6, 7). Small lucencies sometimes seen in the capillary phase correspond to the cysts (5). Splenic vein obstruction due to displacement and compression may be present (3, 5). Angiographic differential diagnosis is with islet cell tumor (5). Cholangiography is usually not done as microcystic adenomas usually do not cause jaundice. Pancreatography may show nonspecific blunt obstruction of the main pancreatic duct or duct displacement (5).

Mucinous Cystic Neoplasm

Clinical Findings. The mode of presentation of mucinous cystic neoplasms is similar to that of microcystic adenomas—nonspecific abdominal symptoms, weight loss, and/or palpable mass of days to years in duration, or incidental finding at laparotomy or autopsy (3, 5–7). An overwhelming percentage of these tumors are in the tail or body and tail (85%) (5), so that jaundice is rare. There is a 9:1 female to male preponderance (4–6). Mucinous cystic tumors have been reported at any adult age (20–82) but 50% are in the 40–60 year age group (4–6). These tumors are uncommon but not rare—cystadenocarcinoma represented about 1% of pancreatic malignancies in a large Memorial Hospital series (13). Rupture, infection, and bleeding varices from splenic vein obstruction are rare complications of mucinous cystic neoplasms (6, 14). Reported association with diabetes, extrapancreatic tumors, and various miscellaneous ailments may be chance findings (4).

The distinction between mucinous cystadenoma and mucinous cystadenocarcinoma does not seem to be warranted because these large tumors cannot be sampled sufficiently to exclude carcinoma (4). All must be treated as at least potentially malignant by local, complete excision (4). In the absence of distant metastases this is potentially curative (4). If incompletely resected or treated by cystoenterostomy, recurrence is almost inevitable even in apparently benign tumors and malignant behavior may occur as late as 12 yr after the initial operation (4, 15). Even if frankly malignant and unresectable, the prognosis is better than with pancreatic duct cell adenocarcinoma (13).

The most common clinical preoperative diagnosis in a series of 30 operative cases of mucinous cystic tumors prior to 1978 was pancreatic pseudocyst (4). The correct diagnosis should be suggested nearly always by sonography or CT.

Pathology. Mucinous cystic neoplasms vary from 5 to 33 cm in largest diameter and average about 12 cm (4, 6, 7, 9). Their external surface is smooth and they are composed of unilocular or multilocular large (>5 cm) cysts (Fig. 22.10A) (4, 6, 7, 9). The cyst wall is usually 1 mm to 2 cm thick and may contain gross calcification (4). Smaller cysts (1–4 cm in diameter) may be present inside the principal cavity (4). Solid papillary excrescences (1–7 cm in diameter) sometimes protrude from the wall into the interior of the tumors (Fig. 22.10B) (4, 5). They denote a relatively poor prognosis as all eight neoplasms with gross excrescences in one series were frankly malignant and were likely to be metastatic at the time of clinical presentation (5). The absence of excrescences does not exclude frank malignancy or metastases, but it appears to diminish the likelihood (5).

The large cystic spaces are lined by mucin-producing columnar cells similar to the cells lining the large pancreatic ducts (4). Mucinous cystic neoplasms are thought to be neoplasms of the epithelium of the large pancreatic ducts (4). The configuration of the lining cells (Fig. 22.11) can range from single, orderly rows through stratification and papillary formation to frank adenocarcinoma (Fig. 22.11A) (4). Frequently, apparently benign and obviously malignant epithelium are found in the same tumor, at times adjacent to each other (Fig. 22.11B) (4). Regions of frank malignant change may be small and isolated (4). Degeneration into anaplastic, adenosquamous or pleomorphic carcinoma may occur with resulting worse prognosis (4, 15). Stains for mucin show substantial amounts of intra and extracellular mucin and no significant amount of glycogen (4, 6, 7, 9). There is a subepithelial connective tissue stroma similar to that of the ovary that may undergo hemorrhage and necrosis (4).

Radiology. Mucinous cystic tumors develop dystrophic peripheral calcification (Fig. 22.12) in their fibrous wall in roughly one-sixth of cases (4, 5). When viewed *en face*, this peripheral calcification can appear to be in the center of the mass. Reports of central, irregular calcification can be explained by failure to obtain films in the proper obliquity.

Small central foci of calcification occur in mucinous cystic neoplasms in areas of subepithelial hemorrhage and necrosis, but are probably too small to be seen on plain films, although conceivably they could be depicted by CT (5).

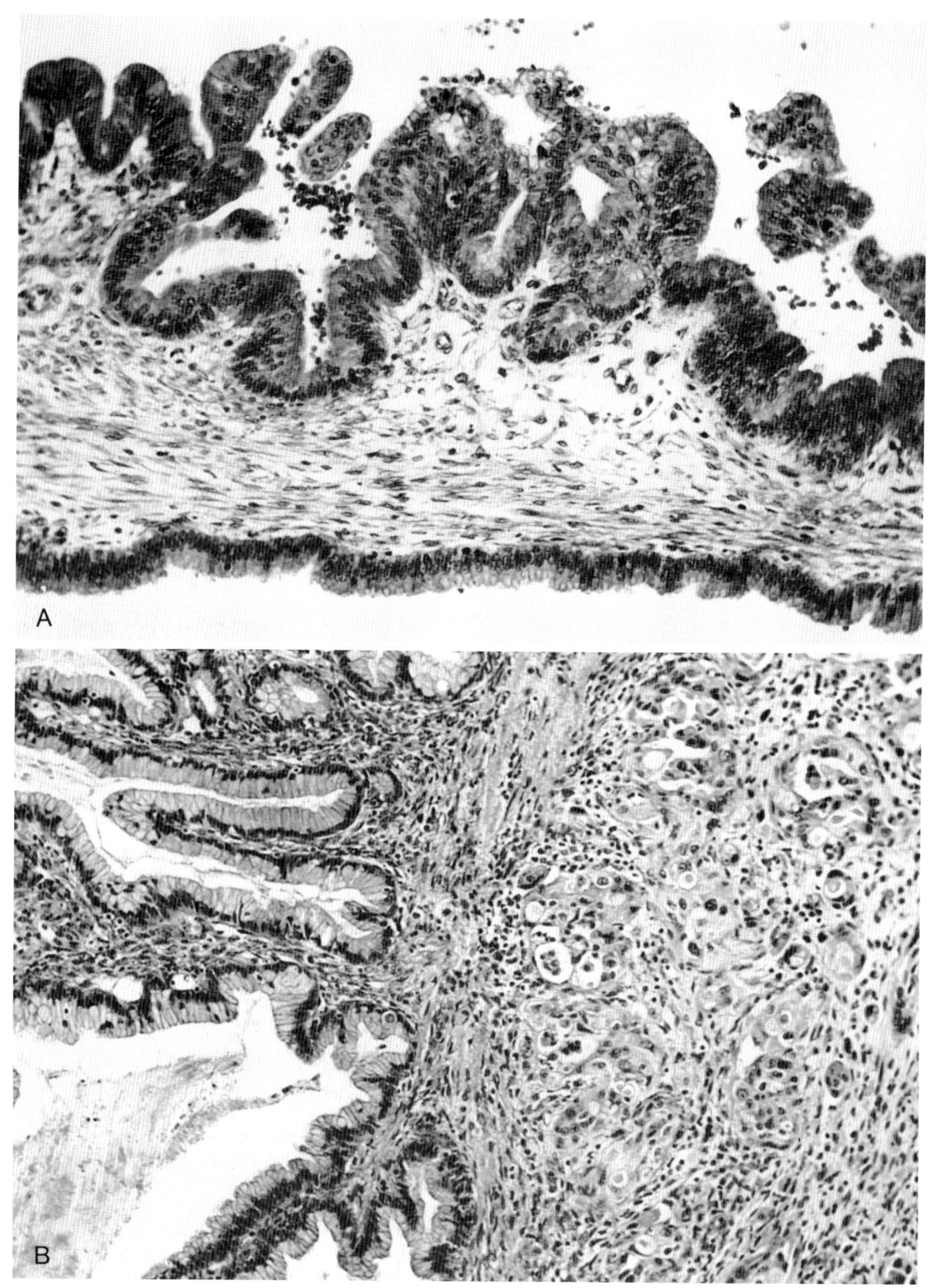

FIGURE 22.11. MUCINOUS CYSTIC NEOPLASM

A: Photomicrograph of a mucinous cystic neoplasm showing single row columnar epithelium at the bottom and papillary formations with atypia at the top. *B:* Photomicrograph of a mucinous cystic neoplasm showing papillary columnar epithelium on the left and frank adenocarcinoma on the right.

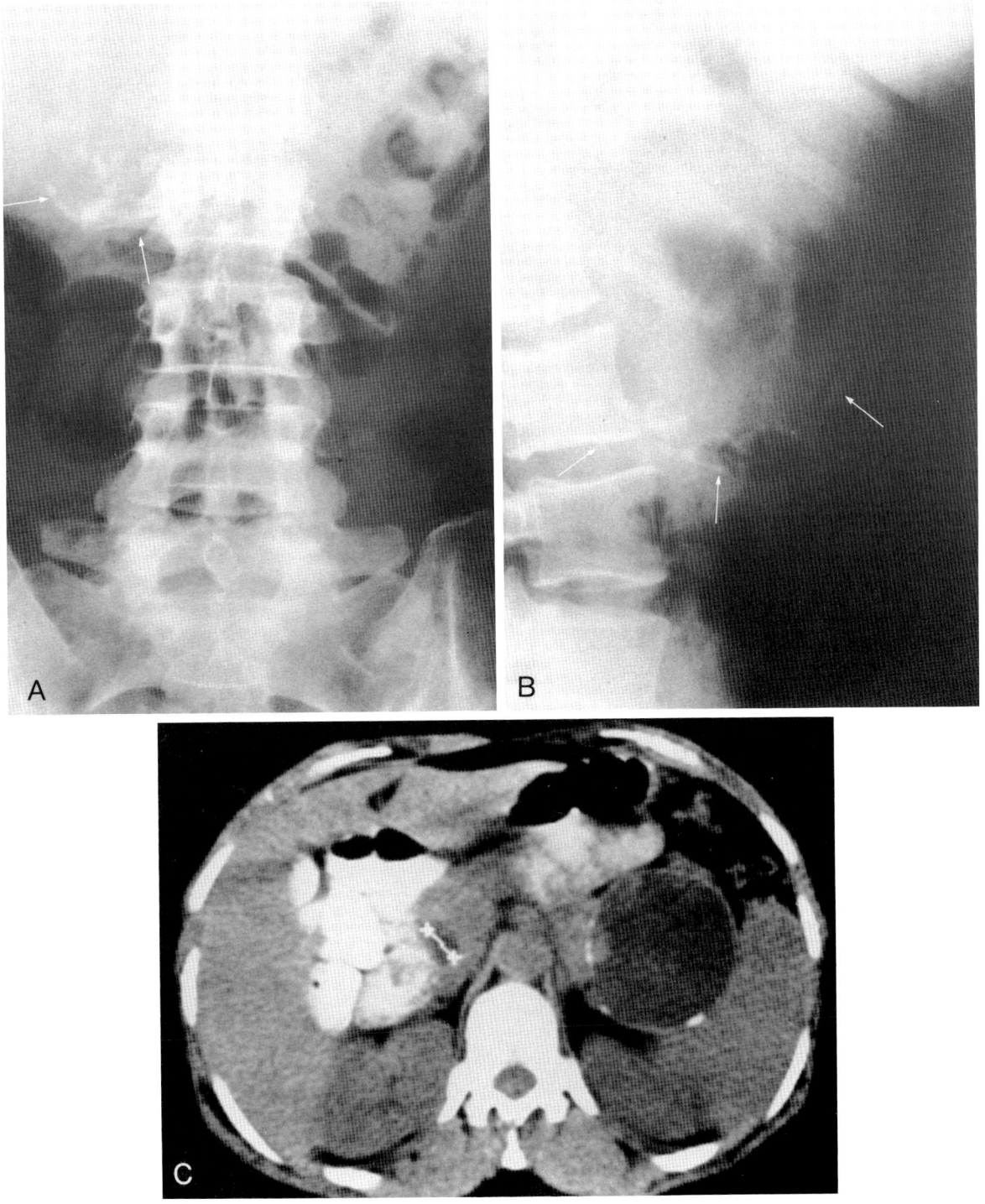

FIGURE 22.12. MUCINOUS CYSTIC NEOPLASM
A: Anteroposterior radiograph of an apparently centrally calcified mucinous cystic neoplasm (*arrows*). *B:* The lateral radiograph of the same patient shows that the calcification is actually peripheral and in the wall (*arrows*) of the neoplasm. *C:* CT of a different patient showing a mucinous cystic neoplasm with peripheral calcification and mural nodularity.

Mucinous cystic neoplasms are depicted as obviously cystic, near water density masses by sonography (Fig. 22.13) and CT (Fig. 22.14) because their cystic regions are large (5 cm or larger) (1, 5, 6, 10, 16). Since the tumors tend to be thick-walled, they are usually well-demar-

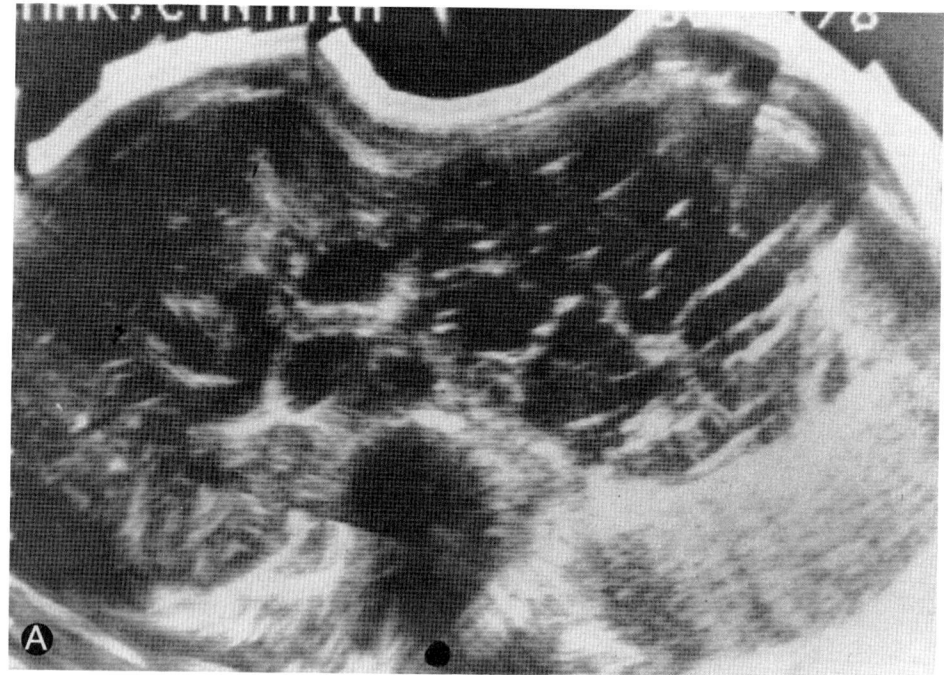

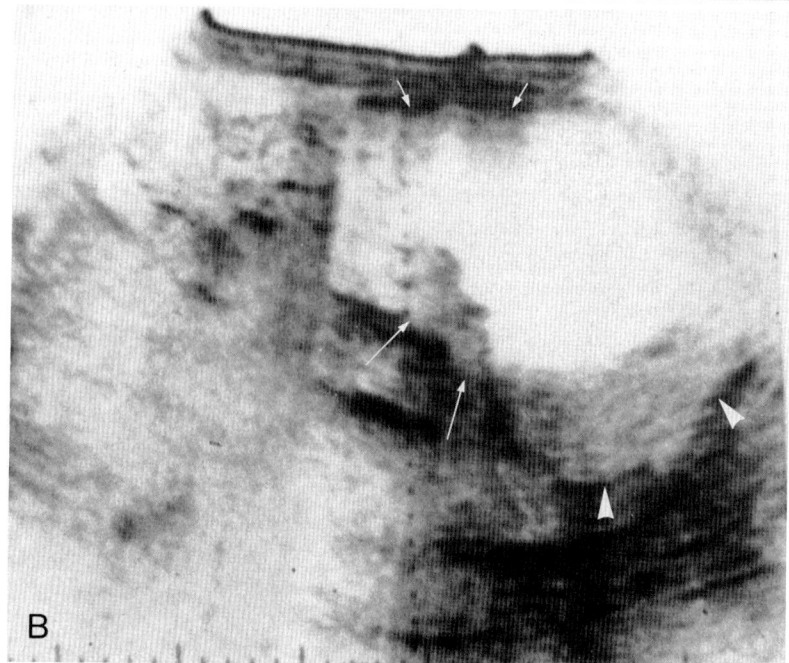

FIGURE 22.13. MUCINOUS CYSTIC NEOPLASM

A: Transverse sonogram of a mucinous cystic neoplasm showing a fairly well demarcated mass composed of multiple, large cysts (same case as seen in Fig. 22.10A). *B:* Transverse sonogram of a mucinous cystic neoplasm showing a large, unilocular cyst with solid excrescences (*arrows*). The mass is growing into the spleen (*arrowheads*).

cated (5). They are round to ovoid with a smooth external surface. The wall, demarcation, and organ of origin tend to be better depicted by CT, whereas ultrasound often shows the septations and solid excrescences to better advantage (5).

Contrast enhancement is usually limited to the wall but may be seen in solid excrescences and septations, especially if bolus, dynamic CT techniques are used (5). The presence of solid excrescences on either ultrasound or CT correlates

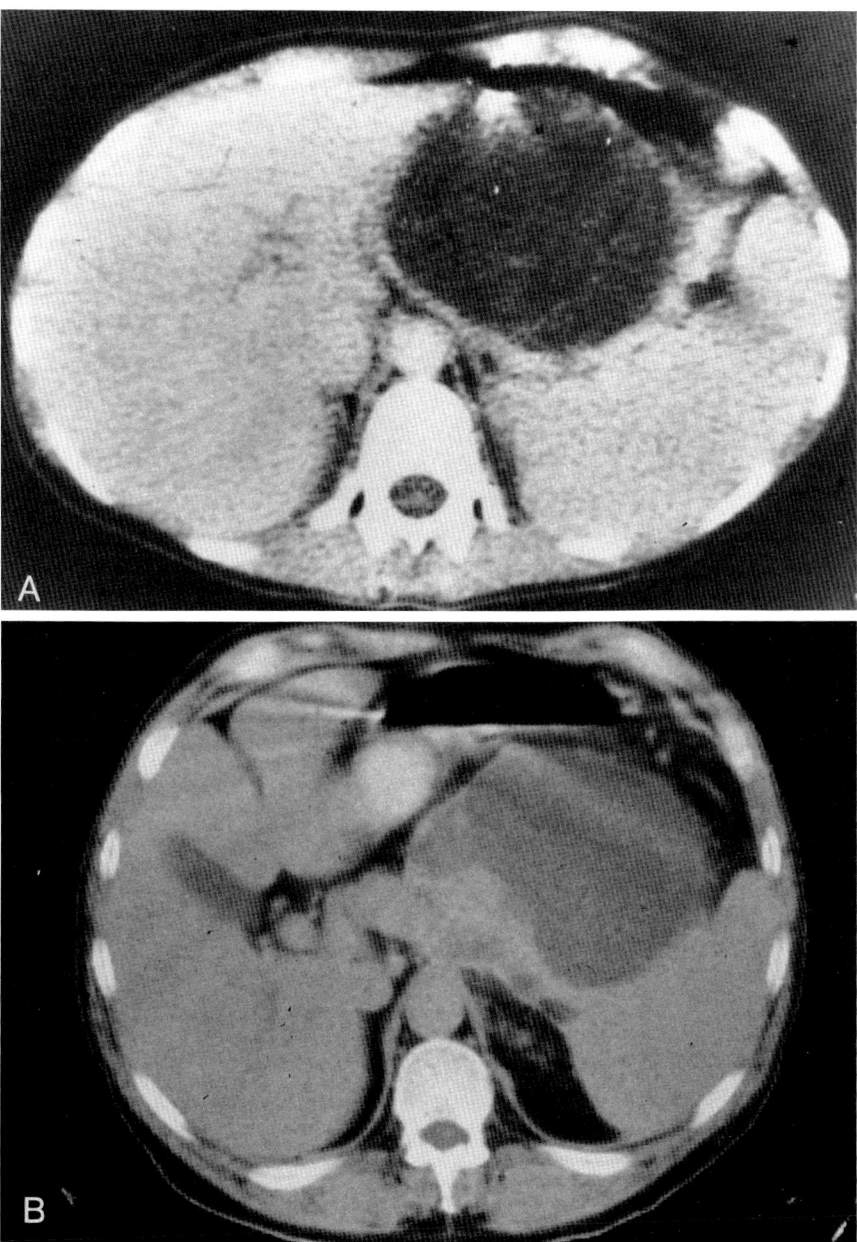

FIGURE 22.14. MUCINOUS CYSTIC NEOPLASM

A: Enhanced CT scan of a mucinous cystic neoplasm showing a large cyst with a thick, slightly enhanced wall. Septations are only faintly seen (same case as seen in Figs. 22.10A and 22.13A). *B:* CT scan of a mucinous cystic neoplasm showing a large water density mass with a solid excrescence (same case as seen in Fig. 22.13B).

with a pathologic diagnosis of frank adenocarcinoma which may still be resectable, however (5). A lack of excrescences and presence of an intact wall with good demarcation does not preclude the diagnosis of frank malignancy, although it diminishes the probability (5). Liver metastases may be indistinguishable from simple liver cysts by ultrasound or CT unless nodular excrescences or thick walls can be demonstrated (Fig. 22.15).

The angiographic appearance (Fig. 22.16) in mucinous cystic neoplasms of vessels surrounding and draping an avascular area correlates with a mass that is mostly cyst (4–7). Small areas of faint blush and minimal neovascularity correlate

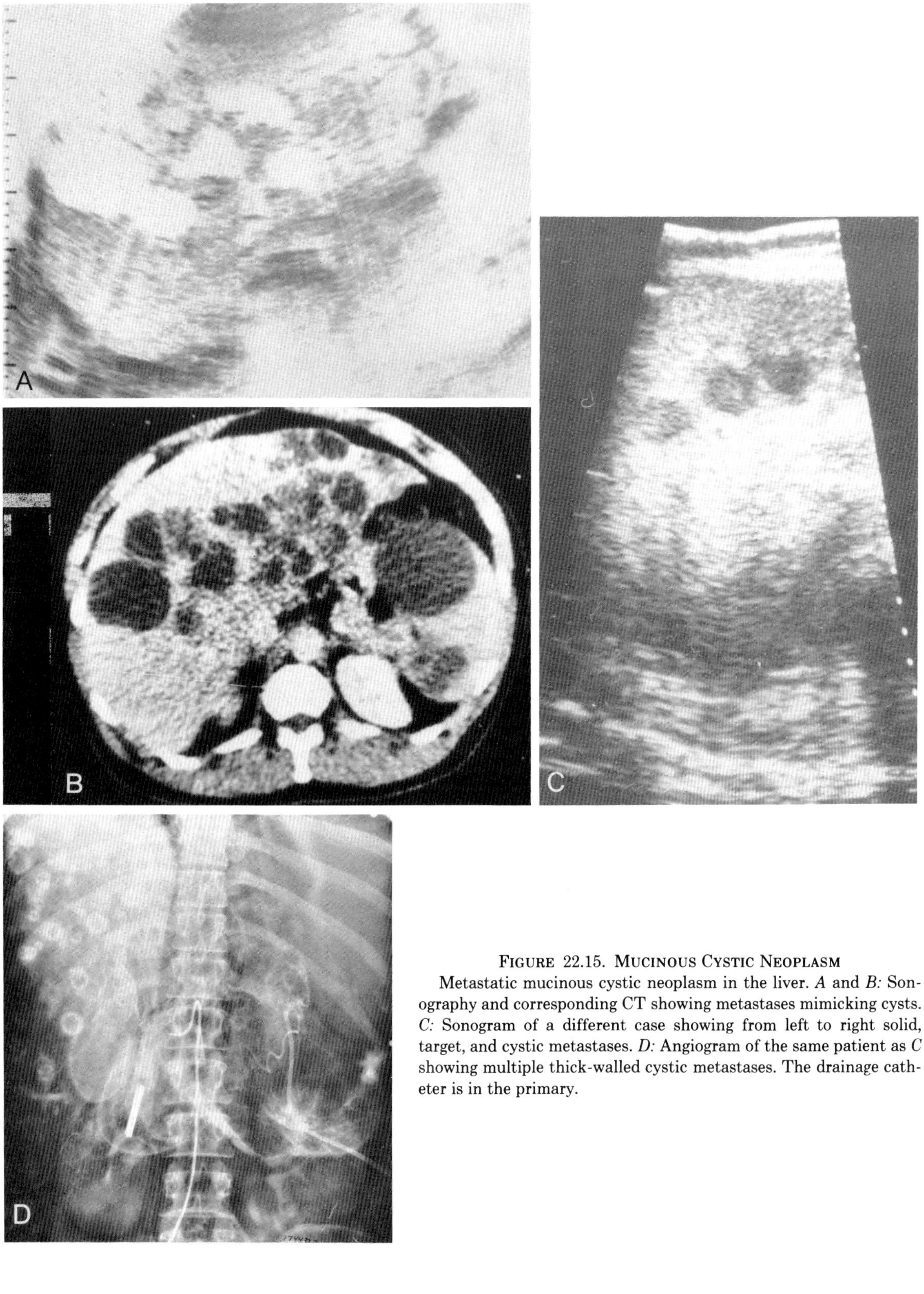

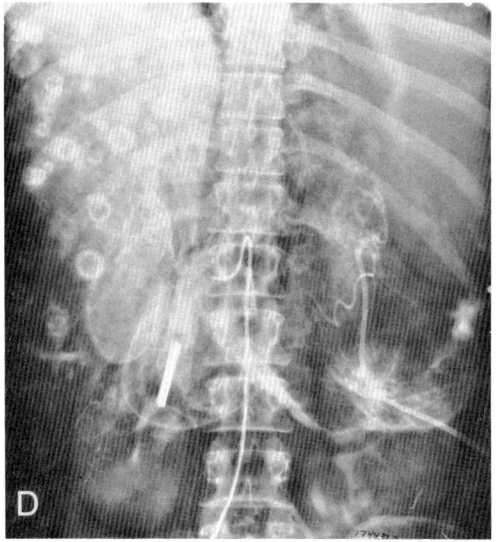

FIGURE 22.15. MUCINOUS CYSTIC NEOPLASM
Metastatic mucinous cystic neoplasm in the liver. *A* and *B:* Sonography and corresponding CT showing metastases mimicking cysts. *C:* Sonogram of a different case showing from left to right solid, target, and cystic metastases. *D:* Angiogram of the same patient as *C* showing multiple thick-walled cystic metastases. The drainage catheter is in the primary.

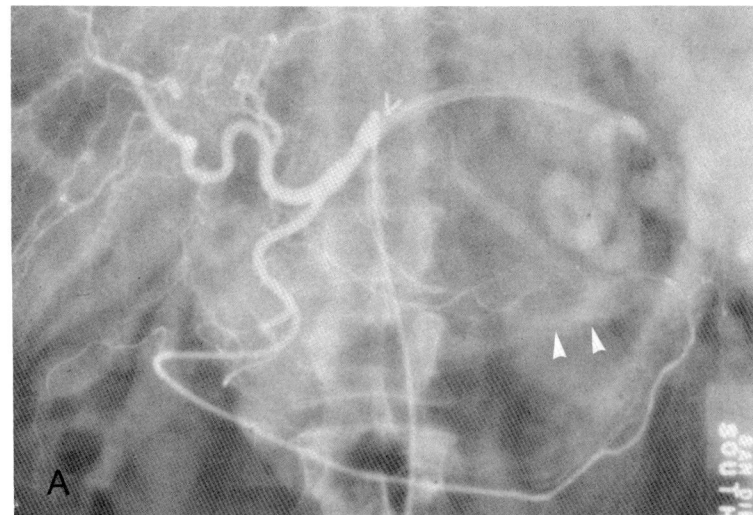
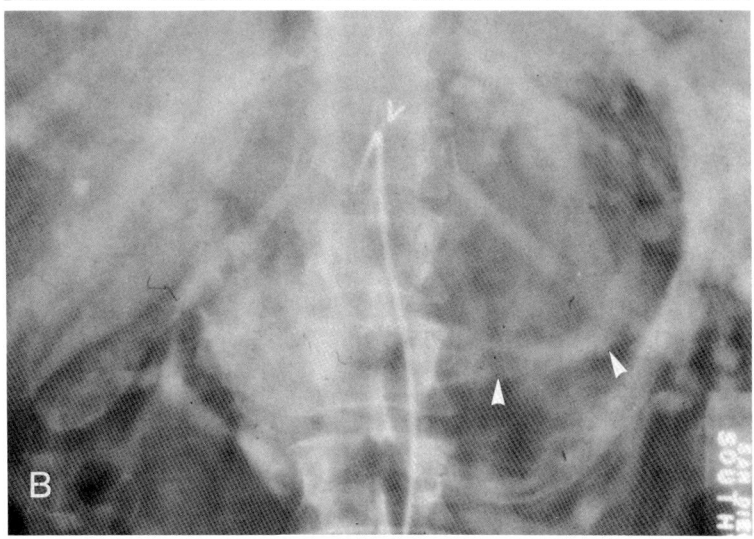

FIGURE 22.16. MUCINOUS CYSTIC NEOPLASM
A and B: Arterial and capillary phases, respectively, of an angiogram of a mucinous cystic neoplasm showing splenic vein obstruction caused by a large hypovascular mass whose only blush is in the thick wall (*arrowheads*); the blush to the right of the spine is the duodenum.

with the cyst wall and/or solid excrescences (5). Vascular encasement, when seen, may correlate with the presence of frank malignancy. The splenic vein is often obstructed, usually by displacement and/or compression (4). Differential diagnosis is pancreatic pseudocyst (5). Cholangiography is rarely done as mucinous cystic neoplasms rarely involve the head of the pancreas. There has been one cholangiogram of a mucinous cystic neoplasm reported in which the bile ducts were obstructed by mucin produced by tumor implants within the ducts (17). Proposed mechanisms were metastasis to the ducts or fistulous communication between a duct and the primary tumor (17). Endoscopic retrograde pancreatography has been reported to show three different appearances: blunt obstruction of the main pancreatic ducts (Fig. 22.17), duct displacement, and filling of the cystic cavity via the main pancreatic duct (5, 18). These appearances are not distinguishable from pseudocyst.

With modern sonography and CT, the recognition of multiple septations or shaggy nongravity dependent excrescences within the cyst should suggest the diagnosis of mucinous cystic neoplasm, not pseudocyst. However, the occasional mucinous cystic neoplasm will be depicted as a thick-walled cyst without internal architecture, leading to a radiologic misdiagnosis of pseudocyst. Uncommonly, chronic pseudocysts will develop enough debris to mimic excrescences and be misdiagnosed as mucinous cystic neoplasms. Clinical correlation and cyst wall biopsies will avoid the serious error of treating a resectable

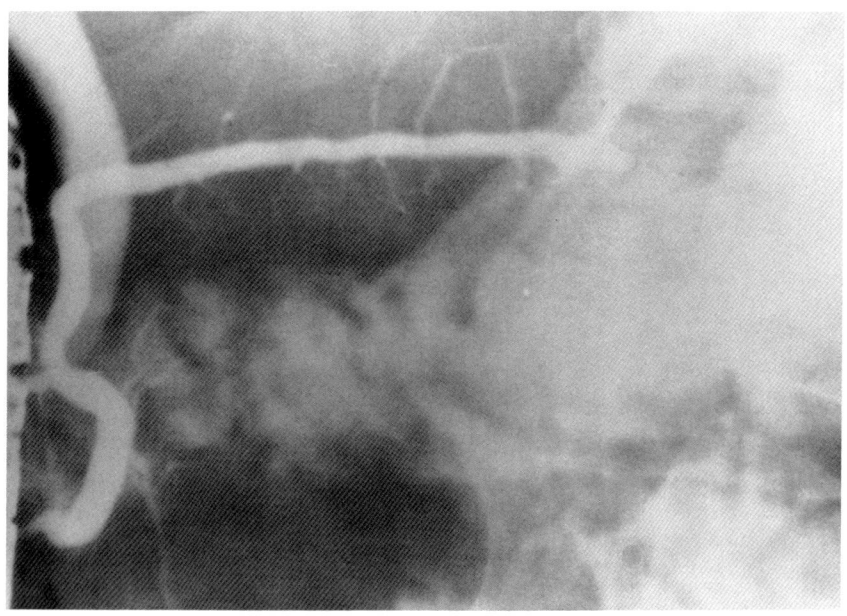

FIGURE 22.17. MUCINOUS CYSTIC NEOPLASM
An ERCP of a mucinous cystic neoplasm shows an obstructed pancreatic duct with a blunt, nonspecific termination.

mucinous cystic neoplasm as one would a pseudocyst by a cyst drainage procedure.

REFERENCES

1. Wolfman NT, Ramquist NA, Karstaedt N, Hopkins MB: Cystic neoplasms of the pancreas. CT and sonography. AJR 138:37–41, 1982.
2. Didolkar MS, Malhotra Y, Holyoke ED, Elias EG: Cystadenoma of the pancreas. Surg Gynecol Obstet 140:925–928, 1975.
3. Compagno J, Oertel JE: Microcystic adenomas of the pancreas (glycogen-rich cystadenomas). Am J Clin Pathol 69:289–298, 1978.
4. Compagno J, Oertel JE: Mucinous cystic neoplasms of the pancreas with overt and latent malignancy (cystadenocarcinoma and cystadenoma). Am J Clin Pathol 69:573–580, 1978.
5. Friedman AC, Lichtenstein JE, Dachman AH: Primary cystic neoplasms of the pancreas: radiologic-pathologic correlation. Radiology 149:45–50, 1983.
6. Hingrat JY, LeNeel JC, Charles JF, Cousin C, Lenne Y: Cystadenomas or rather microcystic adenomas and mucinous cysts of the pancreas. J Chir (Paris) 117:369–375, 1980.
7. Warter J, Walter P, Warter A, Bareiss P, Sibilly A: Cystadenoma of the pancreas. Study of the angiogenesis and the associated diseases. Sem Hop Paris 57:529–537, 1981.
8. Schwerk WB: Ultrasonically guided percutaneous puncture and analysis of aspirated material of cystic pancreatic lesions. Digestion 21:184–192, 1981.
9. Lo JW, Fung CHK, Yonan TN, Martinez N: Cystadenoma of the pancreas. Cancer 39:2470–2474, 1977.
10. Freeny PC, Weinstein CJ, Taft DA, Allen FH: Cystic neoplasms of the pancreas: new angiographic and ultrasonographic findings. AJR 131:795–802, 1978.
11. DeSantos LA, Bernardino ME, Paulus DD, Martin RE: Computed tomography of cystadenoma of the pancreas. J Comput Assist Tomogr 2:222–225, 1978.
12. Parienty RA, Ducellier R, Lubrano JM, Picard JD, Pradel J, Smolarski N: Cystadenoma of the pancreas diagnosis by computed tomography. J Comput Assist Tomogr 4:364–367, 1980.
13. Cubilla AL, Fitzgerald PJ: Classification of the pancreatic cancer (non-endocrine). Mayo Clin Proc 54:449–458, 1979.
14. Sheers R: A pancreatic cystadenoma complicated by varices: case report. Br J Surg 67:144–145, 1980.
15. Logan SE, Voet RL, Tompkins RK: The malignant potential of mucinous cysts of the pancreas. West J Med 136:157–162, 1982.
16. Carroll B, Sample WF: Pancreatic cystadenocarcinoma. CT body scan and gray scale ultrasound appearance. AJR 131:339–344, 1978.
17. Ito Y, Blackstone MO, Frank PH, Skinner DB: Mucinous biliary obstruction associated with a cystic adenocarcinoma of the pancreas. Gastroenterology 73:1410–1412, 1977.
18. Herrera L, Glassmasn CI, Komins JI: Mucinous cystic neoplasm of the pancreas demonstrated by ultrasound and endoscopic retrograde pancreatography Am J Gastroenterol 73:512–515, 1980.

DUCT CELL ORIGIN: SOLID

Duct Cell Adenocarcinoma

Clinical Findings. Duct cell adenocarcinoma represents 75% of nonendocrine malignancies of the pancreas and is a mucinous adenocarcinoma, probably arising from duct cell epithelium (1). It is the fourth or fifth most common cause of cancer death and its incidence is said to have tripled over the last 40 yr (4). The peak age is the seventh decade of life and the male to female ratio is 1.5:1 (2). The validity of epidemiologic statistics has been questioned since 40–50% of cases of cancer of the pancreas in tumor registries have been signed out without histologic confirmation (3). Articles have appeared recently linking carcinoma of the pancreas to coffee consumption (4–6). Although correlation has been shown in two studies (4, 6), there are confounding variables, especially cigarette smoking, and cause and effect cannot be inferred (6). Cigarette smoking appears to increase the risk of pancreatic carcinoma by a factor of 1.5–3 (6, 7), and alcohol intake is probably insignificant except as possibly a co-carcinogen with tobacco (7). No other occupational or environmental factors are known (8), although the high calorie, high fat, high protein U.S. diet has been implicated (7). Chronic calcific alcoholic pancreatitis probably does not predispose toward pancreatic cancer (9), whereas familial pancreatitis does (7). There is a high incidence of diabetes mellitus in patients with carcinoma of the pancreas and the duration of the diabetes is bimodal—40% greater than 2 yr and 60% less than 1 yr (7). This suggests both that long-standing diabetes may be a predisposing factor and that the onset of diabetes may be a prodromal sign (7, 9). Diabetes is a presenting sign in 25–50% of patients and may be the sole initial clinical manifestation of carcinoma of the tail of the pancreas (10). *Streptococcus bovis* septicemia occurs in patients with gastrointestinal tract neoplasms and may also occur in patients with carcinoma of the pancreas (11).

Presenting symptoms and signs of carcinoma of the head of the pancreas include loss of appetite, weight loss, pain, fatigue, jaundice, nausea and vomiting, and diabetes (2, 3, 12, 13). Cancer of the body and tail is more likely to present with abdominal pain that radiates to the back and is relieved by bending forward, and/or weight loss and anorexia (2, 3, 12, 13). In one large series, 13% of cases of cancer of the pancreas presented as metastatic adenocarcinoma of unknown primary. Of these, 70% were in the body and tail and 30% in the head (2). Occasionally, superficial thromboembolic phenomena or psychiatric problems, especially depression, are prominent clinical features (2, 14). Physical examination may reveal hepatomegaly, a palpable gallbladder, jaundice, or heme-positive stools (3). The mass itself is usually not palpable (2, 3). Eighty-five percent of patients have an elevated alkaline phosphatase, 67% elevated SGOT, 60% elevated fasting blood sugar, 38% elevated lipase, and only 9% an elevated amylase (3). Anemia from chronic gastrointestinal blood loss may be present in two-thirds of patients with cancer of the head of the pancreas (13).

The cancer is localized to the head in about 60% of cases, the body in about 10% of cases, the tail in about 5%, combination head and body about 5%, combination body and tail 10%, and the entire gland about 10% (2, 8). Prognosis is grim. In a series of 317 histologically proven cases, mean and median survival from time of diagnosis was 4 months and there were only three 5-yr survivors, who eventually died of their disease at 60, 63, and 90 months (1). When all patients (both "resectable" and unresectable) with carcinoma of the pancreas were considered in a literature review, 5-yr survival was less than 1% (3). Of these long-term survivors, 12% had bypass only. Survival is related to stage, site, and size (7). Stage I is localized and confined to the pancreas. Stage II involves the regional nodes, and Stage III is spread beyond the pancreas and the regional nodes (7).

Mean survival with Stage I is twice that of Stage II and thrice that of Stage III (7). Unfortunately, only 5% of patients are Stage I at the time of diagnosis (1). Patients with tumors of the head of the pancreas have longer survivals than those with tumors of the body and tail, since such tumors may encroach on vital structures at a smaller size and thus are usually detected earlier (8). Potentially curable "early" cancers of the ampulla or the head of the pancreas are usually 2 cm or less in diameter (15, 16). Cancer of the body and tail cannot currently be diagnosed at an "early" curable stage by investigating a symptomatic population (15). Sites of spread in descending order of frequency are liver, lymph nodes (superior head, superior body, inferior head, posterior pancreaticoduodenal most common but also inferior body, pyloric, mesenteric, anterior pancreaticoduodenal and midcolic), peritoneum, lungs, and pleura (2, 8). The duodenum is frequently invaded, the stomach less often (1).

Histologic confirmation of the clinical diagnosis should always be sought because there is a significant error in distinguishing between pancreatic carcinoma and pancreatitis by palpation alone even in experienced hands (3). In one large series, one-fourth of tumors in the head of the pancreas region were not pancreatic, instead they were ampullary, duodenal, biliary ductal, metastatic and primary retroperitoneal, and all carried an incorrect clinical diagnosis of carcinoma of the pancreas (7). Fine needle aspiration biopsy is probably the best way to obtain tissue, even intraoperatively (3).

REFERENCES

1. Cubilla AL, Fitzgerald PJ: Cancer (non-endocrine) of the pancreas. A suggested classification. *Monogr Pathol* 21:82–100, 1980.
2. Cubilla AL, Fitzgerald PJ: Pancreas cancer (non-endocrine): a review—part I. *Clin Bull* 8:91–99, 1978.
3. Gudjonsson B, Livstone EM, Spiro H: Cancer of the pancreas. Diagnostic accuracy and survival statistics. *Cancer* 42:2494–2506, 1978.
4. McMahon B, Yen S, Trichopolous D, Warren K, Nardi G: Coffee and cancer of the pancreas. *N Engl J Med* 304:630–633, 1981.
5. Goldstein HR: No association found between coffee and cancer of the pancreas (letter). *N Engl J Med* 306:997, 1982.
6. Benarde MA, Weiss W: Coffee consumption and pancreatic cancer: temporal and spatial correlation. *Br Med J* 284:400–402, 1982.
7. Cubilla AL, Fitzgerald PJ: Pancreas cancer (non-endocrine): a review—part II. *Clin Bull* 8:143–155, 1978.
8. Cubilla AL, Fitzgerald PJ: Classification of pancreatic cancer (nonendocrine). *Mayo Clin Proc* 54:449–458, 1979.
9. Schultz RE, Finkler NJ: Pancreatic calcification and pancreatic carcinoma: the relationship reconsidered. *Mt Sinai J Med* 47:622–626, 1980.
10. Katz LA, Spiro HM: Gastrointestinal manifestations of diabetes. *N Engl J Med* 275:1350–1361, 1966.
11. Herrington P, Finkelman D, Balart L, Hines Jr. C, Ferrante W: Streptococcus bovis septicemia and pancreatic adenocarcinoma (letter). *Ann Intern Med* 92:441, 1980.
12. Malegelada JR: Pancreatic cancer: an overview of epidemiology, clinical presentation, and diagnosis. *Mayo Clin Proc* 54:459–467, 1979.
13. Pollard HM, Anderson WAD, Brooks FP, Cohn I, Copeland MM, Connelly RR, Fortner JG, Kissane JM, Lemon HM, Palmer PES, Thomas LB, Webster PD III, Carter S: Staging of cancer of the pancreas. *Cancer* (Suppl) 47:1631–1637, 1981.
14. Sack GH, Levin JH, Bell WR: Trousseau's syndrome and other manifestations of chronic disseminated coagulopathy in patients with neoplasms: clinical, pathophysiologic, and therapeutic features. *Medicine* 56:1–37, 1977.
15. Moosa AR, Levin B: The diagnosis of "early" pancreatic cancer: the University of Chicago experience. *Cancer* 47:1688–1697, 1981.
16. Cubilla AL, Fitzgerald PJ. Surgical pathology aspects of cancer of the ampulla-head-of-pancreas region. *Monogr Pathol* 21:67–81, 1980.

Pathology. Grossly, adenocarcinoma of the pancreas is a gray-white scirrhous, homogeneous tumor which infiltrates and replaces normal architecture (1). Tumor margins are poorly defined. There are few, if any, foci of hemorrhage and there are only occasionally small regions of necrosis (1–4). Most duct cell adenocarcinomas are characterized by a marked desmoplastic response with disappearance of acinar tissue (2–4). Calcification is rare (2). Adenocarcinomas of the head are frequently fairly small causing little or only moderate enlargement of the head (1). They may be totally inapparent on external examination, causing merely increased consistency and nodularity on palpation (5). The masses sometimes are as large as 8–10 cm in diameter (5). The duodenal wall may be invaded, and a small percentage extend through to the mucosa to produce a fungating mass or ulceration (5). The common bile duct and ampulla are surrounded and compressed, producing biliary tract obstruction, but these structures are not commonly invaded. (Fig. 22.18) (5). Adenocarcinomas of the body and tail tend to be larger than those in the head at the time of discovery (5). Pancreatitis is present grossly in 25–40% of cases of carcinoma and microscopically in virtually all (2, 4). The pancreatitis is usually focal and secondary to duct(ule) obstruction. Carcinoma is often distributed diffusely throughout the gland on histologic examination (4). Carcinoma in situ is present in 24% of cases separate from the main tumor and atypical hyperplasia of duct epithelium is present in 27% (2). The cell of origin is believed to be the duct epithelium (1–5).

Microscopically, duct cell adenocarcinoma resembles the common adenocarcinoma seen in other organs such as the intestinal tract, lung, uterus, etc. (5), except for the frequent presence of biliary and pancreatic ductular type epithelium (3, 5, 6). Large, small, and partially formed glands as well as ductular structures are present (5). Foci of papillary areas and other cell types such as giant cells, adenosquamous cells, acinar cells, and anaplastic areas are present but constitute a small percentage of the total number of cells and less than 20% of the tumor (5). Electron microscopy shows mucinogen granules, without zymogen or islet cell granules, consistent with

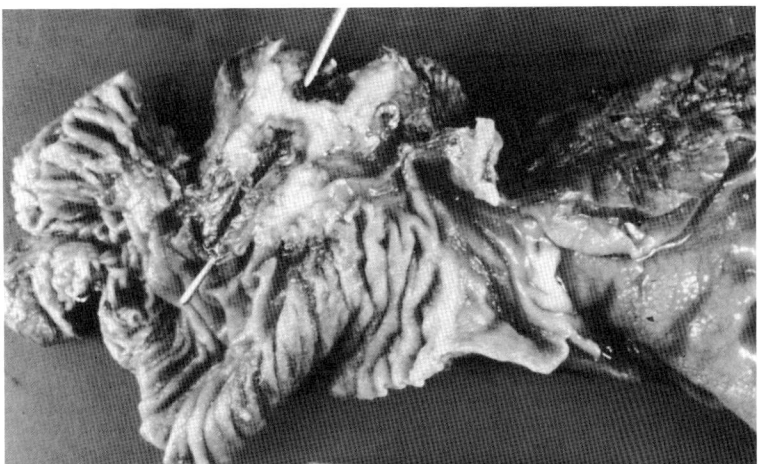

FIGURE 22.18. DUCT CELL ADENOCARCINOMA
Gross specimen of duct cell adenocarcinoma encasing the common bile duct which is probe patent despite being functionally obstructed.

origin from ductal epithelium (5). Recent evidence exists, however, that after losing zymogen granules and decreasing in height, dedifferentiated acinar units appear ductule-like. Acinar cells cannot be eliminated as possible cells of origin of adenocarcinomas that by present criteria are classified as duct cell type (6).

There are three main methods of obtaining tissue diagnosis: open wedge biopsy, transduodenal core needle biopsy, and thin needle aspiration biopsy. The first two are associated with a 5–10% complication rate (7, 8) and a 3–4% false-positive frozen section interpretation (7). Difficulties with frozen section include sampling errors, distinguishing well-differentiated cancer from normal or hyperplastic ducts, distinguishing desmoplastic response to malignancy from pancreatitis, and mistaking accessory pancreatic tissue in the duodenal wall for malignancy (9). Advantages of percutaneous fine needle aspiration are very low complication rate, ability to make multiple passes with impunity, and the possibility of avoiding surgery (8). Aspiration biopsy is 87–100% accurate with no false positives reported (8, 10). Criteria for a cytologic diagnosis of well-differentiated pancreatic adenocarcinoma are cellular pleomorphism, large vesicular nuclei, and prominent nucleoli (8). Criteria for malignancy in general are abnormal nuclear to cytoplasmic ratio, variations in size and number of nucleoli, and abnormal chromatin clumping (8).

Ampullary Carcinoma

Many carcinomas in the ampullary region are relatively large with extensive infiltration, making it difficult or impossible to designate a site of origin. The uncommon localized ampullary carcinoma has a much better prognosis than carcinoma of the head of the pancreas—26% 5-yr survival of patients resected for cure, excluding operative and noncancer caused deaths (11). Division into intraampullary carcinoma, periampullary carcinoma, and mixed is useful. Intraampullary is defined as confined to the ampulla without significant extension into duodenum or pancreas, periampullary involves primarily duodenal mucosa at the ampulla, and mixed is a combination of the two (11). Five-year survival is 33%, 17%, and 0%, respectively. As with carcinoma of the pancreatic head, tumors larger than 2 cm in diameter are almost never curable (11, 12). No one knows if the relatively good prognosis of ampullary cancers vis-à-vis carcinomas of the pancreatic head is due to more frequent detection at a smaller size or an intrinsic biologic difference in the malignancies.

Most ampullary cancers are typical adenocarcinomas. Intraampullary tumors are mucinous with a mix of gastrointestinal, biliary, and pancreatic ductal epithelium present (11). Periampullary cancers contain more gastrointestinal epithelium (11). A few ampullary cancers contain the same unusual cell types as the uncommon pancreatic carcinomas (giant cell, adenosquamous, etc.) (11). The Whipple procedure is appropriate for attempted cure of ampullary carcinoma (11). Care must be taken to resect an adequate amount of bile duct, as tumor extent is often underestimated by cholangiography.

REFERENCES

1. Robbins SL, Cotran SR: *Pathologic Basis of Disease.* Philadelphia, W. B. Saunders, 1979, pp 1104–1107.

2. Cubilla AL, Fitzgerald PJ: Pancreas cancer (non-endocrine): a review, part II. *Clin Bull* 8:143–155, 1978.
3. Cubilla AL, Fitzgerald PJ: Classification of pancreatic cancer (nonendocrine). *Mayo Clin Proc.* 54:449–458, 1979.
4. Frantz VK: Tumors of the pancreas. In *Atlas of Tumor Pathology.* Washington, D.C., Armed Forces Institute of Pathology, Sect. 7 Fasc. 27&28, 1959, pp 36–75.
5. Cubilla AL, Fitzgerald PJ: Cancer (non-endocrine) of the pancreas. A suggested classification. *Mongr Pathol* 21:82–100, 1980.
6. Bockman DE: Cells of origin of pancreatic cancer: experimental animal tumors related to human pancreas. *Cancer* 47:1528–1534, 1981.
7. Lee YN: Tissue diagnosis for carcinoma of the pancreas and periampullary structures. *Cancer* 49:1035–1039, 1982.
8. Beazley RM: Needle biopsy diagnosis of pancreatic cancer. *Cancer* 47:1685–1687, 1981.
9. Rosai J: *Ackerman's Surgical Pathology.* St. Louis, C. V. Mosby, 1981, pp 670–674.
10. Gudjonsson B, Spiro HM: Biopsy techniques in the diagnosis of pancreatic cancer. *Gastroenterology* 75:726–728, 1978.
11. Cubilla AJ, Fitzgerald PJ: Surgical pathology aspects of the ampulla-head of-pancreas region. *Mongr Pathol* 21:67–81, 1980.
12. Moosa AR, Levin B: The diagnosis of "early" pancreatic cancer: the University of Chicago experience. *Cancer* 47:1688–1697, 1981.

Radiologic Features of Duct Cell Adenocarcinoma

Plain Films

Adenocarcinoma of the pancreas is not associated with tumor calcification (1). Coexistent calcification may rarely be present due to pancreatitis, either preexisting or superimposed because of ductal obstruction by the malignancy. Splenomegaly from splenic vein obstruction or enlargement of the gallbladder from cystic duct obstruction is occasionally detected by plain films of the abdomen (Fig. 22.19A). Small bowel ischemia can occur from mesenteric vascular encasement and occlusion (Fig. 22.19B). Adenocarcinoma of the pancreas may metastasize to mediastinal or hilar lymph nodes (Fig. 22.20). Extension of tumor into parenchyma from hilar nodes can mimic bronchogenic carcinoma (1). Lung metastases can be either hematogenous in the form of multiple peripheral nodules or lymphangitic (1). Pleural metastases are uncommon.

Symptomatic bone metastases from adenocarcinoma of the pancreas are relatively rare, although autopsy series show frequencies of skeletal metastases as high as 20% (2). Bone involvement may result from direct posterior extension of the primary tumor (affecting the twelfth thoracic through the third lumbar vertebrae) or hematogenous dissemination (1, 2). Although usually lytic, purely blastic lesions can occur and may be more common than generally believed (2).

Conventional Contrast Examinations

If ultrasound or CT is available, barium studies are no longer the primary screening examinations for patients with suspected pancreatic cancer. The routine upper gastrointestinal series misses almost all adenocarcinomas in the body and tail and detects only about half in the head (3). However, those adenocarcinomas that do not produce jaundice may present with gastrointestinal or genitourinary complaints resulting in a barium study or an excretory urogram being performed initially. Unfortunately, there are no findings to reliably differentiate malignancy from pancreatitis other than pancreatic lithiasis, which almost always indicates pancreatitis (1, 4). When duct cell adenocarcinomas of the pancreas produce abnormalities on conventional examinations, they are unresectable save for localized ampullary tumors.

Upper Gastrointestinal Series

Esophagus. Adenocarcinomas of the pancreas occasionally present with dysphagia, usually due to a mass in the tail, but sometimes one in the body or head (1, 5, 6). Esophageal manifestations are caused either by tumor involvement of lymph nodes in the hiatus and paracardiac area or direct extension of a large adenocarcinoma of the tail. The usual radiologic manifestation is lifting up and straightening of the distal (subdiaphragmatic) esophagus, resulting in an abnormal horizontal course (1, 5, 6). Constriction and ulceration mimicking primary gastric or esophageal carcinoma may occur (1, 5, 6). A radiologic appearance indistinguishable from achalasia with diminished peristalsis, functional obstruction with "beaking" of the distal esophagus and absence of the gastric air bubble may be seen (5, 6). Esophageal and/or gastric varices may be demonstrated when adenocarcinomas of the body and tail obstruct the splenic vein, but significant bleeding from these varices is not common.

Stomach and Duodenum. A commonly cited radiologic finding attributable to pancreatic masses is widening of the retrogastric space (1). Because of a wide range of normal, widening of the retrogastric space is usually an unreliable

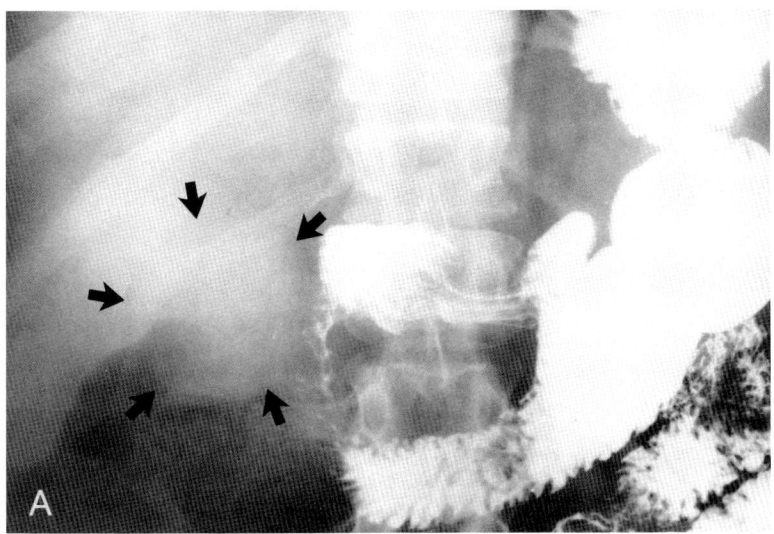

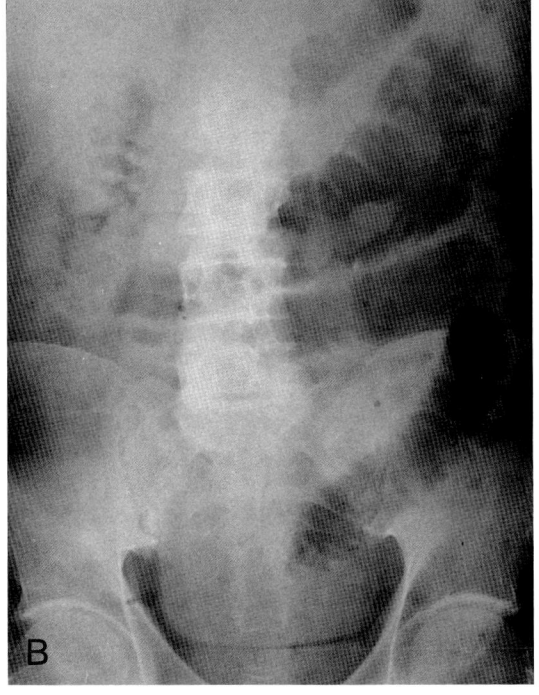

FIGURE 22.19. DUCT CELL ADENOCARCINOMA
A: Film from an upper gastrointestinal tract examination shows a large gallbladder (*arrows*) in a patient with duct cell adenocarcinoma of the pancreas. B: Abdominal film showing ascites and dilated loops of small bowel. The patient died shortly thereafter from extensive gangrene of the small bowel caused by carcinoma of the pancreas occluding the superior mesenteric vein.

sign unless there is an extrinsic mass impression on the posterior gastric wall, which could be caused by an adenocarcinoma in the body or tail (Fig. 22.21A) (1). Adenocarcinomas of the head or head and body can produce "antral padding" which refers to extrinsic indentation of the posteroinferior antrum with splaying of gastric folds (Fig. 22.21B). A smooth indentation of the stomach usually means that the carcinoma has not yet invaded the stomach, whereas irregularity or ulceration indicate invasion (1). Pancreatic adenocarcinoma can present as an intraluminal ulcerated mass mimicking primary gastric carcinoma (1).

Adenocarcinoma of the pancreatic head tends to involve the duodenal sweep, whereas carcinomas of the body and tail affect the distal duodenum and duodenojejunal junction. "Widening of the C-loop" is a nonspecific finding usually produced by fat in a mesomorphic or obese patient. When pathologic, it can be caused by any mass in the region (Fig. 22.22) (1). Changes in the duodenal sweep suggestive of carcinoma include mucosal fold changes, padding, distorted

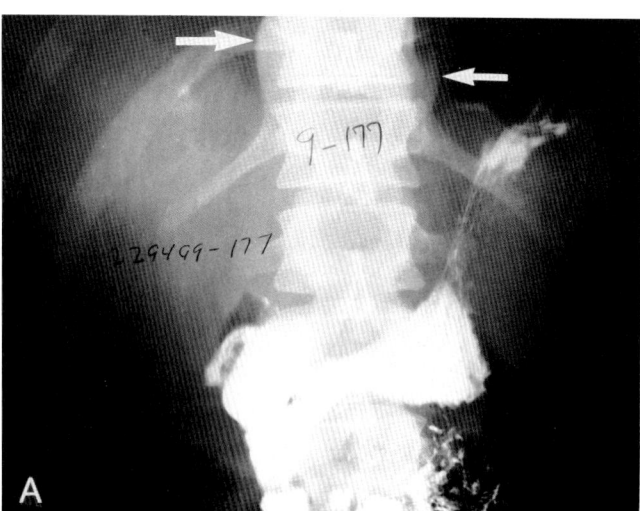
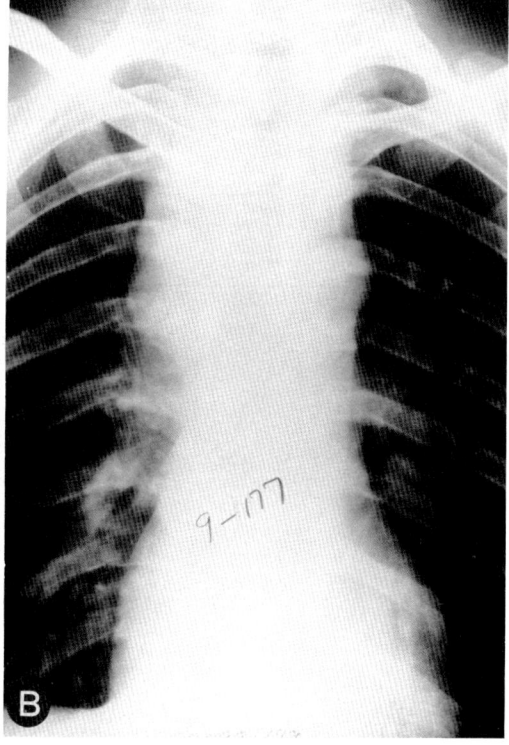

FIGURE 22.20. DUCT CELL ADENOCARCINOMA

A: An upper gastrointestinal radiograph shows posterior mediastinal adenopathy (*arrows*) and displacement of the stomach by an enlarged spleen in a patient with duct cell adenocarcinoma of the pancreas. *B:* A chest x-ray of the same patient shows superior mediastinal adenopathy.

diverticula and the "Frostberg 3 sign" (Fig. 22.23).

Neoplastic infiltration of the duodenal wall and/or desmoplastic response to tumor produces traction on and fixation of folds. This manifests itself as spiculation (sharpening and elongation of barium trapped between folds), blunting or nodularity of folds. These findings must be differentiated from peristalsis which can easily produce false positives on any one or two radiographs (1). (Fig. 22.23A and B). An enlarged gallbladder may indent the superolateral duodenal bulb or second portion of the duodenum (Fig. 22.23C). Padding of the sweep refers to a smooth indentation giving a double contour image. It is a reliable sign of a mass when not transient, but it can be produced by a dilated common bile duct as well as by a mass in the head of the pancreas (Fig. 22.23D) (7, 8). Distortion of a duodenal diverticulum is a rare but valid sign of a mass in the head of the pancreas (Fig. 22.23E) (1). It is more easily appreciated with confidence when serial films are available. Frostberg 3 sign (Fig. 22.23F) refers to an inverted 3 contour to the medial portion of the duodenal sweep. It is an uncommon finding in carcinoma of the pancreas (1). The central limb of the 3 is thought to be the point of fixation of the duodenal wall at the ampulla (1). Spasm, edema, and common bile duct dilatation as well as the actual tumor mass could all contribute to the remainder of the deformity. The occasional far advanced carcinoma of the pancreas will produce an irregular, stenosing, ulcerated mucosal lesion at times indistinguishable from primary duodenal diseases such as post-bulbar ulcer, lymphoma, and carcinoma (Fig. 22.23G–I).

Carcinoma of the ampulla is distinguished radiographically by its location—above the straight segment, within the superior portion of the longitudinal fold and just below the promontory (1). The usual appearance is that of an irregular nodular mass often with mucosal destruction. This corresponds to either a periampullary or a mixed carcinoma. Intraampullary carcinoma can cause a smooth submucosal mass effect with a deceptively benign appearance (Fig. 22.24) (1). The latter has a better prognosis

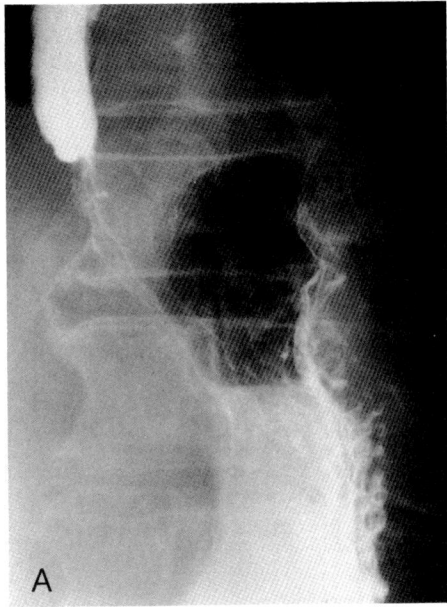
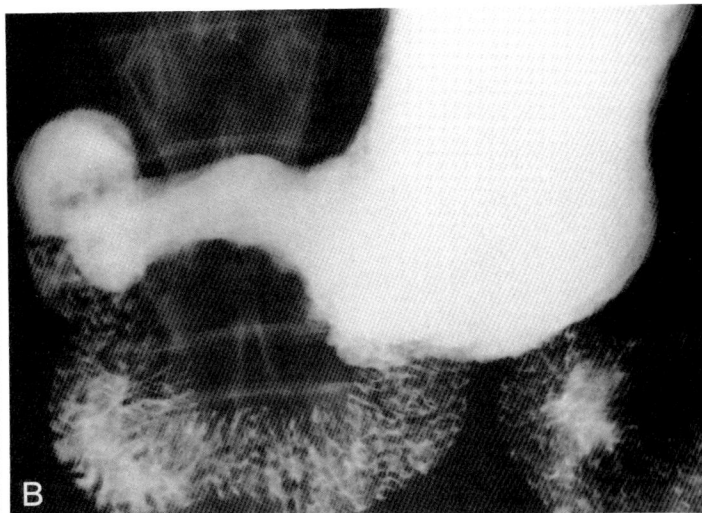
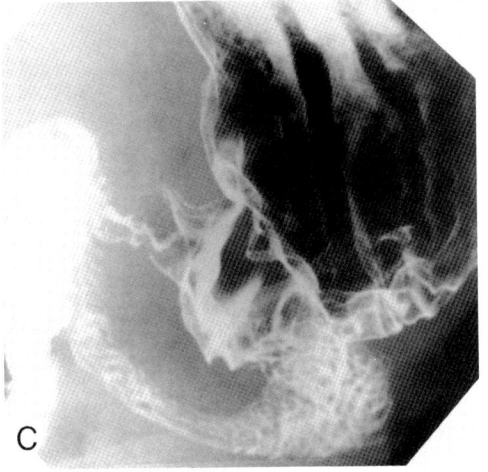

FIGURE 22.21. DUCT CELL ADENOCARCINOMA
A: Right posterior oblique (RPO) film shows indentations of the posterior fundus by duct cell adenocarcinoma of the pancreatic tail. *B:* Antral padding by duct cell adenocarcinoma of the head and body of the pancreas. *C:* Thickened, distorted folds in an encased antrum produced by duct cell carcinoma of the body of the pancreas.

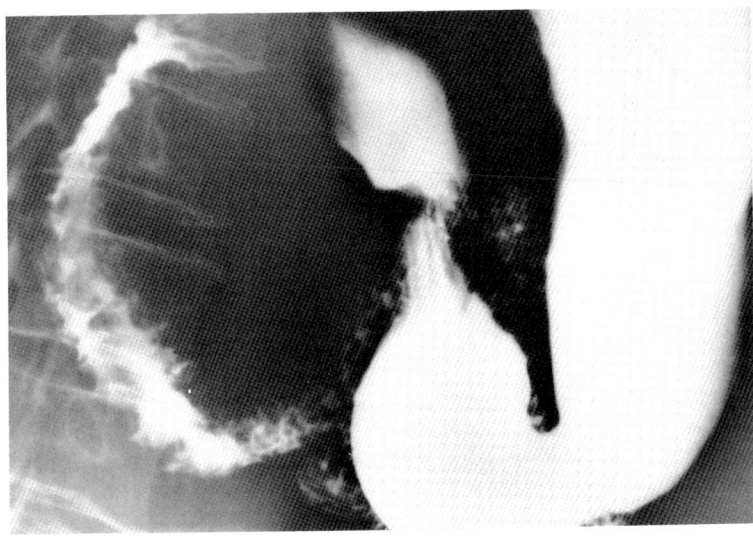

FIGURE 22.22. DUCT CELL ADENOCARCINOMA
Widening of the duodenal sweep with thickened and distorted folds due to duct cell adenocarcinoma. Pancreatitis can produce the same picture.

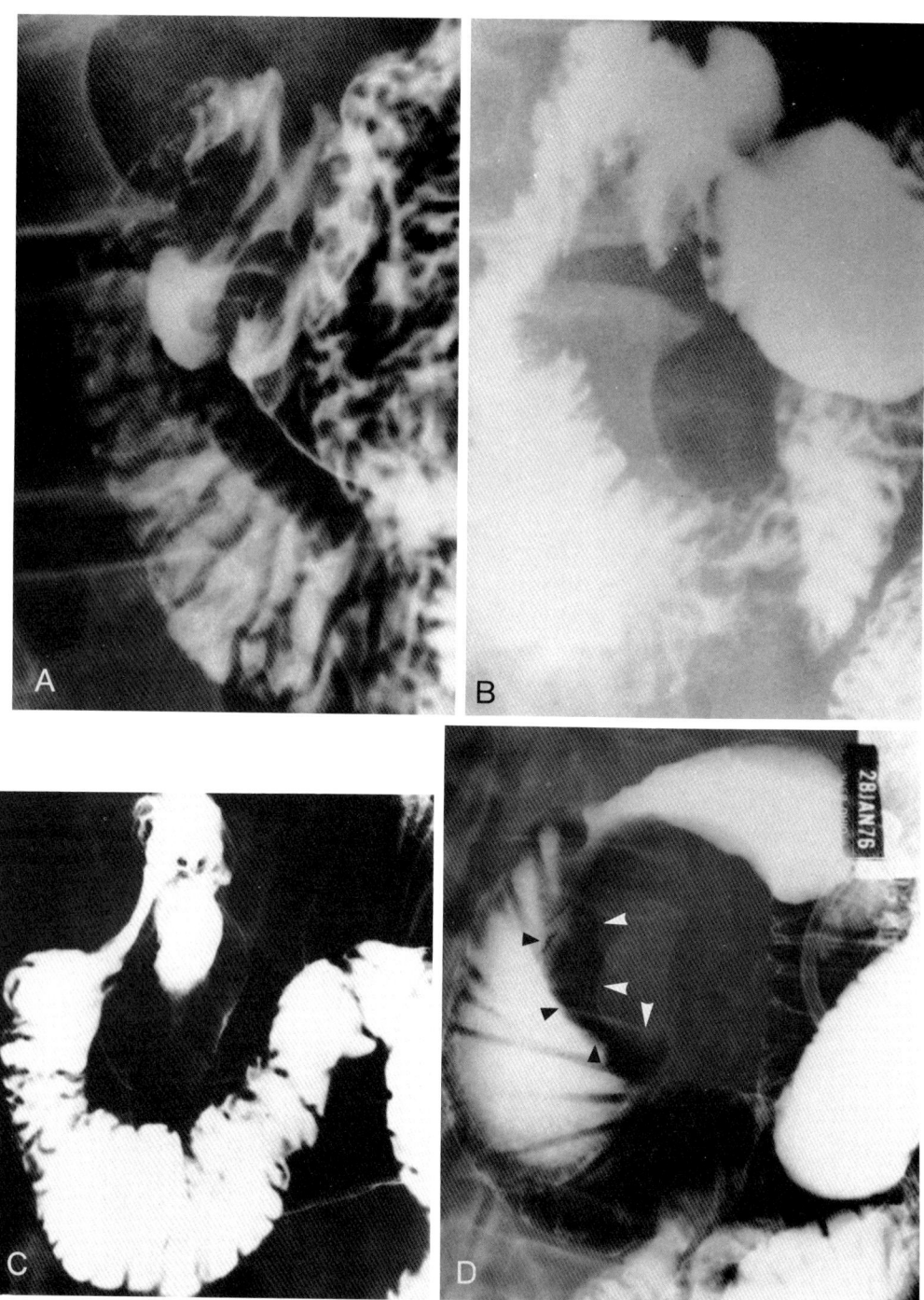

FIGURE 22.23. DUCT CELL ADENOCARCINOMA

A: Spiculation of folds along the medial border of the duodenal sweep in a patient with duct cell adenocarcinoma. *B:* Same patient, same examination, showing normal folds in the same region. The spiculation was a transitory, spurious finding in this case and must be persistent to be real. *C:* Smooth, extrinsic indentation of an enlarged gallbladder in the second portion of the duodenum in a patient with duct cell adenocarcinoma. Anteroposterior projection. *D:* Padding of the medial border of the C-loop (*arrowheads*) by duct cell adenocarcinoma. Right anterior oblique (RAO) projection. *E:* Duct cell adenocarcinoma distorting a duodenal diverticulum (*arrows*). RAO projection. *F:* Frostberg's 3 sign (*arrowheads*) produced by duct cell adenocarcinoma. Note biliary drainage catheter marking common duct and ampulla. *G:* Carcinoma of the head of the pancreas mimicking post bulbar ulcer. (*arrows*). *H:* Carcinoma of the pancreas invading the duodenum producing a large intraduodenal mass. Findings are indistinguishable from primary duodenal lymphoma. *I:* Carcinoma of the body of the pancreas causing a large ulceration in the transverse duodenum. Carcinoma of the duodenum, lymphoma, and leiomyosarcoma would be in the differential.

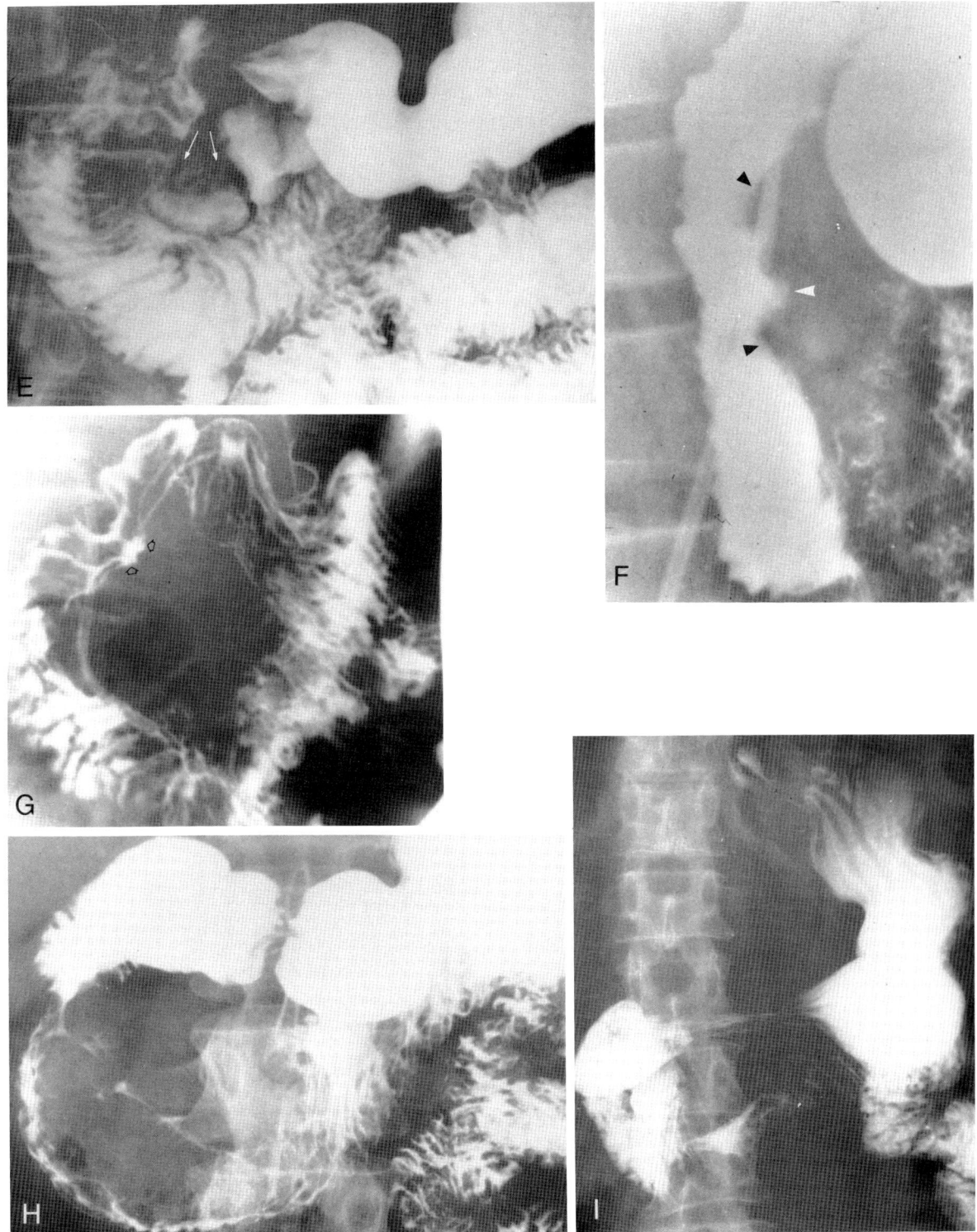

FIGURE 22.23*E–I*

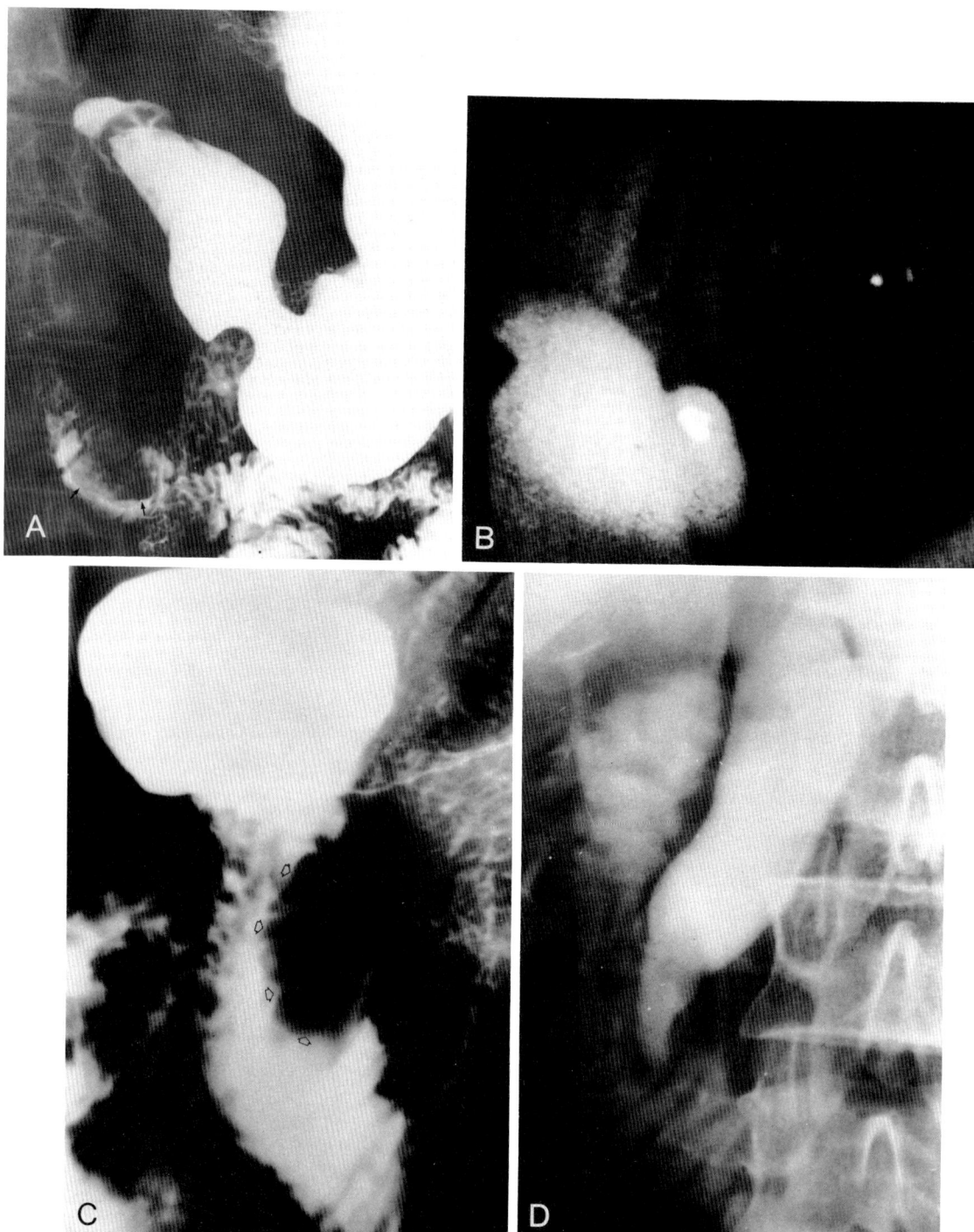

FIGURE 22.24. AMPULLARY CARCINOMA

A: Ampullary carcinoma presenting as a smooth, submucosal duodenal mass (*arrows*). *B:* Endophoto of *A*. *C:* Indentation of anterior portion of C-loop with intact folds (*arrows*) produced by a dilated common duct in a patient with ampullary carcinoma (steep RAO). *D:* Transhepatic cholangiogram of same patient. The neoplasm is the unopacified area between the distal common duct and the duodenum. The bulk of the mass effect is produced by the dilated common duct.

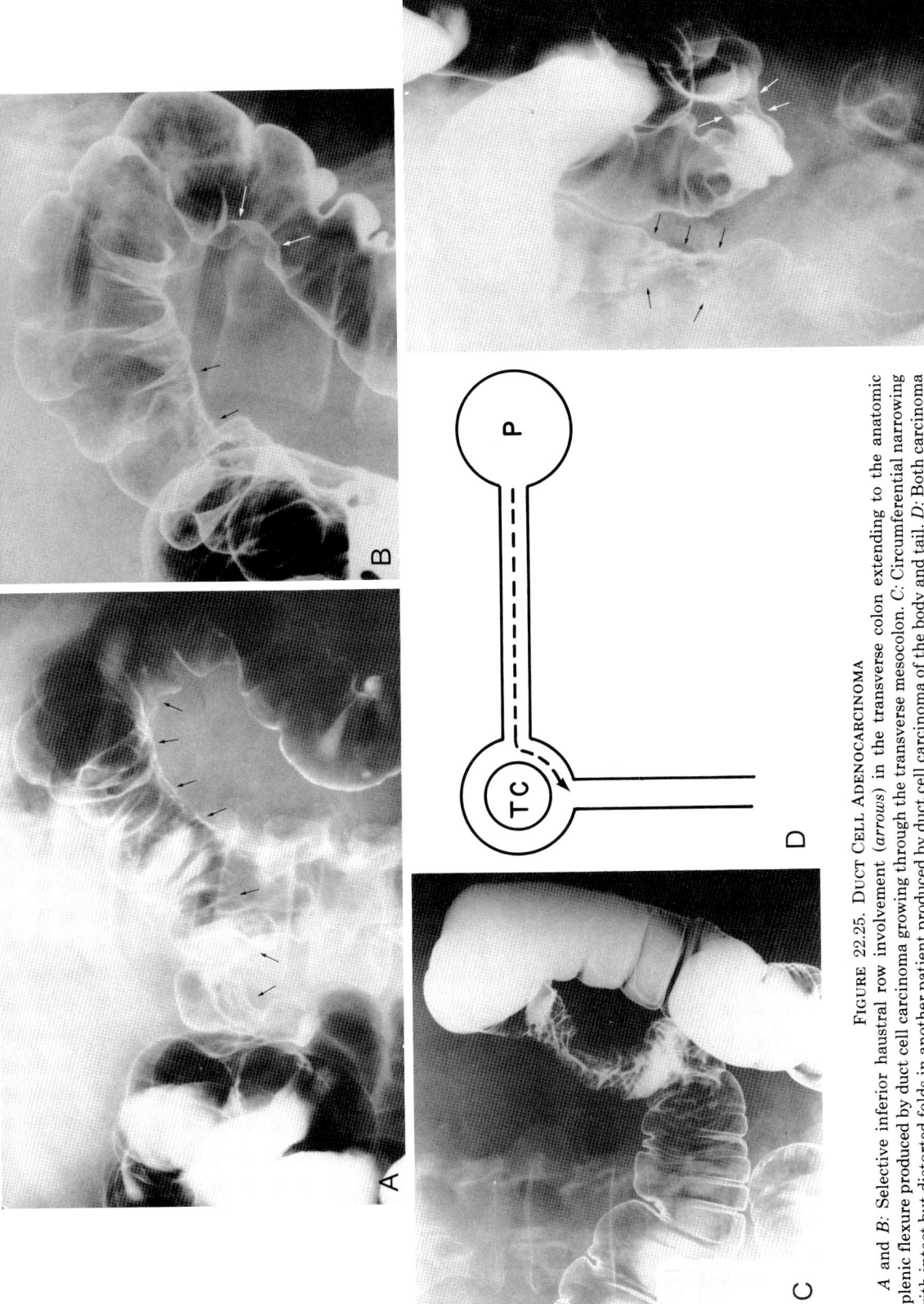

FIGURE 22.25. DUCT CELL ADENOCARCINOMA

A and *B*: Selective inferior haustral row involvement (*arrows*) in the transverse colon extending to the anatomic splenic flexure produced by duct cell carcinoma growing through the transverse mesocolon. *C*: Circumferential narrowing with intact but distorted folds in another patient produced by duct cell carcinoma of the body and tail. *D*: Both carcinoma and pancreatitis preferentially spread to involve the inferior haustral row of the transverse colon via the transverse mesocolon. Barium injected into the mesocolon at the pancreatic border follows the path shown. *P* = pancreas; *TC* = transverse colon. *E*: Luminal narrowing with intact mucosa (*arrows*) in the rectosigmoid and sigmoid from duct cell carcinoma of the pancreas spreading intraperitoneally to the pouch of Douglas and the sigmoid mesocolon.

compared to the former two (see "Ampullary Carcinoma" for definitions).

Carcinomas of the body and tail are quite large by the time they affect the duodenojejunal junction. They produce a posterosuperior or sometimes left-sided mass effect associated with distortion of folds and, at times, ulceration (1).

Colon and Small Bowel. Carcinomas of the

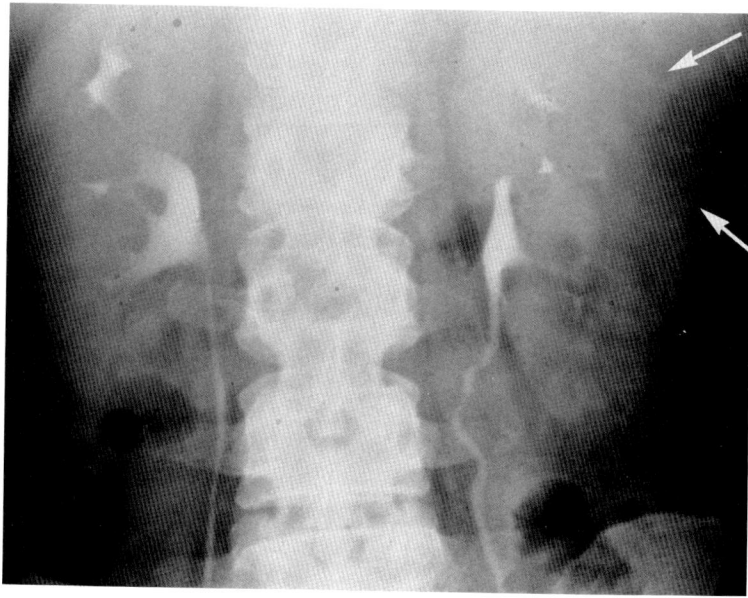

FIGURE 22.26. DUCT CELL ADENOCARCINOMA
Loss of the upper outer cortical margin of the left kidney (*arrows*) from invasion by a carcinoma of the tail of the pancreas.

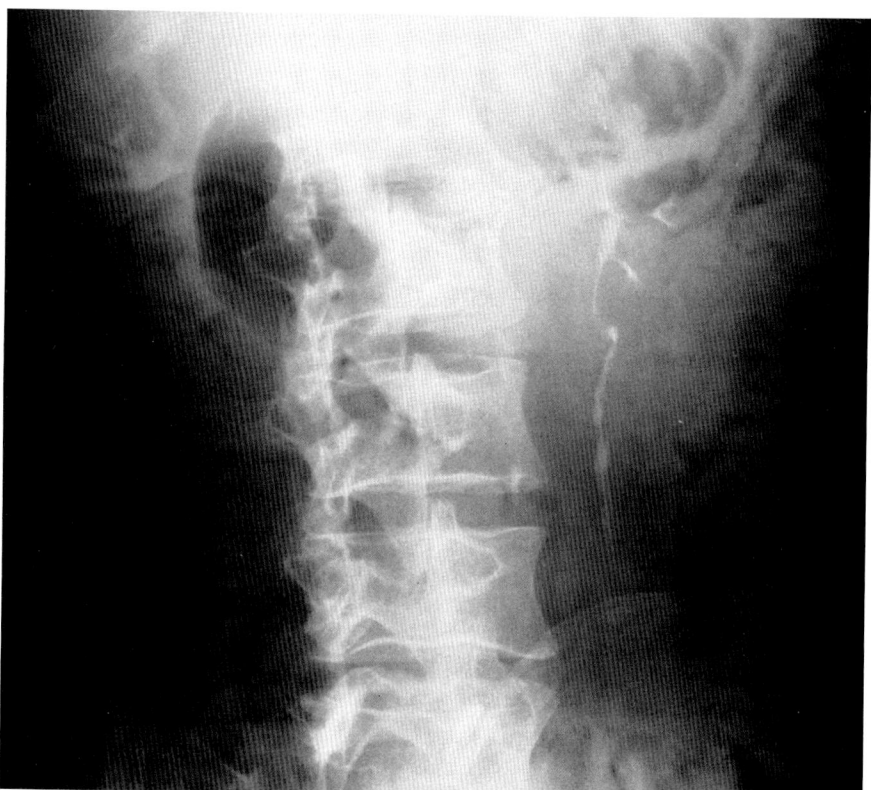

FIGURE 22.27. DUCT CELL ADENOCARCINOMA
Notching of the left pelvis and ureter from renal vein occlusion and collateral veins secondary to encasement by duct cell carcinoma of the pancreas.

body and tail not uncommonly involve the transverse colon and splenic flexure by direct extension via the transverse mesocolon and the splenorenal and phrenocolic ligaments. The inferior haustral row is involved first or predominantly in the transverse colon (Fig. 22.25A and B). This is because of preferential downward extension of the mesenteric plane of the transverse mesocolon (10). Initial findings are localized haustral flattening and padding which may then progress through luminal narrowing with a serrated contour to a circumferential stricture with the latter a late finding (Fig. 22.25C and D) (1, 9, 10). The haustral pattern of a relatively uninvolved superior row may be thrown into pseudosacculation (9, 10).

Adenocarcinomas of the pancreas affect other segments of the colon as well as small bowel by intraperitoneal seeding. Dependent areas tend to be predominantly involved (10). Common areas of pooling and corresponding sites of involvement are: pouch of Douglas—rectosigmoid; lower small bowel mesentery—terminal ileum and cecum; right paracolic gutter—cecum, ascending colon, and small bowel loops; and sigmoid mesocolon—superior border of sigmoid (10). Early findings are fixation, angulation, and mucosal tethering rather than mass effect because of the desmoplastic response to the tumor cells (10). Eventually circumferential narrowing can be produced (Fig. 22.25E) (1, 10).

Excretory Urography

Adenocarcinoma of the pancreas generally does not involve the genitourinary tract until late in the course of the disease, but patients may present with symptoms such as flank pain, hematuria, hypertension from renal artery stenosis, or positive urine cytology (11). The most common urographic abnormality is inferior displacement of the left kidney with lateral displacement of the upper pole caused by a mass in the tail of the pancreas (1, 11). Usually, mass effect is extrinsic with pancaking of the kidney and elongation and thinning of the major calyces (1, 11). However, the tumor can be adherent to or even invade the kidney, closely mimicking an intrarenal mass (Fig. 22.26). The right kidney may be affected by masses in the head of the pancreas in a similar manner (1, 11). Notching of the ureter can be due to adenopathy or renal vein thrombosis (Fig. 22.27) (1, 11). Either the right or the left renal vein can be invaded by a pancreatic carcinoma, as they are in proximity to the gland.

REFERENCES

1. Eaton Jr. SB, Ferrucci Jr. JT: *Radiology of the Pancreas and Duodenum.* Philadelphia, W. B. Saunders, 1973, pp 28–77, 114–124.
2. Joffe N, Antonioli DA: Osteoblastic bone metastases secondary to adenocarcinoma of the pancreas. *Clin Radiol* 29:41–46, 1978.
3. Redman HC: Standard radiologic diagnosis and CT scanning of pancreatic cancer. *Cancer* 47:1656–1661, 1981.
4. Schultz RE, Finkler NJ: Pancreatic calcification and pancreatic carcinoma: the relationship reconsidered. *Mt Sinai J Med* 47:622–626, 1980.
5. Langton L: Dysphagia in carcinoma of the pancreas. *J Faculty Radiol* 6:134–138, 1954.
6. Ward P: Pulmonary and esophageal presentations of pancreatic carcinoma. *Br J Radiol* 37:27–33, 1964.
7. Jaques PF, Bream CA: Barium duodenography as an adjunct to percutaneous transhepatic cholangiography. *AJR* 130:693–696, 1978.
8. Gold RP: Medial indentation of the duodenal sweep by common bile duct dilatation. *AJR* 133:233–237, 1979.
9. Schaudig G: Haustral changes of the colon due to regional processes, especially the pancreas and stomach. *ROFO* 123:542–547, 1975.
10. Meyers MA: *Dynamic Radiology of the Abdomen.* New York, Springer-Verlag, 1976, pp 43, 54–70.
11. Warden SS, Fireash JG, Tynes WV, Shellhammer PF: Urologic aspects of pancreatic adenocarcinoma. *J Urol* 125:265–267, 1981.

Nuclear Medicine

Although a number of radioisotopes have been proposed for pancreatic scanning, only ^{75}Se-selenomethionine has been used in clinical practice in the past. The radiopharmaceutical localizes in organs with active protein synthesis and is therefore seen in both the liver and pancreas. Pancreas scanning was performed after the injection of 250 μCi of ^{75}Se-selenomethionine intravenously with sequential views being obtained at 10-min intervals beginning immediately following injection. The results of the radionuclide pancreas scan have varied with sensitivities for pancreatic disease reported between 50 and 94% and specificities between 79 and 95% (1, 2). The reported sensitivities, although impressive, do not distinguish between pancreatic carcinoma, pancreatitis, and other pancreatic diseases. In a study by Barkin et al. (3), radionuclide scans were abnormal in 96% of patients with carcinoma of the pancreas but were also abnormal in 75% of patients without pancreatic disease. DiMagno et al. (4) showed a low specificity (40%) for the ^{75}Se-selenomethionine pancreas scan. With this lack of specificity and the advent of ultrasound and computerized tomography in the workup of the patients suspected of pancreatic carcinoma, there is no longer a role for the radionuclide scan of the pancreas.

REFERENCES

1. Landman S, Gottschalk A: Pancreas scanning. In Gottschalk A, Potchen EJ (eds): *Diagnostic Nuclear Medicine.* Baltimore, Williams & Wilkins, 1976, pp 456–463.
2. Miale A, Rodriguez-Antunez A, Gill WM: Pancreas scanning after 10 years. *Semin Nucl Med* 2:201–219, 1972.
3. Barkin J, Vining D, Miale A et al: Computerized tomography, diagnostic ultrasound, and radionuclide scanning. Comparison of efficacy in diagnosis of pancreatic carcinoma. *JAMA* 238:2040–2042, 1977.
4. DiMagno EP, Malagelada JR, Taylor WF et al: A prospective comparison of current diagnostic tests for pancreatic cancer. *N Engl J Med* 297:737–742, 1977.

Sonography of Duct Cell Adenocarcinoma

Real-time sonography improves depiction of the pancreas and its duct compared to static B-scanning (1). Most pancreatic duct cell carcinomas are detected as hypoechoic masses enlarging the gland or deforming its contour. As this point they are generally 2–3 cm in diameter or larger, symptomatic, and unresectable. In symptomatic patients, a technically good normal sonogram of the entire pancreas strongly suggests that pancreatic carcinoma is not the cause of the patient's symptoms (2–4). False-negative rates as low as 1% have been reported for technically good scans in which the entire gland is depicted (2). Small carcinomas in the tail are the most difficult to detect. Normal pancreatic echo texture is somewhat greater than the surrounding fibrofatty retroperitoneal tissue and equal to or slightly greater than that of adjacent liver. Evaluation of texture is subjective because of dependence on frequency and focal length of the transducer, setting of gain, output and attenuation and the amount of fatty infiltration present (5). The potential exists for sonographic detection of small intraglandular duct cell carcinomas by virtue of a focal change in echo texture. Unfortunately, this is rarely achieved. Occasionally, potentially resectable tumors are uncovered by ultrasound as biliary and/or pancreatic ductal dilatation without apparent mass.

Technique

Pitfalls in sonographic evaluation for suspected neoplasm relate primarily to technical inadequacy. Delineation of the pancreas is less than optimal in roughly one-fourth of patients, depending on patient population. The most common causes for unsuccessful examinations are overlying bowel gas and excessive intraabdominal fat (2, 6). The tail of the pancreas is the most difficult portion to depict. On routine anterior ultrasonic evaluation, the tail often appears to bend dorsally, rather than continue superolaterally into the splenic hilum. Comparison with CT images has revealed this to be an artifact, the "ghost tail," actually consisting of retroperitoneal fat, with the pancreatic tail not being visualized (7). Another potential pitfall which occurs with static scanning in the prone position is mistaking a feces filled splenic flexure for the pancreatic tail (8).

There are several maneuvers designed to improve visualization of the pancreas, particularly the tail. All of these involve eliminating the problem of bowel gas. Simply repeating the scan after a short time interval will yield a successful examination in 40–50% of patients whose pancreas was obscured by gas at first examination (6). If the gas is fairly well localized, angulation of the scanner or respiratory maneuvers may be helpful. Prone scanning using the upper pole of the left kidney and the spleen as soft tissue acoustic windows was advocated by some (9); however, prone scanning always makes the tail appear larger and is now considered unreliable (7). Distending the stomach and duodenum with water (approximately 300 ml) helps displace gas, providing an aqueous acoustic window (10). A distended stomach also helps shift small bowel and colon caudally, away from the pancreas (10). Water, due to its low attenuation relative to soft tissues, will cause effective amplification of posterior echoes. Meat soup has been shown to have more desirable acoustic properties (11). If the antrum remains air-filled, a right lateral decubitus (10) or erect (12) position will displace the air into the fundus.

The erect position will shift the pancreas caudally with relation to the rib cage. The liver and fluid filled stomach will shift caudally to an even greater extent and will act as acoustic windows (12). Deep inspiration will also shift the abdominal viscera away from the rib cage, and facilitate use of the left hepatic lobe as an acoustic window. Persistent gastric motility, especially if solid food particles or gas bubbles remain in the stomach, may hinder pancreatic visualization. In these cases, intravenous glucagon may be helpful (12). In spite of these manuvers, the normal tail of the pancreas will not be seen in many cases (7). Fortunately, failure to visualize the normal tail will seldom lead to a misdiagnosis, since most cases of pancreatitis or carcinoma involve the head and body and an enlarged tail will usually be detected.

Recently, intraoperative high resolution real time ultrasonic scanning has been performed for tumor localization and staging, as well as for guidance of intraoperative biopsy (13). Since only a few cm. of penetration by the sound beam is needed, a 7.5 MHz transducer can be used yielding resolution of approximately 1 mm. As opposed to the hypoechoic appearance of pancreatic carcinoma when lower frequency transducers are used, the echogenicity of tumors relative to normal parenchyma was unchanged in 6, increased in 6, and decreased in only 1 of 13 pancreatic carcinomas scanned intraoperatively in a recent series (13). These results are questionable, however. In our experience, pancreatic carcinomas are still hypoechoic when scanned intraoperatively. A distinctive common bile duct termination was seen in obstructing lesions, with either a tumor shelf or tapering noted (13).

Sonographic Findings

The fundamental sonographic finding in duct cell carcinoma of the pancreas is a focal pancreatic mass (Fig. 22.28) (2, 3, 5). With commonly used 3.5 MHz transducers, carcinoma is hypoechoic relative to pancreatic parenchyma in nearly all instances (5, 14–16). Varying amounts of coarse echoes are usually present with duct cell carcinomas, differing from the homogeneous, granular appearance of the normal pancreas (7, 14, 15). Sonolucent cystic regions from tumor necrosis are unusual in duct cell carcinomas and if present suggest one of the variant pancreatic carcinomas. However, small sonolucent pseudocysts from tumor induced pancreatitis are difficult to differentiate from tumor necrosis. Transmission of sound through duct cell carcinoma is similar to normal pancreatic parenchyma in most instances (15). The margins of the mass are often irregular. Rounding of the uncinate process suggests a mass (Fig. 22.28A). Anterior compression of the inferior vena cava can be a helpful adjunctive finding (17). When unsuspected pancreatic duct dilatation is detected in addition to biliary dilatation, a pathologic process in the head of the pancreas is usually responsible for the biliary obstruction (Fig. 22.28B and C).

Unfortunately, finding a pancreatic mass with or without pancreatic and/or biliary ductal obstruction is not specific for carcinoma (15, 18). Inflammatory or neoplastic disease of the duodenum and duodenal diverticula can be confused with pancreatic masses on ultrasound. Peripancreatic lymphadenopathy in patients with lymphoma or metastatic disease can mimic a primary pancreatic mass (19). When there are separate focal masses the appearance is distinctive for adenopathy. When the adenopathy is confluent, differentiation from primary pancreatic carcinoma is difficult—both lesions are hypoechoic and often have heterogeneous internal echoes. Smooth lobulation is more characteristic of adenopathy, as are pseudoseptations due to incomplete coalescence (19). Absence of jaundice in the presence of a mass in the region of the head of the pancreas favors peripancreatic adenopathy over duct cell carcinoma (19). Focal pancreatitis without pseudocyst is indistinguishable from duct cell carcinoma unless shadowing echogenicities (calcifications) are present. Lack of a clinical history of pancreatitis, alcohol abuse, or biliary tract disease is highly suspicious for duct cell carcinoma when a noncalcified solid pancreatic mass is detected. Middle-aged or elderly patients presenting with a first attack of pancreatitis with no known predisposing factor should be suspected of harboring a pancreatic carcinoma (18). The bilirubin tends to be higher in carcinoma than in pancreatitis. Carcinoma of the head of the pancreas can lead to diffuse glandular enlargement from secondary pancreatitis or atrophy of the body and tail from chronic obstruction (18).

Effects on the Pancreatic Duct

Pancreatic duct cell carcinoma often produces sonographically visible main pancreatic duct obstruction, especially tumors of the head. Using high resolution real-time equipment, the normal pancreatic duct can be frequently identified (84% in one series) as a thin, anechoic tube with parallel, echogenic walls (1, 16, 20). Sometimes it is seen only as an echogenic line. Sonographic limits of normal (internal diameter) have been reported as high as 3 mm and as low as 0.8 mm (1, 16, 19). The higher measurements were from the duct in the head, whereas the lower ones were from the body and tail. The normal pancreatic duct has been shown to enlarge with age by autopsy pancreatography (21); one would expect a similar trend to be demonstrable by ultrasound. In addition to dilatation, other sonographic signs of a pancreatic duct obstruction that may be due to carcinoma are loss of parallelism of the walls and outward convexity (beading or focal dilatation) (1). Unfortunately, both smooth dilatation and irregular dilatation (beading) can be seen in either carcinoma or pancreatitis (Fig. 22.29A–C) (6, 16).

Effects on the Biliary Tract

Carcinoma of the head of the pancreas nearly always causes biliary tract obstruction and dilatation (22–25). Currently 4–5 mm is considered

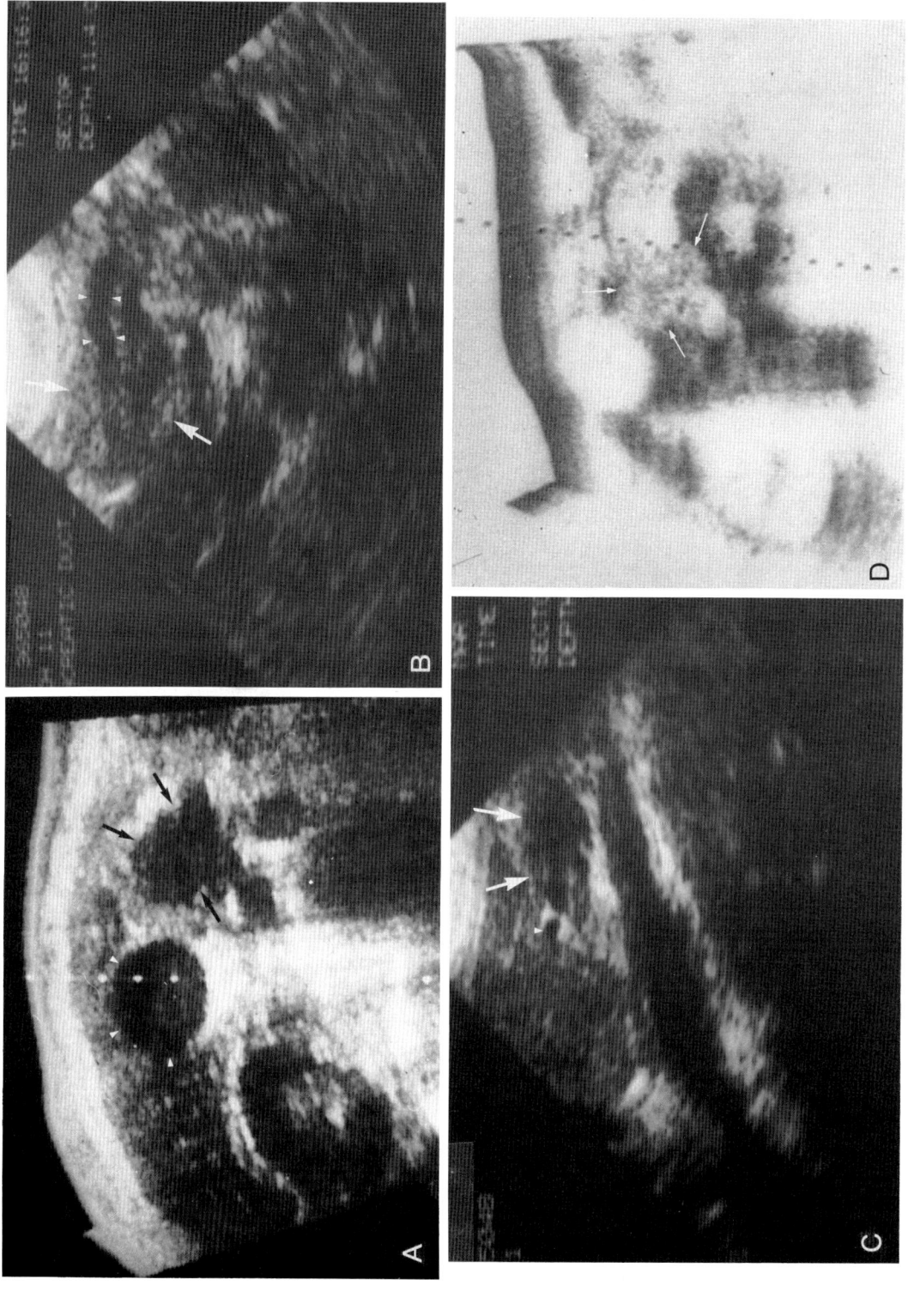

FIGURE 22.28. DUCT CELL ADENOCARCINOMA

A: Transverse scan of a hypoechoic duct cell carcinoma causing enlargement and rounding of the uncinate process (*arrows*). Note the distended gallbladder (*arrowheads*) containing a fluid-debris level. *B* and *C:* Transverse and sagittal sonograms of a duct cell carcinoma in the head of the pancreas (*arrows*) with dilatation of pancreatic and biliary ducts (*arrowheads*). *D:* Duct cell carcinoma of the head of the pancreas deforming and enlarging the contour of the gland (*arrows*). *E* and *F:* Transverse and sagittal sonograms showing an approximately 3 cm. hypoechoic duct cell carcinoma of the body of the pancreas (*arrows*). *G* and *H:* Transverse and sagittal sonograms of a duct cell carcinoma of the tail of the pancreas (*arrows*).

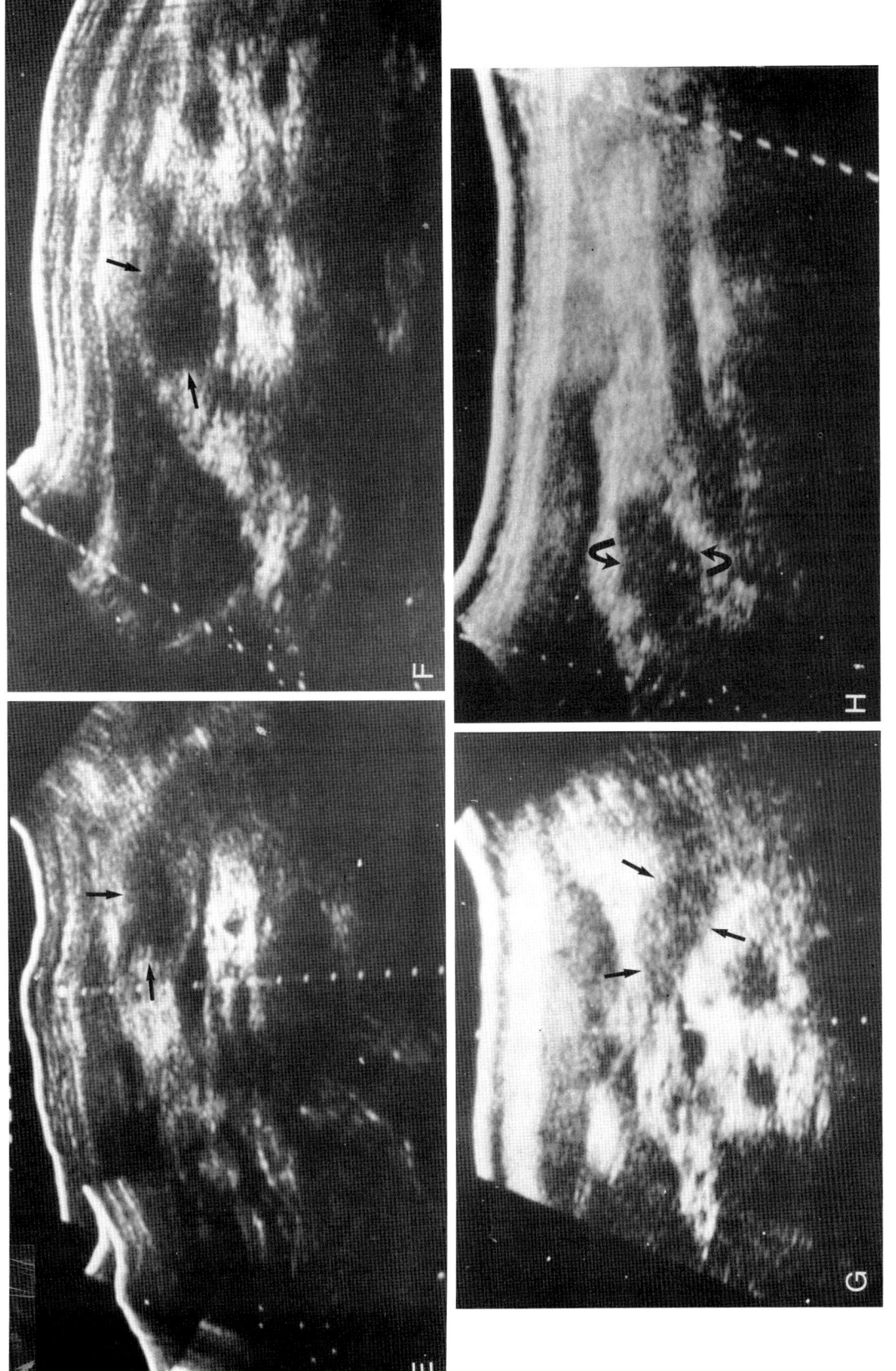

FIGURE 22.28*E–H*

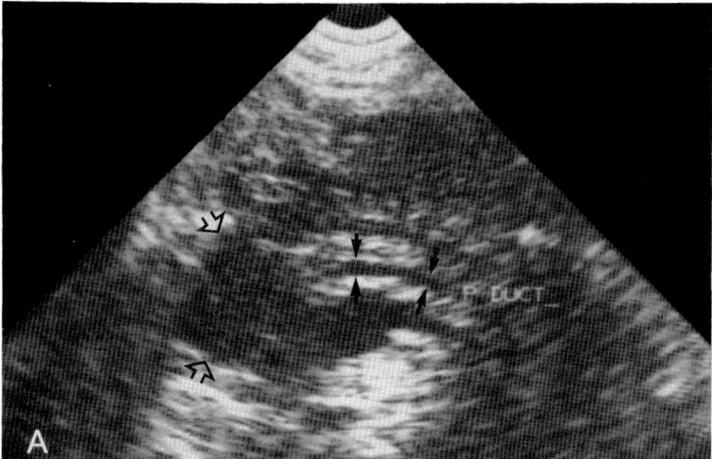
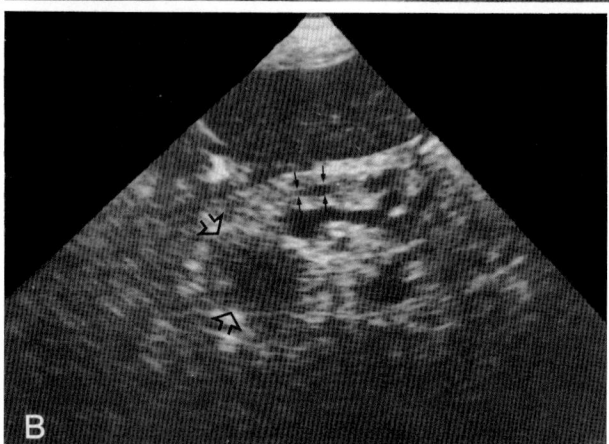
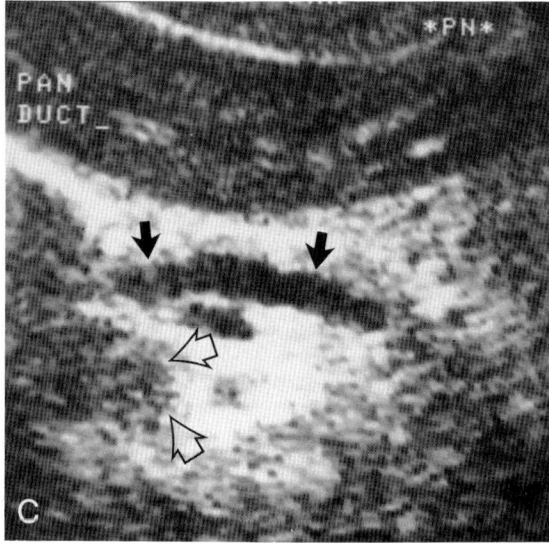

FIGURE 22.29. DUCT CELL ADENOCARCINOMA
A and B: Transverse sonogram showing a smoothly dilated main pancreatic duct (*closed arrows*) caused by a hypoechoic duct cell carcinoma in the head and uncinate process (*open arrows*). C: Irregularly dilated main pancreatic duct (*closed arrows*) distal to an obstructing duct cell carcinoma (*open arrows*).

the upper limits of normal of the common duct in the nonoperated patient. The level of the obstruction is usually in the head of the pancreas, but it may be in the middle portion of the common duct or at the bifurcation due to tumor extension and/or nodal metastasis. Rarely intrahepatic duct obstruction occurs due to hepatic metastases. Although ultrasound is quite sensitive in detecting biliary dilatation, it is less successful in identifying the actual site or cause of obstruction (18, 24). It is our impression that the biliary tree tends to be more dilated in carcinoma of the pancreas than in benign disease and that the serum bilirubin tends to be higher and increase more relentlessly. Abrupt termination of the distal duct at or near the pancreas suggests a malignant etiology of the obstruction (26). Although the etiology will be carcinoma of the pancreas in most of these cases, failure to depict a mass in the head when that region is not obscured by gas in the duodenum suggests the possibility of bile duct or ampullary carcinoma. The presence of an obstructing calculus results in sharp transition between the lumen of the obstructed duct and the calculus but not in abrupt termination of the distal duct per se (26). For optimal depiction of the distal duct it is necessary to scan along its longitudinal axis, find its distal end, and then scan from side to side to determine that the duct is abruptly terminated (26). When the common duct becomes massively dilated, it can become transversely oriented and redundant, so that when scanned in an axial plane many round sonolucencies will be depicted mimicking pancreatic pseudocysts. Potential for confusion with venous structures exists as well (27). Identification of cholelithiasis in a jaundiced patient cannot be interpreted as evidence for choledocholithiasis as the cause of the obstruction; biliary stasis by itself leads to cholelithiasis and cholelithiasis is a common incidental finding in the elderly. Even choledocholithiasis can coexist with a malignant obstruction, so that the point of obstruction should be identified and a mass searched for in all cases.

Ancillary ultrasonic findings suggesting malignancy are present in many patients with pancreatic duct cell carcinoma (15, 18). Nearly half of patients with pancreatic duct cell carcinoma have sonographically detectable hepatic metastases at initial evaluation (15, 18). These liver metastases are usually hypoechoic but may be mixed, isoechoic or hyperechoic. Paraaortic adenopathy is seen as iso or hypoechoic masses surrounding the aorta and inferior vena cava (18). A right coronal scan at the level of the aorta and inferior vena cava is often helpful in evaluating the paraaortic area. Normally, only the right crus of the diaphragm lies between the aorta and inferior vena cava (18). Nonvisualization of the splenic vein in a technically adequate examination, occurring in nearly half of patients with pancreatic carcinoma in one series, should be considered suspicious of venous encasement (15). Varices due to splenic, portal, or superior mesenteric occlusion may be detected, as can vascular displacement (i.e., superior mesenteric artery). Loss of peripancreatic tissue planes may indicate extrapancreatic extension, but may also be caused by secondary pancreatitis or cachexia (18).

REFERENCES

1. Lawson TL, Berland LL, Foley WD, Stewart ET, Geenan JE, Hogan WJ: Ultrasonic visualization of the pancreatic duct. Radiology 144:865–871, 1982.
2. Pollock D, Taylor KJW: Ultrasound scanning in patients with clinical suspicion of pancreatic cancer: a retrospective study. Cancer 47:1662–1665, 1981.
3. Cotton PB, Lees WR, Vallon AG, Cottone M, Croker JR, Chapman M: Gray-scale ultrasonography and endoscopic pancreatography in pancreatic diagnosis. Radiology 134:453–459, 1980.
4. Arter PH, Mulhern CB, Bonavita JA: An analysis of pancreatic sonography in suspected pancreatic disease. J Clin Ultrasound 7:91–97, 1979.
5. Freeny PC, Lawson TL: Radiology of the pancreas. In Stephens DH, Ghahremani GG (eds): Syllabus Gastrointestinal Radiology. Presented at the 68th Scientific Assembly of the Radiological Society of North America (809), 1982, pp 11–14.
6. Meire HB, Farrante P: Pancreatic ultrasound—a systematic approach to scanning technique. Br J Radiol 52:652–657, 1979.
7. Suramo I, Lohela P, Lahde S, Myllyla V, Pamilo M: The "ghost tail" of the pancreas in ultrasonography. Eur J Radiol 2:139–140, 1982.
8. Berger M, Smith EH, Bartrum RJ, Holm HH, Mascatello V: False-positive diagnosis of pancreatic tail lesions caused by colon. J Clin Ultrasound 5:343–345, 1977.
9. Goldstein HM, Katragadda CS: Prone view ultrasonography for pancreatic tail neoplasms. AJR 131:231–234, 1978.
10. Crade M, Taylor KJW, Rosenfield AT: Water distention of the gut in the evaluation of the pancreas by ultrasound. AJR 131:348–349, 1978.
11. Vuoria P, Suramo I, Hyvarinen S: Transmission media for ultrasonography. Radiology 135:520–522, 1980.
12. McMahon H, Bowie JD, Beezhold C: Erect scanning of pancreas using a gastric window. AJR 132:587–591, 1979.
13. Sigel B, Ccoelho JCU, Nyhus LM, Velasco JM, Donahue PE, Wood DK, Spigos DG: Detection of pancreatic tumors by ultrasound during surgery. Arch Surg 117:1058–1061, 1982.
14. Kunzmann A, Bowie JD, Rochester D: Texture patterns in pancreatic sonograms. Gastrointest Radiol 4:353–357, 1979.
15. Weinstein DP, Wolfman NT, Weinstein BJ: Ultrasonic characteristic of pancreatic tumors. Gastrointest Radiol 4:245–251, 1979.
16. Ohto M, Saottome N, Saisho H, Tsuchiya Y, Ono T, Okuda K, Karasawa E: Real-time sonography of the pancreatic duct: application to percutaneous pancreatic ductography. AJR 134:647–652, 1980.
17. Walls WJ, Templeton AW: The ultrasonic demonstration of inferior vena caval compression: a guide to pancreatic head enlargement with emphasis on neoplasm. Radiology 123:165–167, 1977.
18. Freeny PC, Lawson TL: Radiology of the Pancreas. New York, Springer-Verlag, 1982, pp 408–427.
19. Schnur MJ, Hoffman JC, Koenigsberg M: Gray-scale ultrasonic demonstration of peripancreatic adenopathy. J Ultrasound Med 1:139–143, 1982.
20. Hadidi A: Pancreatic duct diameter: sonographic measurement in normal subjects. J Clin Ultrasound 11:17–22, 1983.
21. Kreel L, Sanding B: Changes in pancreatic morphology associated with aging. Gut 14:962–970, 1973.
22. Weinstein DP, Weinstein BJ, Brodmerkel GJ: Ultrasonography of biliary tract dilatation without jaundice. AJR 132:729–734, 1979.
23. Muhletaler CA, Gerlock AM Jr, Fleischer AC, James AE Jr: Diagnosis of obstructive jaundice with nondilated bile ducts. AJR 134:1149–1152, 1980.
24. Honickman SP, Mueller PR, Wittenberg J, Simeone JF, Ferrucci JT, Cronan JJ, VanSonnenberg E: Ultrasound in obstructive jaundice: prospective evaluation of site and cause. Radiology 147:511–515, 1983.
25. Conrad MR, Landay LA, Filly RA: Sonographic "parallel channel" sign of biliary tree enlargement in mild to moderate obstructive jaundice. AJR 130:279–286, 1978.
26. Jones JB, Dubuisson RL, Hughes JJ, Robinson AE: Abrupt termination of the common bile duct: a sign of malignancy identified by high resolution real-time sonography. J Ultrasound Med 2:345–348, 1983.
27. Jacobson JB, Brodey PA: The transverse common duct. AJR 136: 91–95, 1981.

Computed Tomography of Duct Cell Adenocarcinoma

Technique

Computed tomographic examination of the pancreas reveals more useful information than any other imaging modality currently available, and is reliable and reproducible. Fast scanning has improved diagnostic accuracy. In one series comparing 3 sec with 18 sec scanning, technically unsuccessful examinations decreased from 7% to 1%, false-positive examinations from 25% to 6%, while false-negative examinations remained less than 1% (1).

Diagnostic information may best be obtained if the examination is tailored to the pancreas. While 5 mm collimation increases frequency of pancreatic duct visualization (2–4), 10 mm collimation should be sufficient to detect all but the smallest lesions and involves less radiation dosage to the patient (5). Choosing a small pixel diameter, such as 0.8 or 1.1 mm instead of 1.3 mm may improve resolution (2, 3) but in some patients may preclude full evaluation of the liver due to decreased field size.

Optimal use of intravenous and oral contrast also improves evaluation of the pancreas. Because duct cell carcinoma is hypovascular, it does not undergo contrast enhancement to the same degree as does the normal pancreas. Dense opacification of nearby vascular structures also helps define the border of the pancreas, and allows evaluation for vascular encasement or occlusion. The pancreatic and common bile ducts are best seen when the pancreas is enhanced. Theoretically, finely stippled pancreatic calcifications may be obscured, however.

Enhancement of the pancreas with urographic contrast is maximum during the arterial phase of the bolus injection, when arterial levels are much higher than venous levels (6, 7). Peak enhancement of the pancreas follows that of the aorta by just 3 sec, declining rapidly as enhancement of the inferior vena cava is increased (6). While enhancement of most other tissues is mostly a function of interstitial contrast, pancreatic enhancement appears to be more dependent on the concentration of intravascular contrast (7). Optimal use of these pharmacokinetics requires fast scan times, preferably less than 4 sec (7, 8). Slower scan times, such as 18 sec scan times in older units, average the various phases of distribution (9).

Enhancement of the pancreas may best be obtained by a rapid intravenous bolus injection of 50–100 ml of 60% contrast followed by dynamic scanning with table incrementation (7, 8). A rapid infusion immediately following the bolus injection will help maintain high arterial levels and is necessary if the scan sequence lasts more than 45 sec. To take advantage of the maximum arterial levels present at the beginning of the examination, scanning should be tailored to the clinical situation. In a patient presenting with jaundice, a potentially resectable carcinoma of the pancreatic head can best be detected by optimally enhancing the parenchyma in this region. This is best accomplished by beginning the scanning sequence at the caudal margin of the pancreas, usually the L2–3 interspace, and then proceeding cephalad through the remainder of the pancreas and liver. If pain and weight loss are the presenting complaints, unresectable carcinoma of the body or tail is more likely, and vascular involvement should be documented, if possible, to obviate angiography. The scan sequence should begin at the level of the splenic artery and celiac axis, usually the T12–L1 interspace, and proceed caudally through the pancreatic head, and then finally cephalad through the remainder of the liver. The liver must always be completely scanned, since between one fourth and one half of patients with pancreatic carcinoma have detectable liver metastases at the time of initial examination (10–12). Enhancement of the pancreas by multiple boluses throughout the examination has also been advocated (6). Scanning at 10-mm intervals, by requiring less time for the examination, will facilitate contrast enhancement.

Adequate delineation of the duodenum and small bowel aids greatly in accurately defining pancreatic borders. Oral contrast, whether barium suspension or water soluble, should be dilute enough to avoid beam hardening and motion artifacts. With slow scan times, glucagon will help in this regard. Even with a fast scan time, glucagon may help by dilating the duodenum, allowing better filling of the C-loop which facilitates better identification of the pancreatic head (2). The right lateral decubitus position may also help fill the C-loop (13). Alternatively, air from effervescent granules or tablets may be used to fill the stomach and duodenum eliminating some problems with contrast induced artifacts. Biliary stones are also less likely to be obscured when this method is used. Scanning in the left lateral decubitus position may help fill the C-loop with air, especially if glucagon has been given. At our institution, however, we have found that the supine position is easiest for most patients to maintain, and do most of our scanning in this position.

Regarding the use of glucagon, nausea has been reported to be especially frequent when concurrent intravenous contrast has been administered (2). Giving the glucagon a few minutes before beginning the contrast bolus may decrease the frequency of this problem (2). However, glucagon is rarely necessary with newer scanners using 2–5-sec scan times.

Delineation of the pancreatic body and tail

can be impaired by noncontrast-filled loops of jejunum. Complete small bowel opacification will obviate this problem and also increase the accuracy of the detection of adenopathy. Efforts to fully distend the stomach with contrast, water, or air will displace jejunal loops inferiorly, away from the tail of the pancreas (14). The tail of the pancreas may also be displaced somewhat by this maneuver, attaining a more horizontal course, which is more amenable to CT evaluation (14). All efforts should be made to eliminate avoidable sources of artifact. Surgical clips, of course, cannot be removed from the patient, but a nasogastric tube should always be removed or retracted into the esophagus while the patient is being scanned. If nondiluted barium is present within the area to be scanned, the examination should be postponed unless it is clinically urgent.

Other techniques such as administering oral cholecystographic agents (15) or performing ERCP (16, 17) prior to CT help define the biliary and pancreatic ducts but have not received widespread acceptance.

Findings (Tables 22.1–22.3)

The most common CT finding in duct cell adenocarcinoma is a focal mass (1, 11, 12). However, nonfocal enlargement has been reported in 5–27% of cases (10, 12, 18). As is the case with sonography, most duct cell carcinomas are not detected until they are 2–3 cm in size, large enough to alter the size and shape of the gland, and unresectable. Exceptions are small tumors in the head with bile and/or pancreatic duct obstruction (Fig. 22.30) and the rare duct cell carcinoma found incidentally. If abdominal symptoms are present, a normal CT suggests strongly that they are not due to duct cell carcinoma of the pancreas as overall detection rates with current equipment are about 95% (19).

The focal mass representing a duct cell carcinoma enlarges a region of the pancreas and produces either an abrupt or gradual change of contour. Even when the entire gland is enlarged the shape may be distorted in addition (19).

Early reports using slow scan time and large pixel size were discouraging with regard to tissue characterization of the pancreas, stressing that the only reliable sign of a pancreatic mass was an abnormal contour (9). Using current equipment this is no longer true. In the elderly, or the obese, the pancreatic parenchyma often becomes marbled due to fatty infiltration. Focal loss of this marbling should be considered suspicious for a mass. Small intraglandular masses are hardest to detect in the head or within the center of the gland. Small peripheral masses may be detected by virtue of disruption of the normal surface lobularity caused by peripancreatic areolar tissue dipping in between parenchymal lobules (19, 20). Although some investigators have attempted to define normal limits of pancreatic size (21, 22), we feel that these are unreliable due to normal variations in size and shape of the pancreas. In fact, a "normal-sized" head suggests a carcinoma when there is atrophy of the body and tail (Fig.

TABLE 22.1.
LOCATION OF 100 PANCREATIC ADENOCARCINOMAS: JOHNS HOPKINS HOSPITAL, 1978–1981[a]

Location	Number
Head	67
Head and body	7
Body	13
Body and tail	2
Tail	11

[a] Modified from E. K. Fishman and S. S. Siegelman: CT of pancreatic carcinoma. In S. S. Siegelman (ed.): Computed Tomography of the Pancreas. New York, Churchill Livingstone, 1983, pp. 125–126.

TABLE 22.2.
TUMOR ATTENUATION IN 100 CASES (50 ml 60% RENOGRAFIN ENHANCED) OF PANCREATIC ADENOCARCINOMA[a]

Characteristics	Number
Same as normal parenchyma	41
Slightly decreased (5–10 HU) compared to normal parenchyma	35
Moderately decreased (10–20 HU) below normal parenchyma	18
Markedly decreased (water density)	6

[a] Modified from E. K. Fishman and S. S. Siegelman: CT of pancreatic carcinoma. In S. S. Siegelman (ed.): Computed Tomography of the Pancreas. New York, Churchill Livingstone, 1983, pp. 125–126.

TABLE 22.3.
CT FEATURES RESPONSIBLE FOR THE DIAGNOSIS OF ADENOCARCINOMA OF THE PANCREAS IN 100 CASES[a]

Finding	Number
Localized pancreatic mass	17
Mass in pancreatic head and common bile duct obstruction	27
Pancreatic mass with direct extension outside the gland (18 had lymphadenopathy also)	34
Pancreatic mass with liver metastases	22

[a] Modified from E. K. Fishman and S. S. Siegelman: CT of pancreatic carcinoma. In S. S. Siegelman (ed.): Computed Tomography of the Pancreas. New York, Churchill Livingstone, 1983, pp. 125–126.

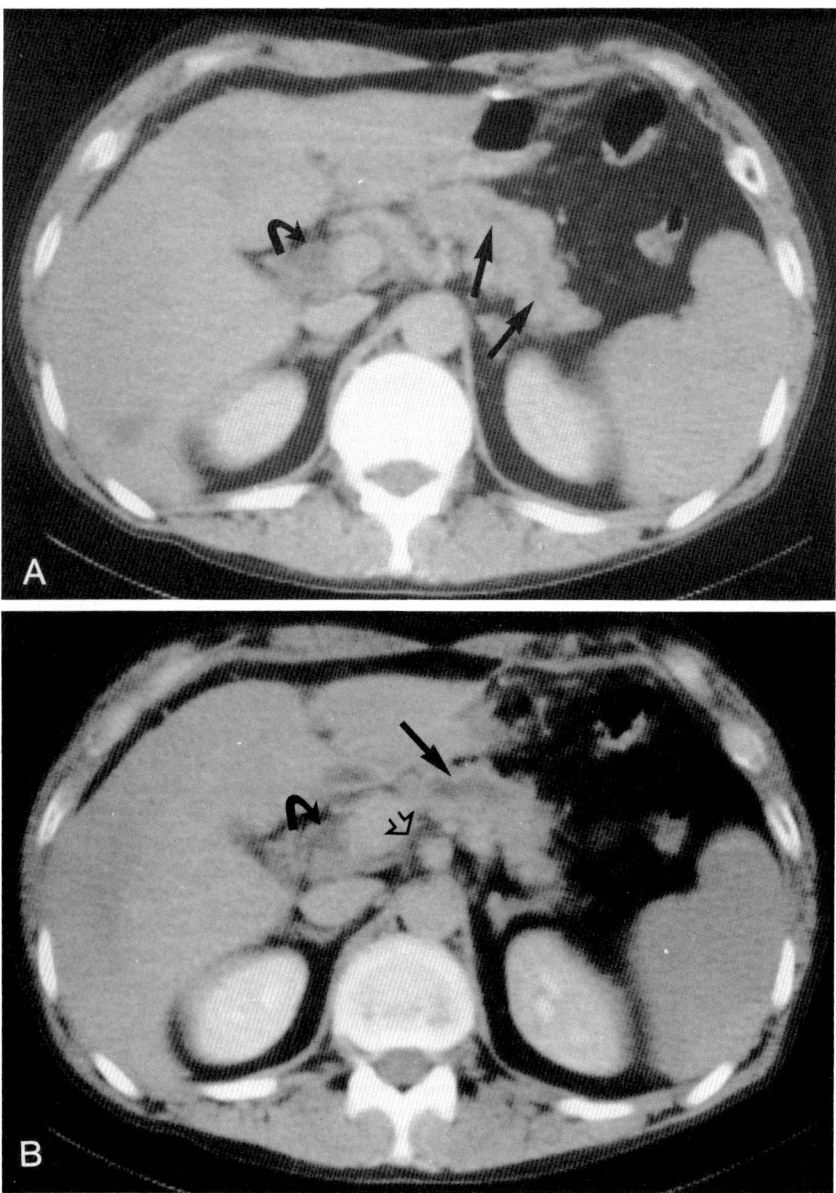

FIGURE 22.30. DUCT CELL ADENOCARCINOMA

Small carcinoma in the head of the pancreas. *A:* Dilated pancreatic (*arrows*) and bile ducts (*curved arrow*). *B:* Dilated ducts as in (*A*). Even though no mass was seen, the tumor was still unresectable. Note invasion of retropancreatic fat around the superior mesenteric artery (*open arrow*).

22.31). Rounding of the normally wedge-shaped uncinate process must be viewed with suspicion (Fig. 22.31). Masses in the tail may, on occasion, extend behind the splenic vein mimicking an adrenal mass (23). Ancillary findings associated with nonresectability may be detected when the mass itself is inapparent. These are discussed further under staging. Finally, biliary and/or pancreatic ductal dilatation may be caused by an inapparent duct cell carcinoma (Figs. 22.30 and 22.32).

Some decreased attenuation of pancreatic carcinoma relative to the normal gland is found in at least half the cases when bolus enhancement and fast scan times are used (10–12, 19) and nearly all when dynamic scanning with table incrementation is used (Fig. 22.33) (7, 24). Duct cell carcinomas are usually isodense on noncon-

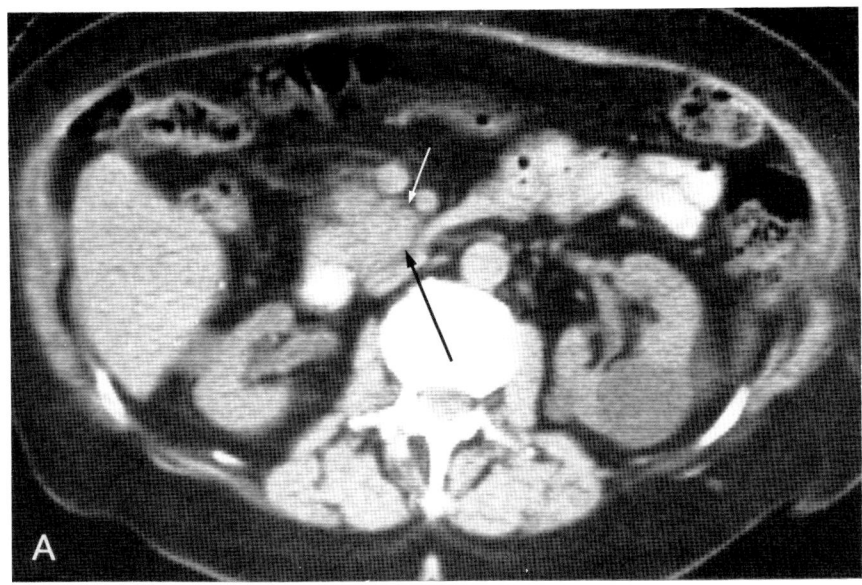

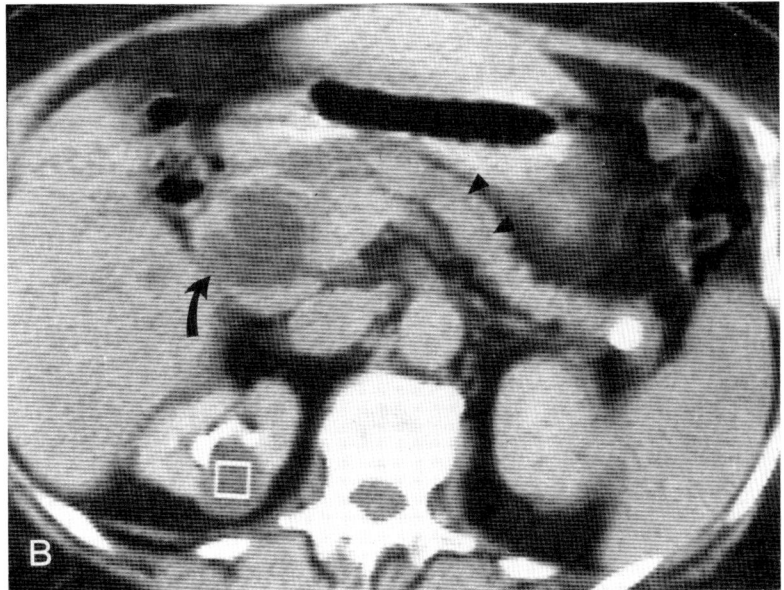

FIGURE 22.31. DUCT CELL ADENOCARCINOMA

A: Subtle carcinoma in the uncinate process: rounding and mild prominence (*arrows*). *B:* Enlargement is better appreciated when compared to the atrophy in the remainder of the gland. Note the massively dilated common bile duct (*curved arrow*) and the barely visible dilated pancreatic duct (*arrowheads*).

trast scans but slightly decreased attenuation has been occasionally noted (Fig. 22.33) (10, 12, 19). Occasionally, more lucent areas within the mass are identified which are invariably smaller than the tumor itself (10–12, 18, 19, 25). Their density is typically slightly higher than that usually seen in pancreatic pseudocysts (10). Although usually ascribed to necrosis, the only actual pathological correlation reported described a "necrotic anaplastic adenocarcinoma" (25); pancreatic duct cell carcinoma rarely includes areas of frank hemorrhage or necrosis. The precise explanation for these low attenuation areas has not yet been found but it may be related to secondary pancreatitis (26) or irregular desmoplastic reaction.

Pancreatic Duct. The upper limits of normal duct diameter on CT is considered to be 2 mm in the body, and 5 mm in the head (3, 27). The duct may lie centrally within the pancreas or closer to either the ventral or dorsal margins of

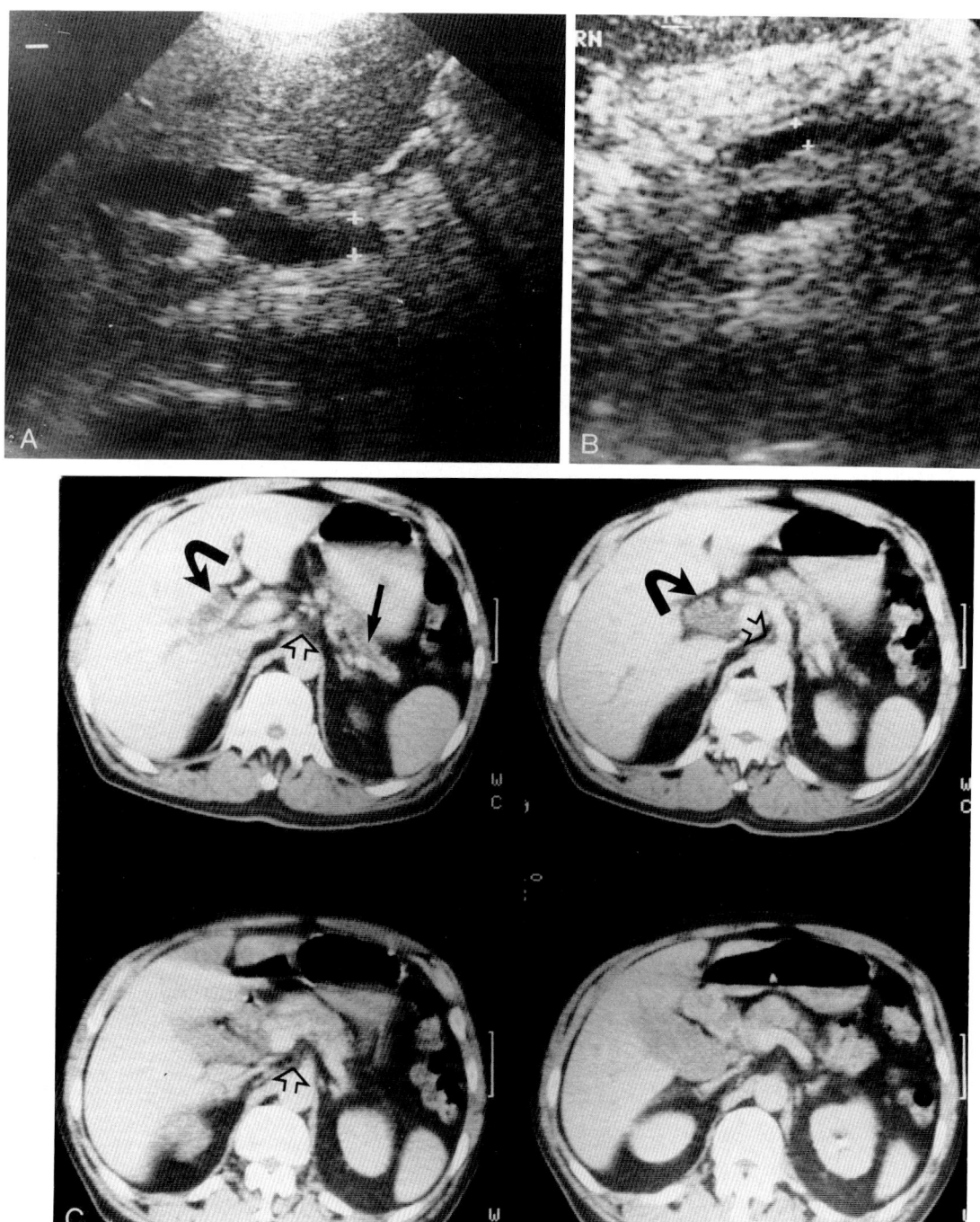

FIGURE 22.32. DUCT CELL ADENOCARCINOMA
Inapparent carcinoma of the neck of the pancreas despite dilated biliary and pancreatic ducts. *A:* Parasagittal sonogram: dilated common duct (*cursors*). *B:* Transverse sonogram: dilated pancreatic duct (*cursors*). *C:* Despite dilated biliary tree (*curved arrows*) and pancreatic duct (*arrow*), no apparent mass. Subtle retropancreatic extension (*open arrows*) into fat around the celiac artery was confirmed at surgery. *D:* Pancreatogram: high grade narrowing with normal distal ducts and dilated main pancreatic duct highly suggestive of carcinoma.

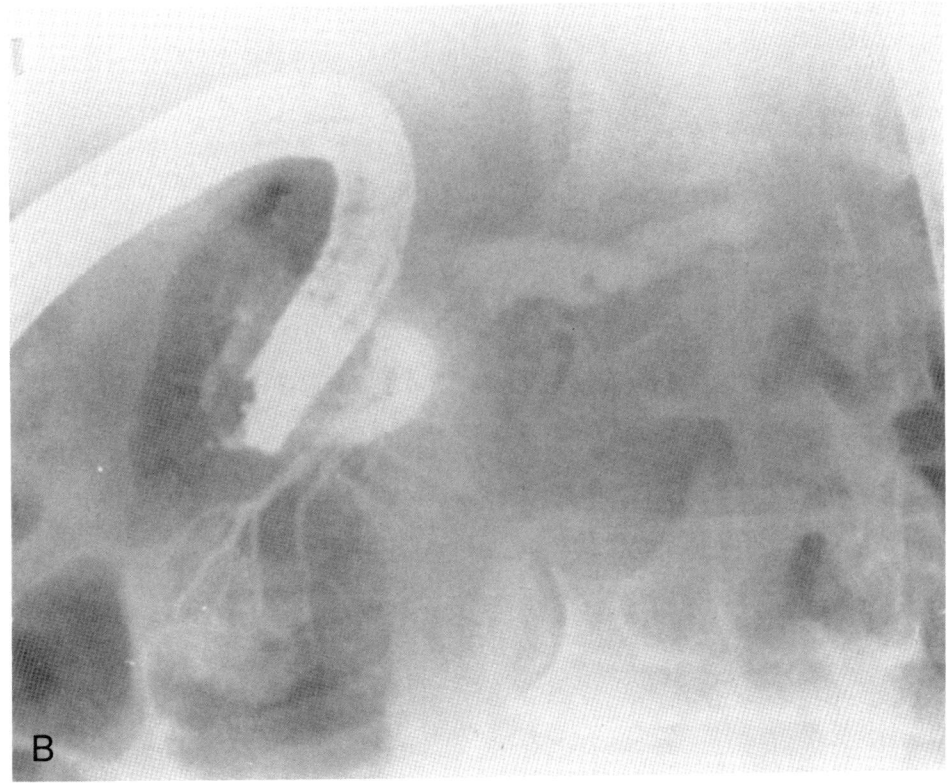

FIGURE 22.32D

the gland (3). The "pseudoduct" consisting of the fat plane between the splenic vein and the pancreas (28) should not present problems if proper contrast enhancement is used and if this potential pitfall is kept in mind during interpretation. The splenic vein should be traced to its junction with the superior mesenteric vein to form the portal vein posterolateral to the pancreatic head.

Dilation of the main pancreatic duct proximal to the obstructing tumor (Figs. 22.30–22.32, 22.34, 22.35 and 22.38) is detected in between 20 and 50% of cases of pancreatic duct cell carcinoma (11, 12), although this finding is somewhat more frequent when 5 mm collimation is used (29, 30). With 5 mm collimation, 56% of pancreatic carcinomas were found to have dilated ducts, 70% if only those tumors of the head and body were considered (29). A dilated main pancreatic duct can be the only abnormal finding in small duct cell carcinomas in the head of the pancreas (<3 cm) (29).

The presence of a dilated duct in and of itself is nonspecific, caused by either chronic pancreatitis or carcinoma. Pseudocysts are more likely to be seen in pancreatitis although retention cysts proximal to ductal obstruction can be seen in carcinoma. A smooth or beaded appearance of the dilated duct is more typical of duct cell carcinoma, as opposed to an irregularly dilated duct in chronic pancreatitis (10, 29). Unfortunately, there is considerable overlap so that in an individual case this distinction is rarely helpful. A dilated duct may be seen within a mass produced by focal pancreatitis but not within a neoplastic mass (10). Approximately 50% of dilated ducts associated with chronic pancreatitis will contain calcification, whereas intraductal calcification coexisting with carcinoma is highly unusual in our experience (11, 29). An increased frequency of carcinoma in patients with chronic calcific pancreatitis has been reported in one series (31), but has not been found by others (30, 32), and probably occurs only in familial hereditary pancreatitis.

Biliary Tree. Patients with duct cell adenocarcinoma of the pancreas frequently have biliary dilatation detected by CT at initial evaluation (10–12). According to LaPlace's law, the segment of a closed system with the largest diameter should be the earliest dilate. In addition, support by the hepatic parenchyma may inhibit dilatation of intrahepatic ducts. Accordingly, bil-

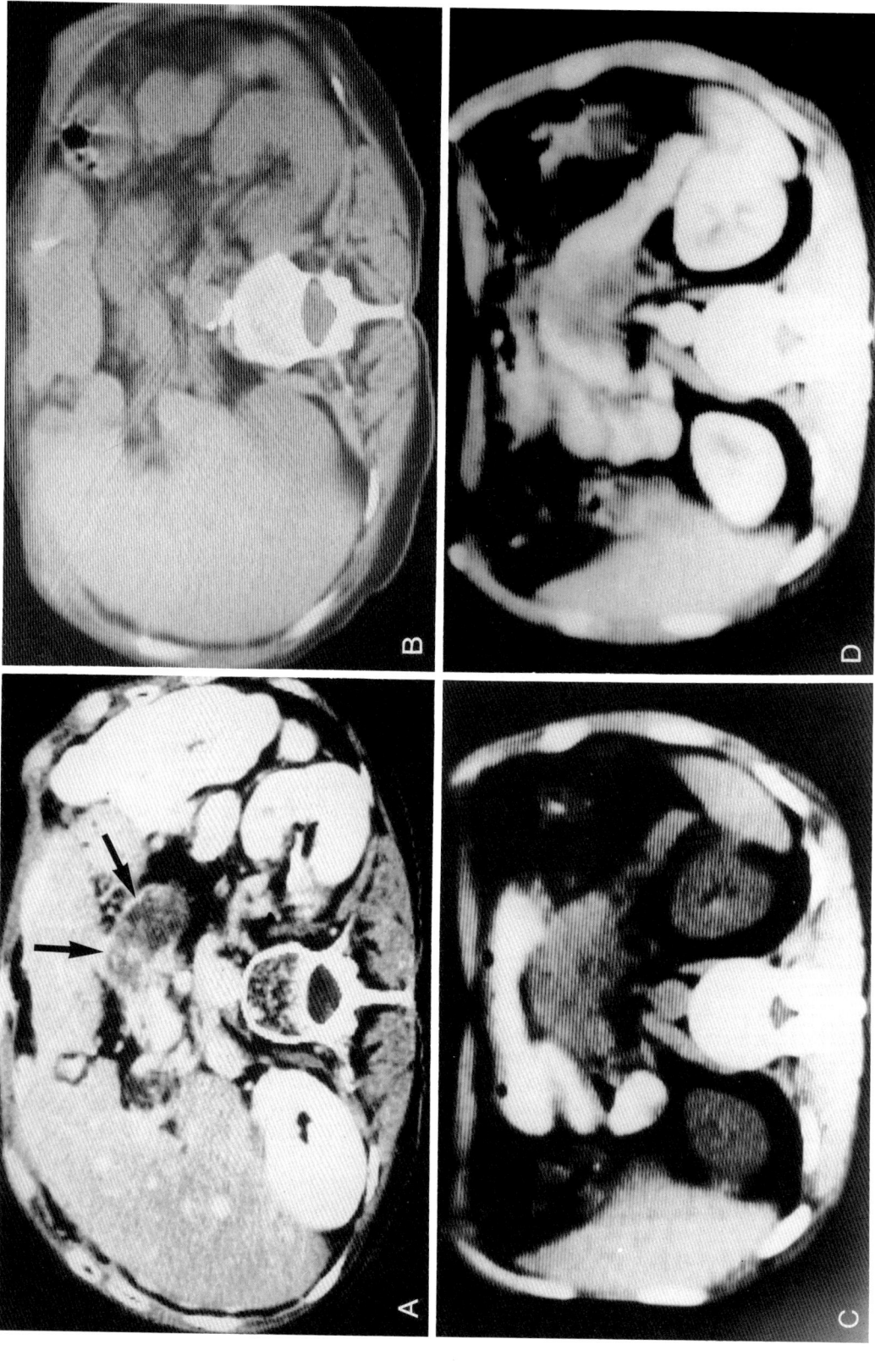

FIGURE 22.33. DUCT CELL ADENOCARCINOMA

A: Bolus dynamic scan: very decreased attenuation in this carcinoma of the body of the pancreas (arrows) due to lack of enhancement. B: Noncontrast scan of the same patient during biopsy: mass is isodense without evidence of necrosis. C and D: Different patient with carcinoma of the body. Noncontrast seen (C) shows an isodense mass, which is unenhancing and better separated from the enhanced normal parenchyma on the bolus enhanced scan (D).

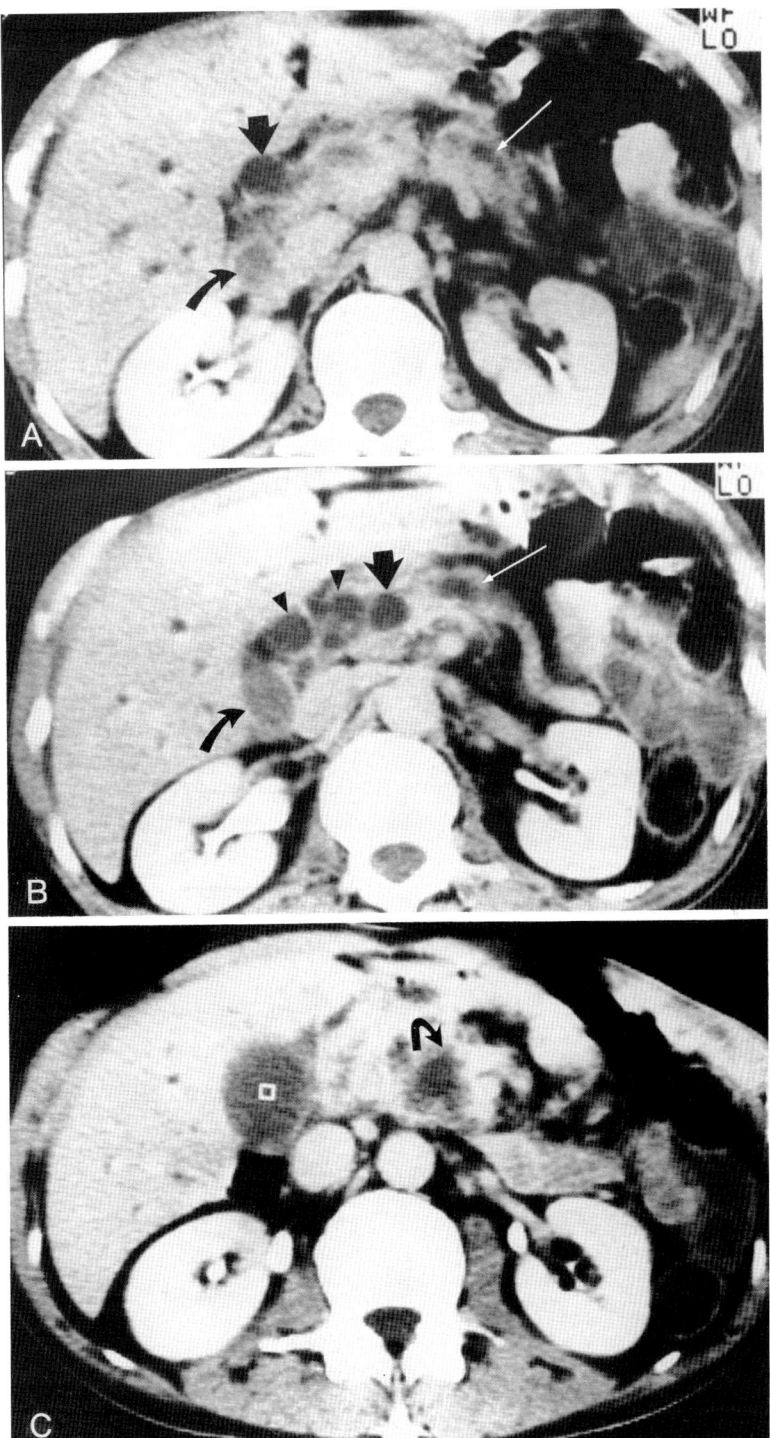

FIGURE 22.34. DUCT CELL ADENOCARCINOMA

Carcinoma of the head and uncinate process causing massive ductal dilatation and abrupt cutoff. Transverse duct orientation causing confusion with pseudocyst. *A:* Dilated intrahepatic ducts seen as lucencies anterior to enhanced portal veins. Dilated common hepatic duct (*arrow*) and neck of gallbladder (*curved arrow*). Dilated pancreatic duct (*white arrow*). *B:* 10 mm caudad to (*A*): same structures and arrows as (*A*) with the addition of the dilated cystic duct (*arrowheads*). *C:* 10 mm caudad to (*B*): Dilated gallbladder (*cursor*). Transverse dilated common bile duct mimicking pseudocyst (*curved arrow*). *D:* 10 mm caudad to (*C*): Abruptly terminating obstructed duct (*arrow*). Next slice showed no duct. *E:* Corresponding transhepatic cholangiogram: transverse common bile duct with abrupt, rounded obstruction.

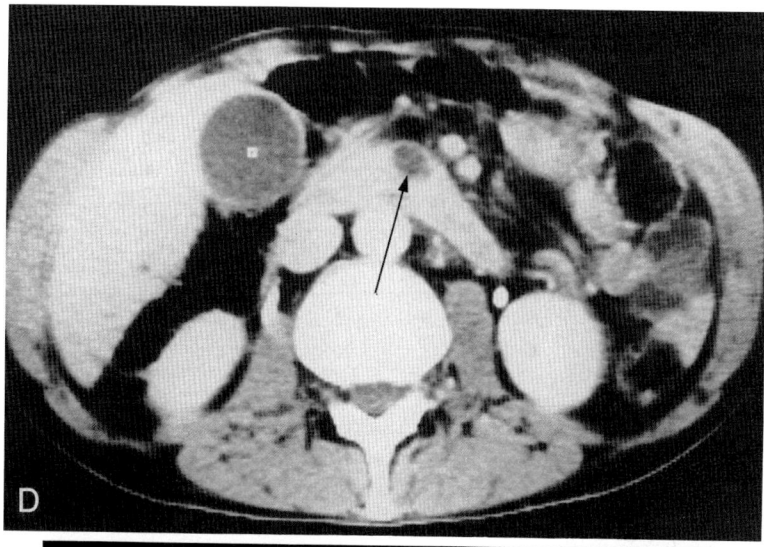

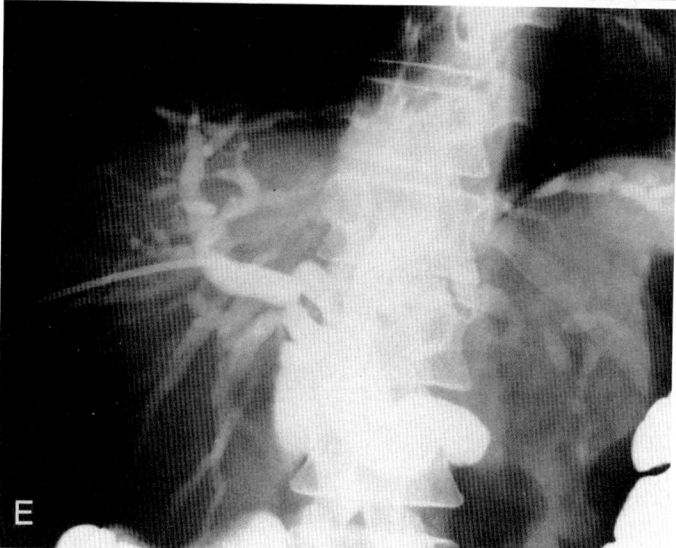

FIGURE 22.34D and E

iary dilatation is most frequently manifested as dilatation of the common bile duct, with intrahepatic dilatation being present somewhat less frequently (11).

The upper limit of normal for the intrapancreatic common bile duct diameter measured by CT is considered to be 7 mm (15), although higher values (9 mm) are accepted by most investigators for patients with prior cholecystectomy (15). Major intrahepatic ducts measuring more than 2–3 mm should be considered abnormal (10). The normal bile duct can frequently be identified as a round lucency within the head of the pancreas, especially if intravenous contrast has been given. Preliminary investigation in 97 patients given oral cholecystographic agents prior to CT allowed the distal common bile duct to be identified in 87% (15). In 30% of these, identification of the common bile duct was considered necessary to differentiate pancreatic head from the adjacent duodenum; no pancreatic tissue is normally found lateral to the duct (15). In this series, mild common bile duct dilatation was the only abnormal finding in four asymptomatic patients; two of these were later proved to have pancreatic carcinoma, the other two remaining asymptomatic (15). Unexplained biliary dilatation may be of no clinical significance, particularly in the elderly, but it deserves follow-up. Duct cell adenocarcinoma of the pancreas almost always but not invariably causes obstructive jaundice and dilatation of both intrahepatic

FIGURE 22.35. DUCT CELL ADENOCARCINOMA

A and *B:* Extension of carcinoma of the neck of the pancreas to the fat around the celiac axis and the diaphragmatic crura. The patient presented with pain and weight loss and these were the only findings. Drip infusion scan (*A*) shows a soft tissue mass anterior to the aorta and thickening of the crura (*arrows*). Bolus dynamic scan clearly shows encased celiac artery (arrow). Percutaneous needle biopsy of the perivascular mass confirmed carcinoma of the pancreas. *C:* Nonenhancing carcinoma of the head and body engulfing the left renal vein, superior mesenteric artery and vein (these structures should be seen at this level during this bolus dynamic scan). Note dilated pancreatic duct (*white arrow*), extension into porta hepatis (*curved arrow*) and collateral vein (*arrow*). Fat plane anterior to the aorta is obliterated.

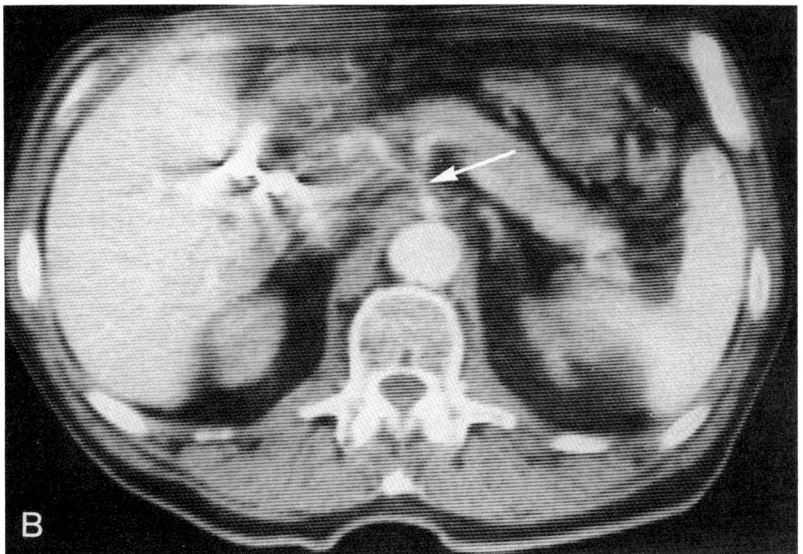

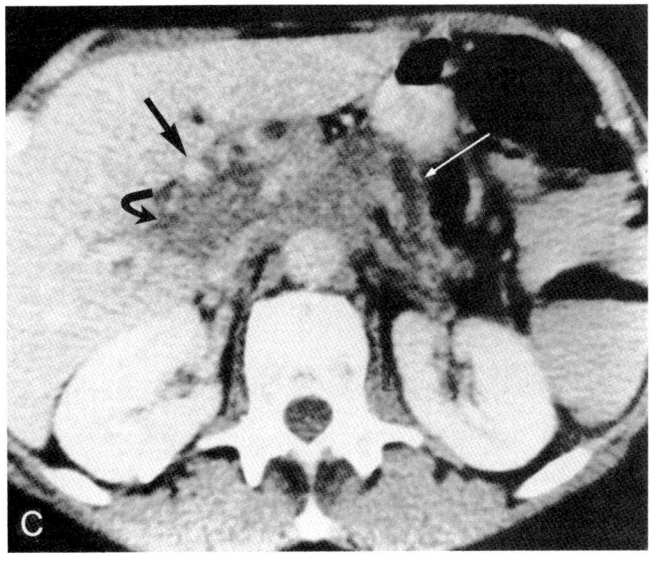

and extrahepatic ducts when the head of the pancreas is affected (19). Early or incomplete obstruction may be limited to the extrahepatic ducts. The gallbladder is often but not always distended when the level of obstruction is distal to the cystic duct. Absence of gallbladder dilatation can be explained by coexisting cholecystitis and scarring. Main pancreatic duct obstruction is frequently also present. CT typically shows abrupt obstruction of the common bile duct usually at the level of the pancreatic head (33, 34). Abrupt obstruction is a sudden transition from a dilated duct to no duct or normal duct; in contrast, tapered, gradual obstruction on CT is seen as a series of progressively smaller rings and is suggestive of benign diseases such as pancreatitis or stricture (33). An associated mass is usually detected in addition to the abrupt obstruction; absence of a mass with abrupt obstruction suggests ampullary carcinoma, a small pancreatic carcinoma, carcinoma of the common duct or a calculus (33, 34). The former can sometimes be depicted as a smooth bulge into the opacified duodenum, mimicking a choledochocoele (34). The latter is usually seen on CT as a round radiodensity. At times, the most caudal portion of the obstructed duct will be an irregular ring on CT in cases of duct cell adenocarcinoma (33). Advanced duct cell carcinoma can obstruct at the level of the suprapancreatic common bile duct or the bifurcation by direct extension or lymphatic spread. Rarely, the level of obstruction will be intrahepatic from metastases.

Sometimes the juxtapancreatic common duct assumes a transverse course and is depicted longitudinally by CT. The horizontal configuration is unreliable for differentiating benign from malignant obstruction and can even be a normal variant (34). Care must be taken by evaluating serial slices not to confuse a dilated transverse common bile duct with a pseudocyst (Fig. 22.34).

Staging

Staging pancreatic duct cell carcinoma involves detecting retroperitoneal extension, vascular encasement, invasion of contiguous structures, lymphadenopathy, and distant metastases. All of these can be accomplished with abdominal CT.

Retroperitoneal extension is present in roughly 40–60% of patients at initial evaluation (10, 11, 20) and is strongly indicative of unresectability (12, 20). Extension often occurs into the fat which normally surrounds and clearly outlines the celiac axis and superior mesenteric artery (Fig. 22.35) (19). Either or both can be engulfed by mass. Soft-tissue density streaks and strands in the retroperitoneal fat in the region of the mass suggests extension (Fig. 22.36) (19). Thickening of Gerota's fascia in association with a mass in the body or tail strongly suggests unresectable duct cell carcinoma (Fig. 22.36) (12). Theoretically, thickening of Gerota's fascia could be caused by pancreatitis due to a resectable obstructing carcinoma of the head. Obliteration of the fat between a mass in the dorsal pancreas and the inferior vena cava or aorta also suggests unresectability (Figs. 22.35C and 22.36D) (10). Evaluation of peripancreatic fat planes can be difficult in the cachectic patients who comprise a significant number of those patients suspected to have pancreatic cancer.

A subtle finding, which may be present in the absence of a conspicuous pancreatic mass (35, 36), is thickening of the celiac axis or superior mesenteric artery. The normal vessel is smooth and tapered, whereas the thickened vessel is irregular and may be bulbous or "club-shaped" distally (Figs. 22.37 and 22.38A) (35). This appearance is thought to be due to malignant invasion of perivascular lymphatics and indicative of unresectability (10, 12, 35). The "thick vessel sign" is somewhat more frequent with carcinoma involving the pancreatic body and tail, in part due to the relatively advanced stage of most of these tumors but also due to lymphatic drainage of the pancreatic head predominantly into the periduodenal lymphatics (35). It is seen prior to angiographically visible "encasement," since narrowing and irregularity of the vascular lumen is a later occurrence (20, 35). Vascular encasement manifests itself on CT as narrowing or obliteration of the lumen and is best evaluated by dynamic techniques (Fig. 22.35B) (12). Encasement of the hepatic, splenic, or superior mesenteric artery or the portal, splenic or superior mesenteric vein indicates unresectability (Fig. 22.38) (10, 12). Variceal dilatation of tributary veins proximal to venous occlusions may be depicted by CT (Figs. 22.35C and 22.36). Collateral veins at the splenic hilus or behind the stomach from splenic vein obstruction were seen fairly frequently in one series (Figs. 22.36A and 22.39) (12). The fat in the mesentery should be searched for round or tubular densities which would suggest dilated veins from superior mesenteric vein obstruction (Fig. 22.40).

Invasion of contiguous structures occurs with unresectable advanced disease, most commonly involving the stomach or duodenum. This can be assessed by CT, but is often better evaluated by

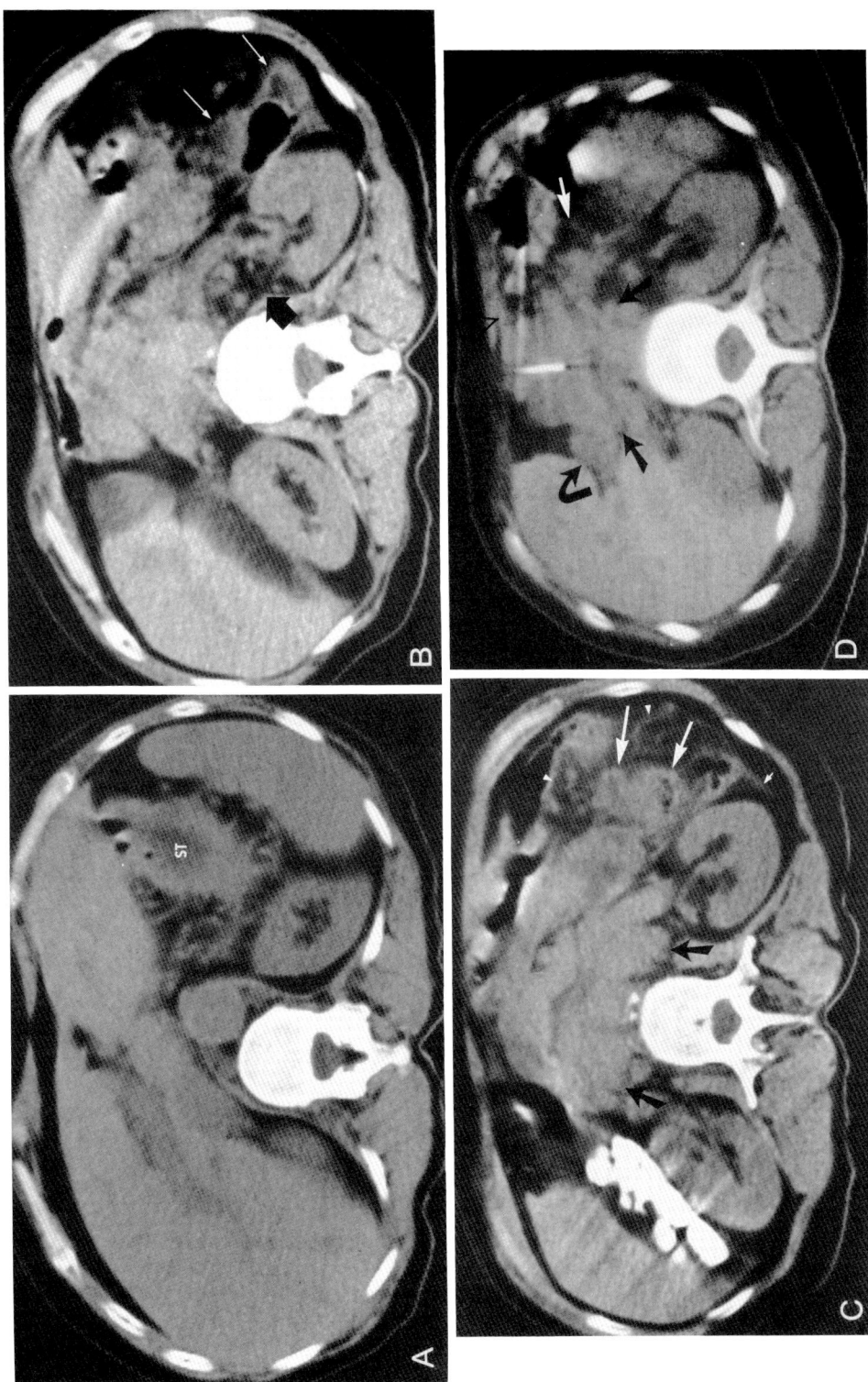

FIGURE 22.36. DUCT CELL ADENOCARCINOMA

Noncontrast CT (allergy) in a patient with carcinoma of the entire pancreas and extensive retroperitoneal disease. *A*: Splenomegaly and perigastric collateral veins from splenic vein occlusion (*ST*=stomach). *B*: Serpiginous densities in the left renal hilum from renal vein occlusion (*arrow*). Mass engulfs superior mesenteric artery and fat anterior to aorta is obliterated. Invasion of mesenteric fat around the colon (*white arrows*) and streaky densities in mesentery (*arrowheads*). Marked adenopathy (*arrows*). Thickened Gerota's and lateroconal fascia (*small white arrow*). Colonic involvement confirmed by barium enema. *D*: Different patient showing obliteration of fat around the aorta and inferior vena cava (*arrows*), extension into the porta hepatis (*curved arrow*) and retroperitoneal fat (*white arrow*). The mass in the body (surrounding biopsy needle) extends into the anterior abdominal wall (*open arrow*).

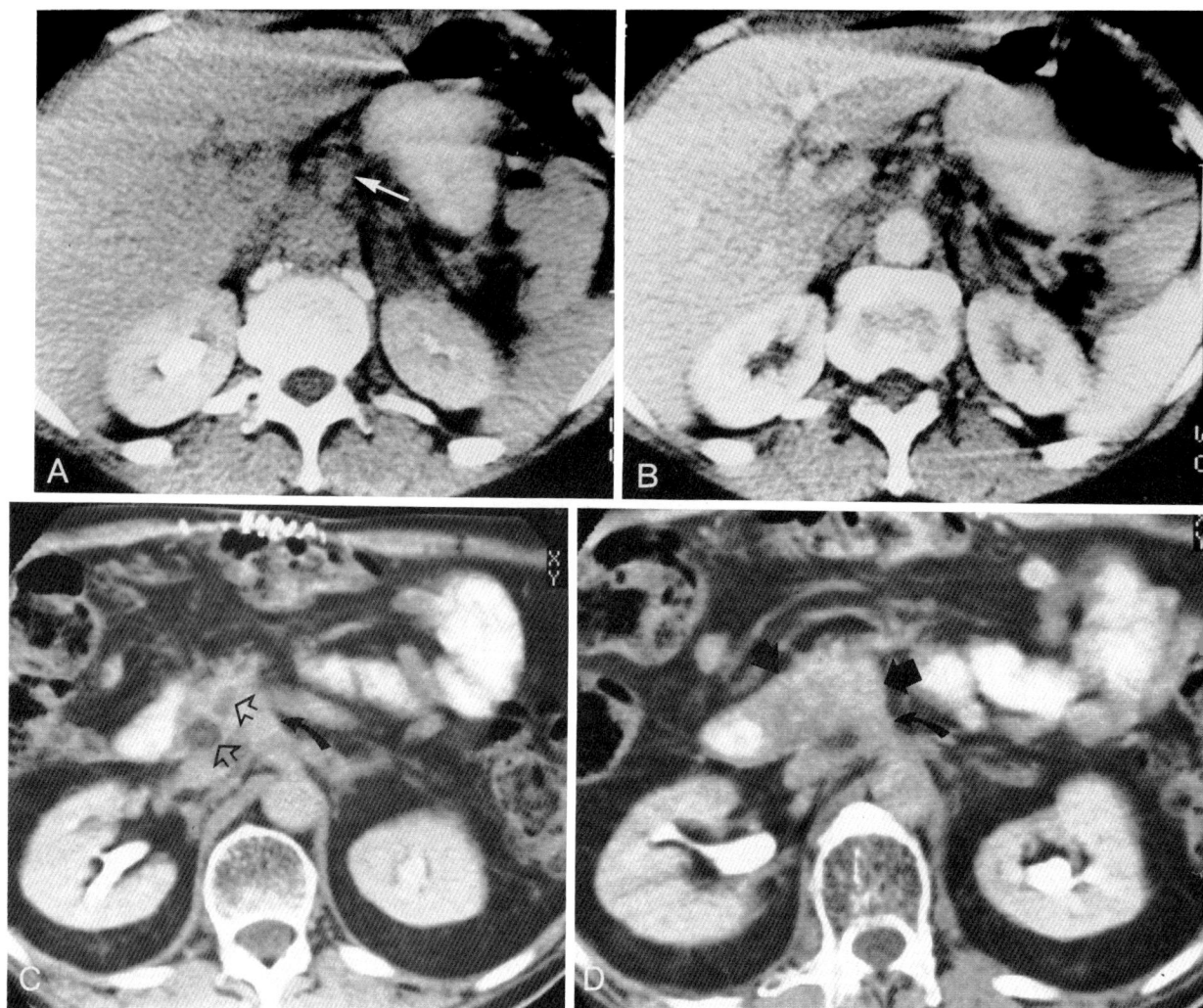

FIGURE 22.37. DUCT CELL ADENOCARCINOMA

A and *B:* "Thickening" of celiac artery (*arrow*) on a drip infusion scan (*A*) confirmed by a bolus injection (*B*) due to carcinoma of the body (same patient as seen in Fig. 22.35*C*). *C* and *D:* Similar findings (*curved arrows*) in another patient in which the superior mesenteric artery is affected by a contiguous carcinoma in the uncinate process (*arrows*). Note dilated common bile duct (*open arrows*).

conventional barium studies (Fig. 22.36*D*) (10). Carcinoma of the body or tail may also invade the aorta, inferior vena cava, kidney, spleen, or even the spine (Figs. 22.39 and 22.40) (11).

Involvement of peripancreatic nodes is demonstrated by CT in roughly 15–25% of patients with duct cell carcinoma (Fig. 22.36*C*) (10–12). Nodes may be confluent with the primary mass. Involvement of contiguous lymph nodes is a poor prognostic sign (10), but resectability is theoretically possible provided the affected nodes and the pancreas can be removed en bloc without leaving residual disease (26, 36). It is often difficult to differentiate by CT peripancreatic adenopathy of nonpancreatic etiology from a duct cell carcinoma (with or without contiguous adenopathy). The former tends to displace the pancreas anteriorly and fat planes are sometimes maintained between the pancreas and the enlarged nodes. A normal ERCP in association with a "pancreatic mass" on CT also suggests peripancreatic adenopathy of nonpancreatic etiology (37).

The liver represents the first capillary bed which pancreatic venous drainage encounters and is thus by far the most common site of distant metastases. Hepatic metastases are present on CT at initial evaluation in 20–50% of

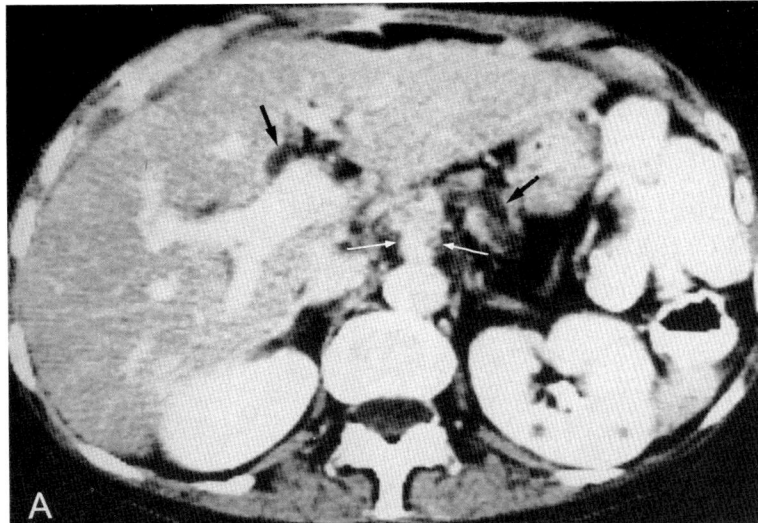
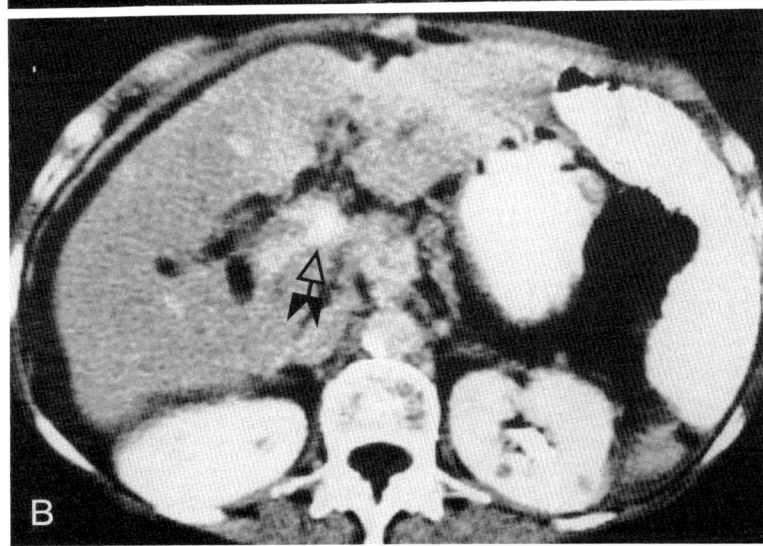

FIGURE 22.38. DUCT CELL ADENOCARCINOMA
Carcinoma of pancreas occluding portal vein. *A:* Baseline scan: celiac artery thickening (*white arrows*) but intact portal vein. Note dilated biliary and pancreatic (*black arrow*) ducts and minimal ascites around liver edge. *B:* Scan at same level 2½ months later does not demonstrate normal portal vein enhancement; collaterals (*arrow*) seen beneath dilated bile ducts. Larger amount of ascites around liver from portal hypertension or peritoneal implants.

cases (10–12) and are hypodense hepatic masses (Fig. 22.40). Detectable ascites is a late finding, present on CT in 9% in one series (10). Ascites may be secondary to portal vein obstruction, but is most often due to diffuse peritoneal metastases too small to be detected by CT (Fig. 22.38*B*) (10).

Other Uses of CT

CT is the most accurate guidance method for percutaneous biopsy of pancreatic duct cell carcinoma. The likelihood of a positive biopsy when duct cell carcinoma is present is high, but failure to obtain malignant cells does not exclude the diagnosis. False positives are almost nonexistent in the hands of experienced cytopathologists. CT is also useful for palliative radiotherapy planning and percutaneous splanchnic and celiac plexus nerve block guidance (38). CT is considered the procedure of choice for evaluation of metastatic adenocarcinoma of unknown primary, increasing the diagnostic yield of conventional radiography (8–9%) to 33% (39). The most common primary detected is pancreatic, representing one third of those detected (39).

Differentiation of Carcinoma and Pancreatitis

Focal Mass. The presence of a focal pancreatic mass is generally indicative of a neoplasm, but chronic pancreatitis not infrequently causes a focal pancreatic mass on sonography and CT (17, 18, 40). Clinical data are usually, but not always, helpful in differentiation. The best imaging differential is the presence of foci

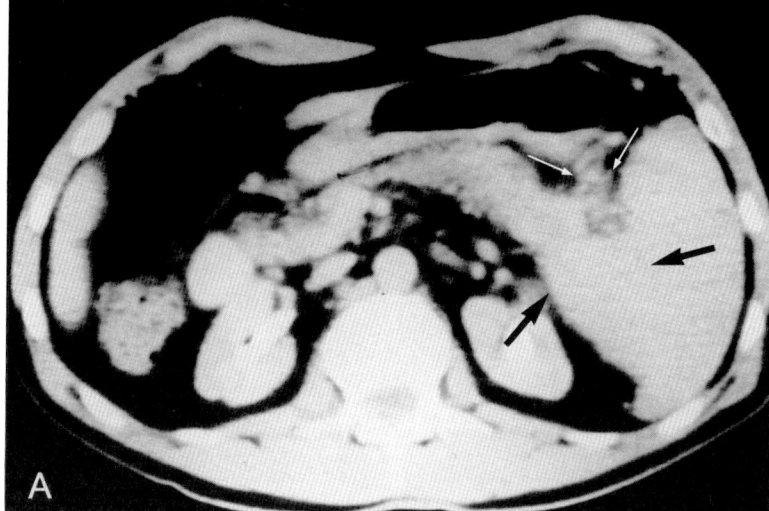
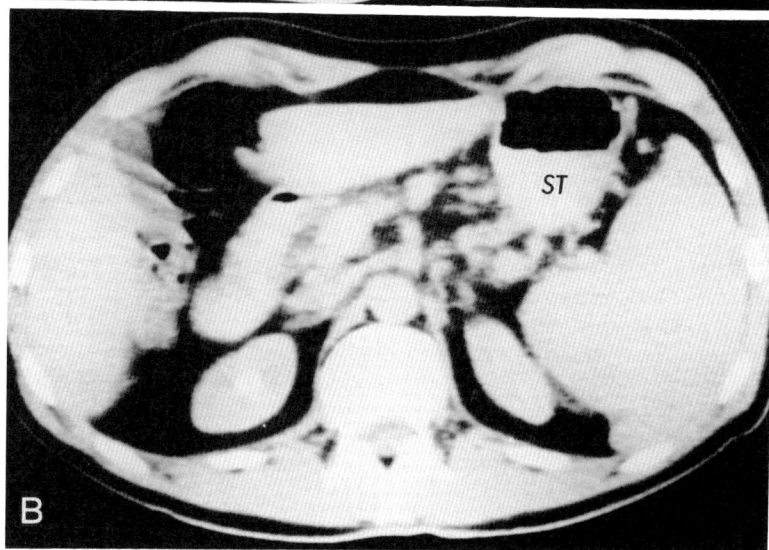

FIGURE 22.39. DUCT CELL ADENOCARCINOMA
Carcinoma of the tail with splenic vein occlusion. *A:* Large mass in tail inseparable (*black arrows*) from spleen. Splenic vein not seen in its expected position behind the pancreas. Extension into retrogastric fat (*white arrows*). *B:* Multiple tubular perigastric collaterals (*ST*=stomach). Splenomegaly (same case as in Fig. 22.67).

of calcification within the mass, which almost never occurs in duct cell carcinoma in our experience. Microcystic adenoma and mucinous cystic neoplasm have larger central and peripheral calcifications, respectively. If there is calcification in the rest of the gland but not in the mass, chronic pancreatitis is still the most likely diagnosis, although it is difficult to exclude a superimposed neoplasm (Fig. 22.41). We have not found the pattern of pancreatic duct dilatation (beaded, irregular, or smooth) helpful, although presence of a dilated duct within the mass indicates inflammatory disease (10).

Pancreatic duct dilatation tends to be more prominent with carcinoma (29). The size of the surrounding gland tends to be larger with chronic pancreatitis, due either to inflammatory change with pancreatitis or atrophy associated with carcinoma or both (12, 29). A "duct/gland" ratio of greater than 0.5 is suggestive of carcinoma but there is significant overlap regarding this measurement (29). Pseudocysts are detected in 8–10% of cases of pancreatic carcinoma by CT (12, 41), although the frequency of pseudocysts at autopsy is approximately 15%, most of which are small (41, 42). Pseudocysts occurring proximal to an obstructing neoplasm are typically intrapancreatic, located along the course of the ductal system, and seldom extend beyond the pancreas (24). Their appearance is otherwise identical to those associated with inflammatory pancreatitis. Pseudocysts associated with carcinoma do not opacify on ERCP, as do many of those of inflammatory origin, because the former are in the body

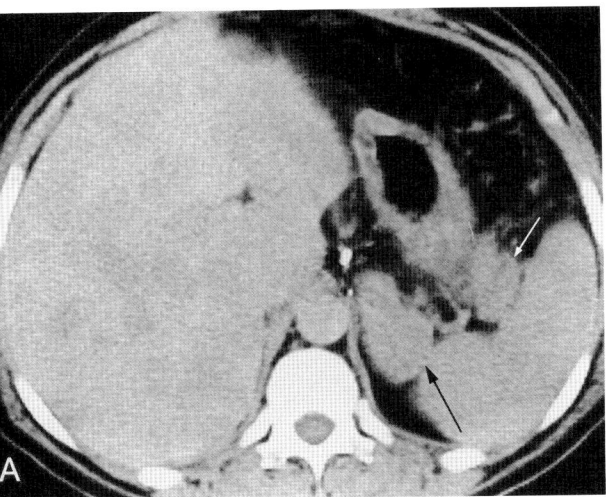 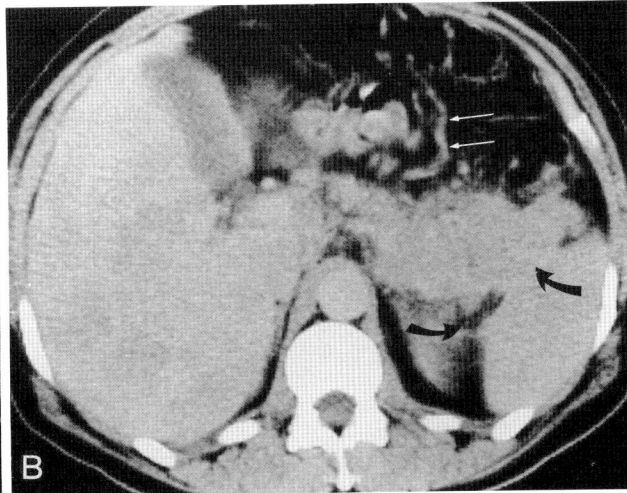

FIGURE 22.40. DUCT CELL ADENOCARCINOMA

Carcinoma of the tail invading spleen, adrenal, mesenteric fat, and metastasizing to liver. *A:* Multiple hypodense liver metastases, mass in splenic hilum (*white arrow*) and adrenal (*black arrow*) and splenomegaly. *B:* Large mass in tail invading spleen and perisplenic fat (*curved arrows*). Collateral vein in mesentery (*white arrows*). Liver metastases less obvious on this cut.

or tail and proximal to a tumor obstructing pancreatic drainage (41).

Intrahepatic biliary duct dilatation is less likely to occur with focal pancreatitis in the head than with carcinoma (11). The double duct sign on sonography or CT is nonspecific. Although a smooth, long segment tapered obstruction suggests pancreatitis, and a short segment abrupt obstruction suggests carcinoma, these criteria are not absolute (40). Mild jaundice with severe dilatation suggests focal pancreatitis, high bilirubin levels that advance relentlessly suggest carcinoma.

The direction of retroperitoneal extension associated with pancreatitis is predominantly anterior, as opposed to the predominantly retropancreatic direction of malignant invasion (10, 35). Detecting thickening of the celiac axis or superior mesenteric artery or obliteration of the fat surrounding these vessels strongly favors carcinoma over pancreatitis. Infiltration of the periaortic or pericaval regions, although reported in focal pancreatitis (40), favors carcinoma. The presence of hepatic metastases or adenopathy indicates neoplasm.

Diffuse Enlargement. Secondary pancreatitis is a nearly universal histologic finding with pancreatic duct cell carcinoma, and is often present grossly when the tumor involves the pancreatic head (26). This pancreatitis is subclinical in most cases, although 3% of pancreatic carcinomas present as acute pancreatitis, and 1–2% of cases of acute pancreatitis are due to pancreatic carcinoma (26, 42). Symptoms of acute pancreatitis may antedate carcinoma by as much as 2 yr (26). Diffuse enlargement of the pancreas by carcinoma may be mostly secondary to inflammation and fibrosis with tumor cells scattered throughout the gland (18). Pancreatic carcinoma should be suspected if a middle-aged or elderly patient presents with acute pancreatitis for the first time with no apparent cause, or if the body and tail are diffusely enlarged with a normal head, an unusual pattern for pancreatitis (26). Carcinoma is extremely unlikely in a diffusely enlarged gland if intraductal calcifications can be demonstrated.

Computed Pancreatography

Computed tomography immediately after ERCP has been utilized to obtain information not available with either modality alone. It is imperative that all delays between the two examinations are avoided; when ERCP was followed by CT within 30 min only one-half of patients studied had contrast remaining within the pancreas (16). Another report concerning this technique was successful in visualizing contrast within peripheral radicals not seen with plain film radiography, resulting in diffuse opacification of normal pancreatic tissue (17). Areas of chronic pancreatitis were seen as patchy opacification, whereas carcinoma demonstrated no

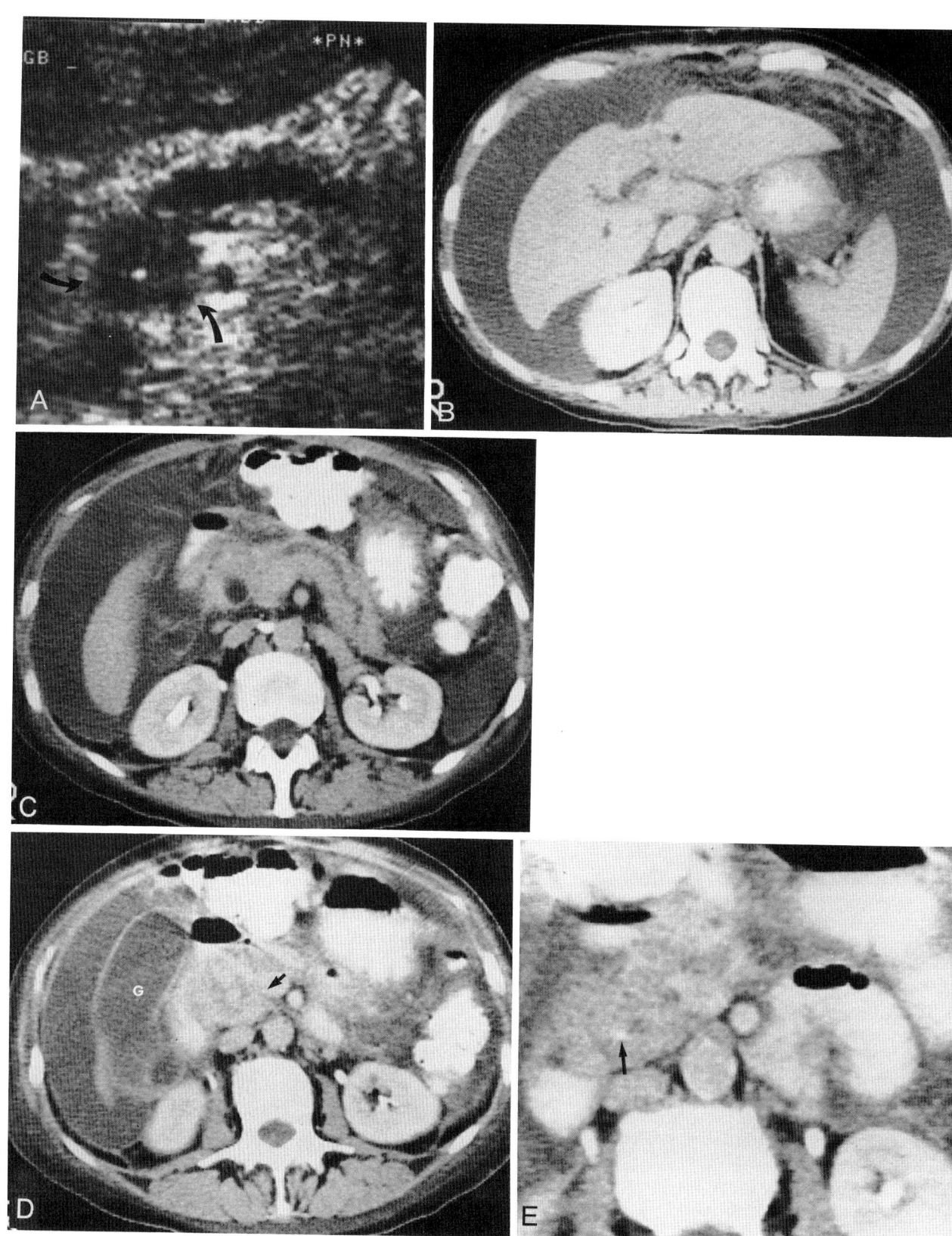

FIGURE 22.41. DUCT CELL ADENOCARCINOMA OR PANCREATITIS?
A: Carcinoma of the uncinate process superimposed on chronic alcoholic pancreatitis. Transverse sonogram shows a hypoechoic mass in the uncinate process (*curved arrows*) engulfing a preexisting calcification (shadowing echogenicity in the center of mass). Note dilated pancreatic duct (*arrows*) obstructed by the mass, not the calcification, which was verified by CT.

CT versus Other Methods

While in some cases other examinations provide information not obtainable by CT, CT is the best single examination for pancreatic carcinoma. The results of one early series suggested that ERCP and ultrasound are more sensitive in detecting early or resectable carcinoma (43), but CT is more sensitive in detecting and staging nonresectable carcinoma (43, 44). However, high resolution CT with bolus enhancement technique should have improved sensitivity for early carcinoma compared to earlier reports. While ultrasound may still be of value in screening and in following a known lesion, CT is usually more sensitive and specific, and is more frequently technically satisfactory (44). When the two exams disagreed, CT was correct in 85% of cases in one series (44). Reserving ERCP (45, 46) or angiography (21, 45) for indeterminate CT evaluations can drastically reduce the frequency of these invasive modalities with little if any reduction in diagnostic accuracy. If successful, accuracy of ERCP in experienced hands is comparable to CT (46). When the two examinations agree, diagnostic accuracy is higher than for either alone; when they disagree the abnormal examination is usually correct (46). ERCP will exclude pancreatic disease if normal in a patient with an apparently enlarged gland on sonographic or CT (37, 46). Angiography is most helpful in staging by detecting vascular encasement (45). Pancreatic carcinoma should be considered unresectable if any major vessel other than the gastroduodenal artery is involved (19, 47). If only the gastroduodenal artery is involved, the tumor may be resected for palliation although survival is not likely to be prolonged (48). CT is more sensitive in detecting involvement of the celiac axis or superior mesenteric artery but it is inferior to angiography in detecting involvement of other vessels (20).

REFERENCES

1. Levitt RG, Stanley RJ, Sagel SS, Lee JKT, Weyman PJ: Computed tomography of the pancreas: three second scanning versus 18 second scanning. *J Comput Assist Tomogr* 6:259–267, 1982.
2. Berland LL, Lawson TL, Foley WD: Dynamic pancreatic scanning. In Siegelman SS (ed): *Computed Tomography of the Pancreas.* New York, Churchill Livingstone, 1983, pp 33–60.
3. Berland LL, Lawson TL, Foley WD, Geenan JE, Stewart T: Computed tomography of the normal and abnormal pancreatic duct: correlation with pancreatic ductography. *Radiology* 141:715–724, 1981.
4. Callen PW, London SS, Moss AA: CT evaluation of the dilated pancreatic duct. *Radiology* 134:253–255, 1980.
5. Seeram E: *Computed Tomography Technology.* Philadelphia, W. B. Saunders, 1982, pp 139–152.
6. Rossi P, Baert A, Marchal W, Tipaldi L, Wilms W, Pavone P: Multiple bolus technique vs. single bolus or infusion of contrast medium to obtain prolonged contrast enhancement of the pancreas. *Radiology* 144:929–931, 1982.
7. Hosoki T: Dynamic CT of pancreatic tumors. *AJR* 140:959–965, 1983.
8. Marchal G, Baert L, Wilms G: Intravenous pancreaticography in computed tomography. *J Comput Assist Tomogr* 10:727–732, 1979.
9. Kivisaari L, Kormano M, Rantakokko V: Contrast enhancement of the pancreas in computed tomography. *J Comput Assist Tomogr* 3:722–726, 1979.
10. Freeny PC, Lawson TL: *Radiology of the Pancreas.* New York, Springer-Verlag, 1982, pp 427–449.
11. Fishman EK, Siegelman SS: CT of pancreatic carcinoma. In Siegelman SS (ed): *Computed Tomography of the Pancreas.* New York, Churchill Livingstone, 1983, pp 123–156.
12. Ward EM, Stephens DH, Sheedy PF: Computed tomographic characteristics of pancreatic carcinoma: an analysis of 100 cases. *Radiographics* 3:547–565, 1983.
13. Donovan PJ: Technique of examination and normal pancreatic anatomy. In Siegelman SS (ed): *Computed Tomography of the Pancreas.* New York, Churchill Livingstone, 1983, pp 1–32.
14. Stuck KJ, Kuhns LR: Improved visualization of the pancreatic tail after maximum distention of the stomach. *J Comput Assist Tomogr* 5:509–512, 1981.

Very unusual case-calcification of this type almost always would indicate focal pancreatitis. Large "duct/gland" ratio (there is almost complete absence of parenchyma in body and tail) suggests the correct diagnosis of carcinoma. Patient presented with abdominal pain initially though to be an exacerbation of his pancreatitis. B–E: Middle-aged woman presenting with ascites and weight loss. Clues to the correct diagnosis of chronic pancreatitis are subtle calcification, preserved fat around the superior mesenteric artery, and lack of jaundice despite quite dilated bile ducts. B: Dilated bile ducts and massive ascites. Note bare area of spleen (posteromedial surface). C: Dilated pancreatic duct and dilated common duct in the head of the pancreas. Note intact fat around the superior mesenteric artery, suggesting benign disease. D: Large mass in the uncinate process and head of the pancreas. Tiny calcification (*arrow*). Dilated gallbladder (*G*). E: Enlargement of adjacent section shows another subtle calcification (*arrow*). Preserved fat around the superior mesenteric artery in both D and E.

15. Greenberg M, Greenberg BM, Rubin JM, Greenberg IM: Computed tomographic cholangiography. *Radiology* 144:363–368, 1982.
16. Jaffe MH, Glazer GM, Amendola MA, Nostrant T, Wilson JAP: Endoscopic retrograde computed tomography of the pancreas. *J Comput Assist Tomogr* 8:63–66, 1984.
17. Frick MP, O'Leary JF, Salomonowitz E, Stoltenberg P, Hutton S, Gedgaudas E: Pancreas imaging by computed tomography after endoscopic retrograde pancreatography. *Radiology* 150:191–194, 1984.
18. Wittenberg J, Simeone JF, Ferrucci JT: Non-focal enlargement in pancreatic carcinoma. *Radiology* 144:131–135, 1982.
19. Stephens DH: Pancreatic Neoplasms. Syllabus for the Categorical Course on Computed Body Tomography with MRI Correlation. Presented at the Annual Meeting of The American Roentgen Ray Society, Las Vegas, Nevada, April, 1984.
20. Jafri SZ, Aisen AM, Glazer GM, Weiss CA: Comparison of CT and angiography in assessing resectability of pancreatic carcinoma. *AJR* 142:535–539, 1984.
21. Haaga JR, Alfidi RJ: Computed tomographic scanning of the pancreas. *Radiol Clin North Am* 15:367–376, 1977.
22. Kreel L, Maertel M, Katz D: Computed tomography of the normal pancreas. *J Comput Assist Tomogr* 1:290–299, 1977.
23. Callen PW, Breiman RS, Korobkin M, DeMartini WJ, Mani JR: Carcinoma of the tail of the pancreas: an unusual CT appearance. *AJR* 133:135–137, 1979.
24. Stephens DH, Sheedy PF II, James EM: Neoplastic lesions of the pancreas. In Margulis AR, Burhenne AJ (eds): *Alimentary Radiology*. St. Louis, C. V. Mosby, 1983, pp 1316–1345.
25. Kaplan JO, Isikoff MB, Barkin J, Livingstone AS: Necrotic carcinoma of the pancreas: "the pseudo-pseudocyst." *J Comput Assist Tomogr* 4:166–167, 1980.
26. Levine E: Carcinoma of the pancreas as acute pancreatitis: CT diagnosis. *Gastrointest Radiol* 6:29–33, 1981.
27. Hauser H, Battikha JG, Wettstein P: Computed tomography of the dilated main pancreatic duct. *J Comput Assist Tomogr* 4:53–58, 1980.
28. Seidelmann FE, Cohen WN, Bryan PJ, Brown J: CT demonstration of the splenic vein-pancreatic relationship: The pseudodilated pancreatic duct. *AJR* 129:17–21, 1977.
29. Karasawa E, Goldberg HI, Moss AA, Federele MP, London SS: CT pancreatogram in carcinoma of the pancreas and chronic pancreatitis. *Radiology* 148:489–493, 1983.
30. Johnson JR, Zintel HA: Pancreatic calcification and cancer of the pancreas. *Surg Gynecol Obstet* 117:585–588, 1963.
31. Paulino-Netto A, Dreiling DA, Baronofsky ID: The relationship between pancreatic calcification and cancer of the pancreas. *Ann Surg* 151:530–537, 1960.
32. Schultz RE, Finkler NJ: Pancreatic calcification and pancreatic carcinoma: the relationship reconsidered. *Mt Sinai J Med* 47:622–626, 1980.
33. Pedrosa CS, Casanova R, Rodriguez R: Computed tomography in obstructive jaundice. *Radiology* 139:627–645, 1981.
34. Baron RL, Stanley RJ, Lee JKT, Koehler RE, Levitt RG: Computed tomographic features of biliary obstruction. *AJR* 140:1173–1178, 1983.
35. Megibow AJ, Bosniak MA, Ambos MA, Beranbaum ER: Thickening of the celiac axis and/or superior mesenteric artery: a sign of pancreatic carcinoma on computed tomography. *Radiology* 141:449–453, 1981.
36. Itai T, Araki T, Tasaka A, Maruyama M: Computed tomographic appearance of resectable pancreatic carcinoma. *Radiology* 143:719–726, 1982.
37. Frick MP, Feinberg SB, Goodale RL: The value of endoscopic retrograde cholangiopancreatography in patients with suspected carcinoma of the pancreas and indeterminate computed tomographic results. *Surg Gynecol Obstet* 155:177–182, 1982.
38. Berg JN, Moss AA, Singler RC: CT guided celiac plexus and splanchnic nerve neurolysis. *J Comput Assist Tomogr* 6:315–319, 1982.
39. Karsell PR, Sheedy PF, O'Connell MJ: Computed tomography in search of cancer of unknown origin. *JAMA* 248:340–343, 1982.
40. Neff CC, Simeone JF, Wittenberg J, Mueller PR, Ferrucci JT Jr: Inflammatory pancreatic masses. Problems in differentiating focal pancreatitis from carcinoma. *Radiology* 150:35–38, 1984.
41. Itai Y, Moss A, Goldberg HI: Pancreatic cysts caused by carcinoma of the pancreas: A pitfall in the diagnosis of pancreatic carcinoma. *J Comput Assist Tomogr* 6:772–776, 1982.
42. Niccolini DG, Graham JH, Banks PA: Tumor-induced acute pancreatitis. *Gastrointest Radiol* 71:142–145, 1976.
43. Moossa AR, Levin B: The diagnosis of "early" pancreatic cancer: The University of Chicago experience. *Cancer* 47:1688–1697, 1981.
44. Hessel SJ, Siegelman SS, McNeil BJ, Sanders R, Adams DF, Alderson PO, Finberg ML, Adams HL: A prospective evaluation of computed tomography and ultrasound of the pancreas. *Radiology* 143:129–133, 1982.
45. Freeny PC, Marks WM, Ball TJ: Impact of high-resolution computed tomography of the pancreas on utilization of endoscopic retrograde cholangiopancreatography and angiography. *Radiology* 142:35–39, 1982.
46. Moss AA, Federle M, Shapiro HA, Ohto M, Goldberg H, Korobkin M, Clemett A: The combined use of computed tomography and endoscopic retrograde cholangiopancreatography in the assessment of suspected pancreatic neoplasms: a blind clinical evaluation. *Radiology* 134:159–163, 1980.
47. Hemmingsson A, Jacobson G, Lindgren PG, Lonnerholm T, Lorelius LE, Nordgren CE: Radiologic assessment of resectability of carcinoma of the head of the pancreas. *Acta Radiol Diagn* 23:127–130, 1982.
48. Tylen U, Arnesjo B: Resectability and prognosis of carcinoma of the pancreas by angiography. *Scand J Gastroenterol* 8:691–697, 1973.

##سonography and CT of Ampullary Carcinoma

Sonography is usually unable to show the mass in cases of ampullary carcinoma. On occasion, with optimal duodenal opacification, CT can depict the mass (Fig. 22.42). Ampullary carcinoma must be considered when sonography and CT show unexplained biliary obstruction with or without pancreatic duct dilation, and cholangiography is usually indicated.

Cholangiography of Pancreatic Adenocarcinoma

No matter what its cholangiographic appearance, any complete or near-complete stricture/

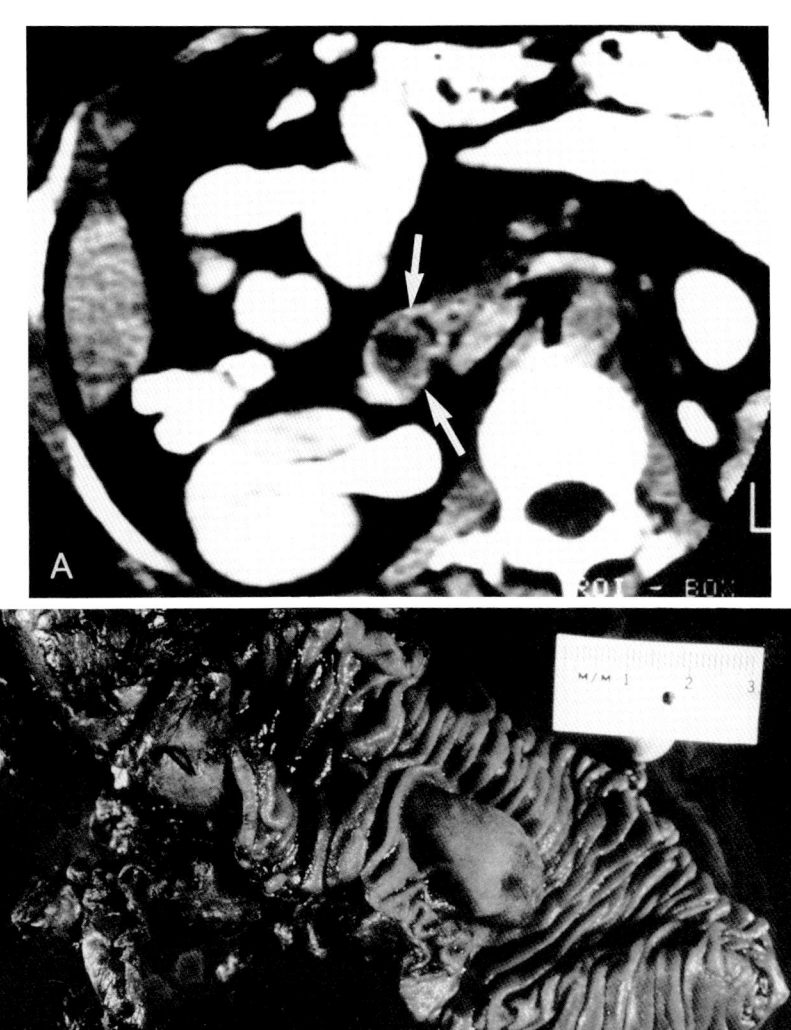

FIGURE 22.42. AMPULLARY CARCINOMA

A: CT scan of an ampullary carcinoma shows the soft tissue mass (*arrows*) indenting the contrast in the duodenum. The central lucency is the distal common duct which is irregular. *B:* Corresponding gross specimen, view from the intraluminal side of the duodenum.

obstruction in the mid or distal common duct is highly suspicious for carcinoma of the head of the pancreas. Most commonly the point of encasement or obstruction is in the distal third of the common duct (the intrapancreatic portion). Proximal to the obstruction the ducts are usually moderately or markedly dilated. Although a rat-tailed obstruction is deemed typical (Fig. 22.43), the configuration of the terminus may be smoothly and symmetrically tapered, conical, or only slightly eccentric and irregular (1–4). A nipple or beak at the point of obstruction is especially characteristic of carcinoma of the pancreas (Fig. 22.44). A nonspecific rounded appearance is quite common and is sometimes due to pooling of contrast and nonfilling of the beak (Fig. 22.45). Although complete obstruction to the flow of contrast is frequent, the duct is usually patent although encased by tumor and guide wires for drainage can almost always be passed

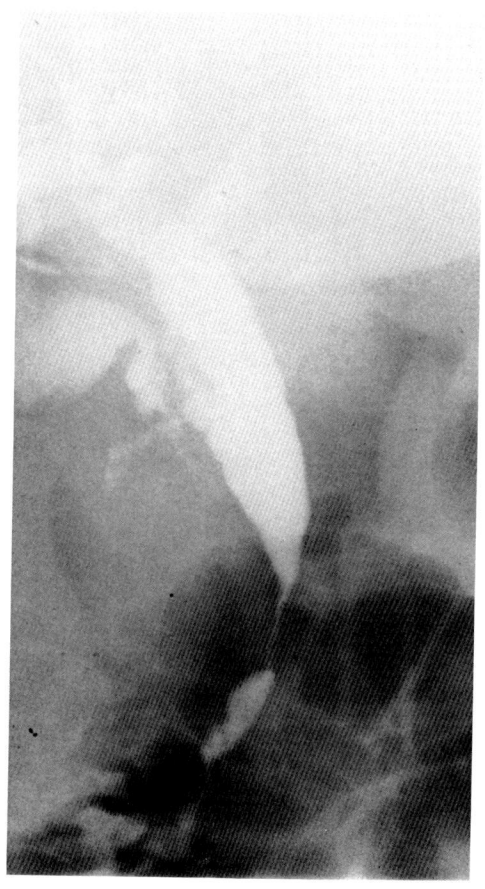

FIGURE 22.43. PANCREATIC ADENOCARCINOMA
Carcinoma of the head of the pancreas producing a rat-tailed encasement of the distal third of the common duct.

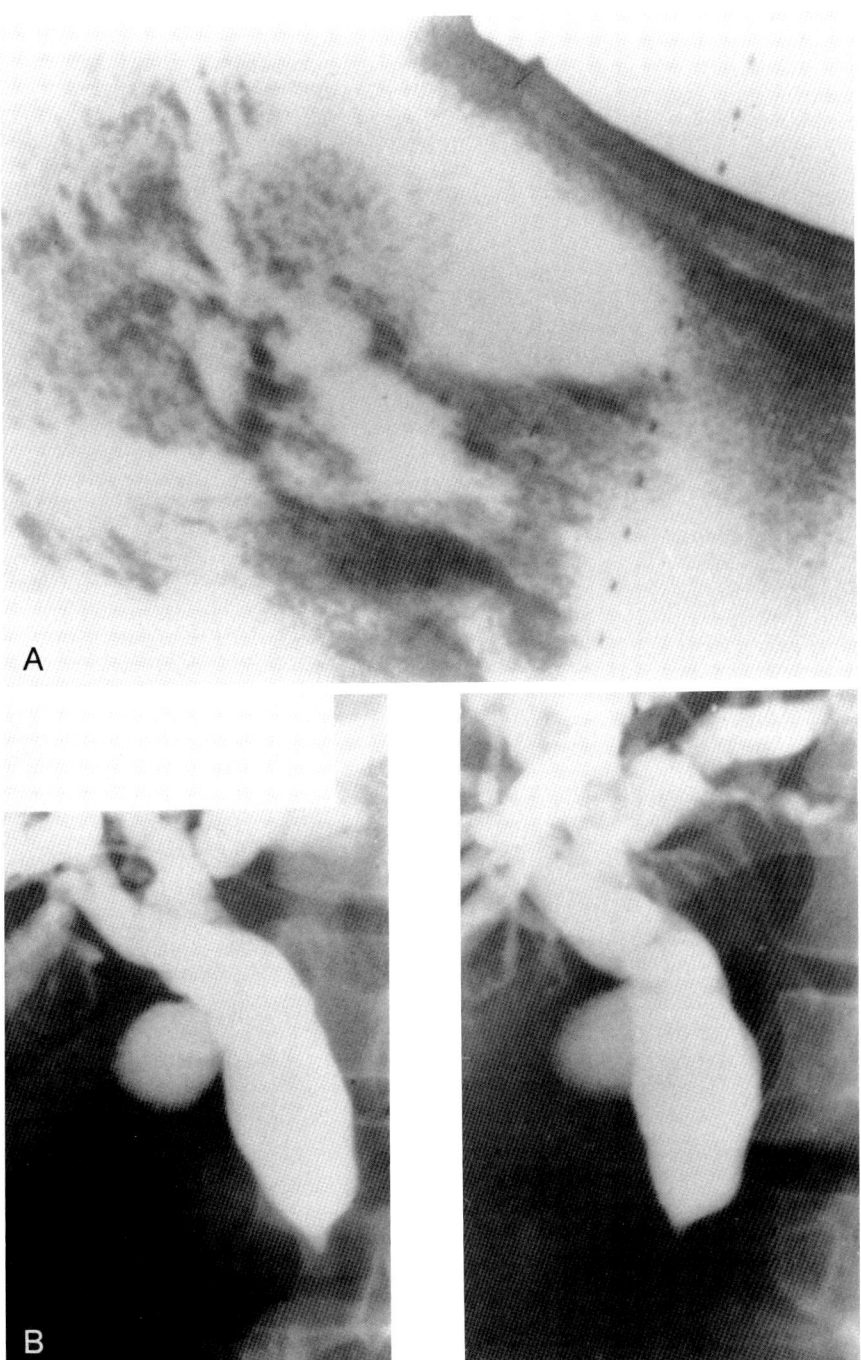

FIGURE 22.44. PANCREATIC ADENOCARCINOMA
A: Dilated bile ducts with a sonographic nipple and a surrounding mass from carcinoma of the head of the pancreas. *B:* Corresponding transhepatic cholangiogram showing the nipple or beak configuration and a complete obstruction to the flow of contrast (semierect).

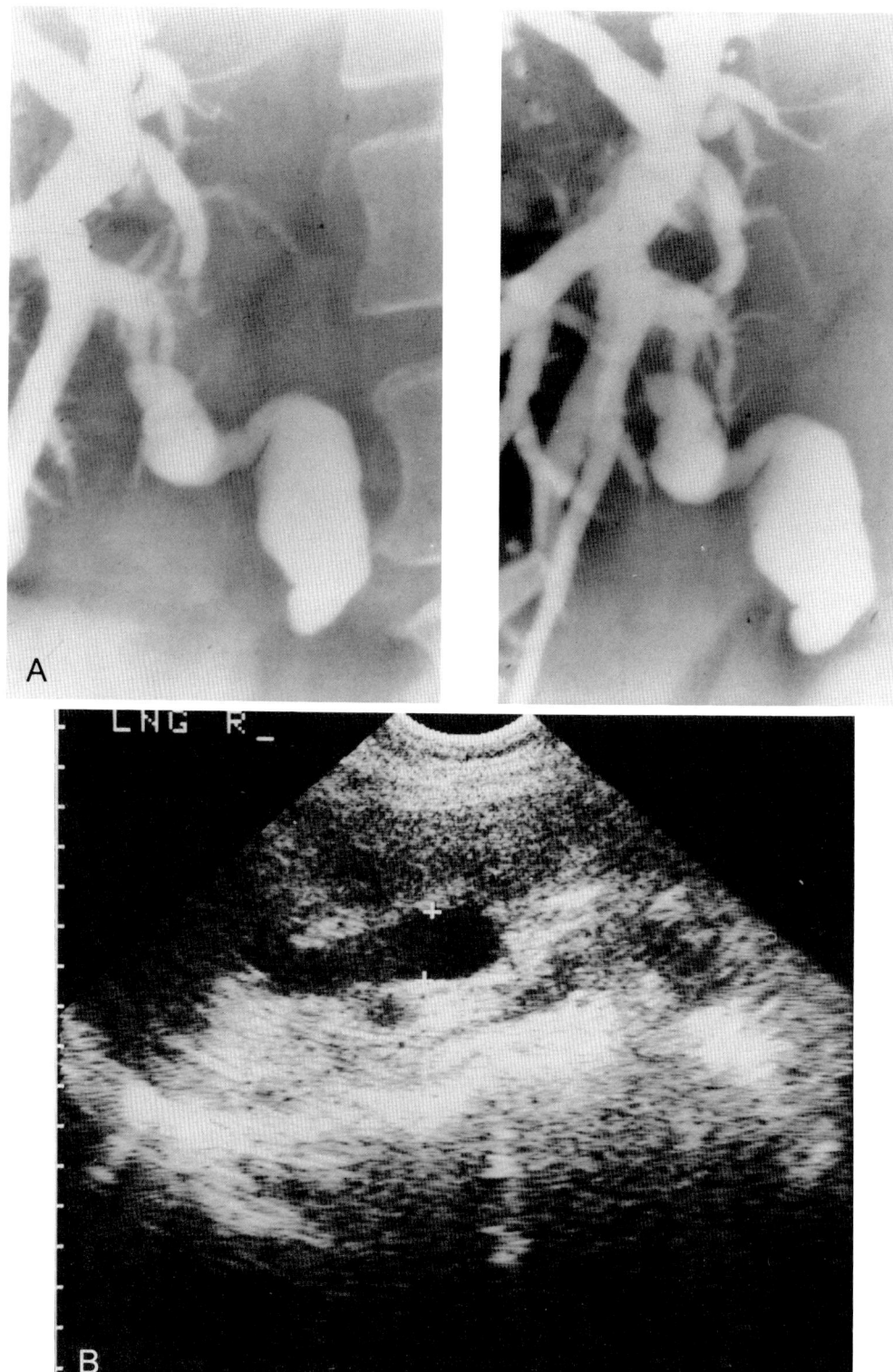

FIGURE 22.45. PANCREATIC ADENOCARCINOMA
Nonspecific blunt obstruction due to carcinoma of the head of the pancreas. Erect film from a transhepatic cholangiogram (A) and corresponding sagittal sonogram (B).

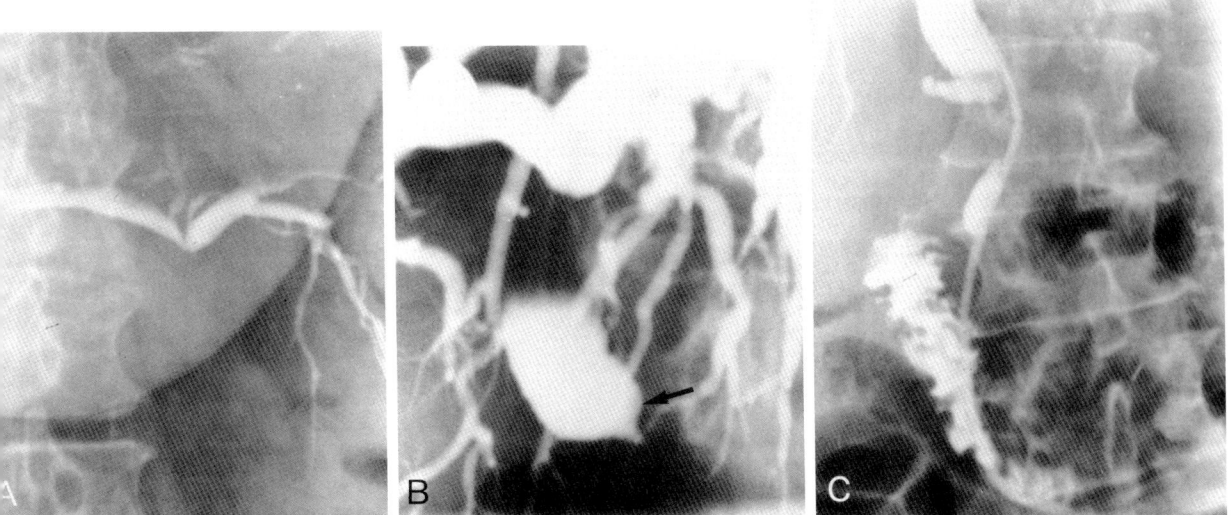

FIGURE 22.46. PANCREATIC ADENOCARCINOMA

A: Supine film during transhepatic cholangiography shows a pseudoobstruction at the level of the porta. *B* and *C:* An erect film causes the contrast to fall to the true level of obstruction, just above the cystic duct. Note the nipple suggesting the correct diagnosis of carcinoma of the pancreas. The route to the duodenum was at the *arrow*, not through the nipple.

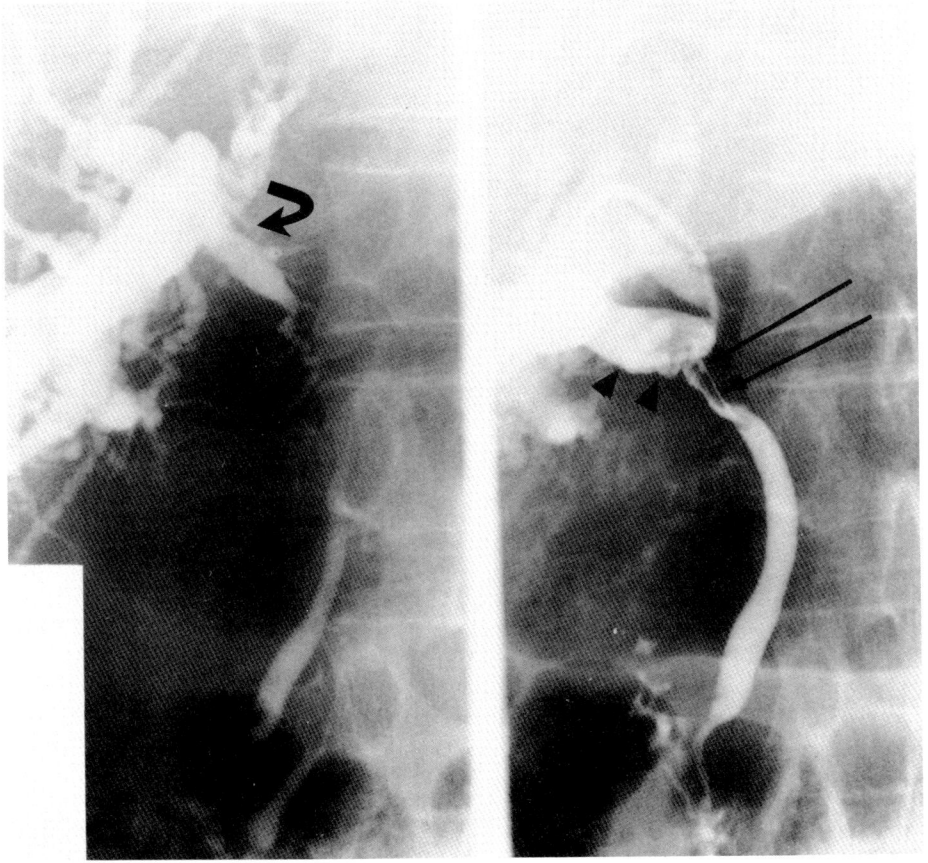

FIGURE 22.47. PANCREATIC ADENOCARCINOMA

Carcinoma of the pancreas obstructing the common hepatic duct just above the cystic duct. The film on the left shows the tip of a cobra catheter at the point of obstruction (*curved arrow*). The obstructed segment appears long. The film on the right, taken during injection, opacifies a minute tract through the obstruction (*arrows*) which is really short segment. Note filling of the cystic duct and gallbladder (*arrowheads*). Internal drainage was achieved.

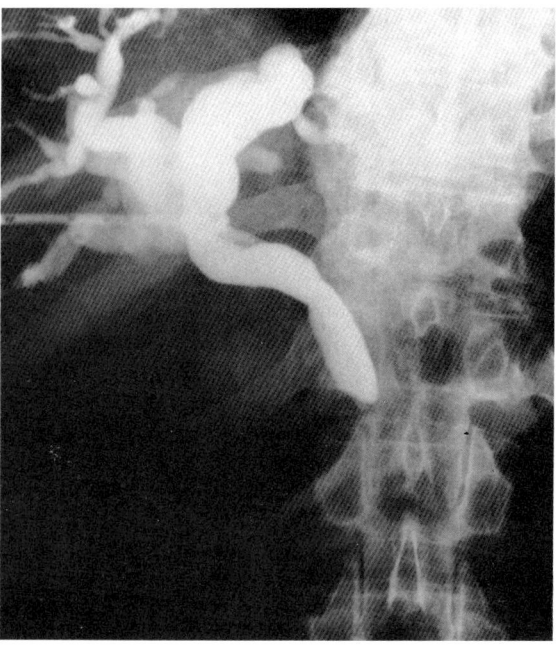

FIGURE 22.48. PANCREATIC ADENOCARCINOMA
Carcinoma of the pancreatic neck producing a short segment biliary obstruction and medial deviation of the duct.

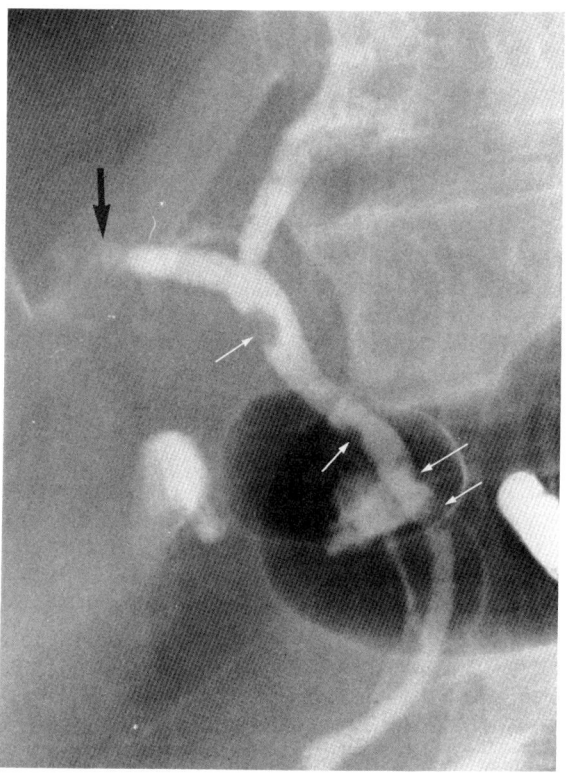

FIGURE 22.50. PANCREATIC ADENOCARCINOMA
ERCP showing intrahepatic obstruction of the right main hepatic duct (*black arrow*). Multiple intrabiliary metastases are present in the common duct (*white arrows*). Carcinoma of the pancreas, metastatic to the liver with biliary drop metastases.

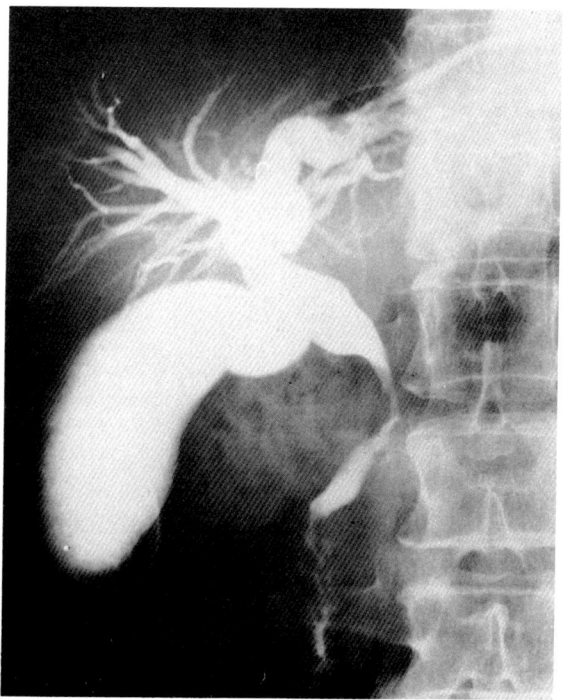

FIGURE 22.49. METASTATIC DISEASE
Metastases from carcinoma of the colon indistinguishable from carcinoma of the pancreas.

(Fig. 22.46). Interestingly, the route through the obstruction is usually not through the nipple (Fig. 22.46B). When the obstruction is bypassed and the distal normal duct is opacified or if the initial cholangiogram is retrograde, the length of the encased segment can be shown and it is usually short (Fig. 22.47) (5). When the site of involvement is at the superior margin of the head of the pancreas, the suprapancreatic duct may assume a medially directed near horizontal course as if it were retracted by the carcinoma (Fig. 22.48) (1). Rarely, metastatic disease near head of the pancreas causes common bile duct obstruction or encasement that is indistinguishable from primary pancreatic malignancy (Fig. 22.49). Carcinoma of the pancreas can produce biliary tract obstruction at higher levels: the common hepatic duct at any level up to the porta hepatis by virtue of direct extension or nodal compression (Fig. 22.47), or less commonly, intrahepatic duct(s) by liver metastases (liver me-

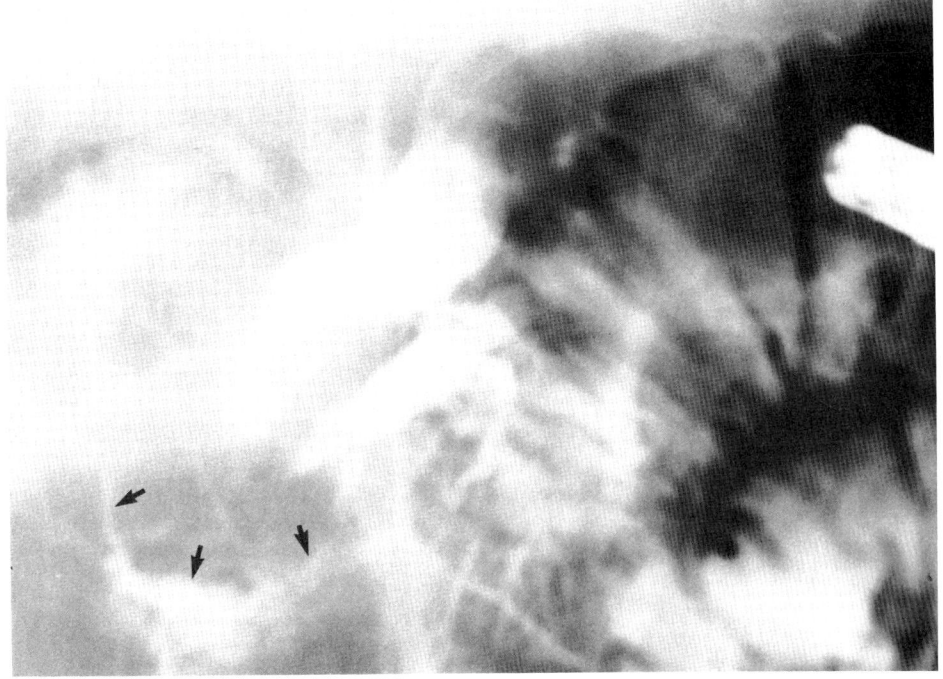

FIGURE 22.51. AMPULLARY CARCINOMA
ERCP of an ampullary carcinoma obstructing both ducts and padding the duodenum (*arrows*).

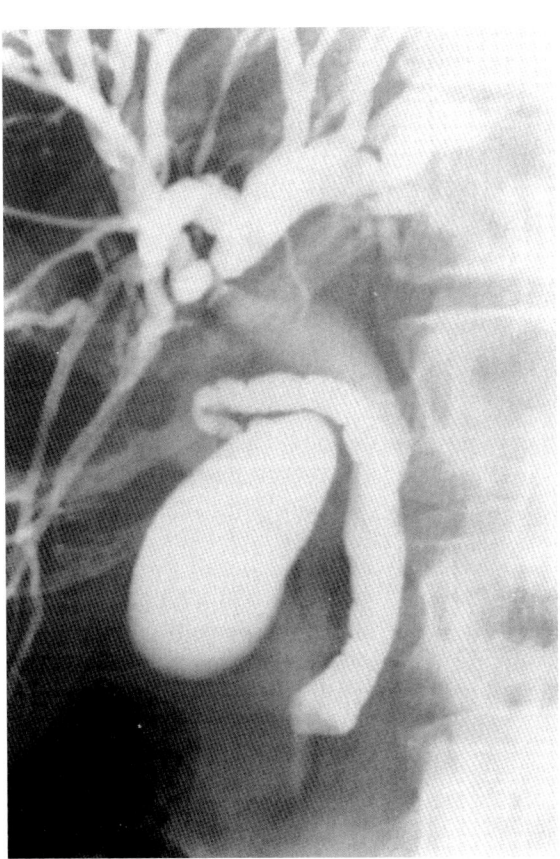

FIGURE 22.52. AMPULLARY CARCINOMA
Carcinoma of the ampulla producing a complete obstruction with an irregular terminus and expansion of the duct at the level of the obstruction.

Ampullary Carcinoma

Classically, ampullary carcinoma is an irregular polypoid intraluminal mass partially obstructing the very distal common bile duct (Fig. 22.51). Local expansion of the duct at the level of the mass when present is a very helpful feature favoring ampullary carcinoma over stone (Fig. 22.52) (1). Ampullary carcinoma can present as an irregularly tapered stricture or a squared off, flattened termination of the contrast column just above the duodenum indistinguishable from carcinoma of the head of the pancreas and hard to differentiate from ampullary stenosis (1, 5). The endoscopic retrograde examination has the advantage of visual inspection and biopsy in the diagnosis of ampullary carcinoma, but the diagnostic capability of the percutaneous transhepatic approach may be improved by the use of intravenous glucagon and simultaneous duodenography (Fig. 22.53) (1).

REFERENCES

1. Ferrucci JT Jr, Mueller PR, vanSonnenberg E: Transhepatic cholangiography. In Berk RN, Ferrucci JT Jr, Leopold GR (eds): *Radiology of the Gallbladder and Bile Ducts, Diagnosis and Intervention.* Philadelphia, W. B. Saunders, 1983, pp 334–336, 342–345.
2. Eaton SB Jr, Ferrucci JT Jr: *Radiology of the Pancreas and Duodenum.* Philadelphia, W. B. Saunders, 1973, pp 345–347.
3. Lang EK: Percutaneous transhepatic cholangiography. *Radiology* 112:283–290, 1974.
4. Freeny PC, Lawson TL: *Radiology of the Pancreas.* New York, Springer-Verlag, 1982, pp 462–465.
5. Rosen RJ, McLean GK: Short segment involvement of the common bile duct in pancreatic carcinoma. *Gastrointest Radiol* 8:151–154, 1983.
6. Stewart ET, Geenen JE: Endoscopic retrograde cholangiography. In Berk RN, Ferrucci JT Jr, Leopold GR (eds): *Radiology of the Gallbladder and Bile Ducts, Diagnosis and Treatment.* Philadelphia, W. B. Saunders, 1983, pp 373–375, 383.

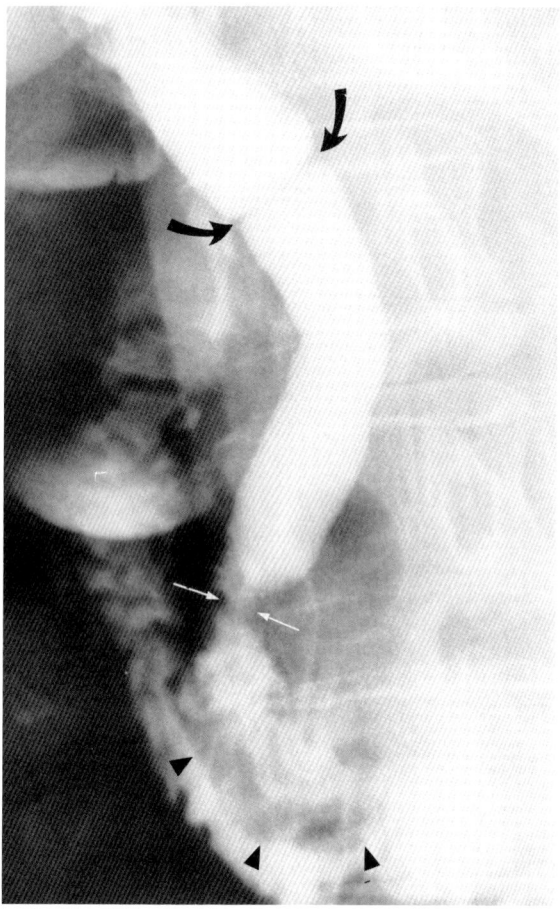

FIGURE 22.53. AMPULLARY CARCINOMA
Transhepatic cholangiogram with intravenous glucagon and simultaneous barium duodenography shows short segment narrowing of the distal common bile duct (*white arrows*) and a smooth submucosal mass in the duodenum (*black arrowheads*) from ampullary carcinoma. (Note the incidental common duct web (*curved arrows*) which is probably congenital. It was able to be traversed for drainage.)

tastases are usually missed by cholangiography) (Fig. 22.50). Erect, semierect, or prone filming may be critical to avoid placing the obstruction at an erroneously high level (Fig. 22.46A and B). Endoscopic retrograde cholangiography has the advantage of inspection of the ampulla, but has a disadvantage vis-à-vis percutaneous cholangiography in that the upper level of the obstruction may not be defined (information vital to the surgeon), since complete filling of the biliary tree in the presence of high grade obstruction is relatively contraindicated (increased risk of sepsis). Both endoscopic retrograde and percutaneous methods permit biliary drainage and brush cytology or guidance for percutaneous biopsy (6).

Pancreatography of Pancreatic Adenocarcinoma

ERCP is quite useful in confirming a suspected diagnosis of carcinoma of the pancreas with specificity reported in successful studies to exceed 88% (1–6). When ERCP is used in conjunction with ultrasound and/or CT and disagreement among studies exists, one should assume that the abnormal examination is correct.

Obstruction of the main pancreatic duct is the most common pancreatographic finding in carcinoma (Figs. 22.54 and 22.55) (4). To differentiate obstruction due to carcinoma from that due

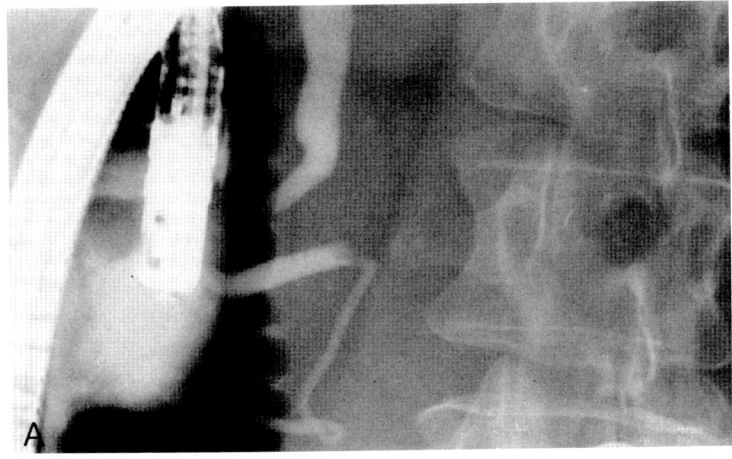
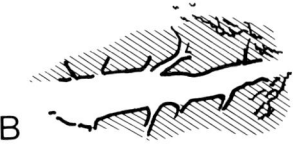

FIGURE 22.54. PANCREATIC ADENOCARCINOMA: ERCP
A: Complete obstruction with an irregular configuration of the terminus. The duct distal to the obstruction is normal. Good filling of the branch to the uncinate process is seen. *B:* Stylized drawing of complete obstruction due to carcinoma.

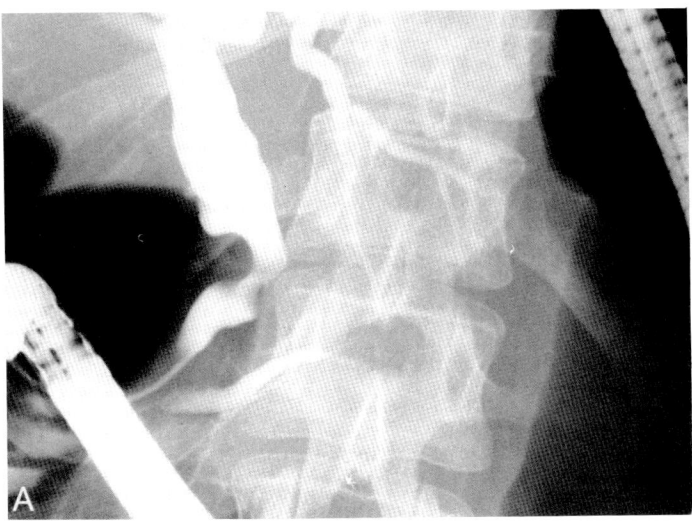
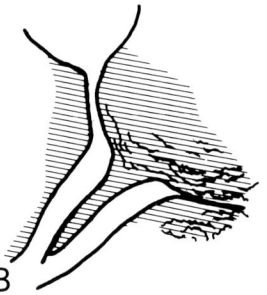

FIGURE 22.55. PANCREATIC ADENOCARCINOMA: ERCP
A: Complete obstruction of the pancreatic duct with an irregular, tapered configuration. Double duct sign with encased common bile duct. Either obstruction alone is consistent with carcinoma of the pancreas. *B:* Stylized drawing of double duct sign.

to pancreatitis, one must evaluate the morphology of the main duct and side branches between the ampulla and the obstruction (distal to the obstruction) as well as the configuration of the terminus. The ducts distal to the obstruction may show some prestenotic dilatation but they are otherwise normal in carcinoma, whereas changes consistent with pancreatitis are usually present in obstruction due to pancreatitis (4, 7). The terminus is usually irregular, nodular, rat-tailed or eccentric in carcinoma and smooth or blunt in inflammatory obstruction (4). Therefore, a normal duct distal to an irregular, nodular, rat-tailed or eccentric obstruction indicates neoplasia (metastatic disease or lymphoma can mimic any of the findings of primary carcinoma on pancreatography). The major differentials are focal inflammatory disease and incomplete filling. Focal inflammatory disease can rarely mimic tumor perfectly (conversely tumor may mimic pancreatitis) and accurate preoperative diagnosis will not always be possible (8). Good filling of side branches with or without acinarization indicates adequate filling. Incomplete side branch filling and subtle fading or feathering of the main duct terminus suggests incomplete filling rather than true obstruction (see Fig. 21.34) (4).

The next most common appearance is localized encasement of the main pancreatic duct (Figs. 27.56 and 22.57) (4, 9). The encasement is generally 1–2 cm long and irregular. The distal duct (papillary side) is normal or minimally dilated and transition is abrupt. The proximal main duct is dilated as are its side branches and they may have the appearance of pancreatitis (indeed, pancreatitis is often present due to the obstructing carcinoma) (Fig. 22.57). The small side branches around the encased segment are frequently compressed and/or obstructed by tu-

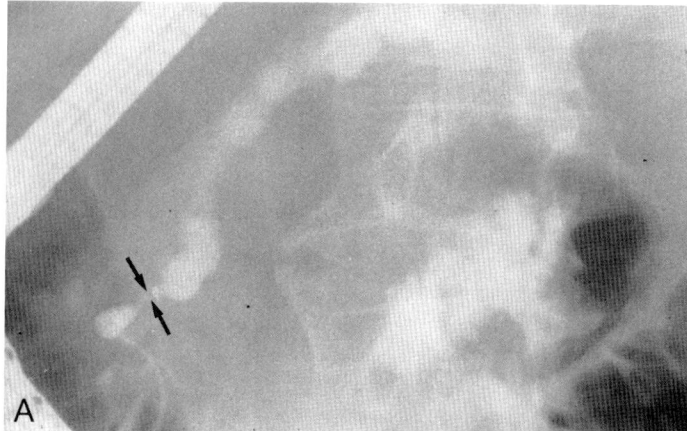

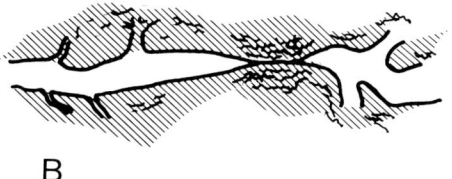

FIGURE 22.56. PANCREATIC ADENOCARCINOMA: ERCP
A: Short segment encasement of the pancreatic duct (*arrows*) from carcinoma of the pancreas. Distal duct is slightly dilated. Proximal duct is markedly dilated with dilution of contrast. *B:* Stylized drawing of encasement by carcinoma.

FIGURE 22.57. PANCREATIC ADENOCARCINOMA: ERCP
Short segment encasement by pancreatic carcinoma (*arrows*). Note normal distal duct and markedly dilated proximal duct with dilated side branches. The dilated proximal system looks like pancreatitis, and, in fact, the patient presented with pancreatitis.

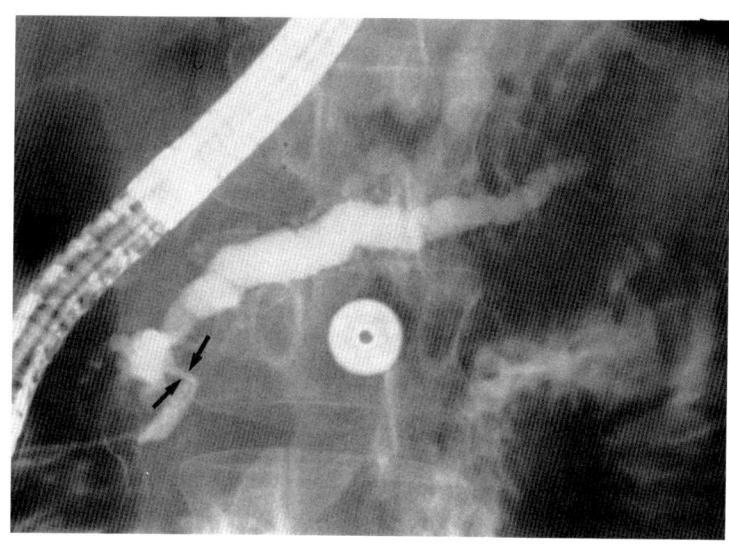

mor, and therefore, do not fill (4, 9). When the proximal duct is very dilated, contrast material can be diluted by retained secretions (Fig. 22.56) (10). The "double duct sign" (obstruction of both the many pancreatic duct and the common bile duct) (Fig. 22.55) has been reported by different authors to be strongly suggestive of carcinoma and nonspecific in differentiating carcinoma from pancreatitis (see Fig. 21.35) (10). In our experience, when there is contiguous obstruction and/or encasement of the common bile duct and main pancreatic duct (10 mm or less separation) and the configuration of both obstructions suggest carcinoma when analyzed individually, the likelihood of malignancy is exceedingly high, with metastatic disease or lymphoma the only serious alternatives to adenocarcinoma of the pancreas (or ampulla of Vater). The following are unusual findings in carcinoma of the pancreas: field defect, excavated tumor, and diffuse infiltration (4). Small peripheral carcinomas can focally obliterate small lateral side branches and cause a focal defect in parenchymal acinarization (field defect) (Fig. 22.58) (4). Good filling of the entire system is necessary to demonstrate field defects, which are, however, not specific for carcinoma of the pancreas. Any neoplastic mass or pancreatitis can cause a field defect. If a field defect is associated with a normal or an encased main pancreatic duct, carcinoma is the likely etiology (4). If contiguous ductal changes of chronic pancreatitis are present, the field defect is probably secondary to fibrosis, calculi or intraductal noncalcified precipitates in pancreatitis (4) (see Fig. 21.37).

When a necrotic tumor cavity communicates with the ductal system, pancreatography can opacify the cavity which has an irregular configuration as opposed to the smooth appearance of a pseudocyst (Fig. 22.59) (4, 11, 12). Excavated tumors are probably more likely to be the variant carcinomas of the pancreas discussed elsewhere

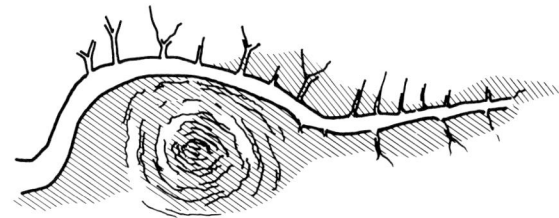

FIGURE 22.58. PANCREATIC ADENOCARCINOMA
Stylized drawing of carcinoma causing a field defect. Note absent branches in region of tumor.

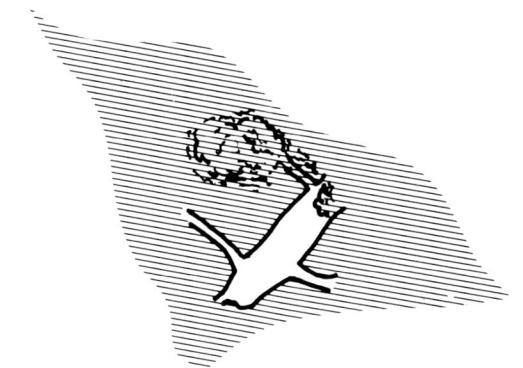

FIGURE 22.59. PANCREATIC ADENOCARCINOMA
Stylized drawing of excavating tumor. Cavity is irregular.

as opposed to duct cell adenocarcinoma, judging by their gross morphology.

Rarely, adenocarcinoma of the pancreas produces a diffuse infiltrating pancreatographic appearance with obliteration of the lateral side branches and a gradual tapering, stiff, rigid, irregular main pancreatic duct (9, 10). Poor demarcation exists between normal and abnormal regions (13, 14).

Finally, a normal pancreatogram may be seen if the tumor does not involve the main pancreatic duct or its larger branches (10, 15). The uncinate process can be a blind spot on pancreatography because of difficulty filling the branches leading to it.

Additional aids to the diagnosis of pancreatic carcinoma during pancreatography are aspiration of ductal juice for cytology and carcinoembryonic antigen measurement (11, 15–19). Abrasive cytologic brushing can also be performed (11, 18, 19).

REFERENCES

1. Moossa AR, Levin B: The diagnosis of "early" pancreatic cancer: The University of Chicago experience. *Cancer* 47:1688–1697, 1981.
2. Hall PJ, Blackstone MO, Cooper MJ, Hughes RG, Moossa AR: Prospective evaluation of ERCP in the diagnosis of periampullary cancers. *Ann Surg* 187:313–317, 1978.
3. Silvis SE, Rohrmann CA, Vennes JA: Diagnostic accuracy of endoscopic retrograde cholangiopancreatography in hepatic, biliary, and pancreatic malignancy. *Ann Intern Med* 84:438, 1976.
4. Freeny PC, Ball TJ: Evaluation of endoscopic retrograde cholangiopancreatography and angiography in diagnosis of pancreatic carcinoma. *AJR* 130:683–691, 1978.
5. Suramo I, Lehtola J, Leinonen A, Kairaluoma M: The diagnostic accuracy of gray scale ultrasonography compared with ERP and arteriography in the detection of pancreatic cancer. *Scand J Gastroenterol* 14:993–966, 1979.
6. Cotton PB, Lees WR, Vallon AG: Gray scale ultrasonography and endoscopic pancreatography in pancreatic diagnosis. *Radiology* 134:453–459, 1980.
7. Hiddell J, Aspelin P, Wehlin L: Gray scale ultrasound and endoscopic ductography in the diagnosis of pancreatic disease. *Acta Chir Scand* 145:239–245, 1979.
8. Ralls PW, Halls J, Renner I, Juttner H: Endoscopic retrograde cholangiopancreatography (ERCP) and pancreatic disease. *Radiology* 134:347–352, 1980.
9. Short WF: Pancreatography. In Eaton SB, Ferrucci JT Jr (eds): *Radiology of the Pancreas and Duodenum.* Philadelphia, W. B. Saunders, 1973, pp 261–275.
10. Bilbao M, Katon RM: Neoplasms of the pancreas. In Stewart ET, Vennes JA, Geenen JE (eds): *Atlas of Endoscopic Retrograde Cholangiopancreatography.* St. Louis, C. V. Mosby, 1977, pp 181–192.
11. Salmon PR: Re-evaluation of ERCP as a diagnostic method. *Clin Gastroenterol* 7:651, 1978.
12. Swensen T, Osnes M, Sarck-Hanssen A: Endoscopic retrograde cholangiopancreatography and primary and secondary tumors of the pancreas. *Br J Radiol* 53:760, 1980.
13. Fukumoto K, Nakajima M, Murakami K, Kawai K: Diagnosis of pancreatic cancer by endoscopic pancreaticocholangiography. *Am J Gastroenterol* 62:211–213, 1974.
14. Takemoto T, Kasugai T: *Endoscopic Retrograde Cholangiopancreatography.* New York, Igaku-Shoin, 1979, pp 159–176.
15. Cotton PB: Progress report: ERCP. *Gut* 18:316, 1977.
16. Okuda K, Someya N, Goto A et al: Endoscopic retrograde cholangiopancreatography. *AJR* 117:437, 1973.
17. Siegel JH: ERCP update; diagnostic and therapeutic applications. *GI Radiol* 3:311, 1978.
18. Goodale RL, Condie RM, Gajl-Peczalska K: Cytologic studies for the diagnosis of pancreatic cancer. *Cancer* 47:1652, 1981.
19. Endo Y, Morii T, Tamura H: Cytodiagnosis of pancreatic malignant tumors by aspiration under direct vision using a duodenal fiberscope. *Gastroenterology* 67:944–951, 1974.

Pancreatography of Ampullary Carcinoma

Endoscopic retrograde pancreatography is often impossible in patients with ampullary carcinoma because of inability to cannulate the pancreatic duct. When successful, obstruction or stenosis at the level of the ampulla with proximal dilatation is seen (see Fig. 22.51) (1, 2).

REFERENCES

1. Short WF: Pancreatography. In Eaton SB, Ferrucci JT Jr (eds): *Radiology of the Pancreas and Duodenum.* Philadelphia, W. B. Saunders, 1973, pp 261–265.
2. Bilbao M, Katon K: Neoplasms of the pancreas. In Stewart ET, Vennes JA, Geenen JE (eds): *Atlas of Endoscopic Retrograde Cholangiography.* St. Louis, C. V. Mosby, 1977, pp 181–192.

Angiography of Pancreatic Duct Cell Carcinoma

Since the early and mid-1950s, when selective celiac and superior mesenteric arteriography were first developed, angiography of the pancreas has evolved into a highly accurate method for detecting and evaluating pancreatic disease. In the mid-1960s it supplanted splenoportography as the primary diagnostic modality, and became even more valuable with the development of superselective techniques and pharmacoangiography in the early 1970s. Following the development of ERCP, ultrasound, and CT in the mid- to late 1970s, however, the role of angiography has been drastically altered. Although no longer indicated for initial evaluation of pancreatic disease, angiography remains an important means for assessing vascular involvement by pancreatic disease processes. Angiography is occasionally helpful in differential diagnosis, but is most useful for preoperative evaluation of a potentially resectable lesion.

Technique

For optimal detection and characterization of pancreatic disease, adequate depiction of both arterial and venous structures of the pancreas is essential. The major arteries and veins of the pancreas lie on the surface of the gland, and will only be affected by pancreatic carcinoma which has extended beyond the confines of the gland. Superselective catheterization of the dorsal pancreatic, inferior pancreaticoduodenal, and pancreaticoduodenal arcades will depict the intraparenchymal arterial network and yield a parenchymal stain in the capillary phase. Small arterial irregularities and lucent parenchymal defects are findings detectable with small resectable carcinomas less than 2 cm in diameter (1–3). Injection of 15–20 cm over 3 sec is recommended for superselective catheterization (1).

Superselective techniques are thought to improve the diagnostic value of pancreatic arteriography (Fig. 22.60) (4–8). In one study, however, although superselective technique was considered necessary prospectively for adequate evaluation of greater than 50% of true positive cases, retrospective blind analysis revealed it to be necessary in only 14% (4). While complications relating to superselective catheterization are unusual, they do occur (4), and superselective techniques are recommended only if doubts persist after standard techniques.

In certain instances, superselective catheterization will not be possible and in these cases pharmacologic manipulation will be especially valuable. Vasoconstrictors such as epinephrine (1, 5, 9) or vasopressin (6, 9, 10) reduce splanchnic blood flow thereby redirecting contrast distribution to pancreatic vessels. Flow is also redistributed to abnormal vessels and collaterals which are not subject to pharmacologic control. Epinephrine (5–15 mg) acts by its α-adrenergic effect (9). Vasopressin (angiotensin) stimulates smooth muscle directly and has a duration of 1–2 min if 0.5–5 mg are injected intraarterially (9). Vasoconstrictors should be used only if a previous injection has been ineffective since transient arterial irregularities may be induced which can mimic pathology (9). While some investigators have found epinephrine unnecessary for gastroduodenal artery injections (5), others have found the resulting decreased flow to the right gastroepiploric artery helpful (1). Tolazoline (Priscoline) is a vasodilator which acts by adrenergic blockade. By augmenting pancreatic arterial flow, it may improve depiction of intrapancreatic arteries if high volumes of contrast are injected (5, 6). Vasodilators are usually used to augment the venous phase of celiac and superior mesenteric artery injections, and are given in a dose of 25–50 mg intra-arterially 30 sec prior to contrast injection. Several other vasodilators have been studied (9, 11), but tolazoline remains the preferred agent. It is fairly safe and its effects are usually transient, but it is contraindicated in the setting of unstable cerebrovascular disease, coronary artery disease, and recent myocardial infarction due to its hypotensive effect (9). Most important in obtaining an adequate venous phase, however, is the use of a high contrast material volume, such as 50–60 ml, given at a slow enough flow rate, such as 8 ml per sec (9, 12). Filming must be continued for at least 30 sec (9, 12).

Secretin, in a dose of 1–1.5 mg per kg acts directly on pancreatic parenchymal cells to intensify the parenchymal phase (9). The importance of this agent has not been adequately assessed, however.

While tailoring of the arteriographic examination to obtain optimal arterial and venous depiction yields high sensitivity and specificity, the high dose required will usually preclude op-

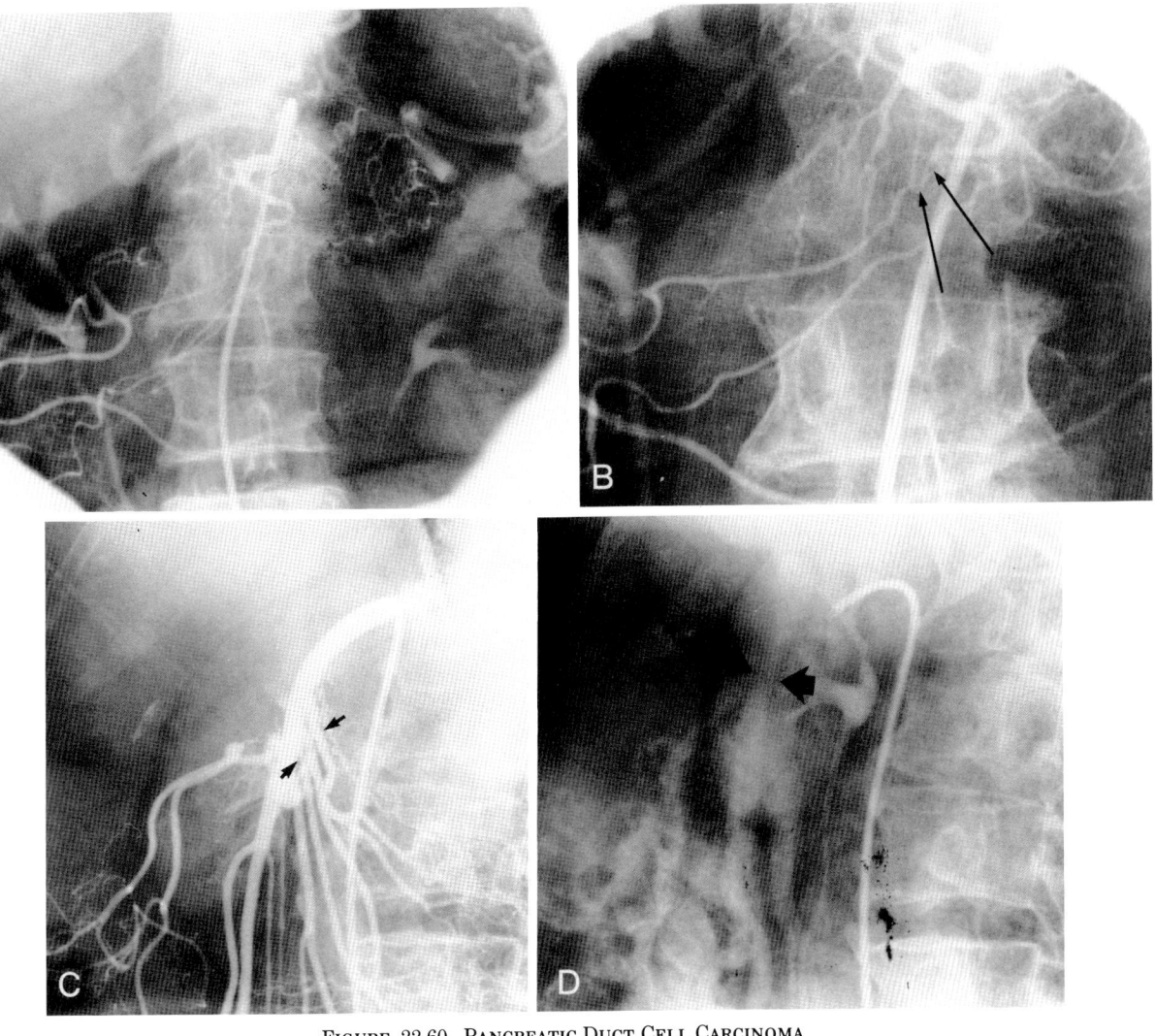

FIGURE 22.60. PANCREATIC DUCT CELL CARCINOMA

Cancer of the head and body of the pancreas demonstrating the advantages of selective magnification arteriography. *A:* Selective dorsal pancreatic arteriogram appears normal. *B:* Selective dorsal pancreatic arteriogram, magnification technique: encasement of the transverse pancreatic artery (*arrows*). *C:* Superior mesenteric arteriogram: encasement of the origin of the first three jejunal arteries (*arrows*). *D:* Venous phase of superior mesenteric arteriogram: smooth encasement of the superior mesenteric vein (*arrows*).

timal evaluation of the liver for metastases. Without hepatic artery infusion technique (approximately 50 ml of contrast material infused into the hepatic artery), angiography is insensitive in this regard (6, 13). Simultaneous celiac and superior mesenteric arteriography is a valuable technique for looking at the junction of the superior mesenteric and portal veins in cases of pancreatic head neoplasms. Since both splenic and superior mesenteric veins are opacified, no question exists that a portal vein narrowing might be a flow defect from unopacified blood (Fig. 22.61). The excellent hepatogram obtained is useful in detecting metastases (Fig. 22.61).

Also helpful in maximally depecting pancreatic vascular morphology are magnification techniques and subtraction (6). Abdominal compression is advocated by some (1). Performing angiography in conjunction with simultaneous hypotonic duodenography has been studied (14), but has not received wide acceptance.

Findings

The angiographic manifestation of pancreatic duct cell carcinoma reflect its growth characteristics. It is an infiltrative, hypovascular, desmoplastic tumor, and its angiographic appearance

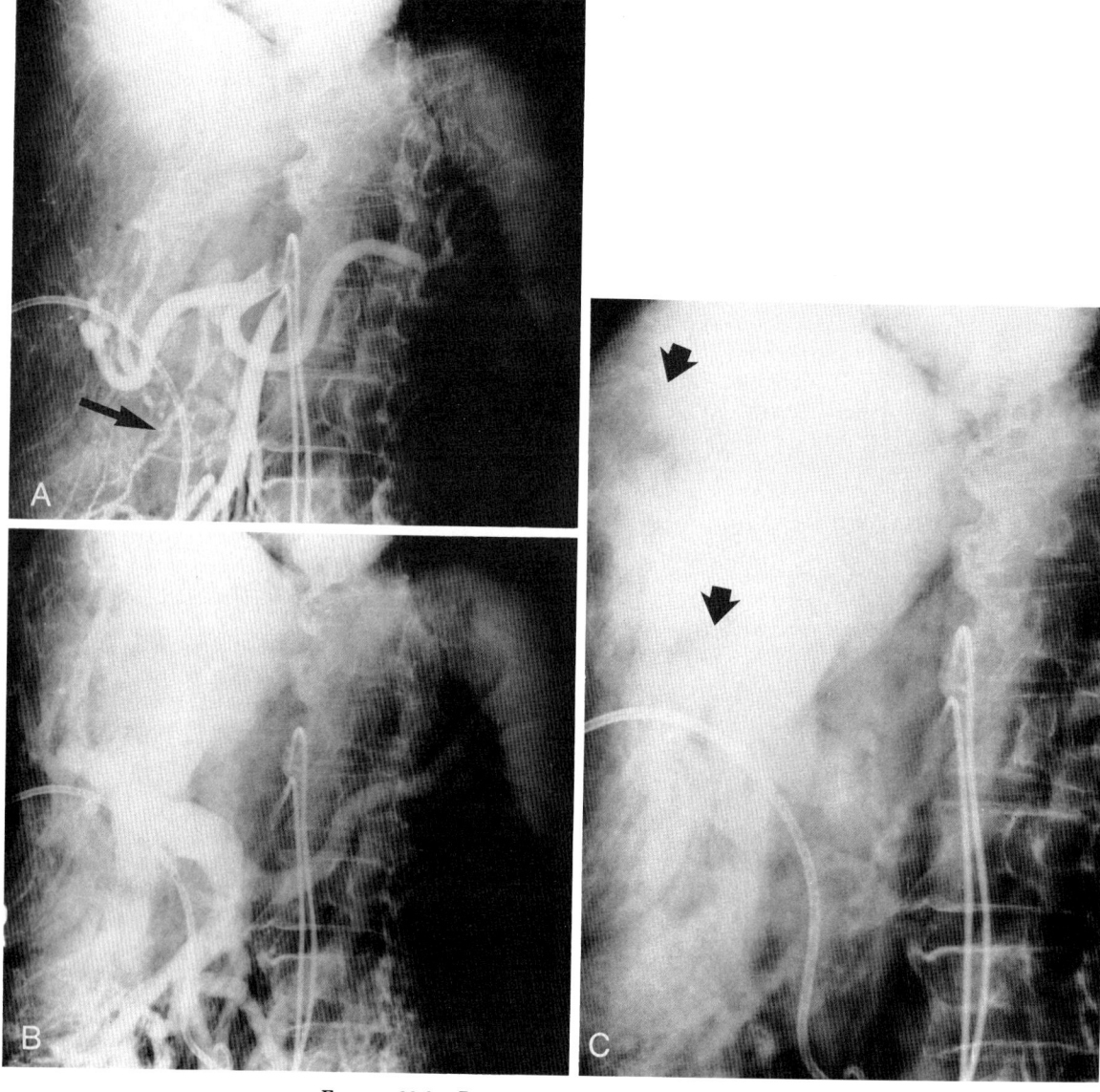

FIGURE 22.61. PANCREATIC DUCT CELL CARCINOMA

Carcinoma of the head of the pancreas: simultaneous celiac and superior mesenteric arteriography, right posterior oblique (RPO) projection, 60 mg papaverine was injected into the superior mesenteric artery. *A:* Arterial phase: encased gastroduodenal artery *(arrow)*. *B:* Early venous phase: nice demonstration of normal splenic, superior mesenteric and portal veins. *C:* Late portal phase: hypovascular metastases in right lobe of the liver *(arrows)*, easily seen in the dense portal hepatogram.

is dominated by encasement of existing vessels rather than by pronounced displacement or neovascularity. Frequently involved arteries include the celiac axis and its major branches (common hepatic, left gastric, and splenic arteries), gastroduodenal artery, pancreaticoduodenal arcades, and the superior mesenteric artery. The major components of the portal venous system, (portal, splenic, and superior mesenteric veins), are frequently involved as well. Carcinoma of the uncinate process in its early stages leaves the celiac axis unaffected but involves the superior mesenteric artery and vein (15).

The angiographic hallmark of pancreatic carcinoma is serrated or serpiginous arterial encasement, present in approximately 85% of cases (1, 6, 16). Serrated encasement refers to an irregular, saw-toothed appearance, and is the arteriographic sign most valuable in diagnosing carcinoma (1, 6, 16, 17), especially when seen in extrapancreatic arteries (17). Serpiginous encasement is sometimes used synonymously, but is used by others to refer to abrupt angulation (1, 16). It is present in approximately 40% of cases and is also a reliable sign of malignancy (16). These two findings may appear similar, and are thus frequently confused (Figs. 22.60–22.67). Smooth encasement is also frequently present in carcinoma (Fig. 22.68) (1, 6, 17, 18), but by itself is a nonspecific finding frequently seen in pancreatitis; this is perhaps the most frequent cause of a false positive diagnosis of carcinoma (16, 17).

Abrupt arterial occlusion is present in approximately 40% of cases of carcinoma of the pancreas in most series (6, 16), although a frequency as high as 60% has been recorded (Figs. 22.69 and 22.70) (17). Occlusion of the intrapancreatic arteries occurs most frequently and reliably indicates malignancy, especially if the occlusion is abrupt and the changes are confined to a focal portion of the pancreas (Fig. 22.71) (6, 16, 17).

Displacement of arteries is difficult to evaluate due to normal variation and is noticeable in less than 30% of cases (Fig. 22.72) (6, 16, 17). It is a nonspecific finding, but if present out of proportion to encasement it is more indicative of pancreatitis (6, 16) or lymphoma (19).

If with superselective and/or pharmacoangiographic techniques a parenchymal phase is depicted, duct cell carcinoma may be seen as a hypovascular defect in approximately 40% of cases due to encasement and obstruction of small intrapancreatic vessels (6, 16, 17). Hypervascular areas are mentioned in occasional tumors (17, 20), but were absent in all duct cell carcinomas in other series (Fig. 22.73) (6). None of the "hypervascular carcinomas" have been well documented pathologically, and they may represent small areas of secondary pancreatitis or a mistaken diagnosis. Some of these pancreatic tumors are described as having highly vascular walls with large areas of cystic degeneration (20), and these probably represent other histologies such as mucinous cystic neoplasms or pleomorphic giant cell tumors.

The possible presence of neovascularity in pancreatic duct cell carcinoma is poorly understood. These small, irregular vessels have been observed in approximately 30% of cases (16), ranging from 20–25% (6, 13) to 65% (21) depending upon the criteria used for differentiation from encased arteries. While the presence of these vessels appears specific for carcinoma (6, 13), their nature remains conjectural. Angiography of surgical specimens as well as microscopic examination failed to reveal any newly formed vessels (22). More likely, most of these pathologic vessels represent encased arteries and/or collaterals arising secondary to arterial occlusion (see Fig. 22.73). As expected, these vessels are unaffected by pharmacologic manipulation (21).

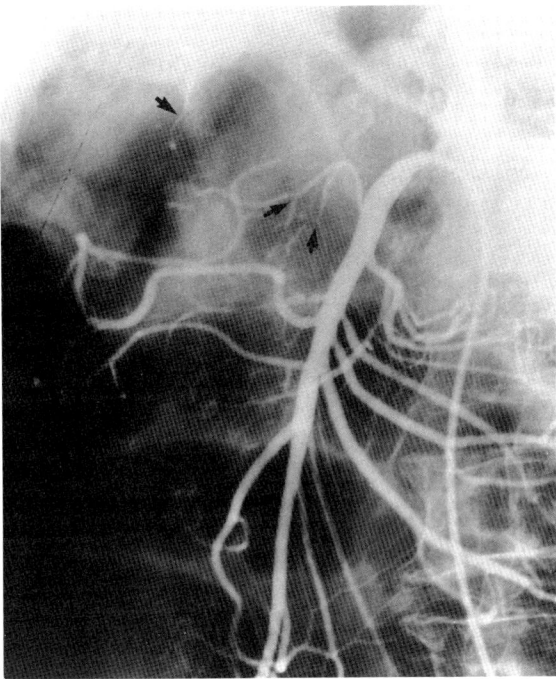

FIGURE 22.62. PANCREATIC DUCT CELL CARCINOMA
Encasement of the inferior pancreaticoduodenal artery and pancreaticoduodenal arcade (*arrows*) in carcinoma of the uncinate process. The superior mesenteric vein was also occluded (note shown).

Venous Phase

Venous abnormalities are seen in approximately two-thirds of the cases of pancreatic carcinoma (16, 17). The yield can be increased to as high as 90% if the examination is tailored to display venous morphology optimally (6, 12). In one series, venous involvement was seen in 98% of carcinomas in which adequate visualization of the splenic, portal, and superior mesenteric veins was obtained (12). The changes may consist of encasement or displacement but in most series occlusion is more frequent (Figs. 22.60, 22.63, 22.65–22.68, and 22.73) (6, 16). The venous lesions tend to be more obvious than the often subtle arterial lesions, and cannot be accounted for by atherosclerosis. While involvement of either arteries or veins alone is more suggestive of pancreatitis, involvement of both is indicative of carcinoma, especially if localized or regional involvement is present (6). A normal vein adjacent to an apparently encased artery virtually

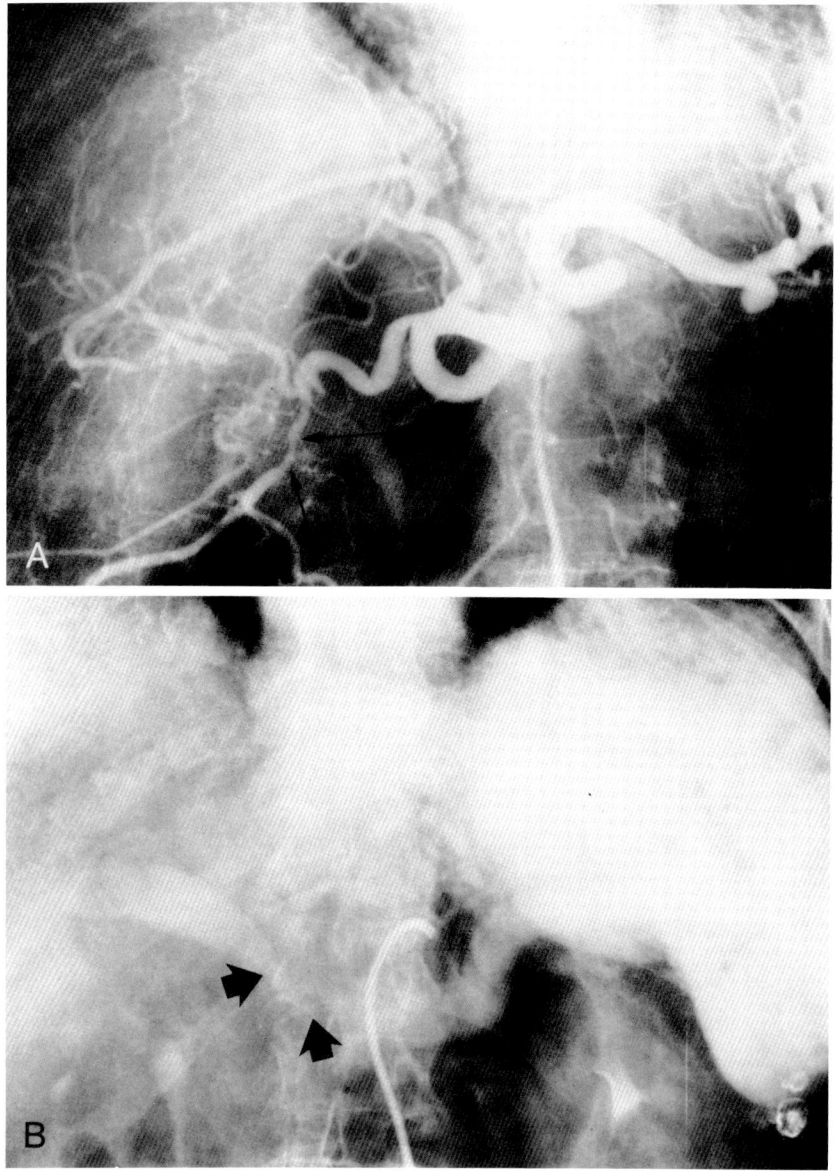

FIGURE 22.63. PANCREATIC DUCT CELL CARCINOMA
Carcinoma of the head of the pancreas, celiac arteriogram. *A:* Right posterior oblique projection: serpiginous encasement of the gastroduodenal artery (*arrows*). *B:* Encasement of the distal splenic vein and the portal vein (*arrows*).

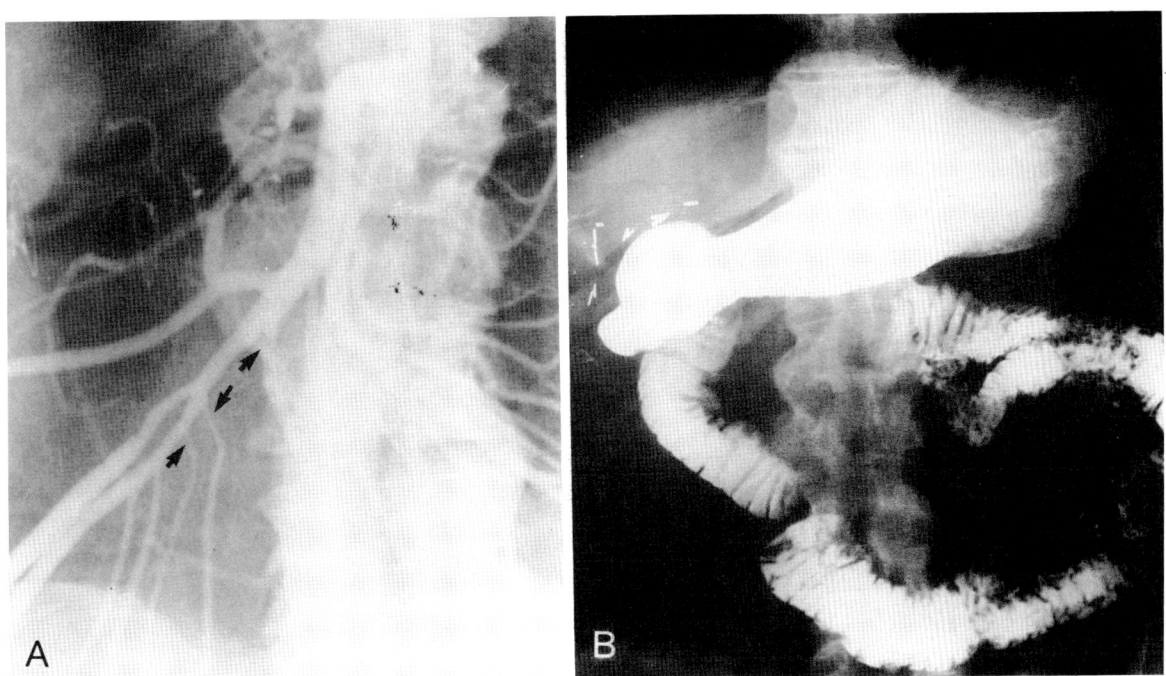

FIGURE 22.64. PANCREATIC DUCT CELL CARCINOMA

Large carcinoma of the head and body of the pancreas obstructing the transverse portion of the duodenum and invading the mesentery. *A:* Arterial phase of a superior mesenteric arteriogram: encasement of the 5th, 6th and 7th jejunal arteries (*arrows*), indicating invasion of the mesentery. *B:* Partial obstruction of the transverse duodenum.

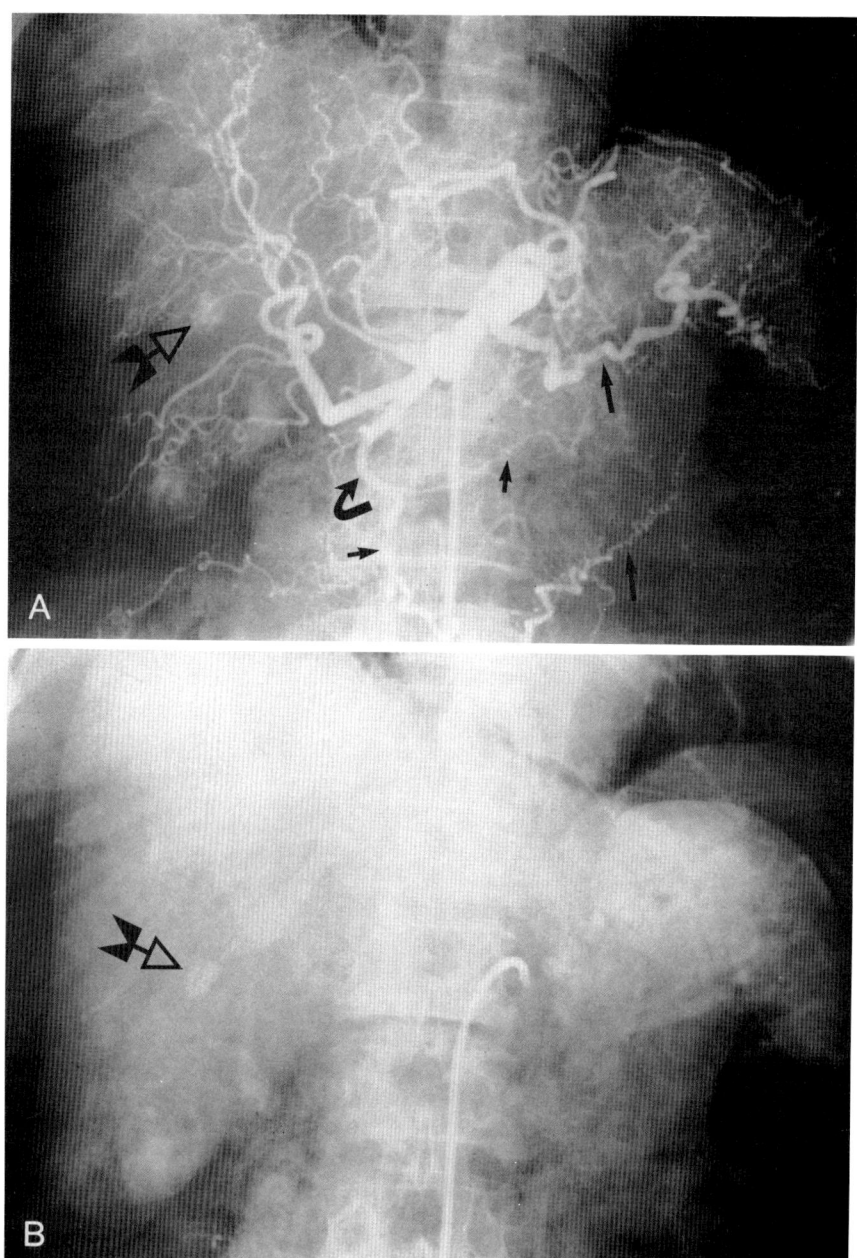

FIGURE 22.65. PANCREATIC DUCT CELL CARCINOMA
Large carcinoma of the body and tail of the pancreas, incidental hemangioma of the liver, celiac arteriogram. *A:* Arterial phase: serpiginous encasement of the splenic, transverse pancreatic, and right gastroepiploic arteries (*straight arrows*). Lateral bowing of the proximal gastroduodenal artery (*curved arrow*). Note hemangioma (*feathered arrow*). *B:* Venous phase: splenic vein obstruction with gastric varices. Note hemangioma (*feathered arrow*) and ascites (displaced liver and spleen).

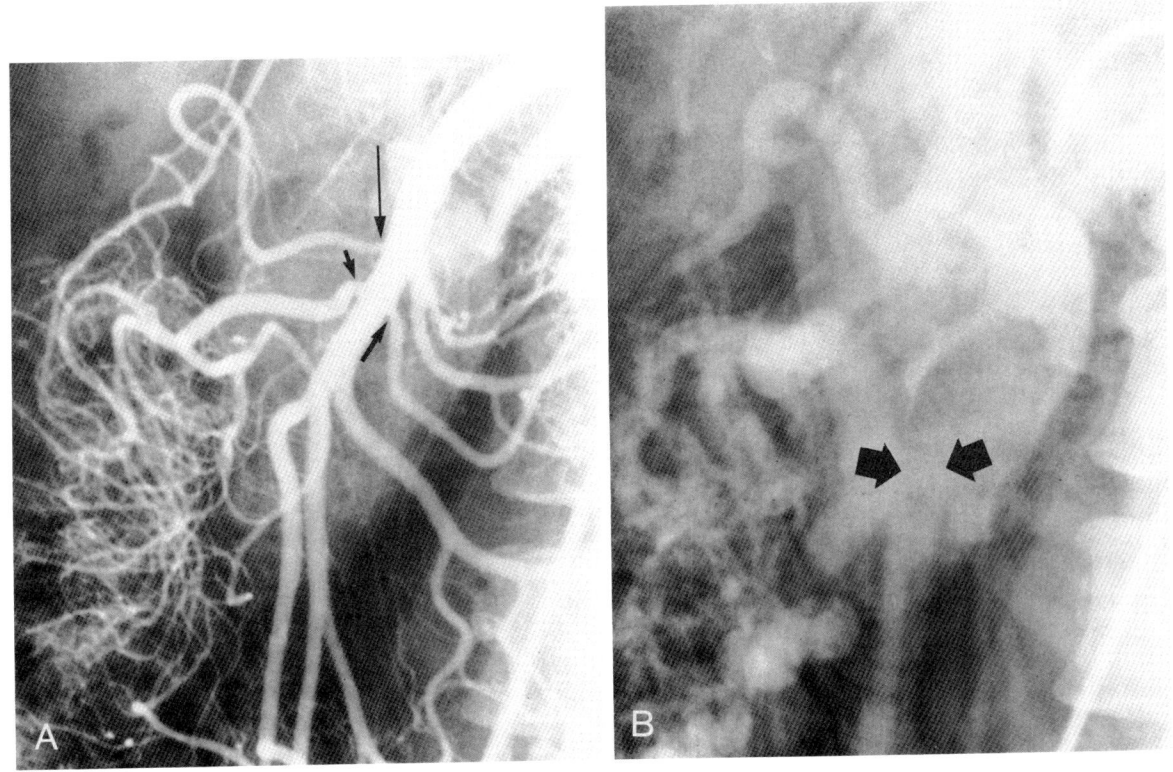

FIGURE 22.66. PANCREATIC DUCT CELL CARCINOMA

Invasion of the mesentery by pancreatic carcinoma, superior mesenteric arteriography. *A:* Arterial phase: subtle narrowing of the origins of the second jejunal, middle colic and right colic arteries (*arrows*). *B:* Venous phase: obstruction of the superior mesenteric vein (*arrows*).

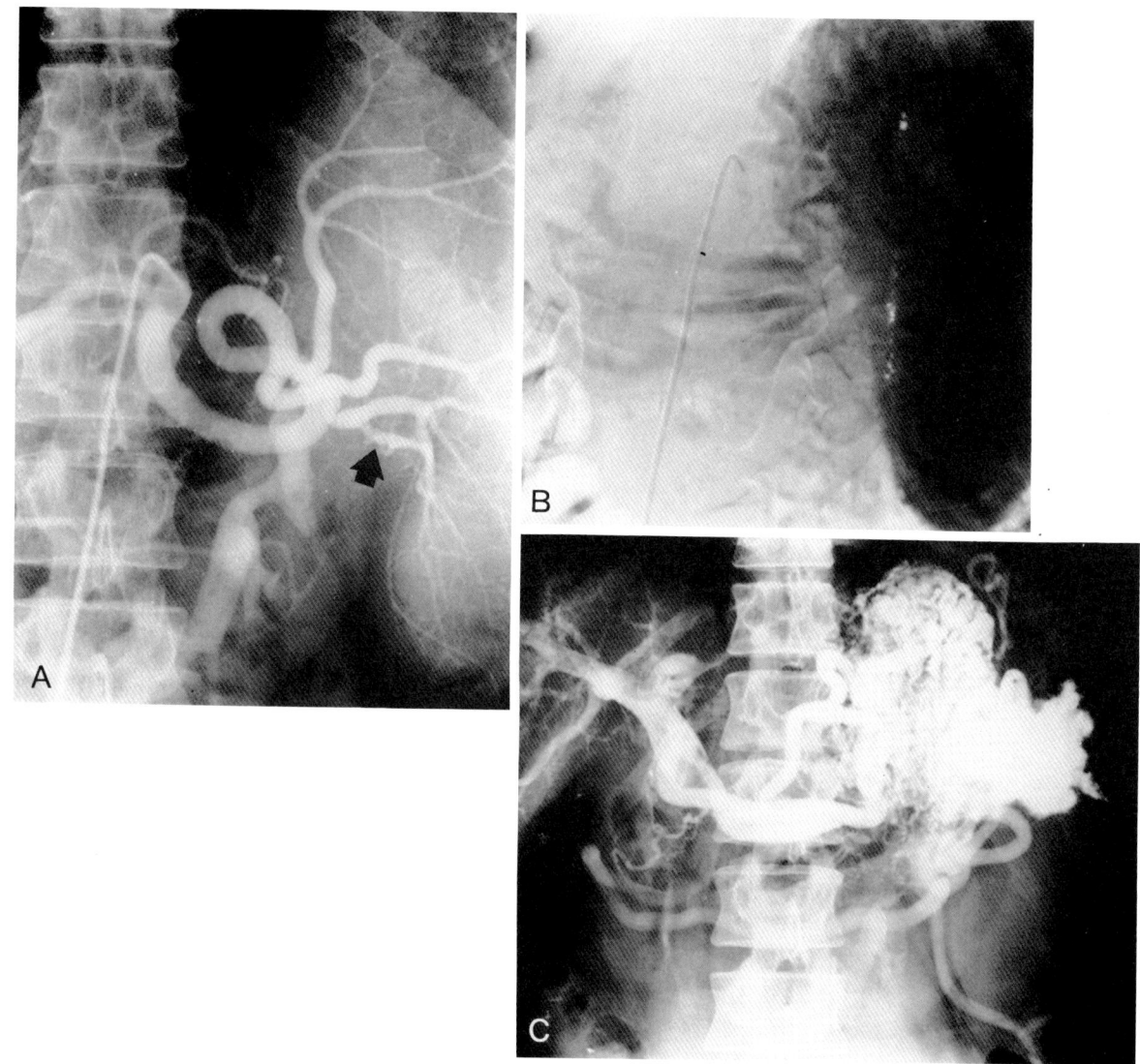

FIGURE 22.67. PANCREATIC DUCT CELL CARCINOMA
Carcinoma of the tail of the pancreas presenting with upper gastrointestinal bleeding, splenomegaly and endoscopic diagnosis of fundal gastritis. *A:* Arterial phase, celiac injection: subtle encasement of a distal lower pole branch of the splenic artery (*arrows*). *B:* Venous phase: patent mid and distal splenic vein and gastric varices implying proximal splenic vein occlusion. *C:* Splenoportogram: occlusion of proximal splenic vein with large gastric varices. (Same case as seen in Fig. 22.39.)

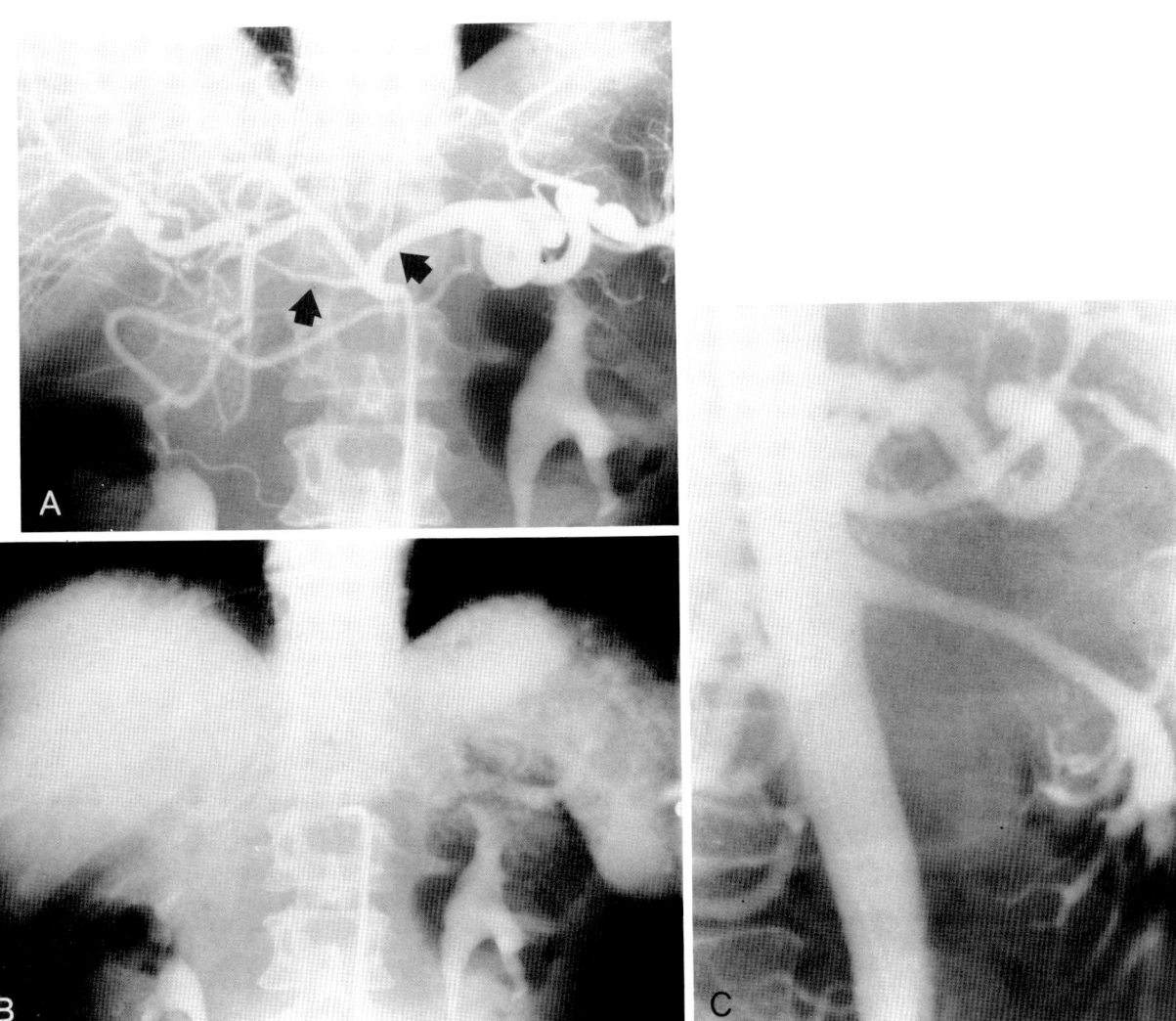

FIGURE 22.68. PANCREATIC DUCT CELL CARCINOMA

Large carcinoma of the head and body of the pancreas with infiltration of the mesentery. *A:* Arterial phase, celiac arteriogram: smooth encasement of the proximal splenic and the right hepatic arteries (*arrows*). *B:* Venous phase: splenic vein obstruction and gastric varices. Note the dilated gallbladder. *C:* Lateral aortogram: stretching and draping of the superior mesenteric artery.

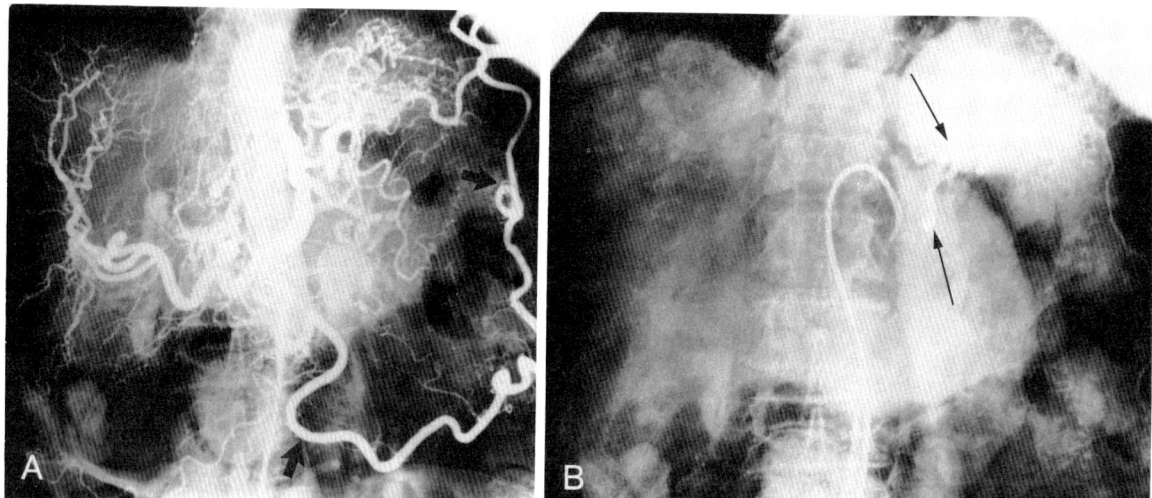

FIGURE 22.69. PANCREATIC DUCT CELL CARCINOMA

Arterial occlusion by carcinoma of the pancreas, celiac arteriography. *A:* Arterial phase: splenic artery occlusion. Right to left gastroepiploic collaterals (*arrows*) and the left gastric artery reconstitute the distal splenic artery. *B:* Late arterial phase: reconstitution of the mid portion of the splenic artery (*arrows*). The splenic vein was also occluded.

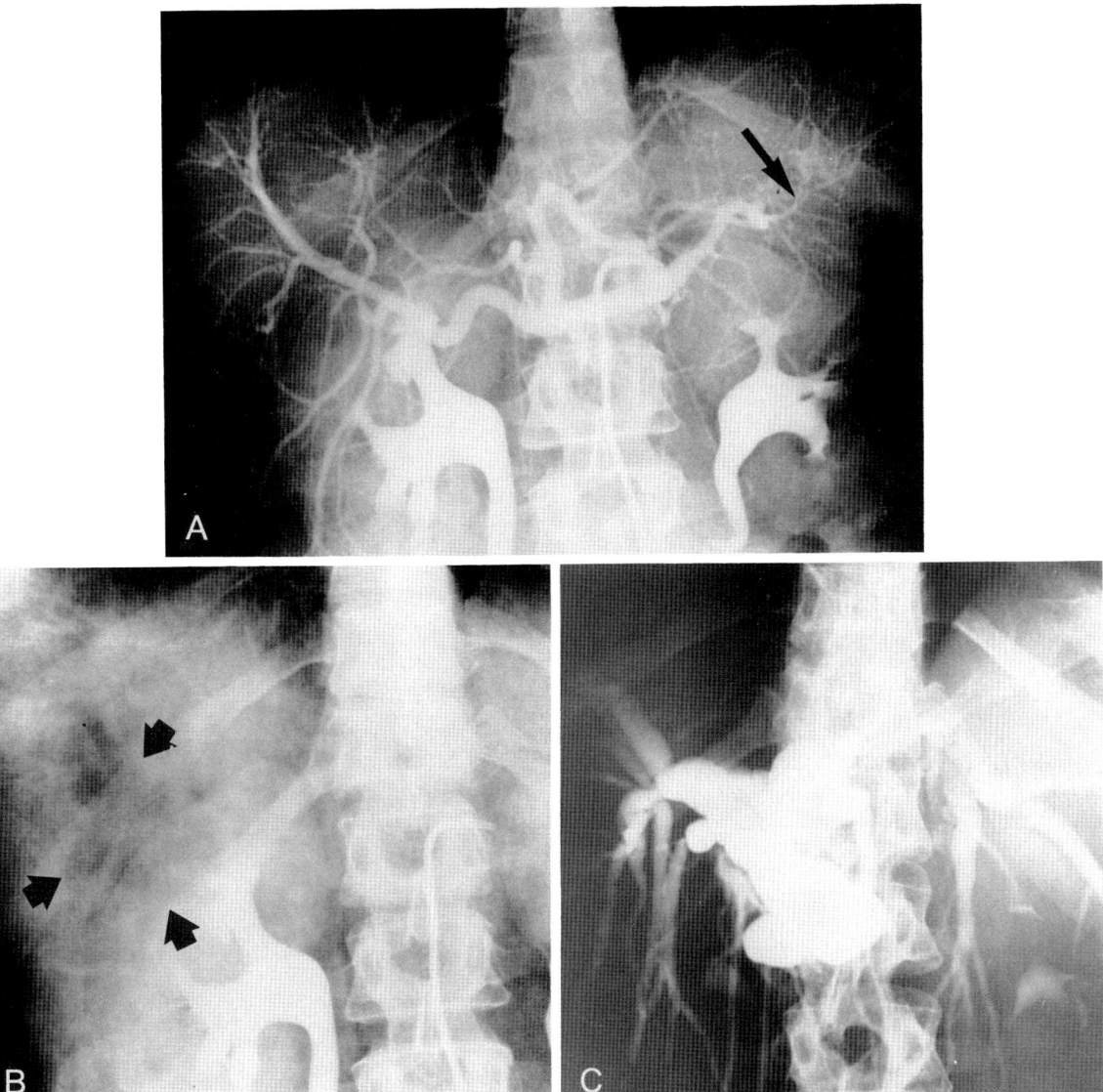

FIGURE 22.70. PANCREATIC DUCT CELL CARCINOMA
Carcinoma of the tail of the pancreas with nodal metastases causing biliary obstruction. Celiac arteriogram. *A:* Arterial phase: occlusion of the distal splenic artery (*arrow*). The splenic vein was also occluded in the splenic hilum (not shown). *B:* Parenchymal phase: the central lucency in the hepatogram represents dilated ducts (*arrows*). *C:* Transhepatic cholangiogram: dilated ducts and obstruction.

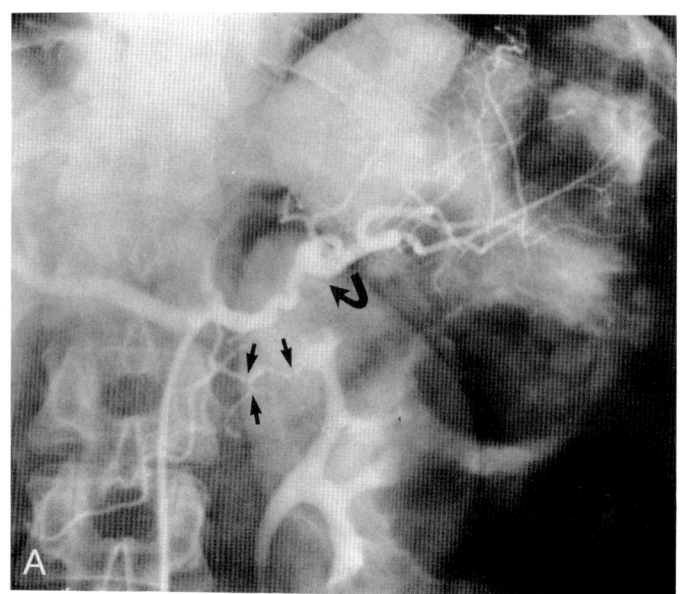
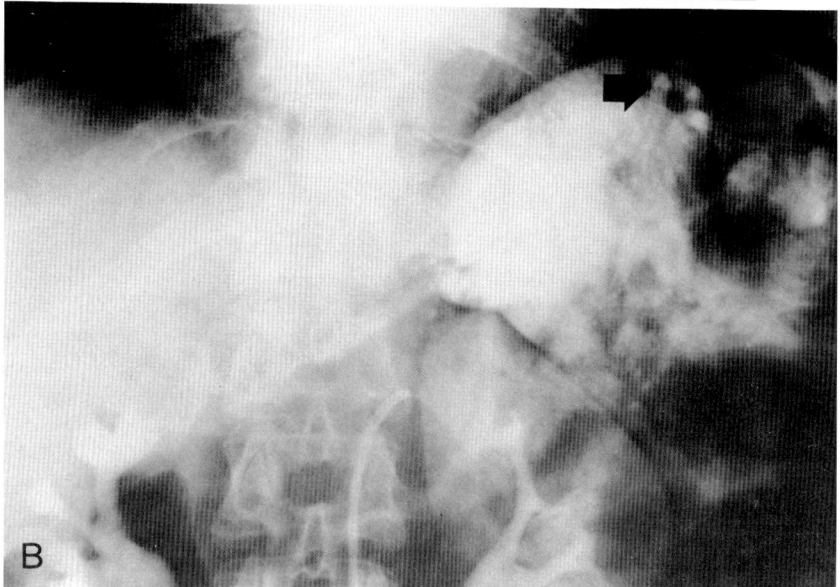

FIGURE 22.71. PANCREATIC DUCT CELL CARCINOMA
A: Celiac arteriogram: occlusion of the pancreatica magna artery at its origin (*curved arrow*) and encasement with occlusion of branches of the dorsal pancreatic artery (*arrows*). *B:* Splenic vein occlusion with varices (*arrow*) on the venous phase.

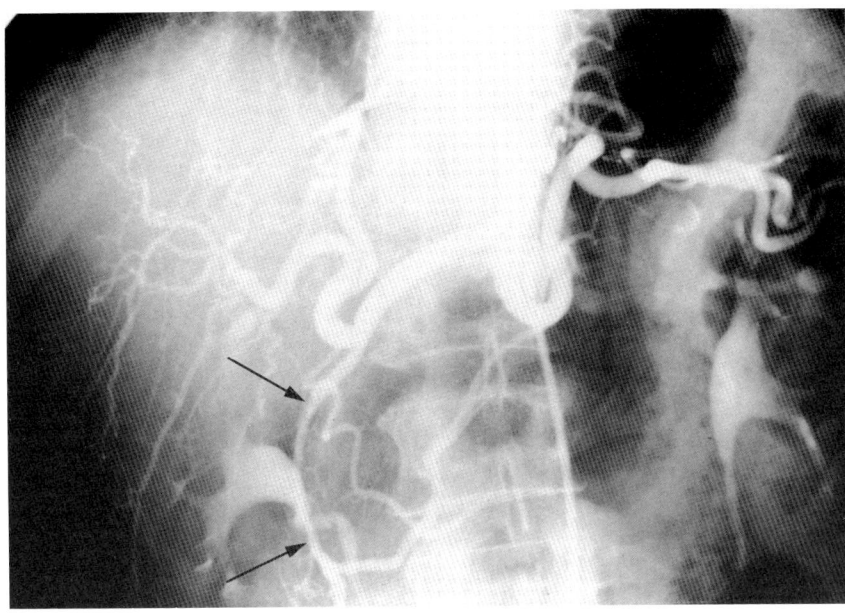

FIGURE 22.72. PANCREATIC DUCT CELL CARCINOMA

Lateral bowing of the gastroduodenal artery by carcinoma of the pancreas (*arrows*). Prospectively, the finding was noted but its significance was thought questionable.

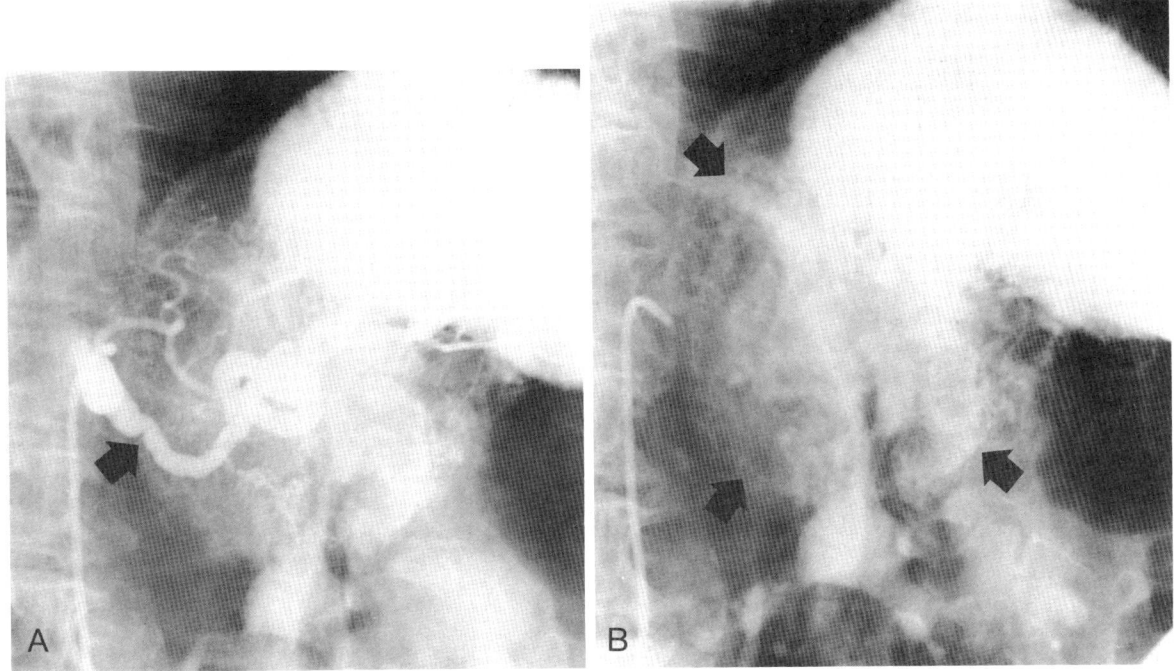

FIGURE 22.73. PANCREATIC CARCINOMA

Unusual arteriographic findings in carcinoma of the pancreas, histologic variant(?), splenic arteriogram. *A:* Arterial phase: encased splenic artery (*arrow*) with encased branches and a large tumor blush. Encasement of small branches is difficult to distinguish from neovascularity. *B:* Early venous phase: large tumor blush (*arrows*) with obstruction of the splenic vein. Findings suggest one of the variant carcinomas of the pancreas.

rules out carcinoma as the cause for the arterial abnormality (6, 12), since veins are affected prior to arteries in neoplastic disease because of their thinner walls. If abnormal small veins can be seen, this is felt by some to be a better indicator of malignancy than changes confined to small arteries (23).

Differential Diagnosis

The primary consideration in the angiographic differential diagnosis of pancreatic duct cell carcinoma is acute or chronic pancreatitis. Mass effect due to pseudocyst manifests itself as smooth, arc-like arterial or venous displacement, unusual in carcinoma. Pseudocysts do, however, occur occasionally in conjunction with carcinoma, and are identical to pseudocysts occurring with pancreatitis. Abrupt, rather than smooth, angulation of vessels may result from desmoplastic response to carcinoma, and is less likely in pancreatitis. Pronounced hypervascular reaction indicates either acute pancreatitis or a less common vascular neoplasm, but pancreatitis secondary to an obstructing carcinoma may theoretically result in a hypervascular reaction. Tumor hypervascularity has never been documented in association with pancreatic duct cell carcinoma.

Any of the vascular changes associated with carcinoma can be found in cases of chronic pancreatitis, but if all findings are correlated, an angiographic diagnosis is usually but not always possible (Figs. 22.74 and 22.75). The hallmark of carcinoma is localized arterial and venous encasement, angulation and/or occlusion, with an absence of comparable vascular changes elsewhere. A normal vessel adjacent to an abnormal vessel suggests pancreatitis. Pseudoaneurysms of the gastroduodenal or splenic arteries strongly suggest pancreatitis. Even as an isolated finding, serrated or serpiginous encasement is likely to represent carcinoma (Fig. 22.61), especially if it involves extrapancreatic arteries (6), but confidence is increased if additional changes are present. Smooth encasement is helpful in detecting any abnormality, but by itself is not helpful in differential diagnosis. False positive diagnoses of carcinoma may result from mistaking vascular irregularities due to inflammation for arterial encasement, difficult at times for even experienced interpreters. Optimal technique, experience, and scrutiny of all pancreatic and peripancreatic vessels is essential if arteriography is to be a reliable technique for diagnosing pancreatic disease.

Dilated intrahepatic ducts can be seen as branching central lucencies in the portal hepatogram but are not specific for carcinoma over pancreatitis (Fig. 22.70). Liver metastases, of course, strongly suggest carcinoma (Fig. 22.61).

Atherosclerosis is commonly found in patients being evaluated for suspected pancreatic neoplasm, and may produce arterial changes mimicking those of carcinoma (Fig. 22.76). Atheromatous narrowing tends to present as a single plaque within a vessel rather than as a sawtooth narrowing, and will involve vessels removed from the pancreas as well (Fig. 22.77) (24). Most important is the demonstration of associated venous abnormalities, absent in atherosclerosis.

Less common diagnostic difficulties concern other malignancies involving the pancreas secondarily. Invasive carcinoma of the ampulla of Vater or common bile duct has a pattern of growth similar to that of pancreatic carcinoma, and may be indistinguishable angiographically (18). Similarly, gastric carcinoma involving the pancreas may be indistinguishable from pancreatic carcinoma involving the stomach, especially since the pyloric artery which continues from the termination of the gastroduodenal artery may have a course similar to that of the anterior pancreaticoduodenal arcade (18). Primary duodenal carcinoma may be differentiated from pancreatic carcinoma by medial displacement of the gastroduodenal artery seen in the former (25). Both duodenal and pancreatic branches may be involved with both primaries, but feeding arteries to the pancreas such as the dorsal pancreatic and proximal superior mesenteric artery tend not to be involved by duodenal primaries (25). Lymphoma involving peripancreatic nodes will produce displacement out of proportion to encasement (Fig. 22.78) (19). Metastases to peripancreatic nodes, most commonly from gastric colonic or biliary carcinoma, may invade the pancreas producing changes indistinguishable from primary carcinoma (18), although vascular displacement is likely to be more pronounced. Many of these difficulties will be resolved by correlation with ERCP, ultrasound, CT and/or conventional barium examinations.

Technical artifacts such as catheter-induced spasm have resulted in false-positive diagnoses (Fig. 22.79) (1, 17). Irregularities mimicking encasement may result from the use of vasoconstrictors, and must be carefully compared with films obtained without the use of such agents (9).

Prognosis and Surgical Planning

The value of angiography in staging pancreatic

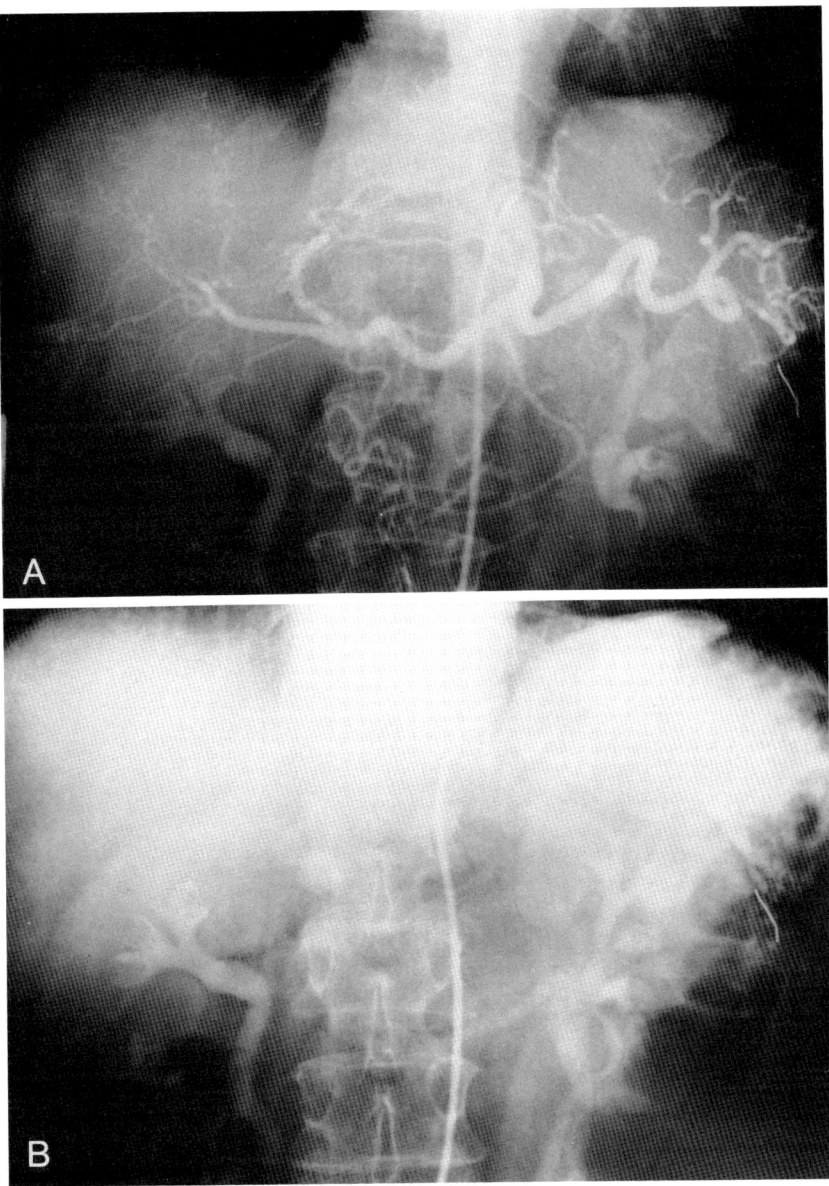

FIGURE 22.74. PANCREATITIS OR CARCINOMA?
Pancreatitis or carcinoma? Celiac arteriogram. *A:* Arterial phase: normal splenic artery except for stretched intrasplenic branches due to splenomegaly. *B:* Venous phase: splenic vein occlusion with gastric varices. Diagnosis: carcinoma of the tail of the pancreas; pancreatitis could look the same.

carcinoma for surgical planning depends to a large extent on the approach of the surgeon. While most surgeons rely heavily on radiographic data for decisions regarding resectability, others believe that the only value of angiography is to detect the approximately 25% of cases with foregut vascular anomalies (13). Almost 90% of these involve the hepatic arterial supply, and the inadvertent ligation of these vessels may result in fatal hepatic necrosis, especially in the presence of jaundice (13). Angiography may also warn the surgeon regarding portal hypertension (2). Thus, preoperative angiography can be helpful whether or not it influences the decision to operate.

Before proceeding further, it is necessary to define some frequently confused terms pertaining to surgical planning. The prognosis for any pancreatic cancer is dismal; although there are isolated case reports of surgical cures, it is unrealistic to speak of "curable" lesions in most cases. "Early carcinomas" are considered poten-

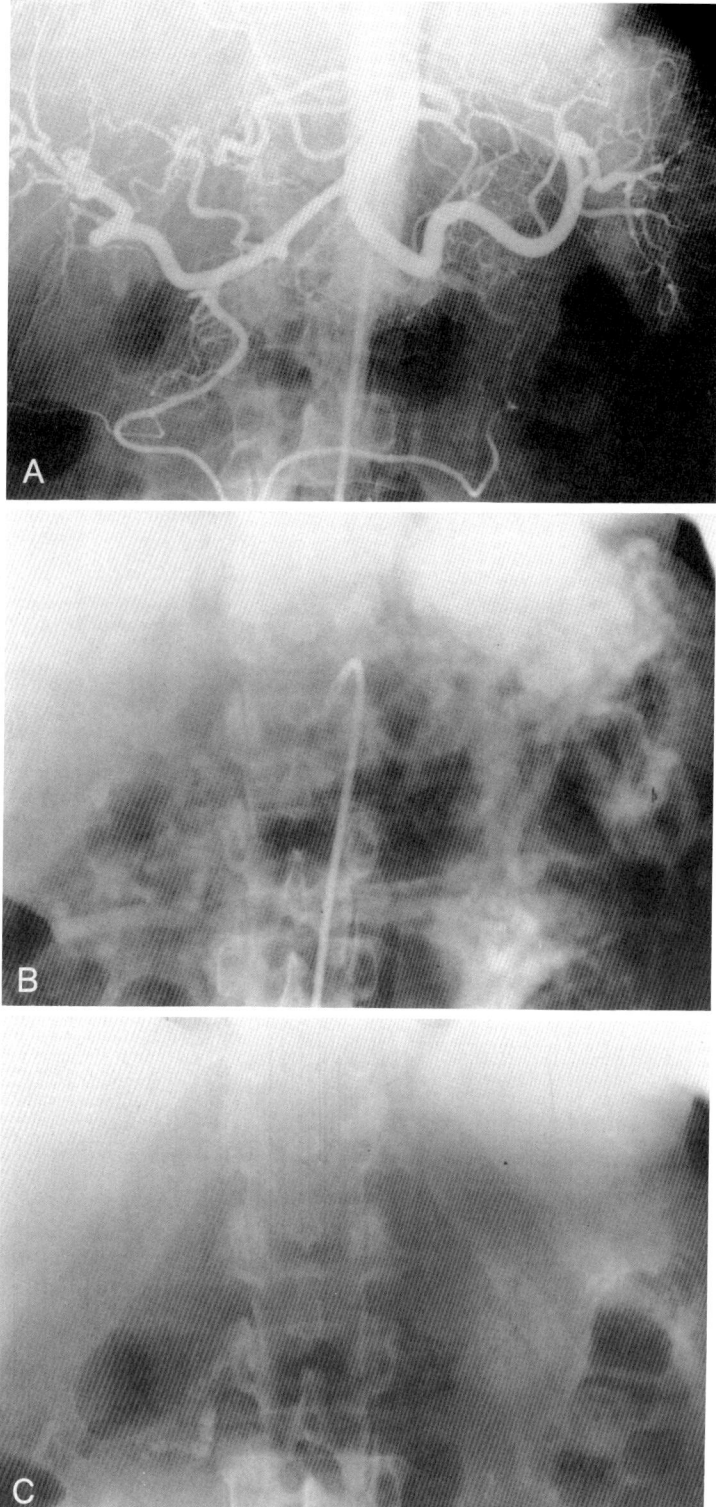

FIGURE 22.75. PANCREATITIS OR CARCINOMA?
Celiac arteriogram. *A:* Arterial phase: normal. *B:* Venous phase: splenic vein occlusion with portal filling via gastroepiploic and omental collaterals. *C:* Plain film: diagnosis is chronic pancreatitis with extensive calcification in the head of the pancreas.

FIGURE 22.76. ATHEROSCLEROSIS OF SPLENIC ARTERY MIMICKING TUMOR ENCASEMENT
Celiac arteriogram. *A:* Arterial phase: irregularity of the splenic artery (*arrow*). *B:* Venous phase: normal splenic vein, suggesting atherosclerosis.

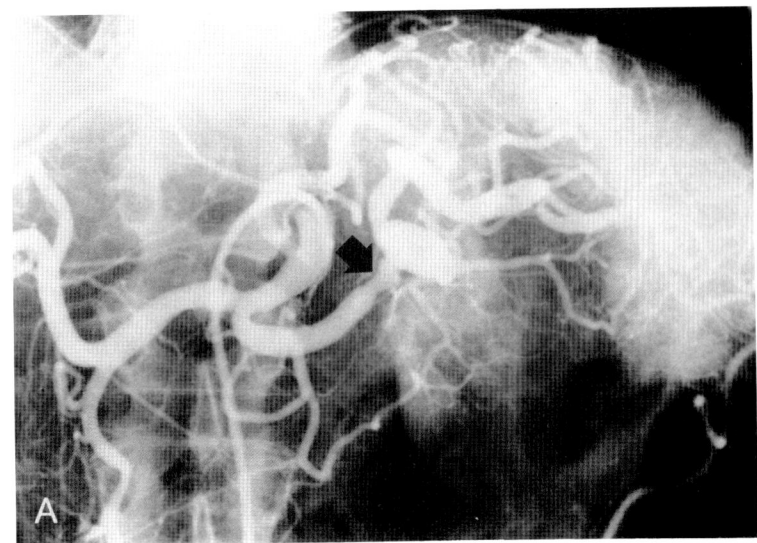
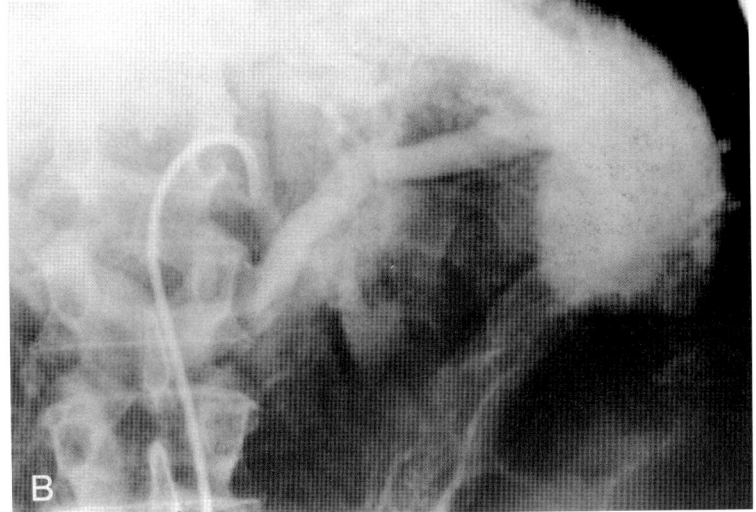

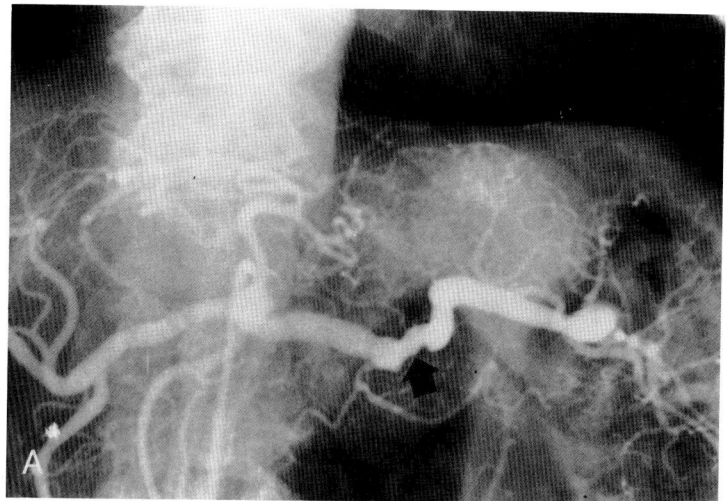
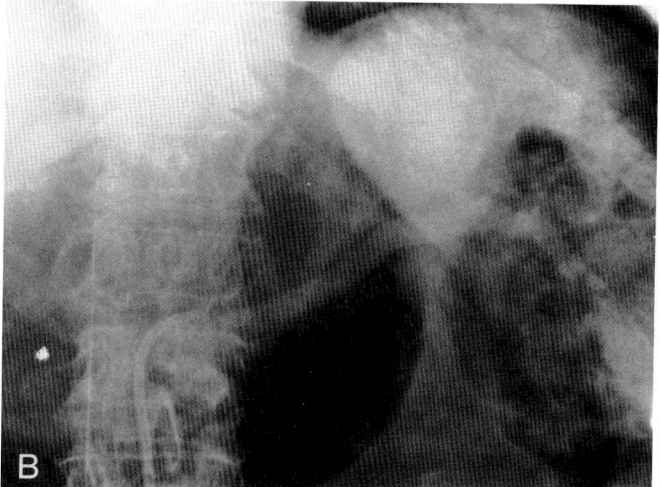
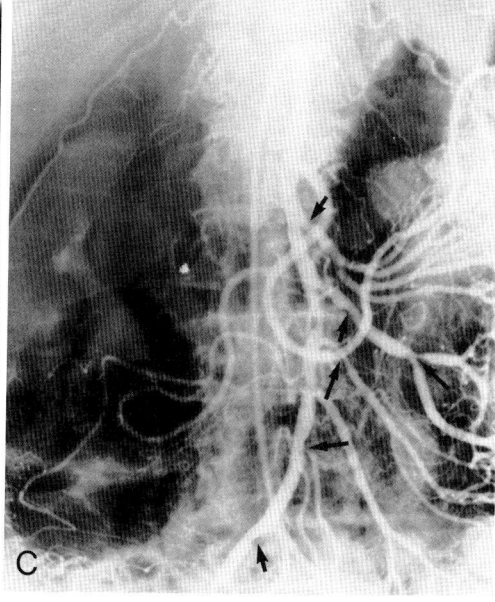
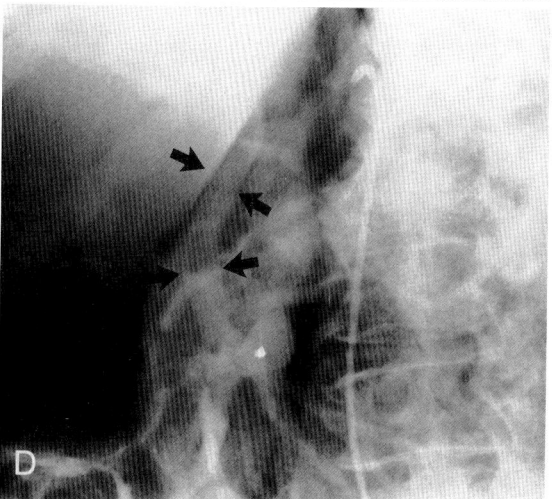

FIGURE 22.77. EXTENSIVE ATHEROSCLEROSIS MIMICKING ENCASEMENT

A: Celiac arteriogram, arterial phase: irregularity of the midportion of the splenic artery mimicking encasement (*arrow*). *B:* Venous phase: normal splenic vein. *C:* Superior mesenteric arteriogram, arterial phase: multiple areas of narrowing in jejunal branches and the ileocolic artery (*arrows*). *D:* Venous phase: normal superior mesenteric vein (*arrows*) and branches.

FIGURE 22.78. PANCREATIC LYMPHOMA

Peripancreatic lymphoma, celiac arteriography. *A:* Arterial phase: stretching and displacement of splenic, common hepatic, dorsal pancreatic, and transverse pancreatic arteries and the pancreaticoduodenal arcade. No encasement. *B:* Venous phase: stretching and displacement of the splenic vein. Vascular displacement out of proportion to encasement favors lymphoma. Superior mesenteric artery and vein were normal.

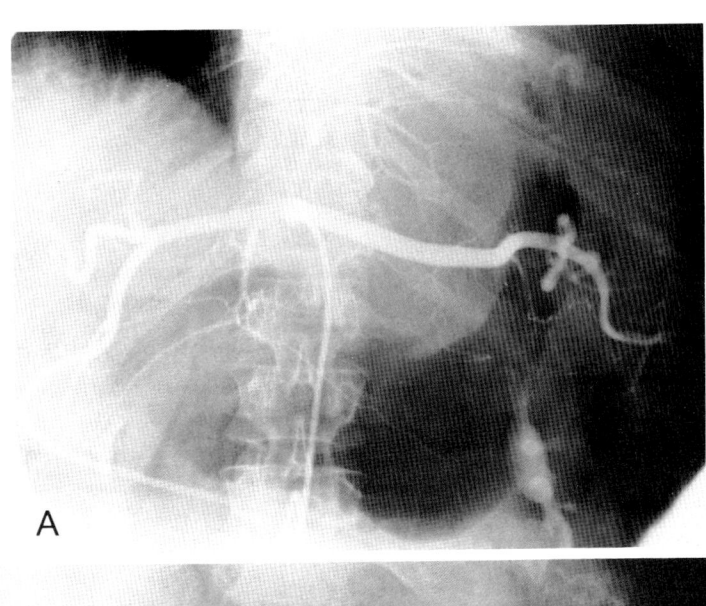
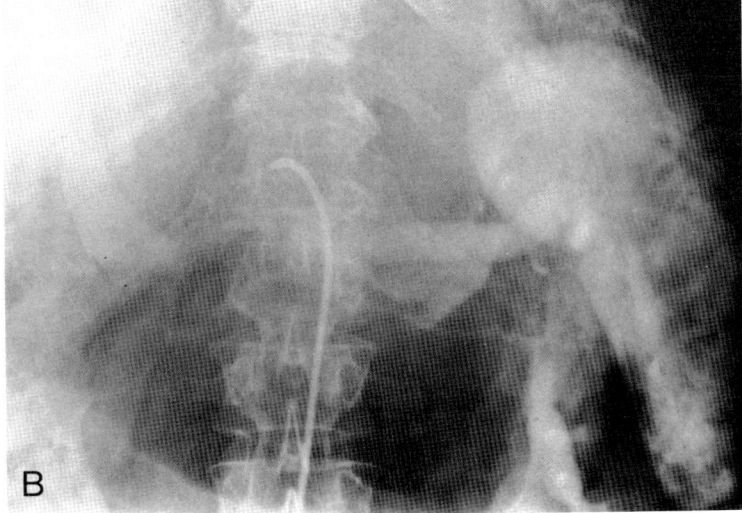

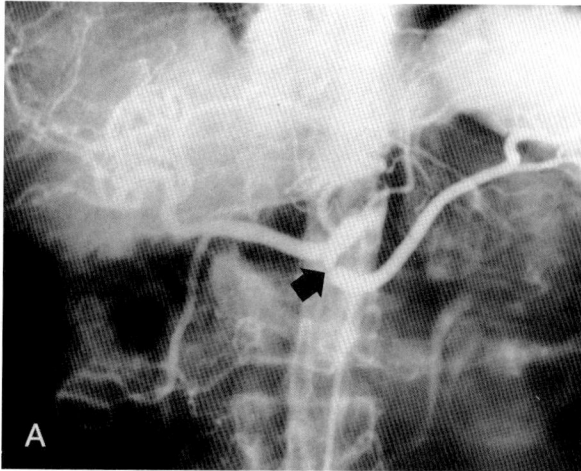 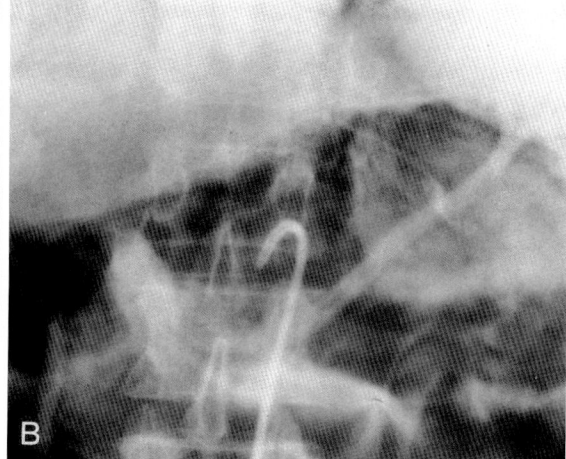

FIGURE 22.79. CATHETER-INDUCED SPASM OF SPLENIC ARTERY MIMICKING ENCASEMENT
Celiac arteriogram. *A:* Arterial phase: band-like narrowing at the origin of the splenic artery (*arrow*). The catheter had entered the splenic artery prior to the injection and had been repositioned in the celiac artery. *B:* Venous phase: normal splenic vein, mitigating against tumor.

tially curable, and consist of lesions of less than 2 cm in diameter which on surgical inspection do not involve the surface of the gland and are unassociated with hepatic or lymphatic metastases (2). In one series 17 of 64 resected carcinomas were considered early, and 5 of these survived 5 yr after surgery for a 5-yr survival rate of 29% among the "early" carcinomas (2). Only with superselective catheterization and/or pharmacological manipulation can these cancers be detected angiographically.

The most important contribution the angiographer can make regarding staging of pancreatic carcinoma is to judge whether the lesion is resectable. Resectability refers to the ability of the surgeon to remove the tumor en bloc, leaving no macroscopic evidence of tumor behind. While cures are unusual, resection is undertaken to delay the almost inevitable death from carcinoma. Perioperative mortality has decreased markedly from the 1950s but remains near 10% (2, 26). The criteria for resectability varies according to the approach of the referring surgeon. This can be as radical as the "regional resection" advocated by some, which involves en bloc removal of the superior mesenteric artery, celiac axis, portal vein, and the base of the transverse mesocolon along with the entire pancreas (27). Knowledge of the referring surgeon's philosophy is necessary to best predict resectability of pancreatic carcinoma.

A term often confused with resectability is called "operability," which is a clinical decision based on the patient's likelihood of surviving surgery. Palliative surgery may be performed to relieve gastrointestinal obstruction in a patient with unresectable disease (26). Surgery to relieve obstructive jaundice frequently results in little if any true palliation and may even shorten survival (26).

The most frequently accepted angiographic criteria for unresectability include hepatic metastases and involvement of major extrapancreatic arteries or veins (26, 28). These include the superior mesenteric artery, major branches of the celiac axis, portal vein, superior mesenteric vein, and splenic vein. Upon inspection at laparotomy, the surgeon may decide that cancer is resectable in spite of angiographic evidence to the contrary, and the cancer is thus, by definition "resectable," but patients with major vessel involvement invariably die within 1 yr, usually within 4-6 months (26, 29, 30). Involvement of the gastroduodenal artery in some centers is unrelated to resectability (26, 31), but is highly correlated in others (29). If the gastroduodenal artery is affected, resection is unlikely to prolong survival (26, 29), although palliation of pain is reported by some (6). Involvement of the anterior pancreaticoduodenal arcade is compatible with survival in excess of 1 yr, while posterior arcade involvement is associated with less frequent resectability (33% in one series) and death within months (29). Surprisingly, the presence of hepatic metastases appears almost unrelated to the degree of vascular involvement (29). Angiography tailored to the pancreas detects liver metastases in less than two-thirds of those cases in which hepatic metastases are visible at surgery (6, 13), but not infrequently liver metastases are the only angiographic evidence of unresectability (28, 29).

Angiography is no longer indicated in the majority of cases of pancreatic carcinoma, since the diagnosis can almost invariably be made by ultrasound, CT, and/or ERCP with confirmation by percutaneous biopsy (2, 3, 32, 33). The majority are found unresectable by CT, which is more sensitive in detecting hepatic metastases and involvement of peripancreatic fascia (28). CT is also more sensitive in detecting encasement of the celiac trunk and proximal superior mesenteric artery, since early encasement may not encroach upon the lumen, and angiography is limited by radiographic projection (unless lateral projections are obtained) and by catheter placement (28, 34). In two series, only 14 of 26 (54%) encased proximal vessels seen by CT were detected angiographically (28, 34). The converse is true of major branches of these vessels, as well as major veins, where angiography is considerably more sensitive (28). Thus, occasional patients without CT signs of resectability may be spared from surgery by angiographic demonstration of encasement of major arteries or veins (28).

Accuracy

Angiography is a highly accurate method for detecting and staging pancreatic carcinoma. When standard superior mesenteric artery and celiac injections are relied upon, diagnostic accuracy is approximately 70% in most reports (8, 13, 16, 35). If superselective catheterization is attempted in all cases in which positive diagnosis of carcinoma has not been established, diagnostic accuracy is consistently above 90% (6, 8, 16, 36). The small carcinomas not detected tend to be within the gland and resectable, and are easily detected by ERCP (37). However accurate angiography may be, the rapid development of ERCP, ultrasound, and CT during the past decade has all but eliminated the need for pancreatic angiography as a diagnostic procedure other than for preoperative planning. Recent reports advocating a primary role for angiography must be interpreted carefully; CT may have been used only in a minority of cases (36), or early generation equipment may have been used (31, 32). At one center, the use of CT as the primary diagnostic procedure for suspected pancreatic carcinoma resulted in a 55% decrease in arteriograms performed and a 47% decreased cost of radiologic evaluation, without affecting diagnostic accuracy (33). With newer generation equipment and increasing confidence of CT diagnosis, the frequency of pancreatic arteriography should continue to decrease. In the past, angiography has been the accepted gold standard for preoperative staging, correctly predicting unresectability in approximately 90% of unresectable lesions (6, 28, 31). High resolution CT with bolus injection appears as accurate, however (28), and can provide guidance for percutaneous biopsy to establish definitive diagnosis.

REFERENCES

1. Herlinger H, Finlay DBL: Evaluation and follow-up of pancreatic arteriograms. A new role for angiography in the diagnosis of carcinoma of the pancreas. *Clin Radiol* 29:277–284, 1978.
2. Moossa AR, Levin B: The diagnosis of "early" pancreatic cancer: the University of Chicago experience. *Cancer* 47:1688–1697, 1981.
3. Ariyama J, Shirakabe H, Ikenobe H, Kurosawa A, Owman T: The diagnosis of the small resectable pancreatic carcinoma. *Clin Radiol* 28:437–444, 1977.
4. Sigstedt B, Boijsen E, Lunderquist A, Tylen U: Angiography in pancreatic disease reevaluated. *Acta Radiol (Diagn)* 22:235–244, 1981.
5. MacGregor AMC, Hawkins IF Jr: Selective pharmacodynamic angiography in the diagnosis of carcinoma of the pancreas. *Surg Gynecol Obstet* 137:917–921, 1973.
6. Goldstein HM, Neiman HL, Bookstein JJ: Angiographic evaluation of pancreatic disease. *Radiology* 112:275–282, 1974.
7. Rosch J, Keller FS: Pancreatic arteriography, transhepatic pancreatic venography, and pancreatic venous sampling in diagnosis of pancreatic cancer. *Cancer* 47:1679–1684, 1981.
8. Rosch J, Holman DC: Superselective arteriography of the pancreas. In Anacker M (ed): *Efficiency and Limits of Radiologic Examination of the Pancreas*. Stuttgart, Georg Thieme, 1975, pp 169–167.
9. Freeny PC, Lawson TL: *Radiology of the Pancreas*. New York, Springer-Verlag, 1982, pp 51–97.
10. Boijsen E, Gothlin J: Abdominal angiography after intraarterial injection of vasopressin. *Acta Radiol (Diagn)* 21:523–533, 1980.
11. Legge D: The use of prostaglandin $F_{2\alpha}$ in selective pancreatic and left gastric angiography. *Clin Radiol* 29:285–288, 1978.
12. Buranasiri S, Baum S: The significance of the venous phase of celiac and superior mesenteric arteriography in evaluating pancreatic carcinoma. *Radiology* 102:11–20, 1972.
13. Mackie CR, Lu CT, Noble HG, Cooper MJ, Collins P, Block GE, Moossa AR: Prospective evaluation of angiography in the diagnosis and management of patients suspected of having pancreatic cancer. *Ann Surg* 189:11–17, 1979.
14. Suzuki T, Uchida K, Tani T, Honjo I: Selective arteriography combined with hypotonic duodenography for pancreatic lesions. *AJR* 122:398–405, 1974.
15. Suzuki T, Manabe T, Tani T, Uchida K: Manifestations of carcinoma of the uncinate process by means of superior mesenteric arteriography. *Surg Gynecol Obstet* 152:163–170, 1981.

16. Freeny PC, Lawson, TL: *Radiology of the Pancreas.* New York, Springer-Verlag, 1982, pp 465–475.
17. Gortenuti G, Cavallini G, Vantini I, Angelini A, Piubello W, Frasson F, Dobrilla D: Angiography in chronic pancreatitis and pancreatic cancer. *Am J Gastroenterol* 70:620–626, 1978.
18. Reuter SR, Redman HC, Bookstein JJ: Differential problems in the angiographic diagnosis of carcinoma of the pancreas. *Radiology* 96:93–99, 1970.
19. Nelman HL, Goldstein HM, Silverman PH, Bookstein JJ: Angiographic features of peripancreatic malignant lymphoma. *Radiology* 115:589–592, 1975.
20. Tylen U: Angiographic differentiation between inflammatory disease and carcinoma of the pancreas. *Acta Radiol (Diagn)* 14:257–272, 1973.
21. Tylen U: Accuracy of angiography in the diagnosis of carcinoma of the pancreas. *Acta Radiol (Diagn)* 14:449–466, 1973.
22. Marions O: Radiologic investigation in jaundice. *Opusc Med (Stockh)* Suppl No 34, 1974.
23. Uden R: Secretin and epinephrine combined in celiac angiography. *Acta Radiol (Diagn)* 17:17–40, 1976.
24. Boijsen E: Pancreatic angiography. In Abrams ML (ed): *Angiography: Vascular and Interventional Radiology,* Ed. 3. Boston, Little, Brown, 1983, pp 1441–1446.
25. Olssen O: Angiography in the diagnosis of duodenal lesions. I. Differentiation between primary duodenal carcinoma and carcinoma of the head of the pancreas including the duodenum. *Acta Radiol (Diagn)* 12:49–58, 1972.
26. Tylen U, Arnesjo B: Resectability and prognosis of carcinoma of the pancreas evaluated by angiography. *Scand J Gastroenterol* 8:691–697, 1973.
27. Fortner JG: Surgical principles for pancreatic cancer: regional total and subtotal pancreatectomy. *Cancer* 47:1712–1718, 1981.
28. Jafri SZH, Aisen AM, Glazer GM, Weiss CA: Comparison of CT and angiography in assessing resectability of pancreatic carcinoma. *AJR* 142:525–529, 1984.
29. Suzuki T, Tani T, Honjo I: Appraisal of arteriography for angiography of operability in periampullary cancer. *Ann Surg* 182:66–71, 1975.
30. Suzuki T, Kawabe K, Imamara M, Honjo I: Survival of patients with cancer in relation to findings on arteriography. *Ann Surg* 176:37–41, 1972.
31. Hemmingsson A, Jacobson G, Lindgren PG, Lonnerholm T, Lorelius LE, Nordgren CE: Radiologic assessment of resectability of carcinoma of the head of the pancreas. *Acta Radiol (Diagn)* 23:127–130, 1982.
32. Mackie CR, Blackstone MO, Dhorajiwala J, Bowie J, Moossa AR: Value of new diagnostic aids in relation to the disease process in pancreatic cancer. *Lancet* 2:385–389, 1979.
33. Freeny PC, Marks WM, Ball TJ: Impact of high-resolution computed tomography of the pancreas on utilization of endoscopic retrograde cholangiopancreatography and angiography. *Radiology* 142:35–39, 1982.
34. Megibow AJ, Bosniak MA, Ambos MA, Beranbaum ER: Thickening of the celiac axis and/or superior mesenteric artery: a sign of pancreatic carcinoma on computed tomography. *Radiology* 141:449–453, 1981.
35. Suzuki T, Kawabe K, Nakayasu A, Takeda H, Kobayashi K, Kubota N, Honjo I: Selective arteriography in cancer of the pancreas at a resectable stage. *Am J Surg* 122:402–407, 1971.
36. Freeny PC, Ball TJ, Ryan J: Impact of new diagnostic imaging methods on pancreatic angiography. *AJR* 133:619–624, 1979.
37. Suzuki T, Imamura M, Katsuhiro T, Sumiyoshi A, Sakanashi S, Nishimura Y, Tobe T: Correlative evaluation of angiography and pancreatoductography in relation to surgery for cancer of the pancreas. *Surgery* 85:644–651, 1979.

Arteriography of Ampullary Carcinoma

The scirrhous pattern of growth of ampullary carcinoma is identical to that of pancreatic duct cell adenocarcinoma (1). Thus, arteriographic findings, if present, are identical, consisting of arterial and venous encasement, angulation, and/or obstruction as described previously (1–3). Hypervascularity is not seen, but could theoretically be present if secondary pancreatitis is prominent. When only standard superior mesenteric and celiac injections are used, the majority are normal arteriographically (2), and even with superselective technique, there may be no abnormality visualized (1).

REFERENCES

1. Herlinger H, Finlay DBL: Evaluation and follow-up of pancreatic arteriograms. A new role for angiography in the diagnosis of carcinoma of the pancreas. *Clin Radiol* 29:277–284, 1978.
2. Suzuki T, Kawabe K, Nakayasu A, Takeda M, Kobayashi K, Kubota N, Honjo I: Selective arteriography in cancer of the pancreas at a resectable stage. *Am J Surg* 122:402–407, 1971.
3. Reuter SR, Redman MC, Bookstein JJ: Differential problems in the angiographic diagnosis of carcinoma of the pancreas. *Radiology* 96:93–99, 1970.

Pancreatic Venography

From the early 1950s until the mid 1960s when pancreatic arteriography was developed, splenoportography and barium examination were the primary radiologic means for evaluation pancreatic disease. Splenoportography consisted of percutaneous injection of contrast into the splenic parenchyma which resulted in filling of the splenic and portal veins (1). These structures, as well as the superior mesenteric vein and smaller pancreatic veins, can be seen with arterial portography as described previously. Splenoportography is no longer performed in most centers.

If arterial portography does not adequately display pancreatic venous morphology or if venous sampling is desired, selective retrograde pancreatic venography is possible, via the transjugular or transhepatic approach (2). Transjugular catheterization of the portal venous system is accomplished by puncturing the internal jugular vein using the Seldinger technique. The catheter is guided into the main right hepatic vein, and a modified Ross transseptal needle is inserted through the catheter and advanced into the liver parenchyma. Small test doses of contrast are injected to evaluate needle position and when the portal vein has been entered a guide wire is inserted and selective catheterization of the desired portal tributary is attempted (3).

A somewhat easier technique for accomplishing selective pancreatic venous catheterization is transhepatic portography (2, 4, 5). The liver is punctured percutaneously and when venous blood is obtained, a test dose of contrast is given to verify position. A guide wire is then inserted and selective venous catheterization proceeds. While venous morphology is better depicted than by arterial portography, the sensitivity of pancreatic venography is limited by venous anatomy. All major veins lie on the surface of the gland, and there are multiple anastomoses between them (4–7). Due to these anastomoses and the retrograde nature of the injection, nonfilling of a venous tributary may be due either to pathology or technical artifacts (4, 5). Inability to catheterize the pancreaticoduodenal veins has been found indicative of obstruction due to carcinoma (4), but in most hands this is unlikely to be a reliable finding.

Venous abnormalities are identical to those described with arterial portography, most frequently involving venous obstruction. Tumors smaller than 3 cm are unlikely to be detected (4–6) and the technique is clearly less sensitive than superselective arteriography, where both arteries and veins can be assessed. The complication rate is significant, especially in inexperienced hands (4). The technique is usually reserved for venous sampling, and may become important in evaluating duct cell carcinoma if a specific tumor marker can be isolated.

REFERENCES

1. Rosch J, Herfort K: Splenoportographic diagnosis of pancreatic diseases. *Geriatrics* 19:725–735, 1964.
2. Freeny PC, Lawson TL: *Radiology of the Pancreas.* New York, Springer-Verlag, 1982, pp 87–97.
3. Rosch J, Dotter CT: Retrograde pancreatic venography. An experimental study. *Radiology* 114:275–279, 1975.
4. Reichardt W. Selective phlebography in pancreatic and peripancreatic disease. *Acta Radiol (Diagn)* 21:513–522, 1980.
5. Rosch J, Keller FS: Pancreatic arteriography, transhepatic pancreatic venography, and pancreatic venous sampling in diagnosis of pancreatic cancer. *Cancer* 47:1679–1684, 1981.
6. Reichardt W, Cameron R: Anatomy of the pancreatic veins: a post-mortem and clinical phlebographic investigation. *Acta Radiol (Diagn)* 21:33–41, 1980.
7. Keller FS, Niles AR, Rosen J, Dotter CT, Stenzel-Poore M: Retrograde pancreatic venography: autopsy study. *Radiology* 135:285–293, 1980.

Variant Carcinomas

Giant Cell Carcinoma (Epulis-Osteoid Type)

Clinical Findings. This is a very rare neoplasm with a better prognosis than duct cell adenocarcinoma. Two patients with apparently successful resection have been reported, a third succumbed to metastatic disease after 4 yr (1).

Pathology. These are large neoplasms (largest diameter 7–13 cm) with well-defined margins and large areas of hemorrhage and necrosis (1, 2). Microscopically, they are composed of benign appearing multinucleated giant cells resembling osteoclasts, bizarre malignant giant cells, and spindle cells ranging from benign appearing to sarcoma-like (1, 2). Multiple foci of osteoid are present (1, 2). Glandular elements, if present at all, are sparse (1).

Radiology. Barium contrast studies show soft tissue masses displacing or extending into adjacent organs. Although we have no experience with CT and ultrasound of these tumors, these modalities most likely would show fairly well-marginated, partially necrotic solid masses judging from the neoplasm's gross morphology. It is conceivable that CT might show small, high density areas corresponding to mineralized osteoid.

REFERENCES

1. Cubilla AL, Fitzgerald PJ: Cancer (non-endocrine) of the pancreas. A suggested classification. *Monogr Pathol* 21:88–89, 1980.
2. Rosai J: Carcinoma of the pancreas simulating giant cell tumor of bone. *Cancer* 22:333–344, 1968.

Giant Cell Carcinoma (Pleomorphic)

Clinical Findings. This unusual neoplasm has a similar age distribution and sex ratio to duct cell adenocarcinoma (1–3). Location is about evenly distributed between the head and the body/tail. Prognosis is poor with median survival from time of diagnosis of 2 months, although an apparent cure of an 8-cm pleomorphic giant cell carcinoma in the head has been reported (1).

Pathology. Pleomorphic giant cell carcinomas tend to be large masses (mean largest dimension 11 cm) with frequent central hemorrhagic necrosis and consequently are often described as hemorrhagic cysts (Fig. 22.81C) (1–3). Histologically, these neoplasms are composed of large, often bizarre mono- or multinucleated giant cells and obviously malignant spindle cells. The former tend to be more prevalent (1). Small foci of mucin-producing adenocarcinoma can be found if sought for diligently. A few osteoclast-like cells are seen, but there is no osteoid (1). Pathologic diagnosis is difficult, especially if made from limited biopsy material. Possible misdiagnoses include spindle cell sarcomas, malignant fibrous histocytoma and angiosarcoma, among others (2).

Radiology. Plain films and barium contrast examinations show a nonspecific soft tissue mass (Fig. 22.80A). Sonography and CT will depict this neoplasm as a large thick-walled cyst with a ragged inner margin (Fig. 22.81A and B) when hemorrhagic necrosis predominates. CT numbers of the cystic component are compatible with old blood. Otherwise pleomorphic carcinomas are solid or mixed, usually well-demarcated masses that may have dystrophic calcification (Fig. 22.82). Lymphadenopathy is, at times, striking (Fig. 22.83). Angiographic experience is very limited, but the solid portions of these neoplasms seem to be more vascular than duct cell carcinomas (Fig. 22.80B).

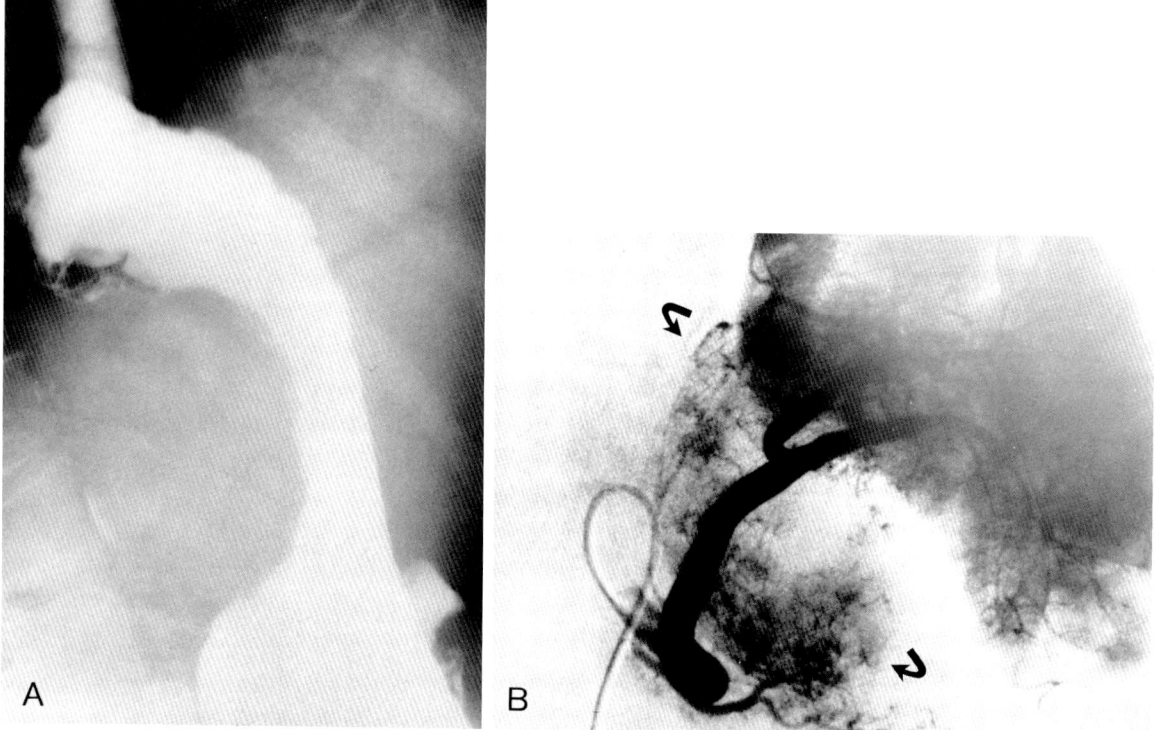

FIGURE 22.80. GIANT CELL CARCINOMA (PLEOMORPHIC)
A: Pleomorphic giant cell carcinoma producing a retrogastric mass. The calcification is vascular. *B:* Arteriogram of the same patient showing hypervascularity in the solid regions of the tumor (*arrows*).

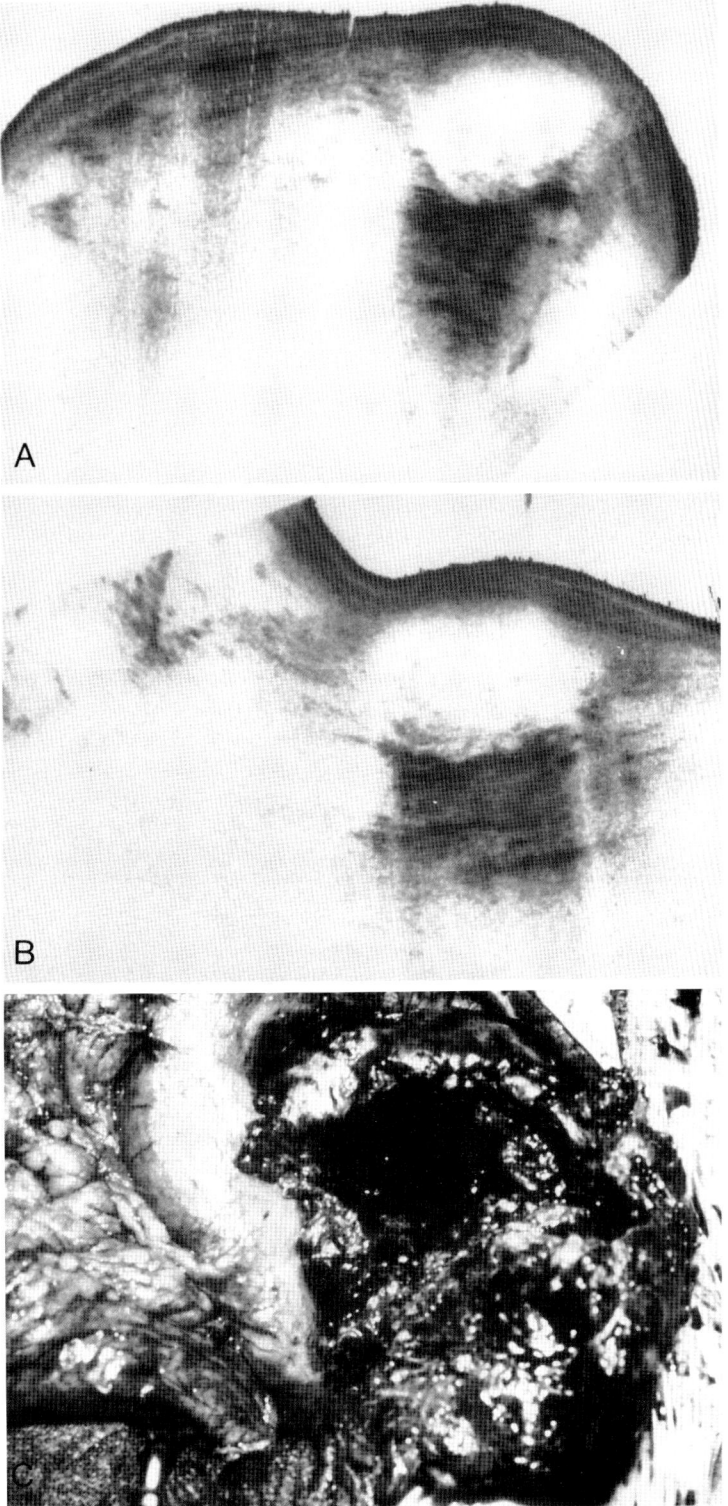

FIGURE 22.81. GIANT CELL CARCINOMA (PLEOMORPHIC)
A and *B:* Transverse and longitudinal sonograms showing a mostly cystic mass with a thick irregular back wall, some internal echoes and good sound transmission in the left upper quadrant. *C:* Operative photograph of the same case showing a blood-filled cystic mass with a thick, nodular wall.

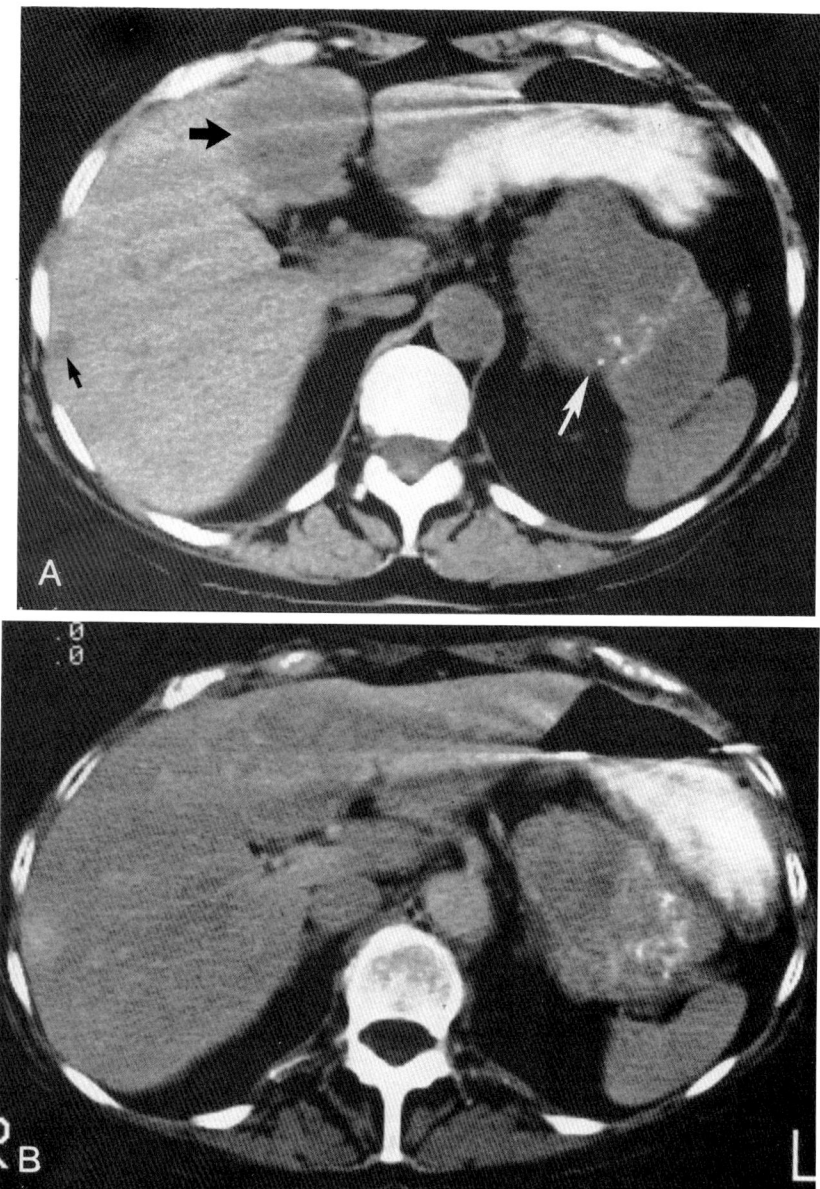

FIGURE 22.82. GIANT CELL CARCINOMA (PLEOMORPHIC)
Slowly progressive pleomorphic giant cell carcinoma with calcification. *A:* Large, well-defined tail of pancreas mass (*white arrow*) with small central calcifications. Liver metastases (*arrows*). *B:* Somewhat different level a year later: not much change in the size of the mass. Patient succumbed to cardiac disease.

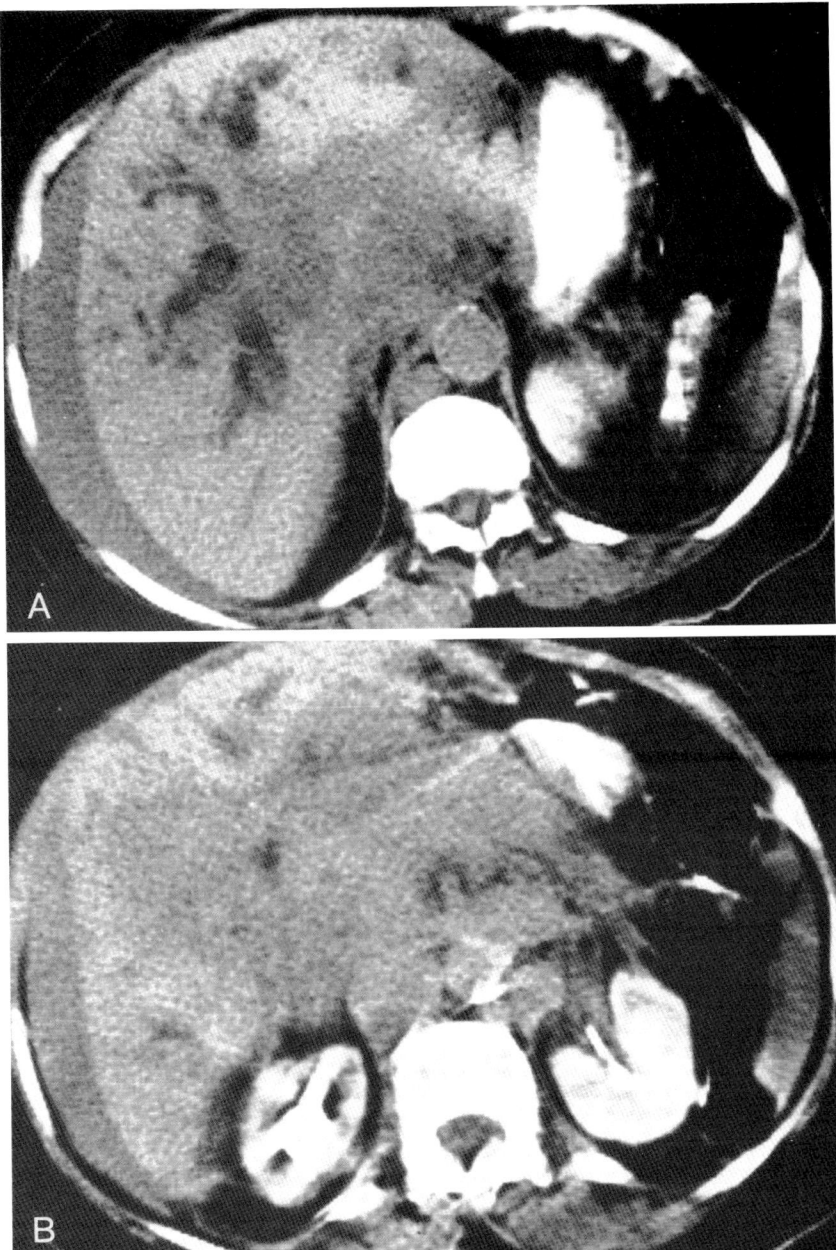

FIGURE 22.83. GIANT CELL CARCINOMA (PLEOMORPHIC)

A and B: Massive pleomorphic carcinoma invading the porta hepatis with prominent retrocrural and paraaortic adenopathy and biliary obstruction.

REFERENCES

1. Cubilla AL, Fitzgerald PJ: Cancer (non-endocrine) of the pancreas. A suggested classification. *Monogr Pathol* 21:86–87, 1980.
2. Alguacil-Garcia A, Weiland LH: The histologic spectrum, prognosis and histogenesis of the sarcomatoid carcinoma of the pancreas. *Cancer* 39:1181–1189, 1977.
3. Guillan RA: Pleomorphic adenocarcinoma of the pancreas. An analysis of five cases. *Cancer* 21:1072–1079, 1968.

Adenosquamous Cancer (Adenoacanthoma, Mucoepidermoid Carcinoma, Squamous Carcinoma)

Clinical Findings. Although rare, this neoplasm which is a mixture of adenocarcinoma and squamous cell carcinoma is well known and found in many organs (1, 2). Clinical behavior is similar to duct cell adenocarcinoma (2).

Pathology. There is a mixture of adenocar-

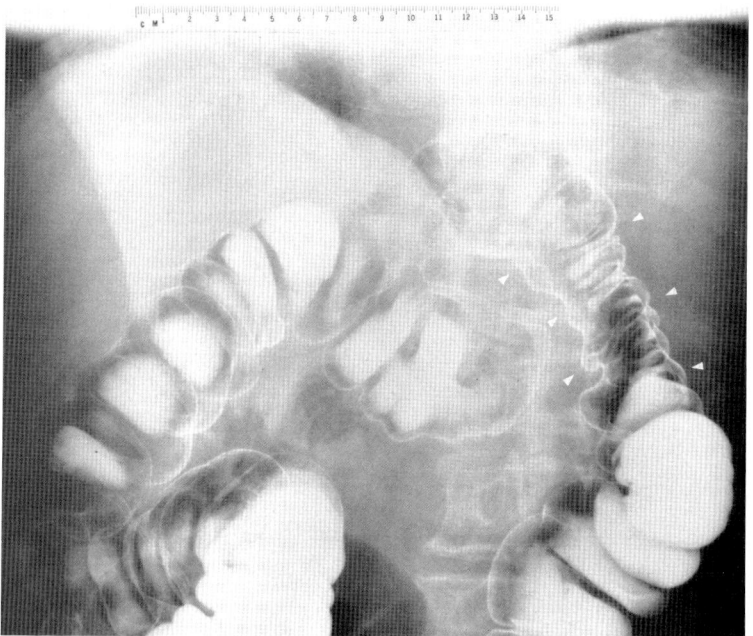

FIGURE 22.84. PANCREATIC ADENOSQUAMOUS CANCER
Mild narrowing with distorted but intact folds in the anatomic splenic flexture caused by adenosquamous carcinoma (*arrowheads*).

cinoma and squamous cell carcinoma. Either component may predominate (2). Desmoplastic response is prominent but hemorrhage and necrosis are not (2).

Radiology. The findings should be indistinguishable from duct cell adenocarcinoma (Fig. 22.84).

REFERENCES

1. Cihak RW, Kawashima, T, Steer A: Adenocanthoma (adenosquamous carcinoma) of the pancreas. *Cancer* 29:1133–1140, 1972.
2. Cubilla AL, Fitzgerald PJ: Cancer (non-endocrine) of the pancreas. A suggested classification. *Monogr Pathol* 21:91, 1980.

Mucinous Adenocarcinoma (Colloid Carcinoma)

This well-recognized, although uncommon, tumor is characterized by the presence of an extraordinary amount of mucin (1). Excess mucin production has caused biliary obstruction and renal tubular obstruction in these patients. Pseudomyxoma peritonei from peritoneal metastases can occur. Otherwise, clinical manifestations and tumor location are similar to duct cell carcinoma (1).

Mucinous adenocarcinomas are larger and softer than duct cell adenocarcinoma and grossly have a gelatinous appearance. Histologically, there are large cystic spaces filled with mucin and surrounded by connective tissue septa. Suspended in the mucin lakes are clumps of malignant columnar glandular epithelium, foci of mucinous carcinoma or signet ring adenocarcinoma cells. The malignant cells may be difficult to find (1).

Radiologic descriptions are sparse (2, 3). CT may demonstrate low density regions consistent with necrosis or mucin pools in the primary and show the associated pseudomyxoma peritonei if present (2). Calcification may occur in the primary and/or metastases after chemotherapy (3).

REFERENCES

1. Cubilla AL, Fitzgerald PJ: Cancer (non-endocrine) of the pancreas. A suggested classification. *Monogr Pathol* 21:92–95, 1980.
2. Gustafson KD, Karnaze GC, Hattery RR, Scheithauer BW: Pseudomyxoma peritonei associated with mucinous adenocarcinoma of the pancreas: CT findings and CT guided biopsy. *J Comput Assist Tomogr* 8:335–338, 1984.
3. Dastur KJ, Lewin JR: Computed tomography demonstration of tumor calcification after chemotherapy in a case of pancreatic carcinoma. *Comput Tomogr* 5:351–354, 1981.

Microadenocarcinoma

Epidemiology and clinical behavior and tumor location are not significantly different from duct cell carcinoma in this very rare type of pancreatic cancer (1). Microadenocarcinomas are relatively large (median diameter 14 cm) with more necrosis and less desmoplastic response than duct cell carcinoma. They are composed of glands smaller than those of duct cell carcinoma surrounded by solid foci of small cells. Electron microscopy shows an absence of zymogen and islet cell granules consistent with duct cell origin. Radiologic findings have not been described. We have seen one case in which CT demonstrated a large mass in the body with small low density areas consistent with necrosis that did not invade the retroperitoneum (Fig. 22.85). Angiography showed a hypervascular mass without major vessel encasement, findings suggesting that the mass was not duct cell adenocarcinoma (Fig. 22.86). Examination of the resected specimen showed pushing margins and absence of desmoplastic response, and a complete resection was thought to be accomplished.

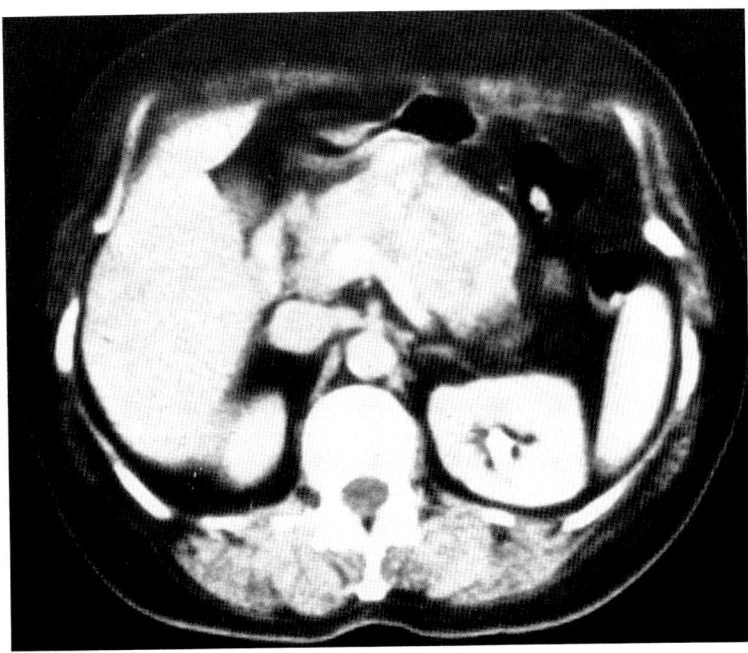

FIGURE 22.85. PANCREATIC MICROADENOCARCINOMA
CT scan showing a homogeneous, well-demarcated large mass in the body of the pancreas without evidence of extrapancreatic spread.

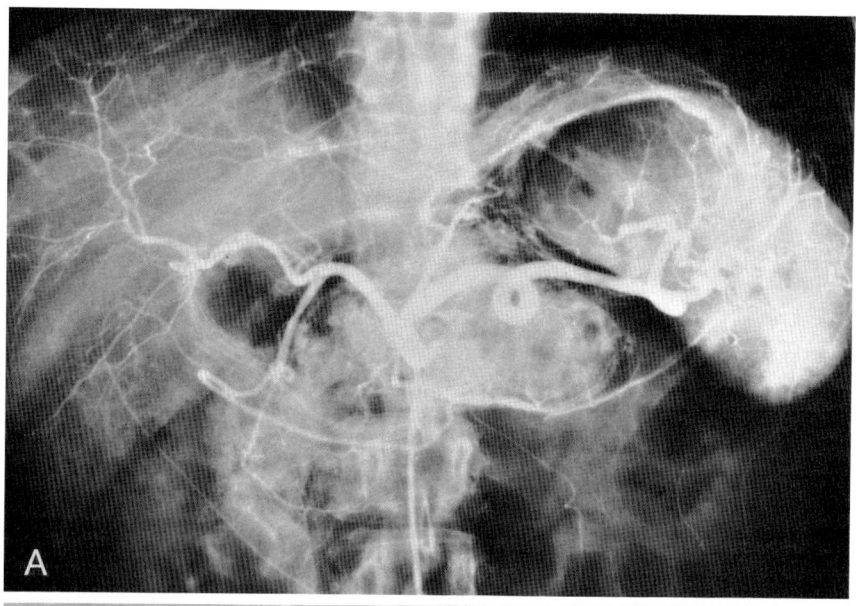
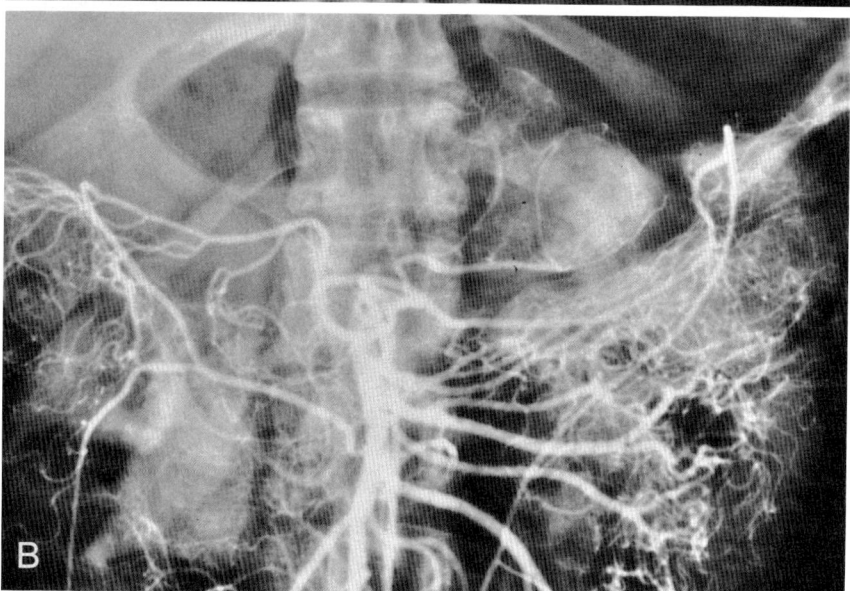

FIGURE 22.86. PANCREATIC MICROADENOCARCINOMA
Celiac and superior mesenteric arteriograms demonstrate a hypervascular mass in the body of the pancreas.

REFERENCES

1. Cubilla AL, Fitzgerald PJ: Cancer (non-endocrine) of the pancreas. A suggested classification. *Monogr Pathol* 21:92, 1980.

Anaplastic Carcinoma

This is a group of malignant neoplasms (about 5% of pancreatic cancers) that are undifferentiated. Clinical features are similar to duct cell adenocarcinoma and prognosis is very poor. Hemorrhage and necrosis are not prominent. Histologically, there are large cell, small cell and clear cell varieties in descending order of frequency (1). The small cell variety is hard to distinguish from poorly differentiated lymphoma, and clear cell tumors are similar in appearance to carcinomas of the kidney or adrenal (1).

Radiologically, anaplastic carcinomas are large, aggressive solid masses similar in appearance to duct cell adenocarcinomas (Figs. 22.87 and 22.88).

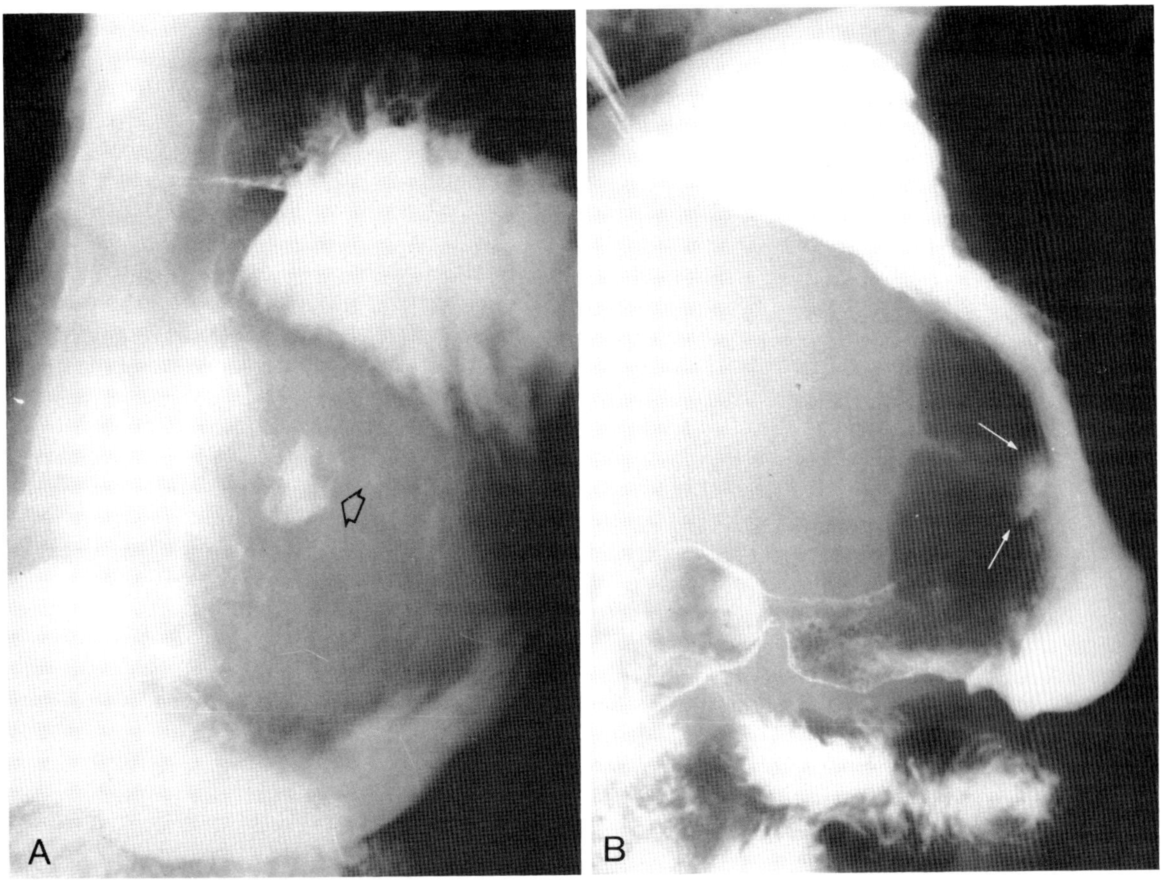

FIGURE 22.87. PANCREATIC ANAPLASTIC CARCINOMA
A and *B:* Anteroposterior and lateral views of the stomach showing a large retrogastric mass invading the stomach producing ulceration (*arrows*).

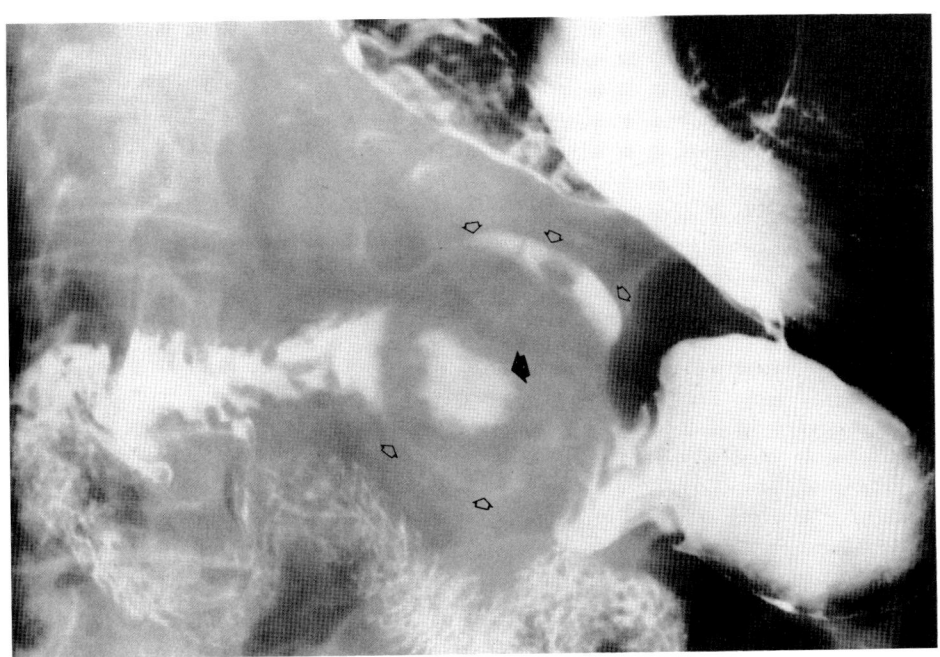

FIGURE 22.88. PANCREATIC ANAPLASTIC CARCINOMA
Anaplastic carcinoma of the pancreas pancaking the duodenal bulb (*open arrows*) and invading, causing a large ulcer (*arrow*).

REFERENCE

1. Cubilla AL, Fitzgerald PJ: Cancer (non-endocrine) of the pancreas. A suggested classification. *Monogr Pathol* 21:104, 1980.

Solid and Papillary Epithelial Neoplasm

(This lesion is also referred to as papillary and cystic neoplasm, papillary cystic carcinoma, or papillary epithelial neoplasm.)

Clinical Findings. First characterized by Hamoudi in 1970 (1), this is an uncommon tumor found chiefly in young females (2). The mean age is 24 and one-third occur in adolescents (3). Presenting symptoms and signs are progressive abdominal discomfort and enlarging abdominal mass, frequently in the left upper quadrant (there is a predilection for the tail). These neoplasms are often first noted in teenagers after abdominal trauma (3). Only 3 instances of metastases after resection have been documented in a series of 74 cases (3) and 1 case of a nonfatal recurrence after incomplete resection has been reported (4). Duration of follow-up is limited and this tumor is currently considered to be a low grade malignancy which is curable in most cases by complete resection (3).

Pathology. Solid and papillary epithelial neoplasms of the pancreas are large, encapsulated masses (mean 10 cm diameter) (2). The vessels within the tumor are thin-walled with little connective tissue support, resulting in frequent hemorrhage (3). Focal necrosis leading to cystic change is common (3). Microscopically, there is limited, if any, evidence of aggressive behavior consisting of capsular invasion, extension into adjacent parenchyma and vascular invasion. The neoplastic cells are polygonal to somewhat elongated, slightly eosinophilic with small ovoid nuclei (3). They are arranged in both a solid pattern and a papillary pattern with a fibrovascular core (Fig. 22.89) (2, 3). Stains for mucin are negative (3). These neoplasms are often misclassified as islet cell tumors and mucinous cystic neoplasms (2). Electron microscopy reveals an absence of zymogen and islet cell granules and the presence of features suggesting a small duct origin in most cases reported to date (3, 4).

Radiology. Plain films and barium contrast studies demonstrate a nonspecific soft tissue mass (Fig. 22.91*A* and *B*). Calcification is uncommon but is peripheral when present (Fig. 22.90*A* and *B*). Sonography will depict a well demarcated echogenic mass with hypoechoic areas of varying number and size depending on the degree of hemorrhage and necrosis (Figs. 22.91*C* and *F*, 22.92*A* and *C*, and 22.93*A*). CT shows a well-demarcated muscle density mass containing low density areas of variable size corresponding to hemorrhage and necrosis (Figs. 22.91*D* and *F*, 22.92*B* and *C*, and 22.93*B* and *C*). In extreme instances of hemorrhage both modalities will depict a thick-walled "cyst" with a ragged inner margin (Fig. 22.92). The CT numbers in the "cysts" may be higher than water, correctly suggesting old blood and necrotic debris. Angiography generally shows a mildly vascular mass on celiac injections and a moderately vascular mass on superselective injections (Fig. 22.91*E*). Avascular areas will be present if there has been sufficient hemorrhage and/or necrosis. Splenic artery encasement can occur but is unusual.

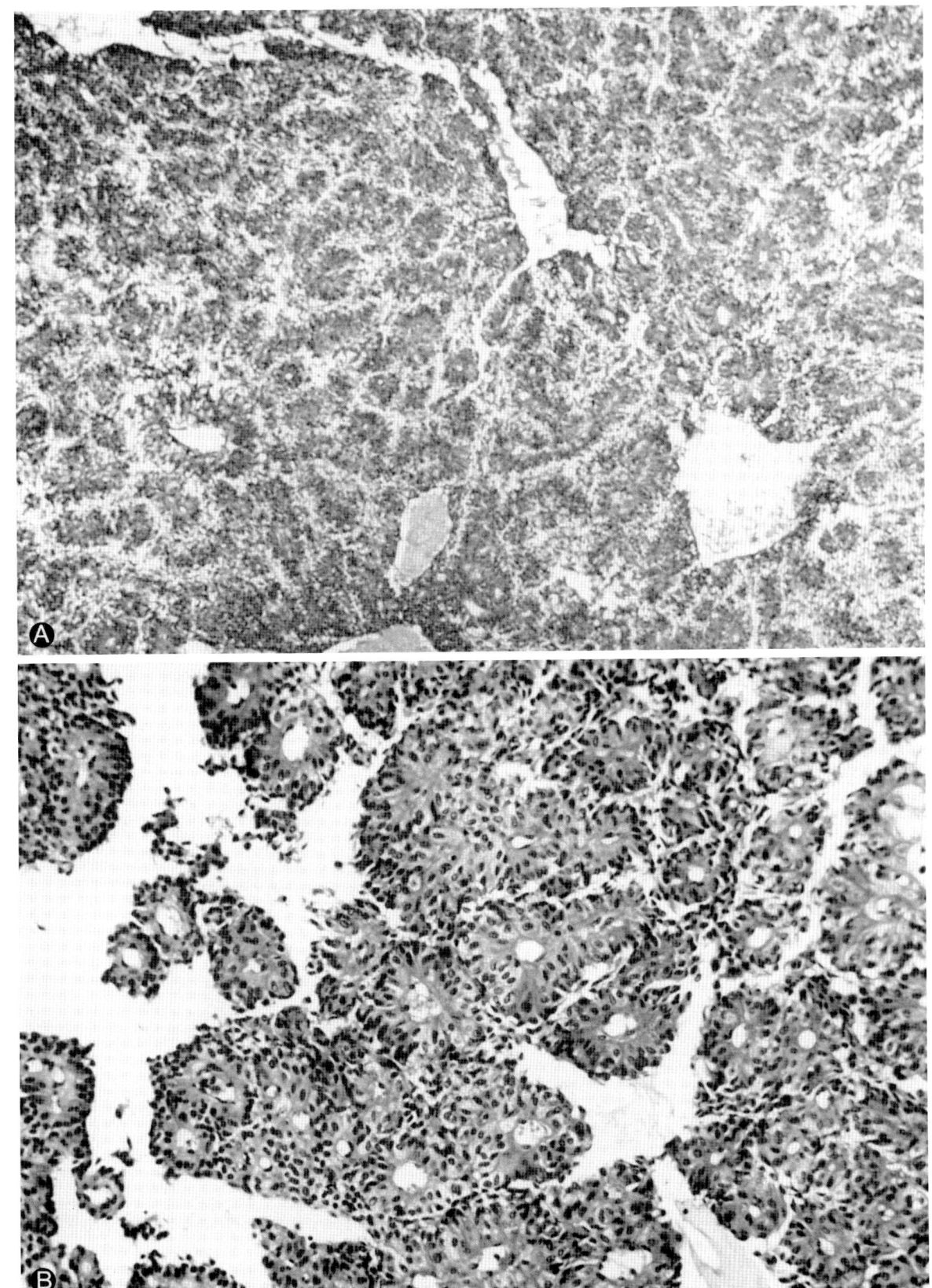

FIGURE 22.89. SOLID AND PAPILLARY EPITHELIAL NEOPLASM
A and *B:* Microscopy of a solid and papillary epithelial neoplasm showing a predominantly solid pattern (*A*) and a papillary pattern (*B*) in two different fields. The clear spaces are clefts where cells have died.

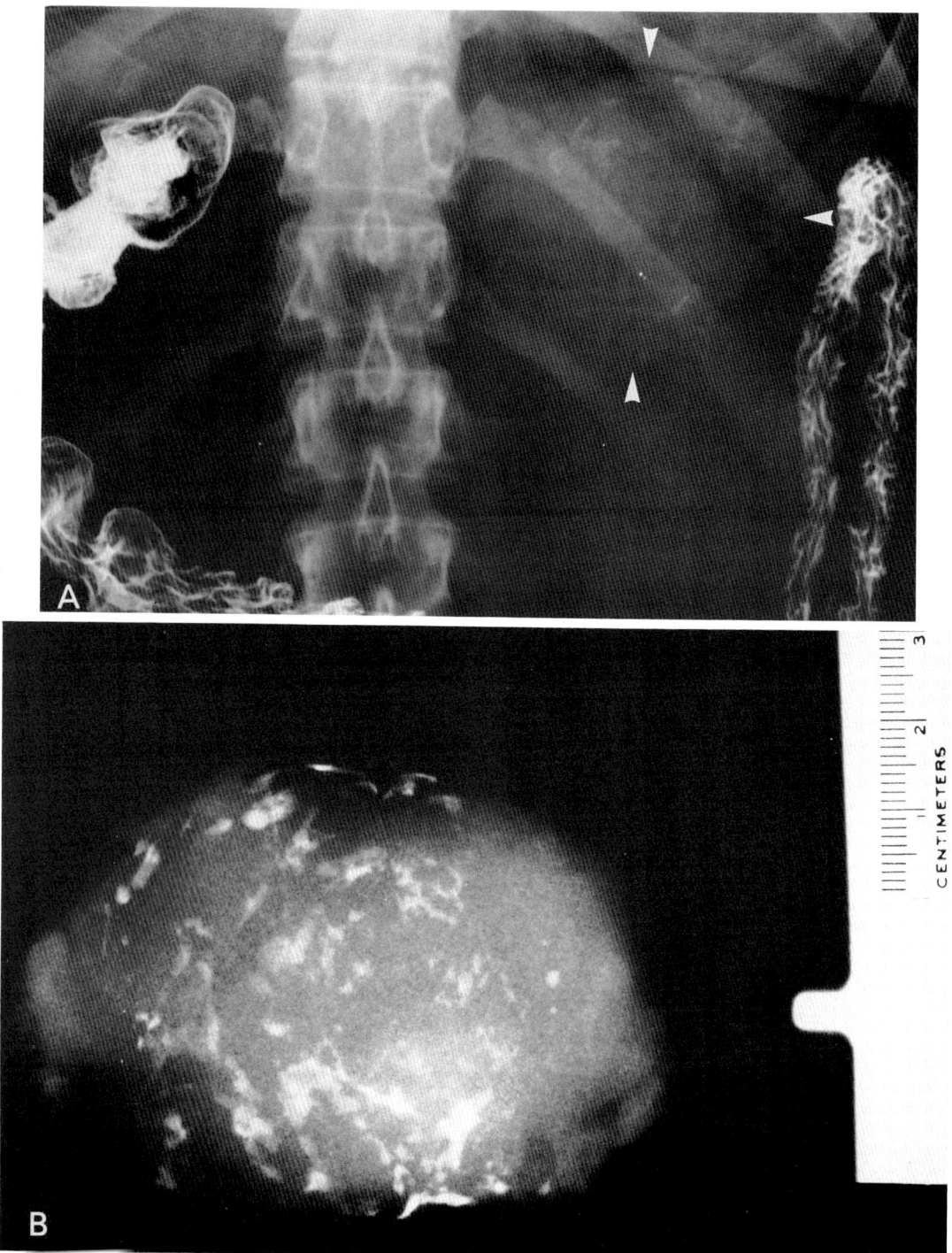

FIGURE 22.90. SOLID AND PAPILLARY EPITHELIAL NEOPLASM
A: Evacuation film from a barium enema showing a peripherally calcified left upper quadrant mass (*arrowheads*): solid and papillary epithelial neoplasm. *B:* Specimen radiograph.

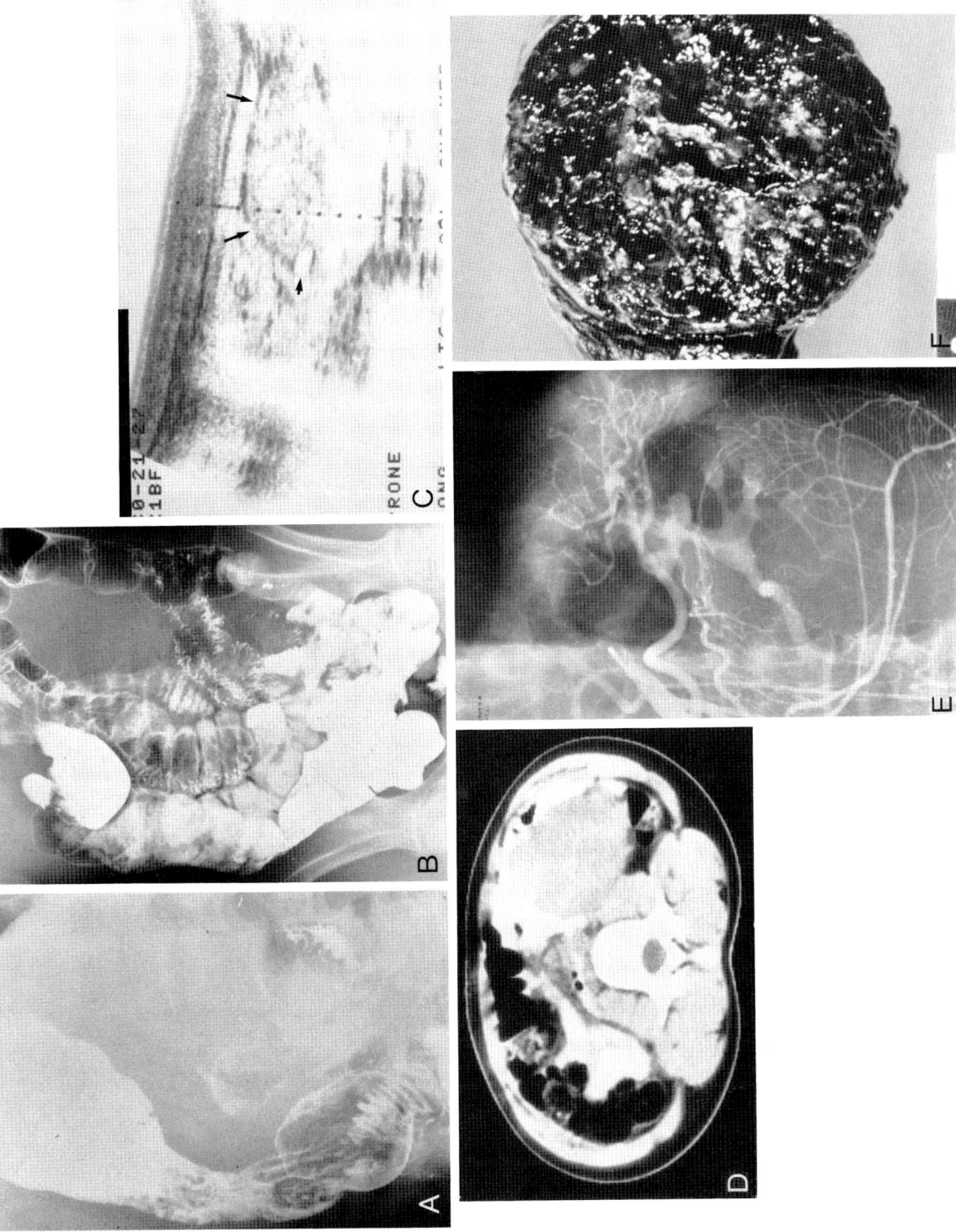

FIGURE 22.91. SOLID AND PAPILLARY EPITHELIAL NEOPLASM

A and *B*: Gastrointestinal contrast examinations showing a large retrogastric mass indenting the colon and no evidence of invasion. *C*: Parasagittal sonogram of the same patient showing a well-demarcated solid mass (*large arrows*) with a small hypoechoic region (*small arrow*). *D*: CT scan of the same patient showing a well-demarcated homogenous mass approximately muscle density. *E*: Moderately vascular mass on angiography. *F*: Gross specimen showing an encapsulated well-demarcated large mass with small areas of hemorrhage, one of which was probably the small sonolucency. The CT was homogenous because the blood had the same attenuation as the solid portion.

849

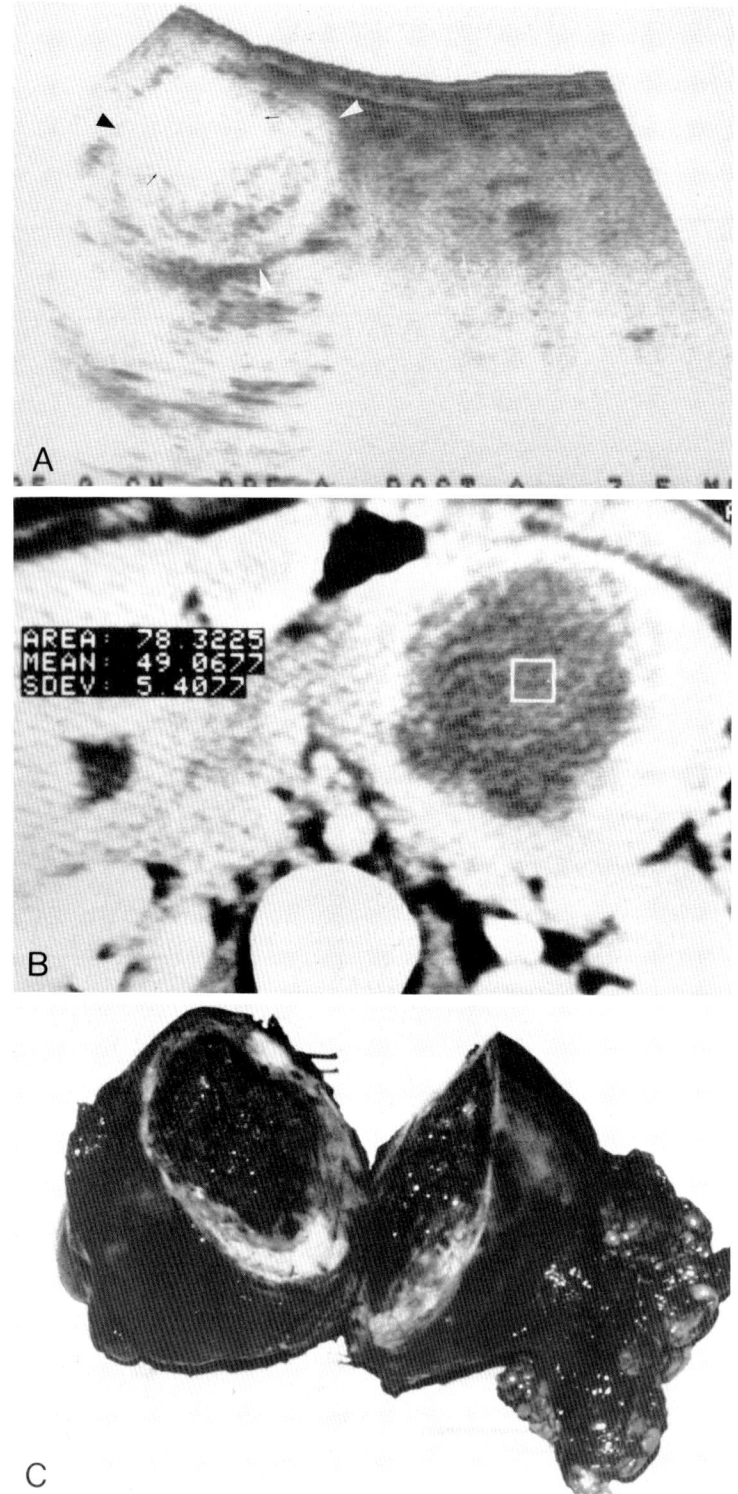

FIGURE 22.92. SOLID PANCREATIC AND PAPILLARY EPITHELIAL NEOPLASM
A: Parasagittal sonograms 5 cm to the left of midline of a solid and papillary epithelial neoplasm (*arrowheads*) with a large sonolucent component (*small arrows*). *B:* CT scan of the same patient showing a thick-walled "cyst" in the pancreatic tail. The low density component measures 49 HU, consistent with blood. *C:* Gross specimen showing a thick-walled cystic mass with a ragged lining. The blood filling the cavity was evacuated prior to photography.

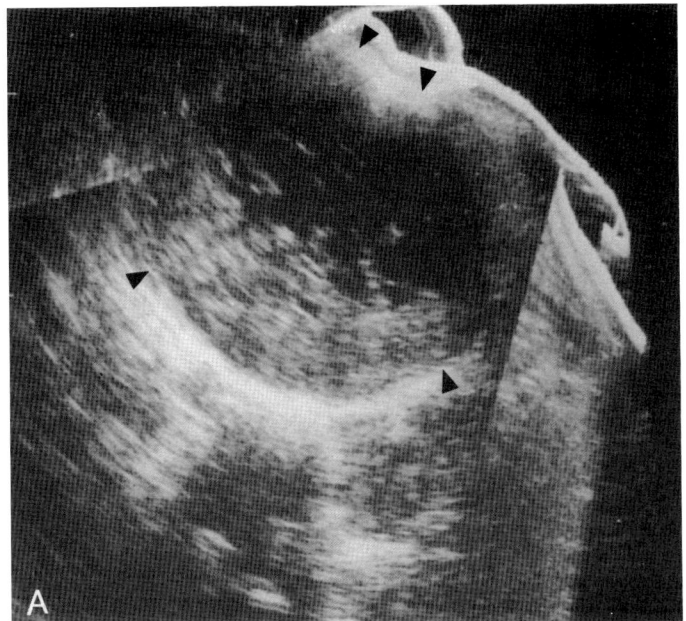
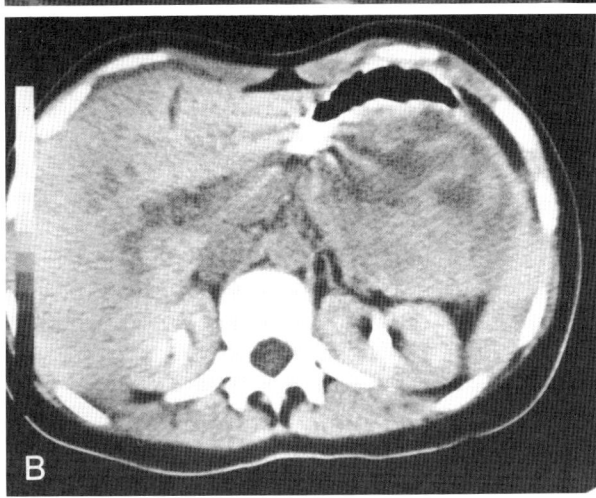
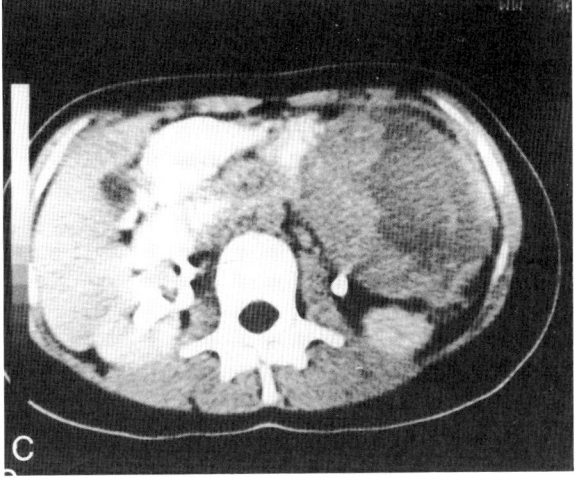

FIGURE 22.93. SOLID AND PAPILLARY EPITHELIAL NEOPLASM
A: Transverse sonogram in a left-upper decubitus position showing a partially necrotic solid and papillary epithelial neoplasm (*arrowheads*) in the tail. *B:* and *C:* CT scans of the same patient showing a low density region corresponding to the sonolucencies representing necrosis. The mass displaces stomach and bowel without appearing to invade.

REFERENCES

1. Hamoudi AB, Misugi K, Grosfeld JL, Reiner CR: Papillary epithelial neoplasm of pancreas in a child. *Cancer* 26:1126–1134, 1970.
2. Compagno J, Oertel JE, Krezmar M: Solid and papillary epithelial neoplasm of the pancreas, probably of small duct origin: a clinicopathologic study of 52 cases (abstract). *Lab Invest* 40:248–249, 1979.
3. Oertel JE, Mendelsohn G, Compagno J: Solid and papillary epithelial neoplasms of the pancreas. In Humphrey GB (ed): *Pancreatic Tumors in Children.* The Hague, Martinus Nijhoff, 1982, pp 167–171.
4. Cubilla AL, Fitzgerald J: Cancer (non-endocrine) of the pancreas. A suggested classification. *Monogr Pathol* 21:102–104, 1980.

ACINAR CELL ORIGIN

Acinar Cell Carcinoma (1)

This uncommon tumor is usually indistinguishable from duct cell adenocarcinoma clinically (Fig. 22.94). However, subcutaneous fat necrosis and polyarthralgia have been reported in lipase-secreting acinar cell carcinomas. Necrosis is a prominent feature of these tumors. Microscopically, the tumors are composed of solid nests of cells which in their better differentiated forms closely resemble those found in normal acini. Differentiation from islet cell tumor may require immunoperoxidase staining and/or electron microscopy. Radiologic findings are not de-

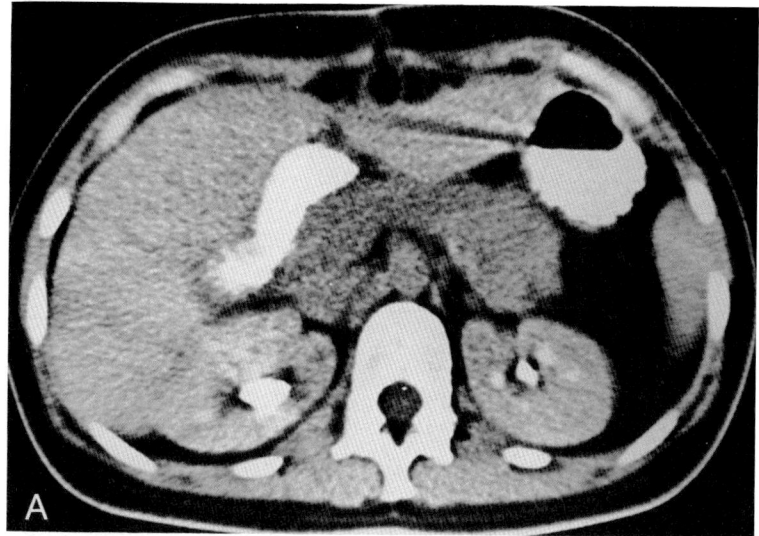

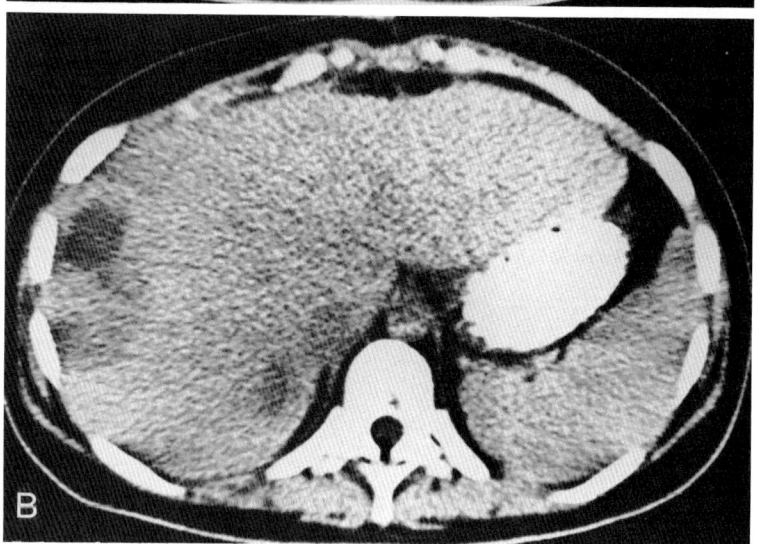

FIGURE 22.94. ACINAR CELL CARCINOMA
A: and *B:* Nonspecific mass in the tail of the pancreas in a 28-yr-old woman: acinar cell carcinoma (*A*). Liver metastases were present (*B*).

scribed, but should correlate with gross pathology.

Acinar Cell Cystadenocarcinoma (1, 2)

One case with radiologic findings has been reported in a 64-yr-old man of a 35-cm multiloculated cystic mass in the body and tail of the pancreas of acinar cell origin. Cyst size varied from microscopic to 7 cm in diameter. Metastases were present in the peritoneal cavity and liver. Most cysts were lined with a single layer of flattened cuboidal epithelium, but regions of columnar epithelium were present. Acini were present, as were papilla projecting into the cysts. Stains for mucin and glycogen were negative, but a histochemical stain for trypsin was positive. Electron microscopy showed intracytoplasmic zymogen granules. The patient survived for 7 months after surgery.

Sonography and CT in this case demonstrated a mixed cystic and solid mass, probably indistinguishable from a mucinous cystic neoplasm.

REFERENCES

1. Cubilla AL, Fitzgerald PJ: Cancer (non-endocrine) of the pancreas. A suggested classification. *Monogr Pathol* 21:99–100, 1980.
2. Cantrell BB, Cubilla AL, Erlandson RA, Fortner J, Fitzgerald PJ: Acinar cell cystadenocarcinoma of human pancreas. *Cancer* 47:410–416, 1981.

INDETERMINATE ORIGIN

Pancreaticoblastoma (Infantile Carcinoma of the Pancreas)

This is a rare neoplasm whose uniqueness is based on age (patients younger than 7 yr old), location (head of the pancreas), and histopathology (1). It arises in the ventral pancreas and is thought to be caused by a disturbance in organogenesis due to failure of the duct of Wirsung to communicate with the duct of Santorini and the ampulla (1). Prognosis is good if the tumor is discovered prior to metastasis (1, 2).

Grossly, pancreaticoblastomas are generally large (4–11 cm in largest diameter) (1, 2), encapsulated masses with considerable hemorrhage and necrosis and some cystic degeneration (2).

Pancreaticoblastomas are composed of sheets of small cells with clear cytoplasm and larger acinar cells with zymogen granules (1, 2). There are regions of spindle cells and chondroid, osteoid or bone tissue (1, 2), indicating a hamartoblastomatous nature (1, 2). Potential misdiagnoses are islet cell tumor and neuroblastoma (1–3).

Plain films and barium contrast studies have shown nonspecific soft tissue masses displacing but not invading the duodenum and antrum (1–3). Sonography and CT would be expected to depict a well-demarcated mixed solid and cystic tumor on the basis of the gross morphology (Fig. 22.95) (4).

REFERENCES

1. Horie A, Yano Y, Kotoo Y, Miwa A: Morphogenesis of pancreaticoblastoma, infantile carcinoma of the pancreas. *Cancer* 39:247–254, 1977.
2. Cubilla AL, Fitzgerald PJ: Cancer (non-endocrine) of the pancreas. A suggested classification. *Monogr Pathol* 21:100, 1980.
3. Frable WL, Still WJS, Kay S: Carcinoma of the pancreas. Infantile type. *Cancer* 27:667–673, 1971.
4. Robey G, Daneman A, Martin DJ: Pancreatic carcinoma in a neonate. *Pediatr Radiol* 13:284–286, 1983.

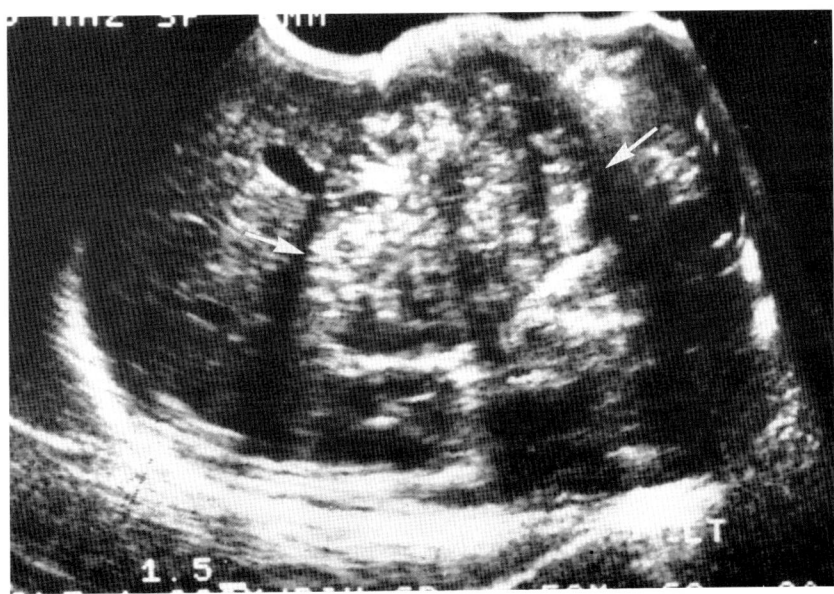

FIGURE 22.95. PANCREATICOBLASTOMA
Transverse sonogram showing a large round, echogenic mass (*arrows*) in the region of the pancreas.

Ductuloinsular Tumors

The neoplastic proliferation of both duct cells and islet cells in a single tumor can be explained by recalling the embryologic development of islets from ducts. Because of the small number of these tumors reported to date, definite statements about clinical associations and behavior cannot be made. Based on histologic evidence of infiltrative growth and nodal metastasis, these tumors are likely to be slowly progressive low grade malignancies. Microscopically, both mucin-producing duct cells and cells indistinguishable from those in islet cell tumors are present (1). Islet cell granules are present by immunoperoxidase stains and electron microscopy, but clinical symptoms from excess hormones are lacking (1).

Ultrasound, CT, cholangiography, and pancreatography have shown findings indistinguishable from duct cell adenocarcinoma or nonfunctioning islet cell tumor (1).

REFERENCES

1. Reid JD, Yuh S, Petrelli M, Jaffe R: Ductuloinsular tumors of the pancreas. *Cancer* 49:908-915, 1982.

CONNECTIVE TISSUE TUMORS

Benign mesenchymal tumors have been described in the pancreas, but are extremely rare and are comparable to those lesions found elsewhere (1).

Primary sarcomas of the pancreas are reported in older literature, but since giant cell carcinomas and anaplastic carcinomas are easily confused with spindle cell sarcomas, the diagnosis of primary pancreatic sarcoma must be viewed with skepticism (2, 3).

REFERENCES

1. Robbins SL, Cotran SR: *Pathologic Basis of Disease.* Philadelphia, W. B. Saunders, 1979, p. 1113.
2. Rosai J: *Ackerman's Surgical Pathology.* St. Louis, C. V. Mosby, 1981, p 89.
3. Cubilla AL, Fitzgerald PJ: Cancer (non-endocrine) of the pancreas. A suggested classification. *Mongr Pathol* 21:107, 1980.

METASTASES, LYMPHOMA, AND LEUKEMIA

Metastases

The pancreas is infrequently clinically involved by metastatic disease and such involvement is usually from direct extension from a contiguous organ (1). Distant metastasis to the pancreatic parenchyma is quite uncommon but involvement of peripancreatic nodes is not (1). It is often difficult to distinguish true metastasis to the pancreas from metastatic disease of adjacent nodes with secondary extension into the pancreas (1). Breast, lung, and melanoma are the most common primary cancers to metastasize to the pancreas (Figs. 22.96-22.98) (2).

Radiologic findings will be similar to pancreatic adenocarcinoma or lymphoma depending on whether the metastatic tumor is unifocal or multifocal. If the metastatic tumor produces pancreatic ductal obstruction, both the clinical and radiologic findings may be those of pancreatitis (Figs. 22.96 and 22.97).

REFERENCES

1. Robbins SL, Cotran SR: *Pathologic Basis of Disease.* Philadelphia, W. B. Saunders, 1979, p 1113.
2. Cubilla AL, Fitzgerald PJ: Cancer (non-endocrine) of the pancreas. A suggested classification. *Monogr Pathol* 21:108, 1980.

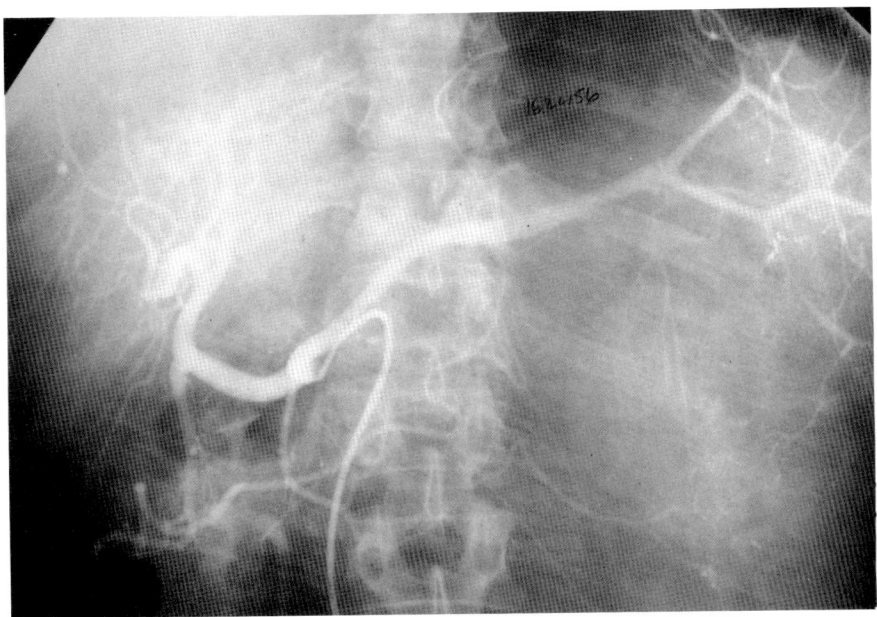

FIGURE 22.96. METASTASIS TO PANCREAS

Celiac angiogram in a patient with lung carcinoma presenting with abdominal pain and a large, palpable mass. The splenic artery and its branches are straightened and stretched. At surgery the pancreas was enlarged and replaced by metastatic carcinoma. There was evidence of pancreatitis as well.

FIGURE 22.97. METASTASIS TO PANCREAS

ERCP in a patient with oat cell carcinoma and common bile duct and obstruction of the main pancreatic duct from metastases to the head of the pancreas.

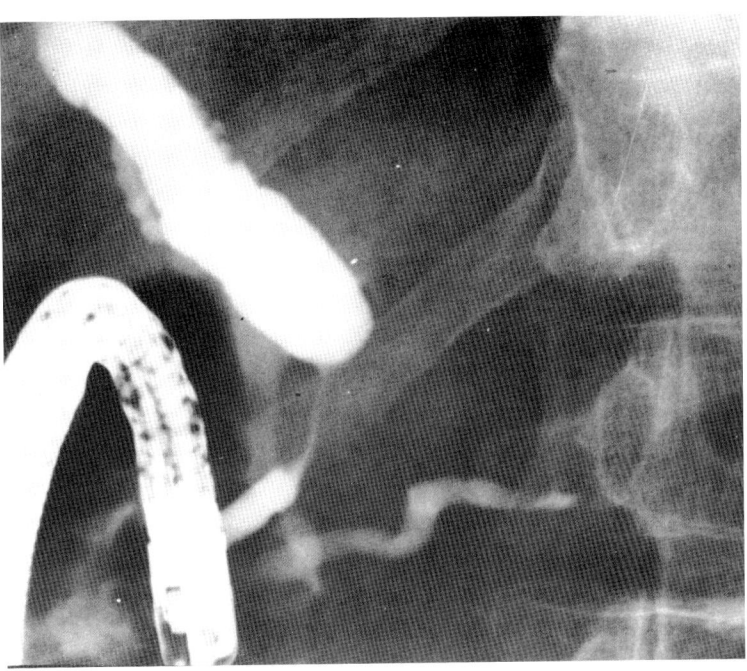

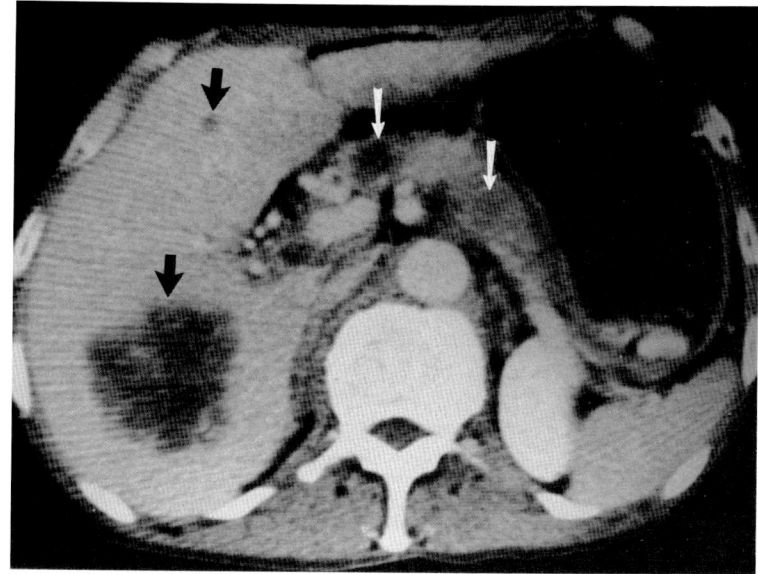

FIGURE 22.98. METASTASIS TO PANCREAS: CONTRAST ENHANCED CT
Gastric carcinoma with two intrapancreatic metastases (*white arrows*) noted as incidental findings in an examination performed to rule out liver metastases, two of which are shown (*black arrows*). The metastases are unenhanced filling defects in the enhanced pancreatic parenchyma.

Lymphoma and Leukemia

Intrinsic pancreatic involvement is extremely rare in Hodgkin disease, although occasionally present in non-Hodgkin lymphoma (1% at staging) (1). However, the incidence of peripancreatic/pancreatic involvement is markedly increased in histiocytic lymphoma and American Burkitt lymphoma compared to other non-Hodgkin lymphomas (2, 3). It is difficult to distinguish peripancreatic nodal disease from intrinsic pancreatic lymphoma because of the absence of a well-defined capsule around the pancreas (1). Adding to the difficulty is the possibility of invasion of the pancreas by tumor in adjacent nodes. Localized intra-abdominal histiocytic lymphoma simulating a pancreatic mass on both upper gastrointestinal series and CT was found in 9% of a large series of histologic lymphoma patients at staging (2). At autopsy the pancreatic/peripancreatic area was involved in approximately 30%.

American Burkitt lymphoma commonly involves the pancreatic region (82% in one autopsy series) (3). The usual gross appearance is multifocal masses. Diffuse pancreatic enlargement is not uncommon and can be due to diffuse pancreatic tumor, tumor-induced pancreatitis (from ductal obstruction) or pancreatitis associated with tumor lysis from chemotherapy (3).

Leukemia involves the pancreas at autopsy in 10–20% of cases, but does not produce clinical pancreatic disease (1).

Radiology. Since peripancreatic nodal masses cannot always be distinguished from intrapancreatic masses and duct cell adenocarcinoma can cause lymph node enlargement, differentiation of peripancreatic lymphoma from carcinoma of the pancreas is difficult. Features favoring lymphoma are massive and/or widespread adenopathy, multifocality and the presence of a very hypoechoic mass which is solid on CT (Figs. 22.99 and 22.100). The diffuse pancreatic involvement of American Burkitt lymphoma cannot be differentiated from pancreatitis except by needle biopsy (Fig. 22.101) (3). Data regarding radiologic appearances of leukemia in the pancreas are not available (1). On angiography, vascular displacement and stretching out of proportion to encasement and obstruction favors lymphoma, although the distinction is difficult (Fig. 22.102).

REFERENCES

1. Castellino RA, Marglin S, Blank N: Hodgkin disease, the non-Hodgkin lymphomas and the leukemias in the retroperitoneum. *Semin Roentgenol* 15:288–301, 1980.
2. Burgener FA, Hamlin DG: Histiocytic lymphoma of the abdomen: radiographic spectrum. *AJR* 137:337–342, 1981.
3. Francis IR, Glazer GM: Burkitt's lymphoma of the pancreas presenting as acute pancreatitis. *J Comput Assist Tomogr* 6:395–397, 1982.

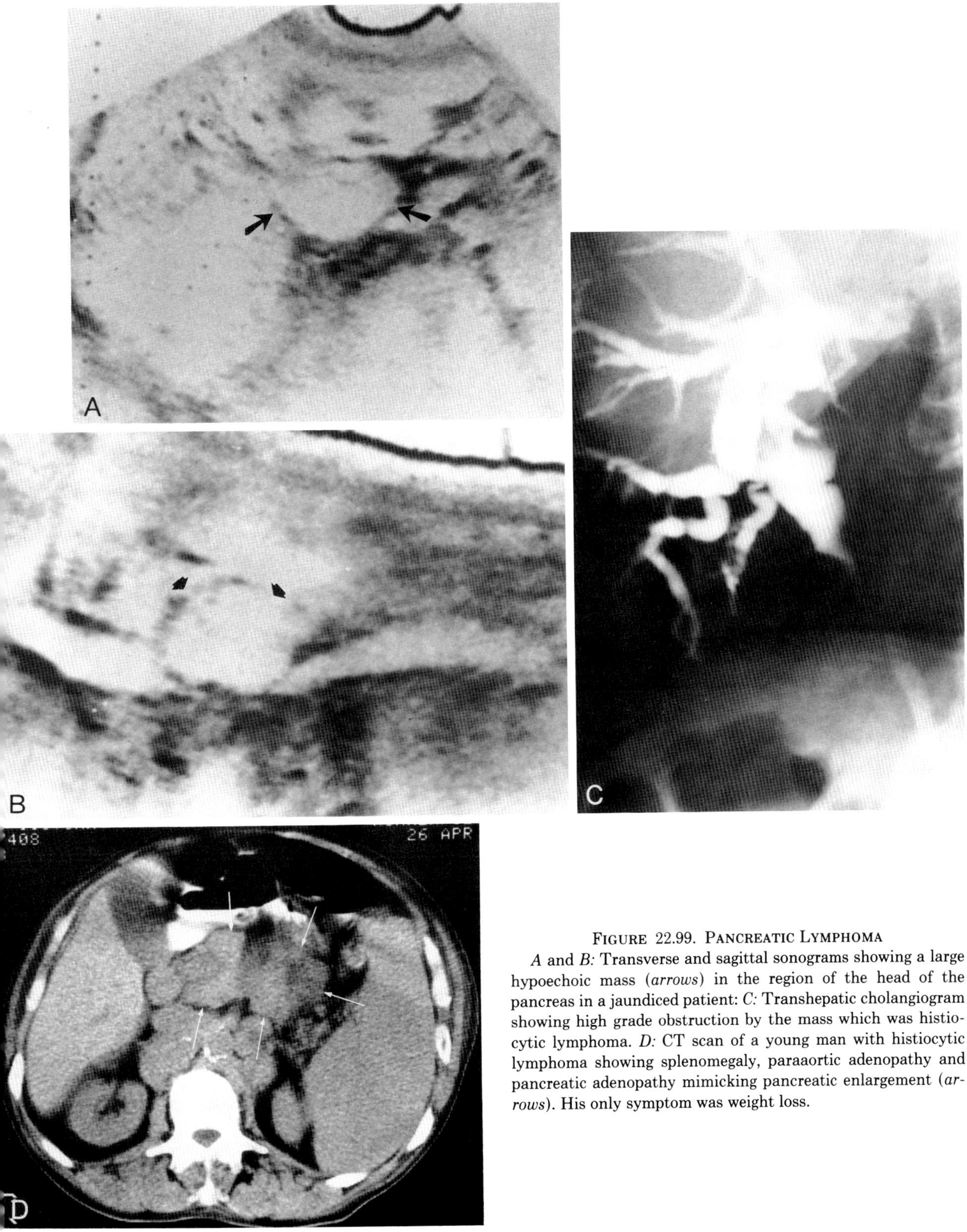

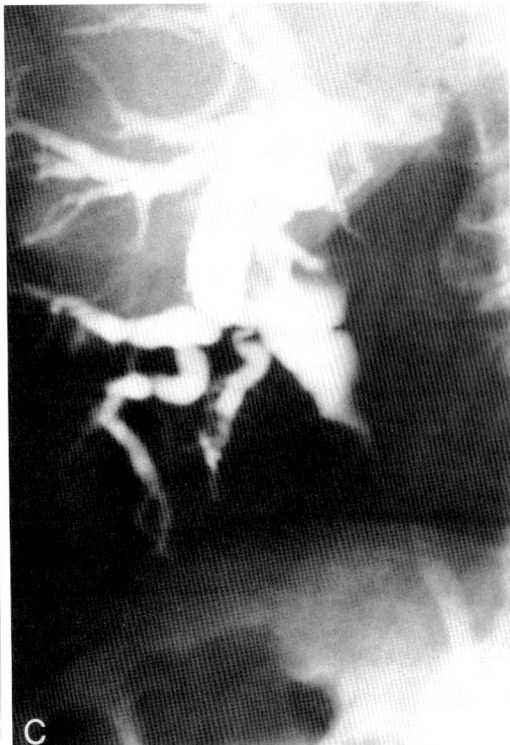
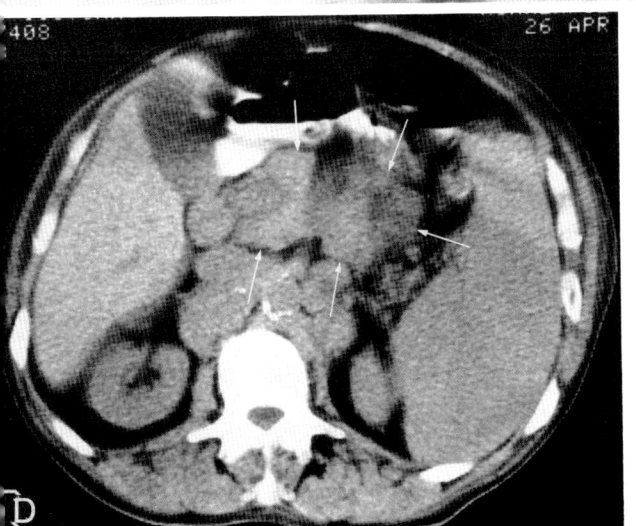

FIGURE 22.99. PANCREATIC LYMPHOMA

A and *B:* Transverse and sagittal sonograms showing a large hypoechoic mass (*arrows*) in the region of the head of the pancreas in a jaundiced patient: *C:* Transhepatic cholangiogram showing high grade obstruction by the mass which was histiocytic lymphoma. *D:* CT scan of a young man with histiocytic lymphoma showing splenomegaly, paraaortic adenopathy and pancreatic adenopathy mimicking pancreatic enlargement (*arrows*). His only symptom was weight loss.

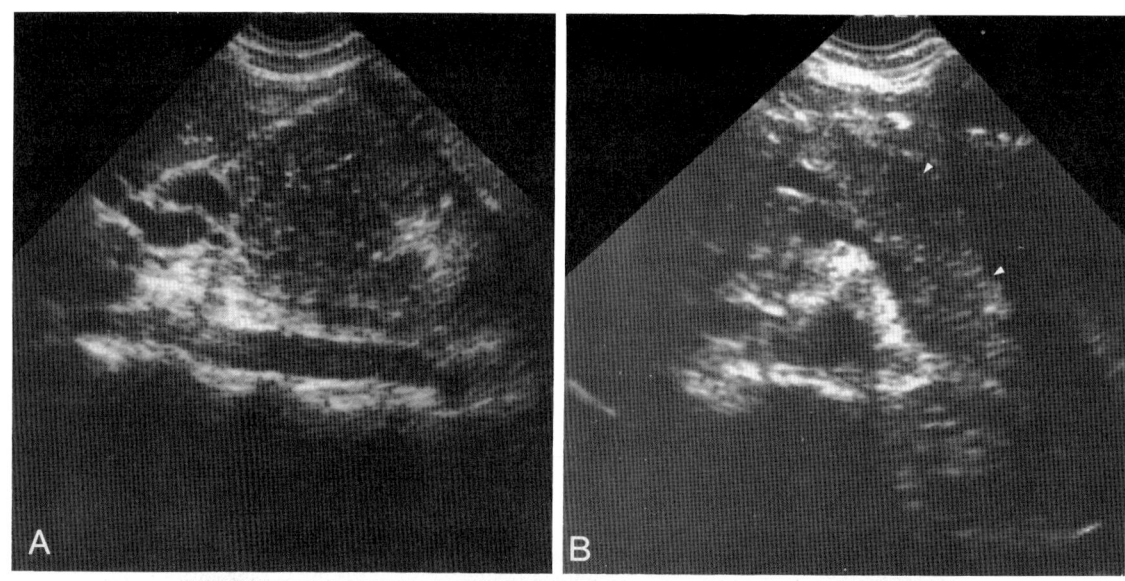
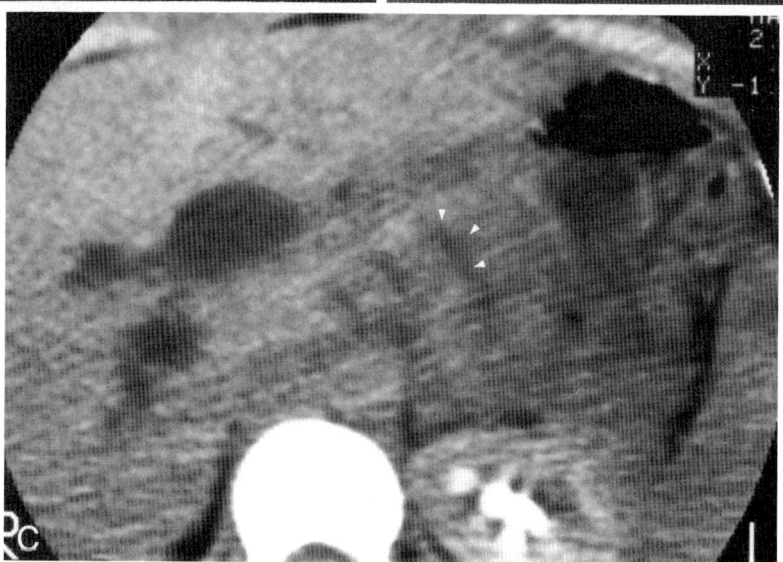
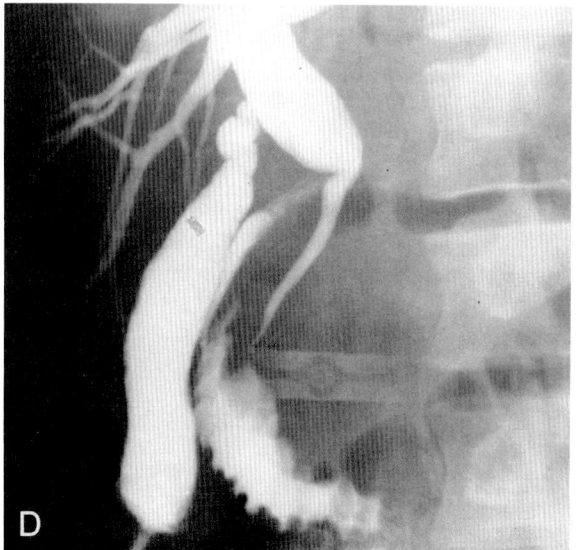

FIGURE 22.100. PANCREATIC LYMPHOMA
A–D: Young man with histiocytic lymphoma presenting with jaundice, fever chills, pain, and elevated amylase. Sagittal sonography shows a huge peripancreatic mass obstructing the common duct (*A*). The tail of the pancreas (*arrowheads*) is enlarged from pancreatitis on a transverse scan (*B*). CT shows biliary obstruction and a dilated pancreatic duct (*arrowheads, C*). *D:* Emergency cholecystostomy was done. A tube cholangiogram 2 days later shows a long segment narrowing of the distal common duct and widening of the duodenal sweep with padding from peripancreatic adenopathy and pancreatitis. The patient improved with chemotherapy.

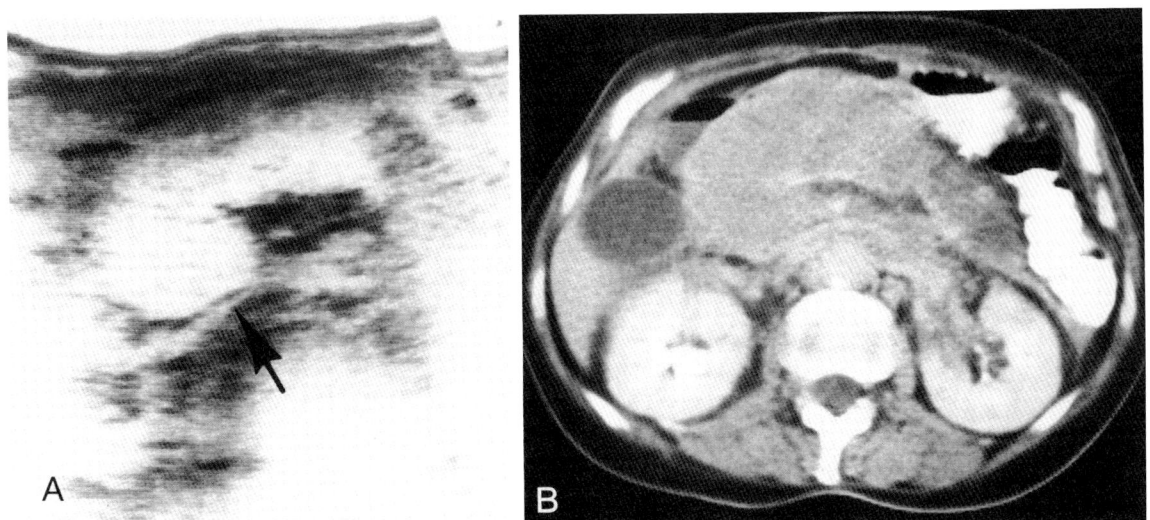

FIGURE 22.101. PANCREATIC LYMPHOMA

Burkitt's lymphoma in the head of the pancreas causing pancreatitis. *A:* Transverse sonogram in a patient with American Burkitt's lymphoma and acute pancreatitis clinically showing diffuse pancreatic enlargement, most marked in the head and uncinate process (*arrow*). *B:* CT of the same patient shows anterior pararenal effusion in addition to the enlarged pancreas. Biopsy of the head of the pancreas showed Burkitt's lymphoma. (Case courtesy of Gary M. Glazer, M.D.; reprinted from Kent et al., 1981).

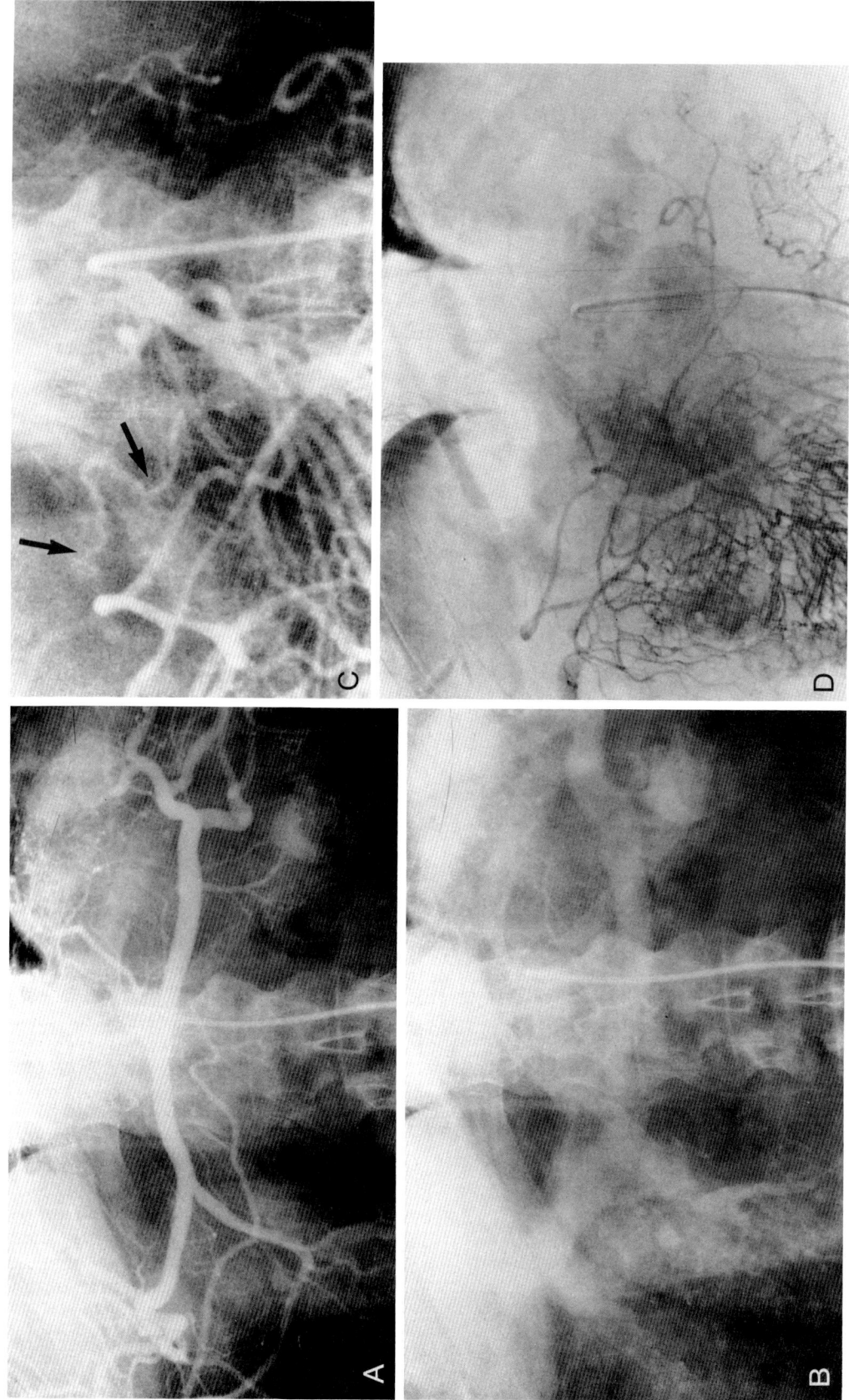

FIGURE 22.102. PERIPANCREATIC LYMPHOSARCOMA

A: Celiac arteriogram: stretching of splenic and common hepatic arteries. No encasement. *B*: Stretching of the splenic vein without encasement. *C*: Superior mesenteric arteriogram: encasement of inferior pancreaticoduodenal artery (*arrows*). *D*: Large peripancreatic tumor blush is against duct cell carcinoma.

ISLET CELL TUMORS

Although islet cell tumors are rarer than exocrine tumors of the pancreas, their detection and localization are important because they are more amenable to treatment. Careful autopsy can reveal islet cell adenomas in up to 1.57% of the population—most of these are not manifest clinically. Islet cell carcinoma has an incidence of about 1 in 100,000. Approximately 85% of clinically manifest islet cell tumors are hormonally active as they probably arise from multipotential stem cells in ductal epithelium, the same cell line that produces the islets of Langerhans (1-3). The exact origin of this cell line is unknown but it is presumed to be neuroectodermal. These cells are referred to as the APUD system and are characterized by cytochemical attributes of *a*mine *p*recursor *u*ptake and *d*ecarboxylation. This concept was introduced in 1968 by Pearse (4) who observed that endocrine cells of the gastrointestinal tract had cytochemical characteristics similar to centrally located neural ganglion cells. A common origin of these cells with similar histochemical and biochemical properties from the neuroectoderm was postulated. The potential for the secretion of multiple hormones is thought to be a common feature of APUD cells which is manifest with neoplastic transformation. The APUD system also partially explains the multicentric and multiorgan origin of tumors in the multiple endocrine neoplasia (MEN) syndromes in which multiple tumors arising in a single organ or in multiple organs can secrete different polypeptides (5). As a consequence of the hormone activity of islet cell tumors, patients will present with a characteristic clinical syndrome and appropriately elevated hormone levels. Metastases usually, but not always, secrete the same hormone as the primary. Currently, based on the predominant hormone produced, at least six varieties of islet cell tumors are recognized. The tumor is named after the hormone it produces. Often, multiple hormones are produced by the same tumor. Usually, only one hormone produces symptoms and the tumor is named accordingly. Otherwise the tumor is classified as multiple (2). Nonfunctional (or hypofunctional) islet cell tumors have no clinical symptoms related to excess hormone production.

Common Pathologic Features of Islet Cell Tumors

Islet cell tumors are evenly distributed over the gland without predilection for the tail as previously thought (1, 2). Gross clinical symptoms are uncommon in tumors of less than 5 g, otherwise size is not related to the severity of symptoms (2). There are three growth patterns: trabecular (ribbon-like) closely resembling normal islets with rows of cells bordering a rich capillary network, a rosette-like arrangement of cells around capillaries (acinar), and a solid pattern. The amount of vascular stroma and connective tissue varies. Islet cell hyperplasia is often present in the rest of the pancreas. Necrosis, hemorrhage, and calcification are more prominent in larger, malignant tumors (2, 6). The cells are usually well-differentiated with pale staining, round to oval nuclei and frequently a granular cytoplasm. Benign islet cell tumors are frequently incompletely or poorly encapsulated. Signs of local invasion and/or growth into blood vessels must be interpreted cautiously. Cytologic features are unreliable in distinguishing benignity from malignancy. Benign adenomas commonly have abundant mitoses and nuclear aberrations. Only dissemination is indisputable evidence of malignancy. Even the malignant varieties are usually slow growing and rarely spread beyond regional nodes and the liver. Electron microscopy and immunocytochemistry are needed to differentiate the varieties of islet cell tumor histologically (6).

Functional Islet Cell Tumors

Functioning islet cell tumors secrete abnormal amounts of polypeptide hormone and at least five clinical syndromes have been described due to physiological abnormalities caused by hormonal excess (Table 22.4). These include 1) hypoglycemia (insulin), 2) Zollinger-Ellison syndrome (gastrin), 3) glucagonoma syndrome (glucagon), 4) somatostatinoma syndrome (somatostatin), and 5) watery diarrhea hypokalemia achlorhydria (WHDA) or Verner-Morrison syndrome (vasoactive intestinal polypeptide). In addition, islet cell tumors are also capable of secreting adrenal corticotropic hormone (ACTH) melanocyte-stimulating hormone (MSH), a polypeptide with parathyroid hormone-like activity or a combination of several polypeptides (5). A polypeptide called pancreatic polypeptide whose physiologic role is unclear can also be found in certain islet cell tumors and also in asymptomatic individuals who are members of families of multiple endocrine neoplasia syndrome (Type 1) patients (5).

Tumor detection and localization frequently requires the most sophisticated imaging tech-

TABLE 22.4.
CLINICAL SYNDROMES ASSOCIATED WITH FUNCTIONING ISLET CELL TUMORS

Type	Syndrome	Tumor	Hormone	Pancreatic Cell of Origin	Percentage Malignant
1	Hypoglycemia	Insulinoma	Insulin	Beta	10
2	Zollinger-Ellison	Gastrinoma	Gastrin	Non-beta	60–70 (or higher)
3	Glucagonoma syndrome	Glucagonoma	Glucagon	Alpha	50
4	Watery diarrhea, hypokalemia, Achlorhydria (WDHA) (Verner-Morrison syndrome)	Vipoma	Vasoactive intestinal hormone	Non-Beta, ?delta	60
5	Somatostatinoma syndrome	Somatostatinoma	Somatostatin	Delta	50–60

niques available including angiography with venous sampling, dynamic CT scanning, and ultrasound. Since the initial "diagnosis" is based on the clinical syndrome and the elevated hormone level, basically the role of diagnostic imaging is to confirm that a functioning islet cell tumor is present, define its location, judge the extent of its dissemination, and assist in postoperative follow-up. While most pancreatic islet cell tumors are eventually located, in some instances no tumor can be found. In these cases, very small pancreatic tumors, ectopic extrapancreatic neoplasms, or in a few cases, islet cell hyperplasia alone without an actual tumor may be responsible for symptoms (7). Once a tumor is located, treatment consists of tumor excision. If surgical excision is incomplete or is not possible, medical therapy is used which consists of drugs to counteract the effects of the abnormally high hormone levels, and in those instances where the islet cell tumor is malignant, chemotherapeutic agents such as streptozotocin to destroy tumor. Streptozotocin is especially effective against liver metastases when given intra-arterially (7). Hepatic arterial embolization is palliative in advanced metastatic disease.

Common Radiologic Features of Functioning Islet Cell Tumors

Plain Radiographs. Routine abdominal films are most often negative. About 10% of primary malignant islet tumors have detectable calcification on either plain films or computed tomography (8). Calcification is typically focal, coarse, and nodular in character, as opposed to the calcification of chronic pancreatitis which tends to be smaller and more diffuse. Calcification is so infrequent in benign islet cell tumors that the presence of calcification strongly suggests malignancy (8) (Fig. 22.103). Similar calcifications may occur in hepatic metastases (Fig. 22.103).

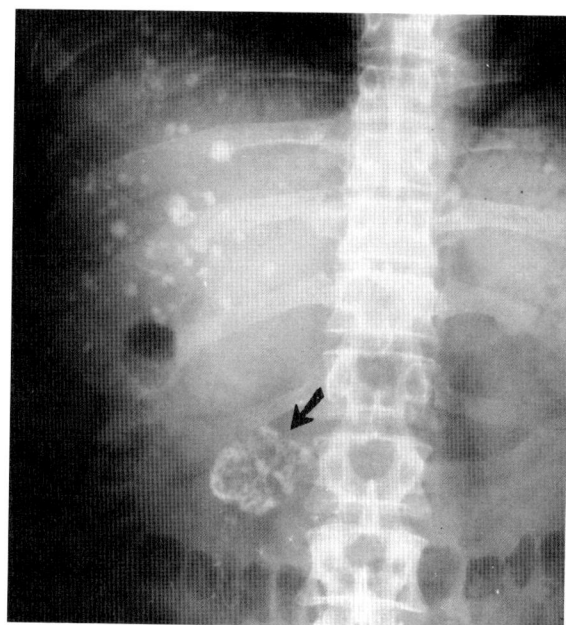

FIGURE 22.103. ISLET CELL TUMOR
Calcified malignant glucagon secreting islet cell tumor of the head of the pancreas (*arrow*) with multiple calcified hepatic metastases. The primary tumor was calcified at presentation and the hepatic calcifications appeared following chemotherapy. This patient did not manifest the "glucagonoma syndrome."

Barium Examination. With the exception of gastrinomas, small functioning tumors of the pancreas usually cause no visible alterations on upper gastrointestinal examinations. When islet tumors become larger, they may show evidence of mass effect on adjacent stomach or duodenum. When malignant, these lesions may occlude the splenic vein and give rise to gastric varices. Frank invasion of adjacent mucosa of small bowel, colon or stomach may occur, changes which are indistinguishable radiographically from pancreatic carcinoma. Ectopic submucosal tumors in the duodenum or stomach may be manifest as defects in the barium column.

Sonography. The effectiveness of ultrasound and CT in the investigation of islet cell tumors and their value compared to angiography and venous sampling is not totally known. This is both because of the relative rarity of islet cell tumors which has made it difficult to assemble a comprehensive case series and because of the rapid changes in imaging technology which has made it difficult to compare detection rates. It is certain, however, that the gray scale display of the current generation of ultrasound scanners is capable of distinguishing subtle differences in pancreatic texture and recent reports have shown that gray scale ultrasound can image small islet cell tumors especially those located in the pancreatic head and body (9–14). Islet cell tumors located in the pancreatic tail probably cannot be detected with the same degree of accuracy as those in the pancreatic head or body since this area is less accessible to ultrasound imaging. The technique for the ultrasound study does not differ from routine pancreatic ultrasound scanning. A good gray scale display and high frequency transducers are mandatory. Because of their good resolution and ease of use, real-time scanners have supplanted static units and are the instruments of choice at present. In general on ultrasound examination, functional pancreatic islet cell tumors tend to appear as homogeneous, solid masses, usually of low echo amplitude with some tendency toward higher echo amplitude in the larger lesions. They also tend to be spherical and well-marginated with little evidence of local invasion. Tumor calcification, central fluid, and large size are indicators of probable malignancy. Hepatic metastases are variable in appearance, but there is a predilection toward high echo amplitude nodules which may get quite large. As in the primary pancreatic neoplasms, central cavitation with fluid and calcification is occasionally encountered in the hepatic metastases. All of the malignant varieties of islet cell tumors are likely to be seen on ultrasound examination. The most difficult types of islet cell tumors to detect with ultrasound are the insulinomas and the small gastrinomas. Intraoperative ultrasound, however, using high frequency transducers directly on the surgically exposed pancreas (Fig. 22.104) should, in the future, have a major role for detecting small lesions and be of special importance in those cases where preoperative tumor localization has failed (15, 16). Surgical localization by palpation is difficult as islet cell tumors often are texturally similar to normal pancreatic parenchyma.

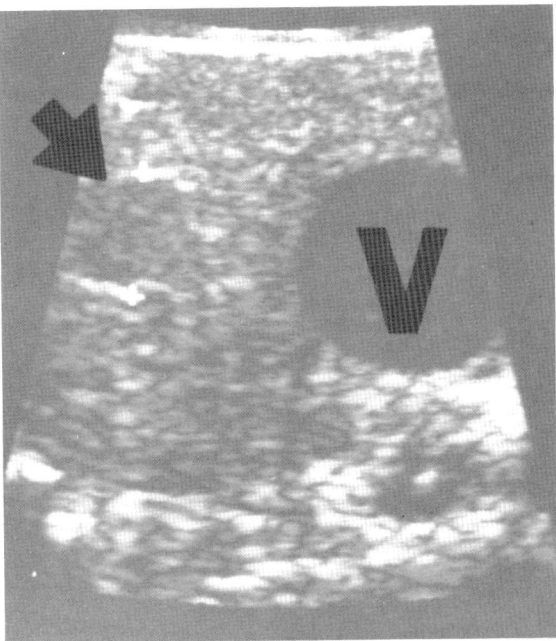

FIGURE 22.104. INSULINOMA
Intraoperative ultrasound with a 10 MHz transducer shows an 8-cm insulinoma (*arrow*) within the pancreatic head (*V*=superior mesenteric vein, cross-section).

Computed Tomography. Optimal CT demonstration of small tumors requires intravenous bolus contrast and dynamic scanning, thin, closely spaced slices (5 mm), and reproducible respirations. By virtue of demonstrating their homogeneous vascular blush, CT with optimal technique can demonstrate a significant percentage of functional islet cell tumors. Malignant islet cell tumors tend to be larger than benign ones on CT. Additional signs of malignancy are calcification, central necrosis, liver metastases and retroperitoneal invasion. Liver metastases are hypodense compared to the liver, and contrast enhancement and central necrosis are frequently demonstrated. A potential source of false positives is mistaking a portion of a tortuous splenic artery or vein for a small islet cell tumor.

Arteriography. All varieties of islet cell tumor look alike angiographically. Unless metastases are seen, malignancy is hard to determine, although the index of suspicion is increased in tumors 5 cm or larger in diameter (17, 18). Small lesions (2–3 cm in diameter or less) manifest themselves as well circumscribed round areas of homogeneous staining superimposed on a less densely staining pancreas, with few or no abnormal vessels (17, 19, 20). The tumor blush persists for 2–6 sec (20). A helpful finding in detecting a small tumor, when present, is demonstration of an artery or draining vein partially or completely encircling the tumor (Fig. 22.105). Seen less commonly are radiating vessels within the tumor or overlying its surface (19). Larger lesions often have more abnormal vessels and dilatation of feeding arteries with visualization of draining veins and may have radiolucent centers corresponding to necrosis (17, 18) (Fig. 22.106). Splenic artery encasement may be seen in islet cell carcinomas. Abnormalities involving the splenic, superior and inferior mesenteric, pancreatic, and portal veins are rare with small islet cell tumors but may be common in tumors 6 cm in size or larger. These include venous occlusion, venous encasement, and intravascular extension

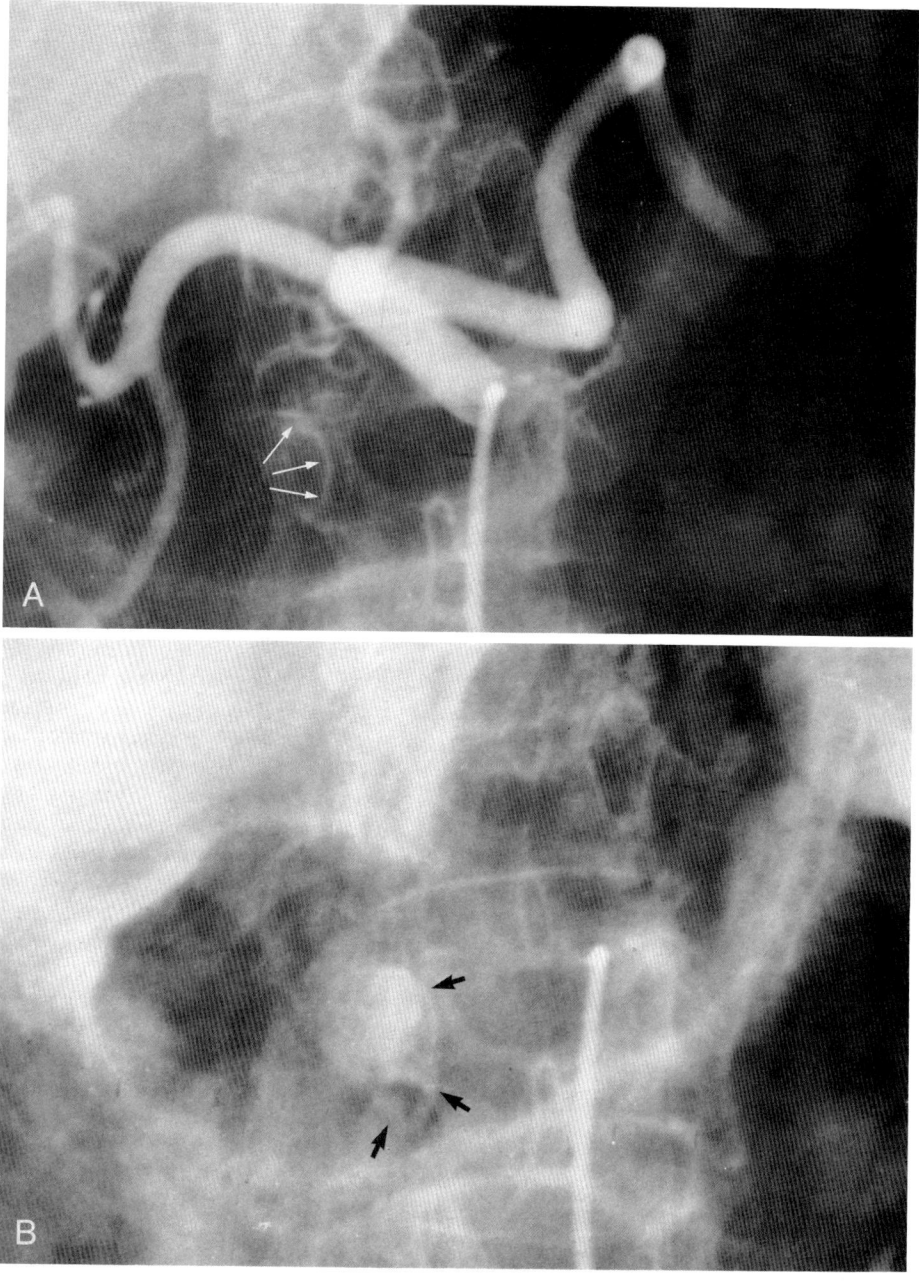

FIGURE 22.105. INSULINOMA

A and *B:* Arterial and capillary phases of a celiac arteriogram showing a small insulinoma with a circumscribing artery (*A, arrows*) and vein (*B, arrows*).

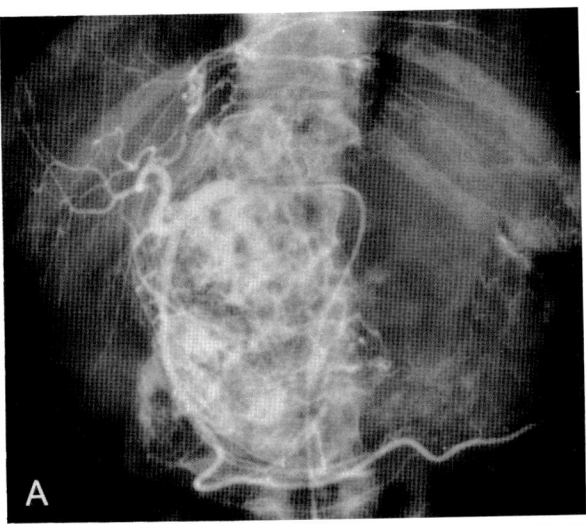 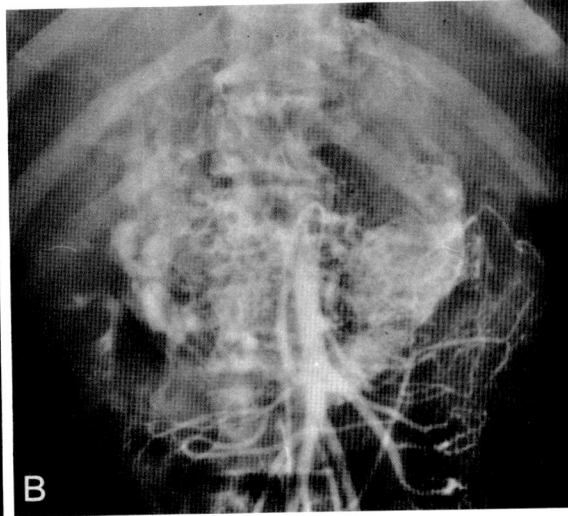

FIGURE 22.106. INSULINOMA

A and *B:* Hepatic and superior mesenteric artery injections, respectively, showing a large hypervascular insulinoma. Although there was vascular invasion and splenic vein occlusion, there were no metastases and the patient was cured by surgery.

of tumor (18). The latter two suggest malignancy and occur in conjunction with liver metastases. Intravenous tumor extension is manifested by fine and/or coarse streaky channels appearing in the arterial phase arising from the tumors and running in the expected course of the venous system (18). Venous occlusion can be produced by either compression or invasion and does not connote malignancy or unresectability in islet cell tumors as it does in duct cell adnocarcinoma of the pancreas (18). Metastases are nodules of variable size identical in appearance to the primary seen in the liver and regional nodes. False-positive diagnosis of small adenomas can be caused by hypervascular lymph nodes (either hyperplastic or involved by hypervascular metastases), accessory spleen, or normal parenchymal blush in the distal third of the pancreas (17, 18, 20). Lymph nodes are in the peripancreatic area, not in the pancreas itself, and their stain is usually not as dense or persistent as that of islet cell tumors. The rounded blush of the distal third of the pancreas seen end-on in the frontal projection can be recognized by profiling the distal third in the left anterior oblique (LAO) projection (17, 18, 20).

Pancreatic Venous Sampling (21–23). This technique has been reported to detect functioning islet cell tumors with nearly 100% accuracy. It is most helpful in detecting small insulinomas which are difficult to localize by other methods. At the National Institutes of Health venous sampling has been of little clinical value in detecting gastrinomas. Transhepatic portography is performed using standard techniques and peripancreatic venous samples are obtained from multiple points along the splenic vein, superior and inferior mesenteric veins, and main portal trunk. Whenever possible, subselective sampling is done from veins draining the head, body, and tail. Sampling should be done either prior to contrast injection or after the contrast has cleared, as contrast medium disturbs the radioimmunoassay. As hormone production is typically variable from moment to moment, simultaneous sampling of the inferior vena cava or right atrium is needed as a control. Phlebography is nearly always normal, but may show draping around a mass. Samples from the right hepatic vein may be helpful in detecting liver metastases. The blood specimens are sent for radioimmunoassay of the appropriate hormone. Local step-ups indicate adenomas, multiple step-ups suggest multiple adenomas, and lack of localization suggests hyperplasia, although the technique is most accurate so far in cases of solitary adenoma. Pancreatic venous sampling is indicated after noninvasive attempts at localization have failed and arteriography is negative or equivocal.

Insulinoma

Clinical Findings

Insulinomas are the most common type of functioning islet cell tumor. They occur at any age although rarely below eighteen and usually in the fourth through sixth decades (1). Symptoms are insidious in onset and may mimic a variety of neuropsychiatric disorders.

Typical symptoms of hypoglycemia include headaches, confusion, seizures, drowsiness, fainting spells, weakness, sweating, and personality changes. The diagnosis is based on demonstrating that the patient's symptoms occur with fasting or exercise; at the time of symptoms, the serum glucose is 40 mg/dl or less; and the hypoglycemic symptoms are relieved by the administration of glucose (Whipple's triad) (24). There is a higher than normal serum proinsulin to insulin ratio (25). Patients are frequently obese because they have unconsciously learned to eat to relieve their symptoms. Infrequently, malignant insulinomas present with symptoms due to mass before hypoglycemia is clinically manifest (1).

Pathology

Insulinomas are usually small (70% are 1.5 cm diameter or less) at presentation since even very small lesions can produce significant hypoglycemia (1, 25–27). It is thought that the tumor has the ability to synthesize hormone and react to stimuli with appropriate hormonal discharge, but lacks the ability to store hormone when it is not needed (2). About 80–90% of insulinomas are solitary adenomas, 5–10% are multiple adenomas, and 5–10% are malignant (25). From 5 to 10% of patients with hypoglycemia have islet cell hyperplasia and 10% have multiple endocrine neoplasia Type 1 (25). Insulinomas are rarely ectopic (26, 27), and hypoglycemia may rarely be caused by extrapancreatic non-islet cell tumors such as hepatoma or retroperitoneal fibrosarcoma (26).

Radiology

Ultrasound. Insulinomas are probably the most difficult of all islet cell tumors to detect with ultrasound because they are usually small, averaging 1.5 cm in diameter (28). Another difficulty for ultrasonography is patient obesity. In one series of 10 patients with proven insulinomas, adequate pancreatic visualization could be

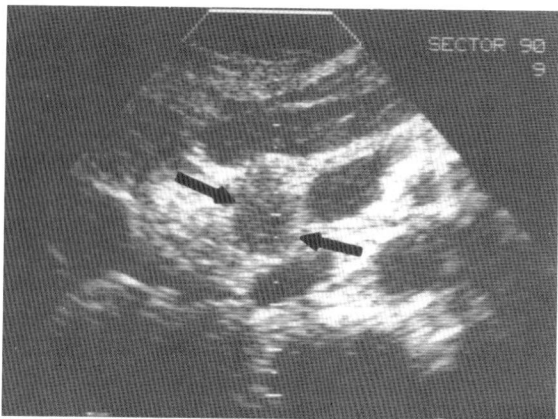

FIGURE 22.107. INSULINOMA
Transverse ultrasound scan shows a 2-cm diameter insulinoma (*arrows*) in the head of the pancreas. Even with imaging during a rapid bolus of contrast material, the CT study of this patient was negative for tumor.

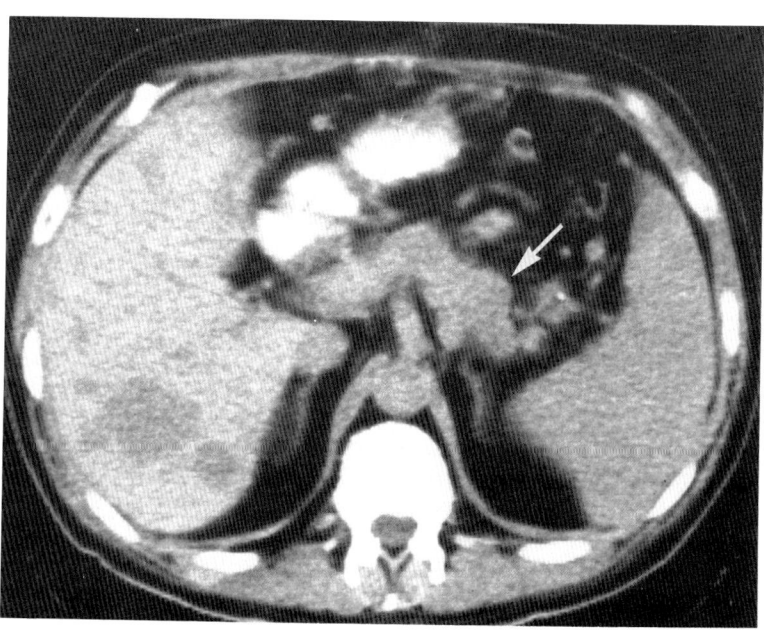

FIGURE 22.108. INSULINOMA
Small malignant insulinoma in tail of pancreas evident as local bulge (*arrow*). Multiple hepatic metastases are evident.

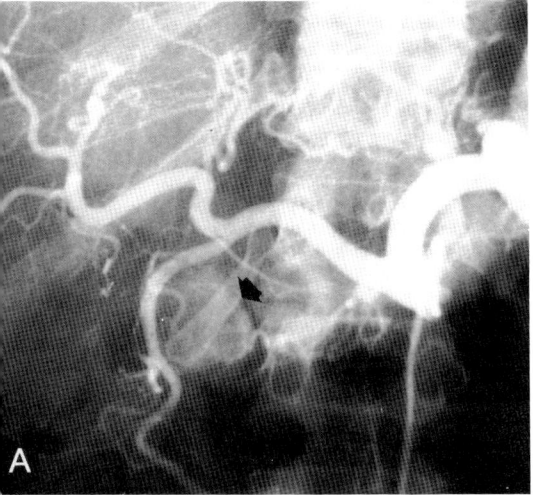
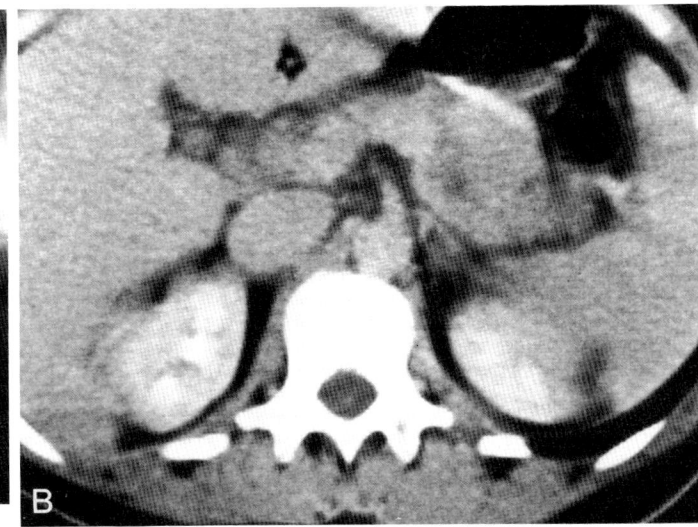
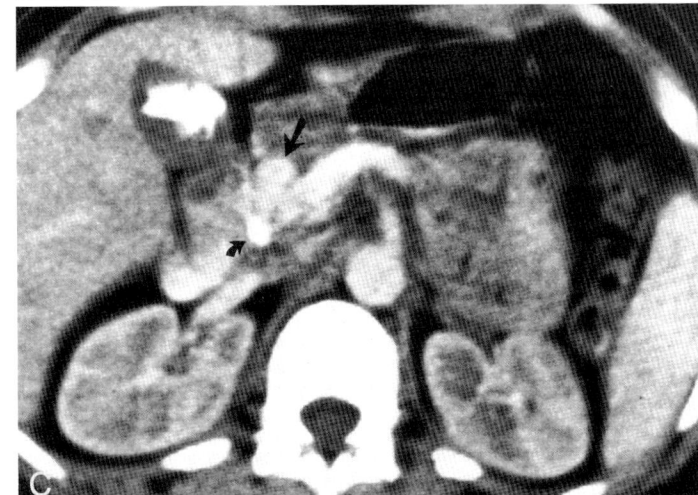

FIGURE 22.109. INSULINOMA
A: A 2-cm insulinoma in the head of pancreas (*arrow*) seen on celiac arteriogram. *B:* Insulinoma not visible on routine CT scan. *C:* Dynamic CT with intravenous bolus demonstrates insulinoma (*large arrow*) lying anterior to common duct (*small arrow*) which has been opacified with intravenous iodipamide.

achieved only in 6 primarily because of obesity, and tumors could be located only in 3 of the 10 (27). At the present time, ultrasound is less sensitive than angiography. It can be helpful for those patients with equivocal angiograms or for those with malignant insulinomas. The ultrasound appearance of insulinomas is one of a solid, homogeneous, low echo amplitude mass with no calcification or cavitation (Fig. 22.107). Insulinomas detected by ultrasound have ranged from 7 mm to 6 cm in diameter (10, 13). In general, the larger the tumor, the more likely it is to be malignant and the easier it is to detect. Metastatic tumor to the liver from malignant insulinomas has been reported in one case and described as small, high echo amplitude lesions (10). Although experience is limited with these tumors, it appears that unlike CT, ultrasound can detect small (<1 cm) islet cell tumors by imaging the change in pancreatic texture.

Computed Tomography. Due to their small size, insulinomas are the most difficult islet cell tumor to detect by CT examination. Dunnick et al. (27) detected only 6 of 14 tumors using an EMI 5005 scanner. In another CT study, only 1 of 10 tumors was detected (21). Small insulinomas will not be visible on routine CT scans unless they deform or extend beyond the pancreatic contours since they are usually not sufficiently different in their attenuation value from normal pancreatic tissue (Fig. 22.108), although Fricke et al. (29) reported insulinomas as visible due to high attenuation values. Insulinomas are better detected by virtue of their angiographic blush on dynamic CT scanning using intravenous bolus technique (Fig. 22.109) (30, 31). Guenther et al. (14) detected 7 of 16 small (<2 cm) islet cell tumors (13 of which were insulinomas) using intravenous bolus dynamic CT scanning and 5-mm slices. None of these lesions

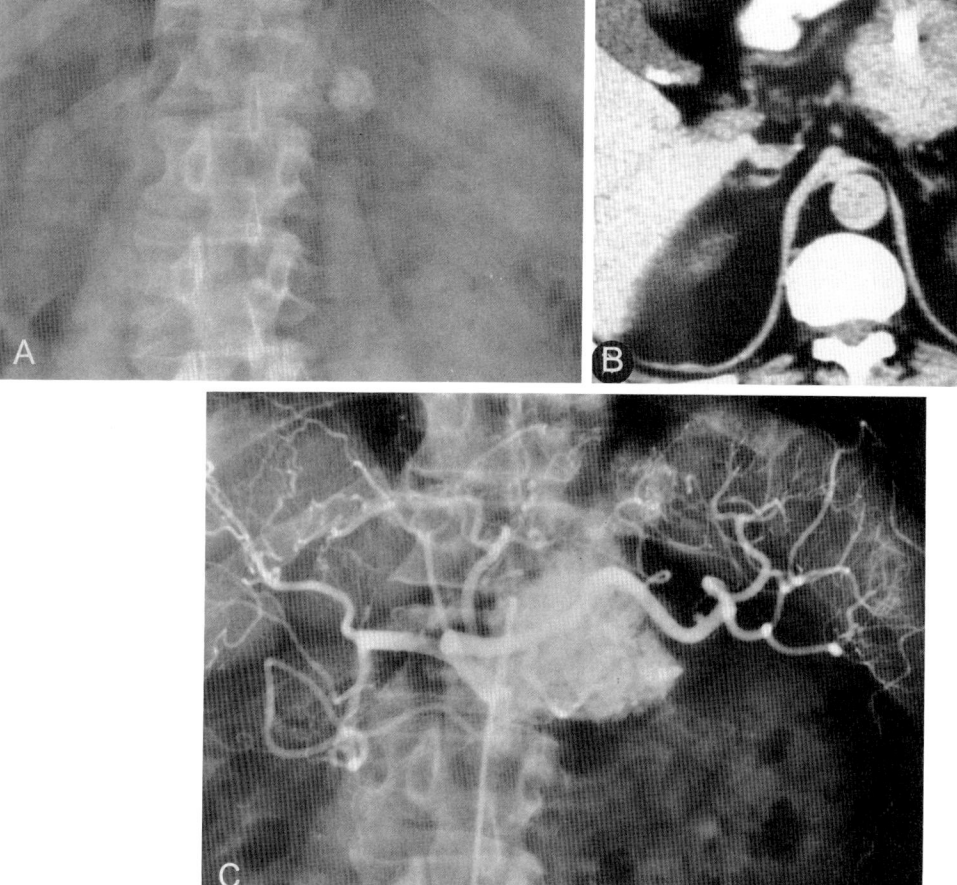

FIGURE 22.110. INSULINOMA

A–C: Dense nodular calcification in malignant insulinoma is visible on plain film (*A*) and CT scan (*B*). Dense capillary staining is visible on celiac arteriogram (*C*).

was visible on precontrast studies. Stark et al. (32) detected 21 of 27 islet cell tumors using similar dynamic CT technique, and detected 4 of 8 insulinomas whose average size was 1.5 cm. Angiography missed 2 of the 4 insulinomas detected by CT and did not detect those insulinomas missed by CT. The latter were identified by venous sampling (32). The major limitations of intravenous bolus dynamic CT is the number of levels that may be examined before a contrast load limit is reached. This may be partially overcome by performing dynamic CT scanning with contrast injection through an arterial catheter in the celiac axis. Malignant insulinomas tend to be larger in size on CT than their benign counterparts, and may have hepatic metastases (32). Although there is little CT experience with malignant insulinomas, calcification suggests malignancy (Fig. 22.110). The adrenal glands should be carefully scrutinized for evidence of concomitant adrenal pathology (hyperplasia or cortical tumors) which occurs with multiple endocrine neoplasia Type 1.

Angiography and Venous Sampling. The success rate of arteriography in the localization of insulinoma has varied in recent reports from 17 to 84% (21, 22, 27, 32). False positives may occur. Arteriography is still currently the best test for insulinoma although initial reports using dynamic CT are encouraging. Pancreatic venous sampling is successful in 95–100%, has few if any false positives, and may correctly suggest the diagnosis of islet cell hyperplasia (21, 22). However, pancreatic venous sampling is riskier and more technically demanding than arteriography and should be undertaken only if the latter is negative or equivocal. Local step-ups of insulin levels correspond to sites of adenomas, and multiple step-ups are found in islet cell hyperplasia or nesidioblastosis (21). Insulin concentrations in the main draining vein of an insulinoma are 7–35 times higher than peripheral levels (32). Arteriography seems superior to venous sampling in the diagnosis of liver metastases (21, 22).

Gastrinomas and the Zollinger-Ellison Syndrome

Gastrin is normally produced by the G-cells of the gastric antrum in response to the mechanical distention and the rise in pH caused by ingested food. Circulating gastrin that reaches the fundus and body of the stomach causes histamine release which in turn causes gastric acid secretion. Emptying of the stomach and dropping of the pH from acid secretion lower the rate of gastrin secretion. Gastrin also lowers the pressure of the lower esophageal sphincter.

Clinical Findings

Gastrinomas are the second most common islet cell tumors after insulinomas, occur mostly in adults, and are almost always responsible for the Zollinger-Ellison (Z-E) syndrome. Antral-G cell hyperplasia is probably the cause in some instances but islet cell hyperplasia is doubtful as an etiology (1, 2). Although the full-blown syndrome consists of diarrhea and multiple gastroduodenal and postbulbar ulcers, roughly two-thirds present as solitary duodenal or gastric ulcer (1, 33). A significant percentage of patients (18–25%) may have no ulceration at the time of diagnosis (1, 33); diarrhea or reflux may be the chief complaint. Z-E syndrome is an important cause of marginal ulceration occurring after partial gastrectomy. About 20–40% of Z-E patients have multiple endocrine neoplasia Type 1 (26, 33). The diagnosis of Z-E is etablished by gastric fluid analysis (high acid levels and large volumes) and measurement of an elevated serum gastrin level (1, 33).

Antral G-cell hyperplasia (pseudo Z-E syndrome) is clinically identical to Z-E syndrome and is caused by a pathologic increase in the number of G-cells in the antrum resulting in hypergastrinemia. It is distinguished from Z-E by a lack of gastrin elevation after secretin injection and an exaggerated gastrin elevation after a test meal (34). Antral G-cell hyperplasia is curable by antrectomy. Other causes of hypergastrinemia that should be excluded clinically are: chronic atrophic gastritis and other causes of achlorhydria, renal failure, gastric outlet obstruction, retained antrum, massive small bowel resection and pheochromocytoma (25).

Treatment of Z-E syndrome is controversial and evolving. Complete cure is rare and recurrence can be late and either from malignancy or another adenoma. H_2 blockers (cimetidine, ranitidine) are competitive blockers of the H_2 receptor site for histamine on the parietal cell. They are effective in controlling gastric hypersecretion thus reducing or eliminating the need for total gastrectomy; unfortunately they do not affect tumor growth (35). Drug resistance resulting in the need for higher and higher doses can be a problem. Surgery is probably warranted in good risk patients. Highly selective vagotomy can decrease acid production and drug dosage. Extirpation of tumors especially in the duodenal wall or pancreatic tail offers the hope of cure. Debulking is useful in cases of metastatic spread. Intolerance of H_2 blockers, drug resistance, or patient unreliability are indications for total gastrectomy. Malignant gastrinomas are slow growing, spread beyond the liver is unusual and survival with liver metastases can be prolonged.

Pathology

Less than 25% of Z-E patients have solitary adenomas and the rate of malignancy, usually quoted at about 60%, is probably higher (1, 2, 33). Of the malignancies, three-fourths are metastatic or otherwise unresectable (1). Multiple adenomas occur in about 20% and are especially common in multiple endocrine neoplasia patients (1, 33). Seven to 33% of gastrinomas are ectopic, most commonly in the duodenal wall or peripancreatic nodes but occasionally in the stomach or omentum (2, 22, 33). The cell of origin, at times thought to be the alpha or delta cell, is currently unknown although probably part of the APUD system (2, 6, 25). The adult human pancreas is practically devoid of gastrin-producing cells, although they are found in the fetus. Although the tumor cells in gastrinoma resemble antral cells, gastrinomas are currently in search of a corresponding normal cell. Gastrinomas appear to be defective in their ability to store their hormone as are insulinomas (2).

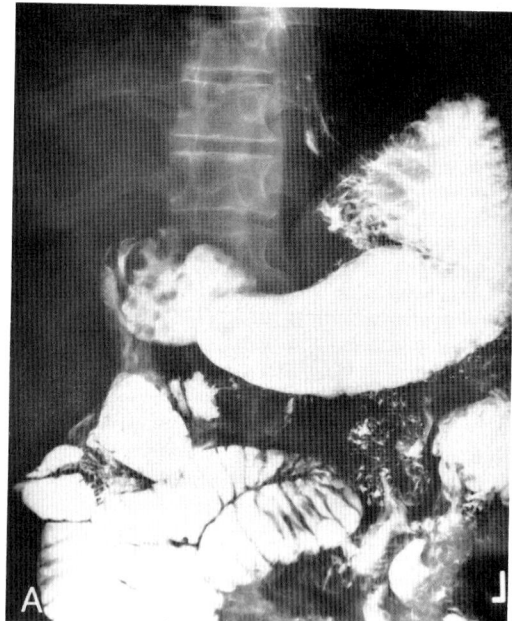
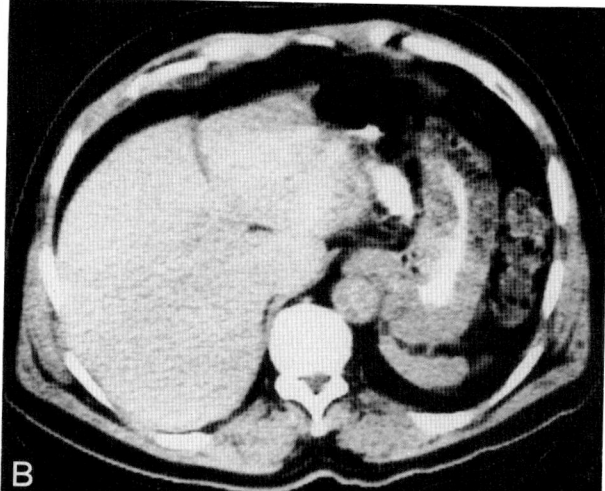
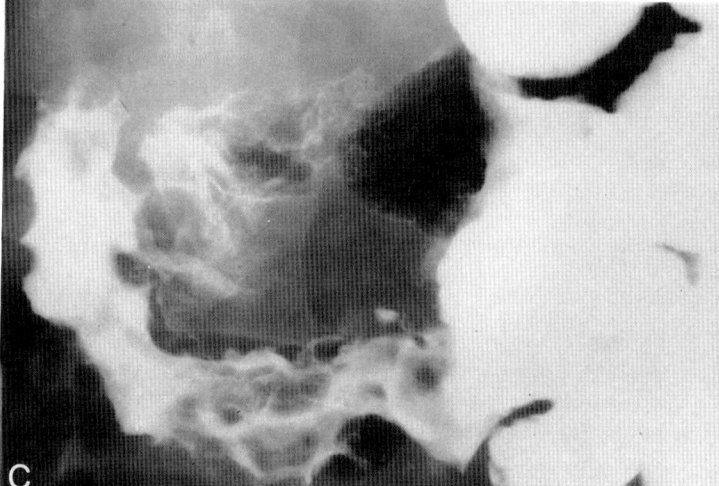
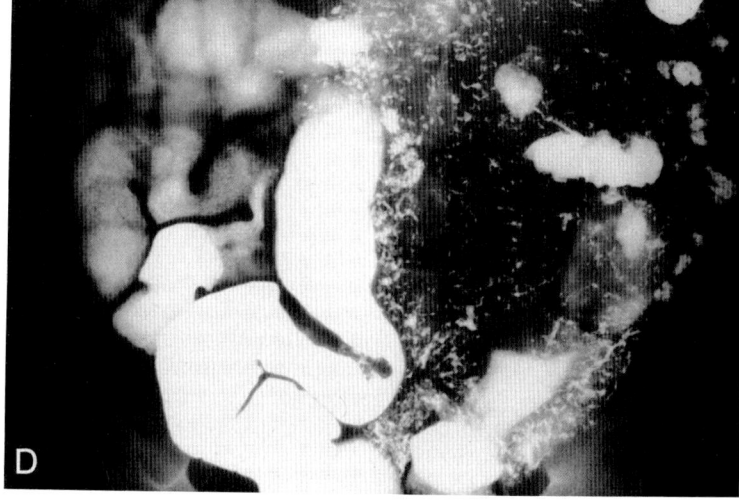

FIGURE 22.111. GASTRINOMA
A: Upper gastrointestinal study in a patient with Zollinger-Ellison syndrome. Note thickened folds in stomach and duodenum as well as mild dilatation of jejunum. *B:* Thickening of gastric wall in the same patient as in *A*, evident on CT scan due to mucosal hypertrophy. *C:* Edematous folds and multiple small ulcerations throughout the duodenum in another Z-E patient. *D:* Small bowel series in the same patient as in *C* shows flocculation, dilatation, and a wet pattern.

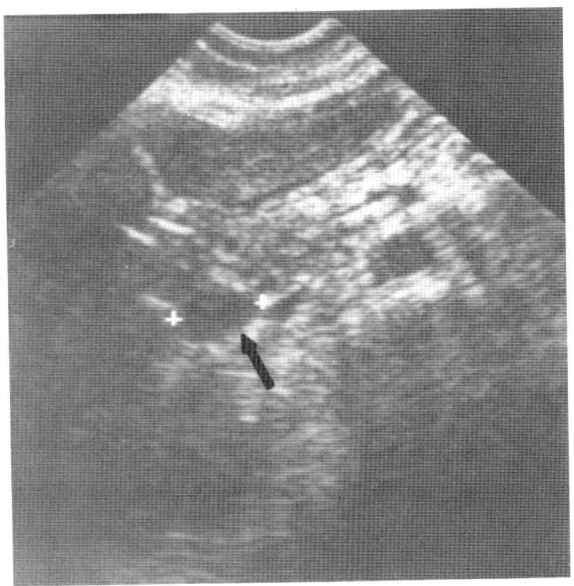

FIGURE 22.112. GASTRINOMA

A 2.5-cm gastrinoma (arrow) is evident positioned posterior and lateral to the head of the pancreas. This tumor was located in the duodenal wall, at the junction of the second and third portions.

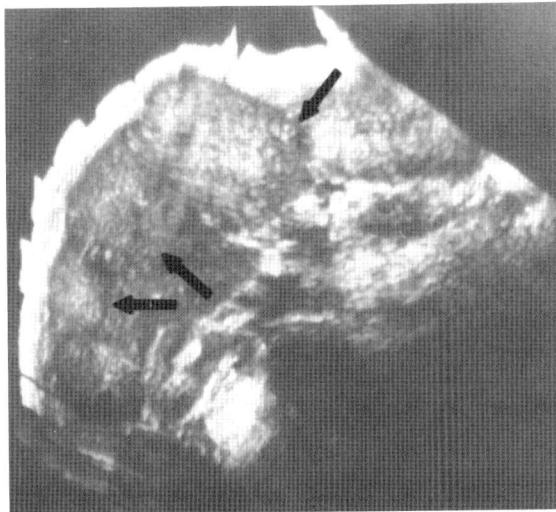

FIGURE 22.113. GASTRINOMA

Typical appearance of gastrinoma metastatic to the liver. Large, high amplitude nodules (arrows) are seen.

Radiology

Plain Films. Bone metastases are extremely rare, occur late in the course of the disease, and can be osteoblastic or lytic (36).

Upper Gastrointestinal Tract and Small Bowel. Gastrinomas, even when small, may cause alterations on upper gastrointestinal study (37–41). Excess gastrin causes antral cell hyperplasia and gastric hypersecretion. This may appear as gastric rugal enlargement and/or prominence of area gastricae (Fig. 22.111A and B) as well as increased secretions in the stomach and small bowel, with or without thickening of small bowel mucosa (Fig. 22.111A, C, and D). In addition to simple duodenal or gastric ulcer, postbulbar duodenal, jejunal, or multiple ulcers may be present. Reflux esophagitis is frequent and may be severe and intractable. Duodenal dilatation may be present, associated with edema of the mucosa which can extend into the jejunum (39) (Fig. 22.111A, C, and D). In patients with diarrhea, there is evidence of excessive fluid in the bowel causing dilution and flocculation of barium (Fig. 22.111A, C, and D). Marginal ulceration may be seen in partial postgastrectomy patients along with edema of the jejunal folds. Unfortunately, many of these changes are suggestive but nonspecific and the diagnosis needs to be confirmed by appropriate serum gastrin measurements.

Ultrasound. In one series of 15 patients with gastrinomas, a tumor was detected with ultrasound in 4 (9). In another larger series of 29 patients, tumor was successfully identified in 14, with tumor sizes ranging from 1.5 to 8 cm in diameter (10). This detection rate by ultrasound compares favorably with reported localization rates for either angiography or CT scanning (10). Ectopic locations outside of the pancreas, as for instance tumors primary in the duodenum (Fig. 22.112), or hyperplasia alone without evidence of frank neoplasm presents diagnostic difficulties for all imaging systems (42). Sonographically, gastrinomas are generally homogeneous and of low echo amplitude compared to the surrounding pancreas. Shadowing from calcification or central sonolucency due to necrosis may be encountered suggesting malignancy. Hepatic metastases are characteristically of high echo amplitude (Fig. 22.113) although an occasional target pattern or low amplitude lesion may also be seen. Like the primary pancreatic tumor, calcification or central fluid may be present within the hepatic metastases.

Computed Tomography. Small gastrinomas within the pancreas are invisible on noncontrast scans unless they project beyond the pancreas and distort its contour. Both intra- and extrapancreatic gastrinomas can be better visualized by virtue of their angiographic blush with dynamic CT scanning and bolus technique, and multiple tumors can be detected (Fig. 22.114) (32, 43). When malignant, these lesions tend to be larger (Fig. 22.115) and may calcify (Fig.

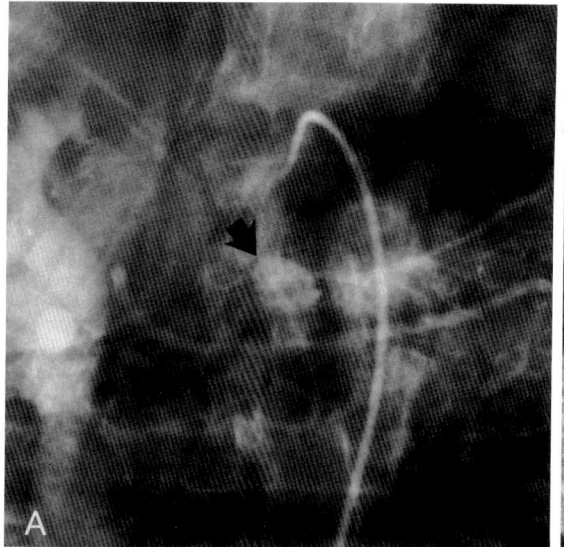
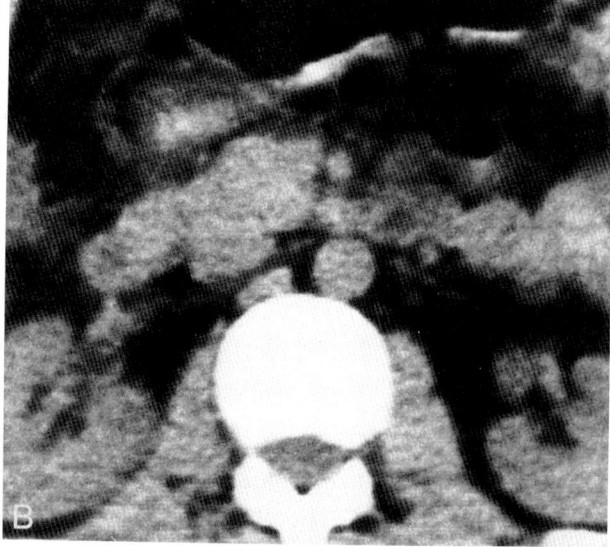
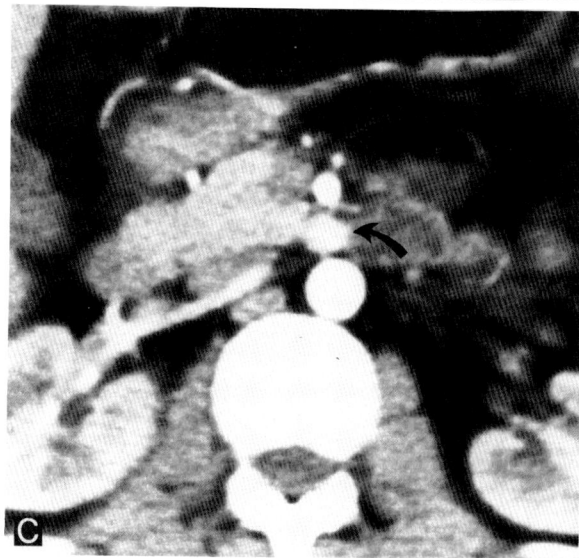

FIGURE 22.114. GASTRINOMA
A–C: Small surgically confirmed gastrinoma (*arrow*) in the uncinate process shown on superior mesenteric arteriogram (A). Gastrinoma is not visible on routine CT scan (B), but is shown by dynamic CT (C) as a brightly enhancing structure (*arrow*) between superior mesenteric artery and aorta.

22.103). As with other endocrine neoplasms (44) malignant gastrinomas may extend into venous structures, such as the renal vein or inferior vena cava, or obstruct the splenic vein (Fig. 22.116B, E, and F). Liver metastases appear as areas of low attentuation within normal liver parenchyma (Figs. 22.115B and 22.117). Retroperitoneal adenopathy or local recurrence following initial resection may be evident (Fig. 22.118). In the late stages, hepatic metastases may grow to a large size (Fig. 22.117) and distant bony metastases can occur (Fig. 22.119). Dunnick et al. (45) reported detecting 4 of 18 gastrinomas on an EMI 5005 scanner. More recently, Deveney et al. (46) demonstrated 7 of 10 gastrinomas (2 of which were missed by superselective arteriography) in the pancreas using an 8800 GE scanner with thin 5-mm sections in association with dynamic scanning. The 3 lesions missed were all less than 1 cm in size. Four hepatic metastases were correctly diagnosed in 16 patients. In 6 additional cases no tumor was found by CT or at surgery. It remains to be seen if this excellent localization rate will hold up in larger series using dynamic CT. Another finding on CT scans is thickening of the wall of the stomach due to mucosal hypertrophy caused by gastrin stimulation (Fig. 22.111B). Normally in the distended state the stomach wall is less than 1 cm in thickness in 90% of patients (47).

Arteriography and Venous Sampling. Success rates for angiographic localization in

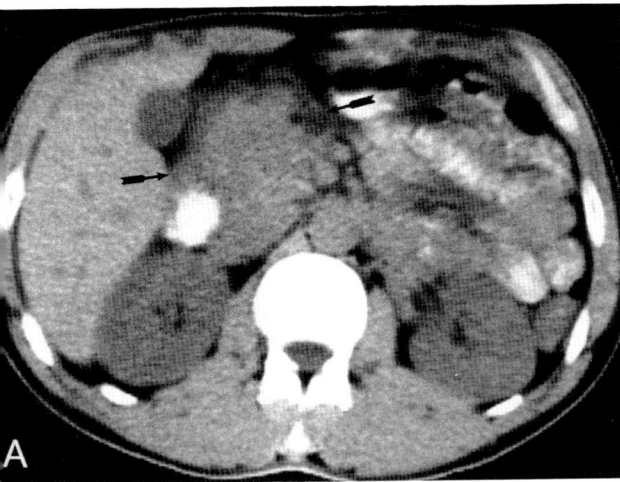 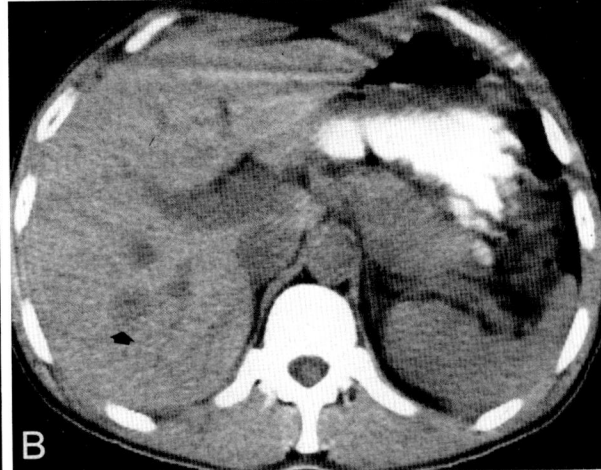

FIGURE 22.115. GASTRINOMA
A: Large malignant gastrinoma in head of pancreas (*arrows*). *B:* Liver metastasis visible on noncontrast CT scan (*arrow*).

Z-E syndrome (Figs. 22.114A and 22.116A and B) are reported to be 13–15% (22, 48), but an unpublished review of 33 cases at the National Institutes of Health showed a 70% success rate. Liver metastases can be demonstrated as small hypervascular masses with great sensitivity even when the primary is not detected (48). Venous sampling was correct in tumor localization in 93% in one series of 16 patients. Half of these tumors were less than 1 cm in size and impalpable at surgery. Gastrin levels in the main draining vein were 1.5–21 times higher than peripheral levels (22). In the National Institutes of Health experience, in contrast to that of Roche et al. (22), venous sampling has been of almost no clinical value in localizing gastrinomas. Venous sampling is not particularly accurate in detecting liver metastases (22), and is of no value in multiple endocrine adenomatosis patients (21).

Glucagonoma

Clinical Findings

This is a very uncommon tumor derived from the pancreatic alpha cell which secretes abnormal amounts of glucagon. Clinically, these lesions may be silent or present as a "glucagonoma syndrome" which consists of a necrolytic migratory erythematous rash, mild diabetes, and anemia (25, 49, 50). The skin lesions tend to occur on the lower extremities, groin, buttocks, and face and are characterized by erythematous macules or papules that later become oozing erosive bullae (50). Other symptoms that may be present include stomatitis, diarrhea, and weight loss.

Glucagonomas may also present as part of the multiple endocrine neoplasia syndrome (49, 51, 52). Laboratory tests are remarkable for extremely elevated sedimentation rates and high levels of plasma glucagon. The rash is a useful marker for the tumor; it regresses when the tumor is resected and reappears with recurrence.

Pathology

These lesions tend to be larger in size (mean 6.4 cm in a series of 29 tumors reported by Stacpoole (51)) and occur more frequently in the pancreatic body and tail. Very few lesions are extrapancreatic in location. A high percentage of lesions have proven to be malignant most having metastases at initial surgery (25, 49). Recurrence is frequent and long-term cures have not been reported.

Radiology

Conventional Examinations. As with other malignant islet cell tumors, calcification of the primary and/or hepatic metastases may occur (Fig. 22.103). Thickened small bowel folds are sometimes observed, possibly due to a toxic effect on intestinal epithelium (Fig. 22.120).

Ultrasound. Ultrasound experience is extremely limited. Glucagonomas are usually malignant and, like most islet cell tumors when malignant, tend to be large and therefore easily visible on ultrasound (Fig. 22.121). The appearance of two glucagonomas has been described, namely solid masses averaging 3–4 cm, in the pancreatic head and body (10). In one of these

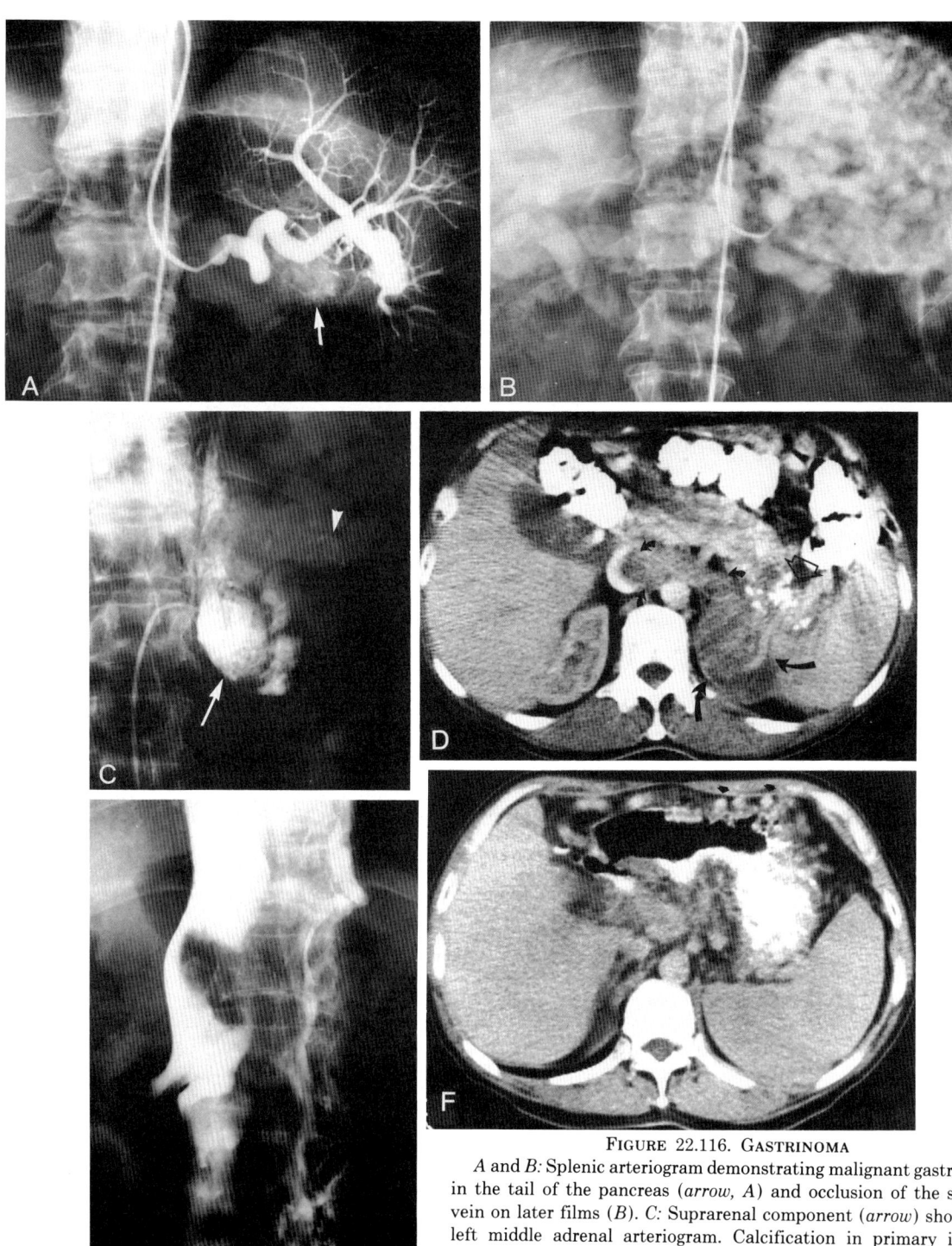

FIGURE 22.116. GASTRINOMA

A and *B:* Splenic arteriogram demonstrating malignant gastrinoma in the tail of the pancreas (*arrow, A*) and occlusion of the splenic vein on later films (*B*). *C:* Suprarenal component (*arrow*) shown on left middle adrenal arteriogram. Calcification in primary is also evident (*arrowhead*). *D* and *E:* CT scan (with pedal injection) shows calcified gastrinoma in the tail of the pancreas (*open arrow*) invading the splenic hilum with a left suprarenal mass (*large arrows, D*). There is extension of tumor into the left renal vein and inferior vena cava (*small arrows*) confirmed by inferior vena cavagram (*E*). *F:* Splenomegaly and gastric varices (*arrows*) due to splenic vein occlusion seen on higher CT scan.

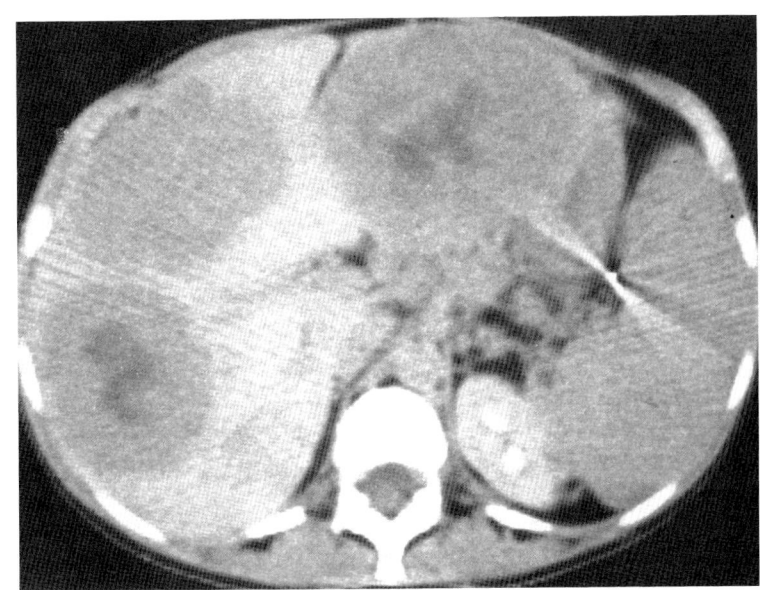

FIGURE 22.117. GASTRINOMA
Massive centrally necrotic gastrinoma metastatic to liver.

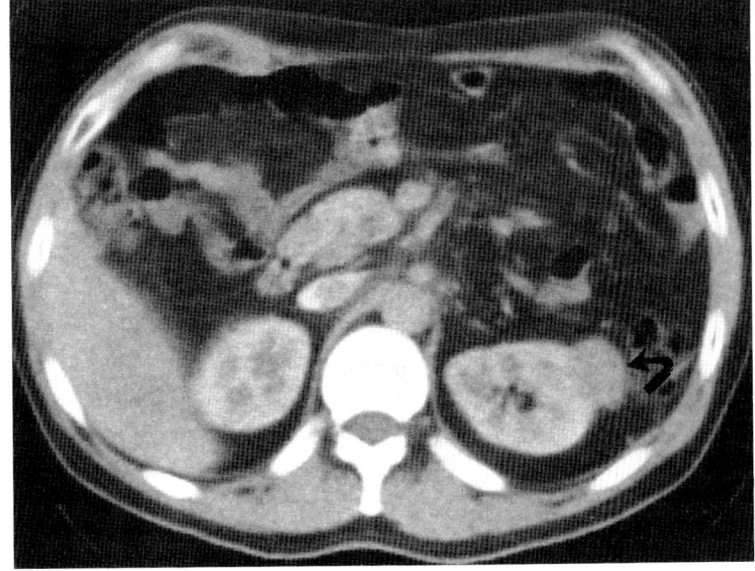

FIGURE 22.118. GASTRINOMA
Surgically proven locally recurrent malignant gastrinoma (*arrow*) adjacent to left kidney following distal pancreatectomy.

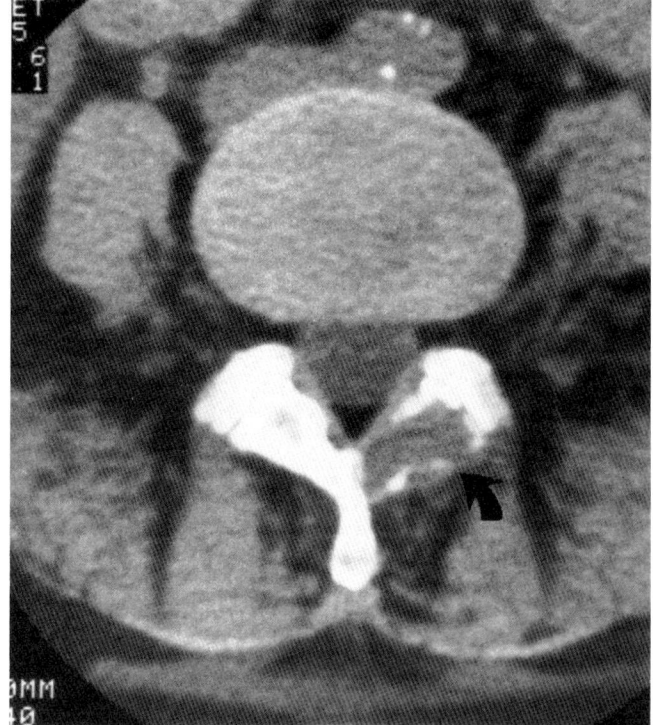

FIGURE 22.119. GASTRINOMA
Late bony metastasis of gastrinoma (*arrow*) to spinal lamina.

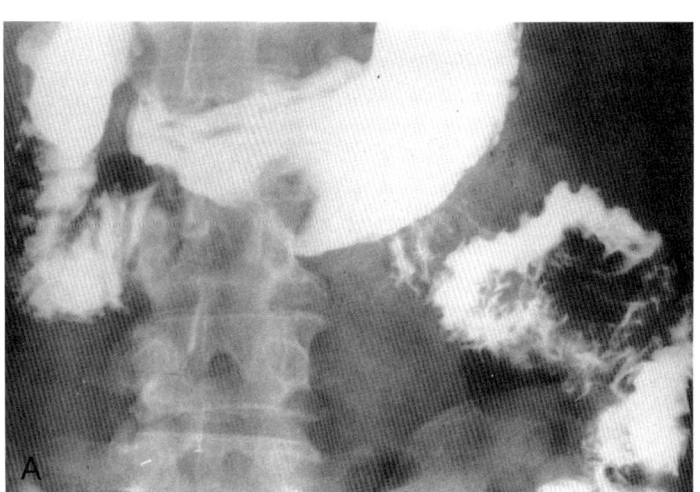

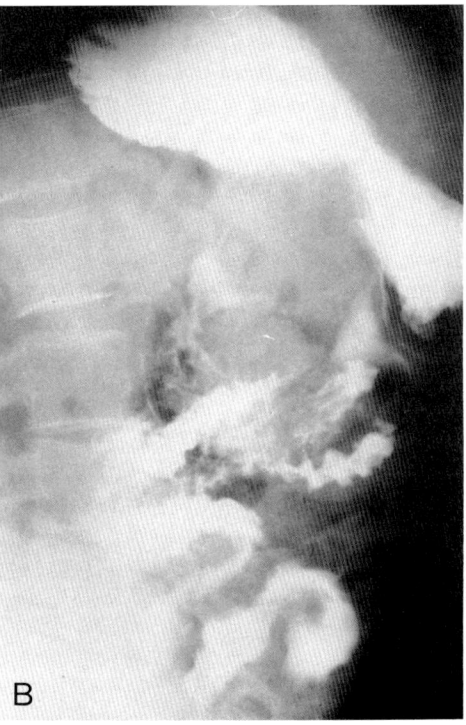

FIGURE 22.120. GLUCAGONOMA
A and *B:* Anteroposterior and lateral views of a barium meal showing a small retrogastric glucagonoma indenting the greater curvature and thickened small bowel folds.

cases, portal vein invasion by tumor was evident. This same malignancy showed a gradual tumor enlargement over a 4-yr period with development of central fluid from tumor necrosis demonstrating the protracted clinical course of patients with malignant islet cell tumors.

Computed Tomography. Few examples of CT scans of glucagonomas have appeared in the literature (32, 45, 49) and they are indistinguishable from other islet cell tumors. They appear as solid pancreatic masses with or without calcifications, necrosis, and metastases. Size has varied from 2.5 to 25 cm (Fig. 22.122).

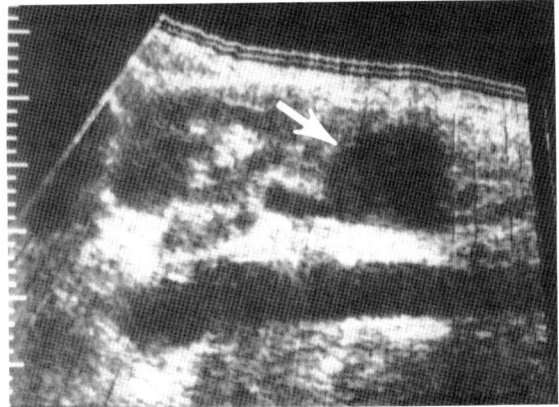

FIGURE 22.121. GLUCAGONOMA
Longitudinal ultrasound scan shows a 4-cm homogeneously solid low amplitude glucagonoma (*arrow*) in the pancreas.

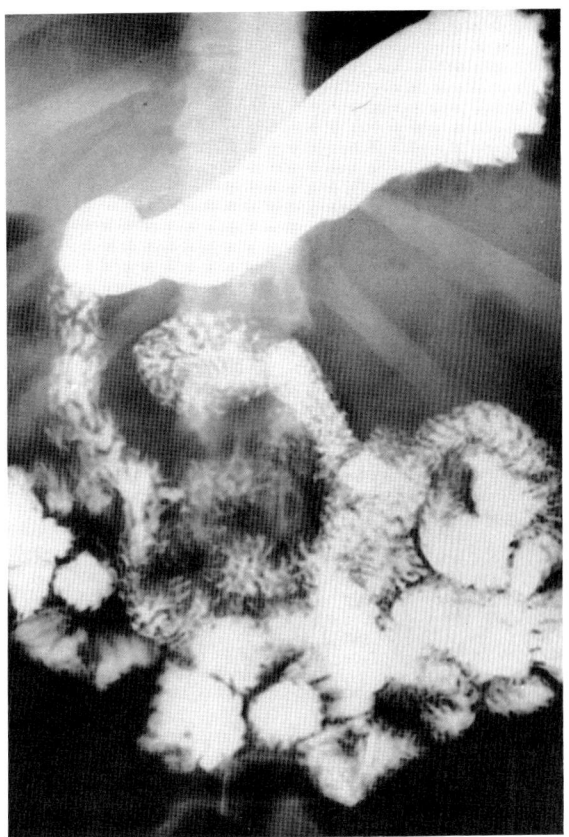

FIGURE 22.123. VIPOMA
Large vipoma in the left upper quadrant displacing the duodeno-jejunal junction. Note the normal small bowel pattern.

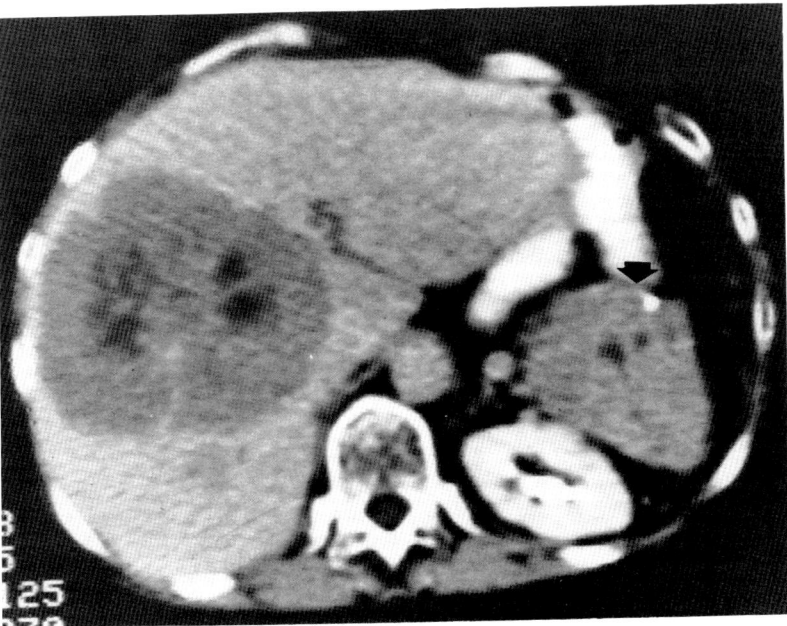

FIGURE 22.122. GLUCAGONOMA
Large calcified partially necrotic recurrent malignant glucagonoma in the retroperitoneum (*arrow*) with necrotic liver metastases. (Courtesy of Dr. David Allison, Hammersmith Hospital, London, England.)

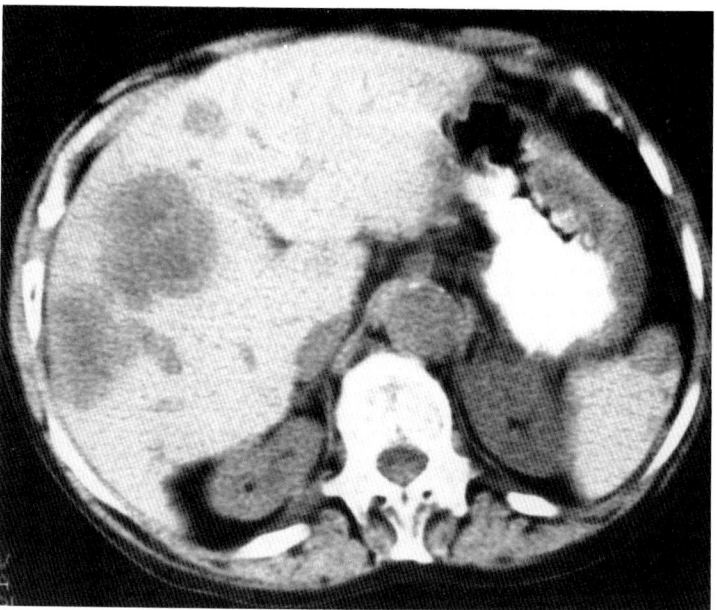

FIGURE 22.124. VIPOMA
Liver metastases from pancreatic vipoma.

Arteriography and Venous Sampling. Glucagonomas are quite vascular and are well shown by arteriography (53). Localization by portal venous sampling for glucagon has also been reported (54).

Vipoma (WDHA Syndrome)

Vipomas are rare tumors originating from delta islet cells that produce *v*asoactive *i*ntestinal *p*olypeptide (VIP) which causes a syndrome of *w*atery *d*iarrhea, *h*ypokalemia, and *a*chlorhydria (WDHA, also called Verner-Morrison syndrome or pancreatic cholera) (55–59). The cells of this tumor secrete a 28 amino acid VIP which is normally present in the central and peripheral nervous system, as well as the gastrointestinal tract (55).

Clinical Findings

Excess production of VIP is thought to be the cause of WDHA syndrome. Continuous or intermittent, profuse, watery diarrhea occurs with consequent loss of potassium and resultant hypokalemia. Hypo- or achlorhydria in the stomach is also commonly present, distinguishing this syndrome from Z-E (55). Flushing of the skin or dilatation of the gallbladder may occur. The latter is thought to be due to a secretin-like effect of VIP. Gallstones may or may not be present (25). Mild hyperglycemia is often present (25).

Pathology

More than 60% of WDHA patients have malignant pancreatic vipomas with metastases usually present at the time of diagnosis (25, 55). Most of the remaining patients have adenomas with an occasional case of islet cell hyperplasia (25, 60). Sympathetic nervous system tumors such as ganglioneuromas and ganglioneuroblastomas are rare causes of WDHA (25, 55). Multicentricity and/or association with multiple endocrine neoplasia occurs rarely (55). Pancreatic vipomas have ranged in size from 1 to 10 cm (55). It is thought that pancreatic vipomas are more common in the body and tail than in the head (25).

Radiology

Small Bowel. Curiously, patients with WDHA often will not have an abnormal wet small bowel pattern (Fig. 22.123).

Ultrasound. Hancke (9) detected a 3-cm tumor in the pancreatic tail, subsequently confirmed by him using ultrasound-directed biopsy. In another series of islet cell tumors, a 6-cm vipoma was detected by ultrasound in the pancreatic tail (10). In this same series, liver metastases present in three patients appeared echogenic in two instances and hypoechoic in one case.

Computed Tomography. Few examples of CT scans of these rare tumors have appeared in the literature (59), and in general they are iden-

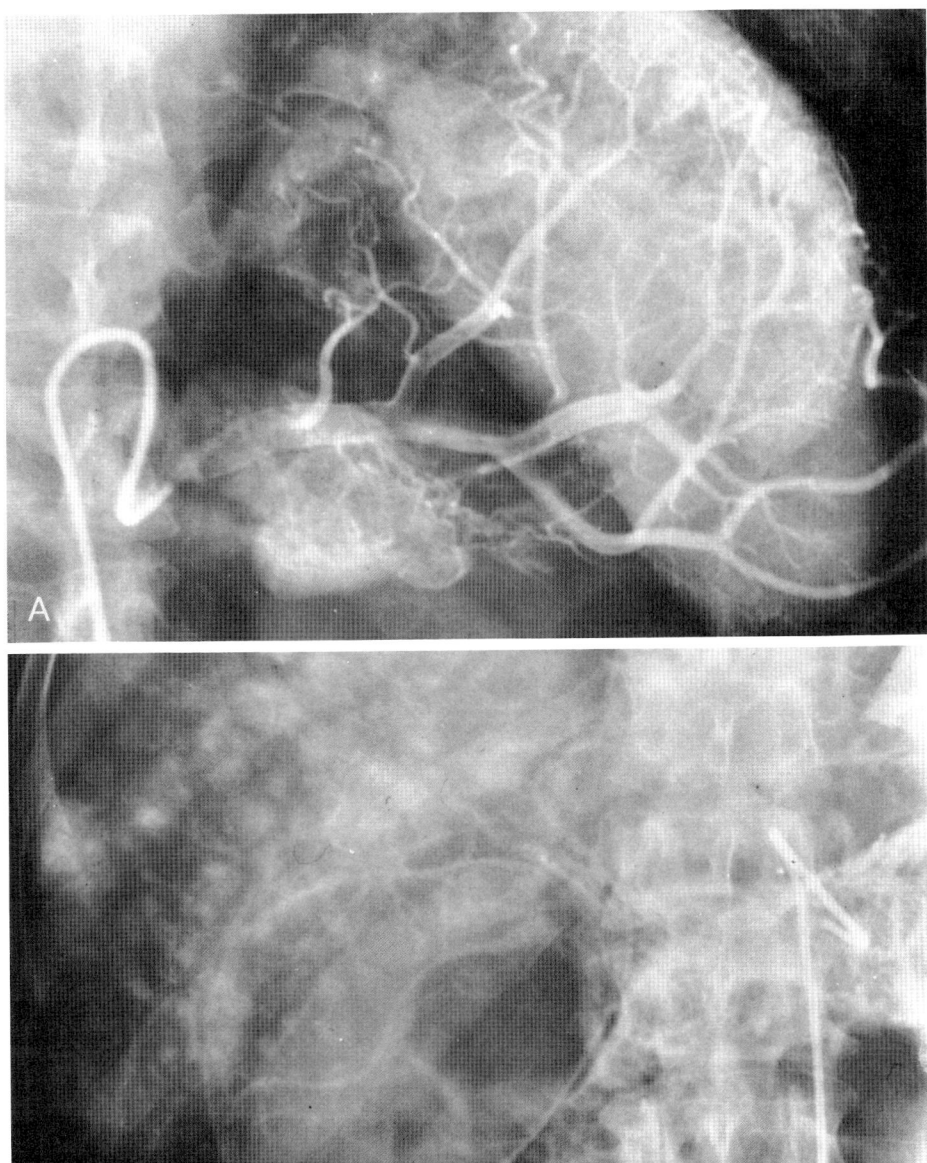

FIGURE 22.125. VIPOMA

A and *B:* Splenic arteriogram showing a hypervascular vipoma (*A*) and a hepatic arteriogram showing small, hypervascular liver metastases in the same patient.

tical to other islet cell tumors. Metastases appear as low density lesions in the liver (Fig. 22.124). Accurate delineation of the primary and metastases is important since surgical resection can result in clinical palliation or cure, even with recurrent disease (61). The adrenals should be scrutinized in this syndrome since it may be caused by a VIP secreting extrapancreatic neurogenic tumor.

Arteriography and Venous Sampling. Localization of vipomas by arteriography is generally successful because of hypervascularity and relatively large size (62) (Fig. 22.125). If necessary, venous sampling can be successful (63).

Somatostatinoma

This very rare tumor arises from the delta cells of the pancreas and elaborates a polypeptide hormone which resembles the hypothalamic growth hormone release inhibiting hormone, somatostatin (64–67). Somatostatin also suppresses release of TSH, insulin, glucagon, gastric acid, pepsin, secretin, and pancreatic exocrine enzymes, and inhibits gallbladder and intestinal motility (2). The associated clinical syndrome is poorly defined, but mild diabetes, hypochlorhydria, steatorrhea, and cholelithiasis have been observed, although the clinical manifestations vary considerably (68–70). In a recent review, a total of 13 patients with this entity were known (70). Eleven of the lesions were intrapancreatic and two occurred in the duodenum. The size ranged from 0.6 to 20 cm. Nine out of 13 had evidence of metastases within the liver. In 7 out of 13 patients there was biochemical evidence of secretion of other hormones including pancreatic polypeptide (3), calcitonin (3), vasoactive intestinal peptide (2), glucagon (2), ACTH (1), insulin (1), and prostaglandin GE_2 (1). Immunocytochemistry of somatostatinomas has demonstrated the presence of other peptide hormones giving rise to a more recent theory that suggests these tumors may function as mixed-cell neoplasms (70).

A 5-cm diameter pancreatic head somatostatinoma has been imaged with ultrasound, and CT findings have been described in a few patients (10, 65). Somatostatinomas resemble other islet cell tumors radiologically.

Carcinoid Tumors

Carcinoid tumors of the gastrointestinal foregut share similar cytochemical characteristics with APUD cells and may secrete a variety of polypeptides (5, 71). These lesions comprise a small percentage (4–6%) of all carcinoid tumors and most often occur in the stomach, duodenum, or very rarely the pancreas (72–77). The classic carcinoid syndrome, produced by midgut carcinoids, is associated with hepatic metastases, overproduction of serotonin and elevated urine 5-hydroxyindoleacetic acid (5-HIAA). In addition to the classic syndrome, foregut carcinoids (stomach and duodenum more so than pancreas) are also capable of producing an atypical carcinoid syndrome in which there is more severe and prolonged flushing or cutaneous vasodilatation, periorbital edema, and lacrimation, which is thought to result from histamine release (5). A lesion can be considered a pancreatic carcinoid if it is of pancreatic origin, has histopathological features found in other carcinoid tumors and secretes 5-hydroxytryptophan or 5-hydroxytryptamine (serotonin) (77). The histological differentiation of islet cell tumor and carcinoid may be difficult or impossible (77). Carcinoid tumors frequently also secrete a variety of other hormones including gastrin, insulin, calcitonin, ACTH, VIP, somatostatin, glucagon, or pancreatic polypeptide (5, 73, 75, 78). Due to their rarity, the exact incidence of malignancy is difficult to ascertain but any pancreatic lesion probably should be treated as potentially malignant since 70–82% of carcinoids of the bowel greater than 2 cm have been malignant in past experience (74). There are no reliable histologic criteria to determine the degree of malignancy (25). Pancreatic carcinoids are often multicentric and disseminated at the time of diagnosis, so that primary surgical excision is rarely feasible. Drugs (serotonin antagonists), chemotherapy, and embolization of liver metastases are often successful for palliation (25).

Very few descriptions of radiologic findings of pancreatic carcinoids have appeared (79). In our experience these neoplasms resemble other islet cell tumors (Fig. 22.126).

Multihormonal Tumors

Pancreatic islet cell tumors can secrete multiple peptide hormones either synchronously or metachronously (5, 71, 78–82). When carefully examined immunohistochemically, islet cell tumors previously thought to be secreting only one peptide can show evidence of multihormonal production so that this phenomenon may be more common than previously suspected (83, 84). The clinical manifestations of patients with such tumors ultimately depend on the predominate polypeptide present and the usual syndromes associated with functioning tumors may overlap. Many of the multihormonal tumors described in the literature have been malignant (78–82). Radiographically these neoplasms will be identical to and indistinguishable from other islet cell tumors.

Nesidioblastosis

Nesidioblastosis is an uncommon cause of neonatal hyperinsulinism, to be considered after the more frequent maternal diabetes has been excluded. It is characterized by diffuse islet cell hyperplasia and possibly microadenomatous transformation of the pancreas (2). The cause is thought to be an inappropriately controlled de-

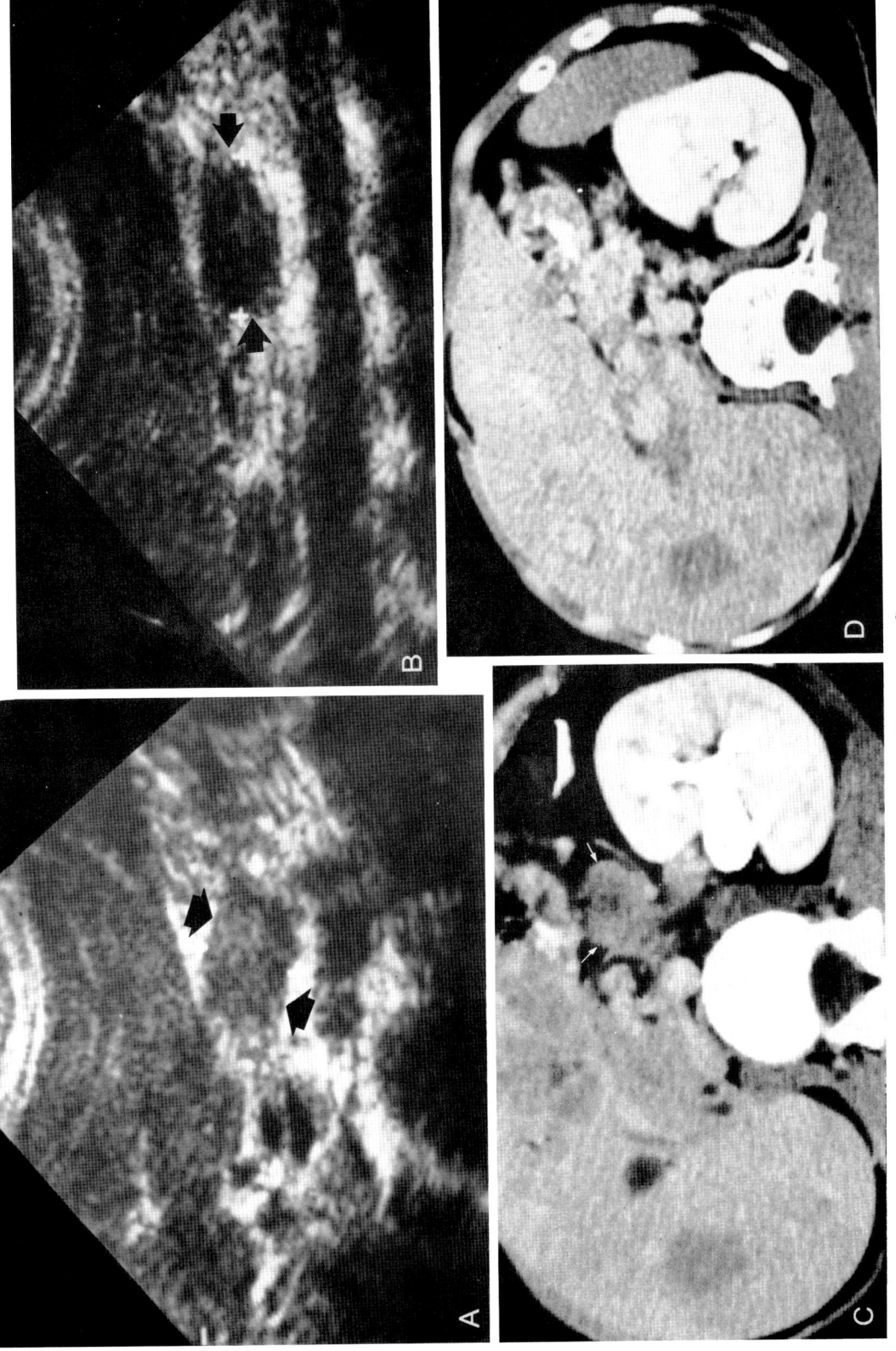

FIGURE 22.126. PANCREATIC CARCINOID

A and B: Transverse and sagittal sonograms respectively, showing a pancreatic carcinoid 3.2 cm in largest diameter (*arrows*). C: Corresponding CT scan showing a tiny lucency probably from necrosis within the tumor (*arrows*). Multiple liver metastases are seen. D: A slightly higher cut showing liver metastases, some of which are enhancing. Other cuts showed retroperitoneal invasion.

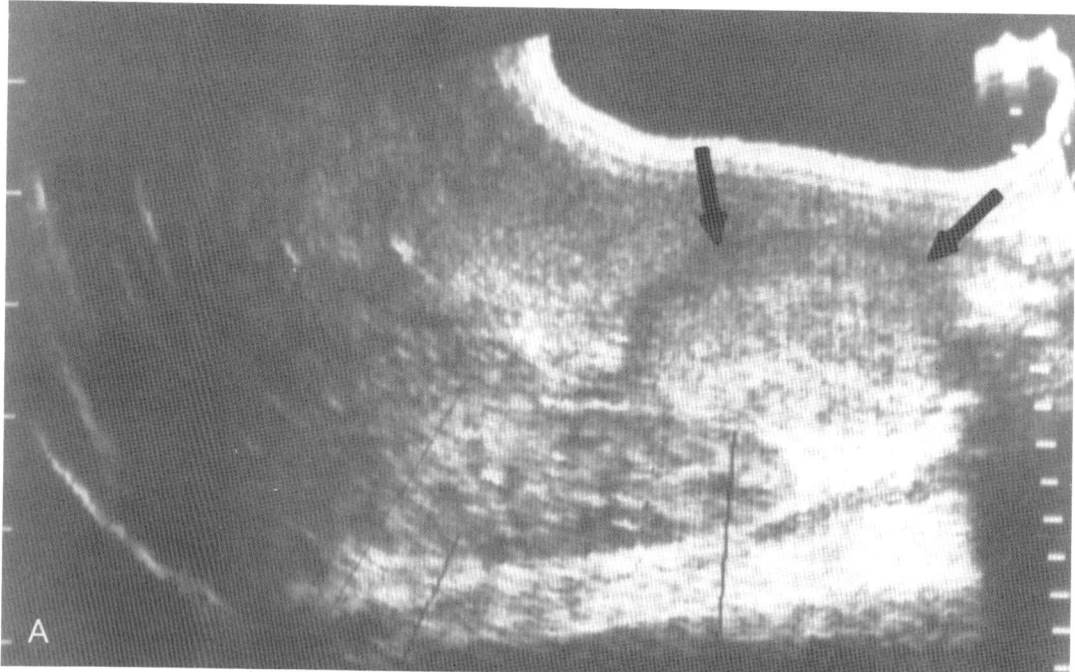
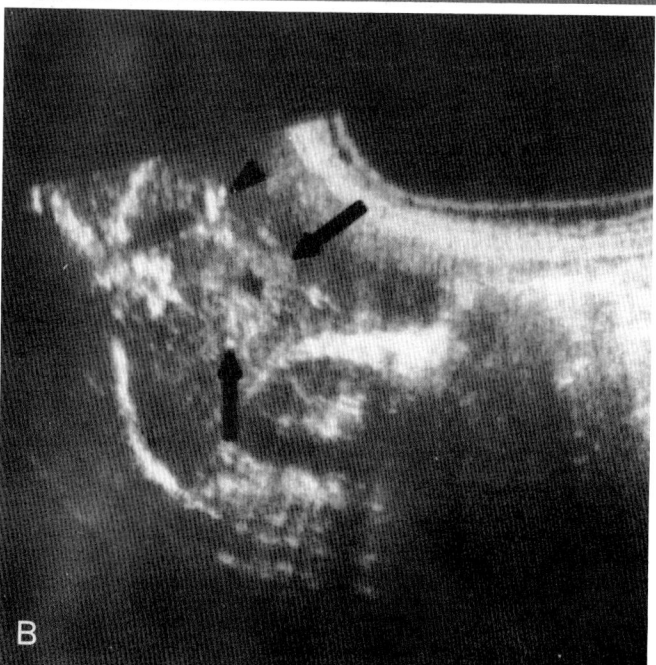

FIGURE 22.127. NONFUNCTIONING ISLET CELL CARCINOMA
A: Longitudinal ultrasound scan shows a large, solid mass. *B:* The liver ultrasound of this patient shows a high echo-amplitude nodule (*arrows*) with central fluid and an additional calcified nodule (*arrowhead*) representing metastases.

velopment of the endocrine pancreas (85). Although there is increased secretion of multiple hormones, insulin hypersecretion predominates clinically (2). Unlike the hypoglycemia in infants of diabetic mothers, that seen in nesidioblastosis does not remit spontaneously or even with medical management in many cases (2, 86). There is a high incidence of neurologic damage because clinical diagnosis is more difficult than in hypoglycemic adults (2). Associated are cardiomyopathy and septal hypertrophy (86). Even after substantial (80–90%) pancreatectomy, medical management (glucose, diazoxide) may be necessary (2, 86).

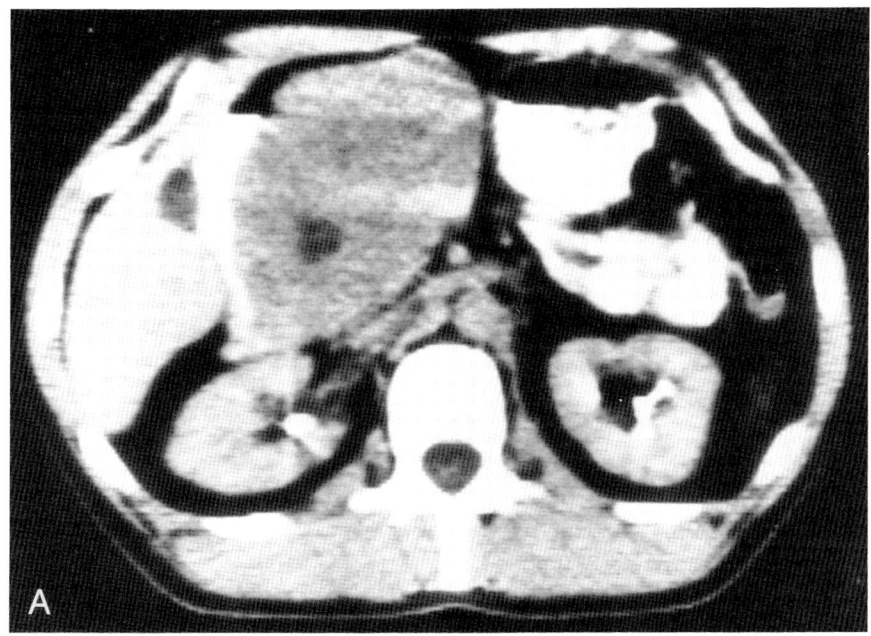
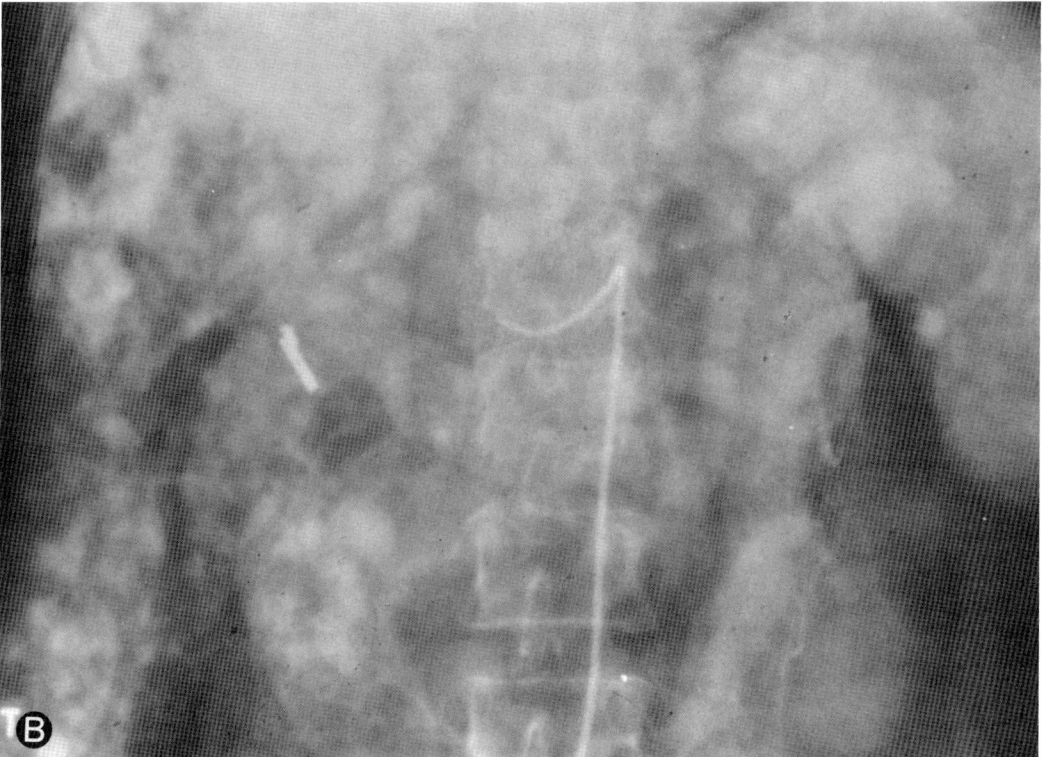

FIGURE 22.128. NONFUNCTIONING ISLET CELL CARCINOMA

A: CT scan shows a mass in the uncinate process. Clinical presentation was indistinguishable from duct cell adenocarcinoma, but large size and central necrosis suggested other histology. *B:* Angiogram shows multiple, small hypervascular liver metastases in another patient with nonfunctioning islet cell carcinoma. CT of the liver (enhanced only) was negative (EMI 5005 scanner).

Radiology

There tends to be a measurable excess of subcutaneous fat in newborn infants of diabetic mothers and in infants with nesidioblastosis, neonatal insulinoma or other causes of neonatal hyperinsulinism, or leucine sensitivity (86). Measured on plain films at the level of T10, the widths of the right and left subcutaneous fat layers are added together; 8.6 mm for term babies and 5.1 mm for 34–35 weeks of gestation are two standard deviations above the mean. Most, if not all, infants with nesidioblastosis will have abnormal fat measurements because of the severe hyperinsulinism in this condition (86).

Nonfunctioning Islet Cell Tumors

Clinical Findings

Nonfunctional tumors comprise about 15–25% of the islet cell neoplasms and are the most common islet cell tumors after insulinomas and gastrinomas (3). Although histologically identical to functioning tumors, they differ in clinical manifestations and behavior (6). As more sensitive hormone assays are developed, it is becoming apparent that most clinically nonfunctioning islet cell tumors do produce some hormone(s). These tumors are only rarely associated with the multiple endocrine neoplasia syndrome in contrast to the functioning variety. Because there is subclinical hormone production, their clinical presentation is identical to adenocarcinoma of the pancreas with jaundice and abdominal pain the predominant clinical symptoms. Delay in detection is common and it is usual for them to be large at the time of initial presentation (87). Age range is 29–72 yr, with most occurring in the fourth and fifth decades (87). Although widespread disease is common at presentation (11), these tumors are frequently slow growing with a 5-yr survival of about 40% in one series (3).

Pathology

Size is usually 6–20 cm in diameter with a slight predominance in the head (3, 81). One large series reported greater than 72% larger than 5 cm in diameter (3). About 80–90% are malignant (3, 11) and 40% have liver metastases at presentation (87). Regional lymph nodes may also be involved. Histology is identical to functioning islet cell tumors (6).

Radiology

Plain Films and Barium Contrast Examination. Plain films are usually nondiagnostic but may show a soft tissue mass or hepatomegaly due to extensive metastases. Although malignant islet tumors calcify in about 10% of cases, most instances of plain film calcification have been in functioning tumors (8). Similar calcifications may occur in hepatic metastases.

A barium meal may show displacement of the stomach and the duodenum depending on the size of the primary lesion.

Ultrasound. All nonfunctioning islet cell tumors visualized with ultrasound have been greater than 5 cm in diameter (10, 11). Most have been uniformly solid neoplasms (Fig. 22.127A), although in one reported case (11) irregular cystic cavities were present within a large primary tumor. This latter case may, in fact, have been a solid and papillary epithelial neoplasm. Hepatic metastases have been varied in appearance, ranging from high amplitude to low amplitude, including target nodules (Fig. 22.127B).

Computed Tomography. Nonfunctional islet cell tumors are large pancreatic masses and about 25% had calcification(s) demonstrable by CT in one series of 24 cases (88). On unenhanced scans about 40% are isodense with the pancreas and 60% had inhomogeneity consistent with necrosis or hemorrhage (Fig. 22.128A) (88). Partial or diffuse contrast enhancement was shown in 75%, and most large masses have central regions that do not enhance (88). Hepatic metastases and nodal enlargement are frequent (53, 88). The former may be shown with greater sensitivity by angiography (Fig. 22.128B). Nonfunctional islet cell tumors tend to be larger than duct cell adenocarcinomas and demonstrate hemorrhage or necrosis and calcification much more frequently. Encasement of the celiac axis or superior mesenteric artery on CT favors duct cell adenocarcinoma versus nonfunctional islet cell tumor (88).

Angiography. Nonfunctional islet cell tumors, both primary and metastatic, are hypervascular with enlarged feeding arteries, a rich arterial bed, and a dense homogeneous capillary stain (11, 87, 89). A minority of cases show pathologic vessels, arteriovenous shunting or vascular encasement (11, 87). Presence of metastases is the best criterion to differentiate malignant lesions from benign ones; venous encasement or intravenous tumor extension are highly suggestive of malignancy (18).

REFERENCES

1. Schein PS, De Lillis RA, Kahn CR, Gorden P, Kraft AR: Islet cell tumors: current concepts and management. *Ann Intern Med* 79:239–257, 1973.

2. Creutzfeld W: Endocrine tumors of the pancreas: clinical, chemical and morphologic findings: *Monogr Pathol* 21:208-230, 1980.
3. Kent RB, van Heerden JA, Weiland LH: Non-functioning islet cell tumors. *Ann Surg* 193:185-190, 1981.
4. Pearse AGE: Common cytochemical and ultrastructural characteristics of cells producing polypeptide hormones (the APUD series) and their relevance to thyroid ultimobranchial C cells and calcitonin. *Proc R Soc Lond [Biol]* 170:71-80, 1968.
5. Freisen SR: Tumors of the endocrine pancreas. *N Engl J Med* 306:580-590, 1982.
6. Larsson LI: Endocrine pancreatic tumors. *Hum Pathol* 9:401-416, 1978.
7. Fajans SS, Floyd JC: Diagnosis and medical management of insulinomas. *Annu Rev Med* 30:313-329, 1979.
8. Imhof M, Frank P: Pancreatic calcifications in malignant islet cell tumors. *Radiology* 122:333-337, 1977.
9. Hancke S: Localization of hormone-producing gastrointestinal tumors by ultrasonic scanning. *Scand J Gastroenterol* (14 Suppl) 53:115-116, 1979.
10. Shawker TH, Doppman JL, Dunnick NR, McCarthy DM: Ultrasonic investigation of pancreatic islet cell tumors. *J Ultrasound Med* 1:193-200, 1982.
11. Gold J, Rosenfield AT, Sostman D: Non-functioning islet cell tumors of the pancreas: radiographic and ultrasonographic appearance in two cases. *AJR* 131:715-717, 1978.
12. Raghavendra BN, Glickstein ML: Sonography of islet cell tumor of the pancreas: report of two cases. *J Clin Ultrasound* 9:331-333, 1981.
13. Kuhn FP, Gunther R, Ruckert K, Beyer J: Ultrasonic demonstration of small pancreatic islet cell tumors. *J Clin Ultrasound* 10:173-175, 1982.
14. Guenther RW, Klose JK, Ruckert K, Kuhn FP, Beyer J, Klotter H, Cordes U: Islet-cell tumors: detection of small lesions with computed tomography and ultrasound. *Radiology* 148:485-488, 1983.
15. Sigel B, Duarte B, Coelho JC, Nyhus LM, Baker RJ, Machi J: Localization of insulinomas of the pancreas at operation by real-time ultrasound scanning. *Surg Gynecol Obstet* 156:145-147, 1983.
16. Charboneau JW, James EM, van Heerden JA, Grant CS, Sheedy PF: Intraoperative real-time ultrasonographic localization of pancreatic insulinomas: initial experience. *J. Ultrasound Med* 2:251-254, 1983.
17. Reuter SR, Redman HC: *Gastrointestinal Angiography.* Philadelphia, W. B. Saunders, 1977, pp 169-174.
18. Bok EJ, Cho KJ, Williams DM, Brady TM, Weiss CA, Forrest ME: Venous involvement in islet cell tumors of the pancreas. *AJR* 142:319-322, 1984.
19. Doppman JL, Brennan MF, Kahn CR, Marx SJ: Circumscribing or peridenomal vessel: a helpful angiographic finding in certain islet cell and parathyroid adenomas. *AJR* 136:163-165, 1981.
20. Robins J, Bookstein JJ, Oberman HA, Fajans SS: Selective angiography in localizing islet-cell tumors of the pancreas. *Radiology* 106:525-528, 1973.
21. Cho KJ, Vinik AI, Thompson NW, Shields JJ, Porter DJ, Brady TM, Cadavid G, Fajans SS: Localization of the source of hyperinsulinism: percutaneous transhepatic portal and pancreatic vein catheterization with hormone assay. *AJR* 139:237-245, 1982.
22. Roche A, Raisonnier A, Gillon-Savouret MC: Pancreatic venous sampling and arteriography in localizing insulinomas and gastrinomas. Procedure and results in 55 cases. *Radiology* 145:621-627, 1982.
23. Doppman JL, Brennan MF, Dunnick NR, Kahn CR, Gorden P: The role of pancreatic venous sampling in the localization of occult insulinomas. *Radiology* 133:557-562, 1981.
24. Kaplan EL, Lee CH: Recent advances in the diagnosis and treatment of insulinomas. *Surg Clin North Am* 59:119-129, 1979.
25. Modlin IM: Endocrine tumors of the pancreas. *Surg Gynecol Obstet* 149:751-768, 1979.
26. Rosai J: *Ackerman's Surgical Pathology.* St. Louis, C.V. Mosby, 1981, pp 674-684.
27. Dunnick NR, Long JA, Krudy A, Shawker TH, Doppman JL: Localizing insulinomas with combined radiographic methods. *AJR* 135:747-752, 1980.
28. Service FJ, Dale AJD, Elveback LR, Jiang NS: Insulinoma. Clinical and diagnostic features of 60 consecutive cases. *Mayo Clin Proc* 51:417-429, 1976.
29. Fricke M, Zick R, Mitzkat HJ: Computed tomography of insulinomas. *Radiology* 118:252-254, 1978.
30. Rossi P, Baert A, Marchal W, Tipaldi L, Wilrus W, Pavone P: Multiple bolus technique vs single bolus or infusion of contrast medium to obtain prolonged contrast enhancement of the pancreas. *Radiology* 144:929-931, 1982.
31. Hosoki T: Dynamic CT of pancreatic tumors. *AJR* 140:959-965, 1983.
32. Stark DD, Moss AA, Goldberg HI, Deveney CW: CT of pancreatic islet cell tumors. *Radiology* 150:491-494, 1984.
33. Jensen RT, Gardner JD, Raufman JP, Pandol SJ, Doppman JL, Collen MJ: Zollinger-Ellison syndrome: current concepts and management. *Ann Intern Med* 98:59-75, 1983.
34. Friesen ST, Tomita T: Pseudo-Zollinger-Ellison syndrome. *Ann Surg* 194:481-483, 1981.
35. McCarthy DM: Report on the United States experience with cimetidine in Zollinger-Ellison syndrome and other hypersecretory states. *Gastroenterology* 74:453-458, 1978.
36. Pederson RT, Haidak DJ, Ferris RA, MacDonald JS, Schein PS: Osteoblastic bone metastasis in Zollinger-Ellison syndrome. *Radiology* 118:63-64, 1976.
37. Schlaeger R, Lemay M, Wermer P: Upper gastrointestinal tract alterations in adenomatosis of the endocrine glands. *Radiology* 75:517-530, 1960.
38. Missakian MM, Carlson HC, Huizenga KA: Roentgenographic findings in Zollinger-Ellison syndrome. *AJR* 94:429-437, 1965.
39. Zboralske FF, Amberg JR: Detection of the Zollinger-Ellison syndrome: the radiologist's responsibility. *AJR* 104:529-543, 1968.
40. Meyers WC, Thompson WM, Kelvin FM et al: A reappraisal of the radiologic diagnosis of Zollinger-Ellison syndrome. *Clin Surg* 1:99-105, 1982.
41. Christoforidis AJ, Nelson SW: Radiological manifestations of ulcerogenic tumors of the pancreas. The Zollinger-Ellison syndrome. *JAMA* 198:511-516, 1966.
42. Bonfils S, Landor JH, Mignon M, Hervoir P: Results of surgical management in 92 consecutive patients with Zollinger-Ellison syndrome. *Ann Surg* 194:692-697, 1981.
43. Krudy AG, Doppman JL, Jensen RT et al: Localization of islet cell tumors by dynamic CT: Comparison with plain CT, arteriography, sonography, and venous sampling. *AJR* 143:585-589, 1984.
44. Dunnick NR, Doppman JL, Geelhoed GW: Intravenous extension of endocrine tumors. *AJR* 135:471-476, 1980.
45. Dunnick NR, Doppman JL, Mills SR, McCarthy DM: Computed tomographic detection of non-beta pancreatic islet cell tumors. *Radiology* 135:117-120, 1980.
46. Deveney CW, Deveney KE, Stark D, Moss AA, Stein S, Way LW: Resection of gastrinomas. *Ann Surg* 198:546-553, 1983.
47. Balfe DM, Koehler RE, Karstaedt N, Stanley RJ, Sagel SS: Computed tomography of gastric neoplasms. *Radiol-*

ogy 140:431–436, 1981.
48. Mills SR, Doppman JL, Dunnick NR, McCarthy DM: Evaluation of angiography in Zollinger-Ellison syndrome. *Radiology* 113:317–320, 1979.
49. Montenegro-Rodas F, Samaan NA: Glucagonoma tumors and syndrome. *Curr Probl Cancer* 6(6):1–54, 1981.
50. Lokich J, Anderson N, Russini A et al: Pancreatic alpha cell tumors: case report and review of literature. *Cancer* 45:2657–2683, 1980.
51. Stacpoole PW: The glucagonoma syndrome: clinical features, diagnosis and treatment. *Endocr Rev* 2:347–361, 1981.
52. Stacpoole PW, Jaspan J, Kasselberg AG, Halter SA, Polonsky K, Cluck FW, Liljenquist JE, Rabin D: A familial glucagonoma syndrome: genetic, chemical and biochemical features. *Am J Med* 70:1017–1026, 1981.
53. Cho KJ, Wilcox CW, Reuter SR: Glucagon-producing islet cell tumor of the pancreas. *AJR* 129:159–161, 1977.
54. Ingemansson S, Holst J, Lars-Inge I, Lunderquist A: Localization of glucagonomas by catherization of the pancreatic veins and with glucagon assay. *Surg Gynecol Obstet* 145:509–516, 1977.
55. Long, RG, Bryant MC, Mitchell SJ, Adrian TE, Polak JM, Blood SR: Clinicopathological study of pancreatic and ganglioneuroblastoma tumors secreting vasoactive intestinal polypeptide (vipomas). *Br Med J* 282:1767–1771, 1981.
56. Ebeid AM, Murray PD, Fischer JE: Vasoactive intestinal peptide and the watery diarrhea syndrome. *Ann Surg* 187:411–416, 1978.
57. Gold RP, Black TJ, Rotterdam H, Casarella WJ: Radiologic and pathologic characterization of the WDHA syndrome. *AJR* 127:397–401, 1976.
58. Thomas LE, Lamb GHR, Barraclough MA: Angiographic demonstration of a pancreatic "vipoma" in the WDHA syndrome. *AJR* 127:1037–1039, 1976.
59. Shenoy SS: Case of fall season: vipoma of body pancreas with hepatic metastases: *Semin Roentgenol* 13:301–302, 1978.
60. Verner JV, Morrison AB: Endocrine pancreatic islet disease with diarrhea. Report of a case due to diffuse hyperplasia of non-beta islet tumor with a review of 54 additional cases. *Arch Intern Med* 133:492–500, 1974.
61. Nagorney DM, Bloom SR, Polak JM, Blumgart LH: resolution of recurrent Verner-Morrison syndrome by resection of metastatic vipoma. *Surgery* 93:348–353, 1983.
62. Imamoto K, Yoshino F, Nakao N, et al: Angiographic diagnosis of a pancreatic islet cell tumor in a patient with WDHA syndrome. *Gastrointest Radiol* 5:259–261, 1980.
63. Kingham JGC, Dick R, Bloom SR, Frankel RJ: Vipoma: localization by percutaneous portal venous sampling. *Br Med J* 2:1682–1683, 1978.
64. Ganda OP, Weir GC, Soeldner JS et al: "Somatostatinoma," a somatostatin containing tumor of the endocrine pancreas. *N Engl J Med* 296:963–967, 1977.
65. Unger RH: Somatistatinoma. *N Engl J Med* 296:998–1000, 1977.
66. Axelrod L, Bush MA, Hirsch HJ, Loo SWH: Malignant somatostatinoma: clinical features and metabolic studies. *J Clin Endocrinol Metab* 52:886–896, 1981.
67. Gerlock A, Muhletaler CA, Halter S, Goncharenko V: Pancreatic somatostatinoma: histologic, clinical and angiographic features. *AJR* 133:939–943, 1979.
68. Krejs GJ, Orci L, Conlon SM et al: Somatostatinoma syndrome. *N Engl J Med* 301:285–292, 1979.
69. Pipeleers D, Couturier E, Gepts W, Reynders J, Somers G: Five cases of somatostatinoma: clinical heterogeneity and diagnosis usefulness of basal and tolbutamide induced hypersomatostatinemia. *J Clin Endocrinol Metab* 56:1236–1242, 1983.
70. Stacpoole PW, Kasselberg AG, Berelowitz M, Chey WY: Somatistatinoma syndrome: does a clinical entity exist? *Acta Endocrinol* 102:80–87, 1983.
71. Friesen SR, Hermreck AS, Mantz FA: Glucagon, gastrin and carcinoid tumors of the duodenum, pancreas, and stomach: polypeptide "apudomas" of the foregut. *Am J Surg* 127:90–101, 1974.
72. Wareing TH, Sawyers JL: Carcinoids and the carcinoid syndrome. *Am J Surg* 145:769–772, 1983.
73. Zeitels J, Naunheim K, Kaplan EL, Strauss F: Carcinoid tumors. A 37 year experience. *Arch Surg* 117:732–737, 1982.
74. Godwin JD: Carcinoid tumors. An analysis of 2837 cases. *Cancer* 36:560–569, 1975.
75. Balthazar EJ, Megibow A, Bryk D, Cohen T: Gastric carcinoid tumors: radiographic features in eight cases. *AJR* 139:1123–1127, 1982.
76. Lasson A, Alwmark A, Nobin A, Sundler F: Endocrine tumors of the duodenum. Clinical characteristics and hormone content. *Ann Surg* 197:393–398, 1983.
77. Gordon DL, Lo MC, Schwartz MA: Carcinoid of the pancreas. *Am J Med* 51:412–415, 1971.
78. Belchetz PE, Brown CL, Makin HLJ et al: ACTH glucagon and gastrin production by a pancreatic islet cell carcinoma and its treatment. *Clin Endocrinol* 2:307–316, 1973.
79. Scheiber W: Insulin-producing Zollinger-Ellison tumor. *Surgery* 54:448–450, 1963.
80. Law DH, Liddle GW, Scott WH, Tauber SD: Ectopic production of multiple hormones (ACTH, MSH, and gastrin) by a single malignant tumor. *N Engl J Med* 273:292–296, 1965.
81. Heintz PH, Steiner H, Walter F, Egli F, Kapp JP: Multihormonal amyloid-producing tumor of the islets of Langerhans in a twelve year old boy. *Virchows Arch Pathol Anat* 353:312–324, 1971.
82. O'Neal LW, Kipnis DM, Luse SA, Lacy PE, Jarett L: Secretion of various endocrine substances by ACTH-secreting tumors—gastrin, melanotrophin, norepinephrine, serotonin, parathormone, vasopressin, glucagon. *Cancer* 21:1219–1232, 1968.
83. Yang K, Ulich T, Cheng L, Lewin KJ: The neuroendocrine products of intestinal carcinoids. An immunoperoxidase study of 35 carcinoid tumors stained for serotonin and eight polypeptide hormones. *Cancer* 51:1918–1926, 1983.
84. Larsson LI, Grimelius L, Hakanson R, Rehfeld JF, Stadil F, Holst J, Angervall L, Sundler F: Mixed endocrine pancreatic tumors producing several peptide hormones. *Am J Pathol* 79:271–279, 1975.
85. Heitz PU, Kloppel G, Hacki WH, Polak JM, Pearse AG: Neisioblastosis: the pathologic basis of persistent hyperinsulinemic hypoglycemia in infants. *Diabetes* 26:632–642, 1977.
86. Oestrich AE, Opperman HC: Abnormal fat thickness in newborns with neisioblastosis. *Radiology* 141:679–680, 1981.
87. Adler O, Kaftori JK, Rosenberger A, Arieh JB: Non-functioning islet cell tumors of the pancreas. A review of the literature and a report of two cases. *ROFO* 127:559–563, 1977.
88. Eelkema EA, Stephens DH, Sheedy PF: Islet cell carcinoma of the pancreas: CT characteristics. Presented at the Society of Gastrointestinal Radiology, Bermuda, October, 1983.
89. Mills SR, Doppman JL, Kahn RE: Metastatic islet cell carcinoma to the liver visualized after intra-arterial epinephrine. *AJR* 132:664–665, 1979.

23

Magnetic Resonance Imaging of the Pancreas

ARNOLD C. FRIEDMAN, M.D.

NORMAL ANATOMY

The normal pancreas can be depicted in three planes by state-of-the-art MRI scanners (Fig. 23.1). As with CT, the pancreas is seen best in those patients who are endowed with abundant retroperitoneal fat. When retroperitoneal fat is sparse, it is difficult to separate pancreatic pa-

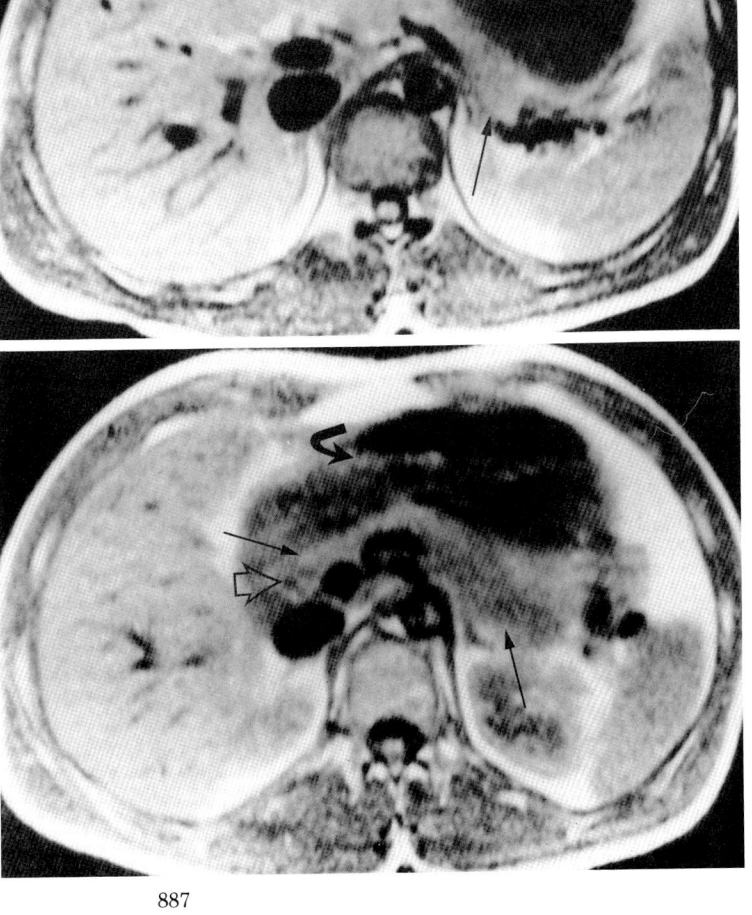

FIGURE 23.1 NORMAL ANATOMY OF PANCREAS
Axial MRI, TE = 28 TR = 500, normal anatomy: even in this thin patient, the pancreas is fairly well-depicted. *Top and bottom:* Medium intensity pancreas (*arrows*) outlined by excellent vascular anatomy and gas/fluid in distended stomach. The latter was distended with gas-producing granules (note air-fluid level, *curved arrow*). The normal common bile duct is shown (*open arrow*). Jejunum (*bottom, straight arrow*), anterior to the left kidney has lower intensity than the pancreatic tail.

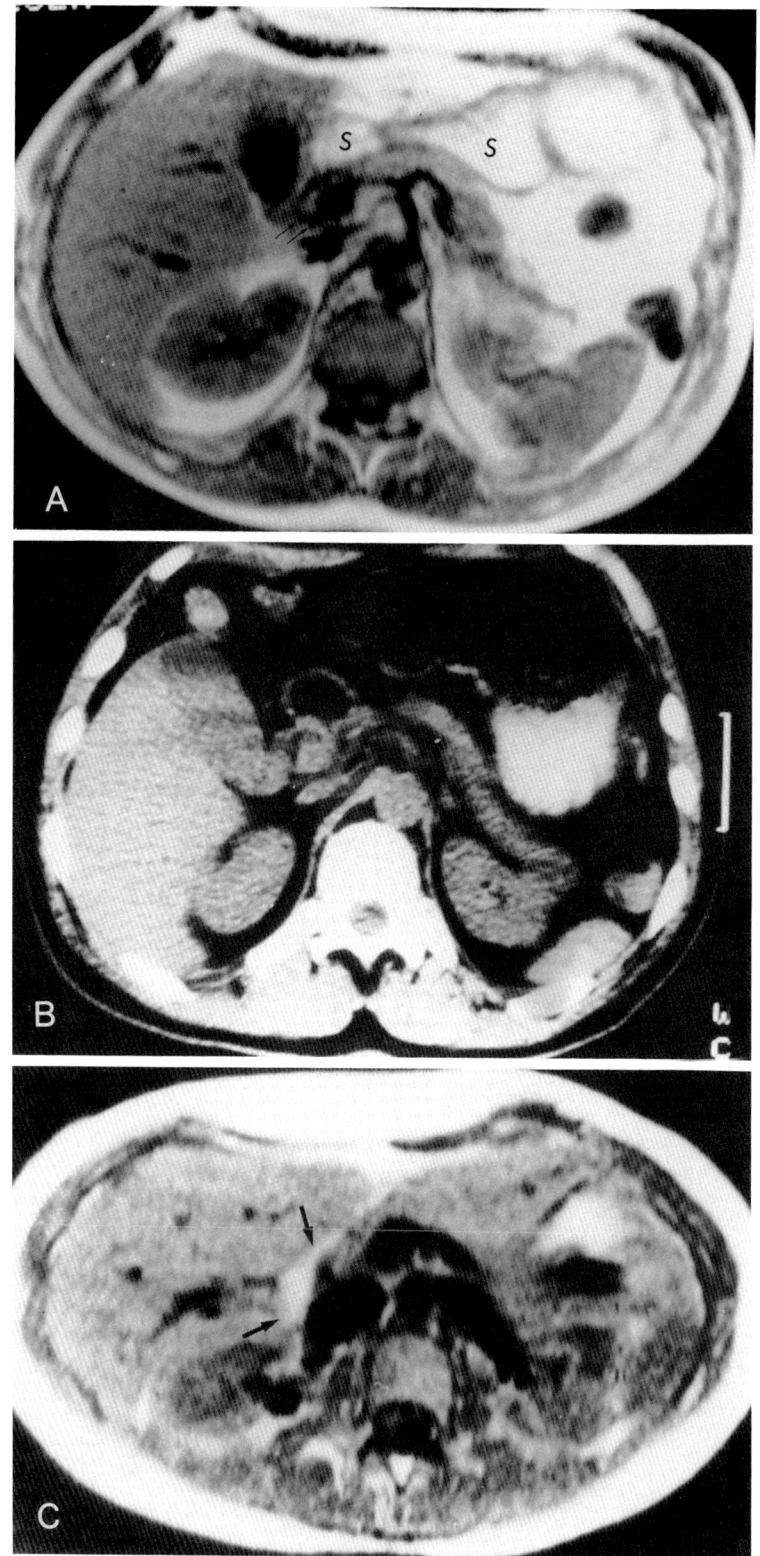

FIGURE 23.2. NORMAL ANATOMY OF PANCREAS

A: Axial MRI, TE = 28, TR = 500: medium intensity pancreas is well-delineated by retroperitoneal fat and high intensity oral contrast in the stomach (*S*). Note excellent vascular anatomy as well as the normal common bile duct and main pancreatic duct (*arrows*). *B:* Corresponding CT on the same patient. *C:* The pancreas would not be seen in this thin patient were it not for high intensity contrast (*arrows*) in the duodenum outlining the head.

renchyma from contiguous stomach, duodenum, and small bowel. This distinction is facilitated if the adjacent viscus is fortuitously or intentionally distended with gas or intestinal fluids. We have had success delineating pancreatic borders using oral ferric ammonium citrate for positive contrast (Fig. 23.2) and gas-producing granules for negative contrast (Fig. 23.1). Degradation of MRI of the pancreas by respiratory and/or peristaltic motion varies from patient to patient. The peripancreatic vasculature is generally superbly depicted by MRI without the need for intravenous contrast agents. The signal intensity of normal pancreatic parenchyma is moderate, similar to that of the liver on both spin echo and inversion recovery sequences (1, 2). Pancreatic intensity is less than that of the kidney and spleen on spin echo images with long TRs or TEs, but it is greater than that of kidney and spleen on inversion recovery images (1). This intensity can be enhanced after intravenous administration of gadolinium-DTPA, but the clinical usefulness of pancreatic enhancement remains to be determined (3). Calculated T1 and

TABLE 23.1.
RELAXATION TIMES OF NORMAL PANCREAS AND SOME NEOPLASTIC AND INFLAMMATORY DISEASES

Condition (Ref.)	T1 (msec)	T2 (msec)	Field Strength (T)
Normal (1)	448 ± 131	52 ± 6	0.35
Normal (5)	180–200		0.04
Normal (4)	190		0.04
Normal (4)	290	60	0.20
Normal (4)	572	189	0.47
Normal (4)	320		0.57
Normal (4)	605		2.35
Pancreatitis (5)	200–275		0.04
Pancreatitis (1)	961 ± 461	265 ± 17	0.35
Pseudocyst (5)	800–1000		0.04
Abscess (5)	400–440		0.04
Adenocarcinoma (1)	625 ± 128	62 ± 2	0.35
Islet cell carcinoma (1)		80 ± 3	0.35

T2 relaxation times will vary with field strength and may not be comparable between different scanners at the same field strength (4). Published values are given in Table 23.1.

INFLAMMATORY DISEASE

In patients with acute pancreatitis, MRI is able to demonstrate pancreatic enlargement and effacement of tissue planes (Fig. 23.3). Changes in intensity of the gland itself due to T1 prolongation may or may not be present and, if present, could be obscured by peripancreatic fluid or phlegmon which also tend to have prolonged T1 (1, 6). Because of relatively prolonged T1 and T2, pancreatic parenchyma in chronic pancreatitis may be hyperintense at long TR or TE on spin echo images and hypointense on inversion recovery images compared to the liver (1). Calcifications and dilated pancreatic ducts are not seen as well with MRI as with CT (1, 2). Calcifications are ill-defined low intensity regions and the contents of a dilated duct are depicted as a high intensity line within the pancreas on long TR spin echo images (1). Pseudocysts are low intensity masses at short TE/TR that show marked intensity increases compared to liver at long TE/TR because of the prolonged relaxation times of cyst fluid. Currently CT detects more pseudocysts than MRI and is better at delineating their margins (1). Pancreatic atrophy and fatty replacement causes increased pancreatic intensity because of the the short T1 and long T2 of fat (Fig. 23.4).

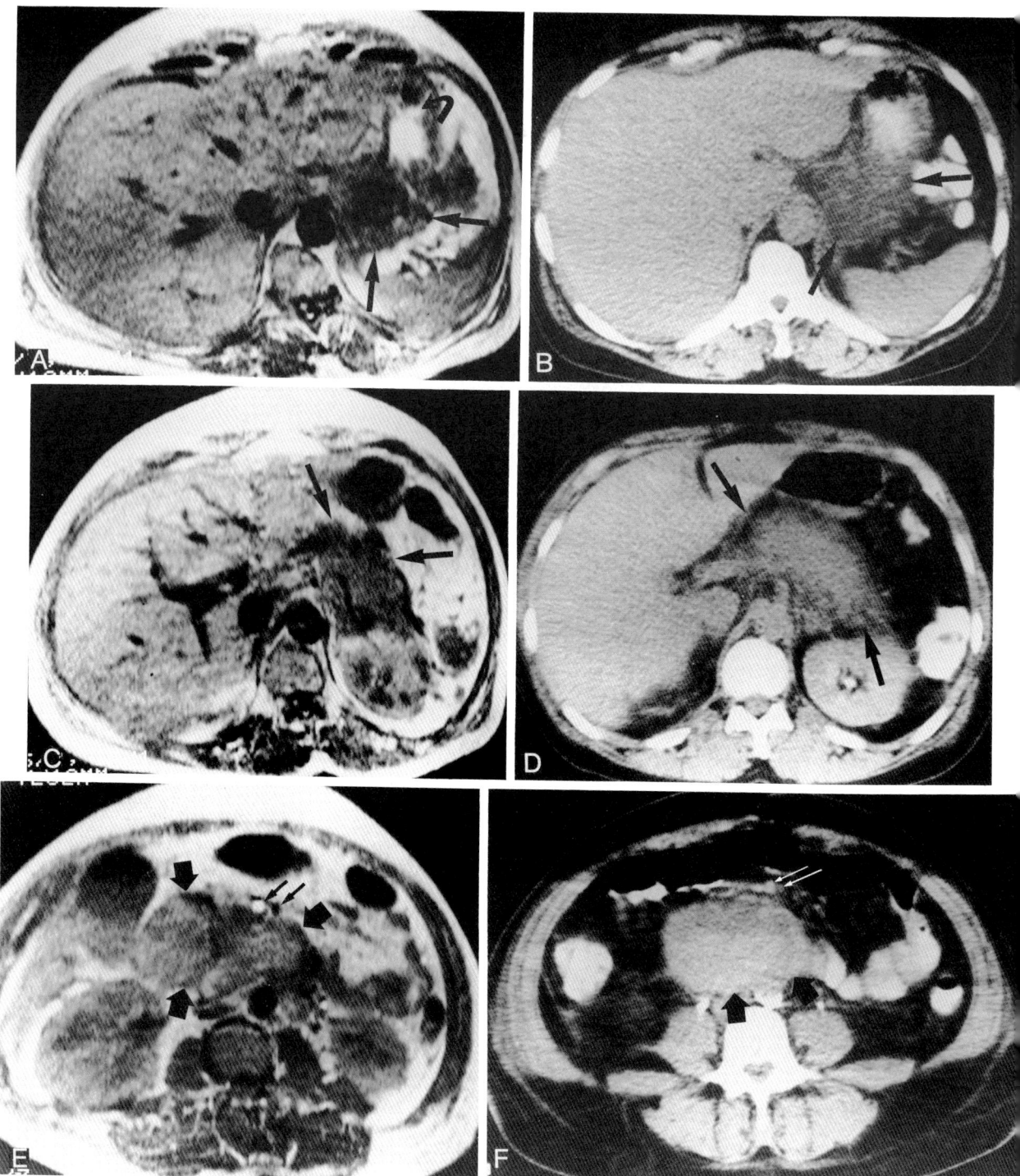

FIGURE 23.3. PANCREATITIS

MRI compared to CT. MR is spin echo, TE = 28/TR = 500, 0.3T *A* and *B:* Retrogastric phlegmon (*arrows*). High signal intensity in the stomach (*curved arrow*) is from ingested ferric ammonium citrate. Tissue planes are better delineated by CT. *C* and *D:* Phlegmon in body and tail (*arrows*). Vascular anatomy is shown better by MRI. *E* and *F:* Hemorrhagic fluid collection (*arrows*) displacing duodenum anteriorly, causing partial obstruction. The blood and the relationship to bowel is shown better by CT. The effects of the mass on the superior mesenteric artery and vein (entrance artifact) are shown better by MRI (*small arrows*).

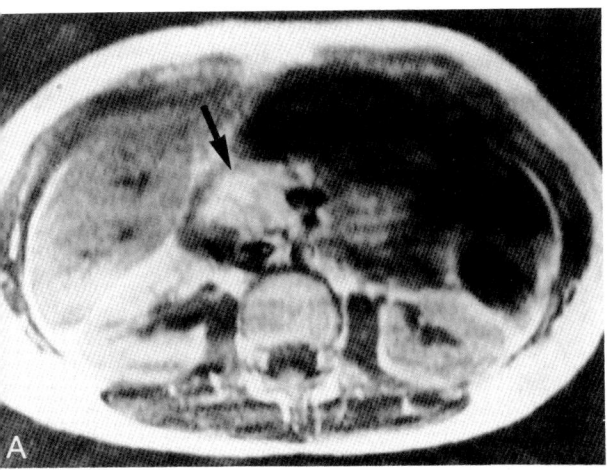
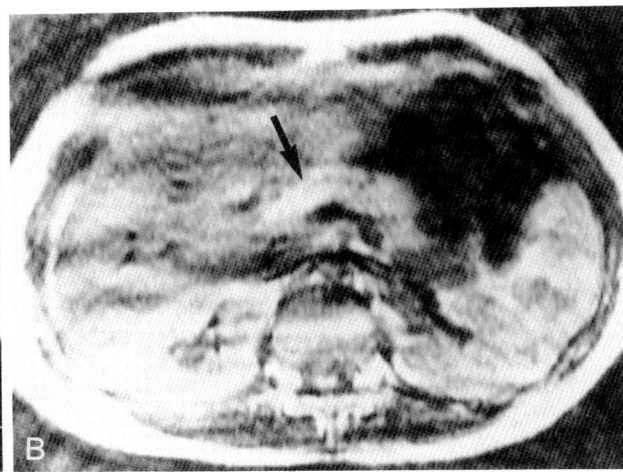
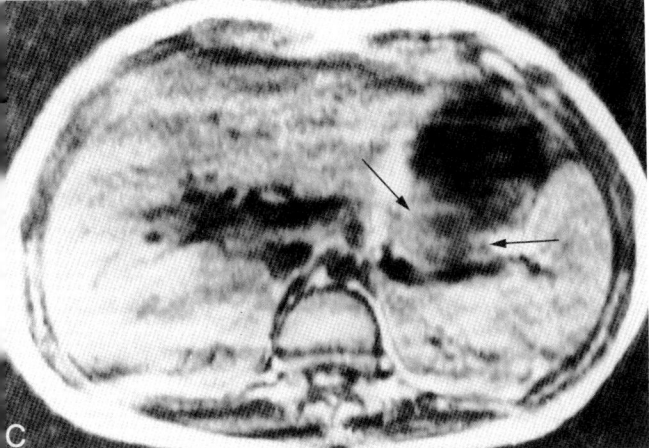

FIGURE 23.4. FATTY REPLACEMENT OF PANCREAS IN CYSTIC FIBROSIS

MR vs. ultrasound, TE = 28/TR = 1000, 0.3T. *A* and *B:* High intensity in the head and body (*arrows*). *C:* Inhomogeneous medium intensity in the tail (*arrows*). Stomach is very low intensity because of ingested effervescent granules. *D* and *E:* Transverse sonography: high echo amplitude in head and body (*arrows*, *D*). Mixed, coarse echo texture in tail (*black arrows*, *E*) and small cyst (*white arrow*) seen through a water-filled stomach (*S*). Little or no additional information gained by MRI compared to ultrasound, although the interpretation of the latter is more subjective.

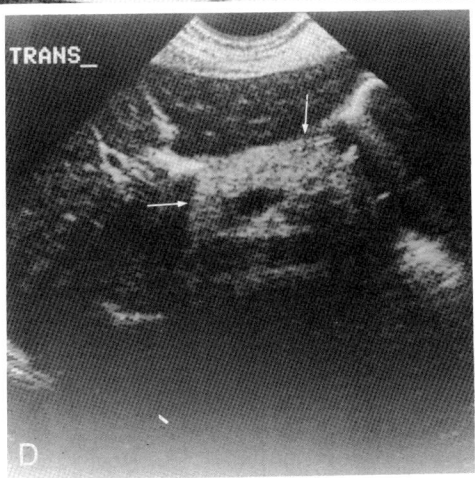
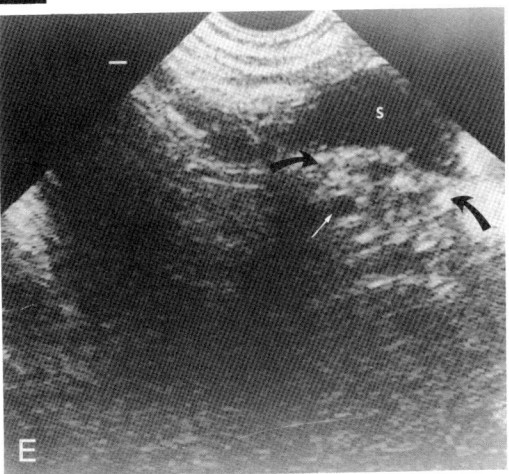

HEMOCHROMATOSIS

Liver biopsy and CT are useful in measuring hepatic iron levels in the diagnosis and treatment of hemochromatosis, but it has not hitherto been feasible to measure pancreatic levels during life. Pathologic studies have shown pancreatic iron levels 20–80% of those in the liver (7). Spin-echo MRI in patients with hemochromatosis has shown decreases in pancreatic and liver intensity of 26 and 90%, respectively (1). Paramagnetic iron shortens both T1 and T2 but the latter effect seems to predominate in hemochromatosis. Calculation of T1 and T2 may be impossible because of the low signal to noise ratio. The decrease in signal intensity should be proportional in some way to parenchymal iron levels and MRI could be used for quantitation once the necessary curves are generated.

NEOPLASMS

Adenocarcinoma of the pancreas can be diagnosed on MRI (Fig. 23.5 and 23.6) using standard morphologic criteria, but signal intensity differences between tumor and normal parenchyma

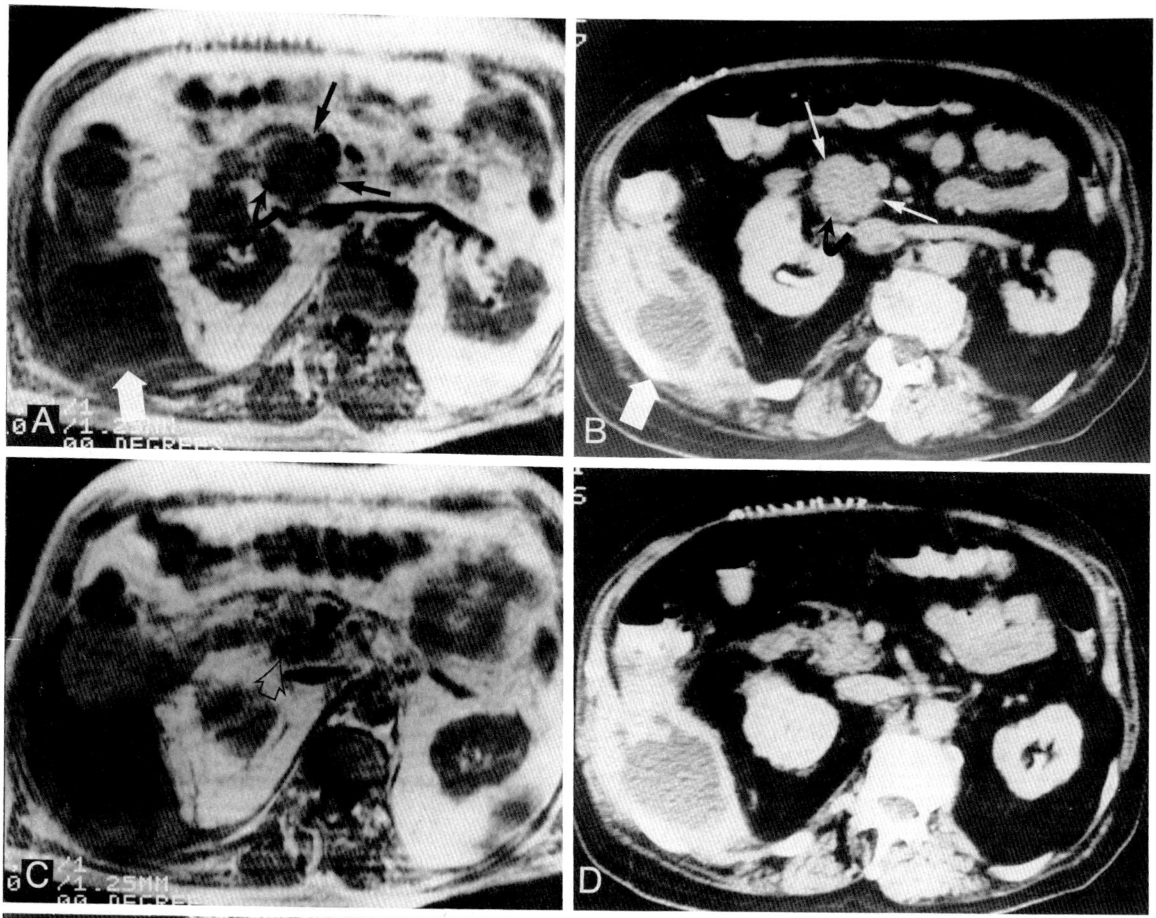

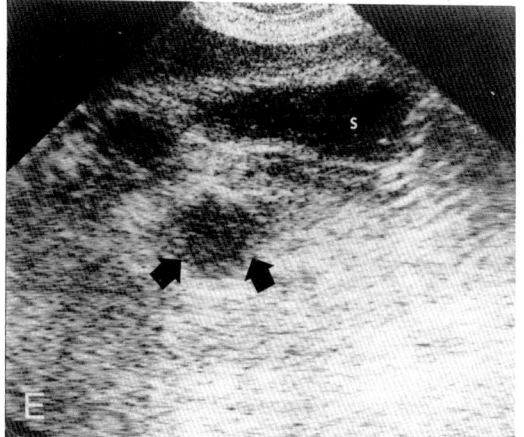

FIGURE 23.5. PLEOMORPHIC GIANT CELL CARCINOMA

Pleomorphic giant cell carcinoma of the pancreas discovered incidentally in the workup of a subhepatic abscess. MRI (TE = 28/TR = 500, 0.3T) vs. CT. *A* and *B:* Mass in the uncinate process (*arrows*). Nonobstructed distal common bile duct (*curved arrow*). Subhepatic abscess (*large white arrows*). Equivalent information on both modalities. Diagnosis of abscess somewhat more specific on CT because of enhancing rind. *C* and *D:* One slice cephalad to A and B through normal pancreas. Distal nondilated common duct seen somewhat better by MRI (*arrow*). *E:* Mass (*arrows*) is also obvious on transverse sonography through a water-filled stomach (*S*).

are not usually detected (1, 2). A focal subtle intensity difference can be the only MRI abnormality seen in patients with adenocarcinoma of the pancreas, but this finding is not specific for neoplasm (1, 5, 6). Vascular compromise by carcinoma can be delineated without intravenous contrast material and invasion of retroperitoneal structures as well as liver metastases and lymphadenopathy can be detected. Pancreatic and biliary ductal dilatation is seen better with CT and ultrasound (Fig. 23.6). Intravenous MRI contrast agents facilitate the differentiation of dilated intrahepatic ducts from vessels (3).

In a small series, islet cell carcinomas showed markedly increased intensity relative to normal pancreas because of prolonged T2 (Fig. 23.7) (1). This contrast is accentuated at long TEs. Although the above seems promising, much further work is needed to determine what role MRI will play in the evaluation of islet cell tumors.

As with CT, peripancreatic lymphoma is difficult to differentiate from an intrinsic pancreatic mass on MRI because of isointensity (1). The associated presense of extensive adenopathy favors lymphoma over pancreatic carcinoma.

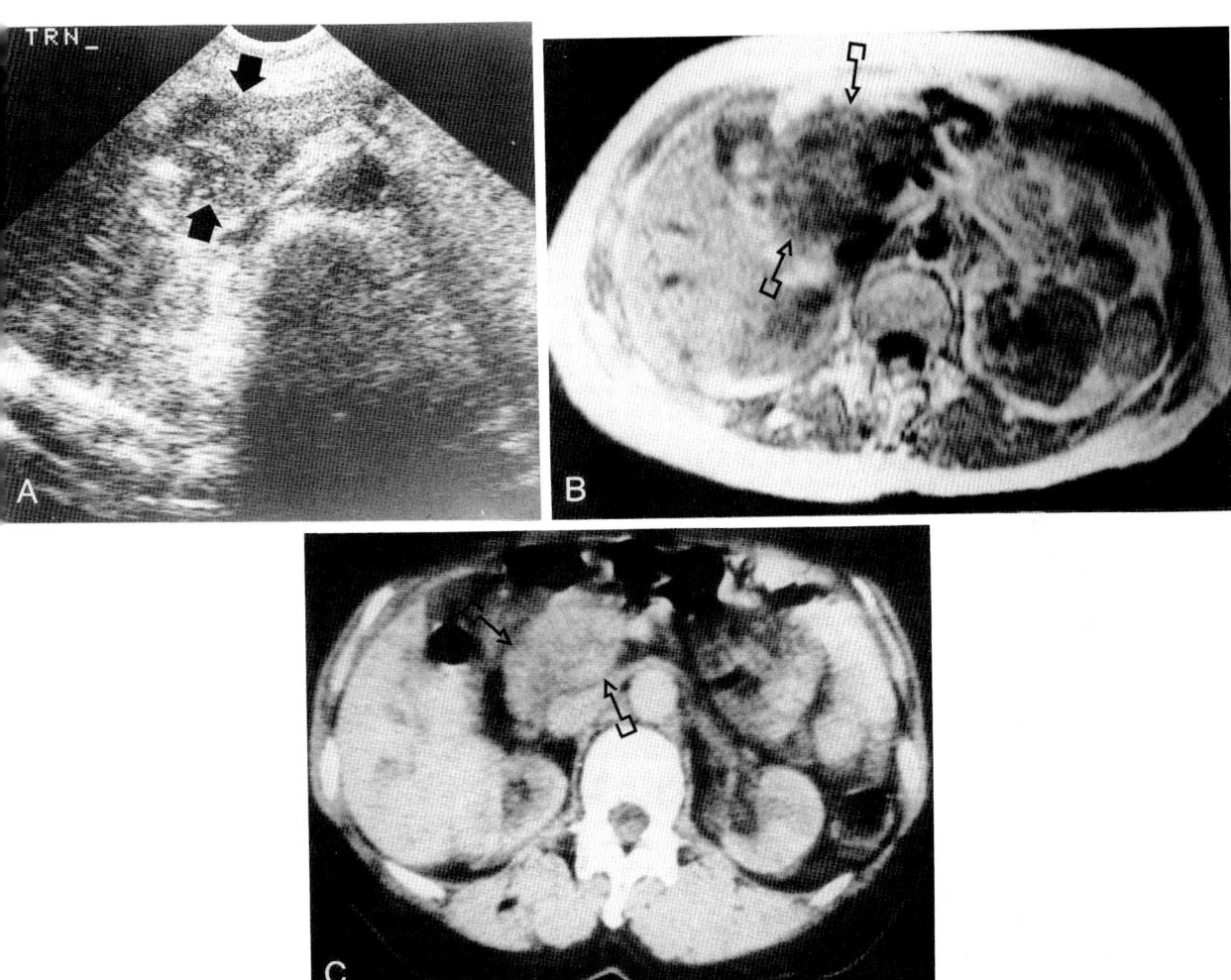

FIGURE 23.6. PANCREATIC CARCINOMA

Advanced carcinoma of the head of the pancreas: MRI vs. CT and ultrasound. *A:* Transverse sonogram: mass (*arrows*) in the head of the pancreas. *B–E:* MRI and CT at nearly the same levels: pancreatic mass (*arrows*). Dilated bile ducts are seen on CT, but not MRI. *F* and *G:* Sagittal sonography of the common duct and transverse sonography of the pancreatic duct, respectively (*cursors*). Dilated ducts are seen best with ultrasound.

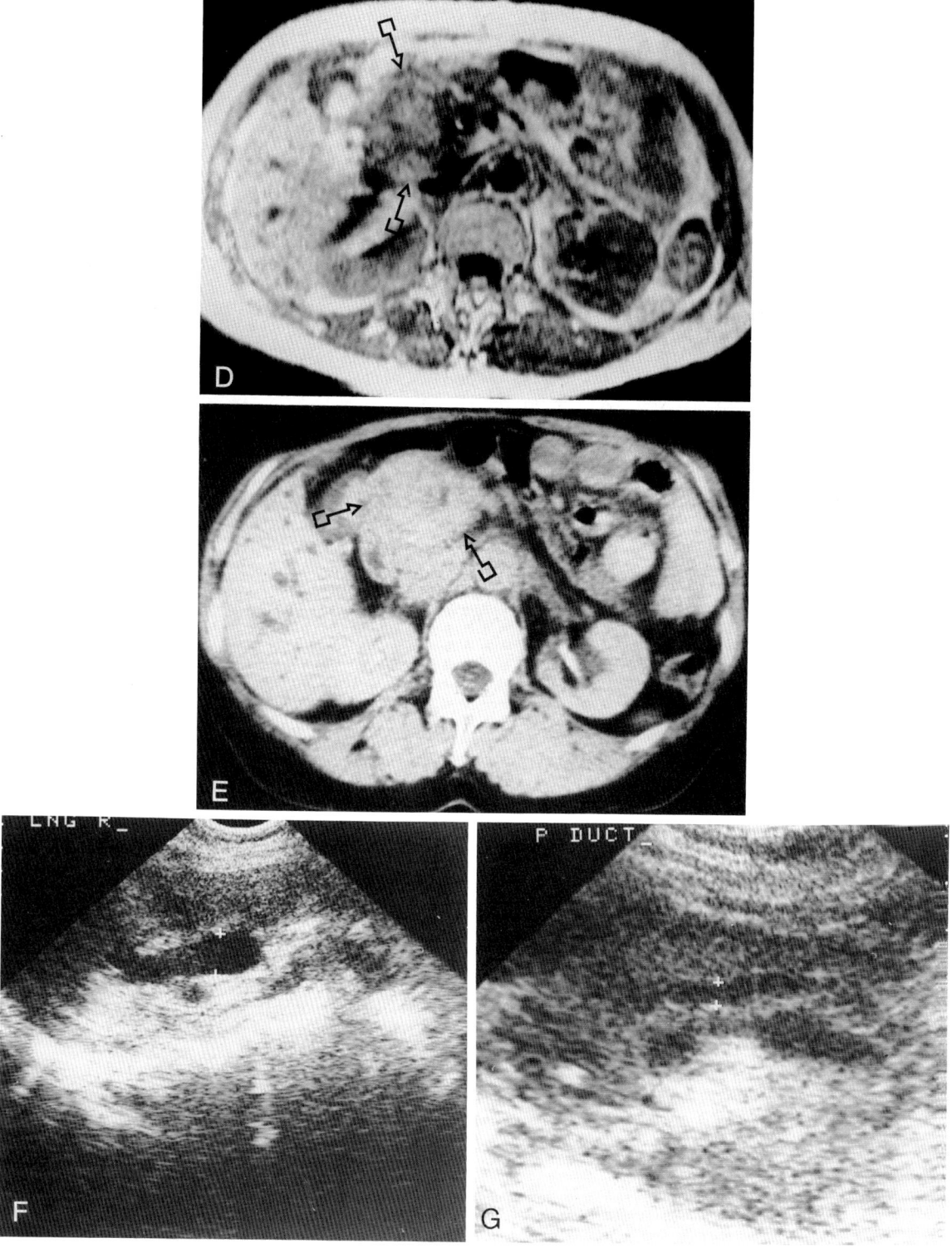

FIGURE 23.6D–G

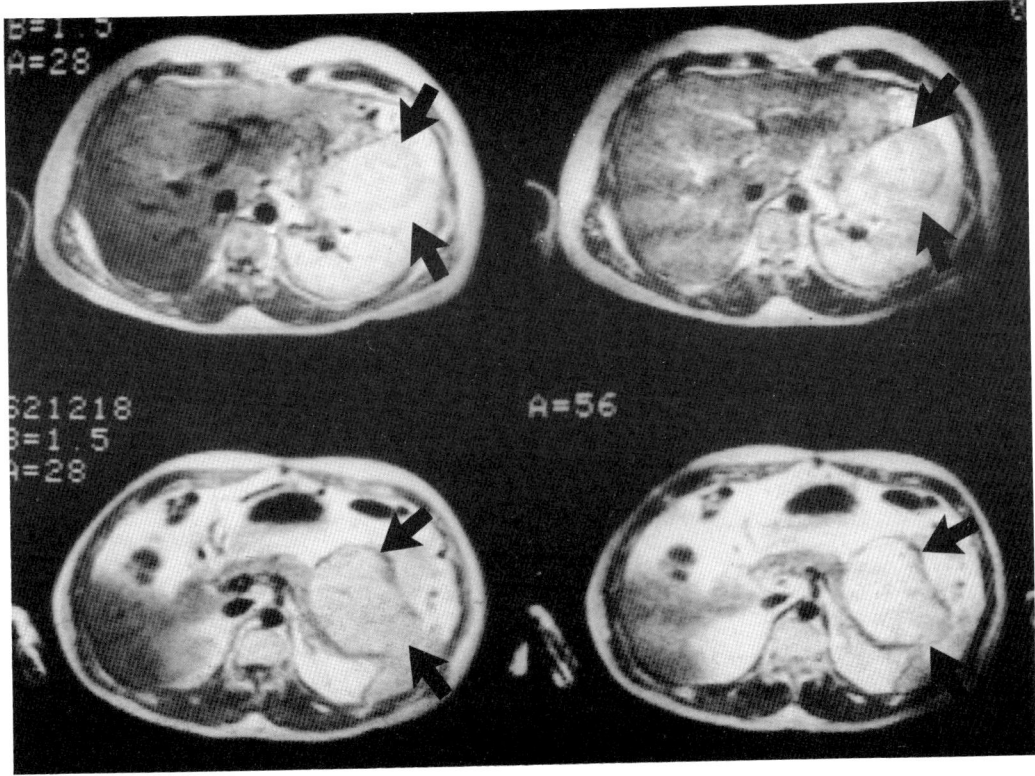

FIGURE 23.7. PANCREATIC GASTRINOMA

MRI of a pancreatic gastrinoma. (Courtesy of Henry Goldberg, M.D., David Stark, M.D., Albert Moss, M.D., Peter L. Davis, M. D., and Michael Federle, M.D., Department of Radiology, University of California, San Francisco.) *Top and bottom left:* TE = 28/TR = 1500; *top and bottom right:* TE = 56/TR = 1500, all at 0.35T. Hyperintense mass in the tail of the pancreas (*arrows*). The normal body of the pancreas can be seen in the bottom two images.

SUMMARY

Regional anatomy is usually demonstrated best on spin echo images with short TE and long TR but multiple sequences are need at every level to avoid missing pathology. Currently MRI of the pancreas is hampered by long examination time, motion induced blurring and poor spatial resolution compared to CT. Its major advantage is its excellent depiction of regional vascular anatomy without the need for contrast material. We have not found the multiplanar capability of MR to be a significant asset in pancreatic imaging (Fig. 23.8).

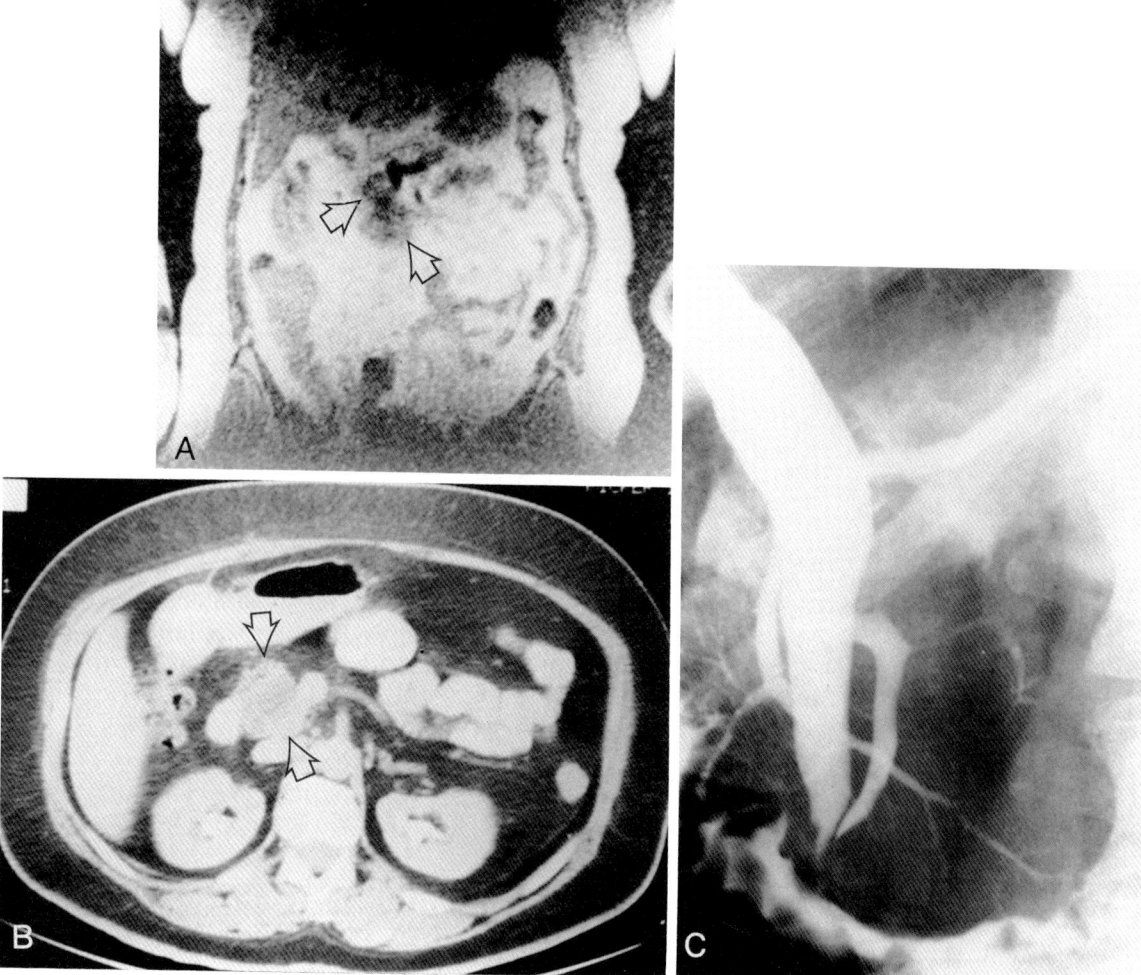

FIGURE 23.8. PANCREATIC MICROCYSTIC ADENOMA

Microcystic adenoma: MRI, CT, and ERCP. *A:* Coronal MRI shows a hypointense mass (*arrows*) in the head and uncinate process on a T1-weighted image, suggesting a fluid-filled mass as a possibility. Coronal projection did not offer any advantage. *B:* CT shows a nonspecific mass in the head and uncinate process (*arrows*). *C:* ERCP: stretching and straightening of the main pancreatic duct and its branches without any obstruction or narrowing, suggesting a benign mass.

REFERENCES

1. Stark DD, Moss AA, Goldberg HI, Davis PL, Federle MP: Magnetic resonance and CT of the normal and diseased pancreas: a comparative study. *Radiology* 150:153–162, 1984.
2. Davis PL, Moss AA, Goldberg HI, Stark DD, Margulis AR: Nuclear magnetic resonance imaging of the liver and pancreas. *Radiographics* 4:159–169, 1984.
3. Carr DH, Brown J, Bydder GM, Steiner RE, Weinmann HJ, Speck U, Hall AS, Young IR: Gadolinium-DTPA as a contrast agent in MRI: initial clinical experience in 20 patients. *AJR* 143:215–224, 1984.
4. Bottomley PA, Foster TH, Argersinger RE, Pfiefer LM: A review of normal tissue hydrogen NMR relaxation times and relaxation mechanisms from 1–100 MHz: dependence on tissue type, NMR frequency, temperature, excision, and age. *Med Phys* 11:425–448, 1984.
5. Smith FW, Reid A, Hutchison JMS, Mallard JR: Nuclear magnetic resonance imaging of the pancreas. *Radiology* 142:667–680, 1982.
6. Young IR, Bailes DR, Burl M, Collins AG, Smith DT, McDonnell MJ, Orr JS, Banks LM, Bydder GM, Greenspan RH, Steiner RE: Initial clinical evaluation of a whole body nuclear magnetic resonance (NMR) tomograph. *J Comput Assist Tomogr* 6:1–18, 1982.
7. Charlton RW, Abrahams M, Bothwell TH: Idiopathic hemochromatosis in young subjects. Clinical, chemical and pathological findings in four patients. *Arch Pathol* 83:132–140, 1967.

SECTION IV
The Spleen

INTRODUCTION

The spleen has long been a mysterious organ whose function was unknown. In medieval times, it was thought to be the seat of humor and laughter. Anatomic descriptions of the spleen are found in the works of Aristotle, Hippocrates, and in the Talmud (1). Surgical splenectomy is documented by Zaccarrelli in 1549 and Zambeccari in 1680 (2), but is alluded to in the Bible (1).

Until the 1950s when Spirer observed the role of the spleen in protecting against infection, the organ was considered unimportant (3). Since then, greater attention has been paid to splenic diseases and trauma, since conservation of splenic tissue is desirable. The spleen is an "orphan" organ in radiology as it is not studied in detail by any one subspecialty. Computed tomography, sonography, and possibly NMR have supplanted much, but not all of the traditional role of nuclear scintigraphy and angiography in the radiologic evaluation of the spleen. The recent resurgance of splenic aspiration biopsy has also rekindled the interest of the radiologist in splenic pathology (4). We hope this section will acquaint the radiologist with the spectrum of splenic pathology that can be diagnosed radiologically and stimulate further study of the splenic manifestations of disease.

REFERENCES

1. Rosner F: *Medicine in the Bible and the Talmud.* New York, Ktav Publishing House Inc., Yeshiva University Press, 1977, pp 86–90.
2. Moynihan B: *The Spleen and Some of Its Diseases.* Philadelphia, W. B. Saunders, 1921, p 5.
3. Spirer Z: The role of the spleen in immunity and infection. *Adv Pediatr* 27:55–88, 1980.
4. Van Sonnenberg E, Quinn SF, Wittich GR, Casola G: Interventional radiology in the spleen: feasability and safety. *Radiology* 157(P):112, 1985.

24
Normal Anatomy and Radiology

ABRAHAM H. DACHMAN, M.D.

EMBRYOLOGY

The spleen develops in the 8-mm embryo when mesenchymal cells aggregate between the two leaves on the dorsal mesogastrium (1). Aggregates from several adjoining areas fuse to form a lobulated spleen. When the stomach rotates, the left aspect of the mesogastrium fuses with the peritoneum over the left kidney (Fig. 24.1A and B). This fusion explains why the lienorenal ligament fuses dorsally and why the course of the splenic artery is to the left behind the peritoneum as it enters the lienorenal ligament in the adult.

The capsule, connective tissue framework, and parenchyma of the spleen form from differentiated mesenchymal cells (1). Until late fetal life the spleen serves a hematopoietic function. Lymphocyte and monocyte production, however, continue throughout life.

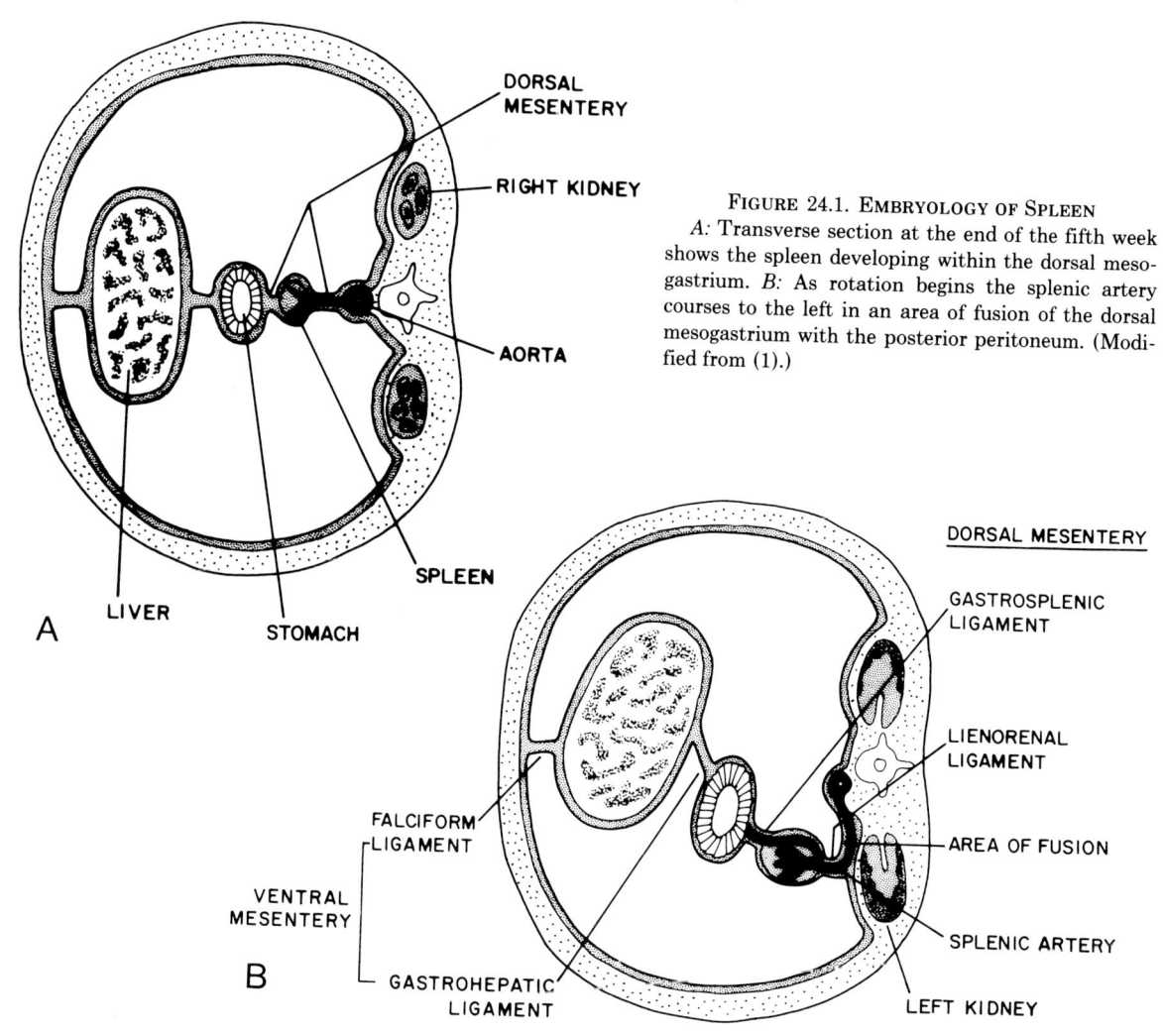

FIGURE 24.1. EMBRYOLOGY OF SPLEEN
A: Transverse section at the end of the fifth week shows the spleen developing within the dorsal mesogastrium. *B:* As rotation begins the splenic artery courses to the left in an area of fusion of the dorsal mesogastrium with the posterior peritoneum. (Modified from (1).)

GROSS AND MICROSCOPIC ANATOMY

The adult spleen weighs 75–100 g and is located in the left upper quadrant with its long axis along the line of the 10th rib (2, 3) (Fig. 24.2). The superior convex surface fits into the concavity of the diaphragm and thus it is closely related to the posterior costophrenic recess and left lung base. The posterior extremity of the spleen lies adjacent to the left adrenal or left kidney, and the anterior extremity is related to the splenic flexure of the colon and connected to it via the splenocolic ligament. The splenophrenic, splenorenal, and gastrosplenic ligaments also fix the spleen in its position. The visceral or concave surface is related to the stomach and tail of the pancreas in addition to left kidney and colon.

The spleen is surrounded by visceral peritoneum which is reflected at its hilum to form two "pedicles." One is reflected over the gastrosplenic ligament, the other reflected posteriorly over the tail of the pancreas and lienorenal ligament (Fig. 24.3). The tail of the pancreas lies within the lienorenal ligament along with the splenic vessels, lymphatics, and nerves.

The splenic artery, a branch of the celiac axis, runs a transverse and often tortuous course along the upper border of the pancreas to reach the splenic hilum where it divides into five or more major branches (4). The splenic vein is formed at the splenic hilum and runs in the lienorenal ligament in front of the left kidney, left diaphragmatic crus, and aorta in a groove in the back of the pancreas. It joins with the inferior mesenteric vein and then joins the superior mesenteric vein behind the head of the pancreas to form the portal vein. The spleen provides 40% of the

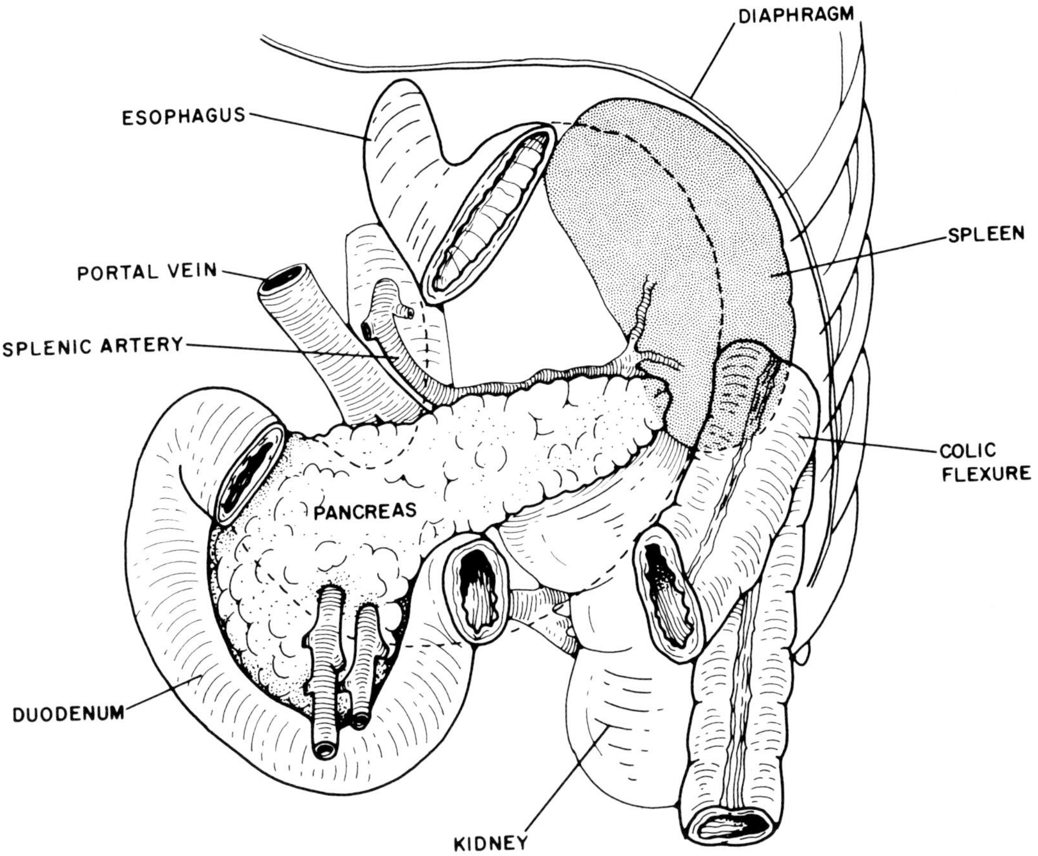

NORMAL SPLEEN

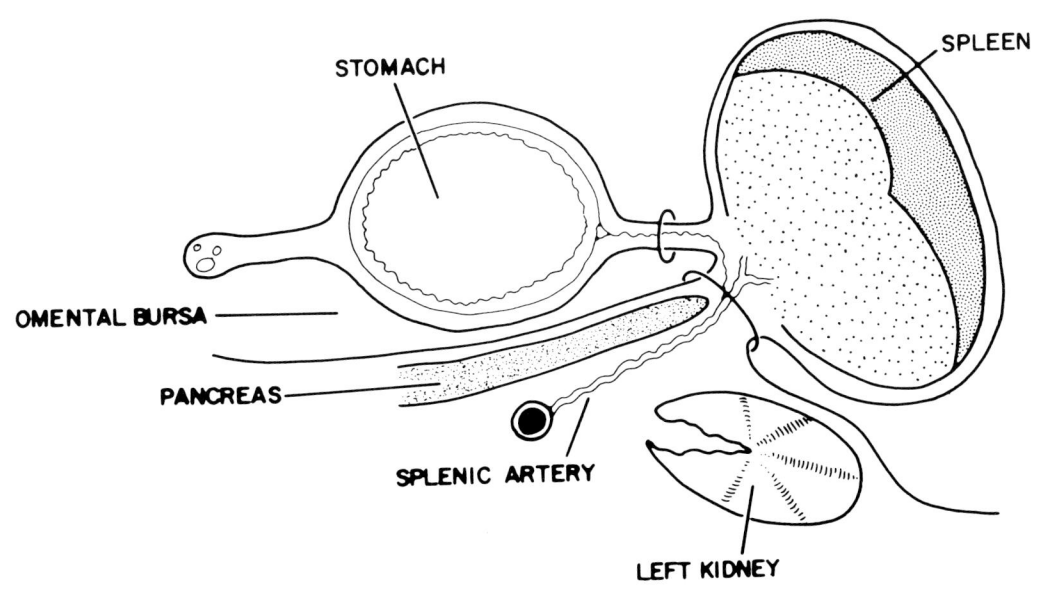

FIGURE 24.2. GROSS ANATOMY
The upper pole of the spleen is related to the diaphragm and the stomach. The lower pole is related to the pancreatic tail, colon, left kidney, and adrenal. (Modified from (3).)

FIGURE 24.3. LIGAMENTS OF SPLEEN
Diaphragmatically, the spleen is shown to have two "pedicles," the gastrosplenic and lienorenal ligaments. (Modified from (3).).

portal circulation's blood. The lymphatic vessels are subcapsular and are formed by the drainage of large trabecular tributaries. These vessels drain into the pancreaticolienal nodes at the splenic hilum.

The connective tissue framework of the spleen consists of collagenous fibrous and elastic tissue forming the capsule, trabeculae and reticular fibers. The splenic arteries ramify along the trabeculae (3, 5). Central (white pulp) arteries have lymphatic sheaths which expand in some places to form follicles called Malpighian bodies. The lymphatic sheaths and follicles make up the white pulp of the spleen. The blood vessels transport blood to sinusoids in the red pulp. Capillaries may open directly into sinusoids or first pass through spaces in the red pulp. The red pulp performs the phagocytic function of the spleen.

Vascular territories have been described in the spleen (3, 6), each of which is separated by a relatively avascular plane running parallel to the short axis of the spleen. This may explain cases of splenic rupture with minimal bleeding (3).

The splenic nerve supply is derived from the celiac plexus. It is located along the splenic artery. It sends postganglionic sympathetic fibers to the smooth muscle of the capsule, trabeculae, and vasculature within the splenic pulp. Few sensory fibers are present (7).

PHYSIOLOGY

About 350 liters of blood pass through the spleen each day and at any one moment about 1% of the total blood volume is in the spleen (8, 9). This blood flow rate (150 ml per min) is approximately 4% of the cardiac output. Under normal conditions, transit time of blood in the spleen is 20–25 sec. The spleen discriminates between normal and abnormal cells and selectively sequesters abnormal and aged red or white blood cells and platelets. The microcirculation of the spleen is thought to direct 10% of splenic arterial blood directly into the venous sinuses and 90% through the red pulp whose endothelial pores and macrophages remove abnormal particles. Abnormal red blood cells, viruses, bacteria, nuclear remnants (Howell-Jolly bodies), and parasites may be removed. Normal erythrocytes are left intact. It is not certain what factors sensitize an aged blood cell to splenic destruction. Biophysical properties including enzyme and metabolic activity of the cell and delay in the transit through the spleen probably play a role (3).

About 30% of platelets are normally sequestered within the spleen. When splenomegaly is present, up to 80% of platelets are sequestered.

The spleen's role in the immune response is incompletely understood. It is important in the initiation of humoral and cellular immune responses (3). The lymphatic tissue in the spleen is unique in that the Malpighian corpuscle is perfused by blood rather than lymph. Thus, this tissue is able to respond rapidly to antigens introduced into the blood stream. The spleen produces a tetrapeptide known as tuftsin (discovered at Tufts University), that coats leukocytes and facilitates phagocytosis. The absence of tuftsin in splenectomized patients may contribute to the increased incidence of infection reported in these patients by impairing opsinization of bacteria.

Tuftsin may have a weak antitumor effect and some experimental evidence suggests that splenectomy may adversely affect survival in cancer patients.

During gestation, the spleen functions as a hematopoietic organ. It produces red blood cells, lymphocytes, etc. At birth, this function ceases and is taken over by the bone marrow. When the bone marrow cannot maintain an adequate volume of formed blood elements (i.e., thalassemia major or bone marrow fibrosis in myeloid metaplasia), multipotential cells within the spleen hypertrophy and function as hematopoietic cells.

The spleen also serves as a reservoir for formed blood elements. There are enough red blood cells within the spleen to maintain red cell volume in the face of bleeding unless the blood loss is marked. The spleen contracts by the actions of postganglionic fibers to the capsule and trabeculae thereby releasing stored red blood cells into the circulation. Platelets and white blood cells are also stored within the spleen. In splenomegaly (increased storage), a pancytopenia can occur; in asplenia (no storage) one may see a panthrombocythemia.

RADIOLOGIC ANATOMY AND TECHNIQUE

There are numerous ways to assess splenic size and morphology: palpation, plain film, nuclear scintigraphy, ultrasonography, computed tomography, angiography, and magnetic resonance imaging. Clinical palpation should always be attempted, but in order for the spleen to be palpable, it must be about 2–3 times normal in size. In individuals with a large body habitus, it may not be palpable, and 10% of normal children do have palpable spleens.

Plain Film

The spleen is outlined by perisplenic fat in the greater omentum and distal transverse mesocolon (10). The spleen was well visualized in less than 100 of 500 abdominal radiographs reviewed by Rosenbaum (10). The long axis of the spleen usually parallels the posterior ribs. The spleen normally does not project below the costal margin (10). Due to the variation in its size, and shape, only marked splenomegaly can be appreciated on plain film. Accessory spleens are not usually seen on plain films and are discussed along with congenital disorders in Chapter 25.

Plain film radiography is useful for detecting moderate or massive splenomegaly, splenic calcifications as commonly seen in granulomatous disease (tuberculosis, histoplasmosis), chronic hematoma, healed abscess, and cysts. Thorotrast deposition is also detectable as increased radiodensity. These are discussed in detail in their respective chapters.

Spleen Scintigraphy—Historical Perspective

Spleen scintigraphy began in 1950, when Gray and Sterling (11) developed the in vitro method of labeling red blood cells with chromium-51. Chromium-51 binds to the β-polypeptide chain of hemoglobin. In 1955, Jandahl and others realized that radiolabeled cells needed to be damaged in order for the spleen to be able to cull sufficient numbers (12). Techniques employed included red blood cell sensitization with anti-D antibodies, in vitro treatment with metabolic protein complexes, and heat. In 1962, Wagner developed the optimal technique for damaging red blood cells—the gentle heating method (Fig. 24.4) (12). The cells are heated for 15 min at 50°C and the red blood cell membrane becomes noncompliant, causing the cell to be culled out of the peripheral circulation. Little hemolysis occurs with this "gentle" technique, thus, uptake within the liver and bone marrow is minimized. Currently, the chromium-51 label has been replaced by technetium-99m. The 140 kev γ-ray is optimal for imaging, and its short half-life (6 hr) results in minimal patient radiation exposure. Chromium-51 has a 322 kev γ-ray emission and a $T_{1/2}$ of 28.7 days (12–14). Red blood cell scanning can yield functional as well as morphologic information. If splenic function is to be studied, some authors recommend ^{51}Cr labeling of cells heated in saline or ^{99m}Tc tagged cells heated as packed cells for 20 min at 49.5°C. Heating red blood cells in plasma for 20 min did not sufficiently damage the cells to study splenic function accurately (15, 16).

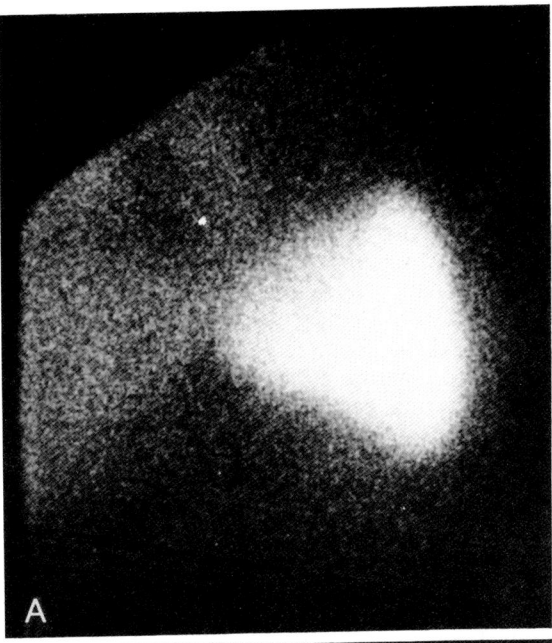

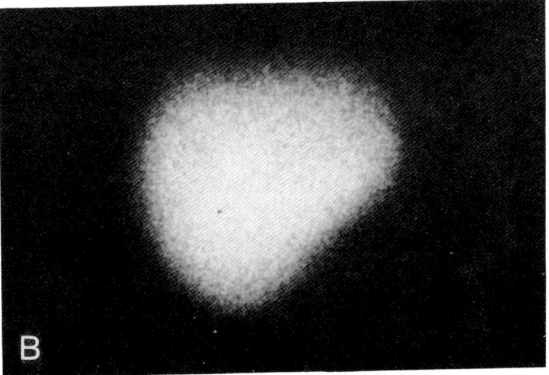

FIGURE 24.4. TAGGED DAMAGED RED BLOOD CELL SCAN
A: Anterior view and *B:* posterior view.

Technetium-99m sulfur colloid was introduced in 1965 by Harper et al. for liver-spleen scintigraphy (17). Technetium-99m sulfur colloid is a suspension of radiolabeled particles, each ranging in size from approximately 100 nm to 1 µm. The particles are "foreign" to the body, and thus are filtered out and trapped by the reticuloendothelial cells of the liver, spleen, and bone marrow. Eighty to ninety percent are trapped by the liver, 5–10% by the spleen, and a smaller amount by the bone marrow. The colloid has a blood $T_{1/2}$ of approximately 2 min. Essentially all particles are cleared by the reticuloendothelial system within 20–30 min. Once within these cells, there is no biological turnover and the colloid remains indefinitely. Radiation exposure from 1 mCi of ^{99m}Tc-sulfur colloid is minimal: 0.1–0.2 rad to the liver and 0.01 rad total body. Three to 5 mCi of ^{99m}Tc-sulfur colloid is employed for adult liver-spleen scintigraphy and 50 µCi per kg body weight for children (14, 17, 18).

Technetium-99m sulfur colloid liver-spleen scintigraphy is simple to perform. No patient preparation is necessary, and no adverse reactions to the radiopharmaceutical have been reported. Following the intravenous administration of the radiopharmaceutical, 20-min delayed anterior, posterior, right and left lateral scintiscans are obtained with a standard or large field of view gamma camera (Fig. 24.5). Thirty and sixty degree anterior and posterior oblique images are performed if an intrasplenic abnormality (trauma, infarct, etc.) is suspected. An identical technique is employed if ^{99m}Tc gently heat-damaged red blood cells are used. The dose, however, is 2 mCi. There is evidence that the mechanisms of uptake of radiocolloid (technetium sulfur colloid) and damaged red blood cells are different and reflect distinct splenic functions. This is currently under investigation (19–22).

Other methods include gallium scanning and indium-111 platelet scanning. Gallium is not an agent of choice to study the spleen specifically but can give incidental information. Injection of autologous platelets labeled with indium-111 can measure splenic blood flow and intrasplenic platelet transit time (23, 24). This technique may have application in studying disorders such as immune complex disease (24).

The Normal Spleen Scan

The normal spleen scan should reveal a homogeneous distribution of radiocolloid and/or heat-damaged red blood cells throughout the spleen (Figs. 24.4 and 24.5). It should be located within the left upper quadrant in close approximation to the costal portion of the diaphragm (15% are not juxtaposed) and adjacent to the lateral body wall at the 9th through the 11th ribs. The hilum is usually located toward the lower pole of the spleen, but may be identified superiorly, i.e., a normal anatomic variant, the "upside down" spleen (Fig. 24.6). The upper pole of the spleen may not be well visualized on the anterior scintiscan, as its location is more posterior than the remainder of the spleen. The posterior vertical height of 95% of normal adult spleens ranges between 7 and 14 cm. In children, the maximal posterior vertical dimension is equal to 5.7 + 0.3 multiplied by the age in years. Spleen shapes are varied (semicircular, triangular, lentiform, ovoid), and fetal lobulations may be present. These, however, are usually only seen in enlarged spleens. They manifest themselves as linear areas of decreased activity. Care must be taken to recognize these as normal variants and not confuse them with splenic infarcts and/or lacerations (13, 14, 17) (see Chapter 26).

Splenic configuration has been anatomically classified as: (a) a compact spleen with a narrow hilus and (b) a widespread or "distributed" hilus with a notched anterior boarder to the spleen, a thumb-like inferior pole extension and a "tubercle" at the upper medial pole (25). This medial tubercle has been reported to cause a potential pitfall in radionuclide cardiac ventriculography with blood pool activity in the spleen mimicking abnormal cardiac wall motion (26). Redundant tissue at the lower pole of the spleen can cause a relative "hot spot" (without an accessory spleen being present) (27). The spleen may have a semilunar configuration with draping of the hilus around the gastric fundus resulting in an apparent superior pole defect on posterior view and wide separation between the liver and spleen on the anterior view (28). Retained barium in the gastrointestinal tract, particularly the splenic flexure of the colon, may cause a false focal splenic defect (29). A large congenital fissure may mimic a defect or hematoma (30). If the left lobe of the liver is significantly enlarged, it may cause an apparent splenic defect on the posterior (prone) view which "disappears" if the posterior view is repeated with patient standing up (31). In 1 of 10 reported cases the pseudodefect of an enlarged left lobe of the liver was also seen on the anterior view (31). Likewise, the left lobe of the liver may mimic normal or accessory spleen following splenectomy (32).

If a liver-spleen scan image shows an equivocal

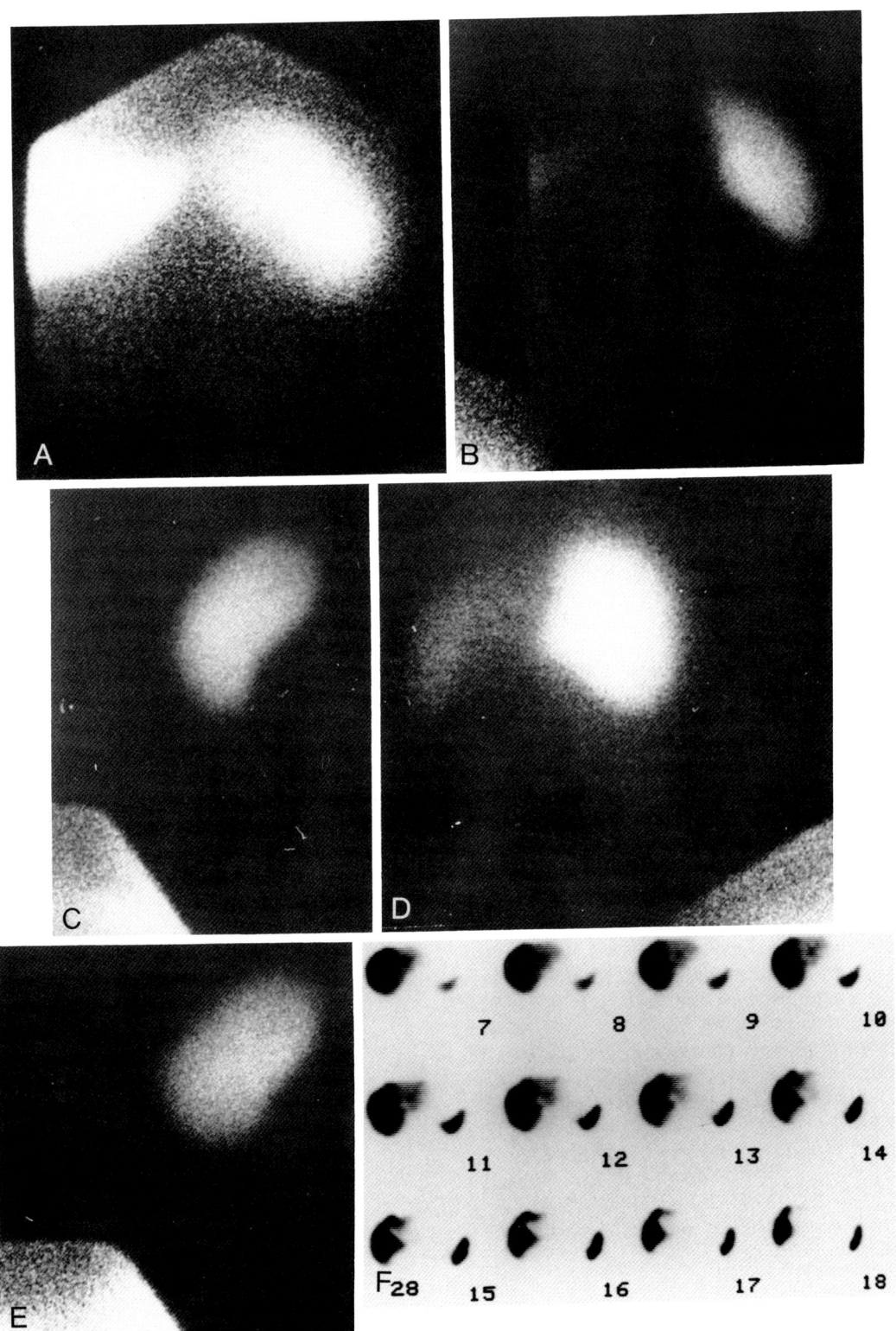

FIGURE 24.5. ^{99m}Tc-Sulfur Colloid Scan
A: Anterior; *B:* 60° left anterior oblique; *C:* 45° left posterior oblique; *D:* left lateral; and *E:* posterior views. *F:* Axial SPECT of a normal liver and spleen.

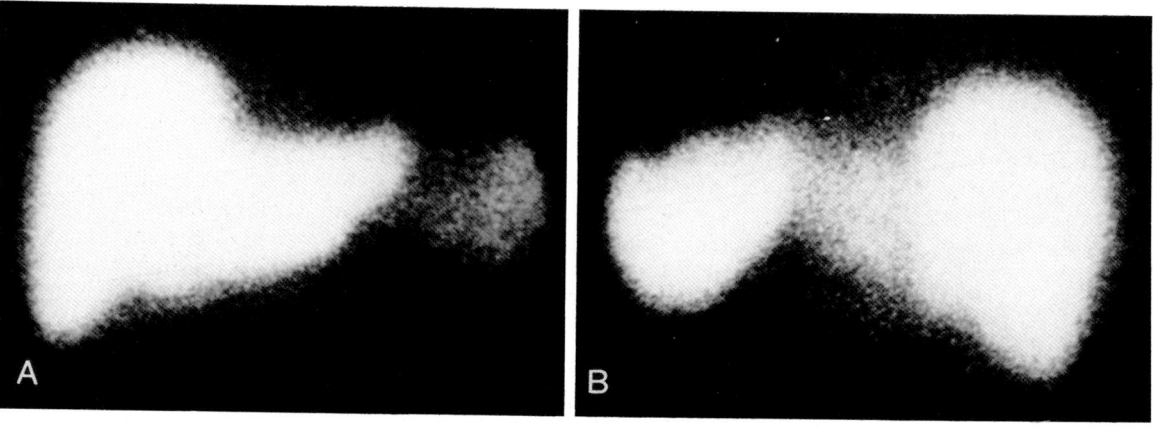

FIGURE 24.6. ^{99m}Tc-Sulfur Colloid Scan, "Upside-Down" Spleen
A normal variation in splenic contour. There was no infarction present. A: Anterior; B: posterior views.

defect, selective scanning with damaged red blood cells as described above often clarifies the problem (23). The red cell scan may show the spleen to be normal with the equivocal defect on technetium scan caused by technique or an enlarged left lobe of the liver, or it may show an abnormality not previously detected (33). The use of single photon emission computed tomography (SPECT) may improve the sensitivity and specificity of the sulfur colloid scan in evaluating the spleen (Fig. 24.5F).

The amount of ^{99m}Tc-sulfur colloid within the spleen should always be less than that of the liver. If there is a reversal of colloid distribution (spleen greater than the liver) hepatocellular disease and/or an intrasplenic abnormality must be considered.

Parameters to be evaluated when interpreting a spleen scan should include size, position, configuration, and amount and distribution of colloid uptake. A search for ectopic and/or accessory splenic tissue should always be undertaken, especially in congenital, postsurgical, and asplenic patients.

Clinical Indications for Spleen Scintigraphy

Clinical indications for spleen scintigraphy include detecting congenital abnormalities of the spleen (34), assessing splenic size, evaluating splenic trauma, evaluating the underlying etiology of a palpable left upper quardrant mass and/or left upper quadrant pain, evaluating asplenic states, and detecting space-occupying lesions within the spleen. They are applicable both to adults and children (35).

Angiography

The splenic artery is a branch of the celiac axis about 13 cm long (range 8–32 cm) which usually originates just distal to the left gastric artery (Fig. 24.7) (36). In 25% of cases all three branches of the celiac trunk arise at the same point (37). Normal variations include origin of the splenic artery from the ventral or right surface of the celiac axis, and origin from the aorta or superior mesenteric artery (36). A branch supplying the upper splenic pole may originate separately from the celiac axis giving the appearance of a double splenic artery (37). The splenic artery can be divided into suprapancreatic, pancreatic, prepancreatic, and prehilar segments (37). Its tortuosity is variable and increases with age (see Chapter 29). The most tortuous segment is usually the pancreatic segment which runs along the dorsal surface of the pancreas and gives off small pancreatic branches. The prepancreatic runs along the anterior surface of pancreatic tail and the prehilar is defined as the segment between the spleen and the tail of the pancreas. Michels analyzed the anatomy of the splenic blood supply in the 1940s (25, 38) and showed its variability. There are two basic configurations (25, 37) of the spleen as described above: the distributed type and the compact type. The vasculature of the "distributed" spleen (70% of cases) consists of a short splenic artery with numerous small branches coming off the trunk which penetrate in a distributed fashion over the medial splenic surface. The "compact" spleen (30% of cases), with a narrow hilus and smooth surface, is supplied by a long splenic artery which gives off a few branches at the hilus which penetrate focally at the medial splenic surface.

The splenic artery gives off branches to the pancreas and stomach. The dorsal pancreatic artery arises from the suprapancreatic segment (i.e., the first 1–3 cm of the splenic artery) in 40% of cases (36). Other pancreatic feeding vessels, the caudal pancreatics, originate along the pancreatic segment, the largest of which is sometimes named separately as the pancreatica magna artery coming off the distal two-thirds of the splenic artery and supplying the tail of the pancreas (37). Another branch, the artery of Buhler, may descend to communicate with the superior mesenteric artery (37). The short gastric arteries and the left gastroepiploic artery arise from the splenic artery. The left gastroepiploic artery usually arises just proximal to the first division of the splenic artery (36).

The parenchymal phase of the splenic angiogram may be homogeneous or slightly speckled and its density depends on the volume of spleen in addition to the contrast volume and selectivity of the injection site (36). The splenic vein opacifies about 7 sec after arterial injection (Fig. 24.8). Immediate filling of the vein suggests an arteriovenous shunt (see Chapter 29).

Splenoportography

Abrams (37) provides an extensive description of splenoportography with an extensive bibliography. It has been employed in patients with signs of portal obstruction, i.e., varices, gastrointestinal hemorrhage with a negative workup, splenomegaly of unknown etiology, for evaluation of portacaval shunts (37), and in some cases of cirrhosis and hepatomegaly. Current indications are limited and its use has diminished markedly. Conventionally, the spleen is punctured with a 16-gauge cannula or catheter and a rapid injection of at least 30 ml or more of contrast is made (Fig. 24.9). Splenoportography performed with a 22-gauge needle, lesser volumes of contrast and digital subtraction has been advocated in lieu of transhepatic portography.

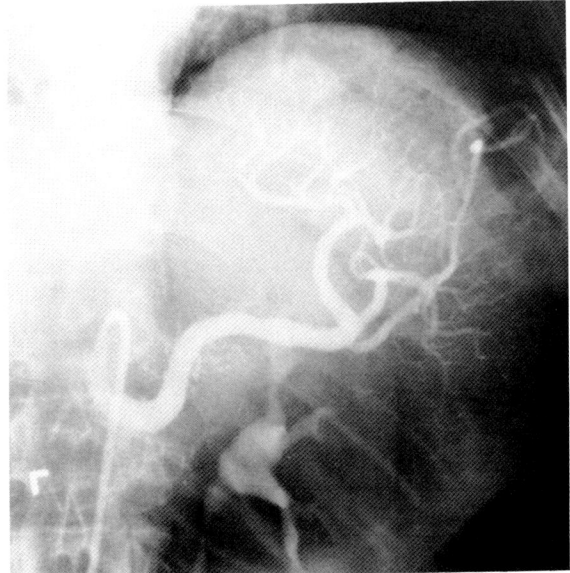

FIGURE 24.7. NORMAL SELECTIVE SPLENIC ARTERIOGRAM
The "distributed" spleen shows three branches penetrating the splenic hilus.

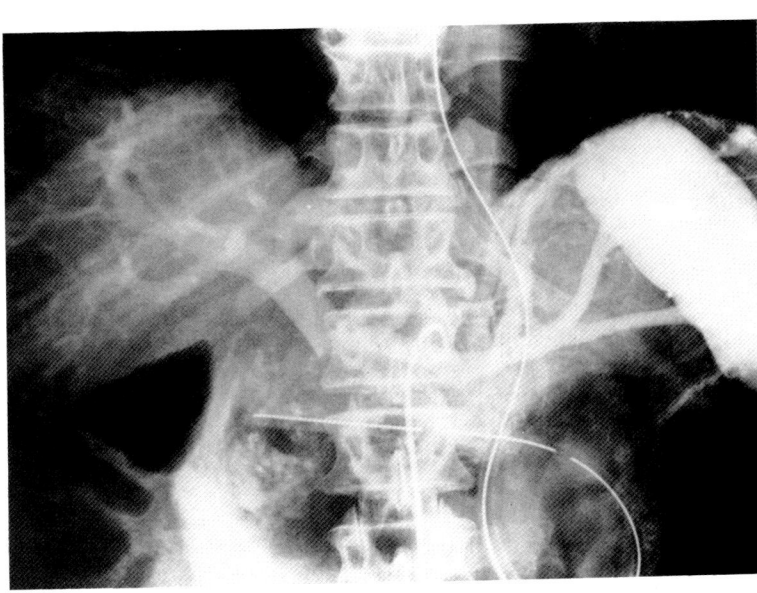

FIGURE 24.8. VENOUS PHASE, SELECTIVE SPLENIC ANGIOGRAM

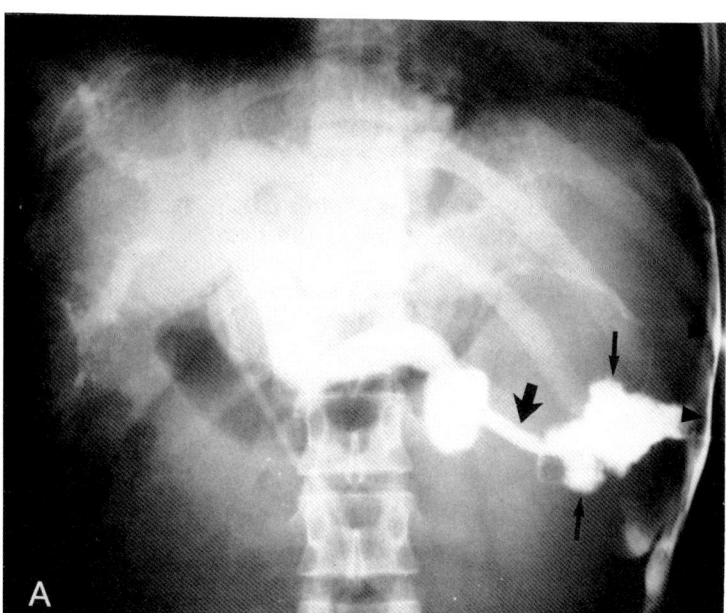
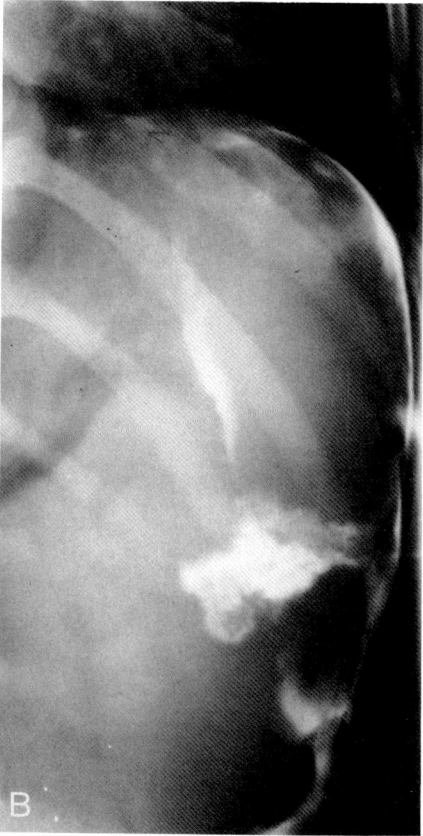

FIGURE 24.9. SPLENOPORTOGRAM

A: A 16-gauge needle enters the lateral lower pole pulp opacifying the parenchyma (*arrows*), splenic vein (*large arrow*) with some subcapsule leakage (*arrowheads*). *B:* Coned view after injection. The vein is cleared of contrast and the parenchymal stain and subcapsular collections are still seen.

Ultrasound

A detailed description of the technique of splenic ultrasound scanning is available (39, 40). Ribs and air-filled stomach and colon may obscure the spleen. Although the spleen may be visualized in the supine position by scanning transversely or intercostally, the best images are usually obtained in the left anterior oblique, left side up decubitus, or prone position using realtime instruments. When possible, subcostal scans are generally better than intercostal scans. Both transverse and longitudinal (coronal) views should be obtained (Fig. 24.10). Varying degrees of inspiration will improve visualization of the paradiaphragmatic portion of the spleen which is the most difficult to image. Another sometimes useful maneuver is filling the stomach with fluid when scanning in a supine position. The transducer may be moved in an arc along the intercostal space or in a sector motion. A 3.5 MHz medium-internally focused transducer is generally used. A convex transducer may improve visualization of the "blind areas" adjacent to the dome of the diaphragm (41).

The splenic parenchyma should produce a homogeneous fine texture of echoes with occasional bright echoes representing blood vessels. Splenic echogenicity is about the same as that of the liver. The size and shape of the spleen, and position of the hilum and its relationship to adjacent organs (diaphragm, stomach, pancreas, left kidney) should be identified. Often the splenic vein can be identified in the hilus.

Computed Tomography

Computed tomography is exquisite in its ability to demonstrate the size, shape, and location of the normal spleen and in demonstrating intrasplenic abnormalities (Fig. 24.11). Technical artifacts may occur due to motion, beam hardening, or dynamic scanning. The spleen's hilum with its vasculature is seen, as well as its relationship

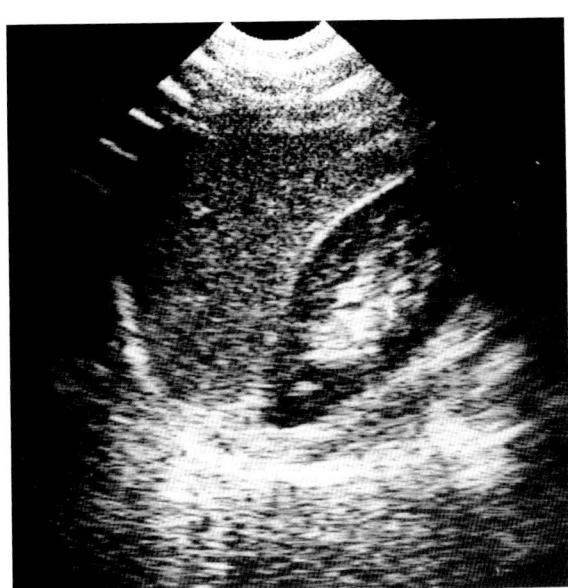

FIGURE 24.10. NORMAL SPLENIC SONOGRAM, CORONAL VIEW
This spleen has a broad renal surface.

to adjacent organs particularly the pancreatic tail, left lobe of the liver, diaphragm, left adrenal, left kidney, stomach, splenic flexure, and adjacent mesenteric and omental fat. The posterior surface of the spleen abutting on the pleural space is called the "bare" area and has a constant relation to Gerota's fascia (Fig. 24.12) (42). This portion of the spleen is about 2–3 cm long and may be outlined by air in the posterior costophrenic sulcus. The point of reflection of the splenorenal ligament at the bare area is thought to correspond to the intermediate ridge of the spleen (42). The bare area may be useful in differentiating ascites from pleural effusion since ascites cannot reach the bare area (42).

There is significant variation in the size, shape, and position of the spleen which is well shown on CT (Fig. 24.13) (43). Positional change was seen in 34 of 38 patients with ventral and caudal shift of both the liver and spleen seen in the prone position compared to the supine position (44). This is significant if CT is used to map areas for radiotherapy although precise volume measurements are difficult to make (see below, "Splenic Volume Measurements"). Without contrast enhancement the spleen is homogeneous and is slightly less radiodense than the liver (45, 46). The omental and mesenteric fat surrounding much of the spleen often permits sharp demarcation of its capsule and hilar vasculature even without contrast enhancement. The splenic artery may wander and appear curvilinear, round or oval on different cuts (see Chapter 29). Contrast enhancement is generally indicated when looking for splenic pathology and separating splenic from pancreatic or adrenal abnormalities. Experimental contrast agents are discussed below. Bolus intravenous injection of urographic contrast will cause dense enhancement of the hilar vasculature and is useful in equivocal cases (47). Slow contrast enhancement will give a uniform increase in parenchymal density whereas rapid infusion will cause an initial heterogenous blush (Fig. 24.14) (43, 47). This is thought to be due to variable rates of flow through the red pulp (47). A homogeneous splenic blush should be seen within 2 min after a bolus injection (47). A detailed analysis of the patterns of inhomogeneity after bolus injection suggests that a mottled pattern is due to uneven enhancement in the capillary phase and curvilinear low densities correspond to intrasplenic veins (48). Also, if at bolus injection the aortic enhancement is compared to that of the spleen, these authors suggest that inhomogeneities lasting longer than 40 sec after the peak aortic enhancement are likely to represent true pathology, whereas those lasting less than 40 sec represent normal hemodynamically caused inhomogeneities (48, 49). A few minutes after bolus injection (or after slow infusion) of contrast, the homogeneous enhancement of the normal spleen is slightly less than that of liver. Although variations exist due to technique, equipment and subjects, with some individuals having higher mean CT numbers and others lower, there is a general concordance between liver and spleen enhancement (50, 51). Thus, if the liver exhibits CT density lower than that of spleen a liver abnormality such as fatty infiltration should be suspected (or, less likely, diffuse splenic calcification) (50).

Experimental Contrast Agents for CT

Lipoid contrast material has been used at the National Institutes of Health since 1978 (52, 53). A 1984 review of 225 examinations indicates the utility of this agent (54). An aqueous emulsion of iodinated esters of poppyseed oil called ethiodized oil emulsion-13 (EOE-13) was used. The complication rate was 3.6% (ascending cholangitis, bronchospasm, hypersensitivity reaction, lumbar pain, or elevated liver function tests). Side effects included primarily fever, rigor, headache, and foul taste. No permanent morbidity resulted, however. There is no nephrotoxicity.

Splenic density was increased by EOE-13 (mostly at 0.25 ml/kg) by an average of 52 HU.

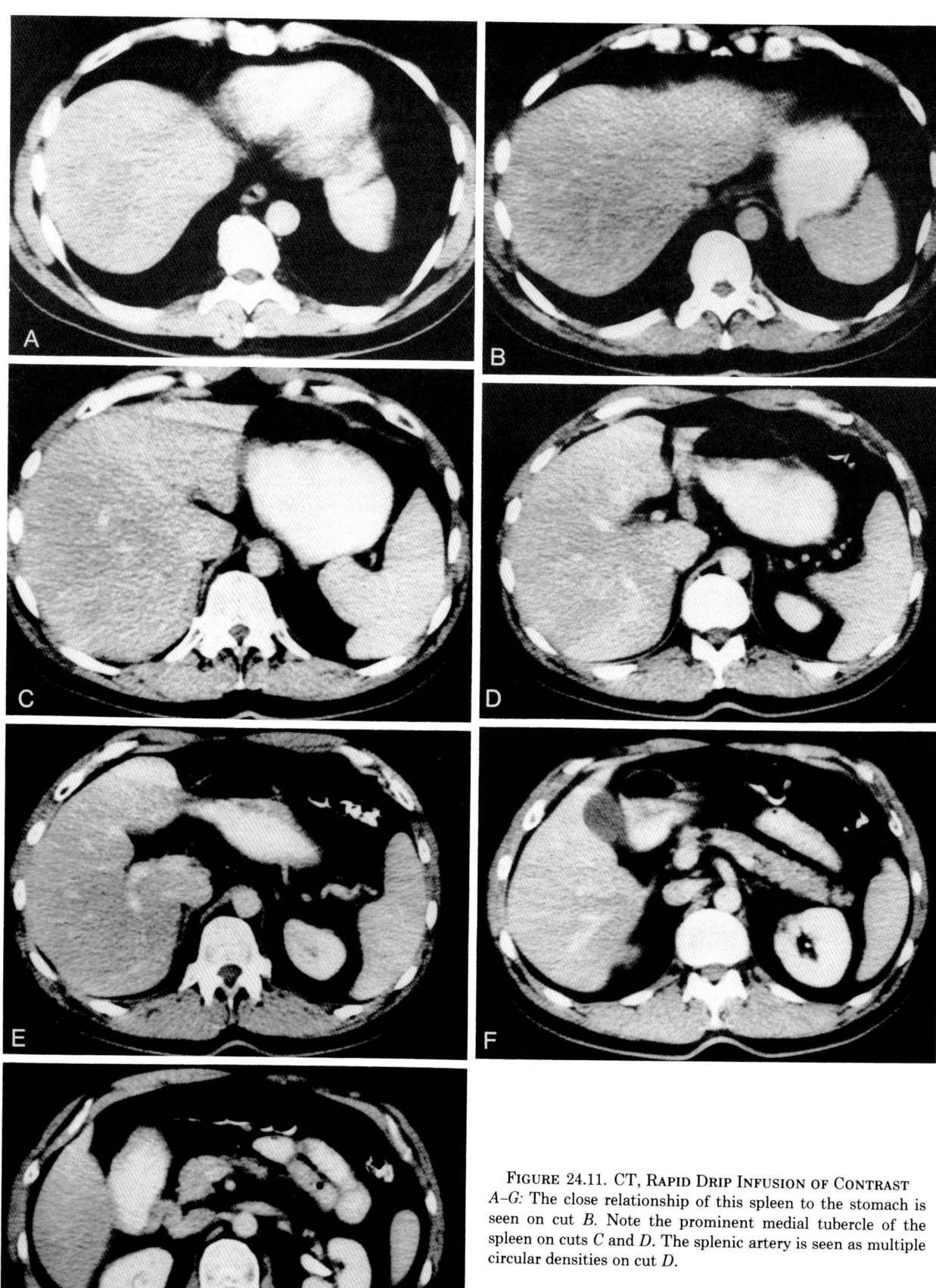

FIGURE 24.11. CT, RAPID DRIP INFUSION OF CONTRAST *A–G:* The close relationship of this spleen to the stomach is seen on cut *B.* Note the prominent medial tubercle of the spleen on cuts *C* and *D.* The splenic artery is seen as multiple circular densities on cut *D.*

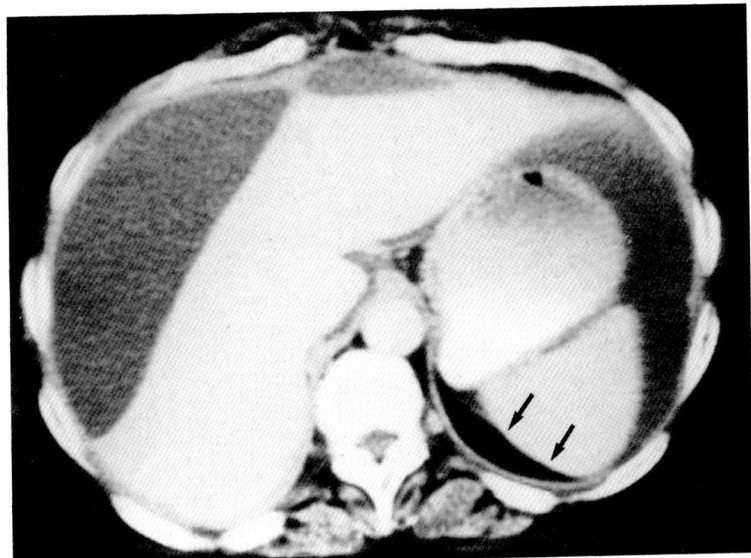

FIGURE 24.12. BARE AREA OF SPLEEN
A: CT shows the bare area of the spleen along the posterior costophrenic sulcus (*arrows*). The bare area continues along Gerota's fascia on lower cuts.

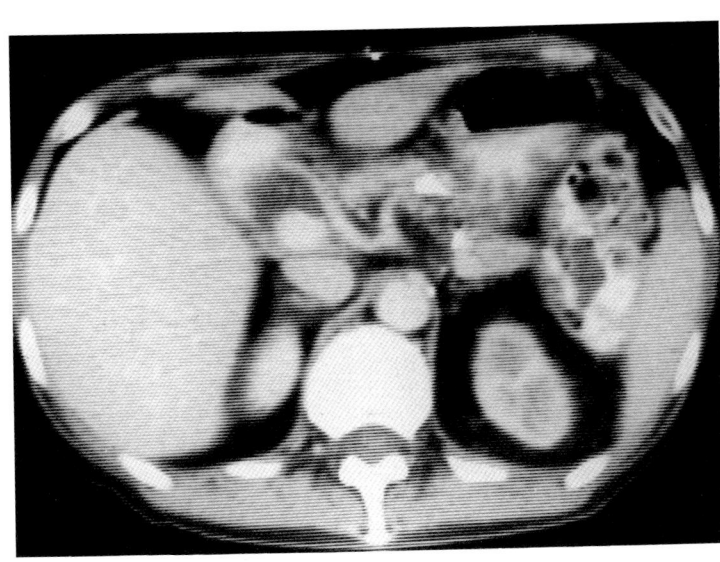

FIGURE 24.13. CT: A VARIATION IN SPLENIC CONFIGURATION
This is a long thin spleen with a long area of contact to the colon but not the stomach.

Tumors in the spleen (or liver) increased an average of only 2.6 HU, making them easily detectable. No bolus injections are needed to increase detection and the enhancement remains for hours should additional scans be needed. Thus, the utility of lipoid contrast lies in its ability to enhance normal liver and spleen to a much greater degree than tumor. Smaller lesions can be detected without loss of accuracy (54). Splenic abnormalities such as regenerating accessory spleens, metastatic disease and lymphomas have been demonstrated by EOE-13 (54). EOE-13 can clearly separate left kidney from the spleen in otherwise equivocal cases (54).

Another experimental approach has been to encapsulate water soluble material inside lipid vesicles. Liposomes are phospholipid vesicles which can trap a variety of materials including contrast agents (55). Liposomes are taken up by the reticuloendothelial system and then cleared over hours to days (55). Havron et al. (55) have used liposomes carrying diatrizoic acid salts (Renografin) to opacify the liver and spleen in rats. Seltzer et al. (56) have used liposomes carrying Iosefamate (a hepatobiliary contrast agent) to opacify the liver and spleen in dogs. Work thus far indicates that these may be safe agents for human use. Application may include not only imaging the liver and spleen but the gallbladder, bile ducts, and gastrointestinal tract as well (56).

Research has also been done with perfluorocarbons such as perfluoroctylbromide which will opacify the reticuloendothelial system and may enhance tumors (57). The future of this and

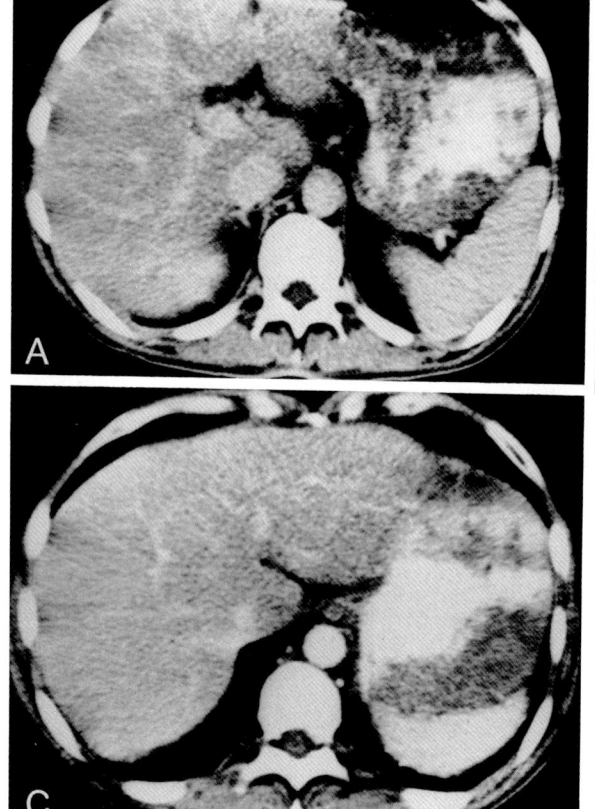
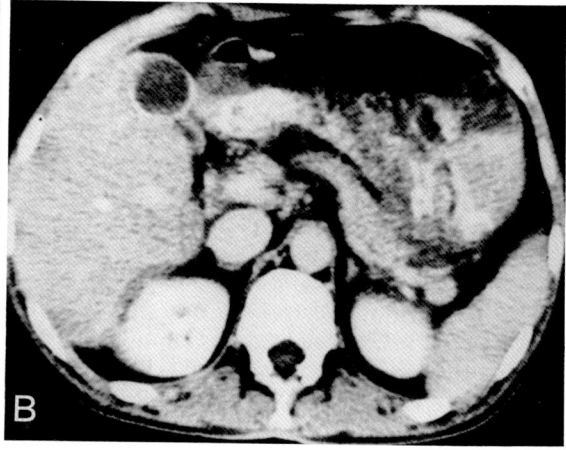

FIGURE 24.14. CT: RAPID BOLUS WITH DYNAMIC SCANNING
A–C: Splenic parenchyma is more heterogenous than usual. Sometimes the pattern is even more marked mimicking defects.

other experimental contrasts agents is promising.

Magnetic Resonance Imaging

See Chapter 31.

Splenic Volume Measurements

Due to the difficulty in establishing criteria for the diagnosis of mild splenomegaly, attempts have been made to produce splenic volume calculations. None have achieved widespread use but they are worthy of consideration and further study.

Plain films cannot accurately determine splenic volume (58). Rough estimates of splenic weight are possible, however, correlating with enlarged spleens by pathologic criteria (59).

Early nuclear scintigraphy measured the spleen in various projections on static scans (60). Mattsson (60) obtained special views on technetium scans, measured the central axis of the spleen using a soft bent ruler and assumed the spleen to be an ellipsoid. He obtained three measured values multiplied by a correction factor. The method is not excessively cumbersome and is reasonably accurate for clinical use (60). More recent data show that, to a small extent, splenic volume changes with exercise (61). Splenic radioactivity, after tagged red cell injection, is reduced with exercise and then increases gradually to normal. This is important when calculating cardiac ventricular volumes by scintigraphy (61).

There were early ultrasound methods of measuring splenic volume by producing multiple scans at 2-cm intervals and measuring them with an electric pencil connected to a computer (60). Recently, a rapid method was devised by measuring the maximum breadth, thickness and height of the spleen. These values are multiplied by each other and the product divided by 27 yielding a splenic volume index which was 8–34 in 95% of normal subjects (based on 45 normal subjects) (62). The method is quick (10 min) and probably useful, but its accuracy is not proven. It is certainly useful in following splenic size in a particular patient without the use of ionizing radiation.

Computed tomographic techniques also started with computer analysis of parallel sections (60, 63–65). This method was refined by Breiman et al. (65) using scans at 2-cm intervals using a summation-of-areas technique. The technique is reproducible and may be more accurate than sonography since the scanning is automated and their are no "blind" areas (65). A simplification of the CT method was described by Cook et al. (66) using simple linear measurements of length, width, and thickness. This method was compared to the more complex summation-of-areas method. While accuracy needs to be proven by a large number of cases, it is a simple method that can be applied to everyday use.

Splenic Aspiration

Splenic aspiration dates to the mid 1800s but was first used in large numbers of patients in India in the early 1900s to diagnose kala azar (67, 68). Core biopsies for tissue were done in the 1950s (69). A detailed history of the early use of splenic puncture is described by Kager and Rees (67). Splenic aspiration for cytologic diagnosis was developed in Scandinavia (67). Today, the technique is used extensively in Kenya for the diagnosis of kala azar (70). The technique uses a rapid insertion and removal of a 21-gauge needle attached to suction. Complications mentioned in the literature are pain, infection, puncture of other viscera and hemorrhage (67). In Kager's series of over 2,000 aspirations only one fatal hemorrhage occurred in a 50 year old male with lymphoma (diagnosed at post-mortem) who had a platelet count of 66,000 cu mm, was cachectic and not considered a candidate for laporatomy (70). In 1983 Jansson et al. (71) reported 180 patients with malignancy and a normal liver and spleen by sonography who underwent splenic and liver aspiration to detect clinically silent disease. They do not discuss any complications and conclude that aspiration was most useful for detecting non-Hodgkin's lymphoma. However, there was no long-term pathologic follow-up to determine accuracy (71). While the technique has not gained popularity in the United States, another report in 1983 from Italy described splenic biopsy in eight cases using a sonographic probe with a central aperture guide (72). A Chiba needle was used and no complications resulted. The diagnoses in these patients included pseudocyst, congenital cyst, hemangioma, hemangiosarcoma, non-Hodgkin's lymphoma, and metastatic hepatocellular carcinoma. In one "simple cyst," the cyst was evacuated on 1200 ml of clear fluid and the defect disappeared completely on follow-up. Solbiati et al. (72) mentions their experience of 45 splenic aspirations in cases of diffuse or focal pathology without any adverse reactions. Recently, there has been renewed interest in splenic puncture for diagnosis and for therapy (73).

Thus, the experience of aspiration in infection (i.e., kala azar) is extensive, the experience in neoplasm is less extensive but equally as encouraging in terms of safety. The data on accuracy in diffuse splenic diseases is not clear.

An approach to splenic disease was proposed by Shirkhoda et al. (74) and modified by Abrams (37). Any algorithm is a guideline and must be modified to the specific clinical situation, relative availability of the modalities, and expertise of the interpreter. If trauma is suspected, CT is usually the best study (see discussion Chapter 26). If a focal abnormality is highly suspected, ultrasound or CT is probably the best study. If diffuse versus focal disease is suspected, nuclear scintigraphy is a good screening procedure. Angiography may be needed as a preoperative guide or in selected difficult cases. When searching for accessory splenic tissue or splenosis nuclear scintigraphy is the best approach. If abscess is suspected on CT or ultrasound, a gallium or tagged white blood cell scan may be useful although percutaneous aspiration is often both diagnostic and therapeutic. Follow up studies for known focal lesions (i.e., hemorrhage) should be done in the least invasive fashion, i.e., ultrasound. The role of MRI and CT with experimental contrast agents is not yet clear.

REFERENCES

1. Moore KL: *The Developing Human*. Philadelphia, W. B. Saunders, 1973.
2. Warwick R, Williams PL (eds): *Gray's Anatomy*, 35th British Ed. Philadelphia, W. B. Saunders, 1973.
3. Coetzee T: Clinical anatomy and physiology of the spleen. *S Afr Med J* 62:746–757, 1982.
4. Anson BJ, McVay CB: *Surgical Anatomy*, Ed 5. Philadelphia, W. B. Saunders, 1971, pp 633–639.
5. Defiore MSH: *Atlas of Human Histology*, Ed 2. Philadelphia, Lea & Febiger, 1963.
6. Huu N, cited by Barnett CH, Lewis OJ: In: Goldby F, Harrison RJ (eds): *Recent Advances in Anatomy*, 2nd series. London, J. & A. Churchill, 1961, pp 388–392.
7. Garner E, Gay D, Rahilly O: *Anatomy—A Regional Study of Human Structure*, Ed 4. Philadelphia, W. B. Saunders, 1975.
8. Harvey AM, Johns RJ, McKusick VA, Owens AH, Ross RS: *The Principles and Practice of Medicine*, Ed 20. New York, Appleton-Century-Crofts, 1980.
9. MacPherson AIS, Richmond J, Stuart AE: *The Spleen*. Springfield, Ill., Charles C Thomas, 1973.
10. Sinner WN, Chirasthivat S: Plain film diagnosis of dis-

eases of the liver and spleen. In Serafini AN, Guter M (eds): *Medical Imaging of the Liver and Spleen*. Norwalk, Conn., Appleton-Century-Crofts, Ch 2, pp 9–21, 1983.
11. Gray SJ, Sterling K: The tagging of red blood cells and plasma proteins with radioactive chromium (abstract). *J Clin Invest* 29:818, 1950.
12. Gottschalk A, Potchen J: *Golden's Diagnostic Radiology Section to Diagnostic Nuclear Medicine*. Baltimore, Williams & Wilkins, 1976.
13. Spencer RP, Pearson HH: *Radionuclide Studies of the Spleen*. Cleveland, CRC Press, 1975.
14. Freeman LM, Johnson P: *Clinical Scintillation Imaging*, Ed 2. New York, Grune & Stratton, 1969.
15. Valk PE, Guille J: Measurement of splenic function with heat-damaged RBC's: effect of heating conditions: concise communication. *J Nucl Med* 25:965–968, 1984.
16. Atkins HL, Goldman AG, Fairchild RO, Oster ZH, Sam P, Richards P, Meinken GE, Srivastava SC: Splenic sequestration of ^{99m}Tc-labeled, heat treated red blood cells. *Radiology* 136:501–503, 1980.
17. Gottschalk A, Potchen J: *Golden's Diagnostic Radiology Section to Dignostic Nuclear Medicine*. Baltimore, Williams & Wilkins, 1976.
18. Sty JR, Starshak RJ, Miller J: *Pediatric Nuclear Medicine*. Norwalk, Conn., Appleton-Century-Crofts, 1983.
19. Spencer RP: Role of radiolabeled erythrocytes in evaluation of splenic function (editorial). *J Nucl Med* 21:450–489, 1981.
20. Klausner MA, Hirsh LJ, Lebbond PF et al: Contrasting splenic mechanisms in the blood clearance of red blood cells and colloid particles. *Blood* 46:965–976, 1975.
21. Frank MM, Hamburger MI, Lawley TJ et al: Defective reticuloendothelial system Fc-receptor function in lupus erythematosus. *N Engl J Med* 300:518–523, 1979.
22. Williams BD, Russell BA, Lockwood CM et al: Defective reticuloendothelial system function in rheumatoid arthritis. *Lancet* 1:1311–1314, 1979.
23. Peters AM, Klonizakis I, Lavender JP, Lewis SM: Use of indium-111-labeled platelets to measure spleen function. *Br J Hematol* 46:587–593, 1980.
24. Peters AM, Walport MJ, Bell RN, Lavender JP: Methods of measuring splenic blood flow and platelet transit time with ^{111}In-labeled platelets. *J Nucl Med* 25:86–90, 1984.
25. Michels NA: The variation anatomy of the spleen and splenic artery. *Am J Anat* 70:21, 1942.
26. Vincent LM, McCartney WH, Hicks R, Sheperd L: Medial splenic tubercle: potential radionuclide ventriculography pitfall. *Clin Nucl Med* 9:294, 1984.
27. Spencer RP: Splenic "hot spot" due to redundant tissue. *Clin Nucl Med* 8:239–240, 1983.
28. Nov AA, Smith GR, McMillin T: Splenic draping: clarification by gastric and splenic scintigraphy. *AJR* 142:323–324, 1984.
29. Rao BR, Winebright JW, Dresser TP: Splenic artifact caused by barium in the colon. *Clin Nucl Med* 4:249, 1979.
30. Smidt KP: Splenic scintigraphy: a large congenital fissure mimicking splenic hematoma. *Radiology* 122:169, 1977.
31. Chaudhuri TK, Bobbitt JV: Marked enlargement of the left lobe of the liver causing a false positive spleen image. *Radiology* 119:169–170, 1976.
32. Noel A, Harbert JC: Splenic simulation by left hepatic lobe following splenectomy. *Clin Nucl Med* 9:147–148, 1984.
33. Van Nostrand D, Corley JH, Kyle RW, Statler RE: Value of selective spleen scintigraphy when liver/spleen image shows equivocal spleen defects: concise communication. *J Nucl Med* 24:559–562, 1983.
34. Piepsz A, Viart P, Szymusik B, Jeghers O: A real clinical indication for selective spleen scintigraphy with 99m-Tc labeled red blood cells. *Radiology* 123:407–408, 1977.
35. Ehrlich CP, Papanicolaou N, Treves S, Horwitz RA, Richards P: *J Nucl Med* 23:209–213, 1982.
36. Reuter SR, Redman HC: *Gastrointestinal Angiography*, Ed 2. Philadelphia, W. B. Saunders, 1977.
37. Abrams HL: *Abrams Angiography: Vascular and Interventional Radiology*, Ed 3. Boston, Little, Brown, 1983, pp 1531–1604.
38. Michels NA: *Blood Supply and Anatomy of the Upper Abdominal Organs*. Philadelphia, J. B. Lippincott, 1955.
39. Cooperberg P: Ultrasound of the spleen. In Sarti DA, Sample WF (eds): *Diagnostic Ultrasound*. Boston, G. K. Hall Medical Publishers, 1980, pp 244–267.
40. Cosgrove DO, McCready VR: *Ultrasound Imaging: Liver, Spleen, Pancreas*. New York, John Wiley & Sons, 1982.
41. Nakanishi T, Ogawa H, Kawamura T, Nakano S, Miura T, Watanabe K, Honjo N: Comparison of conves and linear transducers for sonographic assessment of the liver, spleen and pancreas. *AJR* 143:1110–1112, 1984.
42. Wibhakar SD, Bellon EM: The bare area of the spleen: a constant CT feature of the ascitic abdomen. *AJR* 141:953–955, 1984.
43. Koehler RE: Spleen. In Lee JKT, Sagel SS, Stanley RJ (eds): *Computed Body Tomography*. New York, Raven Press, 1983, pp 243–256.
44. Ball WS, Wicks JD, Medttle FA Jr.: Prone-supine change in organ position: CT demonstration. *AJR* 136:815–820, 1980.
45. Mategrano VC, Petasnick J, Clark J, Bin JC, Weinstein R: Attenuation values in computed tomography of the abdomen. *Radiology* 125:135–140, 1977.
46. Stephens DH, Sheedy PF, Hattery RR, MacCarthy RL: Computed tomography of the liver. *AJR* 128:579–590, 1977.
47. Glazer GM, Axel L, Goldberg HI, Moss AA: Dynamic CT of the normal spleen. *AJR* 137:343–346, 1981.
48. Partanen K, Soimakallio S, Kivimaki T, Syrjanen K, Kormano M: Dynamic topography of the contrast enhancement of the spleen. *Eur J Radiol* 4:101–106, 1984.
49. Kormano M, Partanen K, Soimakallio S, Kivimaki T: Dynamic contrast enhancement of the upper abdomen: effects of contrast medium and body weight. *Invest Radiol* 18:364–367, 1983.
50. Piekarski J, Federle MP, Moss AA, London SS: Computed tomography of the spleen. *Radiology* 135:683–689, 1980.
51. Kaufman RA: Liver-spleen computed tomography: a method tailored for infants and children. *J Comput Tomogr* 7:45–57, 1983.
52. Vermess M, Doppman JL, Sugarbaker P, Fisher RI, Chatterji DC et al: Clinical trials with a new intravenous liposoluble contrast material for computed tomography of the liver and spleen. *Radiology* 137:217–222, 1980.
53. Vermess M, Doppman JL, Sugarbaker PH, Fisher RI et al: Computed tomography of the liver and spleen with intravenous lipid contrast material: review of 60 examinations. *AJR* 138:1063–1071, 1982.
54. Miller DL, Vermess M, Doppman JL, Simon RM et al: CT of liver and spleen with EOE-13: review of 225 examinations. *AJR* 143:235–243, 1984.
55. Havron A, Seltzer SE, Davis MA, Shulkin P: Radiopaque lipsomes: a promising new contrast material for computed tomography of the spleen. *Radiology* 140:507–511, 1981.

56. Seltzer SE, Shulkin PM, Adams DF, Davis MA et al: Usefulness of liposomes carrying Iosefamate for CT opacification of liver and spleen. *AJR* 143:575–579, 1984.
57. Mattrey RF, Long DM, Multer F, Mitten R, Higgins CB: Perfluoroctylbromide: a reticuloendothelial—specific and tumor-imaging agent for computed tomography. *Radiology* 145:755–758, 1982.
58. Riemenschneider PA, Whalen JP: The relative accuracy of estimation of enlargement of the liver and spleen by radiologic and clinical methods. *AJR* 94:462, 1965.
59. Whitley JE, Maynard CD, Rhyne AL: A computer approach to the prediction of spleen weight from routine films. *Radiology* 86:73, 1966.
60. Mattson O: Scintigraphic spleen volume calculation. *Acta Radiol Diag* 23:471–477, 1982.
61. Sandler MP, Kronenberg MW, Forman MB, Wolfe OH et al: Dynamic fluctuations in blood and spleen radioactivity: splenic contraction and relation to clinical radionuclide volume calculations. *J Am Coll Cardiol* 3:1205–1211, 1984.
62. Pietri H, Boscaini M: Determination of a splenic volumetric index by ultrasound scanning. *J Ultrasound Med* 3:19–23, 1984.
63. Heymsfield SB, Fulenwider T, Nordlinger B, Barlow R, Sones P, Kutner M: Accurate measurement of liver, kidney and spleen volume and mass by CT. *Ann Intern Med* 90:185–187, 1979.
64. Henderson JM, Hymsfield SB, Horowitz J, Kutne MH: Measurements of liver and spleen volume by CT. *Radiology* 141:525–527, 1981.
65. Breiman RS, Beck JW, Korobkin M, Glenny R et al: Volume determinations using CT. *AJR* 138:329–333, 1982.
66. Cook L, Osteaux M, Divano L, Jeanmart L: Prediction of splenic volume by simple CT measurement: a statistical study. *J Comput Assist Tomogr* 7:426–430, 1983.
67. Kager PA, Rees PH: Splenic aspiration: review of the literature. *Trop Geogr Med* 35:111–124, 1983.
68. Napier LE: Technique of spleen puncture. *Lancet* 2:126–129, 1936.
69. Block M, Jacobson LO: Splenic puncture. *JAMA* 142:641–647, 1956.
70. Kager PA, Rees PH, Manguyu FM, Bhatt KM, Bhatt SM: Splenic aspiration: experience in Kenya. *Trop Geogr Med* 35:125–131, 1983.
71. Jansson SE, Bondestam S, Heinonen E, Grohn P, Vupio P: Value of liver and spleen aspiration biopsy in malignant diseases when these organs show no signs of involvement in sonography. *Acta Med Scand* 213:279–281, 1983.
72. Solbiati L, Bossi MC, Bellotti E, Ravetto C, Montali G: Focal lesions in the spleen: sonographic patterns and guided biopsy. *AJR* 140:59–65, 1983.
73. van Sonnenberg E, Quinn SF, Wittich GR: Interventional radiology in the spleen: feasibility and safety. *Radiology* 157(P):112, 1985. (Abstracts at the RSNA, Nov. 17–22, 1985.)
74. Shirkhoda A, McCartney WH, Staab E, Mittelstaedt CA: Imaging of the spleen: a proposed algorithm. *AJR* 135:195–198, 1980.

25
Anomalies and Congenital Disorders

ABRAHAM H. DACHMAN, M.D.

WANDERING SPLEEN/SPLENIC TORSION

Wandering spleen is the most common term applied to an abnormal position of the spleen. It has also been referred to as ectopic spleen, aberrant spleen, splenic ptosis, and floating spleen (1). One should not confuse accessory spleen with wandering spleen.

Wandering spleen is a rare but well known entity. Reports date back to 1889 (2). In 1933 Abell reported a series of 95 cases of wandering spleen with torsion (3). A large Mayo Clinic series (4) of 1003 splenectomies found 2 cases; Eraklis (5) found 4 cases in 1413 splenectomies. There are scattered case reports in the modern literature, the largest recent series being eight cases reported by Gordon et al. (1). The incidence is probably less than 0.2%.

There is controversy regarding the etiology. Most authors favor a congenital origin related to factors such as abnormal fusion of the posterior mesogastrium (6, 7). The splenic ligaments may not fuse or develop with adequate support for the spleen (1). In some cases the splenorenal and gastrosplenic ligaments were absent (8–10).

Wandering spleen may be acquired. One theory is that the hormonal effects of pregnancy and the abdominal laxity associated with pregnancy result in a higher incidence of wandering spleen in multiparous women (11). Similarly it has been suggested that prune-belly syndrome is a risk factor (8, 12). The case reports of wandering spleen with other diseases, such as splenic cyst (8, 13), malaria, Hodgkin's disease, and other conditions (14), suggest that intrinsic splenic enlargement may play a role.

Most cases are diagnosed in adults, often multiparous women (3). The age range in Abell's series was 6–80 yr with most between 20 and 40 yr. It is rarely found in children (3, 8, 15, 16). The youngest reported case is in a 5½-month-old (17). In children it is likely that developmental factors predispose to splenic laxity (8, 15).

Polysplenia syndrome was associated with torsed wandering spleen in one 7½-month-old (18).

Clinical Findings

Patients may be asymptomatic with the incidental finding of a "mass" on physical examination or radiograph. Classically a firm, moveable mass with a "notch" is described (19). Symptoms when present are due to pressure on the vascular pedicle of the spleen or varying degrees of frank torsion. Mild discomfort may be due to splenic congestion (1). Persistent torsion of greater than 180° will lead to splenic infarction and an acute abdomen (3, 15, 20–22). However, torsion may be chronic or recurrent and this may explain vague abdominal pain with an evanescent mass (8, 23). Intermittent torsion may cause hypersplenism (3, 20, 21). Splenomegaly may be present (24). Chronic torsion with venous congestion may cause fundal gastric varices (8). As of 1969 there were 175 cases of torsion of a wandering spleen (25). Physical examination is difficult in the presence of torsion due to acute pain and the splenic engorgement may obscure the classic "notch" (19). Since many patients are female, the clinical impression is often that of a twisted ovarian cyst, appendicitis, or cholecystitis (24). The distal pancreatic tail may be incorporated into the torsed splenic hilum (7) and this may be accompanied by an elevated amylase and ascites.

Rarely, wandering spleen may be complicated by bowel obstruction (3, 24, 26). Abell attributed his 7 cases of bowel obstruction with wandering spleen to splenic adherence or compression (3). In the case reported by Keidar et al. (26), sigmoid volvulus accompanied obstruction of the ascending colon by a wandering spleen. They theorize that since both colon and spleen develop from the dorsal mesogastrium, a single embryonic anomaly could explain both wandering spleen and hypermobility of the colon. In one case small bowel was caught in the twisted splenic pedicle (24).

Radiology

Supine and erect plain films demonstrate a mobile mass in the left or central abdomen (1, 8, 24) which may be confused with a renal or bowel mass. The normal splenic contour in the left upper quadrant is absent and bowel loops fill this location (1). In only seven cases in Abell's series was the spleen in the left upper quadrant (3). A torsed spleen may appear as a notched mass with the notch pointing medially and upward (10).

On excretory urography the left kidney may be elevated and lack the usual splenic impression or hump (Fig. 25.1) (1). The "mass" is seen to be anterior to the kidney. Extrinsic compression on colon may be seen on plain film or barium enema. The splenic flexure is often medial and anterior to its usual location, which may be an indication of early ligamentous laxity (1). Alternately, the splenic flexure may be interposed between the diaphragm and the spleen (24). The elongated pedicle of the spleen may cause a linear defect across bowel in the region of the splenic flexure (1). The stomach may be displaced into the splenic fossa and thus appear "inverted" and ligamentous laxity may contribute to the gastric mobility (1). Solitary gastric varices may be present due to splenic vein compression (27).

Nuclear scintigraphy is the time-honored method for diagnosing wandering spleen (28). It shows the abnormal location of the spleen which may migrate on sequential studies (29, 30). Absence of uptake in a previously demonstrated wandering spleen indicates torsion (31).

Angiography definitively shows the spleen and splenic artery location. Gordon found three cases in the literature diagnosed preoperatively by angiography (1, 32). Splenic vein occlusion was shown in splenoportography in a torsed wandering spleen (27). Thus, angiography can show the exact site of torsion, define the abdominal vasculature preoperatively and may demonstrate gastric varices in chronic torsion.

Ultrasound shows absence of the spleen in its usual location and an echogenic "mass" representing the spleen may be found in the left mid abdomen or flank (Fig. 25.2) (1, 8, 33, 34). A peripheral indentation on the "mass" representing the hilar vasculature helps identify it as spleen (8). When the "mass" on plain film is thought to be renal, ultrasound shows that it is separate from the kidney. Engorged splenic hilar

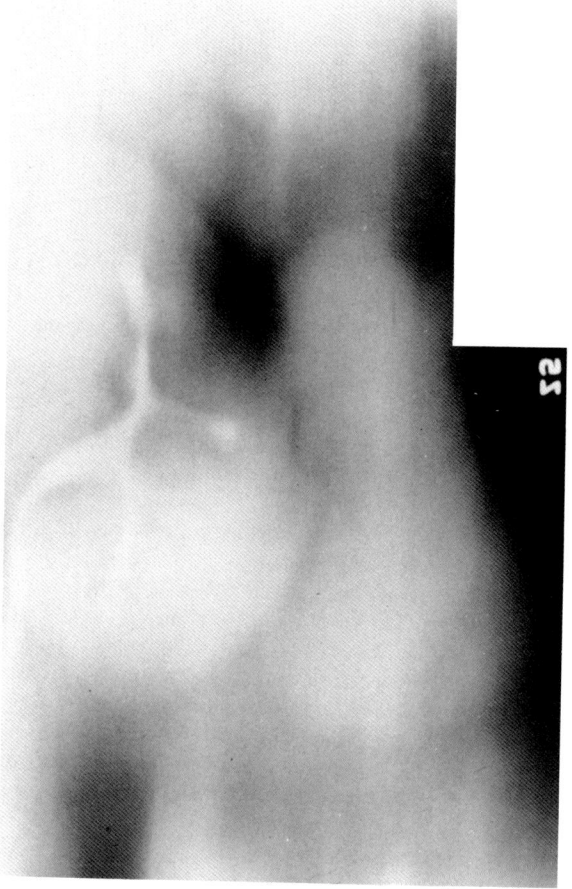

FIGURE 25.1. WANDERING SPLEEN, EXCRETORY UROGRAM
A tomographic cut shows the spleen to be anterolateral to the mid- and lower-pole of the left kidney. There was no splenic tissue in the splenic fossa. The diagnosis was confirmed at autopsy for unrelated disease.

vessels are seen if some degree of torsion is present (8). Involvement of pancreatic tail in a torsion has also been shown sonographically (7). Splenic infarction with necrosis may cause the spleen to appear less echogenic than normal. Superimposed infection in an infarcted, torsed spleen may appear as a thick walled complex mass (9).

CT has been used to show the wandering spleen in an abnormal location (7, 35), preferably using intravenous contrast enhancement. CT has also shown an enlarged wandering spleen in "normal" location (Fig. 25.2) (8). If torsion is present with resultant infarction, a portion of the spleen or the entire organ may appear to be low density (36).

If a wandering spleen is suspected, a ^{99m}Tc-sulfur colloid scan or a sonogram are the studies of choice (7). Diminished uptake on nuclear scan

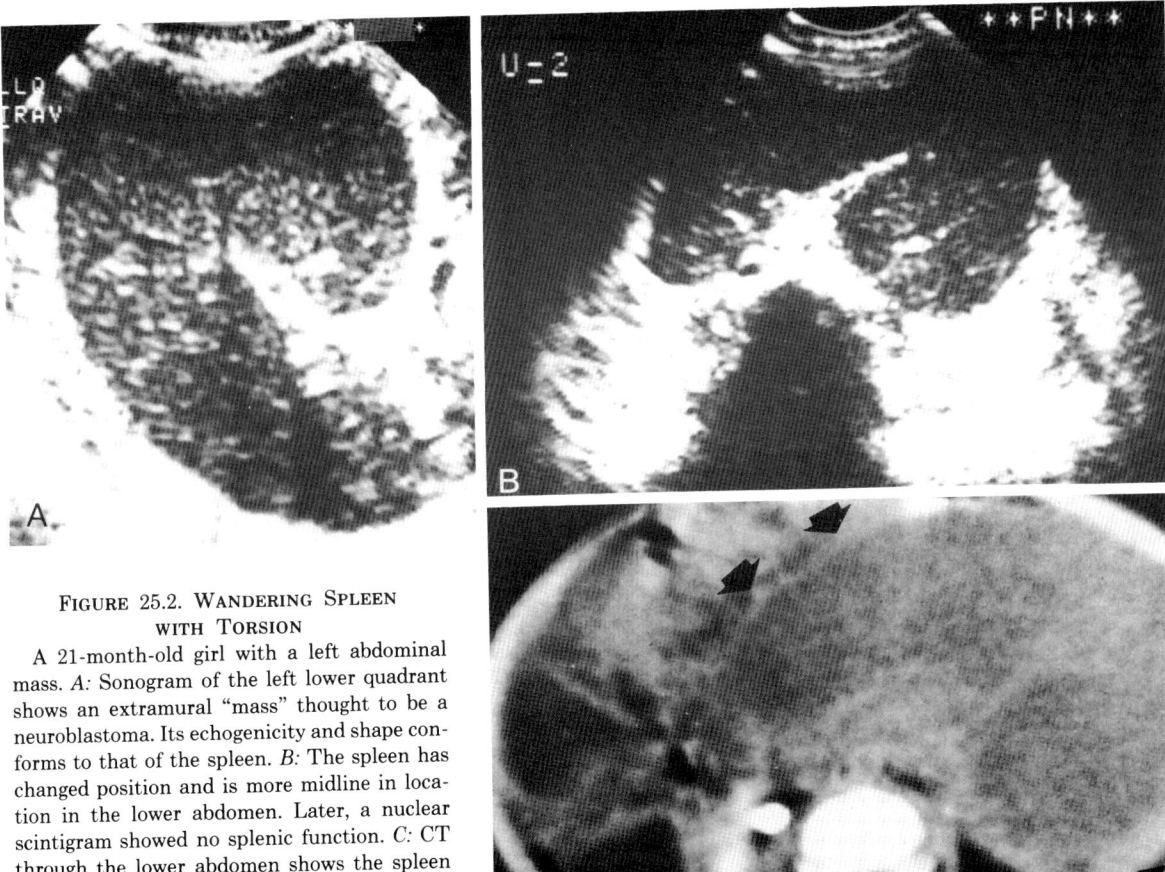

FIGURE 25.2. WANDERING SPLEEN WITH TORSION

A 21-month-old girl with a left abdominal mass. *A:* Sonogram of the left lower quadrant shows an extramural "mass" thought to be a neuroblastoma. Its echogenicity and shape conforms to that of the spleen. *B:* The spleen has changed position and is more midline in location in the lower abdomen. Later, a nuclear scintigram showed no splenic function. *C:* CT through the lower abdomen shows the spleen in an abnormal location (*arrows*) with marked low density throughout. At surgery, it had torsed and infarcted.

suggests torsion. If there is no uptake at all, ultrasound and CT will identify the spleen. (Clinical correlation should exclude autosplenectomy due to sickle cell disease.) CT is particularly useful if bowel gas obscures the spleen on sonography. Angiography should be reserved for cases where diagnosis is uncertain (7).

Traditionally, splenectomy was the treatment of choice (20). With the recognition of postsplenectomy sepsis, splenopexy is now advocated for all cases of wandering spleen (15, 19). Only if splenic torsion has taken place with resultant infarction of the spleen, should splenectomy be done.

ACCESSORY SPLEEN

Accessory spleen is the term used to indicate ectopic splenic tissue of congenital origin. Ectopic tissue due to trauma is termed splenosis and is discussed in Chapter 26. The etiology is probably failure of embryologic splenic buds to unite within the dorsal mesogastrium. Extreme lobulation of the spleen pinching off splenic tissue is also theorized (37).

The incidence of accessory spleens in autopsy series ranges from 10 to 30% (38–40). In a series of 1413 splenectomies in the pediatric age group, Eraklis found 16% had accessory spleens (41). The higher incidences are reported in association with hematologic disease (42). Most are small nodules of splenic tissue located in or near the splenic hilus or ligaments (39, 43), but about 20% may be found anywhere in the abdomen or retroperitoneum, particularly around the tail of the pancreas (38). They are usually located on the left side of the body, above the renal pedicle

(44). Paratesticular, diaphragmatic, gastric and pararenal sites are reported (45–47). The morphology is identical to normal spleen and the accessory tissue is usually supplied by a branch of the splenic artery and drains into splenic veins (38, 48).

Single foci are found in 88%, two foci in 9% and more than two foci in 3% (38). When multiple, they are clustered in a single location (48).

Symptoms may be produced by compression of adjacent organs, but most patients are asymptomatic with the accessory spleen found incidentally at surgery, autopsy or radiologic examination (49). After a splenectomy, accessory tissue will hypertrophy. If theraputic splenectomy was performed for thrombocytopenic purpura, the hypertrophy of accessory spleens may cause recurrence of disease (37, 38, 50). Splenic neoplasms may also involve the accessory tissue (38, 51), especially recurrent lymphoma (38, 51).

Rare complications which may cause acute symptoms include spontaneous rupture (52), infarction (53), or torsion of an accessory spleen (54, 55). Torsion of an accessory spleen may be intermittent causing recurrent pain and torsion of an accessory spleen with a long vascular pedicle has mimicked acute appendicitis (55).

The radiologic interpretation will depend on the site of the tissue. Nuclear scintigraphy, sonography, CT, or angiography may show the accessory tissue, especially if hypertrophied due to splenectomy.

When not hypertrophied, accessory tissue is usually small. In Beahrs' review of 8000 abdominal CT examinations, no accessory spleens

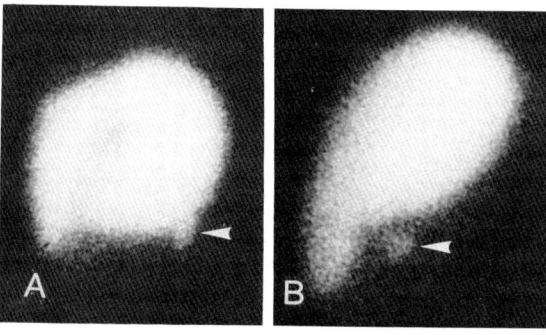

FIGURE 25.4. ACCESSORY SPLEEN: ^{99m}Tc-SULFUR COLLOID SCAN
A: Left lateral and B: left posterior oblique views, show a single small accessory spleen (*white arrowhead*).

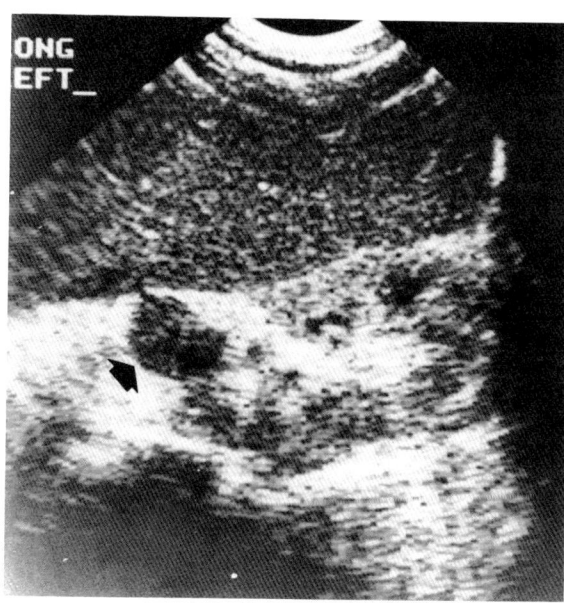

FIGURE 25.5. ACCESSORY SPLEEN: SONOGRAM
A single 2-cm accessory spleen (*arrow*), is seen abutting the normal spleen.

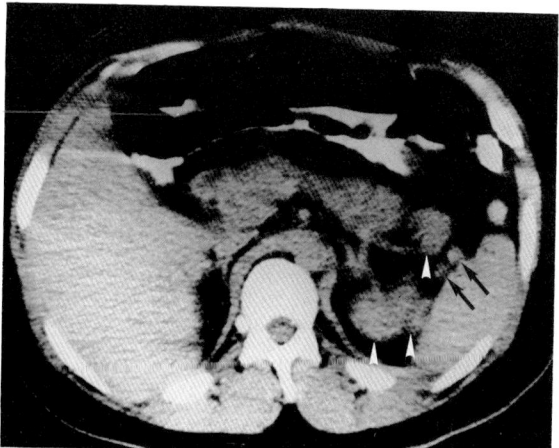

FIGURE 25.3. ACCESSORY SPLEENS: CT
Three large (*white arrowheads*) and two small (*black arrows*) accessory spleens are seen. At this level, two splenic veins are seen draining two of the larger accessory spleens.

larger than 2.5 cm were observed (Fig. 25.3) (46). If the accessory spleen compresses the stomach, a primary gastric mass may be simulated (56–58). Diagnostic studies are performed when a neoplasm is simulated. Although arteriography was often used in these cases (59, 60), nuclear scintigraphy should be done if accessory spleen is suspected (Fig. 25.4) (49). In cases of gastrointestinal bleeding, accessory spleen has been known to cause a false-positive bleeding scan (61). The clue is that the size, shape and location of the accessory spleen will not change whereas a true bleeding site will vary in appearance on sequential scans (61).

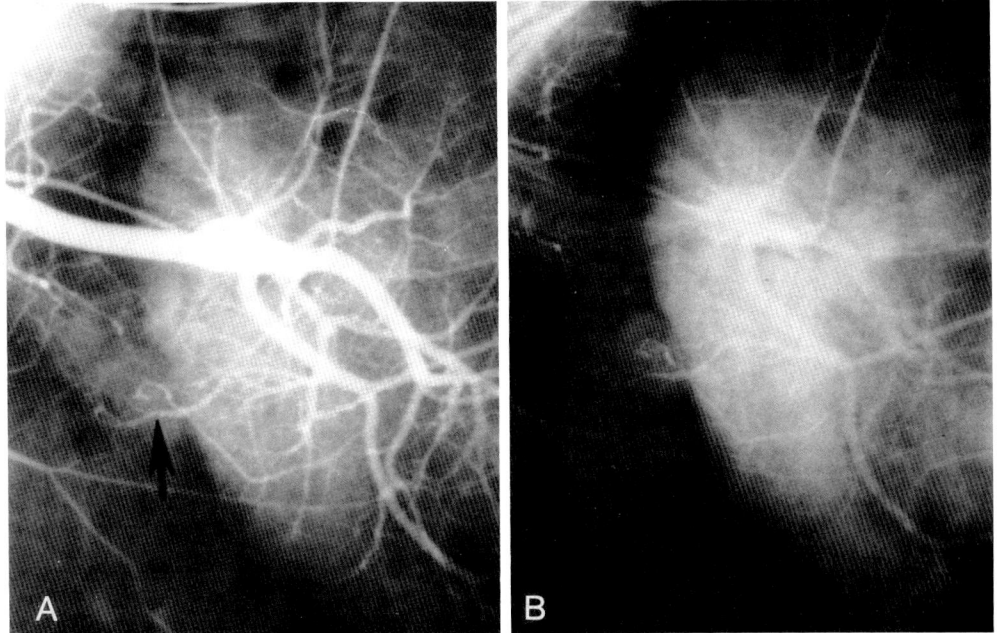

FIGURE 25.6. ACCESSORY SPLEEN: ARTERIOGRAM

A: Arterial phase shows a small branch (arrow) off a secondary splenic artery supplying the accessory spleen. B: Parenchymal phase shows a blush in the main and accessory spleens.

Subramanyam et al. (48) used sonography to detect 20 accessory spleens in 19 patients with intact spleens, although splenomegaly was present in 7 and 2 had areas of infarction within enlarged spleens. The accessory spleens were all less than 2.5 cm, corresponding to Beahrs' findings (48). They were separable from adjacent structures and their echogenicity was the same as the main spleen (Fig. 25.5). The locations were: the splenic hilus (15 cases), splenocolic ligament (3 cases), and anterior to tail of pancreas (2 cases). While CT may fortuitously show the relationship of the accessory spleen to the splenic artery, sonography can establish the relationship to the splenic artery or vein, and this was possible in 90% of Subramanyam's cases (48). In 6 cases, a single branch came off the splenic artery near the hilum to supply the accessory spleen and in 1 case, two small vessels fed the accessory spleen (Fig. 25.6). A single straight vein draining the accessory spleen was demonstrated in 12 cases (48). Previous sonographic reports have also demonstrated a parenchymal bridge between the main spleen and accessory spleen (62).

Beahrs et al. (46) reported six cases with hypertrophied splenic tissue demonstrated on CT at various sites in the left upper quadrant, from near the diaphram to the level of L3. The "mass" was separable from surrounding structures and its nature was confirmed by uptake on ^{99m}Tc-sulfur colloid scans. The tissue varied in size from 3–5 cm in these patients, all of whom were asymptomatic postsplenectomy with nonruptured spleens. One case was discovered incidentally in excretory urography, mimicking an adrenal tumor.

The differential diagnoses will depend on the location: when asymptomatic and located in the splenic hilus there is no confusion. An exogastric location mimics leiomyoma or other submucosal gastric masses. Peripancreatic locations mimic pancreatic mass or pseudocyst. Renal, adrenal, or primary retroperitoneal mass are additional possible misdiagnoses. Nuclear scintigraphy is generally diagnostic.

SPLENIC BAND

While lobulation or fissure in the spleen is considered a normal feature of splenic anatomy, an abnormally deep fissure may give the appearance of a "band" (Fig. 25.7) (63). If the fissure traverses the entire spleen, a "waist" is created which may mimic a laceration (63, 64). Peritoneum may be embedded on this waist. If peripheral, the deep fissure may mimic a hematoma or infarct (65). This is particularly confusing when a history of trauma is present. These deep fissures tend to occur on the superior border or less frequently on the inferior border where normal lobulation is known to be more prominent (65). This represents an extreme in the spectrum of normal lobulation.

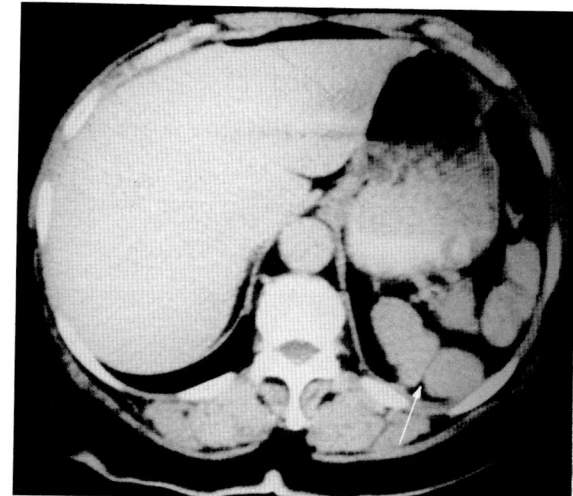

FIGURE 25.7. SPLENIC BAND: CT
A deep fissure traverses the splenic parenchyma appearing as a sharp line (arrow).

SPLENIC-GONADAL FUSION

Splenic-gonadal fusion is a rare congenital anomaly with an abnormal connection between the left gonad and the spleen or with ectopic splenic gonadal tissue. It was first reported in 1889 by Pommer (66). Under 100 cases have been reported in the literature (67, 68).

Two forms are described: continuous and noncontinuous (69). If a strand of tissue connects the main spleen to the left gonad, it is classified as continuous. This strand of tissue may arise anywhere on the surface of the spleen, but usually originates from the upper pole and, less often, the hilus or lower pole (67). It consists of a combination of fibrous and splenic tissue in varying degrees, often with a beaded appearance. If there is no connection between the main spleen and the gonadal splenic tissue, it is classified as discontinuous splenogonadal fusion. This should not be confused with accessory spleen, although it has been referred to as "scrotal or paratesticular accessory spleen." The two types occur in about equal frequency (68), usually in males with only four cases reported in females (67), all of the continuous type. The left gonad is virtually always involved (68) with only one case report of right-sided involvement (70).

The age at presentation varies from newborn to 69 yr with one case report in a stillborn. Most patients have been Caucasian, but blacks and Orientals may be affected. It usually presents as an incidental finding of a scrotal mass at physical examination or at surgery for hernia or autopsy (71, 72). Some patients present with scrotal tenderness after systemic infections such as mononucleosis, malaria, leukemia, or marching (68, 73). Up to 25% of cases, particularly the continuous type, are associated with other abnormalities, the most common of which is cryptorchism (68). Other associations include malformed limbs, micrognathia, anal atresia, skull asymmetry, and abnormal fissures of lung or liver (67, 74). In one case, microgastria and multiple accessory spleens in the inguinal area were associated (75). One patient presented with bowel obstruction due to compression of the transverse colon by the cord connecting the spleen and gonadal tissue (76).

One embryologic explanation is that the gonadal and splenic anlagen are in proximity prior to the 6th week of gestation and they fail to separate normally (69, 77). This may be due to adhesions between the anlagen (78). The gonadal precursor tissue is the mesonephros which is near the left dorsal mesogastrium (the splenic precursor). Descent of gonadal tissue usually begins at 8 weeks of gestation. The rare association with microgastria is reasonable since both originate from the dorsal mesogastrium, although association of microgastria with asplenia is more common. Why peromelus is associated is unexplained, but the limb bud does differentiate at about the 6th week, nearly simultaneous with the onset of gonadal descent (79). One case of associated cardiac anomalies is also explained by a simultaneous teratogenic insult (80).

The splenic tissue may be within or outside of the tunica albuginea, in the epididymis or along the spermatic cord (68, 81). It is microscopically separate from mesoephric-gonadal tissue (67).

The diagnosis should be suspected if swelling or mass on the left gonad has been present chronically, especially in association with an undescended testes (67). The gonadal mass, if palpable, is firm and rubbery and may feel poorly delineated from the testes, thus a primary neoplasm is the usual preoperative diagnosis (67). At least one case was correctly diagnosed preoperatively (82).

The first study performed in analysis of a scrotal mass is generally ultrasound. The mass would probably have characteristics similar to splenic tissue as found in accessory spleens (vide supra).

The key to diagnosis is nuclear scintigraphy with ^{99m}Tc-sulfur colloid which shows uptake in the inguinal or scrotal area (75, 83). If functioning tissue is present in the cord of the continuous type, uptake may be seen along the cord, although this has not been reported.

Although the entity is rare, with the increased availability of ultrasound, case reports are sure to appear.

While therapy is indicated only if symptomatic, surgery is usually performed because the diagnosis is not suspected or confirmed. Removal of the cord in the continuous type is unnecessary, thus only local inguinal surgery need be done, assuming the testes are intrascrotal (67, 84).

One case of associated anaplastic seminoma in an intra-abdominal testes with continuous splenic-gonadal fusion is reported (85).

ASPLENIA

Absence of the spleen is virtually always accompanied by a variety of congenital malformations, particularly cardiovascular and is thus referred to as asplenia syndrome (86) or Ivemark syndrome after Ivemark who studied it extensively (87). The description of the association dates back to 1826 (88).

Many of its features are those of a right isomerism, e.g., situs ambiguus with bilateral right-sidedness. While solitary absence of the spleen is reported (89), it is thought to be due to postnatal rather than prenatal factors (90).

Asplenia syndrome occurs in 1 in 40,000 live births (91), but reports ranged from 1:1,750 (92) to 1:40,000 (93). It occurs predominantly in males (90, 93).

The etiology is uncertain. Teratogens and genetic factors do not seem to be involved (90). For example, in one case report of monozygotic twins, only one twin had asplenia syndrome (94). This does not preclude genetic or teratogenic factors in some cases (95, 96). An altered timing in the development of embryonic body curvature has been postulated to explain the visceroatrial situs abnormalities: delay in curvature causing asplenia, accelerated curvature causing polysplenia (97). Monie (90) found one case with miniscule spleen suggesting that pressure of adjacent structures may have interfered with the splenic blood supply.

The diagnosis of asplenia syndrome is defined by a spectrum of multi-system abnormalities only some of which represent a dextroisomerism. The cardiac abnormalities (present in about half the cases (98), include mesocardia, dextrocardia, single ventricle, single atrioventricular valve, ventricular septal defect, atrial septal defect, transposition of the great vessels, pulmonary stenosis or atresia, absent coronary sinus, bilateral superior vena cavae, and total (or less often, partial) anomalous venus return.

In a review of 39 cases, Rose et al. (93) found the intracardiac and great vessel anomalies to be most common. Pulmonary anomalies include an abnormal distribution of lobes, usually represented by bilateral trilobed lungs. Common gastrointestinal abnormalities are situs inversus (total or partial) and rarely, imperforate anus, annular pancreas, ectopic liver, esophageal varices, duplication and hypoplasia of the stomach, agenesis of the gallbladder, Hirschsprung disease, and hindgut duplication (93, 94). Genitourinary anomalies seen in about 15% of cases (93) include horseshoe kidney, double collecting system, bilobed urinary bladder, hydroureter, and cystic kidney. Other reported associations are cleft palate, cleft lip, fused or horseshoe adrenal, absent left adrenal, bicornuate uterus, scoliosis, single umbilical artery, and lumbar myelomeningocele (93, 94).

In Rose's series nearly 80% of the patients died by the end of the first year of life due to

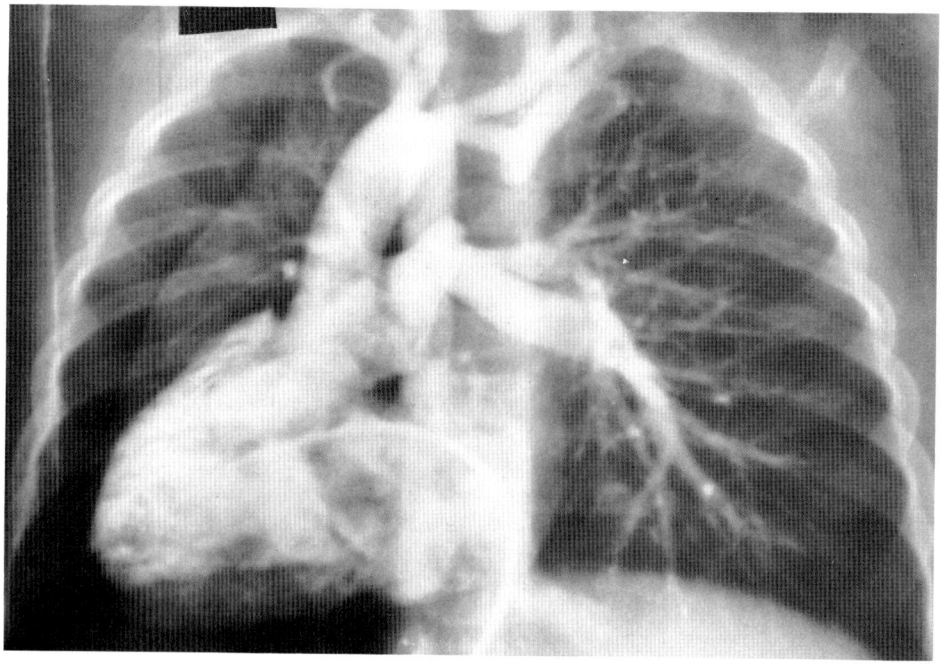

FIGURE 25.8. ASPLENIA: VENTRICULOGRAM

No splenic tissue was present on nuclear scintigram or CT. A ventriculogram shows dextrocardia and simultaneous opacification of the aorta and pulmonary artery. A single atrium and a single ventricle was present.

cardiac failure or postoperative complications. If the cardiac anomalies are mild, symptoms due to gastrointestinal abnormalities may predominate causing a delay in diagnosis (94). A retrospective review of 36 autopsied cases by Mishalany et al. showed that 83% presented with cardiopulmonary disease, but 17% presented with intestinal obstruction without obvious cardiopulmonary disease (94). Some patients may be asymptomatic (93).

Because of the increased risk of sepsis, prophylactic antibiotics are recommended (98).

The radiographic manifestations are as protean as those of the syndrome (Figs. 25.8 and 25.9). Plain film may show situs solitus, situs ambiguus or inversus (99–101). Analysis of the bronchial configuration may show a bilateral right-sided pattern and a minor fissure may be present bilaterally. The lateral chest film may show both pulmonary arteries to project anterior to the trachea (100). The inferior vena caval

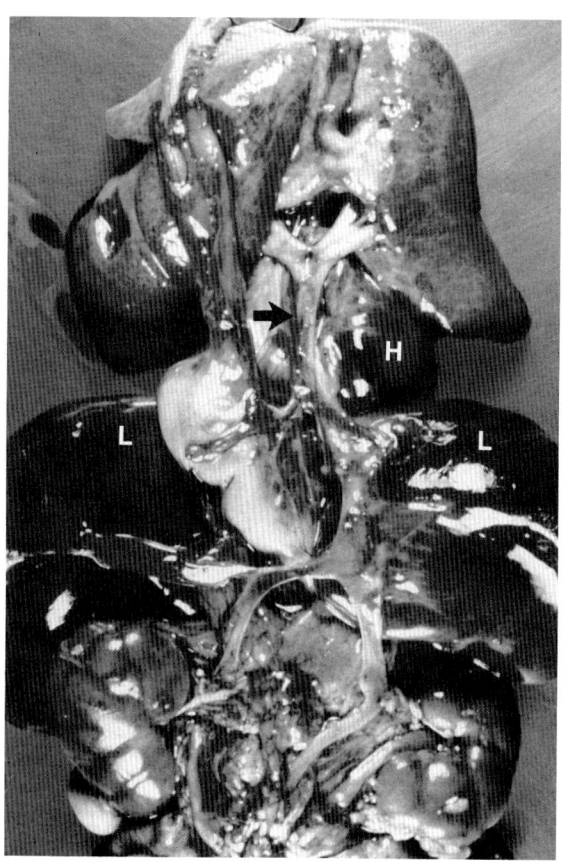

FIGURE 25.9. ASPLENIA, GROSS SPECIMEN, POSTERIOR VIEW

Autopsy specimen of a patient with asplenia, infracardiac anomalous pulmonary venous return, atrial septal defect, and pulmonic atresia. The liver (L) straddles the midline. The heart (H) and the vertical vein (arrow) are seen from a posterior view.

shadow is present but may be difficult to see in infants (100). Bilateral superior vena cavae may widen the superior mediastinum. The liver may be symmetric with no distinct splenic contour visible (101, 102).

Angiography is necessary to define the nature and extent of the cardiac anomalies. Virtually all the anomalies described above may be demonstrated angiographically and will not be detailed here. Abdominal aortic arteriography may show absence of the splenic artery or the entire celiac axis with the hepatic artery arising from the superior mesenteric artery (103). The abdominal aorta and inferior vena cava are on the same side (a nearly pathognomonic finding, usually on the right side of the abdomen (104).

Bronchography, while usually unnecessary, may show a bilateral eparterial right-sided pattern. The pattern may vary and actually not be that of a normal right or left lung, but show bilateral tracheal bronchi (105). This may complicate endotracheal intubation especially if an aberrant bronchus is also present (105).

Nulcear scintigraphy has been used to diagnose asplenia with a variety of agents including ^{99m}Tc-sulfur colloid, iminodiacetic acid agents and tagged red blood cells (101, 103, 106, 107). These show absence of the spleen and hepatic symmetry or a prominent left lobe. The iminodiacetic acid agents also may show the gallbladder to the left of the common bile duct (103). This is particularly useful since absence of the spleen may be difficult to prove on ^{99m}Tc-sulfur colloid scan when a large left lobe of the liver is present. Also, functional rather than anatomic splenic absence is possible in a variety of disease states such as vascular occlusion or thrombosis, thalassemia, polycythemia, and infiltrative processes (103). Thus, comparison of the hepatobiliary and ^{99m}Tc-sulfur colloid scan is useful where the ^{99m}Tc-sulfur scan alone is equivocal (103).

Sonography and CT are useful in demonstrating abnormalities of situs by location of the heart, liver, gallbladder or bowel and absence of the spleen. Sonography is particularly useful in a acutely ill infant. It may show location of the inferior vena cava and inferior vena cava-atrial communication (108). While vascular anatomy is well seen on CT with intravenous contrast enhancement, sonography can locate the abdominal aorta and inferior vena cava (108). Rarely will interruption of the vena cava with azygous continuation be present in asplenia syndrome (100, 109). If both the aorta and inferior vena cava are seen on the same side of the spine, this suggests asplenia syndrome (104). Using these signs, Tonkin diagnosed visceroatrial situs abnormalities on sonography and CT in 20 patients, 8 of whom had asplenia syndrome.

POLYSPLENIA

Polysplenia syndrome is a multisystem, congenital abnormality characterized by multiple small splenic masses and features of bilateral left-sidedness; it is often referred to as situs ambiguus with left isomerism. Descriptions of the syndrome date to the 1960s (110–112). In contrast to asplenia, there is a female predilection to polysplenia (93). Familial occurrence is rare but is reported in both polysplenia and asplenia (93). The etiology of polysplenia has been explained in a manner analogous to asplenia: an abnormality of embryonic body curvature, with accelerated curvature causing polysplenia (97).

The characteristic features of the syndrome are bilateral morphologic left lung, infrahepatic interruption of the inferior vena cava with azygous continuation (110), atrial or ventricular septal defects and abdominal situs ambiguus.

The spectrum of reported findings are extensive and have been recently reviewed and tabulated by Peoples et al. (113). The number of splenic masses vary from 2 to 16, located in the right and left upper quadrants (113). Abdominal heterotaxy is present in 57% of cases, usually with a symmetrical liver and midgut malrotation of varying degrees (113), (usually a nonrotation or reverse rotation) (114). Less often there is abdominal situs solitus or situs inversus. One should not exclude polysplenia merely on the basis of situs solitus (113). The lungs are bilaterally morphologic left lungs in 58%, normal in 18% and right-sided lungs in 7% of cases.

The majority of patients have some cardiovascular anomaly. Azygous continuation is seen in 65% of cases, transposition of the great vessels or double outlet right ventricle are each found in 13% of cases, pulmonic valvar stenosis in 23% of cases and subaortic stenosis or atresia is rarely present (113). Some patients lack any cardiac abnormality (113, 115–117).

Uncommon associated gastrointestinal abnormalities include esophageal atresia, tracheoesophageal fistula, gastric duplication, semiannular pancreas, duodenal webs or atresia, short bowel, mobile cecum, biliary atresia, absent gall-

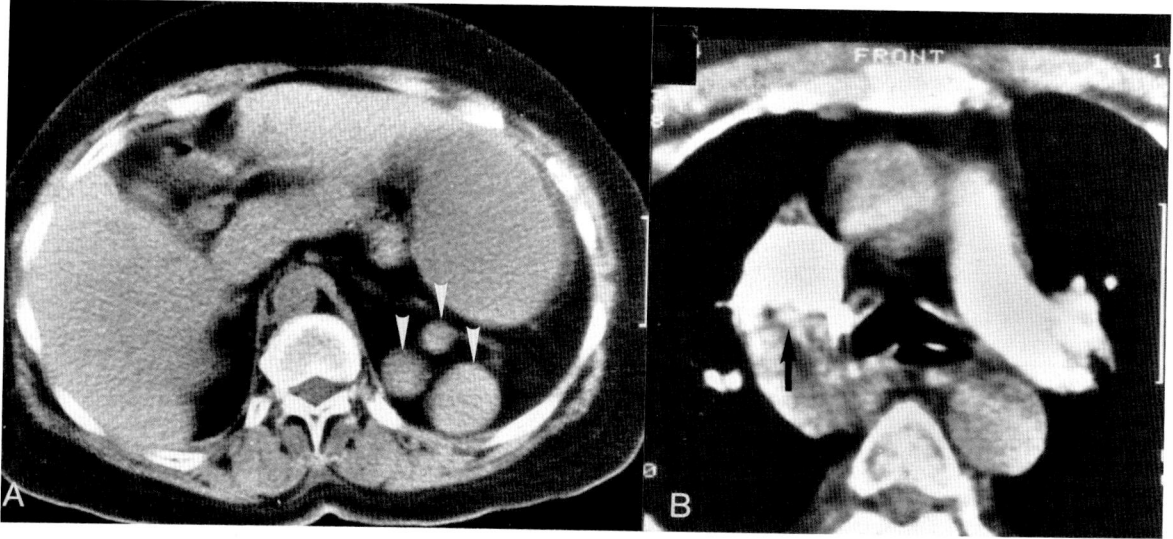

FIGURE 25.10. POLYSPLENIA WITH AZYGOUS CONTINUATION: CT SCAN
A: Abdominal CT shows multiple small spleens (*white arrowheads*) and a splenic vessel to the largest splenule. The inferior vena cava is absent. *B:* Bolus CT with dynamic scanning of the chest at the level of the azygous vein shows a markedly enlarged azygous vein (*arrow*) due to absence of the infradiaphragmatic inferior vena cava with azygous continuation.

bladder, and preduodenal portal vein (113, 118–123). An interesting association is polysplenia and abnormal cilia—reported as part of Kartagener syndrome (polysplenia, sinusitis, and bronchiectasis) in two siblings (124) and also seen in association with extrahepatic biliary atresia (118). The pathogenesis of this association is unclear. Renal anomalies were associated in 15% of cases in Rose's series (93), but their nature was not specified.

Since there are fewer cardiac and pulmonary anomalies in polysplenia compared with asplenia, the mortality is lower—about 50–60% within the first year of life (93, 119). In Peoples' review, however, only 25% of patients were alive by 5 yr of age and only 10% were alive to midadolescence (113). The cause of death is usually the cardiac disease (113). Since patients without cardiac disease may be asymptomatic, the true incidence and mortality is uncertain (113).

The clinical presentation is usually related to the cardiac disease; however, bowel malrotation may cause obstruction (113), pain due to infarction (125) or it may be an incidental finding in childhood or adulthood (108). In distinction from asplenia, prophylactic antibiotics are not needed in polysplenia (108).

The radiographic findings are as variable as the components of the syndrome. Plain films of the chest show the cardiac abnormalities, most commonly absence of the inferior vena cava on lateral view and paratracheal soft tissue prominence due to a dilated azygous or hemiazygous vein on frontal view (83, 108, 126, 127). This venous prominence due to interruption of the inferior vena cava may mimic a mediastinal mass in adults (108, 126). Sonography, CT, and angiography can confirm this diagnosis by showing the absence of the inferior vena cava between the renal and hepatic veins with independent drainage of the hepatic veins into the right atrium and a prominent azygous or hemiazygous vein (Fig. 25.10) (128, 129). Bilateral hyparterial bronchi are seen on frontal view and both pulmonary arteries project posterior to the trachea on lateral view (100).

Angiography can demonstrate the multiple spleens with a common splenic (or celiac) artery (Fig. 25.11) (130) and inferior vena caval interruption (93).

Liver-spleen radionuclide scan shows multiple spleens (131); however, there may be false negatives (108). Hepatobiliary imaging delineates the liver and not the spleen, and may therefore, help differentiate hepatic from adjacent splenic tissue and also show the presence and position of the gallbaldder (132).

Sonography and CT can demonstrate the size, position and number of spleens and simultaneously demonstrate position of the liver and bowel (108, 133). They are probably the best noninvasive studies for showing the multiple features of polysplenia syndrome. CT has also demonstrated polysplenia complicated by infarction of the

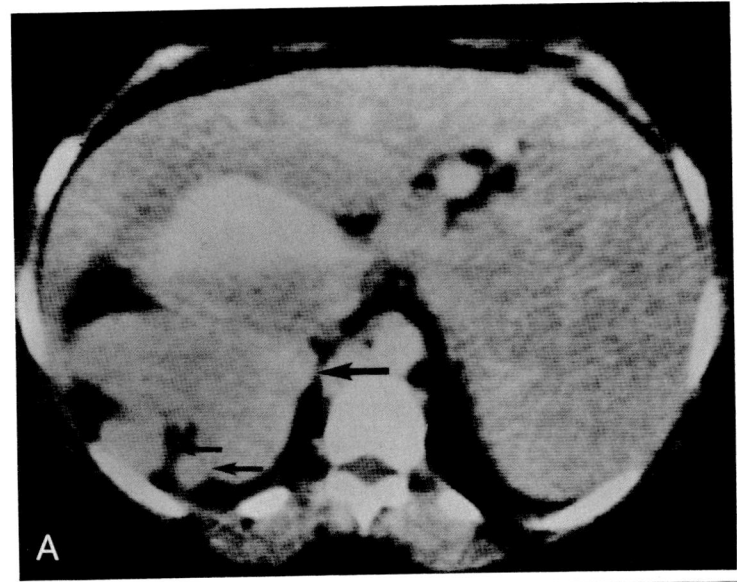

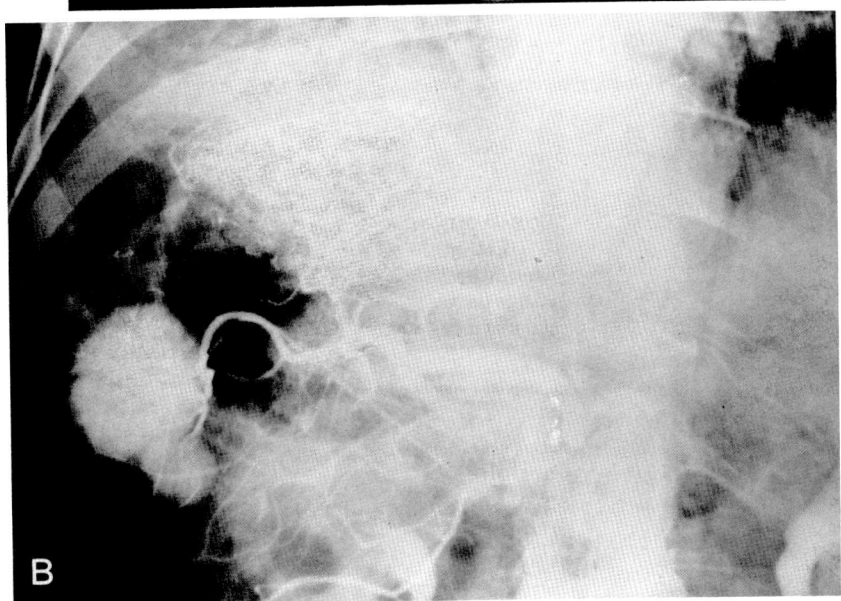

FIGURE 25.11. POLYSPLENIA WITH ABDOMINAL SITUS INVERSUS
A: CT shows multiple right-sided spleens (*arrows*) and the liver is on the left side. The azygous vein is enlarged and the inferior vena cava is absent. *B:* Selective splenic artery arteriogram shows multiple right-sided spleens supplied by a right-sided splenic artery.

spleen (125). The etiology in that case report was not determined, but torsion of the spleen in polysplenia has been reported (18) and might lead to infarction.

REFERENCES

1. Gordon DH, Burrell MI, Levin DC, Mueller CF, Becker JA: Wandering spleen—the radiological and clinical spectrum. *Radiology* 125:39–46, 1977.
2. Bond YH: Splenectomy for floating spleen with strangulated pedicle. *Weekly Med Rev* 19:393, 1889.
3. Malins E: Rotation of the spleen; removal; recovery. *Lancet* 2:627, 1894.
4. Pugh HL: Collective review, splenectomy, with special reference to historical background; indications and rationale, and comparison of reported mortality. *Int Abstr Surg* 83:209–224, 1946.
5. Eraklis AJ, Filler RM: Splenectomy in childhood: a review of 1,413 cases. *J Pediatr Surg* 7:382–388, 1972.
6. Michaels L: Spontaneous torsion of the spleen involving the tail of the pancreas. *Lancet* 2:23, 1954.
7. Sheflin JR, Chung ML, Kretchmar KA: Torsion of the

wandering spleen and distal pancreas. *AJR* 142:100–101, 1984.
8. Vermylen C, Lebecque P, Claus D, Otte JB, Cornu G: The wandering spleen. *Eur J Pediatr* 140:112–115, 1983.
9. Kelly KJ, Chusid MJ, Camitta BM: Splenic torsion in an infant associated with secondary disseminated Hemophilus influenzae infection. *Clin Pediatr* 21:365–366, 1982.
10. McClain GH, Lebherz TB: Radiographic evidence of splenic torsion: report of a case. *Obstet Gynecol* 29:475–478, 1967.
11. Simpson, A, Ashby EC: Torsion of the wandering spleen. *Br J Surg* 52:344–346, 1965.
12. Teramoto, N, Opas LM, Andrassy R: Splenic torsion with Prune-Belly syndrome. *J Pediatr* 98:91–92, 1981.
13. Dachman AH, Ros P, Murari P, Olmsted WW, Lichtenstein JE: Splenic cysts: a report of 52 cases with radiologic pathologic correlation (in press).
14. Carswell JW. Wandering spleen: 11 cases from Uganda. *Br J Surg* 61: 495–497, 1974.
15. Siplovich L, Mares AJ, Bar-Ziv J: Splenopexy for the wandering spleen. *Isr J Med Sci* 20:170–172, 1984.
16. Woodward DAK: Torsion of the spleen. *Am J Surg* 114:953–955, 1967.
17. Gotlieb, DE, Hanukoglu A, Geisler P et al: Torsion of the spleen in a five-and a-half month old infant. *Isr J Med Sci* 15:35–37, 1979.
18. Ackerman NB Jr, Smith MD, Strobel CT, Wheller JJ: Splenic torsion in the polysplenia syndrome. *South Med J* 75:897–898, 1982.
19. Stringel G, Soucy P, Mercer S: Torsion of the wandering spleen: splenectomy or splenopexy. *J Pediatr Surg* 17:373–375, 1982.
20. DeBartolo HM, Van Heerden JA, Lynn HB, Norris DG: Torsion of the spleen. *Mayo Clin Proc* 48:783–786, 1973.
21. Pollak EW, Tesluk H: Volvulus of the spleen. *JAMA* 237:469–470, 1977.
22. Weinreb N, Bauer J, Dikman S, Forte FA: Torsion of the spleen as a rare cause of hypersplenism. *JAMA* 230:1015–1016, 1974.
23. Van Dorp J: Bowel obstruction due to torsion of the spleen (letter). *N Engl J Med* 303:1002, 1980.
24. Salomonowitz E, Frick MP, Lund G: Radiologic diagnosis of wandering spleen complicated by splenic volvulus and infarction. *Gastrointest Radiol* 9:57–59, 1984.
25. Maingot R: Wandering spleen. *Abdominal Operations,* Ed 5. New York. Appleton-Century-Crofts, 1969, pp 615–616.
26. Keidar S, Freud M, Rosenchein S, Meir J, Rothfeld H: Intestinal obstruction due to a wandering spleen. *Am J Gastroenterol* 69:701–704, 1978.
27. Smulewicz JJ, Clemett AR: Torsion of the wandering spleen. *Dig Dis* 20:274–279, 1975.
28. McArdle C: Case of the winter season. *Semin Roentgenol* 15:7–8, 1980.
29. Barnett SM, Poole JR, Briggs RC: Sequential liver-spleen scanning for documentation of wandering spleen. *Clin Nucl Med* 6:528–531, 1981.
30. Isikoff MB, White DW, Diaconis JN: Torsion of the wandering spleen, seen as a migratory abdominal mass. *Radiology* 123:36, 1977.
31. Rosenthall L, Lisbona R, Banerjee K: A nucleographic and radioangiographic study of a patient with torsion of the spleen. *Radiology* 110:427–428, 1974.
32. Bosniak MA, Byck W: Wandering spleen diagnosed preoperatively by intravenous aortography. *AJR* 84:898–901, 1960.
33. Hunter TB, Haber K: Sonographic diagnosis of a wandering spleen. *AJR* 129:925–926, 1977.
34. Lee TG, Brickman FE, Satterwhite GR, Avecilla LS: Ultrasound demonstration of wandering spleen. *Arch Surg* 114:13–15, 1979.
35. Leeman M, Struyven J: Case report: wandering spleen in supra-hepatic position. *J Belge Radiol* 67:25–27, 1984.
36. Toback AC, Steece DM, Kaye MD: Case report: splenic torsion: an unusual cause of splenomegaly. *Dig Dis Sci* 29:868–871, 1984.
37. Blaustein A: *The Spleen.* New York, McGraw-Hill, 1963, p 45.
38. Halpert B, Gyorkey F: Lesions observed in accessory spleens of 311 patients. *Am J Clin Pathol* 32:165–168, 1959.
39. Curtis GM, Moritz D: The surgical significance of the accessory spleen. *Ann Surg* 123:276–298, 1946.
40. Wadham BM: Incidence and location of accessory spleens. *N Engl J Med* 304:111, 1981.
41. Eraklis AJ, Filler RM: Splenectomy in childhood: a review of 1413 cases. *J Pediatr Surg* 7:382–388, 1972.
42. Olsen WR, Beaudoin DE: Increased incidence of accessory spleens in hematologic disease. *Arch Surg* 98:762–763, 1969.
43. Schwartz SI, Adams J, Bauman AW: Splenectomy for hematologic disorders. *Curr Probl Surg* 48–49, 1971.
44. Voet D, Afschrift M, Nachtegaele P, Delbeke MJ, Schlestrate K, Benoit Y: Sonographic diagnosis of an accessory spleen in recurrent idiopathic thrombocytopenic purpura. *Pediatr Radiol* 13:39–41, 1983.
45. Wick MR, Rife CC: Case report: paratesticular accessory spleen. *Mayo Clin Proc* 56:455–456, 1981.
46. Beahrs JR, Stephens DH: Enlarged accessory spleens: CT appearance in postsplenectomy patients. *AJR* 135:483–486, 1980.
47. Rosenthal CL, Bishop MC: Accessory spleen presenting as a retroperitoneal tumour. *Eur Urol* 7:314–316, 1981.
48. Subramanyam BR, Balthazar EJ, Horii SC: Sonography of the accessory spleen. *AJR* 143:47–49, 1984.
49. Joshi SN, Wolverson MK, Cusworth RB, Nair SG, Perrillo RP: Case report: complementary use of computerized tomography and technetium scanning in the diagnosis of accessory spleen. *Dig Dis Sci* 25:888–892, 1980.
50. Verheyden CN, Beart RW, Clifton MD, Phyliky RL: Accessory splenctomy in management of recurrent idiopathic thrombocytopenic purpura. *Mayo Clin Proc* 53:442–446, 1978.
51. Jacobson JM, Reynolds, RD: Accessory spleen in Hodgkin's disease. *JAMA* 240:2081, 1978.
52. Texeira MB, Hardin WJ: Spontaneous rupture of an accessory spleen. *Am Surg* 40:491–493, 1974.
53. Babcock TL, Cocker DD, Haynes JL, Conklin HB: Infarction of an accessory spleen causing an acute abdomen. *Am J Surg* 127:336–337, 1974.
54. Bass RT, Yao ST, Freeark RJ: Torsion of an accessory spleen of the cecum presenting as an acute appendicitis. *N Engl J Med* 277:1190–1191, 1967.
55. Grunspan M: Torsion of an accessory spleen simulating acute appendicitis. *Isr J Med Sci* 17:458–459, 1981.
56. Das Gupta TK, Busch RC: Accessory splenic tissue producing indentation of the gastric fundus resembling gastric neoplasm. *N Engl J Med* 263:1360–1361, 1960.
57. Hargrove MD Jr, Kilpatrick ZM: Pseudotumor of the gastric fundus caused by an accessory spleen. *J La State Med Soc* 121:386–387, 1969.
58. Brown RB, Dobbie RP: Splenic indentation of the gastric fundus resembling gastric neoplasm. *AJR* 81:599–602, 1959.
59. Clark RE, Korobkin M, Palubinskas AJ: Angiography of accessory spleens. *Radiology* 102:41–44, 1972.
60. Kaude J: Accessory spleens as demonstrated by celiac angiography. *Radiology* 13:53–56, 1973.

61. Heyman S, Sunaryo FP, Ziegler MM: Gastrointestinal bleeding: an accessory spleen causing a false-positive ^{99m}Tc-sulfur colloid study. Clin Nucl Med 7:38–40, 1982.
62. Bagni P, Belloir A, Rhomer P, Weill F: Accessory spleens: scanographic and ultrasonic study. J Radiol (Paris) 64:43–46, 1983.
63. Wilson DG, Lieberman LM: Unusual splenic band appearance on liver-spleen scan. Clin Nucl Med 8:270, 1983.
64. Hansen RM, Spiegelhoff DR: Marked congenital fissure masquerading as splenic laceration: report of a case. J Nucl Med 22:151–152, 1981.
65. Smidt KP: Splenic scintigraphy: a large congenital fissure mimicking splenic hematoma. Radiology 122:169, 1977.
66. Pommer G: Verwachsung des linken kryptorchishen Hodens und Nebenhodens mit der Milz in einer Missgeburt mit zahlreichen Bildungsdefecten. Ber Naturwmed Ver Innsbruck 18:144, 1888–1889.
67. Bearss RW: Splenic-gonadal fusion. Urology 16:277–279, 1980.
68. Ceccacci L, Tosi S: Splenic-gonadal fusion: case report and review of the literature. J Urol 126, 1981.
69. Putschar WG, Manion WC: Splenic-gonadal fusion. Am J Pathol 32:15, 1956.
70. Halvorsen JF, Stray O: Splenogonadal fusion. Acta Paediatr Scand 67:379, 1978.
71. Finbeiner AE, DeRidder DA, Ryden SE: Splenic-gonadal fusion and adrenal cortical rest associated with bilateral cryptorchism. Urology 10:337, 1977.
72. Settle E: The surgical importance of accessory spleens with report of two cases. Am J Surg 50:22–26, 1940.
73. Pendse AK, Mathur PN, Sharma MM: Splenic-gonadal fusion. Br J Surg 62:624, 1975.
74. Warkany J: Congenital Malformations. Chicago, Year Book, 1971, pp 749–750.
75. Mandell GA, Heyman S, Alvai A, Ziegler MM: A case of microgastria with splenic-gonadal fusion. Pediatr Radiol 13:95–98, 1983.
76. Hines JR, Eggum PR: Splenic-gonadal fusion causing bowel obstruction. Arch Surg 83:887, 1961.
77. Putschar WGJ, Manion WC: Congenital absence of the spleen and associated anomalies. Am J Clin Pathol 26:429, 1956.
78. Sneath WA: An apparent third testicle consisting of a scrotal spleen. J Anat Physiol 47:340, 1913.
79. Almenoff IA: Splenic-gonadal fusion. NY J Med 66:1679, 1966.
80. Loomis KF, Moore GW, Hutchins GM: Unusual cardiac malformations in splenogonadal fusion-peromelia syndrome: relationship to normal development. Teratology 25:1–9, 1982.
81. Keizur, LW: Accessory spleen in scrotum: report of two cases. J Urol 68:759, 1952.
82. Kadlic T: Nebenmilz in einer angeborenen Skrotalhernie. Zentralbl Allg Pathol 81:49, 1943.
83. Guarin U, Dimitrieva Z, Ashley S: Splenogonadal fusion—a rare congenital anomaly demonstrated by ^{99m}Tc-sulfur colloid imaging. J Nucl Med 16:922, 1975.
84. Dhall JC, Singla S: Splenogonadal fusion. Br J Surg 69:348, 1982.
85. Falkowski WS, Carter MF: Splenogonadal fusion associated with an anaplastic seminoma. J Urol 124, 563–564, 1980.
86. Polhemus DW, Schafer WB: Congenital absence of the spleen. Syndrome with atrioventricularis and situs inversus. Case reports and review of literature. Pediatrics 9:696–708, 1952.
87. Ivemark BI: Implications of agenesis of the spleen on the pathogenesis of cono-truncus anomalies in childhood. An analysis of the heart malformations in the splenic agenesis syndrome with fourteen new cases. Acta Paediatr 44(Suppl 104): 1–110, 1955.
88. Breschet G: Memoire sur l'ectopie de l'appareil de la circulation, et particulierment sur celle due coeur. Repert Gen Anat Physiol Pathol (Paris) 2:1–39, 1826.
89. Honigman R, Lanzkowsky P: Isolated congenital asplenia: an occult case of overwhelming sepsis. Am J Dis Child 133:552, 1979.
90. Monie IW: The asplenia syndrome: an explanation for absence of the spleen. Teratology 25:215–219, 1982.
91. Abrams HL: Abrams Angiography: Vascular and Interventional Radiology, Ed 3, Vol II. Boston, Little, Brown, 1983, pp 1544–1547.
92. Majeski JA, Upshur JK: Asplenia syndrome: a study of congenital anomalies in sixteen cases. JAMA 140:1508–1510, 1978.
93. Rose V, Izukawa T, Moes CAF: Syndromes of asplenia and polysplenia: a review of cardiac and non-cardiac malformations in 60 cases with special reference to diagnosis and prognosis. Br Heart J 37:840–852, 1975.
94. Wilkinson JL, Holt PA, Dickinson DF, Jivani SK: Asplenia syndrome in one of mono-zygotic twins. Eur J Cardiol 10:301, 1979.
95. Cox DR, Martin L, Hall BD: Asplenia syndrome after fetal exposure to warfarin. Lancet 2:1134, 1977.
96. Katcher AL: Familial asplenia, other malformations, and sudden death. Pediatrics 65:633, 1980.
97. Hutchins GM, Morre GW, Lipford EH, Haupt HM, Walker MC: Asplenia and polysplenia malformation complexes explained by abnormal embryonic body curvature. Pathol Res Pract 177:60–76, 1983.
98. Biggar WD, Ramirez RA, Rose V: Congenital asplenia: immunologic assessment and a clinical review of eight surviving patients. Pediatrics 67:548–551, 1981.
99. Randall PA, Moller JH, Amplatz K: The spleen and congenital heart disease. AJR 119:551–559, 1973.
100. Soto B, Pacifico AD, Souza AS Jr, Bargeron LM Jr, Ermocilia R, Tonkin IL: Identification of thoracic isomerism from the plain chest radiograph. AJR 131:995–1002, 1978.
101. Freedom RM, Fellows KE Jr: Radiographic visceral patterns in the asplenia syndrome. Radiology 107:387–391, 1973.
102. Forde WJ, Finby N: Roentgenographic features of asplenia, a teratological syndrome of visceral symmetry. AJR 86:523–533, 1961.
103. Rao BK, Shore RM, Lieberman LM, Polcyn RE: Dual radiopharmaceutical imaging in congenital asplenia syndrome. Radiology 145:805–810, 1982.
104. Elliott LP, Cramer, GG, Amplatz K: The anomalous relationship of the inferior vena cava and abdominal aorta as a specific angiocardiographic sign in asplenia. Radiology 87:859–863, 1966.
105. Fernbach SK: Case of the fall season. Semin Roentgenol 16:239–240, 1981.
106. Fitzer PM: An approach to cardiac malposition and the heterotaxy syndrome using ^{99m}TC-sulfur colloid imaging. AJR 127:1021–1025, 1976.
107. Piepsz A, Viart P, Szymusik B, Jeghers O: A real clinical indication syndrome using ^{99m}Tc-labeled red blood cells. Radiology 123:407–408, 1977.
108. Tonkin ILD, Tonkin AK: Visceroatrial situs abnormalities: sonographic and computed tomographic appearance. AJR 138:509–515, 1982.
109. Bussatt PL, Bopp P, Duchosal PW: Congenital heart disease with the Ivemark syndrome and absence of the inferior vena cava. Radiology 84:657–659, 1965.
110. Moller JH, Nakib A, Anderson RC, Edwards JE: Congenital cardiac disease associated with polysplenia. A

developmental complex of bilateral "left-sidedness." *Circulation* 36:789–799, 1967.
111. Rahimtoola SH, Marshall HJ, Edwards JE: Anomalous connection of pulmonary veins to right atrium associated with anomalous inferior vena cava, situs inversus and multiple spleens: developmental complex. *Mayo Clin Proc* 40:609–613 1965.
112. VanMierop LHS, Gessner JH, Schieber GL: Asplenia and polysplenia syndromes. *Birth Defects* 8:36–44, 1972.
113. Peoples WM, Moller JH, Edwards JE: Reviews: polysplenia, a review of 146 cases. *Pediatr Cardiol* 4:129–137, 1983.
114. Moller HH, Amplatz K, Wolfson J: Malrotation of the bowel in patients with congenital heart disease associated with splenic anomalies. *Radiology* 99:393–398, 1971.
115. Ivemark BI: Implications of agenesis of the spleen on the pathogenesis of conotruncus anomalies in childhood, an analysis of the heart malformations in the splenic agenesis syndrome with 14 new cases. *Acta Paediatr Scand* 44 (Suppl 104):7–110, 1955.
116. Majeski JA, Upshur JK: Polysplenia associated with a congenital diaphragmatic defect. *South Med J* 68:1263–1265, 1975.
117. Sugiura M, Okada R, Hiraoka K: Isolated levocardia with polysplenia in an aged with special reference to minor cardiac abnormalities. *Jpn Heart J* 9:603–608, 1968.
118. Teichberg S, Markowitz J, Silverberg M, Aiges H, Schneider K, Kahn E, Daum F: Abnormal cilia in a child with polysplenia syndrome and extrahepatic biliary atresia. *J Pediatr* 100:399–401, 1982.
119. Paddock RJ, Arensman RM: Polysplenia syndrome: spectrum of gastrointestinal congenital anomalies. *J Pediatr Surg* 17:563–566, 1982.
120. Chandra RS: Biliary atresia and other structural anomalies in the congenital polysplenia syndrome. *J Pediatr* 85:649–655, 1974.
121. Raff LJ, Schwartz ST: Polysplenia complex and duodenal atresia. A case report. *Arch Pathol Lab Med* 107:202–203, 1983.
122. Dimmick, VE, Bone KE, McAdames AJ: Extrahepatic biliary atresia and the polysplenia syndrome. *J Pediatr* 86:644, 1975.
123. Taybi H: *Radiology of Syndromes and Metabolic Disorders*, Ed 2. Year Book, Chicago, 1983, p 315.
124. Schidlow DV, Katz SM, Turtz MG, Donner RM, Capasso S: Polysplenia and kartagener syndromes in a sibship: association with abnormal respiratory cilia. *J Pediatr* 100:401–403, 1982.
125. Shadle CA, Scott ME, Ritchie DJ, Seliger G: Case report: spontaneous splenic infarction in polysplenia syndrome. *J Comput Assist Tomogr* 6:177–179, 1982.
126. Heller RM, Dorst JP, James AE Jr, Rowe RD: a useful sign in the recognition of azygos continuation of the inferior vena cava. *Radiology* 101:519–522, 1971.
127. Floyd GD, Nelson WP: Developmental interruption of the inferior vena cava with azygos and hemiazygos substitution. *Radiology* 119:55–57, 1976.
128. Garris JB, Kangarloo H, Sample WF: Ultrasonic diagnosis of infrahepatic interruption of the inferior vena cava with azygos (hemiazygos) continuation. *Radiology* 134:179–183, 1980.
129. Train JS, Henderson MR, Smith AP: Sonographic demonstration of left-sided inferior vena cava with hemiazygos continuation. *AJR* 134:1056–1057, 1980.
130. Vaughn TJ, Hawkins IF Jr, Elliott LP: Diagnosis of polysplenia syndrome. *Radiology* 101:511–518, 1971.
131. Baert AL, Myle J: Polysplenia. *Br J Radiol* 48:496–499, 1975.
132. Polga JP, Spencer RP: Interesting images: hepatobiliary imaging as an aid in determining situs in a case of polysplenia. *Clin Nucl Med* 9:159–160, 1984.
133. De Maeyer P, Wilms G, Baert AL: Case report: polysplenia. *J Comput Assist Tomogr* 5:104–105, 1981.

26
Trauma and Nontraumatic Rupture

ABRAHAM H. DACHMAN, M.D.

TRAUMA

Splenic injury may follow blunt or penetrating trauma, or be spontaneous or iatrogenic. In blunt abdominal trauma the spleen is the most commonly injured organ (1). The concern in cases of splenic injury is mainly that of splenic rupture which is associated with a >75% mortality if surgery is not performed (2). Thus splenic injury was previously considered an absolute indication for surgical intervention. Recent data indicates an increased incidence of life-threatening infection in splenectomized patients, thus a trend toward conservative management has evolved. Accurate grading of splenic injury has become an important part in managing the traumatized patient. Radiographic evaluation is thus important in diagnosing the nature and extent of injury.

Historically, the operative mortality for splenic rupture was over 50% at the turn of the century. Currently the overall mortality for splenic rupture is 10–15% which is partly attributable to associated injuries (2). In one large series, 71% of patients with penetrating splenic injury had associated injuries and 63% of patients with blunt abdominal trauma had associated injuries (3). In a pediatric series, 80% of patients with blunt abdominal trauma had associated extraabdominal injuries and 56% of penetrating abdominal trauma patients had concomitant extra-abdominal injuries. This underscores the need for complete evaluation and diagnosis when following a course of conservative therapy (4). The most common cause of blunt splenic injury is automobile accidents (50–80%) which may account for the high association between splenic and hepatic lacerations (2).

Iatrogenic splenic injury is not uncommon during abdominal surgery (5). Between 10–40% of adult splenectomies are done for iatrogenic injury, usually caused by traction on the splenic peritoneal attachments with resultant capsular tear. The splenic peritoneal attachments are relatively avascular and accessible, however the spleno-omental ligament may be hidden by the gastrosplenic ligament, and traction on the ligament may cause a capsular tear. Other less known iatrogenic causes of splenic injury are thoracentesis and renal biopsy (6). Although rare, the incidence is probably under-reported because pain may be transient and attributed to the procedure and bleeding may be contained to the subcapsular or perisplenic region. Rauch et al. (6) reported three cases, one which required emergency splenectomy.

Splenic injuries have been classified in a variety of ways. A useful scheme is: (*a*) contusion, (*b*) subcapsular hematoma, (*c*) parenchymal injury with small capsular tear, and (*d*) rupture with hemoperitoneum (2). Others add (*e*) splenic root and hilar injury and (*f*) late complications (7).

The clinical manifestations depend on the severity of the splenic and associated injuries. Pain may be referred to the left shoulder. One must determine if there is hemoperitoneum which might indicate splenic laceration or rupture. There may be signs of shock or peritoneal fluid and traditionally, peritoneal lavage is performed to diagnose hemoperitoneum. One must judge the severity of injury in each particular case; if there is time for performing a radiologic examination, peritoneal lavage may be omitted, since not only can hemoperitoneum be diagnosed radiologically, but the severity and extent of other abdominal organ injury can be obtained. Where urgent surgery seems necessary and there is no time for imaging the abdomen, peritoneal lavage may be useful to confirm hemoperitoneum although there may be false positives. If CT is done after peritoneal lavage, one may be uncertain whether the intraperitoneal blood is due to the initial trauma or the lavage. Thus if CT may be used, peritoneal lavage should be delayed or omitted.

Plain Film

When bleeding is confined to the parenchyma or subcapsular region a plain film may show splenic enlargement with resultant displacement of the stomach, splenic flexure, and elevation of the left hemidiaphragm. Associated rib fracture(s) or pleural effusion may be present.

While capsular tear or splenic rupture may obscure or distort the splenic outline, this is not a reliable finding since the spleen may normally not be visualized (8) and fetal lobulation may distort its contour. The presence of rib fracture(s), pleural effusion, or severe gastric dilatation should suggest significant splenic injury. Massive hemoperitoneum may be demonstrated in the same manner as ascites on a plain film. Theoretically, even smaller amounts of free fluid can be detected on an abdominal radiograph if the colon is distended, by noting fluid in the paracolic gutter on a supine film, which moves on a decubitus view (9). Chronically, hematomas may resolve with residual calcification (Fig. 26.1).

Plain film findings thus are suggestive at best and are necessary primarily to evaluate for evidence of free peritoneal air, retroperitoneal air, pneumothorax, and other associated injuries.

Nuclear Medicine

Prior to CT and sonography, scintigrams were frequently used to evaluate for splenic injury. If one is aware of the pitfalls of interpretation, nuclear scintigraphy can still be a useful screening study in selected cases.

In 1967, the first scintigraphic diagnosis of a surgically proven splenic hematoma was made using ^{51}Cr-tagged damaged red blood cells (10). ^{99m}Tc-sulfur colloid scanning using a gamma camera with multiple views was developed later. Dynamic flow scanning has been added to define avascular areas, and the caudally angulated view was devised to separate the left lobe of the liver from the spleen. The sensitivity of sulfur colloid scanning was sufficient to give it the role of procedure of choice (11). With time, awareness of pitfalls increased; heart-shaped or "upside-down" spleen (12), congenital fissures (13), and accessory spleens could mimic post-traumatic fragments and barium in the splenic flexure can stimulate a defect (11).

The scintigraphic signs of splenic trauma as described by Nesbesar et al. (14) include linear, wedge-shaped, or stellate defects within the splenic parenchyma (Fig. 26.2). Concave defects along the contour or an indistinct margin ("dou-

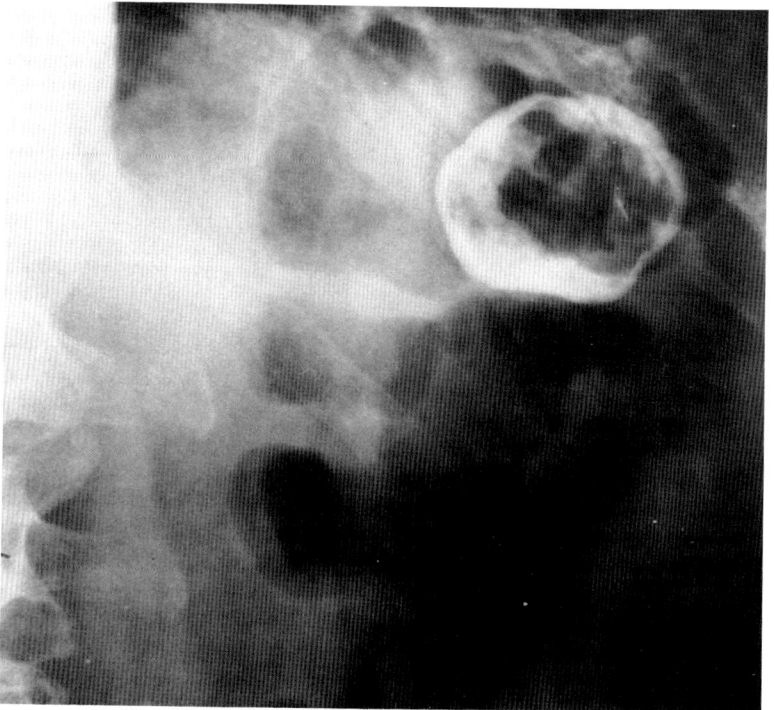

FIGURE 26.1. SPLENIC HEMATOMA
Plain film of old splenic hematoma with thick rim calcification.

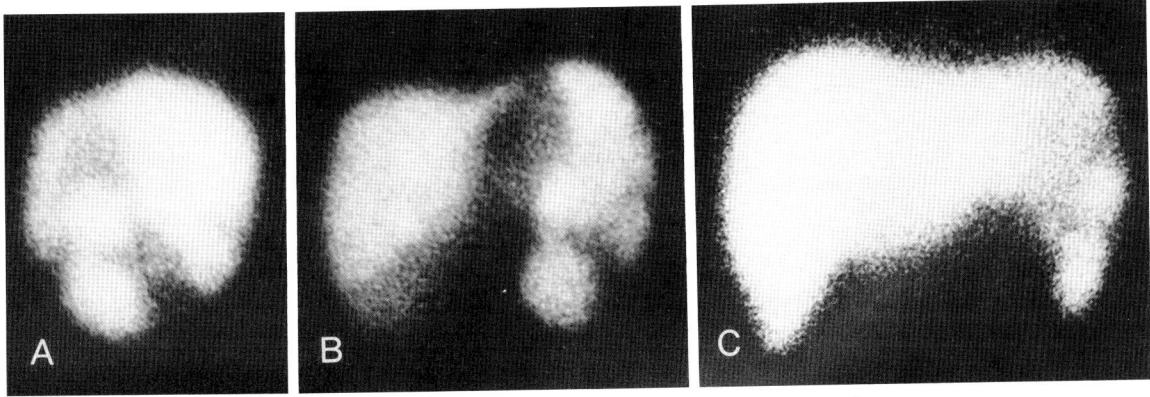

FIGURE 26.2. FRAGMENTED SPLEEN: ^{99m}Tc-SULFUR COLLOID SCAN
The spleen was traumatized during an automobile accident. A: Anterior; B: left anterior oblique; and C: left lateral views show linear and wedgeshaped defects representing hematoma and actual shattering of splenic parenchyma.

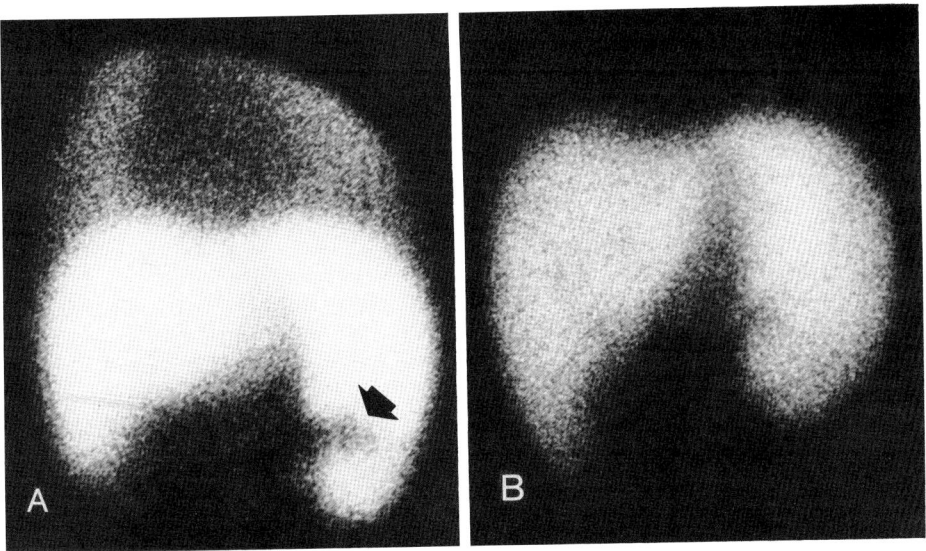

FIGURE 26.3. RESOLVING HEMATOMA, ^{99m}Tc-SULFUR COLLOID SCAN
A: Left anterior oblique view immediately following the trauma shows a defect (arrow) representing hematoma. B: Same view taken 3 months later shows near complete resolution.

ble density sign") may represent subcapsular hematoma. Displacement of the spleen from the body wall may also be seen ("splenic crowding sign"). As recently as 1982, Froelich et al. (15) recommended nuclear scan as the primary screening examination for liver-spleen trauma. However, sonographic equipment has improved, CT has proven highly accurate and both have become widely available. Nevertheless, the specificity of properly performed nuclear studies is documented (15, 16). When sonography or CT are inadequate due to technique problems, e.g., patient pain or skin injury for sonography and contrast allergy and patient motion for CT then a nuclear study may be more convenient. If splenic injury is found, a renal scan should be done as well to look for associated renal injury.

The follow-up of patients managed conservatively may be done with scintigraphy (Fig. 26.3) (17–19). Twenty-two children with splenic trauma were followed by repeat Tc-sulfur colloid scan over a period ranging from 1 week to 2 yr. Follow-up revealed complete resolution or slowly resolving or stable defects.

Angiography

In analyzing a group of 102 cases of splenic trauma, Fisher et al. (20) developed a detailed angiographic classification of splenic injury. "Massive" injury includes: splenic fragmentation and transection of major arterial branches. "Major" injury includes: large intra- or extrasplenic extravasations, extrasplenic or subcapsular hematoma, or large avascular areas (Figs. 26.4 and 26.5). "Minor" injury includes small avascular areas, small extravasations with a "snowstorm" appearance or "Seurat pattern" (small discrete punctate collections of contrast). Fisher's analysis concluded that the radiologist could not always make an accurate diagnosis of splenic laceration, thus lacerations after blunt injury may be suspected whenever any abnormality is seen on an angiogram. However, the presence or absence of laceration was not always crucial. At least three patients with lacerations were managed without surgery and did well. He recommends surgery for "massive" lesions. "Major" lesions constitute a grey zone where management may include therapeutic embolization, conservative therapy or surgery depending on the extent of bleeding. "Minor" injuries can usually be managed without surgery.

The specific angiographic signs of splenic injury in order of reliability as described by Delany and Jason (2) are:

1. Extravasation. This is a reliable sign of injury if the extravasation is large. It may be intra- or extrasplenic, amorphous and ill-defined, or localized and well-defined due to surrounding hematoma or pseudoaneurysm formation. It usually appears early in the arterial phase and remains until late in the venous phase.

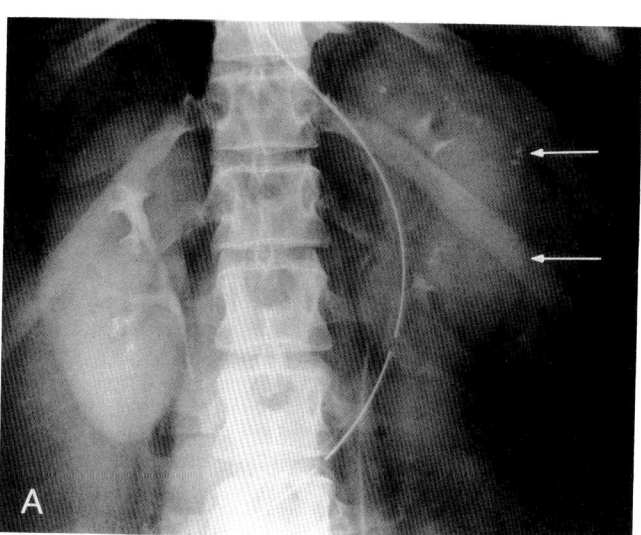
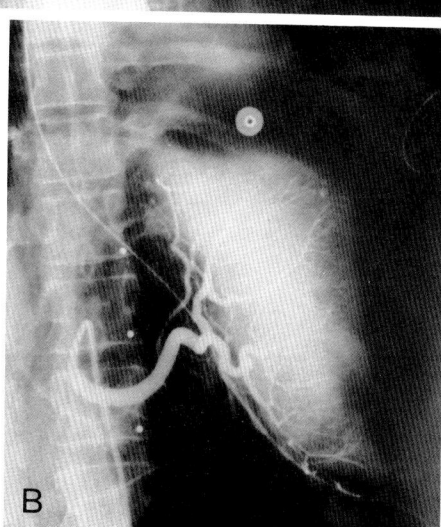
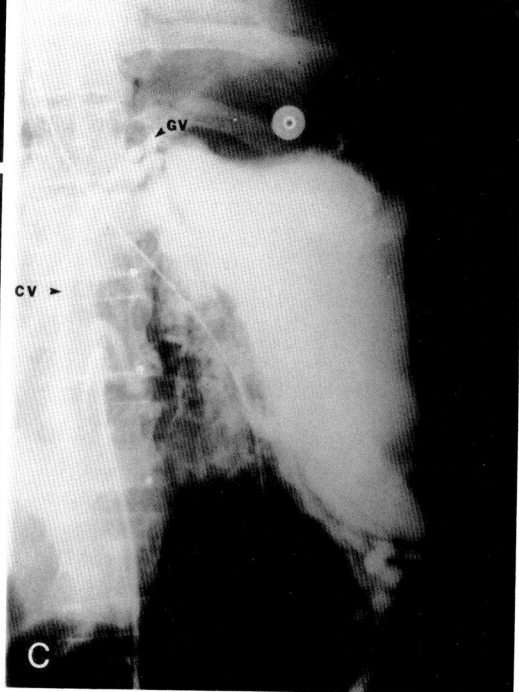

FIGURE 26.4. SUBCAPSULAR HEMATOMA
A: Excretory urogram, 10-min films: mass effect (*arrows*) on the lateral margin of the left kidney and medial displacement of the nasograstric tube. *B* and *C:* Arterial (*B*) and capillary (*C*) phases of a splenic arteriogram demonstrate a superolateral subcapsular splenic hematoma compressing and displacing the spleen. There is nonfilling of the splenic vein and collateral opacification due to a chronic splenic vein occlusion secondary to chronic pancreatitis.

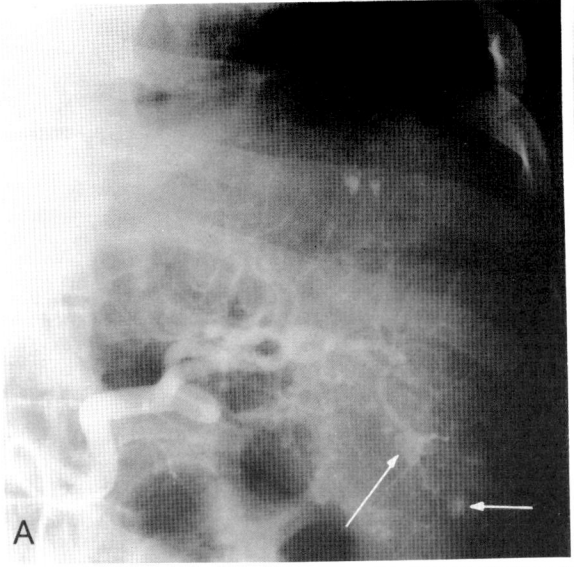
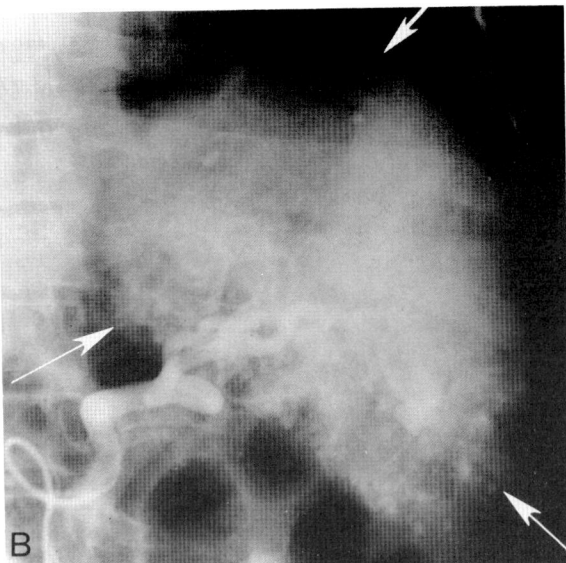
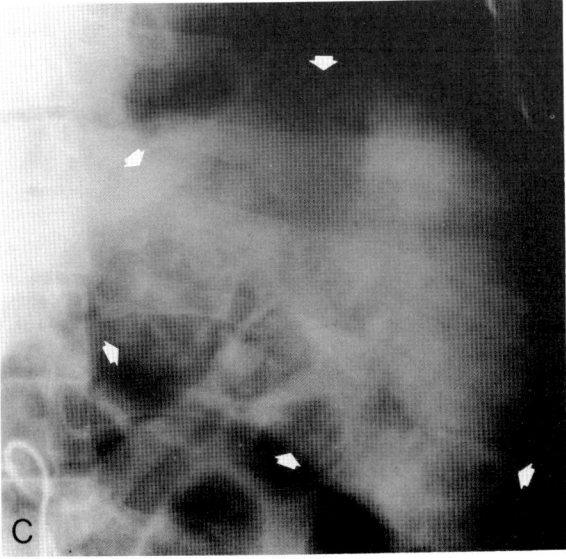

FIGURE 26.5. SPLENIC HEMATOMA WITH ACTIVE BLEEDING
A and *B:* Early and late arterial phase films from a splenic arterial injection show multiple sites of extravasation (*small arrows*) and attenuated, stretched arteries within the relatively lucent inferomedial portion of the spleen (*large arrows*). *C:* Capillary phase: large lucent intrasplenic hematoma (*arrows*) responsible for the regional arterial changes. (Figs. 26.4 and 26.5: Courtesy of the Center for Devices and Radiological Health, FDA, and The American College of Radiology from The Learning File, Gastrointestinal Section, GI-804, 805 and Dr. Francis F. Ruzicka, Bethesda, Md.)

2. **Venous Shunting.** Either early venous filling (i.e., venous channels seen at ≤3 sec) or direct visualization of an arteriovenous shunt.

3. **Mottled Parenchymal Phase.** A coarse irregular parenchymal phase is due to multiple small areas of arterial extravasation or disrupted sinusoids.

4. **Amputated Vessel or Thrombosis.** The pathophysiology of apparent abrupt termination of a vessel includes: spasm, partial or complete transection, thrombosis, or acute angulation of a vessel giving a false appearance of transection. A filling defect in a vascular channel indicates thrombus.

5. **Mass Effect.** If bowing, stretching, or crowding of vessels is seen surrounding an avascular area, this is reliable for hematoma. If no avascular area is seen, these findings alone are unreliable and may be projectional or due to normal surrounding structures.

6. **Splenic Artery.** Adjacent hematoma may encase the artery, displace it, or cause reflex vasospasm. The artery may be lacerated, arteriovenous fistula may form, or a pseudoaneurysm may form. A pseudoaneurysm, which may form around any damaged artery, represents an organized hematoma with fibrous capsule that is attached to the vessel wall. It may form in as little as 48 hr and is more prone to rupture than true aneurysm. Rupture of a pseudoaneurysm may result in ischemia of the distal spleen or an arteriovenous fistula. If bacteremia is present, a

pseudoaneurysm may become infected (mycotic aneurysm).

7. Linear or Wedge Defects. These may be due to laceration, ischemia distal to arterial injury, or false defects due to fetal lobulation or poor filling of peripheral vessels. Poor filling can generally be excluded if the defects are present on both flush aortogram and selective splenic artery injections. Fetal lobulation defects are linear and have sharper margins than lacerations.

8. Splenic Displacement. Displacement from the lateral thoracic wall with a lenticular defect peripherally is suggestive of a subcapsular hematoma (21). Otherwise, splenic displacement alone is unreliable due to the wide variation in normal.

In cases of penetrating injury angiography is not as useful since the organs damaged may be known by analysis of the wound vector. The angiographic pattern is characterized by vascular occlusion and parenchymal defects rather than extravasation (7).

Of the late complications of splenic injury, angiography may demonstrate pseudoaneurysm formation, rupture or arteriovenous fistula. Rupture of a pseudoaneurysm into the pancreatic duct ("hemosuccus pancreaticus") is a rare complication which causes intermittent pancreaticointestinal hemorrhage (7, 22).

The classification of splenic injury is now done primarily by CT rather than angiography in most, but certainly not all cases. Angiography can detect exact sites of bleeding, arteriovenous fistulae and pseudoaneurysm formation. More importantly, angiographic occlusion of bleeding sites is an important mode of nonsurgical therapy which can decrease the need for splenectomy. Vasopressin infusion, steel-coil embolization and gelfoam or other small particle embolization are some methods which have been tried. Sclafani (23) advocates temporary vasoconstriction and occlusion of large vessels to control bleeding, rather than small particle embolization. This is also supported by experimental evidence.

Sonography

In 1976 Asher studied the accuracy of sonographic diagnosis of splenic injury and described its sonographic signs (24). While his data are often quoted in comparing the accuracy of various radiographic modalities, they are not applicable to the 1980s. His description of sonographic findings includes: irregular splenic border, change in splenic contour, splenomegaly especially if progressive, a double contour, and free peritoneal fluid. Currently, with real time sonography we can detect splenic hematoma, subcapsular hematoma and rupture, as well as associated liver, gallbladder, or renal injuries (Fig. 26.6). If sonography can be performed in the emergency room setting, the detection of free intraperitoneal fluid is presumptive evidence of blood and peritoneal lavage may not be necessary (25). The sonographic appearance of hematoma in solid viscera has been studied experimentally

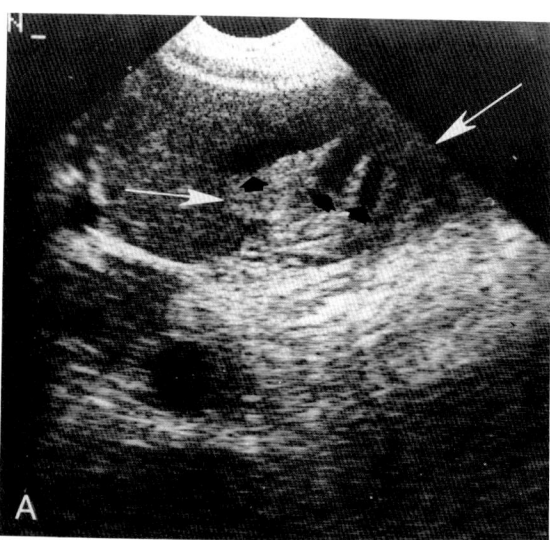
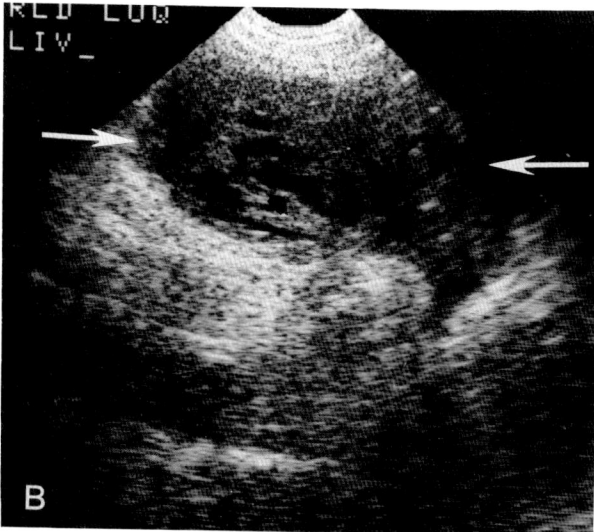

FIGURE 26.6. SPLENIC HEMATOMA: SONOGRAM
A: Transverse and *B:* right side down longitudinal scan. Hypoechoic foci (*black arrows*) within a large hematoma (*white arrows*).

(26). Injection of fresh blood into cadaver organs yielded echogenic foci which were linear if <2 ml were injected and rounded if larger quantities of blood were injected. Margins of the collection became poorly defined with injections >10 ml.

Ultrasound can also be used to follow patients managed conservatively. Lupien and Sauerbrei (27) studied 16 cases of splenic trauma with a mean follow-up time of 4.4 months. One group demonstrated healing within 2–4 weeks. This included subcapsular hematoma, intraperitoneal fluid, or left pleural effusion. Intrasplenic hematomas and contusion (manifested initially as splenic inhomogenity) usually resolved over a period of months. One patient with a laceration which transected the spleen (also had perisplenic fluid) rebled at 6 weeks and required splenectomy. Of 8 patients with contusion, evolution was seen in 4 from an inhomogeneous pattern to anechoic fluid collections which decreased in size and either disappeared or left an echogenic line. Of 11 patients with perisplenic fluid, one became infected (this was the only case whose splenic injury was surgical in origin). Of note is the fact that only two patients became symptomatic during follow-up; the patient requiring splenectomy and the patient with postoperative infection. There were four cases with fluid collection (two intrasplenic, two perisplenic) who demonstrated an increase in size of the fluid collection, but remained asymptomatic and did not require splenectomy. Thus an increase in size of a fluid collection without clinical abnormality (i.e., pain or anemia) is probably not significant.

Computed Tomography

The usefulness of CT in the diagnosis of splenic injury was established by early experimental and clinical studies (28, 29). The changing appearance of hematoma with time was studied in experimentally produced splenic hematomas. An initially isodense collection was inseparable from normal spleen unless the contour of spleen was deformed, or if normal spleen was enhanced by the intravenous administration of contrast material (Fig. 26.7). Some hematomas will be partially hyperdense initially on noncon-

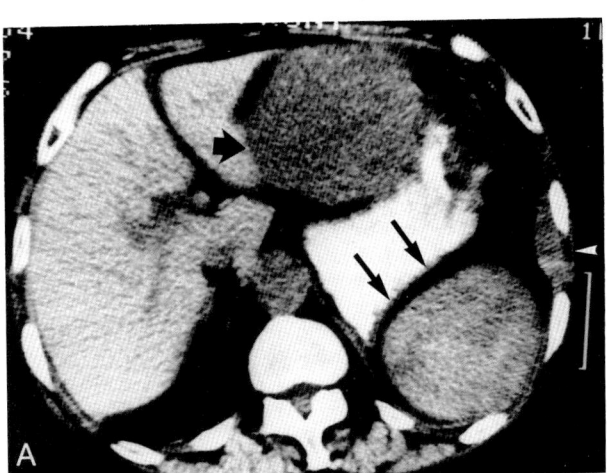
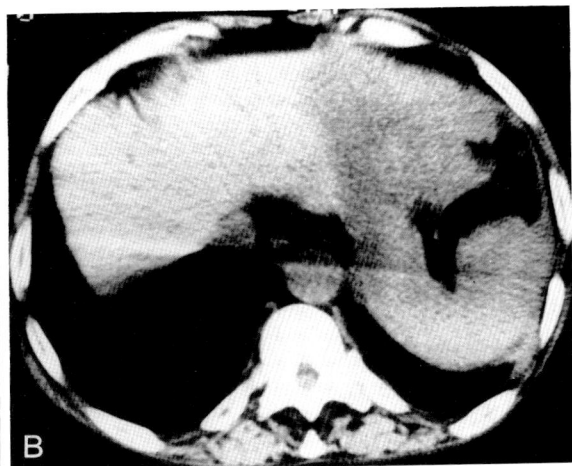
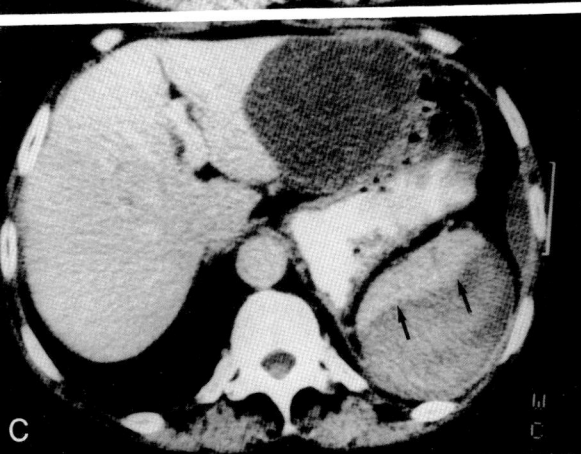

FIGURE 26.7. SPLENIC HEMATOMA: CT

Same patient as seen in Figure 26.6. Unenhanced CT (*A* and *B*) shows a splenic hematoma extending around the stomach. The posterolateral fresher component compresses the stomach (*arrows*), and is nearly isodense to the spleen. The ventral older component is lower density (*short arrow*). A small chest wall hematoma (*white arrowhead*) was associated with a rib fracture. *C:* After contrast enhancement, differentiation of the denser, more recent hematoma from the enhancing spleen (*arrows*) is easier.

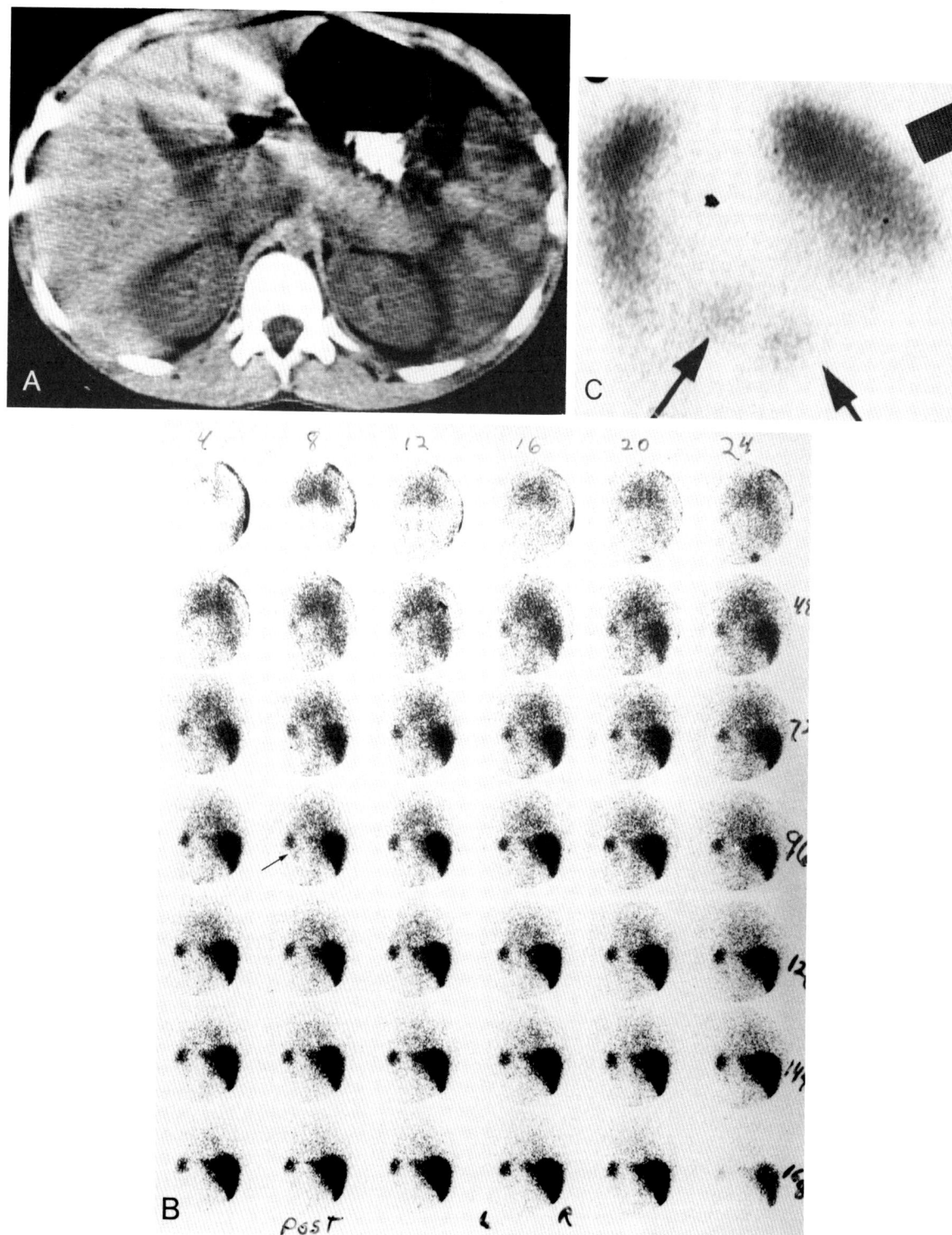

FIGURE 26.8. LACERATED SPLEEN
An 11-yr-old boy fell off his bicycle. *A:* CT scan. Multiple low density lines traverse the spleen representing lacerations. Free peritoneal blood and hemothorax were present. *B:* A nuclear scintigraphic flow study shows little uptake in the spleen. A laceration is discernible (*arrow*), but is better seen on the static scan (*C*), after shielding the liver. *Arrows* point to lacerated pieces of inferior pole separated from the larger splenic body by hematoma.

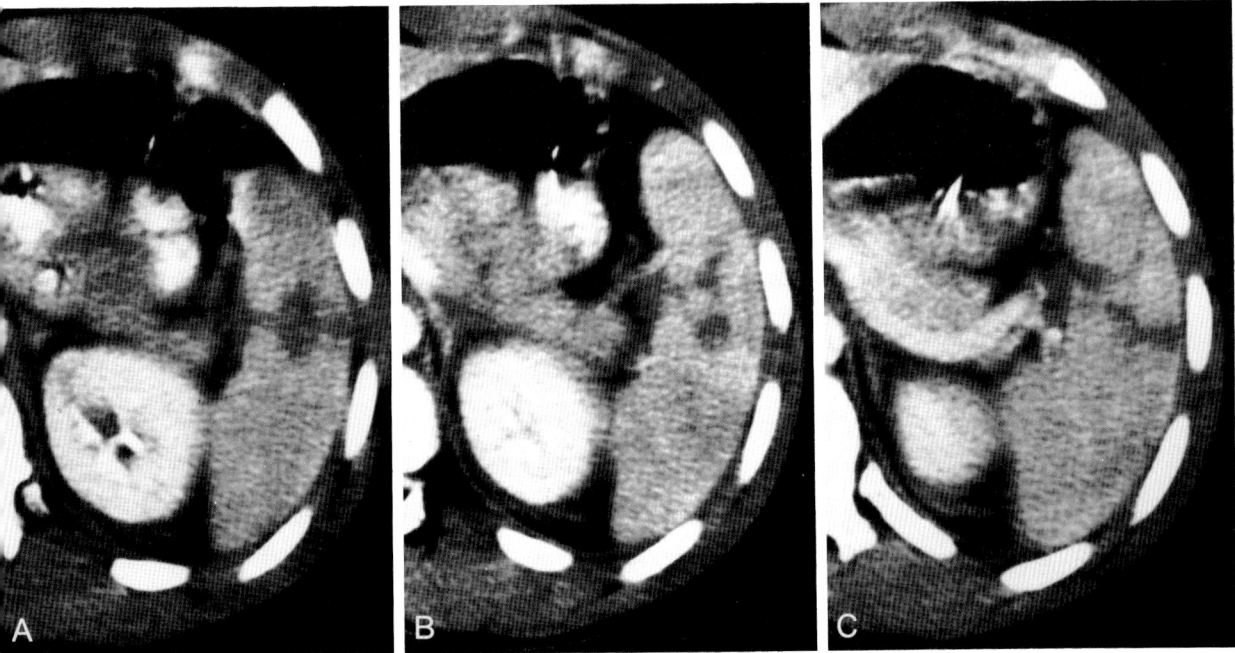

FIGURE 26.9. LACERATED SPLEEN
Sequential cuts (A–C) through the spleen after contrast enhancement show a fractured spleen with intrasplenic hematoma. (Courtesy of Drs. Potter and Markle, Children's Hospital, Washington, D.C.)

trast scans due to clot retraction. With time the hematoma became hypodense, initially at the periphery and then throughout. This correlated with a decrease in hemoglobin content within the hematoma. These studies indicated the need for contrast enhanced CT when evaluating acute splenic injuries. Mall and Kaiser (30) described five cases of splenic laceration diagnosed by CT; hematoma adjacent to the spleen with free intraperitoneal fluid and in some cases a fracture through the spleen could be identified (Figs. 26.8 and 26.9). They advocated omitting noncontrast CT and performing only postcontrast CT.

In a large prospective series of 50 patients, Jeffrey et al. (31) showed a 96% accuracy for CT in diagnosing splenic injury (21 out of 22 surgically proved injuries). There was one false negative due to motion and streak artifacts, and one false positive in a 4-yr-old (follow-up scan 2 days later showed no abnormality). Subcapsular hematomas (10 cases) were peripheral low density lesions that flattened the contour of the spleen (Fig. 26.10). Low density bands producing parenchymal defects within the spleen were diagnosed as splenic lacerations. All lacerations involved the lateral aspect of the spleen and had associated free intraperitoneal fluid; only one subcapsular hematoma was associated with free fluid.

The role of CT has now been established as a primary means of evaluating splenic trauma in the stable patient. High resolution scanning and fast scanning for patients unable to hold their breath have increased the utility and accuracy of CT. Potential pitfalls are caused primarily by technically inadequate examinations and by anatomic variants. Splenic clefts may be differentiated from true laceration by the lack of contour deformity, lack of free fluid, and by their thin linear configuration (31). A normal CT thus virtually excludes a significant injury (31). The capability of CT to define the extent of injury which might guide the surgeon's decision between splenorrhaphy vs. splenectomy, as well as its ability to detect multiorgan injury give it a primary role in all abdominal trauma (31, 32).

Since there is some controversy regarding conservative surgical management of splenic injury, a prospective study of patients undergoing splenic surgery for trauma has been established at the Naval Hospital at San Diego (32). The prospective accumulation of data commenced in 1977 and is ongoing. The registry encourages collaboration with other institutions (33).

The late complications of splenic trauma are pseudocyst formation and splenosis. Pseudocysts are discussed in Chapter 27. Residual calcification in a hematoma may also been seen on CT (Fig. 26.11).

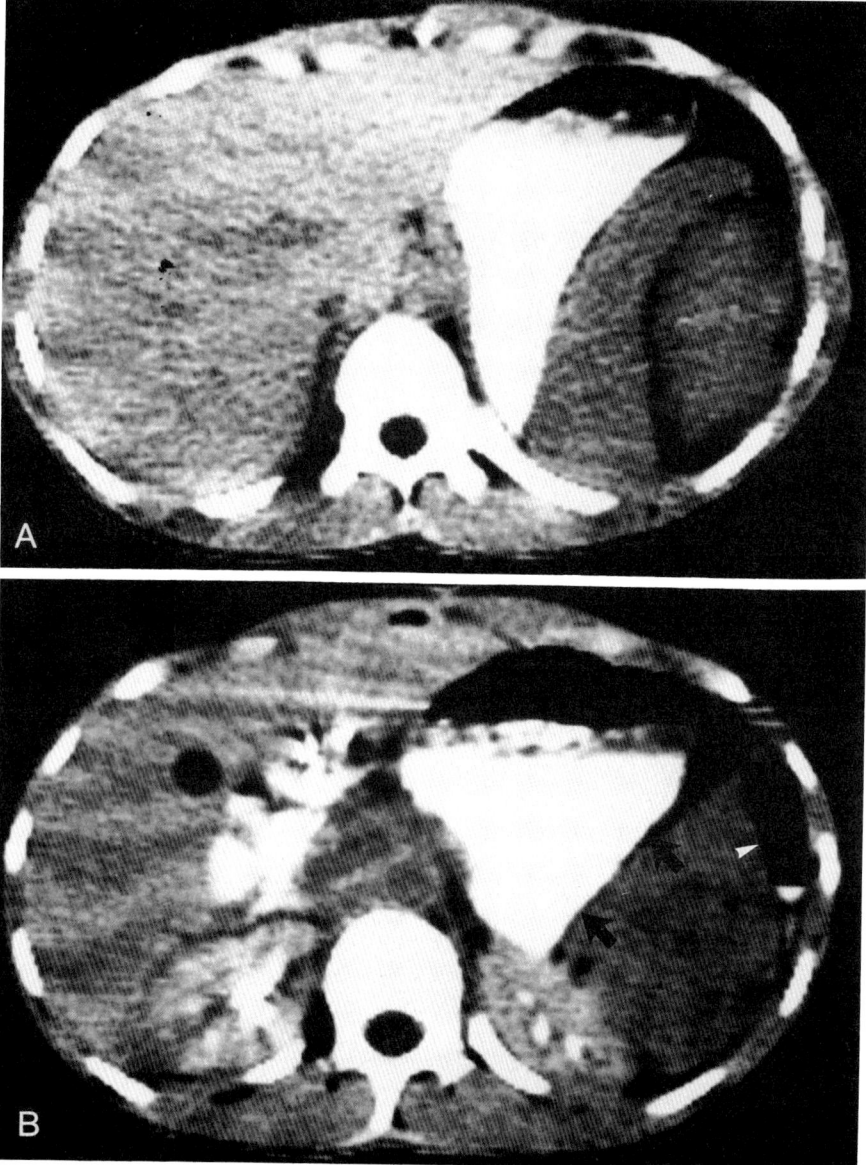

FIGURE 26.10. SUBCAPSULAR HEMATOMA: CT
A and B: A large subacute subcapular hematoma compresses the spleen on cut (*A*), and on lower cut (*B*) shows some inhomogeneity and compresses the stomach (*arrows*) and splenic flexure (*white arrowhead*).

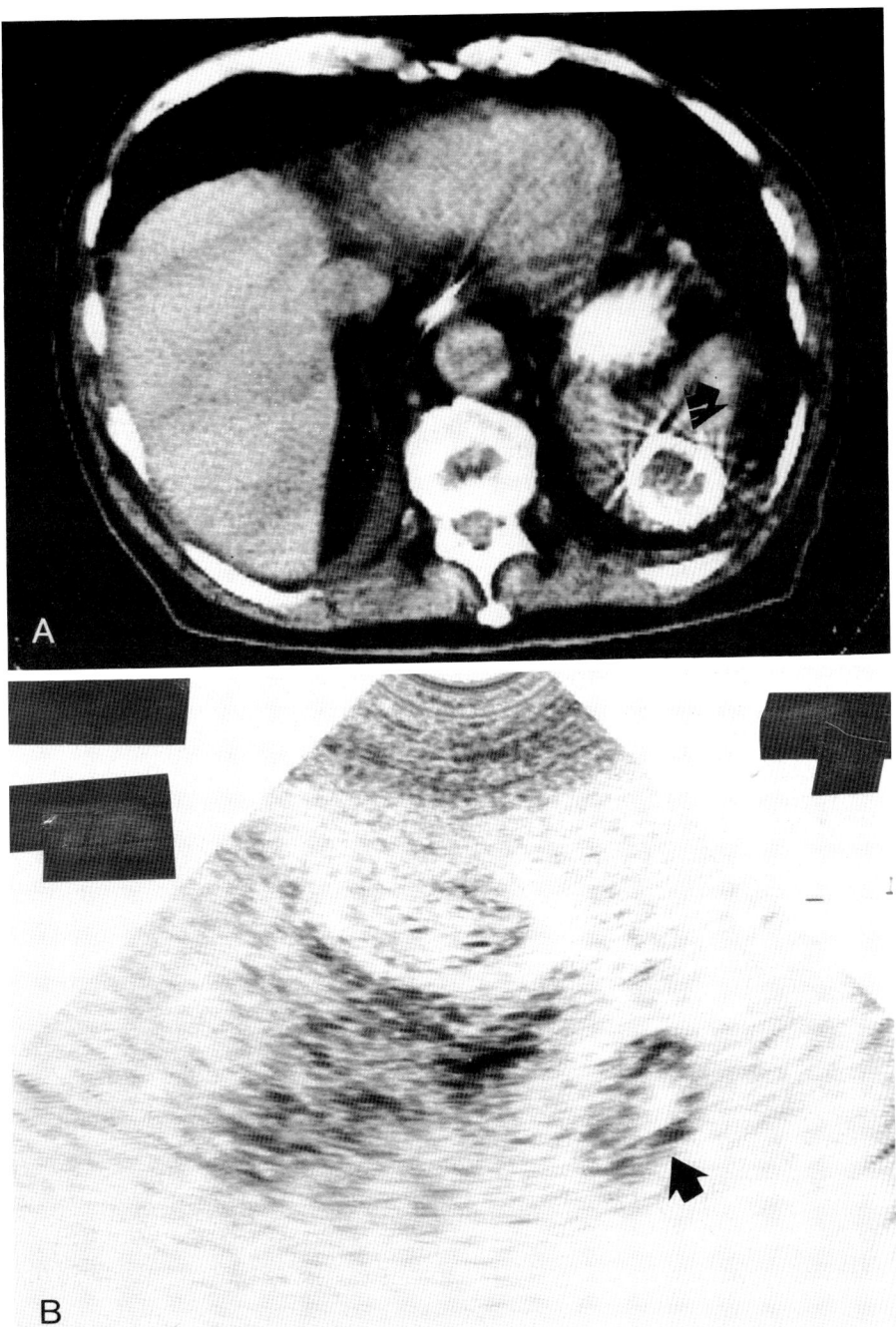

FIGURE 26.11. CALCIFIED HEMATOMA
(Same case as seen in Fig. 26.1.) *A:* CT shows a thick rim of calcium within the splenic parenchyma (*arrow*). The density within the calcification is similar to normal spleen rather than low density as would be seen in a post-traumatic cyst. *B:* Prone oblique sonogram shows the calcification correlating to the CT (*arrow*).

SPLENOSIS

The term "splenosis" was coined by Buckfinder and Lipkoff (34). It represents autotransplantation of splenic tissue usually after traumatic rupture of the spleen. The nodules may implant on any intraperitoneal structure although most implant on the mesentery of the small bowel. If a diaphragmatic tear has occurred or if the diaphragm is penetrated, thoracic splenosis may occur (35–37).

The true incidence is unknown and variably reported as 30–67% based on uptake by ^{99m}Tc-sulfur colloid or heat damaged tagged red blood cells on nuclear scintigraphy. The latter method is said to be more sensitive (38, 39).

At surgery, the implants are multiple, small, usually 2–7 mm up to several centimeters and reddish-blue without a hilum. This differentiates them from accessory spleens which do have a hilum and derive their blood supply from the splenic artery. Also, splenotic nodules lack muscle and elastin fibers in their capsules and are rarely larger than 3 cm (36).

The differential diagnosis at surgery may include metastasis, endometriosis, hemangiomas, and accessory spleens. Metastases differ in color and appear imbedded in the serosa. Hemangiomas are soft and compressible but refill with blood (40).

The patients are virtually all asymptomatic with splenosis detected incidentally at surgery, autopsy, or during radiologic evaluation for another problem. Rarely intestinal obstruction may occur due to adhesions, which in some cases are documented to be occur at the site of splenosis (41, 42). In two cases torsion of a nodule of splenosis with resultant infarction of the nodule produced acute abdominal pain and required surgery (43, 44). Recurrence of hematologic disease such as idiopathic thrombocytopenic purpura (45), or Felty's syndrome, has been attributed to splenosis (44). The pathophysiology of splenic autotransplantation has been studied experimentally in a variety of animals (46–50). Homogenized or cut up pieces of spleen will implant on vascular surfaces. They then undergo a partial necrosis followed by vascularization and growth after a few weeks.

There is controversy regarding the function of these nodules. While they have reticuloendothelial properties, the incidence of postsplenectomy infection in these patients is variable. Most data indicate a lower infection rate compared to the totally splenectomized patient. Nevertheless, certain indicators of immunologic function do not return to normal. IgG levels generally remain depressed (51–56). The volume of transplanted tissue and integrity of its blood supply may be important variables in resistance to infection (51, 57).

When the spleen must be removed due to severe trauma, some surgeons intentionally leave some splenic tissue in order to produce splenosis with the assumption that this will afford protection from postsplenectomy infection. This is usually done in the form of an omental pouch (58–60).

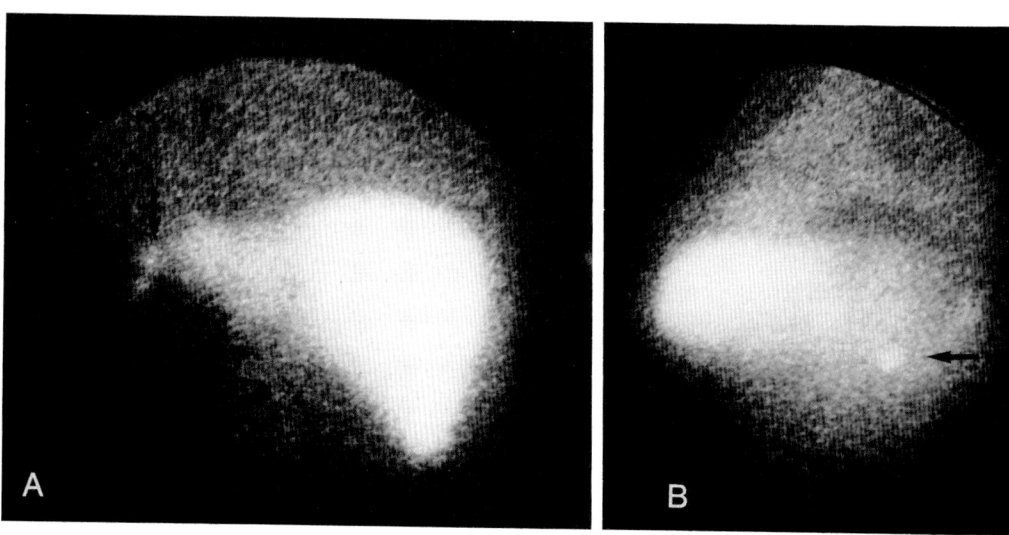

FIGURE 26.12. SPLENOSIS: ^{99m}TC-SULFUR COLLOID SCAN
The patient is postsplenectomy. A: Posterior and B: left lateral views show activity in the splenic bed (arrows).

Radiology

Radiographically, the gastrointestinal tract usually appears normal in splenosis, though large implants may mimic submucosal or extrinsic mass(es). In one case, splenosis simulated a fundal gastric mass (61).

Splenosis is usually detectable on ^{99m}Tc-sulfur colloid scan (35, 41) or tagged damaged red cell scan (Fig. 26.12) (62). The uptake may not correlate with normal immunologic function (55). Nevertheless it is the best gross test of integrity and functional potential of the implants.

There have been CT reports of presumptive splenosis. Gentry et al. (63) report a case with presumptive splenosis appearing as multiple 1-4 cm masses which were adherent to stomach, small bowel, omentum, diaphragm, and lateral parietal peritoneum. They were round or ovoid but sometimes cresentic or irregular in shape. Scalloped and lobulated margins suggested coalescent nodules. Some were sharply demarcated while others were inseparable from their attachment site. They showed a uniform enhancement pattern similar to accessory spleens present in the same individual. Mendelson et al. (64) also reported one presumptive case of splenosis on CT with multiple soft tissue masses in splenic bed, porta hepatis, and along the left lobe of the liver. In both cases, the nodules correlated with areas of uptake on ^{99m}Tc-sulfur colloid scan. Thoracic splenosis may be depicted by CT as multiple pleural-based soft tissue nodules.

When multiple small masses are seen in the abdominal or thoracic cavity on CT in a patient with a history of splenic trauma or surgery, splenosis should be suspected and confirmed with a radionuclide scan.

NONTRAUMATIC SPLENIC RUPTURE

Splenic rupture may be due to (a) trauma, (b) an underlying disease or rarely, (c) spontaneous rupture of a normal spleen. The term "spontaneous" is often used loosely to refer to all nontraumatic rupture, although strictly speaking it should be reserved for rupture of apparently normal spleens. Predisposing diseases modified from Hyun et al. (65) include: (a) infectious or inflammatory disease: malaria, infectious mononucleosis, typhoid fever, typhus, influenza, relapsing fever, viral hepatitis, kala azar, tuberculosis, sarcoidosis, Crohn's disease, actinomycosis, subacute bacterial endocarditis, brucellosis, tularemia, syphilis, aspergillosis, rheumatoid arthritis, and yaws; (b) neoplastic disorders: leukemias, lymphoma, myeloproliferative disease, plasma cell leukemia, and metastatic carcinoma; (c) hematologic disorders: hemolytic disease of the newborn, autoimmune hemolytic anemia, congenital hemolytic anemia, hemophilia, and Felty's syndrome; (d) cardiovascular disorders: congestive splenomegaly, splenic infarcts, and splenic vein thrombosis; and (e) miscellaneous: Gaucher's disease, amyloidosis, ceroid storage disease, ectopic pregnancy and splenic peliosis. Spontaneous rupture of apparently normal spleens may occur in adults, newborn infants, or during labor.

In Smith and Cluster's classic review in 1946 of 46 cases from the Armed Forces Institute of Pathology (AFIP), malaria and infectious mononucleosis were the most common causes of nontraumatic rupture (66). Today the most common causes are probably infectious mononucleosis and hematologic malignancies (67, 68).

It is possible that trauma plays a role in the rupture of a diseased spleen, since minor trauma may not be recalled by the patient.

In infectious mononucleosis the incidence of splenic rupture is probably low; York (69) found only 1 case out of 940 patients with infectious mononucleosis. Rutkow (68) distinguishes cases with no trauma from those with probable or possible trauma and found only 18 cases of "true" spontaneous rupture out of 107 reported cases of splenic rupture in infectious mononucleosis reported in the world's literature as of 1978. This strict definition is probably unwarranted. It does however, bear on the mortality rate quoted; in Smith's series it is reported to be as high as 30% (70), but applying the strict definition was zero in the 18 cases reviewed by Rutkow. While excessive palpation of the enlarged spleen should be avoided, there is no evidence that this is a factor in rupture (68, 69). Abdominal pain is usually absent in uncomplicated infectious mononucleosis, but present in cases with rupture and is thus an important clue. Tachycardia of greater than 100 beats per min and a reversal of the differential WBC count are also clues (68). The event usually occurs between 1 and 4 weeks after diagnosis, but may occur later, thus avoidance of physical activity is advised for 2-3 months (68, 71). There is evidence that fragmentation of the fibrous capsule of the spleen by infiltrating atypical lymphocytes predisposes to rupture (65, 69). There are three reported cases of sonographic diagnosis of rupture in infectious mononucleosis (71) and one of CT diagnosis (72). The findings included splenomegaly, areas of decreased echogenicity within the splenic parenchyma, subcapsular hematoma, perisplenic hematoma, and/or free intraperitoneal blood (71). Johnson found that early hematoma may be indistinguishable from splenomegaly, thus if there is clinical suspicion, follow-up scans should be done. The perisplenic and subcapsular hematomas may remain unchanged for weeks. In one case after 4 weeks of monitoring, the hematoma was aspirated percutaneously under sonographic guidance yielding old blood and serous fluid, which did not reaccumulate. In one case the diagnosis was made by scintigraphy (73).

Of the hematologic malignancies, acute leukemia is the most common cause of spontaneous splenic rupture although this is a rare event. In a review of the English literature in 1981, Bauer et al. (67) reported 53 cases, virtually all of whom presented with abdominal pain and the initial diagnosis was usually not splenic rupture. Abdominal pain may be mild however (74). Without surgery, the mortality was 48% vs. 22% mortality in those undergoing surgery (67). Rarely, rupture may be the presenting feature especially in lymphoma (75). The factors contributing to rupture are thought to be (a) infiltration of the capsule, (b) splenic infarction, and (c) coagulopathy (63, 65).

The rare occurrence of splenic rupture in infective endocarditis is probably preceded by splenic infarction and/or abscess. Splenic infarction or abscess from embolized vegetations or bacteremia occurs in 40-60% of patients (76). Mycotic aneurysms may form as well, also predisposing to splenic rupture (77).

In the solitary case report of Crohn's disease with splenic rupture, there was perforation of the splenic flexure with evidence of fistulous tracts extending to the splenic hilum (78).

In Henderson and Keeping's (79) review of splenic rupture in pregnancy, there were 59 cases reported in the English literature as of 1979; 67% occurred in the third trimester and there was a high mortality. Splenic enlargement with increased blood flow and superimposed trauma are implicated.

There is one example of CT diagnosis of spontaneous splenic rupture without underlying pathology or recognized trauma (28). CT showed a subcapsular hematoma confirmed at surgery.

Although reports of sonographic and CT diagnosis are sparse, with the recognized role of these modalities in traumatic rupture, one can expect to see a greater role in nontraumatic rupture especially since these modalities are often employed in cases of abdominal pain not accounted for by the patient's known underlying disease process.

REFERENCES

1. Stivelman RL, Glaubitz JP, Crampton RS: Laceration of the spleen due to nonpenetrating trauma. One hundred cases. *Am J Surg* 106:888-891, 1963.
2. Delany, Harry M, Jason, Robert S: *Abdominal Trauma: Surgical and Radiological Diagnosis*. New York, Springer-Verlag, 1981.
3. Steele M, Lim RC: Advances in management of splenic injuries. *Am J Surg* 130:159-169, 1975.
4. Traub AC, Perry JF: Injuries associated with splenic trauma. *J Trauma* 10:840-847, 1981.
5. Pachter HL, Hofstetter SR, Spencer FC: Evolving concepts in splenic surgery. Splenography versus splenectomy and postsplenectomy drainage: experience in 105 patients. *Ann Surg* 194:262-267, 1981.
6. Rauch RF, Korobkin M, Silverman PM, Moore AV: CT dectection of iatrogenic percutaneous splenic injury. *J Comput Assist Tomogr* 7:1018-1021, 1983.
7. Haertel M, Ryder D: Radiologic investigation of splenic trauma. *Cardiovasc Radiol* 2:27-33, 1979.
8. Wyman AC: Traumatic rupture of the spleen. *AJR* 72:51-63, 1954.
9. Cimmino CV, Southworth LE: Further refinements in the plain radiologic diagnosis of splenic rupture: the air enema. *Radiology* 127:649-653, 1978.
10. Wener L, Boyle CD: Splenic scintiscanning in the preoperative diagnosis of subcapsular hematoma. *N Engl J Med* 277:35-37, 1967.
11. Lutzker L, Koenigsberg M, Meng C-H et al: The role of radionuclide imaging in spleen trauma. *Radiology* 110:419-425, 1973.
12. Westcott JI, Krufky EL: The upside-down spleen. *Radiology* 105:517, 1972.
13. Smidt KP: Splenic scintigraphy: a large congenital fissure mimicking splenic hematoma. *Radiology* 122:169, 1977.
14. Nebesar RA, Rabinov KR, Potsaid MS: Radionuclide imaging of the spleen and suspected splenic injury. *Radiology* 110:609-614, 1974.
15. Froelich JW, Simeone JF, McKusick KA, Winzelberg GG, Strauss HW: Radionuclide imaging and ultrasound in liver/spleen trauma: a prospective comparison. *Radiology* 145:457-461, 1982.
16. Gilday DL, Alderson PO: Scintigraphic evaluation of liver and spleen injury. *Semin Nucl Med* 4:357-370, 1974.
17. Fischer KC, Eraklis A, Rosello P, Treves S: Scintigraphy in the followup of pediatric splenic trauma treated without surgery. *J Nucl Med* 19:3-9, 1978.
18. Howman-Giles R, Gilday DL, Venugopal S, Shandling B, Ash JM: Splenic trauma—nonoperative and long-term follow-up by scintiscan. *J Pediatr Surg* 13:121-126, 1978.
19. Mishalany HG, Miller JH, Wooley MM: Radioisotope spleen scan in patients with splenic injury. *Arch Surg* 117:1147-1154, 1982.
20. Fisher RG, Foucar K, Estrada R, Ben-Menachem Y: Splenic rupture in blunt trauma. *Radiol Clin North Am* 19:141-165, 1981.

21. Osborn DJ, Glickman MG, Graja V, Ramsby G: The role of angiography in abdominal nonrenal trauma. *Radiol Clin North Am* 11:579-592, 1973.
22. Sandblom P. Gastrointestinal hemorrhage through the pancreatic duct. *Ann Surg* 17:61-66, 1970.
23. Sclafani SJA. The role of angiographic hemostasis in salvage of the injured spleen. *Radiology* 141:645-650, 1981.
24. Asher WM, Parvin S, Virgilio RW, Haber K: Echocardiographic evaluation of splenic injury. *Radiology* 118:411-415, 1976.
25. Hauenstein KH, Wimmer B, Billmann P, Noldge G, Zavisic: The role of sonography in blunt abdominal trauma (in German). *Radiologe* 22:106-111, 1982.
26. vanSonnenberg E, Simeone JF, Mueller PR, Wittenberg J, Hall DA, Ferrucci JT: Sonographic appearance of hematoma in liver, spleen, and kidney: a clinical, pathologic, and animal study. *Radiology* 147:507-510, 1983.
27. Lupien C, Sauerbrei EE: Healing in the traumatized spleen: sonographic investigation. *Radiology* 151:181-185, 1984.
28. Korobkin M, Moss AA, Callen PW, DeMartini WJ, Kaiser JA: Computed tomography of subcapsular splenic hematoma. *Radiology* 129:441-445, 1978.
29. Moss AA, Korobkin M, Price D, Brito AC: Computed tomography of splenic subcapsular hematomas: an experimental study in dogs. *Invest Radiol* 1:60-64, 1979.
30. Mall JC, Kaiser JA: CT diagnosis of splenic laceration. *AJR* 134:265-269, 1980.
31. Jeffrey RB, Laing FC, Federle MP, Goodman PC: Computed tomography of splenic trauma. *Radiology* 141:729-732, 1981.
32. Federle MP: Progress in clinical radiology. *Invest Radiol* 16:260-268, 1981.
33. Fridlund PH, Shackford SR: Establishment of a registry for patients undergoing splenic surgery for trauma. *Milit Med* 149:137-138, 1984.
34. Jacobson SJ, De Nardo GL: Splenosis demonstrated by splenic scan. *J Nucl Med* 12:570-572, 1971.
35. Dillion ML, Koster JK, Coy J et al: Intrathoracic splenosis. *South Med J* 70:112, 1977.
36. Nielsen JL: Splenosis on the right kidney and the diaphragmatic surface following traumatic rupture of the spleen. *Acta Chir Scand* 147:721-724, 1981.
37. Dalton ML Jr, Strange WH, Downs EA: Intrathoracic splenosis: case report and review of the literature. *Am Rev Respir Dis* 103:827-830, 1971.
38. Pearson HA, Johnston MT, Smith KA, Touloukian RJ: The born-again spleen; Return of splenic function after splenectomy for trauma. *N Engl J Med* 298:1389-1392, 1978.
39. Kiroff GK: Splenosis following splenectomy. *Arch Surg* 119:351, 1984.
40. Brewster DC: Splenosis; report of two cases and review of the literature. *Am J Surg* 126:14-19, 1973.
41. Trimble, C, Eason FJ: A complication of splenosis. *J Trauma* 12:358-361, 1972.
42. Moinuddin M: Splenosis: first scintigraphic demonstration of extensive splenic implants. *Clin Nucl Med* 7:67-68, 1982.
43. Sirinek KR, Livingston CD, Bova JG, Levine BA: Bowel obstruction due to infarcted splenosis. *South Med J* 77:764-767, 1984.
44. Fleming CR, Dickson ER, Harrison EG: Splenosis: autotransplantation of splenic tissue. *Am J Med* 61:414-419, 1976.
45. Mazur EM et al: Idiopathic thrombocytopenic purpura occurring in a subject previously splenectomized for traumatic splenic rupture. *Am J Med* 65:843-846, 1978.
46. Stubenrauch E: Verlust und regeneration der milz beim menschen. *Beitr Klin Chir* 118:285-305, 1919.
47. Calder RM: Autoplastic splenic grafts: their use in the study of the growth of splenic tissue. *J Pathol* 49:351-362, 1939.
48. Kreuter E: Experimentelle untersuchungen uber die entstehung der sogennannten nebenmilzen, insbesondere nach milzverletzungen. *Bruns Beitr Klin Chir* 118:76, 1920.
49. Manley OT, Marine D: The transplantation of splenic tissue into the subcutaneous fascia of the abdomen in rabbits. *J Exp Med* 25:619-628, 1917.
50. Perla D: The regeneration of autoplastic splenic transplants. *Am J Pathol* 126:14-19, 1936.
51. Orda R, Barak J, Baron J, Spirer Z, Wiznitzer T: Postsplenectomy splenic activity. *Ann Surg* 194:771-774, 1981.
52. Church JA, Mahour GH, Lipsey AI: Antibody responses after splenectomy and splenic autoimplantation in rats. *J Surg Res* 31:343-346, 1981.
53. Livingston CD, Levine BA, Sirinek KR: Intraperitoneal splenic autotransplantation. *Arch Surg* 118:458-461, 1983.
54. Livingston CD, Levine BA, Sirinek KR: Improved survival rate for intraperitoneal autotransplantation of the spleen following pneumococcal pneumonia. *Surg Gynecol Obstet* 156:761-766, 1983.
55. Smidt N, Laufer N, Grover NB, Freund HR, Charuzi I: The influence of splenic tissue implantation upon platelet population in rabbits after splenectomy. *Surg Gynecol Obstet* 153:717-720, 1981.
56. Moore GE, Stevens RE, Moore EE, Argon GE: Failure of splenic implants to protect against fatal postsplenectomy infection. *Am J Surg* 146:413-414, 1983.
57. Vega A, Howell C, Krasna I, Campos J, Heyman S, Ziegler M, Koop CE: Splenic autotransplantation: optimal functional factors. *J Pediatr Surg* 16:898-904, 1981.
58. Patel J, Williams JS, Naim JO, Hinshaw JR: Protection against pneumococcal sepsis in splenectomized rats by implantation of splenic tissue into an omental pouch. *Surgery* 91:638-641, 1982.
59. Williams JS, Patel JM, Hinshaw JR: Omental pouch technique for reimplantation of the spleen. *Surg Gynecol Obstet* 155:731, 1982.
60. Kusminsky RE, Chang H, Hossino H, Zekan SM, Boland JP: An omental implantation technique for salvage of the spleen. *Surg Gynecol Obstet* 155:407-408, 1982.
61. Kutzen BM, Levy N: Splenosis simulating an intramural gastric mass. *Radiology* 126:45-46, 1978.
62. Spencer GR, Bird C, Prothero DL, Brown TR, MacKenzie FAF, Phillips MJ: Spleen scanning with ^{99m}Tc-labelled red blood cells after splenectomy. *Br J Surg* 68:412-414, 1981.
63. Gentry LR, Brown JM, Lindgren RD: Splenosis: CT demonstration of heterotopic autotransplantation of splenic tissue. *J Comput Assist Tomogr* 6:1184-1187, 1982.
64. Mendelson DS, Cohen BA, Armas RR: CT appearance of splenosis. *J Comput Assist Tomogr* 6:1188-1190, 1982.
65. Hyun BH, Varga, CF, Rubin RJ: Spontaneous and pathologic rupture of the spleen. *Arch Surg* 104:652-657, 1972.
66. Sakulsky SB, Wallace RB, Silverstein MN, Dockerty MB: Ruptured spleen in infectious mononucleosis. *Arch Surg* 94:349-352, 1967.
67. Bauer TW, Haskins GE, Armitage JO: Splenic rupture in patients with hematologic malignancies. *Cancer* 48:2729-2733, 1981.
68. Rutkow IM: Rupture of the spleen in infectious mononucleosis; a critical review. *Arch Surg* 113:718-720, 1978.

69. York WH: Spontaneous rupture of the spleen: report of a case secondary to infectious mononucleosis. *JAMA* 179:170–171, 1962.
70. Smith EB, Custer RP: Rupture of the spleen in infectious mononucleosis; a clinicopathologic report of seven cases. *Blood* 1:317–333, 1946.
71. Johnson MA, Cooperberg PL, Boisvert J, Stoller JL, Winrob H: Spontaneous splenic rupture in infectious mononucleosis: sonographic diagnosis and follow-up. *AJR* 136:111–114, 1981.
72. Stiris MG: Computed tomography of the spleen. *Radiology* 140:249, 1981.
73. Howman GR, Gilday DL, Venugopal S, Shandling B, Ash JM: Splenic trauma—nonoperative management and long-term follow-up by scintiscan. *J Pediatr Surg* 13:121–126, 1978.
74. Karakousis CP, Elias EG: Spontaneous (pathologic) rupture of spleen in malignancies. *Surgery* 76:674–677, 1974.
75. Dobrow RB: Spontaneous (pathologic) rupture of the spleen in previously undiagnosed Hodgkin's disease; report of a case with survival. *Cancer* 39:354–358, 1977.
76. Baron JM, Weinshelbaum EI, Block GE: Splenic rupture associated with bacterial endocarditis and sickle cell trait. *JAMA* 205:102–104, 1968.
77. Vergne R, Selland B, Gobel FL, Hall WH: Rupture of the spleen in infective endocarditis. *Arch Intern Med* 135:1265–1267, 1975.
78. Nichols TW, Wright FM, Pyeatte JC, O'Connell JP: Spontaneous rupture of the spleen; an unusual complication of Crohn's disease. *Am J Gastroenterol* 75:226–228, 1981.
79. Henderson PR, Keeping P: Spontaneous rupture of the spleen in late pregnancy. *Aust NZ J Obstet Gynaecol* 19:116–117, 1979.

27

Focal Diseases

ABRAHAM H. DACHMAN, M.D., AND DONNA MAGID, M.D.

CYSTS

Splenic cysts represent a heterogeneous group of lesions that have been classified in various ways (1–4). Most classifications represent modifications of that given by Fowler (2) in 1940. Excluding cystic neoplasms and parasitic cysts, splenic cysts can be classified as "true" cysts (also called primary, epithelial, epidermoid or congenital cysts) containing an epithelial lining and "false" or pseudocysts without an epithelial lining. False cysts are probably post-traumatic in origin and may be hemorrhagic or serous although some are reportedly inflammatory (i.e., acute necrosis in infection) or degenerative (i.e., secondary to emboli) (1).

Garvin and King (5) reviewed 102 splenic cysts. Excluding two which were echinococcal, 80% were post-traumatic (false) cysts and 20% were true cysts most of which contained a squamous epithelial lining (the "epidermoid cyst"). Most authors consider false or post-traumatic cysts more common but as Doolas (6) noted, careful review of the histology indicates that up to 60% may be true cysts with small islands of cellular lining. Inadequate sampling may also contribute to the underdiagnosis of true cysts.

The male to female ratio in the Armed Forces Institute of Pathology (AFIP) series was 2:1 (5). In most series (which include parasitic cysts) the female to male ratio is 6:4. Greater than 80% are solitary (7). Most occur in the 2nd to 3rd decade (7) with 60% in the <40-yr-old age group (3, 6, 7).

Splenic cysts have also been diagnosed in children (8, 9) and may even be present at birth (6). Both true and false cysts are reported (10, 11).

There is one case report of three siblings with multicystic spleens consistent with epidermoid cysts without other organ involvement. One must exclude polycystic kidney disease since 2% of these patients will have splenic involvement (12).

Clinical Findings

The natural history of splenic cysts is probably one of slow growth (13–15). There are numerous documented cases of slow growth over a number of years. In patients with post traumatic cysts, a history of trauma is present in about one-fourth to one-half of cases (5, 7), but the trauma may be in the distant past and not recalled. Up to 50% of false cysts are said to be diagnosed within 3 yr of the initial injury (16). Symptoms are usually vague: epigastric fullness, dull pain, post prandial pain, and slow left upper quadrant enlargement (3, 18). A mass is palpable in about 40% (17). Renal colic may be simulated due to pressure on the renal pelvis or ureteropelvic junction kinking (3). With further enlargement, pressure on the stomach, diaphragm, and kidney may cause nausea, vomiting, cough, dyspnea, dysuria (18), and rarely respiratory infection or pyelonephritis (3). Reversible hypertension may occur if there is renal artery compression (3, 13). The cyst may present acutely after rapid increase in size (19). Some may be discovered incidentally at surgery, radiologic examination, or autopsy.

Patients may present acutely with complications due to trauma, rupture or infection of a cyst (20, 21).

Laboratory data are usually normal except if infection or hypertension is present. One case of hypersplenism in association with splenic cyst is reported (22).

Preferred treatment is surgical removal of the symptomatic cyst. Needle aspiration of splenic cysts for diagnosis has been done in the past but

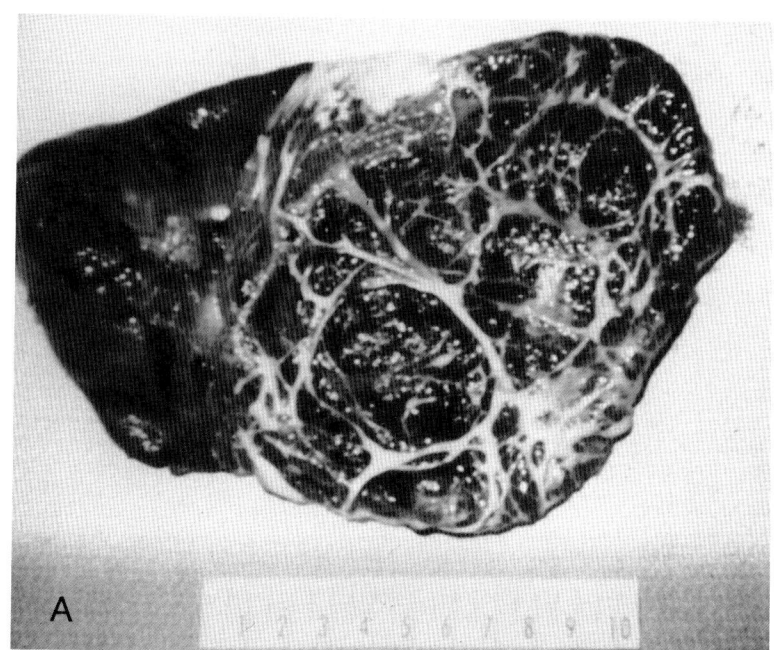

FIGURE 27.1. SPLENIC CYSTS
A: Gross specimen, false splenic cyst. The cyst is open and the fluid removed. Trabeculation of the cyst wall is seen in both true and false cysts. When prominent, they appear as septations. *B:* Microscopy, true splenic cyst (×160). The fibrous wall is lined by stratified squamous epithelium with intracellular bridges seen at higher magnification.

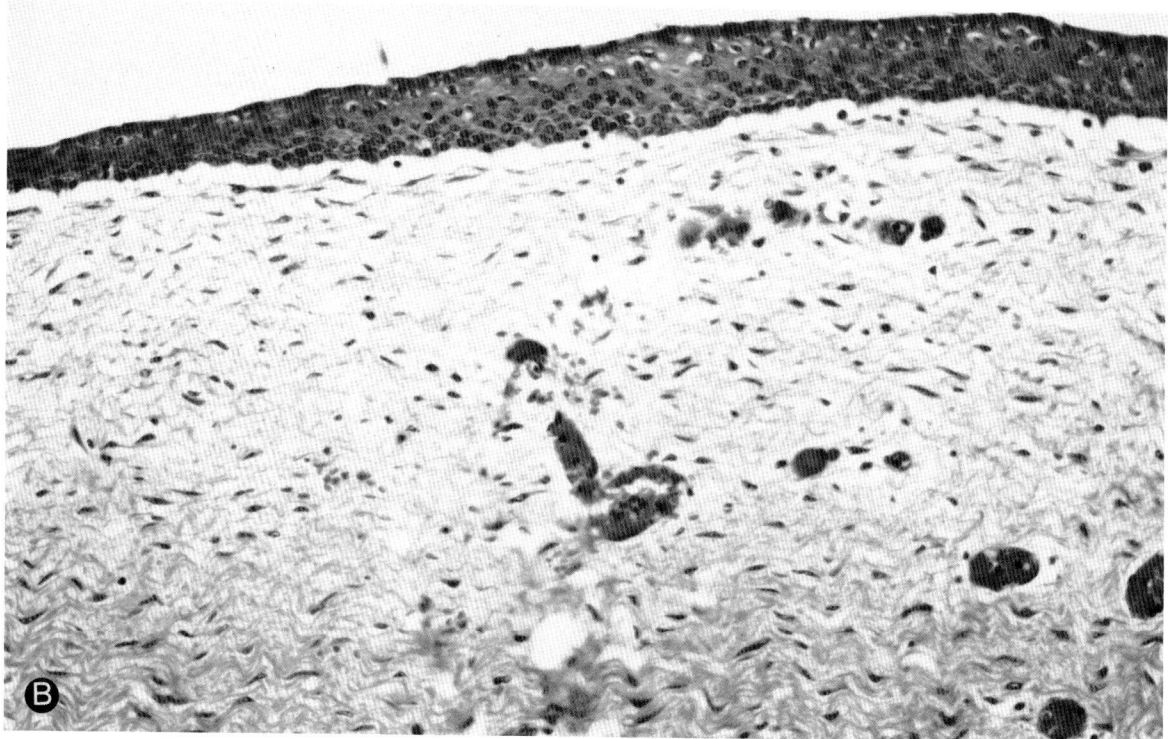

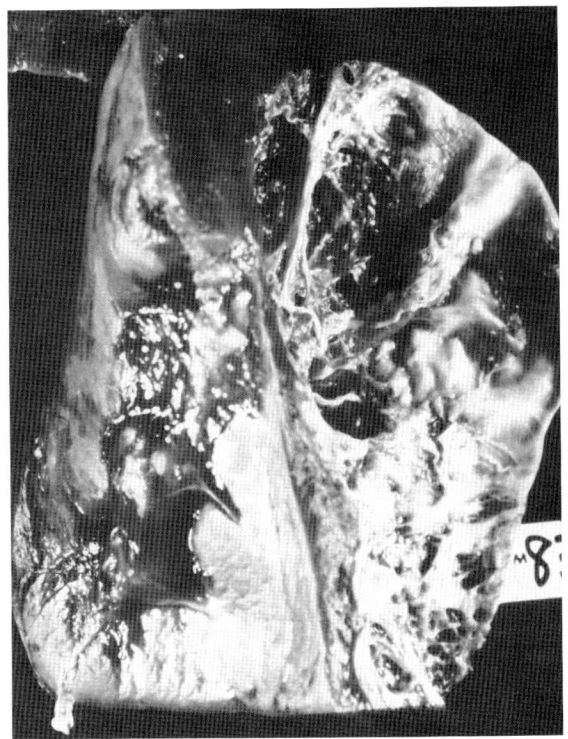

FIGURE 27.2. CUT GROSS: FALSE CYST
The cyst contains organizing hematoma. This may represent a "missing link" or transition between hematoma and false cyst.

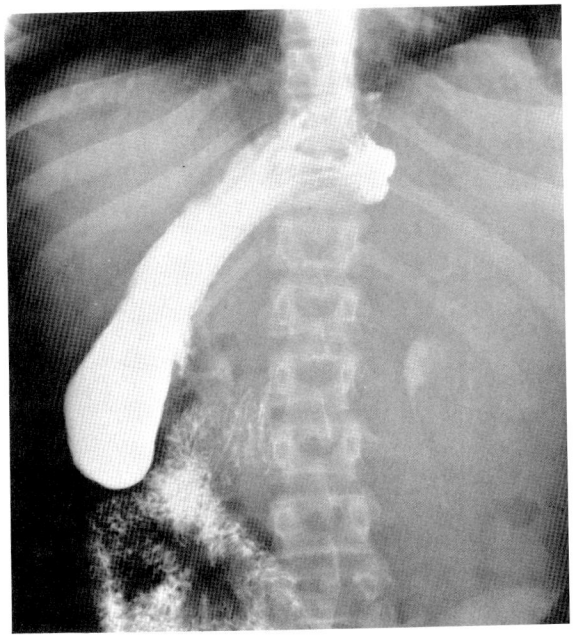

FIGURE 27.3. FALSE CYST: UPPER GASTROINTESTINAL SERIES
These cysts are often large and may displace the stomach to the right of the midline.

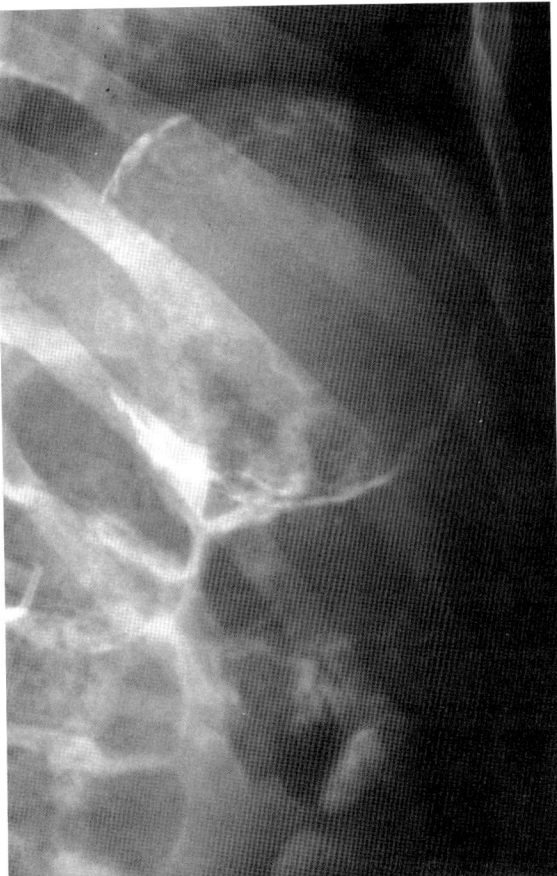

FIGURE 27.4. SPLENIC CYST: PLAIN FILM
Rim calcification may be seen indicating a focal lesion, usually a cyst, rather than merely splenomegaly.

did not gain favor in the United States. Recently, thin needle puncture has once again been advocated for diagnosis and therapy. There is some concern for the remote possibility of echinococcal cyst with false negative serology. Splenectomy should be avoided if possible to reduce the risk of subsequent infection. Laparoscopic cyst puncture and creation of a cyst-peritoneal window under general anesthesia has been successfully performed in one case with an 8-month follow-up (23). There is evidence that, if left alone, cysts may rarely rupture into the peritoneal cavity or chest with subsequent empyema or pleural effusion (24).

Pathogenesis and Pathology

About 80% are solitary and unilocular, and 20% are multiple or multilocular. They are usually subcapsular but one-third are located deep in the splenic tissue (6). Most are large; the average size in Garvin's series was 10 cm. The

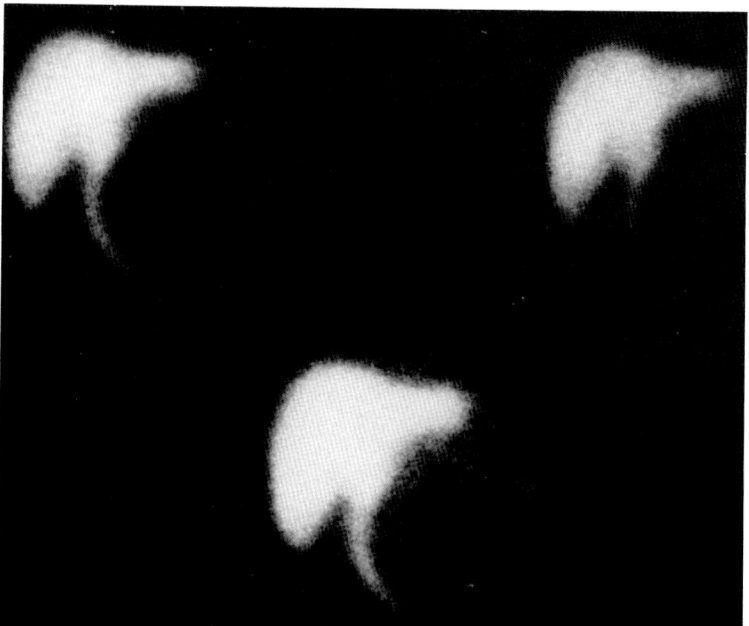

FIGURE 27.5. FALSE CYST: NUCLEAR SCINTIGRAPHY
The lesion is large and round with compressed splenic tissue surrounding a portion of the cyst.

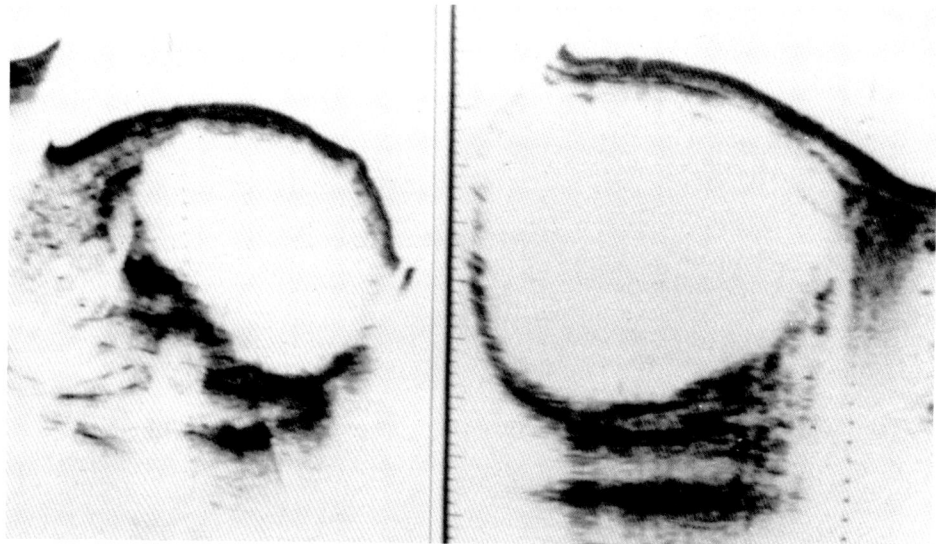

FIGURE 27.6. FALSE CYST: TRANSVERSE AND LONGITUDINAL SONOGRAM
The lesion is anechoic with good thorough transmission.

cyst contents may be clear or turbid with cholesterol crystals, fat, and blood. The cyst wall consists of a fibrous lining sometimes dense, with a trabeculated appearance, grossly resembling the chordae tendonae of the heart (25) (Fig. 27.1A). Post-traumatic cysts may also have this gross appearance but may also be smooth.

Histologically the true cyst will be lined by stratified squamous epithelium with intercellular bridges (Fig. 27.1B). Smaller cysts may be embedded in the wall of a large epidermoid cyst (15). Some mesothelial lining may be seen in continuity with or separated from the epithelial lining (9). The differentiation of true cyst from false cyst thus depends on both history, adequate sampling and careful histologic evaluation of multiple sections of the cyst wall.

True cysts are thought to be congenital in

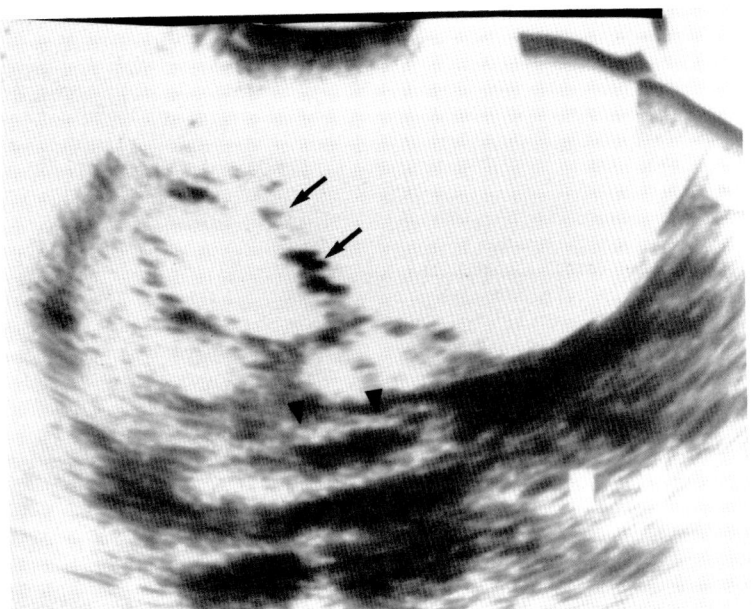

FIGURE 27.7. FALSE CYST: SONOGRAM
The lesion is anechoic with a few thick septations (*arrows*). The right kidney is being compressed (*arrowheads*).

origin. Theories of origin include: (*a*) infolding of peritoneal mesothelium following rupture of the splenic capsule (26), or (*b*) collections of peritonal mesothelial cells being trapped in splenic sulci (27), or (*c*) origin from normal lymph spaces (28).

False cysts may be due to a post-traumatic hematoma in the subcapsular region which leaves the capsule intact. The resolving hematoma may form a fibrous wall with the blood being resorbed (18). Dachman et al. (29) demonstrated three cases with resolving hematoma within a false cyst suggesting a "transition" case between hematoma and false cyst or possibly hemorrhage into a cyst (Fig. 27.2).

Roentgen Findings

Roentgen findings are those of a splenic mass, usually large in size. Plain film may show a left upper quadrant mass with elevation of the left hemidiaphragm with left lower lobe atelectasis (7, 30). Barium studies will show displacement of the stomach to the right sometimes crossing the midline (Fig. 27.3) and inferior displacement of the splenic flexure. The left kidney is usually displaced caudad although cephalic displacement may occur (20, 31). Severe renal compression may cause diminished renal function (14).

Curvilinear or plaque-like calcification may be present on plain film (Fig. 27.4). This is said to occur in 9-25% of post-traumatic cysts (5, 32), but is less common in true cysts (33). With the rare pedunculated lesion, the mass and calcification may present in an unusual location, even in the pelvis (15). Splenic cysts may occur in a wandering spleen (29, 34).

Angiography demonstrates an avascular mass with stretched vessels around it. Large cysts may displace the aorta (29). The caliber of the splenic artery is normal. On the splenogram phase, the parenchyma is compressed. There is no neovascularity (35, 36). Occasionally the cyst wall may appear thickened on the venous phase, which reportedly suggests inflammation (35). With the advent of sonography and CT, angiography is probably superfluous for diagnosis (37).

Liver-spleen scans show a nonspecific photopenic mass (Fig. 27.5). If a splenic cyst develops in ectopic splenic tissue within the pancreas, the sonographic and CT appearance would mimic a pancreatic pseudocyst (37).

Ultrasound is the simplest noninvasive diagnostic modality. It can demonstrate the splenic origin of the lesion as well as its cystic nature (24) (Fig. 27.6). If the cyst is hemorrhagic it may demonstrate layering of two fluids within the cyst with the dependent one being relatively echogenic as reported in two cases by Propper et al. (33). Faint trabeculation of the wall, or less often more obvious trabeculation may be discernable (29) (Fig. 27.7). Bright wall echoes with

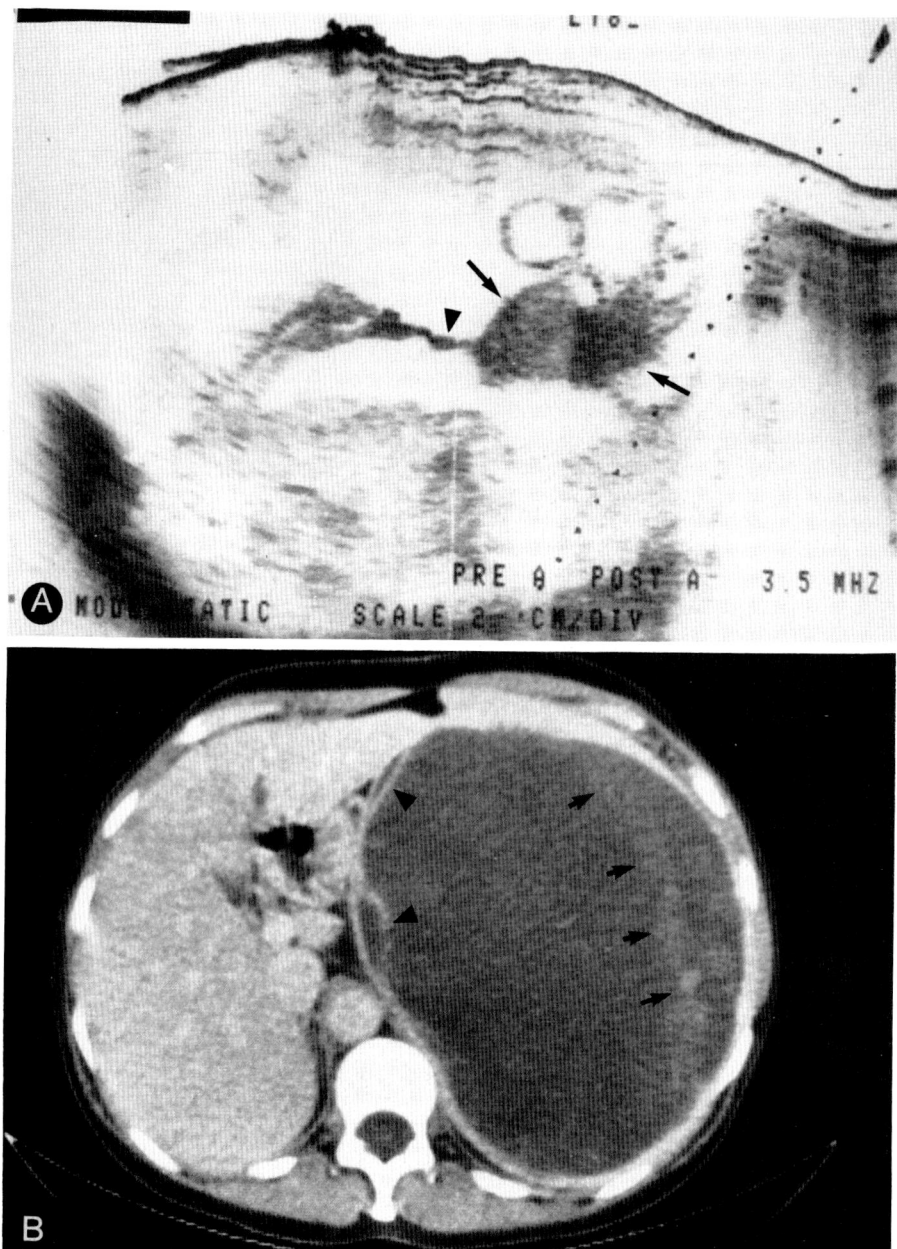

FIGURE 27.8. TRANSITION BETWEEN HEMATOMA AND FALSE CYST
A: Sonogram: A complex lesion with anechoic areas and solid components (*arrows*) with septations (*arrowhead*). *B:* CT: A large low density false cyst with areas of increased density representing organizing hematoma (*arrows*) and septation (*arrowheads*).

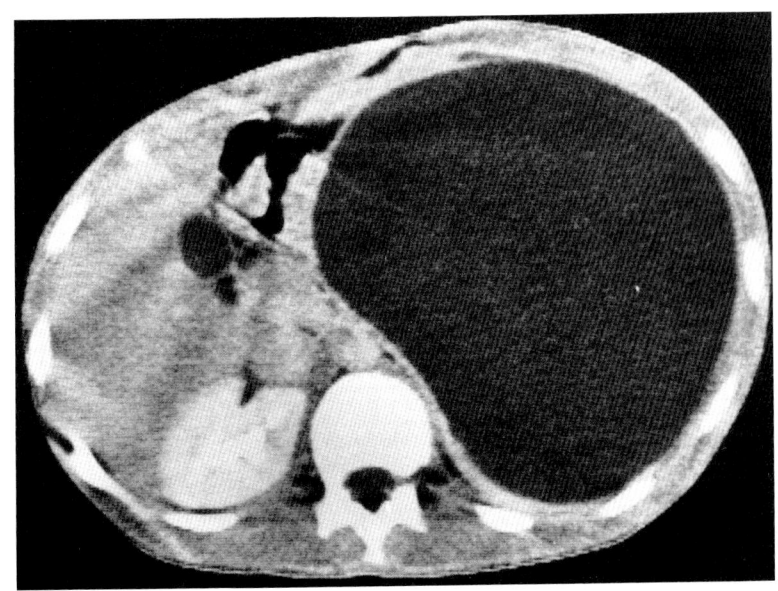

FIGURE 27.9. FALSE CYST: CT
Classic appearance as a large, homogeneous low density intrasplenic lesion without internal debris. The left kidney was deviated caudad.

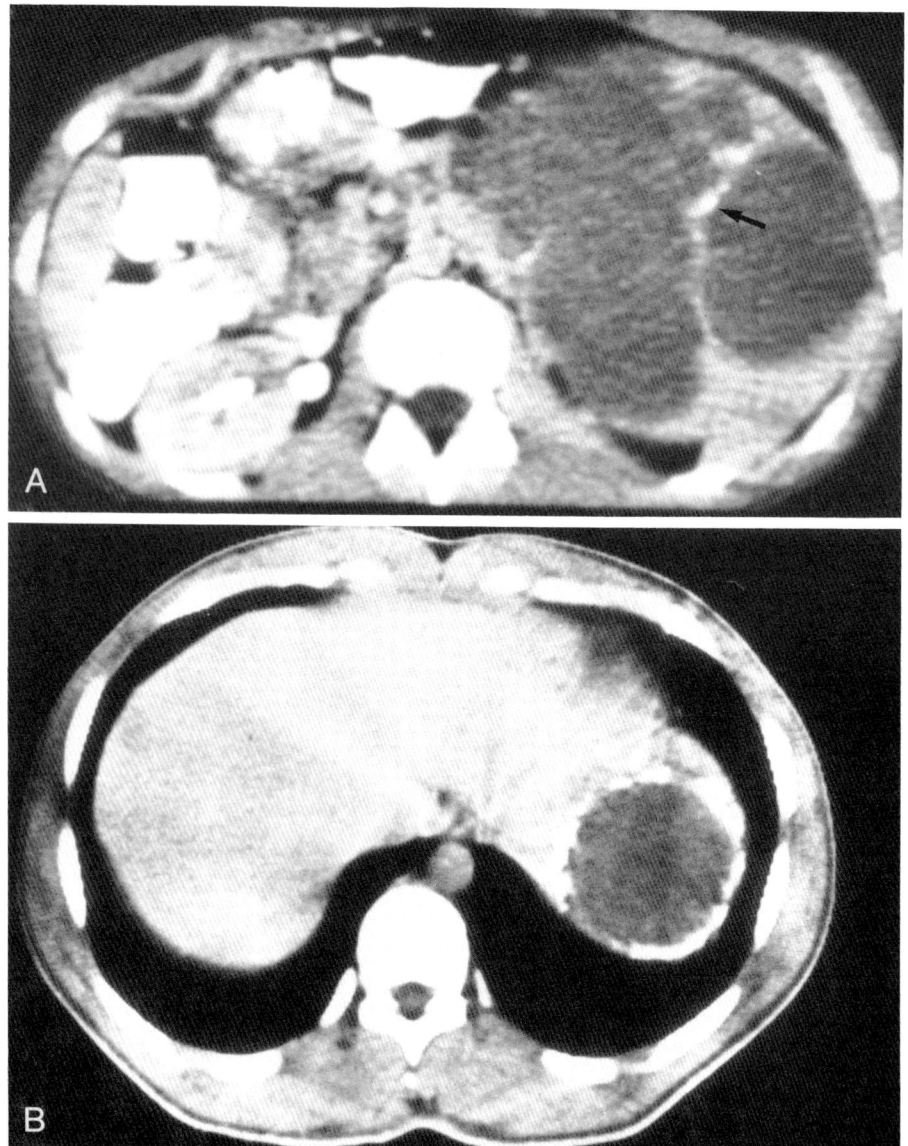

FIGURE 27.10. TRUE SPLENIC CYST: CT
A: Septations, although infrequently this prominent, can be seen in false or true cysts. There is calcification within a septation *(arrow)*. *B:* Dense calcification of the cyst wall is evident.

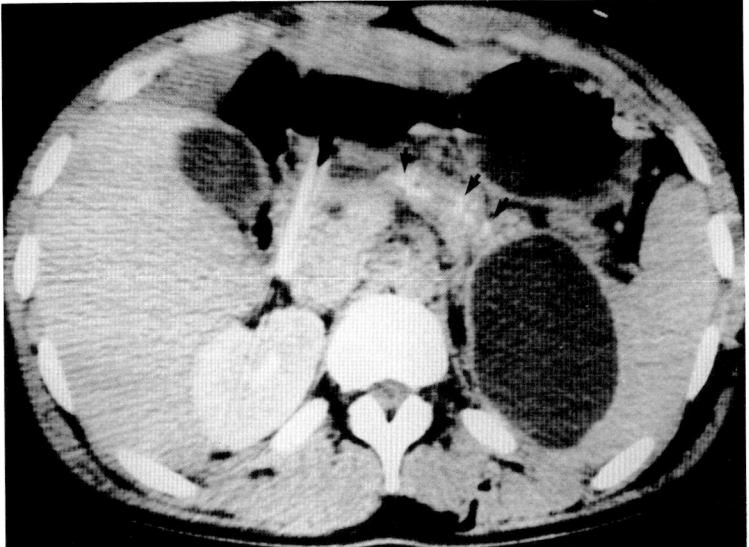

FIGURE 27.11. PANCREATIC PSEUDOCYST
A rare mimic of splenic cyst is intrasplenic extension of a pancreatic pseudocyst. Note the pancreatic calcification (*arrows*) due to chronic pancreatitis.

shadowing indicate wall calcification (29). While a complex mass with solid components is atypical, this may be seen with false cysts due to organizing hematoma within the cyst (29) (Fig. 27.8*A*).

CT reports of splenic cysts are rare showing smooth walled, near water density large lesions which do not enhance (37–40) (Fig. 27.9). Thirteen cases with CT were included in a review by Dachman et al. (29) indicating that CT can show the trabeculated or septated nature of the cyst wall, as well as wall calcification (Fig. 27.10*A* and *B*). The "transition" cases, with organizing hematoma, may have a complex internal structure on CT as well (Fig. 27.8*B*). The CT differential diagnosis would include echinococcal cyst which is usually multiseptated, large solitary abscess or hematoma (clinical context is usually diagnostic), and rarely intrasplenic pancreatic pseudocyst (Fig. 27.11) or cystic neoplasms. These neoplasms include cytic hamartoma and vascular lesions such as hemangioma and lymphangioma.

In summary, once a mass is localized to the spleen and is demonstrated by sonography or CT to be a single large cystic lesion with a relatively thin wall, if echinococcus is excluded, a false (post-traumatic) or true (epidermoid) cyst is the likely diagnosis.

SPLENIC ABSCESS

Although splenic abscess was first mentioned by Hippocrates, it is only recently that such a diagnosis could be made with confidence prior to surgery or autopsy. Early correct diagnosis is critical. The natural history includes complications such as rupture into the peritoneal cavity, bowel, or chest; formation of fistulas, bowel obstruction, generalized sepsis, and nearly inevitably, death; while with early diagnosis and intervention, the survival rate reverses to greater than 93% (41, 42). As a rule, treatment requires surgery and antibiotics, with appropriate attention to the underlying predisposing condition. Emergency splenectomy following splenic rupture carries a mortality rate of 43%, which drops to less than 13% if surgery can be performed electively and prior to rupture (42).

Splenic abscess is relatively rare, with an incidence ranging from 0.14 to 0.70% of 20th century autopsy series (41, 42). Without surgery, mortality may reach 60% (43). The tendency of antibiotics to reduce the incidence of splenic abscess has been countered by the increasing survival of the chronically debilitated or immunosuppressed host such as patients with malignancies, collagen vascular disease, hematological disease, endocarditis, diabetes, the premature, and the elderly.

There appear to be three overlapping mechanisms and subsequently three characteristic patterns of splenic infection (41, 42, 44, 45). Normally, the spleen's efficient phagocytosis and antibody functions offer sufficient protection against infection. Most commonly (75% of splenic abscess patients), multiple small abscesses are caused by overwhelming hematological seeding from a distant focus, as may be seen in the immunocompromised host or the patient with embolizing endocarditis (46). Far less commonly (10–15), a solitary, large abscess may represent the hematogenous seeding of a predisposing splenic infarct or hematoma, such as may be seen in the patient with sickle cell or other hematological disease, or with inadvertent iatrogenic embolization of the spleen. Third, the spleen may undergo direct inoculation and subsequent abscess formation due to penetrating trauma, bowel perforation, surgery, dissecting pancreatic pseudocyst or penetration by adjacent perinephric or subphrenic abscess. Such a mechanism both introduces the infecting agent and creates a receptive medium for it (41–43).

Clinically, the symptoms may be nonspecific, obscuring the correct diagnosis and therefore deferring appropriate treatment (42, 45, 47). Ninety-five percent of patients show such nonspecific symptoms as chills, fever, nausea, vomiting, and leukocytosis. About 60% complain of abdominal pain, which only occasionally is localized to the left upper quadrant or left shoulder (due to diaphragmatic irritation termed "Kehr's sign"). A prolonged course may be accompanied by malaise and weight loss. More localized left upper quadrant symptoms such as focal pain and tenderness, left upper quadrant friction rub, left chest space dullness, and splenomegaly are helpful but less common. Blood culture may be positive (47). Up to 70% may show plain roentgenogram findings, but they again frequently are nonspecific (41, 42, 48).

Prior to 1970, diagnosis was predominantly clinical with a limited contribution from diagnostic imaging—primarily through plain films, barium studies, and radionuclide liver-spleen scan. In the 1970s, angiography, gallium scanning, ultrasound, and CT were added. The combination of relatively noninvasive imaging and increased imaging specificity in the 1980s should allow earlier diagnosis and more effective treatment of splenic abscess.

Plain Films

The routine posteroanterior (PA) and lateral chest, with left side-down lateral decubitus views as indicated, may be positive in up to 70% of patients with splenic abscess. Unfortunately, the pathology is reflected in nonspecific findings such as left lower lobe atelectasis or infiltrates, left pleural effusion, or left hemidiaphragm elevation (42, 49) (Fig. 27.12). These are common

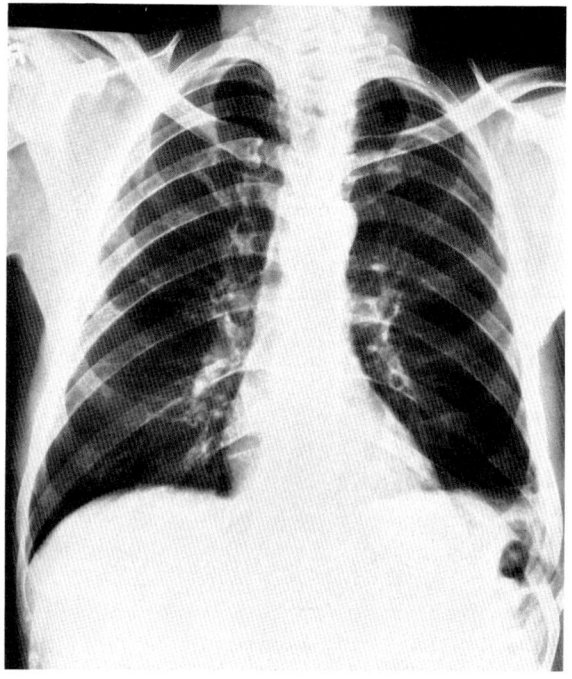

FIGURE 27.12. SPLENIC ABSCESS: PLAIN FILM
A 42-yr-old white man with splenic abscess. Left costophrenic angle blunting is noted, compatible with small pleural effusion, and there is minimal focal atelectasis or infiltrates near the left costophrenic angle. Minimal left hemidiaphragm elevation is noted. Left lateral decubitus view showed a mobile left pleural effusion.

findings and generate long differentials, including (in terms of abdominal pathology), pancreatitis, pancreatic or perinephric abscess, perforated colon, subphrenic abscess, or gastric lesion.

Slightly more specific findings on a chest x-ray or an abdominal film would include left upper quadrant mass or left upper quadrant gas. The normal presence in the left upper quadrant of the air and feces-filled splenic flexure, or of fluid-filled stomach, may limit interpretation of these signs when present. There may be focal ileus in the left upper quadrant. Splenomegaly may be appreciated on the chest or the abdominal film, but is nonspecific and frequently associated with the underlying systemic disease (malignancy, hematogenous disorder, etc.), seen in this population. A specific diagnosis may be suggested when gas or gas-fluid levels are seen within the spleen; this is not common (Fig. 27.13).

Complications such as splenic rupture may alter the plain film findings, with more widespread ileus, evidence of bowel obstruction, free air due to the formation of fistula and/or bowel penetration, generalized or local bowel edema and displacement, and free fluid in the abdomen

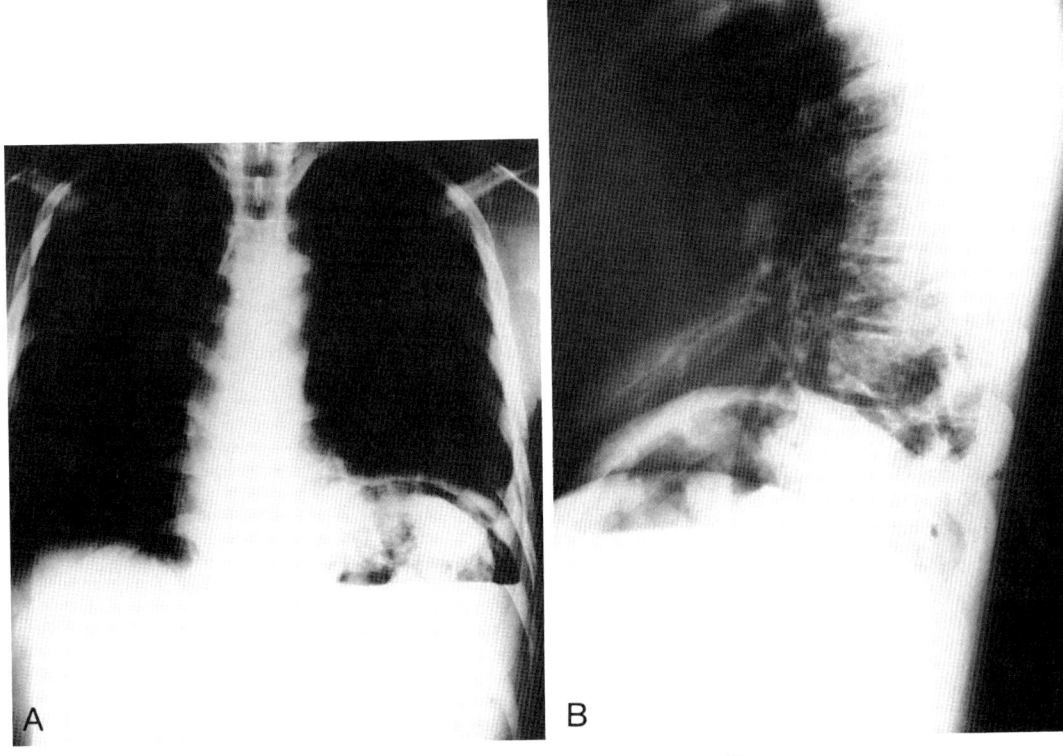

FIGURE 27.13. SPLENIC ABSCESS: PLAIN FILM
A: Frontal and *B:* lateral chest x-rays show a gas/fluid level and elevation of the left hemidiaphragm. Although initially confused for bowel gas, CT proved its intrasplenic location.

and pelvis. Again, these are nonspecific in terms of localizing pathology to a splenic process.

Barium Studies

Barium studies help visualize pathology in the left upper quadrant only indirectly, in that the barium-filled stomach or colon may be indented or displaced by splenic enlargement from any cause. Perisplenic involvement may be secondary to extension from ruptured splenic abscess or may represent the primary pathway through which direct extension from an extrasplenic location involves the spleen. In either case, secondary involvement of the stomach and splenic flexure may be seen, with displacement and mass effect, or less commonly, focal edema, spasm or local ileus. Later, as with the plain roentgenogram of the abdomen, complications and advancing disease create more widespread abnormalities in both the barium enema and the upper GI series. When splenic pathology is suspected, ultrasound or computed tomography (CT) provide more specific screening examinations and in fact, doing the barium studies first may interfere with the quality of these higher-yield examinations. Barium studies are most useful in eliminating stomach and colon as the cause of abnormal left upper quadrant gas collections seen on plain films.

Radionuclide Studies

Splenomegaly is a common, although not invariable, finding with splenic abscess. The patient with multiple diffuse abscesses may show diffuse patchy alterations in uptake and subtle changes in splenic contour (Figs. 27.14 and 27.15). A solitary abscess may present as a single photon deficient defect within the spleen (Fig. 27.16A), and the differential diagnosis must include cyst, trauma, metastatic or primary neoplasm, infarct, abscess, hamartoma, extramedullary hematopoiesis, dissecting pseudocyst, hemangioma, etc. (50). Lesions under 2 cm may be missed, making this a poor screening examination early in the workup when intervention could make the greatest impact. Patients with underlying splenic dysfunction (e.g., myelofibrosis, functional asplenia with sickle cell disease, splenic irradiation) may lack sufficient general uptake to outline focal defects. Prolonging im-

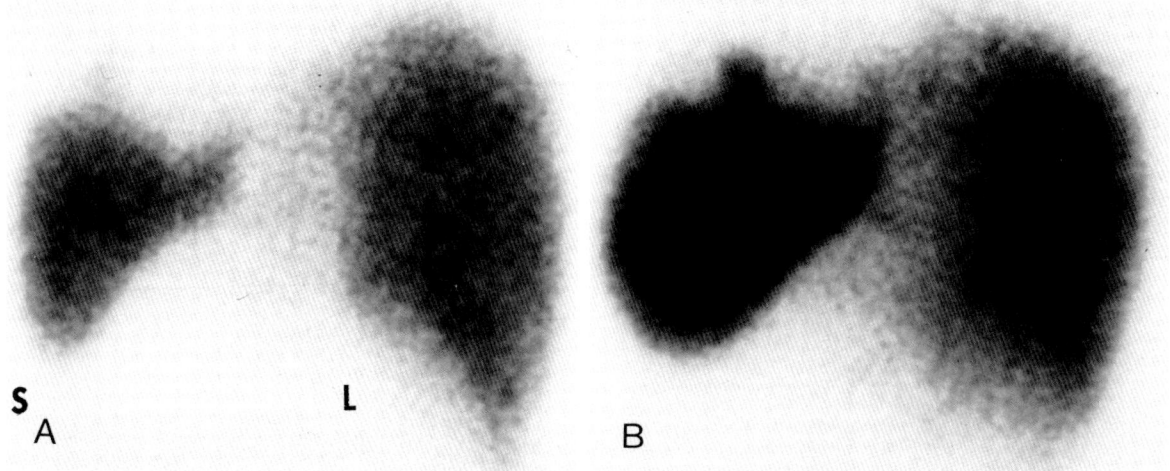

FIGURE 27.14. SPLENIC ABSCESS: ^{99m}Tc-SULFUR COLLOID SCAN
A: Irregular lobulated defects are present at the dome of the spleen, seen best on posterior and posterior oblique views. B: In order to enhance visualization of these defects, a second left posterior oblique view was done for 1 million counts.

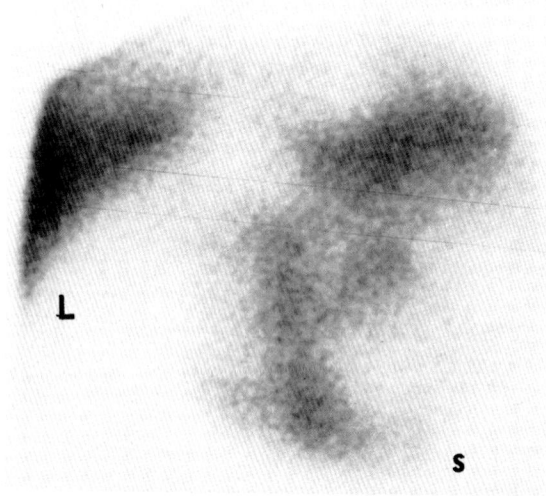

FIGURE 27.15. MULTIPLE ABSCESSES: ^{99m}Tc-SULFUR COLLOID SCAN
A 40-yr-old white woman with fever and abdominal pain. Left anterior oblique view shows minimal enlargement of the spleen, with several photon deficient defects compatible with the multiple small abscess confirmed by surgery.

aging for a higher number of counts may help to delineate focal processes better in the spleen with compromised function (Fig. 27.13).

Gallium-67 Citrate

Gallium-67 citrate is a relatively nonspecific agent usually used as a secondary study to increase the specificity of preceding exams (Fig. 27.15B) (51). Occasionally, gallium-67 citrate will reveal a focus of infection of abnormality not previously detected on the technetium-99m sulfur colloid studies (52). However, conversely, abscesses may be galliopenic, especially in infected infarcts (see Fig. 27.23).

Left upper quadrant gas, fluid collections, and recent surgery usually do not interfere with abscess localization. Since gallium is also a tumor seeking agent, clinical information and correlation will be needed to make the distinction between abscess and neoplasm.

Arteriography

Since the advent of computed tomography and ultrasound, angiography plays little role in the diagnosis of splenic abscess. Selective celiac injection allows visualization of the spleen, with filming sequences timed to produce images of arterial, capillary, and venous phases. There is no single observation diagnostic of splenic abscess, and it may be impossible to distinguish between avascular lesions such as abscess, infarct, cyst, or metastases (53). Splenomegaly and irregular, avascular intrasplenic mass are the two most common findings; the mass effect may stretch or displace splenic branches. As a rule, hypervascularity, arterial encasement, and contrast puddling are not seen and splenic venous drainage remains normal. Large abscesses may lead to splenic rupture, with extravasation of contrast confined by or spilling from the splenic capsule, and avascular areas marking the disruption of splenic tissues.

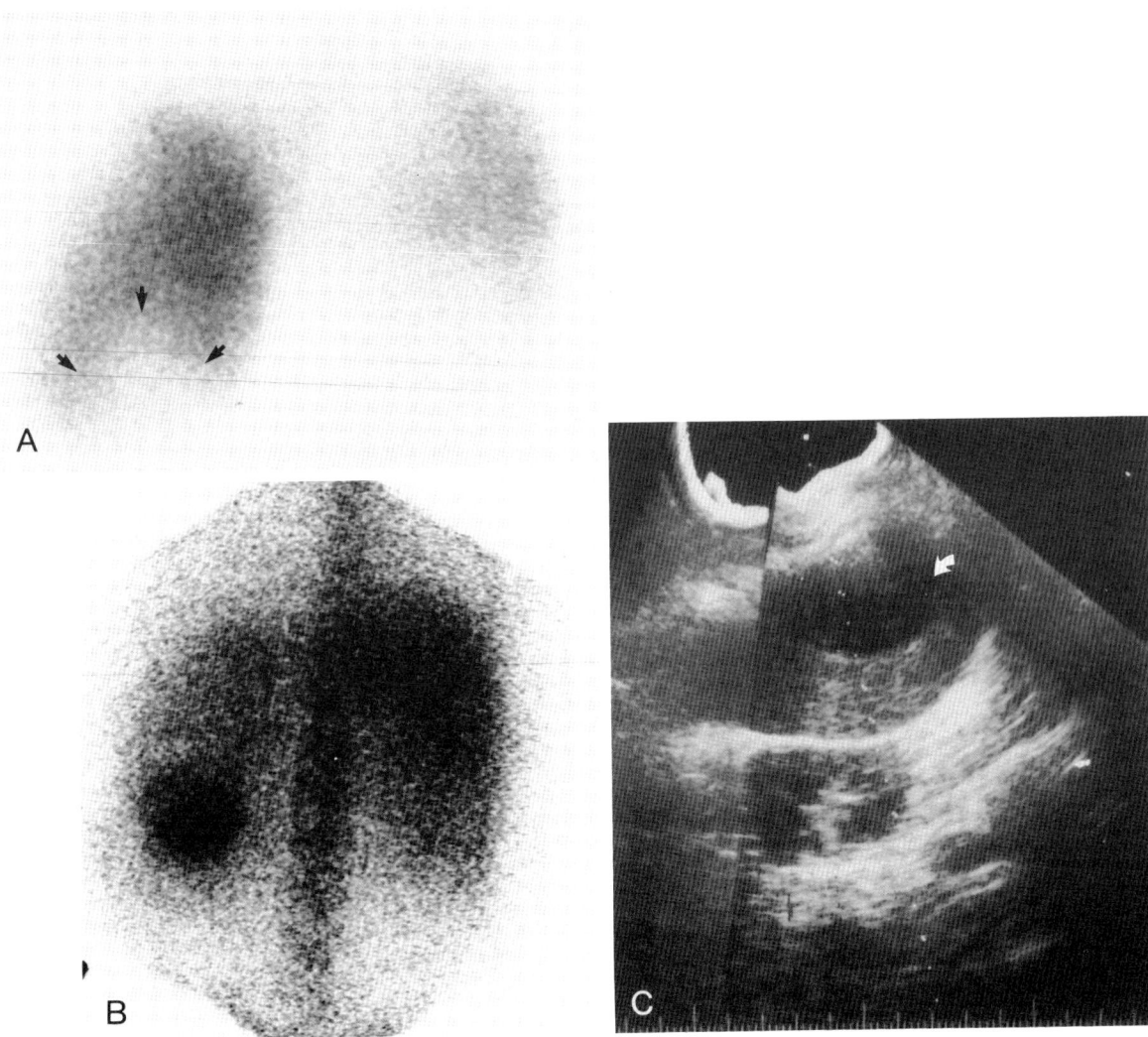

FIGURE 27.16. SPLENIC ABSCESS

Solitary abscess in a 47-yr-old black woman with fever post extraction of abscessed tooth. A: ^{99m}Tc-sulfur colloid scan. Left posterior oblique view shows a solitary photopenic defect in the lower pole of the spleen (arrows). B: ^{67}Ga-citrate study performed 48 hr later, posterior view, confirms splenomegaly and shows the photon-deficient area from the liver-spleen scan to be a focus of markedly uptake of gallium on this study. This was a surgically proven splenic abscess. C: Sonogram: Splenomegaly was noted, with a relatively echopenic area noted centrally in the spleen (arrow), compatible with a fluid collection. Some internal echoes and only moderate back wall enhancement were noted, compatible with hemorrhage or abscess rather than simple cyst.

Ultrasound

Early splenic abscess may produce a subtle alteration in echogenicity, diffuse or focal, with ill-defined areas of increased and decreased echogenicity, particularly in the patient with multiple small abscesses. A focal abscess may be demonstrated as an irregular, echopenic area with scattered internal echoes, septations and eased through transmission less than that of a simple cyst (49, 54) (Fig. 27.16C). These internal echoes should help distinguish abscess from cyst, but do not rule out hematoma. Marked alterations in sonogenic texture may be noted secondary to rupture, and subdiaphragmatic, perinephric or perisplenic fluid may be detected. Realtime imaging may be useful in the peridiaphragmatic regions. Gas within the abscess will appear intensely echogenic and will limit the exam by blocking through-transmission (Fig. 27.17A and B). Increased left upper quadrant gas due to ileus or to aerophagia can also interfere with the ex-

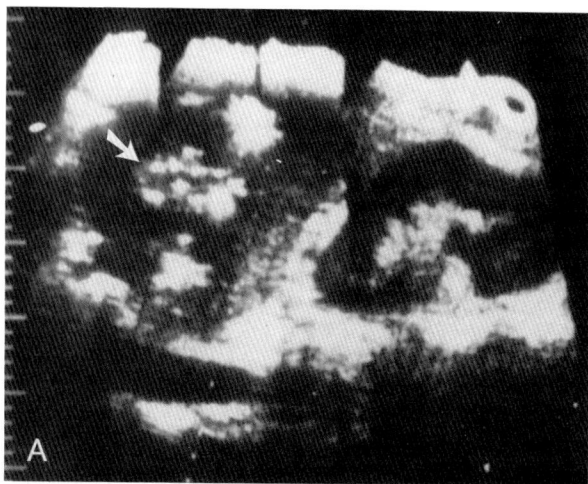 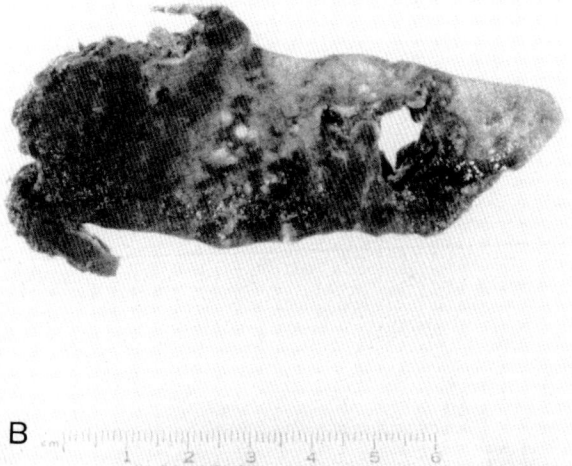

FIGURE 27.17. SPLENIC ABSCESS
A: 42-yr-old white man (see Fig. 27.12). Ultrasound showed moderate to marked splenomegaly, with patchy echogenic foci (*arrow*) with some shadowing, compatible with abscesses and with air within the abscesses. *B:* Gross specimen: At splenectomy, multiple areas of recent infarction and thrombosis with foci of abscess were seen with markedly necrotic tissue corresponding to the air collections noted at CT and ultrasound.

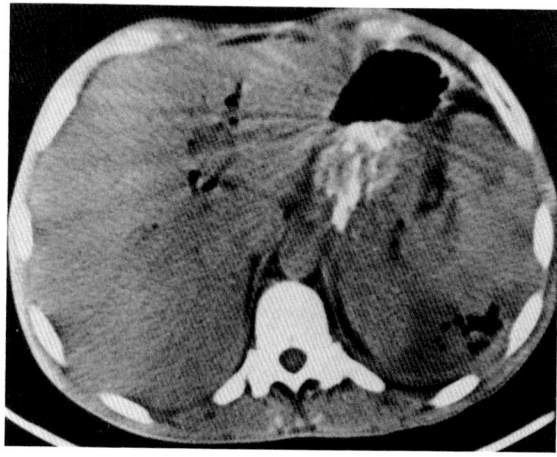

FIGURE 27.18. SPLENIC ABSCESS
A 33-yr-old black man with abdominal pain. CT scan through the level of the liver and spleen shows marked splenomegaly, with a large, irregular low attenuation area posterior in the spleen, with air distributed throughout the low attenuation areas. This was a surgically proven splenic abscess. There do not appear to be air fluid levels in this collection. Scans at lower levels showed thickening of Gerota's fascia on the left side, compatible with spread of inflammation.

amination in the patient with abscess (55). Very small lesions are likely to be missed, as are lesions in the superior portion of the normal or enlarged spleen.

Computed Tomography

Although air is present only in a small percent of splenic abscesses, it is readily visualized on CT and unlike ultrasound, will not interfere with visualization or regions deep to such a collection (Fig. 27.18). Air-fluid or fluid-fluid levels may also be detected within the spleen (Fig. 27.19A–C). Rarely, air may enter the splenic vein and portal venous system (Fig. 27.20A and B). A focal low density abscess may be inhomogeneous and poorly defined (Fig. 27.21). The use of narrower "liver" windows (e.g., window width 108, center 43), in addition to conventional window settings (e.g., window width 420, window width 36) and intravenous contrast, will accentuate subtle differences in CT attenuation (Fig. 27.22). Abnormalities of 5 mm or less may be identified. Adequate opacification of stomach and small bowel aids in the assessment of the perisplenic spaces and limits false positive interpretation. The evolution of high resolution rapid scanners has also eliminated the problems of cardiac and diaphragmatic motion which limited resolution on early scanners (56); but a juxtadiaphragmatic lesion may still be difficult to localize precisely. In such cases, selective sagittal or coronal reconstruction may provide valuable information.

Perisplenic fluid or inflammation, or clinically unsuspected splenic rupture may be seen (Fig. 27.23A–C). In the case of hematogenous seeding of infection from distant foci, either the source (e.g., mycotic aneurysm) or other secondary affected organs (e.g., liver, kidney) may be discovered. Definition of adjacent pancreatic pseudocyst or perinephric abscess, or trauma may help in determining the etiology of infection, as may findings associated with systemic or hematological disease.

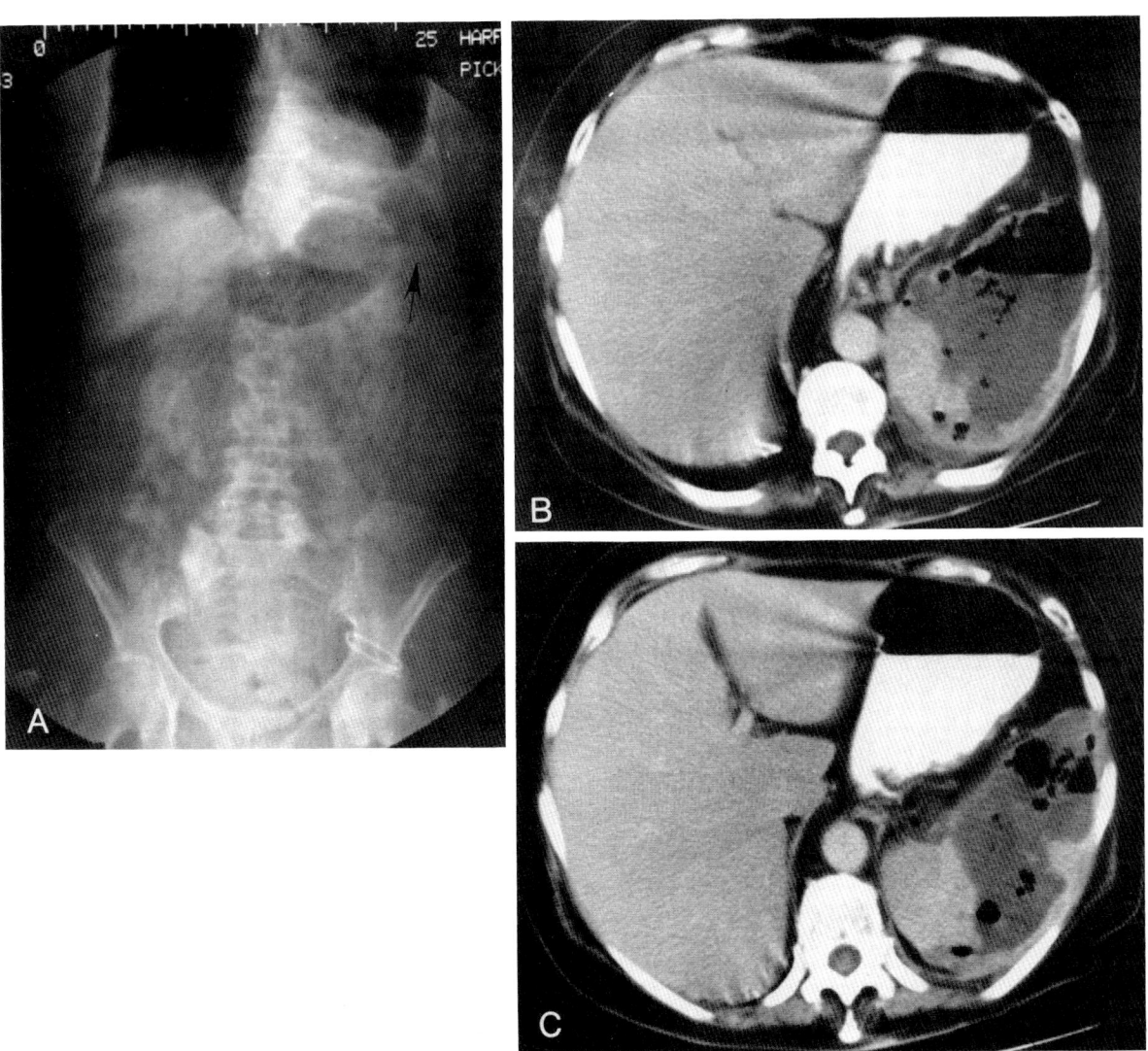

FIGURE 27.19. SPLENIC ABSCESS

A 43-yr-old white woman with a history of subacute bacterial endocarditis, fever, and left upper quadrant pain. *A:* Localizing topogram shows an air collection lateral to the stomach under the left hemidiaphragm, and some left costophrenic angle blunting (*arrow*). *B* and *C:* CT at the level of the spleen and liver shows marked splenomegaly, with replacement of most of the normal splenic parenchyma with areas of low attenuation and many loculated air collections. A large air-fluid level can be seen in the spleen at one level (*B*), and several smaller air-fluid levels can be seen at another level (*C*). This was a surgically proven splenic abscess, believed to be secondary to septic emboli from cardiac valve disease.

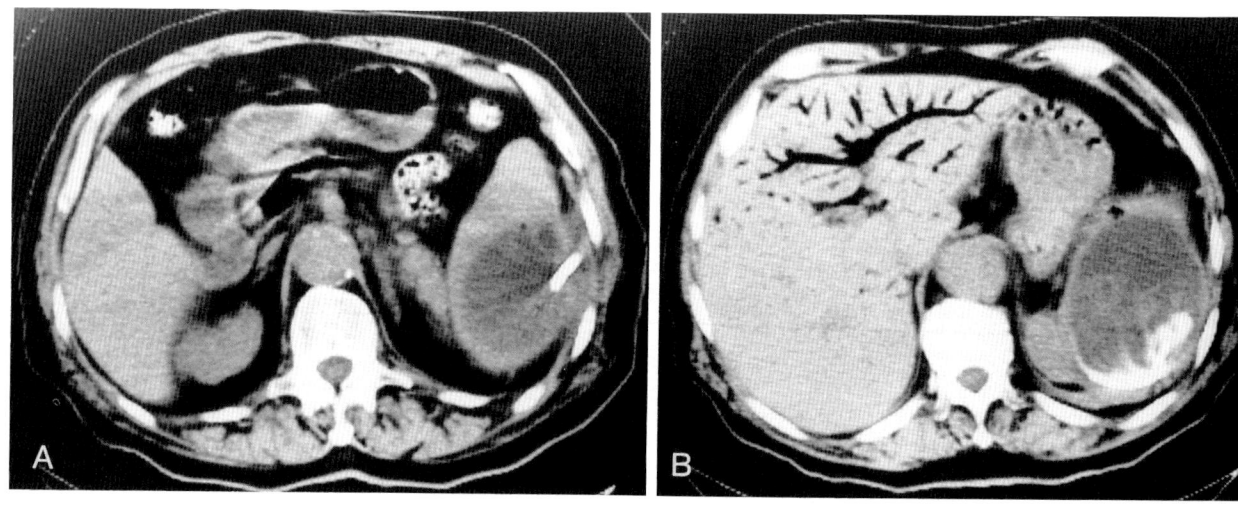

FIGURE 27.20. SPLENIC ABSCESS WITH VENOUS AIR: CT

A large abscess is being drained percutaneously under CT guidance. Before intervention, as well as on these cuts, air is seen in the venous system. *A:* Gas is seen in the splenic vein and confluence of splenic and superior mesenteric vein. *B:* A higher section showing gas in the intrahepatic portal venous system. Contrast was introduced via percutaneous needle into the abscess prior to catheter placement.

FIGURE 27.21. SPLENIC ABSCESS

Same patient as Figure 27.16. CT scan through the level of the spleen shows splenomegaly, displacing and compressing the left kidney, and a large, irregular low attenuation area in the middle of the spleen. This is measured about 10 HU, and was a surgically proven splenic abscess.

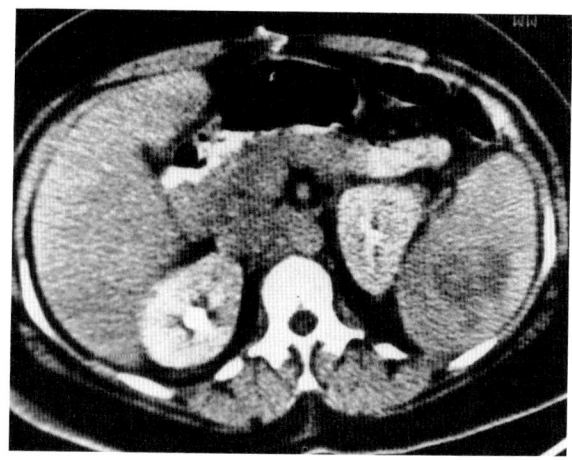

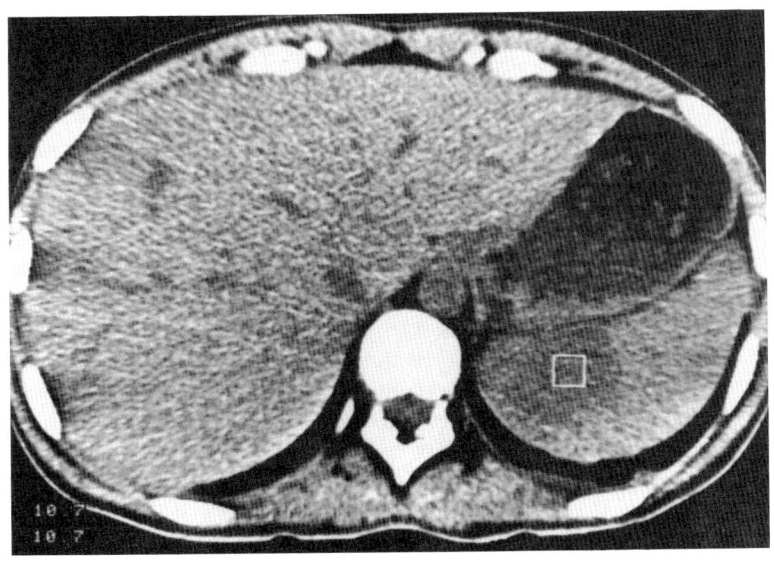

FIGURE 27.22. SPLENIC ABSCESS
A 21-yr-old woman with a 2-week history of nausea, vomiting, leukocytosis, and fever. Patient had a normal ultrasound. CT scan through the level of the spleen shows minimal enlargement of the spleen, with a large, low attenuation area in the medial half of the spleen (*cursor*). Narrow windows are used to accentuate attenuation differences between the abscess and the surrounding normal spleen.

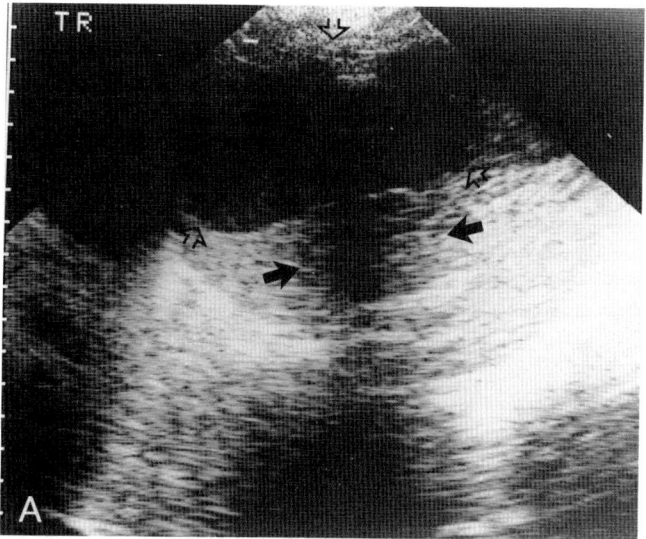
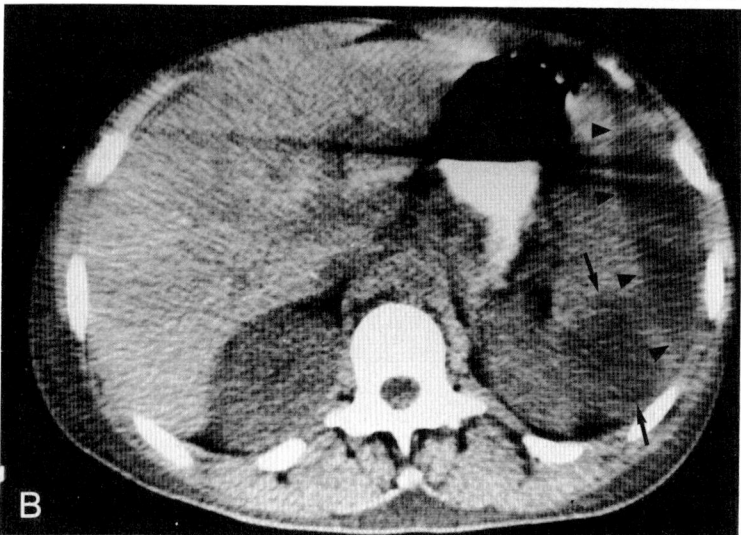
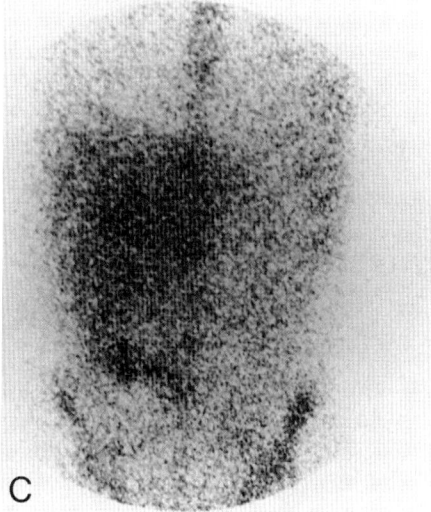
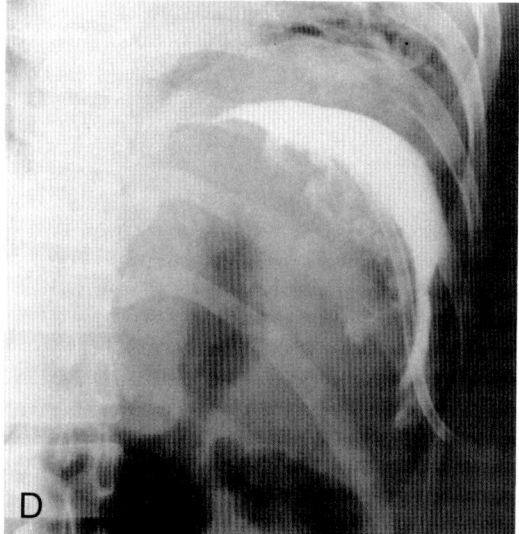

FIGURE 27.23. SPLENIC ABSCESS

Ruptured splenic abscess in a splenic infarct. *A:* Sonogram shows an inhomogeneous spleen with hypoechoic lesion (*arrows*) and a large extrasplenic anechoic fluid collection (*open arrows*). *B:* CT confirms the intrasplenic lesion (*arrows*) and extrasplenic collections (*arrowheads*). At surgery, both areas were infected. The intrasplenic lesion was a ruptured abscess, probably in a previously infarcted area. *C:* Gallium scan. Due to the antecedent infarction, the gallium scan was falsely negative for abscess. *D:* Initially, the large extrasplenic fluid was drained percutaneously.

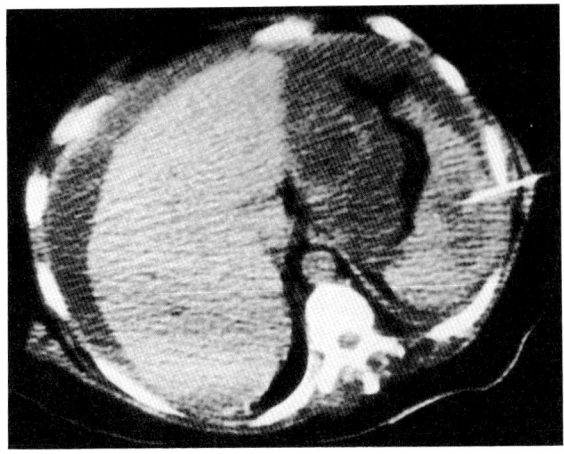

FIGURE 27.24. SPLENIC ABSCESS: NEEDLE ASPIRATION
CT demonstrates a low density area in the spleen consistent with abscess. This is confirmed with a needle aspiration and treated with percutaneous drainage. (Courtesy Dr. Eric Van Sonnenberg.)

Although splenic abscess traditionally is considered a surgical disease, either computed tomography or ultrasound can be used to guide percutaneous drainage of an abscess when it is deemed advisable to avoid or to defer surgery (Figs. 27.20, 27.23D, and 27.24). Where surgery is anticipated, CT confirms the diagnosis and can focus subsequent intervention. CT provides a pathoanatomical "road map" which can simplify surgery, decrease postoperative complications, and where possible, help avoid splenectomy with the goal of preserving the immunological role of the spleen (55). Finally, CT provides a relatively noninvasive, reliable, and repeatable means to follow-up in an inpatient or outpatient setting.

LYMPHOMA

Splenic lymphoma is a common entity which is usually a manifestation of generalized lymphoma. In a large autopsy and postsurgical series only two primary splenic lymphomas were found (57). The malignant lymphomas characteristically involve the white pulp and usually appear as nodules (58). When advanced, the entire spleen may be replaced by tumor, especially in the large cell variety (59). However, in some cases, notably in poorly differentiated lymphocytic lymphoma, the spleen may appear normal with small cleaved tumor cells visible only on high power microscopy (58). The red pulp involvement microscopically represents confluence of white pulp disease. In Hodgkin's disease the periarteriolar lymphoid sheath is initially involved and later a small solitary nodule (59) or miliary nodules develop (60).

Ahmann classified the gross pathologic appearance of splenic lymphoma into four categories (61): (a) homogeneous enlargement without masses, (b) miliary masses, (c) 2–10-cm masses, and (d) a large solitary mass. On this basis one could predict the potential difficulty in accurate radiographic diagnosis of splenic lymphoma which exists. Conventional methods such as physical examination, plain film, nuclear scintigraphy (62), gallium scan (63), arteriography (64), sonography (65), and CT (66), have not proven accurate. Nevertheless, the role of splenectomy as part of the staging laparotomy remains controversial (67, 68). Asplenic patients are prone to infection and thus there is a continued search for noninvasive radiologic splenic evaluation particularly for stage I and II clinical disease so that splenectomy can be avoided. Some studies have shown that in stage III Hodgkin's disease, splenic involvement did not affect survival but did affect the recurrence free intervals (69).

At the time of presentation, the spleen is uninvolved in 30% of patients with non-Hodgkin's lymphoma. Over 67% of patients with nodular, poorly differentiated lymphocytic lymphoma have splenic involvement at presentation (70). In Hodgkin's disease the spleen is involved in 40% at initial staging and almost 70% have splenic involvement in autopsy series (71).

While an enlarged spleen in a patient with non-Hodgkin's lymphoma usually indicates splenic involvement, up to one-third of patients with splenomegaly will not have splenic lymphoma at histologic examination (65). Up to one-third of lymphoma patients (Hodgkin's and non-Hodgkin's) without splenomegaly do have histologic involvement. Thus, as a rule, splenic size is not a reliable indicator of disease although it is suggestive of involvement in non-Hodgkin's lymphoma. While evaluation of spleen size by sonography or CT has limited usefulness, splenomegaly in conjunction with hilar adenopathy or focal defects does correlate with histologic disease (72). Therefore, although, sonography and CT cannot exclude splenic lymphoma, they do have clinical utility in strongly suggesting the diagnosis.

Sonography

In addition to evaluating splenic size and hilar adenopathy, sonography can evaluate splenic texture (Fig. 27.25). Claims that diminished echogenicity of the spleen in association with

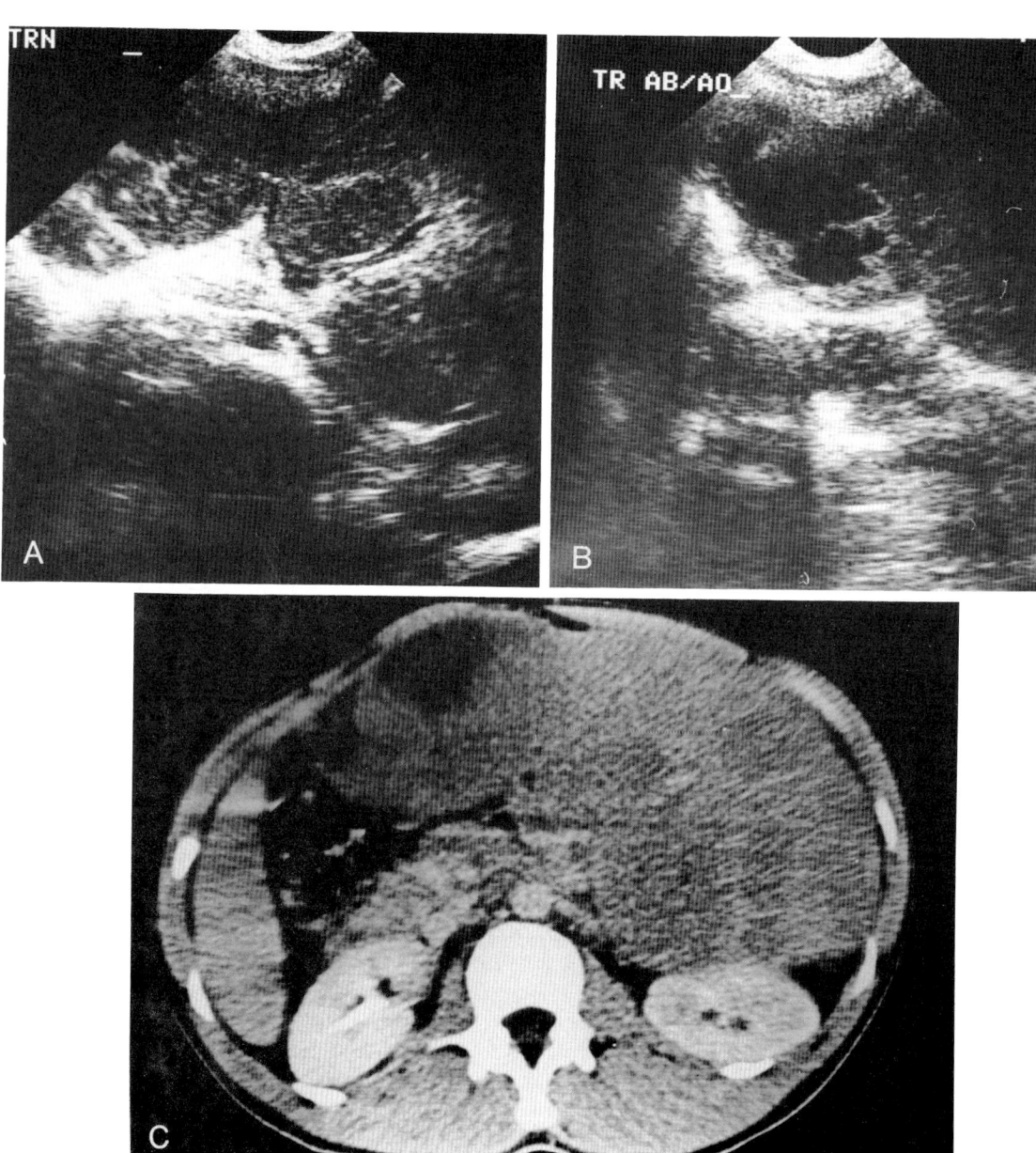

FIGURE 27.25. LYMPHOMA
A and *B:* Sonography shows inhomogeneous, hypoechoic masses throughout the spleen, (*A*), and necrosis in one mass (*B*). *C:* This corresponded to the inhomogeneous, decreased density masses on contrast enhanced CT and a lower density focus anteriorly, respectively. The left kidney is compressed by splenic enlargement. Note that the low density focus could mimic an abscess on sonography and CT.

splenomegaly may correlate with lymphomatous involvement have not been verified (72). Carroll points out that while splenic hilar nodes may be detected particularly with the use of a left coronal or lateral decubitus view, splenic lobulations and accessory spleen can be confused with hilar adenopathy (72). Technetium sulfur colloid scans may help in demonstrating accessory spleen(s) in confusing cases. Hilar nodes were demonstrated in 10 out of 18 patients with splenomegaly (65, 72). The adenopathy may be more echogenic than the spleen or focal splenic defects (65, 72). Of 18 cases with splenomegaly, 4 had focal poorly marginated 3 mm to 3 cm lesions, 3 had relatively hypoechoic lesions, and 1 had a relatively hyperechoic lesion (65, 72). Focal anechoic defects have been known to mimic an abscess (64, 73, 74). This is particularly important because the clinical features of lymphoma and splenic abscess may also overlap (Fig. 27.25). One such case turned out to be a diffuse histiocytic lymphoma (73) and another, lymphocyte depleted type of Hodgkin's disease (74). If sonography (or other modalities) can prove liver involvement, it is highly likely that the spleen is involved even if it appears normal radiologically (65).

Computed Tomography

In general, CT is least effective in early lymphoma because normal or borderline enlargement of nodes cannot be discerned as abnormal. In advanced disease it may replace lymphangiography and gallium-67 imaging.

As with other modalities, the spleen is often the site of occult disease (60). In 18 patients with histologic splenic lymphoma, 14 had normal CT and radionuclide scans (75). Zornoza's detection rate of 22% using CT with intravenous water soluble contrast enhancement is similar to the results of precontrast CT scans done by Thomas who detected only one case of splenic lymphoma. Breiman et al. (76) detected nodules, all >0.9 cm in diameter in 5 of 10 spleens with proven lym-

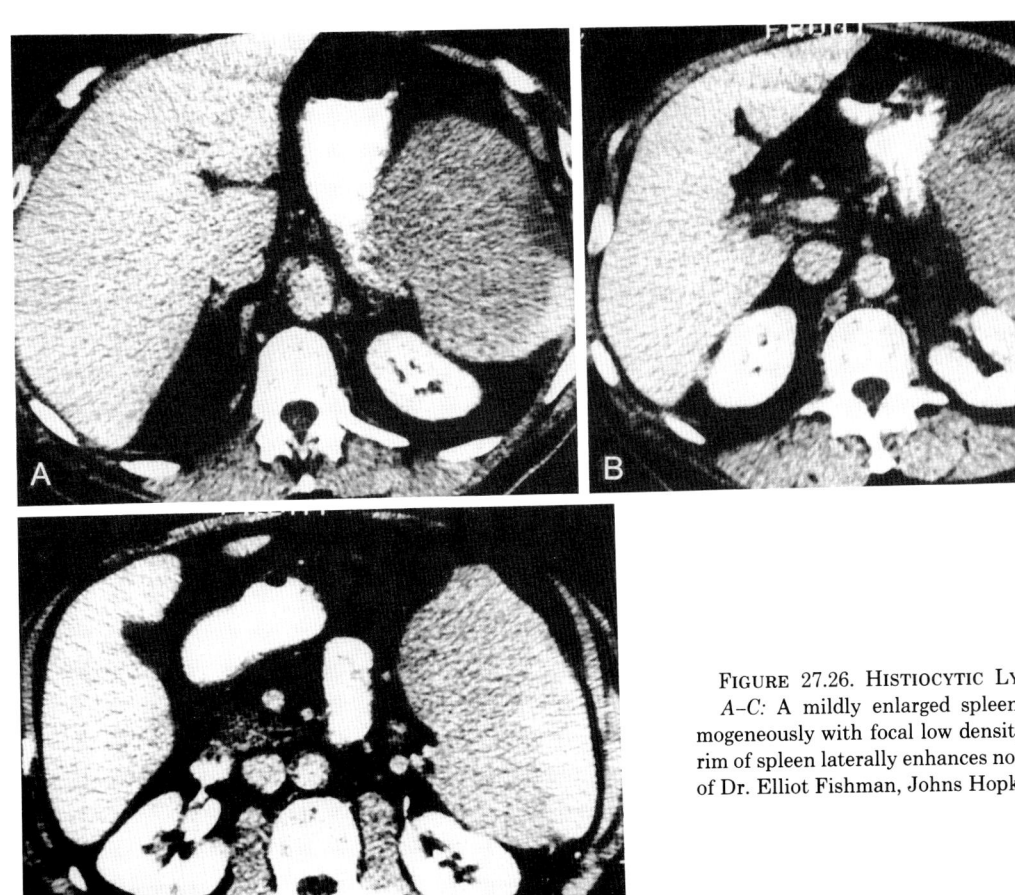

FIGURE 27.26. HISTIOCYTIC LYMPHOMA: CT A–C: A mildly enlarged spleen enhances inhomogeneously with focal low density areas within. A rim of spleen laterally enhances normally. (Courtesy of Dr. Elliot Fishman, Johns Hopkins Hospital.)

phoma nodules. Another 5 spleens had nodules less than 0.9 cm in diameter which were not detected on CT. Focal low density lesions in diffusely involved spleen might be due to inhomogeneous involvement, focal infarcts, or hematoma (Figs. 27.26–27.28). Another 8 spleens were normal by CT and gross pathology, one of which was positive for lymphoma on microscopic examination. Nodes in the splenic hilus are seen in 50% of non-Hodgkin's disease patients (77), but are uncommon in Hodgkin's disease (60).

Although many authors do not separate their CT data on Hodgkin's vs. non-Hodgkin's, some claim that a splenic abnormality on CT is more likely in non-Hodgkin's (78). This is probably the case, because the early periarteriolar involvement or late miliary nodules usually seen in Hodgkin's disease may be too small to be detected by CT.

In a study of Burkitt's lymphoma, 4 of 29 patients had splenomegaly and a low attenuation focal mass was seen in one case with a normal-sized spleen. However, this is not clinically significant in determining therapy which is dependent more on tumor volume than on site of involvement since the treatment of choice is chemotherapy (79).

Recent studies using CT with ethiodol-oil-

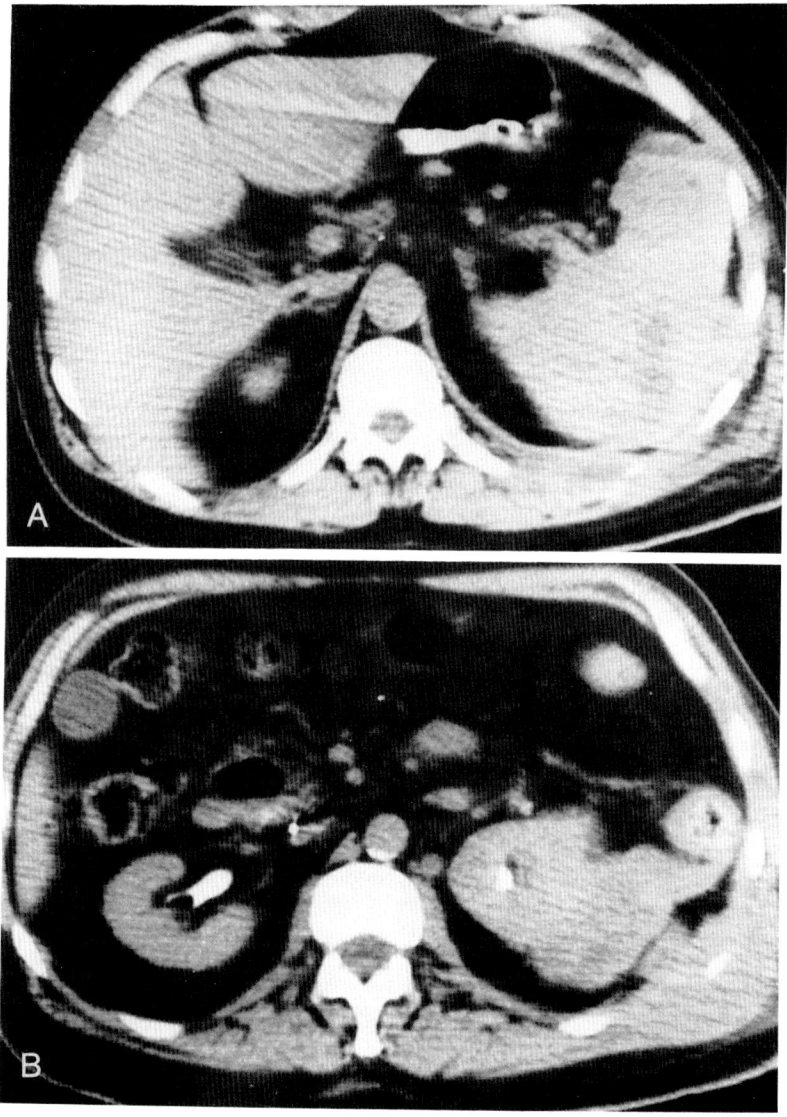

FIGURE 27.27. LYMPHOMA: CT
A and *B:* The spleen is enlarged with lymphoma involving the spleen and adjacent kidney and descending colon. (Courtesy of Dr. Elliot Fishman, Johns Hopkins Hospital.)

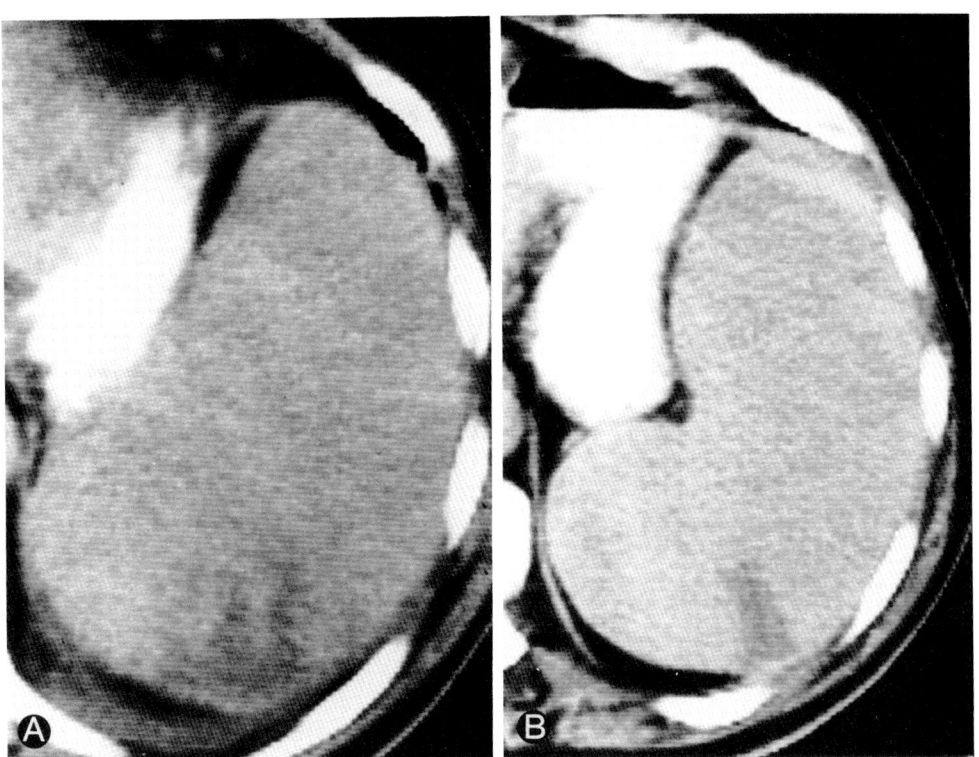

FIGURE 27.28. LYMPHOMA: PRESUMPTIVE INFARCT
A and *B:* CT shows an enlarged spleen with a wedge-shaped defect peripherally, presumably an infarction.

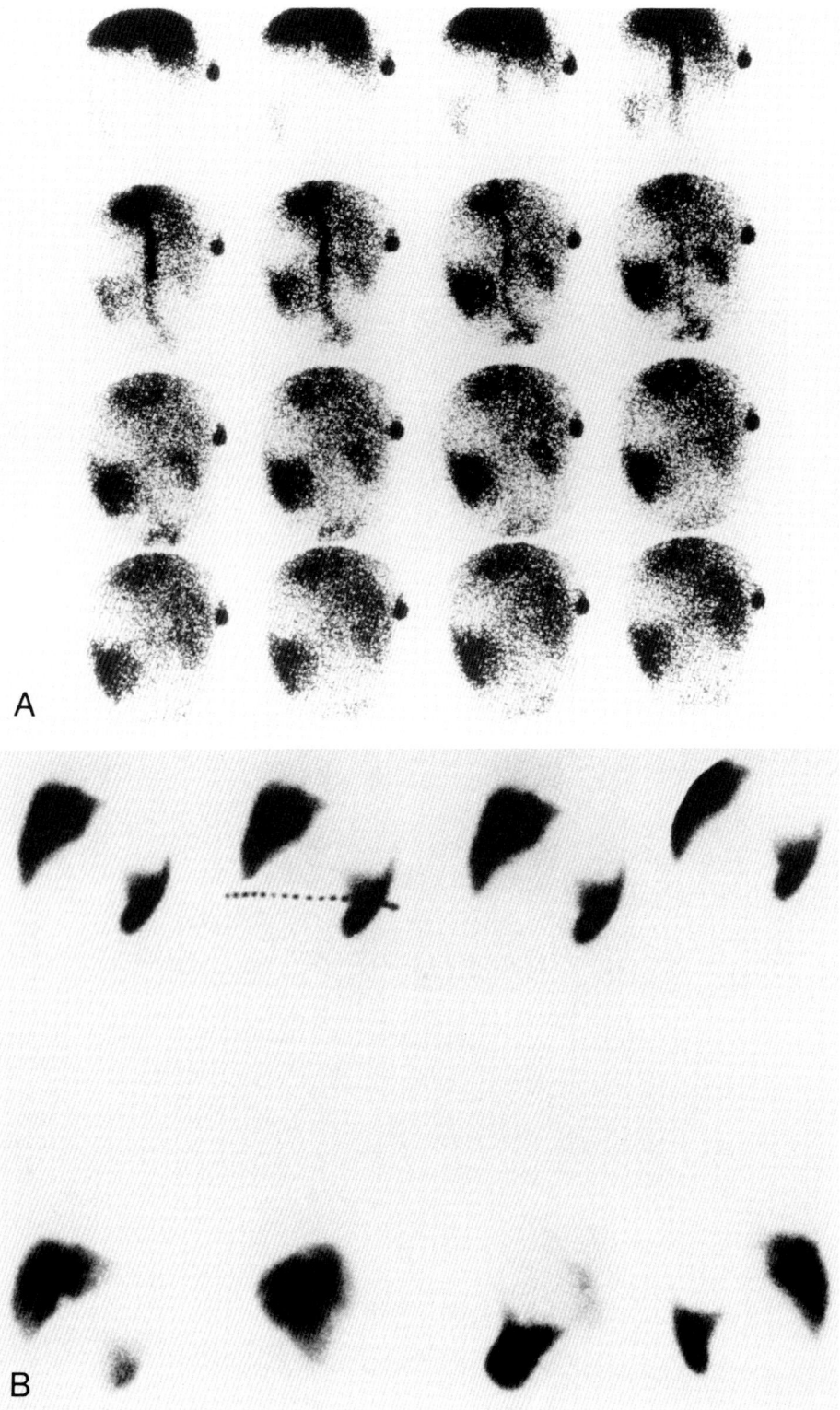

FIGURE 27.29. LYMPHOMA: ^{99m}TC-SULFUR COLLOID SCAN
A: Dynamic study (posterior) shows normal flow to an enlarged spleen with an upper pole defect better seen in (*B*), the static scan. This corresponds to lymphoma presenting as a single large splenic mass.

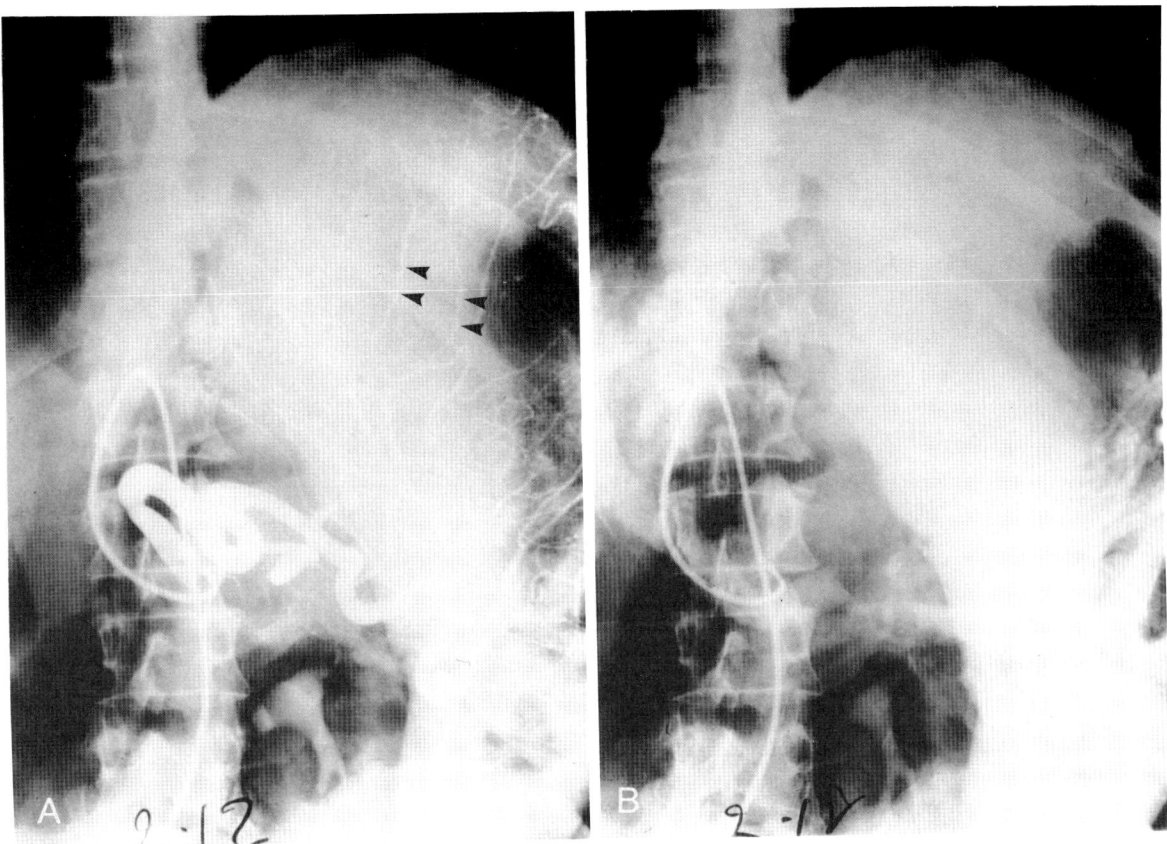

FIGURE 27.30. LYMPHOMA: ANGIOGRAM
A: Arterial phase showing splenomegaly with stretched vessels which are irregular in the upper pole, representing encasement (*arrowheads*). *B:* Parenchymal phase shows upper pole involvement as a large defect.

emulsion-13 (EOE-13) contrast enhancement have shown a detection rate of 92% in splenic lymphoma using focal defect(s) as the criterion of involvement vs. a noncontrast detection rate of 8% (80). There was only one false negative in the series of 12 cases with histologically proven splenic lymphoma (excluding one additional reader error). This case showed multiple nodules 0.5 cm or less in diameter at laparotomy. There were no false positives.

Other Imaging Modalities

Technetium sulfur colloid scans are not routinely performed for lymphoma as they usually add no additional information (Fig. 27.29). It has been shown that the bone scanning agent technetium-MDP may accumulate in splenic lymphoma possibly representing areas of necrosis (81). Angiography may show tumor encasement of vessels, neovascularity or masses in malignant lymphomas (Fig. 27.30) (82), but studies show that both normal and diseased spleens may show a nonhomogeneous capillary phase (64, 83). Thus angiography is unreliable and not useful in determining splenic involvement.

HEMANGIOMA

Splenic hemangioma is the most common benign splenic tumor with an incidence of 0.03–14% in autopsy series (84). The exact incidence is uncertain because some autopsies did not distinguish between hemangioma and hamartoma (85). Also, lymphangiomas may be confused with hemangiomas (86). Most patients are 20–50 yr of age. There is a slightly higher incidence in males than females (84), and the lesion is also reported in children.

The solitary splenic hemangioma is usually asymptomatic, associated with splenomegaly

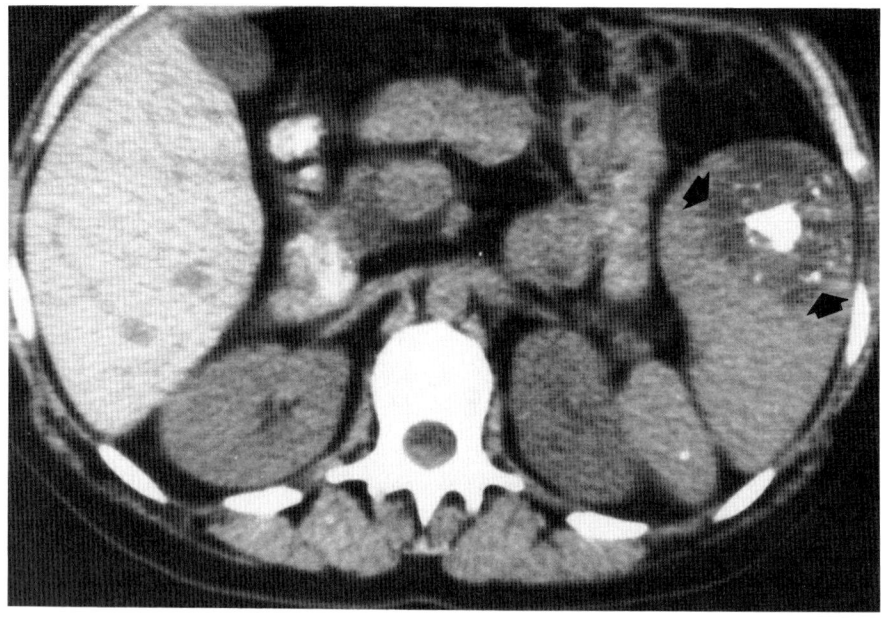

FIGURE 27.31. HEMANGIOMA
CT shows dense solid and punctuate calcifications within a low density mass (*arrows*). (Courtesy of Dr. Elliot Fishman, Johns Hopkins Hospital.)

(45%) or found at autopsy (30%) (84). About 25% may present acutely due to rupture or less often with symptoms secondary to hypersplenism. Malignant transformation has been claimed but these may represent cases of primary hemangiosarcoma. Multisystem hemangiomatosis has been reported (86–88) and may present with a consumptive coagulopathy, although this has rarely been reported with solitary splenic hemangioma as well (88).

Pathologically, they are similar to hemangiomas elsewhere in the body (86), consisting of a proliferation of vascular channels with endothelial lining (86, 89, 90). They are usually of the cavernous type (84), but may also be capillary or mixed (91). Calcification is usually not present but has been reported rarely (84).

There is a paucity of radiologic reports of solitary splenic hemangioma. The radiologic appearance is similar to hemangiomata elsewhere. Plain films demonstrate splenomegaly as a discrete mass (92). Calcification (reported in three cases) were either peripheral and rim-like, diffuse and punctate (Fig. 27.31) (92), or stellate (93). Scintigrams show a single or less often multiple defects surrounded by normal spleen on sulfur colloid scan (92). In one case, there was uptake of Tc-diphosphonate by a calcified tumor (93). On sonography, the lesions are either echogenic, rarely with small anechoic foci representing areas of necrosis or large vascular spaces, or alternatively are composed of multiple large anechoic areas (92). On CT, the solid portion is isodense with normal spleen and enhances similarly to spleen except for the large vascular spaces (92). There is one case report of peripheral enhancement with delayed central enhancement similar to hepatic hemangioma (94). The angiographic pattern is variable: it may be vascular with pooling of contrast or have avascular area within (92, 93).

ANGIOSARCOMA

Angiosarcoma of the spleen may represent a solitary primary lesion or be associated with lesions elsewhere especially in the liver. Defining the primary site is usually based on lesion size which may be a fallacy. By strict definition only solitary splenic lesions are primary. Many hepatic angiosarcomas are associated with exposure to thorium, vinyl chloride, or arsenic, whereas primary splenic angiosarcoma is generally not (95, 96). The relative rarity of solitary splenic angiosarcoma in toxic exposures has not been explained (97). Congenital hemangiomata were associated in one case (98).

Primarily splenic angiosarcoma is a rare lesion with about 64 reported cases (95, 98–100), and an additional 30 cases from the AFIP, some of which may have been previously reported (101). The entity was first reported in 1879 by Langhans (102). In fact, Langhans' case and 39 of the 55 cases reviewed by Chen (95) had hepatosplenic involvement. In Locker's review of 103 cases of hepatic angiosarcoma, although multicentric lesions were excluded, in fact 16% had splenic involvement at autopsy which was presumed to be metastatic (103). The male-to-female ratio is about equal with a slight male predominance. The age range is from infancy to adult but the vast majority of cases are in the 50–60-yr-old age group. Symptoms include: abdominal pain, left upper quadrant mass, fever, malaise, weight loss, and anemia. Major complications include rupture of the spleen with often fatal hemoperitoneum (17 out of 55 cases reviewed by Chen up to 1979), and a consumptive coagulopathy (99). There is no correlation between spleen size, age or anemia and splenic rupture (97). Metastasis may occur, primarily to liver, to bone, and lymph nodes (96). Weakness or dyspnea may predominate if lung metastases or pleural effusion is present (97). The survival rate has been uniformly poor with a six month survival rate of about 20% (95), but the diagnosis is typically delayed which may be a factor in poor prognosis (5). If splenectomy is performed before hemoperitoneum is present, the survival is 14.4 months compared to 4.4 months. If splenectomy is done after splenic rupture, survival is 4.4 months (96). Multiagent chemotherapy has been employed (95, 97).

Grossly, the lesion consists of solid and cystic components (101). Microscopically there is a proliferation of anastomosing vascular channels often with a sarcomatous appearing stroma (90, 96, 101). Spindle cell, papillary, and undifferentiated varieties are described (90, 101).

Radiographic evaluation is usually nonspecific. Splenomegaly is evident and Tc-sulfur colloid scan may show splenomegaly with multiple cold defects (95, 100). The kidney and ureters may be deviated by splenomegaly or para-aortic adenopathy (95) as demonstrated on excretory urography. Angiography will show vascular lesions similar to angiosarcomas or hemangiomas elsewhere (95, 100). There are vascular lakes supplied by dilated arterial branches with or without tumor vessels (99). Ultrasound described in one case showed a mildly enlarged spleen, and CT in that case showed varying-sized nodules in the spleen (and the liver) (99). In Smith's case CT showed an irregular diffuse low attenuation lesion.

The paucity of radiographic data reflects the rarity of this lesion as well as its high complication rate and rapidly fatal course. The diagnosis should be suspected, particularly in adults over 50 yr of age with hematologic abnormalities such as anemia or consumptive coagulopathy in conjunction with splenomegaly or splenic mass. It should also be suspected if there is a history of irradiation, congenital hemangiomas or other vascular abnormalities (95) (See "Thorotrast" for an example of angiosarcoma on CT).

HAMARTOMA

Splenic hamartoma has been called by a variety of names including splenoma, splenoadenoma, fibrosplenoma, and nodular hyperplasia of the spleen (104). They occur slightly more commonly in females (104) and have been reported in all age groups including young children (105), although most patients are adults.

Iozzo reviewed the literature in 1980 and found that 74 of 91 reported cases were incidental findings at laparotomy or autopsy. Morgenstern reported an additional 12 cases in 1984, 3 of which were symptomatic (106). Large hamartomas or multiple confluent hamartomas may become symptomatic, usually with vague pain or left upper quadrant mass. Rarely, there may be associated hematologic abnormalities including hypersplenism with anemia, thrombocytopenia and bone marrow hyperplasia (104, 107, 108). In these cases, complete recovery from the hematologic abnormalities usually occurs after splenectomy. One case presented with spontaneous rupture (106).

Splenic hamartoma has been associated with growth retardation accompanied by frequent infections, hepatosplenomegaly, anemia, leukopenia, and thrombocytopenia in two children. Examples of associated hamartomas in other organs is rare (104). Two such cases have been reported in tuberous sclerosis (104) and one in a patient with Wiskott-Aldrich syndrome (104).

The lesions are usually solitary, but may be multiple. Two types have been described: a white pulp type composed of lymphoid tissue and a red pulp type composed of sinuses and structures similar to red pulp. Usually there is a mixture of both types (104). In Morgenstern's series nine were of the red pulp type and three were mixed (106). The wide vascular channels are lined by a single layer of plump endothelial cells and filled with lymphoreticular cells. Foci of hemoside-

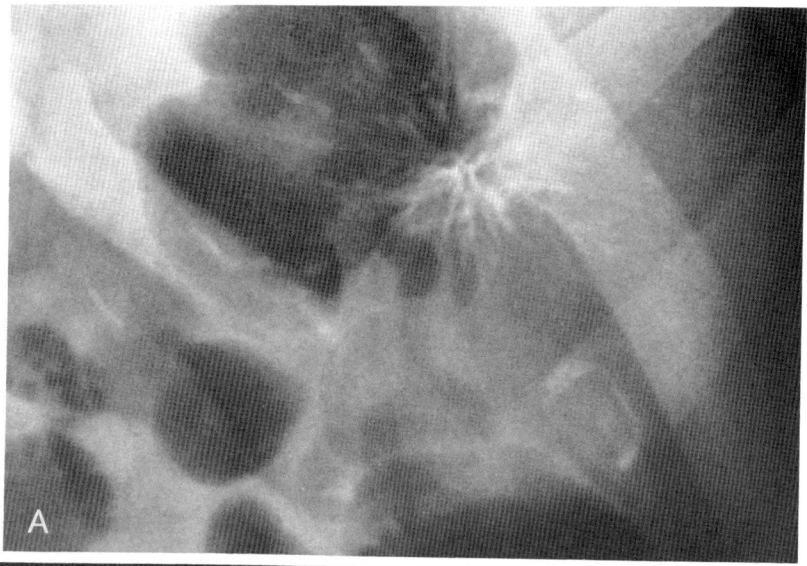
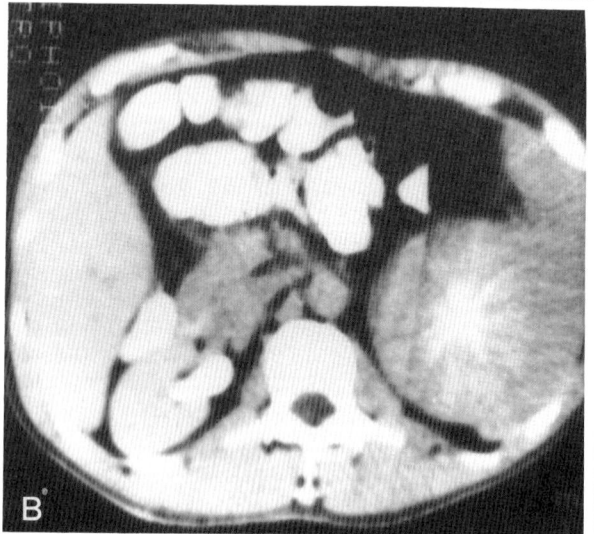
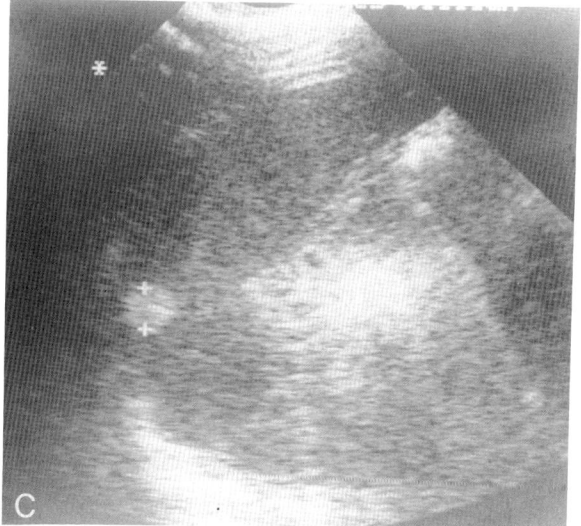
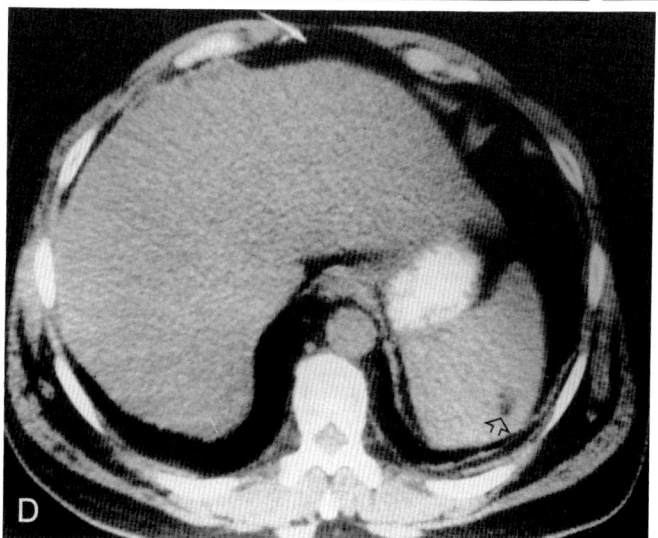

FIGURE 27.32. HAMARTOMA
A: Plain film showing a stellate calcification which is seen on CT (*B*), to be within a splenic mass. (Courtesy of Dr. E. Parsek, Mercy Hospital, Pittsburgh, Pa.) *C* and *D:* Probable angiomyolipoma or lipoma of the spleen that might be classified by some as a hamartoma. The coronal sonogram shows a densely echogenic mass (*cursors, C*). The contrast-enhanced CT reveals a hypodense mass (*arrow*) most of which measured −25HU, diagnostic of fat.

rosis, calcification, and fibrosis are seen. The lesion compresses adjacent normal spleen, thus it appears sharply demarcated, but no true capsule is present. Trabeculae extended from the splenic capsule into the hamartoma in three of Morgenstern's cases (106).

Plain films are either normal or show splenomegaly. Punctate calcification has been reported in one case and a central stellate scar in another (Fig. 27.32) (102). Histologically, the calcifications were in the fibrotic parts of the lesion, not within the vascular channels and were thought to be due to areas of ischemia and hemorrhage.

Angiography, while said to be characteristic is not diagnostic. The lesion is well demarcated with prominent tumor vascularity, aneurysmal dilatation, occasional vascular lakes, or arteriovenous shunting (105, 109, 110). Similar findings have been reported in splenic angiosarcoma (111). Uncommonly, the lesion is avascular as it was in the case with punctate calcification, probably due to tumor necrosis.

In one case a technetium pertechnetate flow study showed the lesion to be vascular, and ^{51}Cr-labeled red blood cells were sequestered in a red pulp type hamartoma (112). Excretory urogram demonstrated the lesion as a defect in the spleen due to total body opacification effect in one case and less dense than adjacent spleen in another case with central stellate calcification (Fig. 27.32) (113).

On contrast-enhanced CT the lesion was nearly isodense with the spleen in one case (113). The only other case with CT and sonography was a cystic hamartoma where CT showed a cystic and a solid component, the solid component of which was almost isodense with spleen and sonography showed the lesions to be relatively hypoechoic with respect to the spleen (114). To date, accurate differentiation from other splenic neoplasms including malignant ones is not possible with reliability, although CT and sonographic data may prove useful.

LYMPHANGIOMATOSIS

Lymphangioma of the spleen was first reported by Fink in 1885 (115). Fowler reported 27 cases in his review of splenic tumors in 1953 (116). The lesion is characterized by a single or classically by multiple macroscopic and microscopic cysts lined by flat endothelium and filled with proteinaceous fluid (117–119). If only a single large cyst is present, the appearance will mimic a focal cyst of the spleen of congenital or traumatic etiology (118, 120). Classic splenic lymphangiomatosis is a diffuse process involving the entire spleen (117, 121, 122).

The etiology is controversial. Some authors (119) have proposed that lymphangiomatosis is identical in pathogenesis to cystic hygroma. Both are due to congenital obstruction to a localized area of lymphatic drainage and differ only morphologically, reflecting the character of surrounding tissue. Others (122) support Willis' theory (123) that the accumulation of fluid, opening of collaterals and thrombosis in already formed lymphatic channels leads to cystic dilatation. They claim that finding cases with solitary splenic involvement associated with cysts and fibrosis suggest progression during life rather than a purely congenital process.

Clinical Findings

When symptoms are present in splenic lymphangioma they are usually nonspecific due to compression of adjacent viscera. Pain or discomfort in the left upper quadrant is most common. Disseminated lymphangiomatosis may also present with consumptive coagulopathy (124), although this is more likely to occur in hemangiomatosis (125). Other symptoms may occur related to the specific organ system involved, such as respiratory distress, neck or skin masses or blebs on mucous membranes of the mouth. Secondary mycotic infection of the skin or mucous membrane lesions may occur (119).

Pathology

Microscopically, lymphangiomas are classified as simple, cavernous and cystic (126). The simple type is composed of capillary-sized, thin-walled channels, the cavernous type consists of dilated lymphatic channels often with fibrous adventitial coats, and the cystic type is composed of cysts ranging from a few millimeters to several centimeters in diameter. The spaces must be lined by flattened endothelial cells or the diagnosis is suspect. Even when a large cyst is present, there often are other small cysts, in the splenic parenchyma or in the subcapsular region (118, 127). The spaces are filled with fluid which may contain amorphous eosinophilic debris, cholesterol crystals, calcium, hemosiderin, and lipid-laden macrophages. Occasionally, lymphangiomas with secondary hemorrhage may be confused with hemangiomas (128).

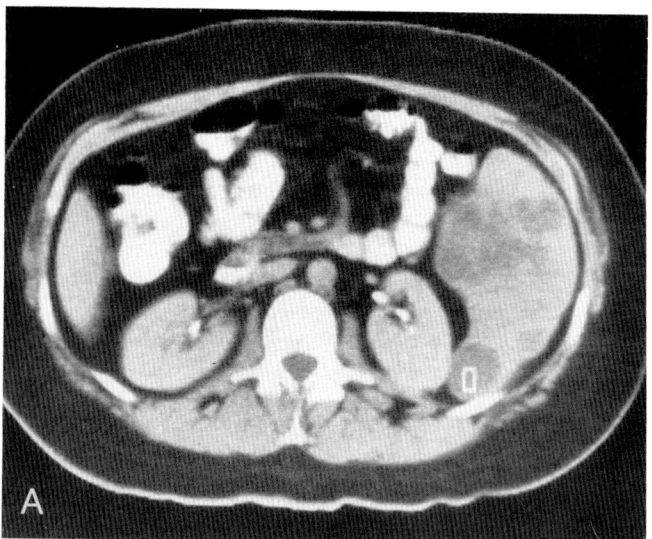 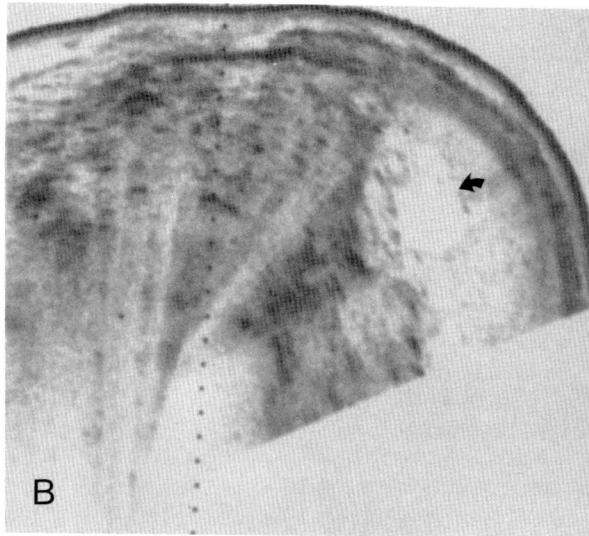

FIGURE 27.33. LYMPHANGIOMATOSIS
A 44-yr-old woman with 6 weeks of left upper quadrant pain. A: CT showed an enlarged spleen with multiple low density masses throughout, deforming the contour of the spleen. B: Sonogram shows the masses to be cystic (arrow). (Courtesy Robert S. Pyatt, M.D., Bethesda Naval Medical Center, previously published in (128)).

If the lesion is limited to the spleen, surgery is curative, and is recommended in the presence of hypersplenism or symptoms due to extrinsic compression of adjacent organs (121). If the disease involves multiple organ systems, such as liver, bone, lungs, or kidneys, the prognosis is guarded (117). This has been termed "cystic angiomatosis" in the past. When multiple organs are involved, the spleen is often involved as well (117).

Radiology

Plain films of the abdomen may show an enlarged spleen. No calcification is seen. The left kidney and splenic flexure may be depressed by the spleen (113). The mass may be evident on total body opacification phase of an excretory urogram (113). Tc-sulfur colloid scan shows single or multiple defects (113).

Sonographically, the spleen may be enlarged. Depending on the size and macroscopic morphology of the lesion, its sonographic appearance will vary. A single well defined cyst similar to a post-traumatic cyst can be seen. In diffuse lymphagiomatosis multiple variably-sized sonolucent areas are depicted (Fig. 27.33) (127). Septations are sometimes seen. A central stellate echogenic scar (non-calcified) was seen in one case (113).

CT will show single or multiple low density cystic areas, some of which may be subcapsular in location and deform the splenic contour (Fig. 27.33) (127). CT numbers range from 15 to 33 HU, depending mostly on the protein content of the fluid. The thin wall and sharp margination of the lesion should suggest lymphangioma rather than other neoplasms which may be of low density due to necrosis or lipid content (127). An alternate appearance is an inhomogeneous low density mass without macroscopic cysts which may not show significant enhancement (113).

Angiography shows splenomegaly with stretched intrasplenic arteries and numerous lucent areas varying from one millimeter to a few centimeters in diameter. The appearance is reminiscent of renal polycystic disease (121), and has been described as a "Swiss cheese" pattern (121, 129). Some are hypovascular, however (113).

METASTASES

The incidence of metastases to the spleen as reported in the literature varies greatly from rare to greater than 50% (130, 131). There are no recent large series dealing with splenic metastasis. Patients with splenic metastasis generally have multiorgan involvement suggesting that splenic involvement is a late event in the natural history of most metastatic tumors. Thus, one would expect the incidence to vary depending on the type of series studied, i.e., surgical vs. autopsy. Microscopic lesions are found in 33% and grossly visible lesions in up to 67% (132, 133). Solitary splenic metastases without other organ involvement have been reported (131). There are case reports of rupture due to splenic metastasis (134).

The primary sites of origin in approximate decreasing order include: lung, breast, prostate, colon, stomach, malignant melanoma, ovary, and pancreas (130, 131). Malignant melanoma is probably more common than previously thought however; according to Robbins and Cotran (135), 50% of malignant melanomas metastasize to the spleen and melanoma may be the most common splenic metastasis (136, 137). Case reports include other tumors such as chondrosarcoma, endometrial carcinoma (138), thymoma (138), and invasion by pseudomyxoma peritonei (140).

Most metastases are hematogenous in origin. In Marymount's large series there were 93 of presumed hematogenous origin and 14 which involved the spleen by direct extension or peritoneal seeding (133). Carcinoma of the stomach, pancreas, left colon, and left kidney may involve the spleen by direct extension. In general, the splenic capsule acts as a barrier against direct invasion (136). Marymount analyzed the location of the microscopic lesions (31 cases) and divided them into five groups: venous sinusoids, red pulp, white pulp, trabecular vessels and multiple sites. Most were located in venous sinusoids alone or in multiple sites. He also presented evidence that splenic sinusoidal metastases are not always preterminal events in the natural history of the carcinomas involved. In particular, not all cases had multiorgan involvement. The one example of microscopic tumor limited to the white pulp raises the possibility of lymphatic dissemination of tumor. Grossly visible tumor (62 cases in Marymount's series) may be nodular or diffuse. Large nodules were more likely to exhibit necrosis. Splenic trabeculae were often incorporated into larger nodules with tumor in the vascular channels as well. With diffuse metastases the overall spleen size is increased, but its contour is preserved (133).

Roentgen Findings

Plain films are usually normal, unless there is splenomegaly. The contour of the spleen is normal. Liver spleen scan will show photopenic areas if metastatic foci of sufficient size are present (Fig. 27.34). Extensive splenic involvement may cause non-visualization, essentially an "autosplenectomy," probably by encasing the splenic vasculature (Fig. 27.35).

Sonography may show hypoechoic or echodense lesions (Fig. 27.36A and B). In a series of three cases of metastatic melanoma to the spleen, all demonstrated splenomegaly with a densely echogenic splenic architecture and multiple 2–4 cm lesions which were relatively hypoechoic in two cases and echogenic in one case (141). Interestingly, one of the cases had a nor-

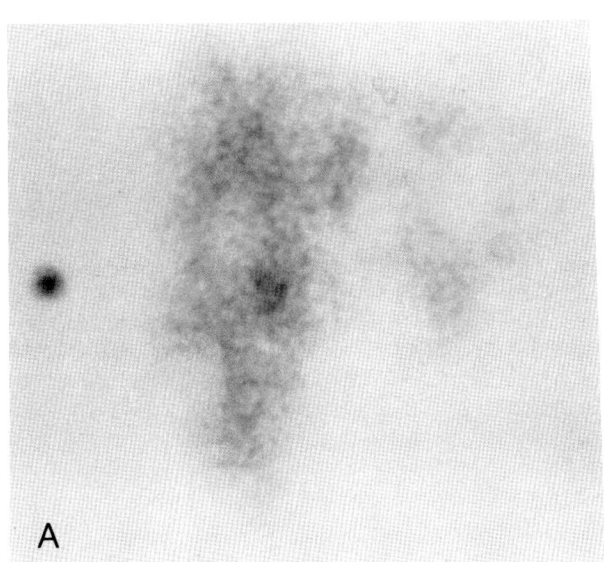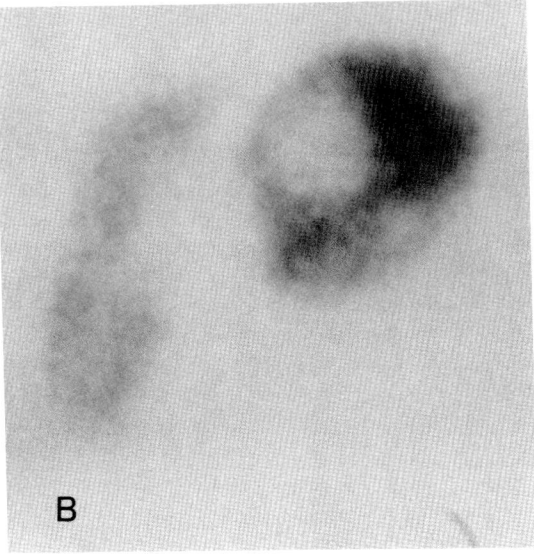

FIGURE 27.34. METASTATIC BREAST CARCINOMA: ^{99m}Tc-SULFUR COLLOID SCAN
A: Anterior view and B: lateral view show multiple defects.

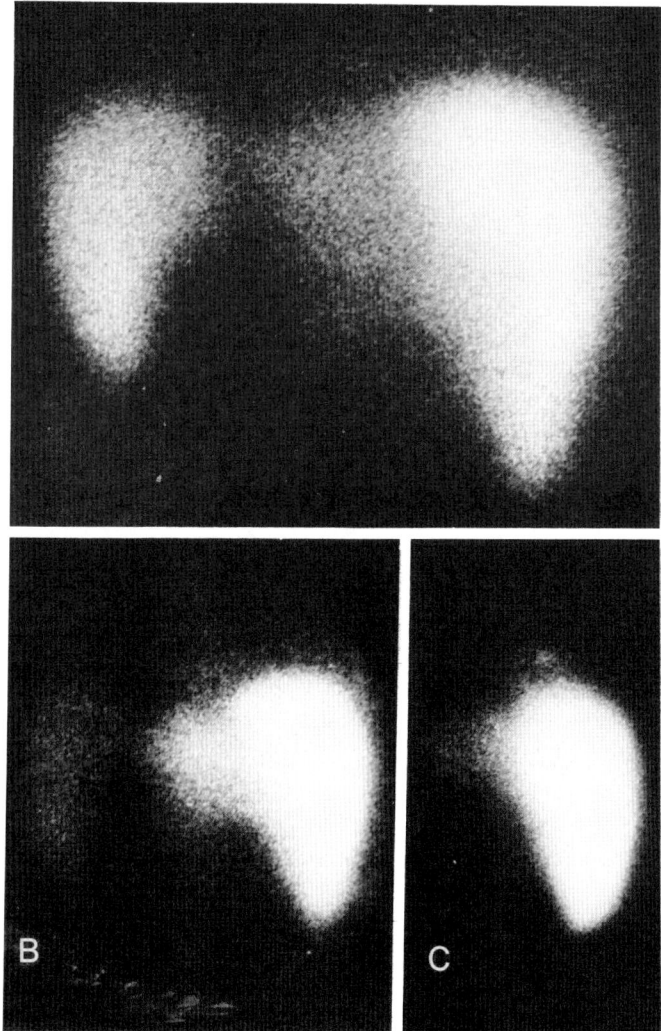

FIGURE 27.35. METASTATIC BREAST CARCINOMA: ^{99m}TC-SULFUR COLLOID SCANS, POSTERIOR VIEWS
A: September 1977, *B:* April 1980, and *C:* April 1982. There is decreasing visualization of the spleen over time, progressing to complete nonvisualization.

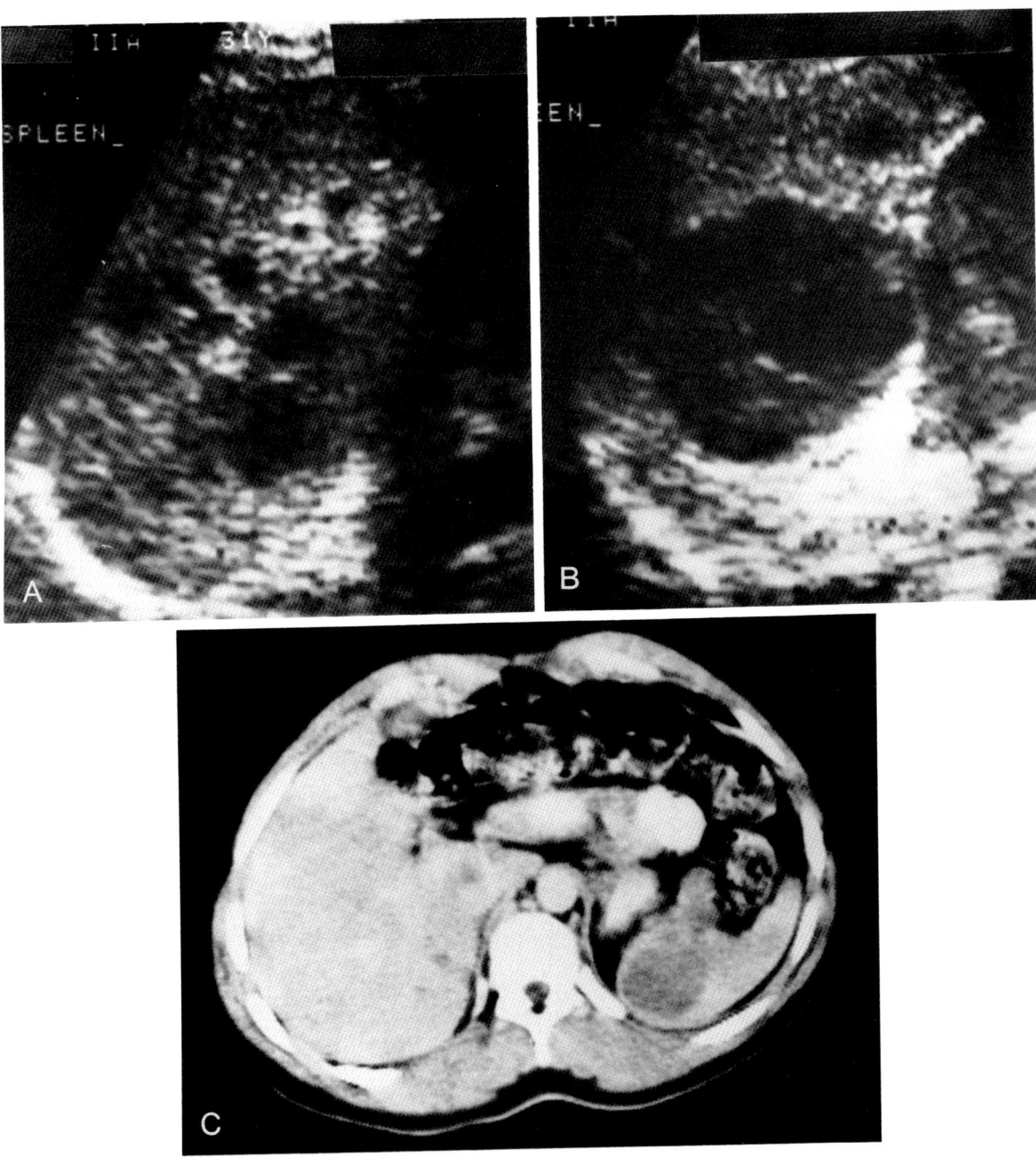

FIGURE 27.36. METASTATIC ADENOCARCINOMA: SONOGRAM
A–C: A 41-yr-old man with an unknown primary neoplasm, diffusely metastatic. *A* and *B:* Sonogram shows hypoechoic masses. *C:* CT shows a large low attenuation mass corresponding to the sonogram.

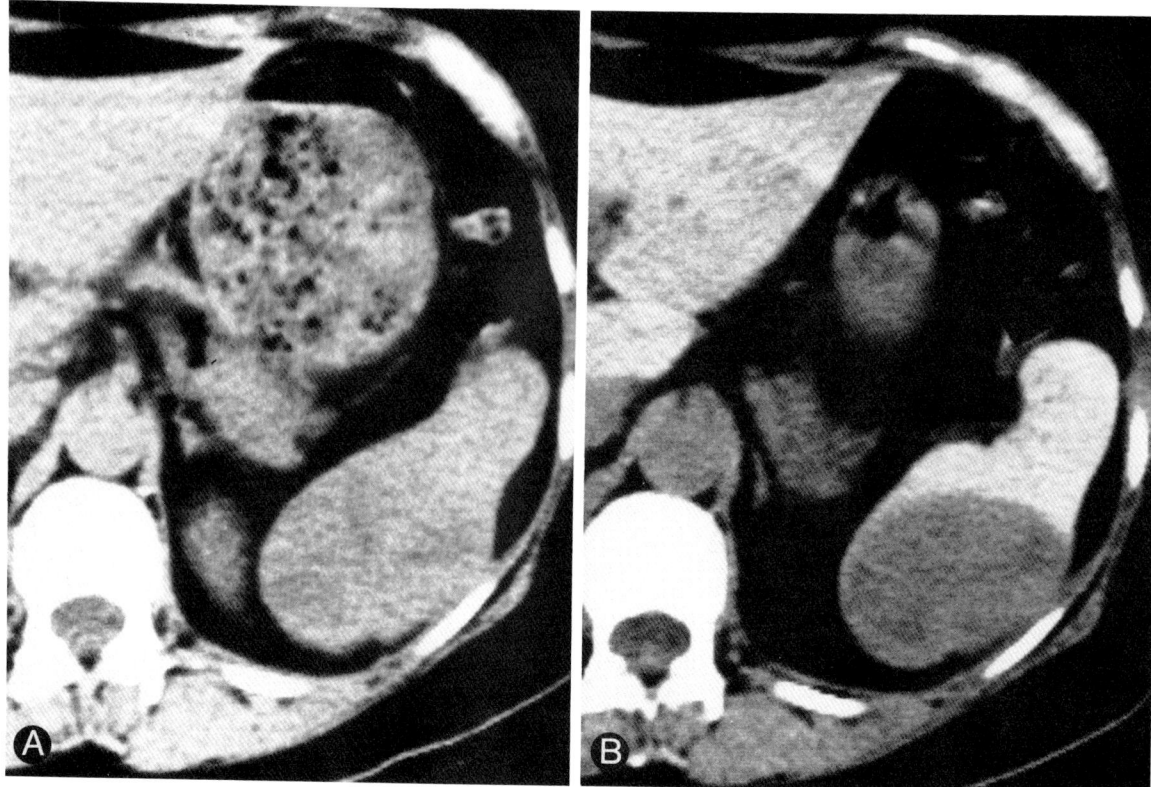

FIGURE 27.37. METASTATIC OVARIAN CARCINOMA: CT WITH EOE
A: Unenhanced CT shows subtle inhomogeneity. B: Enhanced CT clearly shows a well-demarcated, low attenuation mass.

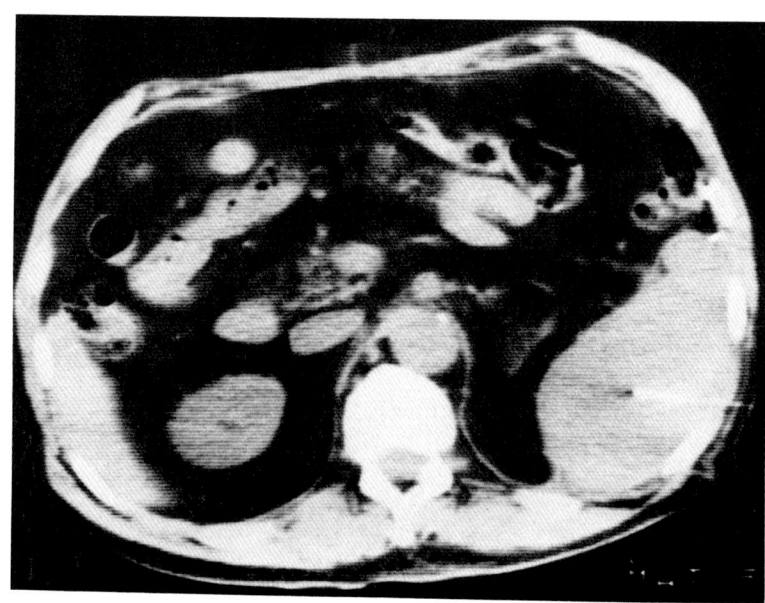

FIGURE 27.38. METASTATIC MELANOMA: CT, NEEDLE BIOPSY
An aspiration biopsy done under CT guidance diagnosed metastatic melanoma. The procedure was performed without complication (Courtesty of Dr. Eric Van Sonnenberg, San Francisco, Calif.)

mal liver-spleen radionuclide scan. Mittelstaedt demonstrated a focal sonodense lesion due to metastatic ovarian carcinoma (in the absence of hepatic metastasis) (142).

Piekarski et al. (138) reported 10 cases of splenic metastasis on computed tomography (Fig. 27.36C); 8 of 10 had no hepatic lesions on CT (4 of which had surgical or autopsy confirmation) and only 1 had associated retroperitoneal adenopathy. All lesions were of lower attenuation than surrounding spleen (average 25 HU lower) prior to contrast infusion. Two had cystic metastases with attenuation values near zero. In 2 of 10 the lesions were seen only after injection of intravenous contrast (Fig. 27.37). Seven were multiple and 3 single or confluent. Although only 4 of 10 had confirmation by surgery or autopsy, the lack of hepatic involvement in the majority of cases suggests that Marymount was correct in assuming that splenic metastasis need not be a preterminal event.

Metastatic nodules can exhibit irregular shapes probably due to regions of necrosis (78). Areas of water density also probably represent necrosis with liquefaction (78). This would correspond to the pathologic findings described by Marymount above; only large nodular metastases showed evidence of necrosis.

With the advent of percutaneous splenic needle biopsy, CT guided diagnostic studies can be performed (Fig. 27.38).

Given the varied sonographic and CT appearances, it would be interesting to correlate the radiologic findings with the microscopic locations described by Marymount, but such pathologic-radiologic correlation studies have not yet been done. In evaluating patients for metastatic disease, the spleen is often glanced over once hepatic metastases have been excluded. The reported cases of solitary splenic metastases indicate that the spleen deserves full attention in the metastatic workup.

REFERENCES

1. McClure RD, Altemeier WA: Cysts of the spleen. *Ann Surg* 116:98–102, 1942.
2. Fowler RH: Collective review: nonparasitic benign cystic tumors of the spleen. *Int Abstr Surg* 96:209–227, 1953.
3. Qureshi MA, Hafner CD: Clinical manifestations of splenic cysts: study of seventy-five cases. *Am Surg* 31:605–608, 1965.
4. Martin JW: Congenital splenic cysts. *Am J Surg* 96:302–308, 1958.
5. Garvin DF, King FM: Cysts of the nonlymphomatous tumors of the spleen. *Pathol Annu* 16:61–80, 1981.
6. Doolas A, Nolte M, McDonald OG, Economou SG: Splenic cysts. *J Surg Oncol* 10:369–387, 1978.
7. Sirinek KR, Evans WE: Nonparasitic splenic cysts: case report of epidermoid cyst with review of the literature. *Am J Surg* 126:8–13, 1973.
8. Montgomery AH, McEnery ET, Frank AA: Epidermoid cysts of the spleen. *Ann Surg* 108:877, 1938.
9. Griscom NT, Hargreaves HK, Schwartz MZ, Reddish MJ, Colodny AH: Huge splenic cyst in a newborn: comparison with 10 cases in later childhood and adolescence. *AJR* 129:889–891, 1977.
10. Allen RP, Condon VR: Epidermoid cysts of the spleen in children. *Am J Surg* 99:242, 1960.
11. Griscom NT: High splenic cysts. *Am J Dis Child* 109:224, 1965.
12. Gilmartin MB: Familial multiple epidermoid cysts of the spleen. *Conn Med* 42:295–300, 1978.
13. Ross ME, Ellwood R, Yang SS, Lucas RJ: Epidermoid splenic cysts. *Arch Surg* 112:596–599, 1977.
14. Lambie RW, Rubin S, Halperin PH: Epidermoid cyst of the spleen. *Missouri Med* 60:27, 1963.
15. Blank E, Campbell JR: Epidermoid cysts of the spleen. *Pediatrics* 51:75–83, 1973.
16. Park JY, Song KT: Splenic cyst: a case report and review of literature. *Am Surg* 37:544–547, 1971.
17. Qureshi MA, Hafner CD: Clinical manifestations of splenic cysts: study of seventy-five cases. *Am Surg* 31:605, 1965.
18. Economides NG, Benton BF, Fortner TM, Miles RM: Splenic pseudocysts: report of two cases and review of the literature. *Am Surg* 46:644–648, 1980.
19. Dibble JB, Weigent CE: Epidermoid cyst of the spleen presenting as an abdominal emergency. *JAMA* 194:1144–1146, 1965.
20. Bhimiji SD, Cooperberg PL, Naiman S, Morrison RT, Shergill P: Ultrasound diagnosis of splenic cysts. *Radiology* 122:787–789, 1977.
21. Tsakraklides T, Hadley TW: Epidermoid cysts of the spleen. *Arch Pathol* 96:251–254, 1973.
22. Steidl RM, Cardy JD: Solitary cyst of spleen associated with hypersplenism: report of case. *Lancet* 77:45, 1957.
23. Salky B, Zimmerman M, Bauer J, Gelernt I, Kneel I: Splenic cyst—definitive treatment by laparoscopy. *Gastrointest Endosc* 31:213–215, 1985.
24. Wright FW, Williams EW: Large post-traumatic splenic cyst diagnosed by radiology, isotope scintigraphy and ultrasound. *Br J Radiol* 47:454, 1974.
25. Cave RH, Garvin DF, Doohen DJ: Metaplastic mesodermal cyst of the spleen. *Am Surg* 37:97, 1971.
26. Beneke J: Cited by Fowler RH, in cystic tumors of the spleen. *Int Abstr Surg* 70:213, 1940.
27. Pepere A: Sui i'origine della cesti multiple della milza. *Policlin Roma* 19:335, 1912.
28. Frank LW: Solitary cysts of the spleen. *South Med J* 23:212–216, 1930.
29. Dachman AH, Ros PR, Murari PJ, Olmstead WW, Lichtenstein JE: Nonparasitic splenic cysts: a report of 52 cases with pathologic radiologic correlation. *AJR* (in press).
30. King MC, Glick BW, Freed A: The diagnosis of splenic cysts. *Surg Gynecol Obstet* 127:509–512, 1968.
31. Lewis H: Epidermoid cyst of the spleen. *Am J Surg* 99:242, 1960.
32. Dennen EV: Hemorrhagic cyst of the spleen. *Ann Surg* 116:103–108, 1942.
33. Propper RA, Weinstein BJ, Skolnick ML, Kisloff B: Ultrasonography of hemorrhagic splenic cysts. *J Clin Ultrasound* 7:18–20, 1979.
34. Spencer GR: A wandering cystic spleen. *J R Coll Surg Edinb* 27:183–185, 1982.
35. Bron KM, Hoffman WJ: Preoperative diagnosis of splenic cysts. *Arch Surg* 102:459–461, 1971.
36. Shanser JD, Moss AA, Clark RE, Palubinskas AJ: Angiographic evaluation of cystic lesions of the spleen. *AJR* 119:166–174, 1973.
37. Davidson ED, Campbell WG, Hersh T: Epidermoid splenic cyst occurring in an intrapancreatic accessory spleen. *Dig Dis Sci* 25:964–967, 1980.
38. Faer MJ, Lynch RD, Lichtenstein JE, Madewell JE, Feigin DS: RPC from the AFIP. *Radiology* 134:371–376, 1980.
39. Shin MS, Ho K: Mesodermal cyst of the spleen: computed tomographic characteristics and pathogenetic

considerations. *J Comput Tomogr* 7:295–299, 1983.
40. Piekarski J, Federle MP, Moss AA: Computed tomography of the spleen. *Radiology* 135:683–689, 1980.
41. Lawhorne TW, Zuidema GD: Splenic abscess. *Surgery* 79:686–689, 1976.
42. Freund R, Pichl J, Heyder N, Rdl W, Reiman JF: Splenic abscess—clinical symptoms and diagnostic possibilities. *Am J Gastroenterol* 77:35–38, 1982.
43. Miller FJ, Rothermel FJ, O'Neil MF, Shochat SJ: Clinical and roentgenographic findings in splenic abscess. *Arch Surg* 111:1156–1159, 1976.
44. Simson JNL: Solitary abscess of the spleen. *Br J Surg* 67:106–110, 1980.
45. Chulay JD, Lankerani MR: Splenic abscess: report of 10 cases and review of the literature. *Am J Med* 61:513–522, 1976.
46. Blumer G: Subacute bacterial endocarditis. *Medicine* 2:105, 1923.
47. Gangahar DM, Delany HM: Intrasplenic abscess: two case reports and review of the literature. *Am Surg* 47:488–491, 1981.
48. Abu-Dallo KI, Manny Y, Penchas S, Eyal Z: Clinical manifestations of splenic abscess. *Arch Surg* 110:281–283, 1975.
49. Pawar S, Kay CJ, Gonzaley R, Taylor KHW, Rosenfield AT: Sonography of splenic abscess. *AJR* 138:259–262, 1982.
50. Freeman MH, Tarkin AK: Focal splenic defects. *Radiology* 121:689–692, 1976.
51. Henkin RE: Selected topics in inter-abdominal imaging via nuclear medicine techniques. *Radiol Clin North Am* 17:39–54, 1975.
52. Coopersmith A, Richey AK, Zinkham WH: Fever of unknown origin and the value of gallium-67 and technetium-99m for defining abnormality of the spleen. *Johns Hopkins Med J* 137:51–54, 1975.
53. Jacobs RP, Shanser JE, Lawson DL, Palubinskas AJ: Angiography of splenic abscess. *AJR* 122:419–424, 1974.
54. Ralls PW, Quinn MF, Collitti P, Lapin SA, Halls J: Sonography of pyogenic splenic abscess. *AJR* 138:523–525, 1982.
55. Moss M, Kirschner L, Peerebaum G, Ferris RA: CT demonstration of a splenic abscess not evident at surgery. *AJR* 135:159–160, 1980.
56. Chiu LC, Young CS, Yiu VS, Shapiro RL: Computed tomographic scanning of the left upper quadrant and left flank: advantages and pitfalls. *Comput Tomogr* 3:220–238, 1979.
57. Bostick WL: Primary splenic neoplasms. *Am J Pathol* 21:1143–1165, 1945.
58. Burke JS: Surgical pathology of the spleen: an approach to the differential diagnosis of splenic lymphomas and leukemias. *Am J Surg Pathol* 5:551–563, 1961.
59. Kim H, Dorfman RF: Morphological studies of 84 untreated patients subjected to laparotomy for the staging of non-Hodgkin's lymphomas. *Cancer* 33:557–647, 1974.
60. Kadin ME, Glatstein E, Dorfman RF: Clinicopathologic studies of 117 untreated patients subjected to laparotomy for the staging of Hodgkin's disease. *Cancer* 27:1277–1294, 1971.
61. Ahmann DL, Kiely JM, Harrison EG Jr, Payne WS: Malignant lymphoma of the spleen. A review of 49 cases in which the diagnosis was made at splenectomy. *Cancer* 19:461–469, 1966.
62. Milder MS, Larson SM, Bagley CM, DeVitta VT, Johnson RE, Johnston GS: Liver-spleen scan in Hodgkin's disease. *Cancer* 31:826–834, 1973.
63. Richman SD, Levenson SM, Jones AE, Johnston GS: Radionuclide studies in Hodgkin's disease. *Semin Nucl Med* 5:103–118, 1975.
64. Castellino RA, Silverman JF, Glatstein E, Blank N, Wexler L: Splenic arteriography in Hodgkin's disease: a roentgenotogic-pathologic study of 33 consecutive untreated patients. *AJR* 114:574–582, 1972.
65. Carroll BA: Ultrasound of lymphoma. *Semin Ultrasound* 3:114–122, 1982.
66. Glazer GM, Axel K, Goldberg HI, Moss AA: Dynamic CT of the normal spleen. *AJR* 137:343–346, 1981.
67. Glatstein E, Guernsey JM, Rosenberg SA, Kaplan HS: The value of laparotomy and splenectomy in the staging of Hodgkin's disease. *Cancer* 24:709–718, 1969.
68. Slanina J, Wannenmacher M, Heidmann S: Risk of infection following iatrogenic asplenia—a study of the indications for exploratory laparotomy with splenectomy for Hodgkin's disease (German, English abstract). *Strahlentherapic* 158:395–404, 1982.
69. Worthy TS: Evaluation of diagnostic laparotomy and splenectomy in Hodgkin's disease. *Clin Radiol* 32:523–525, 1981.
70. Stein RS: Saturday conference: Hodgkin's lymphoma. *South Med J* 71:1261–1268, 1978.
71. Kaplan HS: *Hodgkin's Disease*, Ed 2. Cambridge, Mass., Harvard University Press, 1980, pp 114, 282.
72. Carroll BA, Ta HN: The ultrasonic appearance of extranodal abdominal lymphoma. *Radiology* 135:419–425, 1980.
73. Cunningham JJ: Ultrasonic findings in isolated lymphoma of the spleen simulating splenic abscess. *J Clin Ultrasound* 6:412–414, 1978.
74. Bloom RA, Freund U, Perkes EH, Weiss Y: Acute Hodgkin's disease masquerading as splenic abscess. *J Surg Oncol* 17:279–282, 1981.
75. Zornoza J, Ginaldi S: Computed tomography in hepatic lymphoma. *Radiology* 138:405–410, 1981.
76. Breiman RS, Castellino RA, Harell GS, Marshall WH, Glatstein E, Kaplan HS: CT-pathologic correlations in Hodgkin's disease and non-Hodgkin's lymphoma. *Radiology* 126:159–166, 1978.
77. Goffinet DR, Castellino RA, Dorfman L: Staging laparotomies in un-selected patients with non-Hodgkin's lymphoma. *Cancer* 32:672–681, 1973.
78. Koehler RE: Spleen. In Lee JK, Sagal SRJ (eds): *Computed Body Tomography*. New York, Raven Press, 1983, Ch 9, pp 243–256.
79. Krudy AG, Dunnick NR, Magrath IT, Shawker TH, Doppman JL, Speigel R: CT of American Burkitt lymphoma. *AJR* 136:747–754, 1981.
80. Thomas JL, Bernardino ME, Vermess M, Barnes PA et al: EOE-13 in the detection of hepatosplenic lymphoma. *Radiology* 145:629–634, 1982.
81. Birch SJ, Garvie NW: Splenic accumulation of technetium 99m methyl diphosphonate in non-Hodgkin's lymphoma. *Br J Radiol* 53:161–163, 1980.
82. Kishikawa T, Numaguchi Y, Watanabe K, Matsuura K: Angiographic diagnosis of benign and malignant splenic tumors. *AJR* 130:339–344, 1978.
83. Johnson K, Lunderquist A: Angiography of the liver and spleen in Hodgkin's disease. *AJR* 121:789–792, 1974.
84. Hushi EA: The clinical course of splenic hemangioma. *Arch Surg* 83:681–685, 1961.
85. Fowler RH: Collective review: non-parasitic benign cystic tumors of the spleen. *Int Abstr Surg* 96:209–227, 1953.
86. Garvin DF, King FM: Cysts and nonlymphomatous tumors of the spleen. *Pathol Annu* 16(Part I):61–80, 1981.
87. Pitlik S, Cohen L, Hadar H, Srulijes B, Rosenfeld JB:

Portal hypertension and esophageal varices in hemangiomatosis of the spleen. *Gastroenterology* 72:937–940, 1977.
88. Dadash-Zadeh M, Czapek EE, Schwartz AD: Skeletal and splenic hemangiomatosis with consumptive coagulopathic response to splenectomy. *Pediatrics* 57:803–806, 1976.
89. Segal I, Fancourt MN, Decker GAG, Hodkinson KJ: Cavernous hemangioma of the spleen. *S Afr Med J* 51:637–638, 1977.
90. Enzinger FM, Weiss SW (eds): *Soft Tissue Tumors*. St. Louis, C. V. Mosby, 1983.
91. Macpherson AIS: The spleen: cysts and tumors. *Br J Hosp Med* 24:413–416, 1980.
92. Ros PR, Murari P, Dachman AH: Hemangioma of the spleen (in preparation).
93. Halgrimson CG, Rustad DG, Zeligman BE: Calcified hemangioma of the spleen. *JAMA* 252:2959–2960, 1984.
94. Paivansalo M, Siniluoto T: Cavernous hemangioma of the spleen. *Fortschr Rontgenstr* 142:228–230, 1985.
95. Chen KTK, Bolles JC, Gilbert EF: Angiosarcoma of the spleen. *Arch Pathol Lab Med* 103:122–124, 1979.
96. Mahony B, Jeffrey RB, Federle MP: Spontaneous rupture of hepatic and splenic angiosarcoma demonstrated by CT. *AJR* 138:965–966, 1982.
97. Smith VC, Eisenberg BL, McDonald EC: Primary splenic angiosarcoma: case report on literature review. *Cancer* 55:1625–1627, 1985.
98. Sordillo EM, Sordillo PP, Hajdu SI: Primary hemangiosarcoma of the spleen: report of four cases. *Med Pediatr Oncol* 9:314–324, 1981.
99. Arbona GL, Lloyd TV, Lucas J, Sharma HM: Computed tomographic demonstration of angiosarcoma of the spleen. *South Med J* 75:348–350, 1982.
100. Kiskikawa T, Numaguchi Y, Tokunaga M, Matsuura K: Hemangiosarcoma of the spleen with liver metastasis: angiographic manifestations. *Radiology* 123:31–35, 1977.
101. Garvin DF, King FM: Cysts and nonlymphomatous tumors of the spleen. *Pathol Annu* 16 (Part I): 61–80, 1981.
102. Langhans T: Pulsating cavernous neoplasm of spleen with metastatic nodules to the liver. *Virchows Arch [Pathol Anat]* 75:273–291, 1879.
103. Locker GY, Doroshow JH, Zwelling LA, Chabner BA: The clinical features of hepatic angiosarcoma: a report of four cases and a review of the English literature. *Medicine* 58:48–64, 1979.
104. Iozzo RV, Haas JER, Chard RL: Symptomatic splenic hamartoma: a report of two cases and review of the literature. *Pediatrics* 66:261–265, 1980.
105. Wexler L, Abrams HL: Hamartoma of the spleen: angiographic observations. *AJR* 92:1150–1155, 1964.
106. Morgenstern L, McCafferty L, Rosenberg J, Michel SL: Hamartomas of the spleen. *Arch Surg* 119:1291–1293, 1984.
107. Shalev O, Ariel I: Hamartoma of the spleen. *Isr J Med Sci* 14:862–864, 1978.
108. Rappaport H: The pathologic anatomy of the splenic red pulp. In Lennert K, Harms D (eds): *Spleen: Structure, Function, Pathology, Clinical Aspects, Therapy*. Berlin, Springer-Verlag, 1970, pp 24–41.
109. Teats CD, Seale DL, Allen MS: Hamartoma of the spleen. *AJR* 116:419–422, 1972.
110. Komaki S, Gombas OF: Angiographic demonstration of a calcified splenic hamartoma. *Radiology* 121:77–78, 1978.
111. Kishikawa T, Numagudi Y, Watanabe K, Matsuura K: Angiographic diagnosis of benign and malignant splenic tumors. *AJR* 130:339–344, 1978.
112. Spalding RM, Jennings CV, Yam LT: Splenic hamartoma. *Br J Radiol* 53:1197–120, 1980.
113. Dachman AH, Murari P, Ros P: Lymphangioma and hamartoma of the spleen (in preparation).
114. Brinkley AA, Lee JKT: Cystic hamartoma of the spleen: CT and sonographic findings. *J Clin Ultrasound* 9:136–138, 1981.
115. Fink F: Zur Kenntuis der geschwulstbildungen in der milz. *Z Heilk* 6:399, 1885.
116. Fowler RH: Nonparasitic benign cystic tumors of the spleen. *Int Abstr Surg* 96:209–227, 1953.
117. Asch MJ, Cohen AH, Moore TC: Hepatic and splenic lymphangiomatosis with skeletal involvement: report of a case and review of the literature. *Surgery* 76:334–339, 1974.
118. Pearl GS, Nassar VH: Cystic lymphangioma of the spleen. *South Med J* 72:667–669, 1979.
119. Bill AH, Sumner DS: Unified concept of lymphangioma and cystic hygroma. *Surg Gynecol Obstet* 120:79–86, 1965.
120. Cornaglia-Ferraris P, Perlino GF, Barabino A, Soave F, Oliva L: A pediatric case of cystic lyphangioma of the spleen. *J Comput Assist Tomogr* 5:449–450, 1981.
121. Avigad S, Jaffe R, Frand M, Izhak Y, Rotem Y: Lymphangiomatosis with splenic involvement. *JAMA* 236:2315–2317, 1976.
122. Tuttle RJ, Minielly JA: Splenic cystic lymphangiomatosis. *Radiology* 126:47–48, 1978.
123. Willis RA: *Pathology of Tumors*. London, Butterworth, 1948, p 712.
124. Dietz WH, Stuart MJ: Splenic consumptive coagulopathy in a patient with disseminated lymphangiomatosis. *J Pediatr* 90:421–423, 1977.
125. Shauberge JN, Tanaka K, Gruhl MC: Chronic consumption coagulopathy due to hemangiomatous transformation of the spleen. *Am J Clin Pathol* 56:723–729, 1971.
126. Landing BH, Farber S: Tumors of the cardiovascular system. In: *Atlas of Tumor Pathology*. Washington, D.C., Armed Forces Institute of Pathology, 1956.
127. Enzinger FM, Weiss SW (eds): *Soft Tissue Tumors*. St. Louis, C. V. Mosby, 1983, p 485.
128. Pyatt RS, Williams ED, Clark M, Gaskins R: CT diagnosis of splenic cystic lymphangiomatosis. *J Comput Assist Tomogr* 5:446–448, 1981.
129. Uflacker R: Cystic lymphangioma of the spleen. A cause of splenomegaly. *Br J Radiol* 52:148–149, 1979.
130. Anderson WAD, Kissone JM (eds): *Pathology*, Ed 7. St. Louis, C. V. Mosby, 1977, vol 2, p 1504.
131. Federle M, Moss AA: Computer tomography of the spleen. *CRC Crit Rev Diagn Imaging* 19:1–16, 1983.
132. Warren S, Davis AH: Studies on tumor metastasis: the metastases of carcinoma to the spleen. *Am J Cancer* 21:517, 1934.
133. Marymont JH Jr, Gross S: Patterns of metastatic cancer in the spleen. *Am J Clin Pathol* 40:58–66, 1963.
134. Rydell WB Jr, Ellis R: Spontaneous rupture of the spleen from metastatic carcinoma. *JAMA* 240:53–54, 1978.
135. Robbins SL, Cotran RS (eds): *Pathologic Basis of Disease*, Ed 2. Philadelphia, W. B. Saunders, 1979.
136. Shawker TH: Tumor invasion and dissemination. In Brascho DJ, Shawker TH (eds): *Abdominal Ultrasound in the Cancer Patient*. New York, John Wiley & Sons, 1980, pp 49–92.
137. Freeman MH, Tonkin AK: Focal splenic defects. *Radiology* 121:689–692, 1976.

138. Piekarski J, Federle MP, Moss AA, London S: Computed tomography of the spleen. *Radiology* 135:683–689, 1980.
139. Ibrahim NBN, Briggs JC, Jeyasingham K, Owen JR: Metastasizing thymoma. *Thorax* 37:371–373, 1982.
140. Mets T, Van Hove W, Louis H: Pseudomyxoma peritonei: report of a case with extraperitoneal metastasis and invasion of the spleen. *Chest* 72:792–794, 1977.
141. Murphy JF, Bernardino ME: The sonographic findings of splenic metastases. *J Clin Ultrasound* 7:195–197, 1979.
142. Mittelstaedt CA, Partain CL: Ultrasonic-pathologic classification of splenic abnormalities: gray-scale patterns. *Radiology* 134:697–705, 1980.

28

Diffuse Diseases

ABRAHAM H. DACHMAN, M.D., AND DONNA MAGID, M.D.

SPLENOMEGALY

Normal spleen size and shape is variable and presents a difficulty in defining splenomegaly. One formula used for approximate normal splenic size in children is $L = 5.7 + 0.31A$ where L is the length of the spleen in centimeters and A is the age in years (1). Maximum splenic weight and size is reached at puberty. In adults, average splenic weight is 150 g, but is related somewhat to body weight and decreases slightly with increasing age. Splenomegaly can be divided into mild (less than 500 g), moderate (500–1000 g) or massive (greater than 1000 g) (21).

The diagnosis of splenomegaly is not always obvious. A normal spleen may be palpable, and a mildly enlarged diseased spleen is not necessarily palpable. In one study, 3% of normal young adults had palpable spleens (3). In children, the spleen is palpable in 10% (4). Splenomegaly may present acutely in splenic crisis due to malaria with blackwater fever and in sickle cell anemia (5). Spontaneous rupture may occur with marked splenomegaly (see Chapter 26). Conversely, splenomegaly may be relatively asymptomatic, for example, when due to portal hypertension or in congestive splenomegaly due to splenic vein thrombosis (6). "Adhesive splenomegaly" is reported as a rare cause of colon obstruction reported in a patient with chronic lymphocytic leukemia who developed perisplenic adhesions, probably due to a previous subcapsular hematoma (7).

The differential diagnosis of splenomegaly is extensive and can be categorized in a variety of ways (5). Table 28.1 lists some examples of splenomegaly. Many of these entities, such as splenic neoplasms and infarcts, usually show focal or inhomogeneous lesions in the spleen and are discussed in Chapters 27 and 29. Other diseases usually manifest with nonspecific splenomegaly and the diagnosis is made on clinical or laboratory data.

Once splenomegaly is suspected, the history, physical examination, and peripheral blood smear will direct the diagnostic approach. An algorithm for the workup of splenomegaly has been suggested by Eichner (6, 8).

The radiographic methods of measuring splenic size and volume discussed in Chapter 24 include the use of nuclear scintigraphy, sonography, and CT. In some cases of splenomegaly, there may be increased uptake of ^{99m}Tc-sulfur colloid in the spleen (a "reversed ratio") (9). Massive splenomegaly ("giant splenomegaly," i.e., 10 times normal weight (10)) helps limit the differential diagnosis. Some causes of giant splenomegaly include: myeloproliferative disorders, hairy cell leukemia, chronic myelogenous leukemia, Gaucher's disease, Niemann-Pick's disease, chronic malaria, leishmaniasis, congenital syphilis, long-standing thalassemia major, sarcoid, and chronic congestive splenomegaly (2, 9).

The therapy for splenomegaly will depend on the underlying etiology. Splenectomy may be done to stage the disease (e.g., lymphoma), control the disease (e.g., hereditary spherocytosis), and control hypersplenism or disease-related symptoms (e.g., varices due to splenic vein thrombosis). In considering splenectomy, one must evaluate the severity, chronicity and progression of hypersplenism, age of the patient, concurrent illness and therapeutic alternatives (11). Data on the effectiveness of splenectomy must be evaluated individually for each disease. For example, splenectomy is preferred for hairy cell leukemia (12), whereas splenectomy for Felty's syndrome is controversial (6).

Myeloproliferative Disorders/Leukemia

Myeloproliferative disorders associated with massive splenomegaly include chronic myelogenous leukemia and myelofibrosis (agnogenic myeloid metaplasia). Acute leukemia is common in children, whereas chronic leukemia is more common in adults. Chronic lymphocytic leuke-

TABLE 28.1.
SPLENOMEGALY

I. *Congestive Splenomegaly* 　Heart failure 　Portal hypertension 　Cirrhosis 　Cystic fibrosis 　Banti syndrome 　Splenic vein obstruction I. *Neoplasms* 　Leukemia 　Lymphoma 　Rare splenic neoplasms 　Metastases III. *Storage Disease* 　Gaucher's disease 　Neimann-Pick 　Amyloid 　Diabetes 　Gargoylism 　Histiocytosis 　Hemochromatosis IV. *Infections* 　Hepatitis 　Malaria 　Infectious mononucleosis 　Leishmaniasis 　Tuberculosis 　Typhoid 　Syphilis 　Echinococcus	V. *Hemolytic Anemias* 　Hemoglobinopathies 　Hereditary spherocytosis 　Primary neutropenia 　Thrombotic thrombocytopenic purpura VI. *Collagen Vascular* 　Systemic Lupus 　Rheumatoid 　Felty's syndrome VII. *Extramedullary Hematopoiesis* 　Osteopetrosis 　Myelofibrosis VIII. *Non-neoplastic Mass* 　Hematomas 　Abscess 　Congenital cyst 　Post-traumatic cyst IX. *Miscellaneous* 　Hypersensitivity state 　Porphyria 　Sarcoid 　Hemodialysis

mia (CLL) is the commonest form of adult leukemia in the United States. The diagnosis is made on examination of peripheral blood smears and bone marrow smears. The major radiologic manifestations are osseous. Splenomegaly may be seen on ^{99m}Tc-sulfur colloid scan (Fig. 28.1). The configuration of massive splenomegaly is variable, possibly due to the extensive variation in shape of the normal spleen (Figs. 28.2 and 28.3). Erythroleukemia (Fig. 28.3), is a rare variant of acute myelogenous leukemia which infrequently produces splenomegaly. It occurs with increased frequency following radiation or administration of cytotoxic drugs (11).

Passive Hyperemia/Fibrocongestive Splenomegaly

The common causes of chronic passive congestion are portal hypertension and congestive heart failure. Marked splenomegaly may accompany portal hypertension. The term "Banti's syndrome" was originally used to describe fibrosis of the malpighian corpuscles due to cirrhosis. It is now used to describe fibrocongestive splenomegaly with hypersplenism in association with gastrointestinal hemorrhage, with no pathologic findings in the liver, portal and splenic veins. The condition is also referred to as "idiopathic portal hypertension" (13).

The spleen is enlarged but uniform in texture (Fig. 28.4A–C). One should look for dilation of the splenic vein or associated varices (Fig. 28.5).

Sarcoidosis

Sarcoid is a disease with protean manifestations. About one-quarter of cases have hepatomegaly and splenomegaly and one-fifth of those with splenomegaly develop hypersplenism. Splenomegaly may occur even with a paucity of lesions elsewhere (Fig. 28.6) (14). Reports of focal defects on Tc-sulfur colloid scan may be due to infarcts and a pattern of multifocal defects due to sarcoid granulomas have been reported (15).

Gaucher's Disease

The two important lipid storage diseases are Niemann-Pick disease (sphingomyelin is stored) and Gaucher's disease (glucocerebroside is stored). They are due to hereditary absence of lysosomal enzymes necessary for glycolipid deg-

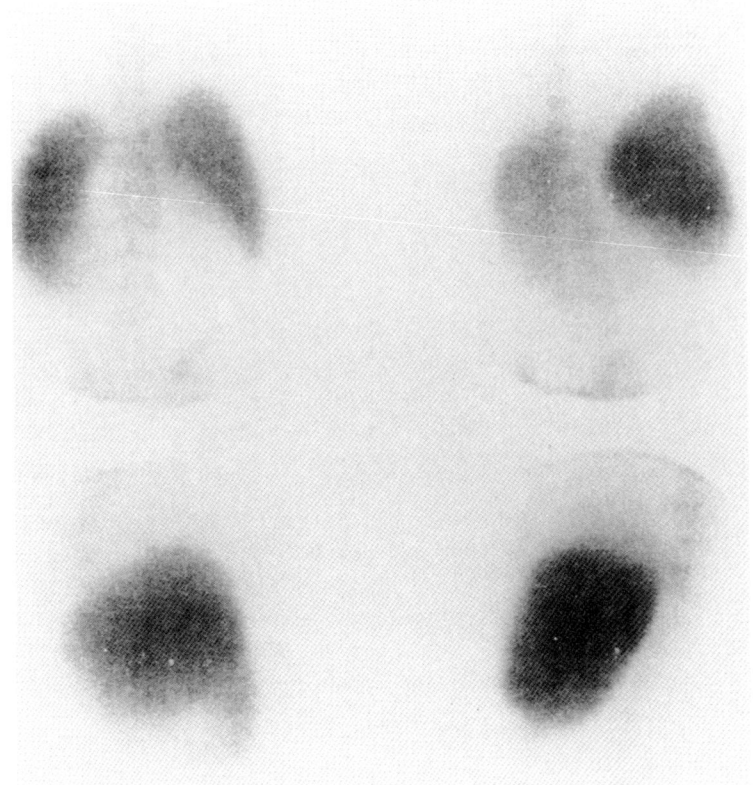

FIGURE 28.1. CHRONIC LYMPHOCYTIC LEUKEMIA: ^{99m}Tc-SULFUR COLLOID SCAN

Top row: Anterioposterior and left posterior oblique views. *Bottom row:* Left lateral and posterior views. Marked splenomegaly is present with a "colloid shift" causing visualization of the bones.

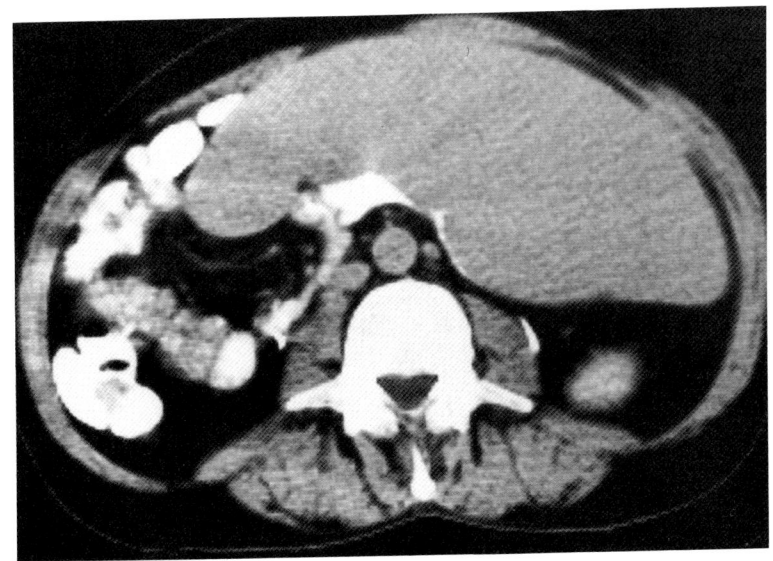

FIGURE 28.2. ACUTE LYMPHOCYTIC LEUKEMIA

CT scan shows a massively enlarged spleen, oriented predominantly transversely, crossing the midline and compressing adjacent contrast filled loops of bowel.

radation. Gaucher's disease may be of the chronic adult form (type 1) or rarely of the acute infantile neuronopathic form (type 2) which is fatal, or a juvenile form (type 3). The adult type has an increased frequency in Ashkenazic (European) Jews (16).

Glucocerebroside-laden macrophages accumulate predominantly in the spleen, liver and bone marrow resulting in massive hepato-splenomegaly, yellow-brown skin pigmentation, and widespread skeletal lesions ("Erlenmeyer flask" deformity, patchy demineralization with small

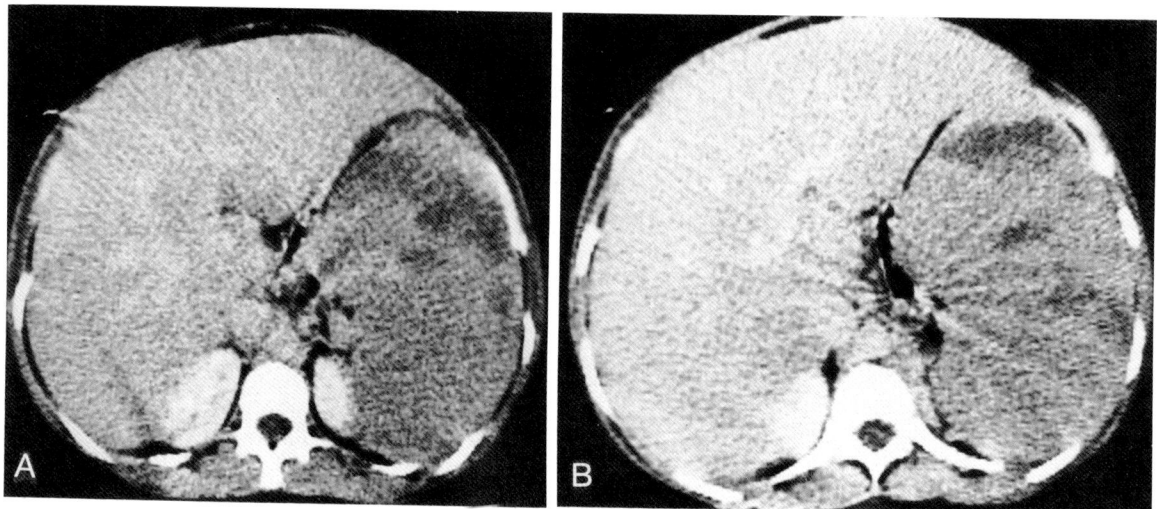

FIGURE 28.3. ERYTHROLEUKEMIA

A and *B:* A 23-yr-old patient with erythroleukemia, CT scan. Splenomegaly, oriented predominantly in an anterior-posterior fashion. The stomach and left kidney are compressed. Low attenuation foci probably represent infarcts.

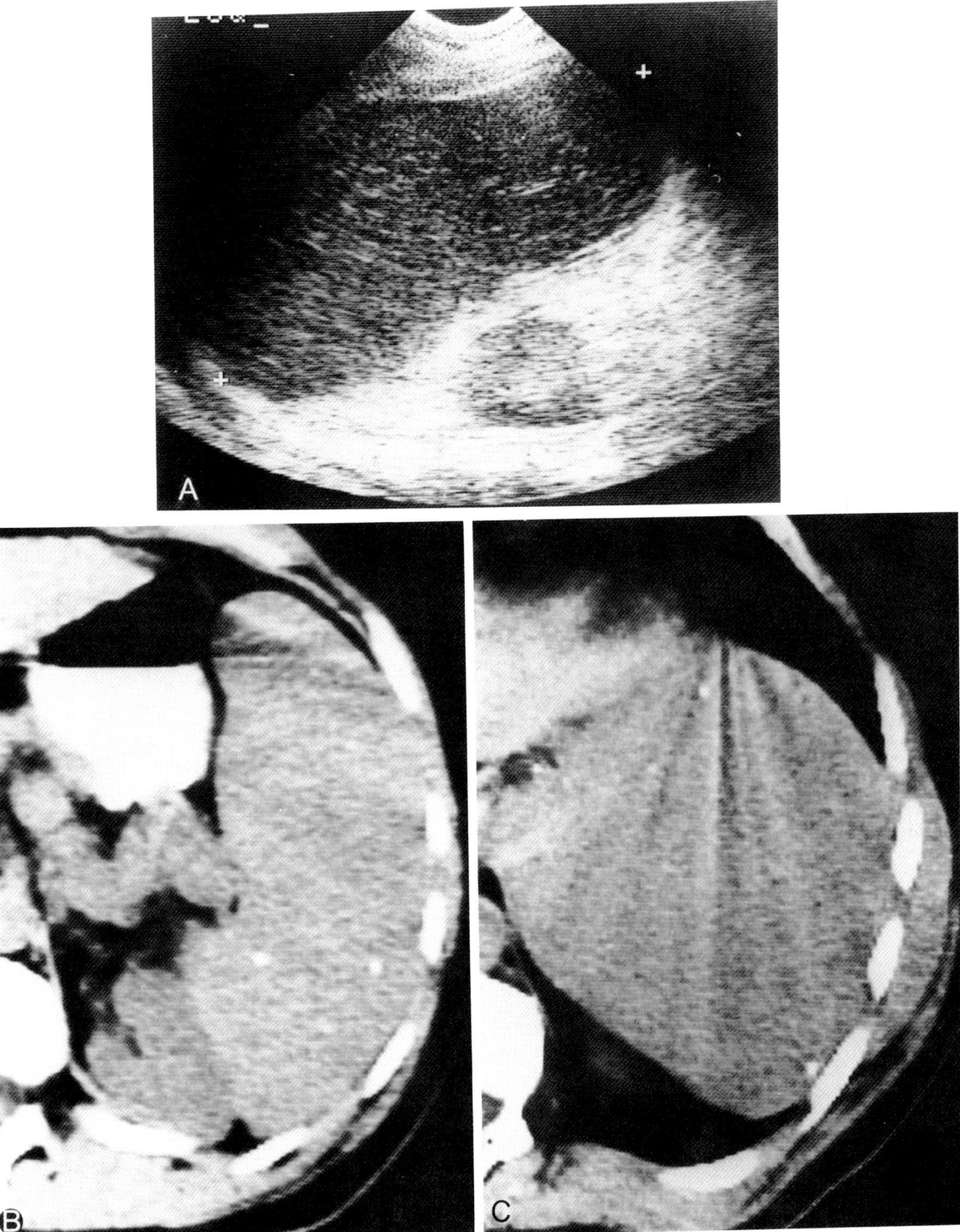

FIGURE 28.4. SPLENOMEGALY CURSORS

Portal hypertension with congestive splenomegaly. *A:* Sonogram: *Cursors* measure a 19 cm spleen in largest diameter (coronal view). *B* and *C:* Different patient with splenomegaly and a few incidental calcific granulomata on CT. Note orientation of the spleen in this patient causes marked renal compression, but the stomach is only minimally affected.

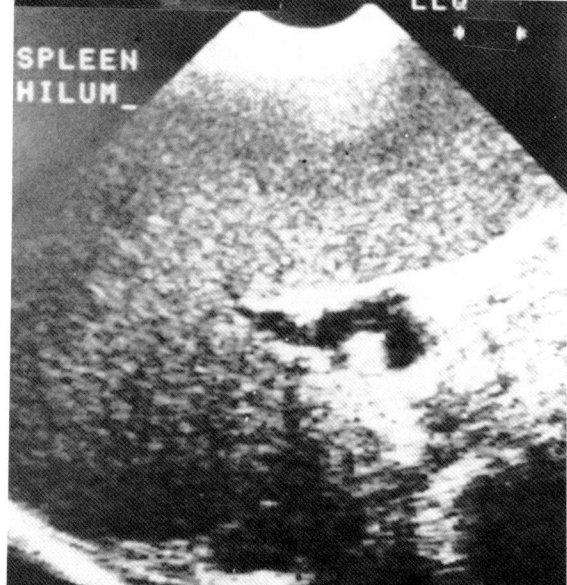

FIGURE 28.5. CONGESTIVE SPLENOMEGALY: SONOGRAM
The splenic hilus shows a prominent but patent splenic vein.

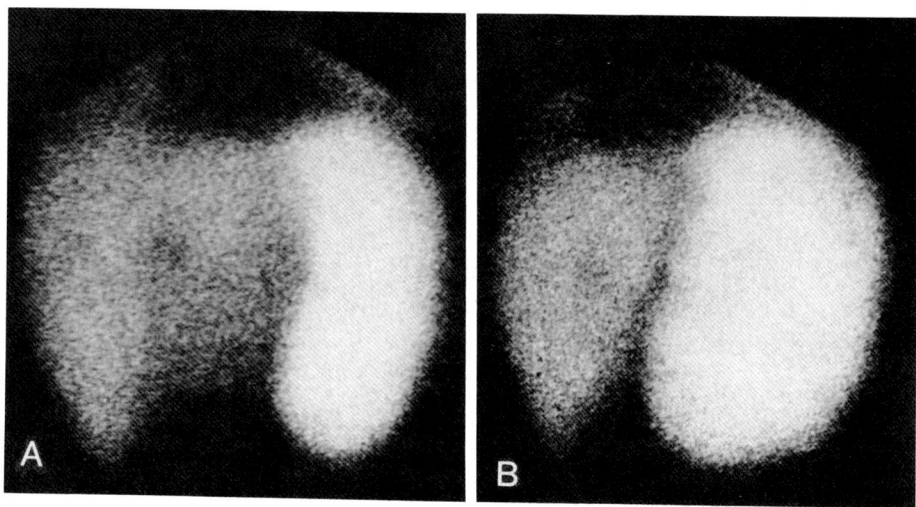

FIGURE 28.6. SARCOIDOSIS
^{99m}Tc-sulfur colloid scan shows splenomegaly with a colloid shift to the spleen. The liver is not significantly enlarged. *A:* Anterior; *B:* left posterior oblique views.

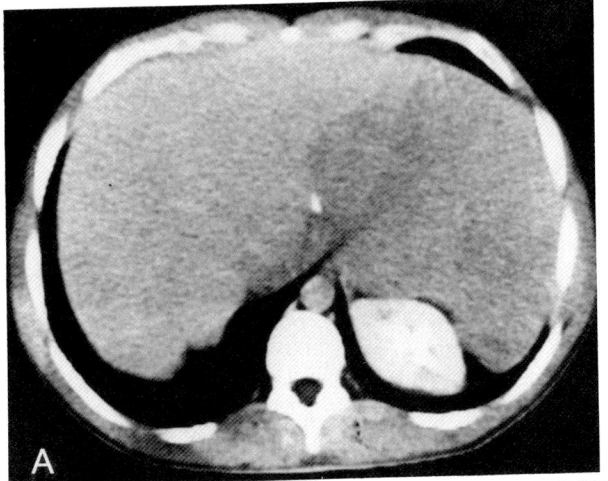
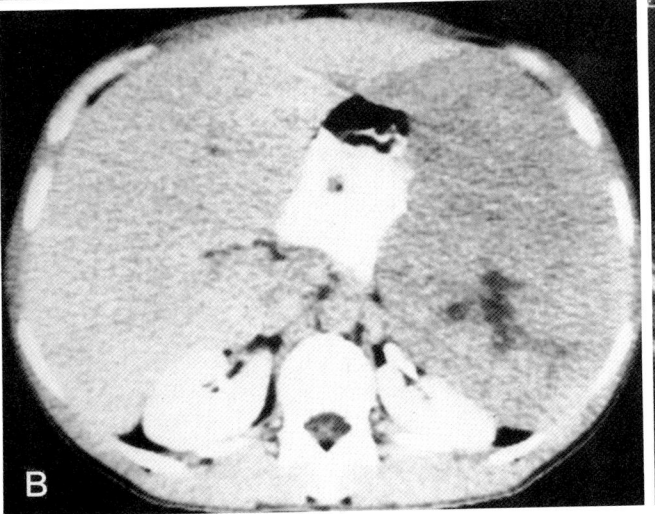
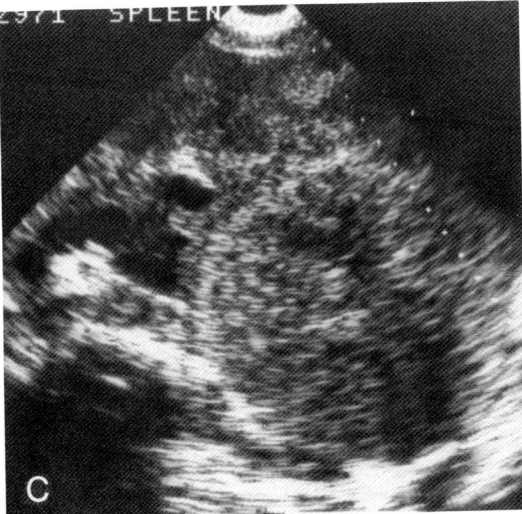

FIGURE 28.7. GAUCHER'S DISEASE, TYPE 1
A and *B:* Contrast-enhanced CT shows hepatosplenomegaly compressing bowel and both kidneys. Focal low attenuation defect in the spleen might represent an area of infarction. *C:* Sonogram: Hypoechoic foci correspond to low attenuation areas on CT.

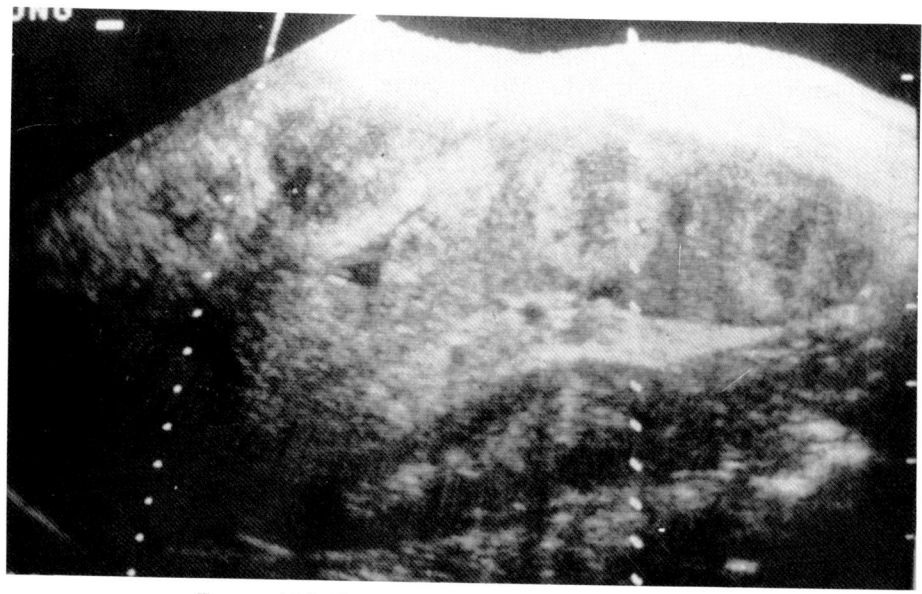

FIGURE 28.8. GAUCHER'S DISEASE TYPE 1: SONOGRAM
A different patient than seen in Figure 28.7. The spleen is enlarged, with focal inhomogenous echogenic foci. No pathologic correlation was available. (Courtesy of Dr. Leora Sachs.)

sharply demarcated lytic lesions, bone infarcts, fractures and in some chronic stages, bone sclerosis). Pulmonary involvement is uncommon, but may manifest as interstitial or diffuse reticulonodular disease (17). Splenectomy, which will alleviate the hypersplenism, has been reported to accelerate disease elsewhere, particularly the destructive bone lesions (18).

We have seen focal splenic defects in Gaucher's disease (Figs. 28.7 and 28.8). The intrasplenic defects are usually hypoechoic on sonography and less often hyperechoic (19). On pathologic examination, the lesions correspond to areas of accumulation of glucocerebroside (seen on cut gross as yellow deposits) as well as areas of infarction, fibrosis and occasionally extramedullary hematopoiesis with calcification (19). Factor IX deficiency and thrombocytopenia known to occur commonly in these patients (even without severe liver disease), as well as glucocerebroside deposition might predispose to splenic infarcts.

INFECTIONS

A variety of organisms can cause focal splenic abscess which is discussed in Chapter 27. Some infections may cause multiple microabscesses, granulomata or result in splenomegaly.

Infections causing splenomegaly include: malaria, infectious mononucleosis, leishmaniasis, trypanosomiasis (Chaga's disease), histoplasmosis, schistosomiasis, echinococcus, and congenital syphilis. "Tropical splenomegaly," also referred to as "big spleen syndrome," may be related to malarial infection (20). Diffuse microabscess formation is generally due to fungal infection, (usually candida), in immunocompromised hosts. Diffuse calcific granulomata are caused by tuberculosis and histoplasma. Some specific examples are discussed below.

Malaria

Malaria is a common cause of splenomegaly in endemic areas. The manifestations of the disease vary with the strain of *Plasmodium* infection. Typically hepatosplenomegaly is seen in chronic infection. Acute intravascular hemolytsis ("blackwater fever") is a rare complication of infection with *Plasmodium falciparium* which will cause acute splenomegaly (21). Anemia may be accompanied by leukopenia and thrombocytotopenia, and jaundice develops in some cases. When severe symptoms secondary to splenomegaly are present, splenectomy has been performed.

Infectious Mononucleosis

This acute infection caused by the Epstein-Barr virus usually affects young adults and manifests with fever, adenopathy, pharyngitis and splenomegaly. While marked splenomegaly may occur, it is the exception rather than the rule. Mild splenomegaly occurs around the second week of clinical illness in about 75% of patients (Fig. 28.9) (21). One of the rare complications of the disease is splenic rupture which may cause a fatal hemoperitoneum (22). Rupture may be preceded by minor subcapsular or focal perisplenic hemorrhage. CT or sonography are useful modalities to evaluate suspected rupture. Clinical signs such as tachycardia, hypotension, severe pain, peritoneal irritation and shifting dullness should strongly indicate rupture and a need for surgical intervention (21).

Schistosomiasis

Flukes such as schistosomiasis produce splenomegaly due to cirrhosis, perisplenic vein fibrosis and splenic vein thrombosis (21). Ultrasound has been used in these patients to evaluate the portal hypertension by measuring portal and splenic vein size (23). There is a positive correlation between portal pressures and sonographic measurements: In 13 patients studied, mean splenic vein diameter was 1.1 ± 0.22 cm (mean portal pressure 34.5 ± 12.7 cm saline) compared to normal control group showing splenic vein diameter of 0.75 ± 0.14 cm (pressure 10 ± 5 cm saline) (23). Ultrasound can detect splenic or portal vein thrombosis (24). A recent large series using ultrasound to study 103 patients with hepatosplenic *Schistosoma mansoni* showed splenomegaly in all cases and an echogenic nodular pattern throughout the spleen in 7 cases correlating with siderotic nodules (fibrosis around Gamna-Gandy bodies) (25). Ultrasound also commonly shows periportal fibrosis, hypertrophy of the left lobe of the liver with associated atrophy of the right lobe, thickening of the gallbladder wall, and echogenic hepatic nodules (25). Rarely, a large granuloma will appear as a solitary echogenic hepatic nodule.

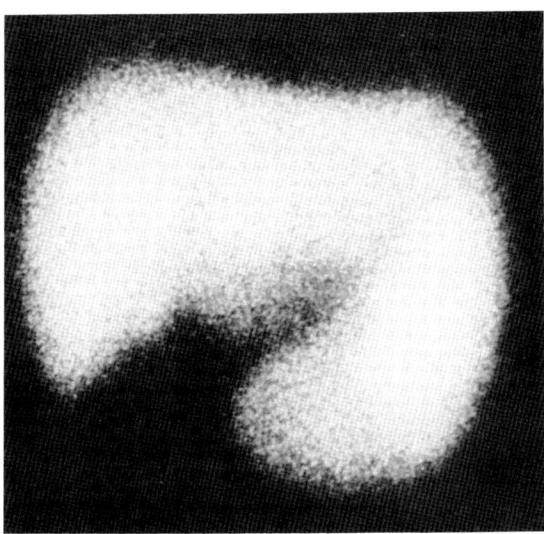

FIGURE 28.9. INFECTIOUS MONONUCLEOSIS: ^{99m}Tc-SULFUR COLLOID SCAN
Anterior view shows moderate splenomegaly without a colloid shift in a 17-yr-old male patient.

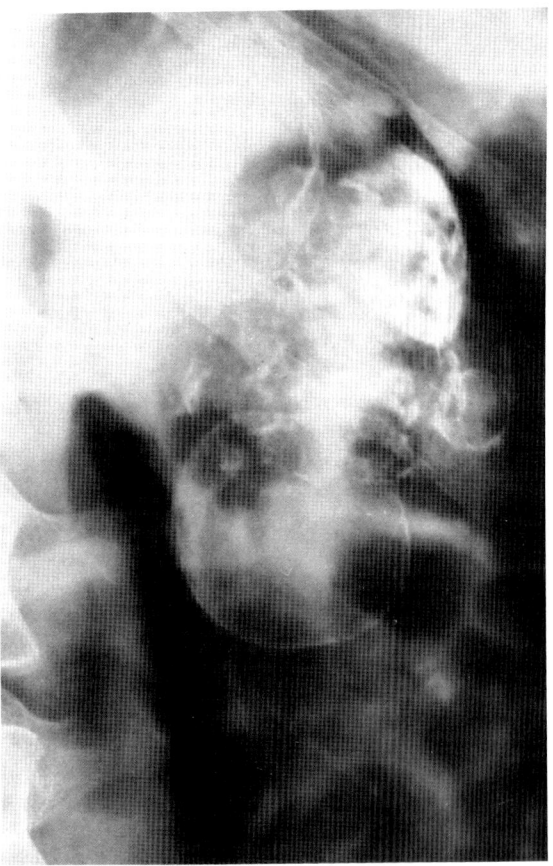

FIGURE 28.10. ECHINOCOCCUS: PLAIN FILM
Twenty-year-old patient. Multiple varied size calcified splenic cysts, typical of echinococcus. No calcification was present in the liver, however.

Echinococcus

Hydatid disease may be due to *Echinococcus granulosus* or *Echinococcus multilocularis*, more commonly the former. Solitary splenic infection is rare (26); it is usually associated with liver and/or lung involvement.

It is the only parasite which produces splenic cysts. Splenic infection may be due to systemic dissemination ("primary"), or intraperitoneal spread from a ruptured liver cyst ("secondary"). Solitary or multiple cysts may enlarge the spleen or produce focal mass effect. Rarely it presents as splenomegaly with or without portal hypertension (27).

Plain film may show splenomegaly or splenic mass(es) which may calcify peripherally producing ring-like calcifications similar to true or posttraumatic false cysts (see Chapter 21) (28). A clue to diagnosis is multiplicity of cysts or the appearance of daughter cysts within a large cyst (Fig. 28.10). Nuclear scintigrams show photopenic defects due to the cyst(s). Ultrasound may show a solitary cyst or multiple cysts with a cyst-within-a-cyst pattern (26). The cysts may contain internal debris, scolices and brood capsules, sometimes producing extensive echoes throughout (29). This may also occur in "infected" hydatid cysts (30–32). The debris may layer within the cyst and the germinal layer may detach, causing a "floating-water lily sign" on sonogram (26, 30). Computed tomography would show a similar morphologic spectrum and may show concomitant liver and renal cysts.

Granulomatous Disease: Tuberculosis, Histoplasmosis

Tuberculosis of the spleen is usually a manifestation of generalized disease. The spleen is almost always involved in miliary tuberculosis. Primary tuberculosis of the spleen is rare, with about 100 reported cases (20, 33). Splenomegaly may be mild or marked, and calcifications may or may not be present. Anemia, leukopenia, thrombocytopenia and rarely, jaundice, ascites and hematemesis may be present (19).

Histoplasmosis is usually clinically silent and may also produce splenic calcifications. As with tuberculosis, the calcifications are small and round or punctate in appearance (Fig. 28.11*A*). On sonography, they produce small bright echogenic foci, with shadowing (Fig. 28.11*B*). This may be accompanied by similar calcifications in the lungs.

Microabscesses/Candida

Splenic abscess is usually a solitary focal lesion and is discussed as such in Chapter 27. Microabscesses, however, are diffuse and usually occur in spleens enlarged due to underlying disease, commonly leukemia (34). *Candida albicans* is the most common cause of microabscesses, but other organisms, notably *Aspergillus* and *Streptococcus*, are reported to produce microabscesses (35, 36). The spleen is usually involved without concomitant hepatic infection. If the underlying disease causing compromise of the immune system

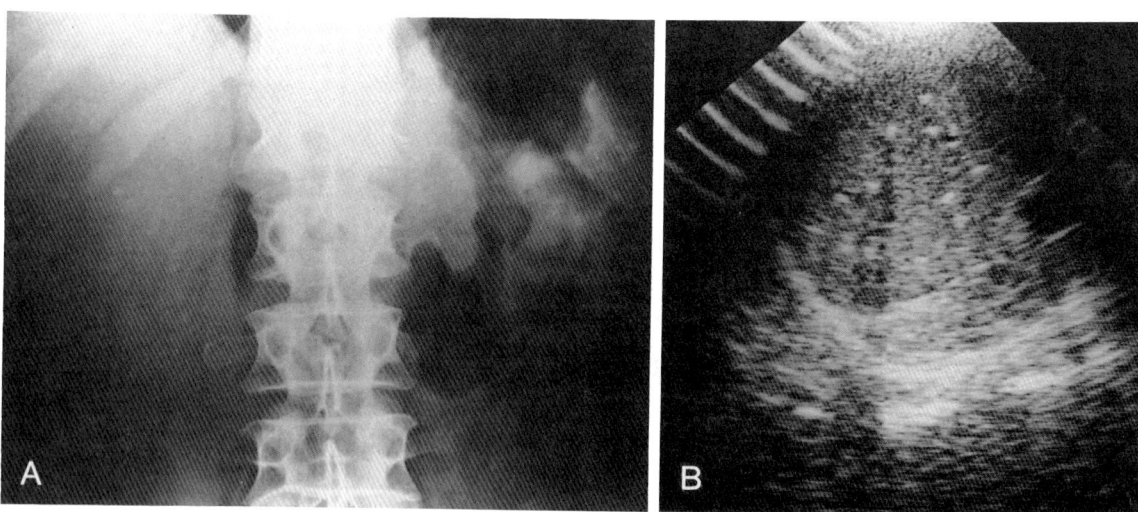

FIGURE 28.11. HISTOPLASMOSIS
A: Plain film; Solid, punctate, calcifications are scattered in the liver and spleen, typical of histoplasmosis or TB. *B:* A sonogram shows multiple, shadowing echogenicities corresponding to calcifications.

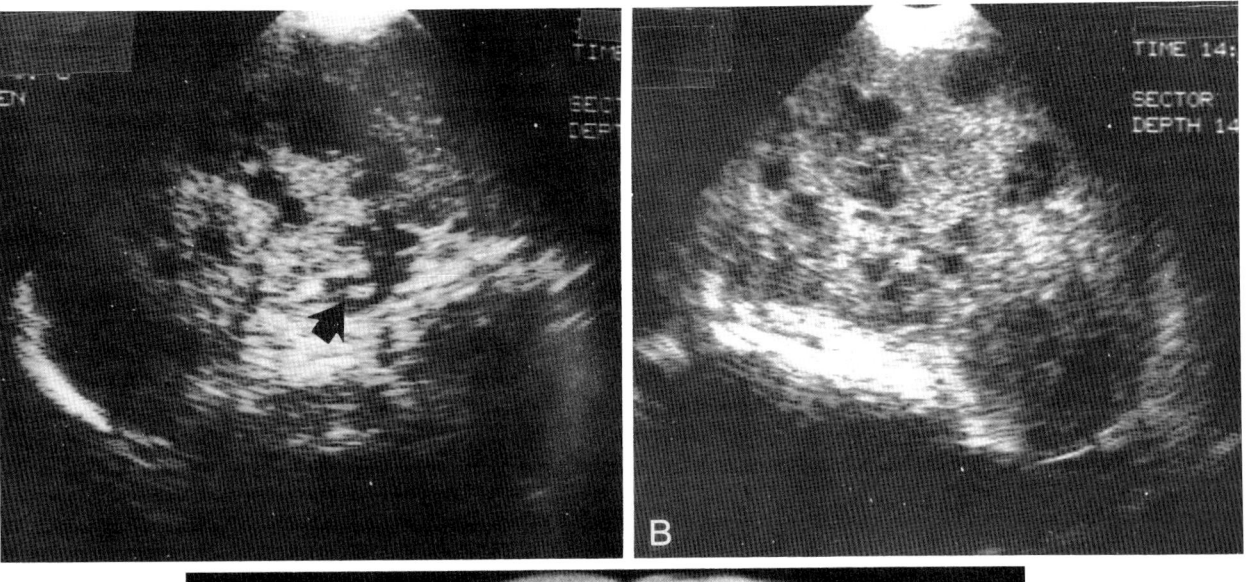
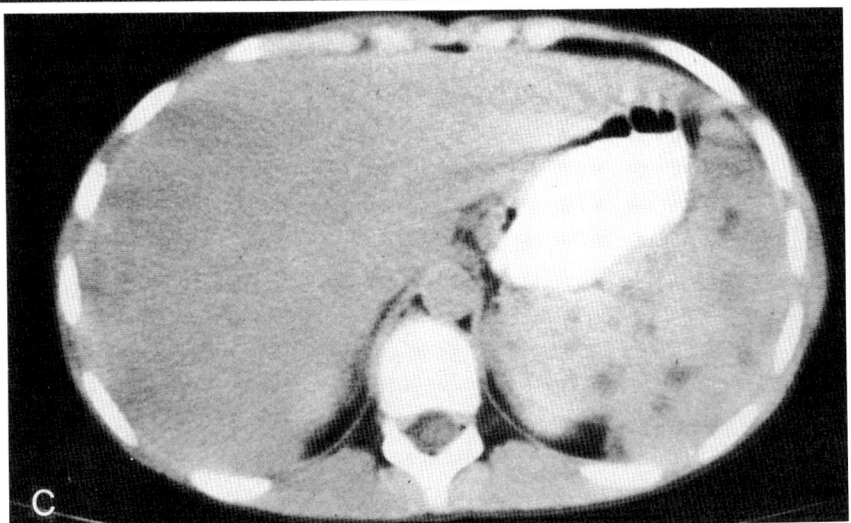

FIGURE 28.12. SPLENIC CANDIDIASIS WITH MICROABSCESSES
A and *B:* Sonogram coronal and transverse: Multiple hypoechoic and anechoic foci, a few of which have echogenic centers, or "target" appearance (*arrow*). *C:* CT: Unenhanced scan shows multiple small target low density microabscesses in an enlarged spleen. (Case courtesy of Dr. Leora Sachs.)

has not been previously diagnosed, the presentation may be one of fever, pain, tenderness in the left upper quadrant, splenomegaly, and hepatomegaly (37). Early diagnosis and medical therapy may obviate the need for surgery, which historically was the preferred treatment (37).

^{99m}Tc-sulfur colloid scan shows hepatosplenomegaly and small defects in the spleen. The lesions are variably "hot" or "cold" on gallium scan (37).

Ultrasound may show hepatosplenomegaly, a hypoechoic spleen, focal hypoechoic splenic lesions, and echogenic or "target" lesions (hypoechoic with small echodense center) in the liver or spleen (Fig. 28.12*A* and *B*) (37, 38). These central echogenic foci may represent growing fungus within the microabscess or granuloma (37, 38).

CT shows focal low density areas with or without a target appearance (Fig. 28.12*C*). The lesions do not enhance with contrast (35–37). Serial CT scans may be used to evaluate the response to antifungal therapy (39).

REFERENCES

1. Spencer RP, Pearson HA, Lange RC: Human spleen: scan studies on growth and response to medications. *J*

Nucl Med 12:466, 1971.
2. DeGowin EL, DeGowin RL: *Bedside Diagnostic Examination.* Ed 4. New York, Macmillan, 1981, pp 505–511.
3. McIntyre OR, Ebauch FG Jr: Palpable spleens in college freshman. *Ann Intern Med* 66:301, 1967.
4. Sty JR, Conway JJ: The spleen: development and functional evaluation. *Semin Nucl Med* 15:276–298, 1985.
5. Crosby HW: Hypersplenism. In Williams WJ, Beutler E, Erslev AJ, Lictman MA (eds): *Hematology*, Ed 3. New York, McGraw-Hill, 1983, pp 242, 660–666.
6. Eichner ER, Whitfield CL: Splenomegaly: an alogrithmic approach to diagnosis. *JAMA* 246:2858–2861, 1981.
7. Walsh M: Diagnosis of splenomegaly (letter). *JAMA* 247:2096, 1982.
8. Didlake RH, Pass HI, Raju S: Journal MSMA (Mississippi Medical Center). November 1980, pp 237–239.
9. Burt RW, Kuhl DE: Giant splenomegaly in sarcoidosis demonstrated by radionuclide scintigraphy. *JAMA* 215:2110, 1971.
10. Eichner ER: Splenic function: normal, too much, and too little. *Am J Med* 66: 311–320, 1979.
11. Henderson ES: Acute myelogenous leukemia. In Williams WJ, Beutler E, Erslev AJ, Lictman MA (eds): *Hematology*, Ed 3. New York, McGraw-Hill, 1983, pp 239–243.
12. Bouza E, Burgaleta C, Golde DW: Infection in hairy-cell leukemia. *Blood* 51:851, 1978.
13. Anderson WAD, Kissane JM: *Pathology*, Ed 7. St. Louis, C. V. Mosby, 1972, pp 1489–1513.
14. Longscope WT, Freiman DG. Study of sarcoidosis. *Medicine* 31:1, 1952.
15. Iko BO, Chunwuba C, Anderson JE et al: Multifocal defects and splenomegaly in sarcoidosis: a new scintigraphic pattern. *J Natl Med Assoc* 74:739–741, 1982.
16. Groen JJ: Present status of knowledge of Gaucher's disease. *Isr J Med Sci* 1:507, 1965.
17. Fisher MR, Sider L: Diffuse reticulonodular infiltrate associated with splenomegaly (case of the month). *Chest* 84:609–610, 1983.
18. Rose JS, Grabowski GA, Barnett SH, Desnick RJ: Accelerated skeletal deterioration after splenectomy in Gaucher's type I disease. *AJR* 139:1202–1204, 1982.
19. Dr. Susan Hill, National Institute of Health, Department of Radiology (by personal communication).
20. Crane GG et al: Tropical splenomegaly syndrome in New Guinea. *Trans R Soc Trop Med Hyg* 66:724–733, 1972.
21. Wintrobe MM, Lee GR, Boggs DR, Bithell TC, Foerster J, Athens JW, Lukins JN: *Clinical Hematology*, Ed 7. Philadelphia, Lea & Febiger, 1981, pp 94–95, 1426–1446.

22. Penman HG: Fatal infectious mononucleosis: a critical review. *J Clin Pathol* 23:765, 1970.
23. Abdel-Latif Z, Abdel-Wahab F, El-Kady NM: Evaluation of portal hypertension in cases of hepatosplenic schistosomiasis using ultrasound. *J Clin Ultrasound* 9:409–412, 1981.
24. Mousa AH, Atta AA, Cel-Rooby A et al: Hepatosplenic schistosomiasis. In Mostofi FK (ed): *Bilharziasis*. New York, Springer-Verlag, 1967, p 15.
25. Cerri GG, Alves VAF, Magalhaes A: Hepatosplenic schistosomiasis mansoni: ultrasound manifestations. *Radiology* 153:777–780, 1984.
26. Wurtele LH, Tondrea RL, Pllack H: Ultrasonic appearance of splenic echinococcal cyst. *Pa Med*, pp 55–56, Oct 1982.
27. Varghese C, Balakrishnan V: Hydatid cyst of the spleen-an unusual presentation. *J Assos Physicianc India* 27:1039–1041, 1979.
28. Soler-Bechara J, Soscia JL: Calcified echinococcus (hydatid) cyst of the spleen. *JAMA* 187:162, 1964.
29. Schulman A, Van Jaarsveld J, Loxton AJ, Grove WH: Pseudosolid appearance of simple and echinococcal cysts in ultrasonography. *SAfr Med J* 63:905–906, 1983.
30. Niron EA, Ozer H: Ultrasound appearances of hydatid disease. *Br J Radiol* 54:335–338, 1981.
31. Haddi A: Ultrasound findings in liver hydatid cysts. *J Clin Ultrasound* 7:365–368, 1975.
32. Itzchak Y, Rubinstein Z, Heyman Z, Gerzof S: Role of ultrasound in the diagnosis of abdominal hydatid disease. *J Clin Ultrasound* 8:341–345, 1980.
33. Chapman AZ et al: Neutropenia secondary to tuberculous splenomegaly. *Ann Intern Med* 41:1225, 1954.
34. Bodey GP: Fundal infections complicating acute leukemia. *J Chronic Dis* 19:667–687, 1966.
35. Kulkarni R, Murray DL, Gupta S et al: Multiple splenic aspergillomas in a patient with acute lymphoblastic leukemia. *Am J Pediatr Hematol Oncol* 4:141–145, 1982.
36. Belinke SA, Chandra-Narayanan N, Russel JC, Becker DR: Splenic abscess associated with streptococcus bovis septicemia and neoplastic lesions of the colon. *Dis Colon Rectum* 3:825–824, 1983.
37. Miller JH, Greenfield LD, Wald BR: Candidiasis of the liver and spleen in childhood. *Raidology* 142:375–380, 1982.
38. Sumner TE, Volberg FM, Chauvenet AR et al.: Radiologic case of the month: hepatic and splenic candidiasis in acute leukemia. *Am J Dis Child* 137:1193–1194, 1983.
39. Berlow ME, Spirt BA, Weil L: CT follow-up of hepatic and splenic fungal microabscesses. *J Comput Assist Tomogr* 8:42–45, 1984.

29
Vascular Disease

ABRAHAM H. DACHMAN, M.D.

ARTERIOSCLEROSIS AND OCCLUSION OF SPLENIC ARTERY

The splenic artery is affected by arteriosclerosis in a manner similar to other abdominal arteries; by intimal and medial calcification and tortuosity which may be evident on plain film, sonography, or CT (Fig. 29.1). Tortuosity or ectasis increases with age and may involve the main splenic artery and its divisions (1). Extrinsic mass effect on the stomach due to splenic artery ectasia may occur anywhere from the cardia to the incisura along the posteromedial wall (2). The defect is broad and may involve a focal or long segment of stomach. The etiology may be suggested at fluoroscopy by noticing transmitted pulsations of the artery on the stomach or calcification in the artery wall. If the extrinsic impression is broad or multilobular in configuration, an ulcer may be mimicked (2).

The artery may be sclerotic but severe stenosis is unusual and is virtually always asymptomatic (1). Complete thrombosis of the splenic artery or aneurysm formation may occur (1). Thrombosis of the splenic artery has been reported in sickle cell anemia (3), leukemia, polyarteritis nodosa, arteritis, splenic torsion (4), and Ménétrièr's disease (5). Cohen reported one case of total occlusion due to a pancreatic carcinoma in the tail of the pancreas (4).

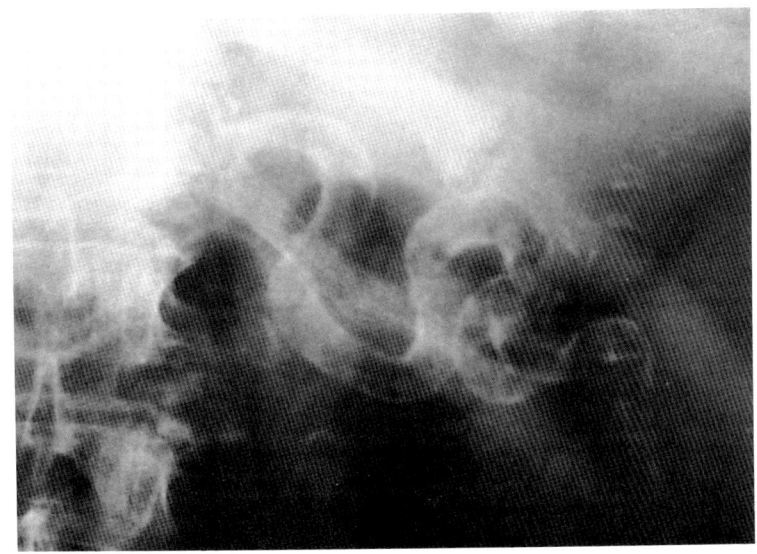

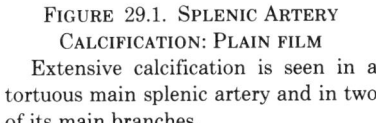

FIGURE 29.1. SPLENIC ARTERY CALCIFICATION: PLAIN FILM
Extensive calcification is seen in a tortuous main splenic artery and in two of its main branches.

FIBROMUSCULAR HYPERPLASIA

In 1964, Palubinskas and Ripley (6) reported that fibromuscular hyperplasia may involve extrarenal arteries, including the splenic artery. The appearance is similar to renal artery involvement with a string of beads or septa-like configuration. A case of fibromuscular dysplasia has been reported as an incidental finding in a 9-yr-old boy (7). Fibromuscular hyperplasia is also found in some females with splenic artery aneurysms (see below).

SPLENIC ARTERY ANEURYSM

Although visceral artery aneurysms are rare, the splenic artery is the one most often affected (8). The incidence is unknown since it is usually asymptomatic, but based on clinical and autopsy series the incidence range is 0.07–10% with females more often affected than males. The etiology in males may be atherosclerotic. Other etiologies include: congenital defects, infection, trauma, syphillis, pancreatitis and Ehlers-Danlos syndrome. Dilation and tortuosity of the splenic artery may accompany the splenomegaly caused by malaria or Gaucher's disease (9). Although atherosclerosis is present in many cases of splenic artery aneurysm (SAA), this does not explain why about three-fourths of celiac axis aneurysms involve the splenic artery selectively (10). In women, there is a significant correlation with pregnancy and multiparity (11). The factors predisposing pregnant women to SAA may include: preexisting weakness of the artery, connective tissue changes related to pregnancy, splenic arteriovenous shunting, and mechanical stress by increased blood flow and direct pressure (8). Portal hypertension has also been linked to SAA. In one series 8.8% of cirrhotic patients with portal hypertension have a SAA (12), and up to 2.6% of pregnant women with SAA have portal hypertension (13). This association may be related to a chronically increased blood flow through the splenic artery (10). Multiple visceral artery aneurysms including SAA, have been reported as a sporadic finding as well as part of Ehlers-Danlos syndrome (14).

Most patients are asymptomatic, but up to 20% may have symptoms referrable to the aneurysm. Epigastric pain, left upper quadrant pain which may radiate to the left shoulder or lower quadrant, or nausea are the common symptoms. A large aneurysm may be palpable as a pulsatile mass and may cause a bruit (11). In some series splenomegaly is the most common finding, especially for intrasplenic SAA (10). An enlarging or ruptured SAA often produces focal peritoneal signs. There may be an episode of bleeding which stops, followed by free rupture shortly thereafter ("double rupture") (10).

Rupture may occur into the anterior pararenal space (15) or into the lesser sac (10). Less often rupture is into a viscus (i.e., stomach), into the splenic vein creating an arteriovenous fistula, or into the pancreatic duct (so-called hemosuccus pancreaticus or hemoductal pancreatitis (10, 16, 17). The mortality from rupture is about 25% except in pregnancy it rises to >75% for mother and fetus (11, 16). In chronic pancreatitis there is an increased incidence of aneurysm formation in the peripancreatic arteries, sometimes classified as pseudoaneurysms. These patients have a history of recurrent pancreatitis, usually alcoholic, often with pancreatic pseudocyst formation. Involvement of the splenic artery by pancreatic enzymes or surrounding pseudocyst may lead to pseudoaneurysm of the main splenic artery. This has been diagnosed by ultrasound, CT, and MRI (18, 19). The pseudoaneurysm is cystic on sonography and enhances with contrast on CT (18). On MRI with spin-echo technique, it has been seen as a low signal area compatible with flowing blood (19). It may be partly filled with blood clot. If the wall ruptures, the classic triad of pancreatitis, bile duct obstruction and gastrointestinal hemorrhage may be present, however, the diagnosis is usually delayed. Harper et al. (20) reviewed the literature and found an average delay in correct diagnosis of 2.3 yr, with multiple hospital admissions for recurrent gastrointestinal hemorrhage and unnecessary surgery in some cases.

The radiologic diagnosis of SSA is usually made on the basis of a ring calcification in the right upper quadrant (Fig. 29.2A–D). Some may be incidentally detected on CT or sonography. Noncalcified aneurysms may be detected incidentally on angiography or Tc sulfur colloid abdominal flow study. Real-time sonography generally cannot identify pulsations in a splenic artery aneurysm, however pulsed Doppler sonography can prove the vascular nature of the lesion (21).

Angiography can demonstrate multiple intrasplenic and extrasplenic aneurysms and can evaluate for rupture, fistulization, portal hypertension and splenomegaly (9). When aneurysms are multiple, they often occur at the convexities of the bends in the vessel in an eccentric and fusiform shape (Fig. 29.3A and B) (9). Aneurysm size diminishes in the peripheral and intrasplenic vessels (9). A bleeding aneurysm may be treated with transcatheter embolization or, as preferred by some, embolization of the feeding vessel alone (22, 23). The use of steel coils to embolize the feeding vessel is probably the safest approach especially in association with pancreatitis (23).

Asymptomatic splenic artery aneurysms should probably be treated with embolization or resection electively only if found in pregnant women, women of childbearing age, or if the aneurysm is greater than 2.5 cm in diameter (10).

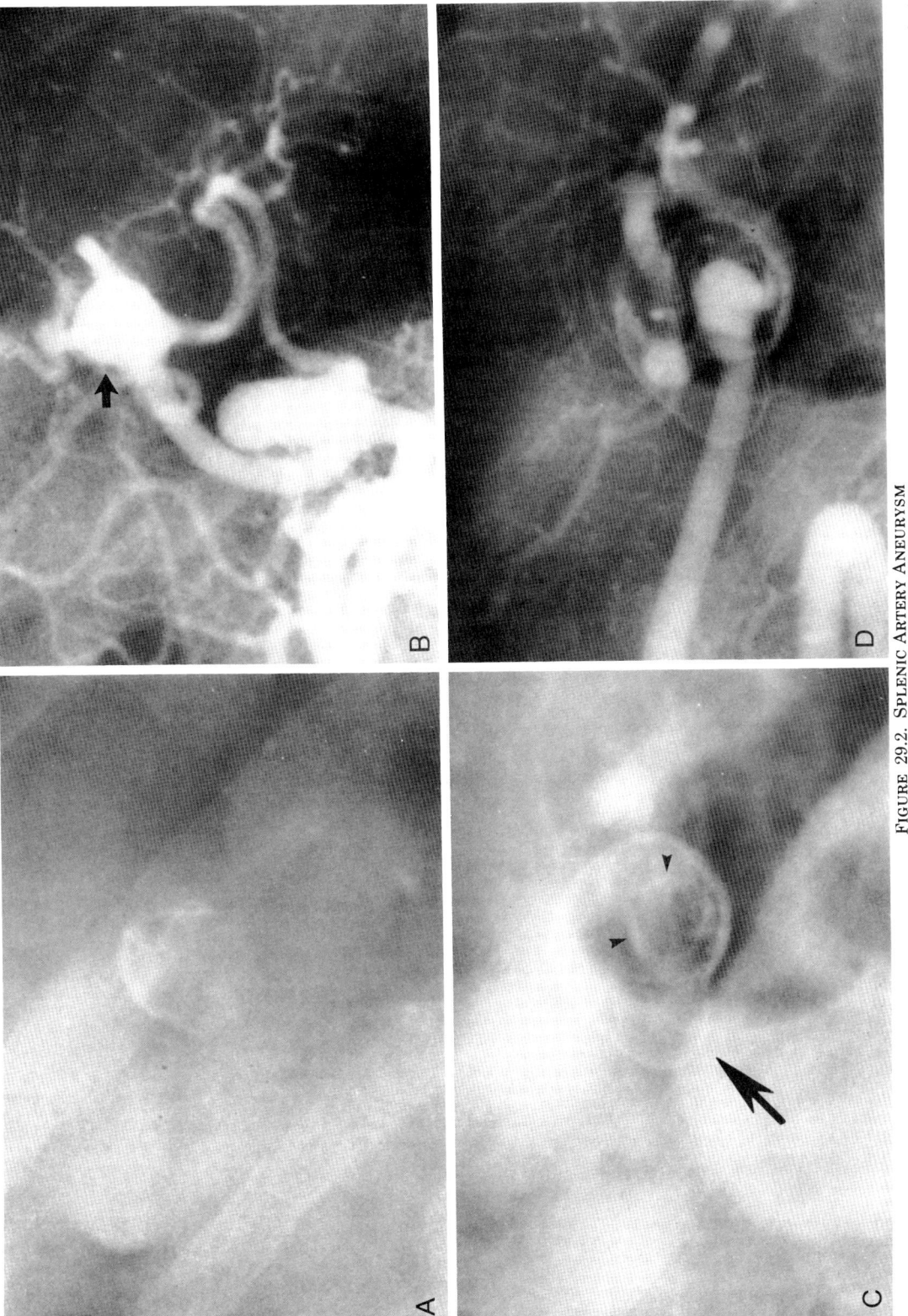

FIGURE 29.2. SPLENIC ARTERY ANEURYSM

A: Curvilinear calcification which is seen on arteriogram (*B*) to represent a splenic artery aneurysm (*arrow*). *C* and *D*: Splenic artery aneurysm. *C*: A large ring-like calcification is seen in a splenic artery aneurysm (*arrow*). Within this a second ring calcification is seen (*arrowheads*) which represents calcification in the wall of the residual lumen as seen on arteriogram (*D*).

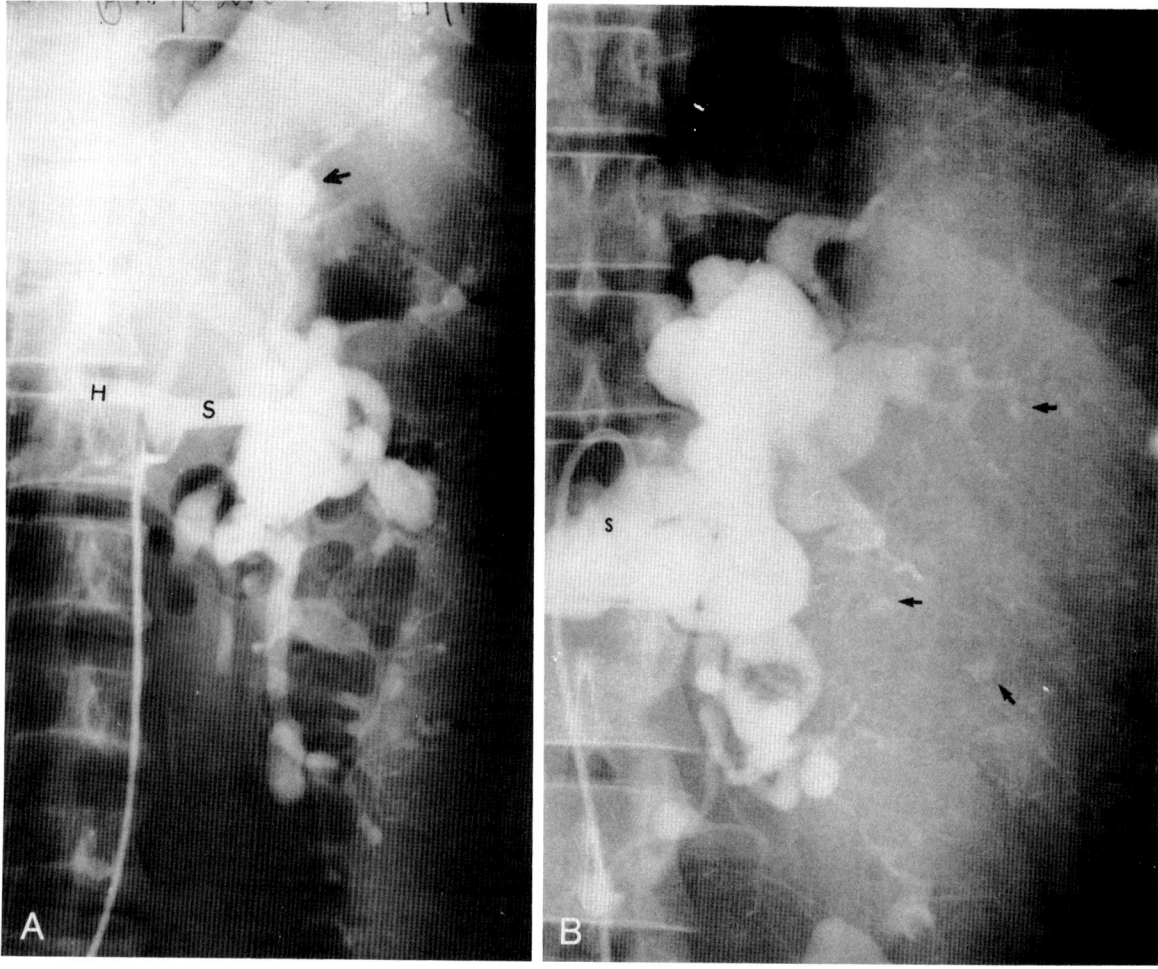

FIGURE 29.3. MULTIPLE SPLENIC ARTERY ANEURYSMS

A: A 23-yr old woman with early cirrhosis and splenomegaly. Multiple intra- and extrasplenic aneurysms are opacified (*arrow*). Note the increase in size as the aneurysms progress distally from the splenic hilus. H = hepatic artery, S = splenic artery. *B:* A 28-yr-old woman with splenomegaly and esophageal varices whose liver biopsy showed some fibrosis with preservation of the portal architecture. Large extrasplenic and multiple smaller intrasplenic (*arrows*) aneurysms are present. S = splenic artery. (From Feist JH, Gajaraj A: Extra- and intrasplenic artery aneurysms in portal hypertension. *Radiology* 125:331–334, 1977.)

ARTERIOVENOUS FISTULA

This is a rare condition representing a complication of splenic artery aneurysm rupture (vide supra). Rarely it occurs postsplenectomy, congenitally, as a result of a penetrating wound (i.e., stab or gunshot), or as a complication of splenoportography. This excludes shunting associated with cirrhosis or hepatocellular carcinoma (see Chapter 5). In 1971, Van Way (24) reviewed arteriovenous (AV) fistula in the portal circulation and found 59 cases, 21 of which were splenic in location. Thus, about one-third of portal AV fistulas are splenic. More recently, Bredfeldt and O'Laughlin (25) reviewed the literature and found 7 additional cases bringing the total to 29. While most portal AV fistulas are traumatic in origin, most of those in the splenic vasculature are due to a ruptured aneurysm. AV fistula is more common in women, reflecting the predilection of splenic artery aneurysms for women.

As with other portal AV fistulas, the predominant clinical manifestation is portal hypertension presenting as an upper gastrointestinal bleed from esophageal varices and/or ascites. Abdominal pain or a bruit may be present (24). The key to the diagnosis is the abdominal bruit, which if absent will delay diagnosis. The bruit may be heard best in left upper quadrant, but sometimes is located in the epigastrum, left lower chest or posterior left abdomen (25). Splenomegaly is present and the hepatic venous pressure gradient when measured is normal or slightly elevated (26).

If chronic, the AV fistula causes "arterialization" of the portal venous system involved (27) and eventually hepatoportal sclerosis results. It is unknown how often this occurs with splenic AV fistula specifically.

The definitive diagnosis of splenic AV fistula is established on angiography by selective splenic artery injection. The splenic artery is usually tortuous and a splenic artery aneurysm may be visualized in conjunction with early splenic venous filling (25, 27). The splenic vein may be dilated and bulbous in configuration (27). Venous collaterals and gastroesophageal varices may be visualized. Retrograde flow into the superior mesenteric vein may be present (25).

The treatment of choice is said to be surgical resection of the AV fistula (25), however depending on its location, splenectomy, splenic artery ligation or conceivably transcatheter embolization may be performed. Resection generally cures the patient of variceal bleeding unless the surgery is complicated by portal venous thrombosis (28).

SPLENIC ARTERY EMBOLIZATION

Madison (29) described embolic therapy for hypersplenism in 1973. Since then a variety of techniques have been employed experimentally or clinically including detachable balloons (30), Gelfoam (31, 32), dextran, polystyrene, silicone (33), and Bucrylate (34). These nonsurgical techniques have been dubbed "medical splenectomy." The procedure has been employed in a variety of clinical situations including trauma (33) and hypersplenism of a variety of etiologies. In hypersplenism the goal is to alleviate the thrombocytopenia and anemia of hypersplenism. This may alleviate abdominal discomfort, reduce the risk of surgery and the transfusion requirements (35). It is also desirable to avoid splenectomy in patients with cirrhosis because this would eliminate the possibility of a splenorenal shunt (34). In trauma cases the goal is to reduce or stop bleeding while preserving splenic function and thus avoid the risk of postsplenectomy sepsis. The major problem with embolization is the complication rate (36, 37). Complications of splenic and subphrenic abscess have been high in some series and low in others (34): the complications generally occur when extensive small particle embolization is used (i.e., Gelfoam). Main splenic artery occlusion is considered safer. Embolization with steel coils or detachable balloons causes occlusion of the main trunk of the splenic artery but collateral flow generally reconstitutes the circulation (33, 38, 39) primarily via the left gastric, gastroepiploic and right gastric arteries. Total or major infarction may also occur (especially with small particle embolization) (36), but this alone is not a significant complication unless accompanied by splenic rupture (37).

In an attempt to reduce the complication rate, partial splenic embolization was attempted. Costansda et al. (40) observed a lower complication rate in experimental partial embolization.

Vujic and Lauver (31) had severe complications in three patients who underwent partial splenic embolization. Others describe encouraging results. In 1977 Spigos et al. (32) used Gelfoam to ablate about two-thirds of the spleen in 13 cases. All these patients were renal transplant patients where splenectomy improved the tolerance to azathioprine. No significant complications (such as abscess) occurred. This was attributed to the partial embolization, aseptic technique, and postembolization care. The partial nature of the embolization preserves flow in the splenic circulation, whereas total embolization causes reversal of flow in the splenic vein which may allow portal blood draining the gastrointestinal tract which may contain bacteria to contaminate the infarcted spleen (32). Gerlock et al. (41) confirmed Spigos' results in six patients with hypersplenism in renal failure using the same technique.

Bucrylate (isobutyl 2-cyanoacrylate) has been used successfully for "medical splenectomy" in the treatment of gastric varices due to splenic vein thrombosis, or portal hypertension, or in patients with hypersplenism (34). Of 13 patients, only one developed an abscess. This patient's splenic arterial collateral pathways were occluded whereas in the other twelve patients the left gastric, gastroepiploic and pancreatic collaterals continued to supply the spleen; in effect a partial "medical splenectomy."

Splenic embolization remains the treatment of choice in severe hypersplenism, especially if steel coils are used to occlude the main splenic artery.

SOLITARY SPLENIC VEIN THROMBOSIS

When Sutton reviewed the literature through 1968 there were only 53 cases of isolated splenic vein thrombosis (SVT) without portal vein involvement (42). The number of reported cases has since more than doubled (43–45) but is still probably underdiagnosed and underreported. It is a cause of chronic abdominal pain, weight loss and upper gastrointestinal bleeding from gastric varices. The diagnosis is often delayed, thus an increased awareness is deserving in the appropriate clinical settings.

The etiology of SVT in the majority of patients is pancreatic carcinoma and chronic pancreatitis. Other etiologies include lymphoma, abdominal trauma, pancreatic pseudocyst, penetrating gastric ulcer, splenic artery aneurysm, polycythemia, retroperitoneal fibrosis (46, 47), and idiopathic SVT. The pathophysiology involves either compression, encasement or inflammation around the splenic vein. The splenic vein courses along the superior-posterior margin of the pancreas which explains why pancreatic conditions represent the most common etiology. Theoretically, any upper retroperitoneal neoplasm could cause SVT. Cirrhosis, a common cause of portal vein thrombosis rarely causes SVT (and never causes solitary SVT) (44, 48).

If SVT is part of general mesenteric venous thrombosis, the presentation is related to the generalized condition and has a high mortality (49). Clinically, a large percentage of SVT patients will be asymptomatic (50). The "classic" presentation of solitary SVT is chronic abdominal pain, weight loss, iron deficiency anemia, and bleeding from gastric varices. The incidence of acute gastric variceal bleeding is between 16 and 65% (45). Variceal bleeding which is often the first clinical manifestation, may also present as hematemesis, or melena. Clinical evidence of splenomegaly may be lacking, thus a normal sized spleen does not exclude splenic vein thrombosis (44, 45). Itzchak reported 19 cases of SVT, eleven of which had normal sized spleens. In Muhletaler's series only 6 of 18 had splenomegaly.

Endoscopy may also give false negative results. Endoscopy was suggestive of gastric varices in 4 of 10 cases in one series (45), and in only 2 of 31 in another (51). Prominent folds may be seen or the varices may appear beaded, nodular, or mimic a fundal submucosal mass on endoscopy (52). Clues to the correct diagnosis are a bluish hue and compressability of the lesion. This underscores the usefulness of the upper gastrointestinal series.

Roentgen Findings

Findings may relate to the SVT per se or its underlying etiology: patients with chronic pancreatitis may have pancreatic calcifications on plain film. Pancreatic pseudocyst or neoplasm will produce mass effect on the duodenum or stomach. Retroperitoneal masses are best seen on CT and splenomegaly may or may not be present. Lymphadenopathy may be a clue to lymphoma.

The principal finding is the demonstration of solitary gastric varices. The varices are usually fundal or cardiac in location corresponding to the vasa breva draining from the splenic hilus to the coronary vein. They were demonstrated on barium study in 10 of 11 patients with solitary SVT in Cho and Martel's series and 15 of 18 patients in Muhletaler's series (43, 45). Their appearance is variable; broad varicoid defects, clusters of polyps, thick folds or a polypoid fundal mass may be seen (43, 45). Lymphoma, adenocarcinoma or leiomyoma may be considered in the differential diagnosis. Varices are best demonstrated by double contrast (43, 53), however, theoretically overdistention could efface varices, thus views of the stomach with varying degrees of distention should be obtained. In differentiating prominent folds from varices, a clue is subtle undulation of the margins of the fold causing a variation in its thickness (43). In the case of a polypoid mass, hyperdistention of the stomach may demonstration some decrease in the size of the mass indicating its soft consistency.

Gastric varices need not be limited to the fundus, but may occur in the body and antrum particularly along the greater curvature (44). Itzchak also found duodenal varices on upper gastrointestinal series in two cases and in another three cases prominent duodenal folds were seen only in retrospect (44). This may relate to the site of thrombosis being within the splenic vein, which will affect the collateral pathways used. In that series the site of obstruction was at the splenic hilum in eight and near the junction of the splenic and portal veins in 3 of 11 patients with SVT without splenomegaly. In those with splenomegaly, the obstruction was hilar in 3 and near the portal vein in 5. Esophageal varices are usually absent unless there is associated portal or superior mesenteric venous thrombosis. Esophageal varices were present in 2 cases of solitary SVT reported in one series however (53).

Angiographic evaluation may be done with high dose celiac or splenic artery arteriography, transhepatic portography or historically splenoportography. Nonopacification of the splenic vein in its entirety or in part, with opacification of venous collaterals is diagnostic (Figs. 29.4 and 29.5). Three major collateral pathways are: (a) the short gastric veins to the coronary or left gastric vein, (b) short gastric veins to the esophageal plexus to the azygous system, and (c) left gastroepiploic to right gastroepiploic to gastroduodenal to portal vein (this may give duodenal and omental varices). Note that superior mesenteric artery injection will not demonstrate splenic vein opacification as is usually the case in portal hypertension. Thus solitary SVT flow physiology has been referred to as "left sided" or sinistral portal hypertension. The exact flow pattern will depend on the degree of collateral flow, reduction in arterial flow and compensatory splenomegaly (44).

A potential pitfall in the angiographic diagnosis of SVT occurs in the presence of portal hypertension when portal vein pressure exceeds splenic vein pressure. This will cause reversal of flow in the splenic and superior mesenteric veins (blood is directed toward the spleen and the bowel). In this case, a splenic artery injection may fail to opacify the splenic vein and might be confused with SVT.

Ultrasound has been used to diagnose portal and splenic venous thrombosis on rare occasion and is probably underused (54–56). In 1982, Weinberger et al. (55) demonstrated a dilated splenic vein with an echogenic rim which on follow-up examination showed increasing echogenicity within the splenic vein with autopsy confirmation of splenic and portal venous thrombosis. In a case report by Goldberg et al. (57) in 1984, CT demonstrated enlarged retroperitoneal veins and a thickened gastric cardia in a patient with SVT confirmed by splenic arteriogram. Dense calcification in intra- and extrasplenic venous and portal thrombosis has also been shown on CT (58). Of course sonography and CT also aid in evaluating underlying etiologies such as pancreatic or other retroperitoneal disease.

The treatment of choice for SVT is splenectomy (59, 60), which will cure the gastrointestinal bleeding and other symptoms. If the patient is asymptomatic, therapy should probably be directed only to the underlying etiology. Without surgical intervention, SVT is thought to be a chronic condition. However, Hershfield and Morrow (61) reported a case of "narrowed" splenic vein in a patient with chronic pancreatitis and gastric varices whose varices resolved spontaneously. If surgery is done to drain a pancreatic pseudocyst, Rouex-en-y cystojejunos-

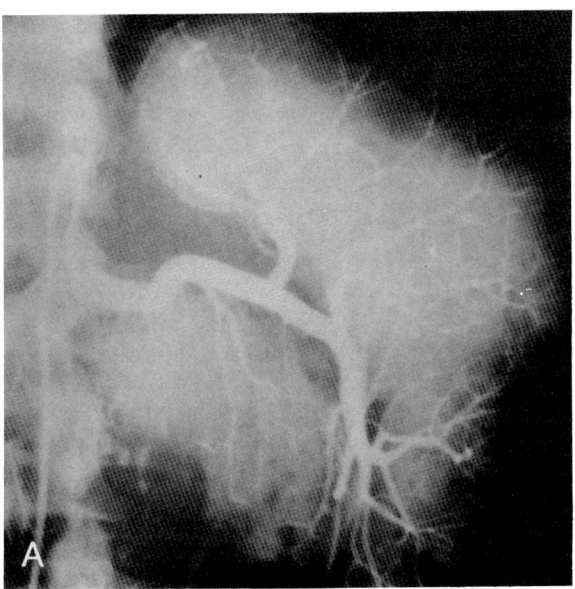 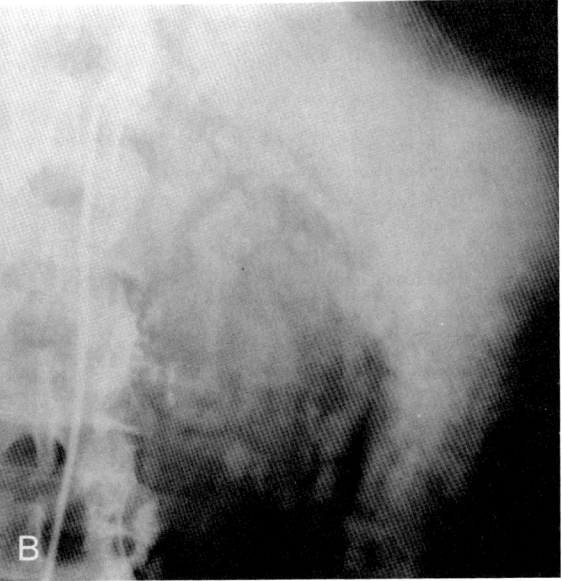

FIGURE 29.4. SPLENIC VEIN OCCLUSION

A: Arterial phase shows patent arteries in a selective splenic artery injection. B: Venous phase shows absence of splenic vein filling with extensive perisplenic collateral flow (varices).

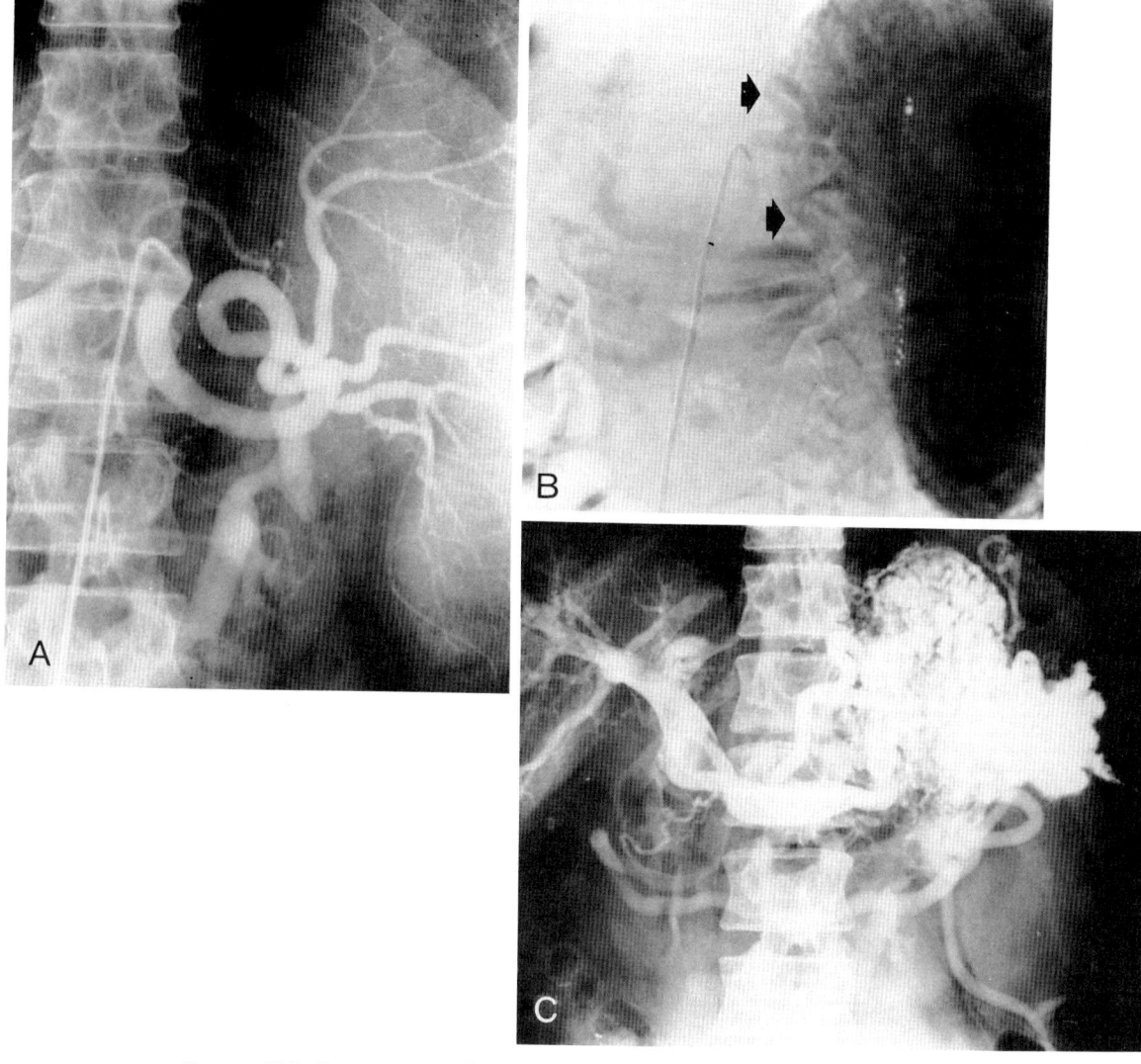

FIGURE 29.5. CARCINOMA OF TAIL OF PANCREAS WITH SPLENIC VEIN THROMBOSIS
A: Selective splenic artery injection and *B:* late phase subtraction films show congestive splenomegaly and lack of splenic vein opacification with some venous collaterals seen on the subtraction film (*arrows*). *C:* Splenoportogram in the same patient shows extensive venous collaterals draining mainly into the distal splenic vein or portal vein. The proximal splenic vein is thrombosed and was invaded by tumor.

tomy should be done rather than cystogastrostomy since surgical manipulation of the stomach may cause bleeding from gastric varices (62). Likewise, if percutaneous drainage is used, a path avoiding areas of collateral pathways should be used.

An alternate to surgical splenectomy is transcatheter embolization of the splenic artery. This has been done in poor risk patients with hypersplenism, pancreatitis (62) and pancreatic carcinoma. The success rate is best with main splenic artery occlusion by steel coils.

RUPTURE OF SPLENIC VEIN

Excluding cases of major abdominal trauma, there are four case reports of spontaneous rupture of the splenic vein due to hepatic cirrhosis. In 1983, Almgren and Bowald (63) published two cases and found two additional cases reported in the 1920s. The symptoms are acute severe abdominal pain with nausea, vomiting, and diarrhea. In one case, the patient was previously asymptomatic, although cirrhosis was found at autopsy in all cases. Rapid blood loss causes shock and signs of peritonitis. In one case bleeding ceased briefly and then recurred ("double rupture"). The pathophysiology of the rupture is not understood. In one case there may have been preexisting splenic vein thrombosis with recanalization. This diagnosis should be considered in a cirrhotic patient with hemoperitoneum. Spontaneous rupture has been reported in one case with no underlying pathology (63).

SPLENIC INFARCT

Occlusion of the splenic artery or one of its branches may lead to ischemia since parenchymal branches are end arteries which do not intercommunicate (64). Any cause of splenic artery occlusion (especially if acute) can therefore cause ischemia: sickle cell disease or its variants, embolic disease particularly from the left heart (i.e., mitral valve disease), myeloproliferative disease, atherosclerosis, arteritis, splenic artery aneurysm, and rarely pancreatitis, pancreatic mass, bacteremia and splenic torsion (4, 65, 66).

Pathologically, infarcts may be hemorrhagic or anemic although most are probably hemorrhagic initially then become anemic and eventually are replaced by fibrotic tissue (66). The chronic fibrotic infarct may also cause a depressed scar resulting in a contour defect on the splenic surface (65, 66). The infarct may be wedge-shaped, less often irregular and even multiple (66). Multiple areas of irregular necrosis diffusely was originally described in uremia and termed "Fleckmilz" or spotted spleen. It may also occur in systemic infection, arteritis and arteriolitis (64, 66).

Splenic infarct may be symptomatic with left upper quadrant pain, fever, left shoulder pain and occasionally a friction rub is heard (65). Many patients are asymptomatic.

Plain film findings which are rarely present, include splenomegaly, elevated left hemidiaphragm and left pleural effusion (65).

Nucear scintigraphy was, and may still be, the best screening test for splenic infarct. The infarcted area produces a photopenic defect on liver spleen scan but may or may not have the classic wedge shape (Fig. 29.6) (67–69). Freeman found six examples of splenic infarct; patterns included focal defect and in one case multiple

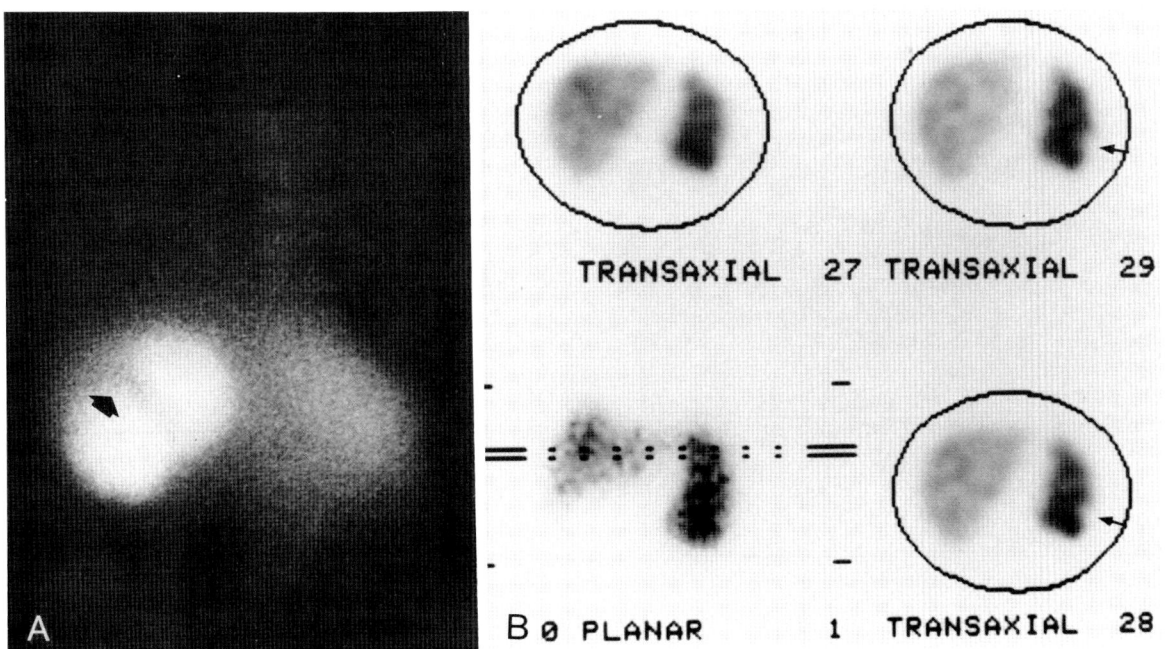

FIGURE 29.6. SPLENIC INFARCT: ^{99m}TC SULFUR COLLOID SCAN
A: Posterior view demonstrated a peripheral based wedge-shaped defect typical of infarct (*arrow*). *B:* Splenic infarct with SPECT. In this patient the planar image (routine ^{99m}Tc-sulfur colloid scan) fails to show the infarct. The SPECT images show a peripheral wedge-shaped area of absent uptake (*arrow*).

defects. The etiologies in these cases were subacute bacterial endocarditis (2 cases), pancreatitis (3 cases) and sarcoid (1 case). The wedge appearance with the apex of defect pointing toward the splenic hilum, is virtually diagnostic when present (68). Other shapes or the less common appearance of multiple lesions is nonspecific (67, 69). When the defect is in the upper pole of the spleen, the splenic configuration may resemble that of a heart, the so-called "spleen of hearts" (70). SPECT (single photon emission computed tomography) may be a useful tool in equivocal cases (Fig. 29.6B).

Angiography may demonstrate occlusion of the splenic artery or one of its branches with a triangular ischemic zone (Fig. 29.7) (71). While this appearance is fairly specific, infarct due to venous occlusion in sickle cell disease may produce splenomegaly with stretched vessels and avascularity mimicking a subcapsular hemorrhage (3).

There is a paucity of sonographic data on

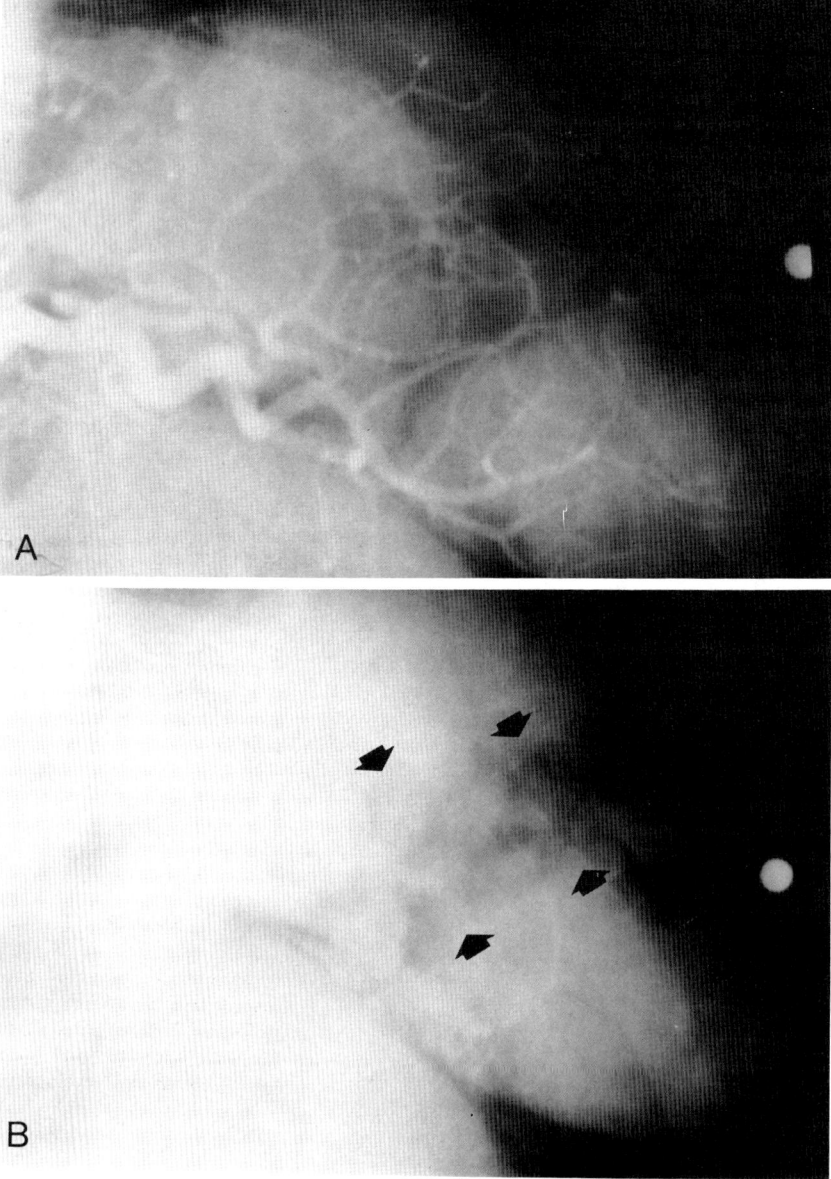

FIGURE 29.7. SPLENIC INFARCT: ANGIOGRAM
A: Arterial phase shows peripheral defect which becomes more visible on parenchymal phase (B, arrows). Although not wedge-shaped, it is based at the capsular surface.

splenic infarct. Although no cases are listed among the 40 patients with splenic abnormalities on sonography reported by Mittelstaedt and Partain (72), or the 13 cases reported by Siler et al. (73), it is likely that in some of the patients with myeloproliferative disorder or hemaglobinopathies infarction was present. Yeh et al. (74) reported a pathologically proven sonographic example of a splenic infarct. The infarct was a sharply demarcated hypoechic area in an enlarged spleen which pathologically correlated with necrosis and edema within a large infarct. The wedge-shaped nature was not apparent due to the plane of scanning (as shown by Yeh) (Fig. 29.8). Thus one would expect the echogenicity to vary with the stage of infarction. Weingarten et al. (75) reported six cases of splenic infarct after transcatheter therapeutic embolization. All were peripheral, sharply demarcated, hypoechoic lesions, four of which had the characteristic triangular shape with the apex pointing toward the splenic hilus. These six cases also had cold defects on ^{99m}Tc-sulfur colloid scans but the wedge shape could not be appreciated (75).

On CT the appearance also depends on the phase of infarction. In 1984, Balcar et al. (65) studied experimentally produced splenic infarction in dogs (using a previously described technique (76)) showing four phases: hyperacute (day 1), acute (2–4 days), subacute (4–8 days), and chronic (studied 15–28 days). In the hyperacute phase there are two patterns: a decrease in density compared to normal spleen which enhanced in a diffuse mottled pattern or large focal hyperdense lesions without contrast enhancement. This correlated with microscopic congestion and only focal redness on gross inspection. The acute and subacute phase showed discrete focal low densities which became progressively more well demarcated and did not enhance. In the chronic phase the splenic density may return to normal homogeneity on both pre- and postcontrast with

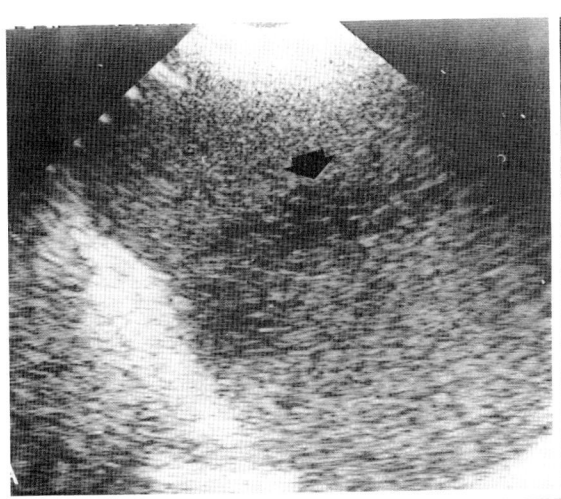
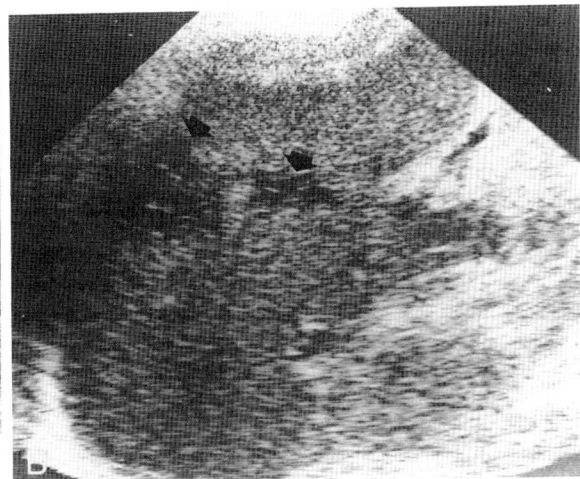
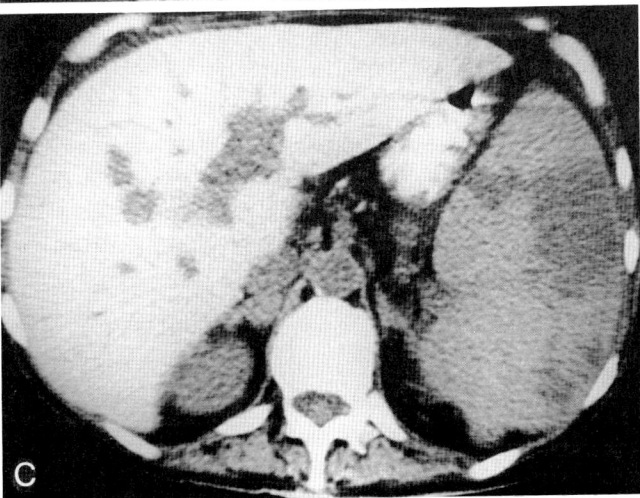

FIGURE 29.8. SPLENIC INFARCT

A: Transverse and B: Coronal views of the spleen show an ill-defined hypoechoic focus (arrows). C: CT shows that this is in fact multifocal peripheral lesions which were presumptive infarcts in a patient with sideroblastic anemia, hemosiderosis, and myelophthisis.

residual scarring seen as contour notching in the area of infarction (65). The patterns seen included wedge shaped defects (Fig. 29.9), multiple heterogeneous lesions or a massive hypodense lesion (Fig. 29.10). A massive hypodense lesion was also reported by Cohen et al. (4) and one of the four cases reported by Maier in 1982 shows the same pattern with two-thirds of the spleen involved by a hypodense, sharply demarcated non-enhancing infarct (77). A thin rind of

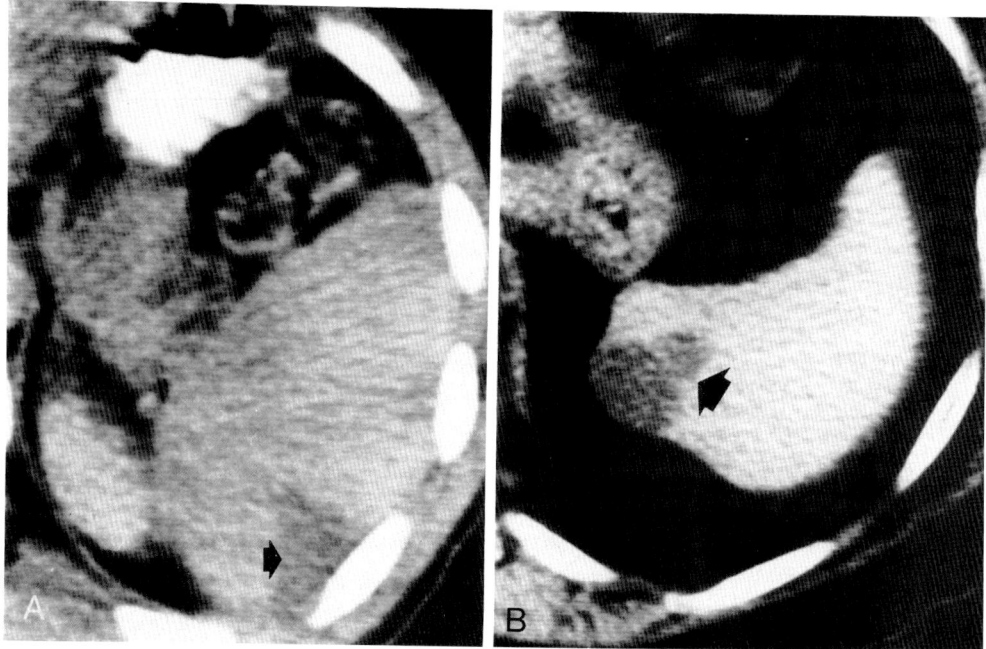

FIGURE 29.9. SPLENIC INFARCT
A: and *B:* Two different patients with typical wedge-shaped low attenuation splenic infarcts (*arrows*).

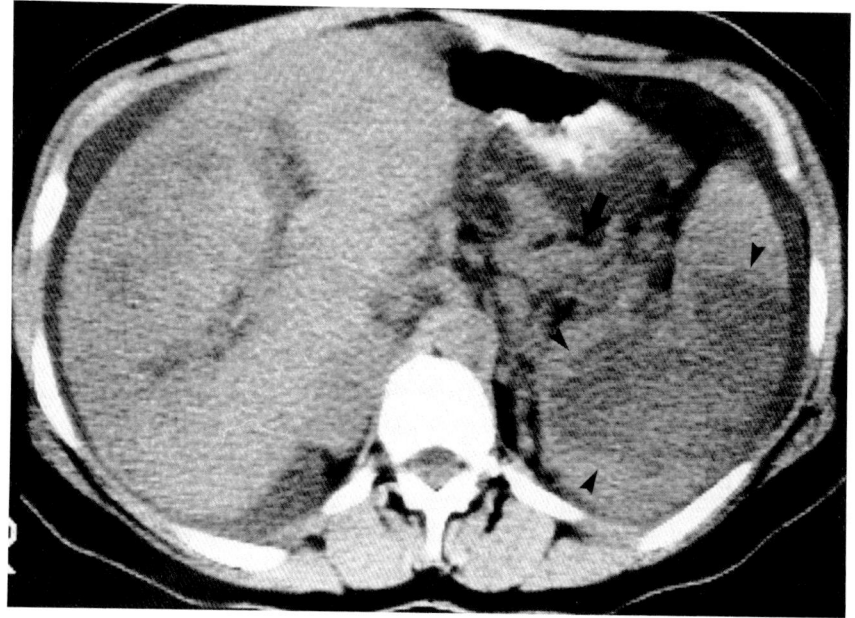

FIGURE 29.10. MASSIVE SPLENIC INFARCT: CT
A patient with polycythemia vera and a large splenic infarct (*arrowheads*). Portal hypertension and varices (*arrows*) were also present due to superimposed Budd-Chiari.

splenic capsule was seen possibly due to residual blood supply to the capsule and subcapsular tissue (77). As Cohen points out, a similar CT appearance has been reported in renal infarction.

Three of the 12 cases reported by Balcar had multiple irregular defects; in one the etiology was presumably therapeutic embolization of a hepatoma and the etiology was not specified in the others. He also claims that in 3 other cases nonenhanced CT alone would have missed the diagnosis. It would be interesting to know if they were acute or chronic infarcts. Nevertheless, in most clinical situations abdominal CT is performed with contrast enhancement.

Perisplenic hematoma accompanied a small splenic infarct in one of Maier's patients with chronic myeloid leukemia, representing a splenic rupture confirmed on autopsy (77). Maier claims that splenic rupture may occur as a complication of infarction, however this remains to be proven

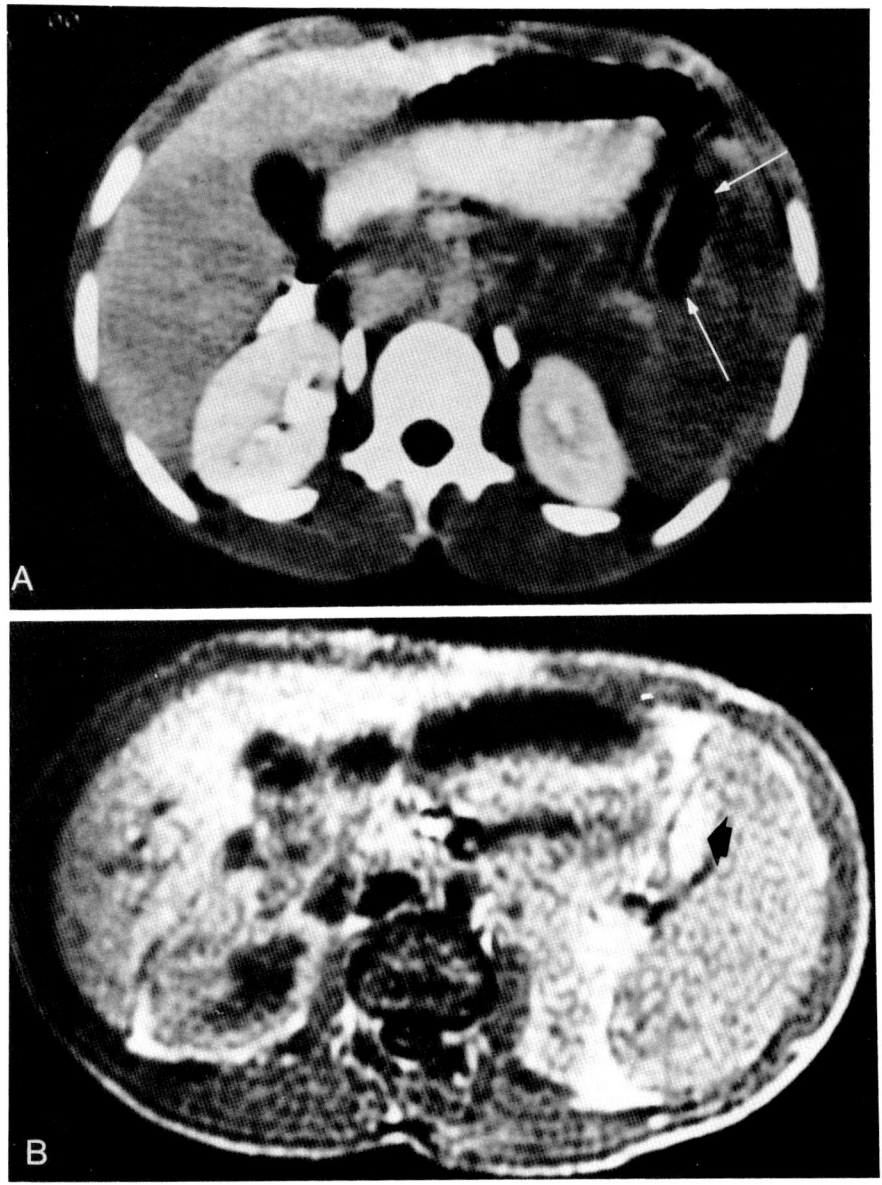

FIGURE 29.11. SPLENIC INFARCT: MRI

Sickle cell disease and a high fetal hemoglobin. *A:* The CT scan showed a hypodense lesion (*arrows*), but an abscess could not be excluded, thus an MRI was performed. *B:* The inversion recovery scan (TI = 310, TR = 1500) shows a hypertense lesion (*arrow*), probably due to hemorrhage in the infarct. (An abscess would give a low signal.)

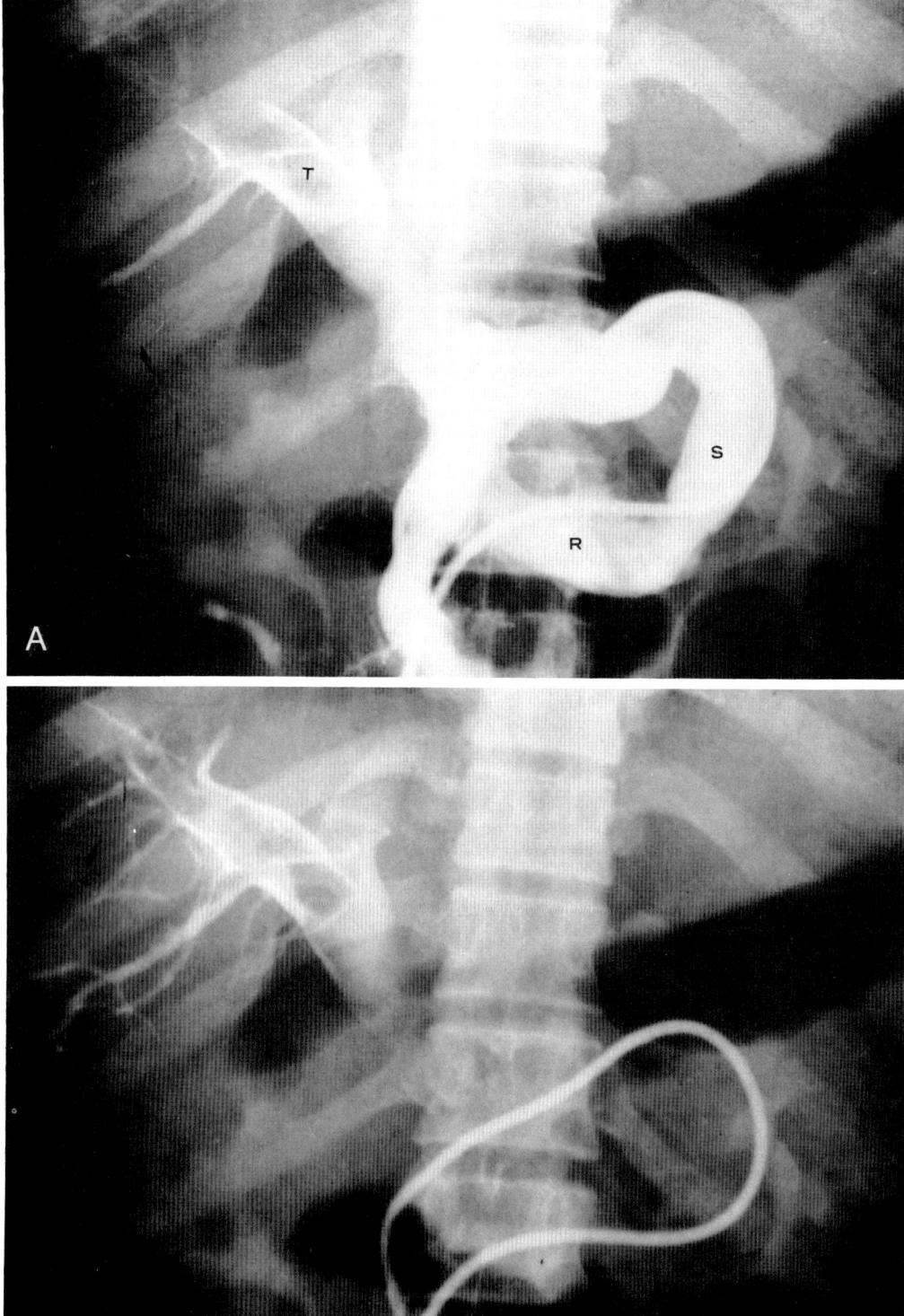

FIGURE 29.12. SPLENORENAL SHUNT
A patient with portal hypertension secondary to schistosomiasis treated with splenorenal shunt. *A:* The catheter passes up the IVC into the renal vein (R), through the splenorenal shunt(s) with the tip in the superior mesenteric vein. Contrast outlines this vascular anatomy and shows a thrombosis (T) in the portal vein better seen on (*B*), a delayed film from the same study.

since his case did have leukemic infiltration of the spleen which may cause rupture.

Shadle et al. (78) reported a CT demonstration of situs inversus in polysplenia with infarction in one of the spleens presenting as right flank pain. The lesion was a sharply demarcated low density lesion with a thick crescent of preserved splenic tissue around it in spite of complete occlusion of the supplying artery on arteriography.

A clinical study analogous to Balcar's experiment is exhibited by the five splenic infarcts as a complication of hepatic arterial embolization for liver malignancy reported by Takayasu et al. (79). All had multiple low density lesions on CT of varied shape. In 3 cases the lesions enhanced markedly in the immediate post embolization period corresponding to the hyperacute phase in Balcar's experiment. Takayasu performed follow-up CT on some cases to 3 months. He showed that the natural history is one of a gradual decrease in size of the infarct and in two cases the infarct disappeared completely. Only two showed the typical contour indentation or scar at site of infarction on follow-up.

While air bubbles in a solid organ generally imply abscess, nonsuppurative gas formation after transcatheter embolization has been reported in the liver, kidney, and the spleen (80). One theory is that infarcted tissue allows oxyhemaglobin to release its oxygen (81). The appearance on CT is one of numerous small gas bubbles diffusely with a central predominance.

New modalities such as NMR and SPECT scanning have also demonstrated splenic infarcts (Figs. 29.6B, 29.11, and 29.12).

SPLENORENAL SHUNT

Splenorenal shunts are reported in patients with chronic portal hypertension usually due to cirrhosis. Small splenorenal shunts are probably not rare but are often undetected. These patients generally present with signs and symptoms of severe cirrhosis. Hepatic encephalopathy is usually present (82). The diagnosis is made definitively by splenoportography (83, 84). Since flow is reversed in the splenic vein, one sees dilated collaterals which communicate with the left renal vein with opacification of the inferior vena cava (84). Note that this is in contrast to splenic vein thrombosis where the portal vein generally fills via collateral flow (85). Sonography or CT was used in five cases reported by Takayasu (86) from Japan. Sonography showed winding tubular structures near the splenic hilus measuring 17–32 mm in diameter, splenomegaly, and in two cases a dilated left renal vein. While not diagnostic, the splenic vein is usually less than 15 mm in diameter in portal hypertension without splenorenal shunt (86). CT also shows dilated perisplenic veins and an enlarged renal vein which enhance with contrast injection.

Some authors theorize that since blood is shunted to the renal vein, upper gastrointestinal bleeding from esophageal varices is less likely to occur in these patients (87).

Splenorenal shunts may be created surgically to treat portal hypertension. This allows pressure in the portal system to approximate that of the inferior vena cava. The Warren shunt is a distal splenorenal shunt (Fig. 29.12). Postoperative patency may be evaluated by celiac or selective splenic and superior mesenteric angiogram (88) or direct catheterization of the shunt. Recently, nuclear magnetic resonance has proved reliable in proving patency except when steel coils are in place from a prior embolization (88). With time, angiography may demonstrate development of collateral flow between the superior mesenteric or portal veins and the gastric veins. Reuter and Redman demonstrate a Warren shunt with hemorrhoidal vein dilation due to failure to ligate the middle colic vein allowing collateral flow via the middle colic to the internal iliac veins (89).

Rarely, arteriovenous shunt may occur as a complication of splenectomy (90).

SPLENIC VASCULAR CHANGES IN PANCREATIC DISEASE

Pancreatic masses or pancreatitis will often cause changes in the splenic artery or vein. For a detailed discussion of the roentgen findings in pancreatic disease see Chapters 21 and 22.

A mass (i.e., pseudocyst) in the distal portion of the pancreas may cause a nonspecific displacement of the splenic artery and vein cephalad. Carcinoma may incase the splenic artery and cause an irregular stenosis or even complete occlusion (91). This finding suggests malignant rather than benign pancreatic disease. The encasement may be smoother and tapered over a larger segment than usually seen with atherosclerosis or may mimic an atherosclerotic stenosis (1). Encasement may be due to desmoplasia associated with a neoplasm rather than neoplasm per se (91). Since differentiation of atherosclerotic from malignant arterial narrowing may be difficult, splenic vein evaluation is useful. If the vein is normal, atherosclerosis is the likely diagnosis. If the splenic vein is obstructed, pancreatic carcinoma is most likely. Pancreatitis should be excluded as well since it too can cause fibrosis with narrowing of the pancreatic arteries and occasionally splenic artery.

Pseudoaneurysms of the splenic artery due to pancreatitis are discussed above under splenic artery aneurysm.

PELIOSIS OF THE SPLEEN

Peliosis is a rare condition usually involving the liver, characterized by numerous varying sized blood filled cysts diffusely throughout the organ. Splenic involvement is even rarer with at least 13 cases reported, none with radiographic data (92, 93). In all cases the liver was involved. Numerous purple nodules fill the red pulp of the spleen and produce an irregularity to the splenic contour. They are thought to be due to a progressive dilatation of the sinuses. There is an association with the use of anabolic steroids. They may undergo thrombosis and fibrosis. The clinical significance lies in blood loss due to rupture of the cyst which can cause pancytopenia or fatal hemorrhage. Although not reported in the radiologic literature, the appearance might mimic diffuse hematogenous abscesses or lymphangioma/hemagioma or metasases.

REFERENCES

1. Abrams HL: Splenic arteriography. In Abrams HL (ed): *Abrams Angiography: Vascular and Interventional Radiology*. Boston, Little, Brown, 1983.
2. Childress MH, Cho KJ, Newlin N, Martel W: Arterial impression on the stomach. *AJR* 132:769–772, 1972.
3. Fishbone G, Nunez D Jr, Leon R, Paz G, Isturiz P, McLoughlin C: Massive splenic infarction in sickle cell-hemoglobin C disease: angiographic findings. *AJR* 129:927–928, 1977.
4. Cohen BA, Mitty HA, Mendelson DS: Case report: computed tomography of splenic infarction. *J Comput Assist Tomogr* 8:167–168, 1984.
5. Scharschmidt BF: The natural history of hypertrophic gastropathy (Ménétriêr's disease). *Am J Med* 63:644, 1977.
6. Palubinskas AJ, Ripley HR: Fibromuscular hyperplasia in extrarenal arteries. *Radiology* 82:451, 1964.
7. Garti LJ, Meiraz D: Fibromuscular dysplasia of the splenic artery in a child; case report. *Vasa* 8:83, 1979.
8. Cobos JM, Hisano K, Matsumori M, Okada M, Nakamura K: Multiple calcified aneurysms of splenic artery, hypersplenism and concomitant cholelithiasis. *Jpn J Surg* 12:448–452, 1982.
9. Feist JH, Gajaraj A: Extra- and intrasplenic artery aneurysms in portal hypertension. *Radiology* 125:331–334, 1977.
10. de Vries JE, Schattenkerk ME, Malt RA: Complications of splenic artery aneurysm other than intraperitoneal rupture. *Surgery* 91:200–204, 1982.
11. Barrett JM, Caldwell BH: Association of portal hypertension and ruptured splenic artery aneurysm in pregnancy. *Obstet Gynecol* 57:255–257, 1981.
12. Puttini M, Aseni P, Brambilla G, Belli L: Splenic artery aneurysms in portal hypertension. *J Cardiovasc Surg* 23:490–493, 1982.
13. Cheng Y: Pregnancy in liver cirrhosis and/or portal hypertension. *Am J Obstet Gynecol* 128:812, 1977.
14. Haynes CD, Smith RB III, Dempsey RL, Darden WA Jr: Multiple congenital aneurysms associated with spontaneous vascular rupture. *Surgery* 92:910–912, 1982.
15. Margulis AR, Burhenne HJ: *Alimentary Tract Radiology*, Ed 3. St. Louis, C. V. Mosby, 1983, p 1825.
16. Mayefsky E, Kaynan A, Waxman J, Kim U: Acute intraabdominal hemorrhage from ruptured aneurysms of the splenic artery. *Mt Sinai J Med (NY)* 49:487–491, 1982.
17. Bodine JA, Hunt TH: Splenic artery-colonic fistula due to pancreatitis. *South Med J* 76:1187–1189, 1983.
18. Nino-Murcia M, Kurtz A, Brennan RG, Shaw E et al: CT diagnosis of splenic artery pseudoaneurysm: a complication of chronic pancreatitis and pseudocyst formation. *J Comput Assist Tomogr* 7:527–529, 1983.
19. Martin KW, Morian JP Jr, Lee JKT, Scharp DW: Demonstration of a splenic artery pseudoaneurysm by MR imaging. *J Comput Assist Tomogr* 9:190–192, 1985.
20. Harper PC, Gamelli RL, Kaye MD: Recurrent hemorrhage into the pancreatic duct from a splenic artery aneurysm. *Gastroenterology* 87:417–420, 1984.
21. Derchi LE, Biggi E, Cicio GR, Bertoglio C, Neumaier CE: Aneurysms of the splenic artery: noninvasive diagnosis by pulsed doppler sonography. *J Ultrasound Med* 3:41–44, 1944.
22. Probst P, Castaneda-Zuniga WR, Gomes AS, Yonehiro EG, Delaney JP, Amplatz K: Nonsurgical treatment of splenic-artery aneurysms. *Radiology* 128:619–623, 1978.
22. Uflacker R, Diehl JC: Successful embolization of a bleeding splenic artery pseudoaneurysm secondary to necrotizing pancreatitis. *Gastrointest Radiol* 7:379–382, 1982.
24. Van Way CW, Crane J, Riddell DH, Foster JH: Arteriovenous fistula in the portal circulation. *Surgery* 70:876–890, 1971.
25. Bredfeldt JE, O'Laughlin JC: Portal hypertension secondary to a congenital splenic arteriovenous fistula. *J Clin Gastroenterol* 2:355–358, 1980.
26. Donovan AJ, Reynolds TB, Mikkelsen WP, Peters RL: Systemic-portal arteriovenous fistulas: pathologic and hemodynamic observations in two patients. *Surgery* 66:474–482, 1969.
27. Pasternak BM, Cohen H: Arteriovenous fistula and forward hypertension in the portal circulation. *Angiology* 29:367–373, 1978.
28. Trede M, Linder R, Vollmar J, Krumhaar D: Arteriove-

nous fistula of the portal system. *J Cardiovasc Surg* 10:254–257, 1969.
29. Madison FE: Embolic therapy of hypersplenism. *Invest Radiol* 8:280–281, 1973.
30. Anderson JH, Buban A, Wallace S, Hester JP, Burke JS: Transcatheter splenic arterial occlusion: an experimental study in dogs. *Radiology* 125:95–102, 1977.
31. Vujic I, Lauver JW: Severe complications from partial splenic embolization in patients with liver failure. *Br J Radiol* 54:492–495, 1981.
32. Spigos DG, Jonasson O, Mozes M, Clark V: Partial splenic embolization in the treatment of hypersplenism. *AJR* 132:777–782, 1979.
33. Guilford WB, Scatliff JH: Transcatheter embolization of the spleen for control of splenic hemorrhage and in situ splenectomy: an experimental study using silicone spheres. *Radiology* 119:549–553, 1976.
34. Goldman ML, Philip PK, Sarrafizadeh MS, Sarfeh IJ, Salam AA, Galambos JT, Powers SR, Balint JA: Intra-arterial tissue adhesive for medical splenectomy in humans. *Radiology* 140:341–349, 1981.
35. Steinherz PG, Exelby PR, Young J, Watson RC: Splenectomy after angiographic embolization of the splenic artery in patients with massive splenomegaly and severe thrombocytopenia in juvenile subacute myelomonocytic leukemia. *Med Pediatr Oncol* 12:28–32, 1984.
36. Owman T, Lunderquist A, Alwmark A, Borjesson B: Embolization of the spleen for treatment of splenomegaly and hypersplenism in patients with portal hypertension. *Invest Radiol* 14:457–464, 1979.
37. Wholey MH, Chamorro H, Rao G et al: Splenic infarction and spontaneous rupture of the spleen following therapeutic embolization. *Cardiovasc Radiol* 1:249, 1978.
38. Pabst R, Kamran D, Creutzig H: Splenic regeneration and blood flow after ligation of the splenic artery or partial splenectomy. *Am J Surg* 147:382–386, 1984.
39. Johnson PM, Spencer RP, Grossbard L: Return of splenic function after intragenic occlusion of the splenic artery. *Clin Nucl Med* 516, 1980.
40. Castaneda-Zuniga WR, Hammerschmidt DE, Sanchez R, Amplatz K: Nonsurgical splenectomy. *AJR* 129:805–811, 1977.
41. Gerlock AJ Jr, MacDonell RC Jr, Mohletaler CA et al: Partial splenic embolization for hypersplenism in renal transplantation. *AJR* 138:451, 1982.
42. Sutton YP, Yarbrough DY, Richards JT: Isolated splenic vein occlusion. *Arch Surg* 100:623–626, 1970.
43. Cho KJ, Martel W: Recognition of splenic vein occlusion. *AJR* 131:439–443, 1978.
44. Itzchak Y, Glickman MG: Splenic vein thrombosis in patients with a normal size spleen. *Invest Radiol* 12:158–163, 1977.
45. Muhletaler C, Gerlock AJ Jr, Goncharenko V, Avant GR, Flexner JM: Gastric varices secondary to splenic vein occlusion: radiographic diagnosis and clinical significance. *Radiology* 132:593–598, 1979.
46. Lavender S, Lloyd-Davies RW, Lea Thomas M: Retroperitoneal fibrosis causing localized portal hypertension. *Br Med J* 3:627–628, 1970.
47. Walter J, Chuang VP, Bookstein JJ, Reuter SR, Cho KR, Pulmano CM: Angiographic of massive hemorrhage secondary to pancreatic disease. *Radiology* 124:337–342, 1977.
48. Johnston FR, Myers RT: Etiologic factors and consequences of splenic vein obstruction. *Ann Surg* 177:736, 1973.
49. Verbanck JJ, Rutgeerts LJ, Haerens MH, Tytgat JH, Segaert MF, Tytgat HJ, Afschrift MB: Partial splenoportal and superior mesenteric venous thrombosis: early sonographic diagnosis and successful conservative management. *Gastroenterology* 86:949–952, 1984.
50. Bunt TJ, Hackler MT, Greene FL: Isolated splenic vein thrombosis: the curable variceal hemorrhage. *South Med J* 76:936–938, 1983.
51. Neimann HL, Goldstein HM, Silverman PJ, Bookstein JJ: Angiographic features of peripancreatic malignant lymphoma. *Radiology* 115:589, 1975.
52. Rice RP, Thompson WM, Kelvin FM, Driner AF, Garbutt JT: Gastric varices: enhanced radiologic visualization by anticholinergic drugs. *Am J Dig Dis* 17:703–712, 1972.
53. Itzchak Y, Glickman MG: Duodenal varices in extrahepatic portal obstruction. *Radiology* 124:619–624, 1977.
54. Merritt CRB: Ultrasonographic demonstration of portal vein thrombosis. *Radiology* 133:425, 1979.
55. Weinberger G, Mitra SK, Yoeli G: Case report: ultrasound diagnosis of splenic vein thrombosis. *J Clin Ultrasound* 10:345–346, 1982.
56. Jeanty P, Brion JP, Van Gossum A, Struyven J: Case report: portal and splenic vein thrombosis: ultrasonic demonstration. *J Belge Radiol* 65:45–47, 1982.
57. Goldberg S, Katz S, Naidich J, Waye J: Isolated gastric varices due to spontaneous splenic vein thrombosis. *Am J Gastroenterol* 79:304, 1984.
58. Hadar H, Sommer R: Calcification in the portal venous system demonstrated by computed tomography. *Eur J Radiol* 3:187–188, 1983.
59. Little A, Moosa A: Gastrointestinal hemorrhage from left sided portal hypertension. *Am J Surg* 141:153–158, 1981.
60. Salam A, Warren D, Tyras D: Splenic vein thrombosis: a diagnosable and curable form of portal hypertension. *Surgery* 74:961–972, 1973.
61. Hershfield N, Morrow I: Gastric bleeding due to splenic vein thrombosis. *Can Med Assoc J* 98:649–652, 1968.
62. Jones KB, Thur de Koos P: Postembolization splenic abscess in a patient with pancreatitis and splenic vein thrombosis. *South Med J* 77:390–393, 1984.
63. Almgren B, Bowald S: Spontaneous rupture of the splenic vein secondary to hepatic cirrhosis. *Acta Chir Scand* 149:109–111, 1983.
64. Macpherson AIS, Richmond J, Stuart AE: *The Spleen.* Springfield, Ill., Charles C Thomas, 1973, p 101.
65. Balcar I, Seltzer SE, Davis S, Geller SC: CT patterns of splenic infarction: a clinical and experimental study. *Radiology* 151:723–729, 1984.
66. Anderson WAD, Kissone JM (eds): *Pathology,* Ed 7. St. Louis, C. V. Mosby, 1977, vol 2, pp 1489–1513.
67. Freeman MH, Tonkin AK: Focal splenic effects. *Radiology* 121:689–692, 1976.
68. Lin MS, Donati RM: Wedged appearance of splenic infarcts on scans. *Clin Nucl Med* 11:556, 1981.
69. Polga JP, Spencer RP: Menetrier's disease with occlusion of splenic and brachial arteries. *Clin Nucl Med* 8:335–336, 1983.
70. Spencer RP, Sziklas JJ, Rosenberg R: The "spleen of hearts" in upper pole infarction. *Clin Nucl Med* 6:278, 1981.
71. Abrams HL (ed): *Abrams Angiography: Vascular and Interventional Radiology.* Boston, Little, Brown, 1983, p 1551.
72. Mittelstaedt CA, Partain CL: Ultrasonic-pathologic classification of splenic abnormalities: gray-scale patterns. *Radiology* 134:697–705, 1980.
73. Siler J, Hunter TB, Weiss J et al: Increased echogenicity of the spleen in benign and malignant disease. *AJR* 134:1011, 1980.
74. Yeh H-C, Zacks J, Jurado RA: Ultrasonography of

splenic infarct. *Mt Sinai J Med NY* 48:446–448, 1981.
75. Weingarten MJ, Fakhry J, McCarthy J, Freeman SJ, Bisker JS: Sonography after splenic embolization: the wedge shaped acute infarct. *AJR* 141:957–959, 1984.
76. Anderson JH, VuBan A, Wallace S, Hester JP, Burke JS: Transcatheter splenic arterial occlusion: an experimental study in dogs. *Radiology* 125:95–102, 1977.
77. Maier W: Computer tomography of splenic infarction. *Eur J Radiol* 2:202–204, 1982.
78. Shadle CA, Scott ME, Ritchie DJ, Seliger G: Spontaneous splenic infarction in polysplenia syndrome. *J Comput Assist Tomogr* 6:177–179, 1982.
79. Takayasu K, Moriyama N, Muramatso V. Suzuki M et al: Splenic infraction, a complication of transcatheter hepatic arterial embolization for liver malignancies. *Radiology* 151:371–375, 1984.
80. Levy JM, Wasserman PI, Weiland DE: Nonsuppurative gas formation in the spleen after transcatheter splenic infarction. *Radiology* 139:375–376, 1981.
81. Rankin RN: Gas formation after renal tumor embolization without abscess: a benign occurrence. *Radiology* 130:317–320, 1979.
82. Lam KC, Juttner HU, Reynolds TB: Spontaneous portosystemic shunt. Relationship to spontaneous encephalopathy and gastrointestinal hemorrhage. *Dig Dis Sci* 26:346–352, 1981.
83. Nunez D Jr, Russell E, Yrizarrt J, Pereiras R, Viamonte M: Portosystemic communication studied by transhepatic portography. *Radiology* 127:75–79, 1978.
84. Redman HC, Reuter SR: Angiographic demonstration of protocaval and other decompresive liver shunts. *Radiology* 92:790, 1969.
85. Reuter SR, Redman HC (eds): *Gastrointestinal Angiography*, Ed 2. Philadelphia, W. B. Saunders, 1977, p 336.
86. Takayasu K, Moriyama N, Shima Y, Yamada T, Kobayashi C, Musha H, Okuda K: *Br J Radiol* 57:565–570, 1984.
87. Wexler MW, MacLean L: Massive spontaneous portalsystemic shunting without varices. *Arch Surg* 110:995–1002, 1975.
88. Bernardino ME, Steinberg, HV, Pearson TC et al: Shunts for portal hypertension: MR and angiography for determination of patency. *Radiology* 158:57–61, 1986.
89. Freeman MH, Tonkin AK: Focal splenic effects. *Radiology*, 121:348.
90. Lacombe M, Hannoun L: Arteriovenous fistula of splenic vessels after splenectomy. *J Chir* 121:159–162, 1984.
91. Abrams HL (ed): *Abrams Angiography: Vacular and Interventional Radiology*. Boston, Little, Brown, 1983, p. 1540.
92. Lacson A, Berman L, Neiman R: Case reports: peliosis of the spleen. *Am J Clin Pathol* 586–590, 1979.
93. Garcia RL, Kahn MK, Berlin RB: Peliosis of the spleen with rupture. *Hum Pathol* 13:177–179, 1982.

30
Miscellaneous Disorders

ABRAHAM H. DACHMAN, M.D.

DENSE OR OPACIFIED SPLEEN

A variety of conditions are discussed separately in this chapter because of their unique or varied manifestations. Only sickle cell anemia is discussed in detail since it is one of the most common of these "miscellaneous disorders" encountered by the radiologist.

Thorotrast

Thorotrast is a radiographic contrast agent introduced commercially in 1930 and used extensively for various contrast studies, particularly angiography. It contains thorium dioxide in colloidal solution. The ^{232}Th decays to ^{208}Pb by emitting α, β and γ rays. Because of the high radiation dose, especially the α rays, and the fact that Thorotrast has negligible excretion with a biologic half-life of 400 yr, its use was discontinued. The radiation dose is highest to the spleen followed by liver and bone marrow, where reticuloendothelial cells phagocytose the Thorotrast particles (11). There is an increased incidence of hepatic angiosarcoma, hepatocellular carcinoma, cholangiocarcinoma, and assorted other tumors in patients who have received Thorotrast.

The spleen undergoes fibrous replacement and shrinks markedly in size and functional asplenia may result (2, 3). Splenic neoplasms are rare, probably because most of the splenic tissue is destroyed or fibrosed by the radiation, with little splenic mass remaining to potentially undergo malignant change (4). There are rare reports of Thorotrast-induced splenic angiosarcoma (2, 4, 5). When liver angiosarcoma is present as well, the splenic lesions are thought to be secondary (2). (See Chapter 27 for a detailed discussion of splenic angiosarcoma.)

Plain films show a small, dense spleen with punctate opacities throughout (Fig. 30.1). Hepatic, lymphatic and peripancreatic nodal opacification is also seen. Splenic masses may be visible as filling defects in a dense spleen and this may be confirmed with CT (4). See Chapter 4 for a more detailed discussion of thorotrast-induced disease.

Hemochromatosis

Abnormal iron deposition in body tissues or hemochromatosis may be "primary," i.e., an inherited disorder causing increased intestinal absorption of iron, or "secondary." Secondary hemochromatosis may occur in chronic anemias or any cause of chronic red blood cell destruction, or repeated blood transfusions (6, 7).

Increased density is noted particularly in the liver, spleen, pancreas, lymph nodes, adrenal glands, and cardiac muscle. This may result in dysfunction of the involved organ, especially causing cirrhosis and diabetes. The spleen may be spared in primary hemochromatosis (6), and may be more severely involved than liver in transfusion-related hemochromatosis (7). Increased density may be detected on CT. Attenuation values in Hounsfield numbers are markedly elevated and sometimes correlate with iron concentration in biopsy specimens (8, 9), but are also affected by the degree of cirrhosis and hepatic fibrosis (9). There may be significant variation in CT numbers obtained at different kVp values (10–12). Plain film will rarely detect the increased density as depicted on CT (9).

Lymphangiogram Contrast

In one case report, a patient with nodular sclerosing Hodgkin's disease with splenic involvement demonstrated extensive hepatic and splenic opacification after a lymphangiogram (13). There was lymphatic obstruction in the upper lumbar area with filling of paralumbar lymphatics which do not normally opacify. The liver was histologically normal and paraduodenal nodes were diseased. It was postulated that the volume of lymphangiogram contrast entering the liver via lymphoportal communications caused a

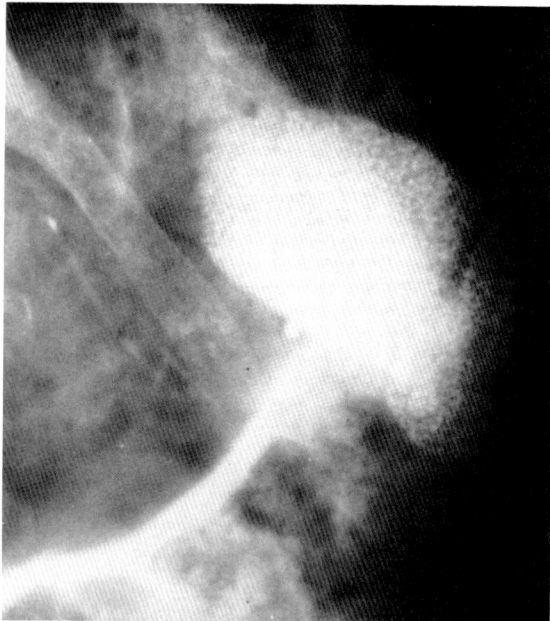

FIGURE 30.1. CALCIFIED SPLEEN
Thorotrast, plain film. Dense mottled calcification in a small spleen. The density is usually more marked than in other causes of splenic calcification.

transient rise in portal venous pressure allowing hepatofugal flow into the splenic vein. Since the spleen has little lymphatic tissue, and no perisplenic or perihepatic lymph ducts opacified, the proposed mechanism is a reasonable explanation in this case.

Splenic Calcification

A densely calcified spleen may occur in diffuse splenic infarction, especially due to sickle cell disease (see below) (14). The pattern may mimic Thorotrast, but will be less dense and will be limited to the spleen, without nodal or hepatic density. The density may be apparent on plain film or CT. ^{99m}Tc-diphosphonate may be taken up by a calcified spleen (15).

Other causes of multiple splenic calcifications include: tuberculosis, histoplasmosis (Chapter 28), multiple infarcts (16), arterial calcification (Chapter 29), and focal lesions, including cysts, abscess, hematoma, and neoplasms (Chapter 27).

Hyposplenism (Functional Asplenia)

The term hyposplenism was introduced in 1913 by Eppinger (17) to describe the hematologic findings after splenectomy. Dameshek (18) further defined the meaning of hyposplenism and broadened it to include diseases causing auto- splenectomy. The term now includes all causes of splenic atrophy with resultant defective splenic function (19).

Hematologic findings in functional asplenia include: lymphocytosis, monocytosis, thrombocytosis, Howell-Jolly bodies, acanthocytes, siderocytes, and pitting of red blood cells. In hyposplenism due to surgical splenectomy, some acute changes such as the thrombocytosis, may return to near normal levels with other hematologic abnormalities persisting chronically (20).

The key confirmatory test is nuclear scintigraphy. The best method is use of heat-damaged red blood cells (see Chapter 25) (21). A variety of erythrocyte labeling and damaging techniques can be used (i.e., chemical or thermal damage). Marsh et al. (22) used heat-damaged chromium-51-labeled red blood cells and showed that asplenic patients had a $t_{1/2}$ (blood clearance halftime) of 35 min to several hours, compared with 10–16 min for normal subjects.

The pathophysiology of functional asplenia may involve (23): (a) interruption of the splenic artery, vein or microscopic vasculature, or (b) altered reticuloendothelial activity (e.g., radiation damage, tumor, sprue, anoxia, or bone marrow transplant).

Diseases associated with hyposplenism with splenic atrophy include: ulcerative colitis, Crohn disease, celiac disease, tropical sprue, dermatitis herpetiformis, thyrotoxicosis, hemorrhagic thrombocythemia, and Thorotrast (19, 20). Hyposplenism with a normal or enlarged spleen may be seen in sarcoidosis, amyloidosis, sickle cell anemia (unless the spleen is totally infarcted), and possibly in association with high dose corticosteroids (20).

Of these, the conditions most commonly associated with hyposplenism are sickle cell disease (see below), celiac sprue (or idiopathic steatorrhea), dermatitis herpetiformis, and ulcerative colitis. Up to 40% of patients with the latter three conditions show evidence of hyposplenism on peripheral blood smear (20). In ulcerative colitis, the hyposplenism waxes and wanes with the activity of the colitis and tends to be severe if pancolitis is present (24).

The pathogenesis of hyposplenism in these disorders is unknown, but the current favored theory is that of an autoimmune mechanism (20).

There is an increased risk of infection and fatal bacteremia when severe hyposplenism is present. Thus, total splenectomy (i.e., in trauma), should be avoided if possible. Hyposplenic patients probably should receive vaccines for pneumococcus, influenza, and meningococcus.

SICKLE CELL ANEMIA

Sickle cell (SC) disease was first recognized in 1920, and in the United States affects predominantly blacks. A slight ambiguity is found in the literature; for the purposes of this chapter "sickle cell anemia" will refer to homozygous SS disease, while "sickle cell disease" may refer to homozygous (HbSS) or to heterozygous (HbAS, SC-Thal, etc.) disease. Sickle cell anemia affects 1 in 600 black children at birth. Heterozygous trait disease (HbAS) is found in 8 to 10% of the black population. The disease is multisystemic, with recurrent episodes of crisis and a high incidence of infections, particularly of lung, bone, and brain. In the child with homozygous disease, 40 to 100% of the hemoglobin can be Hemoglobin S (HBS), while the trait patient may have only 20 to 40% HBS (25–27).

Sickle cell hemoglobin substitutes valine for glutamic acid in the beta chain, rendering the erythrocyte subject to drastic alterations in shape and plasticity. Areas of slow flow, such as the spleen, liver, and renal medulla, or areas of rapid metabolism, such as brain, muscle or fetal placenta, can also sickle the erythrocyte. In the spleen, partial phagocytosis can be corrective, removing particles of sickled cells.

These deformed red cells are rigid and may impact and lodge in end-arteries, resulting in the so-called "log-jam" occlusion of small blood vessels, and can cause infarction in every organ system. The resultant regions of necrotic tissue can predispose to bacterial superinfection (25–27).

Repetitive local infarctions tend to cause autoinfarction of the spleen in most SS patients, with splenic function being lost by age 5. Prior to total loss of function, sickle cell patients may be subject to episodes of splenic sequestration. It is a common cause of death in the young homozygous patient, and is, in effect, a functional splenic drainage obstruction. Sequestration may be temporary (transfusion-reversible) or persistent. The sudden vascular pooling causes an acute onset and progression of symptoms.

At one time, splenectomy was the treatment of choice, but it is now reserved only for the intractable cases of recurrent sequestration. This is both because in the known association of splenectomy with immune deficiency and infection, and because in the sickle cell patient anesthesia and surgery impose increased risks.

Sickle Cell Trait

Patients with sickle cell trait (HbAS), form erythrocytes containing less than 50% HbS (usually closer to 45%), and may have near-normal blood counts and smears (26, 27). As a rule, sickling is elicited only under conditions of extreme stress (flight in unpressurized aircraft, anoxia associated with congenital heart disease, prolonged anesthesia, marathon running) (26, 27, 29–32). Trait patients tend to have far milder disease, with fewer episodes of crisis and infection than their HbSS counterparts. With fewer and less severe episodes of vaso-occlusion, the spleen is damaged but not functionally destroyed. Unlike the autosplenectomized organ of the homozygous patient, the partially functioning sickle cell trait spleen continues to provide a site of potential pathology, including splenic abscess, infarcts, hemorrhage and rupture.

SC Disease

Three percent of the black population in this country are believed to be carriers of the gene HbC, and HbSC disease is about one-fourth as common as HbSS (27). There are abnormalities of splenic size and function; the risk of infection exceeds normal, but does not approach that of the homozygous patient (33, 34). Various sorts of deoxygenating stress can elicit sickling and vaso-occlusion; therefore, complications such as painful vaso-occlusive crisis, avascular necrosis and pulmonary infarctions and infection are not rare.

Sickle-Thal Disease

Sickle cell thalassemia patients with β-0-thalssemia genes have no normal adult hemoglobin, and as a result clinically resemble SS patients. Like the sickle cell trait or thalassemia minor patient, they have hemolytic anemia and persistent splenomegaly (26, 27).

Splenic Imaging in Sickle Cell Disease

In the homozygous population, the spleen tends to be of active clinical interest only in early childhood, prior to autosplenectomy. Most heterozygous disease is clinically milder, with at least partial splenic function persisting into adulthood. In these groups, therefore, the spleen remains the site of potential pathology. Both homozygous and heterozygous patients may be high profile consumers of medical care, presenting frequently with episodes of crisis, abdominal pain, and/or fever. It is important to consider the benefits and limitations of any diagnostic imaging exam being considered in the workup of such patients.

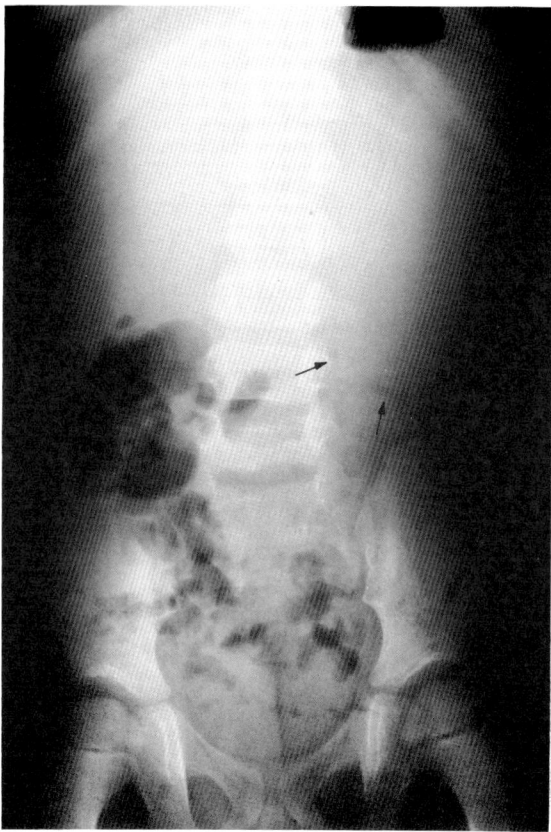

FIGURE 30.2. SICKLE CELL DISEASE
A 3-yr-old black boy with abdominal pain and drop in hematocrit. Upright examination of abdomen shows a large radiodensity in the left upper quadrant (*arrows*) displacing the splenic flexure inferiorly and medially. This was compatible with enlarged spleen during sequestration crisis, a diagnosis is confirmed at surgery.

Plain Film

In the homozygous patient, splenomegaly most commonly is seen only until about 5 yr of age, although it can be seen at any age in the heterozygous population. Plain film will show an enlarged spleen displacing the stomach medially and splenic flexure inferiorly. Splenic sequestration crisis may be marked by a rapid increase in size (Fig. 30.2). Infarction or abscess may cause splenic enlargement and perisplenic inflammation, reflected in posteroanterior and lateral chest films as left pleural effusion, left hemidiaphragm elevation, or left lower lobe atelectasis or infiltrates; and in the abdominal series as splenomegaly, focal ileus, gastric distention, or local edema of bowel wall.

The autoinfarcted and fibrotic end-stage spleen in the older homozygous patients may show diffuse or patchy calcification on plain film (Figs. 30.3 and 30.4). This correlates with the microscopic perivascular and parenchymal calcifications, and increased iron deposition, first demonstrated in 1935 (35). As a rule, by the time such an appearance is noted on plain film, splenic function has been greatly impaired or lost, and this may be seen in up to 31% of patients with sickle cell anemia. Diffuse punctate or stippled calcifications are most common (55%), creating a "pseudothorotrast" appearance. Larger, more amorphous calcifications may be seen in 32%, occurring in a slightly older population and believed to represent the natural progression of fibrosis and contraction in a stippled spleen. Rarely, diffuse or focal curvilinear densities are noted (36).

Also to be noted on chest and abdominal films are other common stigmata of sickle cell disease, such as cardiomegaly, "Lincoln log" or "fish" vertebrae, patchy bony sclerosis, cholelithiasis, and avascular necrosis of the femoral heads (37).

Angiography

With CT and ultrasound readily available in most institutions, angiography rarely is required in a workup of abdominal pain and/or fever in the patient with sickle cell disease. Although computed tomography is faster and less invasive, angiography may be used to define suspected splenic rupture, which may follow splenic infarction or abscess. It will also define whether a splenic rupture or laceration is contained by the capsule, or whether the capsule also has been disrupted (Fig. 30.5). One patient in a series at Johns Hopkins Medical Center came to angiography as part of a prolonged workup for chronic left upper quadrant pain of no definable etiology (Fig. 30.6).

Liver-Spleen Radionuclide Scan

The liver-spleen ^{99m}Tc-sulfur colloid scan is dependent on a homogeneous distribution of normally functioning reticuloendothelial cells for organ visualization. Prior to autosplenectomy, the homozygous spleen will show decreasing uptake commensurate with declining function. At least partial uptake usually persists into adulthood in heterozygous patients, but may be markedly impaired proportional (as is the clinical severity of disease) to the percent of abnormal hemoglobin and to the presence or absence of protective fetal hemoglobin (Fig. 30.6*B*). In order to enhance visualization and to assess size and contour in any patient with impaired splenic

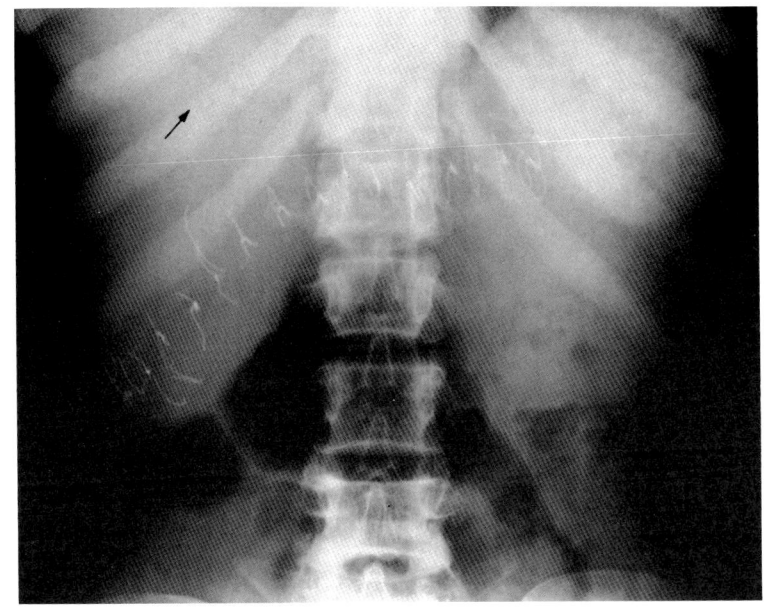

FIGURE 30.3. SICKLE CELL DISEASE
A 27-yr-old black woman with HbSS. Supine radiograph of the abdomen shows a 7 × 8 cm speckled radiodensity in the left upper gradrant compatible with a densely calcified spleen. There has been surgery with prior cholecystectomy, and reflux of air is seen into the biliary tree (*arrow*).

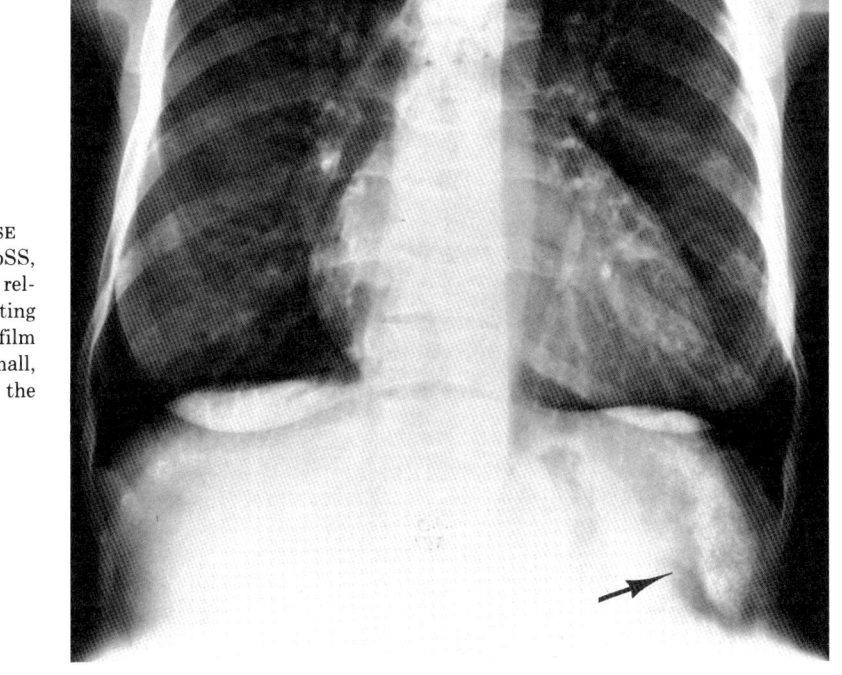

FIGURE 30.4. SICKLE CELL DISEASE
A 50-yr-old black woman with HbSS, apparently clinically modified by the relatively high level (3.4%) of persisting fetal hemoglobin, HbF. Upright film shows cardiomegaly and a very small, densely calcified spleen just under the left hemidiaphragm (*arrow*).

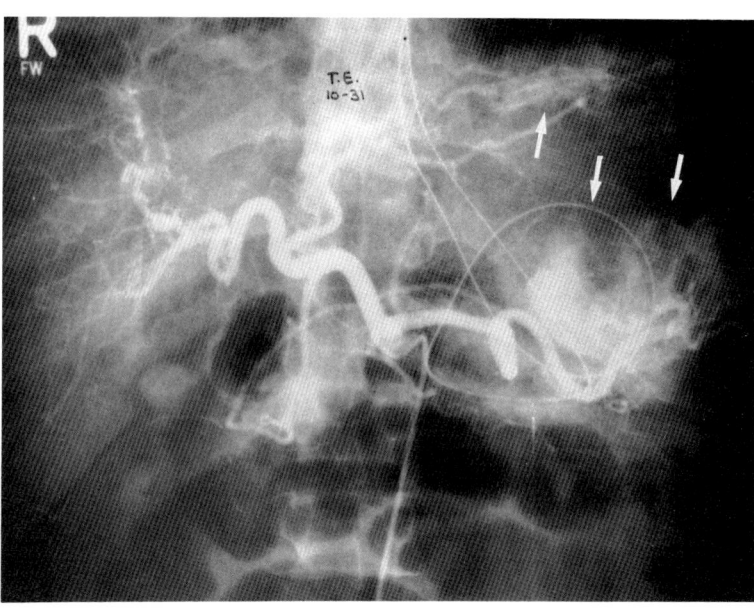

FIGURE 30.5. SICKLE CELL DISEASE
A 30-yr-old black man with HbSA and acute abdominal pain. Selective catheterization of the celiac axis shows patent hepatic and splenic arteries. There has been a spontaneous splenic rupture (arrows), with no evidence of extravasation outside of the splenic capsule. This was confirmed at surgery.

function, splenic imaging may be prolonged until a certain number of emitted counts have been recorded. An assessment of function can be made by comparing this image to a similarly positioned image obtained during the routine imaging interval (Fig. 30.7A and B). When imaging "for counts," a small field of view is used to exclude the more normal and therefore, "hotter" liver.

Focal splenic abnormalities such as infarct, abscess or hemorrhage may be seen as focal photon-deficient areas or contour irregularities. Imaging "for counts" will help to enhance visualization of such lesions, but in general lesions less than 2 cm in size will not be detected reliably.

Technetium-99m Bone Scan

Radionuclide bone agents such as ^{99m}Tc-methylene diphosphonate (MDP) may accumulate in a calcified spleen, as they accumulate in other calcified soft tissues. On first glance, this may mimic osteomyelitis in an overlying rib. Such splenic accumulation may be seen on bone scan prior to the appearance of calcifications on plain film and corresponds with microscopic tissue deposits of calcium (Fig. 30.7C). This also corresponds with increased splenic density on the CT scan, which is more sensitive to small density differences. The infarcted spleen showing low density areas on CT scan may also accumulate radionuclide bone agents, which is less readily understood. Probably this parallels the documented accumulation of bone agents in infarcted brain and myocardial tissue even in the absence of calcifications under light microscopy. This is believed to be due to altered cell membranes and organelles, allowing an enhanced calcium-phosphate flux into the cell. This creates subcellular crystals seen only via electron microscopy, which in time may advance microscopically and ultimately become radiographically detectable calcifications (38, 39).

Ultrasound

As in other clinical conditions, the sickle cell patient with splenomegaly is more likely to get an adequate exam of the left upper quadrant than the patient with either a normal or atrophic spleen, since the enlarged organ provides a better acoustic window. Even with splenomegaly, the region of the dome of the spleen and of the left hemidiaphragm can be difficult to sort out, and in this case, real time may help. As noted earlier, it is the heterozygous population which tends to have persisting splenomegaly and splenic function, and therefore, to demonstrate active splenic disease such as infarction or abscess; and this population may benefit from ultrasound more than the homozygous population. Intrasplenic foci of altered echogenicity may be noted with focal infarction or abscess. These usually appear as echopenic areas with scattered internal echoes and irregular borders, distinguishing such lesions from simple splenic cysts (Fig. 30.8A and B). Infarction can lead to hemorrhage, which may be echogenic, and with large infarctions, necrosis, air collection, and rupture may be noted. Air

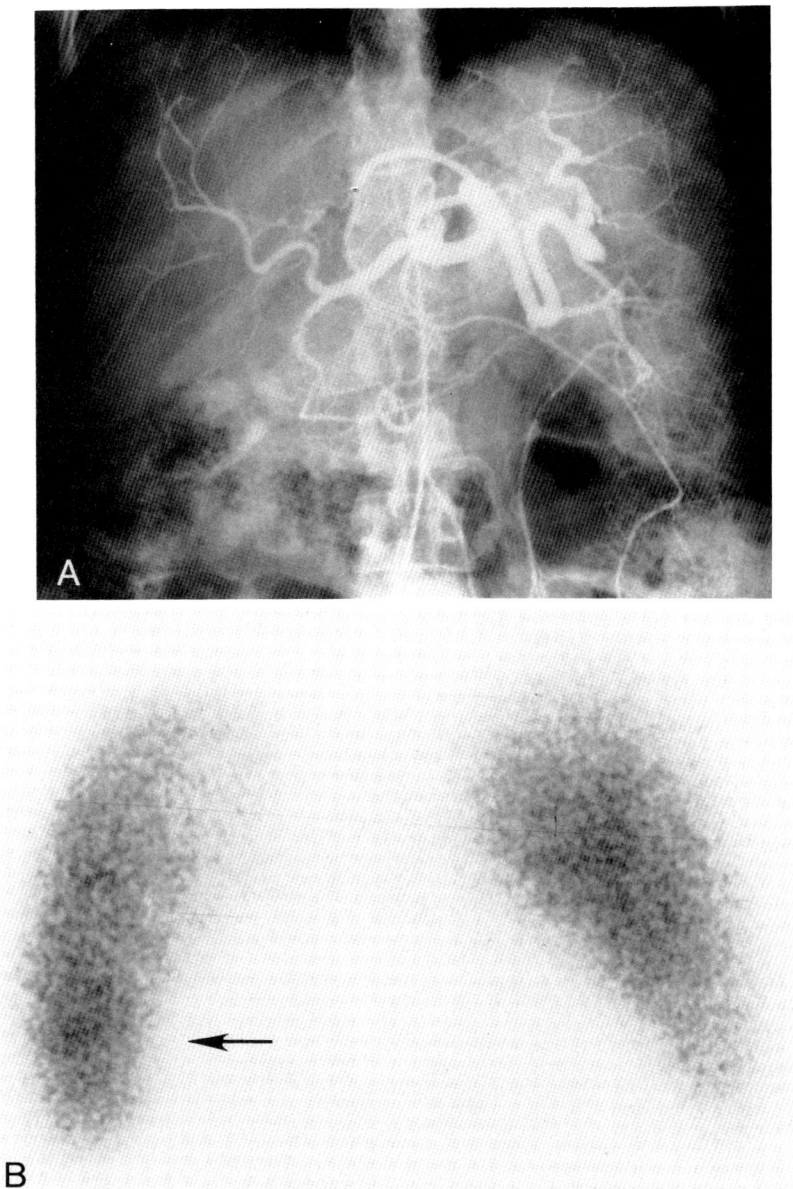

FIGURE 30.6. SICKLE CELL DISEASE

A 49-yr-old black woman with HbSC and a long history of vague left upper quadrant pain of uncertain etiology. *A:* Selective catheterization of the celiac axis shows patent hepatic and splenic arteries, with diffuse splenomegaly. No focal abnormalities or irregularities in contour were noted. Focal tortuosity of proximal splenic vessels was noted, but was of unclear clinical significance. *B:* ^{99m}Tc-sulfur colloid liver spleen scan, posterior view, shows marked enlargement of a spleen with near-normal function (*arrow*). No focal defects or abnormalities are noted; the contour appeared normal on all views.

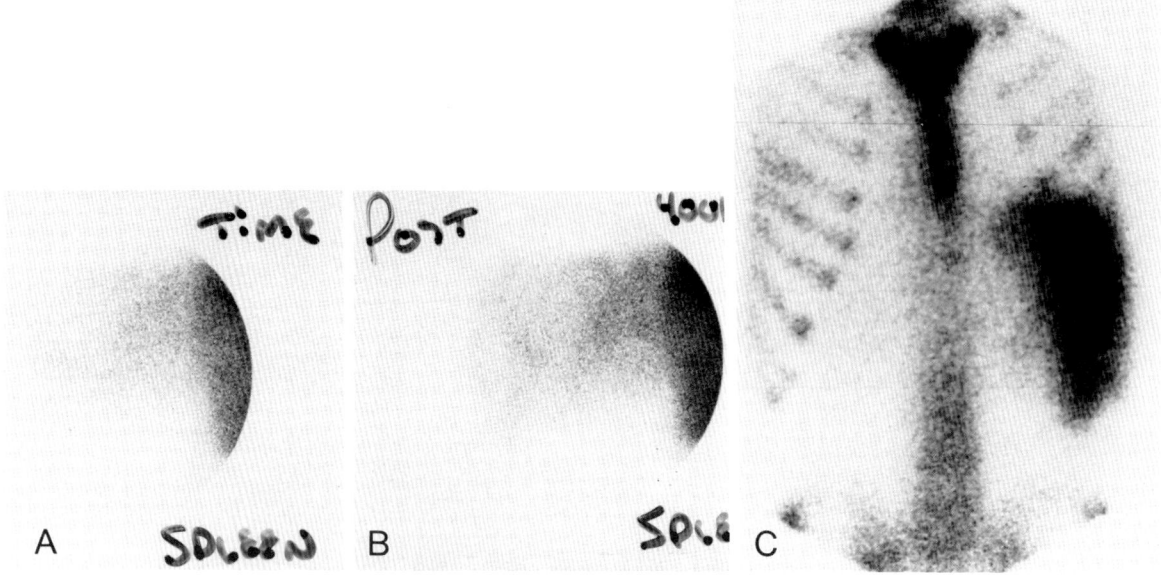

FIGURE 30.7. SICKLE CELL DISEASE

A 17-yr-old black male patient with HbSS, with abdominal pain and fever. ^{99m}Tc-sulfur colloid liver spleen scan failed to show any evidence of splenic uptake on conventional views. Posterior views were repeated with small field view collimator, with one image done for time (A) and one for 400,000 counts (B). An enlarged, poorly functioning spleen was seen. A ^{99m}Tc-MDP bone scan (C) was subsequently performed on the same patient, and showed marked localization of radionuclide bone agent in an enlarged spleen. No definite contour abnormalities or focal defects were noted.

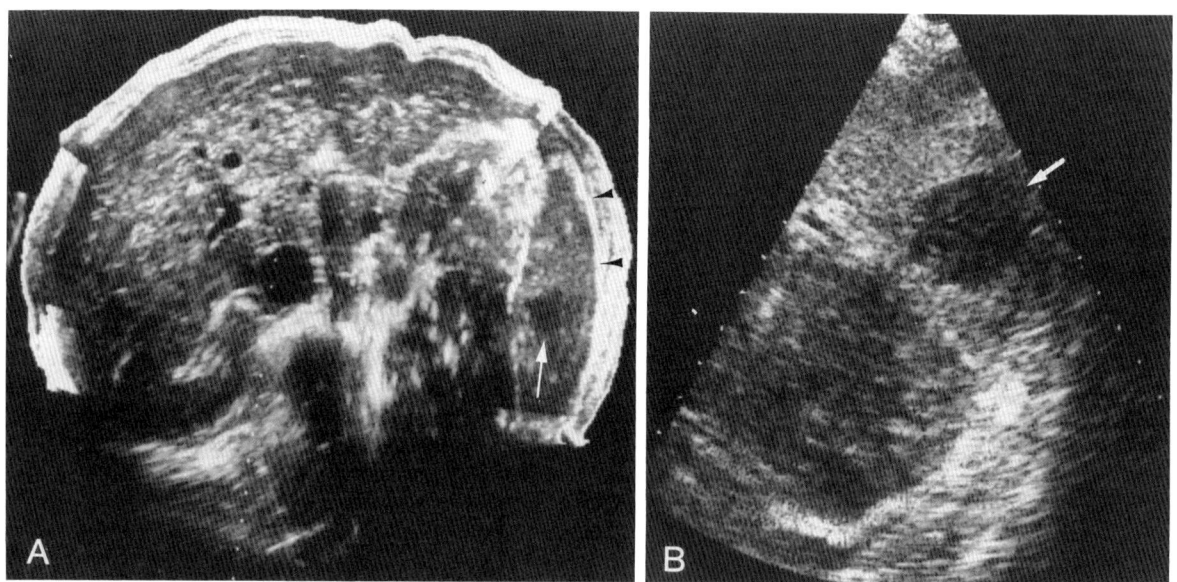

FIGURE 30.8. SICKLE CELL DISEASE

A 12-yr-old black boy with HbSS, with vague upper abdominal pain and fever. Chest x-rays showed some left lower lobe infiltrates and small pleural effusion. A: Static transverse image shows hepatomegaly and an enlarged spleen (*arrowheads*) projecting anteriorly well past the anterior border of the aorta at the same level. A central 3 × 3 cm focal splenic defect is defined (*arrow*), with minimally irregular walls and no definite internal echoes on this one view. B: A left oblique real-time view confirms this 3 cm focal echopenic area in the spleen (*arrow*), which was found on multiple images to have a few ill-defined internal echoes and no definite increase through transmission. The walls appeared relatively smooth. This was felt to be compatible with splenic infarct, although abscess or hemorrhage could not be ruled out.

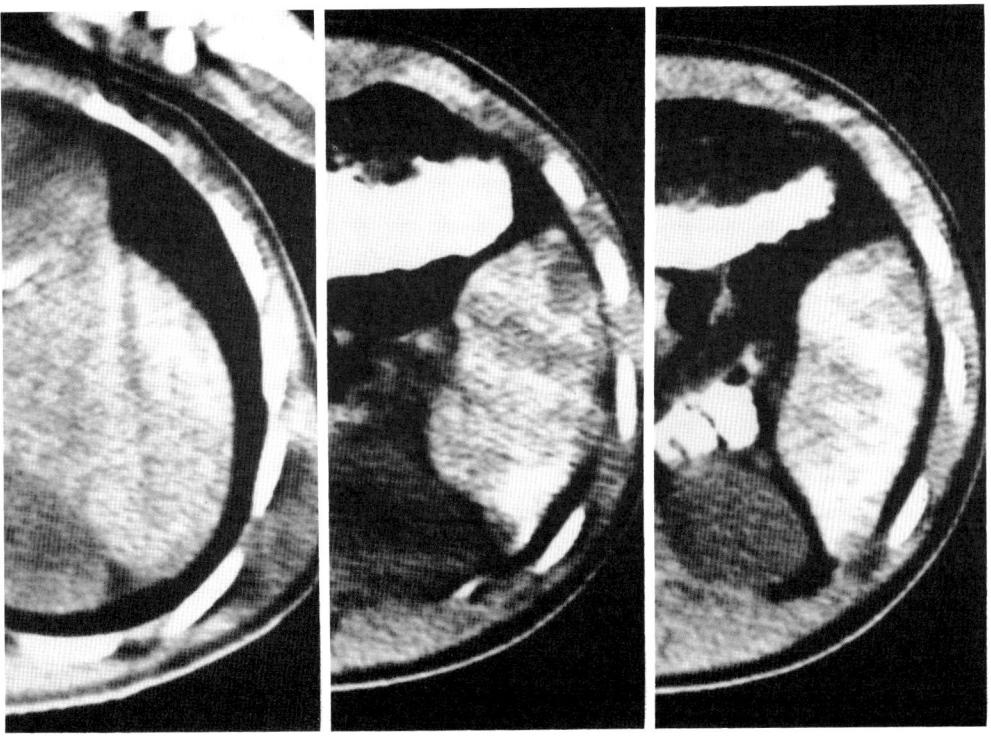

FIGURE 30.9. SICKLE CELL DISEASE
A 17-yr-old black boy with HbSS and nonfunctioning enlarged spleen. Splenomegaly with diffuse mottled calcifications noted on CT scan.

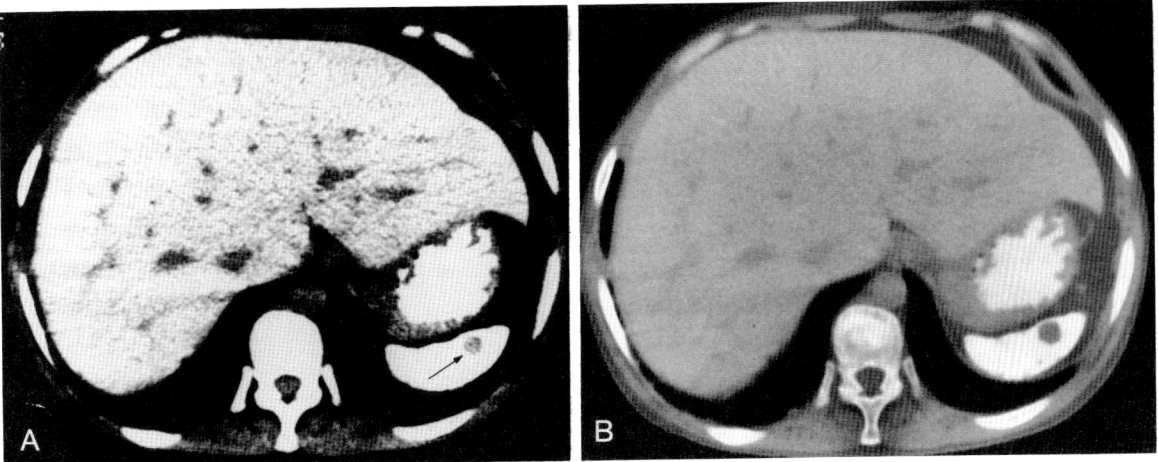

FIGURE 30.10. SICKLE CELL DISEASE
A 31-yr-old black man with HbSS and abdominal pain. *A:* Normal-sized but densely calcified spleen seen, with one area of central sparing (*arrow*). Liver is also noted to be unusually dense at about 110 HU, compatible with biopsy-proven transfusion hemochromatosis. *B:* Same section, at wide "bone" windows, demonstrating density of splenic calcification.

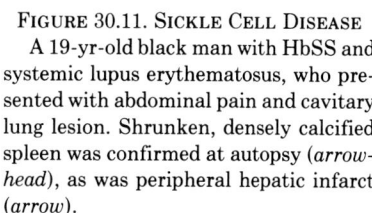

FIGURE 30.11. SICKLE CELL DISEASE
A 19-yr-old black man with HbSS and systemic lupus erythematosus, who presented with abdominal pain and cavitary lung lesion. Shrunken, densely calcified spleen was confirmed at autopsy (*arrowhead*), as was peripheral hepatic infarct (*arrow*).

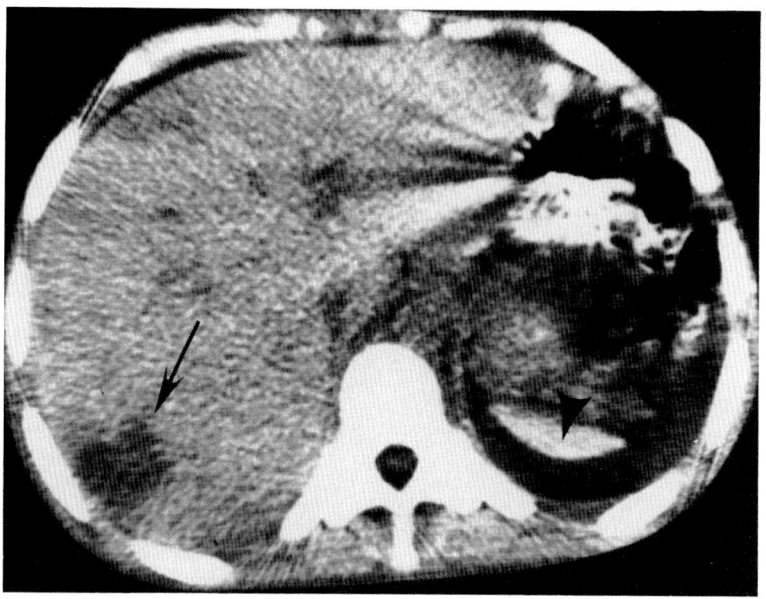

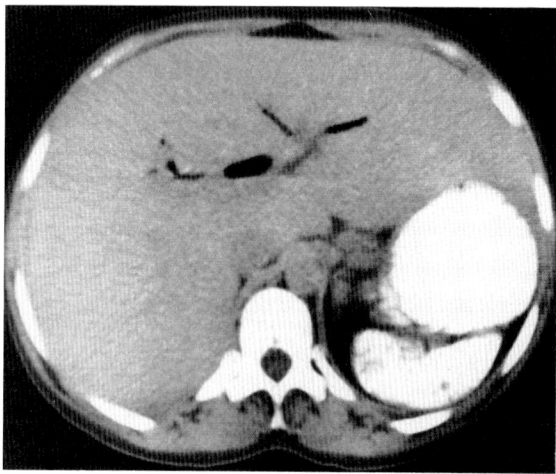

FIGURE 30.12. SICKLE CELL DISEASE
A 27-yr-old black woman with HbSS. The spleen is near-normal size and densely calcified with a few areas of mottling. Air in the biliary tree is compatible with surgery. Hepatomegaly is also noted.

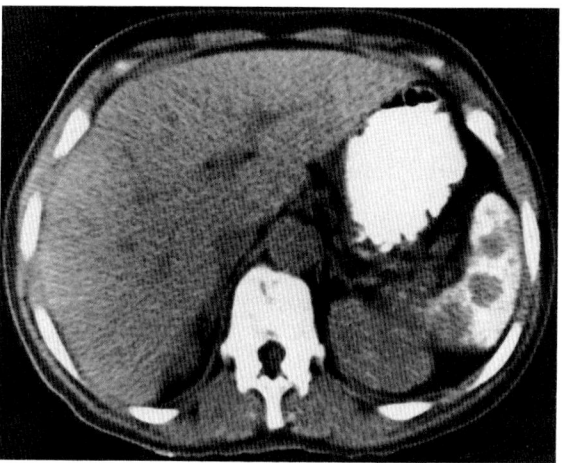

FIGURE 30.13. SICKLE CELL DISEASE
A 54-yr-old black woman with homozygous disease and 3.4% hemoglobin F, who presented with abdominal pain. Normal-sized but calcified sleen with several islands of more-normal splenic attenuation.

is more common in abscess than in infarction, and as is the case with air in any tissue, will prevent through-transmission of the beam. Perisplenic abnormalities may be noted, particularly perisplenic or left pleural fluid collections.

The high incidence of diffuse calcifications in the homozygous population creates a major pitfall for sonography. The image may be subtly compromised, becoming grainy and with loss of resolution; or the beam may be reflected to an extent where adequate imaging becomes impos-

sible. The small, fibrotic spleen may also be impossible to visualize adequately as it retreats through atrophy to a position well under the ribs, lacking adequate acoustic access. Sickle cell patients may be referred frequently to the ultrasound department in search of cholelithiasis or another common complication as an explanation for recurrent abdominal pain and/or fever. Inability to obtain an adequate splenic exam may not be crucial in the homozygote, in whom active splenic disease is unlikely. However, it may be

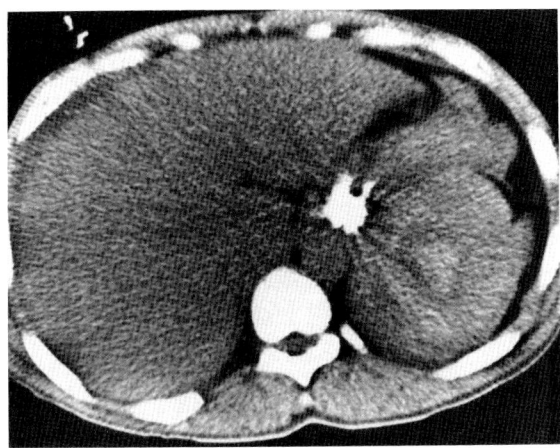

FIGURE 30.14. SICKLE CELL DISEASE
A 36-yr-old black man with trait disease, HbAS. Patient was an alcoholic and presented with abdominal pain suggesting pancreatitis. Splenomegaly with central area of increased attenuation consistent with splenic hemorrhage, confirmed by surgery.

that in the heterozygous group populations, where adequate assessment of the spleen specifically is in question, CT may provide a more appropriate screening exam.

Computed Tomography

The examination initially is performed without intravenous contrast in order to assess splenic density and calcifications. Each scan must be reviewed at both conventional abdominal windows and at narrower "liver-spleen" windows to avoid missing subtle alterations in attenuation. Intravenous contrast may be given later as necessary to further characterize splenic texture, function, or focal defects (39).

Homozygous patients tend to be functionally asplenic although near-normal or even enlarged splenic sizes occasionally are seen into adulthood. Even the enlarged spleens may be dense and clinically nonfunctional (Fig. 30.9). CT is more sensitive to attenuation differences than plain radiographs, and the frequently-seen higher density spleen in sickle cell disease is believed to represent both calcification and increased iron deposition due to hemolysis and frequent transfusion (Fig. 30.10A and B). Calcifications may be finely reticular and diffuse, amorphous and patchy (Fig. 30.9), or dense (Figs. 30.10A, 30.11, and 30.12) corresponding to plain film findings. Occasionally, small islands of near-normal density tissue may be seen within an otherwise calcified spleen (Fig. 30.13). The origin of these "spared" areas is unclear, but does not appear to reflect a clinically significant difference in functional status.

Many heterozygous patients do not present clinically until later childhood or even adulthood. The spleen more frequently is normal or enlarged in size. Distinct focal calcifications are far less common in this group, although splenic density may also be increased. Infancy aside, this group is far more likely to have active splenic disease than the homozygotes. Infarctions will be seen on CT as low density areas with a wedge or irregular contour; and can be solitary or multiple. Frequently they are seen to have higher density areas corresponding to hemorrhage, confirmed at splenectomy (Fig. 30.14). Infarction may produce perisplenic irritation leading to perisplenic or left pleural fluid collections (40). Large infarctions can necrose before they can fibrose, with occasional air collections or even spontaneous splenic rupture being seen later in the clinical course (Fig. 30.15A and B). Splenic hemorrhage or sequestration may be seen, with focal areas of increased attenuation which on subsequent studies are seen to resolve or to progress into low density areas (Fig. 30.16A and B). As described earlier, sickle cell patients are prone to increased infection both because of niches created by focal tissue necrosis and systemic alterations in immunity; as a result, these patients may develop splenic abscesses. At CT, an abscess may be solitary or multiple, and is usually seen to be an irregular, low attenuation area which may have scattered higher density foci of presumed hemorrhage. Air is seen rarely in such lesions but air, when seen, tends to indicate abscess far more often than infarction. With time, the abscess may expand; in the past, with deferred diagnosis and treatment, splenic rupture with intraperitoneal spill was frequently detected at surgery or at autopsy.

CT is probably the most reliable and repeatable method to image the sickle cell spleen. Since these patients frequently are referred because of abdominal pain and/or fever of uncertain etiology, and because their disease leaves them prone to multiple complications, CT provides the extra advantage of imaging the entire abdomen at once. There is a high incidence of hepatic, biliary, renal, and osseous complications in these patients. CT can provide an overview of the entire abdomen, and may be the only imaging method reliably demonstrating the spleen, whether or not clinical information seems to localize the problem to the left upper quadrant.

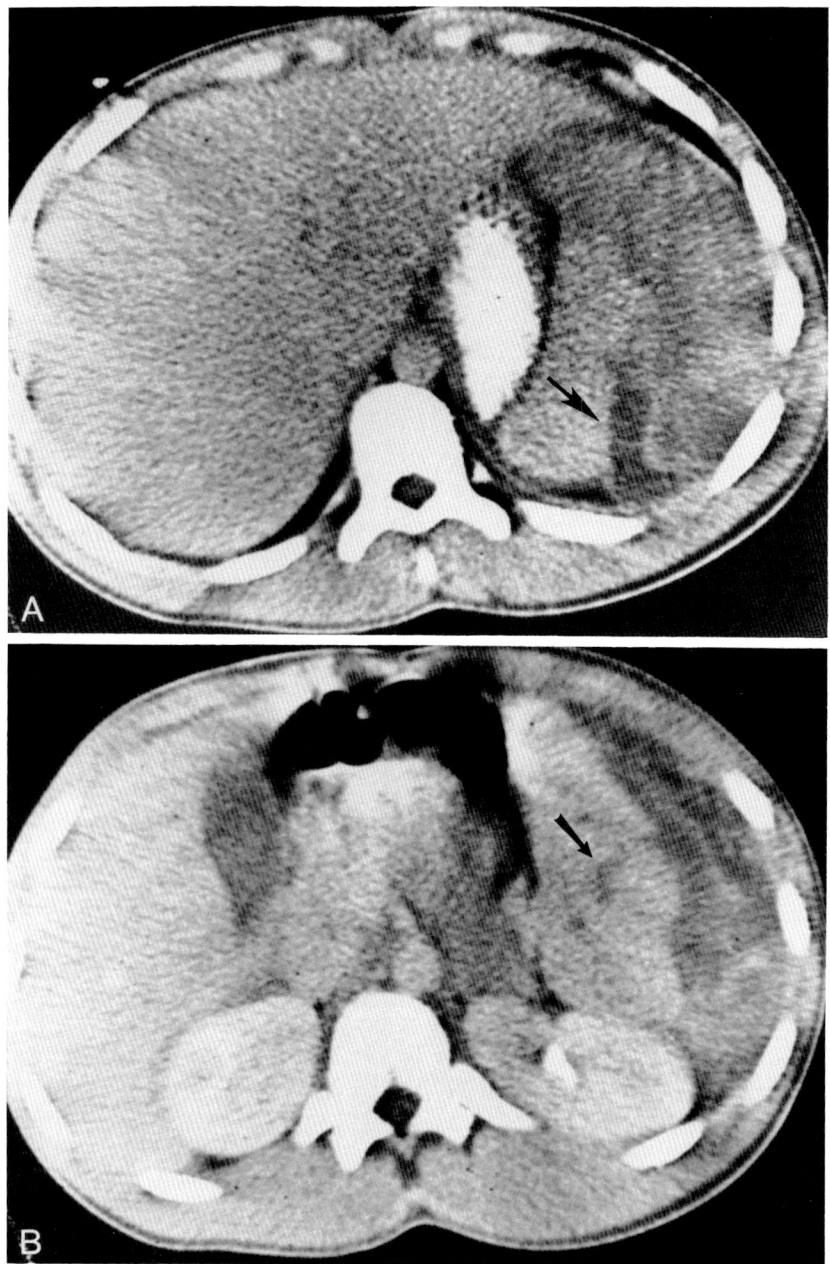

FIGURE 30.15. SICKLE CELL DISEASE

A 15-yr-old black boy with HbSC and acute left upper quadrant pain. *A:* Marked hepatosplenomegaly with laceration and rupture of spleen (*arrow*). *B:* Enlarged spleen with laceration (*arrow*). Perisplenic fluid is noted laterally, near the left lateral colic gutter.

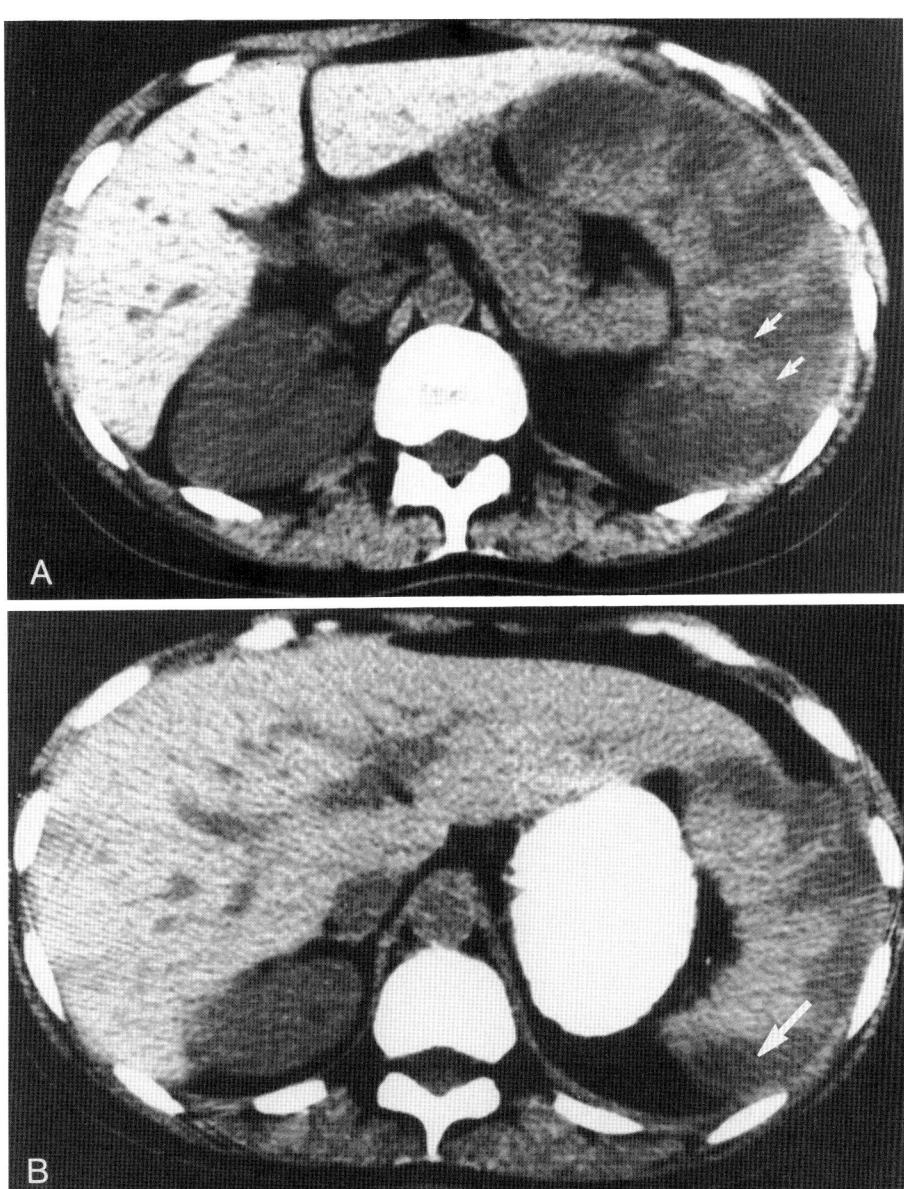

FIGURE 30.16. SICKLE CELL DISEASE

A 43-yr-old female patient with sickle-thalassemia presented with acute left upper quadrant pain and precipitous hematocrit drop of 20 units. *A:* CT at level of pancreas. Diffuse splenomegaly. Patchy low densities represent splenic infarction. A few smaller foci of increased density in spleen are consistent with splenic hemorrhage (*arrows*). *B:* CT 8 weeks later. Decrease in splenic size, subcapsular fluid collection is consistent with resolving hematoma. Patchy areas of infarction (*arrow*) against background of more normal splenic tissue.

DIAPHRAGMATIC HERNIATION

Large diaphragmatic defects, either congenital or acquired, may allow abdominal contents to herniate into the chest. Occasionally the spleen, either alone or with other organs, comprises the contents of a hernia. It may mimic a mass in the left lower lobe or loculated fluid at the left base. The diagnosis may be suspected by absence of a normal splenic outline on abdominal film and confirmed with a ^{99m}Tc-sulfur colloid scan (41).

GASTRIC ULCERS PENETRATING INTO SPLEEN

Benign gastric ulcers may perforate the stomach but be enclosed by surrounding fibrous adhesions. If the penetration is deep and loculated, adjacent organs may be involved. The pancreas is the most common organ to be involved, but gastrohepatic ligament, liver, mesocolon or other structures may be involved depending on the ulcer site (42). The spleen is rarely involved, probably because benign gastric ulcers are relatively less common along the proximal greater curvature (43). At least five cases of splenic penetration by a benign gastric ulcer are reported (43–45). In one case, hematoma and splenic rupture resulted (45).

Radiographically, the ulcer is located along the fundal portion of the greater curvature. The crater is deep and may simulate a diverticulum (43, 44). Unlike a diverticulum, it does not change size or shape, lacks a narrow neck, and will not occur in the classic location for gastric diverticulum (on the posterior wall of the cardia near the gastroesophageal junction). The appearance of a confined gastric perforation has been referred to as an accessory pocket (43) or pseudodiverticulum. The large size and irregular shape of the ulcer may raise the possibility of leiomyosarcoma or lymphoma in the differential diagnosis. In one case, the diagnosis was confirmed preoperatively by demonstrating splenic tissue in the endoscopic biopsy specimen (43).

INFLAMMATORY PSEUDOTUMOR

Two cases of "inflammatory pseudotumor" of the spleen were reported, one of which was detected as a mass on CT (46). The pathogenesis and significance of this lesion is uncertain, but its gross and radiologic appearance could not be distinguished from malignancy.

REFERENCES

1. Kaul A, Noffz W: Tissue dose in thorotrast patients. *Health Phys* 35:113–121, 1978.
2. Burroughs AK, Bass NA, Wood J, Sherlock S: Absence of splenic uptake of radiocolloid due to thorotrast in a patient with thorotrast-induced cholangiocarcinoma. *Br J Radiol* 55:598–600, 1982.
3. Rao BR, Winebright JW, Dresser TP: Functional asplenia after thorotrast administration. *Clin Nucl Med* 4:437–438, 1979.
4. Levy DW, Rindsberg S, Friedman AC, Fishman EK, Ros PR et al: Thorotrast-induced hepatosplenic neoplasia: CT identification. *AJR* 146:997–1004, 1986.
5. Gardner DC, Ogilvie RF: The late results of injection of thorotrast: 2 cases of neoplastic disease following contrast angiography. *J Pathol Bacteriol* 78:133–144, 1959.
6. Finch SC, Finch CH: Idiopathic hemochromatosis, an iron storage disease. *Medicine* 34:381, 1955.
7. Shanbram E, Zhevtlin N: Radiologic signs in hemosiderosis. *JAMA* 168:33, 1958.
8. Mills SR, Doppman JL, Nienhuis AW: Computed tomography in the diagnosis of disorders of excessive iron storage of the liver. *J Comput Assist Tomogr* 1:101–104, 1977.
9. Mitnick JS, Bosnick MA, Megibow AJ et al: CT in B-thalassemia: iron deposition in the liver, spleen, and lymph nodes. *AJR* 136:1191–1194, 1981.
10. Houang MTW et al: Correlation between computed tomographic values and liver iron content in thalassemia major with iron overload. *Lancet* 1:1322–1323, 1979.
11. Long JA Jr et al: Computed tomographic analysis of beta-thalassemic syndromes with hemochromatosis: pathologic findings with clinical and laboratory correlations. *J Comput Assist Tomogr* 4:159–165, 1980.
12. Stephens DH, Sheedy PF: The liver. In Haaga Jr, Alfeidi RF (eds): *Computed Tomography of the Whole Body.* St. Louis, C. V. Mosby, 1983, p 585.
13. Schulman A, Fataar S, Tidbury I, Rad FF: Case report: lymphographic opacification of liver and spleen. *Br J Radiol* 51:389–391, 1978.
14. McCall LW, Vaidya S, Serjeant GR: Splenic opacification in homozygous sickle cell disease. *Clin Radiol* 32:611–615, 1981.
15. Perlmutter S, Jacobstein JG, Kazam E: Splenic uptake of Tc-diphosphonate in sickle cell disease associated with increased splenic density on computerized axial tomography. *Gastrointest Radiol* 2:77–79, 1977.
16. Felson B, Reeder M: *Gamuts In Radiology.* Audiovisual Radiology of Cincinnati, Inc. 1975 (Gamut G-84, G-85).
17. Eppinger H: Zur pathologie der milzfunktion. *Berl Klin Wochenschr* 2:1509–1512, 1571–1576, 1913.
18. Daneshek WJ: Hyposplenism. *JAMA* 157:613, 1955.
19. Corozza GR, Gasbarrini G: Defective splenic function and its relation to bowel disease. *Clin Gastroenterol* 12:651–669, 1983.

20. Eichner ER: Splenic function: normal, too much and too little. *Am J Med* 66:311–320, 1979.
21. Armas RR: Clinical studies with spleen-specific radiolabelled agents. *Semin Nucl Med* 15:260–275, 1985.
22. Marsh GW, Lewis SM, Szor L: The use of ^{51}Cr-labelled heat-damaged red cells to study splenic function. I. Evaluation of the method. *Br J Hematol* 12:161–166, 1966, and II. Splenic atrophy in thrombocystopenia. *Br J Hematol* 12:167–171, 1966.
23. Spencer RP: Spleen imaging. In Alavi A, Arger PH (eds): *Multiple Imaging Procedures; Abdomen.* Orlando, Fla., Grune & Stratton, 1980, p 72.
24. Morowitz DA, Allen LW, Kirsner JB: Thrombocytosis in chronic inflammatory bowel disease. *Ann Intern Med* 68:1013, 1968.
25. Spirer A: The role of the spleen in immunity and infection. *Adv Pediatr* 17:55–88, 1980.
26. Williams WS, Beutler D, Ensler AJ, Rundle RW: *Hematology.* New York, McGraw-Hill, 1977.
27. Beesan PB, McDermott W, Wyngaarden JB: *Cecil Textbook of Medicine,* Ed 15. Philadelphia, W. B. Saunders, 1974.
28. Barrett-Conner E: Bacterial infection and sickle cell anemia. *Medicine* 50:97–112, 1971.
29. Overturf G, Powars D: Multi-institutional study group of pneumococcal vaccine in sickle cell disease: infections in sickle cell anemia: pathogenesis and control. *Tex Rep Biol Med* 40:283–292, 1980.
30. King DT, Lindstrom RR, State D, Hirose FM, Schwartz JA: Unusual cause of acute abdomen-sickle cell trait and nonhypoxic splenic infarction. *JAMA* 238:2173–2174, 1977.
31. O'Brien RT, Pearson HA, Godley JA et al: Splenic infarction and sickle-(cell)-trait. *N Engl J Med* 287:720, 1972.
32. Sears DA: The morbidity of sickle cell trait: a review of the literature. *Am J Med* 64: 1021, 1978.
33. Buchanan GR, Smith SJ, Holtkamp CA, Fuseler JP: Bacterial infection and splenic reticuloendothelial function in the abdomen with hemoglobin SC disease. *Pediatrics* 72:93–98, 1983.
34. Topley JM, Cupidore L, Vaidya S et al: Pneumococcal and other infections in children with sickle-cell hemoglobin C (SC) disease. *J Pediatr* 101:176–416, 1982.
35. Diggs LW: Sidero fibrosis of the spleen in sickle cell anaemia. *JAMA* 104:538–541, 1935.
36. McCall IW, Vaidya S, Serjeant GR: Splenic opacification in homozygous sickle cell disease. *Clin Radiol* 31:611–615, 1981.
37. Karayalcin G, Dorfman J, Rosner F, Abolli AJ: Radiological changes in 127 patients with sickle cell anemia. *Am J Med Sci* 271:131–144, 1976.
38. Fischer KC, Shapiro S, Treves S: Visualization of the spleen in a bone-seeking radionuclide in a child with sickle-cell anemia. *Radiology* 122:398, 1977.
39. Magid D, Fishman EK, Siegelman SS: Computed tomography of the spleen and liver in sickle cell disease. *AJR* 143:245–249, 1984.
40. Yeung K-Y, Lessin LS: Splenic infarction in sickle cell-hemoglobin C disease. *Arch Intern Med* 136:905–911, 1976.
41. Gonzalez G. Isotope scanning for diagnostic lesions projecting into the lower chest. *JAMA* 218:590, 1971.
42. Haubrich WS: In Bockus HC (ed): *Gastroenterology,* Ed 3. Philadelphia, W. B. Saunders, 1976, pp 720–759.
43. Jaffe N, Antoniol DA: Penetration into spleen by benign gastric ulcers. *Clin Radiol* 32:177–181, 1981.
44. Stoica T, Dragomir T, Gabrovescu D, et al: Ulcer al fornexului perforatin splina imilind un diverticul gastric. *Chirurgia (Bucur)* 22:509–512, 1973.
45. Immelman EJ: Rupture of a subcapsular hematoma of the spleen resulting from a penetrating gastric spleen. *S Afr J Surg* 13:261–263, 1975.
46. Cotelingam JD, Jaffe ES: Inflammatory pseudotumor of the spleen. *Am J Surg Pathol* 8:375–380, 1984.

31
Magnetic Resonance Imaging of the Spleen

ARNOLD C. FRIEDMAN, M.D.

NORMAL ANATOMY

Compared to the liver, the spleen is normally somewhat hypointense or isointense on very T1-weighted images (either short TE spin echo or inversion recovery), and hyperintense on T2-weighted spin echo sequences (Fig. 31.1). On mixed spin echo sequences it is nearly isointense. Calculated in vivo values for relaxation times of the spleen have been published and reviewed (1); these suffer from the fact that calculations from intensity measurements compound the errors present in the latter (2). Some representative data are: T1 = 250–290 ms, 0.04T (3), T1 = 440–580 ms, 0.15T (4, 5), T1 = 780 ms, T2 = 59 ms, 0.35T (6). In general, both T1 and T2 of the spleen are longer than those of the liver, possibly because of a higher water content in the spleen (7).

MRI demonstrates both the splenic artery and vein quite nicely in the splenic hilum as low intensity tubular structures surrounded by high intensity fat (Fig. 31.1*A*, *B*, *F*, and *G*). The spleen itself often is outlined by a thin hypointense rim that appears to be a capsule, but in fact is probably a chemical shift artifact.

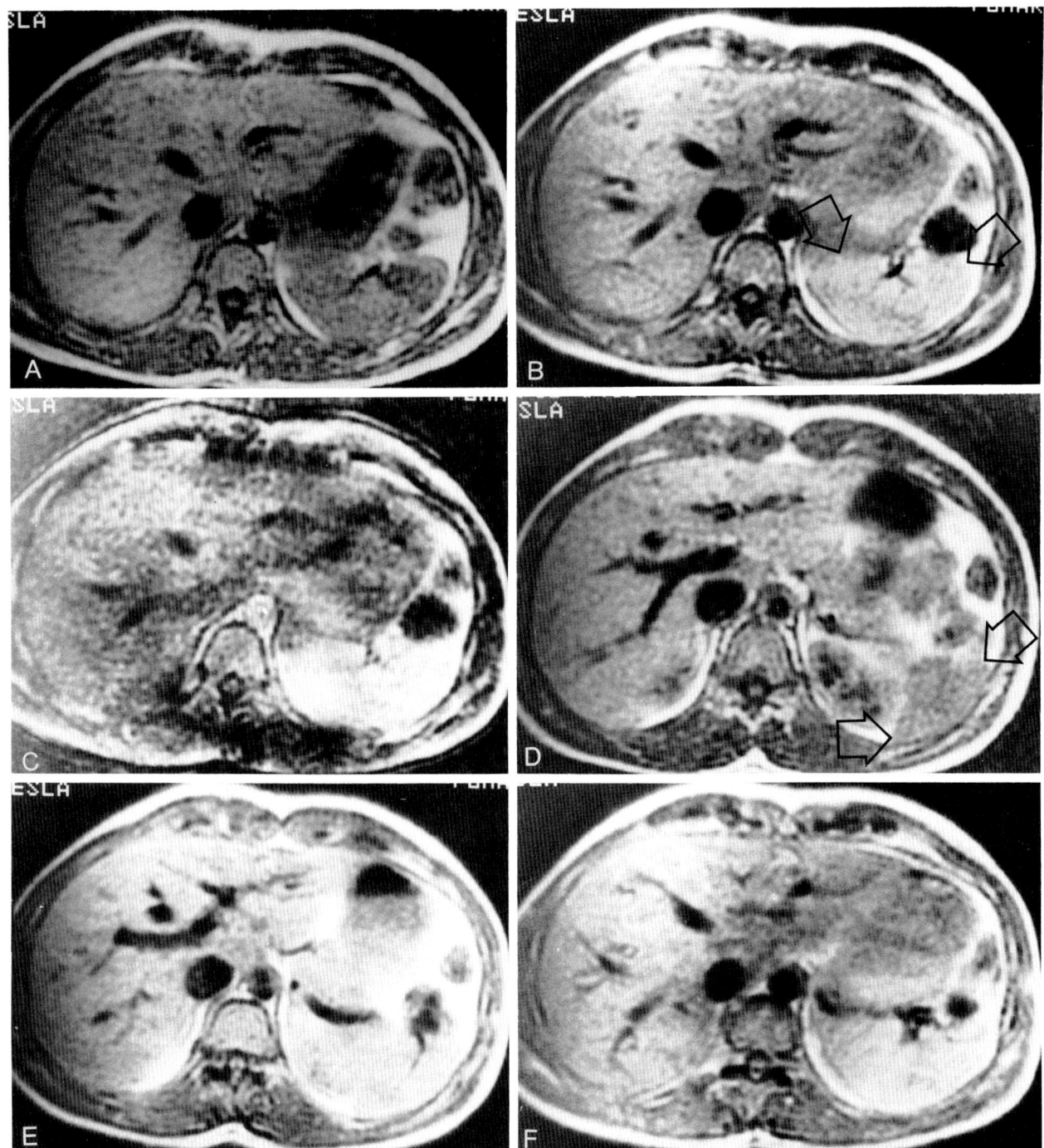

FIGURE 31.1. NORMAL ANATOMY OF SPLEEN

A–C: Inversion recovery TI 310, TR-1500, TE-28, spin echo 28/1000 and 56/1000, respectively, in the same patient at a level just above the left kidney. The spleen becomes progressively more intense with increasing T2 dependence. Its borders are seen best at this level on SE 28/1000 (*arrows*). The hilar vasculature is black on all sequences. *D–G:* Same patient, through the left kidney and upper pole of the right kidney. IR 310/1500/28, SE 28/1000, SE 28/2000, SE 56/2000, respectively. The borders of the spleen are well delineated from the left kidney and surrounding fat at this level only on inversion recovery (*arrows*). Splenic vessels are seen posterior to the pancreas on all sequences. Note again increasing splenic intensity with increasing T2-dependence.

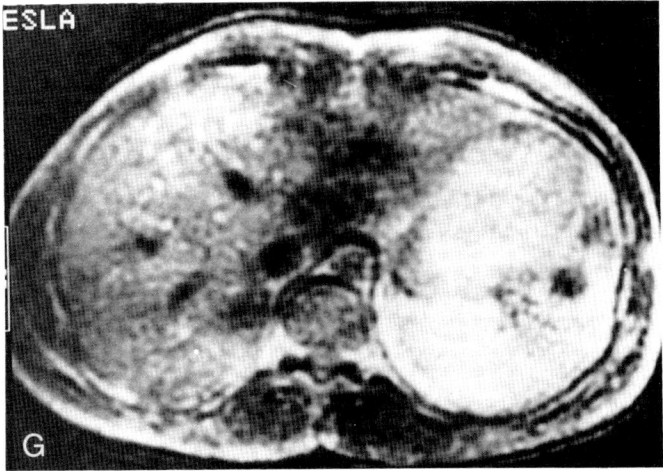

FIGURE 31.1G

SPLENIC PATHOLOGY

Splenomegaly is readily appreciated by MRI, and the ability to scan in a coronal plane in addition to the axial plane aids in the evaluation of spleen size compared to CT. More important, splenic intensity is altered by conditions such as portal hypertension or splenic vein thrombosis/compression that increase spleen water content by virtue of venous congestion (3, 6). Both T1 and T2 relaxation times are prolonged, therefore splenic intensity is diminished on T1-weighted images and increased on T2-weighted images (Fig. 31.2). Splenic hematomas and intrasplenic metastases can be detected by MRI. The former are usually quite intense on T1-weighted images when older than one day, probably because of T1 shortening by the paramagnetic effect of the ferric ion in methemoglobin (Fig. 31.3), whereas the latter are usually hypointense on T1-weighted images because of T1-prolongation in neoplastic tissue, suggesting a potential role for MR in differential diagnosis. Very fresh hematomas will be hypointense on T1-weighted images, however (Fig. 31.3). Hemorrhagic splenic infarcts may have an appearance similar to that of hematoma (Figs. 31.4 and 31.5). However, the greatest potential role for MRI in the spleen, in my opinion, is the detection of intrasplenic lymphoma.

Neither radionuclide scanning, sonography or CT can detect lymphoma of the spleen with sufficient sensitivity to spare patients the expense and discomfort of a staging laparotomy and splenectomy, the results of which are often negative. If MRI can detect splenic lymphoma by virtue of superior soft-tissue contrast discrimination with a high sensitivity, negative laparotomy and splenectomy might be avoided in a large number of patients, both improving their quality of care and saving health care dollars.

Although splenic involvement with Hodgkin's disease may be quite bulky and easily imaged late in the course of uncontrolled disease, proven involvement of the spleen at presentation often is in the form of one or more scattered foci of tumor less than 1 cm. in greatest dimension (8). Splenic involvement in patients with Hodgkin's disease may be present in 39% of patients at presentation and increases to 69% at autopsy (9). Splenic involvement occurs in 32% of patients with non-Hodgkin's lymphoma at initial staging (9). Focal defects within the spleen have a high degree of correlation with the presence of

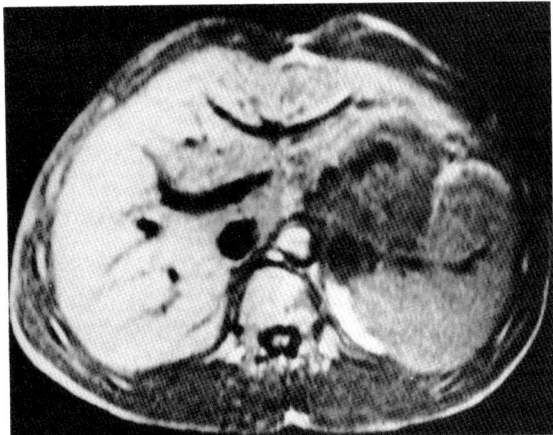

FIGURE 31.2. SPLENIC VEIN THROMBOSIS
Spin echo (SE) 28/500: Slightly enlarged and very hypointense spleen (compared to liver) due to splenic vein thrombosis.

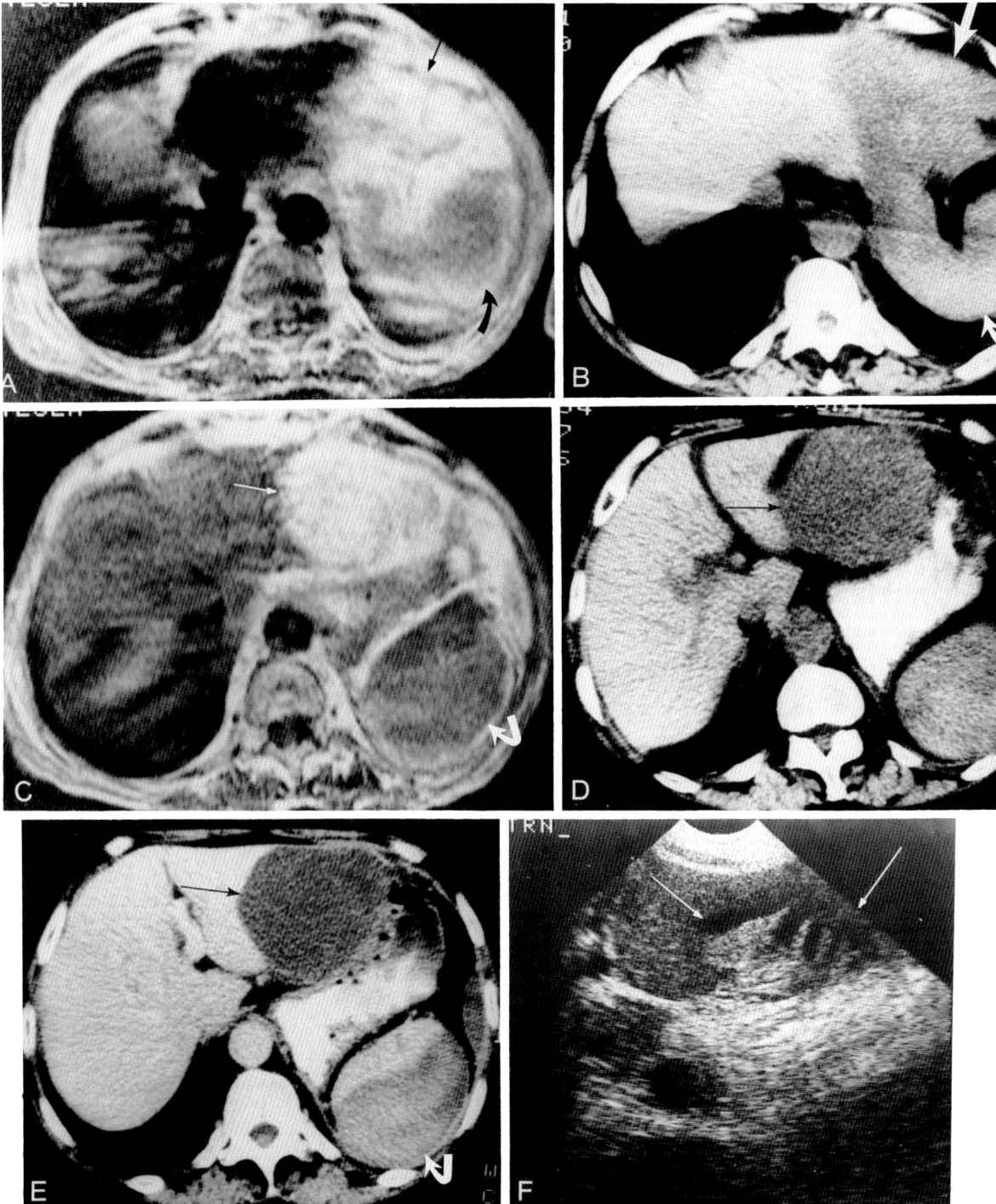

FIGURE 31.3. ACUTE AND CHRONIC SPLENIC HEMATOMA

A and B: (SE) 28/500 MRI and noncontrast CT beneath left hemidiaphragm. Fresh hematoma posteriorly (*curved arrows*) is hypointense and hyperdense. Anterior older hematoma is hyperintense and hypodense (*straight arrows*). Low density fat surrounded by the hematoma is obvious on the CT but masked on the MRI. C–E: Spin echo (SE) 28/500 MRI, noncontrast CT and contrast-enhanced CT through the spleen. The anterior older hematoma (*straight arrows*) is hyperintense and hypodense and the fresh subcapsular hematoma (*curved arrows*) is hypointense and hyperdense. F: Transverse scan through the left lobe of the liver and the older hematoma shows an organized clot with complex architecture (*arrows*).

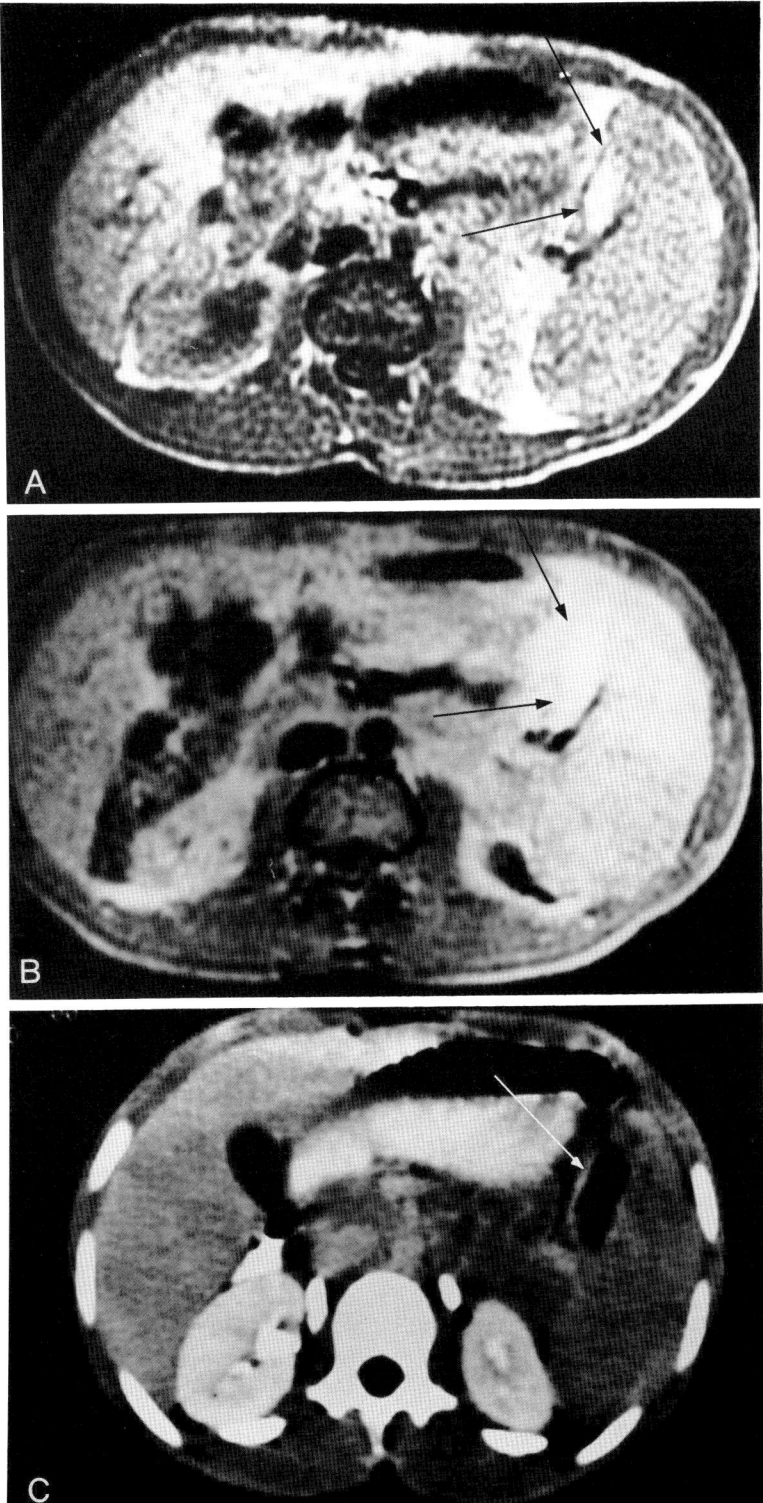

FIGURE 31.4. SPLENIC INFARCT

Splenic infarct in a febrile 14-yr-old with sickle cell disease and high fetal hemoglobin. CT was consistent with abscess, but MR findings prompted conservative management. *A* and *B:* Inversion recovery 310/1500/28 and SE 28/2000 MRI both show a peripheral very high intensity region (*arrows*) within the spleen suggesting hemorrhagic infarct. *C:* Corresponding low density area (*arrow*) on CT.

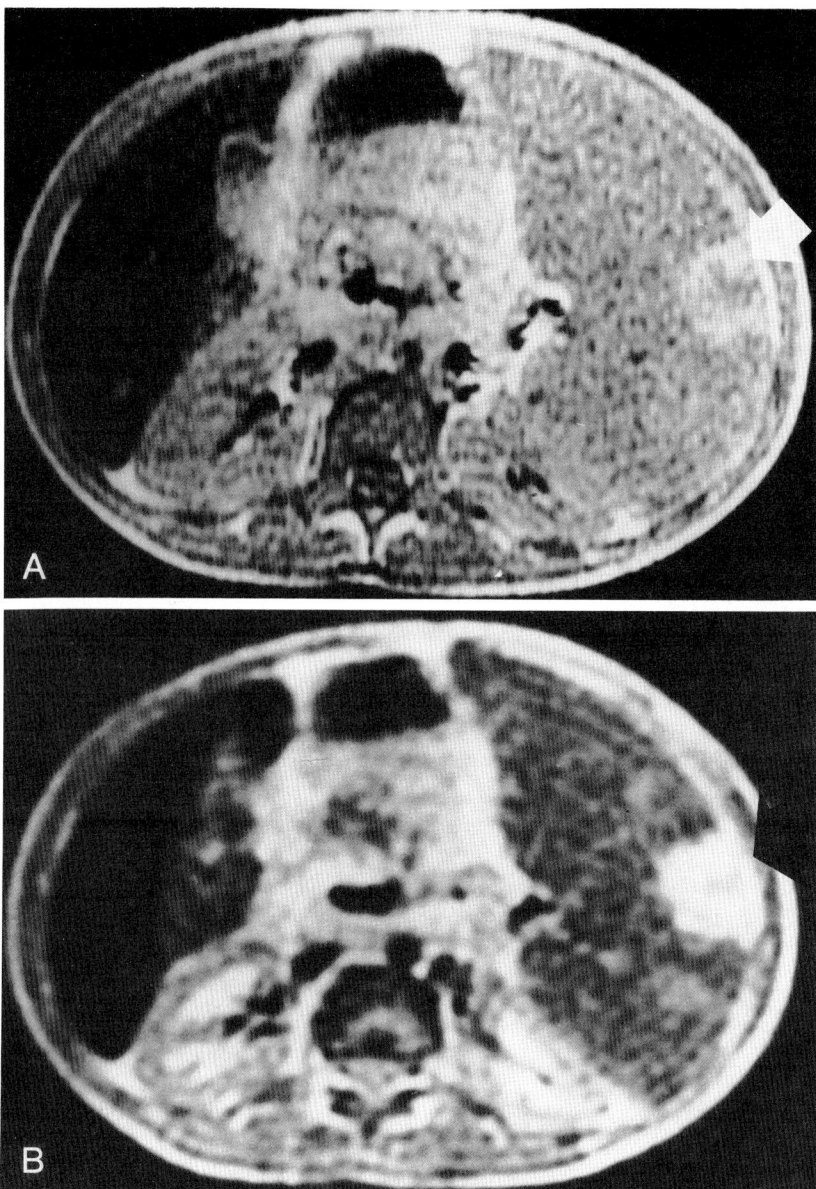

FIGURE 31.5. HEMOSIDEROSIS

Hemosiderosis in the liver and spleen and high intensity splenic infarct in a patient with sickle cell disease. *A* and *B:* SE 28/500 and 56/2000 MRI show a heterogeneous peripheral high intensity region (*arrow*) suggesting an infarct. Note the abnormally low hepatic intensity consistent with transfusion overload hemosiderosis. Splenic intensity decreases as the imaging parameters become more T2-weighted, the opposite of normal, suggesting increased iron storage in the spleen as well (short T2 predominating over a short T1). The liver spleen scan in this patient showed functional asplenia.

lymphoma, however, they are usually not detected by CT with or without conventional contrast material, ultrasound, or radionuclide scanning (8, 9). In one series, CT detected only 22% of lymphomatous spleens (3). Splenomegaly, by itself, unless massive, is a poor predictor of the presence of splenic Hodgkin's disease or non-Hodgkin's lymphoma (8, 9). Thus, a large percentage of patients with lymphoma must undergo a staging laparotomy with splenectomy to detect splenic lymphoma, a procedure which could be modified or eliminated if a reliable method of non-invasively detecting splenic lymphoma were available (10). CT using the reticuloendothelial specific contrast agent, EOE-13, was shown to be very sensitive in detecting

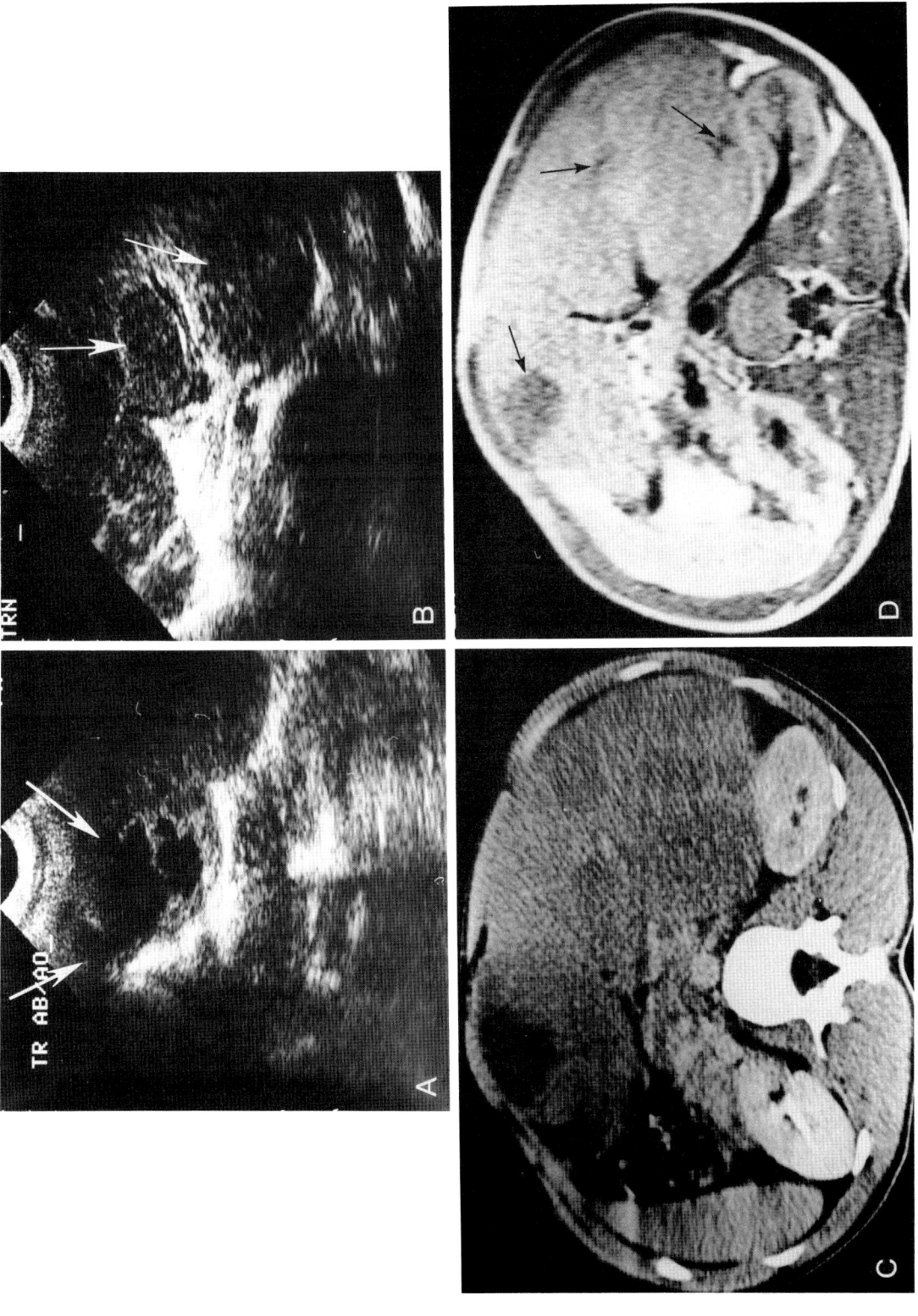

FIGURE 31.6. HISTIOCYTIC LYMPHOMA

Histiocytic lymphoma, MRI with CT and sonographic correlation. *A*: Transverse sonogram: splenomegaly and complex medial mass (*arrows*). *B*: At the same axial level there are multifocal solid nearly isoechoic masses (*arrows*) posterolaterally. *C*: CT scan: medial necrotic mass and multiple posterolateral hypodense masses. *D*: MRI, SE 28/500: Splenomegaly with poorer depiction of focal masses (*arrows*).

splenic lymphoma, however nodules 0.5 cm. or less in diameter are probably undetectable despite EOE-13 (9).

MRI of the spleen may be able to detect splenic lymphoma with greater sensitivity than any other imaging modality and do so without any contrast agents because of its inherently superb contrast discrimination. By virtue of its longer T1 and T2 compared to splenic parenchyma, a lymphomatous nodule should be imaged as a region of increased relative intensity on T2-weighted sequences and decreased relative intensity on T1-weighted sequences (4). Histologically normal areas in neoplastically involved organs have been shown to possess longer T1 and T2 than normal parenchyma (11–14), thus by accurate measurements of relaxation times of proven normal and lymphomatous spleens microscopic lymphoma may be detectable by MRI. To date, using mildly T1-weighted spin echo and inversion recovery techniques without cardiac or respiratory gating, we have not been able to demonstrate splenic lymphoma with greater sensitivity than CT (Fig. 31.6). We hope that with improved T2-weighted images and/or short TE spin echo sequences with or without gating we will have more success.

SECTION V
Biopsy and Drainage Procedures in the Upper Abdomen

INTRODUCTION

The availability of flexible and precise three-dimensional imaging techniques (CT and ultrasound) has spurred the growth of percutaneous diagnosis and treatment of diseases in the upper abdomen. A precise preoperative histologic diagnosis facilitates surgical planning, precludes surgery in some cases, and dramatically diminishes the number of exploratory laparotomies. Percutaneous aspiration and drainage of fluid collections has decreased health care costs both by shortening hospital stays and avoiding surgery. The indications for guided percutaneous procedures continue to expand as these techniques are applied to new problems and as new equipment is developed.

32

Percutaneous Abscess and Fluid Drainage in the Upper Abdomen

DEAN L. GAIN, M.D., AND ROGER C. SANDERS, M.D.

Untreated abdominal abscesses present a significant and sometimes fatal complication of intraabdominal surgery, trauma, or spontaneous rupture of an infected hollow viscus. With the exception of some forms of pelvic inflammatory disease, focal renal abscess, and hepatic ameboma, medical management is not generally considered adequate care. Surgical inspection, irrigation, and drainage were until recently regarded as definitive. Interventional radiology bridges the gap between closely supervised medical management and a trip to the operating room for the patient who may have generalized sepsis and multiorgan system failure. Ultrasound and computed tomography permit early identification and localization of abscesses, allow the mapping of satellite lesions, and enable avoidance of uninvolved sterile potential spaces. Using any one of a variety of percutaneous puncture techniques described in this seciton, the abscess may be effectively treated and surgery avoided.

BACKGROUND

The word abscess is believed to be derived from the latin word abscessus meaning *ab* — "away from" plus *cedere* — "to go" (1, 2). An abscess is an infection in the "act of going away." It is defined as a localized collection of pus surrounded by hyperemic inflamed tissue with marked leukocytic infiltration (3). Abscesses are characterized by local destruction of parenchymal and stromal cells. The suppurative process may be limited to the tissue, organ, or confined space (4).

According to Ariel and Kazarian (5) in their book devoted to abscesses, Hippocrates first described drainage tubes for abscess drainage; he designed them for the treatment of pleural empyemas. Celsus was the first to drain abdominal fluid using conical metal tubes. (Petit published a necropsy result in 1753 where a subphrenic abscess was the result of a perforated colon (6)). In 1890, Penrose, a name still recognized by physicians of all specialties, described the ideal drainage tube: "Theoretically, an aseptic, unirritating drainage tube ought never to become shut off by adhesions from the general peritoneal cavity since adhesions imply more or less irritation" (5).

Although a chemist's water pump was described by Heaton in 1898, a syphon drain was needed for human use. In the 1940s, a surgical sump drain was developed which had a built-in air vent (5).

Since the 1930s, Ochsner and others have written extensively concerning the necessity of surgical cure for abscesses. He stated, "diagnostic aspirations should never be attempted, and in those cases in which the diagnosis remains doubtful, exploratory operation preferably should be undertaken" (7).

Not only was surgery advocated for all abscesses, Ochsner concluded the following concerning liver abscess drainage, "The employment of that type of drainage which completely avoids the slightest possibility of contamination of the peritoneal or pleural cavity is of paramount importance" (8). Ironically, this argument can now be used to defend percutaneous abscess drainage (PAD).

Perhaps one of the most significant landmarks in intraabdominal abscess therapy came from Hong Kong. In 1953, McFadzean published a series of 14 consecutive cases of solitary pyogenic liver abscesses which were successfully treated with percutaneous needle aspiration and antibiotics (9). This concept was conceived by that author only after antibiotics made it possible to treat minor spillage of abscess contents across "sterile" body spaces.

IMAGING

The diagnosis of abdominal abscess may be made on plain film examination when a mottled gas density is seen within the abdomen in a location atypical for bowel. Early on, decubitus views, barium studies, and intravenous urography were all that were available. Today patients who are at increased risk for abscess formation are examined by the complementary imaging modalities of ultrasound (US), computed tomography (CT), and nuclear medicine (NM).

Ultrasound is portable and inexpensive. It is usually successful in recognizing fluid-filled masses such as abscesses. Ultrasound is most useful in imaging the upper abdomen and the anatomic pelvis (10). Successful examination is most likely accomplished when a good hepatic, splenic, gastric, or urinary bladder sonographic window is present. Static scans, much like multiplanar computed tomography scans, yield an overview of the abdomen including organ situs, size, and relationships. On the other hand, real-time sonography permits tens of thousands of images to be viewed and selected scans photographed. It is quite similar to real-time fluoroscopy except that no ionizing radiation is used. Physiologic motion in abscess look-alikes such as partially distended gut permits one to dismiss such a finding as a pseudoabscess.

On the other hand, demonstration of a sonolucent mass with irregular, poorly defined, or thickened borders exhibiting some enhanced through transmission suggests an abscess is present. Additional characteristics such as internal echoes suggesting pus, blood, or gas, are helpful (11). Distal shadowing suggests the latter entity (12). Unless the clinical and ultrasound findings are definitive, further evaluation is indicated prior to any drainage procedure (Fig. 32.1).

Computed tomography is usually the next procedure performed. Rapid, precise transverse axial scans may be obtained regardless of overlying surgical dressings, residual barium, bone, and pathologic (or nonpathologic) intraabdominal gas. Well described CT signs include a low density soft tissue mass (0–25 Hounsfield units (HU), sometimes higher) surrounded by edematous tissue planes, presence of gas or of an air fluid level within the mass, and the "rind sign" (13). The latter finding is produced following intravenous contrast infusion and represents the enhancing ill-defined periphery caused by hypervascularity of the inflamed abscess wall (14).

Nuclear medicine also plays an important role in the radiologic workup of abscess. Gallium-67 and indium-111 white blood cell scans offer high sensitivity—both in the 90% range (15, 16). The former may require 48 to 72 hours plus bowel preparation (because of colonic excretion and accumulation). Indium-111 WBC scans are more rapid with as little as 6–12 hr between onset of white cell tagging and final scan interpretation. Drawbacks include nonspecific uptake of radiogallium by noninfected healing wounds and possible failure of indium 111-WBC scans to dem-

FIGURE 32.1. DIAGNOSTIC IMAGING
Diagnostic imaging is usually performed by the US, CT, and NM sections, resectively. However, at Johns Hopkins Hospital, any possible aspiration, biopsy, or drainage procedure is performed by the US section team. When no safe access is available by multiplanar real-time US guidance, CT is obtained and the procedure performed either with (a) utilizing the CT scan as a guide for US or (b) directly under CT guidance. In either case, fluoroscopy is necessary for safe guide-wire and catheter manipulation. Surgical backup is recommended in case of catastrophic complication, i.e., vessel or diaphragm laceration. NM is usually reserved for stable equivocal cases where diagnostic skinny needle (20–22-gauge) aspiration cannot be performed.

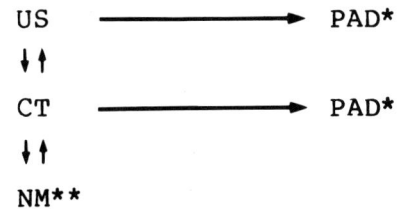

COMMON SEQUENCE OF EVENTS AT JHH

US ⟶ PAD*
⇅
CT ⟶ PAD*
⇅
NM**

*OBTAIN FLUOROSCOPY AND SURGICAL BACKUP.
**SUITABLE ONLY FOR THOSE PATIENTS WITH SIGNIFICANT RISKS TO DIAGNOSTIC NEEDLE ASPIRATION, I.E. STABLE PATIENT WITH ABNORMAL BLEEDING.

onstrate an older, mature, abscess without leukocyte infiltration of its thick wall. Both agents may be used to survey the entire body (17). This is most important when localizing signs are absent.

TECHNIQUE

The radiologic findings of an abscess already described in the imaging section are rarely specific. The differential diagnosis may include normal gut, hematoma, seroma, lymphocele, biloma, urinoma, or cyst depending upon the history and location of the fluid collection. A sample of the abnormal fluid obtained by puncture is necessary to be certain an abscess is present. The referring physician may be contacted and puncture arranged. Surgical consultation is usually warranted. This way, there is no delay of surgery or risk of doing an invasive procedure without having informed surgical standby. Quite often the patient is severely ill and a poor surgical risk. The procedure is suitable as a temporizing measure even if not curative in the moribund patient (18).

Finally, the patient or legal guardian must want PAD performed. The patient must understand the procedure, risks, indications, and alternatives *and* consent to the procedure.

The patient should be sedated and, when the causative organisms are known, it is best to administer appropriate antibiotics immediately. In very ill patients, antibiotics may be started empirically prior to the procedure. One may administer standard normal doses of Demerol, Benadryl, and Valium 30 min prior to anticipated catheter manipulation. Patient consent must be obtained prior to administration of drugs. An initial 5 ml sample of abscess fluid should be sent to the laboratory for Gram stain, culture, and sensitivity. An abscess should not be drained with the diagnostic tap. A collapsed collection will not permit introduction of a catheter.

If the patient is not allergic, local and systemic analgesia will be used as needed. This allows one to inform the patient of progress and ask for his assistance in turning, etc. Generally, the patient is very interested in knowing when the collection has been entered and when the fluid is draining.

Localization for Needle Placement

Ultrasound Technique

The patient is scanned with a real-time sector scanner over the area of interest using previous ultrasound and CT studies for comparison. When a bowel-free route is found, the preferred entry site is marked on the skin by applying pressure on an inverted capped needle hub. Acoustic couplant (gel or mineral oil) is removed by wiping the skin with acetone. The basic tray (Fig. 32.2) is opened on a movable cart next to the patient. The skin is prepared by wiping the needle entry site from the center outwards in a spiral fashion three times with betadine swabs and once with alcohol. A sterile drape is then placed with the fenestration over the skin marker and taped at the edge if necessary, i.e., when the patient is in the semi-upright position.

Lidocaine 1% without epinephrine is used for superficial and deep local anesthesia, if the patient has no allergy. The 25-gauge needle is perfect for raising a generous wheal followed by deeper numbing through the same needle hole with the 22-gauge needle. At this point, the patient is instructed to request more analgesia if needed throughout the procedure. A number 11 scalpel blade is then held with the dominant thumb and index finger and advanced in one rapid motion parallel to Langer's Lines, perpendicular to the long axis of the body. The dermatotomy has been described as being 4 mm in length. However, a longer dermatotomy with blunt spreading with a mosquito clamp and a second dermatotomy parallel to the long axis of the body forming an "x" facilitate large catheter placement. The scalpel blade can be effectively shielded from patient sight by resting the nondominant hand above the entry site. This has the combined effect of providing a steady entry and reducing the possibility of rapid patient movement countering the thrust.

The depth of the lesion can easily be measured on the frozen ultrasound image on the screen (Fig. 32.3). A line of dots (regular scale marker) is superimposed directly through the lesion in the anticipated approach angle. From this row of 1 cm spaced dots, the depth of the skin's surface to the leading edge of the fluid collection, as well as the thickness of the collection, can be easily determined.

Using the ruler as a guide, a metal or plastic needle stop is placed along the 18-gauge needle so that the needle cannot be advanced beyond the midportion of the abscess cavity. Sterile tape may be used as a substitute needle stop. How-

BASIC STERILE TRAY

BASIN OF BETADINE
BASIN OF ALCOHOL, 70%
SCRUB SWABS, -4
DRAPE, FENESTRATED LARGE
NEEDLE 25G x 5/8 IN.
  22G x 1.5 IN.
  22G x 20 cm
  18G x 20 cm
RULER
NEEDLE STOP
SCALPEL BLADE #11

GAUZE 4 4-4
  2 2-2

SYRINGE, 5 cc
(WITH LIDOCAINE 1%)
SYRINGES, 60 cc
EXTENSION TUBING, K-50
STOPCOCK
ANAEROBIC CULTURE VIAL
STERILE TEST TUBES x 4

A

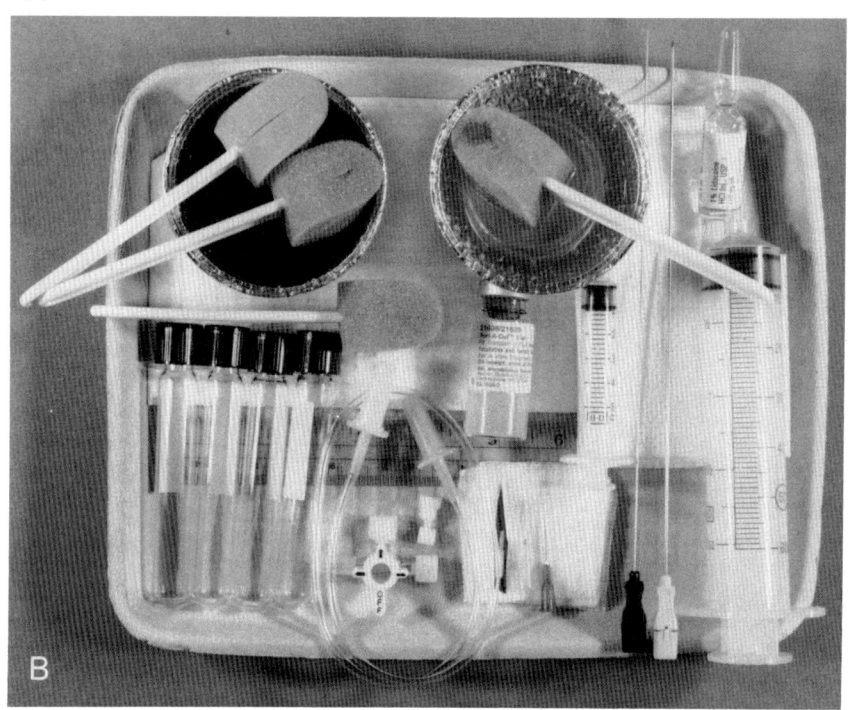

FIGURE 32.2. DRAINAGE EQUIPMENT

A: This table lists all of the sterile items normally used during PAD. Nonsterile acetone is used initially to remove mineral oil or other acoustic couplant from the patient's skin surface. Various complete catheter sets, an anaerobic culture vial, and irrigating saline are held on standby alongside the patient stretcher. If not included in the catheter sets, angiographic/fascial dilators, 3 mm 0.038 J guide-wire, and external biliary drainage bag systems are placed nearby for rapid access. *B*: A photograph of the basic tray is shown.

ever, a rubber tipped hemostat is preferred if advancing a large stiff trocar system (vide infra).

With the patient temporarily suspending respiration, rapidly advance the needle in as straight a fashion as possible up to the needle stop. The patient may now take shallow breaths. The needle stylet is removed and an attempt is made to aspirate 5 ml of fluid for immediate Gram stain, culture, and sensitivity.

The ultrasound unit chosen primarily depends upon availability (Table 32.1). It may be easiest to scan under the sterile drape outside of the sterile field (Fig. 32.4). This is perhaps the most common and easiest to perform method of ultrasound guidance. However, simultaneous imaging may be achieved with special needle biopsy transducers. Real-time sector scanners are available with special biopsy guides so that a selected

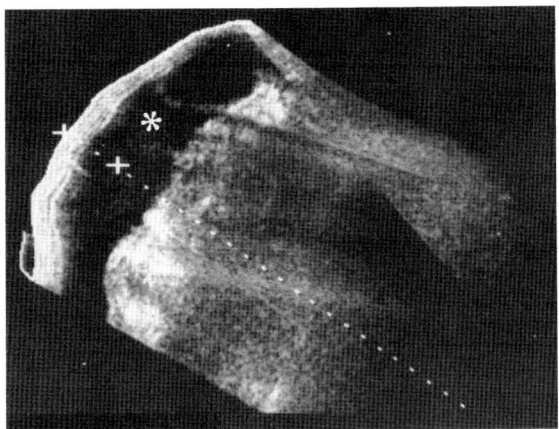

FIGURE 32.3. Localization for Needle Placement: Ultrasound
A typical frozen static ultrasound image is shown with a superimposed 1 cm scale marker. This 57-yr-old ethanol abuser with spontaneous bacterial peritonitis had ascites documented one month earlier. A tap was requested to evaluate new internal echoes within the abdominal fluid (*asterisk*). The caliper measurement on the screen suggests that a needle depth of 3.1 cm would place the needle tip in the center of a large pocket of fluid. A 20-gauge needle aspiration yielded 135 ml of grossly bloody fluid.

TABLE 32.1.
ULTRASOUND GUIDANCE OPTIONS

Ultrasound Approach	Indications
B-scan guidance by transducer angle	Large collection
Sector scanner at right angles to needle	Liver lesions pelvic collections with vaginal needle approach
Sector transducer with biopsy guide	Limited access Intraoperative Renal Spine Common bile duct Neurologic Between ribs
A-mode aspiration transducer	Respiratory motion (i.e., kidneys, pleural lesions, high liver lesions)
Linear array transducer with biopsy guide	Obstetrics Intraoperative liver

needle angle permits visualization of the needle tip at a predetermined depth. A high resolution linear array real-time biopsy transducer may be used for a variety of collections ranging from thoracocentesis to amniocentesis (Fig. 32.5). Sterilizable B-mode capable transducers are also available with the key-hole slit (Fig. 32.6). This simple transducer can be useful in puncturing large superficial collections (such as a loculated pleural effusion) by A-mode alone. However, the needle tip is not as readily seen. Articulated B-mode scanning may also be of use. The mechanical arm is left in the best scan angle (if other than perpendicular to the horizontal). The arm may then be used as a guide while introducing the needle or covered with a sterile bag for extra scanning when necessary. Sometimes, an assistant standing at the foot of the patient comparing the angle formed with the actual locked mechanical arm or the frozen image on the screen is helpful. Angle adjustment is performed until the proper alignment has been achieved. No matter which system is utilized, needle position within the fluid collection should be documented on at least one image.

Computed Tomography Technique

Obtain a digital scout radiograph (Topogram, Deltaview, Scoutview, etc.) with a taped capped needle or an array of radioopaque catheters spread 1 cm apart over the area of interest. Using previous studies as a guide only, several scans may be required to find the best path and entry site for the needle. Additional scans may be obtained above and below the believed path to double check. A comfortable patient breath-holding pattern should be practiced so that the transverse scan plane is reproducible.

If the proper entry site is not directly under the needle or one of the opaque catheters, simply measure the distance to the right or left using the CT console and mark the position on the skin appropriately (Fig. 32.7). Most CT tables are now equipped with a laser guide for ease in positioning the patient. This light guide is helpful for needle localization by CT since the typical laser marker may be turned on when the patient has been advanced to the proper table position determined from previous images.

Using the same technique described in the ultrasound section, the needle is advanced within the scan plane preferably at a 90° angle to the horizontal. However, its path may be angled identical to the best path determined from the CT console. When the needle has been advanced to the proper depth determined from the console screen, a repeat scan should be obtained to confirm the position of the needle tip within the fluid collection. One can be certain of the position of the tip when distal shadowing is clearly seen on the image (Fig. 32.7).

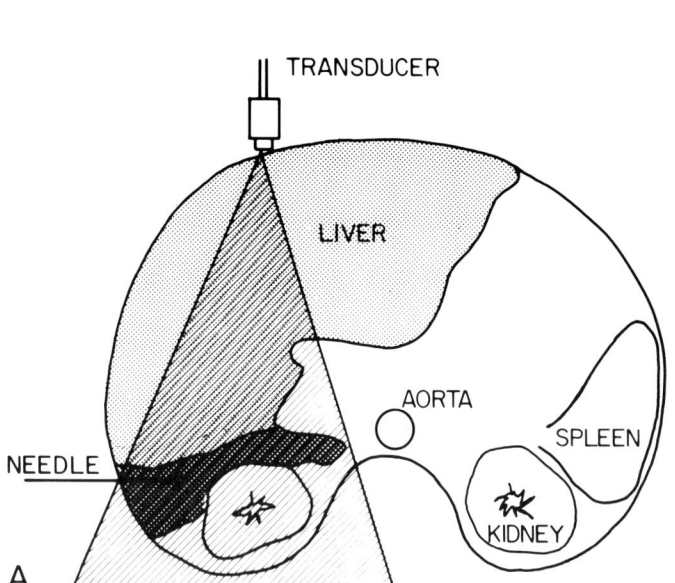 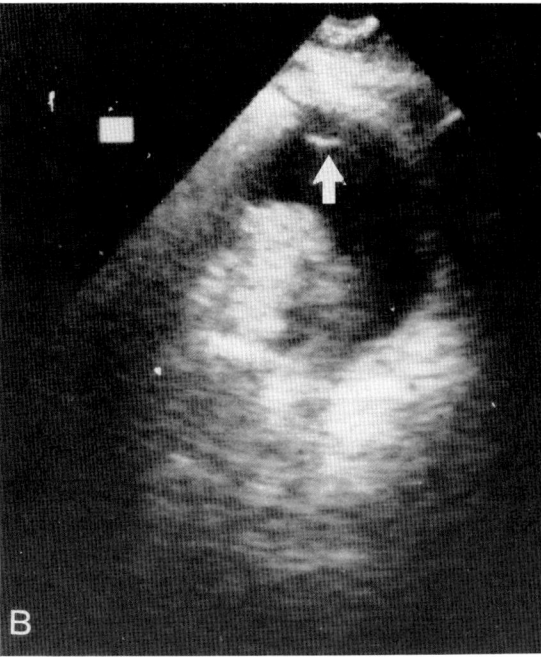

FIGURE 32.4. LOCALIZATION FOR NEEDLE PLACEMENT: ULTRASOUND
Although special biopsy transducers are available, punctures may be performed with a wide variety of US transducers. The interventionalist may observe from a nonsterile position, i.e., vertically (A). A needle may be introduced from a sterile field horizontally as in this illustration. The needle, fluid collection, and surrounding anatomy may be visualized simultaneously during the course of the procedure. For documentation of needle position, a single real-time image (B) clearly shows the needle tip (arrow) within the pocket of ascites of a 74-yr-old white man with colon carcinoma metastatic to the liver.

Catheter Placement

Trocar Method

A wide variety of trocar introduction systems are available (Argyle, Cook-Cope type Loop and Elecath-Sacks, and vanSonnenberg Sump). The trocar stylet method is considered a form of direct puncture. It is generally reserved for superficial large collections with a wide bowel-free path.

Since the diagnosis of abscess must be made prior to the introduction of a catheter, a tandem needle approach is utilized. Using the previously described needle placement localization, the diagnostic needle is left in place. Alongside and parallel to the initial needle tract, the catheter and central trocar are inserted as a single unit through a large dermatotomy following fascial dilatation with a mosquito clamp. The central trocar is removed when the catheter is at the appropriate depth and a small sample of fluid is aspirated for confirmation. A blunt central cannula through which the trocar passed may be removed with the catheter tip returning to its preformed curve. Fenestrated straight catheters, pigtail catheters, and loop-forming catheters are typical variants. The Cope type loop catheter anchors when a string is tightened so that the catheter remains where it is placed. However, the Malecot catheter, which will be described in the next section, has an expanding mushroom type tip so it cannot be moved by an uncooperative patient prone to removing catheters. The vanSonnenberg catheter has the distinct advantage of having a second lumen through which air may pass to prevent tissue encroachment on the catheter from the vacuum effect of suction. A microbial filter caps the ingress sump orifice. This latter catheter comes in straight and curved tip sets to match the shape of the collection. Many side holes assist with drainage of viscous collections.

Modified Angiographic Dilatation Approach

Since Seldinger first described a technique of guide-wire exchange placement of a catheter in a human artery (19, 20), many variations of this technique have been tried. Of the catheter sets which permit this technique, some are used with the strict purpose of guide-wire exchange and

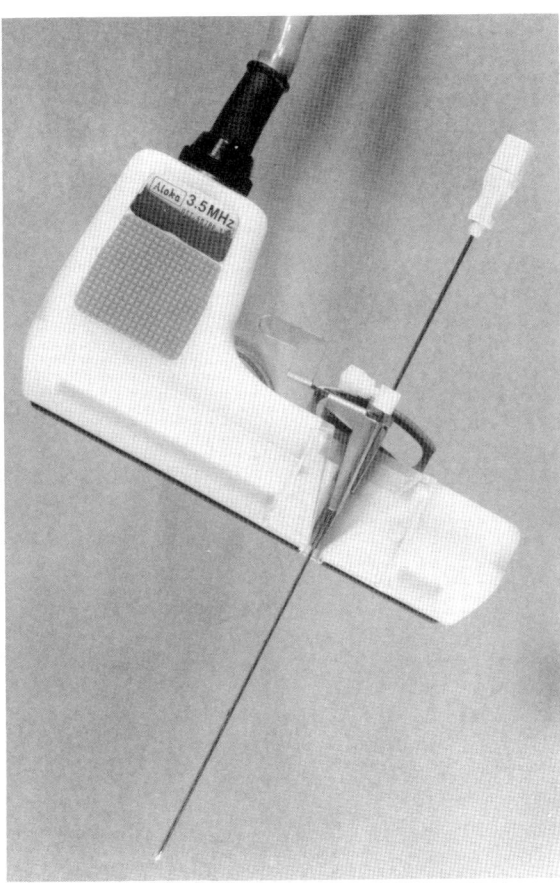

FIGURE 32.5. BIOPSY TRANSDUCER
High resolution linear-array real-time biopsy transducer (Aloka). A side exit or key-hole component for the needle is present as well as a built-in angling device for puncturing at other than 90°.

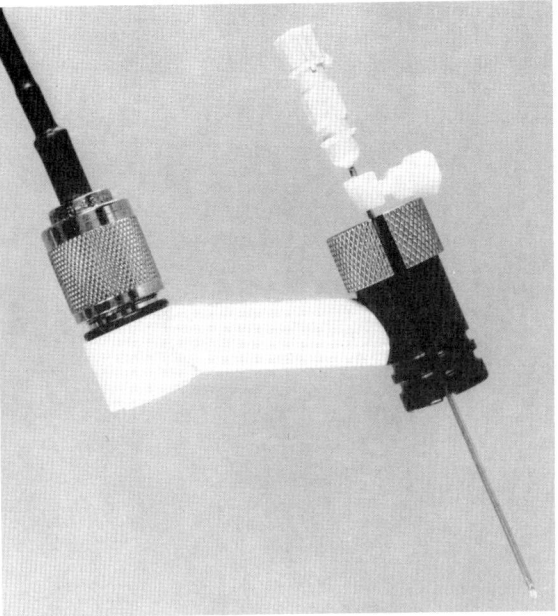

FIGURE 32.6. BIOPSY TRANSDUCER
A typical slotted biopsy transducer (Picker) is illustrated. The usefulness of this type of simple transducer is that the needle may remain in place once the fluid collection has been localized and the transducer may be slipped off. A transducer with only a central hole and no exit path for the needle requires that the needle be removed to take away the transducer from the skin and should be avoided.

the remainder may be introduced by both this method and the previously described trocar method (i.e., vanSonnenberg sump). One advantage to this technique is the possibility of using the diagnostic needle as the pathway through which the catheter will be placed.

A typical system is the Malecot nephrostomy system which may be used for percutaneous abscess drainage. A guide-wire is placed through the stationary needle after the needle tip has been confirmed to lie within the fluid collection. With the guide-wire coiled within the lesion, the needle is removed and a series of fascial dilators are passed to facilitate passage of the catheter. The catheter is ultimately passed with a central stiffening cannula so that the preformed tip is straight and easily introduced. A soon as the catheter is confirmed to be within the collection, the central hollow cannula is removed as with the trocar system. This technique is preferable when a very narrow ultrasound or CT window is present and the less delicate trocar technique must be avoided.

A sinogram (abscessogram) is performed through the catheter to confirm the extent of the abscess and imaged with fluoroscopy and computed tomography if necessary. At the very least, plain films can be obtained in at least two projections for confirmation; after which, the fluid contents may be completely evacuated.

Securing the Catheter

Stabilization of a percutaneous catheter is as important as actual catheter placement. As noted, once the collection has been drained, putting a catheter back into the collection site is much more difficult and complications become likely unless the abscess is allowed to reaccumulate. Catheters may be anchored using a variety of techniques.

A secure placement may be achieved with the Stoma wafer (Squibb Stomahesive Wafer) technique (21). Once the surgical drape has been removed, the skin around the catheter is cleaned with the standard skin prep for ostomy appli-

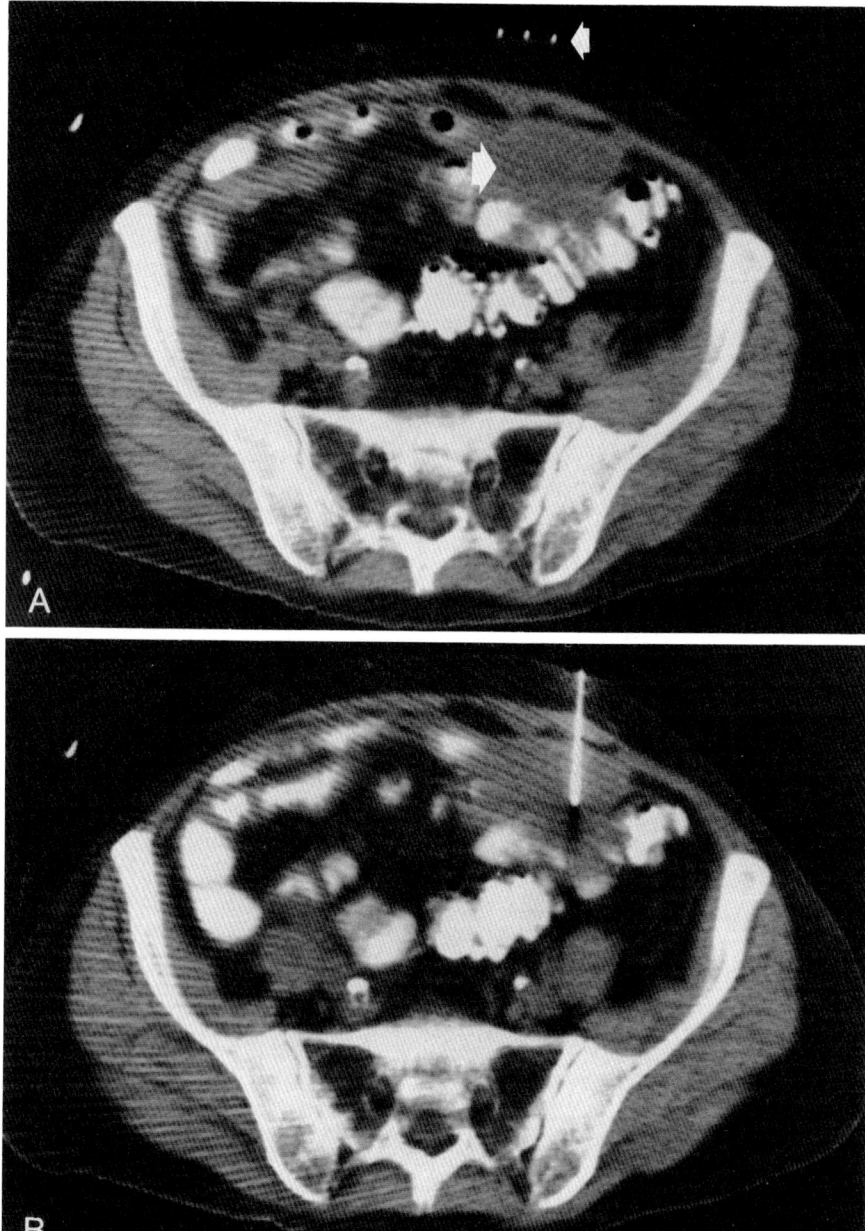

FIGURE 32.7. LOCALIZATION FOR NEEDLE PLACEMENT: CT

A 64-yr-old white man with a history of numerous abdominal procedures including a Whipple presented with a left lower quadrant interloop abscess (*bottom arrow*) (*A*). In this instance, three consecutive radiopaque catheters overlying the anticipated target could be observed (*top arrow*). It was elected to place the diagnostic needle along the third or lateral most radiopaque marker (*B*). The position was satisfactory and an 8.3 French pigtail catheter drained the abscess.

ances (United Skin-Prep) or alcohol. Once this has dried, Aerozoin skin conditioner spray is applied to the area and allowed to dry. If the outer attachment of the catheter will not permit passage through the central hole in the stoma wafer, the hole is expanded with a single cut extending from the inner hole to the outer perimeter. Although the catheter may be sutured to the flange on the stoma wafer, it is preferable to actually place the 38 mm Sur-Fit retention disk inside the wafer. Choose a disc with the appropriate hole diameter, i.e., 10 French size. This

TABLE 32.2.
SUBPHRENIC ABSCESS CASES

Series Authors (Ref.) Year	Subphrenic/ Total (%)	Percutaneous Abscess Drainage Successful	Complications
Altemeier et al. (23) 1973	27/540 (5%)	Surgery only	
Gerzof et al. (25) 1979	4/24 (17%)	4	1—empyema
Kleinhaus and Rosenberger (24) 1981	4/8 (50%)	4	1—violated pleura 2—pain
Johnson et al. (28) 1981	7/27 (26%)	6	1—empyema
Clark and Towbin (27) 1982	12/57 (21%)	10	2—violated pleura

disk may then be secured by suturing to the wafer flange and the catheter anchored by pulling the single plastic drawstring at the disk hub.

Alternatively, a finger-trap method (22) may be used to avoid tension over any short length of the catheter. The easiest method is to place a suture firmly around the base of the catheter and suture this to the skin or stoma wafer.

Location of Upper Abdominal Punctures

Common upper abdominal percutaneous abscess drainage sites and cyst aspiration regions include the subphrenic intraperitoneal space and intravisceral lesions of the liver, gallbladder, pancreas and spleen. Although more detailed information concerning each of these areas may be obtained in other chapters of this text, a summary of each site is included to assist in puncture of these areas.

Subphrenic Collection

Historically, two general patterns of intraperitoneal abscess formation were observed. The first is one of diffuse peritonitis seeding all areas lined by the peritoneum. The most dependent regions such as the anatomic pelvis, Morison's pouch, pericolic gutters, and subphrenic zones were commonly involved by one or more abscesses (23). The second pattern of intraperitoneal abscess formation is that of a localized process without generalized peritonitis. This latter form may occur in any of the above-mentioned zones and is believed to be partly explained by a sufficiently rapid body defense mechanism to prevent spreading peritonitis.

The subphrenic abscess is a good model for intraabdominal abscess drainage since it is a common abscess site. On the right, it is a perihepatic intraperitoneal space which is continuous with the subhepatic space and communicates freely with the general peritoneal cavity. However, with its repetitive net negative pressure in the suprahepatic region, the pleuroperitoneal pressure gradient has been theorized as a possible etiology for frequent subdiaphragmatic abscesses (7). In addition, the close proximity to the diaphragm requires the utmost accuracy in catheter placement to avoid complications involving the thorax. The risk of pneumothorax and empyema may be of greater consequence than the more common puncture complications such as hemorrhage or infection.

Of 35 drainage procedures performed by the ultrasound section at Johns Hopkins Hospital in a single calendar year, 13 cases (37%) involved the chest and 22 cases (63%) involved the abdomen. Of the abdominal cases, 4 (18%) were subdiaphragmatic collections. From published reports (Table 32.2), the incidence of subphrenic collections amongst abdominal abscesses ranges from a low of 5% (23) to a high of 50% (24). The majority of published reports puts the actual incidence closer to 20% (25–28). Previously, the most common cause of a subphrenic abscess was suppurative lesions of the appendix (30.9% of 3533 collected cases) (7). In the antibiotic era, the most common etiologic factors are gastric and biliary disease with surgical complications accounting for 52% of the abscesses and appendicitis responsible for only 8% of the subphrenic collections (29). The presentation of the subphrenic abscess clinically has also changed from sudden onset of high fever and abdominal pain following an acute event. Widespread use of preoperative and postoperative antibiotics have changed the common symptoms to a low grade fever and less commonly one of abdominal tenderness or pain (29). Because of the close proximity to the thorax, previously noted radiographic findings have been ipsilateral pleural effusion, pneumonitis, and partial atelectasis. There may be an increase in the distance between the apex of the left hemidiaphragm and the gastric air bubble on upright views as may

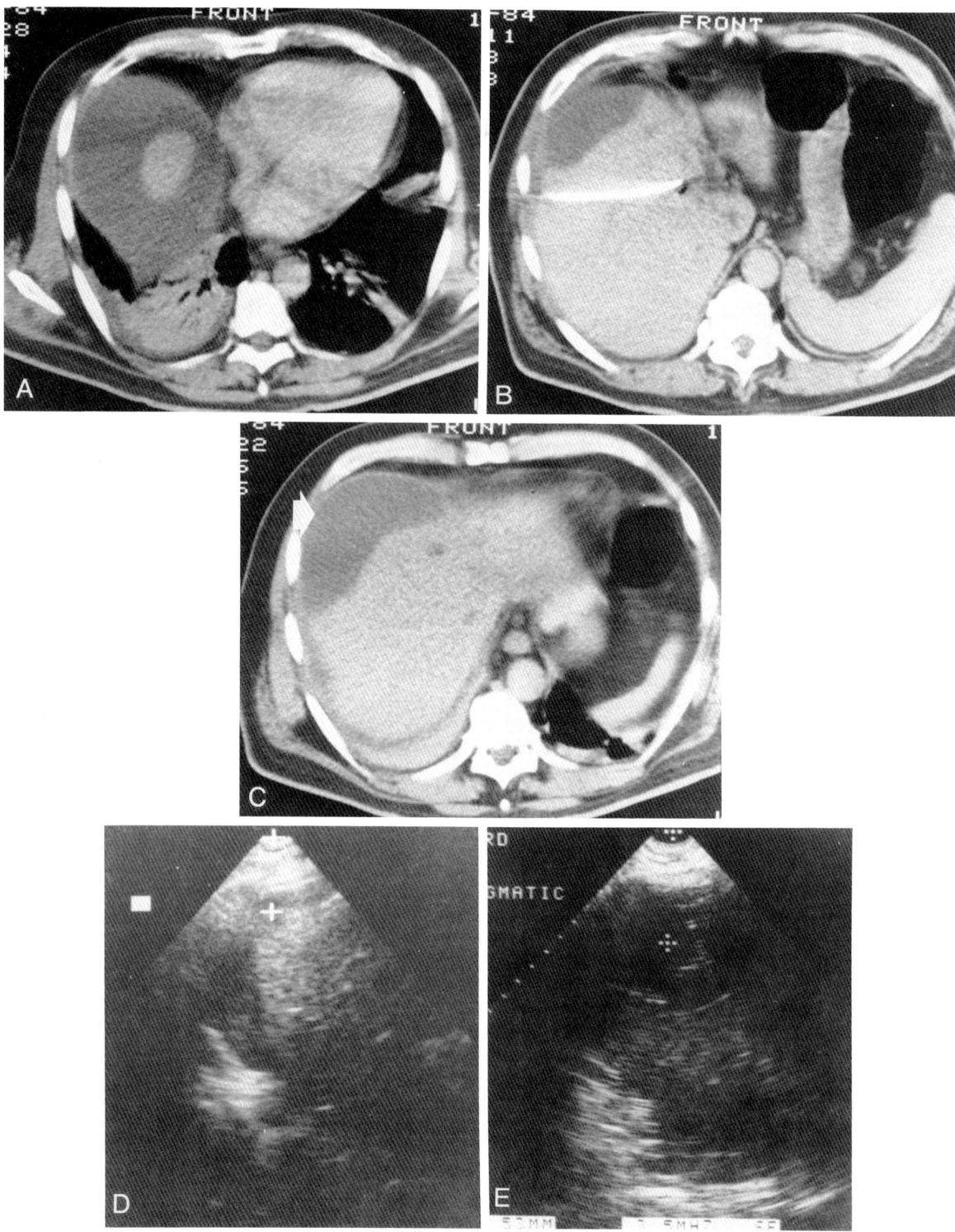

FIGURE 32.8. SUBPHRENIC COLLECTION

This 57-yr-old man with a history of Klatskin tumor and previous right external biliary drainage catheter placement presented with a large right subdiaphragmatic fluid collection (*arrow*) with bilateral lower lobe partial atelectasis and pleural effusions (*A–C*). Using ultrasound guidance, a right subdiaphragmatic tap (*D*) was performed which yielded 50 ml of bilious fluid. Consequently, an 8.3 French pigtail catheter was placed in the subphrenic collection using ultrasound guidance, and 660 ml of turbid bilious fluid were drained (*E*). Anteroposterior and oblique views from a follow-up abscessogram demonstrate subdiaphragmatic placement of the pigtail catheter and bilateral intrahepatic biliary tubes (*F* and *G*).

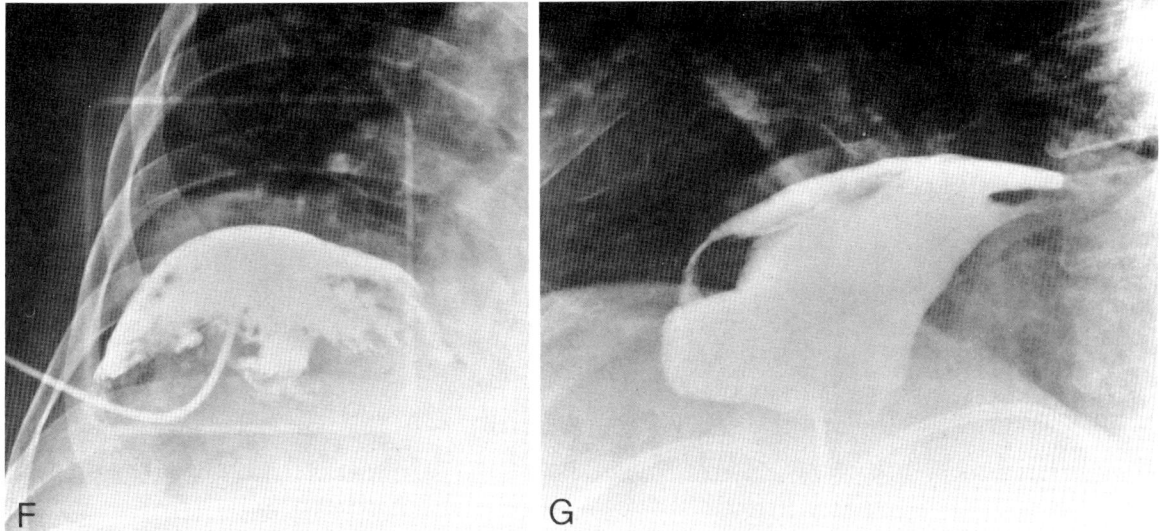

FIGURE 32.8 *F* and *G*

also be seen with subpulmonic fluid. An air-fluid level within the abscess cavity may be seen in only 30% of subphrenic abscesses (6). CT and ultrasound have been helpful in that the true level of the hemidiaphragm on either side can be immediately ascertained and collections identified.

Initial needle placement in the subdiaphragmatic abscess is easily performed using real-time ultrasound guidance. This way, the needle tip may be observed to lie within the fluid collection away from the diaphragm (Fig. 32.8). Alternatively, a triangulation approach for angling the needle localization may be performed utilizing the Pythagorean theorem for right angles (30, 31). A perpendicular or a nearly perpendicular puncture may still be performed anteriorly for large collections (Fig. 32.8). However, the pleura must be avoided so that no pneumothorax, hemothorax, or pyothorax will occur.

Hepatic Puncture

Hepatic puncture may be separated into two categories. The first is cystic disease of the liver. The second is intrahepatic abscess.

Only 150 cases of hepatic cystic disease were observed in a Mayo Clinic review of 88,000 abdominal explorations. Thus, the incidence of hepatic cysts observed at surgery was 17 per 10,000 explorations. This is probably an underestimate of the true number of cysts since small hepatic cysts were probably not observed at surgery (32). Histologically, congenital cysts have cuboidal epithelium. In approximately half of the congenital cysts of this series, the cyst walls contained bile duct tissue. Cysts may be observed in association with polycystic renal disease. When this is the case, the diagnosis is usually straightforward. However, other etiologies such as hydatid cysts, traumatic cysts and inflammatory cysts have been described.

Hepatic cysts are easily observed by ultrasound because of their anechoic internal structure, sharp smooth borders, enhanced through transmission, and circle or oval shape (33). Some may say that the completely echo-free thin walled solitary hepatic cyst may be of no clinical significance. Sometimes, large cysts may cause epigastric pain or mass effect (up to 25% of hepatic cysts may be symptomatic) (32). It is particularly helpful to know whether or not the cyst is infected or whether or not the abnormality could represent a necrotic tumor (34). The diagnosis of hepatic cyst may be confirmed by needle aspiration. It is not necessary to leave a catheter in place. However, therapeutic decompression may sometimes be effective. Avoid unknowingly puncturing hydatid cysts where peritoneal dissemination or anaphylaxis might occur. Travel to endemic areas, eosinophilia, or calcification of the cyst wall may suggest hydatid disease (Fig. 32.9) (35). In this case, obtain serologic tests prior to puncture as a precaution. Evidence exists that hydatid cysts may be safely drained percutaneously (see section on echinococcal disease of the liver in Chapter 5).

A follow-up study of hepatic cyst puncture suggests that although definitive diagnosis may be ascertained, there is not likely to be perma-

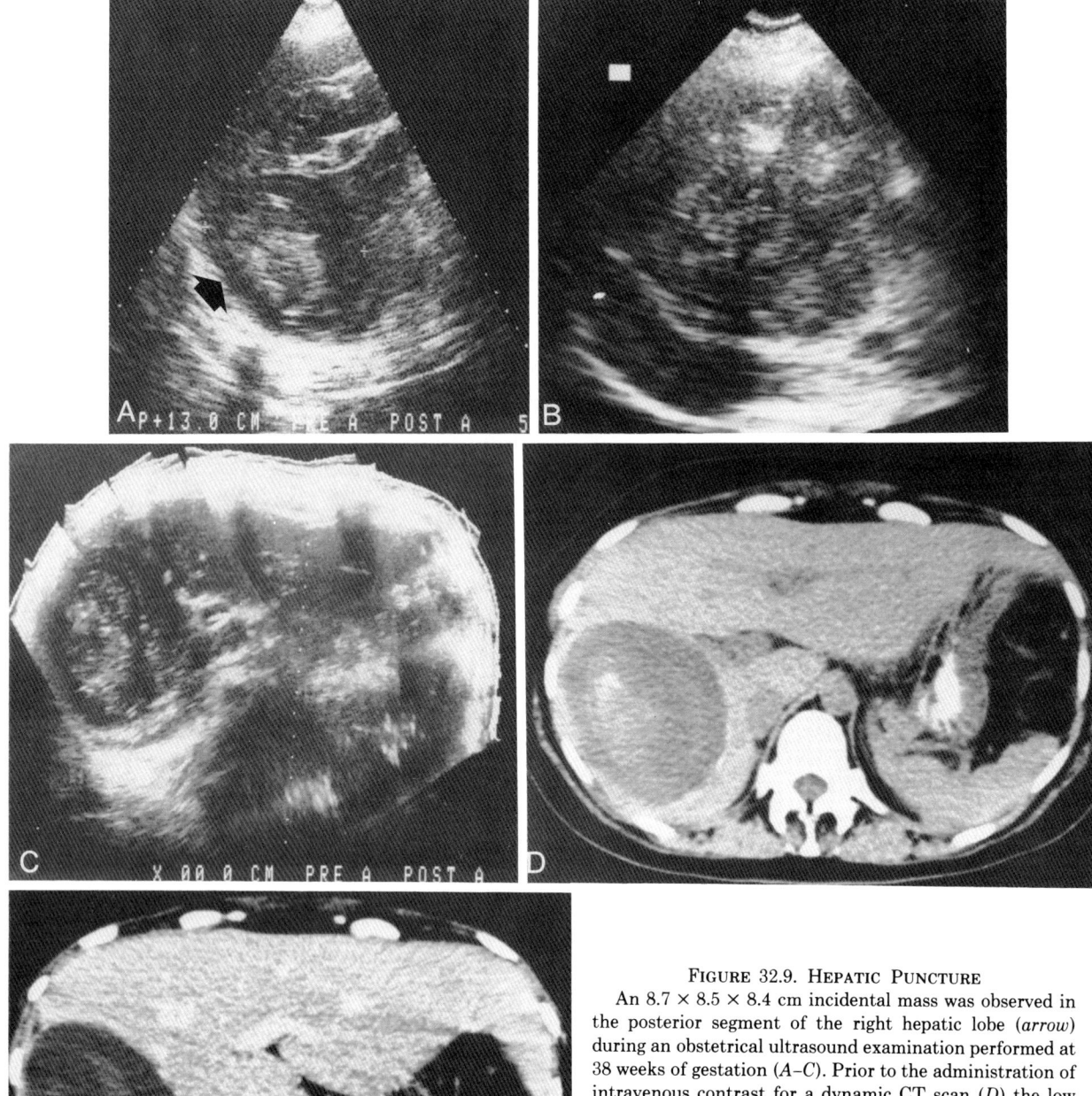

FIGURE 32.9. HEPATIC PUNCTURE

An 8.7 × 8.5 × 8.4 cm incidental mass was observed in the posterior segment of the right hepatic lobe (*arrow*) during an obstetrical ultrasound examination performed at 38 weeks of gestation (*A–C*). Prior to the administration of intravenous contrast for a dynamic CT scan (*D*) the low density rounded mass appears to have an area of high attenuation centrally and along its rim consistent with calcification. No other lesion was observed. No internal enhancement was observed following the intravenous bolus of contrast (*E*). The above findings are most consistent with echinococcal cyst and no percutaneous aspiration was performed.

nent therapeutic benefit from complete aspiration percutaneously (36). However, this study did not examine the possible role of sclerosing agents to determine whether or not they are efficacious. A single report from Goldstein et al. (37) is an example where sclerosis was attempted. An 18-gauge catheter sheath needle was introduced into the hepatic cyst and a double contrast cystogram was performed with instillation of Renografin 60 into the cyst cavity. Since

TABLE 32.3.
DIAGNOSTIC FINDINGS IN HEPATIC PUNCTURE

Entity (Ref.)	White Blood Cells	Red Blood Cells	Chemistry	Remarks
Amebic abscess (38)			—	"Anchovy paste"
Pyogenic abscess (27)		±		Foul smelling, + Gram stain
Biloma (39, 40)	—	—	Bilirubin	+ ^{99m}Tc-HIDA
Pancreatic pseudocyst (41)	—	—	Amylase	History of pancreatitis
Hematoma (42)	±		—	Trauma
Tumor (43)	—	±	—	+ Cytopathology

the internal lining was entirely smooth, a finding previously used to suggest benign disease during renal cyst puncture, Pantopaque was used to initiate a fibrous reaction. At 16 months, the patient was asymptomatic without evidence of a persistent cystic defect.

Hepatic abscesses have been divided into amoebic and nonamoebic abscesses. At the turn of this century, the majority of hepatic abscesses were amoebic in origin (75%) (8). However, amoebic abscesses are often successfully treated noninvasively with metronidazole (Flagyl). The aspirate when performed usually demonstrates numerous white blood cells (Table 32.3) and may have an anchovy paste appearance (38).

Nonamoebic abscesses, in particular pyogenic abscesses, may spread by direct extension from contiguous disease processes such as cholecystitis and peptic ulcer disease. However, other modes of transportation of virulent strains of bacteria are drainage via the portal system, such as necrotic inflamed bowel, trauma with penetrating injuries and direct introduction into the liver, and blood-borne infections via the hepatic arteries (8). As with abdominal abscesses in general, the most commonly isolated bacterium is *Escherichia coli*. However, now that anaerobic culture techniques are being used routinely, up to 60% of intraabdominal abscesses, including liver abscesses, have positive anaerobic cultures. The most common anaerobe is *Bacteroides fragilis* (44).

Similar to subphrenic abscesses, intrahepatic abscess drainage procedures should not involve the gallbladder, portal vein, and hepatic flexure of the colon (45). Real-time sonography is helpful in avoiding all of the above. However, gas within adjacent organs may sometimes cause a problem. Consequently, CT, with or without intravenous, oral, or rectal contrast may be used (Fig. 32.10).

Gallbladder Puncture

Until recently, puncture of the gallbladder and related procedures such as drainage of pericholecystic fluid collections and bilomas have been predominently surgical procedures. Percutaneous fine-needle transhepatic cholangiography has been well described as a fluoroscopic nonsurgical technique (46, 47). Except for the intraoperative manipulation of the human gallbladder, this latter structure has been primarily punctured percutaneously utilizing animal models (48, 49). Ultrasound was shown to be uniquely capable of real-time imaging of the unopacified gallbladder during these animal trials.

Direct gallbladder puncture enables sampling of the biliary tract for Gram stain, culture, sensitivity, and cytology (Fig. 32.11). It also permits opacification of the gallbladder determining cystic and bile duct patency (Fig. 32.12). Unlike radionuclide imaging, it permits closer evaluation of the gallbladder wall confirming the presence of any mass lesion. Finally, utilizing the previously mentioned drainage techniques, a small bore catheter may be introduced as a temporizing measure (50). This is a particularly important alternative to surgery in a patient with severe cardiac, pulmonary, liver, or renal failure.

The reason percutaneous cholecystostomy has been slow to evolve is primarily one of fear of producing bile peritonitis. Although this can occur even after fine-needle transhepatic cholangiography with or without external drainage, in one series of 13 cases, only one patient developed peritonitis and subsequent fatal septic shock and this was only after inadvertent cholecystostomy catheter removal. All of the other patients remained free of sepsis, peritonitis, or other complication related to percutaneous cholecystostomy (51). The other major reason for reluctant acceptance of cholecystostomy is the possibility of a profound vagal reaction resulting in marked hypotension and bradycardia. This appears to be related to extensive manipulation of the gallbladder catheter (52). Consequently, close monitoring of the patient's vital signs and the rapid accessibility of intravenous atropine are necessities.

The most direct method of precisely diagnosing pericholecystic fluid collections is placement

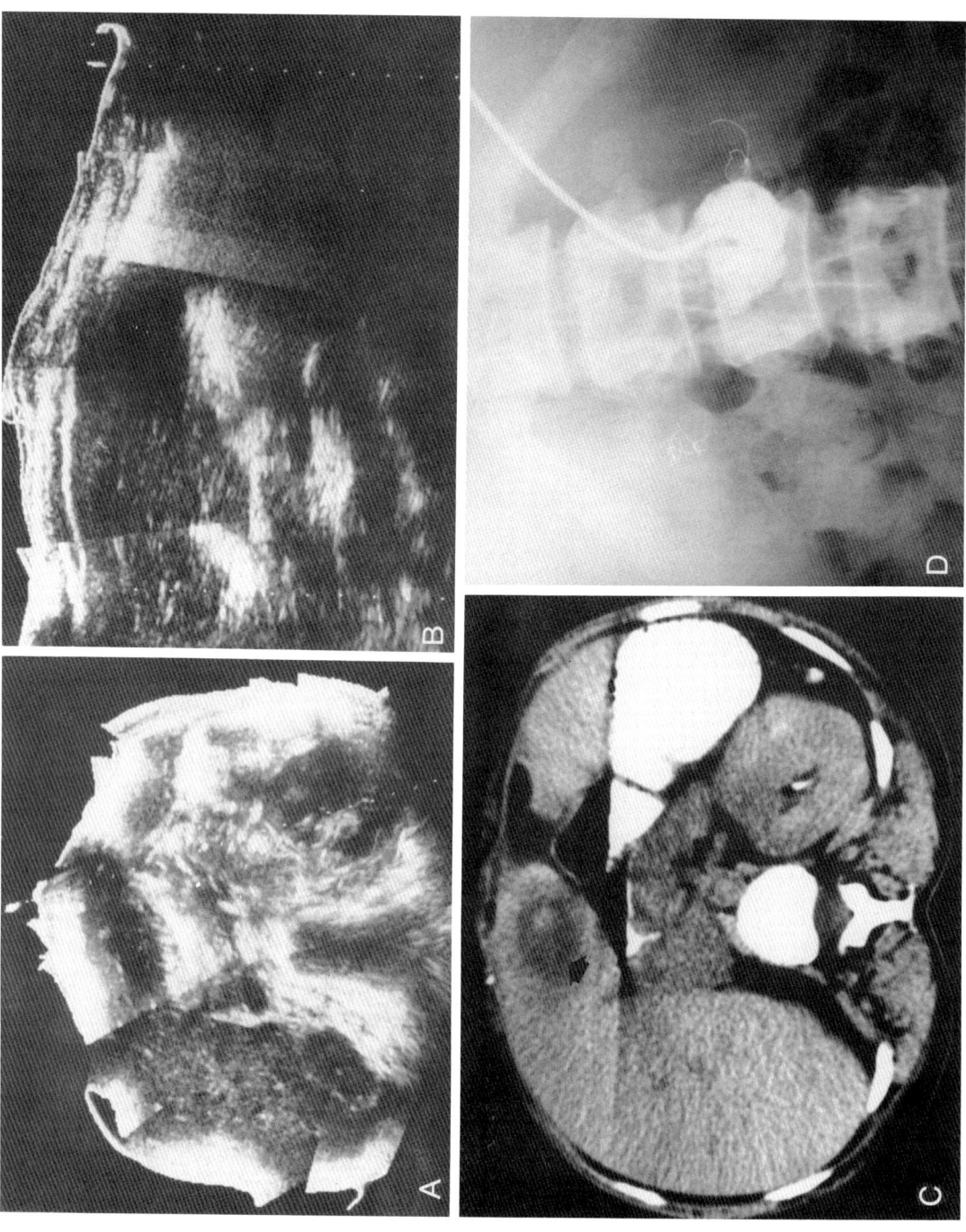

FIGURE 32.10. HEPATIC PUNCTURE

This 28-yr-old black woman with sickle cell disease was noted to have an abnormal left hepatic lobe during ultrasound examination (*A, B*: transverse and sagittal). Computed tomography confirmed a low density lesion (*arrow*) within the lateral segment of the left hepatic lobe (*C*). A preliminary diagnostic aspiration was performed under ultrasound guidance yielding 15 ml of what appeared to represent old blood which was sent for culture and Gram stain which were positive. A sinogram was then performed (*D*) which confirmed the catheter tip was within the intrahepatic abscess.

1054

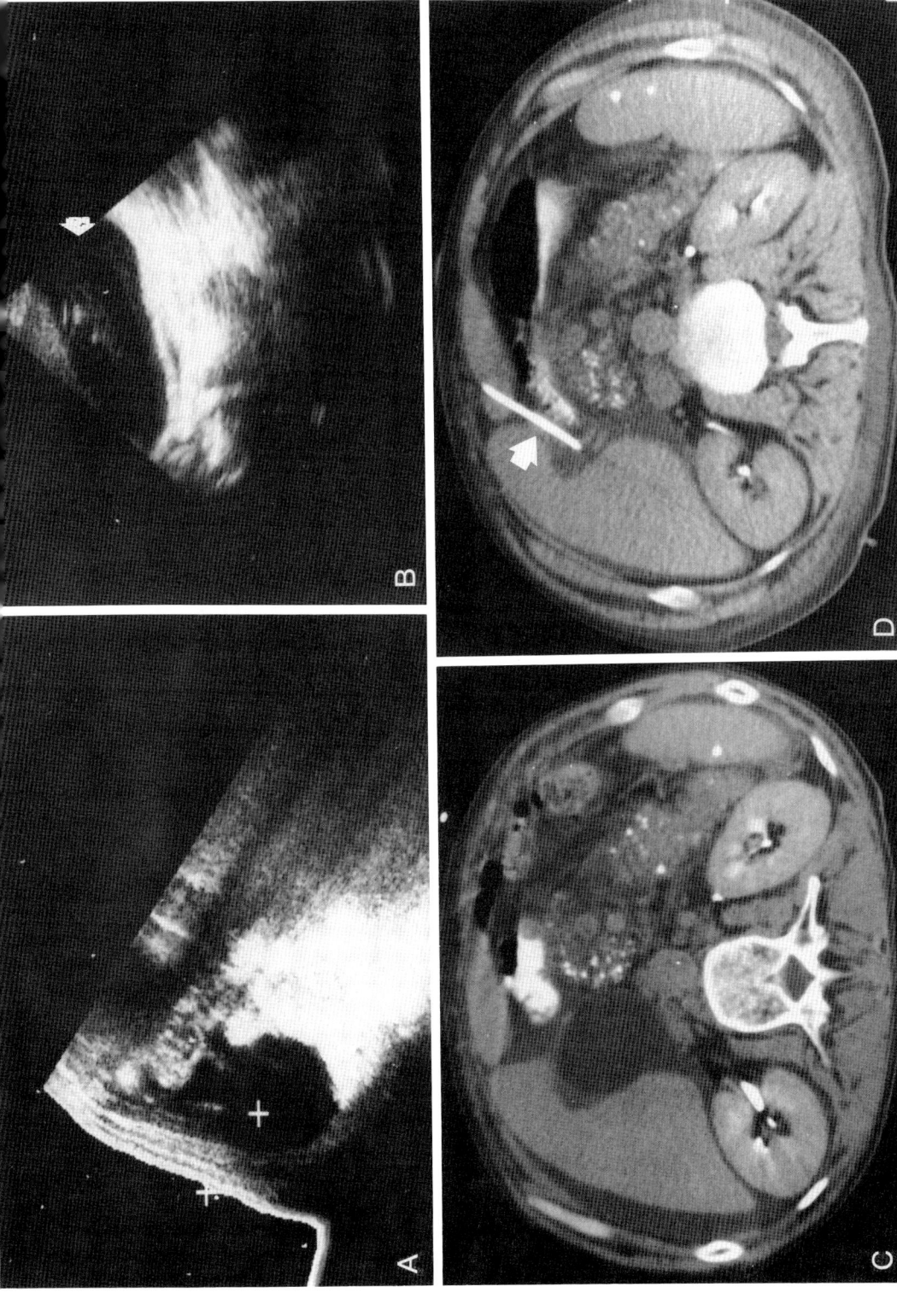

FIGURE 32.11. GALLBLADDER PUNCTURE

This 71-yr-old male alcoholic presented with liver failure. A right US-guided paracentesis was performed which yielded 20 ml of clear yellow fluid (*A*). The gallbladder (*arrow*) was noted to be markedly distended (*B*). CT confirmed the ascites, gallbladder distension, and calcific pancreatitis (*C*). Percutaneous transhepatic puncture was unsuccessful secondary to the nondilated intrahepatic bile ducts. Consequently, using US guidance, a 6.3 French pigtail catheter was placed into the gallbladder lumen, and 300 ml of viscous bile were obtained for Gram stain, culture, and sensitivity. A follow-up CT scan confirmed catheter (*arrow*) placement within the nondilated gallbladder (*D*). Incidental note is made of calcified splenic granulomas.

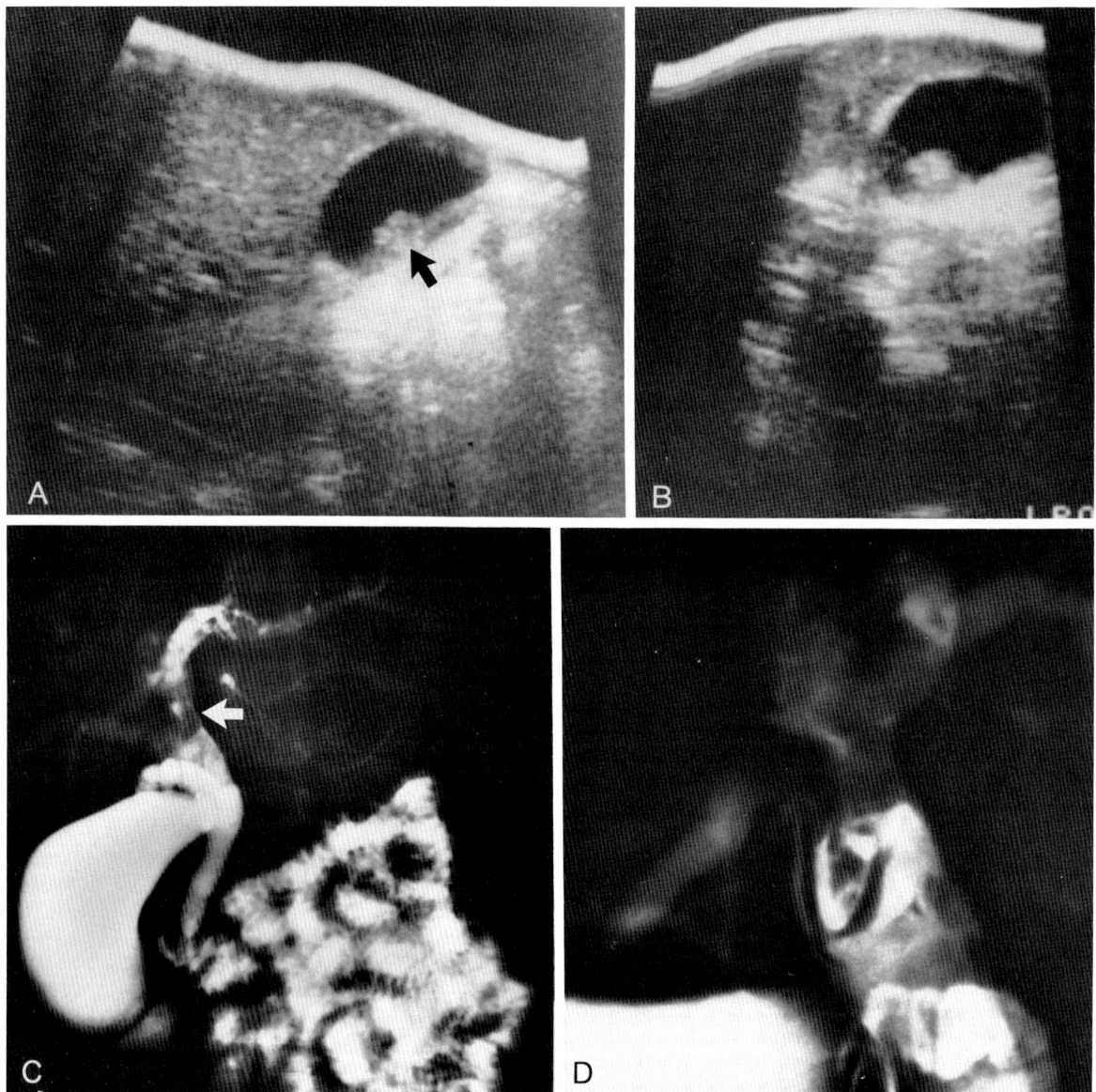

FIGURE 32.12. GALLBLADDER PUNCTURE

A 4½-yr-old Korean orphan brought to the United States was found to have hepatosplenomegaly and elevated liver function tests. Sagittal and transverse US images (*A* and *B*) demonstrate an echogenic dependent mass (*arrow*) without acoustical shadowing within the gallbladder lumen. Using US guidance and sterile technique, a 20-gauge Longdwel (Becton, Dickenson & Co.) was used to puncture the gallbladder. Thirty milliliters of dark green bile were aspirated from the gallbladder. Some of the bile was observed to contain debris. However, subsequent injection of contrast through the Teflon catheter demonstrated multiple serpiginous filling defects compatible with the clinical diagnosis of liver flukes (*C* and *D*). Parasitology examination of the stool confirmed *Fasciola hepatica*. These liver flukes were visualized by percutaneous cholecystography within the gallbladder and at the bifurcation of the right and left bile ducts (*arrow*). The patient responded well to medical therapy.

of a needle (53). Since pericholecystic fluid may simply represent the regional appearance of a more widespread process such as generalized ascites, this finding may require complete evaluation of the abdomen by diagnostic techniques. Other etiologies include frank pus at one end of the spectrum to a localized collection of bile from spontaneous gallbladder rupture or previous surgery (54). A frequent site of infection following biliary surgery is the right anterior subhepatic space known as the gallbladder fossa. Although this was continuous with the other perihepatic intraperitoneal regions, pyogenic septa may form causing loculation of fluid (55). A perihepatic or intrahepatic collection detected by ultrasound or CT (56) may represent bile. A rapid noninvasive procedure to document the presence of a bile leak is a technetium-99m-HIDA cholescintigram. However, the other modalities must still be used in case the intra- or perihepatic bile collection no longer communicates with the biliary tract (57).

Initial evaluation of any aspirate of a bile collection should include identification of the presence of bilirubin with Multistix (Ames Co.) and a preliminary microscopic examination (which yields numerous leukocytes and Gram positive or Gram negative bacteria if an infection is present). Although drainage catheter placement would be straightforward, the presence of a positive ^{99m}Tc-HIDA scan suggests an active bile leak which in the past mandated surgery (57). In our experience, surgery is only undertaken after a trial of PAD.

Some technical points for these drainages include the closed gravity drainage bag for a sterile biloma utilizing a pigtail catheter. The catheter within a sterile collection should be allowed to remain for only the minimal time required for evacuation of the collection (58). The tip of the catheter should be as close as possible to the point of communication with the biliary tree.

Follow-up may be achieved with a sinogram, ultrasound or CT, and ^{99m}Tc-HIDA scan within 24–48 hr. Following prompt definitive diagnosis, drainage, and appropriate intravenous antibiotics, surgery may be either avoided or postponed until the patient is a better surgical risk.

Pancreatic Puncture

Much has been written describing the use of ultrasound and computed tomography in the evaluation of acute pancreatitis and its complications (59, 60). However, the radiologist can play a more active role than just acting as a diagnostician since intervention in this region is becoming increasingly important.

Severe steady epigastric pain with nausea and vomiting accompanying heavy alcohol consumption is a common clinical presentation. The physical findings such as abdominal distension secondary to ileus, tenderness, fever and tachycardia are often not as severe as the patient's subjective status would lead the clinician to expect. Sequential ultrasound studies may demonstrate diffuse enlargement of the entire gland, although alcoholics can have focal pancreatitis more commonly in the region of the head. Echotexture may become uniformly echopenic. The above findings are consistent with frank pancreatic edema. The pancreatic duct which is normally less than 2 mm in size may markedly dilate as well. Computed tomography at this stage confirms enlargement of the pancreas, dilatation of the pancreatic duct, and blurring of the margins of the gland. A halo of edema may surround the pancreas with a resulting increase in attenuation of the peripancreatic fat (59). Sometimes, clinical and laboratory findings become a dominant factor in recognizing pathology related to the pancreas. This is because patients with recurrent or chronic relapsing pancreatitis, such as the alcoholic, may have an episode of acute pancreatitis which has no observable ultrasound or CT findings.

The problem patient who may require intervention is the one who presents several days or more following the episode of acute pancreatitis. An enlarging mass may be palpated within the abdomen and fever may be present. The differential diagnosis is one of pancreatic phlegmon, pseudocyst, or abscess. Surgery and percutaneous intervention can be avoided in the case of phlegmon. An indurated inflamed pancreas is seen without a drainable structure such as a fluid collection (61). However, pancreatic and extrapancreatic fluid collections are amenable to either percutaneous intervention or surgical drainage.

Proteolytic, lipolytic, and elastolytic enzymes result in autodigestion of the pancreatic parenchyma and subsequent accumulation of necrotic debris if this fluid does not escape. However, commonly the thin layer of peripancreatic fibrous connective tissue is not sufficient to prevent passage of the pancreatic enzymes allowing fluid to collect in the anterior pararenal space. The posterior layer of the peritoneum is all that stands between these enzymes and the commonly involved lesser sac (Fig. 32.13) (60). These early extrapancreatic accumulations of fluid may be easily demonstrated as cystic appearing structures by ultrasound. With decompression of the pancreatic ductal system and escape of fluid outside the pancreas the gland may appear remarkably normal (62) as opposed to retention of pancreatic juice in the interstitium of the gland causing persistent intrapancreatic inflammation. Peripancreatic fluid collections are hyperosmolar and may continue to grow in size because of the accumulation of fluid. Fluid may also be spontaneously resorbed. Following the cystic structure by either ultrasound or CT will demonstrate a change in size over a period of days to weeks. Initially, these collections are anechoic by ultrasound and close to water density by computed tomography. Percutaneous fine-needle

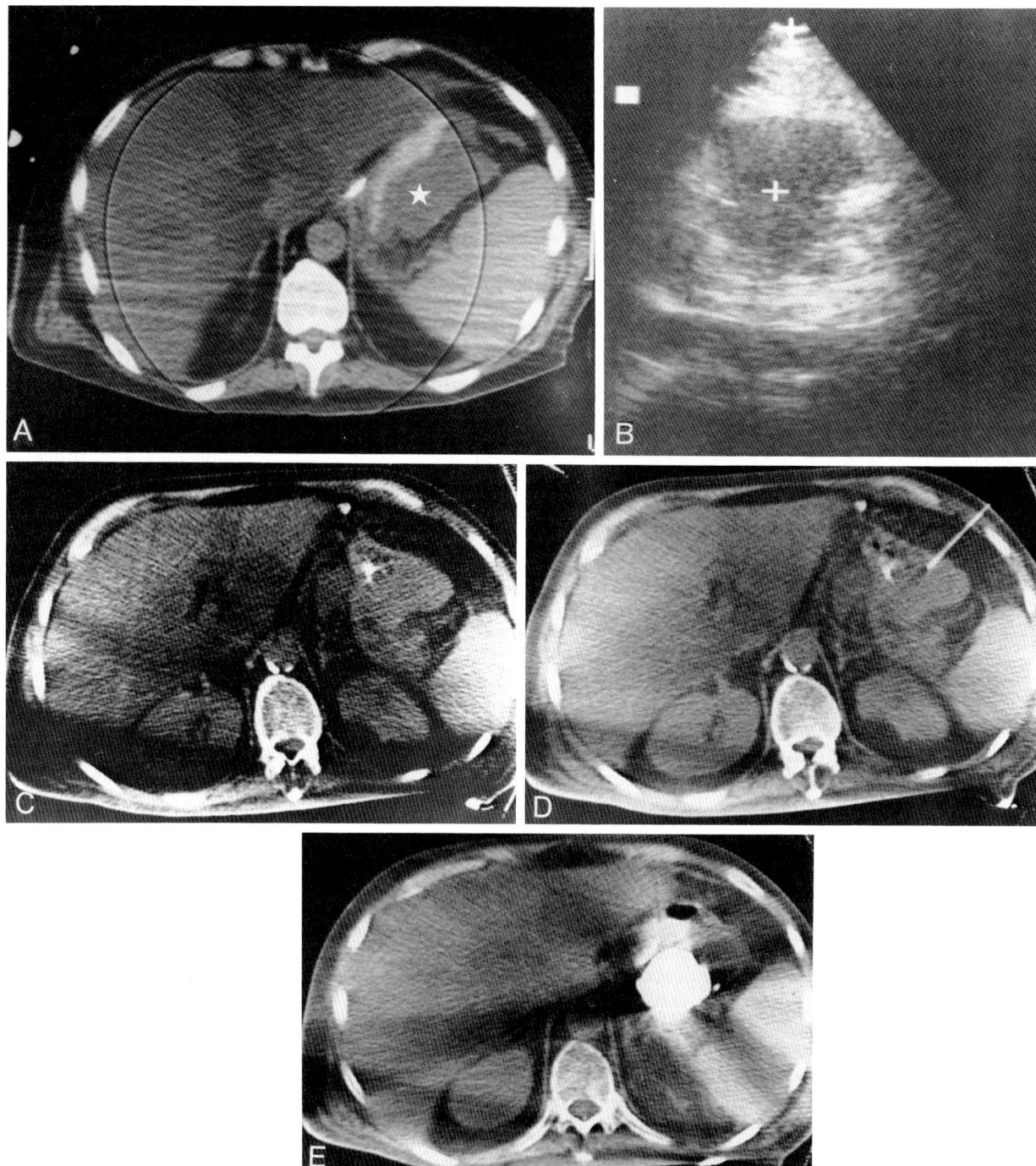

FIGURE 32.13. PANCREATIC PUNCTURE

A 64-yr-old white man following an episode of necrotizing pancreatitis presented with a pancreatic abscess of the lesser sac (*A*). Compression of the minimally opacified gastric body by an abscess (*star*) in the lesser sac is demonstrated. Note the circular CT detector artifact, fatty replaced liver, and enlarged spleen. Percutaneous aspiration by ultrasound (*B*), confirmed the presence of an abscess. Using CT guidance (*C*), a bowel-free route was observed. Note the continued artifact overlying the posterior half of the transverse axial image secondary to the patient's upper extremities remaining alongside the abdomen during this emergency scan. However, more than sufficient detail could be observed to permit passage of an 8.2 French pigtail catheter into the lesser sac collection (*D*). Forty milliliters of thin brownish yellow fluid which formed a coagulum were aspirated. The catheter was then injected with contrast (*E*).

aspiration will be diagnostic when there is an abnormally high amylase value. If there is still communication with the pancreatic ductal system, external drainage is not recommended because of the high incidence of persistent pancreatico-cutaneous fistula (62).

Loculated fluid collections following acute pancreatitis may go on to develop a thick wall of connective tissue which may then be termed a pseudocyst. The name implies absence of a true epithelial lining. The avascularity of the wall is confirmed by intravenous enhanced computed tomography. However, even pseudocysts may become infected at which point the wall may enhance by CT. Internal structure demonstrated by internal echoes by ultrasound and higher attenuation (greater than water density) by CT suggests a complicated pseudocyst. This may be secondary to either infection or hemorrhage. A pancreatic abscess may occur either as a result of secondary infection of the devitalized pancreas or conversion of a pseudocyst into an abscess (61).

Interventional procedures range from cannulation of the pancreatic duct (63) to drainage of pseudocysts and abscesses (41). Any patient who has a pancreatic or peripancreatic fluid collection who is clinically suspected of having an abscess should have a skinny needle percutaneous aspiration (64). If there are many white blood cells and bacteria, a drainage catheter should be placed. It is less important what type of catheter is used initially. Modified trocar (65) or angiographic catheters may be useful. A sinogram should confirm absence of communication with the pancreatic duct (Fig. 32.14). Adequate imaging follow-up should confirm decrease in the size of the pseudocyst or abscess. The next line of percutaneous manipulation could be placement of a sump catheter (i.e., vanSonnenberg sump). Alternatively, two catheters may be placed utilizing paired guide-wires through a single sheath (41). These techniques permit continuous irrigation of the cavity. The catheter should not be removed until fever subsides.

Splenic Puncture

A solitary abscess within the spleen is a distinctly unusual pathologic entity. Although immunosuppressed patients may have multiple abscesses, one of which may involve the spleen, only 10 cases out of 100,000 admissions over a 10-yr period were secondary to solitary abscess of the spleen (66). Prior to the advent of ultrasound and CT, secondary findings of splenic abscess such as nonspecific splenic enlargement, elevation of the left hemidiaphragm, and dispalcement of the gastric bubble were key radiographic findings. Sulfur colloid liver spleen scans and arteriography were used to demonstrate splenic defects. However, gray-scale sonographic examination of the spleen further refined splenic imaging. Instead of looking only for the presence of a cystic structure within the spleen such as hematoma or pancreatic pseudocyst, splenic abscesses could be more easily differentiated appearing as irregular, poorly defined, anechoic masses (67, 68). Internal echoes may sometimes be present and enhanced through transmission is usually observed. However, if there is intravisceral gas, corresponding increased echogenicity and shadowing would be observed. Septations are sometimes noted (69). Gallium nuclear medicine scan activity may be diagnostic, but percutaneous puncture still yields the specific infective organisms and a means for therapy (Fig. 32.15). Fever may be a common clinical feature of both splenic abscess and splenic lymphoma (70). Splenic infarction may also appear this way. This latter entity must always be considered since patients with sickle cell disease may present with either infarction or abscess. However, the most common underlying etiology is infective endocarditis as a cause for splenic abscess (69).

CT will be helpful in some cases to define any underlying pathology such as polycystic disease also involving the liver or kidney (71). Vascular splenic pathology (such as hemangioma and hemangiosarcoma) may be excluded from percutaneous puncture by intravenous enhanced computed tomography (72).

Splenostomy is the procedure of choice when splenectomy is not feasible either secondary to abscess size, adhesions, or patient's poor surgical risk (73). Percutaneous splenostomy may be performed as a less invasive procedure avoiding and thus preserving the large residual splenic rind. This route also permits avoidance of concomitant varices.

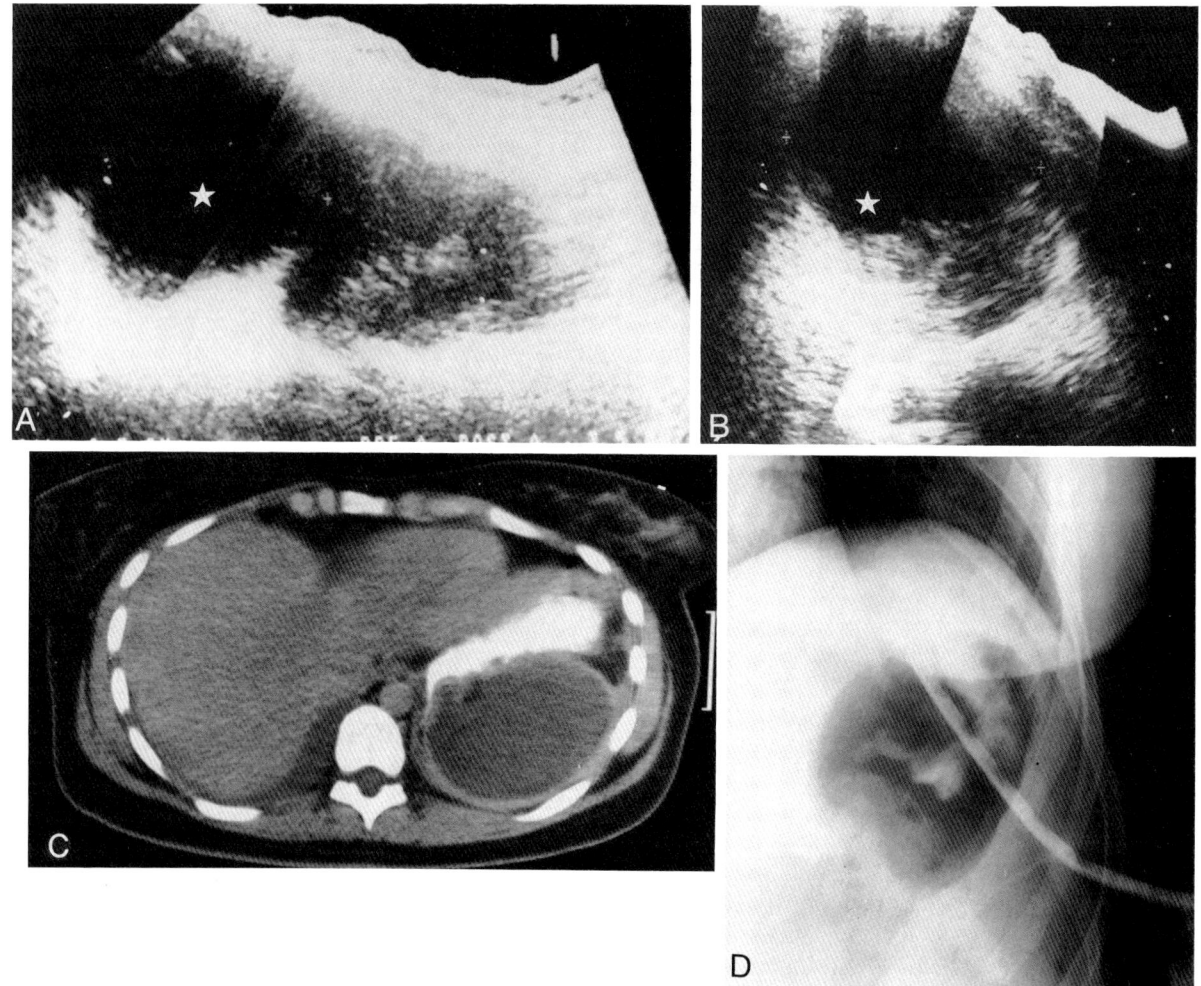

FIGURE 32.14. PANCREATIC PUNCTURE

A 32-yr-old white woman was transfered for evaluation of a post-traumatic pancreatic abscess. She had undergone a previous splenectomy following spouse abuse. A right thoracocentesis by ultrasound guidance was performed to exclude hemothorax. However, longitudinal and transverse (A and B) scans of the upper abdomen demonstrated an 8.7 cm nearly echo-free fluid collection (star) in the left upper quadrant. Computed tomography confirmed the presence of a loculated collection with the presence of a thick wall and mean attenuation coefficient which was higher than water (C). Using ultrasound guidance, a 22-gauge needle diagnostic aspiration was performed which yielded 15 ml of brownish fluid. The fluid had an amylase level of 4920 Caraway U/dl (normal 0–160), Gram-negative rods, and numerous white blood cells (96,000/mm^3). Consequently, a 12 French van Sonnenberg Sump catheter was inserted into the remaining left upper quadrant collection permitting 400 ml of additional brown fluid to be expelled. A sinogram confirms the location and lack of communication with the pancreatic duct in this post-traumatic pancreatic abscess (D).

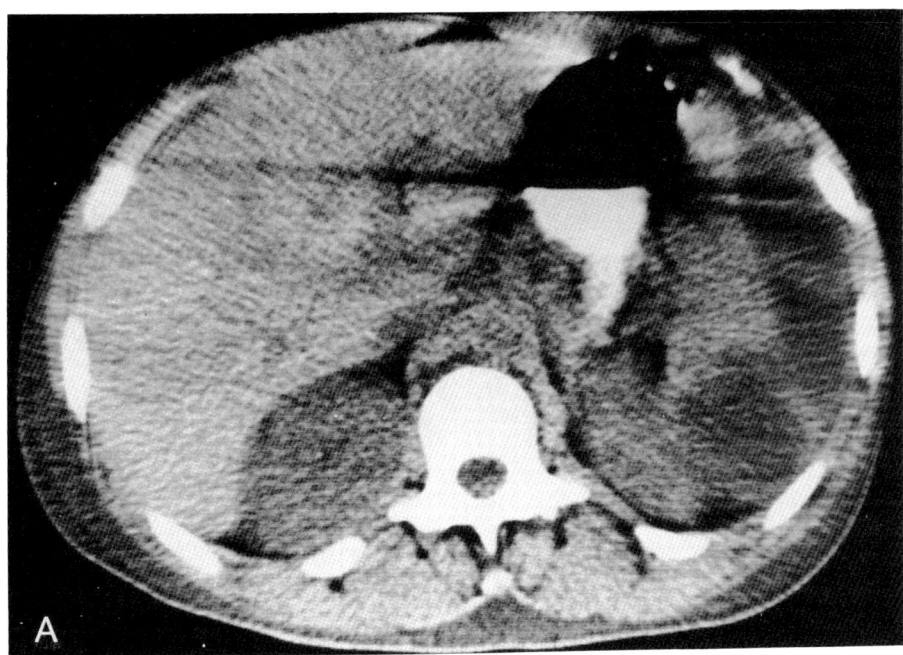
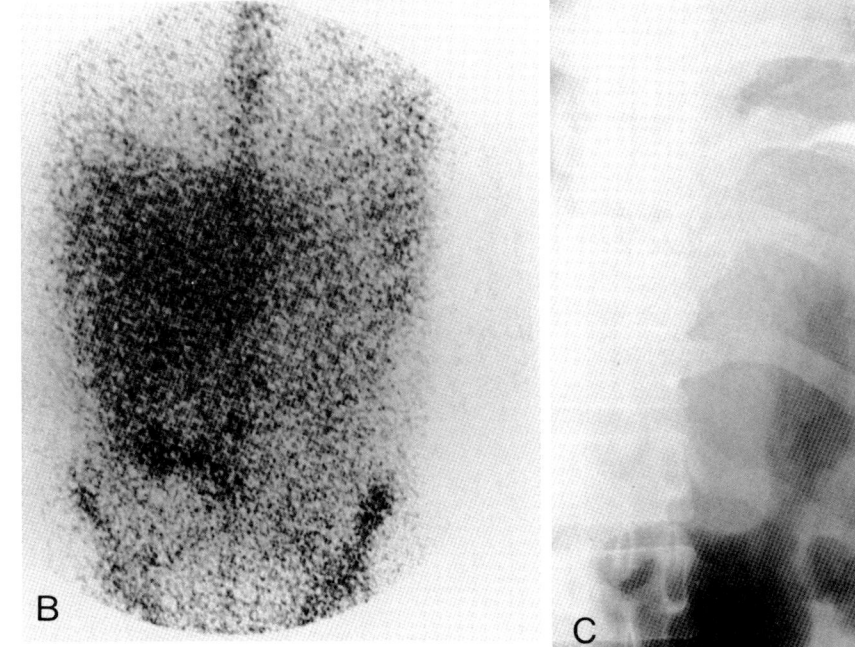
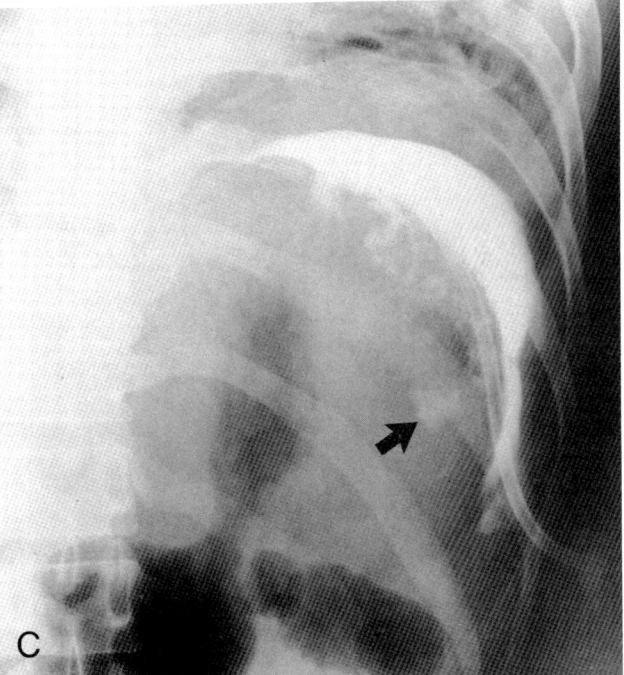

FIGURE 32.15. SPLENIC PUNCTURE
Ruptured splenic abscess in a patient with bacterial endocarditis. *A*: CT scan: round low density mass within spleen and lenticular extrasplenic collection. Abscess vs. infarct vs. hematoma. *B*: Gallium scan: no increased uptake within the spleen. Despite this result, abscess was thought to be the most likely diagnosis. *C*: Percutaneous puncture and drainage was performed successfully under ultrasound guidance. Frank pus was aspirated; only one catheter was needed to drain both the intra- and extrasplenic components. *Arrow* points to intrasplenic component starting to fill on this abscessogram.

CONCLUSION

Abdominal abscesses all required surgical drainage in the past. With the exceptions of appendiceal abscess, diverticulitis, and tuboovarian abscess most can be handled percutaneously. Even in the above exceptional instances, percutaneous drainage is useful in stabilizing an ill patient and may be definitive therapy in selected instances (74, 75). Earlier diagnosis by ultrasound and CT has also improved the patient's chance of going to operating room when indicated. When compared with the best surgical data available, percutaneous drainage in abdominal abscesses has a higher success rate with a decreased hospital stay and correspondingly decreased complication rate, recurrence rate and mortality (76). Since the early stages of ultrasound (77, 78) and CT (79) guided puncture, numerous authoritative articles (80, 81) and chapters (82–84) have chronicled the successes and failures. Previous barriers to percutaneous puncture, i.e., multiseptation, are being eroded (85). Additional targets of puncture, i.e., percutaneous gastrostomy, are being attempted with definite benefits for the patient (86). Most recently, robotic intervention has even been suggested (87). The ultimate role of percutaneous puncture may actually be greater than what is suspected today.

REFERENCES

1. Burriss EE, Casson L: *Latin and Greek in Current Use.* Englewood Cliffs, N.J., Prentice-Hall, 1949, pp 102–103.
2. *Dorland's Illustrated Medical Dictionary.* Philadelphia, W. B. Saunders, 1974, p 5.
3. *Webster's Third New International Dictionary of the English Language Unabridged.* Springfield, Mass., G. C. Merriam, 1971, p 6.
4. Robbins SL; *Pathologic Basis of Disease.* Philadelphia, W. B. Saunders, 1974, p 86.
5. Ariel IM, Kazasian KK: *Diagnosis and Treatment of Abdominal Abscesses.* Baltimore, Williams & Wilkins, 1971, pp 1–20.
6. Sanders RC: The changing epidemiology of subphrenic abscess and its clinical and radiological consequences. *Br J Surg* 57:449–455, 1970.
7. Ochsner A, DeBakey M: Subphrenic abscess. *Int Abst Surg* 66:426–438, 1938.
8. Ochsner A, DeBakey M, Murray S: Pyogenic abscess of the liver. *Am J Surg* 40:292–319, 1938.
9. McFadzean AJS, Chang KPS, Wong CC: Solitary pyogenic abscess of the liver treated by closed aspiration and antibiotics. *Br J Surg* 41:141–152, 1953.
10. Mueller PR, Simeone JF: Intraabdominal abscesses: diagnosis by sonography and computed tomography. *Radiol Clin North Am* 21:425–443, 1983.
11. Doust BD, Quiroz F, Stewart JM: Ultrasonic distinction of abscesses from other intra-abdominal fluid collections. *Radiology* 125:213–218, 1977.
12. Kressel HY, Filly RA: Ultrasonographic appearance of gas-containing abscesses in the abdomen. *AJR* 130:71–73, 1978.
13. Gerzof SG, Spira R, Robbins AH: Percutaneous abscess drainage. *Semin Roentgenol* 16:62–71, 1981.
14. Gerzof SG, Robbins AH, Birkett DH: Computed tomography in the diagnosis and management of abdominal abscesses. *Gastrointest Radiol* 3:287–294, 1978.
15. Hoffer P: Gallium and infection. *J Nucl Med* 21:484–488, 1980.
16. Knochel JQ, Koehler PR, Lee TG, Welch DM: Diagnosis of abdominal abscesses with computed tomography, ultrasound, and ^{111}In leukocyte scans. *Radiology* 137:425–432, 1980.
17. Dutcher JP, Schiffer CA, Johnston GS: Rapid migration of indium-111-labeled granulocytes to sites of infection. *N Engl J Med* 304:586–589, 1981.
18. vanSonnenberg E, Wing VW, Casola G, Coons HG, Nakamoto SK, Mueller PR, Ferrucci JT, Halasz NA, Simeone JF: Temporizing effect of percutaneous drainage of complicated abscesses in critically ill patients. *AJR* 142:821–826, 1984.
19. Seldinger SI: Catheter replacement of the needle in percutaneous arteriography. *Acta Radiol* 39:368–376, 1953.
20. Gronvall J, Gronvall S, Hegedus V: Ultrasound-guided drainage of fluid-containing masses using angiographic catheterizatoin techniques. *AJR* 129:997–1002, 1977.
21. Shoenfeld RB, Lecky D, Ring EJ, McLean GK, Freiman DB: Stabilization of percutaneous catheters. *AJR* 138:972, 1982.
22. Mitchell SE, Clark RA: Finger-trap method of suturing biliary drainage catheters to the skin. *AJR* 137:628, 1981.
23. Altemeier WA, Culbertson WR, Fullen WD, Shook CD: Intra-abdominal abscesses. *Am J Surg* 125:70–79, 1973.
24. Kleinhaus U, Rosenberger A: Computed tomography-guided percutaneous drainage of right upper abdominal abscesses. *Cardiovasc Intervent Radiol* 5:8–13, 1982.
25. Gerzof SG, Robbins AH, Birkett DH, Johnson WC, Pugatch RD, Vincent ME: Percutaneous catheter drainage of abdominal abscesses guided by ultrasound and computed tomography. *AJR* 133:1–8, 1979.
26. Gerzof SG, Robbins AH, Johnson WC, Birkett DH, Nasbeth DC: Percutaneous catheter drainage of abdominal abscesses. A five-year experience. *N Engl J Med* 305:653–657, 1981.
27. Clark RA, Towbin R: Abscess drainage with CT and ultrasound guidance. *Radiol Clin North Am* 21:445–459, 1983.
28. Johnson WC, Gerzof SG, Robbins AH, Nasbeth DC: Treatment of abdominal abscesses. Comparative evaluation of operative drainage versus percutaneous catheter drainage guided by computed tomography or ultrasound. *Ann Surg* 194:510–520, 1981.
29. Wang SMS, Wilson SE: Subphrenic abscess. *Arch Surg* 112:934–936, 1977.
30. vanSonnenberg E, Wittenberg J, Ferrucci JT, Mueller PR, Simeone JF: Triangulation method for percutaneous needle guidance: The angled approach to upper abdominal masses. *AJR* 137:757–761, 1981.
31. Gerzof SG: Triangulation: indirect CT guidance for abscess drainage. *AJR* 137:1080–1081, 1981.
32. Sanfelippo PM, Beahrs OH, Weiland LH: Cystic disease of the liver. *Ann Surg* 179:922–925, 1974.
33. Spiegel RM, King DL, Green WM: Ultrasonography of primary cysts of the liver. *AJR* 131:235–238, 1978.

34. Roemer CE, Ferrucci JT, Mueller PR, Simeone JF, vanSonnenberg E, Wittenberg J: Hepatic cysts: diagnosis and therapy by sonographic needle aspiration. *AJR* 136:1065–1070, 1981.
35. Itzchak Y, Rubinstein Z, Heyman Z, Gerzof SG: Role of ultrasound in the diagnosis of abdominal hydatid disease. *J Clin Ultrasound* 8:341–345, 1980.
36. Saini S, Mueller PR, Ferrucci JT, Simeone JF, Wittenberg J, Butch RJ: Percutaneous aspiration of hepatic cysts does not provide definitive therapy. *AJR* 141:559–560, 1983.
37. Goldstein HM, Carlyle DR, Nelson RS: Treatment of symptomatic hepatic cyst by percutaneous instillation of Pantopaque. *AJR* 127:850–853, 1976.
38. Landay MJ, Setiawan H, Hirsch G, Christensen EE, Conrad MR: Hepatic and thoracic amebiasis. *AJR* 135:449–454, 1980.
39. Weissmann HS, Chun KJ, Frank M, Koenigsberg M, Milstein DM, Freeman LM: Demonstration of traumatic bile leakage with cholescintigraphy and ultrasonography. *AJR* 133:843–847, 1979.
40. Mueller PR, Ferrucci JT, Simeone JF, Cronan JJ, Wittenberg J, Neff CC, vanSonnenberg E: Detection and drainage of bilomas: special considerations. *AJR* 140:715–720, 1983.
41. Karlson KB, Martin EC, Fankuchen EI, Mattern RF, Schultz RW, Casarella WJ: Percutaneous drainage of pancreatic pseudocysts and abscesses. *Radiology* 142:614–624, 1982.
42. Bhatt GM, Jason RS, Delany HM, Rudavsky AZ: Hepatic hematoma: percutaneous drainage. *AJR* 135:1287–1288, 1980.
43. vanSonnenberg E, Ferrucci JT, Mueller PR, Wittenberg J, Simeone JF: Percutaneous drainage of abscesses and fluid collections: technique, results, and applications. *Radiology* 142:1–10, 1982.
44. Saini S, Kellman JM, O'Leary MP, O'Donnell TF, Tally FP, Carter B, Deterling RA, Curtis LE: Improved localization and survival in patients with intraabdominal abscesses. *Am J Surg* 145:136–142, 1983.
45. Haaga JR: CT-guided procedures. In Haaga JR, Alfidi RJ (eds): *Computed Tomography of the Whole Body.* St. Louis, C. V. Mosby, 1983, pp 867–933.
46. Harbin WP, Mueller PR, Ferrucci JT: Transhepatic cholangiography: complications and use patterns of the fine-needle technique. A multi-institutional survey. *Radiology* 135:15–22, 1980.
47. Greenfield AJ: Percutaneus biliary drainage. In Athanasoulis CA, Pfister RC, Greene RE, Roberson GH (eds): *Interventional Radiology.* Philadelphia, W. B. Saunders, 1982, pp 535–556.
48. Hogan MT, Watne A, Mossburg W, Castaneda W: Direct injection into the gallbladder in dogs, using ultrasonic guidance. *Arch Surg* 111:564–565, 1976.
49. Klapdor R, Scherer K, Sepehr H, Kloppel G: The ultrasonically guided puncture of the gallbladder in animals. *Endoscopy* 9:166–169, 1977.
50. Skillings JC, Kumal C, Hinshaw JR: Cholecystostomy: a place in modern biliary surgery? *Am J Surg* 139:865–869, 1980.
51. Shaver RW, Hawkins IF, Soong J: Percutaneous cholecystostomy. *AJR* 138:1133–1136, 1982.
52. vanSonnenberg E, Wing VW, Polland JW, Casola G: Life-threatening vagal reactions associated with percutaneous cholecystostomy. *Radiology* 151:377–380, 1984.
53. Phillips G, Bank S, Kumari-Subaiya S, Kutz LM: Percutaneous ultrasound-guided puncture of the gallbladder (PURG). *Radiology* 145:769–772, 1982.
54. Bean WJ, Calonje MA, Aprill CN, Gashner BS: Percutaneous catheterization of the gallbladder with ultrasound guidance. *South Med J* 72:612–614, 1979.
55. Hillman BJ, Smith EH, Holm HH: Ultrasound diagnosis and treatment of gallbladder fossa collections following biliary tract surgery. *Br J Radiol* 52:390–392, 1979.
56. Blickman JG, Overbosch EH, Falke THM: Computed tomographic demonstration of a biloma. *Eur J Radiol* 4:98–100, 1984.
57. Mueller PR, Ferrucci JT, Simeone JF, Cronan JJ, Wittenberg J, Neff CC, vanSonnenberg E: Detection and drainage of bilomas: specific consideration. *AJR* 140:715–720, 1983.
58. Miller MH, Frederick PR, Tocine I, Bahr AL: Percutaneous catheter drainage of intraabdominal fluid collections including infected biliary ducts and gallbladders. *Am J Surg* 144:660–667, 1982.
59. Lawson TL: Acute pancreatitis and its complications: computed tomography and sonography. *Radiol Clin North Am* 21:495–513, 1983.
60. Siegelman SS: *Computed Tomography of the Pancreas.* New York, Churchill Livingstone, 1983, pp 83–111.
61. Warshaw AL: Inflammatory masses following acute pancreatitis: phlegmon, pseudocyst, and abscess. *Surg Clin North Am* 54:621–636, 1974.
62. Siegelman SS, Copeland BE, Saba GP, Cameron JL, Sanders RC, Zerhouni EA: CT of fluid collections associated with pancreatitis. *AJR* 134:1121–1132, 1980.
63. Gobien RP, Stanley JH, Anderson MC, Vujic I: Percutaneous drainage of pancreatic duct for treating acute pancreatitis. *AJR* 141:795–796, 1983.
64. Hill MC, Dach JL, Barkin J, Isikoff MB, Morse B: The role of percutaneous aspiration in the diagnosis of pancreatic abscess. *AJR* 141:1035–1038, 1983.
65. Mauro MA, Jaques PF: Modified trocar-cannula system for percutaneous pancreatic abscess drainage. *Radiology* 139:227–228, 1981.
66. Dubbins PA: Ultrasound in the diagnosis of splenic abscess. *Br J Radiol* 53:488–489, 1980.
67. Mittelstaedt CA: Ultrasound of the spleen. *Semin Ultrasound* 2:233–239, 1981.
68. Pawar S, Kay CJ, Gonzalez R, Taylor KJW, Rosenfield AT: Sonography of splenic abscess. *AJR* 138:259–262, 1982.
69. Rudick MG, Wood BP, Lerner RM: Splenic abscess diagnosed by ultrasound in the pediatric patient. *Pediatr Radiol* 13:269–271, 1983.
70. Cunningham JJ: Ultrasonic findings in isolated lymphoma of the spleen simulating splenic abscess. *J Clin Ultrasound* 6:412–414, 1978.
71. Solbiati L, Bossi MC, Bellotti E, Ravetto C, Montali G: Focal lesions in the spleen: sonographic patterns and guided biopsy. *AJR* 140:59–65, 1983.
72. Dubuisson RL, Jones TB: Splenic abscess due to blastomycosis: scintigraphic, sonographic, and CT evaluation. *AJR* 140:66–68, 1983.
73. Berkman WA, Harris SA, Bernardino ME: Nonsurgical drainage of splenic abscess. *AJR* 141:395–396, 1983.
74. Welch CE: Catheter drainage of abdominal abscesses. *N Eng J Med* 305:694–695, 1981.
75. Aeder MI, Wellman JL, Haaga JR, Hau T: Role of surgical and percutaneous drainage in the treatment of abdominal abscesses. *Arch Surg* 118:273–280, 1983.
76. Gerzof SG: Percutaneous drainage of abdominal abscesses. *Appl Radiol* 12:77–89, 1983.
77. Smith EH, Bartrum RJ: Ultrasonically guided percutaneous aspiration of abscesses. *AJR* 122:308–312, 1974.
78. Conrad MR, Sanders RC, Mascardo AD: Perinephric abscess aspiration using ultrasound guidance. *AJR* 128:459–464, 1977.

79. Haaga JR, Weinstein AJ: CT-guided percutaneous aspiration and drainage of abscesses. *AJR* 135:1187–1194, 1980.
80. vanSonnenberg E, Mueller PR, Ferrucci JT: Percutaneous drainage of 250 abdominal abscesses and fluid collections; I. Results, failures, and complications. *Radiology* 151:337–341, 1984.
81. vanSonnenberg E, Mueller PR, Ferrucci JT: Percutaneous drainage of 250 abdominal abscesses and fluid collections; II. Current procedural concepts. *Radiology* 151:343–347, 1984.
82. Haaga JR, Alfid RJ: Peritoneal abscesses and other disorders. In Haaga JR, Alfidi RJ (eds): *Computed Tomography of the Whole Body*. St. Louis, C. V. Mosby, 1983, pp 835–866.
83. Gerzof SG: Guided percutaneus catheter drainage of abdominal abscesses. In Athanasoulis CA, Pfister RC, Greene RE, Roberson GH (eds): *Interventional Radiology* Philadelphia, W. B. Saunders, 1982, pp 557–567.
84. Pfister RC, Newhouse JH: Percutaneus catheter drainage of abscesses, urinoma, and other fluid collections. In Athanasoulis CA, Pfister RC, Greene RE, Roberson GH (eds): *Interventional Radiology*. Philadelphia, W. B. Saunders, 1982, pp 497–508.
85. Bernardino ME, Berkman WA, Plemmons M, Sones PJ, Price RB, Casarella WJ: Percutaneous drainage of multiseptated hepatic abscess. *J Comput Asst Tomogr* 8:38–41, 1984.
86. Wills JS, Oglesby JT: Percutaneous gastrostomy. *Radiology* 149:449–453, 1983.
87. Hawkins IF: Robotic intervention: why not? *AJR* 142:1292–1293, 1984.

33

Guided Percutaneous Biopsy in the Upper Abdomen

JOHN C. SCATARIGE, M.D.

Despite an extensive and favorable Scandinavian experience with percutaneous aspiration biopsy of the abdomen (1–4), the American medical community was slower to adopt the technique, probably because of unfamiliarity with cytological interpretation and a concern that such biopsy procedures would disseminate otherwise resectable tumors (5). However, within the past decade, enthusiasm for percutaneous guided aspiration biopsy in North America has expanded and barely kept pace with a burgeoning literature on the subject. The development of the cross-sectional imaging modalities of gray-scale ultrasound and computed tomography, the increasing availability of pathologists familiar with cytological diagnosis in aspiration biopsy, and cost-consciousness in the delivery of diagnostic health care services have all served to fuel this process (5).

While generally reviewing the topic of guided percutaneous biopsy of the hepatobiliary tract, pancreas, and spleen, particular attention will be paid to the relevant recent literature.

CYTOPATHOLOGY

Percutaneous guided aspiration biopsy is primarily a cytological technique, and as such requires, for its success, the availability of personnel trained in the processing of cytological biopsy material and the interest of pathologists familiar with the interpretation of aspiration specimens. Bernardino has stressed the central role of the cytopathologist and the need for cooperation and communication between radiologist and cytopathologist to ensure the success of a biopsy program (6).

At the Johns Hopkins Hospital, the Radiology Department is fortunate to enjoy a good working relationship with superb pathologists who are highly motivated and actively participate in the guided biopsy process. Acknowledging that there are a number of different technical approaches to the handling of biopsy material, the procedure followed at this institution will be briefly reviewed.

Technique

Guided percutaneous biopsies are scheduled in advance with Cytopathology and are generally performed in the early afternoon, to permit attendance of a cytopathologist. The Cytopathology personnel are alerted when the initial target localization begins, and arrive within 5–10 min, bringing a cart which contains a rapid fixation and staining system (DIFF-QUIK—American Scientific Products, McGaw Park, Ill 60885), slides and a light microscope. The apparatus is set up within a few moments, usually in an adjacent room or hallway.

After the first biopsy pass, a small specimen drop from the needle tip is placed at the end of each of 2 slides and evenly spread by the cytotechnologist; while one slide air dries, the other is immediately fixed and stained using the DIFF-QUIK system (Fig. 33.1). In less than 1 min the cytopathologist can assess the adequacy of the submitted material and render a preliminary impression (e.g., positive for tumor cells, normal liver or pancreas, necrotic material, etc.). Meanwhile, the biopsy needle and syringe are disconnected, Hanks' balanced salt solution is drawn directly into the syringe then emptied into a sterile vial, and additional Hanks' solution is flushed through the needle into the vial.

If the first specimen is cellular and diagnostic, the procedure is ended and the patient spared additional passes. If the submitted material is nondiagnostic, additional passes are made into

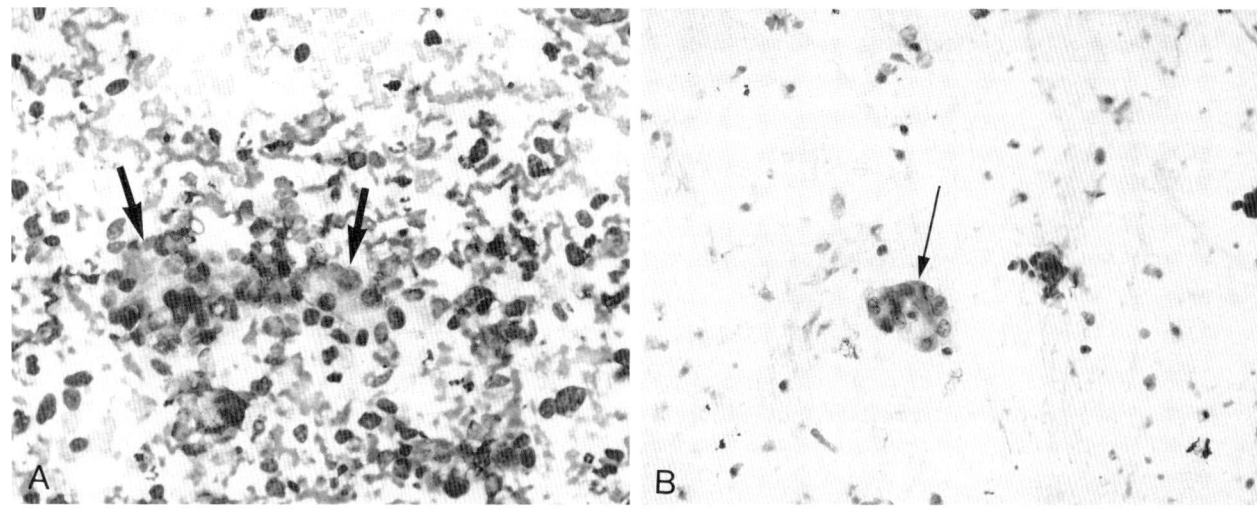

FIGURE 33.1. ASPIRATION STAINING
Comparison of rapid and standard (Papanicolau) staining for aspiration specimens. A 22-gauge needle biopsy of a focal liver mass in an elderly man with weight loss and a small bowel mass. A: Rapid staining system: direct smear of a drop of aspirate. Note the large number of darkly staining nuclei superimposed on a background of red blood cells. There are clumps of abnormal cells (arrows), but the cytoplasmic and nuclear details are indistinct. Preliminary cytopathological diagnosis: definitely malignant, probably adenocarcinoma. B: Routine Papanicolau preparation from a Millipore-filtered specimen, same patient. Note the improved definition of nuclear and cytoplasmic features, and the acinar (glandular) arrangement of cells (arrow). Adenocarcinoma (original magnification, × 75).

other portions of the target mass. The immediate feed back from the cytopathologist is crucial and decreases the number of repeat procedures, particularly important for our outpatients who travel a distance.

Once the procedure is terminated, the material in Hanks' solution and air-dried slides are transported to the Cytopathology Department for routine processing and Papanicolaou staining. Large fragments and cores of tissue are separated and submitted for histology. Depending on the clinical history and biopsy site, the cytopathologist may elect to submit a portion of the specimen for special staining or electron microscopy (EM). The final cytopathology report is available the following morning.

IMAGING MODALITIES AVAILABLE FOR BIOPSY GUIDANCE

Although the early experience with percutaneous fine needle aspiration biopsy of the abdomen was gained by "blind" approach to a mass or organ based on palpation or percussion (1, 2), recent attention has focussed on the application of imaging modalities for direction of the biopsy needle toward a specific target. Although radionuclide liver-spleen scanning, visceral angiography and endoscopic retrograde cholangiopancreatography (ERCP) have been utilized in this way, fluoroscopy, static and real-time gray-scale ultrasound, and computed tomography have emerged as the most important guidance systems. Table 33.1 summarizes the advantages and disadvantages of each.

Fluoroscopy

Available in most radiological facilities, fluoroscopic equipment can guide percutaneous upper abdominal biopsy. Ho et al. (7) described a technique for fluoroscopically guided aspiration liver biopsy which utilized frontal and right lateral radionuclide liver-spleen images for directing needle placements. These investigators reported a 93% true-positive rate for malignant lesions. Using fluoroscopic landmarks and abnormalities noted on ERCP or visceral angiography (8), percutaneous aspiration biopsy of the pancreas has been successfully performed. Others have performed fluoroscopically guided pancreatic head biopsies following peroral administration of carbon dioxide-producing pills to delineate the stomach and duodenum (9). Percutaneous biopsy of abdominal masses displacing contrast-filled stomach or colon has also been described (10, 11).

The use of fluoroscopy for percutaneous upper abdominal biopsy has two distinct disadvantages. First, the target lesion, particularly if

TABLE 33.1.
COMPARISON OF IMAGING MODALITIES FOR PERCUTANEOUS BIOPSY GUIDANCE IN THE UPPER ABDOMEN

Fluoroscopy	Ultrasound		Computed Tomography	
	Static B-Mode	Real-time	Older scanners	Newer units
ADVANTAGES				
Equipment available	Equipment inexpensive	Same as static scanner	Bone, gas, and obesity do not hinder imaging	As for older scanners
Procedure fast	Target position and depth easily determined	Infinite variety of scan planes		Procedures much faster
		Needle placement in target can be confirmed	Needle placement in target unequivocally demonstrated	Anteroposterior, lateral topographic capability
	No radiation	Requires less technical skill than static scanning		
DISADVANTAGES				
Unless opacified, target usually not visible	Cannot confirm needle in target	Limited by bone, gas and obesity	Equipment expensive and may not be available	Equipment very expensive and may not be available
Target depth not known	Considerable technical skill required	Larger transducers may be cumbersome in intercostal biopsy	Procedures very time-consuming	Radiation exposure, but less than older scanners
Ionizing radiation to patient, operator	Obesity, gas, bone may limit target access		Patient exposed to ionizing radiation	

small, is often not visible and its location and depth from the skin surface are not precisely known. Therefore, the operator cannot usually confirm that the biopsy needle has sampled the target volume. Second, fluoroscopy exposes the patient and operator to ionizing radiation.

At this institution, fluoroscopically guided biopsy is reserved for the small, strategically located hepatobiliary or pancreatic mass which narrows or obstructs the biliary tree and is easily identified at cholangiography.

Ultrasound

An extensive literature (3, 4, 8, 10, 12–34) attests to the dominant role diagnostic ultrasound has played in the evolution of guided percutaneous biopsy in the upper abdomen. This role has resulted from the success of ultrasound in visualizing neoplastic masses in the liver, pancreas and spleen, the great flexibility of scan planes offered, and the widespread availability of reliable, relatively inexpensive equipment.

Static B-Mode Guidance

The standard method of sonographically guided biopsy consists of the following steps: (*a*) localization of the suspect mass in sagittal and transverse scan planes, (*b*) choice of a reference point on the patient's skin close to and ideally perpendicular to the target, (*c*) determination of the target's depth from skin surface, and (*d*) following skin preparation, the introduction of a biopsy needle to the desired depth, angled precisely as was the B-mode transducer for the localizing scans. Sterilizable slotted B-mode biopsy transducers may also be used. This technique is simple, fast, and very satisfactory for large or relatively superficial lesions. However, confirmation of needle position is difficult, a particularly troublesome feature when the biopsy target is less than 3 cm in diameter, deep, or requires needle angulation to reach. In this situation, the end point of a successful biopsy may be tactile (gritty sensation or resistance transmitted through the needle) or, simply, a positive cytological result. One author has suggested the introduction of a very small volume of air (0.3–0.5 ml) through the introduced needle prior to aspiration to provide an echogenic marker on subsequent scans (20).

Real-Time Biopsy Guidance

Following the pioneering work of Holm et al. (4) in the 1970s, the recent resurgence of interest in real-time sonographic guidance of percutaneous biopsy largely reflects the development of and improvements in commercially available real-time instruments (25–34). Real-time sonographic biopsy assistance may be rendered in several ways: first, the use of a dedicated biopsy transducer, usually a focused linear array transducer with a built-in biopsy slot or guide (25, 26, 28); second, by attachment of a specially made biopsy guide to an existing, commercially available transducer, usually a sector scanner (27, 31, 32, 34); or finally, simply by monitoring the needle passage toward a target with a nearby sterilized or draped real-time instrument (29, 30, 33). Regardless of which technique is used, real-time biopsy assistance permits visualization of the target while the biopsy needle approaches and enters it, overcoming the major disadvantage of static sonographic biopsy guidance.

Several manufacturers are currently producing dedicated real-time biopsy transducers. The larger focused linear array units, while producing superb images, may be a bit cumbersome when attempting an intercostal or subcostal approach for liver biopsy. Most investigators with real-time experience report success in visualizing the needle tip within the biopsy target (32, 33); some have noted that even when the needle lies outside of the scan plane, slight oscillation of the needle will produce a characteristic visible tissue deformity indicating needle proximity to the target. A few of the biopsy transducer designs offer a variable puncture angle, allowing adjustment for different target depths (27, 31).

Computed Tomography

The enthusiasm for CT-guided biopsy procedures has been reflected in the literature over the past 8 years (35–44). Computed tomography (CT) provides superb spatial and contrast resolution in the transverse plane, permitting visualization of the upper abdominal organs independent of overlying ribs, bowel gas or obesity. Furthermore, CT provides precise delineation of small biopsy targets and confirmation of needle placement within them, preventing sampling errors. CT also provides the opportunity to evaluate the vascularity of a target mass prior to biopsy, permitting a rational choice of needle size (38). Although CT-guided biopsy is usually performed in the transaxial plane with needle perpendicular to skin surface, one group has developed a technique for CT localization and biopsy of subdiaphragmatic masses which require cephalad needle angulation (40).

Despite the many advantages, CT as a biopsy guidance system is not without fault (Table 33.1). CT units are expensive and may not be available in all hospitals or outpatient imaging facilities. The scheduling demands on existing CT facilities are often great, and the time-consuming biopsy procedures are discouraged. Finally, CT-guided biopsy exposes the patient to additional ionizing radiation.

As new CT units with faster scan and reconstruction times, lower radiation dose and topographic localization capability in the frontal and lateral views (44) supplement or replace the existing units, some of the above disadvantages of CT-guided biopsy will no longer apply.

Which Modality Shall I Use?

The eventual choice of guidance modality depends upon (a) the characteristics (size, location, depth, nearby vital structures) of the target; (b) availability of sonographic and CT equipment; (c) the experience and confidence of the operator; and (d) established referral patterns.

In this institution, because of the availability of superb sonographers and sonographic equipment, over 90% of the percutaneous upper abdominal biopsies are attempted under B-mode static or real-time sonographic guidance. CT guidance is reserved for small, deep or strategically located lesions, masses poorly seen on ultrasound, or second attempts after initial unsuccessful sonographic-guided biopsy.

NEEDLE SELECTION

Although the technique of guided percutaneous mass biopsy in the upper abdomen has been described by many authors, the selection of an appropriate needle for a given patient and biopsy target has received relatively little attention. This selection process has become more complicated by an increasing array of commercially available needles and a paucity of comparative studies on biopsy needle success and yields. In this section, basic needle characteristics and recent comparative studies on needle yields will be briefly reviewed.

Diameter

The diameter or gauge of the biopsy needle is the parameter most familiar to radiologists performing percutaneous biopsy. While needles from 14- to 23-gauge are available, the vast majority of biopsies are performed with needles in the 18–22-gauge range. The outer diameter of a needle determines the size of the tract created in tissue, the inner diameter defines the amount of tissue potentially retrievable, and the needle wall thickness contributes to the flexibility of the system. Zornoza has noted that differences in wall thickness exist, even among available needles of the same gauge (e.g., 22-gauge) (45). These differences will alter the needle flexibility and amount of material aspirated.

Table 33.2 presents a simplified but useful comparison of an idealized 22-gauge aspiration and 18-gauge core biopsy needle. While the 22-gauge needle provides safe access to virtually any organ, excessive needle flexibility and scanty aspirated material may limit its usefuless in some cases. On the other hand, the more controllable 18-gauge needle provides a much larger specimen for histology, but may be limited by hypervascularity of the mass or intervening major vascular structures or bowel. As with other situations, advantages and "trade-offs" are inherent in either choice.

Needle Tip Configuration

Bevel

Bevels ranging from acute angles of 25° on the Chiba needle to 90° are commercially available on biopsy needles in the 16–22-gauge size range (46) (Fig. 33.2). Needles with a more acute bevel angle permit easier skin entry and loosen tissue fragments near the needle tip when rotated (45).

Cutting Tips

Several specially machined cutting tips have been designed for percutaneous biopsy (Fig. 33.3). In addition to cytological material, the manufacturers claim that these needles will provide larger tissue fragments and cores for histological preparation. Included in this group are the Greene needle with a 90° sharpened concentric cutting bevel (47) (Cook, Inc., Bloomington, Ind. 47401), tumor mass biopsy (Turner) needle with a 45° sharpened cutting bevel (48, 49)

TABLE 33.2.
IDEALIZED COMPARISON OF 22-GAUGE ASPIRATION AND 18-GAUGE CORE BIOPSY NEEDLE

Factors	22-Gauge	18-Gauge
Specimen	Cytological, with small fragments or cores for histology	Large core for histology
Access limitations	None. May traverse vessels and bowel	Limited access
Number of needle passes	Multiple	Usually one
Needle control	Needle flexible, may be difficult to control for deeper biopsy	Rigid, easy to control
Hypervascular masses	May biopsy	Avoid
Benign disease	Specific diagnosis often not made	Frequently permits definitive diagnosis

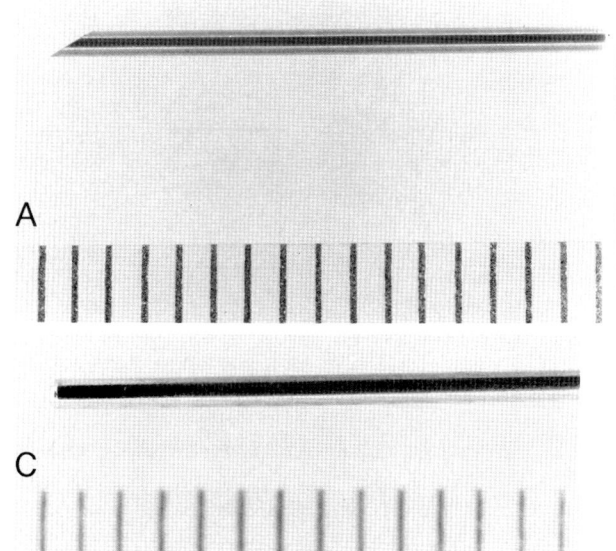

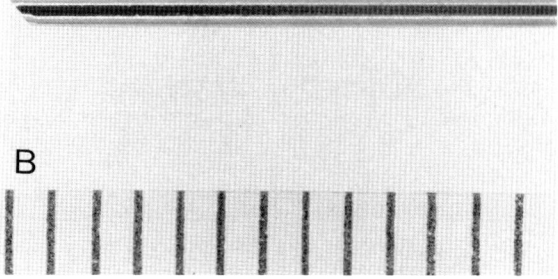

FIGURE 33.2. ANGLES OF BIOPSY NEEDLES
Bevel angles available on commercial biopsy needles. Close up photographs of the tips of (A) Chiba needle, 22-gauge, 25° noncutting bevel; (B) tumor mass (Turner) biopsy needle, 22-gauge, 45° sharpened bevel; and (C) Greene needle, 22-gauge, 90° concentrically sharpened cutting bevel. (Scale divisions = 1 mm.)

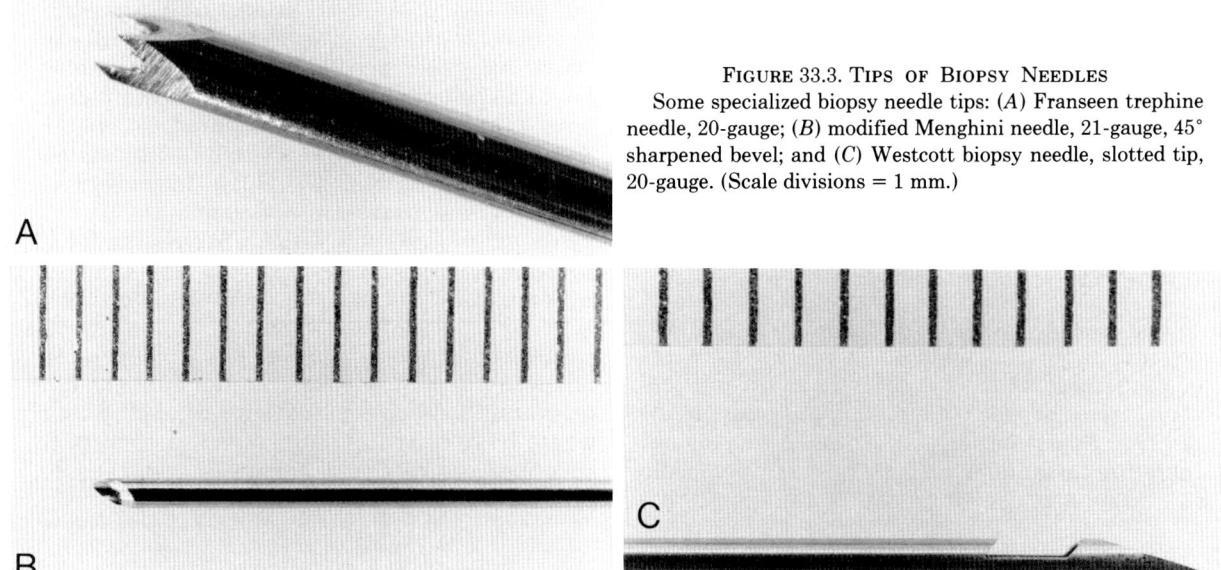

FIGURE 33.3. TIPS OF BIOPSY NEEDLES
Some specialized biopsy needle tips: (A) Franseen trephine needle, 20-gauge; (B) modified Menghini needle, 21-gauge, 45° sharpened bevel; and (C) Westcott biopsy needle, slotted tip, 20-gauge. (Scale divisions = 1 mm.)

(Cook, Inc.), the trephine type Franseen needle (50), available in several diameters, (Cook, Inc), slotted-tip cutting needles (Wescott (51), (Becton Dickinson Co., Rutherford, N.J. 07070) and Tru-cut (Travenol Laboratories, Deerfield, Ill. 60015), and the Modified Menghini needle (Surgimed, Inc., Summerville, S.C. 29483).

Length

Most biopsy needles are manufactured in two lengths, a shorter needle usually 9 cm for more superficial masses, and a longer version, usually 12–15 cm for deeper targets.

Cost

In general, needles of simplest design (Chiba, spinal needles) are the least expensive. Needles possessing sharpened cutting bevels or specialized trephine or slotted cutting tips are more expensive.

Clinical Studies on Needle Design

Some recent studies have examined the relationship of percutaneous biopsy success to the size and tip configuration of the biopsy instrument. In 1982, Lieberman et al. (49) reported favorable results in the diagnosis of malignant lesions using a 20-gauge Turner needle, which has a sharpened 45° bevel. These authors found that the needle consistently yielded long tissue cores for histology as well as cytological material, and suggested that needle design was an important determinant of biopsy success. Comparing a 22-gauge core biopsy needle with an 18-gauge Menghini and 14-gauge Travenol Tru-cut needle in 51 patients, Haaga et al. (52) noted superior results in diagnosing both malignant and benign masses, and more specific tumor cell-type information with the larger cutting needles. Finally Pagani (42) compared 18- and 22-gauge noncutting spinal needles in the CT-guided biopsy of focal hepatic lesions in 100 patients. His results, similar to those of Haaga et al., indicated superiority of the larger needle, with an overall accuracy of 98% for the 18-gauge and 84% for the 22-gauge needle.

In Vitro Comparative Studies of Needle Design

In a study using fresh and preserved cadaver kidneys, Lieberman et al. (49) obtained excellent tissue cores with 20- and 22-gauge Turner needle (45° cutting bevel), but were unable to consistently obtain cores with a 22-gauge Greene (90° cutting bevel). In contrast, Wittenberg et al. (53) found no difference in specimen size retrieved from normal cadaver liver by four different 22-gauge needles (30° noncutting bevel, Greene 90° cutting bevel, Rotex screw tip, and Menghini).

In the most comprehensive in vitro study to date, Andriole et al. (46) assessed the quantity of material, quality for cytological preparation and quality for histological preparation of specimens retrieved from normal postmortem liver by 30 different biopsy needles, utilizing a standard biopsy technique. The study revealed the following: (a) the quantity and quality of biopsy material improved as needle diameter increased; (b) the needle's bevel angle was an important factor, the more acute angles producing larger and better quality specimens; and (c) needles with the slotted-type or trephine cutting tips yielded consistently excellent specimens.

Summary

The needle chosen for any guided biopsy will depend upon the individual circumstances including lesion location and depth, nearby critical structures, the suspected diagnosis, and the interpreting cytopathologist; the radiologist should therefore be familiar with more than one needle (6). Since a major attraction of fine-needle aspiration biopsy is its record of safety, the ideal biopsy needle in any clinical situation should be the safest (smallest) that will provide the necessary (not always maximum) information needed to answer the clinical questions posed. The data of Andriole et al. (46) suggest that significant differences exist among commercially available biopsy needles of the same gauge. Exploitation of these differences by utilizing small (20–22-gauge) needles with acute bevel angles or specialized cutting tips may improve biopsy yield while minimizing patient risk.

In certain cases where fine-needle biopsy has failed to provided adequate material or has not permitted definitive cell-type determination, or where lymphoma (6, 54) or a benign process is suspected, a larger cutting biopsy needle should provide a diagnostic specimen.

INDICATIONS

In this section, the indications, technical considerations and results for percutaneous biopsy of the hepatobiliary region, pancreas, and spleen will be reviewed.

Hepatobiliary

The most frequent indications for percutaneous guided biopsy of the liver and biliary tract in this institution include: (a) confirmation of suspected liver metastasis in a patient with a known primary malignancy; (b) confirmation of suspected hepatocellular carcinoma demonstrated on cross-sectional imaging or suspected bile duct malignancy (either primary or due to porta hepatis metastasis) with stenosis or occlusion of biliary tree demonstrated on cholangiography; (c) diagnosis of an incidental, focal, solid hepatic abnormality demonstrated on imaging for the gallbladder or right kidney; and (d) guidance for large core biopsy by a gastroenterologist in patients with suspected diffuse liver disease (e.g., cirrhosis, hepatitis) in whom anatomic landmarks for standard biopsy are lacking (e.g., small liver, obese patient).

Technical Considerations

General Guidelines. Excellent technical reviews of the performance of percutaneous guided biopsy have been presented by Doherty (5) and Zornoza (45) and will not be repeated here. Variations from the basic technique will depend upon the imaging modality used, the needle selected for biopsy (manipulation of a Chiba needle and Franseen trephine needle differ), and the experience and idiosyncrasies of the operator. At The Johns Hopkins Hospital, guided percutaneous biopsy is generally performed under ultrasound guidance. Patients are fasting or are allowed only clear liquids. Coagulation studies are routinely obtained and coagulation deficits are corrected prior to biopsy. Informed patient consent is mandatory and presents the important opportunity for physician and patient to meet, exchange information and establish rapport. Except in the cases of infants, children or disoriented adults, sedation and/or general anesthesia is unneccessary; cooperative children and adults require only local anesthesia. Outpatients undergoing aspiration biopsy are usually observed for 2–3 hr after biopsy, prior to discharge from the department.

Technique for Liver Biopsy. Focal masses which narrow or obstruct the intrahepatic or common bile ducts may undergo fluoroscopically guided biopsy in the cardiovascular laboratory at the time of transhepatic cholangiography or biliary drainage procedure. Other nonobstructing focal liver masses larger than 3 cm are ordinarily biopsied under B-mode sonographic guidance (Fig. 33.4). The shortest distance from skin surface to target mass is chosen, taking care to avoid the costophrenic angle laterally and gallbladder anteriorly. For high, subdiaphragmatic masses in the right lobe, real-time sector scan biopsy apparatus (32) or CT (40) may be useful. In the case of small, peripheral hepatic masses not visible by sonography, CT will permit successful

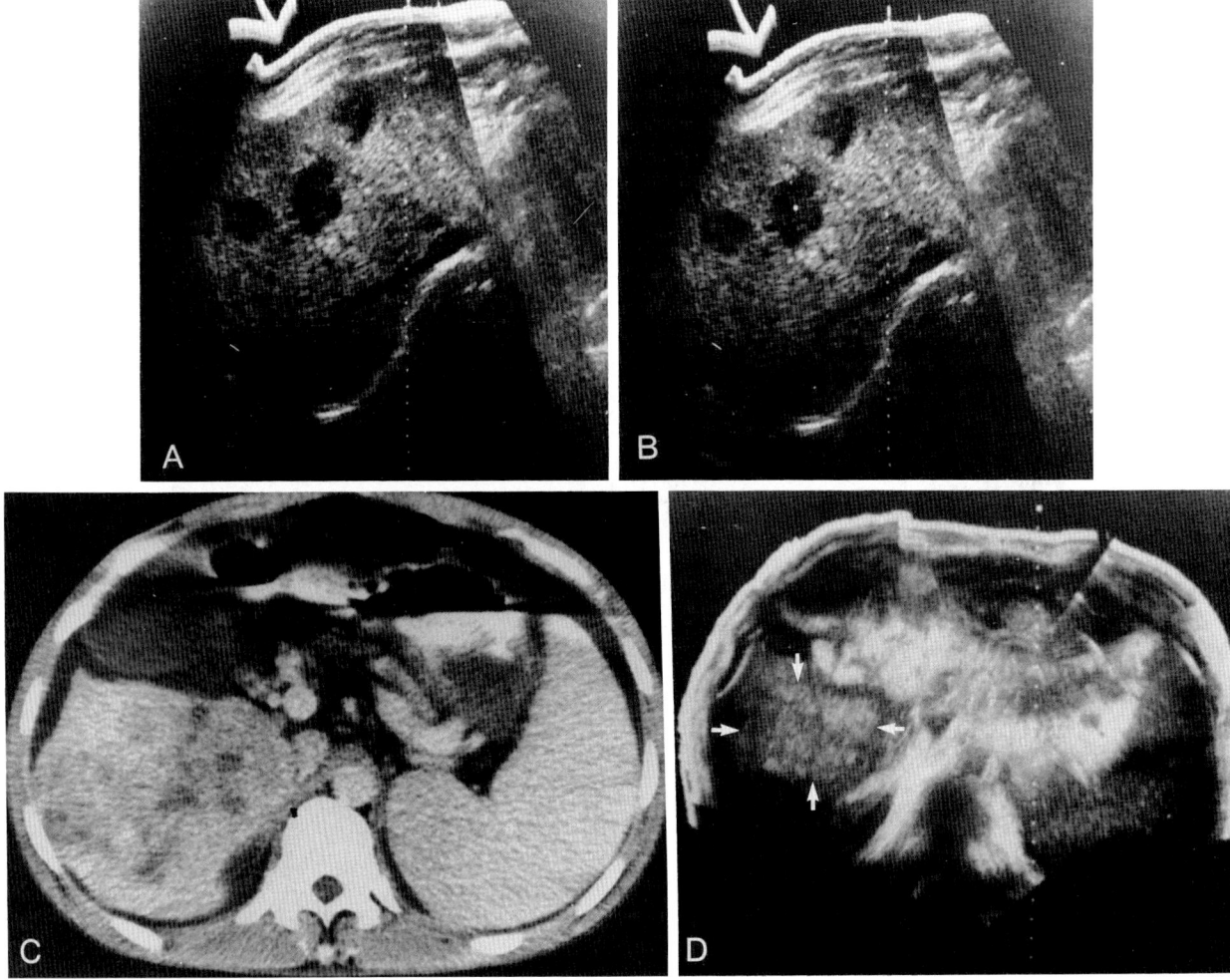

FIGURE 33.4. LIVER BIOPSY
Sonographically guided liver biopsy in malignant disease. A and B: B-mode guidance in patient with known colon cancer and abnormal liver function tests. A: Transverse scan of the liver, angled slightly cephalad, shows 3 hypoechoic masses. The 3-cm central mass was selected and skin entry point indicated by the arrow. B: Placement of scale indicates depth of 7 cm to anterior portion of mass and 8.5 cm to center. Passage of 22-gauge Turner needle in the same axis as the transducer, to the appropriate depth, yielded adenocarcinoma. C and D: B-mode biopsy in suspected hepatoma. C: Contrast enhanced CT in a young man from Southeast Asia complaining of weight loss and abdominal pain shows a poorly defined mass in the right hepatic lobe, splenomegaly and ascites. D: Transverse sonogram reveals corresponding focal increased echogenicity in the right lobe (arrows). B-mode guided aspiration biopsy of this right lobe, using a 22-gauge Turner needle, yielded abundant malignant cells, compatible with hepatocellular carcinoma.

biopsy (Fig. 33.5). A cooperative patient able to control respiration is a definite advantage for biopsying small intrahepatic masses.

The 20- or 22-gauge Turner or Franseen needles are generally selected for initial biopsy of a suspect hepatic metastasis. Care is taken to sample the solid periphery or wall of a mass exhibiting mixed solid/cystic characteristics on sonography (45). Solitary solid hepatic masses discovered in patients with no known primary tumor routinely undergo IV bolus CT examination to exclude hemangioma prior to biopsy.

Results

Very encouraging results for percutaneous liver biopsy in primary and metastatic neoplastic disease have been reported (Table 33.3). Sensitivity (true positive) rates ranging from 87 to 100% have been obtained in several large series reported over the last four years. The results in the series which utilized radionuclide-fluoroscopic, ultrasound, and CT guidance compare favorably with a 78% true positive rate reported for blind biopsy (1). Although larger biopsy

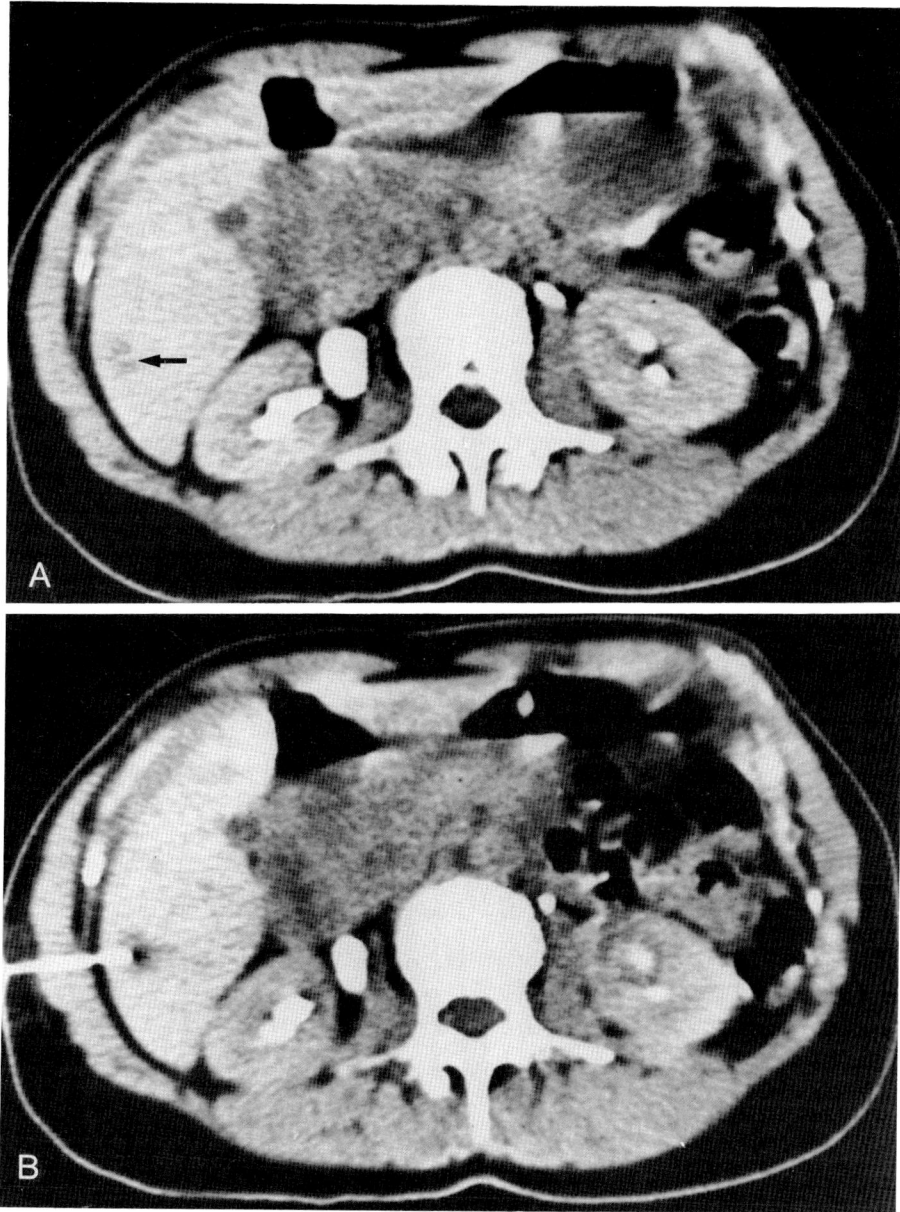

FIGURE 33.5. HEPATIC BIOPSY

CT guidance in biopsy of a peripheral hepatic lesion. *A:* CT in an elderly woman several years post-hysterectomy and bilateral salpingoophorectomy for ovarian malignancy reveals a 1.5-cm low attenuation mass in the lateral right lobe (*arrow*). This lesion could not be visualized on subsequent sonography prior to contemplated biopsy. *B:* A 22-gauge aspiration biopsy was performed easily under CT guidance. Cytology positive for adenocarcinoma.

needles will provide larger specimens (46), comparable excellent results for the diagnosis of malignancy are reported with 22-gauge aspiration (28, 32) and 18–20-gauge (43) needles. One study, in fact, suggests that detection of intrahepatic malignancy may be superior with aspiration-cytologic technique than with core biopsy-histological methods (22).

The record for specific diagnosis of focal, solid benign liver disease by fine needle aspiration is less enviable, however (Table 33.4). Ho et al. (7) established a definitive benign diagnosis with a 22-gauge spinal needle in 57% of a small series, while Rosenblatt et al. (21) could not establish a definite benign diagnosis in any of 6 patients. More recent reports by Pagani (42) and Haaga

TABLE 33.3.
SUMMARY OF PERCUTANEOUS BIOPSY IN MALIGNANT LIVER DISEASE

Series Author (Ref.)	Year	Patients with Proven Malignant Mass	Guidance Modality	Gauge Needle	Patients (%) True Positive	Percent False Negative
Lundquist (1)	1970	57	None (BlindBx)	23	39 (78)	22
Zornoza et al. (13)	1980	18	Sonographic	22 spinal	12 (67)	33
Nosher and Plafker (14)	1980	15	Sonographic	22, 23	14 (93)	7
Ho et al. (7)	1981	30	Radionuclide fluoroscopy	22 spinal	28 (93)	7
Rosenblatt et al. (21)	1982	47	Sonographic	22, 23	41 (87)	13
Montali et al. (28)	1982	92	Real-time sono. (linear array)	22 Chiba	85 (92)	8
Sundaram et al. (41)	1982	84	CT	20, 22	83 (99)	1
Alspaugh et al. (43)	1983	27	CT	18, 20	26 (96)	4
Grant et al. (32)	1983	26	Real-time sono. (sector)	22	26 (100)	0
Jacobsen et al. (22)	1983	48	Sonographic	23	48 (100)	0
				Tru-cut	41 (85)	15
Schwerk et al. (24)	1983	102	Sonographic	20, 22 spinal	94 (92)	8

TABLE 33.4.
GUIDED PERCUTANEOUS LIVER BIOPSY RESULTS FOR SOLID BENIGN ABNORMALITIES

Series Author (Ref.)	Year	Patients with Benign Diagnosis	Guidance Modality	Needle Gauge	Patients (%) Positive	Guided Biopsy Specific Diagnosis Made (Patients)
Ho et al. (7)	1981	7	Radionuclide and fluoroscopy	22 spinal	4/7 (57)	Cirrhosis (1) Hepatitis (2) Fatty infiltrate (1)
Haaga (38)	1979	4	CT	18 Menghini	2/4 (50)	Hepatitis (1) Hemangioma (1)
Rosenblatt et al. (21)	1982	6	Sonographic	22, 23	0/6 (0)	—
Haaga et al. (52)	1983	5	CT	22 Core	1/5 (20)	Fatty infiltrate
				18 Menghini	5/5 (100)	Fatty infiltrate (3) Hemangioma (1) Cirrhosis (1)
Pagani (42)	1983	6	CT	22	3/6 (50)	Focal fatty infiltrate (3)
Pagani (42)	1983	6	CT	18 (noncutting)	6/6 (100)	Hemangioma (1) Focal fatty infiltrate (5)

et al. (52) demonstrate the superiority of guided biopsy with 18-gauge spinal or Menghini needles in benign lesions. Although limited, experience at this institution indicates that in selected cases where initial aspiration biopsy is inconclusive, large bore cutting biopsy will provide a more certain benign diagnosis (Fig. 33.6).

Hepatic Hemangioma

Hepatic hemangiomas are being discovered with increasing frequency in patients undergoing upper abdominal imaging for a variety of indications (29). Correct diagnosis of an incidental hemangioma and accurate discrimination from hepatic malignancy is essential when staging patients with known or suspected extrahepatic malignancy. Although angiography has been the traditional method for diagnosing hemangiomas (55), less invasive modalities have been sought more recently. Several reports have documented the nonspecificity of sonographic patterns of hepatic hemangiomas (29, 55–57). CT with bolus intravenous contrast enhancement has been advocated for definitive diagnosis of hepatic hemangiomas (58). However, several authors have described hemangiomas which did not fulfill the strict bolus-CT criteria (29, 38, 42, 59). Finally, one group has suggested the use of ^{99m}Tc-RBC liver imaging as a safe, simple and effective examination to confirm a hemangioma (60).

In the patient with a mass "not typical" for hemangioma, biopsy or angiography may be needed (42). There is now ample evidence that percutaneous fine needle aspiration biopsy of hemangiomas can be performed safely. Unevent-

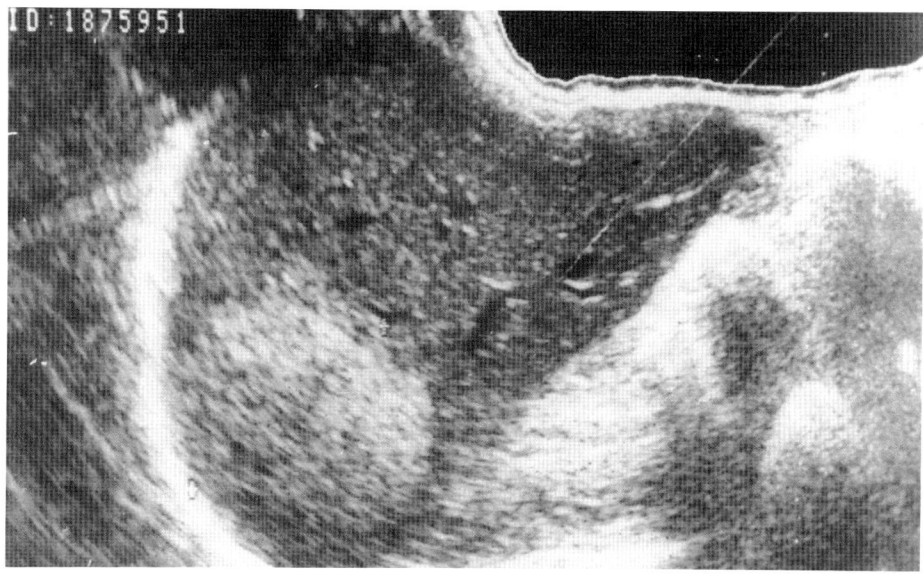

FIGURE 33.6. HEPATIC BIOPSY

Guided biopsy in focal benign hepatic disease. A 47-yr-old woman, 2 yr post-successful renal transplant for chronic renal failure, developed elevation of serum alkaline phosphatase and SGOT. Sagittal hepatic sonogram revealed a 6.5-cm hyperechoic mass in the posterior aspect of the right lobe. IV bolus CT examination (not shown) did not reveal an enhancement pattern typical of hemangioma. A 22-gauge aspiration biopsy under sonographic guidance revealed scattered normal hepatocytes and inflammatory cells, but no neoplasm. Sonographically guided biopsy with a large cutting needle one week later revealed changes compatible with chronic active hepatitis.

ful 22-gauge aspiration biopsies of hemangiomas, performed under ultrasound guidance, have been reported by several authors (24, 28, 29, 32, 33). Fine needle aspiration of a hemangioma generally provides frank blood with no cellular material (32, 59). Bondestam et al. (29), however, noted recovery of scanty cytological material with "small clusters of mesenchymal cells of uniform shape and size arranged in order of polarity" in 2 of 3 hemangiomas aspirated with a 22-gauge needle. No false positives for tumor were reported in any of the hemangioma biopsies.

Haaga (38) biopsied under CT control, without complication, three poorly vascular hemangiomas, utilizing an 18-gauge Menghini needle; diagnostic biopsy material was retrieved in one patient. One instance of serious post-biopsy hemorrhage following 18-gauge Menghini biopsy of a hemangioma has been reported (39). Using 18- and 22-gauge noncutting needles, Pagani (42) biopsied successfully and without complication one hemangioma. In the largest experience reported to date, Sheu and colleagues, employing 22-gauge aspiration and larger Vim-Silverman cutting needles, biopsied without complication 9 hemangiomas smaller than 3 cm in diameter (59). In each case, only blood was aspirated with the smaller needle, and definitive diagnosis required a tissue core.

Pancreas

The most frequent indications for guided percutaneous biopsy of the pancreas are: (a) suspected pancreatic carcinoma in a patient with focal pancreatic enlargement on cross-sectional imaging, (b) mass producing narrowing/occlusion of distal CBD or pancreatic duct noted on cholangiography or ERCP, and (c) suspected recurrent cancer in the pancreatic bed following attempted curative resection.

Technical Considerations

Focal pancreatic masses are approached anteriorly with needle passage perpendicular to skin surface. B-mode or real-time sonographic guidance is preferred (Fig. 33.7) in patients with average and thin body habitus. CT guidance is necessary when marked obesity or gas-filled bowel prevents adequate sonographic visualization (Fig. 33.8). Due to alteration of overlying bowel, the presence of surgical clips, or the ascites that is often present, biopsy experience in patients who have undergone previous subtotal

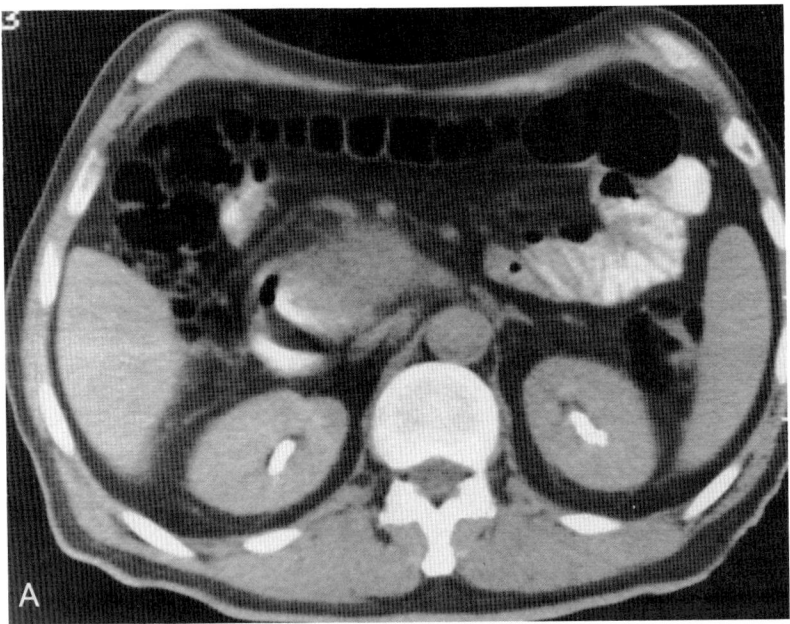

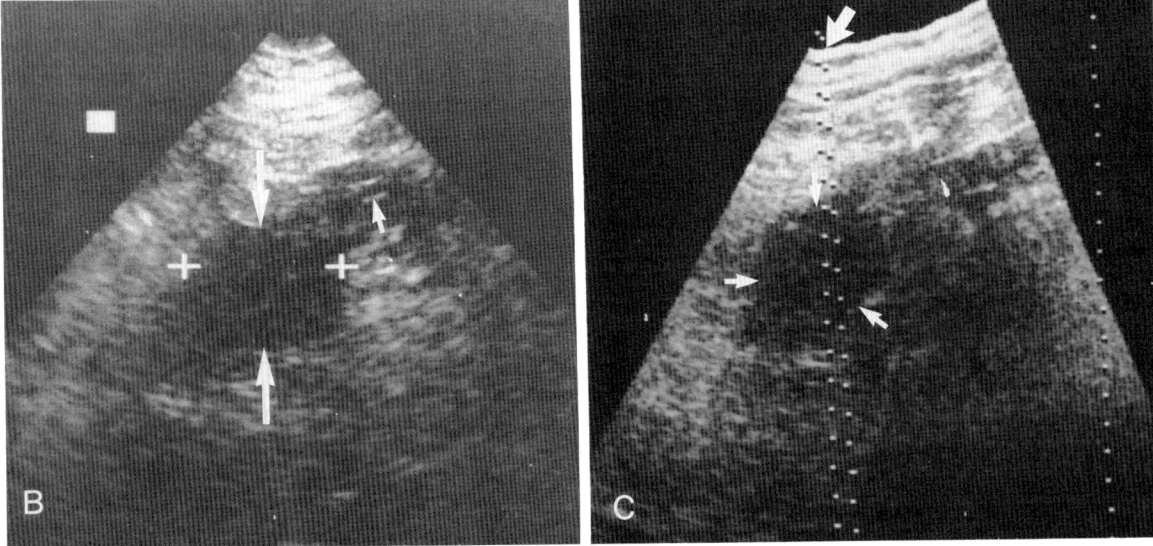

FIGURE 33.7. PANCREATIC BIOPSY

Sonographic biopsy guidance in typical pancreatic neoplasm. *A:* Abdominal CT in a middle-aged man complaining of weight loss reveals a large mass in the pancreatic head. *B:* Transverse, oblique real-time sonographic evaluation revealed a large hypoechoic mass in the pancreatic head (*large arrows*) and a dilated duct in the pancreatic body (*small arrow*). *C:* B-mode biopsy localization image in transverse plane delineates the mass (*small arrows*), the anterior border of which is about 5.5 cm deep to the planned skin entry point (*large arrow*). Biopsy with 20-gauge Franseen needle yielded carcinoma.

pancreatic resection and/or biliary bypass surgery has been more successful with CT guidance (Fig. 33.9). A 20- or 22-gauge Turner, Franseen or Westcott needle is usually employed for pancreatic biopsy. Some pancreatic tumors are sufficiently firm to deflect the smaller, more flexible needles, making a larger more rigid 20-gauge needle necessary. Schwerk et al. (24) attempt to avoid transverse colon during transabdominal puncture of the pancreas.

Results

Table 33.5 presents a summary of the major recent series reporting percutaneous biopsy for pancreatic adenocarcinoma. Sensitivity (true positive) rates for cancer diagnosis have ranged from as low as 62% to as high as 100% in the series of Grant et al. (32), with an average true positive rate of 83%. These sensitivities, disappointing compared to liver biopsy, have been

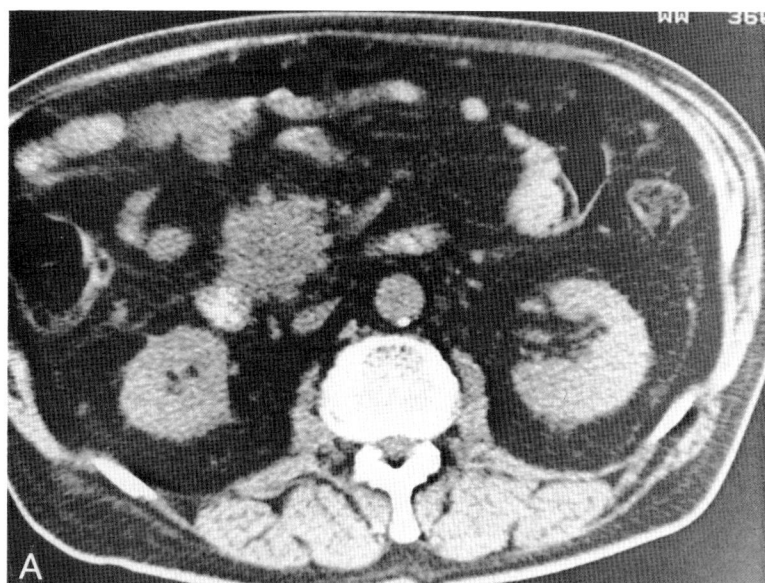
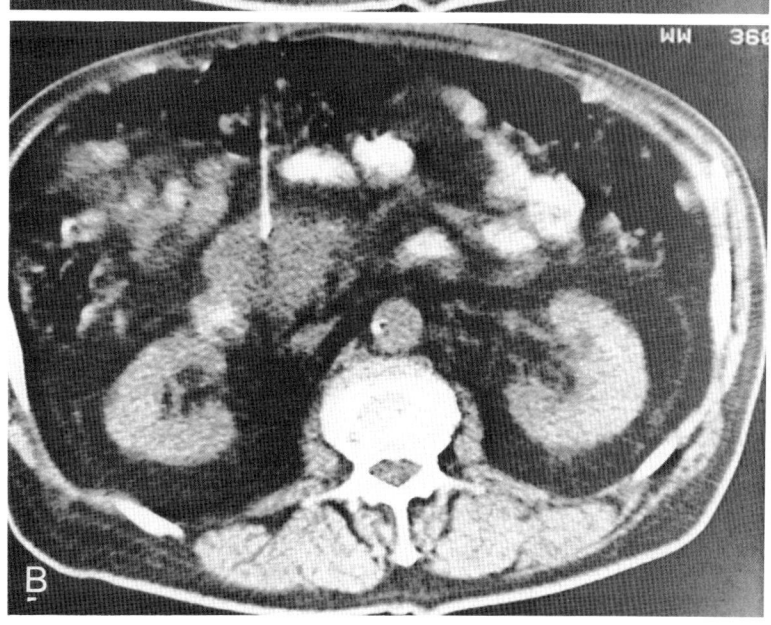

FIGURE 33.8. PANCREATIC BIOPSY
CT-guided pancreatic biopsy. *A:* Focal enlargement of the pancreatic head was incidentally discovered in this elderly gentleman undergoing abdominal CT for other reasons. Sonographic visualization of the pancreatic head was unsuccessful due to abundant mesenteric fat and bowel gas. *B:* Percutaneous 22-gauge Turner needle biopsy of the pancreatic head under CT guidance was positive for adenocarcinoma.

addressed by several authors, and appear to reflect characteristics of the malignant pancreatic mass itself. Zornoza observed that because scirrhous pancreatic tumors contained an extensive connective tissue stroma, recovery of adequate biopsy material may require more passes with a larger needle (45). In four false negative pancreatic biopsies in another series, subsequent surgery revealed "acellular desmoplastic tumors" (17). Bernardino has advocated multiple biopsies at different sites within a pancreatic mass to reduce sampling errors (false negatives) (6). A second difficulty with percutaneous pancreatic biopsy has been identified by Wittenberg et al. (61). In 27% of their proven pancreatic cancer patients, CT evaluation revealed enlargement of three or more pancreatic segments (head, neck, body, tail). In planning percutaneous approach to nonfocal pancreatic enlargement, these authors suggest performing a minimum of six biopsies at several different sites.

Spleen

The paucity of published data on percutaneous guided biopsy of solid splenic masses probably reflects the uncommon discovery of such masses and a general reluctance to percutaneously bi-

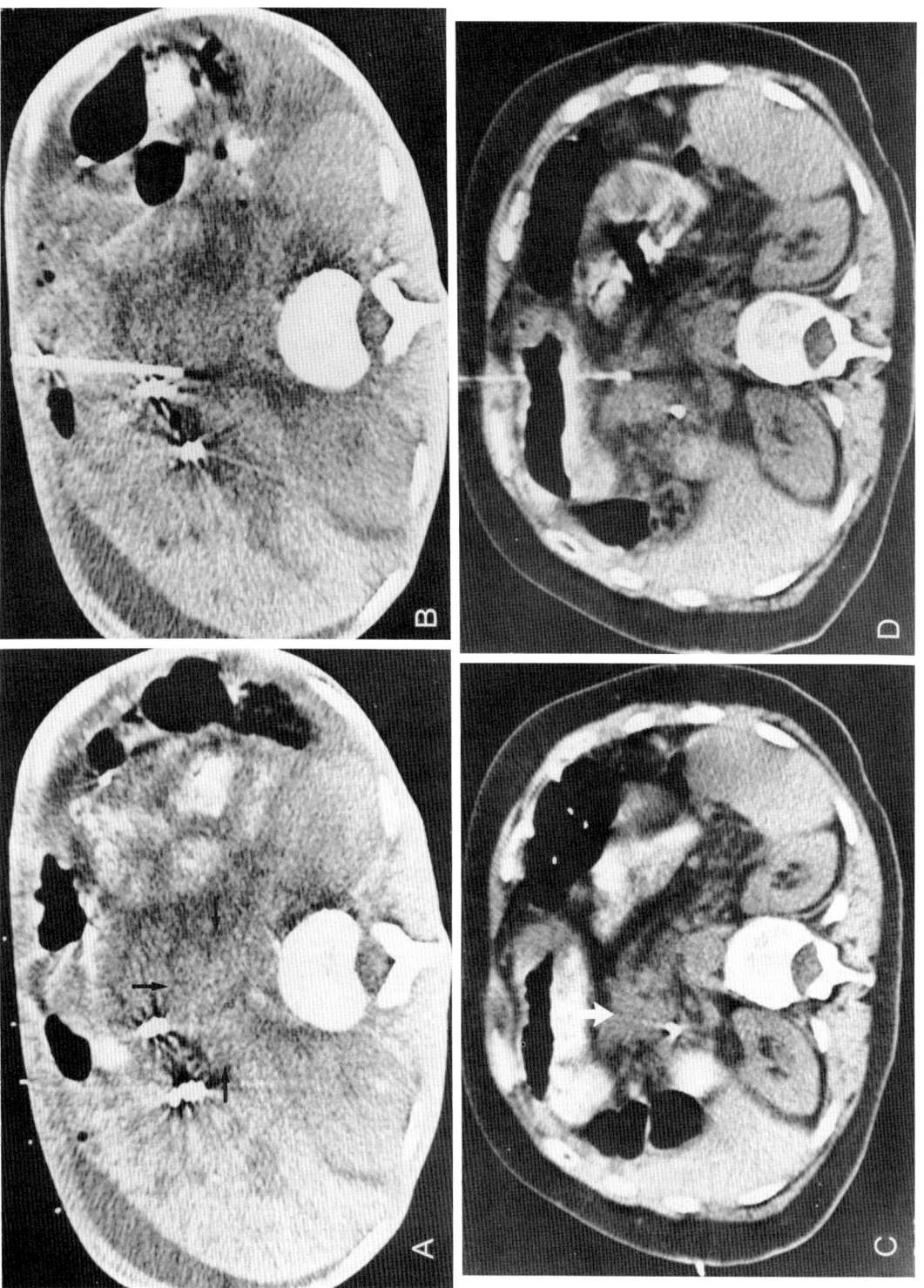

FIGURE 33.9. PANCREATIC BIOPSY

The value of CT-guided biopsy in patients who have undergone previous pancreatic resection and/or biliary bypass surgery. *A:* Localization CT in a 54-yr-old woman status post biliary bypass surgery for a pancreatic head mass reported to be chronic pancreatitis. Note the lobulated mass in the region of the pancreatic head and neck (*arrows*), surgical clips in the porta hepatis, ascites, and cutaneous reference markers. The mass was not well delineated on ultrasound. *B:* CT-guided biopsy with a 22-gauge Turner needle yielded adenocarcinoma on the first pass. *C* and *D:* 64 year old woman who developed jaundice 2-½ yr following partial pancreatic resection for malignant islet cell tumor. Sonographic evaluation of the pancreas was not successful. *C:* Preliminary CT localization reveals a small, focal mass in the pancreatic head (*arrow*). Radiodensity in posterior portion of the pancreatic head represents a biliary drainage catheter. *D:* Placement of a 20-gauge Westcott needle into the mass yielded sufficiently cellular material to allow a diagnosis of recurrent islet cell tumor. Note that the needle traverses stomach. The patient tolerated the procedure well

TABLE 33.5.
SERIES SUMMARY, PERCUTANEOUS BIOPSY OF PANCREATIC CANCER

Series Author (Ref.)	Year	Patients with Proven Cancer	Guidance Modality	Needle Gauge	True Positive (%)	Percent False Negative
Holm et al. (4)	1975	17	Sonographic	22	15/17 (88)	12
Zornoza (45)	1981	52	Sonographic or CT	Not known	32/52 (62)	38
Phillips and Schneider (17)	1981	21	Sonographic	22	17/21 (81)	19
Isler et al. (47)	1981	17	Fluoroscopy, sonographic, CT	22 Greene	15/17 (88)	12
Sundaram et al. (41)	1982	16	CT	20, 22	11/16 (69)	31
Schwerk et al. (24)	1983	52	Sonographic	20, 22	47/52 (90.5)	9.5
Grant et al. (32)	1983	15	Sonographic (sector, real-time)	22	15/15 (100)	0.0

opsy splenic lesions. In 1979, Haaga (38) recovered histiocytic lymphoma cells from an avascular splenic mass biopsied with a 22-gauge needle under CT guidance. More recently, Solbiati and his colleagues (62) reported their experience with percutaneous biopsy of solid splenic lesions in five patients. The aspirations, performed with a single pass and a 22-gauge Chiba needle, were obtained on suspended respiration and guided by a commercially available linear array real-time biopsy transducer. The biopsies were positive for cancer in both patients with non-Hodgkin's lymphoma and in one patient with hepatoma metastatic to spleen, but yielded only blood in one splenic hemangioma and necrotic material from one splenic hemangiosarcoma. There were no complications.

Blind splenic aspiration biopsies (22-gauge needle) have been performed in patients with known Hodgkin's lymphoma, non-Hodgkin's lymphoma or other malignancy but no clinical or radiological evidence of hepatic or splenic disease (18, 63). Jonsson et al. (63) reported a 27% sensitivity for the diagnosis of occult splenic involvement by Hodgkin's lymphoma in 31 patients undergoing subsequent staging procedure. In another series, Jansson et al. (18) noted a 25% positive yield for tumor in non-Hodgkin lymphoma patients who underwent blind 22-gauge aspiration biopsies of the spleen and liver.

CONTRAINDICATIONS

There are only two contraindications to percutaneous fine needle aspiration biopsy of solid masses in the upper abdomen. (a) coagulopathy that cannot be corrected by administration of drugs or infusion of blood products, and (b) suspected echinococcal cystic disease of the upper abdominal viscera (64). Due to the risk of anaphylaxis, percutaneous needle aspiration or biopsy of echinococcal cysts is often avoided. Recent report of a solid, tumor-like sonographic appearance of hydatid liver cysts underscores the need for caution when a patient from an area in which echinococcus is endemic presents with a liver mass of undetermined etiology (65). Such a patient should undergo specific serological studies to exclude hydatid disease prior to biopsy.

As noted in an earlier section, fine needle aspiration biopsy of hepatic hemangiomas has been performed safely, and is not contraindicated in a suspect hemangioma which has not fulfilled the bolus computed tomographic or ^{99m}Tc-RBC blood pool imaging criteria.

MORTALITY AND MORBIDITY

From 1970 to the present, only two fatalities following 22-gauge fine needle aspiration biopsy have been reported in the English language literature. One patient suffered a fatal intraabdominal hemorrhage following successful biopsy of multifocal hepatoma in a cirrhotic liver (66). Another patient developed severe and ultimately fatal necrotizing pancreatitis following a 22-gauge fluoroscopically guided biopsy of an enlarged pancreatic head (67).

Morbidity

Percutaneous fine needle aspiration biopsy has appropriately earned a reputation as a safe diagnostic procedure with a very low complication rate. In two large Scandinavian series, the frequency of minor and major post-biopsy complications was 0.6% in a liver biopsy study (2), and 0.4% in a study group which included aspiration of upper abdominal, renal and retroperitoneal masses (68). In one American series of 100 fine needle abdominal aspiration biopsies, complications, none of which affected patient outcome, occurred in 3% (10).

Specific complications are discussed below.

Bleeding

Despite fine needle passage close to or through vascular structures in the upper abdomen, the risk of clinically significant post-biopsy hemorrhage in patients with normal coagulation status appears to be very low. Following 22-gauge percutaneous biopsy in a large series including over 500 malignant lesions, Holm et al. (68) reported only two incidental hematomas, both discovered at surgery. In a study of 2305 patients who underwent fine needle aspiration liver biopsy, Lundquist (2) reported one patient who developed an intrahepatic hematoma requiring surgical drainage. Intrahepatic hematomas that were self-limited (6) or required a two unit blood transfusion (53) have also been reported. Passage of a blood clot per rectum, presumably due to gastric or transverse colon bleeding, has been reported following percutaneous fine needle pancreatic biopsy (69).

The risk of clinically significant bleeding will be greater in patients undergoing biopsy with a larger diameter needle (70). In a series of 1000 outpatients who underwent non-guided liver biopsy with Tru-cut, JAM-Shidi, or Franklin-Silverman needles, post-biopsy pain and/or hypotension requiring prolonged observation or hospitalization developed in 5.9% (71). However, no complications occurred in 100 patients who underwent CT-guided liver biopsy utilizing 18- and 22-gauge spinal (noncutting) needles, although 2 small intrahepatic and 3 small (50 cc) subcapsular hematomas were incidentally discovered at subsequent surgery (42). An asymptomatic subcapsular hematoma requiring no intervention was recently reported following 20-gauge CT-guided liver biopsy (43). One instance of bleeding which required transfusion and surgery has occurred following 18-gauge Menghini biopsy of an hepatic hemangioma (39).

Tumor Seeding along Needle Tract

Of great theoretical concern, the risk of needle tract seeding following percutaneous fine needle biopsy of a malignant mass appears to be exceedingly small. Only one case of needle tract seeding following 22-gauge aspiration biopsy of a pancreatic cancer has been reported (72). The authors felt that in this, the only such reported case, the larger than usual number of needle passes required to aspirate diagnostic material may have contributed to the complication.

There is currently insufficient data to assess the risk of needle tract seeding when upper abdominal biopsy is performed with larger needles. However, review of a series of 1264 malignant lung masses biopsied with 18–20-gauge needles yielded only one case (0.08%) of documented implantation metastasis at the biopsy site (73).

Infection

One instance of liver abscess developing one month post-percutaneous Menghini needle liver biopsy has appeared in the literature (74). Presumed needle inoculation of enteric flora into the pancreatic bed resulted in one instance of gram negative sepsis occurring after 22-gauge aspiration biopsy of the pancreas (10). Whether a similar mechanism accounts for exacerbations of preexisting pancreatitis and one case of fatal necrotizing pancreatitis reported following fine needle pancreatic biopsy (67) is unclear. In a study of percutaneous 20–23-gauge pancreatic biopsy performed on normal pigs and a group of pigs affected with experimentally induced pancreatitis, Coel and Niwayama found no post-biopsy structural changes in mesentery, stomach or duodenum and no alterations in serum amylase or lipase (75).

Peritonitis

Peritonitis resulting from needle puncture and subsequent spillage of bile or intestinal contents into the peritoneal cavity is a theoretical hazard which appears to be exceedingly rare following percutaneous biopsy. Experimental 23-gauge needle puncture of the abdomen in 4 large anesthetized dogs with subsequent laparotomy up to 48 hours post-biopsy revealed no bowel injury or peritonitis, even when puncture was repeated under direct vision at surgery (8). Sundaram et al. (41) reported no complications following use of 20-gauge spinal needles to perform percutaneous biopsies which required traversing bowel. One instance of transient right upper quadrant pain and a small pneumoperitoneum, requiring no intervention, developed following an 18-gauge CT-directed liver biopsy (43).

Bile peritonitis has been reported following 22-gauge aspiration liver biopsy in an anicteric patient (76), and after intentional 18-gauge percutaneous gallbladder puncture and contrast injection which demonstrated a common duct calculus (68). Both patients recovered after surgery.

Local Pain

Patients not infrequently experience local pain, during and immediately following upper abdominal aspiration biopsy; the former can generally be controlled with local anesthetic. In a large series which included abdominal, retroperitoneal and pelvic biopsies, Zornoza (45) reported that about 15% of patients experienced self-limited local pain at the biopsy site. In a group of over 200 patients undergoing abdominal biopsies and aspirations, Sundaram et al. reported 2 patients (less than 1%) who complained of local pain for several hours after biopsy.

Pneumothorax

Aspiration biopsy of the liver or spleen may result in a pneumothorax if the biopsy needle violates the nearby pleura. One clinically insignificant pneumothorax following fine-needle liver biopsy has been reported (14).

SUMMARY AND FUTURE PROSPECTS

Referring to his 1-sec liver biopsy technique, Menghini (70) observed that "there should be a tolerable relation between the potential danger of a diagnostic method and its diagnostic value." This principle applies equally well to fine needle aspiration biopsy. When guided by an appropriate imaging modality, percutaneous fine-needle biopsy of the liver, pancreas and spleen is a safe, sensitive and inexpensive alternative to surgery in the diagnosis of suspected primary or metastatic malignancy.

For several reasons, utilization of guided percutaneous aspiration biopsy should increase in the coming years. First, the increasing familiarity of radiologists and, perhaps more important, referring physicians with this diagnostic technique will result in expanding demand. Second, improvements in cytological technique and wider availability of pathologists trained in aspiration cytopathology will encourage the establishment of new biopsy programs and services. Finally, as the prospective payment scheme for reimbursement of hospital care is implemented, pressures for rapid, inexpensive and non-surgical diagnosis of suspected malignant disease will mount and promote further utilization of percutaneous guided biopsy (5, 77).

Several trends relating to percutaneous biopsy may emerge in the coming years. As more attention is focused on outpatient diagnostic procedures, an increasing number of well-equipped and staffed hospital-based and free-standing medical imaging facilities will offer percutaneous biopsy to the outpatient population. More extensive use of electron microscopy (EM) to study aspirated materials can also be expected. Percutaneous biopsy provides excellent material for EM analysis (2, 78). In cases of poorly differentiated carcinomas, sarcomas or viral infections where light microscopy is limited, EM, by identifying specific cytoplasmic inclusions or organelles, can suggest a specific diagnosis (78). Finally, novel needle tips or bevels may be designed which provide improved biopsy material retrieval while retaining the safety of the smaller needle diameter.

REFERENCES

1. Lundquist A: Fine-needle aspiration biopsy for cytodiagnosis of malignant tumour in the liver. Acta Med Scand 188:465–470, 1970.
2. Lundquist A: Liver biopsy with a needle of 0.7 mm outer diameter. Safety and quantitative yield. Acta Med Scand 188:471–474, 1970.
3. Rasmussen SN, Holm HH, Kristensen JK, Barlebo H: Ultrasonically-guided liver biopsy. Br Med J 2:500–502, 1972.
4. Holm HH, Pedersen JF, Kristensen JK, Rasmussen SN, Hancke S, Jensen F: Ultrasonically-guided percutaneous puncture. Radiol Clin North Am 13:493–503, 1975.
5. Doherty FJ: Fine-needle percutaneous aspiration biopsy of abdominal mass lesions. In Athanasoulis CA, Pfister RC, Greene RE, Roberson GH (eds): Interventional Radiology. Philadelphia, W. B. Saunders, 1982, pp 568–576.
6. Bernardino ME: Percutaneous biopsy. AJR 142:41–45, 1984.
7. Ho CS, McLoughlin MJ, Tao LC, Blendis L, Evans WK: Guided percutaneous aspiration biopsy of the liver. Cancer 47:1781–1783, 1981.
8. Goldstein HM, Zornoza J, Wallace S, Anderson JH, Bree RL, Samuels BI, Lukeman J: Percutaneous fine-needle aspiration biopsy of pancreatic and other abdominal masses. Radiology 123:319–322, 1977.
9. Yandow DR, Matallana RH: Gas contrast guided needle biopsy of the head of the pancreas. Radiology 137:543–544, 1980.
10. Ferrucci JT, Wittenberg J, Mueller PR, Simeone JF, Harbin WP, Kirkpatrick RH, Taft PD: Diagnosis of abdominal malignancy by radiologic fine-needle aspiration biopsy. AJR 134:323–330, 1980.
11. Pereiras RV, Meiers W, Kunhardt B, Troner M, Hutson D, Barkin JS, Viamonte M: Fluoroscopically guided thin needle aspiration biopsy of the abdomen and retroperitoneum. AJR 131:197–202, 1978.
12. Skolnick ML, Dekker A, Weinstein B: Ultrasound guided fine-needle aspiration biopsy of abdominal masses. Gastrointest Radiol 3:295–302, 1978.
13. Zornoza J, Wallace S, Ordoney N, Lukeman J: Fine-needle aspiration biopsy of the liver. AJR 134:331–334, 1980.

14. Nosher JL, Plafker J: Fine needle aspiration of the liver with ultrasound guidance. *Radiology* 136:177–180, 1980.
15. Bondestam S, Jansson SE, Taavitsainen M, Standertskjold-Nordenstam M: Ultrasound guided fine-needle biopsy of mass lesions affecting the hepatobiliary tract. *Acta Radiol Diag* 22:549–551, 1981.
16. Yeh HC: Percutaneous fine needle aspiration biopsy of intra-abdominal lesions with ultrasound guidance. *Am J Gastroenterol* 75:148–152, 1981.
17. Phillips G, Schneider M: Ultrasonically guided percutaneous fine needle aspiration biopsy of solid masses. *Cardiovasc Intervent Radiol* 4:33–38, 1981.
18. Jansson SE, Bondestam S, Heinonen E, Grohn P, Vuopio P: Value of liver and spleen aspiration biopsy in malignant diseases when these organs show no signs of involvement in sonography. *Acta Med Scand* 213:279–281, 1983.
19. Schwerk WB, Schmitz-Moormann P: Ultrasonically guided fine-needle biopsies in neoplastic liver disease: cytohistologic diagnoses and echo pattern of lesions. *Cancer* 48:1469–1477, 1981.
20. Lee TG, Knochel JQ: Air as an ultrasound contrast marker for accurate determination of needle placement. *Radiology* 143:787–788, 1982.
21. Rosenblatt R, Kutcher R, Moussouris HF, Schrieber K, Koss LG: Sonographically guided fine-needle aspiration of liver lesions. *JAMA* 248:1639–1641, 1982.
22. Jacobsen GK, Gammelgaard J, Fuglo M: Coarse needle biopsy versus fine needle aspiration biopsy in the diagnosis of focal lesions of the liver. *Acta Cytol* 27:152–156, 1983.
23. Elyaderani MK: Ultrasonic guidance of liver biopsy and fine-needle aspiration in difficult cases. *South Med J* 76:850–854, 1983.
24. Schwerk WB, Durr H, Schmitz-Moormann P: Ultrasound guided fine-needle biopsies in pancreatic and hepatic neoplasms. *Gastrointest Radiol* 8:219–225, 1983.
25. Ohto M, Saotome N, Saisho H, Tsuchiya Y, Ono T, Okuda K, Karasawa E: Real-time sonography of the pancreatic duct: application to percutaneous pancreatic ductography. *AJR* 134:647–652, 1980.
26. Ohto M, Karasawa E, Tsuchiya Y, Kimura K, Saisho H, Ono T, Okuda K: Ultrasonically guided percutaneous contrast medium injection and aspiration biopsy using a real-time puncture transducer. *Radiology* 136:171–176, 1980.
27. Buonocore E, Skipper GJ: Steerable real-time sonographically guided needle biopsy. *AJR* 136:387–392, 1981.
28. Montali G, Solbiati L, Croce F, Ierace T, Ravetto C: Fine-needle aspiration biopsy of liver focal lesions ultrasonically guided with a real-time probe. Report on 126 cases. *Br J Radiol* 55:717–723, 1982.
29. Bondestam S, Somer K, Hekali P, Takkunen H: Sonography and computed tomography in hepatic haemangioma. *Acta Med Scand* 668:68–75, 1982.
30. Tasuta M, Yamamoto R, Yamamura H, Okuda S, Tamura H: Cytologic examination and CEA measurement in aspirated pancreatic material collected by percutaneous fine-needle aspiration biopsy under ultrasonic guidance for the diagnosis of pancreatic carcinoma. *Cancer* 52:693–698, 1983.
31. Reid MH: Real-time sonographic needle biopsy guide. *AJR* 140:162–163, 1983.
32. Grant EG, Richardson JD, Smirniotopoulos JG, Jacobs NM: Fine-needle biopsy directed by real-time sonography: technique and accuracy. *AJR* 141:29–32, 1983.
33. Livraghi T: A simple no-cost technique for real-time biopsy. *J Clin Ultrasound* 12:60–62, 1984.
34. Lindgren PG: Ultrasonically guided punctures. A modified technique. *Radiology* 137:235–237, 1980.
35. Haaga JR, Alfidi RJ: Precise biopsy localization by computed tomography. *Radiology* 118:603–607, 1976.
36. Haaga JR, Reich NE, Havrilla TR, Alfidi RJ, Meaney TF: Computed tomography-guided biopsy. 1. Overview. *Comput Tomogr* 2:25–30, 1978.
37. Ferrucci JT, Wittenberg J: CT biopsy of abdominal tumors: Aids for lesion localization. *Radiology* 129:739–744, 1978.
38. Haaga JR: New techniques for CT-guided biopsies. *AJR* 133:633–641, 1979.
39. Haaga JR, Vanek J: Computed tomographic guided liver biopsy using the Menghini needle. *Radiology* 133:405–408, 1979.
40. van Sonnenberg E, Wittenberg J, Ferrucci JT, Mueller PR, Simeone JF: Triangulation method for percutaneous needle guidance: The angled approach to upper abdominal masses. *AJR* 137:757–761, 1981.
41. Sundaram M, Wolverson MK, Heiberg E, Vas WG, Shields JB: Utility of CT-guided abdominal aspiration procedures. *AJR* 139:1111–1115, 1982.
42. Pagani JJ: Biopsy of focal hepatic lesions. Comparison of 18 and 22 gauge needles. *Radiology* 147:673–675, 1983.
43. Alspaugh JP, Bernardino ME, Sewell CW, Sones PJ, Berkman WA, Price RB: CT directed hepatic biopsies: increased diagnostic accuracy with low patient risk. *J Comput Assist Tomogr* 7:1012–1017, 1983.
44. Vogelzang RL, Matalon TA, Neiman HL, Sakowicz BA: Lateral scout radiograph in CT-guided aspiration biopsy. *AJR* 140:164, 1983.
45. Zornoza J: Abdomen. In Zornoza J (ed): *Percutaneous Needle Biopsy.* Baltimore, Williams & Wilkins, 1981, pp 102–140.
46. Andriole JG, Haaga JR, Adams RB, Nunez C: Biopsy needle characteristics assessed in the laboratory. *Radiology* 148:659–662, 1983.
47. Isler RJ, Ferrucci JT, Wittenberg J, Mueller PR, Simeone JF, van Sonnenberg E, Hall DA: Tissue core biopsy of abdominal tumors with a 22 gauge cutting needle. *AJR* 136:725–728, 1981.
48. Turner AF, Sargent EN: Percutaneous pulmonary needle biopsy. An improved needle for a simple direct method of diagnosis. *AJR* 104:846–850, 1968.
49. Lieberman RP, Hafez GR, Crummy AB: Histology from aspiration biopsy: Turner needle experience. *AJR* 138:561–564, 1982.
50. Franseen CC: Aspiration biopsy with a description of a new type of needle. *N Engl J Med* 224:1054–1058, 1941.
51. Westcott JL: Percutaneous needle aspiration of hilar and mediastinal masses. *Radiology* 141:323–329, 1981.
52. Haaga JR, Lipuma JP, Bryan PJ, Balsara VJ, Cohen AM: Clinical comparison of small and large-caliber cutting needles for biopsy. *Radiology* 146:665–667, 1983.
53. Wittenberg J, Mueller PR, Ferrucci JT, Simeone JF, van Sonnenberg E, Neff CC, Palermo RA, Isler RJ: Percutaneous core biopsy of abdominal tumors using 22 gauge needles: further observations. *AJR* 139:75–80, 1982.
54. Zornoza J, Cabanillas FF, Altoff TM, Ordonez N, Cohen MA: Percutaneous needle biopsy in abdominal lymphoma. *AJR* 136:97–103, 1981.
55. Freeny PC, Vimont TR, Barnett DC: Cavernous hemangioma of the liver: ultrasonography, arteriography, and computed tomography. *Radiology* 132:143–148, 1979.
56. Wiener SN, Parulekar SG: Scintigraphy and ultrasonography of hepatic hemangioma. *Radiology* 132:149–153, 1979.
57. Mirk P, Rubaltelli L, Bazzocchi M, Busilacchi P, Candiani F, Ferrari F et al: *J Clin Ultrasound* 10:373–378, 1982.

58. Barnett PH, Zerhouni EA, White RI, Siegelman SS: Computed tomography in the diagnosis of cavernous hemangioma of the liver. *AJR* 134:439–447, 1980.
59. Sheu JC, Sung JL, Chen DS, Yu JY, Wang TH, Su CT, Tsang YM: Ultrasonography of small hepatic tumors using high-resolution linear-array real-time instruments. *Radiology* 150: 797–802, 1984.
60. Engel MA, Marks DS, Sandler MA, Shetty P: Differentiation of focal intraheptic lesions with ^{99m}Tc-red blood cell imaging. *Radiology* 146:777–782, 1983.
61. Wittenberg J, Simeone JF, Ferrucci JT, Mueller PR, van Sonnenberg E, Neff CC: Non-focal enlargement in pancreatic carcinoma. *Radiology* 144:131–135, 1982.
62. Solbiati L, Bossi MC, Bellotti E, Ravetto C, Montali G: Focal lesions in the spleen: sonographic patterns and guided biopsy. *AJR* 1983; 140:59–65, 1983.
63. Jonsson K, Karp W, Landberg T, Mortensson W, Tennvall J, Tylen U: Radiologic evaluation of subdiaphragmatic spread of Hodgkin's disease. *Acta Radiol Diagn* 24:153–159, 1983.
64. Mueller PR, Simeone JF: Intra-abdominal abscess. Diagnosis by sonography and computed tomography. *Radiol Clin North Am* 21:425–443, 1983.
65. Barriga P, Cruz F, Lepe V, Lathrop R: An ultrasonographically solid, tumor-like appearance of echinococcal cysts in the liver. *J Ultrasound Med* 2:123–125, 1983.
66. Riska H, Friman C: Fatality after fine-needle aspiration biopsy of liver. *Br Med J* 1:517, 1975.
67. Evans WK, Ho CS, McLoughlin MJ, Tao LC: Fatal necrotizing pancreatitis following fine-needle aspiration biopsy of the pancreas. *Radiology* 141:61–62, 1981.
68. Holm HH, Als O, Gammelgaard J: Percutaneous aspiration and biopsy procedures under ultrasound visualization. In Taylor KJW (ed): *Clinics in Diagnostic Ultrasound*; Vol 1, *Diagnostic Ultrasound in Gastrointestinal Disease*. New York, Churchill Livingstone, 1978, pp 137–149.
69. Smith EH, Bartrum RJ, Chang YC, D'Orsi CJ, Lokich J, Abbruzzese A, Dantono J: Percutaneous aspiration biopsy of the pancreas under ultrasonic guidance. *N Engl J Med* 292:825–828, 1975.
70. Menghini G: One-second biopsy of the liver—problems of its clinical application. *N Engl J Med* 283:582–585, 1970.
71. Perrault J, McGill DB, Ott BJ, Taylor WF: Liver biopsy: complications in 1000 inpatients and outpatients. *Gastroenterology* 74:103–106, 1978.
72. Ferrucci JT, Wittenberg J, Margolies MN, Carey RW: Malignant seeding of the tract after thin-needle aspiration biopsy. *Radiology* 130:345–346, 1979.
73. Sinner WN, Zajicek J: Implantation metastasis after percutaneous transthoracic needle aspiration biopsy. *Acta Radiol Diagn* 17:473–480, 1976.
74. Klein B, Lewinski UH, Cohen AM, Chaimoff C, Djaldetti M: Liver abscess as a late complication of percutaneous liver biopsy. *Arch Surg* 115:1233–1234, 1980.
75. Coel MN, Niwayama G: Safety of percutaneous fine-needle pancreatic biopsy: A porcine model. *Invest Radiol* 13:547–549, 1978.
76. Schultz TB: Fine-needle biopsy of the liver complicated with bile peritonitis. *Acta Med Scand* 199:141–142, 1976.
77. Mitty HA, Efremidis SC, Yeh HC: Impact of fine-needle biopsy on the management of patients with carcinoma of the pancreas. *AJR* 137:1119–1121, 1981.
78. Ordonez NG: Electron microscopy: the future of percutaneous biopsy. In Zornoza J (ed): *Percutaneous Needle Biopsy*. Baltimore, Williams & Wilkins, 1981, pp 198–203.

Index

Page numbers in *italics* denote figures; those followed by "*t*" denote tables.

A

Abdomen
  displacement, by pancreatic pseudocyst, 723, *724*
  gasless, 663
  mass, and jaundice, 357–358
  pancreatic-enteric fistula, 720, *721*, 721–722
  upper
    biopsy and drainage procedures (*see also* Percutaneous abscess and fluid drainage; Percutaneous biopsy, guided), 1039
  wall, fistula, 447
Abdominal film
  of abscess, splenic, 956
  of lymphangiomatosis, splenic, 976
  of pancreatitis, acute, *661*, 661–664
Abscess (*see also* Microabscess; Percutaneous abscess and fluid drainage)
  abdominal, diagnosis, 1042
  with cholangitis, *551*
  defined, 1041
  formation, intraperitoneal, 1049
  hepatic, 1053
    amebic, 158–163
    cryptogenic, 151
    intrahepatic, 1051
    pyogenic (*see* Pyogenic liver abscess)
    radionuclide imaging, 28
    staphylococcal, 40, *41*
  pancreatic, 713
    clinical findings, 713, 715
    in pancreatitis, 706
    radiology, 714, *715*, 715–719
  pericholecystic, 425, 426, *427*, 428
  splenic, 955–956, 994, 1001, 1025, 1059
    arteriography, 958
    aspiration, 913
    barium studies, 957
    computed tomography, *960*, 960–965
    gallium-67 citrate scan, *958*, 958, 964
    plain film, *956*, 956–957
    radionuclide scan, 957–958, *959*
    ultrasound, *959*, 959–960
  subhepatic, 31
  subphrenic, 31, 1001
  drainage, 1049*t*, 1049–1050
Abscessogram, 1047
Accelerator, cyclotron or linear, 32
Acinar cells, pancreatic, 619, 639, *639*
  in pancreatitis, 682
  tumors, 851–852

Acinarization, in ERCP, 337
Acinus
  hepatic, 6
  pancreas, 639, *639*, 640
    development, 619, *620*
Acoustic enhancement, in cavernous hemangioma, 174
Acute lymphocytic leukemia, associated with splenomegaly, 985, *987*
Adenoacanthoma, pancreatic (*see* Adenosquamous cancer, pancreatic)
Adenocarcinoma (*see also* Cystadenocarcinoma)
  common duct, 536
  gallbladder, 484, 492
  metastases to spleen, *979*
  metastatic, 204–205
  pancreatic duct cell, 603, *604*, 854
    ampullary carcinoma, 767, 770, *774*, *775*, 776
    angiography, microadenocarcinoma, 843, *844*
    cholangiography, 802, 803, *804–810*
    clinical findings, 765–766
    computed tomography, 783–*801*
    contrast examination, 768
    differentiated from pancreatitis, 797, 798, 799, *800*
    metastases, 768, *770*
    microadenocarcinoma, 842–844
    MRI of, 892, 893
    mucinous, 824
    pancreatography, 810–813
    pathology, 766–767
    plain film, *767*, 768, *769*
    sonography, 778–781, *782*
    staging, *793*, 794–797, *798*, *799*
    upper gastrointestinal series, 768, 769, 770, *772*, 773–777
Adenoma (*see also* Cystadenoma; Gastrinoma; Insulinoma)
  biliary, 536, 544
  gallbladder, 472, 479–481
  hepatic, 183, 186, 188
    arteriography, 189, *190*, *191*
    bile duct hamartoma, 193
    clinical findings, 188–189
    computed tomography, 189, *190*, *191*
    in glycogen storage disease, 37, *37*, 38–39
    magnetic resonance imaging, 271
    nuclear medicine, *192*, 192
    pathology, 189
    ultrasound, 189, *190*, *191*
  pancreatic duct cell, microcystic, 751–757, 798, *896*

Adenomatous hyperplasia, gallbladder, 479
Adenomyoma, gallbladder, fundal, *468*, 468, *469*
Adenomyomatosis, gallbladder, 479
  pathology and oral cholecystography, 463–472, *472*
  sonography, 474–477
Adenomyosis, 573
Adenopathy
  in gallbladder carcinoma, 489
  peripancreatic, 796
Adenosquamous cancer, pancreatic, 841–842
Admixture, defects, 528
Adolescents (*see* Liver, congenital disorders and pediatric neoplasms)
Adrenal gland
  effect of hepatomegaly on, 66, 68
  right, tumor, *57*
  in vipoma, 879
Adriamycin (*see* Doxorubicin)
Aerobacter, 40
Aerozoin skin conditioner, 1048
Afferent loop, obstruction, 497, *498*
Aflatoxin, and hepatocellular carcinoma, 220
Air
  of abscess, splenic, *960*, 960, *962*
  bubbles, 532
    vs. stones, *528*, 529
  differentiated from calculi in postcholedochoduodenostomy, 523, *532*
  in fistula, biliary, *449*
  study, of gallstone ileus, 452, *453*
  use in computed tomography, 784
  of sickle cell anemia, 1025
Alagille's syndrome, 361, *361*
Albumin, macroaggregated, 28
Alcohol, alcoholic
  cirrhosis, magnetic resonance imaging of, 268
  fatty liver in, 105, 105*t*, 109, 114
  liver disease
    differentiated from cholecystitis, acute, 421
    nuclear medicine scan of, 148
  pancreatic disease, calcifications, 685
  pancreatitis in, 657–658, 681
Alkaline phosphatase, levels
  in cholangitis, 559
  in cirrhosis, 569
  in jaundice, 499
Alkylating agents, in hepatic artery infusion, 296

1085

Alpha cell, pancreatic, 873
Alpha-fetoprotein (α-fetoprotein), levels
   in hepatoblastoma, 49
   in hepatocellular carcinoma, 221, 246
   in infantile hemangioendothelioma, 44
Alveolar infiltrates, in pancreatitis, 659
Amebic abscess, liver, 158
   clinical findings, 158–159
   pathology, 159
   radiology, 159–*163*
Aminoglycoside antibiotics, 334
Aminophenyl compounds, triiodinated, 393
Ampicillin, 606
Ampulla of Vater, 625
   in adenocarcinoma, 766
   anatomy and physiology, 573
   carcinoma, 767, 770, *774*, *775*, 776, 794, 828
     arteriography, 836
     cholangiography, *809*, *810*, 810
     pancreatography, *809*, 813
     sonography and CT, 805, *803*
   stenosis (*see* Stenosis, papillary)
   stones, 511, *512*, 523
   villous tumors, 545, *545*
Amylase, 641
   isoamylase, 712
   levels
     in pancreatitis, acute, 658, 659, 711, 712*t*, 712
   urine, testing of, 712
Amyloidosis, 132
   nuclear medicine of, 132, *133*
Anaplastic carcinoma, pancreatic, 844, *845*
Anastomosis, biliary-enteric, *328*, 329, 529
   cholangiography, 532, *533*–*535*
     barium reflex, 529, *530*, *531*
     intravenous, 529
   computed tomography (CT), 532, *532*
   plain radiographs, 529, *530*
   scintigraphy, *531*, 531, *532*, 532
   sonography, 529, 531
   for surgical trauma, 579
Anechoic tube, 556
Aneurysm (*see also* Pseudoaneurysm)
   hepatic artery, 134–*136*
   in pancreatitis, 674, 675, 705–706, 708
   splenic artery, 997, 998–1000
Angioblasts, 3
Angiography (*see also* specific type of abscess; Pyogenic liver abscess), 1, *153*, *156*, 156
   of adenoma
     hepatic, of bile duct hamartoma, 193
     pancreatic duct cell, 757
   of angiosarcoma of liver, 262, *263*, 264
   of Budd-Chiari syndrome, 97, *99*, 100, *101*, *102*, 102
   of carcinoma
     gallbladder, 491, 492
     hepatocellular (*see* Angiography, hepatocellular carcinoma)
     pancreatic duct cell (*see* Angiography, pancreatic duct cell carcinoma)

   of Caroli's disease, 367
   of cavernous transformation of portal vein, 91, *92*
   celiac, of annular pancreas, 648
   of cholangiocarcinoma, 542
     intrahepatic, 254, *259*, 260
   of cholecystitis, acute, of complications, *427*, 428
   of cirrhosis, 72–73, 83–87, 148
   of cyst
     hepatic, congenital simple, *172*, *172*
     pancreatic, 751
     splenic, 951
   of cystadenoma and cystadenocarcinoma, biliary, 194, *195*, *198*
   dilatation approach, for catheter placement, 1046, 1047
   of echinococcal disease, hepatic, 167, *170*, 170
   of focal nodular hyperplasia, *184*, *185*, 186, *187*
   of gallbladder and biliary tract, normal, *332*, 332
   of giant cell carcinoma, 838, *838*
   of glycogen storage disease, 39
   of hamartoma, mesenchymal, 43
   of hemangioendothelioma, infantile, 45, *46*, 47
   of hemangioma
     cavernous, 178–181
     splenic, 973
   of hemobilia, 583
   of hepatis, peliosis, 140, *142*
   of hepatoblastoma, 50, *51*, 51
   of hepatocellular carcinoma, 243
     diagnostic features, 237–239
     digital subtraction, 242
     fibrolamellar, 247, *248*, *249*, *250*
     for staging, *223*–*224*, *227*–*228*, *229*–*230*, 239
   of hereditary hemorrhagic telangiectasia, 137, *139*
   of infarction
     hepatic, *144*, 144
     splenic, 1006, *1006*
   infusion, 924
   of insulinoma, 868–869
   of islet cell tumors, nonfunctioning, *883*, 884
   of liver
     of metastatic disease and lymphoma, *203*, 215, 206–220
     of normal liver, 13–15
   of lymphangiomatosis, splenic, 976
   of lymphoma
     pancreatic, 856, *860*
     splenic, 971
   of Mirizzi syndrome, 461
   of mucinous cystic neoplasm, pancreatic duct cell, 761, *763*, 763
   of pancreatic duct cell carcinoma, 814
     accuracy, 835
     differential diagnosis, 828, *829*, *832*–*833*
     findings, *815*, 815–817, *818*–*827*
     prognosis and surgical planning, 828, 829, 834–935

     technique, 814–815, *816*
     venography, 836–837
     venous phase, *815*, 817, *818*–*820*, *827*, 828
   of pancreatitis, 703
     acute, 703
     chronic, 703–709
   of polycystic liver disease, 363
   of portal hypertension, 80
   of pseudocyst, pancreatic, 740, *741*
   radionuclide, 27–28
     of biliary trauma, 581, 582, *584*
   of sarcoma, hepatic, undifferentiated (embryonal), *54*
   of schistosomiasis, 124, 126
   of sickle cell anemia, 1018, *1020*, *1021*
   of spleen, 906–907, *907*, 975
     of asplenia, 925
     of polysplenia, 926
     of wandering spleen, 918
     in splenic artery aneurysm, 998, *1000*
   of splenic vein thrombosis, 1003
   of Thorotrast-induced diseases of liver and spleen, 130
   of trauma
     hepatic, 286, *288*–*289*, 290
     splenic, 934–936
Angioplasty, Gruntzig balloon, 103, 104
Angiosarcoma
   liver, 220, 1015
     clinical findings, 260
     etiology, 260
     pathology, 260, *261*, 261
     radiology, *261*, 261–264
   splenic, 972–973, 1015
   Thorotrast-induced, 126, *128*, 128, 129, 130, 1015
Angiotensin (vasopressin), 814
Annular pancreas (*see* Pancreas, annular)
Antibiotic(s), 606
   for abscess, splenic, 955
   aminoglycoside, 334
   in sphincterotomy, 339
Antibody(ies)
   anti-D, 903
   antimitochondrial, 570
Antral cell hyperplasia, 869, 871
"Antral padding," 769, *771*
Anus, imperforate, 646
Aorta
   celiac axis of, 8, *9*
   in asplenia, 925
   pancreatic, sonography, 631
APUD system, and islet cell tumors, 861
APUDoma, pancreas, treatment, 300
Arterial encasement, in carcinoma of pancreatic duct cell, 815, *816*, 816–817, *818*–*823*
Arterial hepatogram, 13, 15
Arterial occlusion, in carcinoma of pancreatic duct cell, 817, *824*–*826*
Arterial system, abdominal, embryology, 3
Arteriography, arteriogram (*see also* Angiography)
   of adenoma, hepatic, 189, *190*, *191*
   of angiosarcoma, *263*

in Budd-Chiari syndrome, 100, *101*
celiac, of liver, 13, 14–15, 294
for chemotherapy infusion, 294, *295*
of hepatic artery aneurysm, 134, *135, 136*
of portal venous thrombosis, 91
of gastrinoma, *872*, 872, 873
of glucagonoma, 878
of hepatocellular carcinoma, *227, 228, 229*, 234–235, 239
of insulinoma, 868–869
of islet cell tumors, 863–865, *865*
mesenteric, 815
superior, 14–15
of metastatic liver disease, 201, 216, *217, 218*, 219, *219*
of pancreatic duct cell carcinoma, ampullary, 836
in pancreatitis, chronic, 707
of periportal sinusoidal dilatation, 140, *141*
of schistosomiasis, 124
of spleen
of abscess, 958
of accessory spleen, *920*, 920, *921*
of splenic vein thrombosis, 1003
of vipoma, *879*, 879
Arteriohepatic dysplasia, 261
Arteriosclerosis, and splenic artery occlusion, 997, *997*
Arteriovenous fistula, 1000–1001
pancreatic, 643
Arteriovenous shunt, 1011
Artery(ies) (*see also* specific artery)
displacement, in carcinoma of pancreas, 817, *827*
pancreatic
anatomy, computed tomography (CT) of, 638, *639*
in islet cell tumors, 864, *865*
in pancreatitis, 703–704, *705*
Artery of Buhler, 907
Arthralgia, 117
Arthritis, 117
Arthropathy, 117
Artifacts
angiographic, 828, *834*
in computed tomography (CT), 286
liver-spleen scintigraphy, 30
Ascariasis, biliary, 556–558
Ascaris, 552
lumbricoides, 482, 556
Ascites, 72
in cirrhosis, 146
in gallbladder wall thickening, 411, *414*
in pancreatitis, acute, 664
Aseptic necrosis, in pancreatitis, 660
Aspergillus, 40, 994
Aspiration
biopsy
of adenocarcinoma, pancreatic duct cell, 767
of hemangioma, cavernous, 173
transendoscopic, 338
percutaneous
in echinococcal disease, 166
of lymphoma, 206
for pancreatic pseudocyst, 723

in upper abdomen, (*see also* Percutaneous abscess and fluid drainage), 1039
splenic, 913
Asplenia, 922, 923–925
functional, 1016
Atherosclerosis
differentiated from carcinoma of pancreatic duct cell, 828, *831–832*
pancreatitis, chronic, 708
in pancreatitis, chronic, 703
and splenic artery aneurysm, 998
Atherosclerotic aneurysm, in pancreatitis, chronic, 706
Atresia
biliary, 358–359, *359*, 360–361, *361*
intrahepatic (*see* Alagille's syndrome)
related to jaundice, 507, 510
esophageal, 646
Attenuation
in fatty liver, 107, 108, *109*
in pancreatic carcinoma, 786, 787, *790*
values, for metastatic disease of liver, 199
Autoimmune disease, in cirrhosis, 569
Autoimmune markers, in cirrhosis, 570
Avulsion, gallbladder, 589
Azathioprine, 572

B

B-mode sonography, of fatty liver, *107–108*
Bacteremia
in splenic trauma, 935–936
vein, 567, 568
Bacteria (*see also* specific organism)
in abscess, hepatic, 151
Balloon(s), detachable, 1001
Balloon catheter
angioplasty, 610
extraction of common bile duct stones with, 342–344
Balloon dilatation, 346, *346*
for cholangitis, 560
in strictures, biliary, 580
transhepatic, of anastomotic strictures, 532
Bands
echoic, 124
splenic, *922*, 922, 939
"Bare" area, spleen, 909, *911*
Barium, retained, splenic defect from, 904
Barium contrast study, 82, *82*
of abscess, splenic, 957
of carcinoma
gallbladder, 484, *485*
giant cell, 837, 838, *839*
hepatocellular, *222, 223*, 223
of cholecystitis
acalculous, 428
of complications, 424
of cyst
choledochal, 372, *372, 374*
splenic, 949, 951
of fistula, biliary, 447, *448*, 450

of gallstone ileus, *453, 454*, 454–455, 457
gastrointestinal tract, for cystic fibrosis, 652, *653*, 655
of islet cell tumors
functional, 862
nonfunctional, 884
of jaundice, 511, *512–514*
in pancreatitis
acute, *664*, 664–668
chronic, 688–690
in portal hypertension, 82, *82*
of pseudocyst, pancreatic, 725, 729, *729*
Barium enema, of cholecystitis, 410
Barium meal, for schistosomiasis, 124
Barium reflux cholangiography, of anastomoses, biliary-enteric, 529, *530*
Barium sulfate suspension, for computed tomography of pancreas, 633
"Barium on velvet" gallbladder, 328, *328*, 329
Benadryl, 334
Bentoromide test, of pancreatitis, 711
Bezoar, gallstone, *453*
Bicarbonate, pancreatic secretion of, 640, 710
"Big spleen syndrome" (*see* Splenomegaly, tropical)
Bile, 387
composition of, 387–388
calcium, 387
destruction, 571
echogenic, 402, *403*, 404–405
extravasation of, 482
hepatic
T1-weighted spin echo images, 593, *594*
T2-weighted sequence, 593
lakes, 142, 143, *144*, 144
leakage, 542
milk of calcium bile (*see* Milk of calcium bile)
peritonitis, 1080
pigments, 388
precipitation, 380
reflux, 657
salts, 387, 388
white, 446
Bile duct (*see also* Common bile duct; Common duct; Hepatic duct)
anomalies, 353–356
calculi
floating, 526, 528
in nondilated ducts, 523–528
carcinoma
angiography, 542
cholangiography, 537, 540
dilatation, 529, 531
in jaundice, 499–501, 502, 504–510, 511
in papillary stenosis, 573
distensibility, 325
extrahepatic, obstruction, 358–359
hamartoma, 193
intrahepatic, 3
obstruction, 419, *419*
over-distention, 607, *607*

Bile duct (see also Common bile duct; Common duct; Hepatic duct)—continued
  paucity (see Alagille's syndrome)
  proliferation, 184
Bilhemia, 583, 585
Biliary cyst (see Biloma)
Biliary cystadenoma and cystadenocarcinoma, 193, 545
  clinical findings, 193
  pathology, 193–194
  radiology, 194–*198*
Biliary disease, functional, 437
Biliary drainage
  for cholangitis, 549
  in PTC, 607, 608
Biliary-enteric anastomoses (see Anastomoses, biliary-enteric)
Biliary obstruction
  causes, 499
  in gallbladder carcinoma, 491
  hepatocellular carcinoma induced, 241, *241*
  MRI of, 597, *598*
  sphincterotomy for, 341
Biliary obstruction syndrome of the Chinese (see Cholangitis, recurrent pyogenic)
Biliary radiology, interventional (see Interventional biliary radiology)
Biliary surgery, endoscopic
  extraction of common bile stones, 342–345
  retrograde stents and drains, 345–346
  sphincterotomy, 338–342
Biliary tract, 303
  anatomy, 306–308
  biopsy, percutaneous, guided, 1071–1074, *1075*
  cholecystogram of, normal, *310*, 311
  disease, and pancreatitis, 681
  effect of adenocarcinoma of pancreas on, 779, 780–781
  ERCP of (see Endoscopic retrograde cholangiopancreatography)
  histology, 309
  magnetic resonance imaging, (see Magnetic resonance imaging, gallbladder and biliary tract)
  normal imaging (see Gallbladder and biliary tract, normal imaging)
  trauma, 579
    bilhemia, 583, *585*
    biloma, 586–589
    blunt and penetrating, 581–582, *583*, *584*
    hemobilia, 582, 583
    surgical, 579–581
Biliary tree
  bleeding into, 707
  calcification, during cholangiography, 523
  in cirrhosis, 570, *570*
  dilation, 529, 531
    in adenocarcinoma of pancreatic duct cell, 789, 790, *791–792*, 792, 794
    in cholangiocarcinoma, 536

normal, computed tomography (CT) of, 327, *327*
opacification, in ERCP, 337
sarcoma botryoides of, 545, *547*–548
size, related to jaundice, 499–501
Biliary tumors
  benign, 544–545
  malignant (see also Cholangiocarcinoma), 545–548
Bilirubin
  levels
    in adenocarcinoma of pancreas, 779
    in biliary dilatation, 499, 501
    in cirrhosis, 570
    and hepatic artery embolization, 298
    in jaundice, 356–357
  stones, *391*, 393
Biloma (biliary cyst), 586–589
Biopsy (see also Aspiration, biopsy)
  biliary, 610
  brush, 541
  guided percutaneous (see Percutaneous biopsy, guided)
  intraductal forceps, 338
  liver, 568
    of biliary atresia, 359
    blind, 1
    in Budd-Chiari syndrome, 95
    in congenital hepatic fibrosis, 363, 364, 365
    of hemochromatosis, 891
  needle aspiration (see Aspiration, biopsy)
  pancreatic duct, computed tomography (CT) for, 797
  transducer, 1045, *1047*
"Blackwater fever," 992
Bleeding (see also Hemorrhage)
  following guided percutaneous biopsy, 1080
  gastrointestinal, in accessory spleen, 920
  related to angiography, 286, *289*
Blood
  elements, reservoir of, spleen as, 902
  flow rate, through spleen, 902
  supply, spleen, 906
Blood clots, in choledocholithiasis, 528
Blood pool studies
  of cholangiocarcinoma, intrahepatic, 260
  of hemangioma, cavernous, 178
  of hepatocellular carcinoma, 243
  of metastatic disease in the liver, 211
Blood vessel
  amputation, in splenic trauma, 935
  "log-jam" occlusion, 1017
  spleen, 902
Blush
  in islet cell tumor, 863, 865
  splenic, 909
Bone, metastases, from adenocarcinoma of pancreas, 768
Bone marrow, uptake of nuclear medicines, 149
Bone scanning agents, ^{99m}Tc labeled, in hepatocellular carcinoma, 244
Bouveret's syndrome, 454

Bowel (see also Small bowel)
  gas, 57
  inflammatory disease (see Inflammatory bowel disease)
  obstruction
    from pseudocyst, pancreatic, 722–723
    in wandering spleen, 917
Brain, changes, in Wilson's disease, 119–120
Breast tumors, metastases
  to liver, 210, *211*, *219*
  to spleen, 854, *855*–856, 977, *977*, *978*
Bronchography, of asplenia, 925
Brucella
  abortus, 121
  suis, 121
Brucellosis, 121
Bruit, abdominal, in arteriovenous fistula, 1000–1001
Brushes, cytology, 338
Bucrylate, 1001
Budd-Chiari syndrome, 93, 94, 166
  angioplasty and membranes in, 102–104
  clinical features, 94, 95
  pathology, 95
  radiology, 95–102
Bull's eye appearance, 209
  in ascariasis, biliary, 556
"Bull's eye" lesions, 493
Burkitt lymphoma
  pancreatic involvement in, 856, *859*
  splenic involvement in, 968

C

C-loop, 784
Calcification, 281
  in adenoma, pancreatic duct cell, 752, *753*
  in brucellosis, 121
  gallbladder (see Porcelain gallbladder)
  in hemangioma, splenic, 972
  liver
    in cholangitis, 552, *553*
    in echinococcal disease, 166, 167
    in hepatoblastoma, 50
    in hepatocellular carcinoma, 50, 222, 231, 246, 247, *248*
    in metastatic disease, 199, *201*, 203, 214
    related to tuberculosis or histoplasmosis, *123*
  in lymphoma, 207
  in mucinous cystic tumors, 757, *759*
  of pancreas, 601, 702
    in pancreatitis, 698, 699
  plaque-like, 951
  portal vein, 89
  RUQ, 390
  splenic, 1016
    related to tuberculosis or histoplasmosis, *123*
    in sickle cell anemia, *1024*, 1025
Calcium
  content of gallstones, 387

levels, in pancreatitis, 658
Calcium bile (*see* Milk of calcium bile)
Calcium bilirubinate, gallstones, 387, 388
Calcium carbonate
  gallstones, 387
  salts, 439
Calcium ipodate, 328
Calculus, calculi (*see also* Pseudocalculus effect; specific biliary area)
  and adenocarcinoma of pancreas, 782
  extraction, 611, *612*, 612–613, *614*
  common bile duct (*see* Choledocholithiasis)
  in cholangitis, 552, 556
  in choledochal cyst, 383
  differentiated from air, in post-surgical choledochoduodenostomy, 532, *532*
  gallstones (*see* Cholelithiasis)
  jaundice from, 511, *512*
  lucent, *444*
  of pancreatitis, chronic, *684*, 685. *686*, 687, 696
  urinary, 390
Camera(s)
  γ-camera, 313
  SPECT, 32, 33
Canals of Hering, 309
Candida
  albicans, 994
  splenic microabscesses from, 994, 995, *995*
Candidiasis, hepatic, 157–158
Cannulation, in ERCP, failure of, 335, 336, 336t
Capillaries, spleen, 902
Capsule, disruption of, 284
Caput medusa, 73
Carbon dioxide, 640
Carcinoembryonic antigen (CEA), 492, 493
Carcinogen(s), and hepatocellular carcinoma, 220–221
Carcinoid tumors
  biliary, 545, *545*
  gallbladder, 492
  pancreatic islet cell, 880
Carcinoma (*see also* Adenocarcinoma; specific body area)
  of acinar cell origin, 851–852
  ampullary (*see* Ampulla of Vater, carcinoma)
  biliary, 523, 602–*603*
    primary, 610
  cholangiocarcinoma (*see* Cholangiocarcinoma)
  cholangiohepatocellular, 231
  differentiated from cholangitis, 562
  ERCP of, 337
  gallbladder, 425, 439, 483, 536, 602, 603
    angiography, *491*, 492
    cholangiography, *490*, 491–492
    cholecystography, oral, 484, *484*
    clinical findings, 483–484

computed tomography (CT), 489, *489*, 491
  in situ, 479, 481, 484
  MRI of, 595, *596*
  oat cell, 492
  pathology, 484
  plain film and barium studies, 484, *485*
  polypoid intraluminal, 488
  sonography, 484–489, *489*
gastric, 828
  afferent loop obstruction for, 497, *498*
hepatocellular (*see* Hepatocellular carcinoma)
mucoepidermoid (*see* Adenosquamous cancer)
pancreatic (*see also* Pancreatic duct cell, carcinoma), 499, 536, *537*, 545, *546*, 603–604, 646
  diagnosis, 699, 700
  infantile, *853*, 853
  and pancreatitis, 658, 676–677, 702 708
  splenic vascular changes in, 1011–1012
  papillary, 536
  polypoid, *525*, 528, 535, *604*
Cardiac anomalies
  in asplenia, 924
  in polysplenia, 926
Cardiac features, of hemochromatosis, 117
Caroli's disease
  distinguished from hepatic fibrosis, congenital, 364
  evaluation, 510
  interventional radiology, 605, 606
  in neonate, 362, *367*, 367, *368–370*, *371*
Castor oil, polyoxyethylene hydrogenated, 337
Catheter
  angiographic, 612
  balloon (*see* Balloon catheter)
  for chemotherapy infusion, 294
  French Cobra, 608
  French Cope, 608, *609*
  6.5 French Rim, 611
  -induced spasm, 828
  in percutaneous abscess drainage placement, 1046, 1047
    securing of, 1047, 1048, 1049
  Teflon, 338, 608
  toposcopic, 347, *348*
Catheterization
  angiographic
    for hepatocellular carcinoma staging, 239
    for pancreatic angiography, 814
  pancreatic venous system, 836–837
Caudate lobe
  in Budd-Chiari syndrome, 95, 97
  in cirrhosis, 78, *78*, 79, *80*
  papillary process, 22
Cavernous hemangioma, 43, 173
  pathology, 173–174
  radiology, 174–181

Cavography, of Budd-Chiari syndrome, 97, *99*, 100
CCK (*see* Cholecystokinin)
CDDP (*see* Cis-diamminedichloroplatinum)
Celiac angiography, 13, 14–15
Celiac axis
  of aorta, 8, *9*
  involvement in pancreatic carcinoma, 816
  thickening, in adenocarcinoma of pancreas, 794, *796*, 797
  variations in, *10*, *11*
"Celiac" disease (*see also* Cystic fibrosis, 651
Celiac injections, 13, 14, 15
Celiac trunk, branches, 906
Cell cycle, drugs effecting, 296
Cephalosporin, 339
Ceruloplasmin, and Wilson's disease, 119
Chaga's disease, 992
"Chemoembolization," 300
Chemotherapy, chemotherapeutic agents contact time with tumor, 293–294
  for hepatic neoplasms
    dose-response curve, 293
    intra-arterial infusion (*see also* Transcatheter management), 293
    local effectiveness, 293
  types and descriptions, 295–298
Chest
  pancreatic pseudocyst entry into, 723, *725*, 729
  pancreaticopleural fistula, 720
Chest film
  of abscess, splenic, 956
  in asplenia, 924–925
  in hereditary hemorrhagic telangiectasia, 137
  of pancreatitis, acute, 659
  of trauma, hepatic, 284
Children (*see also* Liver, congenital disorders and pediatric neoplasms)
  jaundiced, 507, 510
  trauma, 291
Chinese, biliary obstruction of (*see* Cholangitis, recurrent pyogenic)
Chlorambucil, 572
Chloroma, 209, 215
Chloroquine, 159
Cholangiocarcinoma, 261, 535, 543
  of biliary tree, MRI of, 597
  clinical findings, 535
  diffuse sclerosing, 540, *541*, 559
  gallbladder, 499
  intrahepatic, 231, 253, 537
    clinical findings, 253
    magnetic resonance imaging, 275, *276*, *277*
    pathology, 253–254
    radiology, 254–260
    sclerosing cholangitis type, 253, 254
  pathology, 536
  radiology, 536
    angiography, 542
    cholangiography, 538, *539–541*

Cholangiocarcinoma—*continued*
  computed tomography, 536, 537, *538*
  interventional, 602–*603*
  nuclear medicine, 541, *542*
  ultrasound, 536, *537*
  sclerosing, differentiated from cholangitis, 562
  surgical considerations, 543
  Thorotrast-induced, 128, 129–130
Cholangiography, cholangiogram
  of adenocarcinoma, pancreatic duct cell, 603, *604*, 802, 803, *804–810*
    of ampullary carcinoma, *809*, *810*, 810
  of adenoma, pancreatic duct cell, 752
  of anastomoses, biliary-enteric, 529, *530*, 532, *533–535*
  of ascariasis, biliary, 557, *558*, 558
  barium, 329
  of bile duct tumors, benign, 544, 545
  of biliary tract trauma, surgical, 580
  of biloma, 587
  of carcinoma, gallbladder, *490*, 491–492
  of Caroli's disease, 367, *368*
  of cholangiocarcinoma, intrahepatic, 254
  of cholangitis
    acute, 549
    primary sclerosing, 560, *562*, 562, 563, *564*, 564
    recurrent pyogenic, 556
  of choledocholithiasis, 523–524
  of cirrhosis, 87–88
    primary biliary, 571, *571*
  of cystadenoma and cystadenocarcinoma, biliary, 194, *198*
  of cystic fibrosis, 39, 40
  direct
    of bilhemia, 585
    of choledochocele, *384*, 385
    of choledochal cyst, *372*, 373, *374*, *375*, *377*, *378*, *379*
    of embryonal rhabdomyosarcoma, *548*, 548
  of echinococcal disease, 167, *170*
  of fibrotic papillary stenosis, *575*, 575
  of gallbladder and biliary tract, 303, 328–329
    ampullary sphincters and the pseudocalculus effect, 331
    normal, 329–331
  of hemobilia, 582
  of hepatocellular carcinoma, 241–*242*
  interventional aspects, 542–543
  intravenous, 333
    of anastomoses, biliary-enteric, 529
    of choledochal cyst, 372, *378*
    of cholecystitis, 410–411
    of cholelithiasis, 394, 397, *397*
    of gallbladder and biliary tract, 303
  of jaundice, 497, 501, 502, 504
  of metastatic melanoma in gallbladder, 493, *493*
  of Mirizzi syndrome, 457, 461
  of mucinous cystic neoplasm, pancreatic duct cell, 763
  operative, of choledochal cyst, 373, *379*
  of pancreatitis
    acute, 699, 670
    chronic, *694*, *695*, 697, *697*, *698*, 698
  of polycystic liver disease, 363
  of pseudocyst, pancreatic, *739*, 740
  T-tube
    of biliary anomalies, 355, *355*
    for stone removal, 611, *612*, 612–613
Cholangiohepatitis, oriental (*see* Cholangitis recurrent pyogenic)
Cholangiopancreatography (*see* Endoscopic retrograde cholangiopancreatography)
Cholangitis, (*see also* Pericholangitis), 388, 536, 602
  acute (ascending), 549, 563
    and ERCP, 334
    radiology, 549–551
  following sphincterotomy, 339
  primary sclerosing, 559, 601
    in cirrhosis, 571
    clinical findings, 559–560
    differential diagnosis, 562–564
    nuclear medicine, 564
    pathology, 560
    and pericholangitis, 567
    radiology, 560–562, 564, *565*, *566*
  recurrent pyogenic, 552–556
  sclerosing type of cholangiocarcinoma, 253, 254
  secondary sclerosing, 559, 563, 601
Cholecystectomy, 389
  for cholangitis, 409
  for cholangiocarcinoma, 543
  complications (*see* Choledocholithiasis)
  and endoscopic sphincterotomy, 339
  for milk of calcium bile, 442
  for pancreatitis, 657
  post-cholecystectomy common duct, 324–325
Cholecystitis, 39, 357, 479
  acalculous, 428–431
    chronic, 430
  acute, 434, 447, 484
    in children, related to jaundice, 507, 510
    clinical findings, 409
    complications, 423–428
    computed tomography, 422
    gastrointestinal examination, contrast, 409–410
    hepatobiliary scintigraphy, 416–422
    metastatic melanoma presenting as, *494*, 494–495
    MRI of, 595
    oral cholecystography and intravenous cholangiography, 410–411
    plain film, 409
    "rule out" acute cholecystitis, 415
    ultrasound, 411–416
  chronic, 420, 423, 447, 435–439, 452, 487
    acalculous, 393
    complications (*see* Mirizzi syndrome)
    MRI of, 599
  complicated, 489
  emphysematous, 423, 431–435, 439
  gangrenous, 419–420, 424, *424*
  hemorrhagic, 423
  traumatic, 589
  xanthogranulomatous, *482*, 482, 489
Cholecystography
  gallbladder and biliary tract
    of anomalies, 351
    of ascariasis, 557, *558*, 558
    of carcinoma, 484, *484*
    of hydrops, 446
    of metastatic melanoma, 493, *493*
    of Mirizzi syndrome, 457
    normal, 303, *310*, 310, 311
  intravenous, of gallstone ileus, *453*, *454*, 454–455, 457
  oral
    of adenocarcinoma of pancreas, 792
    of Caroli's disease, 365
    in cholecystitis, acute, 410–411
    in cholecystoses, hyperplastic, 463–472, *472*
    of choledochal cyst, 372
    of cholelithiasis, 389, 390, 391–394, *395–396*, 399, 401
    of porcelain gallbladder, 439, 441
Cholecystokinin (pancreozymin)
  action on biliary tract, 325
  in cholecystitis
    acalculous, 430
    acute, 416, 417
  and cholelithiasis diagnosis, 393
  pancreozymin-secretin test, 710
  release, 641
Cholecystopaque, 401, 423
Cholecystoses
  hyperplastic, 423, 463, 487
    adenomyomatosis, *475*, 476–477, 477
    clinical findings, 472, *473*
    computed tomography, 477
    pathology and oral cholecystography, 463–472, *472*
    scintigraphy, hepatobiliary, 477
    sonography, cholesterolosis, 472, *474*, 474, 475
  MRI of, 595, *596*
  sulfatide, *482*, 483
Cholecystosonography, for cholelithiasis, 398–399
  of floating stones, 401–402, 403
  of sludge, 402, *403*, 404–405
  of type I gallstone, 399–400
  of type II gallstone, 400, 401
  of type III gallstone, 400, 401
Cholecystostomy
  for cholecystitis, 409
  for gallstones, 389
  percutaneous, 615, 1053

Choledochal cyst
  evaluation, 510
  interventional radiology, 605
  in neonate and infant, 362, 371–380
    in jaundice, 357–358
    type I, 381
    type II, 371, 381, *382*
    type III, 371, 383–395
Choledochocele, 605
  neonatal, 383–385
Choledochoduodenal junction,
    embryology, 305
Choledochoduodenostomy, 344
Choledochoenterostomy, 358
Choledochojejunostomy, 344
  Roux-en Y, 371
Choledocholithiasis, 419, 499, 515
  and biliary obstruction, 782, 783
  cholangiography, 523–529
  clinical findings, 515
  computed tomography (CT), 519–523
  differentiated from
    cholangiocarcinoma, 536
    papillary stenosis, 572–573
  ERCP for, 334
  extraction, 342–344
    ERCP for, 342–344
  interventional radiology of, 605
  papillary stenosis associated with, 573
  pathology, 515
  sonography, 515–519
Cholelithiasis, 39, 387, 431, 507
  in cholangitis, 552
  classical gallstones, 399, 399–400
  coexisting with adenomyomatosis,
    472, *473*, *476*
  complications, 447
  confused with cholecystitis,
    emphysematous, 434–435
  floating stones, 401, *402*, 402
  in gallbladder carcinoma, 483, 488,
    491
  and gallbladder hyperplasia, 479
  gallstone ileus (*see* Gallstone ileus)
  movement around gallbladder, 472
  natural history and clinical
    considerations, 388–389
  in neonatal and infant jaundice, 357
  obstructing, 388
  and pancreatitis, acute, 657
  papillary stenosis associated with, 573
  pathophysiology, 387–388
  and porcelain gallbladder, 439, *440*
  radiology, 390
    cholecystography, oral, 391–394,
      395–396
    computed tomography (CT), 406,
      407, 407–409
    plain film, 390, *391*
    sonography (*see*
      Cholecystosonography)
  silent stones, 388
  treatment, 389
Choledcintigraphy
  of cholecystitis
    acalculous, 430
    acute, 411, *412–413*, 416–417, *417*,
      418, 419*t*, 420–421, 421*t*

  chronic, 435, *436*, 436–437
  ^{99m}Tc-DISIDA, *314*, 417, *417*
  ^{99m}Tc-IDA, of complications, 426,
    426
  of jaundice, 505, 506, 507*t*, 507, *508*
Cholestasis
  biochemical, asymptomatic, 567
  in cirrhosis, 570
  intrahepatic, 506
    of neonatal hepatitis, 359
  of pregnancy, 319
Cholesterol
  polyp, gallbladder, 472, *472*, 478, 481,
    482, 488
  stones, 387–388, 393, 394
Cholesterolosis, 468, *471*, 482
  morphologic form, 468, *471*, 472
  polypoid form, 472, *472*
  sonography, 472, *474*
Cholestyramine, 560
Cholograffin, 373, *377*
Chondrocalcinosis, 117
Chromium-51, 903
Cigarette smoking, and
    adenocarcinoma, of pancreatic
    duct cell, 765
Cilia, abnormal, related to polysplenia,
    926
Cirrhosis (*see also* Portal hypertension),
    37, 69, 94, 116, 121
  angiographic characteristics, 83–*87*
  biliary (*see also* Cirrhosis, primary
    biliary), 70, 270, 271
    due to cystic fibrosis, 39, *40*, 40
  cholangiography in, 87–88
  cholestatic, 70
  computed tomography (CT) features,
    78–82
  differentiated from cholecystitis,
    acute, 421
  effect on stomach, *63*, 63
  etiology, 69, 70*t*, 116
  and hepatocellular carcinoma, 220,
    221, 229, 231
  Hereditary hemorrhagic telangiectasia
    with, 137
  interventional radiology of, 605
  magnetic resonance imaging of, 268,
    270
  metastases occurring in, 210
  nuclear medicine of, 149
  pathogenesis, 69
  pathology, 69, 70
  pathophysiology, 70
  primary biliary, 559, 569
    course, 571
    clinical findings, 569–570
    differentiated from cholangitis, 564
    experimental modalities, 572, 573
    pathology, 570
    radiology, 570–571, *571*
    treatment, 571, 572*t*
  radionuclide scanning, 28
  scintigraphic changes in, 146–148
  ultrasound of, 70–78
Cis-diamminedichloroplatinum (CDDP),
    296, 297, 300
Clips, surgical, 519, 580

Clonorchis sinensis, 482, 552, 557
Clostridium
  perfringens, 431
  welchii, 431
Coagulopathy, and percutaneous biopsy,
  guided, 1079
Coils, steel, 998
Colectomy, and pericholangitis, 568
Colic biliary, 388
Colitis, ulcerative, 559
Collagen diseases, 569
Collateral pathways, in portal
    hypertension, 80, *81*
Colloid (*see also* Sulfur-colloid scan)
  hepatic reticuloendothelial clearance
    of, 149
Colon
  abnormalities, in pancreatitis
    acute, 665, 666, 667, 668
    chronic, 690
  adenocarcinoma, metastasis to liver,
    204–205
  carcinoma, 775, 776, 777
    metastasis to liver, 200, *202*, 203,
      210, *212*, *214*, *215*, *218*
  cut-off sign, in pancreatitis, acute,
    661, 661, 662
  displacement, by pancreatic
    pseudocyst, 729, *729*
  hepatic flexure of, 60
    displacement, 65–66
  transverse, in pancreatitis, acute,
    662
Common bile duct (*see also* Common
    duct)
  in adenocarcinoma
    of liver, 792, 794
    of pancreas, 766, *767*
  anatomy, 306, *307*, 307
    vascular and lymphatic, 308
  carcinoma, 828
  cholangiography, 330
  cholecystogram of, *310*, 311, *311*
  computed tomography, 327, *327*, 328,
    633
  dilatation
    cystic, 605
    in jaundice, plain film and barium
      studies, 511, *513–514*
  diverticulum/type II choledochal cyst,
    381, *382*
  duplication, 356
  fistulas, 447
  histology, 309
  obstruction, 536
  reflux of pancreatic secretions into,
    371
  stones (*see* Choledocholithiasis)
  sonography, 625, 627, 631, 632
  villous tumors, 545
Common duct (*see also* Biliary duct;
    Common hepatic duct; Hepatic
    duct)
  and adenocarcinoma of pancreas,
    782
  cancer, 536, 537, 542
  dilatation, 501
  normal, MRI of, *595*

Common duct (*see also* Biliary duct; Common hepatic duct; Hepatic duct)—*continued*
  obstruction, in jaundice, scintigraphy, 505, 507
  sonography, 321, *321, 322,* 322
    post-cholecystectomy, 324–325
    of size of normal duct, 323–324
    using fatty meal, 325
  stones, jaundice from, 511, *512*
  trauma, 581, *583*
Common hepatic artery, 625
Common hepatic duct (*see also* Biliary duct; Common duct; Hepatic duct)
  computed tomography (CT), 327, *327,* 328
  cystadenoma, *198*
Computed tomography (CT), 1
  of abscess
    amebic, 163, *163*
    pancreatic, *718,* 718, *719*
    percutaneous, 1041
    in percutaneous abscess drainage, 1045, *1048*
    pyogenic, 151, 154–156
    splenic, *960,* 960–965
    upper abdominal, 1042
  of adenocarcinoma of pancreatic duct cell, 603, 797, 835
    of ampullary carcinoma, 802, *803*
    computed pancreatography, 799, 901
    differentiating carcinoma and pancreatitis, 798, 799, *800–801*
    findings, 785–794
    of microadenocarcinoma, 843, *843*
    staging, 793, 794–797, *798, 799*
    technique, 783–785
    vs. other methods, 801
  of adenoma
    hepatic, 189, *190, 191*
    pancreatic duct cell, 752, *754, 755*
  of aneurysm
    hepatic artery, 134, *135*
    splenic artery, 998
  of angiosarcoma, of liver, 262, *262*
  of ascariasis, biliary, 558
  of biliary-enteric anastomoses, 532, *532*
  of biloma, 587, *587,* 588
  for biopsy, tumor, 610
  of Budd-Chiari syndrome, 97, *99, 101*
  of candidiasis, hepatic, *158,* 158
  of carcinoma
    gallbladder, 489, *489,* 491
    hepatocellular (*see* Computed tomography (CT), of hepatocellular carcinoma)
  of Caroli's disease, 365, 367, *368*
  of cholangiocarcinoma, 536, 537, *538*
    intrahepatic, 254, *256, 257, 258, 259*
  of cholangitis
    acute, 549
    primary sclerosing, 560, *563*
    recurrent pyogenic, 552, *553,* 556
  of cholecystitis
    acalculous, 431
    acute, 423
    of complications, 426, *427,* 428
    emphysematous, 435
    hyperplastic, 477
  of choledochocele, *384,* 385
  of cholelithiasis, 393, 407–409, 512–523
    chronic, *438,* 439
  of cirrhosis, 78–79, *80*
    in portal hypertension, 79, 80, *81*
  contrast enhanced, of portal venous thrombosis, 91
  of cyst
    choledochal, 372, 373, *374, 379,* 381
    liver, congenital simple, 172, *172*
    pancreatic, 749
    splenic, 955
  of cystadenoma and cystadenocarcinoma, biliary, 194, *195,* 196
  of echinococcal disease, 167, *169,* 170
  of embryonal rhabdomyosarcoma, 548
  emission (*see* Emission computed tomography)
  of epithelial neoplasms, pancreatic, 846, *849, 850, 851*
  of fat replacement of pancreas, 746, *746*
  of fibrosis, hepatic, congenital, 365, *366*
  of fistula
    biliary, 450, *451*
    pancreatic, 722
  of focal nodular hyperplasia, *184, 185,* 186
  of gallbladder and biliary tract, 303, *326,* 327–328
    of anomalies, 351, 353
    of porcelain gallbladder, 441–442
  of gallstone ileus, *456,* 457
  of gas, portal venous, 145, 146, *146*
  of gastrinoma, 871–872, *873, 874*-876
  of giant cell carcinoma, 837
  of glucagonoma, 877, *877*
  of glycogen storage disease, 39
  of hamartoma
    mesenchymal, 43
    splenic, 975
  of hemangioendothelioma, infantile, 45, *46*
  of hemangioma
    cavernous, 174, *175,* 176, *178,* 181, *182*
    splenic, *972,* 972, 973
  of hemobilia, 582, *583*
  of hemochromatosis, 117–118, 891
  of hepatitis, 116
  of hepatoblastoma, *50,* 50
  of hepatocellular carcinoma, *224,* 231–233, 239
    dynamic CT, 234–235, 239, 240
    fibrolamellar, 246, 247, *250, 251, 252,* 252
    Lipiodol-CT studies, 243
    for staging, 233–234
  of hydrops of gallbladder, 446, *447*
  of infarction
    hepatic, *143,* 144
    splenic, 1007, 1008–1009
  of insulinoma, *866, 867,* 867–868
  of islet cell tumor, 862, 863, 893
    nonfunctioning, *883,* 884
  of jaundice, 497, 502–504
    in children, 507
    compared to sonography, 499
  of liver
    compared to magnetic resonance imaging, 281
    of fatty liver, 106–107, 108, *109,* 109, *112, 113*
    of normal liver, 22, 23, *23, 24, 25, 26, 26*
    of polycystic liver disease, 363
  of lymphangiomatosis, splenic, *976,* 976
  of lymphoma
    pancreatic, 856, *857–859*
    splenic, 966, *967–969,* 971, 1036, 1038
  of metastatic disease of the liver, 199–204, 213, 219
  of lymphoma, 207, *208, 209,* 209–210
  of milk of calcium bile, 442
  of Mirizzi syndrome, 457, *459–460,* 461
  of mucinous cystic neoplasm, pancreatic duct cell, 759–761, *762,* 763
  of pancreas
    of anatomy, normal, 632–633
    annular, 646
    of arterial veins and lymphatic anatomy, *637,* 638–639
    of ductal anatomy, 639
    technique of examination, 633–637, 638
  of pancreaticoblastoma, 853, *853*
  of pancreatitis
    acute, 676–680, 1057
    chronic, 696, 699, *700,* 700–702
  of percutaneous biopsy, guided, upper abdomen, 1067t, 1067, 1071, 1072–1073, 1074, *1075,* 1075, *1076,* 1076, *1077,* 1077, 1079
  of pseudocyst, pancreatic, 723, 730, 732, *734,* 734, 735
  role in Thorotrast-induced diseases of liver and spleen, 130–132
  of rupture, splenic, 944, 993
  of sarcoma, hepatic, undifferentiated (embryonal), 54
  scanner, 633
  of schistosomiasis, 124
  of Schwachman-Diamond syndrome, 650, *651*
  of shunt, splenorenal, 1011
  of sickle cell anemia, 1018, 1020, *1023, 1025,* 1025–1027
  single photon emission (*see* Single photon emission computed tomography)
  of spleen, 908, 909, *910, 911, 912*
    of accessory spleen, *919,* 920, 921
    of asplenia, 925
    experimental contrast agents, 909, 911, 912

for measurement, 913
of metastasis, *979, 980*–981
of polysplenia, *926,* 926, 927
of splenomegaly, 994
of splenosis, 943
of wandering spleen, 918, *919,* 919
of splenic vein thrombosis, 1003
of stenosis, papillary, 573, *574*
of stricture, biliary, benign, 601
of trauma
   gallbladder, 590, 591–592
   hepatic, 284, *285,* 286, *287, 288,* 290, 291
   pancreatic, 743, *743, 744,* 745
   splenic, 913, 931, 933, 936, 937–941
   surgical, to biliary tract, 579
of vipoma, *878,* 878, 879
in Wilson's disease, 119–120
Congenital disorders
  gallbladder and biliary tract
   atresia, biliary, 358–359, *359*
   bile duct paucity (Alagille's syndrome), 361, *361*
   biliary tree, interventional radiology, 605–606
   Caroli's disease, 362, 365, 367, *368–370,* 371
   choledochal cyst (*see* choledochal cyst)
   hepatic fibrosis, 362, 363, 364–365, *366, 367*
   hepatitis, neonate, 358, *359,* 360
   jaundice in neonate and infant, 356–358, 361
   polycystic liver disease, 362, 363, *364*
  pancreas
   annular pancreas, 645–650
   cystic fibrosis, 651–655
   pancreas divisum, 643–645
   Schwachman-Diamond syndrome, 650–651
  spleen
   accessory spleen, 919–921
   asplenia, 923–925
   polysplenia, 925–927
   splenic-gonadal fusion, 922–923
   wandering spleen, 917–919
Congestive heart failure (CHF), 94
  in hemangioendothelioma, infantile, 44, 45, *47,* 48
Connective tissue
  pancreas, tumors, 854
  spleen, 902
Contraceptives, oral
  and adenoma, hepatic, 188, 189, *191*
  and focal nodular hyperplasia, 183
  and hepatocellular carcinoma, 220
  infarction from, hepatic, 142
  periportal sinusoidal dilatation from, 140
Contrast enhancement
  in abscess, amebic, 163
  for CT of spleen, 909, *912*
  in gallbladder carcinoma, 491
  of pancreas, 784
Contrast examination
  of adenocarcinoma, pancreatic duct cell, 768

barium (*see* Barium contrast examination)
of gallbladder ileus, 452, *453, 454,* 454–455, 457
gastrointestinal (*see* Gastrointestinal contrast study)
of schistosomiasis, 124
of trauma, pancreatic, *742,* 743
Contrast material
  barium (*see* Barium)
  cholecystographic and cholangiographic, *26,* 26, 520
  entry of biliary tract, 607
  for hepatic computed tomography (CT)
   cholecystographic and cholangiographic, *26,* 26
   for dynamic scanning, 23, 26
   intravenous, 22, 23, *24, 25*
   oral, 22
   for metastatic disease of liver, 203, *203,* 204
  for pancreatic computed tomography (CT), 633–634
  punctate lakes of, 178
  for splenic computed tomography (CT), 909, 911, 912
  water-soluble iodinated, 199, 200
Contusion
  gallbladder, 589, 592
  intrasplenic, 937
  liver, 286
  pancreatic, 743
Copper
  accumulated, 119
  deposition, in liver, 70
  disease states, magnetic resonance imaging of, 270–271
  levels, in cirrhosis, 569
  metabolism, inherited disorders of, 118 (*see also* Wilson's disease)
Coronary ligament, 4, 5, *5*
Coronary vein
  catheterization, 613
  in portal hypertension, 73
Creatinine, clearance, preinfusion, 296
Creatorrhea, 652
Crohn's disease, 388, 559, 944
"Crow-foot" sign, 390, *392*
Cruveilhier-Baumgarten syndrome, 73
CT (*see* Computed tomography)
Cullen's sign, 658
Cycasin, 220
Cyclosporin-A, 572
Cyst(s)
  bile-filled, 142, 143, *144,* 144
  biliary (*see* Biloma)
  choledochal (*see* Choledochal cyst)
  false (*see* Pseudocyst)
  liver, 499, 1051–1053, *1054*
   from amebic abscess, 160
   congenital simple, 171–172
   hydatid (*see* Echinococcal disease)
   mesenchymal hamartoma, 41–43
   peliotic, 261
   puncture, 1051–1053, *1054*
   simple, MRI of, 271, *271*

pancreatic
  of duct cell origin (*see* Pancreatic duct cell, neoplasm, cystic)
  hemorrhagic, 838, *839*
  multiple true, 749, *750*
  pathology, *750,* 750
  radiology, 750–751
  solitary true, 749, 750
  true (congenital), 749, 750, *750*
splenic, 947, 994, 1020
  aspiration, 913
  clinical findings, 947, 949
  pathogenesis and pathology, *948, 949,* 949, 950, 951
  post-traumatic, 947, 949
  roentgen findings, *949, 950, 951,* 951–955
  true, differentiated form false, 950, 951
Cystadenocarcinoma
  acinar cell, 852
  biliary (*see* Biliary cystadenoma and cystadenocarcinoma)
  pancreatic duct cell, 757
Cystadenoma
  biliary (*see* Biliary cystadenoma and cystadenocarcinoma)
  pancreatic, 752, 757
Cystic artery, 8, 307, 308
Cystic diseases, echinococcal, 1079
Cystic duct
  abnormalities, in cholangitis, 562, *564,* 565
  anatomy, *306,* 306
  dilated, 421
  duplication, 356
  obstruction, 428, 439
  stones
   and cholecystitis, *413*
   implantation in, (*see also* Mirizzi syndrome), 457
Cystic fibrosis, 39, 388, 651
  clinical findings, 652
  fatty replacement of pancreas in, *891*
  and pancreatitis, chronic, 681, 682, 685, *687,* 687
  pathology, 39, 651–652, *652*
  radiology, 39–40, 652, *653*–655
  symptomatology, clinical, 39
Cystic malformation, hepatobiliary
  Caroli's disease (*see* Caroli's disease)
  choledochal cyst (*see* Choledochal cyst)
  hepatic fibrosis congenital (*see* Fibrosis, hepatic)
  polycystic liver disease (*see* Polycystic liver disease)
Cystic neoplasm
  metastases to liver, 216
  pancreatic (*see* epithelial neoplasms, pancreatic)
Cystic regions, sonolucent, 779
Cystography, percutaneous, of cystadenoma and cystadenocarcinoma, biliary, 194, *197*
Cystojejunostomy, roux-en-y, 1003, 1004
Cytology, endoscopic, 338

D

Demerol, 606
Densitometry, CT, in pyogenic liver abscess, 154, 155
Density(ies), in pancreatitis, acute, 663
Diabetes
  and adenocarcinoma, pancreatic duct cell, 765
  and gallstone surgery, 389
Diaphragm
  bulge, from hepatocellular carcinoma, 221, 222
  disruption, from amebic abscess, 160, 163
  effect of hepatomegaly on, 61–62
Diatrizoic acid salts, 911
Diazepam (Valium), 337, 600
DIFF-QUIK, 1065
Diffuse diseases
  liver (see Liver, diffuse diseases)
  spleen (see Spleen, diffuse diseases)
Diisopropyl-IDA compound, for gallbladder and biliary tract imaging
  false positive, in cholecystitis, 412
  radiation exposure, 313t, 314
Diisopropylphenylcarbomoyl iminodiacetic acid (Hepatolite), 416
Dilatation
  biliary stenosis, 611
  periportal sinusoidal (see Periportal sinusoidal dilatation)
Dilator, 607, 608
Dimethyl-1-triazeno imidazole carboximide (DTIC), 296
DISIDA (see Diisopropyl-IDA compound)
Diverticulum, diverticula
  in cholangitis, 562, 564, 565
  choledochal, 605
  common bile duct, 381, 382
  intramural, in adenomyomatosis, 474
  -like collection, in gallstone ileus, 452, 454
  Meckel's, 390
DNA, effect of chemotherapeutic agents on, 295, 296
Doppler scanning, 72
  of portal venous thrombosis, 90, 91
Dose-response curve, of chemotherapeutic agents, 293
"Double-arc" shadow, 400, 401
"Double bubble" appearance, in annular pancreas, 646, 647
"Double density sign," 932, 933
"Double dose," 393
"Double duct sign," in adenocarcinoma of pancreas, 811, 812
"Double target sign," 155
Doxorubicin (Adriamycin), 293, 295, 296, 297
Drain
  APD, 611
  endoscopic retrograde, 345–346
Drainage
  biliary (see Biliary drainage)
  percutaneous, of abscess (see also Percutaneous abscess and fluid drainage)
  of spleen, 962, 964, 965
Drainage tubes, for abscess, 1041
DTIC (see Dimethyl-1-triazeno imidazole carboximide)
Dubin-Johnson syndrome, 506
Duct of Santorini (see Pancreas divisum)
  sonography, 627
Duct of Wirsung, 619 (see also Pancreas divisum)
  in pancreatitis, chronic, 693, 695
  sonography, 627
  stenosis, 696
Ductuloinsular tumors, 854
Duodenobiliary reflux, 341, 573
Duodenostomy, 648
Duodenography
  in annular pancreas, 646, 648, 649
  of choledochal cyst, 383, 383, 385
  of embryonal rhabdomyosarcoma, 548
Duodenojejunal junction, 623
Duodenojejunostomy, 648
Duodenoscope, 338
Duodenum, 317
  abnormality, in pancreatitis
    acute, 665, 666
    chronic, 688, 690, 690
  in adenocarcinoma, pancreatic duct cell, 768, 769, 770, 771, 772, 784, 794
  anatomy, 311, 312
  displacement
    by liver, 64, 64
    by pancreatic pseudocyst, 726–728, 729
  distention, 778
  fistulas, 447
  ileus, in pancreatitis, acute, 663
  post-bulbar, 446, 447
  sonographic appearance, 632
  varices, in portal hypertension, 82
Dynamic scanning, 23, 26, 26
  high resolution survey, 23
Dyskinesia, biliary, 338

E

Echinococcal (hydatid) disease, cyst, 170, 949
  clinical findings, 164–166
  epidemiology, 164
  hepatic alveolar, 167, 169, 170
  pathology, 166
  and percutaneous biopsy, guided, 1079
  radiology, 166–167, 168, 169, 170
Echinococcus
  granulosus, 164, 167, 170, 994
  multilocularis, 167, 994
  splenomegaly from, 993, 994
Echo (see Hypoechoic center)
  in abscess
    amebic, 162
    pyogenic liver, 152, 153, 154
  in candidiasis, hepatic, 157, 158
  "comet-tail," 519
  in gas, portal venous, 145
  pattern, in hepatocellular carcinoma, 226, 229
  in porcelain gallbladder, 439
  spin (see Spin echo)
  texture, in cirrhosis, 72
Echodensities, in gallbladder carcinoma, 484
Echogenicity
  of abscess, splenic, 959
  in angiosarcoma of the liver, 262
  in choledocholithiasis, 516
  of liver, 627
    in hepatocellular carcinoma, 223, 224–225
    in metastatic disease, 205, 205
    in pancreatic hemorrhage, 674
    of pancreatic parenchyma, 627
Echoic bands, in schistosomiasis, 124
Ectasia
  of main pancreatic duct, 695, 696
  splenic artery, 997
Edge detection, 31
Elastase, 657
Electrolyte, secretion, pancreatic, 640
Electron microscopy, 1081
Emboli, hepatic parenchyma, 284
Embolization, 290, 293
  Gelfoam, 134
  hepatic arterial, 298–300, 362
  splenic artery, 1001, 1004
  steel-coil, 936
  transcatheter therapeutic, 1007
Emission computer tomography, of liver, 31–32
  positron emission tomography, 32
  single photon emission computed tomography (see also Single photon emission computed tomography), 32–35
Encephalopathy, hepatic, 1011
Endocarditis, infective, and splenic rupture, 944
Endoprosthesis, 345, 345, 346
  biliary, placement, 610–611
Endoscopic retrograde cholangiography, of jaundice, 504
Endoscopic retrograde cholangiopancreatography (ERCP) (see also Cholangiography), 333
  of adenocarcinoma, of pancreas, 796, 801, 810–813, 835
  of anastomoses, biliary-enteric, 532, 535, 535
  of bilhemia, 585
  of cholangiocarcinoma, 540, 541, 542
  of cholangitis
    primary sclerosing, 559, 560, 564
    recurrent pyogenic, 556
  of choledochal cyst, 373, 379
  of choledocholithiasis, 519
  of cirrhosis, primary biliary, 570
  of cystadenoma and cystadenocarcinoma, biliary, 194, 197
  experimental uses
    per oral transducer pancreatochlangioscopy, 347, 347
    toposcopic catheter, 347, 348
  of fistula, pancreatic, 720, 722
  of jaundice, 497, 506
  of mucinous cystic neoplasm, pancreatic duct cell, 763, 764
  in normal patient, 330–331

of pancreas
  anatomy, 634
  annular, 646, 648, *649*
  of fat replacement, 746
  of pancreas divisum, 643, *644*
  in pancreatic function tests, 710, 711
  of pseudocyst, pancreatic, 736–740
of pancreatitis
  acute, 669, *670*, 674
  chronic, 691*t*, 691–696, 699, 711
procedure
  contraindications, 334–335
  endoscopic and radiologic, 336, 337
  failure of cannulation, 335, *336*, 336*t*
  indications, 333–334
  vs. PTC, 335, 336
of stenosis, papillary, 573, *574*, *575*, 575, 576, 578
success rate, 329, 330
as therapeutic procedure, 338
  endoscopic biliary surgery, 338–346
  endoscopic cytology and fluid collection, 338
  sphincter of Oddi manometry, 338
of trauma, pancreatic, *744*, *745*, 745
Endoscopic technique, in ERCP, 336, 337
Endoscopy, in thrombosis, splenic vein, 1002
Entamoeba
  coli, 552
  histolytica, 158, 159
Enterobacteriaceae, 151
Enzymes
  elastolytic, 1057
  lipolytic, 1057
  liver, in pancreatitis, 658
  pancreatic, 640–641, 711–713
  proteolytic, 1057
EOE-13 (*see* Ethionized oil emulsion-13)
Eosinophil count, in echinococcal disease, 166
Epidermoid cyst, 947
Epinephrine, 814
Epithelial cells, gastric, in heterotopias, 481
Epithelial neoplasm, pancreatic, solid and papillary
  clinical findings, 846
  pathology, 846, *847*
  radiology, 846, *848–851*
Epithelium
  cuboidal, 171
  pancreatic duct, 639, 640
ERCP(*see* Endoscopic retrograde cholangiopancreatography)
"Erlenmeyer flask" deformity, 987
Erythroleukemia, splenomegaly from, 986, *988*
Escherichia coli, 151, 335, 431, 549
  bacteremia, 559
Esophageal varices (*see also* Gastroesophageal varices), 82, *82*, 233, 372, 705
  in splenic vein thrombosis, 1003
Esophagus
  abnormalities, in pancreatitis, acute, 664

displacement, by pancreatic pseudocyst, *725*, 729
involvement in adenocarcinoma of pancreas, 768
Ethionized oil emulsion-13 (EOE-13), 909, 911
for lymphoma
  diagnosis, 208, 209
  splenic, 968, 971, 1036, 1038
for metastatic disease of the liver, 203, *203*, 204, 219
side effects, 208
Extrahepatic duct
  cholangiography, 330
  dilatation
    in adenocarcinoma of liver, 794
    in cholangitis, 552
    in jaundice, CT of, 502, 504
  embryology, 305
  histology, 309
  involvement in cholangitis, 560
  trauma, 579, 581
Extravasation, 580
  in splenic trauma, 934

F

Falciform ligament, 4, *5*, 17
Fasciola hepatica, 482, 552, 557
Fasting, and cholecystitis scintigraphy, 421
Fat
  abnormal deposits, 119
  in adenocarcinoma of pancreas, *793*, 794, *795*
  extraperitoneal, 7
  hepatic, 149
  necrosis, in pancreatitis, 658, *659*, 660
  and pancreas echogenicity, 627, *629*
  peripancreatic, 316
  periportal, 8
  replacement of pancreas, 746, *746*, *747*
  MRI of, 889, *891*
  surrounding spleen, 909
Fatty change
  diffuse, in fatty liver, 111
  focal (*see* Focal fatty change)
  in hemochromatosis, 117
Fatty infiltration of liver (steatosis)
  in cirrhosis, 78, 88
  magnetic resonance imaging, 268–270
  in Wilson's disease, 120
Fatty liver, 105
  acute, 105
  clinical disorders associated with, 105, 105*t*
  clinical features, 105
  pathogenesis, 105
  radiological imaging in, 105–108
  significance of, 111–*114*
  "silent," 105, 111
  unusual features and radiologic significance, 108–114
Fatty meal
  and cholelithiasis diagnosis, 393
  in common duct sonography, 325
Feeding tube, French, 611
Fentanyl, 606
Ferritin, 270

α-Fetoprotein (*see* Alpha-fetoprotein)
Fibroma, biliary, 544
Fibromuscular hyperplasia, 997
Fibromyosarcoma, 53
Fibrosarcoma, 52
Fibrosis
  hepatic, 70, 121, 262
    clay-pipestem, 124
    congenital, 362, 363, 364–365, *366*
    hepatoportal, 91, 92, 93, *94*
    magnetic resonance imaging, 270
    periportal (*see also* Schistosomiasis), 124, *125*
  pancreatic, 696–697, 698
  in pericholangitis, 567
  perisinusoidal, 70
  Thorotrast-induced, 128, 129
Fibroxanthogranulomatous inflammation, 481, 482
Filariasis, 482
Filters, Ramp-Hanning, 33
Fissures
  gallbladder
    from gallstones, 390
    main interlobar, 316–317, *319*
  hepatic
    computed tomography of, 22, *24*
    ultrasonography of, 17, 20, *20–21*
  spleen, 904
Fistula
  anterioportal, 610
  arteriovenous, 1000–1001
    angiography of, 286, *289*
    in HHT, 137, *138*
    pancreatic, 643
  biliary, 447–451, 579
  biliohepatic vein, 583, 585
  biliovenous, 608
  hepato-bronchial, 159
  mesenteric, 93
  pancreatic, 334, 720–722
  pancreatic-enteric, 720, *721*, 721–722
  tracheoesophageal, 646
Fistulogram, for surgical trauma to biliary tract, 579
Flagyl (*see* Metronidazole)
"Flashing artery" sign, 707
"Fleckmilz," 1005
Flexure, hepatic (*see also* Colon, hepatic flexure of), 32, *58*, 60
"Floating-water lily" sign, 994
"Floppy duct," 499, 501
Floxuridine (FUDR), 296
Fluid
  collection, 287
    in abscess, pancreatic, 717, 718, *719*
    in ERCP, 338
    in pancreatitis, acute, 678, *679*, 679
    pancreatic/peripancreatic, 722
    pericholecystic, 1053, 1056
    in trauma, splenic, 937
  drainage (*see* Percutaneous abscess and fluid drainage)
Fluoroscopy, 82
  for percutaneous upper abdominal biopsy, 1066, 1067*t*, 1067
5-Fluorouracil (5FU), 296, 297
  intra-abdominal administration, 293
FNH (*see* Focal nodular hyperplasia)

Focal fatty change, in fatty liver, 108, 109, *110*, 111, *111*
Focal fatty infiltration, in liver, magnetic resonance imaging, 268
Focal nodular hyperplasia (FNH), 183, 252
　clinical findings, 183
　distinguished from hepatic adenoma, 189
　magnetic resonance imaging, 271, *273*
　pathology, 183–184, *184*
　radiology, 184, *185–188*
Focal nodular lesions, in lymphoma, 207
Fractures, pancreatic, 743, *744*, 745
"Frostberg 3 sign," 770, *772*
5-FU (*see* 5-Fluorouracil)
FUDR (*see* floxuridine)

G

G-cell, antral, hyperplasia, 869
Gallbladder, 3, 303
　absence, 794
　agenesis, 351
　anatomy, 305–306, 316–317, *319*
　anomalies, 351–356
　ascariasis, 557
　bifid, 353, *354*
　cholecystitis (*see* Cholecystitis)
　congenital diseases (*see* Congenital diseases, gallbladder and biliary tract)
　dilatation, 501
　distention, in cholecystitis, *412*, 414, *415*
　duplication, 351, 353, *354*
　ectopia, 317
　effect of hepatomegaly on, 64, *64*, 65, 65
　embryology, 305
　enlarged, 770, 772
　ERCP of (*see* Endoscopic retrograde cholangiopancreatography)
　fasting, MRI of, 593, *594*
　fossa, 419
　herniation, 353
　histology, 309
　"hydropic," 357
　hydrops of, 446, *446*, 447
　hyperexcretion, 463
　hypoplastic or rudimentary, 351
　left-sided, 353, *355*
　magnetic resonance imaging (*see* Magnetic resonance imaging)
　normal (*see also* Gallbladder and biliary tract, normal imaging)
　　cholecystogram of, *310*, 311
　porcelain, 439–449
　perforation, 424, 425, 426
　in pregnancy, 317, 319
　puncture, 1053, *1055*–1057
　small, differentiated from cholecystitis, acute, 421
　stasis, 388
　strawberry, 468, *471*
　trauma, 589
　　diagnosis, 589
　　radiology, *590, 591*, 591–592
　　treatment, 592
　triple, 351, 353
　tumors (*see also* specific type)
　　benign, 478–483
　　malignant, 492–493
　　secondary, 493–495
　visualization, in cholecystitis, 418
　volvulus, 353
　wall
　　sonolucency, 414, *415*
　　thickening, 411, 414, *414*, 423, 487, 494
"Gallbladder attack," 388
Gallbladder and biliary tract, normal imaging
　angiography, *332*, 332
　cholangiography, 328–331
　computed tomography, 326–328
　normal scan, 315, 315t
　patient preparation, 315
　pharmacology, 313, 314
　radiation exposure, 313t, 314
　radiopharmaceuticals, 312–313
　sonography, 316–325
Gallium, gallium-67 citrate scan, 28, 31
　of abscess
　　amebic, 159
　　pyogenic liver, 155
　　splenic, *958*, 958, 964
　　upper abdominal, 1042
　of angiosarcoma of the liver, 262
　of candidiasis, hepatic, 157, 158
　of cholangiocarcinoma, intrahepatic, 260
　of hepatoblastoma, 49
　of hepatocellular carcinoma, 243, *244*
　of metastatic disease of the liver, 211
　of lymphoma and leukemia, 213
　of pancreatitis, acute, 669
　of spleen, 904
　of tuberculosis, miliary, 121, *121*
Gallstone(s) (*see* cholelithiasis)
Gallstone ileus, 389, 437, 447, 448, 451
　radiology, 451–457
Gamma camera, 932
　Anger, 315
Gangrenous cholecystitis, 424, *424*
Gap phase, drugs acting on, 296
Gas
　in abscess
　　hepatic, 153, *154*, 154
　　pancreatic, 715, 717, 718
　　splenic, 959, 961
　bowel, 57
　bubbles, pericystic, 166
　in cholecystitis, emphysematous, 431, 434, *434*, 435
　collection, pericholecystic, 426, *427*, 428
　duodenal, 321
　in fistula, biliary, 447, *450*
　in gallstone ileus, 452
　portal venous, 145–*146*
"Gasless abdomen," 663
Gastrectomy
　Billroth II, Sohma Papillotome following, 342, 344
　subtotal, and ERCP, 335, *336*
Gastric abnormalities, in pancreatitis
　acute, *664*, 664–665, *665*
　chronic, 688, *689*
Gastric carcinoma, differentiated from pancreatic carcinoma, 828
Gastric ulcers, penetrating into spleen, 1028
Gastric varices
　in portal hypertension, 82, *83*
　in splenic vein thrombosis, 1002
Gastricae, areae, 871
Gastrin, 869
　cells producing, 869
Gastrinoma, 863, 884
　MRI of, *895*
　and Zollinger-Ellison syndrome, 869
　　clinical findings, 869
　　pathology, 869
　　radiology, *870*–873, *874–876*
Gastroduodenal artery, 625
　ultrasonography of, 15
Gastroepiploic artery, right, 625
Gastroepiploic varices, 73
Gastroesophageal varices
　in portal hypertension, 73, *75*, 82, *82*
Gastrohepatic ligament, 5, *5*
Gastrointestinal abnormalities, in polysplenia, 925, 926
Gastrointestinal bleeding, in pancreatitis, chronic, 706, 707–708
Gastrointestinal contrast examination
　of abscess, pancreatic, *715*, 715
　of cysts, pancreatic, *750*, 750–751
　of cholecystitis, acute, 409–410
Gastrointestinal tract
　splenosis, 943
　tumors, metastasis to liver, 210, 211, 214
Gastrosplenic ligament, 900, *901*
Gaucher's disease, 986, 987, *991*, *992*, 992, 998
Gelfoam, 290, 298, 608, 707, 936
　embolization, 134
　plug, 300
Genitourinary anomalies, in asplenia, 923
Genitourinary tract, tumors, metastasis to liver, 210, 211
Gentamicin, 606
Gerota's fascia, 909
　thickening of, 794
Gestation, function of spleen in, 902
Giant cell carcinoma
　epulis-osteoid type, 637
　pleomorphic, 837–841, *892*
Glucagon, 457
　use in computed tomography, 784
Glucagonoma, 873
　clinical findings, 873
　pathology, 873
　radiology, 873, *876–877*, 878
Glucagonoma syndrome, and islet cell tumors, 861, 862t
Glucocerebroside, 986, 987
Glycogen, abnormal deposits of, 119
Glycogen storage disease, 37, 38, 60
　radiology, *37, 38*, 38–39
　Type I (*see* von Gierke's disease)
Gonad-spleen fusion, 922–923
Granular cells, myoblastoma, 544–545
Granule(s), secretory, 640–641

Granulocytopenia, 297
Granuloma (*see also* Granulomatous disease), 571
 in candidiasis, hepatic, 157
 epithelioid, 570
 hepatic, 207
 tuberculosis, 120, 121
Granulomatous diseases of the liver, 120
 in brucellosis, 121
 chronic, 151
  of childhood, 40–41
 in histoplasmosis, 121, *123*
 nuclear medicine of, 149
 pathology, 120
 sarcoidosis, 121, *122*, *123*
 splenomegaly from, 994, *994*
 in tuberculosis, miliary, 120–121, *121*
Granulomatous lesions, gallbladder, 482
Grey Turner's sign, 658

H

HAE, (*see* Hepatic artery, embolization)
Halo, 205, *206*
Hamartoma
 bile duct, 193
 mesenchymal, 41–43, 51, 54
 splenic, 973–975
Hank's balanced salt solution, 1065
Hartmann's pouch, 306
Haustral row, inferior, 777
Hemangioendothelioma, 51
 infantile, 43
  clinical features, 43–44
  pathology, 44–45
  radiology, 45–48
Hemangioma, 44, 45, 239, 943
 cavernous (*see* Cavernous hemangioma)
 distinguished from adenoma, hepatic, 189
 magnetic resonance imaging, 271, 272, *273*, *274*
 percutaneous guided biopsy, 1074–1075
 splenic, 971–972
Hemangiosarcoma (*see* Angiosarcoma, of the liver)
Hematocrit, in PTC, 608
Hematologic abnormalities, in hamartoma, splenic, 973
Hematologic disease, in splenosis, 942
Hematoma
 intrahepatic, 284, *285*
  angiography of, 286
  computed tomography of, 286, *287*
  nuclear medicine of, 290
 perisplenic, 1009
 splenic, 57, 944
  angiography, *934*, *935*, 935
  computed tomography, 937, *937*, *938*, *939*, *940*, *941*
  MRI of, 1033
  plain film of, 932, *932*
  sonography of, 936, *936*, 937
  transition between false cyst, *952*, 955
 subcapsular, 284
  angiography of, 286, *288*

 nuclear medicine, 290
Hematopoiesis, extramedullary, 261
Hemidiaphragm
 effect of liver size on, 61–62
 right, in amebic abscess, *160*, 160, 162, *162*, *163*
Hemiperitoneum, 831, 832
 spontaneous, 130
Hemobilia, 134, 582, 583, 611
 in cholangiocarcinoma, 542
 in cholecystitis, 423
 in choledocholithiasis, 528
 post-PTC, 608, *610*, 610
Hemochromatosis, 116
 clinical features, 116–117
 MRI of, 891–892
 pathology, 117
 primary, 116
 radiology, 117–118
 secondary, 116
 spleen density from, 1015
Hemoperitoneum, 183
 in adenoma, hepatic, 188–189
 in angiosarcoma, 260
 computed tomography of, 285
 plain film of, 284
Hemorrhage (*see also* Bleeding)
 in angiosarcoma of the liver, 262
 echogenicity from, 205
 in focal nodular hyperplasia, 186
 pancreatic, 634
 in pancreatitis
  acute, 658, 674, *675*, 676, 679
  chronic, 706, 707
 from sphincterotomy, endoscopic, 342
Hemosiderosis, 116, *270*, *1036*
Hemostat, biliary tract trauma from, 579
"Hemosuccus pancreaticus," 936
Heparin, 297
 use during chemotherapy infusion, 294, 295
Hepatic artery, 8
 anatomy classification, 294, 294t
 aneurysm, 134–*136*
 cavernous hemangioma, 178, *179*, 180
 common, 8, *9*, 625
 computed tomography of, 633
 embolization, 298–300
 infusion technique, 815
 injury, 283
 left, 8, 10
 middle, 8
 pericholecystic, 419
 proper, 8, *9*, 625
 right, 8
 selective injection into, for chemotherapy, 294
 sonography, 15, 17, *19*, 321, *321*, 322, *322*
Hepatic duct(s) (*see also* Common hepatic duct; Common duct)
 aberrant (accessory), 355, *355*
 anatomy, 306
 cholangiocarcinoma, 536
 obstruction (*see also* Mirizzi syndrome), 499
Hepatic system, left, obstructed, drainage of, 611, *611*
Hepatic vein(s) (*see also* specific vein)

 branching, loss of, 85
 catheterization of, 84
 computed tomography of, 22
 hepatocellular carcinoma invasion of, 229, *230*
 injury, 283
 magnetic resonance imaging of, 265
 occlusion of, 95
  in Budd-Chiari syndrome, 100, *101*
 radionuclide scanning, 29
 thrombosis, in Budd-Chiari syndrome, 101, 102, *103*
 ultrasound of, 20–21
 webs, in Budd-Chiari syndrome, 102, 103, 104
 wedged pressure, 84, 85, *87*
Hepatitis, 115
 acute, 115, 116
 alcoholic, 69
 amebic, 159
 chronic, 116
  active, 115, 119
  hepatitis B virus infection, and hepatocellular carcinoma, 220
  persistent, 115
 computed tomography of, 116
 differentiated from cholecystitis, acute, 421
 neonatal, 358, *359*, 360
  distinguished from biliary atresia, 359, *359*, 360, *360*, 361
 peliosis, 139, 262
  clinical findings, 140
  pathology, 140
  radiology, 140, *142*
  Thorotrast-induced, 128, 130
 ultrasound of, 115–116
 viral, 69
  in gallbladder wall thickening, 411, 414, *415*
 nuclear medicine scan, 148–149
Hepatitis B surface antigen, and ERCP, 334
Hepatoblastoma, 48–49
 clinical features, 49
 cystic, 50
 pathology, 49
 radiology, 49–51
Hepatocellular carcinoma, 49, 51, 220, 221, 261, 536, 602, 603
 angiography, *236*, 237–240
  digital subtraction, 242
 calcifications, 50
 cholangiography, 241–*242*
 clinical findings, 221
 comparison of sulfur colloid scan and IDA scan in, 149
 computed tomography, 231–235
  lipiodol, 243
 development, in hemochromatosis, 117
 diffusing infiltrative, 242, *243*
 distinguished from
  adenoma, hepatic, 189
  cavernous hemangioma, 178
  metastases, 149
 echo texture, 72
 etiology and pathogenesis, 220–221
 fibrolamellar, 185, 231, 246

Hepatocellular carcinoma,
  fibrolamellar—*continued*
  clinical findings, 246
  pathology, 246, 247
  radiology, 246, 247–252
  focal fatty infiltration simulating, *111,
    112*
  frank carcinoma, 221
  hypervascular, *238*
  hypovascular, 15, 240
  icteric, 221
  magnetic resonance imaging, of, 271,
    272, *274*, 275
  metastatic, 221, 913
  multicentric, 239
  nuclear medicine for, 243–246
  occult, 221
  pathology, 221, 222
  radiology, *221*, 222–223
  sclerosing, 231, 246, 247
  staging
    with angiography, *227–228, 229–
      230*, 239
    with ultrasound and CT, 233–234
  Thorotrast-associated, 126, 128, 129
  ultrasound of, 223–231
Hepatocellular degeneration (*see*
  Wilson's disease)
Hepatocellular disease, hepatic uptake
  in, 505, *506*
Hepatocyte, 6–7
  hyperplasia of, 260
  injury, 105
  nodules, 184
  thorium uptake by, 128
Hepatogram
  arterial, 13, 15
  of Budd-Chiari syndrome, 97, *101,
    102*
  mixed, 14–15
  for pancreatic carcinoma metastasis,
    815, *816*
  portal, 14, 15
    of metastatic liver disease, 216, *218*
  Thorotrast, *127*
  types, relevance to space-occupying
    disease, 13–15
Hepatolite (*see*
  Diisopropylphenylcarbamoyl
  iminodiacetic acid)
Hepatoma (*see also* Hepatocellular
  carcinoma)
  treatment, 296
Hepatomegaly, 37, 38, 986
  in abscess, pyogenic, 152
  in candidiasis, 157
  in cirrhosis, 78, 571
  conditions causing, 56, 56*t*, 57*t*
  conditions simulating, 56, 57*t*, *57*
  effect on other structures, 56, 60–68
  in hemochromatosis, 117
  in hepatitis
    peliosis, 140
    viral, 148
  in lymphoma, 207
  in metastatic disease of the liver, 210
  radiography, 55–56, *58–60*
Hepatosplenomegaly, 992, 995
Hepatotomography
  of abscess, amebic, 159

intravenous, in echinococcal disease, 166
Herniation
  diaphragmatic, 1028
  gallbladder, 353
  liver, *58–59*
Heterotopias
  gallbladder, 481
  thyroid and adrenal, 481
Heterozygous trait disease (HbAS), 1017
HHT (*see* Osler-Weber-Rendu disease)
HIDA (*see* Technetium 99m-
  dimethylacetanilido-
  iminodiacetate)
Hilus, hilum
  cholangiocarcinoma, 541, *542*
  hepatic, injuries to, 284
  spleen, 904, *906*
  nodes, in lymphoma, 967, 968
Histoplasma capsulatum, 121
Histoplasmosis, 121, *123*
  splenomegaly from, 994, *994*
Hodgkin's disease, 206, 207
  copper concentrations in, 270
  pancreatic involvement in, 856
  splenic involvement in, 965, 967, 968,
    1015
    MRI of, 1033, 1036
  ultrasound of, 208, 209
Homozygous trait disease (HbAS), 1017
Hot spots, 30
  in angiosarcoma of the liver, 262
  in focal nodular hyperplasia, 186
  in metastatic disease in the liver, 211,
    211
Hounsfield numbers, 1015
Hounsfield units (HU), 22
HU (*see* Hounsfield units)
Hydatid disease (*see* Echinococcal
  disease)
Hydrop(s), 388
  of gallbladder, 446, *446*, 447
Hygroma, cystic, 975
Hyperalimentation-induced liver disease,
  360
Hyperamylasemia, 713
  causes, 334, 712*t*
Hypercalcemia, 681
  pancreatitis in, 658
Hyperemia, passive, 986, *989*
Hyperlipidemia, pancreatitis in, 658
Hyperparathyroidism, pancreatitis in,
  658, 685
Hypersecretion-obstructive theory, of
  pancreatitis, acute, 657
Hypersplenism, 986, 1016
  embolic therapy for, 1001
Hypertriglyceridemia, 658
Hypervascularity, in pancreatitis,
  chronic, 705, 708
Hypoechoic center, in metastatic
  disease in the liver, 205
Hypoglycemia
  in insulinoma, 866
  and islet cell tumor, 861, 862*t*

I

IDA (*see* Iminodiacetic acid)
Ileus
  duodenal, 663
  gallstone (*see* Gallstone ileus)

meconium, 651, 655
Iminodiacetic acid (IDA) (*see also*
  Diisopropyl-IDA compound;
  Technetium-99m-IDA)
  for adenoma, hepatic, 192
  derivatives, for gallbladder and biliary
    tract imaging, 313, 314
  for hepatocellular disease, 244, 245
    compared to sulfur colloid scan,
      149
  for jaundice, neonatal, 510
Immune response, spleen's role in, 902
Immunoglobulin G (IgG), [131]I-
  Antiferritin, for hepatocellular
  carcinoma, 244, 246
Immunoglobulin M (IgM), levels, in
  cirrhosis, 570
Indium-111 white blood cell scan, 31
  for abscess
    differentiation, 155, 156
    upper abdomen, 1042, 1043
  in pancreatitis, acute, 669
Infant (*see* Neonate and infant)
Infarction
  hepatic, 142
    angiography, *144*, 144
    clinical findings, 142
    computed tomography (CT), *143*,
      144
    nuclear medicine, 144
    pathology, 142
    ultrasound, 143, *143*, 144
  pancreatic, *299*
  splenic, *299*, 917, 1005–1009, 1020,
    1025, 1059
Infection
  bacterial, in pancreatitis, acute, 658
  from guided percutaneous biopsy,
    1080
  post-splenectomy, 942
  from PTC, 610
  splenic (*see also* Splenomegaly,
    infections causing)
    aspiration of, 913
Inferior vena cava, 5
  in asplenia, 925
  in Budd-Chiari syndrome, 96, 97, 99,
    100, 102, 103, 104
  hepatocellular carcinoma invasion of,
    229, *230*
  occlusion of, 95
  in polysplenia, 926
Inflammation, in pericholangitis, 567
Inflammatory disease
  bowel
    differentiated from cholangitis, 562,
      563
    pericholangitis associated with (*see*
      Pericholangitis)
    primary sclerosing cholangitis
      associated with, 559
  pancreas, MRI of, 889–*891*
Infusion, intra-arterial (*see also*
  Transcatheter management), 293
Infusion hepatic angiography (IHA), of
  hepatocellular carcinoma, 239,
    240
Injury (*see* Trauma)
Insulinoma, 863, 884
  clinical findings, 865–866

pathology, 866
radiology, *866*, 866–869
Interlobular bile ducts, histology, 309
Interventional biliary radiology, 601
  for cholangitis, 564
  for choledocholithiasis, 605
  of cirrhosis, 605
  of congenital anomalies, 605, *606*
  of strictures
    benign, 601, *602*
    malignant, 602–604, *605*
    post-traumatic, 583
Intraarterial digital subtraction arteriography (IA-DSA), of hepatocellular carcinoma, 242
Intrahepatic ducts
  anatomy, 307, *308*
  biliary obstruction and dilatation, 488, *488*, 489
  in carcinoma of pancreatic duct cell, 828
  cholangiography, 331
  dilatation, 799
    in adenocarcinoma of pancreas, 792, 794
    in cholangitis, 552–556
    in jaundice, 502
  embryology, 305
  histology, 309
  involvement in cholangitis, 560
  MRI of, 593
Iodine, 203, 204
Iodine-131 imaging
  -Antiferritin IgG, for hepatocellular carcinoma, 244, 246
  -diiodofluorescein, of gallbladder and biliary tract, 312
  of metastatic diseases in the liver, 211
  -rose bengal, of gallbladder and biliary tract, 313
  -rose bengal excretion test, of jaundice, neonatal, 507, 510
Iopanoic acid (*see* Telepaque)
Iridium-192 wires, 543
Iron, overload (*see also* Hemochromatosis), 116
  hepatic, magnetic resonance imaging of, 270, *270*
Ischemia, bowel, secondary to pancreatitis, chronic, 707–708
Islet(s), pancreas (*see also* Islet of Langerhans), 639
  development of, 619, *620*
Islet cells, 619
  granules, 854
  hyperplasia, 639
  tumors, 851, 861
    carcinoma, MRI of, 893
    carcinoid, 880, *881*
    functional, 861–865
    gastrinoma and Zollinger-Ellison syndrome, 869–863, 874–876
    glucagonoma, 873, *876*, 877, *877*, 878
    insulinoma, 865–869
    multihormonal, 880
    nesidioblastosis, 880, 882, 884
    nonfunctioning, *882*, *883*, 884
    pathological features, common, 861
    somatostatinoma, 880

vipoma, *878*, 878–879
Islets of Langerhans (*see also* Islet cell), 619
  in cystic fibrosis, 652, *652*
Isoamylase, pancreatic, 712
Ivalon (*see* Polyvinyl alcohol foam)
IVC (*see* Cholangiography, intravenous)

J
Jaundice, 799
  in abscess, pyrogenic liver, 152
  in adenocarcinoma of pancreas, 779
  in cholangiocarcinoma, 535
  cholestatic, 507
  in cirrhosis, primary biliary, 569, 571
  computed tomography of, 502–504
  in cystadenoma and cystadenocarcinoma, biliary, 193
  from hepatic artery aneurysm, 134
  in hepatitis, peliosis, 140
  in neonate and infant, 356–358, *361*
  noncholestatic, 357
  nonobstructive, radiology, 497
  obstructive, radiology, 497, *498*
  plain film and barium studies, 511, *512*–514
  scintigraphy of, 504–507
  of pediatric jaundice, 507, 510
  sonography
    accuracy of, 499
    discrepencies between degree of jaundice and duct size, 494–501
  from surgical trauma, 579

K
Kayser-Fleisher ring, 118, 119, 120
Kidney
  anomalies, in polysplenia, 926
  disease, polycystic, 363, 364–365, *366*, 749
  effect on hepatomegaly on, 60, 66–68
  transplant patient, pancreatitis in, 658
Kinevac (*see* Sincalide)
Klatskin tumor, 536, 602
  cholangiography, 537, *538*, *539*
  surgical considerations, 543
  ultrasound, 536
Kupffer cells, 3, 27
  access of sulfur colloid to, 30
  in cirrhosis, 146, 147
  displacement of, 290
  in fatty liver, 109
  in histoplasmosis, 121
  iron deposition in, 117
  nodules, 184
  sarcoma (*see* Angiosarcoma, of the liver)
  thorium dioxide in, 127, 128
Kwashiorkor, 682, 688, *688*

L
L-asparaginase, 109
Laceration
  gallbladder, 589, 592
  hepatic, 283–284
    angiography, 286, 290
    computed tomography (CT), 286, *287*
    sonography of, 284
    treatment, 283
  splenic, 937

computed tomography (CT) of, *938*–*939*
Lactoferrin, 681
Ladd's bands, 645, 646
Laparoscopy, cyst puncture, 949
Laparotomies, exploratory, 1039
LaPlace's law, 499
Larmor frequency, 265
Lavage, peritoneal, 283, 286
LDH, levels, from hepatic artery embolization, 298
Left anterior oblique (LAO) supine filming, 82
Left upper quadrant, trauma, 284
Leiomyosarcoma, 52, 53
Leptospira icterohemorrhagicae, 122
Leptospirosis, 121, 122, 123
Lesser omentum (*see* Gastrohepatic ligament)
Leukemia
  associated with splenomegaly, 985, 986, *987*, 988
  hepatic involvement in, 209
    cholangiography of, 215, *215*, *216*
    nuclear medicine in, 213
  pancreatic involvement in, 856
  and splenic rupture, 944
Leukocyte, indium 111-labeled (*see* Indium-111 white blood cells)
Leukocytosis
  in abscess, amebic, 158–159
  in cholecystitis, 409
  in echinococcal disease, 166
Leukodystrophy, 482, 483
Life Care Pump, *295*
Ligament(s) (*see also* specific ligament)
  gastrohepatic, 5, *5*
  intrahepatic, ultrasound of, 17, 20, 21
  spleen, 900, *901*
Ligamentum teres, computed tomography (CT) of, 22, *23*
Ligamentum venosum, fissure for, ultrasound of, 17, 20, *21*
Ligature, biliary tract trauma from, 579
Limy bile (*see* Milk of calcium bile)
Linear defects, in splenic trauma, 936
Lienorenal ligament, 900
Lipase
  pancreatic, 712
  serum levels
    following ERCP, 334–335
    in pancreatitis, acute, 658
    testing, 712–713
Lipid, liver content, rapid appearance and disappearance, 109, 111
Lipid storage disease, 936 (*see also* Gaucher's disease; Niemann-Pick disease)
Lipoid contrast material, 909
Lipiodol-CT studies, of hepatocellular carcinoma, 243
Lipolysis, 659, 660
Lipolytic enzymes, 641
Lipoprotein, 105
Liposarcoma, 52
Liposomes, for CT of spleen, 911
Lithiasis, pancreatic, 685, 687
Lithocolic acid, 568
Lithotripsy, for common bile duct stone extraction, 342

Liver, 1
  anatomic variants, 35–36
  anatomy, 4–6
  angiography, normal, 13–15
  biopsy, percutaneous, 1071–1074, *1075*, 1081
  chronic diseases, 567
  computed tomography (CT) of, 784
    emission computed tomography (CT), 31–35
    of normal liver, 22–27
    of size, 26
  congenital disorders and pediatric neoplasms, 37–68
    chronic granulomatous disease of childhood, 40–41
    cystic fibrosis, 39
    focal nodular hyperplasia, 183, 184, *187*
    glycogen storage disease, 37–39
    hepatoblastoma, 48–51
    hepatocellular carcinoma (*see also* Hepatocellular carcinoma), 220–221, 222, 223, 246
    infantile hemangioendothelioma, 43–48
    mesenchymal hamartoma, 41–43
    sarcoma, undifferentiated (embryonal), 52–54
    Wilson's disease, (*see* Wilson's disease)
  diffuse diseases
    alcoholic (*see* alcoholic, liver disease)
    amyloidosis, 132–*133*
    cirrhosis (*see* Cirrhosis)
    fatty liver (*see* Fatty liver)
    granulomatous (*see* Granulomatous diseases, of the liver)
    hemochromatosis (*see* Hemochromatosis)
    hepatitis (*see* Hepatitis)
    hepatocellular, differentiated from metastases, 149
    leptospirosis, 121, 122, 123
    magnetic resonance imaging of, 267–271
    metabolic granulomatous infiltration, 149
    nuclear medicine features, 146–149
    schistosomiasis, 123–126
    Wilson's disease (*see* Wilson's disease)
  dysfunction, in pericholangitis, 566–567
  embryology, 3–4
  fibrosis, congenital, 363–364, 365, *366*
  focal diseases
    amebic abscess, 158–164
    adenoma, 188–192, 193
    candidiasis, 157–158
    carcinoma, hepatocellular (*see* Hepatocellular carcinoma)
    cyst(s), congenital simple, 171–172
    cystadenocarcinoma, biliary, 193–199
    echinococcal, 164–170
    focal nodular hyperplasia, 183–188
    hemangioma, cavernous, 173–*182*
    metastatic (*see* Metastatic diseases, in the liver)
    pyogenic abscess, 151–156
  function, in HHT, 137
  hemangioma, percutaneous guided biopsy, 1074–1075
  histology, 6–7
  infiltrative diseases, nuclear medicine of, 149
  intrinsic disease, differentiated from extrahepatic masses, 30–31
  invasion, by gallbladder carcinoma, 491, 492
  lobes (*see also* Caudate lobe)
    in amebic abscess, 159
    in cirrhosis, 78, *78*, 79, *80*
    congenital abscence, 35, *36*, 36
    enlarged, 904
    hypertrophy, *103*
    Riedel's (*see* Riedel's lobe)
    ultrasound of, 20, *20*
  magnetic resonance imaging of (*see* Magnetic resonance imaging)
  nodules, 35
    parenchymal, 67, 70
    regenerating, 72, *72*, 78, 85
    transformation, 91, 93
  plain film examination, 7–8
  polycystic disease, 362, 363, *364*
  puncture, 1051–1053, *1054*
  radiation injury to, 149, *150*
  radionuclide imaging, 27–31
    of shape, 29
    of size, 29
  size, 55
    in cirrhosis, 70
    decrease, conditions causing, 56
    enlargement (*see* Hepatomegaly)
    measurement, 29, 55
  Thorotrast-induced diseases (*see* Thorotrast-induced diseases in liver and spleen)
  transplantation
    for cholangitis, 560
    jaundice following, 507, *509*
    trauma, 151, 283
    clinical findings, 283
    mortality rate from, 283
    nuclear medicine, 290–291
    pathology, 283–284
    radiology, 284–291
    treatment, 283
  tumors
    computed tomography (CT) of, 26
    conditions mimicking, 56, 57*t*
    radionuclide imaging, 28
    transcatheter management (*see* Transcatheter management of hepatic neoplasms)
  ultrasound of, 15–21, 632
    of size, 21
  vascular anatomy, 8–13
  vascular diseases, 134
    aneurysm, hepatic artery, 134–*136*
    gas, portal venous, 145–146
    infarction, 142–144
    Osler-Weber-Rendu disease (hereditary hemorrhagic telangiectasia), 136–*139*
    periportal sinusoidal dilatation and peliosis, hepatitis, 139–*142*
Liver function tests
  in echinococcal disease, 166
  in hepatocellular carcinoma, 221
  in postembolization syndrome, 298
Liver-spleen scan, of cyst, *950*, 951
Liver-spleen window, 960, *963*, 1025
Lobar arteries, catheterization, 299
Lucent area, in adenocarcinoma of pancreas, 787
Lung
  activity, in cirrhosis, 146
  tumor, metastases
    to liver, *202*
    to pancreas, 854, *855–856*
Luschka ducts, 309
Lymph nodes
  effect of Thorotrast on, 126
  pancreatic, computed tomography (CT) of, 638, *639*, 639
  peripancreatic
    in adenocarcinoma of pancreas, *795*, 796
    in islet cell tumors, 865
Lymphadenopathy, 241, *242*
  in giant cell carcinoma, 838, *841*
  peripancreatic, 779
Lymphangiogram, contrast, of splenic opacification, 1015, 1016
Lymphangioma (*see also* lymphangiomatosis) splenic, 971
Lymphangiomatosis, of spleen, 975
Lymphatic anatomy, pancreas, computed tomography (CT) of, 637, *638*
Lymphatic vessels, spleen, 902
Lymphocytic lymphoma, splenic involvement in, 965, 966
Lymphoma (*see also* specific type)
  biliary, 536, *537*, 537
  hepatic, 186, 206–207
    angiography of, 219, 220
    cholangiography of, 215, *215*, *216*
    computed tomography (CT) of, 207, *208*, *209*, 209–210
    magnetic resonance imaging of, 275
    nuclear medicine for, 213
  pancreatic, 499, 828, 833, 854, 856, *857–860*
    MRI of, 893
  splenic, 965–966, 1079
    angiography, *971*, 971
    computed tomography (CT), 967–*969*, 971
    MRI of, 1033, 1036
    sonography of, 966–967
    technetium sulfur colloid scan, *970*, 971

M

Macroaggregated albumin (MAA), 28
Macroamylasemia, 713
Macrophage(s)
  glucocerebroside-laden, 987
  thorium dioxide in, 127, 128
Magnesium, levels, in pancreatitis, acute, 658
Magnetic resonance imaging (MRI), 1

of gallbladder and biliary tract
of disease, 595–596, *597*
of normal anatomy, 593–594, *595*
of obstruction, 597, *598*
of liver
in cirrhosis, 268
compared to computed tomography (CT), 281
in copper disease states, 270–271
in fatty infiltration (steatosis), 268–270
of fatty liver, 108
in iron overload, 270, *270*
for lymphomatous involvement, 209
of masses, 271–281
of normal anatomy, 265, *266*
of Wilson's disease, 120
of pancreas, 895
of hemochromatosis, 891–892
of inflammatory disease, 889–*891*
of neoplasms, 892–895, *896*
of normal anatomy, 887–889
of spleen
of splenic artery aneurysm, 998
of normal anatomy, 1031, *1032–1033*
of pathology, 1033–1038
of rupture, 1009, 1011
Malaria, 998
splenomegaly from, 992–993
Malpighian bodies, 902
Malpighian corpuscle, 902
Manometry
of papillary stenosis, 575, *576*, 577
of sphincter of Oddi, 338
Marbling, in pancreatic parenchyma, 785
Mass(es) (*see* Cyst; Tumor, specific type)
Mass effect, in splenic trauma, 935
Mebendazole, 166
Meckel's diverticula, 390
Meconium ileus, 651, 655
Mediastinal pseudocysts, 723, *725*, 729
Meglumine diatrizoate, 337
Melanocytes, in gallbladder, 493
Melanoma
breast and lung, metastases to pancreas, 854, *855–856*
metastases
in gallbladder, 493–495
to spleen, 977, *980*, 980
Meniscus sign, in choledocholithiasis, *524*, *525*, 528
"Mercedes-Benz" sign, 390, *392*, *408*, 409
Mesenchyma
liver, hamartoma, 41–43, 51, 54
pancreas, tumors, 854
Mesenchymoma, malignant, 53
Mesenteric artery(ies), superior, 14–15, 624
involvement in pancreatitis, *704*, 704, 705
thickening, in adenocarcinoma of pancreas, 794, *796*, 797
Mesenteric vein(s), 623
thrombosis, 1002
Metabolic diseases, of liver, 149

Metaphyseal infarcts, in pancreatitis, 660
Metastatic disease in the liver
angiography, 215, 216–220
computed tomography (CT), 199–204
differentiated from hepatocellular disease, 149
hypervascular, 181, 216, *217*
hypovascular, 216, *217*, *218*
lymphoma/leukemia
cholangiography of, 215, *215*, *216*
computed tomography (CT) and ultrasound of, 206–209
nuclear medicine for, 213
nuclear medicine for, 210–*212*, 213, 271, 275
of pancreatic tumors
adenocarcinoma, 783, 796, *797*, 797, *799*
duct cell carcinoma, 834–835
of gastrinoma, 872, 873
of islet cell tumors, 863
plain film for, 214–215
screening for, 213
treatment, 296
ultrasound of, 204–*206*
Methylene diphosphate, ^{99m}Tc, of amyloidosis, 132
Metronidazole (Flagyl), 159, 1053
"Mickey Mouse" sign, *19*
Microabscess(es)
liver, 153, 154
in candidiasis, 157
staphylococcal, 154
splenic, 994, *994*, 995
Microadenocarcinoma, pancreatic, 842–844
Milk of calcium bile, 423, 442–446
differentiated from hemobilia, 583
Mirizzi syndrome, 389, 457, 499
radiology, 457–461
Mitomycin C, 296, 297, 300
Mitosis (M phase), 296
Mononucleosis, infectious
and splenic rupture, 943–944
splenomegaly from, 992, 993, *993*
Morphine, 417
Morphine-prostigmine test, 578
Morison's pouch, 5, *5*, 284
MRI (*see* Magnetic resonance imaging)
Mucinous cystic neoplasm, pancreatic, 757–764, 798
Mucosal abnormalities, ERCP of, 336
Mucosal hyperplasia, 479
adenomatous, 479
"Mucosal relief" films, 328
Mud, in cholangitis, 556
Multihormonal tumors, islet cell, 880
Murphy's sign, in cholecystitis, 404, 411
sonographic, 415–416
Muscular dysplasia, 463
Myeloproliferative disorders, associated with splenomegaly, 985, 986, *987*, *988*
Myelosuppression, 296, 297
Myoblastoma
gallbladder, 481
granular cell, 544–545

N

Narcan, 606
Necrosis, focal hepatic, 144
Needle
Chiba, 607, *609*, 610, 913
for percutaneous abscess drainage, localization, 1043–1045, *1046*, *1047*, *1048*
for percutaneous biopsy, guided, 1068–1071
thin-walled 22 gauge, placement of, 607
Needle aspiration (*see* Aspiration)
Neonate and infant (*see also* Liver, congenital diseases and pediatric neoplasms)
jaundice in, 356–358, *361*, 507
Neoplasms (*see* Tumors, specific type)
Nephromegaly, 39
Nephrostomy system, Malecot, 1047
Nesidioblastosis, 880, 882, 884
Neuroblastoma, 51, 210
Neuromatosis, of cholecystosis, hyperplastic, 463
Neuronal hyperplasia, 472
Neuropsychiatric changes, in Wilson's disease, 119
Newborns (*see* Neonate and infants)
Nicotinamide-adenine dinucleotide oxidase, 40
Niemann-Pick disease, 986
Non-Hodgkin's lymphoma, 206, 913
pancreatic involvement in, 856
splenic involvement in, 965, 966, 968, 1079
MRI of, 1033, 1036
ultrasound of, 208
Nuclear medicine (*see also* Scintigraphy)
of abscess, upper abdominal, 1042
of adenocarcinoma of pancreas, 777
of adenoma, hepatic, *192*, 192
of amyloidosis, 132
of angiosarcoma of the liver, *261*, 261–262
of biloma, 586–587
of Budd-Chiari syndrome, 95, 96, *98*, *99*, *100*
of cholangiocarcinoma, 541, *542*
for cholangitis, primary sclerosing, 564
for diffuse liver diseases, 146–*150*
of echinococcal disease, 166–167
of fistula, biliary, 451
of focal nodular hyperplasia, 186, *187*, 188
of hemangioma, cavernous, 176, *176*, *177*, 178
of hemobilia, 583
of hepatocellular carcinoma, 221, 222, 231, 243–246
in infarction, liver, 144
for metastatic disease in the liver, 210–*212*, 213
of pancreatitis, acute, 669
of trauma
gallbladder, *591*, 592
hepatic, 290–291
splenic, 932, *933*, 933

O

Opacification
  arterial, 200
  gallbladder, 410
  in hemangioma, cavernous, 181
Obstruction, biliary (see Biliary obstruction)
Oil emulsions, ethionized (see Ethionized oil emulsion)
Operability, of carcinoma of pancreas, 834
Opisthorchis, 482
  viverrini, 552, 557
Osler-Weber-Rendu disease (hereditary hemorrhagic telangiectasia), 136
  clinical findings, 136–137
  pathology, 137
  radiology, 137–*139*
Osteolysis in pancreatitis, acute, 659, 660
Ostomy appliance, 1047, 1048

P

Padding of the sweep, 770
Pain
  abdominal, ERCP for, 333
  following guided percutaneous biopsy, 1081
  in liver abscess
    amebic, 158
    pyogenic, 152
Palliation, surgical, for cholangiocarcinoma, 543
Pancreas
  anatomy and physiology, 620, *621*, 623, 640, 814
  radiologic (see also Computed tomography; Ultrasound), 623–639
  annular, 645
    clinical presentation, 646
    embryology, 645
    imaging studies, 646–648, *649*
    pathology, 645–646
    treatment, 648
  APUDomas, 300
  calcification, 664
  congenital disorders (see Congenital disorders, pancreas)
  diseases, 601
    splenic vascular changes in, 1011–1012
  divisum
    clinical findings, 643
    and ERCP, 335, *336*
    radiology, 643, 644
  effect of hepatomegaly on, 61
  embryology, 619, *620*
  endocrine, 640
  enlargement, 799
    focal, 676
    in pancreatitis, 663
  enzymes, 711, 712*t*, 712
  exocrine function, 640–641
  fat replacement of, *746*, 746, *747*
  fistula, arteriovenous, 643
  growth, 641
  guided percutaneous biopsy, 1075–1077, *1078*, 1079*t*
  magnetic resonance imaging (see Magnetic resonance imaging)
  obstruction, 549
  pseudocyst (see Pseudocyst, pancreas)
  puncture, 1056, 1059, *1060*
  secretions, reflux into common bile duct, 371
  secretory pressure, 657
  sonographic visualization, 778
  trauma
    clinical findings, 741
    ERCP, *743*, 744, *746*
    pathology, 743
    radiology, *742*, 743–744
    treatment, 741
  tumors, 499, 749
    of acinar cell origin, 851–854
    adenocarcinoma, metastases to liver, 204–205
    carcinoma, 536, *537, 545, 546*
    classification, 749–750
    connective tissue, 854
    cyst(s), 749, 750–751
    cystadenocarcinoma, metastases to liver, *217*
    of duct cell origin (see Pancreatic duct cell, carcinoma; Pancreatic duct cell, neoplasms)
    epithelial, solid and papillary, 846–851
    of indeterminate origin, 853–854
    islet cell (see Islet cell, tumors)
    metastases, lymphoma and leukemia, 854–860
Pancreatectomy, for trauma, 741
Pancreatic artery, dorsal, 8
Pancreatic duct, *630, 631*
  anatomy, *307*, 307
  computed tomography (CT) of, 639
  bleeding into, 707
  computed tomography (CT) of, 633
  diameter, computed tomography (CT) of, 787, 789
  dilatation
    in pancreatitis, chronic, 699, *699*, 702
    in papillary stenosis, 573
  main (see Duct of Wirsung)
  obstruction, from pseudocyst, 736, *738*, 740
  sonography, 631
Pancreatic duct cell, carcinoma
  adenosquamous cancer, 841–842
  anaplastic, 844, *845*
  colloid, 842
  differential diagnosis, 828, *829–830*
  early, 829, 834
  giant cell, 837–841, *841*
  hypervascular, 817, *827*
  MRI of, *893*, 893–894
  prognosis and surgical planning, 828, 829, 834–835
  in situ, 766
Pancreatic duct cell, neoplasms
  carcinoma (see Pancreatic duct cell, carcinoma)
  cystic, 751
    adenoma, microcystic, 751–757
  mucinous, 757–764
  solid
    adenocarcinoma (see Adenocarcinoma, pancreatic duct cell)
    ampullary carcinoma, 767
Pancreatic function testing, for pancreatitis, acute, 710–711
Pancreatic juice, 640
  enzymes, 641
  escape, 722
  pure, collection of, 710, 711
Pancreatic radicles, straightening of, in pancreatitis, acute, 669, *670*
Pancreatica magna artery, 907
Pancreaticoblastoma, 853, *853*
Pancreaticoduodenal artery, 627
  superior, 625
Pancreaticoduodenal nodes, 639
Pancreaticopleural fistula, 720, *721*
Pancreatitis, 388, 481, 646, 657
  acute
    angiography of, 703, 708, 709
    cholangiography of, 669, *671*, 671
    clinical findings, 657
    complications, 671, *672*, 673–676
    computed tomography (CT) of, 676–680
    in cystic fibrosis, 652
    differential diagnosis, 708
    differentiated from cholecystitis, 420–421
    edematous, 658, 671
    endoscopic retrograde pancreatography of, 334, 669, *670*
    etiology and pathogenesis, 657–658
    gangrenous, 663
    hemorrhagic, 658, 671
    interstitial, 671
    necrotizing, 671, 715, *716*, 718
    nuclear medicine for, 669
    pathology, 657
    phlegmonous, 671, 673–674, 677, *677, 678*, 679
    radiology of, 659–668
    sonography of, 671–676, 680
    suppurative, 663, 671
  in adenocarcinoma of pancreatic duct cell, 766
  in cholecystitis, 425
  chronic, 660
    alcoholic, 685
    angiography, 703–709
    calcific, 681, 682, 698, *699*, 706, 765
    cholangiography, 694, *695, 697,* 697, *698,* 698
    clinical findings, 681–682
    complications, 706, 707–708
    computed tomography, *700*, 700–702
    etiology and pathogenesis, 681
    focal, 696
    hereditary, 682, 685
    idiopathic, 687, 680, 682
    obstructive, 682, 683
    pancreatic enzymes in, 711–713
    pancreatic function testing, 710–711
    pancreatography, 690–696, *697*

pathology, 682, 683
radiology, *683, 684, 685,* 685–690
relapsing, 601
sonography, 698–700
splenic artery aneurysm formation in, 998
treatment, 682
tropical (kwashiorkor), *682, 688, 688*
complications
abscess, 713–720
fistula, 720–722
differentiated from
adenocarcinoma of pancreatic duct cell, 797, 798, 799, *800*
carcinoma, 828
and ERCP, 333, 335, 341
fatal, 657
idiopathic recurrent, 643
MRI of, 889, *890*
splenic vascular changes in, 1011, 1012
tumor lysis, 658
Pancreatocholangioscopy, transduodenal, 347, *347*
Pancreatography, pancreatogram, 337
of adenocarcinoma, pancreatic duct cell, *799,* 801, *809,* 813
of fibrotic papillary stenosis, *575,* 575
for pancreas divisum, 643
for pancreatitis, chronic
indications, 690
radiographic findings, 691*t*, 691–696
for pseudocyst, pancreatic, 736–740
Pancreozymin (*see* Cholecystokinin)
Pancytopenia, 902
Papilla of Vater
cholestogram of, oral, 311
stenosis (*see* Stenosis, papillary)
tumors, 573
Papilloma
biliary, 536, 544
gallbladder, 478, 479
Papillomatosis, gallbladder, 479
Papillotome, 576
Sohma (reversal), 344
Papillotomy, 339
endoscopic, 338
for stone impaction, 344
Paragonimus westermani, 482
Parasites, biliary, 556–558
Parasympathomimetic drugs, 641
Parenchyma
liver, 3
abnormalities, 73
attenuation, in fatty liver, 107, 108, *109*
computed tomography (CT), 22
disruption, 284
enhancement, 200
in focal nodular hyperplasia, 186
fragmentation, 286
iron overload, 270
magnetic resonance imaging, 265
nodules, 67, 70, 93
peritumoral lesions, 205
traumatized, 286
ultrasound of, 15, *16*
without portal blood supply, 235

pancreatic, 625, 627
autodigestion of, 1057
fibrosis, 696–697
stain, 669
splenic, ultrasound, 908
Parenchymal phase, of splenic angiogram, 907
mottled, in trauma, 935
Parenchymography, 337
Patient preparation, for PTC, 606
Pediatric diseases and neoplasms, liver (*see* Liver, congenital disorders and pediatric diseases and neoplasms)
"Pedicles," spleen, 900
Peliosis, of the spleen, 1012
Pelvis, sonolucency in, 284
Penicillamine, 572
D-Penicillamine, 560
Percutaneous abscess and fluid drainage, upper abdomen, 1039, 1041, 1062
background, 1041–1042
imaging, 1042–1043
technique, 1043
catheter placement, 1046, 1047
computed tomography (CT), 1045, *1048*
gallbladder puncture, 1053, *1055–1056,* 1056–1057
hepatic puncture, 1051–1053, *1054*
localization for needle placement, 1043–1045, *1046, 1047, 1048*
location of upper abdominal puncture, 1049
pancreatic puncture, 1057–1059, *1060*
securing the catheter, 1047, 1048, 1049
splenic puncture, 1059, *1061*
subphrenic collection, 1049*t*, 1049–1051
Percutaneous cholecystotomy, 615
Percutaneous biopsy, guided, in upper abdomen, 1065, 1081
contraindications, 1079
cytopathology, 1065–1066
future prospects, 1081
imaging modalities available, 1066–1068
indications, 1071
hepatic hemangioma, 1074, 1075
hepatobiliary, 1071–1074, *1075*
pancreas, 1075–1077, *1078*
spleen, 1077, 1079*t*, 1079
mortality and morbidity, 1079–1081
needle selection, 1068–1071
Percutaneous transhepatic cholangiography (PTC), 601
of adenocarcinoma, pancreatic duct cell, 603, *604*
of anastomoses, biliary-enteric, 532, *533*
of bilhemia, 585
of cholangiocarcinoma, 538, *539*–541
of cholangitis
primary sclerosing, 559, 560
recurrent pyogenic, 556
of jaundice, 497

procedures, special, 610–615
of stenosis, fibrotic papillary, *575,* 575
of strictures, biliary, 601, *602*
success rates, 329, 330
technique, 606–610
vs. ERCP, 335, 336
Percutaneous transhepatic drainage, for cholangiocarcinoma, 542
Percutaneous transhepatic portography, 613, *615,* 615
Perfluorocarbons, 911
Perfluoroctylbromide, 205, 911
Pericholangitis, 559
associated with inflammatory bowel disease, 566–567
clinical findings, 567
pathogenesis, 567, 568
pathology, 567
radiology, *568,* 569
treatment, 568
differentiated from cirrhosis, primary biliary, 571, *571*
Pericholecystic vein, enlarged, 73
Periportal sinusoidal dilatation, 139, 140, 262
clinical findings, 140
pathology, 140
radiology, 140, *141*
Perisplenic fluid, 937
Peritoneal cavity, blood in, 284
Peritoneal lavage, in hepatic trauma, 283, 286
Peritoneum
hydatid cyst implantation in, 164, *165*
visceral, spleen, 900
Peritonitis, 1005
biliary, 589
following guided percutaneous biopsy, 1080
Peromelus, 922–923
PET (*see* Positron emission tomography)
Phagocytosis, 149, 902
Phenobarbital, 359, 510
Pheochromocytoma, *57*
Phleboliths, calcified, 173, 174
Phlebosclerosis, 70
Phlegmon, pancreatic, 718
in pancreatitis, acute, 671, 673–674, 677, *677, 678,* 679
Phrygian cap, 468
deformity, 316
Photopenic area, in amebic abscess, 159
Pigment stones
gallstones, 388
intrahepatic (*see* Cholangitis, recurrent pyogenic)
Pixel size, in computed tomography (CT), for pancreatic adenocarcinoma
Plain film examination, 1
abdominal, of hepatomegaly, 55–56, *58,* 60
of abscess
amebic, 159, *160*
pancreatic, *714,* 715, *715, 716*
pyogenic liver, 152
splenic, *956,* 956–957

Plain film examination—*continued*
  of adenocarcinoma, pancreatic duct cell, *767, 768, 769*
  of anastomoses, biliary-enteric, 529
  of angiosarcoma of the liver, *261*, 261
  of carcinoma
    gallbladder, 484, *485*
    giant cell, 838, *839*
  of Caroli's disease, 365
  of cholangitis, recurrent pyogenic, 552, *553, 554–555*
  of cholangiocarcinoma, intrahepatic, 254, *255*
  of cholecystitis
    acalculous, 428
    acute, 409, 424
    emphysematous, 431, *432–433*
  of choledocholithiasis, 519
  of cholelithiasis, 390, *391*
  of cyst
    choledochal, 372, *372, 374*
    liver, congenital simple, 171–172
    pancreatic, *750*, 750–751
    splenic, *949*, 951
  of cystic fibrosis, 652, *653*
  of echinococcal disease, *165*, 166, 169
  of epithelial neoplasms, pancreatic, *846, 848, 849*
  for fatty liver diagnosis, 106, *106*
  of fibrosis, hepatic congenital, 365
  of fistula, biliary, 447, *448–450*
  of gallstone ileus, 451–454
  of gas, portal venous, 145, *145*
  of gastrinoma, 871
  of glycogen storage disease, 38
  of hamartoma
    mesenchymal, 43
    splenic, 975
  of hemangioendothelioma, infantile, 45, *45*
  of hemangioma
    cavernous, 174, *174*
    splenic, 972
  of hepatoblastoma, 49
  of hepatocellular carcinoma, *221*, 222
    fibrolamellar, 246, *247, 248*
  of hydrops of gallbladder, 446
  of infarct, splenic, 1005
  of islet cell tumors
    functional, 862, *862*
    nonfunctioning, 884
  of liver, 7–8
    of metastatic disease in, 214–215
  of lymphangiomatosis, splenic, 976
  of milk of calcium bile, 442, *443–445*
  of Mirizzi syndrome, 457
  of pancreas
    annular, 646, 647
    of pancreaticoblastoma, 853
    of pseudocyst, 723–726, *729*
  of pancreatitis
    acute, *661*, 661–664
    chronic, 683, *684, 685*, 685–688, 696
  of polycystic liver disease, 363
  of porcelain gallbladder, 439, *440, 441*
  of sarcoma, hepatic, undifferentiated (embryonal), 54
  of schistosomiasis, 124
  of sickle cell anemia, *1018*, 1018, 1019
  of spleen, 903
    of asplenia, 924–925
    dense or opacified, 1015, *1016*
    of metastases, 977, *977, 978*
    of polysplenia, 926
    of wandering spleen, 918, *918*
  of splenomegaly, of *Echinococcus*, *993*, 994
  of Thorotrast-induced diseases of liver and spleen, 126–127, *128*
  of trauma
    gallbladder, 591
    hepatic, 284
    spleen, 931, *931*
Planar scintigraphy, 31
  of liver, false-positive studies, 33*t*, 34
Plasmapheresis, 572
Plasmodium falciparum, 992
Pleural effusion
  in amebic abscess, *160*, 160, 162, *162*
  In echinococcal disease, 166
Pleuropulmonary abnormalities, in pancreatitis, acute, 659
Plexus
  nerve, 573
  vascular, 573
Pneumobilia, 145, 146
  in cholangitis, 552
  in echinococcal disease, 166
  indications, 529, *530*
Polycystic kidney disease, 363, 364–365, *366*
Polycystic liver disease, 499
  in neonate, 362, 363, *364*
Polycythemia vera, *101*
Polyhydramnios, 646
Polyp
  biliary, 536
  gallbladder
    adenomatous, 479–481
    benign, 478
    cholesterol, 472, 478, 481, 482, 488
    ERCP of, 333, *334*
    inflammatory and miscellaneous, 481–483
Polypeptide, pancreatic, 861
Polyphosphate compounds, ^{99m}Tc, 28
Polysplenia, 925–927
Polyvinyl alcohol foam (Ivalon), 298, 299–300
Polyvinyl chloride, angiosarcoma of the liver from, 260, 262
Poppel's sign, 666
Porcelain gallbladder, 439
  pathophysiology, 439
  radiology, 439–442
Porta hepatis
  adenopathy, 536
  extension, 488, *488*, 489
  hepatocellular carcinoma, 241
  radionuclide scanning, 29
  sonography, 321, *321*, 322, *322*, 323, 631, 632
  space occupying disease, SPECT imaging of, 34
Portal hepatogram, 14, 15

Portal hypertension
  barium contrast examination in, 82, *82*
  causes, 70, 116, 119, 124, 126, 128
    other than cirrhosis, 88–104
  computed tomography (CT) in, 79–80, *81*
  in focal nodular hyperplasia, 183
  magnetic resonance imaging of, 275, *277–278*, 281
  portosystemic collaterals in, 73–75
  related to hepatocellular carcinoma, 237, *237*
  with sarcoidosis, 121
  ultrasonography of, 72, 73, 74, *74*
Portal pressure, measurement, 84, 85, 87
Portal vein, 9, *11*, 11–13
  aneurysms, 73
  demonstration of (*see also* Portography), 84
  embryology, 900
  in hemangioma, cavernous, *179*, 181
  hepatocellular carcinoma invasion of, 229, *230, 236*, 237, *237*
  injury, 283
  involvement in pancreatitis, *704*, 705
  magnetic resonance imaging of, 265
  obstruction, 91, 92, 93, *94*
  occlusion, 142
  percutaneous transhepatic portography, 613, *615*, 615
  thrombosis, 88–91
  ultrasonography, 15, *16*, 17, 20, 321, *321, 322*, 322
Portal venous gas, 145–*146*
Portal venous system
  catheterization, 836–837
  thrombosis, 702
Portocholecystotomy, 358
Portoenterostomy, 359
Portography (*see also* Splenoportography)
  arterial
    of hepatocellular carcinoma, 239
    in portal hypertension, 81, *81*
  of Budd-Chiari syndrome, 97
  in cirrhosis, 83, 84, 85
  computed tomography (CT), 26
    of hepatocellular carcinoma, 235
  of hemangioma, cavernous, 181
  of metastatic liver disease, 216, *218*, 219
  of splenic vein thrombosis, 1003
  transhepatic
    of islet cell tumors, 865
    of portal hypertension, 91, *93*
    percutaneous, 613, *615*, 615
Positron emission tomography (PET), of liver, 32
Postembolization syndrome, 298, 299
Postevacuation film, in cystic fibrosis, 655
Pregnancy
  gallbladder in, 317, 319
  splenic artery aneurysm during, 998
  splenic rupture during, 944
Priscoline (tolazoline), 814
Prostigmine (*see* Morphine-prostigmine test)

Protein
  hyposecretion and inspissation, in pancreatitis, 681
  secretory, 640
Proteolytic enzymes, 641
Pruritus, in cirrhosis, 569
Prussic acid, 681
Pseudoaneurysm
  in pancreatitis, chronic, 705, 706, *706*, 707, 708
  in splenic trauma, 934, 935–936
Pseudocalculus effect, in cholangiography, *330*, 331
Pseudocyst
  pancreatic, 334, 679, 702, 718, 722, 789, 1003
    angiography, 740, *741*
    barium contrast examination, 725, 729, *729*
    cholangiography, *739*, 740
    clinical findings, 722–723
    computed tomography (CT), 798, 799
    differentiated from aneurysm, 676
    differentiated from carcinoma, 828
    dissection, 735
    MRI of, 889
    in pancreatitis, chronic, 706, 707
    pancreatography, 736–740
    perirenal, 730, *731*
    plain film, 723–726, 729
    septations, 735
    sonography and computed tomography (CT), 732–735
    splenic vascular changes in, 1011
    urography, excretory, *730*, 730, *731*
  splenic, 939, 947, *955*, 955
    computed tomography (CT), *953*
    differentiated from true cyst, 950, 951
    transition between hematoma, *952*, 955
Pseudodiverticula, in cholangitis, 562, *564*, *565*
Pseudomasses, pancreatic, ultrasound of, 632
Pseudomonas, 335
Pseudotumor, of spleen, 1028
Psychiatric disturbances (*see* Neuropsychiatric changes)
PTC (*see* Percutaneous transhepatic cholangiography)
Pulmonary anomalies, in asplenia, 923
Pus, in common duct obstruction, 515
Pyemia, portal, 151
Pyogenic liver abscess, 151
  clinical findings, 152
  etiology and pathogenesis, 151
  pathology, 151–152
  radiology, 152–156, 159
Pyrophosphate, ^{99m}Tc, of amyloidosis, 132

R

"Racemose" appearance, 167
Radiation exposure, in gallbladder and biliary tract imaging, 313t, 314
Radiation injury, to liver, 149, *150*
Radiation therapy, 615
  for cholangiocarcinoma, 543
Radiograph
  digital scout, 1045
  plain (*see* Plain film examination)
Radioimmunoglobulin therapy, for hepatocellular carcinoma, 244–246
Radioisotope scanning, of liver volume, 55
Radiologic technique, in ERCP, 336, 337
"Radiolucent liver sign," 106
Radionuclide scanning (*see also* Nuclear medicine; Scintigraphy)
  in abscess
    pyogenic liver, 151, 155, 156
    splenic, 957–958, *959*
  in cyst, liver, congenital simple, 172, *172*
  of cystadenoma and cystadenocarcinoma, biliary, 194
  of fatty liver, 106, *107*
  liver-spleen
    of polysplenia, 926
    of sickle cell anemia, 1018, 1020, *1021*, *1022*
  of lymphoma, splenic, 967
  of metastatic disease in liver, 199
  of Wilson's disease, 120
Radiopharmaceuticals, for gallbladder and biliary tract imaging, 312–313
Ramp-Hanning filter, 33
Rectal carcinoma, metastasis to liver, *203*
Receiver-operator curve (ROC), 34
Recurrent pyogenic cholangitis (RPC) (*see* Cholangitis, recurrent pyogenic)
Red blood cells
  damage, 903, 906
  scan, spleen in, 906
  sensitization, 903
  ^{99m}Tc-labeled, 27
    in hemangioma, cavernous, 176, 181
Reflux
  biliary, 657
  duodenobiliary, 341, 573
Renal halo sign, 663
Renografin, 911
Resectibility, of pancreatic duct cell carcinoma, 834
Restenosis, 577
Retention disk, Sur-Fit, 1048, 1049
Reticuloendothelial iron overload, 270
Retroperitoneal extension, in pancreatitis, 799
Retroperitoneal perforation, following endoscopic sphincterotomy, 341
Retroperitoneal structures, liver (*see also* specific structure)
  effect of hepatomegaly on, 60, 66
Retroperitoneal tumors, 708
Retroperitoneum, computed tomography (CT) of, 284, *285*
Rhabdomyosarcoma, embryonal, 52, 53, 545, *547*–548
Riedel's lobe, 7, *7*, 35, *35*, 56
Right upper quadrant (RUQ)
  calcifications, 390
  pain, in papillary stenosis, 573
  tumors
    liver metastasis, 214, *215*, 215
    in neonatal and infant jaundice, 357–358
Rigler's triad, 451–452
Rings, in dilated extrahepatic duct, 502, 504
ROC (*see* Receiver-operator curve)
Rokitansky-Aschkoff sinuses, 425, 431, 439
  in cholecystoses, hyperplastic, 463, 464, 468, 474, 477
  in gallbladder carcinoma, 489
  in gallbladder polyp, 482
  and heterotopias, 481
Rose Bengal scan (tetraiodotetrachlorofluorescein)
  of focal nodular hyperplasia, 186
  of gallbladder and biliary tract, 312
Rupture
  in portal hypertension, 73
  spleen (*see* Spleen, rupture)

S

Sarcoidosis
  hepatic, 121, *122*, *123*
  splenomegaly from, 986, *999*
Sarcoma (*see also* Angiosarcoma)
  botryoides, biliary, 545, *547*–548
  gallbladder, spindle cell, 492
  Kupffer cell (*see* Angiosarcoma of the liver)
  hemangioendothelial (*see* Angiosarcoma of the liver
  liver
    mesenteric, 93, *96*
    undifferentiated (embryonal), 52–54
  pancreas, 854
Scan time, in computed tomography (CT) for pancreatic adenocarcinoma, 785
Scar(s)
  echogenic, in hepatocellular carcinoma, fibrolamellar, 252
  fibrotic, in focal nodular hyperplasia, 185, *186*, 186
Schistosoma, 482
  haematobium, 123
  japonicum, 123
  mansoni, 123, 993
Schistosomiasis, 123
  angiography, 124, 126
  clinical findings, 124
  computed tomography (CT), 124
  life cycle and pathophysiology, 123–124
  pathology, 124
  plain film and contrast examination, 124
  splenomegaly from, 993
  ultrasound, 124, *125*
Schwachman-Diamond syndrome, 650, *651*
Scintigraphy (*see also* Cholescintigraphy; Nuclear medicine; Radionuclide scans)

Scintigraphy (*see also* Cholescintigraphy; Nuclear medicine; Radionuclide scans)—*continued*
  of abscess
    amebic, 159, 160, *161*, 163
    pyogenic liver, 155, 156
  of Budd-Chiari syndrome, 95, 96, *98*, *99*, *100*
  of echinococcal disease, 166–167
  of hemangioendothelioma, infantile, 45, *46*
  of hemangioma, splenic, 972
  hepatobiliary
    of anastomoses, biliary-enteric, *531*, 531
    of biliary trauma, 581, 582, *584*
    of cholecystitis, 416–422, 425, 430, *430*, 477
  of hepatoblastoma, 49
  of hepatocellular carcinoma, 243
    fibrolamellar, 247, *248*
  of infarction
    hepatic, 144
    splenic, 1005–1006
  of jaundice, 497, 504–507
    pediatric, 507, 510
  liver, 27
    differentiation of extrahepatic masses from intrinsic hepatic disease, 30–31
    of fatty liver, 106, *107*
    of metastatic disease, 210, *210*, 211, 213
    normal liver scans, 28–30
    techniques, 27–28
  planar (*see* Planar scintigraphy)
  radionuclide, 1
    biliary, of gallbladder, 353
    hepatobiliary, for cholelithiasis, 390
    spleen, 903–904, *905*, *906*, 912
      of accessory spleen, 921
      of asplenia, 925
      clinical indications, 906
      normal scan, 904–906
      of splenomegaly, 994
      of wandering spleen, 918
  of stenosis, papillary, 573, *574*, 575, 576
  of trauma
    gallbladder, 592
    hepatic, 290
    splenic, 932, *933*, 933
    surgical, biliary tract, 579
Scintillation γ-ray, calcium tungstate, 312
Sclerosis
  hepatoportal, 91, 92, 93, *94*
  tuberous, 973
Sclerotherapy, endoscopic, 613, 615
Secretin, 338
  for pancreas divisum diagnosis, 643
  release, 641
  use in angiography, of pancreatic duct cell carcinoma, 814
Secretin test, for pancreatitis, chronic, 682, 711, 711*t*
Secretion, pancreatic, 640–641
  control of, 641
Segmental duct, obstruction, 535
75Se-selenomethionine, 777
Sentinel loop, in pancreatitis, acute, *662*, 662–663

Sepsis, following ERCP, 335
Septa, 70
  arteriovenous anastomoses in, 70
  in hemangioma, cavernous, 174, *178*
  transverse congenital (*see* Phrygian cap)
Septations, in pseudocyst, pancreatic, 735
Septic shock, from PTC, 610
Serratia, 40
"Seurat pattern, " 934
SGOT levels,
  in cholangitis, primary sclerosing, 559
  from hepatic artery embolization, 298
  in hepatic trauma, 283
Shadows, shadowing, acoustic
  in cholangiocarcinoma, 536
  "dirty" distal, 431
  from gallstones, 400, 401, *401*
  in pancreatitis, chronic, 698, 699, *699*
"Shoulder sign," 31
Shunt
  arteriovenous, 1011
  splenorenal, 73, 1010, 1011
Sickle cell anemia, 1017
  angiography, 1018, *1020*, *1021*
  computed tomography (CT) of, *1023*, *1025*, 1025–1027
  liver-spleen radionuclide scan, 1018, 1020, *1021*, *1022*
  plain film of, *1018*, 1018, *1019*
  sickle cell disease, 1017
  sickle cell trait, 1017
  splenic imaging in, 1017
  technetium 99m bone scan, 1020, 1022
  ultrasound of, 1020, *1022*, 1024, 1025
Sincalide (Kinevac), 315, 416
Single photon emission computed tomography (SPECT)
  camera systems, 32, 33
  of liver 32
    of fatty infiltration, 268, *269*, 270
    of hemangioma, cavernous, 178, *182*
    of metastatic disease in, 213
    results, 34–35
  of spleen, 906
    of infarct, *1005*, 1006
  techniques, 33–34
Sinogram (abscessogram), 1047
Sinuses (*see also* Rokitansky-Aschkoff sinuses)
  in adenomyomatosis, 474, 477
Sinusoids, in Budd-Chiari syndrome, 95
Skeletal abnormalities
  in pancreatitis, chronic, 690
  in Schwachman-Diamond syndrome, 650
Skeletal film, of pancreatitis, acute, 659–660
Skin lesions, in glucagonoma, 873
Sludge
  biliary, 402, *403*, 404–405
  in choledochal cyst, Type III, 383
  in gallstones, 388
"Sludge ball," *404*, 405
Small bowel
  abnormalities
    in cystic fibrosis, 655

  in pancreatitis, 665, *667*, 690
  in adenocarcinoma of pancreas, 784
    carcinoma, *775*, *776*, *777*
    pattern, in vipoma, *877*, 878
    study, in gastrinoma, 871
"Snowstorm" appearance, 934
Somatostatinoma, 880
Somatostatinoma syndrome, 862*t*
Sonography (*see* Ultrasound)
Sonolucency
  gallbladder wall, 414, *415*
  ovoid, 284
Sonolucent lesions, 205, *205*
  liver, fatty liver mimicking, *113*
Space-occupying disease, liver
  liver spleen scan for, 28
  in porta hepatis region, SPECT imaging, *34*
  types of hepatogram for, 13–15
Space-occupying processes, 56
Spasm, catheter-induced, 828, *834*
SPECT (*see* Single photon emission computed tomography)
Sphincter of Boyden, 307
  cholangiography, 331
Sphincter of Oddi, 307
  anatomy and physiology, 573
  cholangiography, 331
  disorders (*see also* Stenosis, papillary), 572
  histology, 309
  manometry, 338
Sphincteroplasty, for pancreas divisum, 643
Sphincterotome, 339, 344
Sphincterotomy
  endoscopic electrosurgical
    complications, 339, 340*t*, 341–343
    indications and contraindications, 338–339, 339*t*
    of stenosis, papillary, 576–577
    technique, 339, *340*
  for pancreatitis, acute, 669
Sphingolipids, abnormal accumulation, 482
Sphingomyelin, 986
Spin echo
  in fatty infiltration of liver, 268
  of gallbladder
    T1-weighted images, 539, *594*
    T2-weighted sequences, 593
  in hepatic iron overload, 270
  in hepatocellular carcinoma, 272
  in metastatic disease of liver, 275
  MRI, of hemochromatosis, 891–892
  of normal liver, 265
  in portal hypertension, 275
  T2, in normal spleen, 1031
  TE, 1031
Spine, scalloping of, 60
Spleen, 897
  absence of (*see* Asplenia)
  accessory, 919–921, 943
  autotransplantation, 942
  "compact," 906–907
  congenital disorders (*see* Congenital disorders, spleen)
  coronal scan through, 77
  defects, with SPECT imaging, *33*
  dense or opacified, 1015–1016

diaphragmatic herniation, 1028
diffuse diseases
 infection, 992–995
 splenomegaly, 985–992
displacement, in trauma, 936
embryology, 899, *900*
focal diseases
 abscesses, 955–965
 angiosarcoma, 971–972
 cysts, 947–955
 hamartoma, 973–975
 hemangioma, 971–972
 lymphangiomatosis, 975–976
 lymphoma, 965–971
 metastases, 976–981
gastric ulcers penetrating into, 1028
-gonadal fusion, 922–923
gross and microscopic anatomy, 900–906
guided percutaneous biopsy, 1077, 1079
hematoma, *57*
imaging, in sickle cell disease, 1017
magnetic resonance imaging (*see* Magnetic resonance imaging, spleen)
metastases to, 976–977
 of angiosarcoma, of the liver, 262, *262, 263*
 roentgen findings, 977–981
physiology, 902
pseudotumor, inflammatory, 1028
puncture, 1059, *1061*
radiologic anatomy and technique
 angiography, 906–907, *907*
 aspiration, 913
 computed tomography (CT), 908, 909–912
 normal scan, 904, *905*, 906
 plain film, 903
 scintigraphy, historical perspective, 903–904, *905, 906*
 splenic volume measurement, 912–913
 splenoportography, 907, *908*
 ultrasound, 908, *909*
rupture, 960, *964*, 993, 1009, 1018
 and abscess, 960, *964*
 nontraumatic, 943–944
 in splenomegaly, 985
 splenosis, 942–943
trauma, 913, 931
 angiography, 934–936
 blunt, 931
 classification, 931
 clinical manifestations, 931
 complications, 939
 computed tomography (CT), 937–941
 cyst development following, 947
 iatrogenic, 931
 nuclear medicine of, 932, *933*, 933
 penetrating, 931
 plain film of, 931, *931*
 and rupture, 943
 sonography of 936, *936*, 937
 splenosis, 942–943
tumors, computed tomography (CT), 911
"upside down," 904

vascular diseases
 aneurysm, splenic artery, 998–1000
 arteriosclerosis and occlusion of splenic artery, 997, *997*
 embolization, splenic artery, 1001
 fibromuscular hyperplasia, 997
 fistula, arteriovenous, 1000–1001
 infarct, 1005–1009, 1011
 peliosis, 1012
 rupture, of splenic vein, 1004–1005
 shunt, splenorenal, 1011
 thrombosis, solitary splenic vein, 1001–1004
 vascular changes, in pancreatic disease, 1011–1012
wandering, 917–919
Splenectomy
 for abscess, 955
 for Gaucher's disease, 992
 medical, 1001
 for splenomegaly, 985
 for thrombosis, splenic vein, 1003
 for wandering spleen, 919
Splenic artery, 8, 625, 900, 902, 906, *907*
 aneurysm, 708, 998–1000
 rupture, 1000
 in arteriovenous fistula, 1001
 branches, 907
 computed tomography (CT), 909
 embolization, 1001, 1004
 encasement, in islet cell tumor, 864
 occlusion, and arteriosclerosis, 997, *997*
 rupture, 998
 in trauma, 935
Splenic bands, 922, *922*, 939
Splenic nerve, 902
Splenic tissue, hypertrophied, 921
Splenic vein, 625, 900
 in arteriovenous fistula, 1001
 occlusion, 918
 in pancreatitis, 705
 rupture, 1004–1005
 "double rupture," 1005
 thrombosis, 1002–1004
 MRI of, 1033, *1033*
Splenomegaly, 72, 902, 917, 985, 986*t*
 in abscess, splenic, 956
 in adenocarcinoma, of pancreatic duct cell, 768, *769*
 adhesive, 985
 in angiosarcoma
  of liver, 261–262
  splenic, 973
 diagnosis, splenic volume calculation, 912
 examples, 985, 986*t*
 Gaucher's disease, 986, 987, *991, 992*, 992
 in glycogen storage disease, 37, 38
 in hemangioma, 972
 in hepatitis, viral, 148, 149
 in hepatocellular disease, 149
 infections causing, 992
  Echinococcus, 993, 994
  granulomatous diseases: tuberculosis, histoplasmosis, 994, *994*
  malaria, 992–993
  infectious mononucleosis, 993, *993*

microabscesses/candida, 994, *995*, 995
 schistosomiasis, 993
in lymphoma, 966, 967
MRI of, 1033, 1036
myeloproliferative disorders/leukemia, 985, 986, *987, 988*
passive hyperemia/fibrocongestive splenomegaly, 986, *989*
in sarcoidosis, 986, *990*
in sickle cell anemia, 1017
in splenic vein thrombosis, 1002
tropical, 992
Splenoportography, 84, 907, *908*, 918, 1011
 of carcinoma of pancreatic duct cell, 836
 of hepatis, peliosis, 140
 of portal hypertension, 91, *93*
Splenorenal shunt, 73, 1010, 1011
Splenosis, 942–943
Splenostomy, 1059
Squamous carcinoma (*see* Adenosquamous cancer)
Staphylococcal abscess, 40, 41
 microabscesses, 154
Staphylococcus
 aureus, 40, 151, 153, 154
 epidermidis, 40
 species, 431
Stauffer syndrome, 149
Steatorrhea
 in cystic fibrosis, 652
 in pancreatitis, chronic, 690
Steatosis (*see also* Fatty infiltration of liver
 hepatic, diagnosis, 105
Stenosis
 biliary
  causes, 601
  dilatation, 611
 celiac axis and superior mesenteric artery, 704
 in cholangiocarcinoma, 540, *541*
 papillary (ampullary), 572–573
  anatomy and physiology, 573
  clinical findings, 573
  etiology, 573
  fibrotic, *575*, 575
  radiology, 573–575
  scintigraphy, hepatobiliary, 575, 576
  secondary, 573
  treatment, 576–578
 of main pancreatic duct, 696
 splenic artery, 997
Stent(s), endoscopic retrograde, 345–346
Steroids, 334
Stoma wafer, 1047
Stomach
 abnormalities (*see* Gastric abnormalities)
 displacement
  downward, *57*
  by pancreatic pseudocyst, *726–728*, 729
  in wandering spleen, 918
 distension, for sonography of pancreatic adenocarcinoma, 778
 effect of liver size on, 62–*63*
 involvement in adenocarcinoma of

Stomach—*continued*
    pancreas, 768, 769, 770, *771*, *772*
    sonographic appearance, 632
Stone(s) (*see* Calculus)
Stone basket, 612, 613
    Dormia, 342, 344, 345
"Strawberry gallbladder," 468, *471*
Streptococci, aerobic, 151
Streptococcus, 994
    bovis, 765
    species, 431
Streptomyces
    caespitosus, 297
    peucetius, 296
Streptozoticin, 862
Stricture
    anastomic, 532, *534*, 580
    biliary
        benign, 601, *602*
        iatrogenic, 580, *581*
        malignant, 601, 602–604, *605*
        surgically induced, 579, 580
    and cholangiocarcinoma, 536
    in cholangitis, 560, *564*
    choledochoenterostomy, 611
    dilatation, 564
"Strip sign," 556
Sulfatide, cholecystosis, *482*, 483
Sulfur-colloid scan
    of abscess, amebic, 159, 160
    of adenoma, hepatic, *192*
    of angiosarcoma, of liver, 261–262
    of cholangiocarcinoma, 541, *542*
    for cholangitis, 564
    of choledochal cyst, 372
    of cirrhosis, 146, *147*, 148
    in focal nodular hyperplasia, 186
    in hepatocellular carcinoma,
        fibrolamellar, 247, *248*
    in hepatocellular disease, compared
        to IDA scan, 149
    of liver trauma, 290
    liver-spleen
        of Caroli's disease, 365, *370*
        evaluation, 28, 29–30
        focal defect evaluation, 30
        of jaundice, 497
        of mesenchymal hamartoma, 43
        in radiation injury to the liver, 149
    technetium 99m (*see* Technetium
        99m-sulfur colloid scan)
Sump syndrome, 344, *344*
Surgery
    for annular pancreas, 648
    biliary (*see* Biliary surgery)
    for cholangiocarcinoma, 543
    for cholangitis, primary sclerosing, 560
    for echinococcal disease, 166
    for hepatocellular carcinoma, 233–234
    for pancreatitis, chronic, 682
    planning, for pancreatic duct cell
        carcinoma, 828, 829, 834–835
    for pseudocyst, pancreatic, 723
    trauma to biliary tract from, 579–581
    for trauma
        hepatic, 283
        pancreatic, 741
Suture, for biliary endoprosthesis
    placement, 610
"Swiss cheese" pattern, 976

T

T_1
    in cirrhosis, 268
    in copper disease states, 270, 271
    in fatty infiltration of liver, 268
    in hepatic iron overload, 270
    in hepatic masses, 271, *272*, 272, 275
    in pancreatitis, 889
    prolonged, 267, 268
        in splenic disorders, 1033
    weighted sequences, 265
        in normal spleen, 1031
    in splenic diseases, 1033, 1038
T_2
    in cirrhosis, 268
    in copper disease states, 270
    in fatty infiltration of liver, 268
    in hepatic iron overload, 270
    in hepatic masses, 271, 272, 281
    in pancreatitis, 889
    prolonged, 267
    relaxation time, in splenic disorders,
        1033
    in spleen, normal, 1031
    weighted sequences, 265
"Target" lesions, 493
TE spin echo, 1031
    in hepatic masses, 271
^{99m}TC (*see* Technetium-99^m)
Technetium-99^m, 32
    of biliary atresia, 359
    bone scanning agents, in
        hepatocellular carcinoma, 244
    -dimethylacetanilido-iminodiacetate
        (HIDA), 313
    of Caroli's disease, 365, *370*
    cholescintigram, 1057
    -DISIDA, of cholangitis, acute, 417,
        417
    -iminodiacetic acid, 27, 40
        of adenoma, hepatic, 192
        of atresia, biliary, 359, *359*, 360
        for cholecystitis, 416–417, 419, 420,
            421, 422, 426, 430, 477
        of choledochal cyst, 372
        of cirrhosis, 148
        of fistula, biliary, 451
        of focal nodular hyperplasia, 186
        for gallbladder and biliary tract
            imaging, 312, 313, 314, 315
        of hepatitis, neonatal, 359, *359*
        of hepatocellular carcinoma, 243
        of jaundice, 505, 506, 507, 510
        of stenosis, papillary, 575, 576
    -labeled hepatobiliary agent, for
        gallbladder and biliary tract
        imaging, 313
    -labeled red cell, 27
        in hepatocellular carcinoma, 243
    -methylene diphosphate
        in amyloidosis, 132
        bone scan, of sickle cell anemia,
            1020
    microaggregated albumin, 28
    -penicillamine, for gallbladder and
        biliary tract imaging, 313
    -pertechnetate
        for gallbladder and biliary tract
            imaging, 313, 314
        in hamartoma, splenic, 975
    polyphosphate compounds, 28
    -pyridoxylidene glutamate, 313, 421
    -pyrophosphate scan, of amyloidosis,
        132
    -red cells, 27
        in hamangioma, cavernous, 176, 181
    -sulfur colloid images, 27–28, 30, 33
        of abscess, pyogenic liver, 155, 156
        of accessory spleen, 921
        of asplenia, 925
        of candidiasis, hepatic, 157
        of fatty liver, 106, *107*, 111
        in glycogen storage disease, 38
        of hemangioma, cavernous, 176,
            176, *177*, 178
        of hepatoblastoma, 49
        in infarction splenic, *1005*, 1007
        liver-spleen scan, 315, 904, *905*,
            906, 906
        of lymphoma, splenic, 967, *970*,
            971
        of metastatic disease to the liver,
            210, *211*
        of normal liver, *29*, 29
        of splenic-gonadal fusion, 923
        in splenomegaly, 985, 986, *995*, 995
        of splenosis, 942, 943
        of trauma, splenic, 932, *933*, 933
        of wandering spleen, 918
    tagged cells, 903
Telangiectasia, hereditary hemorrhagic
    (*see* Osler-Weber-Rendu disease)
Telepaque (iopanoic acid), 328
    for cholelithiasis diagnosis, 393
Thalassemia, sickle cell, 1017
"Thick vessel sign," 294
Thorium dioxide (*see* Thorotrast)
Thorotrast (thoriuim dioxide), 126, 1015,
    1016
    -induced diseases of liver and spleen,
        220
    angiosarcoma, 128, 129, 130, 260,
        261, 261, *263*, *264*
    cholangiosarcoma, 129–130, 253
    hepatocellular carcinoma, 130
    pathology, 127, 128, *129*, 129
    plain radiography, 126–127, *128*
    role of computed tomography (CT)
        in, 130–132
    "pseudothorotrast" appearance, 1018
    splenic opacification from, 1015, *1016*
Thrombosis
    mesenteric venous, 1002
    portal vein, 88–91, 702
    of splenic artery, 997
    in splenic traums, 935
    splenic vein, 1002–1004, 1033, *1033*
Thrombus
    development, 294
    echogenic, pancreatic, 700
Tissue diagnosis, of adenocarcinoma, of
    pancreatic duct cell, 767
Tolazoline (Priscoline), 13, 814
Tomogram, excretory urographic, of
    metastatic disease in the liver,
    214, *215*, 215
Toposcopic catheter, 347
Torsion, splenic, 917, 918, *919*, 927
    of accessory spleen, 920
    in splenosis, 942

Tortuosity, splenic artery, 997, 998
Total parenteral nutrition, and
    cholecystitis scintigraphy, 421
Toxic shock syndrome, 115, 116
Toxin(s), hepatic fibrosis from, 70
TR, in hepatic masses, 271, 272
Transcatheter management of hepatic
        neoplasms, 293
    chemotherapy, 295–298
    hepatic artery embolization, 298–300
    radiologic technique, 294–295
    rationale, 293–294
Transducer
    biopsy, 1045, *1047*
    3.5 MHz, 779
    for sonography of pancreas, 630, 631,
        632
Transverse scanning
    of choledocholithiasis, 515, *516*
    of pancreas, 631–632
Trasylol, 335
Trauma
    biliary tract (*see* Biliary tract, trauma)
    gallbladder (*see* Gallbladder, trauma)
    liver (*see* Liver, trauma)
    pancreatic (*see* Pancreas, trauma)
    spleen (*see* Spleen, trauma)
"Tree-in-winter" appearance, 570
Trendelenburg positioning in
    choledocholithiasis scanning, 516
Triglyceride, excessive accumulation, in
    liver (*see also* Fatty liver), 105
Trisegmentectomy, 231
Trocar method, for catheter placement,
    1046
Trypanosomiasis (*see* Chaga's disease)
Trypsin, and pancreatitis, 657
Tubercle, spleen, 904
Tuberculosis
    miliary, liver involvement, 120–121
    splenomegaly from, 994, *994*
Tuftsin, 902
Tumor (*see also* Cyst, specific type)
    biliary (*see* Biliary tumors)
    extrahepatic, differentiation from
        intrinsic hepatic disease, 30–31
    gallbladder (*see* Gallbladder, tumors)
    liver (*see* Liver, tumors)
    localization, by ERCP, 338
    mucinous cystic, 732, *733*
    pancreas (*see* Pancreas, tumors)
    seeding, in guided percutaneous
        biopsy, 1080
Tumor cells, reaction to chemotherapy,
    295
Tunica propria, 309

U

Ulcer, ulceration
    gastric, 481, 1028
    of gastrinoma, 871
Ultrasound, ultrasonography, sonography
    of abdominal mass, in neonatal
        jaundice, 357
    of abscess
        amebic, 160, *162*, 163
        pancreatic, 715, *717*, 717, 718
        percutaneous, 1041
        pyogenic liver, 151, 152, *153*, 154,
            155

splenic, 913, *959*, 959–960, 965
upper abdominal, 1042
of adenocarcinoma, pancreatic duct
    cell, 603, 778
    of ampullary carcinoma, 802, *803*
    effect on biliary tract, 779, 780–781
    effect on pancreatic duct, 779, *782*
    findings, 779, 780–781
    technique, 778–779
of adenoma
    hepatic, 189, *190*, *191*
    pancreatic duct cell, 752, *754*, 754
of aneurysm, splenic artery, 998
of anastomoses, biliary-enteric, 529,
    531
of ascariasis, biliary, 556–558, *558*
of atresia, biliary, 360, 361
of biliary tract, anatomy, 321–325
of biliary tree, 327
of biloma, 587, *587*, 588
for biopsy, tumor, 610
of Budd-Chiari syndrome, 96, 98, *101*
of candidiasis, hepatic, 157–158
of Caroli's disease, 365, *368*
of cholangiocarcinoma, 536, *537*
    intrahepatic, 254, *256*, *257*, 258,
        259
of cholangitis
    acute, 549
    primary sclerosing, 560, *561*
    recurrent pyogenic, 552
of cholecystitis
    acalculous, 428–430
    acute, 411–416, *424*, 424
    chronic, 435, *436*, 436–437
    emphysematous, 431, *434*, 434–435
    hyperplastic, 472, *474*, 474–477
of choledochal cyst, 372, *374*, *379*
    in neonate and infant, 381, 382
of choledocholithiasis, 515–519
of cholelithiasis (*see also*
    Cholecystosonography), 390
of cirrhosis, 70–78
of cystadenoma and
    cystadenocarcinoma,
    biliary, 194, *195*, *196*, *197*, *198*
of cystic fibrosis, 39, *654*, 655
of echinococcal disease, 167, *168*, *169*
    hepatic alveolar
        echinococcus, 169, 170
of embryonal rhabdomyosarcoma, 548
of epithelial neoplasms, pancreatic,
    846, *849*, *850*, *851*
of fatty liver, 106, *107*, *108*, 111
    B-mode ultrasound, *107–108*
of fibrosis, hepatic congenital, 365,
    366
of fistula, biliary, *449*, 450–451
of focal nodular hyperplasia, 185,
    185, 186
of gallbladder
    anomalies, 353
    carcinoma, 484, *486*, 487–489
    technique and anatomy, 316–*320*
of gallstones, in neonate and infant,
    357
of gas, portal venous, 145, *146*
of gastrinoma, 871, *871*
of glucogonoma, 873, 877, *877*
of glycogen storage disease, 38–39

gray scale, 1
of hamartoma, mesenchymal, *42*, 43
of hemangioendothelioma, infantile,
    45, *45*
of hemangioma
    cavernous, 174, *175*, *176*, *178*, 181,
        182
    splenic, 972, 973
of hemobilia, 582
of hemochromatosis, 117
of hepatitis, 115
    peliosis, 140
of hepatoblastoma, 49
of hepatocellular carcinoma, 223–231,
    239
    fibrolamellar, 252
of hereditary hemorrhagic
    telangiectasia, 137, *138*, *139*
of hydrops of gallbladder, 446
of infarction
    hepatic, 143, *143*, 144
    splenic, 1006, 1007, *1007*
of insulinoma, 866, 866, 867
of islet cell tumors
    functional, 862, 863, *863*
    nonfunctioning, 882, 884
of jaundice, 497, 499–501, 504
    in children, 507
of leptospirosis, 122, 123
of liver, 15–21
    of size, 21
    of volume, 55
of lymphoma, splenic, 966–967
of metastatic disease
    gallbladder, 494–495
    liver, 199, 204–209, 213
    splenic, 977, *979*, 980, 981
of milk of calcium bile, 442
of Mirizzi syndrome, 457, *458*, 461
of mucinous cystic neoplasm,
    pancreatic duct cell, 763
of pancreas
    annular, 646, *647*
    of normal anatomy, 623–632
of pancreaticoblastoma, 853, *853*
of pancreatitis
    acute, 671–676, 680, 1057
    chronic, 696, 698–700
in percutaneous abscess drainage,
    1043–1045, *1046*, *1047*
for percutaneous biopsy, guided,
    upper abdomen, 1067*t*, 1067–
    1068, 1071, *1072*, 1075
of polycystic liver disease, 363
of porcelain gallbladder, 439, *441*
of pseudocyst, pancreatic, 732, *732*,
    734, *735*, 735
role in thorotrast-induced diseases of
    liver and spleen, 130
of rupture, splenic, 944
of sarcoma, hepatic, undifferentiated
    (embryonal), 54
of schistosomiasis, 124, *125*
of shunt splenorenal, 1011
of sickle cell anemia, 1018, 1020,
    1022, 1024, 1025
of spleen, 908, *909*
    of accessory spleen, *921*, 921
    of asplenia, 925
    of cysts, 950, *951*, 951, *952*, 955

for measurement, 912
of polysplenia, 926, *927*
of wandering spleen, 918, *919*
of splenomegaly, 993, 994, *994*, *995*, 995
of stricture, biliary, 601
of thrombosis
  portal venous, 89–91
  splenic vein, 1003
transverse, of adenoma, hepatic, 37, *37*, 38–39
of trauma
  gallbladder, 591
  hepatic, 284, *284*, *285*
  pancreatic, *742*, 743
  splenic, 933, 936, *936*, 937
  surgical, to biliary tract, 579
of tuberculosis, miliary, 121
of vipoma, 878
of Wilson's disease, 120
Umbilical vein
  recanalization of, 80, *81*
  recanalized, 73, *76*
Uncinate process, 623, 624
  rounding of, 786, *787*
Unresectibility, in carcinoma of pancreas, 834
Upper abdomen (*see* Abdomen, upper)
Upper gastrointestinal series
  of adenocarcinoma, pancreatic duct cell, 768, 769, 770, *772*, 773–777
  of gastrinoma, 871
  in jaundice, 511, *512*, *513*
Ureter, obstruction, by pancreatic pseudocyst, 730, *731*
Urography, urogram
  in abscess, pyogenic liver, 152, *152*
  excretory
    of adenocarcinoma, of pancreatic duct cell, 768
    of adenoma, of pancreas, *776*, 777
    of Caroli's disease, 365
    of choledochal cyst, 372, *374*, *376*
    of hepatic fibrosis, congenital, 365, *366*
    of mesenchymal hamartoma, 43
    of pseudocyst, pancreatic, *730*, 730, 731
    of polycystic liver disease, 363
    of wandering spleen, 918, *918*

V

Vacuoles, 640
Vagus nerve
  electrical stimulation, 641
  transection, 641
Valium (*see* Diazepam)
Valsalva maneuver, 82
  in Budd-Chiari syndrome, 100, *100*
Variceal, dilatation, *793*, 794

Varices
  duodenal, 82
  esophageal, 82, *82*, 223, 372, 705, 1003
  gastric, 82, *83*, 705, 706, 1002
  gastroepiploic, 73, 705
  gastroesophageal, 73, *75*
Vascular anatomy
  of liver, 8–13
  relationship of pancreas to, 624, 625
Vascular changes (*see also* Venous abnormalities)
  associated with pancreatic carcinoma, 828, 829–830
  in pancreatitis, chronic, 706, 707–708
Vascular disease (*see* specific organ)
Vascular encasement
  in adenocarcinoma of pancreas, *793*, 794
  in mucinous cystic neoplasms, pancreatic duct cell, 763
Vascular landmarks, of pancreas, computed tomography (CT), 633
Vascular structures, opacified, 607
Vascular system, hepatic, embryogenesis, 3
Vascular territories, spleen, 902
Vasculature, of "distributed" spleen, 906
Vasoconstrictors, use in angiography of pancreatic carcinoma, 814
Vasopressin (Angiotensin), 814, 936
Vein(s) (*see also* specific vein)
  bacteremia, 567, 568
  in islet cell tumors, 864, 865
Venography
  of bilhemia, 585
  hepatic
    in Budd-Chiari syndrome, *98*, *100*, 100, *101*
    in cirrhosis, 84, 85, *86–87*
    of sarcoidosis with portal hypertension, 121
    of hepatitis, peliosis, 140
  pancreatic, of carcinoma, 836–837
  percutaneous transhepatic, portal, 613, *615*, 615
  of periportal sinusoidal dilatation, 140
Veno-occlusive disease, hepatic, Thorotrast-induced, 128
Venous abnormalities, in carcinoma of pancreas, *815*, 817–818, *820–821*, *827*, 828
Venous anatomy, pancreas, computed tomography (CT) of, 638, *638*
Venous change, in pancreatitis, chronic, 704, 705
Venous occlusion, in islet cell tumors, 864, 865
Venous sampling, pancreas
  for gastrinoma, 872, 873
  of glucagonoma, 878
  of insulinoma, 868–869
  in islet cell tumors, 865

in vipoma, 879
Venous shunting, in splenic trauma, 935
Venous system, hepatic, embryology, 3, 4
Ventriculogram, of asplenia, *924*
Verner-Morrison syndrome, 861, 862t
Videotape recordings, 82
Villous tumors, biliary, 545, *545*
Vinblastine, 297
Vipoma (WDHA syndrome)
  clinical findings, 878
  gallbladder distention from, 415
  and islet cell tumors, 861, 862t
  pancreatic, 878
  pathology, 878
  radiology, *877*, 878–879
Viscus, gas-filled, 317
Volvulus
  of gallbladder, 353
  in wandering spleen, 917
von Gierke's disease, 37, 188
von Hippel-Lindau disease, 749, 751

W

Warren shunt, *1010*, 1011
Water secretion, pancreatic, 640
Water technique, for sonography of pancreatic anatomy, 632
WDHA syndrome (*see* Vipoma)
Webs, in Budd-Chiari syndrome, 100, 102, 103, 104
Wedge defect, in splenic trauma, 936
Whipple procedure
  in carcinoma, ampullary, 767
  in fistula, biliary, *449*
Whipple's triad, in insulinoma, 866
"White bile," 446
White blood cells, indium-111 labeled (*see* Indium-111 white blood cells)
Wilms' tumor, 210, 220
Wilson's disease, 118–119, 270, 271, 569
  clinical findings, 119
  pathology, 119–120
  radiology, 120
Window
  cyst-peritoneal, 949
  liver, 960, *963*
  liver-spleen, 1025
Wire
  Benson, 607
  Lunderquist, 610
THG, 610, 611
Wiskott-Aldrich syndrome, 973
Worms, *See* Ascariasis

X

Xenon-133 scan, 28, 149
  of fatty liver, 106, *107*, 111

Z

Zollinger-Ellison syndrome, 878
  and gastrinoma (*see* Gastrinoma)
  and islet cell tumors, 861, 862t
  pseudo Z-E syndrome, 869